WHAT'S NEW...

- **NEW!** FREE, 1-year subscription to Davis's Drug Guide Online, powered by Unbound Medicine®. (See inside for more details.)
- **NEW!** Pharmacogenomic content.
- **UPDATED!** Easy-to-use monographs.

Emphasizes **IV administration** with its own subhead in the **Nursing Implications sections**.

Uses **sub-heads** for **Diluent, Concentration,** and **Rate**.

Offers **more patient safety** information than any other drug guide.

Includes extensive **patient/family teaching** information.

Find enhanced Canadian content throughout—in the monographs, appendices, and index.

IS THERE A CD-ROM ON THE INSIDE BACK COVER?

If there isn't, you're missing an outstanding collection of clinical resources that you'll find only on the Davis's Drug Guide Resource Kit CD-ROM—from easily searchable access to nearly 700 drug monographs to a drug dosage calculator.

DAVIS'S
DRUG GUIDE
Online

Activate your FREE subscription today!

You're two steps away from your **FREE**, 1-year subscription to **Davis's Drug Guide Online**, powered by Unbound Medicine®.

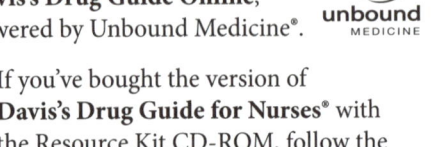

1. If you've bought the version of **Davis's Drug Guide for Nurses®** with the Resource Kit CD-ROM, follow the link on the CD—or simply type the following address into your web browser:

www.drugguide.com/ddo/ub/bookcode

2. Enter your unique, personal code printed on this page.

Davis's Drug Guide Online features the complete **Davis's Drug Guide for Nurses®** database—over 1,100 monographs in all! It's accessible from your desktop, laptop, or any mobile device with a web browser.

WD12-QBDXSFCYJWMPQ

Davis's DRUG GUIDE FOR NURSES®

TWELFTH EDITION

JUDITH HOPFER DEGLIN, PharmD
Consultant Pharmacist
Hospice of Southeastern Connecticut
Uncasville, Connecticut

APRIL HAZARD VALLERAND, PhD, RN, FAAN
Wayne State University
College of Nursing
Detroit, Michigan

CYNTHIA A. SANOSKI, BS, PharmD, FCCP, BCPS
Chair, Department of Pharmacy Practice
Thomas Jefferson University
Jefferson School of Pharmacy
Philadelphia, Pennsylvania

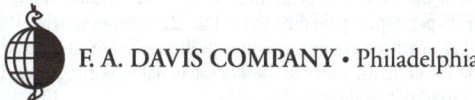

F. A. DAVIS COMPANY • Philadelphia

F. A. Davis Company
1915 Arch Street
Philadelphia, PA 19103
www.fadavis.com

Copyright © 2011 by F. A. Davis Company

Copyright © 1988, 1991, 1993, 1995, 1997, 1999, 2001, 2003, 2005, 2007, 2009 by F. A. Davis Company. All rights reserved. This book is protected by copyright. No part of it may be reproduced, stored in a retrieval system, or transmitted in any form or by any means, electronic, mechanical, photocopying, recording, or otherwise, without written permission from the publisher.

Printed in the United States of America

Last digit indicates print number 10 9 8 7 6 5 4 3 2 1
Editor-in-Chief, Nursing: Patti L. Cleary
Director of Content Development: Darlene D. Pedersen
Publisher, Nursing: Robert G. Martone
Senior Acquisitions Editor: Thomas A. Ciavarella
Project Editor: Meghan K. Ziegler
Director of Production: Michael W. Bailey
Managing Editor: David Orzechowski

NOTE: As new scientific information becomes available through basic and clinical research, recommended treatments and drug therapies undergo changes. The authors and publisher have done everything possible to make this book accurate, up to date, and in accord with accepted standards at the time of publication. However, the reader is advised always to check product information (package inserts) for changes and new information regarding dose and contraindications before administering any drug. Caution is especially urged when using new or infrequently ordered drugs.

Deglin, Judith Hopfer, 1950–
   Davis's Drug Guide for Nurses/Judith Hopfer Deglin,
   April Hazard Vallerand, Cynthia A. Sanoski.--12th ed.
      p. ; cm.
   Other title: Drug guide for nurses
   Includes bibliographical references and index.
   ISBN-13: 978-0-8036-2308-8 (with CD) (pbk.: alk. paper)
   ISBN-10: 0-8036-2308-9 (with CD) (pbk.: alk. paper)
   ISBN-13: 978-0-8036-2309-5 (without CD) (pbk.: alk. paper)
   ISBN-10: 0-8036-2309-7 (without CD) (pbk.: alk. paper)
   1. Drugs—Handbooks, manuals, etc. 2. Nursing—Handbooks, manuals, etc. 3. Clinical pharmacology—Handbooks, manuals, etc. I. Vallerand, April Hazard. II. Title. III. Title: Drug guide for nurses.
[DNLM: 1. Pharmaceutical Preparations—administration & dosage—Handbooks. 2. Pharmaceutical preparations—administration & dosage—Nurses' Instruction. 3. Drug therapy—nursing—Handbooks. 4. Drug therapy—nursing—Nurses' Instruction. 5. Pharmacology, Clinical—methods—Handbooks. 6. Pharmacology, Clinical—methods—Nurses' Instruction. QV 735 D318d 2010]
   RM301.12044 2010
   615'.1024613-dc22

2010003537

Authorization to photocopy items for internal or personal use, of specific clients, is granted by F. A. Davis Company for users registered with the Copyright Clearance Center (CCC) Transactional Reporting Service, provided that the fee of $.25 per copy is paid directly to CCC, 222 Rosewood Drive, Danvers, MA 01923. For those organizations that have been granted a photocopy license by CCC, a separate system of payment has been arranged. The fee code for users of the Transactional Reporting Service is 8036-2308/10 0 (with CD) and 8036-2309/10 0 (without CD) + $.25.

The PERFECT PACKAGE
a comprehensive collection for nurses

Venes
Taber's Cyclopedic Medical Dictionary
Thumb-Indexed Version with Taber'sPlus DVD

To thrive in the ever-changing world of health care, you need a respected, trusted, and cutting-edge cyclopedic resource. Taber's brings meanings to life.

Deglin, Vallerand, & Sanoski
Davis's Drug Guide for Nurses® with Resource Kit CD-ROM

Count on the drug guide that always puts safety first…with all of the guidance you need to administer medications competently and safely across the lifespan.

Van Leeuwen & Poelhuis-Leth
Davis's Comprehensive Handbook of Laboratory and Diagnostic Tests with Nursing Implications

Here's the information you need to understand how laboratory and diagnostic tests work, accurately interpret the test results, and provide quality care for patients—pre-, intra-, and post-test.

Purchase your copies today!

Available in your health science bookstore.

Call 800.323.3555 (US)
800.665.1148 (CAN)
Visit **www.fadavis.com**.

Prefer The Perfect Package on your mobile device or computer? Check out…

 Nursing Central® powered by Unbound Medicine

Nursing Constellation Plus® powered by Skyscape.

Visit **www.fadavis.com/mobile**.

DEDICATION

In loving memory of my older children, Samantha Ann and Randy Eli, both struck and killed by a drinking driver on January 9, 1997. They remain forever in our hearts. The wonder and joy they brought to our lives continue to inspire us.

To Stu, for his continued support and love.

To my daughter Hanna, whose hard work, talent, and grace never cease to amaze me.
To my son Reuben, whose smile warms my heart and whose energy is boundless.
To my parents, Charlotte and Kurt Hopfer, who continue to inspire me.

JHD

To my father, Keith Hazard, whose love and support are always there.
To my mother-in-law, Roberta, who remains a guiding presence in my life.
To my son, Ben, whose sensitivity and sense of humor make even the toughest day easier.
To my daughter, Katharine, whose fearlessness and determination in seeking her goals I admire.
To my husband, Warren, my colleague and friend, whose encouragement and love I have always cherished.

AHV

To my wonderful mother who has provided her continual love, support, and wisdom as I continue to pursue all of my personal and professional goals. To all of my current and former students who have inspired me to undertake this very important project.

CAS

ACKNOWLEDGMENTS

We offer our thanks to the students and nurses who have used our book for over 20 years. We hope our book provides you with the current knowledge of pharmacotherapeutics you need to continue to give quality care in our rapidly changing health-care environment.

Judi and April

CONSULTANTS

Michelle Farkas-Cameron, APRN-PMH, BC
Clinical Nurse Specialist
Sinai-Grace Hospital
Inpatient Psychiatry
Detroit, MI

Jamie Crawley, B.Sc.N., B.A., M.B.A./H.C.M., PhD(c)
Doctoral Student
Wayne State University
Detroit, MI
Lecturer
University of Windsor
Faculty of Nursing
Windsor, ON, Canada

Lisa E. Davis, PharmD, FCCP, BCPS, BCOP
Associate Professor of Clinical Pharmacy
University of the Sciences in Philadelphia
Philadelphia College of Pharmacy
Philadelphia, PA

Wanda Edwards, MSN, APRN, NP
Instructor (Clinical)
Wayne State University
College of Nursing
Detroit, MI

Deborah A. Ennis, RN, MSN, CCRN
Harrisburg Area Community College
Harrisburg, PA

Linda Felver, PhD, RN
Associate Professor
Oregon Health & Science University
School of Nursing
Portland, OR

Charlene C. Gyurko, PhD, RN, CNE
Assistant Professor
Purdue University, Calumet
School of Nursing
Hammond, IN

Althea DuBose Hayes, RD
Renal Dietitian
Greenfield Health System,
a division of Henry Ford Health System
Southfield, MI

Therese Jamison, MSN, APRN-BC, ACNP
Associate Professor
Madonna University
School of Nursing
Livonia, MI

Janeen Kidd, RN, BN
Instructor/School Placement Project Coordinator
University of Victoria
School of Nursing
Victoria, BC, Canada

Wendy Neander, BS, BScN, RN, MN, PhD (student)
Assistant Professor
University of Victoria
School of Nursing
Victoria, BC, Canada
Staff Nurse
Nanaimo Regional Correctional Centre
Nanaimo, BC, Canada
Assistant Professor
Oregon Health & Science University
School of Nursing
Ashland, OR

Norma Perez, BSN, RN
Nursing Faculty & Clinical Coordinator
Ivy Tech Community College
School of Nursing
Valparaiso, IN

Gladdi Tomlinson, RN, MSN
Professor of Nursing
Harrisburg Area Community College
Harrisburg, PA

Linda S. Weglicki, RN, PhD, MSN
Program Director
National Institute of Nursing Research
Office of Extramural Programs
Bethesda, MD

F. A. DAVIS PHARMACOLOGIC PUBLICATIONS ADVISORY BOARD

Tracey Hopkins, BSN, RN
Editorial Consultant and Content Coordinator
Shamim Tejani, PharmD
Pharmacy Clinical Manager
St. Joseph's Hospital & Medical Center
Phoenix, AZ

Debra Abraham, MSN, RN
Lecturer
University of Pennsylvania
School of Nursing
Philadelphia, PA

Gina M. Ankner, RN, MS, ANP, BC
Clinical Instructor & Course Coordinator
University of Massachusetts Dartmouth
College of Nursing
North Dartmouth, MA

Benjamin Barankin, MD, FRCPC
The Dermatology Centre
Toronto, ON, Canada

Angela Ann Boggs, PharmD
Clinical Pharmacist
University of Maryland Baltimore
Springfield Hospital Center
Sykesville, MD

Douglas Lee Boggs, PharmD, MS, BCPP
Research Associate
Maryland Psychiatric Research Center
University of Maryland School of Medicine
Baltimore, MD

Hedy Cohen, RN, BSN, MS
Vice President
Institute for Safe Mediation Practices
Huntingdon Valley, PA

Jane Vincent Corbett, RN, Ed.D
Professor Emerita
University of San Francisco
School of Nursing
San Francisco, CA

Regina S. Cunningham, PhD, RN, AOCN
Senior Director, Oncology
The Tisch Cancer Institute
Mount Sinai Medical Center
New York, NY

Janet Czermak, APRN-BC
Essex County College
Department of Nursing
Newark, NJ

Loretta H. Diehl, MSN, RN
College Associate Professor, Nursing
New Mexico State University Alamogordo
Alamogordo, NM

Chuck DiTrapano, RPh
Pharmacy Supervisor
Reading Hospital and Medical Center
Reading, PA
President
RxToolkit.com

Elizabeth A. Duthie, PhD, RN
Director of Patient Safety
NYU Hospitals Medical Center
New York, NY

Margaret Falahee, APN, BC
Clinical Assistant Professor
Wayne State University
College of Nursing
Detroit, MI

Grant E. Fraser, MD
President
Fraser Consulting, LLC
Bradenton, FL

Linda G. Gooen, PharmD, MS
Certified Geriatric Pharmacist, Certified
Consultant Pharmacist
Adjunct Professor, Rutgers Ernest Mario School
of Pharmacy
President, Gooen Consulting, LLC
Basking Ridge, NJ

F. A. DAVIS PHARMACOLOGIC PUBLICATIONS ADVISORY BOARD

Matthew Grissinger, RPh, FISMP, FASCP
Director, Error Reporting Programs
Institute for Safe Mediation Practices
Huntingdon Valley, PA

Susan M. Hasenau, PhD, RN, CNNP
Professor
Madonna University
School of Nursing
Livonia, MI

Marilyn J. Hehr, RN, MSN
CNCC Nursing Program Director
Colorado Northwestern Community College
Craig, CO

Nadine T. James, RN, BSN, MSN, PhD
Assistant Professor
University of Southern Mississippi
Hattiesburg, MS

Emily Karwacki-Sheff, MS, CMS, RN, FNP-BC
Lecturer and Clinical Instructor
Massachusetts General Hospital
Institute of Health Professions
Charlestown, MA
Clinical Instructor
Boston College
Chestnut Hill, MA

Kathy Kumer, MS, CS, RN
Director of Nurses
Castle Rock Convalescent Center
Green River, WY

Laura G. Leahy, MSN, PMH-CNS/FNP, BC
Psychiatric Advanced Practice Nurse
Clinical Associate Faculty/Lecturer
University of Pennsylvania-
School of Nursing
Philadelphia, PA

Stuart Levine, PharmD
Informatics Specialist
Institute for Safe Medication Practices
Huntingdon Valley, PA

Linda Davis Meseck, RN, BSN, OCN
Providence Tarzana Medical Center
Tarzana, CA

Ginette A. Pepper, PhD, RN, FAAN
Helen Lowe Bamberger Colby Presidential
Endowed Chair in Gerontological Nursing
Associate Dean for Research & PhD Programs
Salt Lake City, UT
Director
University of Utah Hartford Center of Geriatric
Nursing Excellence
Salt Lake City, UT

Rosemary C. Polomano, PhD, RN, FAAN
Associate Professor of Pain Practice
University of Pennsylvania
School of Nursing
Philadelphia, PA

Debbie Richmond, NP-C, ACRN
Wayne State University
Detroit, MI

Noel Dougherty Rosner, MSN, RN, ANP-C, DNP
Nurse Practitioner
Raritan Bay Medical Center
Department of Infectious Diseases
Perth Amboy, NJ
Faculty
University of Medicine and Dentistry
Newark, NJ

Dorie Schwertz, PhD, RN, FAAN, FAHA
Associate Professor
University of Illinois-Chicago College of Nursing
Department of Medical Surgical Nursing and
Adjunct Professor of Pharmacology
Chicago, IL

Sue Seckinger, BSN, RN, CWOCN
Wound Care Specialist
Lower Bucks Hospital
Bristol, PA

Kim Subasic, MSN, RN
The University of Scranton
Scranton, PA

Cynthia Ulreich, RN, NP-C, BSN, OCN
P2 Chemotherapy Nurse Coordinator
Henry Ford Health System
Detroit, MI

Lisa Velazquez-Marsh, RN, BSN, OCN
Community Cancer Center of North Florida
North Florida Regional Medical Center
Gainesville, FL

Kevin Zakrzewski, MD
Internal Medicine
Abington Memorial Hospital
Abington, PA

CONTENTS

HOW TO USE *DAVIS'S DRUG GUIDE FOR NURSES*	1
EVIDENCE-BASED PRACTICE AND PHARMACOTHERAPEUTICS: Implications for Nurses	6
PHARMACOGENOMICS	9
MEDICATION ERRORS: Improving Practices and Patient Safety	12
DETECTING AND MANAGING ADVERSE DRUG REACTIONS	18
Overview of Risk Evaluation and Mitigation Systems (REMS)	22
SPECIAL DOSING CONSIDERATIONS	24
The Pediatric Patient	24
The Geriatric Patient	24
The Patient of Reproductive Age	25
Renal Disease	25
Liver Disease	25
Heart Failure	25
Body Size	25
Drug Interactions	26
EDUCATING PATIENTS ABOUT SAFE MEDICATION USE	27
CLASSIFICATIONS	29
Anti-Alzheimer's agents	29
Antianemics	30
Antianginals	31
Antianxiety agents	32
Antiarrhythmics	34
Antiasthmatics	36
Anticholinergics	37
Anticoagulants	39
Anticonvulsants	40
Antidepressants	42
Antidiabetics	44
Antidiarrheals	46
Antiemetics	47
Antifungals	49
Antihistamines	50
Antihypertensives	52
Anti-infectives	54
Antineoplastics	56
Antiparkinson agents	60
Antiplatelet agents	61
Antipsychotics	62
Antipyretics	65
Antiretrovirals	66
Antirheumatics	67
Antituberculars	69
Antiulcer agents	70
Antivirals	72

Beta blockers	73
Bone resorption inhibitors	76
Bronchodilators	77
Calcium channel blockers	78
Central nervous system stimulants	80
Corticosteroids	82
Diuretics	84
Hormones	86
Immunosuppressants	87
Laxatives	89
Lipid lowering agents	90
Minerals/electrolytes/pH modifiers	91
Natural/Herbal Products	93
Nonopioid analgesics	94
Nonsteroidal anti-inflammatory agents	96
Opioid analgesics	97
Sedative/hypnotics	99
Skeletal muscle relaxants	101
Thrombolytics	102
Vaccines/immunizing agents	104
Vascular headache suppressants	105
Vitamins	107
Weight control agents	108
DRUG MONOGRAPHS IN ALPHABETICAL ORDER BY GENERIC NAME	**109–1316**
LESS COMMONLY USED DRUGS	**1317–1340**
NATURAL/HERBAL PRODUCTS	**1341–1366**
APPENDICES	**1367**
Appendix A. Recent Drug Approvals	1369
Appendix B. Combination Drugs	1378
Appendix C. Ophthalmic Medications	1397
Appendix D. Medication Administration Techniques	1404
Appendix E. Formulas Helpful for Calculating Doses	1407
Appendix F. Body Surface Area Nomograms	1409
Appendix G. Normal Values of Common Laboratory Tests	1411
Appendix H. Commonly Used Abbreviations	1414
Appendix I. Pregnancy Categories	1416
Appendix J. Controlled Substance Schedules	1417
Appendix K. Equianalgesic Dosing Guidelines	1418
Appendix L. Recommendations for the Safe Handling of Hazardous Drugs	1421
Appendix M. Food Sources for Specific Nutrients	1423
Appendix N. Insulins and Insulin Therapy	1425
Appendix O. Canadian and U.S. Pharmaceutical Practices	1427
Appendix P. Routine Pediatric and Adult Immunizations	1429
Appendix Q. Administering Medications to Children	1436
Appendix R. Pediatric Dosage Calculations	1437
Appendix S. Pediatric Fluid and Electrolyte Requirements	1438
Appendix T. Early Management of Anaphylactic Reactions	1439
Appendix U. The Cytochrome P450 System	1440
BIBLIOGRAPHY	**1443**
COMPREHENSIVE GENERIC/TRADE/CLASSIFICATIONS INDEX	**1445**

HOW TO USE *DAVIS'S DRUG GUIDE FOR NURSES*

Davis's Drug Guide for Nurses provides comprehensive, up-to-date drug information in well-organized, nursing-focused monographs. It also includes extensive supplemental material in 18 appendices and the accompanying CD-ROM, thoroughly addresses the issue of safe medication administration, and educates the reader about 50 different therapeutic classes of drugs. In this 12th edition, we have continued the tradition of focusing on safe medication administration by adding a new **Medication Safety Tools** color insert and even more information about health care's most vulnerable patients: children, the elderly, pregnant women, and breastfeeding mothers. Look for more Pedi, Geri, OB, and Lactation headings throughout the monographs. In addition, we've included information relevant to Canadian students and nurses. You'll find an appendix comparing Canadian and U.S. pharmaceutical practices, more Canada-only combination drugs in the Combination Drugs appendix, and additional Canadian brand names in the drug monographs. To help you find this information quickly, we've also added a maple leaf icon (✢) in the index next to each Canadian entry. New to this edition, we have added pharmacogenomic information throughout numerous monographs to guide the nurse in selecting and monitoring various drug therapies. To help you find this information quickly, we've added a double helix icon (⚇) to denote this information as it applies to specific drugs. Use this book to enhance your competence in implementing and evaluating medication therapies. The following sections describe the organization of *Davis's Drug Guide for Nurses* and explain how to quickly find the information you need.

Safe Medication Use Articles

"Medication Errors: Improving Practices and Patient Safety", "Detecting and Managing Adverse Drug Reactions", "Overview of Risk Evaluation and Mitigation Systems (REMS)", Special Dosing Considerations", and "Educating Patients About Safe Medication Use" comprise the safe medication use articles and provide an overview of the medication safety issues that confront practitioners and patients. Leading off this series, the medication errors article familiarizes you with the systems issues and clinical situations repeatedly implicated in medication errors and suggests practical means to avoid them. It also teaches you about *high alert* medications, which have a greater potential to cause patient harm than other medications. "Detecting and Managing Adverse Drug Reactions" explains the different types of adverse reactions and provides guidance on how to detect and manage them. "Risk Evaluation and Mitigation Strategies (REMS)" explains strategies developed by the pharmaceutical industry and required by the FDA to minimize adverse drug reactions from potentially dangerous drugs. "Special Dosing Considerations" identifies the patient populations, such as neonates and patients with renal impairment, who require careful dose adjustments to ensure optimal therapeutic outcomes. "Educating Patients About Medication Use" reviews the most important teaching points for nurses to discuss with their patients and their families. In addition to these safety articles, other critical information is highlighted in red throughout the drug monographs. This allows the reader to quickly identify important information and to see how nursing practice, including assessment, implementation, and patient teaching, relates to it.

Classifications Profile

Medications in the same therapeutic class often share similar mechanisms of action, assessment guidelines, precautions, and interactions. The Classifications Profile provides summaries of the major therapeutic classifications used in *Davis's Drug Guide for Nurses*. It also provides patient teaching information common to all agents within the class and a list of drugs within each class.

Medication Safety Tools

New to this edition is a color insert with tables and charts that nurses can use for a quick but thorough reference to information that will help them avoid making medication errors. It includes lists of drugs

2 DAVIS'S DRUG GUIDE FOR NURSES

that are associated with adverse reactions and falls in the elderly; high alert drugs; sound-alike, look-alike drugs and more.

Drug Monographs

Drug monographs are organized in the following manner:

High Alert Status: Some medications, such as chemotherapeutic agents, anticoagulants, and insulins, have a greater potential for harm than others. These medications have been identified by the *Institute for Safe Medication Practices* as **high alert drugs**. *Davis's Drug Guide for Nurses* includes a high alert tab in the upper right corner of the monograph header in appropriate medications to alert the nurse to the medication's risk. The term "high alert" is used in other parts of the monograph as well, to help the nurse administer these medications safely. See the new **Medication Safety Tools** color insert for a complete list of high alert medications in *Davis's Drug Guide for Nurses*. Refer to ISMP.org for all solutions, groups, and individual high alert drugs.

Generic/Trade Name: The generic name appears first, with a pronunciation key, followed by an alphabetical list of trade names. Canadian trade names are preceded by a maple leaf (✤). Common names, abbreviations, and selected foreign names are also included.

Classification: The therapeutic classification, which categorizes drugs by the disease state they are used to treat, appears first, followed by the pharmacologic classification, which is based on the drug's mechanism of action.

Controlled Substance Schedule: All drugs regulated by federal law are placed into one of five schedules, based on the drug's medicinal value, harmfulness, and potential for abuse or addiction. Schedule I drugs, the most dangerous and having no medicinal value, are not included in *Davis's Drug Guide for Nurses*. (See Appendix J for a description of the Schedule of Controlled Substances.)

Pregnancy Category: Pregnancy categories (A, B, C, D, and X) provide a basis for determining a drug's potential for fetal harm and are included in each monograph. The designation UK is used when the pregnancy category is unknown. (See Appendix I for more information.)

Indications: Medications are approved by the FDA (Food and Drug Administration) for specific disease states. This section identifies the diseases or conditions for which the drug is commonly used and includes significant unlabeled uses as well.

Action: This section contains a concise description of how the drug produces the desired therapeutic effect.

Pharmacokinetics: Pharmacokinetics refers to the way the body processes a medication by absorption, distribution, metabolism, and excretion. This section also includes information on the drug's half-life.

> **Absorption:** Absorption describes the process that follows drug administration and its subsequent delivery to systemic circulation. If only a small fraction is absorbed following oral administration (diminished bioavailability), then the oral dose must be much greater than the parenteral dose. Absorption into systemic circulation also follows other routes of administration such as topical, transdermal, intramuscular, subcutaneous, rectal, and ophthalmic routes. Drugs administered intravenously are usually 100% bioavailable.

> **Distribution:** This section comments on the drug's distribution in body tissues and fluids. Distribution becomes important in choosing one drug over another, as in selecting an antibiotic that will penetrate the central nervous system to treat meningitis or in avoiding drugs that cross the placenta or concentrate in breast milk. Information on protein binding is included for drugs that are >95% bound to plasma proteins, which has implications for drug-drug interactions.

HOW TO USE *DAVIS'S DRUG GUIDE FOR NURSES*

Metabolism and Excretion: Drugs are primarily eliminated from the body either by hepatic conversion to active or inactive compounds (metabolism or biotransformation) and subsequent excretion by the kidneys, or by renal elimination of unchanged drug. Therefore, drug metabolism and excretion information is important in determining dosage regimens and intervals for patients with impaired renal or hepatic function. The creatinine clearance (CCr) helps quantify renal function and guides dosage adjustments. Formulas to estimate CCr are included in Appendix E.

Half-Life: The half-life of a drug is the amount of time it takes for the drug level to decrease by 50% and roughly correlates with the duration of action. Half-lives are given for drugs assuming the patient has normal renal or hepatic function. Conditions that alter the half-life are noted.

Time/Action Profile: The time/action profile table provides the onset of drug action, its peak effect, and its duration of activity. This can aid in planning administration schedules and allows the reader to appreciate differences in choosing one route over another.

Contraindications and Precautions: Situations in which drug use should be avoided or alternatives strongly considered are listed as contraindications. In general, most drugs are contraindicated in pregnancy or lactation, unless the potential benefits outweigh the possible risks to the mother or baby (e.g., anticonvulsants, antihypertensives, and antiretrovirals). Contraindications may be absolute (i.e., the drug in question should be avoided completely) or relative, in which certain clinical situations may allow cautious use of the drug. The precautions portion includes disease states or clinical situations in which drug use involves particular risks or in which dosage modification may be necessary. Extreme cautions are noted separately to draw attention to conditions under which use of the drug results in serious, potentially life-threatening consequences.

Adverse Reactions and Side Effects: Although it is not possible to include all reported reactions, major side effects for all drugs are included. Life-threatening adverse reactions or side effects are **CAPITALIZED**, and the most frequent side effects are underlined. Those underlined generally have an incidence of 10% or greater. Those not underlined occur in fewer than 10% but more than 1% of patients. Although life-threatening reactions may be rare (fewer than 1%), they are included because of their significance. The following abbreviations are used for body systems:

- **CNS:** central nervous system
- **EENT:** eye, ear, nose, and throat
- **Resp:** respiratory
- **CV:** cardiovascular
- **GI:** gastrointestinal
- **GU:** genitourinary
- **Derm:** dermatologic
- **Endo:** endocrinologic
- **F and E:** fluid and electrolyte
- **Hemat:** hematologic
- **Local:** local
- **Metab:** metabolic
- **MS:** musculoskeletal
- **Neuro:** neurologic
- **Misc:** miscellaneous

Interactions: Drug interactions are a significant risk for patients. As the number of medications a patient receives increases, so does the likelihood of drug-drug interactions. This section provides the most important drug-drug interactions and their physiological effects. Significant drug-food and drug-natural product interactions are also noted as are recommendations for avoiding or minimizing these interactions.

Route and Dosage: Routes of administration are grouped together and include recommended doses for adults, children, and other more specific age groups (such as geriatric patients). Dosage units are expressed in the terms in which they are usually prescribed. For example, penicillin G dosage is given in units rather than in milligrams. Dosing intervals also are provided in the manner in which they are frequently ordered. If a specific clinical situation (indication) requires a different dose or interval, this is listed separately for clarity. Specific dosing regimens for hepatic or renal impairment are also included.

Availability: This section lists the strengths and concentrations of available dose forms. Such information is useful in planning more convenient regimens (fewer tablets/capsules, less injection volume) and in determining whether certain dosing forms are available (suppositories, oral concentrates, sustained- or extended-release forms). Flavors of oral liquids and chewable tablets have been included to improve compliance and adherence in pediatric patients. General availability and average wholesale prices of commonly prescribed drugs have also been added as an aid to nurses with prescriptive authority.

Nursing Implications: This section helps the nurse apply the nursing process to pharmacotherapeutics. The subsections provide a step-by-step guide to clinical assessment, implementation (drug administration), and evaluation of the outcomes of pharmacologic therapy.

Assessment: This section includes guidelines for assessing patient history and physical data before and during drug therapy. Assessments specific to the drug's various indications are also included. The **Lab Test Considerations** section provides the nurse with information regarding which laboratory tests to monitor and how the results may be affected by the medication. **Toxicity and Overdose** alerts the nurse to therapeutic serum drug levels that must be monitored and signs and symptoms of toxicity. The antidote and treatment for toxicity or overdose of appropriate medications also are included.

Potential Nursing Diagnoses: The two or three most pertinent North American Nursing Diagnoses Association (NANDA) diagnoses that potentially apply to a patient receiving the medication are listed. Each diagnosis includes the pharmacologic effect from which the diagnosis has been derived. For instance, the patient receiving immunosuppressant drugs should be diagnosed with Risk for Infection. The diagnosis is followed by the term Side Effects in parentheses. Since patient education is fundamental to all nurse-patient interactions, the diagnosis Deficient Knowledge should be assumed to be a nursing diagnosis applicable to all drugs.

Implementation: Guidelines specific for medication administration are discussed in this subsection. **High Alert** information, i.e., information that directly relates to preventing medication errors with inherently dangerous drugs, is included first if applicable. Sound-alike look-alike name confusion alerts are also included here. Other headings in this section provide data regarding routes of administration. **PO** describes when and how to administer the drug, whether tablets may be crushed or capsules opened, and when to administer the medication in relation to food. The **IV** section includes specific information about administering the medication intravenously. It has been thoroughly updated for this edition beginning with a more prominent IV Administration heading that introduces this section. New bold, red headings have been added to highlight the recommended **diluents**, and **concentrations**. These new headings complement the **rate** heading and make this critical information easy to find. Wherever possible, new information has been added about these topics. Several subsections comprise the IV Administration section. The first section, **Direct IV**, which refers to administering medications from a syringe directly into a saline lock, Y-site of IV tubing, or a 3–way stopcock, provides details for reconstitution, concentration, dilution, and rate. **Rate** is also included in both other methods of IV administration, direct or intermittent infusion. **Intermittent Infusion** and **Continuous Infusion** specify standard dilution solutions and amounts, stability information, and rates. In addition, a quick reference for information about dilution amounts in neonates and infants, who are extremely sensitive to excess fluids, is contained in the new **Medication Safety Tools** color insert. **Syringe Compatibility/Incompatibility** identifies compatibile medications when mixed in a syringe. Compatibility of medications in a syringe is usually limited to 15 minutes after mixing. **Y-Site Compatibility/Incompatibility** identifies medications compatible or incompatible with each drug when administered via Y-site injection or 3-way stopcock in IV tubing. **Additive Compatibility/Incompatibility** identifies medications compatible or incompatible when admixed in solution. Compatibility of diluted medications administered through a Y-site for continuous or intermittent infusion is usually limited

HOW TO USE *DAVIS'S DRUG GUIDE FOR NURSES* 5

to 24 hours. **Solution Compatibility/Incompatibility** identifies compatible or incompatible solutions for dilution for administration purposes. Compatibility information is compiled from Trissel's *Handbook of Injectable Drugs*, 14th ed and *Micromedex*. Compatibility and incompatibility information is also located in charts contained in the **Medication Safety Tools** color insert. A printable version of syringe compatibilities is also available at www.drugguide.com.

Patient/Family Teaching: This section includes information that should be taught to patients and/or families of patients. Side effects that should be reported, information on minimizing and managing side effects, details on administration, and follow-up requirements are presented. The nurse also should refer to the **Implementation** section for specific information to teach to the patient and family about taking the medication. **Home Care Issues** discusses aspects to be considered for medications taken in the home setting.

Evaluation: Outcome criteria for determination of the effectiveness of the medication are provided.

EVIDENCE-BASED PRACTICE AND PHARMACOTHERAPEUTICS:
Implications for Nurses

Note: The content below is an excerpt from an article written exclusively for the 12th edition of **Davis's Drug Guide for Nurses**. To access the full article, visit **DavisPlus**, F.A. Davis's online center for student and instructor ancillaries, at http://davisplus.fadavis.com.

The purpose of evidence-based practice is to improve the outcomes of treatment for patients. How pharmacologic agents affect patients is often the subject of research; such research is required by the Food and Drug Administration (FDA) before and after drug approval. Any medication can be the subject of an evidence-based clinical review article. But what does "evidence-based" mean and how does it relate to nursing?

According to Ingersoll, "Evidence-based nursing practice is the conscientious, explicit, and judicious use of theory-derived, research-based information in making decisions about care delivery to individuals or groups of patients and in consideration of individual needs and preferences" (2000, p. 152). Still subject to debate are questions about the sufficiency and quality of evidence. For example, what kind of evidence is needed? How much evidence is necessary to support, modify, or change clinical practice? And, were the studies reviewed of "good" quality and are their results valid?

In general, clinicians use **hierarchy of evidence** schemas to rank types of research reports from the most valuable and scientifically rigorous to the least useful. The hierarchy makes clear that some level of evidence about the effect of a particular treatment or condition exists, even if the evidence is considered weak. Figure 1 illustrates a hierarchy of evidence pyramid with widely accepted rankings: the most scientifically rigorous at the top, the least scientifically rigorous at the bottom. Practitioners and clinicians should look for the highest level of available evidence to answer their clinical questions. However, it is important that clinicians also apply the second fundamental principle of EBP, which is that evidence alone is not sufficient to make clinical decisions. Decision makers must always trade off the benefits and risks, and the costs associated with alternative treatment options, and by doing so, consider the patients' values and preferences.

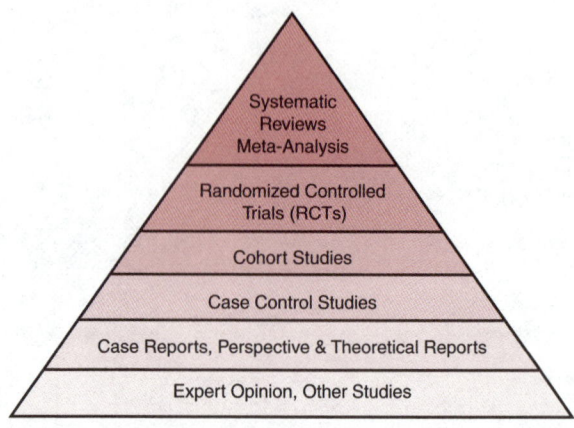

Figure 1: Hierarchy of Scientific Evidence Pyramid

Evidence-Based Practice and Its Importance in Pharmacology

Evidence-based practices in pharmacology generally are derived from well-designed randomized controlled trials (RCTs) or other experimental designs that investigate drugs' therapeutic and nontherapeutic effects. However, although FDA-approved pharmacologic agents have undergone rigorous testing through RCTs, nurses have the responsibility to evaluate the findings for the best scientific evidence available and to determine the most appropriate, safest, and efficacious drugs for their patients.

While numerous databases are available through Internet searches, two valuable and quickly accessible resources for evaluating the current highest level of pharmacologic evidence are 1) the Cochrane Database of Systematic Reviews and the Central Register of Controlled Trials and 2) the National Guidelines Clearinghouse (NGC), supported by the Agency for Healthcare Research and Quality (AHRQ). The Cochrane library and databases provide full text of high-quality, regularly updated systematic reviews, protocols, and clinical trials. The Web address is http://www.cochrane.org/reviews.clibintro.htm.

AHRQ's Evidence-Based Practice Centers (EPCs) provide evidence reports and technology assessments that can assist nurses in their efforts to provide the highest quality and safest pharmacologic health care available. The EPCs systematically review the relevant scientific literature, conduct additional analyses (when appropriate) prior to developing their reports and assessments, and provide guideline comparisons. The Web address is http://www.guideline.gov.

Evidence-based systematic reports and guidelines provide nurses with instantaneous access to the most current knowledge, enabling them to critically appraise the scientific evidence and its appropriateness to their patient population. This is especially important given the need for nurses to keep abreast of the rapidly changing pharmacologic agents in use. New drugs are approved each month, compelling nurses to know these drugs' intended uses, therapeutic effects, interactions, and adverse effects.

Evidence-based practice requires a shift from the traditional paradigm of clinical practice—grounded in intuition, clinical experience, and pathophysiologic rationale—to a paradigm in which nurses must combine clinical expertise, patient values and preferences, and clinical circumstances with the integration of the best scientific evidence in order to make conscientious, well-informed, research-based decisions that affect nursing patient care.

***

Linda S. Weglicki, PhD, RN, MSN
Health Scientist Administrator
Office of Extramural Programs
National Institute of Nursing Research
National Institutes of Health
Bethesda, Maryland

REFERENCES

1. DiCenso, A., Guyatt, G., & Ciliska, D. (2005). *Evidence-based nursing: A guide to clinical practice*. St. Louis, MO: Elsevier Mosby.
2. Guyatt, G., & Rennie, D. (2002). *Users' guide to the medical literature: Essentials of evidence-based clinical practice*. Chicago, IL: American Medical Association Press.
3. Ingersoll, G.L. (2000). "Evidence-based nursing: What it is and what it isn't." *Nursing Outlook*. 48(4), 151-152.

4. Institute of Medicine [IOM]. (2001). *Crossing the quality chasm: A new health system for the 21st century*. Washington, DC: National Academy Press.
5. Leavitt, S.B. (2003). Evidence-based addiction medicine for practitioners: Evaluating and using research evidence in clinical practice. Addiction Treatment Forum, March. Retrieved May, 2007, from http://www.atforum.com/SiteRoot/pages/addiction_resources/EBAM_16_Pager.pdf
6. Melnyk, B.M., & Fineout-Overholt, E. (2005). *Evidence-based practice in nursing & healthcare: A guide to best practice*. Philadelphia, PA: Lippincott Williams & Wilkins.
7. Mitchell, G.J. (1999). "Evidence-based practice: Critique and alternative view." *Nursing Science Quarterly*. 12, 30-35.
8. Polit, D.F., & Beck, C.T. (2008). *Nursing research: Generating and assessing evidence for practice*. (8th ed). Philadelphia, PA: Lippincott Williams & Wilkins.
9. Sackett, D., Rosenberg, W., Gray, J., Haynes, R., & Richardson, W. (1996). "Evidence-based medicine: What it is and what it isn't." *British Medical Journal*. 312, 71-72.

PHARMACOGENOMICS

Introduction
Multiple variables influence the selection and optimization of drug therapy for each individual patient. Pharmacogenomics, the study of the influence of individual genetic variations on drug response in patients, may yield additional information to further enhance safe and effective medication use. Whereas the field originally focused on the effects of specific variants within individual genes on drug response (i.e., pharmacogenetics), efforts increasingly examine the role of multiple variants across the genome and their potential relationship to drug therapy outcomes.

As our understanding of pharmacogenomics and the biological relevance of specific genetic variants in individuals' drug metabolizing enzymes, drug transporter proteins, and drug target receptors to certain drug responses has increased, we have learned that multiple variations across the genome can contribute to significant and relatively predictable treatment outcomes. Virtually every therapeutic area involving medication use includes a drug for which documented genetic variability has the potential to affect drug response. Some of this information is included in the FDA-approved package insert prescribing information. For some agents, the suitability of a specific drug or the determination of an appropriate initial dose for an individual patient based on pharmacogenetic information has been incorporated into dosing algorithms and patient care. As such, it is essential that health care professionals can interpret and utilize this information to facilitate safer and more effective use of medications for individual patients.

Genetic Variation within the Human Genome
The human genome is comprised of approximately 3 billion nucleotide base pair sequences that encode for molecular DNA with, except for identical twins, each individual having his/her own unique human genome sequence. Four nucleotide bases (adenine, guanine, cytosine, and thymine) are responsible for constituting the sequence of each single strand of DNA. Variations in nucleotide sequences can occur, and contribute to alterations in the expression and activities of certain genes. The location of these variations within a DNA sequence on a particular chromosome can have a profound impact on the ultimate biological activity or characteristic of that gene or lead to little or unknown consequences.

Proteins are involved in most enzymatic, structural, and biologic functions associated with drug disposition and effects. The processes involved in DNA replication, RNA transcription, and translation to synthesized proteins are complex. Each of these processes is potentially susceptible to consequences of DNA sequence variations.

Genetic variations can take many forms, including single nucleotide base substitutions (e.g., a cytosine substituted for an adenine), insertions or deletions of a nucleotide base within a sequence, and deletions or extra copies of entire DNA sequences. Variations in DNA that occur at a frequency of greater than 1% in the population are called polymorphisms. The most common genetic variations in humans are referred to as single nucleotide polymorphisms (SNPs) and result from the substitution of one nucleotide base for another. The specific location of a SNP within a gene is important. As mentioned previously, genetic variations can be of unknown or no clinical consequence or they can lead to a truncated, dysfunctional, or complete lack of protein product that is associated with an alteration in drug response.

Clinical Significance of Genetic Polymorphisms
SNPs and other genetic variations influence drug response at different levels through alterations in the activities of enzymes or proteins involved in drug absorption, transport, metabolism, elimination, or at the drug target receptor (site of drug action). Clinically relevant polymorphisms have been identified for genes that encode for most of the common enzymes involved in drug metabolism. Most enzymes

are localized intracellularly throughout a wide variety of tissues in the body, including the enterocytes that line the intestine and within hepatocytes. Variants that cause diminished or absent enzyme activity decrease drug metabolism processes. In this case, if the drug is metabolized to an inactive product, then the prolonged persistence of the parent drug in the body could result in excessive pharmacologic effects and potential toxicities may occur. If the drug requires enzymatic conversion to a pharmacologically active metabolite, drug response may be reduced or absent. In contrast, if the variation is due to extra copies of a gene that results in increased enzymatic activity, opposite effects on drug metabolism and response can occur.

Similar outcomes can be associated with polymorphisms in genes that encode for membrane transporter proteins that are responsible for drug transport into cells (influx), as well as proteins that participate in energy-dependent processes that export drugs out of cells (efflux transporters). Polymorphisms in drug transport proteins can influence drug response by altering drug gastrointestinal absorption, uptake and distribution in tissues, exposure to intracellular drug metabolizing enzymes, and elimination via the bile or urine. Finally, some genes that encode for certain drug receptors are highly polymorphic, resulting in attenuated or exaggerated drug responses. The number of polymorphic genes responsible for variations in drug response at drug receptors is relatively small compared to those associated with drug metabolizing enzymes or transport proteins; however, this area has undergone the least amount of study to date.

Incorporating Pharmacogenomic Information into Clinical Practice

Most drugs are initiated in individual patients based on knowledge about their safety and effectiveness within the general population. Information regarding patient characteristics (e.g., age, ethnicity, renal/hepatic function, concomitant disease, etc.) known to contribute to variability in drug response, when available, is considered at this time. Currently, there are more than 50 drugs with pharmacogenomic information included in the package insert. For selected agents, dosing recommendations based on an individual's genetic information (i.e., genotype) for specific drugs and drug classes are also considered. Genomic biomarkers can play an important role in identifying responders and non-responders, avoiding drug toxicity, and adjusting the dose of drugs to optimize their efficacy and safety. However, the typical strategy for most drug therapy is to monitor the patient's response to treatment and modify regimens as necessary. Patients who develop exaggerated pharmacologic responses or illicit no pharmacologic effect may be expressing a phenotype suggestive of altered drug disposition or target receptor effect that could be associated with an underlying genetic polymorphism. As we continue to learn more about these associations and can incorporate pharmacogenomic information into decisions regarding drug therapy for individual patients, the ultimate goal is to improve therapeutic outcomes by limiting drug exposure to patients that are most likely to derive no therapeutic benefit and/or experience toxic drug effects.

For example, some genetic variants are associated with hypersensitivity reactions to a specific drug. A prescriber who is contemplating initiating that drug for a patient may determine whether the patient possesses that variant in his or her DNA. If that specific variant is present, the prescriber might select an alternate agent, thereby avoiding a potentially life-threatening hypersensitivity reaction. In another example, patients who are determined to have a genetic variant that results in an inactive metabolizing enzyme would not be appropriate candidates for an analgesic drug that requires that enzyme to convert the drug to the active analgesia-producing form. On the other hand, if that metabolizing enzyme is responsible for conversion of an active parent drug to an inactive metabolite, the starting dose of the drug may be reduced or perhaps an alternate drug might be selected.

Several Clinical Laboratory Improvement Amendment (CLIA)-approved laboratories offer pharmacogenetic testing to identify relevant genetic polymorphisms that predict drug response and can be used to initiate appropriate drugs and dosing regimens for individual patients. Some of these tests, while recommended in drug prescribing information, are costly and may not be covered by insurance. Patients may not fully understand the utility of undergoing genetic testing and providing a specimen for DNA analysis, which is typically performed on a blood, saliva, buccal swab, or other tissue collection. On the other hand, patients who are engaged in their medical care may be familiar with the concept of "personalized medicine" and seek information about available tests to "individualize" their own drug therapy. Currently, four drugs are required to have pharmacogenetic testing performed before they are prescribed: cetuximab, trastuzumab, maraviroc, and dasatinib. Other drugs have labeling that include "test recommended" or "for information only". Health care professionals will need to be familiar with pharmacogenetic tests that are recommended for specific drug therapies, how to interpret the results of those tests, and how to incorporate pharmacogenetic data with other clinical information to optimize patient drug therapy and health care outcomes.

Pertinent Resources:

Aquilante CL, Zineh I, Beitelshees AL, Langaee TY. Common laboratory methods in pharmacogenomics studies. *Am J Health-Syst Pharm* 2006;63:2101-10.

Court MH. A pharmacogenomics primer. *J Clin Pharmacol* 2007;47:1087-1103.

Evans WE, McLeod HL. Pharmacogenomics – drug disposition, drug targets, and side effects. *N Engl J Med* 2003;348:538-49.

Evans WE, Relling MV. Moving towards individualized medicine with pharmacogenomics. *Nature* 2004;429:464-8.

NCBI Genetics Primer: http://www.ncbi.nlm.nih.gov/About/primer/genetics_molecular.html

Roden DM, Altman RB, Benowitz NL, et al. Pharmacogenomics: challenges and opportunities. *Ann Intern Med* 2006;145:749-57.

Shin J, Kayser SR, Langaee TY. Pharmacogenetics: from discovery to patient care. *Am J Health-Syst Pharm* 2009;66:625-37.

Weiss ST, McLeod HL, Flockhart DA, et al. Creating and evaluating genetic tests predictive of drug response. *Nat Rev Drug Disc* 2008;7:568-74.

Wilkinson GR. Drug metabolism and variability among patients in drug response. *N Engl J Med* 2005; 352:2211-21.

MEDICATION ERRORS: Improving Practices and Patient Safety

It is widely acknowledged that medication errors result in thousands of adverse drug events, preventable reactions, and deaths per year. Nurses, physicians, pharmacists, patient safety organizations, the Food and Drug Administration, the pharmaceutical industry, and other parties share in the responsibility for determining how medication errors occur and designing strategies to reduce error.

One impediment to understanding the scope and nature of the problem has been the reactive "blaming, shaming, training" culture that singled out one individual as the cause of the error. Also historically, medication errors that did not result in patient harm—near-miss situations in which an error could have but didn't happen—or errors that did not result in serious harm were not reported. In contrast, serious errors often instigated a powerful punitive response in which one or a few persons were deemed to be at fault and, as a result, lost their jobs and sometimes their licenses.

In 1999, the Institute of Medicine (IOM) published *To Err Is Human: Building a Safer Health System*, which drew attention to the problem of medication errors. It pointed out that excellent health care providers do make medication errors, that many of the traditional processes involved in the medication-use system were error-prone, and that other factors, notably drug labeling and packaging, contributed to error. Furthermore, the IOM report, in conjunction with other groups such as the United States Pharmacopeia (USP) and the Institute for Safe Medication Practices (ISMP), called for the redesign of error-prone systems to include processes that anticipated the fallibility of humans working within the system. This initiative is helping shift the way the health care industry addresses medication errors from a single person/bad apple cause to a systems issue.[1]

The National Coordinating Council for Medication Error Reporting and Prevention (NCC-MERP) developed the definition of a medication error that reflects this shift and captures the scope and breadth of the issue:

"A medication error is any preventable event that may cause or lead to inappropriate medication use or patient harm while the medication is in the control of the health care professional, patient, or consumer. Such events may be related to professional practice, health care products, procedures, and systems, including prescribing; order communication; product labeling, packaging, and nomenclature; compounding; dispensing; distribution; administration; education; monitoring; and use."[2]

Inherent in this definition's mention of related factors are the human factors that are part of the medication use system. For example, a nurse or pharmacist may automatically reach into the bin where dobutamine is usually kept, see "do" and "amine" but select dopamine instead of dobutamine. Working amidst distractions, working long hours or shorthanded, and working in a culture where perfection is expected and questioning is discouraged are other examples of the human factors and environmental conditions that contribute to error.

The goal for the design of any individual or hospital-wide medication use system is to determine where systems are likely to fail and to build in safeguards that minimize the potential for error. One way to begin that process is to become familiar with medications or practices that have historically been shown to be involved in serious errors.

High Alert Medications

Some medications, because of a narrow therapeutic range or inherent toxic nature, have a high risk of causing devastating injury or death if improperly ordered, prepared, stocked, dispensed, administered, or monitored. Although these medications may not be involved in more errors, they require special attention due to the potential for serious, possibly fatal consequences. These have been termed **high-alert medications**, to communicate the need for extra care and safeguards. Many of

MEDICATION ERRORS: IMPROVING PRACTICES AND PATIENT SAFETY

these drugs are used commonly in the general population or are used frequently in urgent clinical situations. The Joint Commission (TJC) monitors the use of frequently prescribed high-alert medications, which include insulin, opiates and narcotics, injectable potassium chloride (or phosphate) concentrate, intravenous anticoagulants (such as heparin), sodium chloride solutions above 0.9 percent, and others. See the High Alert Drugs table in the **Medication Safety Tools** color insert, and Table 2 in this article for a complete list of the high alert meds found in *Davis's Drug Guide for Nurses*. (Visit the Institute for Safe Medication Practices at www.ismp.org for more information on high alert drugs.)

Causes of Medication Errors

Many contributing factors and discrete causes of error have been identified, including failed communication, poor drug distribution practices, dose miscalculations, drug packaging and drug-device related problems, incorrect drug administration, and lack of patient education.[3]

Failed Communication: Failed communication covers many of the errors made in the ordering phase, and although ordering is performed by the prescriber, the nurse, the clerk, and the pharmacist who interpret that order are also involved in the communication process.

- *Poorly handwritten or verbal orders.* Handwriting is a major source of error and has led to inaccurate interpretations of the drug intended, the route of administration, the frequency, and dose. Telephone and verbal orders are likewise prone to misinterpretation.
- *Drugs with similar-sounding or similar-looking names.* Similar sounding names, or names that look similar when handwritten, are frequently confused. Amiodarone and amrinone (now renamed inamrinone to help prevent confusion), or Zebeta® and Diabeta® are two examples. The USP has identified over 700 "sound-alike, look-alike" drugs. Mix-ups are more likely when each drug has similar dose ranges and frequencies. Several of the sound-alike/look-alike drugs were targeted for labeling intervention by the FDA, which requested manufacturers of 33 drugs with look-alike names to voluntarily revise the appearance of the established names. The revision visually differentiates the drug names by using "tall man" letters (capitals) to highlight distinguishing syllables (ex.: acetoHEXAMIDE versus acetaZOLAMIDE or buPROPrion versus busPIRone. See the TALL MAN Lettering table in the **Medication Safety Tools** color insert for the list of the pairs of drugs that are commonly confused, often with serious consequences.
- *Misuse of zeroes in decimal numbers.* Massive, ten-fold overdoses are traceable to not using a leading zero (.2 mg instead of 0.2 mg) or adding an unnecessary trailing zero (2.0 mg instead of 2 mg) in decimal expressions of dose. Similar overdosages are found in decimal expressions in which the decimal point is obscured by poor handwriting, stray marks, or lined orders sheets (e.g., reading 3.1 grams as 31 grams). Under-dosing also may occur by the same mechanism and prevent a desired, perhaps life-saving effect.
- *Use of apothecary measures (grains, drams) or package units (amps, vials, tablets) instead of metric measures (grams, milligrams, milliequivalents).* Apothecary measurements are poorly understood and their abbreviations are easily confused with other units of measurement. Use of such measures should be abandoned. Errors also occur when dosage units are used instead of metric weight. For example, orders for 2 tablets, 1½ vials, or 2 ampules can result in overdose or underdose when the medications ordered come in various strengths.
- *Misinterpreted abbreviations.* Abbreviations can be misinterpreted or, when used in the dosage part of the order, can result in incorrect dosage of the correct medication. For example, lower or uppercase "U" for units has been read as a zero, making 10 u of insulin look like 100 units when handwritten. The Latin abbreviation "QOD" for every other day has been misinterpreted as QID (4 times per day). See Table 2 for a list of confusing abbreviations and safer alternatives.
- *Ambiguous or incomplete orders.* Orders that do not clearly specify dose, route, frequency, or indication do not communicate complete information and are open to misinterpretation.

Poor Distribution Practices: Poor distribution includes error-prone storing practices such as keeping similar-looking products next to each other. Dispensing multidose floor stock vials of potentially dangerous drugs instead of unit doses is also associated with error as is allowing non-pharmacists to dispense medications in the absence of the pharmacist.

Dose Miscalculations: Dose miscalculations are a prime source of medication error. Also, many medications need to be dose-adjusted for renal or hepatic impairment, age, height and weight, and body composition (i.e., correct for obesity). Complicated dosing formulas provide many opportunities to introduce error. Often vulnerable populations, such as premature infants, children, the elderly, and those with serious underlying illnesses, are at greatest risk.

Drug Packaging and Drug Delivery Systems: Similar packaging or poorly designed packaging encourages error. Drug companies may use the same design for different formulations, or fail to highlight information about concentration or strength. Lettering, type size, color, and packaging methods can either help or hinder drug identification.

Drug delivery systems include infusion pumps and rate controllers. Some models do not prevent free flow of medication, leading to sudden high dose infusion of potent and dangerous medications. The lack of safeguards preventing free flow and programming errors are among the problems encountered with infusion control devices.

Incorrect Drug Administration: Incorrect drug administration covers many problems. Misidentification of a patient, incorrect route of administration, missed doses, or improper drug preparation are types of errors that occur during the administration phase.

Lack of Patient Education: Safe medication use is enhanced in the hospital and the home when the patient is well informed. The knowledgeable patient can recognize when something has changed in his or her medication regimen and can question the health care provider. At the same time, many issues related to medication errors, such as ambiguous directions, unfamiliarity with a drug, and confusing packaging, affect the patient as well as the health care provider, underscoring the need for careful education. Patient education also enhances adherence, which is a factor in proper medication use.

Prevention Strategies

Since medication use systems are complex and involve many steps and people, they are error-prone. On an individual basis, nurses can help reduce the incidence of error by implementing the following strategies:

- Clarify any order that is not obviously and clearly legible. Ask the prescriber to print orders using block style letters.
- Do not accept orders with the abbreviation "u" or "IU" for units. Clarify the dosage and ask the prescriber to write out the word units.
- Clarify any abbreviated drug name or the abbreviated dosing frequencies q.d., QD, q.o.d., QOD, and q.i.d or QID. Suggest abandoning Latin abbreviations in favor of spelling out dosing frequency.
- Do not accept doses expressed in package units or volume instead of metric weight. Clarify any order written for number of ampules, vials, or tablets (e.g., calcium chloride, 1 ampule or epinephrine, 1 Bristojet).
- Decimal point errors can be hard to see. Suspect a missed decimal point and clarify any order if the dose requires more than 3 dosing units.
- If dose ordered requires use of multiple dosage units or very small fractions of a dose unit, review the dose, have another health care provider check the original order and recalculate formulas, and confirm the dose with the prescriber.
- If taking a verbal order, ask prescriber to spell out the drug name and dosage to avoid sound-alike confusion (e.g., hearing Cerebyx for Celebrex, or fifty for fifteen). Read back the order to the prescriber after you have written it in the chart. Confirm and document the indication to further enhance accurate communication.
- Clarify any order that does not include metric weight, dosing frequency, or route of administration.
- Check the nurse's/clerk's transcription against the original order. Make sure stray marks or initials do not obscure the original order.

- Do not start a patient on new medication by borrowing medications from another patient. This action bypasses the double check provided by the pharmacist's review of the order.
- Always check the patient's name band before administering medications. Verbally addressing a patient by name does not provide sufficient identification.
- Use the facility's standard drug administration times to reduce the chance of an omission error.
- Be sure to fully understand any drug administration device before using it. This includes infusion pumps, inhalers, and transdermal patches.
- Have a second practitioner independently check original order, dosage calculations, and infusion pump settings for high alert medications.
- Realize that the printing on packaging boxes, vials, ampoules, prefilled syringes, or any container in which a medication is stored can be misleading. Be sure to differentiate clearly the medication and the number of milligrams per milliliter versus the total number of milligrams contained within. Massive overdoses have been administered by assuming that the number of milligrams per ml is all that is contained within the vial or ampule. Read the label when obtaining the medication, before preparing or pouring the medication, and after preparing or pouring the medication.
- Educate patients about the medications they take. Provide verbal and written instructions and ask the patient to restate important points. Refer to Educating Patients about Safe Medication Use on page 27 for recommendations on what patients should understand about their medications.

As stated previously, errors are a result of problems within the medication use system and cannot be eliminated by the vigilance of any one group of health care providers. System redesign involves strong leadership from administration and all involved departments. Health care facilities should consider the following when addressing the issue of medication errors:

- Do not provide unit stock of critical, high alert medications. If eliminating these medications from floor stock is not feasible, consider reducing the number available and standardizing the concentrations or forms in which the medication is available.
- Create committees that address safety issues.
- Install a computer physician order entry (CPOE) system to help reduce prescribing orders. Link order entry to pertinent lab, allergy, and medication data.
- Implement bar code technology to ensure the right drug reaches the right patient.
- Develop policies that discourage error-prone prescribing practices such as inappropriate use of verbal orders, use of confusing dosing symbols, and use of abbreviations.
- Develop policies that encourage better communication of medication information such as requiring block-style printing of medications, including indication in prescription, and using both the trade and generic name in prescriptions.
- Ensure a reasonable workload for pharmacists and nurses, and provide a well-designed work area.
- Limit the availability of varying concentrations of high alert medications.
- Provide standard concentrations and infusion rate tables.
- Supply pharmacy and patient care areas with current reference material.
- Cultivate a culture that does not assign blame when medication errors occur but looks for root causes instead.
- Encourage staff to participate in the USP-ISMP-MERP error reporting program.

REFERENCES

1. Kohn, L.T., Corrigan, J.M., and Donaldson, M.S. (eds). *To Err Is Human: Building a Safer Health System.* National Academy Press, Washington, DC (1999).
2. National Coordinating Council for Medication Error Reporting and Prevention. http://www.nccmerp.org/aboutMedErrors.html
3. Cohen, M.R. *Medication Errors: Causes, Prevention, Risk Management.* Jones and Bartlett Publishers, Sudbury (1999).
4. Branowicki, P., et al. "Improving complex medication systems: an interdisciplinary approach." *J Nurs Adm.* (2003) Apr; 33(4):199-200.

5. Burke, K.G. "Executive summary: the state of the science on safe medication administration symposium." *J Infus Nurs.* (2005). Mar-Apr; 28(2 Suppl):4-9.
6. McPhillips, H.A., et al. "Potential medication dosing errors in outpatient pediatrics." *J Pediatr.* (2005) Dec; 147(6):727-8.
7. ISMP. "What's in a name? Ways to prevent dispensing errors linked to name confusion." *ISMP Medication Safety Alert!* 7(12) June 12, 2002. http://www.ismp.org/Newsletters/acutecare/archives/Jun02.asp
8. Santell, J.P., Cousins, D.D., "Medication Errors Related to Product Names." *Joint Commission J Qual Pt. Safety* (2005); 31:649-54.

Table 1: High Alert Medications in Davis's Drug Guide for Nurses

aldesleukin	erlotinib	mitoxantrone
alemtuzumab	esmolol	morphine
alitretinoin	etoposides	nalbuphine
amiodarone	fentanyl (buccal, transmucosal)	nateglinide
amphotericin B cholesteryl sulfate/ lipid complex/liposome	fentanyl (parenteral)	nesiritide
argatroban	fentanyl (transdermal)	nilotinib
arsenic trioxide	fludarabine	nitroprusside
asparaginase	fluorouracil	norepinephrine
azacitidine	fondaparinux	oxaliplatin
bendamustine	gefitinib	oxycodone compound
bevacizumab	gemcitabine	oxymorphone
bivalirudin	gemtuzumab ozogamicin	oxytocin
bleomycin	heparin	paclitaxel
bortezomib	heparins (low molecular weight)	pancuronium
buprenorphine	hydrocodone	panitumumab
busulfan	hydromorphone	pazopanib
butorphanol	hydroxyurea	pegaspargase
capecitabine	hypoglycemic agents, oral	pemetrexed
carboplatin	idarubicin	pentazocine
carmustine	ifosfamide	potassium phosphates
cetuximab	imatinib	potassium supplements
chloralhydrate	insulin mixtures	pramlintide
chlorambucil	insulins (intermediate-acting)	procarbazine
cisplatin	insulins (long-acting)	promethazine (IV)
cladribine	insulins (rapid-acting)	propofol
clofarabine	insulins (short-acting)	propranolol
codeine	irinotecan	repaglinide
colchicine (IV)	ixabepilone	rituximab
cyclophosphamide	labetalol	sodium chloride (hypertonic)
cytarabine	lapatinib	sunitinib
dacarbazine	lepirudin	temsirolimus
DAUNOrubicin hydrochloride	lidocaine	thalidomide
decitabine	magnesium sulfate (IV, parenteral)	thioguanine
digoxin	mechlorethamine	thrombolytic agents
DOBUTamine	melphalan	tirofiban
docetaxel	meperidine	topotecan
DOPamine	methadone	trastuzumab
DOXOrubicin hydrochloride	methotrexate	vinBLAStine
DOXOrubicin hydrochloride liposome	metoprolol	vinCRIStine
epinephrine	midazolam	vinorelbine
epirubicin	milrinone	warfarin
eptifibatide	mitomycin	

Table 2: Abbreviations and Symbols Associated with Medication Errors

Abbreviation/Symbol	Intended Meaning	Mistaken For	Recommendation
AZT	Zidovudine	Azathioprine	Use full drug name
CPZ	Compazine (prochlorperazine)	Thorazine (chlorpromazine)	Use full drug name
HCl	Hydrochloric acid	KCl (potassium chloride)	Use full drug name
HCT	Hydrocortisone	Hydrochlorothiazide	Use full drug name
HCTZ	Hydrochlorothiazide	Hydrocortisone	Use full drug name
MgSO$_4$*	Magnesium sulfate	Morphine sulfate	Use full drug name
MS, MSO$_4$*	Morphine sulfate	Magnesium sulfate	Use full drug name
MTX	Methotrexate	Mitoxantrone	Use full drug name
Nitro drip	Nitroglycerin	Nitroprusside	Use full drug name
Norflox	Norfloxacin	Norflex (orphenadrine)	Use full drug name
PCA	Procainamide	Patient controlled analgesia	Use full drug name
PIT	Pitocin (oxytocin)	Pitressin (vasopressin)	Use full drug name
SSRI	Sliding scale regular insulin	Selective serotonin reuptake inhibitor	Spell out "sliding scale regular insulin"
μg†	Microgram	Mg (milligram)	Use mcg
/ (slash mark)	"per"	"1" (numeral one)	Spell out "per"
HS or hs	Half strength or hour of sleep (at bedtime)	One mistaken for the other	Spell out "half strength" or "bedtime"
D/C	Discharge or discontinue	One mistaken for the other	Spell out "discharge" or "discontinue"
+	Plus sign	"4" (numeral four)	Spell out "and"
Zero **after** a decimal point (e.g., 1.0 mg)*	1 mg	10 mg	DO NOT USE zero after a decimal point
No zero **before** a decimal point (e.g., .1 mg)*	.1 mg	1 mg	ALWAYS USE zero before a decimal point
u or U*	units	0 (zero), 4 (four) or cc	Spell out "units"
I.U.*	International Units	IV or 10	Spell out "units"
q.d. or QD*	Every day	q.i.d. (4 times per day)	Write out "daily"
q.o.d. or QOD*	Every other day	q.i.d. (4 times per day) or qd (daily)	Write out "every other day"
TIW	3 times a week	3 times a day or twice a week	Spell out "3 times weekly"
IN	Intranasal	IM or IV	Spell out "intranasal" or use "NAS"
SC, SQ, sub q	Subcutaneously	SC mistaken as SL (sublingual), SQ as "5 every" or "every"	Use subcut or write out "subcutaneously"
AD, AS, AU	Right ear, left ear, each ear	OD, OS, OU (right eye, left eye, each eye)	Spell out "right ear", "left ear", "each ear"
OD, OS, OU	Right eye, left eye, each eye	AD, AS, AU (right ear, left ear, each ear)	Spell out "right eye", "left eye", "each eye"
Cc†	cubic centimeters	u (units)	Use ml
@†	At	2	Use "at"
>†	Greater than	7 or <	Spell out "greater than"
<†	Less than	L or >	Spell out "less than"
&	And	2	Use "and"
°	Hour	Zero (q 1° seen as q 10)	Use "hr", "h", or "hour"
Drug name and dose run together. Example: Inderal40 mg	Inderal 40 mg	Inderal 140 mg	Leave space between drug name, dose, and unit of measure
Numerical dose and unit of measure run together. Example: 10mg	10 mg	100 mg	Leave space between drug dose and unit of measure

*Appears on TJC's "Do Not Use" list of abbreviations.
†May be considered by TJC for possible inclusion in the "Do Not Use" list in the future.
Modified from The Institute for Safe Medication Practices Safety Alert, Vol 8: Issue 24. Nov 27, 2003.

DETECTING AND MANAGING ADVERSE DRUG REACTIONS

An *adverse drug reaction* (ADR) is any unexpected, undesired, or excessive response to a medication that results in:
- temporary or permanent serious harm or disability
- admission to a hospital, transfer to a higher level of care, or prolonged stay
- death.

Adverse drug reactions are distinguished from adverse drug events, in which causality is uncertain, and side effects, which may be bothersome to the patient and necessitate a change in therapy but are not considered serious.[1] Although some ADRs are the result of medication errors, many are not.

Types of ADRs
The Food and Drug Administration (FDA) classifies ADRs into 2 broad categories: Type A and Type B.[2] Type A reactions are predictable reactions based on the primary or secondary pharmacologic effect of the drug. Dose-related reactions and drug-drug interactions are examples of Type A reactions. Type B reactions are unpredictable, are not related to dose, and are not the result of the drug's primary or secondary pharmacologic effect. Idiosyncratic and hypersensitivity reactions are examples of Type B reactions.

Dose-Related Reactions (Toxic Reactions): In dose related reactions, the dose prescribed for the patient is excessive. Although a variety of mechanisms may interact, reasons for this type of reaction include:
- renal or hepatic impairment
- extremes in age (neonates and frail elderly)
- drug-drug or drug-food interactions
- underlying illness. Dose-related reactions are often the result of preventable errors in prescribing in which physiologic factors such as age, renal impairment, and weight were not considered sufficiently, or in inadequate therapeutic monitoring. Medications with narrow therapeutic ranges (digoxin, aminoglycosides, antiepileptic drugs) and those that require careful monitoring or laboratory testing (anticoagulants, nephrotoxic drugs) are most frequently implicated in dose-related reactions.[3,4] Dose-related reactions usually are managed successfully by temporarily discontinuing the drug and then reducing the dose or increasing the dosing interval. In some instances, the toxic effects need to be treated with another agent (e.g., Digibind for digoxin toxicity or Kayexalate for drug induced hyperkalemia). Appropriately timed therapeutic drug level monitoring, review of new drugs added to an existing regimen that may affect the drug level, and frequent assessment of relevant laboratory values are critical to safe medical management and prevention of dose-related reactions.

Drug-Drug Interactions: Drug-drug interactions occur when the pharmacokinetic or pharmacodynamic properties of an individual drug affect another drug. Pharmacokinetics refers to the way the body processes a medication (absorption, distribution, metabolism, and elimination). In a drug-drug interaction, the pharmacokinetic properties of one drug can cause a change in drug concentration of another drug and an altered response. For example, one drug may block enzymes that metabolize a second drug. The concentration of the second drug is then increased and may become toxic or cause adverse reactions. Pharmacodynamic drug-drug interactions involve the known effects and side-effects of the drugs. For example, two drugs with similar therapeutic effects may act together in a synergistic way. The increased anticoagulant effects that occur when warfarin and aspirin are taken together, or the increased central nervous system (CNS) depression that results when two drugs with CNS depressant effects potentiate each other, are examples of pharmacodymanic drug-drug interactions. Certain classes of drugs are more likely to result in serious drug-drug

DETECTING AND MANAGING ADVERSE DRUG REACTIONS

interactions, and patients receiving these agents should be monitored carefully. The medication classes include anticoagulants, oral hypoglycemic agents, nonsteroidal anti-inflammatory agents, monoamine oxidase inhibitors, antihypertensives, antiepileptics, and antiretrovirals. In addition, specific drugs such as theophylline, cimetidine, lithium, and digoxin may result in serious ADRs.

Idiosyncratic Reactions: Idiosyncratic reactions occur without relation to dose and are unpredictable and sporadic. Reactions of this type may manifest in many different ways, including fever, blood dyscrasias, cardiovascular effects, or mental status changes. The time frame between the occurrence of a problem and initiation of therapy is sometimes the only clue linking drug to symptom. Some idiosyncratic reactions may be explained by genetic differences in drug-metabolizing enzymes.

Hypersensitivity Reactions: Hypersensitivity reactions are usually allergic responses. Manifestations of hypersensitivity reactions range from mild rashes, to nephritis, pneumonitis, hemolytic anemia, and anaphylaxis. Protein drugs (vaccines, enzymes) are frequently associated with hypersensitivity reactions. In most instances, antibody formation is involved in the process and therefore cross-sensitivity may occur. An example of this is hypersensitivity to penicillin and cross-sensitivity with other penicillins and/or cephalosporins. Documenting drugs to which the patient is allergic and the specific hypersensitivity reaction is very important. If the reaction to an agent is anaphylaxis the nurse should monitor the patient during administration of a cross-hypersensitive agent, especially during the initial dose, and ensure ready access to emergency resuscitative equipment.

Recognizing an ADR

Adverse drug reactions should be suspected whenever there is a negative change in a patient's condition, particularly when a new drug has been introduced. Strategies that can enhance recognition include knowing the side effect/adverse reaction profile of medications. Nurses should be familiar with a drug's most commonly encountered side effects and adverse reactions before administering it. (In *Davis's Drug Guide for Nurses*, side effects are underlined, and adverse reactions are CAPITALIZED and appear in second color in the **Adverse Reactions and Side Effects** section.) As always, monitoring the patient's response to a medication and ongoing assessment are key nursing actions. Learn to recognize patient findings that suggest an ADR has occurred. These include:

- rash
- change in respiratory rate, heart rate, blood pressure, or mental state
- seizure
- anaphylaxis
- diarrhea
- fever.

Any of these findings can suggest an ADR and should be reported and documented promptly so that appropriate interventions, including discontinuation of suspect medications, can occur. Prompt intervention can prevent a mild adverse reaction from escalating into a serious health problem. Other steps taken by the health care team when identifying and treating an ADR include:

1. Determining that the drug ordered was the drug given and intended.
2. Determining that the drug was given in the correct dosage by the correct route.
3. Establishing the chronology of events: time drug was taken and onset of symptoms.
4. Stopping the drug and monitoring patient status for improvement (dechallenge).
5. Restarting the drug, if appropriate, and monitoring closely for adverse reactions (rechallenge).[2]

Prevention

Health care organizations have responded to consumer, regulator, and insurer pressures by developing programs that aim to eliminate preventable ADRs. In the inpatient setting, computer systems can display the patient's age, height, weight, and creatinine clearance or serum creatinine concentration and send an alert to the clinician if a prescribed dose is out of range for any of the displayed parameters. Allergy alerts and drug-drug interactions can be presented to the clinician at the time an order is entered.

In the outpatient setting, strategies that increase the patient's knowledge base and access to pharmacists and nurses may help prevent adverse reactions.[5] Outpatient pharmacy computer systems that are linked within a chain of pharmacies may allow the pharmacist to view the patient's profile if the patient is filling a prescription in a pharmacy other than the usual one. Many pharmacy computers have dose limits and drug-drug reaction verification to assist pharmacists filling orders.

Such strategies are a valuable auxiliary to, but cannot replace, conscientious history taking, careful patient assessment, and ongoing monitoring. A thorough medication history including all prescription and nonprescription drugs, all side effects and adverse reactions encountered, allergies, and all pertinent physical data should be available to the prescriber. The prescriber is responsible for reviewing this data, along with current medications, laboratory values, and any other variable that affects drug response.

It is not expected that practitioners will remember all relevant information when prescribing. In fact, reliance on memory is error-fraught, and clinicians need to use available resources to verify drug interactions whenever adding a new drug to the regimen. Setting expectations that clinicians use evidence-based information rather than their memories when prescribing, dispensing, administering or monitoring patients has the potential to reduce the incidence of preventable ADRs.

Food and Drug Administration MedWatch Program

To monitor and assess the incidence of adverse reactions, the FDA sponsors MedWatch, a program that allows health care practitioners and consumers the opportunity to report serious adverse reactions or product defects encountered from medications, medical devices, special nutritional products, or other FDA-regulated items. The FDA considers serious those reactions that result in death, life-threatening illness or injury, hospitalization, disability, congenital anomaly, or those that require medical/surgical intervention.

In addition to reporting serious adverse reactions, health care providers should also report problems related to suspected contamination, questionable stability, defective components, or poor packaging/labeling. Reports should be submitted even if there is some uncertainty about the cause/effect relationship or if some details are missing. This reporting form may be accessed at www.fda.gov/medwatch/report/hcp.htm. Reports also may be faxed to the FDA (1-800-FDA-0178). Reactions to vaccines should be reported to the Vaccine Adverse Event Reporting System (VAERS; 1-800-822-7967). Nurses share with other health care providers an obligation to report adverse reactions to the MedWatch program so that all significant data can be analyzed for opportunities to improve patient care.

REFERENCES

1. Lehmann, J. "Adverse Events - Adverse Reactions." *Drug Intel* (2002-2003) http://www.drugintel.com/public/medwatch/adverse_drug_events.htm (accessed 10 July 2003).
2. Goldman, S., Kennedy, D., Lieberman, R., "Clinical Therapeutics and the Recognition of Drug-Induced Disease." FDA MEDWATCH Continuing Education Article (1995) http://www.fda.gov/medwatch/articles/dig/rcontent.htm#toc (accessed 10 July 2003).
3. Daniels C., Calis K., "Clinical Analysis of Adverse Drug Reactions." Pharmacy Update National Institutes of Health. Sept-Oct 2001. http://www.cc.nih.gov/phar/updates/septoct01/01sept-oct.html (accessed 10 July 2003).
4. Winterstein A., et. al. "Identifying Clinically Significant Preventable Adverse Drug Events Through a Hospital's Database of Adverse Drug Reaction Reports." *Am J Health-Syst Pharm* 59(18):1742-1749, 2002.

5. Ghandi T., Weingart S., Borus J., et. al. "Adverse Drug Events in Ambulatory Care." *New England Journal of Medicine.* Volume 348:1556-1564. Number 16. April 17, 2003.
6. Bennett CL, et al. "The Research on Adverse Drug Events and Reports (RADAR) project." *JAMA.* 2005 May 4;293(17):2131-40.
7. Field TS, et al. "The costs associated with adverse drug events among older adults in the ambulatory setting." *Med Care.* 2005 Dec;43(12):1171-6.
8. Petrone K, Katz P. "Approaches to appropriate drug prescribing for the older adult." *Prim Care.* 2005 Sep;32(3):755-75.
9. Pezalla E. "Preventing adverse drug reactions in the general population." *Manag Care Interface.* 2005 Oct;18(10):49-52.

OVERVIEW OF RISK EVALUATION AND MITIGATION SYSTEMS (REMS)

Over the past several decades, the Food and Drug Administration (FDA) has employed a number of "risk management" programs designed to detect, evaluate, prevent, and mitigate drug adverse events for drugs with the potential for serious adverse drug reactions. Some of the risk management plans used by the FDA over the years have included the use of patient package inserts, medication guides, restricted access programs, and classification of drugs as controlled substances. These programs were acknowledged by the FDA as Risk Minimization Action Plans (RiskMAPS) in 2005. With these programs, the FDA only had the authority to mandate postmarketing commitments from drug manufacturers before the drug was approved; however, these requirements could not be enforced after the drug was approved.

The Food and Drug Administration Amendments Act of 2007 has given the FDA the authority to subject drugs to new risk identification and communication strategies in the postmarketing period. These new strategies, called Risk Evaluation and Mitigation Strategies (REMS), can be required for any drug or drug class that is associated with serious risks. The FDA can require a REMS if it believes that this program is necessary to ensure that the benefits outweigh the potential risks of the drug. The FDA can require a REMS either as part of the drug approval process or during the postmarketing period if new information becomes available regarding potentially harmful effects that are associated with the use of the drug.

Components of the REMS may include a medication guide, a patient package insert, a communication plan, other elements to ensure safe use, and/or an implementation system. A REMS for New Drug Applications or Biologics License Applications requires a timetable for submission of assessment of the REMS. A variety of elements to ensure safe use of drugs can be required as part of the REMS if it is believed that a medication guide, patient package insert, or communication plan are not adequate to mitigate the serious risks associated with a particular drug. These elements may include the following:

- Health care providers who prescribe the drug are specifically trained and/or certified.
- Pharmacies, practitioners, or health care settings that dispense the drug are specifically trained and/or certified.
- The drug is dispensed to patients only in certain health care settings, such as hospitals, or physicians' offices.
- The drug is dispensed only to patients with evidence or other documentation of safe-use conditions, such as laboratory test results.
- Patients using the drug are subject to certain monitoring.
- Patients using the drug are enrolled in a registry.

The FDA maintains an updated list of these REMS programs at http://www.fda.gov/Drugs/DrugSafety/PostmarketDrugSafetyInformationforPatientsandProviders/ucm111350.htm. As of December, 2009, the drugs that have approved REMS programs include the following:

Brand Name	Generic Name
(Actiq)	fentanyl (transmucosal)
(Actoplus Met/Actoplus Met XR)	pioglitazone/metformin
(Actos)	pioglitazone
(Advair Diskus/HFA)	fluticasone/salmeterol
(Amnesteem/Claravis/Sotret)	isotretinoin
(Androgel/Testim)	testosterone
(Aplenzin)	bupropion
(Avandamet)	rosiglitazone/metformin
(Avandaryl)	rosiglitazone/glimepiride
(Avelox)	moxifloxacin
(Banzel)	rufinamide
(Botox/Botox Cosmetic)	onabotulinum toxin A
(Cambia)	diclofenac potassium
(Cimzia)	certolizumab pegol
(Cipro/Proquin XR)	ciprofloxacin
(Clozaril/Fazaclo ODT)	clozapine
(Colcrys)	colchicine
(Creon/Zenpap)	pancrelipase
(Darvon/Darvon-N/Darvocet-N)	propoxyphene

OVERVIEW OF RISK EVALUATION AND MITIGATION SYSTEMS (REMS) 23

(Duetact)	pioglitazone/glimepiride
(Dysport)	abobotulinum toxin A
(Edluar)	zolpidem (sublingual tablets)
(Effexor/Effexor XR)	venlafaxine
(Effient)	prasugrel
(Embeda)	morphine sulfate/naltrexone
(Enbrel)	etanercept
(Entereg)	alvimopan
(Epzicom)	abacavir/lamivudine
(Extavia)	interferon beta-1b
(Factive)	gemifloxacin
(Forteo)	teriparatide
(Infergen)	interferon alfacon-1
(Intron A)	interferon alfa-2a
(Kaletra)	lopinavir/ritonavir
(Keppra/Keppra XR)	levetiracetam
(Lamictal)	lamotrigine
(Lariam)	mefloquine
(Letairis)	ambrisentan
(Levaquin)	levofloxacin
(Lotronex)	alosetron
(Lyrica)	pregabalin
(Metozolv ODT/Reglan)	metoclopramide
(Mifeprex)	mifepristone
(Multaq)	dronedarone
(Myobloc)	rimabotulinum toxin B
(Noroxin)	norfloxacin
(Nplate)	romiplostim
(Nucynta)	tapentadol
(Onsolis)	fentanyl (buccal soluble film)
(Osmoprep/Visicol)	sodium phosphate, dibasic anhydrous and sodium phosphate, mono-basic, monohydrate
(Pegasys)	peginterferon alfa-2a
(PegIntron)	peginterferon alfa-2b
(Plenaxis)	abarelix
(Promacta)	eltrombopag
(Revlimid)	lenalidomide
(Rozerem)	ramelteon
(Sabril)	vigabatrin
(Samsca)	tolvaptan
(Savella)	milnacipran
(Simponi)	golimumab
(Soliris)	eculizumab
(Stelara)	ustekinumab
(Sucraid)	sacrosidase
(Symbicort)	budesonide/formoterol
(Symbyax)	olanzapine/fluoxetine
(Thalomid)	thalidomide
(Tikosyn)	dofetilide
(Topamax)	topiramate
(Tracleer)	bosentan
(Treximet)	sumatriptan/naproxen sodium
(Trilipix)	fenofibric acid
(Trizivir)	abacavir/lamivudine/zidovudine
(Tysabri)	natalizumab
(Tyzeka)	telbivudine
(Vibativ)	telavancin
(Vimpat)	lacosamide
(Viramune)	nevirapine
(Votrient)	pazopanib
(Xenazine)	tetrabenazine
(Xolair)	omalizumab
(Xyrem)	sodium oxybate
(Ziagen)	abacavir
(Zolpimist)	zolpidem (oral spray)
(Zonegran)	zonisamide
(Zyprexa/Zyprexa Zydis)	olanzapine

SPECIAL DOSING CONSIDERATIONS

For many patients the average dose range for a given drug can be toxic. The purpose of this section is to describe vulnerable patient populations for which special dosing considerations must be made to protect the patient and improve clinical outcomes.

The Pediatric Patient

Most drugs prescribed to children are not approved by the Food and Drug Administration (FDA) for use in pediatric populations. This does not mean it's wrong to prescribe these drugs to children, rather it means that the medications were not tested in children. The lack of pediatric drug information can result in patient harm or death, such as what occurred with the drug chloramphenicol. When given to very young children, chloramphenicol caused toxicity and multiple deaths. Referred to as "gray baby syndrome," this toxic reaction was eventually found to be dose dependent. The FDA now requires that new drugs that may be used in children include information for safe pediatric use. For this edition of *Davis's Drug Guide for Nurses*, we have had the pediatric dosing for the top 100 drugs used in children revised and updated by a pediatric pharmacist with a Doctor of Pharmacy (PharmD) degree.

The main reason for adjusting dosages in pediatric patients is body size, which is measured by body weight or body surface area (BSA). Weight-based pediatric drug dosages are expressed in number of milligrams per kilogram of body weight (mg/kg) while dosages calculated on BSA are expressed in number of milligrams per meter squared (mg/m^2). BSA is determined using a BSA nomogram (Appendix F) or calculated by using formulas (Appendix E).

The neonate and the premature infant require additional adjustments secondary to immature function of body systems. For example, absorption may be incomplete or altered secondary to differences in gastric pH or motility. Distribution may be altered because of varying amounts of total body water, and metabolism and excretion can be delayed due to immature liver and kidney function. Furthermore, rapid weight changes and progressive maturation of hepatic and renal function require frequent monitoring and careful dosage adjustments. Gestational age, as well as weight, may be needed to properly dose some drugs in the neonate.

The Geriatric Patient

Absorption, distribution, metabolism, and excretion are altered in adults over 65 years of age, putting the older patient at risk for toxic reactions. Pharmacokinetic properties in the older patient are affected by

- diminished gastrointestinal (GI) motility and blood flow, which delays absorption
- percentage of body fat, lean muscle mass, and total body water, which alters distribution
- decreased plasma proteins, especially in the malnourished patient, which alters distribution by allowing a larger proportion of free or unbound drug to circulate and exert effects
- diminshed hepatic function, which slows metabolism.
- diminished renal function, which delays excretion

Older patients should be prescribed the lowest possible effective dose at the initiation of therapy followed by careful titration of doses as needed. Just as importantly, they should be monitored very carefully for signs and symptoms of adverse drug reactions.

Another concern is that many elderly patients are prescribed multiple drugs and are at risk for polypharmacy. As the number of medications a patient takes increases, so does the risk for an adverse drug reaction. One drug may negate or potentiate the effects of another drug (drug-drug interaction). This situation is compounded by concurrent use of nonprescription drugs and natural products. In general, doses of most medications (especially digoxin, sedative/hypnotics, anticoagulants, nonsteroidal anti-inflammatory agents, antibiotics, and antihypertensives) should be decreased in the

SPECIAL DOSING CONSIDERATIONS 25

geriatric population. The Beers List/Criteria, which appears in the *Medication Safety Tools section*, is a list of drugs to be used with caution in the elderly, and is based on these concerns.

The Patient of Reproductive Age

Generally, pregnant women should avoid medications, except when absolutely necessary. Both the mother and the fetus must be considered. The placenta protects the fetus only from extremely large molecules. The fetus is particularly vulnerable during the first and the last trimesters of pregnancy. During the first trimester, vital organs are forming and ingestion of teratogenic drugs may lead to fetal malformation or miscarriage. Unfortunately, this is the time when a woman is least likely to know that she is pregnant. In the third trimester, drugs administered to the mother and transferred to the fetus may not be safely metabolized and excreted by the fetus. This is especially true of drugs administered near term. After the infant is delivered, he or she no longer has the placenta to help with drug excretion, and drugs administered before delivery may result in toxicity.

Of course, many conditions, such as asthma, diabetes, gastrointestinal disorders, and mental illness affect pregnant women and require long-term medication use. When the medications are used, whether over-the-counter or prescription, prescribing the lowest effective dose for the shortest period of time necessary is the rule.

The possibility of a medication altering sperm quality and quantity in a potential father also is an area of concern. Male patients should be informed of this risk when taking any medications known to have this potential.

Renal Disease

The kidneys are the major organ of drug elimination. Failure to account for decreased renal function is a preventable source of adverse drug reactions. Renal function is measured by the creatinine clearance (CCr), which can be approximated in the absence of a 24-hour urine collection (Appendix E). In addition, dosages in the renally impaired patient can be optimized by measuring blood levels of certain drugs (e.g., digoxin, aminoglycosides).

Patients with underlying renal disease, premature infants with immature renal function, and elderly patients with an age-related decrease in renal function require careful dose adjustments. Renal function may fluctuate over time and should be re-assessed periodically.

Liver Disease

The liver is the major organ of drug metabolism. It changes a drug from a relatively fat-soluble compound to a more water-soluble substance, which means that the drug can then be excreted by the kidneys. Liver function is not as easily quantified as renal function, and it therefore is difficult to predict the correct dosage for a patient with liver dysfunction based on laboratory tests.

A patient who is severely jaundiced or who has very low serum proteins (particularly albumin) can be expected to have some problems metabolizing drugs. In advanced liver disease, portal vascular congestion also impairs drug absorption. Examples of drugs that should be carefully dosed in patients with liver disease include theophylline, diuretics, phenytoin, and sedatives. Some drugs (e.g., enalapril, carisoprodol) must be activated in the liver to exert their effect and are known as prodrugs. In patients with liver dysfunction, these drugs may not be converted to the active component, thereby resulting in decreased efficacy.

Heart Failure

Heart failure results in passive congestion of blood vessels in the gastrointestinal tract, which impairs drug absorption. Heart failure also slows drug delivery to the liver, delaying metabolism. Renal function is frequently compromised as well, adding to delayed elimination and prolonged drug action. Dosages of drugs metabolized mainly by the liver or excreted mainly by the kidneys should be decreased in patients with congestive heart failure.

Body Size

Drug dosing is often based on total body weight. However, some drugs selectively penetrate fatty tissues. If the drug does not penetrate fatty tissues (e.g., digoxin, gentamicin), dosages for the obese patient should be determined by ideal body weight or estimated lean body mass. Ideal body weight may be determined from tables of desirable weights or may be estimated using formulas for lean body mass when the patient's height and weight are known (Appendix E). If such adjustments are not made, considerable toxicity can result.

Body size is also a factor in patients who are grossly underweight. Elderly patients, chronic alcoholics, patients with acquired immune deficiency, and patients who are terminally ill from cancer or other debilitating illnesses need careful attention to dosing. Patients who have had a limb amputated also need to have this change in body size taken into account.

Drug Interactions

Use of multiple drugs, especially those known to interact with other drugs, may necessitate dosage adjustments. Drugs highly bound to plasma proteins, such as warfarin and phenytoin, may be displaced by other highly protein-bound drugs. When this phenomenon occurs, the drug that has been displaced exhibits an increase in its activity because the free or unbound drug is active.

Some drugs decrease the liver's ability to metabolize other drugs. Drugs capable of doing this include cimetidine and ketoconazole. Concurrently administered drugs that are also highly metabolized by the liver may need to be administered in decreased dosages. Other agents such as phenobarbital, other barbiturates, and rifampin are capable of stimulating the liver to metabolize drugs more rapidly, requiring larger doses to be administered. Concurrently administered drugs that are also highly metabolized by the liver may need to be administered in higher dosages.

Drugs that significantly alter urine pH can affect excretion of drugs for which the excretory process is pH dependent. Alkalinizing the urine will hasten the excretion of acidic drugs. An example of this is administering sodium bicarbonate in cases of aspirin overdose to promote the renal excretion of aspirin. Alkalinizing the urine will increase reabsorption of alkaline drugs, which prolongs and enhances drug action. Acidification of the urine will hasten the excretion of alkaline drugs. Acidification of the urine will also enhance reabsorption of acidic drugs, prolonging and enhancing drug action.

Some drugs compete for enzyme systems with other drugs. Allopurinol inhibits the enzyme involved in uric acid production, but it also inhibits metabolism (inactivation) of 6-mercaptopurine, greatly increasing its toxicity. The dosage of mercaptopurine needs to be significantly reduced when coadministered with allopurinol.

The same potential for interactions exists for some foods. Dietary calcium, found in high concentrations in dairy products, combines with tetracycline or fluoroquinolones and prevents their absorption. Foods high in pyridoxine (vitamin B_6) can negate the anti-Parkinson effect of levodopa. Grapefruit juice inhibits the enzyme that breaks down some drugs, and concurrent ingestion may significantly increase drug levels and the risk for toxicity.

Many commonly taken natural products interact with pharmaceutical drugs. St. John's wort, garlic, ephedra, and other natural products can interact with medications and cause known or unpredictable reactions.

Nurses and prescribers should consult drug references and remember that the average dosing range for drugs is intended for an average patient. However, every patient is an individual with specific drug-handling capabilities. Taking these special dosing considerations into account allows for an individualized drug regimen that promotes the desired therapeutic outcome and minimizes the risk of toxicity.

EDUCATING PATIENTS ABOUT SAFE MEDICATION USE

Research has shown that patients need information about several medication-related topics, no matter what the medication. A well-informed patient and/or family can help prevent medication errors by hospital staff and is less likely to make medication errors at home. Adherence to the medication regimen is another goal achieved through patient education.

Before beginning any teaching, however, always assess the patient's current knowledge by asking if he or she is familiar with the medication, how it is taken at home, what precautions or follow-up care is required, and other questions specific to each drug. Based on the patient's current knowledge level and taking into consideration factors such as readiness to learn, environmental and social barriers to learning or adherence, and cultural factors, discuss the following:

1. **Generic and brand names of the medication.** Patients should know both the brand and generic names of each medication for two reasons. It helps them identify their medications when a generic equivalent is substituted for a brand name version, and it prevents patients or health care providers from making sound-alike confusion errors when giving or documenting a medication history. An example of this is saying Celebrex but meaning or hearing Cerebyx.

2. **Purpose of the medication.** Patients have a right to know what the therapeutic benefit of the medication will be but also should be told the consequences of not taking the prescribed medication. This may enhance adherence. For example, a patient may be more likely to take blood pressure medication if told lowering high blood pressure will prevent heart attack, kidney disease, or stroke, rather than saying only that it will lower blood pressure.

3. **Dosage and how to take the medication.** To derive benefit and avoid adverse reactions or other poor outcomes, the patient must know how much of the medication to take and when to take it. Refer to dosages in metric weight (i.e., milligram, gram) rather than dosage unit (tablet) or volume (1 teaspoon). The patient must also be informed of the best time to take the medication, for example, on an empty or a full stomach, before bedtime, or with or without other medications. If possible, help the patient fit the medication schedule into his or her own schedule, so that taking the medication is not difficult or forgotten.

4. **What to do if a dose is missed.** Always explain to patients what to do if a dose is missed. Patients have been reported to take a double dose of medications when a missed dose occurs, putting themselves at risk for side effects and adverse reactions.

5. **Duration of therapy.** It is not uncommon for patients to stop taking a medication when they feel better or to discontinue a medication when they cannot perceive a benefit. For very long term, even lifelong therapy, the patient may need to be reminded that the medication helps maintain the current level of wellness. Patients may need to be reminded to finish short-term courses of medications even though they frequently will feel much better before the prescription runs out. Some medications cannot be discontinued abruptly and patients should be warned to consult a health care professional before discontinuing such agents. Patients will need to know to refill prescriptions several days before running out or to take extra medication if traveling.

6. **Minor side effects and what to do if they occur.** Inform the patient that all medications have potential side effects. Explain the most common side effects associated with the medication and how to avoid or manage them if they occur. An informed patient is less likely to stop taking a medication because of a minor and potentially avoidable side effect.

7. **Serious side effects and what to do if they occur.** Inform the patient of the possibility of serious side effects. Describe signs and symptoms associated with serious side effects, and tell the

patient to immediately inform a physician or nurse should they occur. Tell the patient to call before the next dose of the medication is scheduled and to not assume that the medication is the source of the symptom and prematurely discontinue it.

8. **Medications to avoid.** Drug-drug interactions can dampen drug effects, enhance drug effects, or cause life-threatening adverse events such as cardiac dysrhythmias, hepatitis, renal failure, or internal bleeding. The patient and family need to know which other medications, including which over-the-counter medications, to avoid.

9. **Foods to avoid and other precautions.** Food-drug interactions are not uncommon and can have effects similar to drug-drug interactions. Excessive sun exposure resulting in severe dermal reactions is not uncommon and represents an environmental-drug interaction. Likewise, the patient should be informed of what activities to avoid, in case the medication affects alertness or coordination, for example.

10. **How to store the medication:** Medications must be stored properly to maintain potency. Most medications should not be stored in the bathroom medicine cabinet because of excess heat and humidity. In addition, thoughtful storage practices, such as separating two family members' medications, can prevent mix-ups and inadvertent accessibility by children (or pets). Review storage with patients and ask about current methods for storing medications.

11. **Follow-up care.** Anyone taking medication requires ongoing care to assess effectiveness and appropriateness of medications. Many medications require invasive and noninvasive testing to monitor blood levels; hematopoietic, hepatic, or renal function; or other effects on other body systems. Ongoing medical evaluation may result in dosage adjustments, change in medication, or discontinuation of medication.

12. **What not to take.** Inform patients not to take expired medications or someone else's medication. Warn them not to self-medicate with older, no-longer-used prescriptions even if the remaining supply is not expired. Tell patients to keep a current record of all medications taken and to ask health care providers if new medications are meant to replace a current medication.

As you teach, encourage the patient and the family to ask questions. Providing feedback about medication questions will increase their understanding and help you identify areas that need reinforcement. Also, ask patients to repeat what you have said and return to demonstrate application or administration techniques.

Stress the importance of concurrent therapies. Medications often are only a part of a recommended therapy. Review with the patient and family other measures that will enhance or maintain health. Always consider the cultural context in which health information is provided and plan accordingly. This might include obtaining a same-gender translator or adjusting dosing times to avoid conflict with traditional rituals.

Finally, provide written instructions in a simple and easy-to-read format. Keep in mind that most health care information is written at a 10th grade reading level, while many patients read at a 5th grade level. Tell patients to keep the written instructions, so that they can be reviewed at home, when stress levels are lower and practical difficulties in maintaining the medication plan are known.

CLASSIFICATIONS

• ANTI-ALZHEIMER'S AGENTS

PHARMACOLOGIC PROFILE

General Use
Management of Alzheimer's dementia.

General Action and Information
All agents act by increasing the amount of acetylcholine in the CNS by inhibiting cholinesterase. No agents to date can slow the progression of Alzheimer's dementia. Current agents may temporarily improve cognitive function and therefore improve quality of life.

Contraindications
Hypersensitivity. Tacrine should not be used in patients who have had previous hepatic reactions to the drug.

Precautions
Use cautiously in patients with a history of "sick sinus syndrome" or other supraventricular cardiac conduction abnormalities (may cause bradycardia). Cholingeric effects may result in adverse GI effects (nausea, vomiting, diarrhea, weight loss) and may also increase gastric acid secretion resulting in GI bleeding, especially during concurrent NSAID therapy. Other cholinergic effects may include urinary tract obstruction, seizures, or bronchospasm.

Interactions
Additive effects with other drugs having cholinergic properties. May exaggerate the effects of succinylcholine-type muscle relaxation during anesthesia. May decrease therapeutic effects of anticholinergics.

NURSING IMPLICATIONS

Assessment
- Assess cognitive function (memory, attention, reasoning, language, ability to perform simple tasks) throughout therapy.
- Monitor nausea, vomiting, anorexia, and weight loss. Notify health care professional if these side effects occur.

Potential Nursing Diagnoses
- Disturbed thought process (Indications).
- Imbalanced nutrition: less than body requirements.
- Deficient knowledge, related to disease process and medication regimen (Patient/Family Teaching).

Patient/Family Teaching
- Instruct patient and caregiver that medication should be taken as directed.
- Advise patient and caregiver to notify health care professional if nausea, vomiting, anorexia, and weight loss occur.

Evaluation/Desired Outcomes
- Temporary improvement in cognitive function (memory, attention, reasoning, language, ability to perform simple tasks) in patients with Alzheimer's disease.

Anti-Alzheimer's agents included in *Davis's Drug Guide for Nurses*

donepezil 470
galantamine 624
rivastigmine 1123
tacrine 1181
memantine 819

• ANTIANEMICS

PHARMACOLOGIC PROFILE

General Use
Prevention and treatment of anemias.

General Action and Information
Iron (ferrous fumarate, ferrous gluconate, ferrous sulfate, iron dextran, iron sucrose, polysaccharide-iron complex, sodium ferric gluconate complex) is required for production of hemoglobin, which is necessary for oxygen transport to cells. Cyanocobalamin and hydroxocobalamin (Vitamin B_{12}) and folic acid are water-soluble vitamins that are required for red blood cell production. Darbepoetin and epoetin stimulate production of red blood cells. Nandrolone stimulates production of erythropoetin.

Contraindications
Undiagnosed anemias. Hemochromatosis, hemosiderosis, hemolytic anemia (Iron). Uncontrolled hypertension (darbepoetin, epoetin).

Precautions
Use parenteral iron (iron dextran, iron sucrose, sodium ferric gluconate complex) cautiously in patients with a history of allergy or hypersensitivity reactions.

Interactions
Oral iron can decrease the absorption of tetracyclines, fluoroquinolones, or penicillamine. Vitamin E may impair the therapeutic response to iron. Phenytoin and other anticonvulsants may decrease the absorption of folic acid. Response to Vitamin B_{12} or folic acid may be delayed by chloramphenicol. Darbepoetin and epoetin may increase the requirement for heparin during hemodialysis.

NURSING IMPLICATIONS

Assessment
- Assess patient's nutritional status and dietary history to determine possible causes for anemia and need for patient teaching.

Potential Nursing Diagnoses
- Activity intolerance (Indications).
- Imbalanced nutrition: less than body requirements (Indications).
- Deficient knowledge, related to disease process and medication regimen (Patient/Family Teaching).

Implementation
- Available in combination with many vitamins and minerals (see Appendix B).

Patient/Family Teaching
- Encourage patients to comply with diet recommendations of health care professional. Explain that the best source of vitamins and minerals is a well-balanced diet with foods from the four basic food groups.

- Patients self-medicating with vitamin and mineral supplements should be cautioned not to exceed RDA. The effectiveness of mega doses for treatment of various medical conditions is unproven and may cause side effects.

Evaluation/Desired Outcomes
- Resolution of anemia.

Antianemics included in *Davis's Drug Guide for Nurses*

hormones
darbepoetin 403
epoetin 512

iron supplements
carbonyl iron 736
ferrous fumarate 736
ferrous gluconate 736
ferrous sulfate 736
ferumoxytol 573
iron dextran 736

iron polysaccharide 736
iron sucrose 736
sodium ferric gluconate complex 737

neurokinin antagonists
fosaprepitant 1370

vitamins
cyanocobalamin 1284
folic acid 606
hydroxocobalamin 1284

• ANTIANGINALS

PHARMACOLOGIC PROFILE

General Use
Nitrates are used to treat and prevent attacks of angina. Only nitrates (sublingual, lingual spray, or intravenous) may be used in the acute treatment of attacks of angina pectoris. Calcium channel blockers and beta blockers are used prophylactically in long-term management of angina.

General Action and Information
Several different groups of medications are used in the treatment of angina pectoris. The nitrates (isosorbide dinitrate, isosorbide mononitrate, and nitroglycerin) are available as a lingual spray, sublingual tablets, parenterals, transdermal systems, and sustained-release oral dosage forms. Nitrates dilate coronary arteries and cause systemic vasodilation (decreased preload). Calcium channel blockers dilate coronary arteries (some also slow heart rate). Beta blockers decrease myocardial oxygen consumption via a decrease in heart rate. Therapy may be combined if selection is designed to minimize side effects or adverse reactions.

Contraindications
Hypersensitivity. Avoid use of beta blockers or calcium channel blockers in advanced heart block, cardiogenic shock, or untreated CHF.

Precautions
Beta blockers should be used cautiously in patients with diabetes mellitus, pulmonary disease, or hypothyroidism.

Interactions
Nitrates, calcium channel blockers, and beta blockers may cause hypotension with other antihypertensives or acute ingestion of alcohol. Verapamil, diltiazem, and beta blockers may have additive myocardial depressant effects when used with other agents that affect cardiac function. Verapamil has a number of other significant drug-drug interactions.

ANTIANXIETY AGENTS

NURSING IMPLICATIONS
Assessment
- Assess location, duration, intensity, and precipitating factors of patient's anginal pain.
- Monitor blood pressure and pulse periodically throughout therapy.

Potential Nursing Diagnoses
- Acute pain (Indications).
- Ineffective tissue perfusion (Indications).
- Deficient knowledge, related to disease process and medication regimen (Patient/Family Teaching).

Implementation
- Available in various dose forms. See specific drugs for information on administration.

Patient/Family Teaching
- Instruct patient on concurrent nitrate therapy and prophylactic antianginals to continue taking both medications as ordered and to use SL nitroglycerin as needed for anginal attacks.
- Advise patient to contact health care professional immediately if chest pain does not improve; worsens after therapy; is accompanied by diaphoresis or shortness of breath; or if severe, persistent headache occurs.
- Caution patient to make position changes slowly to minimize orthostatic hypotension.
- Advise patient to avoid concurrent use of alcohol with these medications.

Evaluation/Desired Outcomes
- Decrease in frequency and severity of anginal attacks.
- Increase in activity tolerance.

Antianginals included in *Davis's Drug Guide for Nurses*

beta blockers
atenolol 204
labetalol 759
metoprolol 851
nadolol 892
propranolol 1071

calcium channel blockers
diltiazem 445
felodipine 557
isradipine 746

niCARdipine 915
NIFEdipine 921
verapamil 1275

nitrates
isosorbide dinitrate 742
isosorbide mononitrate 742
nitroglycerin 929

miscellaneous
ranolazine 1099

• ANTIANXIETY AGENTS

PHARMACOLOGIC PROFILE
General Use
Antianxiety agents are used in the management of various forms of anxiety, including generalized anxiety disorder (GAD). Some agents are more suitable for intermittent or short-term use (benzodiazepines) while others are more useful long-term (buspirone, doxepin, fluoxetine, paroxetine, sertraline, venlafaxine).

ANTIANXIETY AGENTS

General Action and Information
Most agents cause generalized CNS depression. Benzodiazepines may produce tolerance with long-term use and have potential for psychological or physical dependence. These agents have NO analgesic properties.

Contraindications
Hypersensitivity. Should not be used in comatose patients or in those with pre-existing CNS depression. Should not be used in patients with uncontrolled severe pain. Avoid use during pregnancy or lactation.

Precautions
Use cautiously in patients with hepatic dysfunction, severe renal impairment, or severe underlying pulmonary disease (benzodiazepines only). Use with caution in patients who may be suicidal or who may have had previous drug addictions. Patients may be more sensitive to CNS depressant effects; dosage reduction may be required.

Interactions
Mainly for benzodiazepines; additive CNS depression with alcohol, antihistamines, some antidepressants, opioid analgesics, or phenothiazines may occur. Most agents should not be used with MAO inhibitors.

NURSING IMPLICATIONS

Assessment
- Monitor blood pressure, pulse, and respiratory status frequently throughout IV administration.
- Prolonged high-dose therapy may lead to psychological or physical dependence. Restrict the amount of drug available to patient, especially if patient is depressed, suicidal, or has a history of addiction.
- **Anxiety:** Assess degree of anxiety and level of sedation (ataxia, dizziness, slurred speech) before and periodically throughout therapy.

Potential Nursing Diagnoses
- Risk for injury (Side Effects).
- Deficient knowledge, related to disease process and medication regimen (Patient/Family Teaching).

Implementation
- Patients changing to buspirone from other antianxiety agents should receive gradually decreasing doses. Buspirone will not prevent withdrawal symptoms.

Patient/Family Teaching
- May cause daytime drowsiness. Caution patient to avoid driving and other activities requiring alertness until response to medication is known.
- Advise patient to avoid the use of alcohol and other CNS depressants concurrently with these medications.
- Advise patient to inform health care professional if pregnancy is planned or suspected.

Evaluation/Desired Outcomes
- Decrease in anxiety level.

Antianxiety agents included in *Davis's Drug Guide for Nurses*

benzodiazepines
alprazolam 138
chlordiazepoxide 314
diazepam 431
lorazepam 799
midazolam 858
oxazepam 961

selective serotonin reuptake inhibitors (SSRIs)
paroxetine hydrochloride 992
paroxetine mesylate 992

miscellaneous
busPIRone 251
doxepin 476
hydrOXYzine 682
venlafaxine 1272

• ANTIARRHYTHMICS

PHARMACOLOGIC PROFILE

General Use
Suppression of cardiac arrhythmias.

General Action and Information
Correct cardiac arrhythmias by a variety of mechanisms, depending on the group used. The therapeutic goal is decreased symptomatology and increased hemodynamic performance. Choice of agent depends on etiology of arrhythmia and individual patient characteristics. Treatable causes of arrhythmias should be corrected before therapy is initiated (e.g., electrolyte disturbances, other drugs). Antiarrhythmics are generally classified by their effects on cardiac conduction tissue (see the following table). Adenosine, atropine, and digoxin are also used as antiarrhythmics.

MECHANISM OF ACTION OF MAJOR ANTIARRHYTHMIC DRUGS

CLASS	DRUGS	MECHANISM
I	moricizine	Shares properties of IA, IB, and IC agents
IA	quinidine, procainamide, disopyramide	Depress Na conductance, increase APD and ERP, decrease membrane responsiveness
IB	tocainide, lidocaine, phenytoin, mexiletine	Increase K conductance, decrease APD and ERP
IC	flecainide, propafenone	Profound slowing of conduction, markedly depress phase O
II	esmolol, propranolol	Interfere with Na conductance, depress cell membrane, decrease automaticity, and increase ERP of the AV node, block excess sympathetic activity
III	amiodarone, dofetilide, ibutilide, sotalol	Interfere with norepinephrine, increase APD and ERP
IV	diltiazem, verapamil	Increase AV nodal ERP, Ca channel blocker

APD = action-potential duration; Ca = calcium; ERP = effective refractory period; K = potassium; Na = sodium.

Contraindications
Differ greatly among various agents. See individual drugs.

Precautions
Differ greatly among agents used. Appropriate dosage adjustments should be made in elderly patients and those with renal or hepatic impairment, depending on agent chosen. Correctable causes (electrolyte abnormalities, drug toxicity) should be evaluated. See individual drugs.

ANTIARRHYTHMICS

Interactions
Differ greatly among agents used. See individual drugs.

NURSING IMPLICATIONS

Assessment
- Monitor ECG, pulse, and blood pressure continuously throughout IV administration and periodically throughout oral administration.

Potential Nursing Diagnoses
- Decreased cardiac output (Indications).
- Deficient knowledge, related to disease process and medication regimen (Patient/Family Teaching).

Implementation
- Take apical pulse before administration of oral doses. Withhold dose and notify physician or other health care professional if heart rate is <50 bpm.
- Administer oral doses with a full glass of water. Most sustained-release preparations should be swallowed whole. Do not crush, break, or chew tablets or open capsules, unless specifically instructed.

Patient/Family Teaching
- Instruct patient to take oral doses around the clock, as directed, even if feeling better.
- Instruct patient or family member on how to take pulse. Advise patient to report changes in pulse rate or rhythm to health care professional.
- Caution patient to avoid taking OTC medications without consulting health care professional.
- Advise patient to carry identification describing disease process and medication regimen at all times.
- Emphasize the importance of follow-up exams to monitor progress.

Evaluation/Desired Outcomes
- Resolution of cardiac arrhythmias without detrimental side effects.

Antiarrhythmics included in *Davis's Drug Guide for Nurses*

class IA
procainamide 1052
quinidine gluconate 1089
quinidine sulfate 1089

class IB
fosphenytoin 616
lidocaine 784
phenytoin 1020

class IC
flecainide 579
propafenone 1064

class II
esmolol 528
propranolol 1071
sotalol 1167

class III
amiodarone 151
dofetilide 467
ibutilide 691
sotalol 1167

class IV
diltiazem 445
verapamil 1275

miscellaneous
adenosine 123
atropine 208
digoxin 439
dronedarone 485
phenytoin 1020

ANTIASTHMATICS

PHARMACOLOGIC PROFILE

General Use
Management of acute and chronic episodes of reversible bronchoconstriction. Goal of therapy is to treat acute attacks (short-term control) and to decrease incidence and intensity of future attacks (long-term control). The choice of modalities depends on the continued requirement for short term control agents.

General Action and Information
Adrenergic bronchodilators and phosphodiesterase inhibitors both work by increasing intracellular levels of cyclic-3', 5'-adenosine monophsphate (cAMP); adrenergics by increasing production and phosphodiesterase inhibitors by decreasing breakdown. Increased levels of cAMP produce bronchodilation. Corticosteroids act by decreasing airway inflammation. Anticholinergics (ipratropium) produce bronchodilation by decreasing intracellular levels of cyclic guanosine monophosphate (cGMP). Leukotriene receptor antagonists and mast cell stabilizers decrease the release of substances that can contribute to bronchospasm.

Contraindications
Inhaled corticosteroids, long-acting adrenergic agents, and mast cell stabilizers should not be used during acute attacks of asthma.

Precautions
Adrenergic bronchodilators and anticholinergics should be used cautiously in patients with cardiovascular disease. Chronic use of systemic corticosteroids should be avoided in children or during pregnancy or lactation. Diabetic patients may experience loss of glycemic control during corticosteroid therapy. Corticosteroids should never be abruptly discontinued.

Interactions
Adrenergic bronchodilators and phosphodiesterase inhibitors may have additive CNS and cardiovascular effects with other adrenergic agents. Cimetidine increases theophylline levels and the risk of toxicity. Coritcosteroids may decrease the effectiveness of antidiabetics. Corticosteroids may cause hypokalemia which may be additive with potassium-losing diuretics and may also increase the risk of digoxin toxicity.

NURSING IMPLICATIONS

Assessment
- Assess lung sounds and respiratory function prior to and periodically throughout therapy.
- Assess cardiovascular status of patients taking adrenergic bronchodilators or anticholinergics. Monitor for ECG changes and chest pain.

Potential Nursing Diagnoses
- Ineffective airway clearance (Indications).
- Deficient knowledge, related to disease process and medication regimen (Patient/Family Teaching).
- Noncompliance (Patient/Family Teaching).

Patient/Family Teaching
- Instruct patient to take antiasthmatics as directed. Do not take more than prescribed or discontinue without discussing with health care professional.
- Advise patient to avoid smoking and other respiratory irritants.
- Instruct patient in correct use of metered-dose inhaler or other administration devices (see Appendix D).

- Advise patient to contact health care professional promptly if the usual dose of medication fails to produce the desired results, if symptoms worsen after treatment, or if toxic effects occur.
- Patients using inhalation medications and bronchodilators should be advised to use the bronchodilator first and allow 5 minutes to elapse before administering other medications, unless otherwise directed by health care professional.

Evaluation/Desired Outcomes
- Prevention of and reduction in symptoms of asthma.

Antiasthmatics included in *Davis's Drug Guide for Nurses*

bronchodilators
albuterol 126
aminophylline 240
epinephrine 504
formoterol 610
ipratropium 732
levalbuterol 780
montelukast 879
salmeterol 1134
tiotropium 1232
terbutaline 1197
theophylline 240

corticosteroids
beclomethasone 365
betamethasone 372
budesonide 365, 372
ciclesonide 1369
cortisone 372
dexamethasone 372
flunisolide 366
fluticasone 366
hydrocortisone 372
methylPREDNISolone 372
mometasone 366
prednisoLONE 372
predniSONE 372
triamcinolone 372

leukotriene antagonists
zafirlukast 1299

monoclonal antibodies
omalizumab 948

• ANTICHOLINERGICS

PHARMACOLOGIC PROFILE

General Use
Atropine—Bradyarrhythmias. **Ipratropium**—bronchospasm (inhalation) and rhinorrhea (intranasal). **Scopolamine**—Nausea and vomiting related to motion sickness and vertigo. **Propantheline and glycopyrrolate**—Decreasing gastric secretory activity and increasing esophageal sphincter tone. Atropine and scopolamine are also used as ophthalmic mydriatics. Benztropine, biperidin, and trihexyphenidyl are used in the management of Parkinson's disease. Oxybutynin and tolterodine are used as urinary tract spasmodics.

General Action and Information
Competitively inhibit the action of acetylcholine. In addition, atropine, glycopyrrolate, propantheline, and scopolamine are antimuscarinic in that they inhibit the action of acetylcholine at sites innervated by postganglionic cholinergic nerves.

Contraindications
Hypersensitivity, narrow-angle glaucoma, severe hemorrhage, tachycardia (due to thyrotoxicosis or cardiac insufficiency), or myasthenia gravis.

Precautions
Geriatric and pediatric patients are more susceptible to adverse effects. Use cautiously in patients with urinary tract pathology; those at risk for GI obstruction; and those with chronic renal, hepatic, pulmonary, or cardiac disease.

ANTICHOLINERGICS

Interactions
Additive anticholinergic effects (dry mouth, dry eyes, blurred vision, constipation) with other agents possessing anticholinergic activity, including antihistamines, antidepressants, quinidine, and disopyramide. May alter GI absorption of other drugs by inhibiting GI motility and increasing transit time. Antacids may decrease absorption of orally administered anticholinergics.

NURSING IMPLICATIONS

Assessment
- Assess vital signs and ECG frequently during IV drug therapy. Report any significant changes in heart rate or blood pressure or increase in ventricular ectopy or angina promptly.
- Monitor intake and output ratios in elderly or surgical patients; may cause urinary retention.
- Assess patient regularly for abdominal distention and auscultate for bowel sounds. Constipation may become a problem. Increasing fluids and adding bulk to the diet may help alleviate constipation.

Potential Nursing Diagnoses
- Decreased cardiac output (Indications).
- Impaired oral mucous membrane (Side Effects).
- Constipation (Side Effects).

Implementation
- **PO:** Administer oral doses of atropine, glycopyrrolate, propantheline, or scopolamine 30 min before meals.
- Scopolamine transdermal patch should be applied at least 4 hr before travel.

Patient/Family Teaching
- Instruct patient that frequent rinses, sugarless gum or candy, and good oral hygiene may help relieve dry mouth.
- May cause drowsiness. Caution patient to avoid driving or other activities requiring alertness until response to medication is known.
- **Ophth:** Advise patients that ophthalmic preparations may temporarily blur vision and impair ability to judge distances. Dark glasses may be needed to protect eyes from bright light.

Evaluation/Desired Outcomes
- Increase in heart rate.
- Decrease in nausea and vomiting related to motion sickness or vertigo.
- Dryness of mouth.
- Dilation of pupils.
- Decrease in GI motility.
- Resolution of signs and symptoms of Parkinson's disease.

Anticholinergics included in *Davis's Drug Guide for Nurses*

atropine 208
benztropine 225
darifenacin 405
dicyclomine 438
difenoxin/atropine 453
diphenoxylate/atropine 453
fesoterodine 574
glycopyrrolate 636
hyoscyamine 684
ipratropium 732
oxybutynin 964
scopolamine 1139
solifenacin 1166
tiotorpium 1232
tolterodine 1238

SYRINGE COMPATIBILITY CHART

C = COMPATIBLE
N = NOT COMPATIBLE
BLANK = CONFLICTING DATA, OR NO DATA AVAILABLE

	atropine	buprenorphine	butorphanol	chlorpromazine	diazepam	diphenhydramine	droperidol	glycopyrrolate	haloperidol	hydromorphone	hydroxyzine	ketorolac	meperidine	metoclopramide	midazolam	morphine	nalbuphine	ondansetron	pentobarbitol	prochlorperazine	promethazine	scopolamine
atropine			C	C		C	C	C		C	C		C	C	C	C	C	C	N	C	C	C
buprenorphine								C	C						C	C						
butorphanol	C			C		C	C			C		C	C		C			N	C	C	C
chlorpromazine	C		C			C	C	C		C	C		C	C	C	C			N	C	C	C
diazepam						N		N		N					N		N					
diphenhydramine	C		C	C	N		C	C	N	C	C		C	C	C	C	C		N	C	C	C
droperidol	C		C	C		C		C			C		C	C	C	C	C	C	N	N	C	C
glycopyrrolate	C	C		C	N	C	C		C	C	C		C		C	C	C	C	N	C	C	C
haloperidol		C				N		C		N	N	N		N	N	N						N
hydromorphone	C			C	N	C		C	N		C	N		C	C	C			C	C	C	C
hydroxyzine	C		C	C		C	C	C	N	C		N	C	C	C	C	C		N	C	C	C
ketorolac									N	N	N			C			N			N	N	
meperidine	C		C	C		C	C	C		C				C	C	C		C	N	C	C	C
metoclopramide	C		C	C		C	C		N	C	C	C	C		C	C		C		C	C	C
midazolam	C	C		C	N	C	C	C	N	C	C		C	C		C	C	C	N	N	C	C
morphine	C	C	C	C		C	C	C	N	C	C		C	C	C			C	N	N	N	C
nalbuphine	C				N	C	C	C		C	N		C		C				N	C	N	C
ondansetron	C					N	C						C	C	C	C						
pentobarbitol	N		N	N		N	N	N		C	N		N		N	N	N			N	N	C
prochlorperazine	C		C	C		C	C	C		C	C	N	C	C	N	N	C		N		C	C
promethazine	C		C	C		C	C	C		C	C	N	C	C	C	N	N		N	C		C
scopolamine	C		C	C		C	C	C	N	C	C		C	C	C	C	C		C	C	C	

Medications combined in a syringe must be administered within 15 minutes. Recommendations may change as new scientific information becomes available.

© 2011, F.A. Davis Company

C1

IV QUICK REFERENCE COMPATIBILITY CHART

MEDICATION SAFETY TOOLS | IV Compatibility Quick Reference Chart

C = COMPATIBLE
N = NOT COMPATIBLE
BLANK = NO DATA AVAILABLE

	amiodarone	Calcium Chloride	calcium gluconate	diltiazem	dobutamine	dopamine	fentanyl	furosemide	heparin	hydromorphone	insulin, regular	lidocaine	lorazepam	magnesium sulfate	meperidine	midazolam	milrinone	morphine	nitroglycerin	nitroprusside	norepinephrine	oxytocin	potassium chloride	sodium bicarbonate	vasopressin
Acyclovir		C	C	N	N	N	C	C	C	C	C	N	C	N	C	N	N		N	C	N		C	C	C
Amikacin	C	C	C	C	C	C	C	N	N	C		C	C	C	C	C		C	C	C	C	C	C	C	C
Amphotericin B Cholesteryl		N	N		N	N	C	C	N	N		N	C	N	N	N		N	C				N	N	
Amphotericin B Colloidal	C	N	N	C	N	N	N	N	N	N	C	N	N	C	N	N	N		N	N	N	N	N	N	N
Amphotericin B Liposome		N	N	N	N	N	C	C	C	C		C	N	N	N	N		N	C	C		C	C	N	C
Ampicillin/Sulbactam	N	N	N	N	N	N	N		C		C		N		C			C		N					
Ampicillin		N	N	N	N	N	N		N	C	C		N	C	C	N		C	N	N	N			N	
Anidulafungin				C	C	C	C	C	C					C	C		C			C	C	N	
Atropine	C	C	C		C	C	C	C	C	C		C		C	C	C		C	C	C	C	C	C	C	C
Azithromycin						C	N	N		N				C		N		N					C	N	C
Aztreonam		C	C	C	C	C	C	C	C	C	C	C	N	C	C		C	C	C	C	C	C	C	C	C
Bumetanide	C	C	C	C	C	C	C	C	C	C	C	C	C	C	C	N	C	C	C	C	C	C	C	C	C
Butorphanol		C	C	C	C	C	C	N	C	N	C	C	C	C			C	C	C	C	C	C	C	N	C
Caspofungin	C	C	C	C	C	C	C	N	N	C	C	N	N	C	C	C	C		C	C	N	C	C	C	C
Cefazolin	N	N	C	C	N	N	C	C	C	C	C	C	C	C	C	C	C	C	C	C	C	C	C	C	C
Cefepime					N	N	C	C	C		C		C	N	N	N		N	C			C	N	C	C
Cefotaxime		C	C	C	N	C	C	C	C	C	C	C	C	C	C		C	C	C	C	C	C	C	N	C
Cefoxitin		C	C	C	N	C	C	C	C	C	N	C	C	C	C		C	C	C	C	C	C	C	N	C
Ceftazidime	N	N	C	C	N	C	C	C	C	C	C	C	C	C	C	N		C	C	N	C	C	C	C	C
Ceftizoxime	C	C	C		C	N	C	C	C	C	C	C	C	C	C			C	C	C	C	C	C	C	C
Ceftriaxone	C	N	C	C	N	C	C	C	C	C	C	C	C	N	C			C	C	C	C	C	C	C	C
Cefuroxime	C	N	C	C	N	C	C	C	C	C	C	C	C	N	C	N		C	C	C	C	C	C	N	C
Chlorpromazine		C	C	C	C	C	C	N	C	C	N	C	C	C	C			C	C	N	C		C	N	C
Ciprofloxacin	C		C	C	C	C		N	N	C		C	C	N	C	C						C	C	N	
Clindamycin	C	C	N	C	C	N	C	C	C	C	C	C	C	C	C	C		C	C	C	C	C	C	C	C
Daptomycin	C	C	C	C	C	C	C	C	C	C	C	C	C	C	C	C	C		C	N	C	C	C	C	C
Dexamethasone		N	N	C	N	C	C	C	C	C	C	C	C	C	N	C	N		C	C	C	C	C	C	C
Diazepam	C	N	N	N	N	N	N	N	N	N	N	N		N	N	N			N	N	N	N	N	N	N
Digoxin	N	C	C	C	C	C	C	C	C	C	N	C	C	C	C	C	C	C	C			C	C	C	C
Diltiazem	C	C	C		C	C	C	N	N	C	N	C	C	C	C	C	C	C	C	C	C	C	C	N	C
Diphenhydramine		C	C	C	C	C	C	N	N	C	N	C	C	C	C	C	C	C	C	N	C	C	C	C	C
Doripenem	C		C	C	C	C	C	C	C	C		C	C	C	C	C		C		C			C	C	
Doxycycline	C	C	C	C	C	C	C	N	C	C	C	C	C	C	C		C	C	C	C	C	C	C	N	C
Droperidol				C		C		N	N	C			C		C	C							C	C	
Enalaprilat		C	C	C	C	C	C	C	C		C	C	C	C	C		C	C	C	C	C	C	C	C	C
Ertepenem	N	C	C	N	C		C	C	C	C	C	C	C	C	C	N		C	C	C	C	C	C	C	C
Erythromycin Lactobionate	C	C	C	C	C	C	C	N	N	C	C	C	C	C	C	C		C	C	N	C	C		C	C
Famotidine	C	C	C	C	C	C	C	N	C	C	C	C	C	C	C	C	C	C	C	C	C	C	C	C	C
Fentanyl	C	C	C	C	C	C		C	C	C	C	C	C	C	C	C	C		C	C	C	C	C	C	C
Fluconazole	C	C	N	C	C	C	C	N	C	C	C	C	C	C	C	C	C		C	C	C	C	C	C	C
Furosemide	N	C	C	N	N	N	C		C	C	C	C	C		N	N	N	N	N	C			C	C	
Ganciclovir		N	C	N	N	N	C	C	C	C	N	C		N	N			N	C	N	C	C	N	C
Gatifloxacin	C	C	C	C	C	C	N	N	C	C	C	C	C	C		C		C	C	C	C	C	C	C	C
Gentamicin	C	C	C	C	N	C	N	N	N	C	C	C	C	C	C	C	C	C	C	C	C	C	C	C	C
Glycopyrrolate		C	C	C	C	C	C	N	C	C		C	C		C	C		C	C	C	C	C	C	C	C
Granisetron	C	C	C	C	C	C	C	C	C	C	C		C	C	C		C		C	C	C	C	C	C	C
Haloperidol		N	N	C	N	N	N	N	N	C		C	C	N	N	C		N		N	C		N	N	
Heparin	N	C	C	N	N	C	C	C		C	C	C	C	C	C	C	C	C	C	C	C	C	C	C	C
Hydralazine		N	N	C	N	C	N	N	N	C	C			N				N	N						

C2

IV QUICK REFERENCE COMPATIBILITY CHART

C = COMPATIBLE
N = NOT COMPATIBLE
BLANK = NO DATA AVAILABLE

	amiodarone	Calcium Chloride	calcium gluconate	diltiazem	dobutamine	dopamine	fentanyl	furosemide	heparin	hydromorphone	insulin, regular	lidocaine	lorazepam	magnesium sulfate	meperidine	midazolam	milrinone	morphine	nitroglycerin	nitroprusside	norepinephrine	oxytocin	potassium chloride	sodium bicarbonate	vasopressin
Hydrocortisone		N	N	N	N	C	C	C	C	C	C	C	C		C	N		C	C	C	C	C	C	C	
Hydromorphone		C	C	C	C	C	C	C	C		C	C	C	C		C	C	C	C	C	C	C	C	N	C
Imipenem/Cilastatin	N	N	N	C	N	C	C	C	C	C	C	C	N	C	N	N	N	C	C		C	C	C	C	C
Insulin, Regular	C	C	C	N	N	N	C	C	C	C		C	C	C	C	C	C	C	C	C	N		C	C	
Ketorolac		N	N	N	N	C	C	C	C	C	C	C	C	C	C	N		C	C	C	C	C	C	C	C
Labetalol	C	C	C	C	C	C	C	N		C	N	C	C	C	C	C	C	C	C	C	C	C	C	C	C
Levofloxacin	N		C	C	C	C	C	N		C	N	C	C	C	C	C		C	N	N		C	C	C	C
Levothyroxine																								N	
Linezolid	C	C	C	C	C	C	C	C	C	C	C	C	C	C	C	C		C	C	C	C	C	C	C	C
Lorazepam	C	C	C	C	C	C	C	C	C	C	C	C		C	N	C	C	C	C	C	C	C	C	C	C
Magnesium Sulfate				C	C	C	C			C	C	C	C		C	C	C	C	C	C	C	C	C	C	C
Mannitol		C	C	C	C	C	C	C		C	C	C	C	C	C	C		C	C	C	C	C	C	C	C
Meperidine	C	C	C	C	C	C	C	N			C	C	N	C		C		C	C	C	C	C	C	N	C
Methylprednisolone	C	N	N	N	C	C	C	C		C	C	C	C	N	C	C		C	C	C	C	C		C	C
Metoclopramide		C	C	C	C	C	C	N	C	C	C	C	C	C	C	C		C	C	C	C	C	C	C	C
Metoprolol		C	C	C	C	C	C	C	C	C	C	C	C	C	C	C		C	C	C	C	C	C	C	C
Metronidazole	C	C	C	C	C	C	C	C	C	C	C	C	C	C	C	C		C	C	C	C	C	C	C	C
Micafungin	N	C	C	N	N	C		C	C	C	N	C	C	C	N	N		N	C	C	C		C		C
Midazolam	C	C	C	C	N	C	C	N	C	C	C	C	C	C		C	C	C	C	C	C	C	N	C
Morphine	C	C	C	C	C	C	C	C	N	C	C	C	C	C	C	C	C		C	C	C	C	C	C	C
Moxifloxacin							N	N														C			C
Nafcillin		C	C	N	C	C	C	C	C	C	N	C	C	C	N	N		C	C	C	C	C	C	C	C
Nalbuphine		C	C	C	C	C	C	N			C	C	C	C	C	C		C	C	C	C	C	C	N	C
Ondansetron		C	C	C	C	C	C	N		C		C	N	C	C	C		C	C	C	C	C	C	N	C
Pantoprazole	N	N		C	N	N	C	N	C		C	C	N	N	C	N	N		C	C		C	C	C	C
Penicillin G Potassium	C	C	C	C	N	C	C	C	C		C	C	C		C	C		C	C	C	C	C	C	C	C
Phenobarbital		C	C	N	N	N	C	C			C		C	C	N	N		N	C	N	C	C	C	C	
Phenylephrine	C	C	C	C	C	C	C	N	C	C	N	C	C	C	C	C		C	C	C	C	C	C	C	C
Phenytoin		N	N	N	N	N	N	N		N	N	N	N	N	N	N		N	N	N	N		N	N	N
Piperacillin/Tazobactam	N	C	C	N	N	C	C	C		C	N	C	C	C	C	N		C	C	C	C	C	C	C	C
Potassium Chloride	C	C	C	C	C	C	C	C	C	C	C	C	C	C	C	C	C	C	C	C	C	C		C	C
Potassium Phosphate	N		N	C	N					C			N	N						C		C	N		C
Prochlorperazine		N	N	C	C	C	C	N		C	N	C	C	C	N	C		C	C	N	C	C	C	N	C
Sodium Bicarbonate	N	N	N	N	N	N	C	C		N	C	C	C	C	N	N	C	C	C	C	N	C	C		C
Sodium Phosphate	N		N										C									C			C
Ticarcillin/Clavulanate		C	C	C	N	C	C	C		C	C	C	C	C	C			C	C	C	C	C	C	C	C
Tigecycline	N	C	C	C	C	C	C	C		C	C	C	C	C	C	C		C	C	C	C	C	C	C	C
Tobramycin	C	C	C	C	C	C	C	C		C	C	C	C	C	C	C		C	C	C	C	C	C	C	C
Trimethoprim/Sulfamethoxazole		N	N	C	N	N	N	N	N	C	N	N	C	N	N	N		N	N	N	N	N	N	N	N
Vancomycin	C	C	C	C	C	C	C	N		C	C	C	C	C	C	C		C	C	C	C	C	C	C	C
Verapamil	C	C	C	C	C	C	C	C		C	C	C	C	C	C	C		C	C	C	C	C	C	N	C
Voriconazole	C	C	C	C	C	C	C	C			C	C	C	C	C	C		C	C	N	C	C	C	C	C

Be aware: New studies may alter the informatin on this chart.

MEDICATION SAFETY TOOLS I IV Compatibility Quick Reference Chart

C3

PEDIATRIC INTRAVENOUS MEDICATION QUICK REFERENCE CHART

Risk of fluid overload in infants and children is always a consideration when administering IV medications. The following table provides maximum concentrations—the smallest amount of fluid necessary for diluting specific medications—and the maximum rate at which the medications be given.

Drug	Maximum Concentration	Maximum Rate
acetazolamide	100 mg/ml	500 mg/min2
acyclovir	10 mg/ml	Give over 1 hr
adenosine	3 mg/ml	Give over 1-2 sec
allopurinol	6 mg/ml	Give over 15-20 min
amikacin	10 mg/ml	Give over 30 min
aminocaproic acid	20 mg/ml	Give over 1 hr
aminophylline	25 mg/ml	25 mg/min
amphotericin B	0.1 mg/ml (peripherally) 0.5 mg/ml (centrally)	Give over 2-6 hr
amphotericin B liposomal	2 mg/ml	Give over 2 hr
amphotericin B colloidal	0.83 mg/ml	Give over 2 hr
ampicillin	100 mg/ml	10 mg/kg/min
ampicillin/sulbactam	30 mg/ml (ampicillin)	Give over 15-30 min
anidulafungin	0.43 mg/ml	1.1 mg/min
atropine	1 mg/ml	Give over 1 min
azithromycin	2 mg/ml	Give over 1 hr
aztreonam	20 mg/ml	Give over 20-60 min
bumetanide	0.25 mg/ml	Give over 1-2 min
caffeine citrate	20 mg/ml	Give over 10-20 min
calcitriol	2 mcg/ml	Give over 15 sec
calcium chloride	100 mg/ml	100 mg/min
calcium gluconate	100 mg/ml	100 mg/min
caspofungin	0.47 mg/ml	Give over 1 hr
cefazolin	138 mg/ml (IVP) 20 mg/ml (Intermittent infusion)	Give over 3-5 min Give over 10-60 min
cefepime	160 mg/ml	Give over 30 min
cefotaxime	200 mg/ml (IVP) 60 mg/ml (Intermittent infusion)	Give over 3-5 min Give over 10-30 min
cefoxitin	200 mg/ml (IVP) 40 mg/ml (Intermittent infusion)	Give over 3-5 min Give over 15-40 min
ceftazidime	200 mg/ml (IVP) 40 mg/ml (Intermittent infusion)	Give over 3-5 min Give over 10-30 min
ceftriaxone	40 mg/ml	Give over 10-30 min
cefuroxime	100 mg/ml (IVP) 30 mg/ml (Intermittent infusion)	Give over 3-5 min Give over 15-60 min
chlorpromazine	1 mg/ml	0.5 mg/min
ciprofloxacin	2 mg/ml	Give over 60 min
clindamycin	18 mg/ml	30 mg/min
cyclosporine	2.5 mg/ml	Give over 2-8 hr
dexamethasone	10 mg/ml	Doses < 10 mg: Give over 1-4 min Doses > 10 mg: Give over 10-20 min
diazepam	5 mg/ml	2 mg/min
diazoxide	15 mg/ml	Give over 30-60 min
digoxin	100 mcg/ml	Give over 5 min
diphenhydramine	50 mg/ml	25 mg/min
doxycycline	1 mg/ml	Give over 1 hr
enalaprilat	1.25 mg/ml	Give over 5 min
erythromycin	5 mg/ml	Give over 20-120 min
ethacrynic acid	2 mg/ml	Give over 5-10 min
famotidine	4 mg/ml	Give over 2-10 min
fentanyl	50 mcg/ml	Give over 1-3 min
fluconazole	2 mg/ml	Give over 1-2 hr
flumazenil	0.1 mg/ml	Give over 15-30 sec
foscarnet	12 mg/ml	60 mg/kg/hr
fosphenytoin	25 mg/ml	3 mg/kg/min
furosemide	10 mg/ml	0.5 mg/kg/min
ganciclovir	10 mg/ml	Give over 1 hr
gentamicin	40 mg/ml	Give over 30 min
glycopyrrolate	0.2 mg/ml	Give over 5-10 sec
granisetron	50 mcg/ml (Intermittent infusion) 1 mg/ml (IVP)	Give over 2-30 min Give over 30 sec
hydralazine	20 mg/ml	5 mg/min or 0.2 mg/kg/min
hydrocortisone sodium succinate	60 mg/ml (IVP) 5 mg/ml (intermittent infusion)	Give over 30 sec Give over 10-30 min

Drug	Maximum Concentration	Maximum Rate
imipenem/cilastatin	7 mg/ml	Give over 15-60 min
inamrinone	5 mg/ml	Give over 2-3 min
indomethacin	1 mg/ml	Give over 20-35 min
kanamycin	5 mg/ml	Give over 20-30 min
ketamine	50 mg/ml (IVP) 2 mg/ml (Intermittent infusion)	2 mg/min or 0.5 mg/kg/min 2 mg/min or 0.5 mg/kg/min
ketorolac	30 mg/ml	Give over 1-5 min
labetalol	5 mg/ml (IVP)	2 mg/min
lansoprazole	0.12 mg/ml	Give over 30 min
levocarnitine	200 mg/ml	Give over 2-3 min
levothyroxine	100 mcg/ml	Give over 2-3 min
linezolid	2 mg/ml	Give over 30-120 min
lorazepam	4 mg/ml	2 mg/min or 0.05 mg/kg over 2-5 min
magnesium sulfate	200 mg/ml	10-20 min
meperidine	10 mg/ml	Give over 5 min
meropenem	50 mg/ml	Give over 15-30 min
methylprednisolone	125 mg/ml (IVP) 2.5 mg/ml (Intermittent infusion)	Give over 1-30 min Give over 20-60 min
metoclopramide	5 mg/ml	Give over 1-2 min
metronidazole	8 mg/ml	Give over 1 hr
micafungin	1.5 mg/ml	Give over 1 hr
midazolam	5 mg/ml	Give over 20-30 sec (5 min in neonates)
milrinone	1 mg/ml	Give over 10 min
morphine	5 mg/ml	Give over 4-30 min
nafcillin	100 mg/ml	Give over 15-60 min
naloxone	1 mg/ml	Give over 30 sec
ondansetron	2 mg/ml	Give over 2-15 min
oxacillin	100 mg/ml (IVP) 40 mg/ml (Intermittent infusion)	Give over 10 min Give over 15-30 min
pancuronium	2 mg/ml (IVP)	Give over seconds
pantoprazole	4 mg/ml	Give over 2-15 min
penicillin g	50,000 units/ml (neonates/infants) 500,000 units/ml (children)	Give over 15-30 min
pentamidine	6 mg/ml	Give over 1-2 hr
pentobarbital	50 mg/ml	Give over 10-30 min
phenobarbital	130 mg/ml	2 mg/kg/min
phenytoin	50 mg/ml	3 mg/kg/min
phytonadione	10 mg/ml	Give over 15-30 min
piperacillin	200 mg/ml (IVP) 70 mg/ml (Intermittent infusion)	Give over 3-5 min Give over 20-60 min
piperacillin/tazobactam	200 mg/ml	Give over 30 min
potassium chloride	80 mEq/L (peripherally) 200 mEq/L (centrally)	1 mEq/kg/hr
promethazine	25 mg/ml	< 25 mg/min
propranolol	1 mg/ml	Give over 10-15 min
protamine	10 mg/ml	5 mg/min
ranitidine	2.5 mg/ml	10 mg/min
rifampin	6 mg/ml	Give over 30 min
tacrolimus	0.02 mg/ml	Give over 4-24 hr
terbutaline	1 mg/ml	Give over 5-10 min
ticarcillin	100 mg/ml	Give over 10-120 min
ticarcillin/clavulanate	100 mg/ml	Give over 10-60 min.
tobramycin	40 mg/ml	Give over 30 min
trimethoprim/sulfamethoxazole	1 ml drug per 10 ml diluent	Give over 1-1.5 hr
valproate sodium	50 mg/ml	2-6 mg/kg/min
vancomycin	5 mg/ml	Give over 60 min
vasopressin	1 unit/ml	Give over 5-30 min
verapamil	2.5 mg/ml (IVP)	Give over 30-60 sec
voriconazole	5 mg/ml	3 mg/kg/hr
zidovudine	4 mg/ml	Give over 60 min

1. Phelps SJ, Hak EB, Crill CM: Pediatric Injectable Drugs, 8th Edition. American Society of Health-System Pharmacists, Bethesda, MD 2007.

BEERS CRITERIA

The Beers criteria for potentially inappropriate medication use in adults 65 and older in the United States is a compilation of drugs and drug classes found to increase the risk of adverse events in older adults. Frequently, older adults are more sensitive to the medications or their side effects. These adverse events have significant economic and quality of life costs for society and individuals and can result in more frequent hospitalizations, permanent injury, or death. Often, the potential for adverse events can be minimized by prescribing safer alternatives or prescribing at the lowest effective dose. The list below appears in Archives of Internal Medicine, volume 163, published in December 2003. It represents an update to the original list, published in 1991 by Mark H. Beers, MD.

alprazolam (Niravam, Xanax)	ethacrynic acid (Edecrin)
amiodarone (Cordarone, Pacerone)	ferrous sulfate (iron, Feosol)
amitriptyline	fluoxetine (Prozac)
amphetamines	flurazepam (Dalmane)
anorexic agents	hydroxyzine (Vistaril)
barbiturates	hyoscyamine (Anaspaz, Levsin)
belladonna alkaloids (Donnatal)	meperidine (Demerol)
bisacodyl (Dulcolax)	meprobamate
carisoprodol (Soma)	metaxalone (Skelaxin)
castor oil	methocarbamol (Robaxin)
chlordiazepoxide (Librium)	methyldopa
chlordiazepoxide-amitriptyline (Limbitrol)	methyldopa-hydrochlorothiazide
chlorpheniramine (Chlor-Trimeton)	methyltestosterone (Android, Testred, Virilon)
chlorpropamide (Diabinese)	mineral oil
chlorzoxazone (Parafon Forte DSC)	naproxen (Aleve, Anaprox, Naprosyn)
cimetidine (Tagamet)	nifedipine (Adalat, Afeditab CR, Procardia)
clidinium-chlordiazepoxide (Librax)	nitrofurantoin (Furadantin, Macrobid, Microdantin)
clonidine (Catapres, Duraclon)	orphenadrine (Norflex)
clorazepate (Tranxene)	oxaprozin (Daypro)
cyclobenzaprine (Amrix, Fexmid, Flexeril)	oxazepam (Serax)
cyproheptadine	oxybutynin (Ditropan, Gelnique, Oxytrol)
dessicated thyroid (Armour Thyroid)	pentazocine (Talwin)
dexchlorpheniramine	piroxicam (Feldene)
diazepam (Valium)	promethazine (Promethegan)
dicyclomine (Bentyl)	propantheline
digoxin (Lanoxin)	propoxyphene (Darvon) and combination products
diphenhydramine (Benadryl)	quazepam (Doral)
dipyridamole (Persantine)	reserpine
disopyramide (Norpace)	temazepam (Restoril)
doxazosin (Cardura)	thioridazine
doxepin (Zonalon)	ticlopidine
ergoloid mesylates (Hydergine)	triazolam (Halcion)
estrogens	trimethobenzamide (Tigan)

Frick DM, et al. Potentially Inappropriate Medications for Use in Older Adults (Beers List). Updating the Beers criteria for potentially inappropriate medication use in older adults: results of a US consensus panel of experts. Arch Intern Med. 2003;163:2716-2724.

DRUGS ASSOCIATED WITH INCREASED RISK OF FALLS IN THE ELDERLY

Many factors are associated with falls in the elderly, including frailty, disease, vision, polypharmacy and certain medications. Below is a list of drugs associated with falls. Assess geriatric patients on these medications for fall risk and implement fall reduction strategies.

ACE Inhibitors
- benazepril (Lotensin)
- captopril (Capoten)
- enalapril (Vasotec)
- fosinopril (Monopril)
- lisinopril (Prinivil, Zestril)
- moexipril (Univasc)
- perindopril (Aceon)
- quinapril (Accupril)
- ramipril (Altace)
- trandolapril (Mavik)

Angiotensin II Receptor Antagonists
- candesartan (Atacand)
- eprosartan (Teveten)
- irbesartan (Avapro)
- losartan (Cozaar)
- olmesartan (Benicar)
- telmisartan (Micardis)
- valsartan (Diovan)

Antiarrhythmics
- digoxin (Lanoxin)
- disopyramide (Norpace)

Anticonvulsants
- carbamazepine (Tegretol)
- ethosuximide (Zarontin)
- felbamate (Felbatol)
- gabapentin (Neurontin)
- lamotrigine (Lamictal)
- levetiracetam (Keppra)
- methsuximide (Celontin)
- phenobarbital (Luminal)
- phenytoin (Dilantin)
- pregabalin (Lyrica)
- primidone (Mysoline)
- tiagabine (Gabatril)
- topiramate (Topamax)
- valproate (Depakene, Depakote, Stavzor)
- zonisamide (Zonegran)

Antidepressants
- amitriptyline (Elavil)
- amoxapine
- bupropion (Aplenzin, Wellbutrin)
- citalopram (Celexa)
- clomipramine (Anafranil)
- desipramine (Norpramin)
- doxepin
- duloxetine (Cymbalta)
- escitalopram (Lexapro)
- fluoxetine (Prozac)
- fluvoxamine (Luvox)
- imipramine (Tofranil)
- isocarboxazid (Marplan)
- maprotiline
- mirtazapine (Remeron)
- nefazodone
- paroxetine (Paxil, Pexeva)
- phenelzine (Nardil)
- protriptyline (Vivactil)
- sertraline (Zoloft)
- tranylcypromine (Parnate)
- trazodone
- trimipramine (Surmontil)
- venlafaxine (Effexor)

Antihistamines/Antinauseants
- dimenhydrinate (Dramamine)
- diphenhydramine (Benadryl)
- hydroxyzine (Vistaril)
- meclizine (Antivert, Bonine)
- metoclopramide (Metozolv ODT, Reglan)
- prochlorperazine (Compro)
- promethazine (Promethegan)
- scopolamine patch (Transderm Scop)

Antiparkinsonian Agents
- amantadine (Symmetrel)
- bromocriptine (Parlodel)
- entacapone (Comtan)
- levodopa/carbidopa (Parcopa, Sinemet)
- pramipexole (Mirapex)
- selegiline (Eldepryl, Zelapar)

Antipsychotics (Atypical)
- aripiprazole (Abilify)
- clozapine (Clozaril, FazaClo)
- olanzapine (Zyprexa)
- paliperidone (Invega)
- quetiapine (Seroquel)
- risperidone (Risperdal)
- ziprasidone (Geodon)

Antipsychotics (Neuroleptics)
- chlorpromazine
- fluphenazine
- haloperidol (Haldol)
- loxapine (Loxitane)
- molindone (Moban)
- perphenazine
- pimozide (Orap)
- thioridazine
- thiothixine (Navane)
- trifluoperazine

Anxiolytics
- buspirone (Buspar)
- meprobamate

Benzodiazepines (Long Acting)
- chlordiazepoxide (Librium)
- clonazepam (Klonopin)
- clorazepate (Tranxene)
- diazepam (Valium)
- flurazepam (Dalmane)
- quazepam (Doral)

Benzodiazepines (Intermediate Acting)
- alprazolam (Niravam, Xanax)
- estazolam (Prosom)
- lorazepam (Ativan)
- oxazepam (Serax)
- temazepam (Restoril)

Benzodiazepines (Short Acting)
- triazolam (Halcion)

Beta Blockers
- acebutolol (Sectral)
- atenolol (Tenormin)
- bisoprolol (Zebeta)
- carvedilol (Coreg)
- labetalol (Trandate)
- metoprolol (Lopressor, Toprol XL)
- propranolol (Inderal, InnoPran XL)
- timolol

Calcium Channel Blockers
- amlodipine (Norvasc)
- diltiazem (Cardizem, Cartia XT, Dilacor XR, Taztia XT, Tiazac)
- felodipine
- isradipine (DynaCirc CR)
- nicardipine (Cardene)
- nifedipine (Adalat CC, Afeditab CC, Procardia XL)
- nisoldipine (Sular)
- verapamil (Calan, Covera HS, Isoptin, Verelan)

Diuretics
- amiloride/HCTZ
- bumetanide
- furosemide (Lasix)
- hydrochlorothiazide (Microzide)
- triamterene/HCTZ (Dyazide, Maxzide)

Opioid Analgesics
- codeine
- fentanyl (Actiq, Duragesic, Fentora, Sublimaze)
- hydrocodone
- hydromorphone (Dilaudid)
- levorphanol (Levo-Dromoran)
- meperidine (Demerol)
- methadone (Dolophine)
- morphine (Avinza, DepoDur, Duramorph, Kadian, MS Contin, Oramorph, Roxanol)
- oxycodone (OxyContin, Roxicodone)
- oxymorphone (Opana)
- pentazocine (Talwin)
- propoxyphene (Darvon)

Skeletal Muscle Relaxants
- Baclofen (Lioresal)

Vasodilators
- doxazosin (Cardura)
- hydralazine
- isosorbide (Dilatrate SR, Imdur, Ismo, Isordil, Monoket)
- nitroglycerin (Minitran, Nitro-Dur, Nitrostat)
- prazosin (Minipress)
- terazosin (Hytrin)

American Geriatrics Society (AGS) Panel on Falls in Older Persons, Guideline for the Prevention of Falls in Older Persons JAGS 49:664–672, 2001.

Keys PA. Preventing Falls in the Elderly: The Role of the Pharmacist. J Pharm Pract. 17(2):149-152, 2004.

Cooper JW, Burfield AH. Medication Interventions for Fall Prevention in the Older Adult. J Am Pharm Assoc. 49:e70-84, 2009.

LOOK-ALIKE, SOUND-ALIKE (LASA) DRUG NAMES

The Joint Commission established a National Patient Safety Goal that requires accredited organizations to identify a list of look-alike or sound-alike drugs used in their organization and, at a minimum, to review the list annually and take action to prevent errors involving the use of these drugs. Organizations must list at least 10 drug combinations from The Joint Commission's list of LASA drugs.

The following are drug pairs that The Joint Commission and others have rated as most problematic. Names in ALL CAPITALS are brand names; those in lowercase are generic names.

ABELCET	amphotericin B (conventional)	idarubicin	daunorubicin
acetazolamide	acetohexamide	idarubicin	doxorubicin
acetohexamide	acetazolamide	KLONOPIN	clonidine
alprazolam	lorazepam	lamivudine	lamotrigine
ADVAIR	ADVICOR	lamotrigine	lamivudine
ADVICOR	ADVAIR	leucovorin calcium	LEUKERAN
AMBISOME	amphotericin B (conventional)	LEUKERAN	leucovorin calcium
AMPHOTEC	amphotericin B (conventional)	lorazepam	alprazolam
amphotericin B (conventional)	ABELCET	metformin	metronidazole
amphotericin B (conventional)	AMBISOME	metronidazole	metformin
amphotericin B (conventional)	AMPHOTEC	morphine	hydromorphone
AVANDIA	COUMADIN	morphine oral liquid concentrate	morphine-non-concentrated oral liquid
AVINZA	EVISTA	MS CONTIN	OXYCONTIN
CARDURA	COUMADIN	NOVOLIN	NOVOLOG
CELEBREX	CELEXA	NOVOLIN	HUMULIN
CELEBREX	CEREBYX	NOVOLIN 70/30	NOVOLOG MIX 70/30
CELEXA	CELEBREX	NOVOLOG	HUMALOG
CELEXA	CEREBYX	NOVOLOG	NOVOLIN
CEREBYX	CELEBREX	NOVOLOG MIX 70/30	NOVOLIN 70/30
CEREBYX	CELEXA	oxycodone	hydrocodone
clonidine	KLONOPIN	oxycodone (immediate-release)	OXYCONTIN (controlled-release)
COUMADIN	AVANDIA	OXYCONTIN	MS CONTIN
COUMADIN	CARDURA	OXYCONTIN (controlled-release)	oxycodone (immediate-release)
daunorubicin	idarubicin	PERCOCET	DARVOCET
DARVOCET	PERCOCET	PRILOSEC	PROZAC
DIABETA	ZEBET-A	PROZAC	PRILOSEC
DIFLUCAN	DIPRIVAN	RETROVIR	ritonavir
DIPRIVAN	DIFLUCAN	ritonavir	RETROVIR
doxorubicin	doxorubicin hydrochloride liposomal	tiagabine	tizanidine
doxorubicin	idarubicin	tizanidine	tiagabine
EFFEXOR	EFFEXOR XL	TOPAMAX	TOPROL XL
EFFEXOR XL	EFFEXOR	TOPROL XL	TOPAMAX
ephedrine	epinephrine	tramadol	trazodone
epinephrine	ephedrine	trazodone	tramadol
EVISTA	AVINZA	vinblastine	vincristine
folic acid	folinic acid (leucovorin calcium)	vincristine	vinblastine
folinic acid (leucovorin calcium)	folic acid	WELLBUTRIN SR	WELLBUTRIN XL
heparin	HESPAN	WELLBUTRIN XL	WELLBUTRIN SR
HESPAN	heparin	XANAX	ZANTAC
HUMALOG	HUMULIN	ZANTAC	XANAX
HUMALOG	NOVOLOG	ZANTAC	ZYRTEC
HUMULIN	HUMALOG	ZEBETA	DIABETA
HUMULIN	NOVOLIN	ZESTRIL	ZETIA
hydralazine	hydroxyzine	ZESTRIL	ZYPREXA
hydrocodone	oxycodone	ZETIA	ZESTRIL
hydromorphone	morphine	ZOCOR	ZYRTEC
hydroxyzine	hydralazine	ZYPREXA	ZESTRIL
		ZYPREXA	ZYRTEC
		ZYRTEC	ZANTAC
		ZYRTEC	ZOCOR
		ZYRTEC	ZYPREXA

Joint Commission. Look-alike/sound-alike Drug Lists. Available at:
http://www.jointcommission.org/NR/rdonlyres/C92AAB3F-A9BD-431C-8628-11DD2D1D53CC/0/lasa.pdf.
Accessed December 12, 2009.

Joint Commission. 2008 National Patient Safety Goals. Available at:
http://www.jointcommission.org/PatientSafety/NationalPatientSafetyGoals/09_hap_npsgs.htm.
Accessed December 12, 2009

DO NOT CRUSH!

Do not crush any oral medication that is labeled as:

Enteric-coated (**EC**)
Extended release
Effervescent tablet (**EVT**)
Irritant (**I**)
Mucous Membrane irritant (**MMI**)
Orally Disintegrating tablets (**ODT**)
Slow-release (**SR**)
Sublingual forms of drugs
Sustained-release

Do not crush any oral medication that ends in the following letters:

CD CR LA SR XL XR XT

MEDICATIONS THAT SHOULD NOT BE CRUSHED:

Accutane Capsule (**MMI**)
Aciphex Tablet (**SR**)
Actiq lozenge (**SR**)
Actonel Tablet (**I**)
Adalat CC tablet (**SR**)
Adderall XR Capsule (**SR**) see code "**C**"
AeroHist Plus Tablet (**SR**)
Afeditab CR Tablet (**SR**)
Afinitor Tablet (**MMI**)
Aggrenox Capsule (**SR**)
Alavert Allergy Sinus 12 Hour Tablet (**SR**)
Allegra-D Tablet (**SR**)
Allfen Jr Tablet (**SR**)
Allfen Jr Capsule (**SR**) see code "**C**"
Alpophen Tablet (**EC**)
Alprazolam ER Tabalet (**SR**)
Altoprev Tablet (**SR**)
Ambien CR Tablet (**SR**)
Amitza Capsule (**SR**)
Amrix Capsule (**SR**)
Aprisor Capsule (**SR**) see code "**C**"
Aptivus Capsule
Aquatab C Tablet (**SR**)
  may break scored tablet only
Aquatab D Tablet (**SR**)
Arthrotec Tablet (**EC**)
Asacol Tablet (**SR**)
Ascriptin A/D Tablet (**EC**)
Aspirin Bayer Enteric coated Caplet (**EC**)
Aspirin Bayer Low Adult Tablet (**EC**)
Aspirin Bayer Regular
  Strength Caplet (**EC**)
Azulfidine EN-tablet (**EC**)
Augmentin XR tablet (**SR**)
  see codes "**A**" and "**B**"
Avinza Capsule (**SR**) see code "**C**"
Avodart Capsule (women of childbearing age should not handle this tablet)
Bellahist –D LA Tablet (**SR**)
Biaxin-XL Tablet (**SR**)
Bidhist Tablet (**SR**)
Bidhist –D Tablet (**SR**)
Biltricide tablet see code "**B**"
Bisa-lax Tablet (**EC**) see code "**D**"

Biohist LA Tablet (SR) see code "**B**"
Bisac-Evac Tablet (EC) see code "**D**"
Bisacodyl Tablet (EC) see code "**D**"
Boniva Tablet (alteration of tablet may cause oropharyngeal irritation)
Bromfed PD Capsule (**SR**)
Budeprion SR Tablet (**SR**)
Calan SR Tablet (**SR**) see code "**B**"
Carbatrol Capsule (**SR**) see code "**C**"
Cardene SR Capsule (**SR**)
Cardizem CD Capsule (**SR**)
Cardizem LA Tablet (**SR**)
Cardura XL Capsule (**SR**)
Cartia XT Capsule (**SR**)
Cefaclor Extended-release Tablet (**SR**)
Ceftin Tablet
Cefuroxime Tablet
CellCept Capsule, Tablet (potential for teratogenic reaction)
Chlor-Trimeton 12 Hour Tablet (**SR**)
Cipro XR Tablet (**SR**)
Claritin-D 12 Hour Tablet (**SR**)
Claritin-D 24 Hour Tablet (**SR**)
Colace Capsule
Colestid Tablet (**SR**)
Concerta Tablet (**SR**)
Commit Lozenge
Cotazym-S Capsule (**EC**) see code "**C**"
Covera-HS Tablet (**SR**)
Creon 5,10,20 Capsule (**SR**) see code "**C**"
Crixivan Capsule see code "**C**"
Cymbalta Capsule (**SR**)
Cytovene Capsule
Dallergy Tablet (**SR**)
  scored tablet may be broken
Dallergy-JR Capsule (**SR**)
Deconamine SR Capsule (**SR**)
Depakene (**SR, MMI**)
Depakote Tablet (**SR**)
Depakote ER Tablet (**SR**)
Detrol LA Capsule (**SR**)
Dilacor XR Capsule (**SR**)
Dilatrate-SR Capsule (**SR**)
Diltiazem **LA, SR, CD, XR**
Ditropan XL Tablet (**SR**)
Divalproex ER Tablet (**SR**)
Doxidan Tablet (**SR**)
Drixoral Cold/Allergy Tablet (**SR**)
Drixoral Nondrowsy Tablet (**SR**)
Drixoral Allergy Sinus Tablet (**SR**)
Droxia Capsule
  (wear gloves to open capsule)
Dulcolax Tablet, Capsule see code "**D**"
DynaCirc CR Tablet (**SR**)
Easprin Tablet (**EC**)
EC-Naprosyn Tablet (**EC**)
E.E.S. 400 Tablet (**EC**)
Effer-K Tablet (**EVT**)
Effexor XR Capsule (**SR**)
Efidac/24 Tablet (**SR**)
Enablex Tablet (**SR**)
Entex LA Capsule (**SR**)
Entocort EC Capsule (**EC**)
Equetro Capsule (**SR**)
Ergomar (Sublingual form)
Ery-Tab Tablet (**EC**)

Erythromycin Stearate Tablet (**EC**)
Erythromycin Base Tablet (**EC**)
Erythromycin Delayed-Release Capsule (pellets) (see code "**C**")
Evista Tablet
  (potential for teratogenic reaction)
Feen-a-mint Tablet (**EC**)
Feldene Capsule (**MMI**)
Fentora Tablet
Feosol Tablet (**EC**)
Feratab Tablet (**EC**)
Fergon Tablet (**EC**)
Fero-Grad 500 mg Tablet (**SR**)
Ferro-Sequels Tablet (**SR**)
Flagyl ER Tablet (**SR**)
Fleet Laxative Tablet (**EC**)
Flomax Capsule (**SR**)
Focalin XR Capsule (**SR**) may be opened and sprinkled on food
Fosamax Tablet (**SR**)
Geocillin Tablet
Gleevec Tablet
Glipizide Tablet (**SR**)
Glucophage XR Tablet (**SR**)
Glucophage XL Tablet (**SR**)
Gluocotrol XL Tablet (**SR**)
Glumetza Tablet (**SR**)
Guaifed Capsule (**SR**)
Guaifenesin Tablet (**SR**)
Guaifenex DM, GP, PSE Tablets (**SR**)
Halfprin 81 Tablet (**EC**)
Hydrea Capsule
  (wear gloves to administer)
Imdur Tablet (**SR**) see code "**B**"
Inderal LA Capsule (**SR**)
Indocin SR Capsule (**SR**)
InnoPran XL Capsule (**SR**)
Intelence Tablet
  (may disperse tablet in water)
Invega Tablet (**SR**)
Isoptin SR Tablet (**SR**)
Isordil Sublingual Tablet
Isorsorbide Dinitrate Sublingual Tablet
Kadian Capsule (**SR**)
  Not to be given thru N/G tubes
Kaletra Tablet
Kaon CL-10 Tablet (**SR**)
Keppra Tablet
Ketek Tablet (**SR**)
Klor-Con Tablet (**SR**)
Klotrix Tablet (**SR**)
K-Lyte CL, DS Tablets (**EVT**)
K-Tab Tablet (**SR**)
Lamictal XR Tablet (**SR**)
Lescol XL Tablet (**SR**)
Levbid Tablet (**SR**)
Levsinex Timecaps Capsule (**SR**)
Lexxel Tablet (**SR**)
Liadal Tablet (**SR**)
Lipram UL Capsule (**EC, SR**) see code "**C**"
Lipram
Lithobid Tablet (**SR**)
Lovaza Capsule (do not put contents of capsule in styrofoam or plastic container)
Luvox CR Capsule (**SR**)
Mestinon Timespan Tablet (**SR**)

C9

DO NOT CRUSH!

MEDICATIONS THAT SHOULD NOT BE CRUSHED:

Metadate ER Tablet **(SR)**
Metadate CD Capsule **(SR)**
Methylin ER Tablet **(SR)**
Metoprolol ER Tablet **(SR)** see code "C"
Micro K Extendcaps Capsule **(SR)** see codes "A" & "C"
Modane Tablet **(EC)** see code "D"
Moxatag Tablet **(SR)**
Morphine Sulfate extended-release tablet **(SR)**
Motrin Tablet
MS Contin Tablet **(SR)** see code "A"
Mucinex Tablet **(SR)**
Mucinex DM Tablet **(SR)**
Myfortic Tablet **(SR)**
Neprelan Tablet **(SR)**
Nasatab LA Tablet **(SR)** see code "B"
Nexium Capsule **(SR)** see code "C"
Niaspan Tablet **(SR)**
Nicotinic Acid Capsule, Tablet **(SR)** see code "B"
Nifedical XL Tablet **(SR)**
Nefedipine extended-release Tablet **(SR)**
NitroQuick Tablet (sublingual only) see code "E"
Nitrostat Tablet (sublingual only) see code "E"
Norpace CR Capsule **(SR)**
**Opana ER (Crushing tablet may be fatal)
Oramorph SR Tablet **(SR)** see code "A"
**OxyContin (Crushing table may be fatal)
Pancrease MT Capsule **(EC)** see code "C"

Pancrecarb MS Capsule **(EC)** see code "C"
Pancrelipase Capsule **(EC)** see code "C"
Paxil CR Tablet **(SR)**
Plendil Tablet **(SR)**
Prevacid Capsule **(SR)**
Prevacid Solu Tablet **(ODT)** may dissolve in water to administer via NG tubes
Prevacid Suspension **(SR)** may mix with water only – **DO NOT** use in NG tubes
Prilosec Capsule **(SR)**
Prilosec OTC Tablet
Procardia XL Capsule **(SR)**
Propecia Tablet (women of child-bearing age should not handle tablet)
Proquin XR Tablet **(SR)**
Proscar Tablet (women of child-bearing age should not handle tablet)
Protonix Tablet **(SR)**
Prozac Weekly Tablet **(EC)**
Ranexa Tablet **(SR)**
Razadyne ER Capsule **(SR)**
Renagel Tablet
Requip XL Tablet **(SR)**
Respa-1st Tablet **(SR)** see code "B"
Respa-DM Tablet **(SR)** see code "B"
Respahist Capsule **(SR)** see code "C"
Respaire 60 SR, 120 SR Capsule **(SR)**
Resperdal M-Tablet **(ODT)**
Revlimid Capsule (potential for teratogenic reaction)
Ritalin LA Capsule **(SR)** see code "C"
Ritalin SR Tablet **(SR)**
Rythmol RS Capsule **(SR)**
Seroquel XR Tablet **(SR)**

Sinemet CR Tablet **(SR)**
Slo-Mag Tablet **(EC)**
Solodyne Tablet **(SR)**
Straterra Capsule
Sudafed 12 hr Capsule **(SR)** see code "A"
Sudafed 24 hr Capsule **(SR)** see code "A"
Sular Tablet **(SR)**
Taztia XT Capsule **(SR)** see code "C"
Tegretol-XR Tablet **(SR)**
Temodar Capsule
Tessalon Perles Capsule
Theo-24 Capsule
Tiazac Capsule **(SR)** see code "C"
Topomax Tablet/Capsule see code "C"
Toprol XLTablet **(SR)** see code "B"
Trental Tablet **(SR)**
Tylenol Arthritis Tablet **(SR)**
Ultram ER Tablet **(SR)** (Crushing tablet may be fatal)
Uniphyl Tablet **(SR)**
Uroxatral Tablet **(SR)**
Valcyte Tablet (potential for teratogenic reaction)
Verapamil SR Tablet **(SR)** see code "B"
Verelan Capsule **(SR)** see code "C"
Verelan PM Capsule **(SR)** see code "C"
VesiCare Tablet **(EC)**
Videx EC Capsule **(SR)**
Voltaren XR Tablet **(SR)**
Wellbutrin SR, XL Tablet **(SR)**
Xanax XR Tablet **(SR)**
Zorprin Tablet **(SR)**
Zyban Tablet **(SR)**
Zyflo CR Tablet **(SR)**

CODES:

A: Liquid forms are available
B: Tablets that are scored may be broken in half
C: Capsule can be opened – contents may be used in pudding or applesauce
D: Do not take with antacids or milk products
E: Disintegrate under the tongue – do not chew

TERATOGENIC REACTION:

An adverse effect to normal cellular development of an embryo or fetus.

C10

TALL MAN LETTERING CHANGES

The Food and Drug Administration has asked manufacturers to update the appearance of 33 look-alike drug names. The changes involve using capital letters ("Tall Man") to minimize medication errors resulting from look-alike confusion.

Acetohexamide Acetazolamide	AcetoHEXAMIDE AcetaZOLAMIDE
Bupropion Buspirone	BuPROPion BusPIRone
Chlorpromazine Chlorpropamide	ChlorproMAZINE ChlorproPAMIDE
Clomiphene Clomipramine	ClomiPHENE ClomiPRAMINE
Cyclosporine Cycloserine	CycloSPORINE CycloSERINE
Daunorubicin Doxorubicin	DAUNOrubicin DOXOrubicin
Dimenhydrinate Diphenhydramine	DimenhyDRINATE DiphenhydrAMINE
Dobutamine Dopamine	DOBUTamine DOPamine
Glipizide Glyburide	GlipiZIDE GlyBURIDE
Hydralazine Hydroxyzine	HydrALAZINE HydrOXYzine
Medroxyprogesterone Methylprednisolone Methyltestosterone	MedroxyPROGESTERone MethylPREDNISolone MethylTESTOSTERone
Nicardipine Nifedipine	NiCARdipine NIFEdipine
Prednisone Prednisolone	PredniSONE PrednisoLONE
Sulfadiazine Sulfisoxazole	SulfADIAZINE SulfiSOXAZOLE
Tolazamide Tolbutamide	TOLAZamide TOLBUTamide
Vinblastine Vincristine	VinBLAStine VinCRIStine

C11

TALL MAN List

MEDICATION SAFETY TOOLS | TALL MAN List

BuPROPion (Wellbutrin®)

- 75 mg
- 100 mg
- 100 mg SR
- 150 mg SR
- 200 mg SR
- 150 mg XL
- 300 mg XL

BuPROPion (Zyban®)

- 150 mg

BusPIRone (Buspar®)

- 5 mg
- 10 mg
- 15 mg
- 30 mg

ChlorproMAZINE

- 10 mg
- 25 mg
- 50 mg
- 100 mg
- 200 mg

ChlorproPAMIDE

- 100 mg
- 250 mg

ClomiPHENE

- 50 mg

ClomiPRAMINE

- 25 mg
- 50 mg
- 75 mg

Copyright © 2010 SFI Images

MEDICATION SAFETY TOOLS | TALL MAN List

DimenhyDRINATE
50 mg

DiphenhydrAMINE
25 mg
50 mg

DOBUTamine

DOPamine

GlipiZIDE (Glucotrol®)
5 mg
10 mg
2.5 mg XL
5 mg XL
10 mg XL

GlyBURIDE (DiaBeta®)
1.25 mg
2.5 mg
5 mg

HydrALAZINE
10 mg
25 mg
50 mg
100 mg

HydrOXYzine
10 mg
25 mg
50 mg

Copyright © 2010 SFI Images

C13

MEDICATION SAFETY TOOLS | TALL MAN List

MedroxyPROGESTERone (Provera®)
- 2.5 mg
- 5 mg
- 10 mg

MethylPREDNISolone (Medrol®)
- 2 mg
- 4 mg
- 8 mg
- 16 mg
- 32 mg

MethylTESTOSTERone
- 10 mg

NiCARdipine
- 20 mg
- 30 mg

NIFEdipine (Adalat® CC)
- 30 mg
- 60 mg
- 90 mg

PrednisoLONE (Orapred®)

PredniSONE
- 1 mg
- 2.5 mg
- 5 mg
- 10 mg
- 20 mg
- 50 mg

TOLAZamide
- 250 mg
- 500 mg

TOLBUTamide
- 500 mg

Copyright © 2010 SFI Images

Additional Drugs

AcetaZOLIMIDE
- 125 mg
- 250 mg

CycloSPORINE
- 25 mg
- 100 mg

Alprazolam (Xanax)
- 0.25 mg
- 0.5 mg
- 1 mg
- 2 mg
- 0.5 mg XR
- 1 mg XR
- 2 mg XR
- 3 mg XR

DOXOrubicin (Adriamycin)

Diltiazem (Cardizem®)
- 120 mg
- 180 mg
- 240 mg
- 300 mg
- 360 mg

Amoxicillin/clavulanate (Augmentin)
- 200 mg
- 400 mg
- 250 mg
- 500 mg
- 875 mg
- 1000 mg XR

Fentanyl oral transmucosal (Actiq)
- 200 mcg

MEDICATION SAFETY TOOLS | Additional Drugs

MEDICATION SAFETY TOOLS | Additional Drugs

Fentanyl transdermal patch

Sertraline (Zoloft)
25 mg • 50 mg • 100 mg

Fentanyl buccal (Fentora)
800 mcg

VinCRISTINE

Glimepiride (Amaryl)
1 mg • 2 mg • 4 mg

Warfarin (Coumadin)
1 mg • 2 mg • 2.5 mg • 3 mg • 4 mg • 5 mg • 6 mg • 7.5 mg • 10 mg

C16

Copyright © 2010 SFI Images

• ANTICOAGULANTS

PHARMACOLOGIC PROFILE

General Use
Prevention and treatment of thromboembolic disorders including deep vein thrombosis, pulmonary embolism, and atrial fibrillation with embolization. Also used in the management of myocardial infarction (MI) sequentially or in combination with thrombolytics and/or antiplatelet agents.

General Action and Information
Anticoagulants are used to prevent clot extension and formation. They do not dissolve clots. The two types of anticoagulants in common use are parenteral heparins and oral warfarin. Therapy is usually initiated with heparin or a heparin-like agent because of rapid onset of action, while maintenance therapy consists of warfarin. Warfarin takes several days to produce therapeutic anticoagulation. In serious or severe thromboembolic events, heparin therapy may be preceded by thrombolytic therapy. Low doses of heparin or heparin-like compounds and fondaparinux are mostly used to prevent deep vein thrombosis after certain surgical procedures and in similar situations in which prolonged bedrest increases the risk of thromboembolism. Argatroban and lepirudin are used as anticoagulation in patients who have developed thrombocytopenia during heparin therapy.

Contraindications
Underlying coagulation disorders, ulcer disease, malignancy, recent surgery, or active bleeding.

Precautions
Anticoagulation should be undertaken cautiously in any patient with a potential site for bleeding. Pregnant or lactating patients should not receive warfarin. Heparin does not cross the placenta. Heparin and heparin-like agents should be used cautiously in patients receiving epidural analgesia.

Interactions
Warfarin is highly protein bound and may displace or be displaced by other highly protein-bound drugs. The resultant interactions depend on which drug is displaced. Bleeding may be potentiated by aspirin or large doses of penicillins or penicillin-like drugs, cefotetan, cefoperazone, valproic acid, or NSAIDs.

NURSING IMPLICATIONS

Assessment
- Assess patient taking anticoagulants for signs of bleeding and hemorrhage (bleeding gums; nosebleed; unusual bruising; tarry, black stools; hematuria; fall in hematocrit or blood pressure; guaiac-positive stools; urine; or NG aspirate).
- Assess patient for evidence of additional or increased thrombosis. Symptoms will depend on area of involvement.
- **Lab Test Considerations:** Monitor prothrombin time (PT) or international normalized ratio (INR) with warfarin therapy, activated partial thromboplastin time (aPTT) with full-dose heparin therapy and hematocrit, and other clotting factors frequently during therapy.
- Monitor bleeding time throughout antiplatelet therapy. Prolonged bleeding time, which is time and dose dependent, is expected.
- **Toxicity and Overdose:** If overdose occurs or anticoagulation needs to be immediately reversed, the antidote for heparins is protamine sulfate; for warfarin, the antidote is vitamin K (phytonadione [AquaMEPHYTON]). Administration of whole blood or plasma may also be required in severe bleeding due to warfarin because of the delayed onset of vitamin K.

Potential Nursing Diagnoses
- Ineffective tissue perfusion (Indications).
- Risk for injury (Side Effects).
- Deficient knowledge, related to disease process and medication regimen (Patient/Family Teaching).

Implementation
- Inform all health care professionals caring for patient of anticoagulant therapy. Venipunctures and injection sites require application of pressure to prevent bleeding or hematoma formation.
- Use an infusion pump with continuous infusions to ensure accurate dosage.

Patient/Family Teaching
- Caution patient to avoid activities leading to injury, to use a soft toothbrush and electric razor, and to report any symptoms of unusual bleeding or bruising to health care professional immediately.
- Instruct patient not to take OTC medications, especially those containing aspirin, NSAIDs, or alcohol, without advice of health care professional.
- Review foods high in vitamin K (see Appendix M) with patients on warfarin. Patient should have consistent limited intake of these foods, as vitamin K is the antidote for warfarin and greatly alternating intake of these foods will cause PT levels to fluctuate.
- Emphasize the importance of frequent lab tests to monitor coagulation factors.
- Instruct patient to carry identification describing medication regimen at all times and to inform all health care professionals caring for patient of anticoagulant therapy before laboratory tests, treatment, or surgery.

Evaluation/Desired Outcomes
- Prevention of undesired clotting and its sequelae without signs of hemorrhage. Prevention of stroke, MI, and death in patients at risk.

Anticoagulants included in *Davis's Drug Guide for Nurses*

active factor X inhibitors
fondaparinux 608

antithrombotics
heparin 654

coumarins
warfarin 1295

thrombin inhibitors
argatroban 193
bivalirudin 234

desirudin 415
lepirudin (rDNA) 773

heparins (low molecular weight)
dalteparin 657
enoxaparin 657
tinzaparin 657

miscellaneous
vigabatrin 1374

• ANTICONVULSANTS

PHARMACOLOGIC PROFILE
General Use
Anticonvulsants are used to decrease the incidence and severity of seizures due various etiologies. Some anticonvulsants are used parenterally in the immediate treatment of seizures. It is not uncommon for patients to require more than one anticonvulsant to control seizures on a long-term basis. Many regimens are evaluated with serum level monitoring. Several anticonvulsants also are used to treat neuropathic pain.

ANTICONVULSANTS

General Action and Information
Anticonvulsants include a variety of agents, all capable of depressing abnormal neuronal discharges in the CNS that may result in seizures. They may work by preventing the spread of seizure activity, depressing the motor cortex, raising seizure threshold, or altering levels of neurotransmitters, depending on the group. See individual drugs.

Contraindications
Previous hypersensitivity.

Precautions
Use cautiously in patients with severe hepatic or renal disease; dose adjustment may be required. Choose agents carefully in pregnant and lactating women. Fetal hydantoin syndrome may occur in offspring of patients who receive phenytoin during pregnancy.

Interactions
Barbiturates stimulate the metabolism of other drugs that are metabolized by the liver, decreasing their effectiveness. Hydantoins are highly protein-bound and may displace or be displaced by other highly protein-bound drugs. Lamotrigine, tiagabine, and topiramate are capable of interacting with several other anticonvulsants. For more specific interactions, see individual drugs. Many drugs are capable of lowering seizure threshold and may decrease the effectiveness of anticonvulsants, including tricyclic antidepressants and phenothiazines.

NURSING IMPLICATIONS

Assessment
- Assess location, duration, and characteristics of seizure activity.
- **Toxicity and Overdose:** Monitor serum drug levels routinely throughout anticonvulsant therapy, especially when adding or discontinuing other agents.

Potential Nursing Diagnoses
- Risk for injury (Indications) (Side Effects).
- Deficient knowledge, related to disease process and medication regimen (Patient/Family Teaching).

Implementation
- Administer anticonvulsants around the clock. Abrupt discontinuation may precipitate status epilepticus.
- Implement seizure precautions.

Patient/Family Teaching
- Instruct patient to take medication every day, exactly as directed.
- May cause drowsiness. Caution patient to avoid driving or other activities requiring alertness until response to medication is known. Do not resume driving until physician gives clearance based on control of seizures.
- Advise patient to avoid taking alcohol or other CNS depressants concurrently with these medications.
- Advise patient to carry identification describing disease process and medication regimen at all times.

Evaluation/Desired Outcomes
- Decrease or cessation of seizures without excessive sedation.

42 ANTIDEPRESSANTS

Anticonvulsants included in *Davis's Drug Guide for Nurses*

barbiturates
pentobarbital 1330
phenobarbital 1015

benzodiazepines
clonazepam 341
clorazepate 347
diazepam 431

hydantoins
phenytoin 1020

valproates
divalproex sodium 1262
valproate sodium 1262
valproic acid 1262

miscellaneous
acetaZOLAMIDE 114
carbamazepine 272
fosphenytoin 616
gabapentin 623
lacosamide 1371
lamotrigine 764
levetiracetam 782
oxcarbazepine 962
pregabalin 1051
rufinamide 1372
tiagabine 1222
topiramate 1240
zonisamide 1315

• ANTIDEPRESSANTS

PHARMACOLOGIC PROFILE

General Use
Used in the treatment of various forms of endogenous depression, often in conjunction with psychotherapy. Other uses include: Treatment of anxiety (doxepin, fluoxetine, paroxetine, sertraline, venlafaxine); Enuresis (imipramine); Chronic pain syndromes (amitriptyline, doxepin, imipramine, nortriptyline); Smoking cessation (bupropion); Bulimia (fluoxetine); Obsessive-compulsive disorder (fluoxetine, fluvoxamine, paroxetine, sertraline); Social anxiety disorder (paroxetine, sertraline).

General Action and Information
Antidepressant activity is most likely due to preventing the reuptake of dopamine, norepinephrine, and serotonin by presynaptic neurons, resulting in accumulation of these neurotransmitters. The two major classes of antidepressants are the tricyclic antidepressants and the SSRIs. Most tricyclic agents possess significant anticholinergic and sedative properties, which explains many of their side effects (amitriptyline, amoxapine, doxepin, imipramine, nortriptyline). The SSRIs are more likely to cause insomnia (fluoxetine, fluvoxamine, paroxetine, sertraline).

Contraindications
Hypersensitivity. Should not be used in narrow-angle glaucoma. Should not be used in pregnancy or lactation or immediately after MI.

Precautions
Use cautiously in older patients and those with pre-existing cardiovascular disease. Elderly men with prostatic enlargement may be more susceptible to urinary retention. Anticholinergic side effects of tricyclic antidepressants (dry eyes, dry mouth, blurred vision, and constipation) may require dosage modification or drug discontinuation. Dosage requires slow titration; onset of therapeutic response may be 2-4 wk. May decrease seizure threshold, especially bupropion.

Interactions
Tricyclic antidepressants—May cause hypertension, tachycardia, and convulsions when used with MAO inhibitors. May prevent therapeutic response to some antihypertensives. Additive CNS depression with other CNS depressants. Sympathomimetic activity may be enhanced when used with other sympathomimetics. Additive anticholinergic effects with other drugs possessing

ANTIDEPRESSANTS 43

anticholinergic properties. **MAO inhibitors**—Hypertensive crisis may occur with concurrent use of MAO inhibitors and amphetamines, methyldopa, levodopa, dopamine, epinephrine, norepinephrine, desipramine, imipramine, reserpine, vasoconstrictors, or ingestion of tyramine-containing foods. Hypertension or hypotension, coma, convulsions, and death may occur with meperidine or other opioid analgesics and MAO inhibitors. Additive hypotension with antihypertensives or spinal anesthesia and MAO inhibitors. Additive hypoglycemia with insulin or oral hypoglycemic agents and MAO inhibitors. SSRIs, bupropion, or venlafaxine should not be used in combination with or within weeks of MAO inhibitors (see individual monographs). Risk of adverse reactions may be increased by almotriptan, frovatriptan, rizatriptan, naratriptan, sumatriptan, or zolmitriptan.

NURSING IMPLICATIONS
Assessment
- Monitor mental status and affect. Assess for suicidal tendencies, especially during early therapy. Restrict amount of drug available to patient.
- **Toxicity and Overdose:** Concurrent ingestion of MAO inhibitors and tyramine-containing foods may lead to hypertensive crisis. Symptoms include chest pain, severe headache, nuchal rigidity, nausea and vomiting, photosensitivity, and enlarged pupils. Treatment includes IV phentolamine.

Potential Nursing Diagnoses
- Ineffective coping (Indications).
- Risk for injury (Side Effects).
- Deficient knowledge, related to disease process and medication regimen (Patient/Family Teaching).

Implementation
- Administer drugs that are sedating at bedtime to avoid excessive drowsiness during waking hours, and administer drugs that cause insomnia (fluoxetine, fluvoxamine, paroxetine, sertraline, MAO inhibitors) in the morning.

Patient/Family Teaching
- Caution patient to avoid alcohol and other CNS depressants. Patients receiving MAO inhibitors should also avoid OTC drugs and foods or beverages containing tyramine (see Appendix M) during and for at least 2 wk after therapy has been discontinued, as they may precipitate a hypertensive crisis. Health care professional should be contacted immediately if symptoms of hypertensive crisis develop.
- Inform patient that dizziness or drowsiness may occur. Caution patient to avoid driving and other activities requiring alertness until response to the drug is known.
- Caution patient to make position changes slowly to minimize orthostatic hypotension.
- Advise patient to notify health care professional if dry mouth, urinary retention, or constipation occurs. Frequent rinses, good oral hygiene, and sugarless candy or gum may diminish dry mouth. An increase in fluid intake, fiber, and exercise may prevent constipation.
- Advise patient to notify health care professional of medication regimen and any herbal alternative therapies before treatment or surgery. MAO inhibitor therapy usually needs to be withdrawn at least 2 wk before use of anesthetic agents.
- Emphasize the importance of participation in psychotherapy and follow-up exams to evaluate progress.

Evaluation/Desired Outcomes
- Resolution of depression.
- Decrease in anxiety.
- Control of bedwetting in children over 6 yr of age.
- Management of chronic neurogenic pain.

Antidepressants included in *Davis's Drug Guide for Nurses*

selective serotonin reuptake inhibitors (SSRIs)
citalopram 320
desvenlafaxine 420
duloxetine 490
escitalopram 526
fluoxetine 587
fluvoxamine 604
paroxetine hydrochloride 992
paroxetine mesylate 992
sertraline 1147

tetracyclic antidepressants
mirtazapine 867

tricyclic antidepressants
amitriptyline 154
desipramine 413

doxepin 476
imipramine 703
nortriptyline 936

monamine oxidase (MAO) inhibitors
isocarboxazid 876
phenelzine 876
tranylcypromine 876

miscellaneous
amoxapine 1318
buPROPion 249
nefazodone 906
selegiline transdermal 1143
trazodone 1251
trimipramine 1338
venlafaxine 1272

• ANTIDIABETICS

PHARMACOLOGIC PROFILE

General Use
Insulin is used in the management of type 1 diabetes mellitus. It may also be used in type 2 diabetes mellitus when diet and/or oral medications fail to adequately control blood sugar. The choice of insulin preparation (rapid-acting, intermediate-acting, long-acting) and source (semi-synthetic, human recombinant DNA) depend on the degree of control desired, daily blood glucose fluctuations, and history of previous reactions. Oral agents are used primarily in type 2 diabetes mellitus. Oral agents are used when diet therapy alone fails to control blood glucose or symptoms or when patients are not amenable to using insulin. Some oral agents may be used with insulin.

General Action and Information
Insulin, a hormone produced by the pancreas, lowers blood glucose by increasing transport of glucose into cells and promotes the conversion of glucose to glycogen. It also promotes the conversion of amino acids to proteins in muscle, stimulates triglyceride formation, and inhibits the release of free fatty acids. Sulfonylureas, nateglinide, repaglinide, and metformin lower blood glucose by stimulating endogenous insulin secretion by beta cells of the pancreas and by increasing sensitivity to insulin at intracellular receptor sites. Intact pancreatic function is required. Miglitol delays digestion of ingested carbohydrates, thus lowering blood glucose, especially after meals. It may be combined with sulfonylureas. Pioglitazone and rosiglitazone increase insulin sensitivity.

Contraindications
Insulin—Hypoglycemia. **Oral hypoglycemic agents**—Hypersensitivity (cross-sensitivity with other sulfonylureas and sulfonamides may exist). Hypoglycemia. Type 1 diabetes. Avoid use in patients with severe kidney, liver, thyroid, and other endocrine dysfunction. Should not be used in pregnancy or lactation.

Precautions
Insulin—Infection, stress, or changes in diet may alter requirements. **Oral hypoglycemic agents**—Use cautiously in geriatric patients. Dose reduction may be necessary. Infection,

ANTIDIABETICS 45

stress, or changes in diet may alter requirements. Use with Sulfonylureas with caution in patients with a history of cardiovascular disease. Metformin may cause lactic acidosis.

Interactions
Insulin—Additive hypoglycemic effects with oral hypoglycemic agents. **Oral hypoglycemic agents**—Ingestion of alcohol may result in disulfiram-like reaction with some agents. Alcohol, corticosteroids, rifampin, glucagon, and thiazide diuretics may decrease effectiveness. Anabolic steroids, chloramphenicol, clofibrate, MAO inhibitors, most NSAIDs, salicylates, sulfonamides, and warfarin may increase hypoglycemic effect. Beta blockers may produce hypoglycemia and mask signs and symptoms.

NURSING IMPLICATIONS

Assessment
- Observe patient for signs and symptoms of hypoglycemic reactions.
- Acarbose, miglitol, and pioglitazone do not cause hypoglycemia when taken alone but may increase the hypoglycemic effect of other hypoglycemic agents.
- Patients who have been well controlled on metformin but develop illness or laboratory abnormalities should be assessed for ketoacidosis or lactic acidosis. Assess serum electrolytes, ketones, glucose, and, if indicated, blood pH, lactate, pyruvate, and metformin levels. If either form of acidosis is present, discontinue metformin immediately and treat acidosis.
- **Lab Test Considerations:** Serum glucose and glycosylated hemoglobin should be monitored periodically throughout therapy to evaluate effectiveness of treatment.

Potential Nursing Diagnoses
- Imbalanced nutrition: more than body requirements (Indications).
- Deficient knowledge, related to medication regimen (Patient/Family Teaching).
- Noncompliance (Patient/Family Teaching).

Implementation
- Patients stabilized on a diabetic regimen who are exposed to stress, fever, trauma, infection, or surgery may require sliding scale insulin. Withhold oral hypoglycemic agents and reinstitute after resolution of acute episode.
- Patients switching from daily insulin dose may require gradual conversion to oral hypoglycemics.
- **Insulin:** Available in different types and strengths and from different species. Check type, species, source, dose, and expiration date with another licensed nurse. Do not interchange insulins without physician's order. Use only insulin syringes to draw up dose. Use only U100 syringes to draw up insulin lispro dose.

Patient/Family Teaching
- Explain to patient that medication controls hyperglycemia but does not cure diabetes. Therapy is long-term.
- Review signs of hypoglycemia and hyperglycemia with patient. If hypoglycemia occurs, advise patient to take a glass of orange juice or 2–3 tsp of sugar, honey, or corn syrup dissolved in water (glucose, not table sugar, if taking miglitol), and notify health care professional.
- Encourage patient to follow prescribed diet, medication, and exercise regimen to prevent hypoglycemic or hyperglycemic episodes.
- Instruct patient in proper testing of serum glucose and ketones.
- Advise patient to notify health care professional if nausea, vomiting, or fever develops; if unable to eat usual diet; or if blood glucose levels are not controlled.
- Advise patient to carry sugar or a form of glucose and identification describing medication regimen at all times.
- Insulin is the recommended method of controlling blood glucose during pregnancy. Counsel female patients to use a form of contraception other than oral contraceptives and to notify health care professional promptly if pregnancy is planned or suspected.

- **Insulin:** Instruct patient on proper technique for administration; include type of insulin, equipment (syringe and cartridge pens), storage, and syringe disposal. Discuss the importance of not changing brands of insulin or syringes, selection and rotation of injection sites, and compliance with therapeutic regimen.
- **Sulfonylureas:** Advise patient that concurrent use of alcohol may cause a disulfiram-like reaction (abdominal cramps, nausea, flushing, headache, and hypoglycemia).
- **Metformin:** Explain to patient the risk of lactic acidosis and the potential need for discontinuation of metformin therapy if a severe infection, dehydration, or severe or continuing diarrhea occurs or if medical tests or surgery is required.

Evaluation/Desired Outcomes
- Control of blood glucose levels without the appearance of hypoglycemic or hyperglycemic episodes.

Antidiabetics included in *Davis's Drug Guide for Nurses*

alpha-glucosidase inhibitors
acarbose 110
miglitol 863

biguanides
metformin 829

dipeptidyl peptidase-4 inhibitors
saxagliptin 1138

enzyme inhibitors
sitagliptin 1158

glucagon-like peptide-1 (GLP-1) receptor agonists
liraglutide 1371

hormone
pramlintide 1046

incretin mimetic agent
exenatide 550

insulins
concentrated regular insulin 714, 1425
insulin aspart protamine suspension/insulin aspart solution mixtures, rDNA origin 712, 1425
insulin aspart, rDNA origin 721, 1425
insulin detemir 719, 1425
insulin glargine 719, 1425
insulin glulisine 721, 1425
insulin lispro protamine suspension/insulin lispro solution mixtures, rDNA origin 712, 1425
insulin lispro, rDNA origin 721, 1425
insulin lispro/protamine insulin lispro mixture, rDNA origin 712, 1425
insulin, regular (injection, concentrated) 714, 1425
NPH insulin (isophane insulin suspension) 717, 1425
NPH/regular insulin mixtures 712, 1425
regular insulin (insulin injection) 714, 1425

meglitinides
nateglinide 903
repaglinide 1103

sulfonylureas
glimepiride 1172
glipiZIDE 1173
glyBURIDE 1173

thiazolidinediones
pioglitazone 1030
rosiglitazone 1128

• ANTIDIARRHEALS

PHARMACOLOGIC PROFILE

General Use
For the control and symptomatic relief of acute and chronic nonspecific diarrhea.

General Action and Information
Diphenoxylate/atropine, difenoxin/atropine, and loperamide slow intestinal motility and propulsion. Kaolin/pectin and bismuth subsalicylate affect fluid content of the stool. Bismuth subsalicylate is also used a part of the management of ulcer disease due to *Helicobacter pylori*. Polycar-

ANTIEMETICS 47

bophil acts as an antidiarrheal by taking on water within the bowel lumen to create a formed stool. Polycarbophil may also be used to treat constipation. Octreotide is used specifically for diarrhea associated with GI endocrine tumors.

Contraindications
Previous hypersensitivity. Severe abdominal pain of unknown cause, especially when associated with fever.

Precautions
Use cautiously in patients with severe liver disease or inflammatory bowel disease. Safety in pregnancy and lactation not established (diphenoxylate/atropine and loperamide). Octreotide may aggravate gallbladder disease.

Interactions
Kaolin may decrease absorption of digoxin. Polycarbophil decreases the absorption of tetracycline. Octreotide may alter the response to insulin or oral hypoglycemic agents.

NURSING IMPLICATIONS
Assessment
- Assess the frequency and consistency of stools and bowel sounds before and throughout therapy.
- Assess patient's fluid and electrolyte status and skin turgor for dehydration.

Potential Nursing Diagnoses
- Diarrhea (Indications).
- Constipation (Side Effects).
- Deficient knowledge, related to disease process and medication regimen (Patient/Family Teaching).

Implementation
- Shake liquid preparations before administration.

Patient/Family Teaching
- Instruct patient to notify health care professional if diarrhea persists; or if fever, abdominal pain, or palpitations occur.

Evaluation/Desired Outcomes
- Decrease in diarrhea.

Antidiarrheals included in *Davis's Drug Guide for Nurses*

bismuth subsalicylate 231
difenoxin/atropine 453
diphenoxylate/atropine 453

loperamide 794
octreotide 941
polycarbophil 1331

• ANTIEMETICS

PHARMACOLOGIC PROFILE
General Use
Phenothiazines, dolasetron, granisetron, metoclopramide, and ondansetron are used to manage nausea and vomiting of many causes, including surgery, anesthesia, and antineoplastic and radiation therapy. Palonosetron and aprepitant are used specifically with emetogenic chemotherapy. Dimenhydrinate, scopolamine, and meclizine are used almost exclusively to prevent motion sickness.

ANTIEMETICS

General Action and Information
Phenothiazines act on the chemoreceptor trigger zone to inhibit nausea and vomiting. Dimenhydrinate, scopolamine, and meclizine act as antiemetics mainly by diminishing motion sickness. Metoclopramide decreases nausea and vomiting by its effects on gastric emptying. Dolasetron, granisetron, palonosetron, and ondansetron block the effects of serotonin at 5-HT$_3$ receptor sites.

Contraindications
Previous hypersensitivity.

Precautions
Use phenothiazines cautiously in children who may have viral illnesses. Choose agents carefully in pregnant patients (no agents are approved for safe use).

Interactions
Additive CNS depression with other CNS depressants including antidepressants, antihistamines, opioid analgesics, and sedative/hypnotics. Phenothiazines may produce hypotension when used with antihypertensives, nitrates, or acute ingestion of alcohol.

NURSING IMPLICATIONS

Assessment
- Assess nausea, vomiting, bowel sounds, and abdominal pain before and following administration.
- Monitor hydration status and intake and output. Patients with severe nausea and vomiting may require IV fluids in addition to antiemetics.

Potential Nursing Diagnoses
- Deficient fluid volume (Indications).
- Imbalanced nutrition: less than body requirements (Indications).
- Risk for injury (Side Effects).

Implementation
- For prophylactic administration, follow directions for specific drugs so that peak effect corresponds to time of anticipated nausea.
- Phenothiazines should be discontinued 48 hr before and not resumed for 24 hr following myelography, as they lower seizure threshold.

Patient/Family Teaching
- Advise patient and family to use general measures to decrease nausea (begin with sips of liquids and small, nongreasy meals; provide oral hygiene; and remove noxious stimuli from environment).
- May cause drowsiness. Advise patient to call for assistance when ambulating and to avoid driving or other activities requiring alertness until response to medication is known.
- Advise patient to make position changes slowly to minimize orthostatic hypotension.

Evaluation/Desired Outcomes
- Prevention of, or decrease in, nausea and vomiting.

Antiemetics included in *Davis's Drug Guide for Nurses*

5-HT$_3$ antagonists
dolasetron 469
granisetron 642
ondansetron 951
palonosetron 981

phenothiazines
chlorproMAZINE 318
prochlorperazine 1056
promethazine 1061

miscellaneous
aprepitant 191
meclizine 811

metoclopramide 847
scopolamine 1139

• ANTIFUNGALS

PHARMACOLOGIC PROFILE

General Use
Treatment of fungal infections. Infections of skin or mucous membranes may be treated with topical or vaginal preparations. Deep-seated or systemic infections require oral or parenteral therapy. New parenteral formulations of amphotericin employ lipid encapsulation technology designed to decrease toxicity.

General Action and Information
Kill (fungicidal) or stop growth of (fungistatic) susceptible fungi by affecting the permeability of the fungal cell membrane or protein synthesis within the fungal cell itself.

Contraindications
Previous hypersensitivity.

Precautions
Because most systemic antifungals may have adverse effects on bone marrow function, use cautiously in patients with depressed bone marrow reserve. Amphotericin B commonly causes renal impairment. Fluconazole requires dosage adjustment in the presence of renal impairment. Adverse reactions to fluconazole may be more severe in HIV-positive patients.

Interactions
Differ greatly among various agents. See individual drugs.

NURSING IMPLICATIONS

Assessment
- Assess patient for signs of infection and assess involved areas of skin and mucous membranes before and throughout therapy. Increased skin irritation may indicate need to discontinue medication.

Potential Nursing Diagnoses
- Risk for infection (Indications).
- Impaired skin integrity (Indications).
- Deficient knowledge, related to disease process and medication regimen (Patient/Family Teaching).

Implementation
- Available in various dosage forms. Refer to specific drugs for directions for administration.
- **Topical:** Consult physician or other health care professional for cleansing technique before applying medication. Wear gloves during application. Do not use occlusive dressings unless specified by physician or other health care professional.

Patient/Family Teaching
- Instruct patient on proper use of medication form.
- Instruct patient to continue medication as directed for full course of therapy, even if feeling better.

50 ANTIHISTAMINES

- Advise patient to report increased skin irritation or lack of therapeutic response to health care professional.

Evaluation/Desired Outcomes
- Resolution of signs and symptoms of infection. Length of time for complete resolution depends on organism and site of infection. Deep-seated fungal infections may require prolonged therapy (weeks–months). Recurrent fungal infections may be a sign of serious systemic illness.

Antifungals included in *Davis's Drug Guide for Nurses*

echinocandins
anidulafungin 186
caspofungin 285
micafungin 857

ophthalmics
natamycin 1398

systemic
amphotericin B cholesteryl sulfate 165
amphotericin B deoxycholate 165
amphotericin B lipid complex 165
amphotericin B liposome 165
fluconazole 581
itraconazole 748
ketoconazole (systemic) 753
posaconazole 1037
terbinafine 1196
voriconazole 1292

topical/local
butenafine 187
butoconazole 187, 190
ciclopirox 187
clotrimazole 187, 190
econazole 187
ketoconazole 187
miconazole 187, 190
naftifine 187
nystatin 187, 190
oxiconazole 187
sertaconazole 1146
sulconazole 187
terbinafine 187
terconazole 190
tioconazole 190
tolnaftate 187

• ANTIHISTAMINES

PHARMACOLOGIC PROFILE

General Use
Relief of symptoms associated with allergies, including rhinitis, urticaria, and angioedema, and as adjunctive therapy in anaphylactic reactions. Topical and ophthalmic antihistamines may immunize systemic side effects. Some antihistamines are used to treat motion sickness (dimenhydrinate and meclizine), insomnia (diphenhydramine), Parkinson-like reactions (diphenhydramine), and other nonallergic conditions.

General Action and Information
Antihistamines block the effects of histamine at the H_1 receptor. They do not block histamine release, antibody production, or antigen-antibody reactions. Most antihistamines have anticholinergic properties and may cause constipation, dry eyes, dry mouth, and blurred vision. In addition, many antihistamines cause sedation. Some phenothiazines have strong antihistaminic properties (hydroxyzine and promethazine).

Contraindications
Hypersensitivity and angle-closure glaucoma. Should not be used in premature or newborn infants.

ANTIHISTAMINES 51

Precautions
Elderly patients may be more susceptible to adverse anticholinergic effects of antihistamines. Use cautiously in patients with pyloric obstruction, prostatic hypertrophy, hyperthyroidism, cardiovascular disease, or severe liver disease. Use cautiously in pregnancy and lactation.

Interactions
Additive sedation when used with other CNS depressants, including alcohol, antidepressants, opioid analgesics, and sedative/hypnotics. MAO inhibitors prolong and intensify the anticholinergic properties of antihistamines.

NURSING IMPLICATIONS

Assessment
- Assess allergy symptoms (rhinitis, conjunctivitis, hives) before and periodically throughout therapy.
- Monitor pulse and blood pressure before initiating and throughout IV therapy.
- Assess lung sounds and character of bronchial secretions. Maintain fluid intake of 1500–2000 mL/day to decrease viscosity of secretions.
- **Nausea and Vomiting:** Assess degree of nausea and frequency and amount of emesis when administering for nausea and vomiting.
- **Anxiety:** Assess mental status, mood, and behavior when administering for anxiety.
- **Pruritus:** Observe the character, location, and size of affected area when administering for pruritic skin conditions.

Potential Nursing Diagnoses
- Ineffective airway clearance (Indications).
- Risk for injury (Adverse Reactions).
- Deficient knowledge, related to disease process and medication regimen (Patient/Family Teaching).

Implementation
- When used for prophylaxis of motion sickness, administer at least 30 min and preferably 1–2 hr before exposure to conditions that may precipitate motion sickness.
- When administering concurrently with opioid analgesics (hydroxyzine, promethazine), supervise ambulation closely to prevent injury secondary to increased sedation.

Patient/Family Teaching
- Inform patient that drowsiness may occur. Avoid driving or other activities requiring alertness until response to drug is known.
- Caution patient to avoid using concurrent alcohol or CNS depressants.
- Advise patient that good oral hygiene, frequent rinsing of mouth with water, and sugarless gum or candy may help relieve dryness of mouth.
- Instruct patient to contact health care professional if symptoms persist.

Evaluation/Desired Outcomes
- Decrease in allergic symptoms.
- Prevention or decreased severity of nausea and vomiting.
- Decrease in anxiety.
- Relief of pruritus.
- Sedation when used as a hypnotic.

Antihistamines included in *Davis's Drug Guide for Nurses*

ophthalmics
azelastine 1397
bepotastine 1397
emedastine 1397
epinastine 1397
ketotifen 1397
olopatadine 1397

systemic
brompheniramine 1322
cetirizine 309
chlorpheniramine 316
cyproheptadine 390

desloratadine 417
diphenhydrAMINE 450
fexofenadine 575
hydrOXYzine 682
loratadine 798
meclizine 811
promethazine 1061

topical
doxepin 476

nasal
olopatadine (nasal spray) 946

• ANTIHYPERTENSIVES

PHARMACOLOGIC PROFILE

General Use
Treatment of hypertension of many causes, most commonly essential hypertension. Parenteral products are used in the treatment of hypertensive emergencies. Oral treatment should be initiated as soon as possible and individualized to ensure adherence and compliance for long-term therapy. Therapy is initiated with agents having minimal side effects. When such therapy fails, more potent drugs with different side effects are added in an effort to control blood pressure while causing minimal patient discomfort.

General Action and Information
As a group, the antihypertensives are used to lower blood pressure to a normal level (<90 mm Hg diastolic) or to the lowest level tolerated. The goal of antihypertensive therapy is prevention of end-organ damage. Antihypertensives are classified into groups according to their site of action. These include peripherally-acting antiadrenergics; centrally-acting alpha-adrenergics; beta blockers; vasodilators; ACE inhibitors; angiotensin II antagonists; calcium channel blockers; and diuretics. Hypertensive emergencies may be managed with parenteral agents, such as enalaprilat or fenoldopam.

Contraindications
Hypersensitivity to individual agents.

Precautions
Choose agents carefully in pregnancy, during lactation, or in patients receiving digoxin. ACE inhibitors and angiotensin II antagonists should be avoided during pregnancy. Alpha-adrenergic agonists and beta blockers should be used only in patients who will comply, because abrupt discontinuation of these agents may result in rapid and excessive rise in blood pressure (rebound phenomenon). Thiazide diuretics may increase the requirement for treatment of diabetics. Vasodilators may cause tachycardia if used alone and are commonly used in combination with beta blockers. Some antihypertensives cause sodium and water retention and are usually combined with a diuretic.

Interactions
Many drugs can negate the therapeutic effectiveness of antihypertensives, including antihistamines, NSAIDs, sympathomimetic bronchodilators, decongestants, appetite suppressants, anti-

ANTIHYPERTENSIVES 53

depressants, and MAO inhibitors. Hypokalemia from diuretics may increase the risk of digoxin toxicity. Potassium supplements and potassium-sparing diuretics may cause hyperkalemia when used with ACE inhibitors.

NURSING IMPLICATIONS
Assessment
- Monitor blood pressure and pulse frequently during dosage adjustment and periodically throughout therapy.
- Monitor intake and output ratios and daily weight.
- Monitor frequency of prescription refills to determine compliance.

Potential Nursing Diagnoses
- Ineffective tissue perfusion (Indications).
- Deficient knowledge, related to disease process and medication regimen (Patient/Family Teaching).
- Noncompliance (Patient/Family Teaching).

Implementation
- Many antihypertensives are available as combination products to enhance compliance (see Appendix B).

Patient/Family Teaching
- Instruct patient to continue taking medication, even if feeling well. Abrupt withdrawal may cause rebound hypertension. Medication controls, but does not cure, hypertension.
- Encourage patient to comply with additional interventions for hypertension (weight reduction, low-sodium diet, regular exercise, discontinuation of smoking, moderation of alcohol consumption, and stress management).
- Instruct patient and family on proper technique for monitoring blood pressure. Advise them to check blood pressure weekly and report significant changes.
- Caution patient to make position changes slowly to minimize orthostatic hypotension. Advise patient that exercise or hot weather may enhance hypotensive effects.
- Advise patient to consult health care professional before taking any OTC medications, especially cold remedies.
- Advise patient to inform health care professional of medication regimen before treatment or surgery.
- Patients taking ACE inhibitors or angiotensin II antagonists should notify health care professional if pregnancy is planned or suspected.
- Emphasize the importance of follow-up exams to monitor progress.

Evaluation/Desired Outcomes
- Decrease in blood pressure.

Antihypertensives included in *Davis's Drug Guide for Nurses*

adrenergics
clonidine 343

aldosterone antagonists
eplerenone 511

ACE inhibitors
benazepril 176
captopril 176
enalapril/enalaprilat 176
fosinopril 176
lisinopril 176
moexipril 176
perindopril 176
quinapril 176
ramipril 176
trandolapril 176

angiotensin II receptor antagonists
candesartan 182
eprosartan 182
irbesartan 182
losartan 182

olmesartan 182
telmisartan 182
valsartan 182

beta blockers (nonselective)
carvedilol 283
labetalol 759
nadolol 892
propranolol 1071
timolol 1229

beta blockers (selective)
atenolol 204
bisoprolol 233
metoprolol 851
nebivolol 905

calcium channel blockers
amlodipine 157
clevidipine 336
diltiazem 445
felodipine 557
isradipine 746
niCARdipine 915
NIFEdipine 921
nisoldipine 926
verapamil 1275

centrally acting antiadrenergics
guanfacine 1326
methyldopa 840

lipoglycopeptides
telavancin 1373

loop diuretics
torsemide 1244

peripherally acting antiadrenergics
doxazosin 475
prazosin 1049
terazosin 1194

renin inhibitors
aliskiren 133

thiazide diuretics
chlorothiazide 458
chlorthalidone (thiazide–like) 458
hydrochlorothiazide 458

thiazide-like diuretics
indapamide 706
metolazone 850

vasodilators
fenoldopam 562
hydrALAZINE 671
minoxidil 1329
nitroprusside 932

• ANTI-INFECTIVES

PHARMACOLOGIC PROFILE

General Use
Treatment and prophylaxis of various bacterial infections. See specific drugs for spectrum and indications. Some infections may require additional surgical intervention and supportive therapy.

General Action and Information
Kill (bactericidal) or inhibit the growth of (bacteriostatic) susceptible pathogenic bacteria. Not active against viruses or fungi. Anti-infectives are subdivided into categories depending on chemical similarities and antimicrobial spectrum.

Contraindications
Known hypersensitivity to individual agents. Cross-sensitivity among related agents may occur.

Precautions
Culture and susceptibility testing are desirable to optimize therapy. Dosage modification may be required in patients with hepatic or renal insufficiency. Use cautiously in pregnant and lactating women. Prolonged inappropriate use of broad spectrum anti-infective agents may lead to superinfection with fungi or resistant bacteria.

Interactions
Penicillins and aminoglycosides chemically inactivate each other and should not be physically admixed. Erythromycins may decrease hepatic metabolism of other drugs. Probenecid increases

ANTI-INFECTIVES 55

serum levels of penicillins and related compounds. Highly protein-bound anti-infectives such as sulfonamides may displace or be displaced by other highly bound drugs. See individual drugs. Extended-spectrum penicillins (ticarcillin, piperacillin) and some cephalosporins (cefoperazone, cefotetan) may increase the risk of bleeding with anticoagulants, thrombolytic agents, antiplatelet agents, or NSAIDs. Fluoroquinolone absorption is decreased by antacids, bismuth subsalicylate, iron salts, sucralfate, and zinc salts.

NURSING IMPLICATIONS

Assessment
- Assess patient for signs and symptoms of infection prior to and throughout therapy.
- Determine previous hypersensitivities in patients receiving penicillins or cephalosporins.
- Obtain specimens for culture and sensitivity prior to initiating therapy. First dose may be given before receiving results.

Potential Nursing Diagnoses
- Risk for infection (Indications).
- Deficient knowledge, related to disease process and medication regimen (Patient/Family Teaching).
- Noncompliance (Patient/Family Teaching).

Implementation
- Most anti-infectives should be administered around the clock to maintain therapeutic serum drug levels.

Patient/Family Teaching
- Instruct patient to continue taking medication around the clock until finished completely, even if feeling better.
- Advise patient to report the signs of superinfection (black, furry overgrowth on the tongue; vaginal itching or discharge; loose or foul-smelling stools) and allergy to health care professional.
- Instruct patient to notify health care professional if fever and diarrhea develop, especially if stool contains pus, blood, or mucus. Advise patient not to treat diarrhea without consulting health care professional.
- Instruct patient to notify health care professional if symptoms do not improve.

Evaluation/Desired Outcomes
- Resolution of the signs and symptoms of infection. Length of time for complete resolution depends on organism and site of infection.

Anti-infectives included in *Davis's Drug Guide for Nurses*

aminoglycosides
amikacin 145
gentamicin 145, 1398
kanamycin 145
neomycin 145
streptomycin 145
tobramycin 145, 1398

carbapenems
doripenem 473
ertapenem 522
imipenem/cilastatin 700
meropenem 823

first-generation cephalosporins
cefadroxil 291
cefazolin 291
cephalexin 291

second-generation cephalosporins
cefaclor 294
cefotetan 294
cefoxitin 294
cefprozil 294
cefuroxime 294

third-generation cephalosporins
cefdinir 300
cefditoren 300

56 ANTINEOPLASTICS

cefixime 300
cefoperazone 300
cefotaxime 300
cefpodoxime 300
ceftazidime 300
ceftibuten 300
ceftizoxime 300
ceftriaxone 300
extended spectrum penicillins
piperacillin/tazobactam 1032
ticarcillin/clavulanate 1224
fluoroquinolones
ciprofloxacin 589
gemifloxacin 589
levofloxacin 589, 1398
moxifloxacin 589, 1398
norfloxacin 589
ofloxacin 589, 1398
macrolides
azithromycin 214, 1397
clarithromycin 334
erythromycin 523, 1398
penicillins
amoxicillin 160
amoxicillin/clavulanate 160
ampicillin 172
ampicillin/sulbactam 172
benzathine penicillin G 1002
dicloxacillin 1005

nafcillin 1005
oxacillin 1005
penicillin G 1002
penicillin V 1002
procaine penicillin G 1002
tetracyclines
bacitracin 1397
doxycycline 1203
minocycline 1203
tetracycline 1203
miscellaneous
besifloxacin 1398
cefepime 287
clindamycin 337
daptomycin 401
drotrecogin 489
gatifloxacin 1398
linezolid 790
metronidazole 854
mupirocin 885
nitrofurantoin 928
quinupristin/dalfopristin 1093
rifaximin 1110
sulfacetamide 1398
temsirolimus 1335
thioguanine 1335
tigecycline 1227
trimethoprim/sulfamethoxazole 1254
vancomycin 1265

• ANTINEOPLASTICS

PHARMACOLOGIC PROFILE

General Use
Used in the treatment of various solid tumors, lymphomas, and leukemias. Also used in some autoimmune disorders such as rheumatoid arthritis (cyclophosphamide, methotrexate). Often used in combinations to minimize individual toxicities and increase response. Chemotherapy may be combined with other treatment modalities such as surgery and radiation therapy. Dosages vary greatly, depending on extent of disease, other agents used, and patient's condition. Some new formulations (daunorubicin, doxorubicin) encapsulated in a lipid membrane have less toxicity with greater efficacy.

General Action and Information
Act by many different mechanisms (see the following table). Many affect DNA synthesis or function; others alter immune function or affect hormonal status of sensitive tumors. Action may not be limited to neoplastic cells.

MECHANISM OF ACTION OF VARIOUS ANTINEOPLASTICS

MECHANISM OF ACTION	AGENT	EFFECTS ON CELL CYCLE
ALKYLATING AGENTS Cause cross-linking of DNA	busulfan carboplatin chlorambucil cisplatin cyclophosphamide ifosfamide mechlorethamine melphalan procarbazine temozolamide	Cell cycle–nonspecific
ANTHRACYCLINES Interfere with DNA and RNA synthesis	daunorubicin doxorubicin epirubicin idarubicin	Cell cycle–nonspecific
ANTITUMOR ANTIBIOTIC	bleomycin	Cell cycle–nonspecific (except bleomycin)
Interfere with DNA and RNA synthesis	mitomycin mitoxantrone	
ANTIMETABOLITES	cytarabine	Cell cycle–specific, work mostly in S phase (DNA synthesis)
Take the place of normal proteins	fluorouracil hydroxyurea methotrexate	
ENZYMES Deplete asparagine	asparaginase pegaspargase	Cell-cycle phase–specific
ENZYME INHIBITORS Inhibits topoisomerase	irinotecan topotecan	Cell-cycle phase–specific
Inhibits kinase	imatinib	Unknown
HORMONAL AGENTS Alter hormonal status in tumors that are sensitive	bicalutamide estramustine flutamide leuprolide megestrol nilutamide tamoxifen testosterone (androgens) triptorelin	Unknown
HORMONAL AGENTS—AROMATASE INHIBITORS Inhibit enzyme responsible for activating estrogen	anastrazole letrozole	Unknown
IMMUNE MODULATORS	aldesleukin alemtuzumab gemtuzumab toremifene trastuzumab	Unknown
PODOPHYLLOTOXIN DERIVATIVES Damages DNA before mitosis	etoposide	Cell-cycle phase–specific
TAXOIDS Interupt interphase and mitosis	docetaxel paclitaxel	Cell-cycle phase–specific
VINCA ALKALOIDS	vinblastine	Cell cycle–specific, work during M phase (mitosis)
Interfere with mitosis	vinCRIStine vinorelbine	
MISCELLANEOUS	aldesleukin altretamine	Unknown Unknown

Contraindications

Previous bone marrow depression or hypersensitivity. Contraindicated in pregnancy and lactation.

Precautions
Use cautiously in patients with active infections, decreased bone marrow reserve, radiation therapy, or other debilitating illnesses. Use cautiously in patients with childbearing potential.

Interactions
Allopurinol decreases metabolism of mercaptopurine. Toxicity from methotrexate may be increased by other nephrotoxic drugs or larger doses of aspirin or NSAIDs. Bone marrow depression is additive. See individual drugs.

NURSING IMPLICATIONS
Assessment
- Monitor for bone marrow depression. Assess for bleeding (bleeding gums, bruising, petechiae, guaiac stools, urine, and emesis) and avoid IM injections and rectal temperatures if platelet count is low. Apply pressure to venipuncture sites for 10 min. Assess for signs of infection during neutropenia. Anemia may occur. Monitor for increased fatigue, dyspnea, and orthostatic hypotension.
- Monitor intake and output ratios, appetite, and nutritional intake. Prophylactic antiemetics may be used. Adjusting diet as tolerated may help maintain fluid and electrolyte balance and nutritional status.
- Monitor IV site carefully and ensure patency. Discontinue infusion immediately if discomfort, erythema along vein, or infiltration occurs. Tissue ulceration and necrosis may result from infiltration.
- Monitor for symptoms of gout (increased uric acid, joint pain, and edema). Encourage patient to drink at least 2 L of fluid each day. Allopurinol may be given to decrease uric acid levels. Alkalinization of urine may be ordered to increase excretion of uric acid.

Potential Nursing Diagnoses
- Risk for infection (Side Effects).
- Imbalanced nutrition: less than body requirements (Adverse Reactions).
- Deficient knowledge, related to disease process and medication regimen (Patient/Family Teaching).

Implementation
- Solutions for injection should be prepared in a biologic cabinet. Wear gloves, gown, and mask while handling medication. Discard equipment in designated containers (see Appendix L).
- Check dose carefully. Fatalities have resulted from dosing errors.

Patient/Family Teaching
- Caution patient to avoid crowds and persons with known infections. Health care professional should be informed immediately if symptoms of infection occur.
- Instruct patient to report unusual bleeding. Advise patient of thrombocytopenia precautions.
- These drugs may cause gonadal suppression; however, patient should still use birth control, as most antineoplastics are teratogenic. Advise patient to inform health care professional immediately if pregnancy is suspected.
- Discuss with patient the possibility of hair loss. Explore methods of coping.
- Instruct patient to inspect oral mucosa for erythema and ulceration. If ulceration occurs, advise patient to use sponge brush and to rinse mouth with water after eating and drinking. Topical agents may be used if mouth pain interferes with eating. Stomatitis pain may require treatment with opioid analgesics.
- Instruct patient not to receive any vaccinations without advice of health care professional. Antineoplastics may decrease antibody response and increase risk of adverse reactions.
- Advise patient of need for medical follow-up and frequent lab tests.

Evaluation/Desired Outcomes
- Decrease in size and spread of tumor.
- Improvement in hematologic status in patients with leukemia.

Antineoplastics included in *Davis's Drug Guide for Nurses*

alkylating agents
busulfan 252
carboplatin 277
carmustine 281
chlorambucil 1322
cisplatin 328
cyclophosphamide 384
dacarbazine 397
ifosfamide 694
mechlorethamine 1328
melphalan 817
oxaliplatin 957
procarbazine 1054

anthracyclines
DAUNOrubicin hydrochloride 408
DOXOrubicin 479
DOXOrubicin liposome 482
epirubicin 508
idarubicin 692

antiandrogens
bicalutamide 228
flutamide 1325

antiestrogens
tamoxifen 1187

antimetabolites
capecitabine 269
cladribine 332
clofarabine 340
cytarabine 392
fludarabine 583
fluorouracil 594
gemcitabine 629
hydroxyurea 1326
mercaptopurine 1328
methotrexate 836
pemetrexed 999

antitumor antibiotics
bleomycin 236
gemtuzumab ozogamicin 633
mitomycin 870
mitoxantrone 872

aromatase inhibitors
anastrozole 175
letrozole 775

enzyme inhibitors
erlotinib 520
gefitinib 628
imatinib 698
irinotecan 734
lapatinib 770
nilotinib 923
romidepsin 1372

enzymes
asparaginase 199
pegaspargase 996

hormones
goserelin 640
leuprolide 778
medroxyPROGESTERone 812
triptorelin 1339

monoclonal antibodies
alemtuzumab 129
bevacizumab 226
cetuximab 311
gemtuzumab ozogamicin 633
ofatumumab 1372
panitumuab 988
rituximab 1121
trastuzumab 1249

podophyllotoxin derivatives
etoposide 546
etoposide phosphate 546

progestins
medroxyPROGESTERone 812
megestrol 814

taxoids
docetaxel 462
paclitaxel 975

vinca alkaloids
vinBLAStine 1278
vinCRIStine 1280
vinorelbine 1282

miscellaneous
anastrozole 175
azacitidine 210
arsenic trioxide 1319
bendamustine 223
bortezomib 239

ANTIPARKINSON AGENTS

decitabine 410
everolimus 1370
ixabepilone 750
oxaliplatin 957
pazopanib 994
raltegravir 1097
sunitinib 1179

• ANTIPARKINSON AGENTS

PHARMACOLOGIC PROFILE

General Use
Used in the treatment of parkinsonism of various causes: degenerative, toxic, infective, neoplastic, or drug-induced.

General Action and Information
Drugs used in the treatment of the parkinsonian syndrome and other dyskinesias are aimed at restoring the natural balance of two major neurotransmitters in the CNS: acetylcholine and dopamine. The imbalance is a deficiency in dopamine that results in excessive cholinergic activity. Drugs used are either anticholinergics (benztropine, biperiden, and trihexyphenidyl) or dopaminergic agonists (bromocriptine, levodopa). Pramipexole and ropinerole are two new nonergot dopamine agonists. Entacapone inhibits the enzyme that breaks down levodopa, thereby enhancing its effects.

Contraindications
Anticholinergics should be avoided in patients with angle-closure glaucoma.

Precautions
Use cautiously in patients with severe cardiac disease, pyloric obstruction, or prostatic enlargement.

Interactions
Pyridoxine, MAO inhibitors, benzodiazepines, phenytoin, phenothiazines, and haloperidol may antagonize the effects of levodopa. Agents that antagonize dopamine (phenothiazines, metoclopramide) may decrease effectiveness of dopamine agonists.

NURSING IMPLICATIONS

Assessment
- Assess parkinsonian and extrapyramidal symptoms (akinesia, rigidity, tremors, pill rolling, mask facies, shuffling gait, muscle spasms, twisting motions, and drooling) before and throughout course of therapy. On-off phenomenon may cause symptoms to appear or improve suddenly.
- Monitor blood pressure frequently during therapy. Instruct patient to remain supine during and for several hours after first dose of bromocriptine, as severe hypotension may occur.

Potential Nursing Diagnoses
- Impaired physical mobility (Indications).
- Risk for injury (Indications).
- Deficient knowledge, related to disease process and medication regimen (Patient/Family Teaching).

Implementation
- In the carbidopa/levodopa combination, the number following the drug name represents the milligram of each respective drug.

Patient/Family Teaching
- May cause drowsiness or dizziness. Advise patient to avoid driving or other activities that require alertness until response to medication is known.
- Caution patient to make position changes slowly to minimize orthostatic hypotension.
- Instruct patient that frequent rinsing of mouth, good oral hygiene, and sugarless gum or candy may decrease dry mouth. Patient should notify health care professional if dryness persists (saliva substitutes may be used). Also notify the dentist if dryness interferes with use of dentures.
- Advise patient to confer with health care professional before taking OTC medications, especially cold remedies, or drinking alcoholic beverages. Patients receiving levodopa should avoid multivitamins. Vitamin B_6 (pyridoxine) may interfere with levodopa's action.
- Caution patient that decreased perspiration may occur. Overheating may occur during hot weather. Patients should remain indoors in an air-conditioned environment during hot weather.
- Advise patient to increase activity, bulk, and fluid in diet to minimize constipating effects of medication.
- Advise patient to notify health care professional if confusion, rash, urinary retention, severe constipation, visual changes, or worsening of parkinsonian symptoms occur.

Evaluation/Desired Outcomes
- Resolution of parkinsonian signs and symptoms
- Resolution of drug-induced extrapyramidal symptoms.

Antiparkinson agents included in *Davis's Drug Guide for Nurses*

anticholinergics
benztropine 225
biperiden 1320
trihexyphenidyl 1338

catechol-O-methyltransferase inhibitors
entacapone 499
tolcapone 1236

dopamine agonists
bromocriptine 1321
carbidopa/levodopa 275
pramipexole 1044
ropinirole 1127

monoamine oxidase type B inhibitors
rasagiline 1100
selegiline 1141

• ANTIPLATELET AGENTS

PHARMACOLOGIC PROFILE

General Use
Antiplatelet agents are used to treat and prevent thromboembolic events such as stroke and MI. Dipyridamole is commonly used after cardiac surgery.

General Action and Information
Inhibit platelet aggregation, prolong bleeding time, and are used to prevent MI or stroke (aspirin, clopidogrel, dipyridamole, ticlopidine). Eptifibatide and tirofiban are used in the management of various acute coronary syndromes. These agents have been used concurrently/sequentially with anticoagulants and thrombolytics.

Contraindications
Hypersensitivity, ulcer disease, active bleeding, and recent surgery.

Precautions
Use cautiously in patients at risk for bleeding (trauma, surgery). History of GI bleeding or ulcer disease. Safety not established in pregnancy, lactation, or children.

Interactions
Concurrent use with NSAIDs, heparin, thrombolytics, or warfarin may increase the risk of bleeding.

NURSING IMPLICATIONS
Assessment
- Assess patient for evidence of additional or increased thrombosis. Symptoms will depend on area of involvement.
- Assess patient taking antiplatelet agents for symptoms of stroke, peripheral vascular disease, or MI periodically throughout therapy.
- **Lab Test Considerations:** Monitor bleeding time throughout antiplatelet therapy. Prolonged bleeding time, which is time- and dose-dependent, is expected.

Potential Nursing Diagnoses
- Ineffective tissue perfusion (Indications).
- Risk for injury (Side Effects).
- Deficient knowledge, related to disease process and medication regimen (Patient/Family Teaching).

Implementation
- Use an infusion pump with continuous infusions to ensure accurate dosage.

Patient/Family Teaching
- Instruct patient to notify health care professional immediately if any bleeding is noted.

Evaluation/Desired Outcomes
- Prevention of stroke, MI, and vascular death in patients at risk.

Antiplatelet agents included in *Davis's Drug Guide for Nurses*

glycoprotein IIb/IIIa inhibitors
eptifibatide 515
tirofiban 1233

platelet adhesion inhibitors
dipyridamole 454

platelet aggregation inhibitors
cilostazol 326
clopidogrel 346
ticlopidine 1225

thienopyridines
prasugrel 1048

• ANTIPSYCHOTICS

PHARMACOLOGIC PROFILE
General Use
Treatment of acute and chronic psychoses, particularly when accompanied by increased psychomotor activity. Use of clozapine is limited to schizophrenia unresponsive to conventional therapy. Selected agents are also used as antihistamines or antiemetics. Chlorpromazine is also used in the treatment of intractable hiccups.

General Action and Information
Block dopamine receptors in the brain; also alter dopamine release and turnover. Peripheral effects include anticholinergic properties and alpha-adrenergic blockade. Most antipsychotics are phenothiazines except for haloperidol, which is a butyrophenone, and clozapine, which is a miscellaneous compound. Newer "atypical" agents such as olanzapine, quetiapine, and risperidone may have fewer adverse reactions. Phenothiazines differ in their ability to produce sedation

ANTIPSYCHOTICS

(greatest with chlorpromazine and thioridazine), extrapyramidal reactions (greatest with prochlorperazine and trifluoperazine), and anticholinergic effects (greatest with chlorpromazine).

Contraindications
Hypersensitivity. Cross-sensitivity may exist among phenothiazines. Should not be used in angle-closure glaucoma. Should not be used in patients who have CNS depression.

Precautions
Safety in pregnancy and lactation not established. Use cautiously in patients with symptomatic cardiac disease. Avoid exposure to extremes in temperature. Use cautiously in severely ill or debilitated patients, diabetic patients, and patients with respiratory insufficiency, prostatic hypertrophy, or intestinal obstruction. May lower seizure threshold. Clozapine may cause agranulocytosis. Most agents are capable of causing neuroleptic malignant syndrome. Should not be used routinely for anxiety or agitation not related to psychoses.

Interactions
Additive hypotension with acute ingestion of alcohol, antihypertensives, or nitrates. Antacids may decrease absorption. Phenobarbital may increase metabolism and decrease effectiveness. Additive CNS depression with other CNS depressants, including alcohol, antihistamines, antidepressants, opioid analgesics, or sedative/hypnotics. Lithium may decrease blood levels and effectiveness of phenothiazines. May decrease the therapeutic response to levodopa. May increase the risk of agranulocytosis with antithyroid agents.

NURSING IMPLICATIONS

Assessment
- Assess patient's mental status (orientation, mood, behavior) before and periodically throughout therapy.
- Monitor blood pressure (sitting, standing, lying), pulse, and respiratory rate before and frequently during the period of dosage adjustment.
- Observe patient carefully when administering medication to ensure medication is actually taken and not hoarded.
- Monitor patient for onset of *akathisia*—restlessness or desire to keep moving—and extrapyramidal side effects; *parkinsonian*—difficulty speaking or swallowing, loss of balance control, pill rolling, mask-like face, shuffling gait, rigidity, tremors; and *dystonia*—muscle spasms, twisting motions, twitching, inability to move eyes, weakness of arms or legs—every 2 mo during therapy and 8–12 wk after therapy has been discontinued. Parkinsonian effects are more common in geriatric patients and dystonias are more common in younger patients. Notify health care professional if these symptoms occur, as reduction in dosage or discontinuation of medication may be necessary. Trihexyphenidyl or diphenhydramine may be used to control these symptoms.
- Monitor for *tardive dyskinesia*—uncontrolled rhythmic movement of mouth, face, and extremities; lip smacking or puckering; puffing of cheeks; uncontrolled chewing; rapid or worm-like movements of tongue. Notify health care professional immediately if these symptoms occur; these side effects may be irreversible.
- Monitor for development of *neuroleptic malignant syndrome*—fever, respiratory distress, tachycardia, convulsions, diaphoresis, hypertension or hypotension, pallor, tiredness, severe muscle stiffness, loss of bladder control. Notify health care professional immediately if these symptoms occur.

Potential Nursing Diagnoses
- Disturbed thought process (Indications).
- Deficient knowledge, related to disease process and medication regimen (Patient/Family Teaching).

ANTIPSYCHOTICS

- Noncompliance (Patient/Family Teaching).

Implementation
- Keep patient recumbent for at least 30 min following parenteral administration to minimize hypotensive effects.
- To prevent contact dermatitis, avoid getting solution on hands.
- Phenothiazines should be discontinued 48 hr before and not resumed for 24 hr following myelography, as they lower the seizure threshold.
- **PO:** Administer with **food**, **milk**, or a full glass of **water** to minimize gastric irritation.
- Dilute most concentrates in 120 mL of distilled or acidified tap water or **fruit juice** just before administration.

Patient/Family Teaching
- Advise patient to take medication exactly as directed and not to skip doses or double up on missed doses. Abrupt withdrawal may lead to gastritis, nausea, vomiting, dizziness, headache, tachycardia, and insomnia.
- Advise patient to make position changes slowly to minimize orthostatic hypotension.
- Medication may cause drowsiness. Caution patient to avoid driving or other activities requiring alertness until response to the medication is known.
- Caution patient to avoid taking alcohol or other CNS depressants concurrently with this medication.
- Advise patient to use sunscreen and protective clothing when exposed to the sun to prevent photosensitivity reactions. Extremes of temperature should also be avoided, as these drugs impair body temperature regulation.
- Advise patient that increasing activity, bulk, and fluids in the diet helps minimize the constipating effects of this medication.
- Instruct patient to use frequent mouth rinses, good oral hygiene, and sugarless gum or candy to minimize dry mouth.
- Advise patient to notify health care professional of medication regimen before treatment or surgery.
- Emphasize the importance of routine follow-up exams and continued participation in psychotherapy as indicated.

Evaluation/Desired Outcomes
- Decrease in excitable, paranoic, or withdrawn behavior. Relief of nausea and vomiting. Relief of intractable hiccups.

Antipsychotics included in *Davis's Drug Guide for Nurses*

phenothiazines
chlorproMAZINE 318
fluphenazine 600
prochlorperazine 1056
thioridazine 1211
trifluoperazine 1337

miscellaneous
aripiprazole 195
asenapine 197

clozapine 349
haloperidol 651
iloperidone 696
olanzapine 943
paliperidone 979
quetiapine 1087
risperidone 1116
ziprasidone 1307

• ANTIPYRETICS

PHARMACOLOGIC PROFILE

General Use
Used to lower fever of many causes (infection, inflammation, and neoplasms).

General Action and Information
Antipyretics lower fever by affecting thermoregulation in the CNS and by inhibiting the action of prostaglandins peripherally. Many antipyretics affect platelet function; of these, aspirin has the most profound effect as compared with other salicylates, ibuprofen, or ketoprofen.

Contraindications
Avoid aspirin, ibuprofen, or ketoprofen in patients with bleeding disorders (risk of bleeding is less with other salicylates). Aspirin and other salicylates should be avoided in children and adolescents.

Precautions
Use aspirin, ibuprofen, or ketoprofen cautiously in patients with ulcer disease. Avoid chronic use of large doses of acetaminophen.

Interactions
Large doses of aspirin may displace other highly protein-bound drugs. Additive GI irritation with aspirin, ibuprofen, ketoprofen, and other NSAIDs or corticosteroids. Aspirin, ibuprofen, ketoprofen, or naproxen may increase the risk of bleeding with other agents affecting hemostasis (anticoagulants, thrombolytic agents, antineoplastics, and certain anti-infectives).

NURSING IMPLICATIONS

Assessment
- Assess fever; note presence of associated symptoms (diaphoresis, tachycardia, and malaise).

Potential Nursing Diagnoses
- Risk for imbalanced body temperature (Indications).
- Deficient knowledge, related to disease process and medication regimen (Patient/Family Teaching).

Implementation
- Administration with food or antacids may minimize GI irritation (aspirin, ibuprofen, ketoprofen, naproxen).
- Available in oral and rectal dosage forms and in combination with other drugs.

Patient/Family Teaching
- Advise patient to consult health care professional if fever is not relieved by routine doses or if greater than 39.5°C (103°F) or lasts longer than 3 days.
- Centers for Disease Control and Prevention warns against giving aspirin to children or adolescents with varicella (chickenpox) or influenza-like or viral illnesses because of a possible association with Reye's syndrome.

Evaluation/Desired Outcomes
- Reduction of fever.

Antipyretics included in *Davis's Drug Guide for Nurses*

acetaminophen 112
aspirin 1131
choline and magnesium salicylates 1131
choline salicylate 1131
ibuprofen, oral 688
ketoprofen 754
magnesium salicylate 1131
naproxen 900
salsalate 1131
sodium salicylate 1131

• ANTIRETROVIRALS

PHARMACOLOGIC PROFILE

General Use
The goal of antiretroviral therapy in the management of HIV infection is to improve CD4 cell counts and decrease viral load. If accomplished, this generally results in slowed progression of the disease, improved quality of life, and decreased opportunistic infections. Perinatal use of agents also prevents transmission of the virus to the fetus. Post-exposure prophylaxis with antiretrovirals is also recommended.

General Action and Information
Because of the rapid emergence of resistance and toxicities of individual agents, HIV infection is almost always managed by a combination of agents. Selections and doses are based on individual toxicities, underlying organ system disease, concurrent drug therapy, and severity of illness. Various combinations are used; up to 4 agents may be used simultaneously. More than 100 agents are currently being tested in addition to those already approved by the FDA.

Contraindications
Hypersensitivity. Because of highly varying toxicities among agents, see individual monographs for more specific information.

Precautions
Many agents require modification for renal impairment. Protease inhibitors may cause hyperglycemia and should be used cautiously in patients with diabetes. Hemophiliacs may also be at risk of bleeding when taking protease inhibitors. See individual monographs for specific information.

Interactions
There are many significant and potentially serious drug-drug interactions among the antiretrovirals. They are affected by drugs that alter metabolism; some agents themselves affect metabolism. See individual agents.

NURSING IMPLICATIONS

Assessment
- Assess patient for change in severity of symptoms of HIV and for symptoms of opportunistic infections throughout therapy.
- **Lab Test Considerations:** Monitor viral load and CD4 counts prior to and periodically during therapy.

Potential Nursing Diagnoses
- Risk for infection (Indications).
- Deficient knowledge, related to disease process and medication regimen (Patient/Family Teaching).
- Noncompliance (Patient/Family Teaching).

Implementation
- Administer doses around the clock.

Patient/Family Teaching
- Instruct patient to take medication exactly as directed, around the clock, even if sleep is interrupted. Emphasize the importance of complying with therapy, not taking more than pre-

scribed amount, and not discontinuing without consulting health care professional. Missed doses should be taken as soon as remembered unless almost time for next dose; patient should not double doses. Inform patient that long-term effects are unknown at this time.
- Instruct patient that antiretrovirals should not be shared with others.
- Inform patient that antiretroviral therapy does not cure HIV and does not reduce the risk of transmission of HIV to others through sexual contact or blood contamination. Caution patient to use a condom during sexual contact and to avoid sharing needles or donating blood to prevent spreading the AIDS virus to others.
- Advise patient to avoid taking any Rx, OTC, or herbal products without consulting health care professional.
- Emphasize the importance of regular follow-up exams and blood counts to determine progress and to monitor for side effects.

Evaluation/Desired Outcomes
- Decrease in viral load and increase in CD4 counts in patients with HIV.

Antiretrovirals included in *Davis's Drug Guide for Nurses*

CCR5 co-receptor antagonists
maraviroc 810

fusion inhibitors
enfuvirtide 1325

interleukin antagonists
tocilizumab 1374

metabolic inhibitors
lopinavir/ritonavir 795

non-nucleoside reverse transcriptase inhibitors
efavirenz 495
etravirine 548
nevirapine 912
stavudine 1334

nucleoside reverse transcriptase inhibitors
abacavir 109
didanosine 1324
emtricitabine 498
lamivudine 762
tenofovir 1193
zidovudine 1303

protease inhibitors
atazanavir 201
darunavir 406
fosamprenavir 612
indinavir 1327
lopinavir/ritonavir 795
nelfinavir 1329
ritonavir 1119
saquinavir 1333
tipranavir 1336

• ANTIRHEUMATICS

PHARMACOLOGIC PROFILE

General Use
Antirheumatics are used to manage symptoms of rheumatoid arthritis (pain, swelling) and in more severe cases to slow down joint destruction and preserve joint function. NSAIDs, aspirin, and other salicylates are used to manage symptoms such as pain and swelling, allowing continued motility and improved quality of life. Corticosteroids are reserved for more advanced swelling and discomfort, primarily because of their increased side effects, especially with chronic use. They can be used to control acute flares of disease. Neither NSAIDs nor corticosteroids prevent disease progression or joint destruction. Disease-modifying antirheumatics drugs(DMARDs, sometimes called slow-acting agents) slow the progression of rheumatoid ar-

thritis and delay joint destruction. DMARDs are reserved for severe cases because of their toxicity. Several months of therapy may be required before benefit is noted and maintained. Serious and frequent adverse reactions may require discontinuation of therapy, despite initial benefit.

General Action and Information
Both NSAIDs and corticosteroids have potent anti-inflammatory properties. DMARDs work by a variety of mechanisms. See individual agents, but most work by suppressing the auto-immune response thought to be responsible for joint destruction.

Contraindications
Hypersensitivity. Patients who are allergic to aspirin should not receive other NSAIDs. Corticosteroids should not be used in patients with active untreated infections.

Precautions
NSAIDs and corticosteroids should be used cautiously in patients with a history of GI bleeding. Corticosteroids should be used with caution in diabetic patients. Many DMARDs have immunosuppressive properties and should be avoided in patients for whom immunosuppression poses a serious risk, including patients with active infections, underlying malignancy, and uncontrolled diabetes mellitus.

Interactions
NSAIDs may diminish the response to diuretics and antihypertensives. Corticosteroids may augment hypokalemia from other medications and increase the risk of digoxin toxicity. DMARDs increase the risk of serious immunosuppression with other immunosuppressants.

NURSING IMPLICATIONS

Assessment
- Assess patient monthly for pain, swelling, and range of motion.

Potential Nursing Diagnoses
- Chronic pain (Indications).
- Deficient knowledge, related to disease process and medication regimen.

Implementation
- Most agents require regular administration to obtain maximum effects.

Patient/Family Teaching
- Instruct patient to contact health care professional if no improvement is noticed within a few days.

Evaluation/Desired Outcomes
- Improvement in signs and symptoms of rheumatoid arthritis.

Antirheumatics included in *Davis's Drug Guide for Nurses*

corticosteroids
betamethasone 372
budesonide 372
cortisone 372
dexamethasone 372
hydrocortisone 372
methylprednisolone 372
prednisolone 372
prednisone 372
triamcinolone 372

DMARDs
adalimumab 121
anakinra 174
certolizumab pegol 308
etanercept 539
golimumab 638
hydroxychloroquine 680
infliximab 710
leflunomide 771
methotrexate 836
penicillamine 1330

NSAIDs
celecoxib 290
ibuprofen 688
indomethacin 708
ketoprofen 754
nabumetone 891
oxaprozin 959
piroxicam 1034
sulindac 1175

miscellaneous
cycloSPORINE 387
desvenlafaxine 420
etodolac 544
sulfasalazine 1171

• ANTITUBERCULARS

PHARMACOLOGIC PROFILE

General Use
Used in the treatment and prevention of tuberculosis. Combinations are used in the treatment of active disease tuberculosis to rapidly decrease the infectious state and delay or prevent the emergence of resistant strains. In selected situations, intermittent (twice weekly) regimens may be employed. Streptomycin is also used as an antitubercular. Rifampin is used in the prevention of meningococcal meningitis and *Haemophilus influenzae* type b disease.

General Action and Information
Kill (tuberculocidal) or inhibit the growth of (tuberculostatic) mycobacteria responsible for causing tuberculosis. Combination therapy with two or more agents is required, unless used as prophylaxis (isoniazid alone).

Contraindications
Hypersensitivity. Severe liver disease.

Precautions
Use cautiously in patients with a history of liver disease or in elderly or debilitated patients. Ethambutol requires ophthalmologic follow-up. Safety in pregnancy and lactation not established, although selected agents have been used without adverse effects on the fetus. Compliance is required for optimal response.

Interactions
Isoniazid inhibits the metabolism of phenytoin. Rifampin significantly decreases saquinavir levels (combination should be avoided).

NURSING IMPLICATIONS

Assessment
- Mycobacterial studies and susceptibility tests should be performed prior to and periodically throughout therapy to detect possible resistance.
- Assess lung sounds and character and amount of sputum periodically throughout therapy.

Potential Nursing Diagnoses
- Risk for infection (Indications).
- Deficient knowledge, related to disease process and medication regimen (Patient/Family Teaching).
- Noncompliance (Patient/Family Teaching).

Implementation
- Most medications can be administered with food or antacids if GI irritation occurs.

70 ANTIULCER AGENTS

Patient/Family Teaching
- Advise patient of the importance of continuing therapy even after symptoms have subsided.
- Emphasize the importance of regular follow-up exams to monitor progress and check for side effects.
- Inform patients taking rifampin that saliva, sputum, sweat, tears, urine, and feces may become red-orange to red-brown and that soft contact lenses may become permanently discolored.

Evaluation/Desired Outcomes
- Resolution of the signs and symptoms of tuberculosis. Negative sputum cultures.

Antituberculars included in *Davis's Drug Guide for Nurses*

ethambutol 541
isoniazid 741

pyrazinamide 1080
rifampin 1112

• ANTIULCER AGENTS

PHARMACOLOGIC PROFILE

General Use
Treatment and prophylaxis of peptic ulcer and gastric hypersecretory conditions such as Zollinger-Ellison syndrome. Histamine H_2-receptor antagonists (blockers) and proton pump inhibitors are also used in the management of gastroesophageal reflux disease (GERD).

General Action and Information
Because a great majority of peptic ulcer disease may be traced to GI infection with the organism *Helicobacter pylori*, eradication of the organism decreases symptomatology and recurrence. Anti-infectives with significant activity against the organism include amoxicillin, clarithromycin, metronidazole, and tetracycline. Bismuth also has anti-infective activity against *H. pylori*. Regimens usually include: a histamine H_2-receptor antagonist, or a proton pump inhibitor, and 2 anti-infectives with or without bismuth subsalicylate for 1–14 days. Other medications used in the management of gastric/duodenal ulcer disease are aimed at neutralizing gastric acid (antacids), decreasing acid secretion (histamine H_2 antagonists, proton pump inhibitors, misoprostol), or protecting the ulcer surface from further damage (misoprostol, sucralfate). Histamine H_2-receptor antagonists competitively inhibit the action of histamine at the H_2 receptor, located primarily in gastric parietal cells, resulting in inhibition of gastric acid secretion. Misoprostol decreases gastric acid secretion and increases production of protective mucus. Proton pump inhibitors prevent the transport of hydrogen ions into the gastric lumen.

Contraindications
Hypersensitivity. Pregnancy.

Precautions
Most histamine H_2 antagonists require dose reduction in renal impairment and in elderly patients. Magnesium-containing antacids should be used cautiously in patients with renal impairment. Misoprostol should be used cautiously in women with childbearing potential.

Interactions
Calcium- and magnesium-containing antacids decrease the absorption of tetracycline and fluoroquinolones. Cimetidine inhibits the ability of the liver to metabolize several drugs, increasing the risk of toxicity from warfarin, tricyclic antidepressants, theophylline, metoprolol, phenytoin, propranolol, and lidocaine. Omeprazole decreases metabolism of phenytoin, diazepam, and warfarin. All agents that increase gastric pH will decrease the absorption of ketoconazole.

ANTIULCER AGENTS 71

NURSING IMPLICATIONS
Assessment
- Assess patient routinely for epigastric or abdominal pain and frank or occult blood in the stool, emesis, or gastric aspirate.
- **Antacids:** Assess for heartburn and indigestion as well as the location, duration, character, and precipitating factors of gastric pain.
- **Histamine H_2 Antagonists:** Assess elderly and severely ill patients for confusion routinely. Notify health care professional promptly should this occur.
- **Misoprostol:** Assess women of childbearing age for pregnancy. Medication is usually begun on 2nd or 3rd day of menstrual period following a negative serum pregnancy test within 2 wk of beginning therapy.
- **Lab Test Considerations:** Histamine H_2 antagonists antagonize the effects of pentagastrin and histamine during gastric acid secretion test. Avoid administration during the 24 hr preceding the test.
- May cause false-negative results in skin tests using allergen extracts. These drugs should be discontinued 24 hr prior to the test.

Potential Nursing Diagnoses
- Acute pain (Indications).
- Deficient knowledge, related to disease process and medication regimen (Patient/Family Teaching).

Implementation
- **Antacids:** Antacids cause premature dissolution and absorption of enteric-coated tablets and may interfere with absorption of other oral medications. Separate administration of antacids and other oral medications by at least 1 hr.
- Shake liquid preparations well before pouring. Follow administration with water to ensure passage to stomach. Liquid and powder dosage forms are considered to be more effective than chewable tablets.
- Chewable tablets must be chewed thoroughly before swallowing. Follow with half a glass of water.
- Administer 1 and 3 hr after meals and at bedtime for maximum antacid effect.
- **Misoprostol:** Administer with meals and at bedtime to reduce the severity of diarrhea.
- **Proton Pump Inhibitors:** Administer before meals, preferably in the morning. Capsules should be swallowed whole; do not open, crush, or chew.
- May be administered concurrently with antacids.
- **Sucralfate:** Administer on an empty stomach 1 hr before meals and at bedtime. Do not crush or chew tablets. Shake suspension well prior to administration. If nasogastric administration is required, consult pharmacist, as protein-binding properties of sucralfate have resulted in formation of a bezoar when administered with enteral feedings and other medications.

Patient/Family Teaching
- Instruct patient to take medication as directed for the full course of therapy, even if feeling better. If a dose is missed, it should be taken as soon as remembered but not if almost time for next dose. Do not double doses.
- Advise patient to avoid alcohol, products containing aspirin, NSAIDs, and foods that may cause an increase in GI irritation.
- Advise patient to report onset of black, tarry stools to health care professional promptly.
- Inform patient that cessation of smoking may help prevent the recurrence of duodenal ulcers.
- **Antacids:** Caution patient to consult health care professional before taking antacids for more than 2 wk or if problem is recurring. Advise patient to consult health care professional if relief is not obtained or if symptoms of gastric bleeding (black, tarry stools; coffee-ground emesis) occur.

72 ANTIVIRALS

- **Misoprostol:** Emphasize that sharing of this medication may be dangerous.
- Inform patient that misoprostol may cause spontaneous abortion. Women of childbearing age must be informed of this effect through verbal and written information and must use contraception throughout therapy. If pregnancy is suspected, the woman should stop taking misoprostol and immediately notify her health care professional.
- **Sucralfate:** Advise patient to continue with course of therapy for 4–8 wk, even if feeling better, to ensure ulcer healing.
- Advise patient that an increase in fluid intake, dietary bulk, and exercise may prevent drug-induced constipation.

Evaluation/Desired Outcomes
- Decrease in GI pain and irritation. Prevention of gastric irritation and bleeding. Healing of duodenal ulcers can be seen by x-rays or endoscopy. Therapy with histamine H_2 antagonists is continued for at least 6 wk after initial episode. Decreased symptoms of GERD. Increase in the pH of gastric secretions (antacids). Prevention of gastric ulcers in patients receiving chronic NSAID therapy (misoprostol only).

Antiulcer agents included in *Davis's Drug Guide for Nurses*

antacids
aluminum hydroxide 140
magaldrate 803
magnesium hydroxide/aluminum hydroxide 803
lansoprazole 767
omeprazole 950
pantoprazole 990
rabeprazole 1095

histamine H_2 antagonists
cimetidine 660
famotidine 660
nizatidine 660
ranitidine 660

proton-pump inhibitors
esomeprazole 530
dexlansoprazole 422

miscellaneous
amoxicillin 158
bismuth subsalicylate 231
clarithromycin 334
metronidazole 854
misoprostol 869
sodium bicarbonate 1159
sucralfate 1169

• ANTIVIRALS

PHARMACOLOGIC PROFILE
General Use
Acyclovir, famciclovir, and valacyclovir are used in the management of herpes virus infections. Acyclovir also is used in the management of chickenpox. Oseltamivir and zanamivir are used primarily in the prevention of influenza A viral infections. Cidofovir, ganciclovir, valganciclovir, and foscarnet are used in the treatment of cytomegalovirus (CMV) retinitis. Vidarabine is used only to treat ophthalmic viral infections. Penciclovir and docosanol are used in the treatment and prevention of oral-facial herpes simplex.

General Action and Information
Most agents inhibit viral replication.

Contraindications
Previous hypersensitivity.

Precautions
All except zanamivir require dose adjustment in renal impairment. Acyclovir may cause renal impairment. Acyclovir may cause CNS toxicity. Foscarnet increases risk of seizures.

Interactions
Acyclovir may have additive CNS and nephrotoxicity with drugs causing similar adverse reactions.

NURSING IMPLICATIONS
Assessment
- Assess patient for signs and symptoms of infection before and throughout therapy.
- **Ophth:** Assess eye lesions before and daily during therapy.
- **Topical:** Assess lesions before and daily during therapy.

Potential Nursing Diagnoses
- Risk for infection (Indications).
- Impaired skin integrity (Indications).
- Deficient knowledge, related to disease process and medication regimen (Patient/Family Teaching).

Implementation
- Most systemic antiviral agents should be administered around the clock to maintain therapeutic serum drug levels.

Patient/Family Teaching
- Instruct patient to continue taking medication around the clock for full course of therapy, even if feeling better.
- Advise patient that antivirals and antiretrovirals do not prevent transmission to others. Precautions should be taken to prevent spread of virus.
- Instruct patient in correct technique for topical or ophthalmic preparations.
- Instruct patient to notify health care professional if symptoms do not improve.

Evaluation/Desired Outcomes
- Prevention or resolution of the signs and symptoms of viral infection. Length of time for complete resolution depends on organism and site of infection.

Antivirals included in *Davis's Drug Guide for Nurses*

acyclovir 118
cidofovir 324
docosanol 465
entecavir 500
famciclovir 555
foscarnet 614
ganciclovir 626
imiquimod 705
lamivudine 762
oseltamivir 956
penciclovir 1001
ribavirin 1107
trifluridine 1399
valacyclovir 1259
valganciclovir 1260
zanamivir 1301

• BETA BLOCKERS

PHARMACOLOGIC PROFILE
General Use
Management of hypertension, angina pectoris, tachyarrhythmias, hypertrophic subaortic stenosis, migraine headache (prophylaxis), MI (prevention), glaucoma (ophthalmic use), congestive

74 BETA BLOCKERS

heart failure (CHF) (carvedilol and sustained-release metoprolol only) and hyperthyroidism (management of symptoms only).

General Action and Information
Beta blockers compete with adrenergic (sympathetic) neurotransmitters (epinephrine and norepinephrine) for adrenergic receptor sites. Beta$_1$-adrenergic receptor sites are located chiefly in the heart where stimulation results in increased heart rate, contractility, and AV conduction. Beta$_2$-adrenergic receptors are found mainly in bronchial and vascular smooth muscle and the uterus. Stimulation of beta$_2$-adrenergic receptors produces vasodilation, bronchodilation, and uterine relaxation. Blockade of these receptors antagonizes the effects of the neurotransmitters. Beta blockers may be relatively selective for beta$_1$-adrenergic receptors (atenolol, betaxolol, esmolol, and metoprolol) or nonselective (carteolol, carvedilol, labetalol, levobunolol, nadolol, penbutolol, pindolol, propranolol, sotalol, and timolol) blocking both beta$_1$- and beta$_2$-adrenergic receptors. Carvedilol and labetalol have additional alpha-adrenergic blocking properties. Acebutolol, carvedilol, penbutolol, and pindolol possess intrinsic sympathomimetic action (ISA) that may result in less bradycardia than other agents. Ophthalmic beta blockers decrease production of aqueous humor.

Contraindications
Uncompensated CHF (most beta blockers), acute bronchospasm, some forms of valvular heart disease, bradyarrhythmias, and heart block.

Precautions
Use cautiously in pregnant and lactating women (may cause fetal bradycardia and hyopoglycemia). Use cautiously in any form of lung disease or underlying compensated CHF (most agents). Use with caution in diabetics and patients with severe liver disease. Beta blockers should not be abruptly discontinued in patients with cardiovascular disease.

Interactions
May cause additive myocardial depression and bradycardia when used with other agents having these effects (digoxin and some antiarrhythmics). May antagonize the therapeutic effects of bronchodilators. May alter the requirements for insulin or hypoglycemic agents in diabetics. Cimetidine may decrease the metabolism and increase the effects of some beta blockers.

NURSING IMPLICATIONS

Assessment
- Monitor blood pressure and pulse frequently during dosage adjustment and periodically throughout therapy.
- Monitor intake and output ratios and daily weight. Assess patient routinely for signs and symptoms of CHF (dyspnea, rales/crackles, weight gain, peripheral edema, jugular venous distention).
- **Angina:** Assess frequency and severity of episodes of chest pain periodically throughout therapy.
- **Migraine Prophylaxis:** Assess frequency and severity of migraine headaches periodically throughout therapy.

Potential Nursing Diagnoses
- Ineffective tissue perfusion (Indications).
- Deficient knowledge, related to disease process and medication regimen (Patient/Family Teaching).
- Noncompliance (Patient/Family Teaching).

Implementation
- Take apical pulse prior to administering. If heart rate is <50 bpm or if arrhythmias occur, hold medication and notify health care professional.

BETA BLOCKERS

- Many beta blockers are available in combination products to enhance compliance (see Appendix B).

Patient/Family Teaching
- Instruct patient to continue taking medication, even if feeling well. Abrupt withdrawal may cause life-threatening arrhythmias, hypertension, or myocardial ischemia. Medication controls, but does not cure, hypertension.
- Encourage patient to comply with additional interventions for hypertension (weight reduction, low-sodium diet, regular exercise, smoking cessation, moderation of alcohol consumption, and stress management).
- Instruct patient and family on proper technique for monitoring blood pressure. Advise them to check blood pressure weekly and report significant changes to health care professional.
- Caution patient to make position changes slowly to minimize orthostatic hypotension. Advise patient that exercising or hot weather may enhance hypotensive effects.
- Advise patient to consult health care professional before taking any OTC medications or herbal/alternative therapies, especially cold remedies.
- Caution patient that these medications may cause increased sensitivity to cold.
- Diabetics should monitor blood glucose closely, especially if weakness, malaise, irritability, or fatigue occurs.
- Advise patient to advise health care professional of medication regimen prior to treatment or surgery.
- Advise patient to carry identification describing disease process and medication regimen at all times.
- Emphasize the importance of follow-up exams to monitor progress.
- **Ophth:** Instruct patient in correct technique for administration of ophthalmic preparations.

Evaluation/Desired Outcomes
- Decrease in blood pressure.
- Decrease in frequency and severity of anginal attacks.
- Control of arrhythmias.
- Prevention of myocardial reinfarction.
- Prevention of migraine headaches.
- Decrease in tremors.
- Lowering of intraocular pressure.

Beta blockers included in *Davis's Drug Guide for Nurses*

beta blockers (nonselective)
carvedilol 283
labetalol 759
nadolol 892
propranolol 1071
sotalol 1167
timolol 1229

beta blockers (selective)
atenolol 204
bisoprolol 233
esmolol 528
metoprolol 851
nebivolol 905

ophthalmics
betaxolol 1399
carteolol 1399
levobunolol 1399
metipranolol 1399
timolol 1399

• BONE RESORPTION INHIBITORS

PHARMACOLOGIC PROFILE
General Use
Bone resorption inhibitors are primarily used to treat and prevent osteoporosis in postmenopausal women. Other uses include treatment of osteoporosis due to other causes, including corticosteroid therapy, treatment of Paget's disease of the bone, and management of hypercalcemia.

General Action and Information
Biphosphonates (alendronate, etidronate, risedronate, and tiludronate) inhibit resorption of bone by inhibiting hydroxyapatite crystal dissolution and osteoclast activity. Raloxifene binds to estrogen receptors, producing estrogen-like effects on bone including decreased bone resorption and decreased bone turnover.

Contraindications
Hypersensitivity. Biphosphonates should not be used in patients with hypocalcemia. Raloxifene should not be used in women with childbearing potential or a history of thromboembolic disease.

Precautions
Use cautiously in patients with renal impairment; some agents should be avoided in moderate to severe renal impairment.

Interactions
Calcium supplements decrease absorption of biphosphonates. Tilundronate's effects may be altered by aspirin or other NSAIDs. Aspirin may increase GI adverse reactions with alendronate. Cholestyramine decreases absorption of raloxifene (concurrent use is contraindicated).

NURSING IMPLICATIONS
Assessment
- Assess patients for low bone density before and periodically during therapy.
- Assess for symptoms of Paget's disease (bone pain, headache, decreased visual and auditory acuity, increased skull size).
- **Lab Test Considerations:** Monitor serum calcium in patients with osteoporosis. Monitor alkaline phosphatase in patients with Paget's disease.

Potential Nursing Diagnoses
- Risk for injury (Indications).
- Deficient knowledge, related to disease process and medication regimen (Patient/Family Teaching).

Patient/Family Teaching
- Instruct patient to take medication exactly as directed.
- Encourage patient to participate in regular exercise and to modify behaviors that increase the risk of osteoporosis.

Evaluation/Desired Outcomes
- Prevention of, or decrease in, the progression of osteoporosis in postmenopausal women. Decrease in the progression of Paget's disease.

Bone Resorption Inhibitors included in *Davis's Drug Guide for Nurses*

biphosphonates
alendronate 130
etidronate 542
ibandronate 687
pamidronate 983
risedronate 1114

zoledronic acid 1309

selective estrogen receptor modulators
raloxifene 1096

• BRONCHODILATORS

PHARMACOLOGIC PROFILE

General Use
Used in the treatment of reversible airway obstruction due to asthma or chronic obstructive pulmonary disease (COPD). Recently revised recommendations for management of asthma recommend that rapid-acting inhaled beta-agonist bronchodilators (not salmeterol) be reserved as acute relievers of bronchospasm; repeated or chronic use indicates the need for additional long-term control agents, including inhaled corticosteroids, mast cell stabilizers, and long-acting bronchodilators (oral theophylline or beta-agonists) and leukotriene modifiers (montelukast, zafirlukast).

General Action and Information
Beta-adrenergic agonists (albuterol, epinephrine, isoproterenol, metaproterenol, pirbuterol, and terbutaline) produce bronchodilation by stimulating the production of cyclic adenosine monophosphate (cAMP). Newer agents (albuterol, metaproterenol, pirbuterol, and terbutaline) are relatively selective for pulmonary (beta$_2$) receptors, whereas older agents produce cardiac stimulation (beta$_2$-adrenergic effects) in addition to bronchodilation. Onset of action allows use in management of acute attacks except for salmeterol, which has delayed onset. Phosphodiesterase inhibitors (aminophylline and theophylline) inhibit the breakdown of cAMP. Ipratropium is an anticholinergic compound that produces bronchodilation by blocking the action of acetylcholine in the respiratory tract. Montelukast, zafirlukast, and zileuton are leukotriene modifiers. Leukotrienes are components of slow-reacting substance of anaphylaxis A (SRS-A), which may be a cause of bronchospasm.

Contraindications
Hypersensitivity to agents, preservatives (bisulfites), or propellants used in their formulation. Avoid use in uncontrolled cardiac arrhythmias.

Precautions
Use cautiously in patients with diabetes, cardiovascular disease, or hyperthyroidism.

Interactions
Therapeutic effectiveness may be antagonized by concurrent use of beta blockers. Additive sympathomimetic effects with other adrenergic (sympathetic) drugs, including vasopressors and decongestants. Cardiovascular effects may be potentiated by antidepressants and MAO inhibitors.

NURSING IMPLICATIONS

Assessment
- Assess blood pressure, pulse, respiration, lung sounds, and character of secretions before and throughout therapy.
- Patients with a history of cardiovascular problems should be monitored for ECG changes and chest pain.

Potential Nursing Diagnoses
- Ineffective airway clearance (Indications).
- Activity intolerance (Indications).
- Deficient knowledge, related to disease process and medication regimen (Patient/Family Teaching).

Implementation
- Administer around the clock to maintain therapeutic plasma levels.

Patient/Family Teaching
- Emphasize the importance of taking only the prescribed dose at the prescribed time intervals.
- Encourage the patient to drink adequate liquids (2000 mL/day minimum) to decrease the viscosity of the airway secretions.
- Advise patient to avoid OTC cough, cold, or breathing preparations without consulting health care professional and to minimize intake of xanthine-containing foods or beverages (colas, coffee, and chocolate), as these may increase side effects and cause arrhythmias.
- Caution patient to avoid smoking and other respiratory irritants.
- Instruct patient on proper use of metered-dose inhaler (see Appendix D).
- Advise patient to contact health care professional promptly if the usual dose of medication fails to produce the desired results, symptoms worsen after treatment, or toxic effects occur.
- Patients using other inhalation medications and bronchodilators should be advised to use bronchodilator first and allow 5 min to elapse before administering the other medication, unless otherwise directed by health care professional.

Evaluation/Desired Outcomes
- Decreased bronchospasm. Increased ease of breathing.

Bronchodilators included in *Davis's Drug Guide for Nurses*

adrenergics
albuterol 126
epinephrine 504
formoterol 610
levalbuterol 780
salmeterol 1134
terbutaline 1197

anticholinergics
ipratropium 732
tiotropium 1232

leukotriene antagonists
montelukast 879
zafirlukast 1299

xanthines
aminophylline 240
theophylline 240

• CALCIUM CHANNEL BLOCKERS

PHARMACOLOGIC PROFILE

General Use
Used in the treatment of hypertension (amlodipine, diltiazem, felodipine, isradipine, nicardipine, nifedipine, nisoldipine, verapamil) or in the treatment and prophylaxis of angina pectoris or coronary artery spasm (amlodipine, diltiazem, felodipine, nicardipine, verapamil). Verapamil and diltiazem are also used as antiarrhythmics. Nimodipine is used to prevent neurologic damage due to certain types of cerebral vasospasm.

CALCIUM CHANNEL BLOCKERS

General Action and Information
Block calcium entry into cells of vascular smooth muscle and myocardium. Dilate coronary arteries in both normal and ischemic myocardium and inhibit coronary artery spasm. Diltiazem and verapamil decrease AV conduction. Nimodipine has a relatively selective effect on cerebral blood vessels.

Contraindications
Hypersensitivity. Contraindicated in bradycardia, 2nd- or 3rd-degree heart block, or uncompensated CHF (verapamil).

Precautions
Safety in pregnancy and lactation not established. Use cautiously in patients with liver disease or uncontrolled arrhythmias.

Interactions
Additive myocardial depression with beta blockers and disopyramide (diltiazem and verapamil). Effectiveness may be decreased by phenobarbital or phenytoin and increased by propranolol or cimetidine. Verapamil and diltiazem may increase serum digoxin levels and cause toxicity.

NURSING IMPLICATIONS

Assessment
- Monitor blood pressure and pulse frequently during dosage adjustment and periodically throughout therapy.
- Monitor intake and output ratios and daily weight. Assess patient routinely for signs and symptoms of CHF (dyspnea, rales/crackles, weight gain, peripheral edema, jugular venous distention).
- **Angina:** Assess frequency and severity of episodes of chest pain periodically throughout therapy.
- **Arrhythmias:** ECG should be monitored continuously during IV therapy and periodically during long-term therapy with verapamil.
- **Cerebral Vasospasm:** Assess patient's neurological status (level of consciousness, movement) before and periodically during therapy with nimodipine.

Potential Nursing Diagnoses
- Ineffective tissue perfusion (Indications).
- Acute pain (Indications).
- Deficient knowledge, related to disease process and medication regimen (Patient/Family Teaching).

Implementation
- May be administered without regard to meals.
- Do not open, crush, or chew sustained-release capsules.

Patient/Family Teaching
- Instruct patient to continue taking medication, even if feeling well.
- Caution patient to make position changes slowly to minimize orthostatic hypotension. Advise patient that exercising or hot weather may enhance hypotensive effects.
- Instruct patient on the importance of maintaining good dental hygiene and seeing dentist frequently for teeth cleaning to prevent tenderness, bleeding, and gingival hyperplasia (gum enlargement).
- Advise patient to consult health care professional before taking any OTC medications or herbal/alternative therapies, especially cold remedies.
- Advise patient to advise health care professional of medication regimen prior to treatment or surgery.

80 CENTRAL NERVOUS SYSTEM STIMULANTS

- Advise patient to carry identification describing disease process and medication regimen at all times.
- Emphasize the importance of follow-up exams to monitor progress.
- **Angina:** Instruct patients on concurrent nitrate therapy to continue taking both medications as directed and using SL nitroglycerin as needed for anginal attacks. Advise patient to contact health care professional if chest pain worsens or does not improve after therapy, or is accompanied by diaphoresis or shortness of breath, or if severe, persistent headache occurs. Caution patient to discuss exercise precautions with health care professional prior to exertion.
- **Hypertension:** Encourage patient to comply with additional interventions for hypertension (weight reduction, low-sodium diet, regular exercise, smoking cessation, moderation of alcohol consumption, and stress management). Medication controls, but does not cure, hypertension.
- Instruct patient and family on proper technique for monitoring blood pressure. Advise them to check blood pressure weekly and report significant changes to health care professional.

Evaluation/Desired Outcomes
- Decrease in blood pressure.
- Decrease in frequency and severity of anginal attacks.
- Decrease need for nitrate therapy.
- Increase in activity tolerance and sense of well-being.
- Suppression and prevention of supraventricular tachyarrhythmias.
- Improvement in neurological deficits due to vasospasm following subarachnoid hemorrhage.

Calcium channel blockers included in *Davis's Drug Guide for Nurses*

amlodipine 157	niCARdipine 915
clevidipine 336	NIFEdipine 921
diltiazem 445	nimodipine 925
felodipine 557	nisoldipine 926
isradipine 746	verapamil 1275

• CENTRAL NERVOUS SYSTEM STIMULANTS

PHARMACOLOGIC PROFILE

General Use
Used in the treatment of narcolepsy and as adjunctive treatment in the management of attention deficit hyperactivity disorder (ADHD).

General Action and Information
Produce CNS stimulation by increasing levels of neurotransmitters in the CNS. Produce CNS and respiratory stimulation, dilated pupils, increased motor activity and mental alertness, and a diminished sense of fatigue. In children with ADHD these agents decrease restlessness and increase attention span.

Contraindications
Hypersensitivity. Should not be used in pregnant or lactating women. Should not be used in hyperexcitable states. Avoid using in patients with psychotic personalities or suicidal/homicidal tendencies. Contraindicated in glaucoma and severe cardiovascular disease.

Precautions
Use cautiously in patients with a history of cardiovascular disease, hypertension, diabetes mellitus, or in elderly or debilitated patients. Continual use may result in psychological dependence or addiction.

Interactions
Additive sympathomimetic (adrenergic effects). Use with MAO inhibitors can result in hypertensive crises. Alkalinizing the urine (sodium bicarbonate, acetazolamide) decreases excretion and enhances effects of amphetamines. Acidification of the urine (ammonium chloride, large doses of ascorbic acid) decreases effect of amphetamines. Phenothiazines may also decrease effects. Methylphenidate may decrease the metabolism and increase effects of other drugs (warfarin, anticonvulsants, tricyclic antidepressants).

NURSING IMPLICATIONS
Assessment
- Monitor blood pressure, pulse, and respiration before administering and periodically during therapy.
- Monitor weight biweekly and inform health care professional of significant loss.
- Monitor height periodically in children; inform health care professional if growth inhibition occurs.
- May produce false sense of euphoria and well-being. Provide frequent rest periods and observe patient for rebound depression after the effects of the medication have worn off.
- **ADHD:** Assess attention span, impulse control, and interactions with others in children. Therapy may be interrupted at intervals to determine if symptoms are sufficient to warrant continued therapy.
- **Narcolepsy:** Observe and document frequency of episodes.

Potential Nursing Diagnoses
- Disturbed thought process (Side Effects).
- Deficient knowledge, related to disease process and medication regimen (Patient/Family Teaching).

Patient/Family Teaching
- Instruct patient not to alter dose without consulting health care professional. These medications have high dependence and abuse potential. Abrupt cessation with high doses may cause extreme fatigue and mental depression.
- Advise patient to avoid intake of large amounts of caffeine.
- Medication may impair judgment. Caution patient to avoid driving or other activities requiring judgment until response to medication is known.
- Inform patient that periodic holidays from the drug may be used to assess progress and decrease dependence.

Evaluation/Desired Outcomes
- Decreased frequency of narcoleptic episodes.
- Improved attention span and social interactions.

Central nervous system stimulants included in *Davis's Drug Guide for Nurses*

amphetamine mixtures 163
caffeine citrate 262
dexmethylphenidate 424
dextroamphetamine 428
methylphenidate 844
modafinil 875

CORTICOSTEROIDS

PHARMACOLOGIC PROFILE

General Use
Used in replacement doses (20 mg of hydrocortisone or equivalent) systemically to treat adrenocortical insufficiency. Larger doses are usually used for their antiinflammatory, immunosuppressive, or antineoplastic activity. Used adjunctively in many other situations, including hypercalcemia and autoimmune diseases. Topical corticosteroids are used in a variety of inflammatory and allergic conditions. Inhalant corticosteroids are used in the chronic management of reversible airway disease (asthma); intranasal and ophthalmic corticosteroids are used in the management of chronic allergic and inflammatory conditions.

General Action and Information
Produce profound and varied metabolic effects, in addition to modifying the normal immune response and suppressing inflammation. Available in a variety of dosage forms, including oral, injectable, topical, and inhalation. Prolonged used of large amounts of topical or inhaled agent may result in systemic absorption and/or adrenal suppression.

Contraindications
Serious infections (except for certain forms of meningitis). Do not administer live vaccines to patients on larger doses.

Precautions
Prolonged treatment will result in adrenal suppression. Do not discontinue abruptly. Additional doses may be needed during stress (surgery and infection). Safety in pregnancy and lactation not established. Long-term use in children will result in decreased growth. May mask signs of infection. Use lowest dose possible for shortest time possible. Alternate-day therapy is preferable during long-term treatment.

Interactions
Additive hypokalemia with amphotericin B and potassium-losing diuretics. Hypokalemia may increase the risk of digoxin toxicity. May increase requirements for insulin or oral hypoglycemic agents. Phenytoin, phenobarbital, and rifampin stimulate metabolism and may decrease effectiveness. Oral contraceptives may block metabolism. Cholestyramine and colestipol may decrease absorption.

NURSING IMPLICATIONS

Assessment
- These drugs are indicated for many conditions. Assess involved systems prior to and periodically throughout course of therapy.
- Assess patient for signs of adrenal insufficiency (hypotension, weight loss, weakness, nausea, vomiting, anorexia, lethargy, confusion, restlessness) prior to and periodically throughout course of therapy.
- Children should have periodic evaluations of growth.

Potential Nursing Diagnoses
- Risk for infection (Side Effects).
- Deficient knowledge, related to disease process and medication regimen (Patient/Family Teaching).
- Disturbed body image (Side Effects).

Implementation
- If dose is ordered daily or every other day, administer in the morning to coincide with the body's normal secretion of cortisol.

CORTICOSTEROIDS

- **PO:** Administer with meals to minimize gastric irritation.

Patient/Family Teaching
- Emphasize need to take medication exactly as directed. Review symptoms of adrenal insufficiency that may occur when stopping the medication and that may be life-threatening.
- Encourage patients on long-term therapy to eat a diet high in protein, calcium, and potassium and low in sodium and carbohydrates.
- These drugs cause immunosuppression and may mask symptoms of infection. Instruct patient to avoid people with known contagious illnesses and to report possible infections. Advise patient to consult health care professional before receiving any vaccinations.
- Discuss possible effects on body image. Explore coping mechanisms.
- Advise patient to carry identification in the event of an emergency in which patient cannot relate medical history.

Evaluation/Desired Outcomes
- Suppression of the inflammatory and immune responses in autoimmune disorders, allergic reactions, and organ transplants.
- Replacement therapy in adrenal insufficiency.
- Resolution of skin inflammation, pruritus, or other dermatologic conditions.

Corticosteroids included in *Davis's Drug Guide for Nurses*

corticosteroids, inhalation
beclomethasone 365
budesonide 365
flunisolide 366
fluticasone 366
triamcinolone 366

corticosteroids, nasal
beclomethasone 369
budesonide 369
ciclesonide 369
flunisolide 369
fluticasone 369
mometasone 369
triamcinolone 369

corticosteroids, ophthalmic
dexamethasone 1400
difluprednate 1400
fluorometholone 1400
loteprednol 1400
prednisolone 1401
rimexolone 1401

corticosteroids, systemic (short-acting)
cortisone 372
hydrocortisone 372

corticosteroids, systemic (intermediate-acting)
methylPREDNISolone 372
prednisoLONE 372
predniSONE 372
triamcinolone 372

corticosteroids, systemic (long-acting)
betamethasone 372
budesonide 372
dexamethasone 372

corticosteroids, topical/local
alclometasone 380
amcinonide 380
betamethasone 380
clobetasol 380
clocortolone 380
desonide 380
desoximetasone 380
diflorasone 380
fluocinolone 380
fluocinonide 380
flurandrenolide 380
fluticasone 380
halcinonide 380
halobetasol 380
hydrocortisone 381
mometasone 381
prednicarbate 381
triamcinolone 381

DIURETICS

PHARMACOLOGIC PROFILE

General Use
Thiazide diuretics and loop diuretics are used alone or in combination in the treatment of hypertension or edema due to CHF or other causes. Potassium-sparing diuretics have weak diuretic and antihypertensive properties and are used mainly to conserve potassium in patients receiving thiazide or loop diuretics. Osmotic diuretics are often used in the management of cerebral edema.

General Action and Information
Enhance the selective excretion of various electrolytes and water by affecting renal mechanisms for tubular secretion and reabsorption. Groups commonly used are thiazide diuretics and thiazide-like diuretics (chlorothiazide, chlorthalidone, hydrochlorothiazide, indapamide, and metolazone), loop diuretics (bumetanide, furosemide, and torsemide), potassium-sparing diuretics (amiloride, spironolactone, and triamterene), and osmotic diuretics (mannitol). Mechanisms vary, depending on agent.

Contraindications
Hypersensitivity. Thiazide diuretics may exhibit cross-sensitivity with other sulfonamides.

Precautions
Use with caution in patients with renal or hepatic disease. Safety in pregnancy and lactation not established.

Interactions
Additive hypokalemia with corticosteroids, amphotericin B, piperacillin, or ticarcillin. Hypokalemia enhances digitalis glycoside toxicity. Potassium-losing diuretics decrease lithium excretion and may cause toxicity. Additive hypotension with other antihypertensives or nitrates. Potassium-sparing diuretics may cause hyperkalemia when used with potassium supplements or ACE inhibitors.

NURSING IMPLICATIONS

Assessment
- Assess fluid status throughout therapy. Monitor daily weight, intake and output ratios, amount and location of edema, lung sounds, skin turgor, and mucous membranes.
- Assess patient for anorexia, muscle weakness, numbness, tingling, paresthesia, confusion, and excessive thirst. Notify health care professional promptly if these signs of electrolyte imbalance occur.
- **Hypertension:** Monitor blood pressure and pulse before and during administration. Monitor frequency of prescription refills to determine compliance in patients treated for hypertension.
- **Increased Intracranial Pressure:** Monitor neurologic status and intracranial pressure readings in patients receiving osmotic diuretics to decrease cerebral edema.
- **Increased Intraocular Pressure:** Monitor for persistent or increased eye pain or decreased visual acuity.
- **Lab Test Considerations:** Monitor electrolytes (especially potassium), blood glucose, BUN, and serum uric acid levels before and periodically throughout course of therapy.
- Thiazide diuretics may cause increased serum cholesterol, low-density lipoprotein (LDL), and triglyceride concentrations.

Potential Nursing Diagnoses
- Excess fluid volume (Indications).
- Deficient knowledge, related to disease process and medication regimen (Patient/Family Teaching).

Implementation
- Administer oral diuretics in the morning to prevent disruption of sleep cycle.
- Many diuretics are available in combination with antihypertensives or potassium-sparing diuretics.

Patient/Family Teaching
- Instruct patient to take medication exactly as directed. Advise patients on antihypertensive regimen to continue taking medication, even if feeling better. Medication controls, but does not cure, hypertension.
- Caution patient to make position changes slowly to minimize orthostatic hypotension. Caution patient that the use of alcohol, exercise during hot weather, or standing for long periods during therapy may enhance orthostatic hypotension.
- Instruct patient to consult health care professional regarding dietary potassium guidelines.
- Instruct patient to monitor weight weekly and report significant changes.
- Caution patient to use sunscreen and protective clothing to prevent photosensitivity reactions.
- Advise patient to consult health care professional before taking OTC medication concurrently with this therapy.
- Instruct patient to notify health care professional of medication regimen before treatment or surgery.
- Advise patient to contact health care professional immediately if muscle weakness, cramps, nausea, dizziness, or numbness or tingling of extremities occurs.
- Emphasize the importance of routine follow-up.
- **Hypertension:** Reinforce the need to continue additional therapies for hypertension (weight loss, regular exercise, restricted sodium intake, stress reduction, moderation of alcohol consumption, and cessation of smoking).
- Instruct patients with hypertension in the correct technique for monitoring weekly blood pressure.

Evaluation/Desired Outcomes
- Decreased blood pressure.
- Increased urine output.
- Decreased edema.
- Reduced intracranial pressure.
- Prevention of hypokalemia in patients taking diuretics.
- Treatment of hyperaldosteronism.

Diuretics included in *Davis's Drug Guide for Nurses*

carbonic anhydrase inhibitors
acetaZOLAMIDE 114

loop diuretics
bumetanide 244
furosemide 620
torsemide 1244

osmotic diuretics
mannitol 808

potassium-sparing diuretics
amiloride 456
spironolactone 456
triamterene 456

thiazide diuretics
chlorothiazide 458
chlorthalidone (thiazide-like) 458
hydrochlorothiazide 458

thiazide-like diuretics
indapamide 706
metolazone 850

HORMONES

PHARMACOLOGIC PROFILE

General Use
Used in the treatment of deficiency states including diabetes (insulin), diabetes insipidus (desmopressin), hypothyroidism (thyroid hormones), and menopause (estrogens or estrogens/progestins). Estrogenic and progestational hormones are used as contraceptive agents in various combinations and sequences. Hormones may be used to treat hormonally sensitive tumors (androgens, estrogens) and in other selected situations. See individual drugs.

General Action and Information
Natural or synthetic substances that have a specific effect on target tissue. Differ greatly in their effects, depending on individual agent and function of target tissue.

Contraindications
Differ greatly among individual agents; see individual entries.

Precautions
Differ greatly among individual agents; see individual entries.

Interactions
Differ greatly among individual agents; see individual entries.

NURSING IMPLICATIONS

Assessment
- Monitor patient for symptoms of hormonal excess or insufficiency.
- **Sex Hormones:** Blood pressure and hepatic function tests should be monitored periodically throughout therapy.

Potential Nursing Diagnoses
- Sexual dysfunction (Indications).
- Disturbed body image (Indications) (Side Effects).
- Deficient knowledge, related to disease process and medication regimen (Patient/Family Teaching).

Implementation
- **Sex Hormones:** During hospitalization, continue to administer according to schedule followed prior to hospitalization.

Patient/Family Teaching
- Explain dose schedule (and withdrawal bleeding with female sex hormones).
- Emphasize the importance of follow-up exams to monitor effectiveness of therapy and to ensure proper development of children and early detection of possible side effects.
- **Female Sex Hormones:** Advise patient to report signs and symptoms of fluid retention, thromboembolic disorders, mental depression, or hepatic dysfunction to health care professional.

Evaluation/Desired Outcomes
- Resolution of clinical symptoms of hormone imbalance including menopause symptoms and contraception.
- Correction of fluid and electrolyte imbalances.
- Control of the spread of advanced metastatic breast or prostate cancer.
- Slowed progression of postmenopausal osteoporosis.

Hormones included in *Davis's Drug Guide for Nurses*

hormones
calcitonin (salmon) 263
danazol 1323
darbepoetin 403
desmopressin 418
epoetin 512
estrogens, conjugated (equine) 535
estrogens, conjugated (synthetic, A) 535
estrogens, conjugated (synthetic, B) 535
fludrocortisone 586
glucagon 634
goserelin 640
leuprolide 778
levothyroxine 1219
liothyronine 1219
liotrix 1219
medroxyPROGESTERone 812
megestrol 814
nafarelin 894
octreotide 1355
oxytocin 972
pramlintide 1046
progesterone 1060
somatropin (recombinant) 645
teriparatide 1199
testosterone buccal system, mucoadhesive 1200
testosterone cypionate 1200
testosterone enanthate 1200
testosterone pellets 1200
testosterone transdermal 1200
thyroid 1219
vasopressin 1271

insulins
insulin aspart protamine suspension/insulin aspart solution mixtures, rDNA origin 712, 1425
insulin aspart, rDNA origin 721, 1425
insulin detemir 719, 1425
insulin glargine 719, 1425
insulin glulisine 721, 1425
insulin lispro protamine suspension/insulin lispro solution mixtures, rDNA origin 712, 1425
insulin lispro, rDNA origin 721, 1425
insulin, regular (injection, concentrated) 714, 1425
NPH insulin (isophane insulin suspension) 717, 1425
NPH/regular insulin mixtures 712, 1425

contraceptive hormones
estradiol acetate 532
estradiol cypionate 532
estradiol topical emulsion 532
estradiol topical gel 532
estradiol transdermal spray 532
estradiol transdermal system 532
estradiol vaginal ring 532
estradiol vaginal tablet 532
estradiol valerate 532
ethinyl estradiol/desogestrel 358
ethinyl estradiol/drospirenone 358
ethinyl estradiol/ethynodiol 358
ethinyl estradiol/etonogestrel 359
ethinyl estradiol/levonergestrel 358
ethinyl estradiol/norelgestromin 359
ethinyl estradiol/norethindrone 358
ethinyl estradiol/norgestimate 358
ethinyl estradiol/norgestrel 358
levonorgestrel 359
levonorgestrel/ethinyl estradiol 359
medroxyprogesterone 359
mestranol/norethindrone 359
norethindrone 359
norethindrone/ethinyl acetate 359
norgestimate/ethinyl estradiol 359
norgestrel 359

• IMMUNOSUPPRESSANTS

PHARMACOLOGIC PROFILE

General Use
Azathioprine, basiliximab, cyclosporine, daclizumab, mycophenolate, sirolimus, and tacrolimus are used with corticosteroids in the prevention of transplantation rejection reactions. Muro-

IMMUNOSUPPRESSANTS

monab-CD3 is used to manage rejection reactions not controlled by other agents. Azathioprine, cyclophosphamide, and methotrexate are used in the management of selected autoimmune diseases (nephrotic syndrome of childhood and severe rheumatoid arthritis).

General Action and Information
Inhibit cell-mediated immune responses by different mechanisms. In addition to azathioprine and cyclosporine, which are used primarily for their immunomodulating properties, cyclophosphamide and methotrexate are used to suppress the immune responses in certain disease states (nephrotic syndrome of childhood and severe rheumatoid arthritis). Muromonab-CD3 is a recombinant immunoglobulin antibody that alters T-cell function. Basiliximab and daclizumab are monoclonal antibodies.

Contraindications
Hypersensitivity to drug or vehicle.

Precautions
Use cautiously in patients with infections. Safety in pregnancy and lactation not established.

Interactions
Allopurinol inhibits the metabolism of azathioprine. Drugs that alter liver-metabolizing processes may change the effect of cyclosporine. The risk to toxicity of methotrexate may be increased by other nephrotoxic drugs, large doses of aspirin, or NSAIDs. Muromonab-CD3 has additive immunosuppressive properties; concurrent immunosuppressive doses should be decreased or eliminated.

NURSING IMPLICATIONS

Assessment
- Monitor for infection (vital signs, sputum, urine, stool, WBC). Notify physician or other health care professional immediately if symptoms occur.
- **Organ Transplant:** Assess for symptoms of organ rejection throughout therapy.
- **Lab Test Consideration:** Monitor CBC and differential throughout therapy.

Potential Nursing Diagnoses
- Risk for infection (Side Effects).
- Deficient knowledge, related to disease process and medication regimen (Patient/Family Teaching).

Implementation
- Protect transplant patients from staff and visitors who may carry infection.
- Maintain protective isolation as indicated.

Patient/Family Teaching
- Reinforce the need for lifelong therapy to prevent transplant rejection. Review symptoms of rejection for transplanted organ and stress need to notify health care professional immediately if they occur.
- Advise patient to avoid contact with contagious persons and those who have recently taken oral polio virus vaccine. Patients should not receive vaccinations without first consulting with health care professional.
- Emphasize the importance of follow-up exams and lab tests.

Evaluation/Desired Outcomes
- Prevention or reversal of rejection of organ transplants or decrease in symptoms of autoimmune disorders.

LAXATIVES 89

Immunosuppressants included in *Davis's Drug Guide for Nurses*

azathioprine 212
basiliximab 220
cyclophosphamide 384
cycloSPORINE 387
methotrexate 836
muromonab-CD3 886
mycophenolate mofetil 887
mycophenolic acid 887
pimecrolimus 1029
sirolimus 1155
tacrolimus (oral, IV) 1182
tacrolimus (topical) 1182
thalidomide 1207

• LAXATIVES

PHARMACOLOGIC PROFILE

General Use
Used to treat or prevent constipation or to prepare the bowel for radiologic or endoscopic procedures.

General Action and Information
Induce one or more bowel movements per day. Groups include stimulants (bisacodyl, sennosides), saline laxatives (magnesium salts and phosphates), stool softeners (docusate), bulk-forming agents (polycarbophil and psyllium), and osmotic cathartics (lactulose, polyethylene glycol/electrolyte). Increasing fluid intake, exercising, and adding more dietary fiber are also useful in the management of chronic constipation.

Contraindications
Hypersensitivity. Contraindicated in persistent abdominal pain, nausea, or vomiting of unknown cause, especially if accompanied by fever or other signs of an acute abdomen.

Precautions
Excessive or prolonged use may lead to dependence. Should not be used in children unless advised by a physician or other health care professional.

Interactions
Theoretically may decrease the absorption of other orally administered drugs by decreasing transit time.

NURSING IMPLICATIONS

Assessment
- Assess patient for abdominal distention, presence of bowel sounds, and usual pattern of bowel function.
- Assess color, consistency, and amount of stool produced.

Potential Nursing Diagnoses
- Constipation (Indications).
- Deficient knowledge, related to disease process and medication regimen (Patient/Family Teaching).

Implementation
- Many laxatives may be administered at bedtime for morning results.
- Taking oral doses on an empty stomach will usually produce more rapid results.
- Do not crush or chew enteric-coated tablets. Take with a full glass of water or juice.
- Stool softeners and bulk laxatives may take several days for results.

Patient/Family Teaching
- Advise patients, other than those with spinal cord injuries, that laxatives should be used only for short-term therapy. Long-term therapy may cause electrolyte imbalance and dependence.
- Advise patient to increase fluid intake to a minimum of 1500–2000 mL/day during therapy to prevent dehydration.
- Encourage patients to use other forms of bowel regulation: increasing bulk in the diet, increasing fluid intake, and increasing mobility. Normal bowel habits are individualized and may vary from 3 times/day to 3 times/wk.
- Instruct patients with cardiac disease to avoid straining during bowel movements (Valsalva maneuver).
- Advise patient that laxatives should not be used when constipation is accompanied by abdominal pain, fever, nausea, or vomiting.

Evaluation/Desired Outcomes
- A soft, formed bowel movement.
- Evacuation of the colon.

Laxatives included in *Davis's Drug Guide for Nurses*

bulk-forming agents
psyllium 1079
opioid antagonists
methylnaltrexone 843
osmotics
lactulose 761
polyethylene glycol 1036
polyethylene glycol/electrolyte 1036
salines
magnesium chloride 804
magnesium citrate 804

magnesium gluconate 804
magnesium hydroxide 804
magnesium oxide 804
phosphate/biphosphate 1025
stimulant laxatives
bisacodyl 230
sennosides 1145
stool softeners
docusate calcium 466
docusate sodium 466

• LIPID-LOWERING AGENTS

PHARMACOLOGIC PROFILE

General Use
Used as a part of a total plan including diet and exercise to reduce blood lipids in an effort to reduce the morbidity and mortality of atherosclerotic cardiovascular disease and its sequelae.

General Action and Information
HMG-CoA reductase inhibitors (atorvastatin, fluvastatin, lovastatin, pravastatin, simvastatin) inhibit an enzyme involved in cholesterol synthesis. Bile acid sequestrants (cholestyramine, colestipol, colesevelam) bind cholesterol in the GI tract. Fenofibrate, niacin, and gemfibrozil act by other mechanisms (see individual monographs).

Contraindications
Hypersensitivity.

Precautions
Safety in pregnancy, lactation, and children not established. See individual drugs. Dietary therapy should be given a 2–3 mo trial before drug therapy is initiated.

Interactions
Bile acid sequestrants (cholestyramine and colestipol) may bind lipid-soluble vitamins (A, D, E, and K) and other concurrently administered drugs in the GI tract. The risk of myopathy from HMG-CoA reductase inhibitors is increased by niacin, erythromycin, gemfibrozil, and cyclosporine.

NURSING IMPLICATIONS
Assessment
- Obtain a diet history, especially in regard to **fat** and alcohol consumption.
- **Lab Test Considerations:** Serum cholesterol and triglyceride levels should be evaluated before initiating and periodically throughout therapy. Medication should be discontinued if paradoxical increase in cholesterol level occurs.
- Liver function tests should be assessed before and periodically throughout therapy. May cause an increase in levels.

Potential Nursing Diagnoses
- Deficient knowledge, related to disease process and medication regimen (Patient/Family Teaching).
- Noncompliance (Patient/Family Teaching).

Implementation
- See specific medications to determine timing of doses in relation to meals.

Patient/Family Teaching
- Advise patient that these medications should be used in conjunction with diet restrictions (**fat**, **cholesterol**, **carbohydrates**, and alcohol), exercise, and cessation of smoking.

Evaluation/Desired Outcomes
- Decreased serum triglyceride and LDL **cholesterol** levels and improved HDL cholesterol ratios. Therapy is usually discontinued if the clinical response is not evident after 3 mo of therapy.

Lipid-lowering agents included in *Davis's Drug Guide for Nurses*

bile acid sequestrants
cholestyramine 322
colesevelam 356
colestipol 357

HMG-CoA reductase inhibitors
atorvastatin 666
fluvastatin 666
lovastatin 666
pitavastatin 666
pravastatin 666
rosuvastatin 666
simvastatin 666

miscellaneous
ezetimibe 552
fenofibrate 559
fenofibric acid 561
gemfibrozil 632
niacin 914
niacinamide 914
omega-3-acid ethyl esters 949

• MINERALS/ELECTROLYTES/pH MODIFIERS

PHARMACOLOGIC PROFILE
General Use
Prevention and treatment of deficiencies or excesses of electrolytes and maintenance of optimal acid/base balance for homeostasis. Acidifiers and alkalinizers are also used to promote urinary excretion of substances that accumulate in certain disease states (kidney stones, uric acid).

92 MINERALS/ELECTROLYTES/pH MODIFIERS

General Action and Information
Electrolytes and minerals are necessary for many body processes. Maintenance of electrolyte levels within normal limits is required for many physiological processes such as cardiac, nerve, and muscle function; bone growth and stability; and a number of other activities. Minerals and electrolytes may also serve as catalysts in many enzymatic reactions. Acid/base balance allows for normal transfer of substances at the cellular and intracellular level.

Contraindications
Contraindicated in situations in which replacement would cause excess or when risk factors for retention are present.

Precautions
Use cautiously in disease states in which electrolyte imbalances are common such as significant hepatic or renal disease, adrenal or pituitary disorders.

Interactions
Depend on individual agents. Alkalinizers and acidifiers can alter the excretion of drugs for which elimination is pH dependent. See specific entries.

NURSING IMPLICATIONS

Assessment
- Observe patient carefully for evidence of electrolyte excess or insufficiency. Monitor lab values before and periodically throughout therapy.

Potential Nursing Diagnoses
- Imbalanced nutrition: less than body requirements (Indications).
- Deficient knowledge, related to medication regimen (Patient/Family Teaching).

Implementation
- **Potassium Chloride:** Do not administer potassium chloride undiluted.

Patient/Family Teaching
- Review diet modifications with patients with chronic electrolyte disturbances.

Evaluation/Desired Outcomes
- Return to normal serum electrolyte concentrations and resolution of clinical symptoms of electrolyte imbalance.
- Changes in pH or composition of urine, which prevent formation of renal calculi.

Minerals/Electrolytes/pH Modifiers included in *Davis's Drug Guide for Nurses*

alkalinizing agents
sodium bicarbonate 1159
sodium citrate and citric acid 1163

calcium salts
calcium acetate (25% Ca or 12.6 mEq/g) 265
calcium carbonate (40% Ca or 20 mEq/g) 265
calcium chloride (27% Ca or 13.6 mEq/g) 265
calcium citrate (21% Ca or 12 mEq/g) 265
calcium gluconate (9% Ca or 4.5 mEq/g) 265
calcium lactate (13% Ca or 6.5 mEq/g) 265
tricalcium phosphate (39% Ca or 19.5 mEq/g) 265

magnesium salts
magnesium chloride (12% Mg; 9.8 mEq Mg/g) 804
magnesium citrate (16.2% Mg; 4.4 mEq Mg/g) 804
magnesium gluconate (5.4 % Mg; 4.4 mEq/g) 804
magnesium hydroxide (41.7% Mg; 34.3 mEq Mg/g) 804

magnesium oxide (60.3% Mg; 49.6 mEq Mg/g) 804
magnesium sulfate (IV, parenteral) 806

potassium phosphates
monobasic potassium phosphate 1332
potassium phosphates 1332
potassium phosphate 1332

potassium and sodium phosphates
potassium and sodium phosphates 1039

potassium salts
potassium acetate 1041
potassium bicarbonate 1041
potassium bicarbonate/potassium chloride 1041
potassium bicarbonate/potassium citrate 1041
potassium chloride 1041
potassium chloride/potassium bicarbonate/potassium citrate 1041
potassium gluconate 1041
potassium gluconate/potassium chloride 1041
potassium gluconate/potassium citrate 1041
trikates (potassium acetate/potassium bicarbonate/potassium citrate) 1041

miscellaneous
sodium chloride 1161
tolvaptan 1239
zinc sulfate 1306

• NATURAL/HERBAL PRODUCTS

PHARMACOLOGIC PROFILE

General Use
These remedies are used for a wide variety of conditions. Prescriptions are not required and consumers have the choice of many products.

General Action and Information
Use of these agents is based on historical and sometimes anecdotal evidence. The FDA has little control over these agents, so currently there is little standardization among products.

Contraindications
Hypersensitivity. Most products are plant extracts that may contain a variety of impurities.

Precautions
Elderly, pediatric, and pregnant or lactating patients should be aware that these agents carry many of the same risks as prescription medications. Patients with serious chronic medical conditions should consult their health care professional before use.

Interactions
These agents have the ability to interact with prescription medications and may prevent or augment a desired therapeutic outcome. St. John's wort and kava-kava have the greatest risk for serious interactions.

NURSING IMPLICATIONS

Assessment
- Assess the condition for which the patient is taking the product.

Potential Nursing Diagnoses
- Deficient knowledge, related to disease process and medication regimen (Patient/Family Teaching).

Patient/Family Teaching
- Discuss with patient the reason for using the product. Encourage patient to choose products with USP label, if possible, to guarantee content and purity of medication.
- Inform patient of known side effects and interactions with other medications.

Evaluation/Desired Outcomes
- Improvement in condition for which medication was taken.

Natural/Herbal Products included in *Davis's Drug Guide for Nurses*

aloe 1341
arnica 1343
billberry 1344
black cohosh 1344
chondroitin 1346
dongquai 1347
echinacea 1348
feverfew 1349
garlic 1350
ginger 1351
ginkgo 1353

ginseng 1354
glucosamine 1356
grape seed extract 1357
green tea 1357
hawthorne 1358
kava-kava 1360
milk thistle 1361
SAMe 1362
saw palmetto 1363
St. John's wort 1364
valerian 1365

• NONOPIOID ANALGESICS

PHARMACOLOGIC PROFILE

General Use
Used to control mild to moderate pain and/or fever. Phenazopyridine is used only to treat urinary tract pain, and capsaicin is used topically for a variety of painful syndromes.

General Action and Information
Most nonopioid analgesics inhibit prostaglandin synthesis peripherally for analgesic effect and centrally for antipyretic effect. Tramadol is a centrally acting agent.

Contraindications
Hypersensitivity and cross-sensitivity among NSAIDs may occur.

Precautions
Use cautiously in patients with severe hepatic or renal disease, chronic alcohol use/abuse, or malnutrition. Tramadol has CNS depressant properties.

Interactions
Long-term use of acetaminophen with NSAIDs may increase the risk of adverse renal effects. Prolonged high-dose acetaminophen may increase the risk of bleeding with warfarin. Hepatotoxicity may be additive with other hepatotoxic agents, including alcohol. NSAIDs increase the risk of bleeding with warfarin, thrombolytic agents, antiplatelet agents, some cephalosporins, and valproates (effect is greatest with aspirin). NSAIDs may also decrease the effectiveness of diuretics and antihypertensives. The risk of CNS depression with tramadol is increased by concurrent use of other CNS depressants, including alcohol, antihistamines, sedative/hypnotics, and some antidepressants.

NURSING IMPLICATIONS
Assessment
- Patients who have asthma, allergies, and nasal polyps or who are allergic to tartrazine are at an increased risk for developing hypersensitivity reactions.
- **Pain:** Assess pain and limitation of movement; note type, location, and intensity prior to and at the peak (see Time/Action Profile) following administration.
- **Fever:** Assess fever and note associated signs (diaphoresis, tachycardia, malaise, chills).
- **Lab Test Considerations:** Hepatic, hematologic, and renal function should be evaluated periodically throughout prolonged high-dose therapy. Aspirin and most NSAIDs prolong bleeding time due to suppressed platelet aggregation and, in large doses, may cause prolonged prothrombin time. Monitor hematocrit periodically in prolonged high-dose therapy to assess for GI blood loss.

Potential Nursing Diagnoses
- Acute pain (Indications).
- Risk for imbalanced body temperature (Indications).
- Deficient knowledge, related to disease process and medication regimen (Patient/Family Teaching).

Implementation
- **PO:** Administer salicylates and NSAIDs after meals or with food or an antacid to minimize gastric irritation.

Patient/Family Teaching
- Instruct patient to take salicylates and NSAIDs with a full glass of water and to remain in an upright position for 15–30 min after administration.
- Adults should not take acetaminophen longer than 10 days and children not longer than 5 days unless directed by health care professional. Short-term doses of acetaminophen with salicylates or NSAIDs should not exceed the recommended daily dose of either drug alone.
- Caution patient to avoid concurrent use of alcohol with this medication to minimize possible gastric irritation; 3 or more glasses of alcohol per day may increase the risk of GI bleeding with salicylates or NSAIDs. Caution patient to avoid taking acetaminophen, salicylates, or NSAIDs concurrently for more than a few days, unless directed by health care professional to prevent analgesic nephropathy.
- Advise patients on long-term therapy to inform health care professional of medication regimen prior to surgery. Aspirin, salicylates, and NSAIDs may need to be withheld prior to surgery.

Evaluation/Desired Outcomes
- Relief of mild to moderate discomfort.
- Reduction of fever.

Nonopioid analgesics included in *Davis's Drug Guide for Nurses*

nonsteroidal anti-inflammatory agents
celecoxib 290
diclofenac potassium 435
diclofenac sodium 435
dicofenac topical 435
etodolac 544
ibuprofen, oral 688
ketoprofen 754
ketorolac 756
meloxicam 815
naproxen 900

salicylates
aspirin 1131
choline and magnesium salicylates 1131
choline salicylate 1131
magnesium salicylate 1131
salsalate 1131
sodium salicylate 1131

NONSTEROIDAL ANTI-INFLAMMATORY AGENTS

miscellaneous
acetaminophen 112
butalbital compounds 255
capsaicin 271
phenazopyridine 1014
pregabalin 1051

• NONSTEROIDAL ANTI-INFLAMMATORY AGENTS

PHARMACOLOGIC PROFILE

General Use
NSAIDs are used to control mild to moderate pain, fever, and various inflammatory conditions, such as rheumatoid arthritis and osteoarthritis. Ophthalmic NSAIDs are used to decrease postoperative ocular inflammation, to inhibit perioperative miosis, and to decrease inflammation due to allergies.

General Action and Information
NSAIDs have analgesic, antipyretic, and anti-inflammatory properties. Analgesic and anti-inflammatory effects are due to inhibition of prostaglandin synthesis. Antipyretic action is due to vasodilation and inhibition of prostaglandin synthesis in the CNS. COX-2 inhibitors (celecoxib) may cause less GI bleeding.

Contraindications
Hypersensitivity to aspirin is a contraindication for the whole group of NSAIDs. Cross-sensitivity may occur.

Precautions
Use cautiously in patients with a history of bleeding disorders, GI bleeding, and severe hepatic, renal, or cardiovascular disease. Safe use in pregnancy is not established and, in general, should be avoided during the second half of pregnancy.

Interactions
NSAIDs prolong bleeding time and potentiate the effect of warfarin, thrombolytic agents, some cephalosporins, antiplatelet agents, and valproates. Prolonged use with aspirin may result in increased GI side effects and decreased effectiveness. NSAIDs may also decrease response to diuretics or antihypertensive therapy. Ibuprofen negates the cardioprotective benefits of low-dose aspirin. COX-2 inhibitors do not negate the cardioprotective effect of low-dose aspirin.

NURSING IMPLICATIONS

Assessment
- Patients who have asthma, allergies, and nasal polyps or who are allergic to tartrazine are at an increased risk for developing hypersensitivity reactions.
- **Pain:** Assess pain and limitation of movement; note type, location, and intensity prior to and at the peak (see Time/Action Profile) following administration.
- **Fever:** Assess fever and note associated signs (diaphoresis, tachycardia, malaise, chills).
- **Lab Test Considerations:** Most NSAIDs prolong bleeding time due to suppressed platelet aggregation and, in large doses, may cause prolonged PT. Monitor periodically in prolonged high-dose therapy to assess for GI blood loss.

Potential Nursing Diagnoses
- Acute pain (Indications).
- Risk for imbalanced body temperature (Indications).
- Deficient knowledge, related to disease process and medication regimen (Patient/Family Teaching).

Implementation
- **PO:** Administer NSAIDs after meals or with food or an antacid to minimize gastric irritation.

Patient/Family Teaching
- Instruct patient to take NSAIDs with a full glass of water and to remain in an upright position for 15–30 min after administration.
- Caution patient to avoid concurrent use of alcohol with this medication to minimize possible gastric irritation; 3 or more glasses of alcohol per day may increase the risk of GI bleeding with salicylates or NSAIDs. Caution patient to avoid taking acetaminophen, salicylates, or NSAIDs concurrently for more than a few days, unless directed by health care professional to prevent analgesic nephropathy.
- Advise patient on long-term therapy to inform health care professional of medication regimen prior to surgery. NSAIDs may need to be withheld prior to surgery.

Evaluation/Desired Outcomes
- Relief of mild to moderate discomfort
- Reduction of fever.

Nonsteroidal anti-inflammatory agents included in *Davis's Drug Guide for Nurses*

nonsteroidal anti-inflammatory agents
celecoxib 290
diclofenac potassium 435
diclofenac sodium 435
diclofenac topical 435
ibuprofen, oral 688
indomethacin 708
ketoprofen 754
ketorolac 756
meloxicam 815
nabumetone 891
naproxen 900
oxaprozin 959
piroxicam 1034
sulindac 1175
tolmetin 1337

ophthalmic NSAIDs
bromfenac 1402
diclofenac 435, 1402
flurbiprofen 1402
ketorolac 756
nepafenac 1402

• OPIOID ANALGESICS

PHARMACOLOGIC PROFILE

General Use
Management of moderate to severe pain. Fentanyl is also used as a general anesthetic adjunct.

General Action and Information
Opioids bind to opiate receptors in the CNS, where they act as agonists of endogenously occurring opioid peptides (eukephalins and endorphins). The result is alteration to the perception of and response to pain.

Contraindications
Hypersensitivity to individual agents.

Precautions
Use cautiously in patients with undiagnosed abdominal pain, head trauma or pathology, liver disease, or history of addiction to opioids. Use smaller doses initially in the elderly and those

with respiratory diseases. Prolonged use may result in tolerance and the need for larger doses to relieve pain. Psychological or physical dependence may occur.

Interactions
Increases the CNS depressant properties of other drugs, including alcohol, antihistamines, antidepressants, sedative/hypnotics, phenothiazines, and MAO inhibitors. Use of partial-antagonist opioid analgesics (buprenorphine, butorphanol, nalbuphine, and pentazocine) may precipitate opioid withdrawal in physically dependent patients. Use with MAO inhibitors or procarbazine may result in severe paradoxical reactions (especially with meperidine). Nalbuphine or pentazocine may decrease the analgesic effects of other concurrently administered opioid analgesics.

NURSING IMPLICATIONS

Assessment
- Assess type, location, and intensity of pain prior to and at peak following administration. When titrating opioid doses, increases of 25–50% should be administered until there is either a 50% reduction in the patient's pain rating on a numerical or visual analogue scale or the patient reports satisfactory pain relief. A repeat dose can be safely administered at the time of the peak if previous dose is ineffective and side effects are minimal. Patients requiring higher doses of opioid agonist-antagonists should be converted to an opioid agonist.
- Opioid agonist-antagonists are not recommended for prolonged use or as first-line therapy for acute or cancer pain.
- An equianalgesic chart (see Appendix K) should be used when changing routes or when changing from one opioid to another.
- Assess blood pressure, pulse, and respirations before and periodically during administration. If respiratory rate is <10/min, assess level of sedation. Physical stimulation may be sufficient to prevent significant hypoventilation. Dose may need to be decreased by 25–50%. Initial drowsiness will diminish with continued use.
- Assess prior analgesic history. Antagonistic properties of agonist-antagonists may induce withdrawal symptoms (vomiting, restlessness, abdominal cramps, and increased blood pressure and temperature) in patients physically dependent on opioids.
- Prolonged use may lead to physical and psychological dependence and tolerance. This should not prevent patient from receiving adequate analgesia. Most patients who receive opioid analgesics for pain do not develop psychological dependence. Progressively higher doses may be required to relieve pain with chronic therapy.
- Assess bowel function routinely. Prevention of constipation should be instituted with increased intake of fluids and bulk, stool softeners, and laxatives to minimize constipating effects. Stimulant laxatives should be administered routinely if opioid use exceeds 2–3 days, unless contraindicated.
- Monitor intake and output ratios. If significant discrepancies occur, assess for urinary retention and inform physician or other health care professional.
- **Toxicity and Overdose:** If an opioid antagonist is required to reverse respiratory depression or coma, naloxone (Narcan) is the antidote. Dilute the 0.4-mg ampule of naloxone in 10 mL of 0.9% NaCl and administer 0.5 mL (0.02 mg) by direct IV push every 2 min. For children and patients weighing <40 kg, dilute 0.1 mg of naloxone in 10 mL of 0.9% NaCl for a concentration of 10 mcg/mL and administer 0.5 mcg/kg every 1–2 min. Titrate dose to avoid withdrawal, seizures, and severe pain.

Potential Nursing Diagnoses
- Acute pain (Indications).
- Disturbed sensory perception (auditory, visual) (Side Effects).
- Risk for injury (Side Effects).
- Deficient knowledge, related to disease process and medication regimen (Patient/Family Teaching).

Implementation
- Do not confuse morphine with hydromorphone or meperidine; errors have resulted in fatalities.
- Explain therapeutic value of medication before administration to enhance the analgesic effect.
- Regularly administered doses may be more effective than prn administration. Analgesic is more effective if given before pain becomes severe.
- Coadministration with nonopioid analgesics may have additive analgesic effects and may permit lower doses.
- Medication should be discontinued gradually after long-term use to prevent withdrawal symptoms.

Patient/Family Teaching
- Instruct patient on how and when to ask for pain medication.
- Medication may cause drowsiness or dizziness. Caution patient to call for assistance when ambulating or smoking and to avoid driving or other activities requiring alertness until response to medication is known.
- Advise patient to make position changes slowly to minimize orthostatic hypotension.
- Caution patient to avoid concurrent use of alcohol or other CNS depressants with this medication.
- Encourage patient to turn, cough, and breathe deeply every 2 hr to prevent atelectasis.

Evaluation/Desired Outcomes
- Decreased severity of pain without a significant alteration in level of consciousness or respiratory status.

Opioid Analgesics included in *Davis's Drug Guide for Nurses*

opioid agonists/antagonists
buprenorphine 246, 1419
butorphanol 257, 1419
pentazocine 1010, 1419

opioid agonists
codeine 351
fentanyl (buccal/transmucosal) 564
fentanyl (parenteral) 567, 1418
fentanyl (transdermal) 570, 1420
hydrocodone 675

hydromorphone 677, 1418, 1420
levorphanol 1418
meperidine 820, 1419
methadone 831, 1418
morphine 880, 1418, 1420
nalbuphine 895, 1419
oxycodone 966, 1418
oxymorphone 969, 1418
propoxyphene 1068
tapentadol 1190

• SEDATIVE/HYPNOTICS

PHARMACOLOGIC PROFILE

General Use
Sedatives are used to provide sedation, usually prior to procedures. Hypnotics are used to manage insomnia. Selected agents are useful as anticonvulsants (clorazepate, diazepam, phenobarbital), skeletal muscle relaxants (diazepam), adjuncts in the management of alcohol withdrawal syndrome (chlordiazepoxide, diazepam, oxazepam), adjuncts in general anesthesia (droperidol), or as amnestics (midazolam, diazepam).

General Action and Information
Cause generalized CNS depression. May produce tolerance with chronic use and have potential for psychological or physical dependence. These agents have NO analgesic properties.

Contraindications
Hypersensitivity. Should not be used in comatose patients nor in those with pre-existing CNS depression. Should not be used in patients with uncontrolled severe pain. Avoid use during pregnancy or lactation.

Precautions
Use cautiously in patients with hepatic dysfunction, severe renal impairment, or severe underlying pulmonary disease. Use with caution in patients who may be suicidal or who may have had previous drug addictions. Hypnotic use should be short-term. Geriatric patients may be more sensitive to CNS depressant effects; dosage reduction may be required.

Interactions
Additive CNS depression with alcohol, antihistamines, some antidepressants, opioid analgesics, or phenothiazines. Barbiturates induce hepatic drug-metabolizing enzymes and can decrease the effectiveness of drugs metabolized by the liver, including oral contraceptives. Should not be used with MAO inhibitors.

NURSING IMPLICATIONS
Assessment
- Monitor blood pressure, pulse, and respiratory status frequently throughout IV administration. Prolonged high-dose therapy may lead to psychological or physical dependence. Restrict the amount of drug available to patient, especially if patient is depressed, suicidal, or has a history of addiction.
- **Insomnia:** Assess sleep patterns before and periodically throughout course of therapy.
- **Seizures:** Observe and record intensity, duration, and characteristics of seizure activity. Institute seizure precautions.
- **Muscle Spasms:** Assess muscle spasms, associated pain, and limitation of movement before and throughout therapy.
- **Alcohol Withdrawal:** Assess patient experience alcohol withdrawal for tremors, agitation, delirium, and hallucinations. Protect patient from injury.

Potential Nursing Diagnoses
- Insomnia (Indications).
- Risk for injury (Side Effects).
- Deficient knowledge, related to disease process and medication regimen (Patient/Family Teaching).

Implementation
- Supervise ambulation and transfer of patients following administration of hypnotic doses. Remove cigarettes. Side rails should be raised and call bell within reach at all times. Keep bed in low position.

Patient/Family Teaching
- Discuss the importance of preparing the environment for sleep (dark room, quiet, avoidance of nicotine and caffeine). If less effective after a few weeks, consult health care professional; do not increase dose. Gradual withdrawal may be required to prevent reactions following prolonged therapy.
- May cause daytime drowsiness. Caution patient to avoid driving and other activities requiring alertness until response to medication is known.
- Advise patient to avoid the use of alcohol and other CNS depressants concurrently with these medications.
- Advise patient to inform health care professional if pregnancy is planned or suspected.

Evaluation/Desired Outcomes
- Improvement in sleep patterns.
- Control of seizures.
- Decrease in muscle spasms.
- Decreased tremulousness.
- More rational ideation when used for alcohol withdrawal.

Sedative/hypnotics included in *Davis's Drug Guide for Nurses*

barbiturates
pentobarbital 1330
phenobarbital 1015

benzodiazepines
chlordiazepoxide 314
clorazepate 347
diazepam 431
flurazepam 603
lorazepam 799
midazolam 858
oxazepam 961
temazepam 1192

triazolam 1253

miscellaneous
chloral hydrate 312
dexmedetomidine 423
droperidol 487
eszopiclone 583
hydrOXYzine 682
promethazine 1061
ramelteon 1098
zaleplon 1300
zolpidem 1313

• SKELETAL MUSCLE RELAXANTS

PHARMACOLOGIC PROFILE

General Use
Two major uses are spasticity associated with spinal cord diseases or lesions (baclofen and dantrolene) or adjunctive therapy in the symptomatic relief of acute painful musculoskeletal conditions (cyclobenzaprine, diazepam, and methocarbamol). IV dantrolene is also used to treat and prevent malignant hyperthermia.

General Action and Information
Act either centrally (baclofen, carisoprodol, cyclobenzaprine, diazepam, and methocarbamol) or directly (dantrolene).

Contraindications
Baclofen and oral dantrolene should not be used in patients in whom spasticity is used to maintain posture and balance.

Precautions
Safety in pregnancy and lactation not established. Use cautiously in patients with a history of previous liver disease.

Interactions
Additive CNS depression with other CNS depressants, including alcohol, antihistamines, antidepressants, opioid analgesics, and sedative/hypnotics.

NURSING IMPLICATIONS

Assessment
- Assess patient for pain, muscle stiffness, and range of motion before and periodically throughout therapy.

102 THROMBOLYTICS

Potential Nursing Diagnoses
- Acute pain (Indications).
- Impaired physical mobility (Indications).
- Risk for injury (Side Effects).

Implementation
- Provide safety measures as indicated. Supervise ambulation and transfer of patients.

Patient/Family Teaching
- Encourage patient to comply with additional therapies prescribed for muscle spasm (rest, physical therapy, heat).
- Medication may cause drowsiness. Caution patient to avoid driving or other activities requiring alertness until response to drug is known.
- Advise patient to avoid concurrent use of alcohol or other CNS depressants with these medications.

Evaluation/Desired Outcomes
- Decreased musculoskeletal pain
- Decreased muscle spasticity
- Increased range of motion
- Prevention or decrease in temperature and skeletal rigidity in malignant hyperthermia.

Skeletal muscle relaxants included in *Davis's Drug Guide for Nurses*

centrally-acting
baclofen 219
carisoprodol 280
chlorzoxazone 321
cyclobenzaprine 383
diazepam 431

metaxalone 828
methocarbamol 835

direct-acting
dantrolene 398

• THROMBOLYTICS

PHARMACOLOGIC PROFILE

General Use
Acute management of coronary thrombosis (MI). Streptokinase and urokinase are used in the management of massive pulmonary emboli, deep vein thrombosis, and arterial thromboembolism. Alteplase is used in the management of acute ischemic stroke.

General Action and Information
Converts plasminogen to plasmin, which then degrades fibrin in clots. Alteplase, reteplase, and urokinase directly activate plasminogen. Streptokinase binds with plasminogen to form activator complexes, which then convert plasminogen to plasmin. Results in lysis of thrombi in coronary arteries, pulmonary emboli, or deep vein thrombosis, or clearing of clots in cannulae/catheters.

Contraindications
Hypersensitivity. Cross-sensitivity with streptokinase may occur. Contraindicated in active internal bleeding, history of cerebrovascular accident, recent CNS trauma or surgery, neoplasm, or arteriovenous malformation. Severe uncontrolled hypertension and known bleeding tendencies.

Precautions
Recent (within 10 days) major surgery, trauma, GI or GU bleeding. Severe hepatic or renal disease. Subacute bacterial endocarditis or acute pericarditis. Use cautiously in geriatric patients. Safety not established in pregnancy, lactation, or children.

Interactions
Concurrent use with aspirin, NSAIDs, warfarin, heparins, ticlopidine, or dipyridamole may increase the risk of bleeding, although these agents are frequently used together or in sequence. Risk of bleeding may also be increased by concurrent use with cefotetan, cefoperazone, and valproic acid.

NURSING IMPLICATIONS
Assessment
- Begin therapy as soon as possible after the onset of symptoms.
- Monitor vital signs, including temperature, continuously for coronary thrombosis and at least every 4 hr during therapy for other indications. Do not use lower extremities to monitor blood pressure.
- Assess patient carefully for bleeding every 15 min during the 1st hr of therapy, every 15–30 min during the next 8 hr, and at least every 4 hr for the duration of therapy. Frank bleeding may occur from sites of invasive procedures or from body orifices. Internal bleeding may also occur (decreased neurologic status; abdominal pain with coffee-ground emesis or black, tarry stools; hematuria; joint pain). If uncontrolled bleeding occurs, stop medication and notify physician immediately.
- Inquire about previous reaction to streptokinase therapy. Assess patient for hypersensitivity reaction (rash, dyspnea, fever, changes in facial color, swelling around the eyes, wheezing). If these occur, inform physician promptly. Keep epinephrine, an antihistamine, and resuscitation equipment close by in the event of an anaphylactic reaction.
- Inquire about recent streptococcal infection. Streptokinase may be less effective if administered between 5 days and 6 mo of a streptococcal infection.
- Assess neurologic status throughout therapy.
- Altered sensorium or neurologic changes may be indicative of intracranial bleeding.
- **Coronary Thrombosis:** Monitor ECG continuously. Notify physician if significant arrhythmias occur. IV lidocaine or procainamide (Pronestyl) may be ordered prophylactically. Cardiac enzymes should be monitored. Radionuclide myocardial scanning and/or coronary angiography may be ordered 7–10 days following therapy to monitor effectiveness of therapy.
- Monitor heart sounds and breath sounds frequently. Inform physician if signs of CHF occur (rales/crackles, dyspnea, S3 heart sound, jugular venous distention, relieved central venous pressure (CVP)).
- **Pulmonary Embolism:** Monitor pulse, blood pressure, hemodynamics, and respiratory status (rate, degree of dyspnea, arterial blood gases).
- **Deep Vein Thrombosis/Acute Arterial Occlusion:** Observe extremities and palpate pulses of affected extremities every hour. Notify physician immediately if circulatory impairment occurs. Computed tomography, impedance plethysmography, quantitative Doppler effect determination, and/or angiography or venography may be used to determine restoration of blood flow and duration of therapy; however, repeated venograms are not recommended.
- **Cannula/Catheter Occlusion:** Monitor ability to aspirate blood as indicator of patency. Ensure that patient exhales and holds breath when connecting and disconnecting IV syringe to prevent air embolism.
- **Acute Ischemic Stroke:** Assess neurologic status. Determine time of onset of stroke symptoms. Alteplase must be administered within 3 hr of onset.
- **Lab Test Considerations:** Hematocrit, hemoglobin, platelet count, fibrin/fibrin degradation product (FDP/fdp) titer, fibrinogen concentration, prothrombin time, thrombin time, and activated partial thromboplastin time may be evaluated prior to and frequently throughout therapy. Bleeding time may be assessed prior to therapy if patient has received platelet aggregation inhibitors. Obtain type and cross match and have blood available at all times in case of hemorrhage. Stools should be tested for occult blood loss and urine for hematuria periodically during therapy.

104 VACCINES/IMMUNIZING AGENTS

- **Toxicity and Overdose:** If local bleeding occurs, apply pressure to site. If severe or internal bleeding occurs, discontinue infusion. Clotting factors and/or blood volume may be restored through infusions of whole blood, packed RBCs, fresh frozen plasma, or cryoprecipitate. Do not administer dextran, as it has antiplatelet activity. Aminocaproic acid (Amicar) may be used as an antidote.

Potential Nursing Diagnoses
- Ineffective tissue perfusion (Indications).
- Risk for injury (Side Effects).
- Deficient knowledge, related to disease process and medication regimen (Patient/Family Teaching).

Implementation
- This medication should be used only in settings in which hematologic function and clinical response can be adequately monitored.
- Starting two IV lines prior to therapy is recommended: one for the thrombolytic agent, the other for any additional infusions.
- Avoid invasive procedures, such as IM injections or arterial punctures, with this therapy. If such procedures must be performed, apply pressure to all arterial and venous puncture sites for at least 30 min. Avoid venipunctures at noncompressible sites (jugular vein, subclavian site).
- Systemic anticoagulation with heparin is usually begun several hours after the completion of thrombolytic therapy.
- Acetaminophen may be ordered to control fever.

Patient/Family Teaching
- Explain purpose of medication and the need for close monitoring to patient and family. Instruct patient to report hypersensitivity reactions (rash, dyspnea) and bleeding or bruising.
- Explain need for bedrest and minimal handling during therapy to avoid injury. Avoid all unnecessary procedures such as shaving and vigorous tooth brushing.

Evaluation/Desired Outcomes
- Lysis of thrombi and restoration of blood flow
- Prevention of neurologic sequelae in acute ischemic stroke
- Cannula or catheter patency.

Thrombolytics included in *Davis's Drug Guide for Nurses*

alteplase 1214	tenecteplase 1214
reteplase 1214	urokinase 1214
streptokinase 1214	

• VACCINES/IMMUNIZING AGENTS

PHARMACOLOGIC PROFILE

General Use
Immune globulins provide passive immunization to infectious diseases by providing antibodies. Immunization with vaccines and toxoids containing bacterial or viral antigenic material results in endogenous production of antibodies.

General Action and Information
Immunity from immune globulins is rapid, but short-lived (up to 3 months). Active immunization with vaccine or toxoids produces prolonged immunity (years).

Contraindications
Hypersensitivity to product, preservatives, or other additives. Some products contain thimerisol, neomycin, and/or **egg protein**.

Precautions
Severe bleeding problems (IM injections).

Interactions
Decreased antibody response to vaccine/toxoids and increased risk of adverse reactions in patients receiving concurrent antineoplastic, immunosuppressive, or radiation therapy.

NURSING IMPLICATIONS

Assessment
- Assess previous immunization history and history of hypersensitivity.

Potential Nursing Diagnoses
- Risk for infection (Indications).
- Deficient knowledge, related to disease process and medication regimen (Patient/Family Teaching).

Implementation
- Measles, mumps, and rubella vaccine, trivalent oral polio virus vaccine, and diphtheria toxoid, tetanus toxoid, and pertussis vaccine may be given concurrently.
- Administer each immunization by appropriate route.

Patient/Family Teaching
- Inform patient/parent of potential and reportable side effects of immunization. Health care professional should be notified if patient develops fever over 39.4°C (103°F); difficulty breathing; hives; itching; swelling of the eyes, face, or inside of nose; sudden severe tiredness or weakness; or convulsions occur.
- Review next scheduled immunization with parent. Emphasize the importance of keeping a record of immunizations and dates given.

Evaluation/Desired Outcomes
- Prevention of diseases through active immunity.

Vaccines/immunizing agents included in *Davis's Drug Guide for Nurses*

immune globulins
$Rh_o(D)$ immune globulin standard dose IM 1105
botulism immune globulin 1320
$Rh_o(D)$ globulin IV 1105
$Rh_o(D)$ globulin microdose IM 1105

miscellaneous
cytomegalovirus immune globulin 1323
human papillomavirus quadrivalent (types 6, 11, 16 and 18) vaccine, recombinant 670

• VASCULAR HEADACHE SUPPRESSANTS

PHARMACOLOGIC PROFILE

General Use
Used for acute treatment of vascular headaches (migraine, cluster headaches, migraine variants). Other agents such as some beta blockers and some calcum channel blockers are used for suppression of frequently occurring vascular headaches.

VASCULAR HEADACHE SUPPRESSANTS

General Action and Information
Ergot derivatives (ergotamine, dihydroergotamine) directly stimulate alpha-adrenergic and serotonergic receptors, producing vascular smooth muscle vasoconstriction. Almotriptan, frovatriptan, naratriptan, rizatriptan, sumatriptan, and zolmitriptan produce vasoconstriction by acting as serotonin (5-HT$_1$) agonists.

Contraindications
Avoid using these agents in patients with ischemic cardiovascular disease.

Precautions
Use cautiously in patients with a history of, or risk for, cardiovascular disease.

Interactions
Avoid concurrent use of ergot derivative agents with serotonin agonist agents; see also individual agents.

NURSING IMPLICATIONS

Assessment
- Assess pain location, intensity, duration, and associated symptoms (photophobia, phonophobia, nausea, vomiting) during migraine attack and frequency of attacks.

Potential Nursing Diagnoses
- Acute pain (Indications).
- Deficient knowledge, related to disease process and medication regimen (Patient/Family Teaching).

Implementation
- Medication should be administered at the first sign of a headache.

Patient/Family Teaching
- Inform patient that medication should be used only during a migraine attack. It is meant to be used for relief of migraine attacks but not to prevent or reduce the number of attacks.
- Advise patient that lying down in a darkened room following medication administration may further help relieve headache.
- May cause dizziness or drowsiness. Caution patient to avoid driving or other activities requiring alertness until response to medication is known.
- Advise patient to avoid alcohol, which aggravates headaches.

Evaluation/Desired Outcomes
- Relief of migraine attack.

Vascular headache suppressants included in *Davis's Drug Guide for Nurses*

alpha-adrenergic blockers
dihydroergotamine 518
ergotamine 518

beta blockers
propranolol 1071
timolol 1229

5-HT$_1$ agonists
almotriptan 136
eletriptan 497
frovatriptan 619

naratriptan 902
rizatriptan 1125
sumatriptan 1177
zolmitriptan 1312

miscellaneous
divalproex sodium 1262
valproate sodium 1262
valproic acid 1262
verapamil 1275

• VITAMINS

PHARMACOLOGIC PROFILE

General Use
Used in the prevention and treatment of vitamin deficiencies and as supplements in various metabolic disorders.

General Action and Information
Serve as components of enzyme systems that catalyze numerous varied metabolic reactions. Necessary for homeostasis. Water-soluble vitamins (B-vitamins and vitamin C) rarely cause toxicity. Fat-soluble vitamins (vitamins D and E) may accumulate and cause toxicity.

Contraindications
Hypersensitivity to additives, preservatives, or colorants.

Precautions
Dose should be adjusted to avoid toxicity, especially for fat-soluble vitamins.

Interactions
Pyridoxine in large amounts may interfere with the effectiveness of levodopa. Cholestyramine, colestipol, and mineral oil decrease absorption of fat-soluble vitamins.

NURSING IMPLICATIONS

Assessment
- Assess patient for signs of vitamin deficiency before and periodically throughout therapy.
- Assess nutritional status through 24-hr diet recall. Determine frequency of consumption of vitamin-rich foods.

Potential Nursing Diagnoses
- Imbalanced nutrition: less than body requirements (Indications).
- Deficient knowledge, related to disease process and medication regimen (Patient/Family Teaching).

Implementation
- Because of infrequency of single vitamin deficiencies, combinations are commonly administered.

Patient/Family Teaching
- Encourage patients to comply with diet recommendations of physician or other health care professional. Explain that the best source of vitamins is a well-balanced diet with foods from the four basic food groups.
- Patients self-medicating with vitamin supplements should be cautioned not to exceed RDAs. The effectiveness of megadoses for treatment of various medical conditions is unproved and may cause side effects and toxicity.

Evaluation/Desired Outcomes
- Prevention of, or decrease in, the symptoms of vitamin deficiencies.

Vitamins included in *Davis's Drug Guide for Nurses*

fat-soluble vitamins
calcitriol 1287
doxercalciferol 1287
ergocalciferol 1287
paricalcitol 1287
phytonadione 1026
vitamin E 1291

water-soluble vitamins
ascorbic acid 1319
cyanocobalamin 1284

108 WEIGHT CONTROL AGENTS

folic acid 606
niacin 914
niaciamide 914
pyridoxine 1083

thiamine 1209
riboflavin 1332
hydroxocobalamin 1284

• WEIGHT CONTROL AGENTS

PHARMACOLOGIC PROFILE

General Use
These agents are used in the management of exogenous obesity as part of a regimen including a reduced-calorie diet. They are especially useful in the presence of other risk factors including hypertension, diabetes, or dyslipidemias.

General Action and Information
Phentermine and sibutramine are anorexiants that are designed to decrease appetite via their action in the CNS. Orlistat is a lipase inhibitor that decreases absorption of dietary fat.

Contraindications
None of these agents should be used during pregnancy or lactation. Phentermine and sibutramine should not be used in patients with severe hepatic or renal disease, uncontrolled hypertension, known CHF, or cardiovascular disease. Orlistat should not be used in patients with chronic malabsorption.

Precautions
Phentermine and sibutramine should be used cautiously in patients with a history of seizures, or angle-closure glaucoma and in geriatric patients.

Interactions
Phentermine and sibutramine may have additive, adverse effects with CNS stimulants, some vascular headache suppressants, MAO inhibitors, and some opioids (concurrent use should be avoided). Orlistat reduces absorption of some fat-soluble vitamins and beta-carotene.

NURSING IMPLICATIONS

Assessment
- Monitor weight and dietary intake prior to and periodically during therapy. Adjust concurrent medications (antihypertensives, antidiabetics, lipid-lowering agents) as needed.

Potential Nursing Diagnoses
- Disturbed body image (Indications).
- Imbalanced nutrition: more than body requirements (Indications).
- Deficient knowledge, related to medication regimen (Patient/Family Teaching).

Patient/Family Teaching
- Advise patient that regular physical activity, approved by healthcare professional, should be used in conjunction with medication and diet.

Evaluation/Desired Outcomes
- Slow, consistent weight loss when combined with a reduced-calorie diet.

Weight control agents included in *Davis's Drug Guide for Nurses*

orlistat 954
phentermine 1017
sibutramine 1150

abacavir (ah-**back**-ah-veer)
Ziagen

Classification
Therapeutic: antiretrovirals
Pharmacologic: nucleoside reverse transcriptase inhibitors

Pregnancy Category C

Indications
Management of HIV infection (AIDS) in combination with other antiretrovirals (not with lamivudine and/or tenofovir).

Action
Converted inside cells to carbovir triphosphate, its active metabolite. Carbovir triphosphate inhibits the activity of HIV-1 reverse transcriptase, which in turn terminates viral DNA growth. **Therapeutic Effects:** Slows the progression of HIV infection and decreases the occurrence of its sequelae. Increases CD4 cell counts and decreases viral load.

Pharmacokinetics
Absorption: Rapidly and extensively (83%) absorbed.
Distribution: Distributes into extravascular space and readily distributes into erythrocytes.
Metabolism and Excretion: Mostly metabolized by the liver; 1.2% excreted unchanged in urine.
Half-life: 1.5 hr.

TIME/ACTION PROFILE (blood levels)

ROUTE	ONSET	PEAK	DURATION
PO	unknown	unknown	unknown

Contraindications/Precautions
Contraindicated in: Hypersensitivity (rechallenge may be fatal); Lactation:Breastfeeding not recommended for HIV-infected patients.
Use Cautiously in: Coronary heart disease; OB: Safety not established; Pedi:Children <3 mo (safety not established).
Exercise Extreme Caution in: Patients positive for HLA-B*5701 allele (unless exceptional circumstances exist where benefits clearly outweigh the risks).

Adverse Reactions/Side Effects
CNS: headache, insomnia. **CV:** MYOCARDIAL INFARCTION **GI:** HEPATOMEGALY (WITH STEATOSIS), diarrhea, nausea, vomiting, anorexia. **Derm:** rashes. **F and E:** LACTIC ACIDOSIS **Misc:** HYPERSENSITIVITY REACTIONS

Interactions
Drug-Drug: Alcohol ↑ blood levels. May ↑ **methadone** metabolism in some patients; slight ↑ in **methadone** dosing may be needed.

Route/Dosage
PO (Adults): 300 mg twice daily.
PO (Children 3 mo–16 yr): 8 mg/kg twice daily (not to exceed 300 mg twice daily).

Availability
Tablets: 300 mg. **Oral solution (strawberry/banana flavor):** 20 mg/mL in 240-mL bottles. *In combination with:* lamivudine (Epzicom); lamivudine and zidovudine (Trizivir). See Appendix B.

NURSING IMPLICATIONS
Assessment
- Assess patient for change in severity of HIV symptoms and for symptoms of opportunistic infections throughout therapy.

- Assess for signs of hypersensitivity reactions (fever; rash; gastrointestinal—nausea, vomiting, diarrhea, abdominal pain; constitutional—malaise, fatigue, achiness; respiratory—dyspnea, cough, pharyngitis). May also cause elevated liver function tests, increased creatine phosphokinase or creatinine, and lymphopenia. Patients who carry the HLA-B*5701 allele are at high risk for hypersensitivity reaction. Discontinue promptly if hypersensitivity reaction is suspected. Regardless of HLA-B*5701 status, permanently discontinue abacavir if hypersensitivity cannot be ruled out, even when other diagnoses are possible. Following a hypersensitivity reaction, never restart abacavir or abacavir-containing products. More severe symptoms may occur within hours and may include life-threatening hypotension and death. Symptoms usually resolve upon discontinuation.

- May cause lactic acidosis and severe hepatomegaly with steatosis. Monitor patient for signs (↑ serum lactate levels, ↑ liver enzymes, liver enlargement on palpation). Therapy should be suspended if clinical or laboratory signs occur.

- *Lab Test Considerations:* Monitor viral load and CD4 cell count regularly during therapy.

✦ = Canadian drug name. = Genetic implication.
*CAPITALS indicates life-threatening; underlines indicate most frequent.

110   acarbose

- ▮ Screen for HLA-B*5701 allele prior to initiation of therapy to decrease risk of hypersensitivity reaction. Screening is also recommended prior to reinitiation of abacavir in patients of unknown HLA-B*5701 status who have previously tolerated abacavir.
- Monitor liver function. May cause ↑ levels of AST, ALT, and alkaline phosphatase, which usually resolve after interruption of therapy. Lactic acidosis may occur with hepatic toxicity, causing hepatic steatosis; may be fatal, especially in women.
- May cause ↑ serum glucose and triglyceride levels.

Potential Nursing Diagnoses
Risk for infection (Indications)
Noncompliance (Patient/Family Teaching)

Implementation
- **PO:** May be administered with or without food. Oral solution may be stored at room temperature or refrigerated; do not freeze. Tablet may be used with children if able to swallow and dose is correctly calculated.

Patient/Family Teaching
- Emphasize the importance of taking abacavir as directed. Must always be used in combination with other antiretroviral drugs. Do not take more than prescribed amount, and do not stop taking without consulting health care professional. Take missed doses as soon as remembered; do not double doses.
- Instruct patient not to share abacavir with others.
- Inform patient that abacavir does not cure AIDS or prevent associated or opportunistic infections. Abacavir does not reduce the risk of transmission of HIV to others through sexual contact or blood contamination. Caution patient to use a condom, and avoid sharing needles or donating blood to prevent spreading the AIDS virus to others. Advise patient that the long-term effects of abacavir are unknown at this time.
- Advise patient of potential for hypersensitivity reactions that may result in death. Instruct patient to discontinue abacavir and notify health care professional immediately if symptoms of hypersensitivity occur. *Medication guide* for patients should be dispensed with prescription. Advise patient to read it thoroughly with each refill. A warning card summarizing symptoms of abacavir hypersensitivity should be provided with each prescription; instruct patient to carry card at all times.
- Emphasize the importance of regular follow-up exams and blood counts to determine progress and monitor for side effects.

Evaluation/Desired Outcomes
- Delayed progression of AIDS, and decreased opportunistic infections in patients with HIV.
- Decrease in viral load and increase in CD4 cell counts.

---

acarbose (aye-kar-bose)
Precose

Classification
Therapeutic: antidiabetics
Pharmacologic: alpha-glucosidase inhibitors

Pregnancy Category B

Indications
Management of type 2 diabetes in conjunction with dietary therapy; may be used with insulin or other hypoglycemic agents.

Action
Lowers blood glucose by inhibiting the enzyme alpha-glucosidase in the GI tract. Delays and reduces glucose absorption. **Therapeutic Effects:** Lowering of blood glucose in diabetic patients, especially postprandial hyperglycemia.

Pharmacokinetics
Absorption: <2% systemically absorbed; action is primarily local (in the GI tract).
Distribution: Unknown.
Metabolism and Excretion: Minimal amounts absorbed are excreted by the kidneys.
Half-life: 2 hr.

TIME/ACTION PROFILE (effect on blood glucose)

ROUTE	ONSET	PEAK	DURATION
PO	unknown	1 hr	unknown

Contraindications/Precautions
Contraindicated in: Hypersensitivity; Diabetic ketoacidosis; Cirrhosis; Serum creatinine >2 mg/dL; OB: Lactation, Pedi: Safety not established.
Use Cautiously in: Presence of fever, infection, trauma, stress (may cause hyperglycemia, requiring alternative therapy).

Adverse Reactions/Side Effects
GI: abdominal pain, diarrhea, flatulence, ↑ transaminases.

Interactions
Drug-Drug: Thiazide diuretics and **loop diuretics, corticosteroids, phenothiazines,** thy-

acarbose

roid preparations, **estrogens (conjugated)**, **progestins**, **hormonal contraceptives**, **phenytoin**, **niacin**, **sympathomimetics**, **calcium channel blockers**, and **isoniazid** may ↑ glucose levels in diabetic patients and lead to ↓ control of blood glucose. Effects are ↓ by **intestinal adsorbents**, including **activated charcoal** and **digestive enzyme preparations (amylase, pancreatin)**; avoid concurrent use. ↑ effects of **sulfonylurea hypoglycemic agents**. May ↓ absorption of **digoxin**; may require dosage adjustment.

Drug-Natural Products: Glucosamine may worsen blood glucose control. **Chromium** and **coenzyme Q-10** may ↑ hypoglycemic effects.

Route/Dosage
PO (Adults): 25 mg 3 times daily; may be increased q 4–8 wk as needed/tolerated (range 50–100 mg 3 times daily; not to exceed 50 mg 3 times daily in patients ≤60 kg or 100 mg 3 times daily in patients >60 kg).

Availability (generic available)
Tablets: 25 mg, 50 mg, 100 mg.

NURSING IMPLICATIONS

Assessment
- Observe patient for signs and symptoms of hypoglycemia (sweating, hunger, weakness, dizziness, tremor, tachycardia, anxiety) when taking concurrently with other oral hypoglycemic agents.
- *Lab Test Considerations:* Monitor serum glucose and glycosylated hemoglobin periodically during therapy to evaluate effectiveness.
- Monitor AST and ALT every 3 mo for the 1st yr and then periodically. Elevated levels may require dose reduction or discontinuation of acarbose. Elevations occur more commonly in patients taking more than 300 mg/day and in female patients. Levels usually return to normal without other evidence of liver injury after discontinuation.
- *Toxicity and Overdose:* Symptoms of overdose are transient increase in flatulence, diarrhea, and abdominal discomfort. Acarbose alone does not cause hypoglycemia; however, other concurrently administered hypoglycemic agents may produce hypoglycemia requiring treatment.

Potential Nursing Diagnoses
Imbalanced nutrition: more than body requirements (Indications)

Noncompliance (Patient/Family Teaching)

Implementation
- Patients stabilized on a diabetic regimen who are exposed to stress, fever, trauma, infection, or surgery may require administration of insulin.
- Does not cause hypoglycemia when taken while fasting, but may increase hypoglycemic effect of other hypoglycemic agents.
- **PO:** Administer with first bite of each meal 3 times/day.

Patient/Family Teaching
- Instruct patient to take acarbose at same time each day. If a dose is missed and the meal is completed without taking the dose, skip missed dose and take next dose with the next meal. Do not double doses.
- Explain to patient that acarbose controls hyperglycemia but does not cure diabetes. Therapy is longterm.
- Review signs of hypoglycemia and hyperglycemia (blurred vision; drowsiness; dry mouth; flushed, dry skin; fruit-like breath odor; increased urination; ketones in urine; loss of appetite; stomachache; nausea or vomiting; tiredness; rapid, deep breathing; unusual thirst; unconsciousness) with patient. If hypoglycemia occurs, advise patient to take a form of oral glucose (e.g., glucose tablets, liquid gel glucose) rather than sugar (absorption of sugar is blocked by acarbose) and notify health care professional.
- Encourage patient to follow prescribed diet, medication, and exercise regimen to prevent hypoglycemic or hyperglycemic episodes.
- Instruct patient in proper testing of serum glucose and urine ketones. Monitor closely during periods of stress or illness. Notify health care professional if significant changes occur.
- Caution patient to avoid using other medications without consulting health care professional.
- Advise patient to inform health care professional of medication regimen before treatment or surgery.
- Advise patient to carry a form of oral glucose and identification describing disease process and medication regimen at all times.
- Emphasize the importance of routine follow-up examinations.

✱ = Canadian drug name. ▌ = Genetic implication.
*CAPITALS indicates life-threatening; underlines indicate most frequent.

Evaluation/Desired Outcomes
- Control of blood glucose levels without the appearance of hypoglycemic or hyperglycemic episodes.

acetaminophen
(a-seet-a-**min**-oh-fen)

♣Abenol, Acephen, Aceta, Aminofen, Apacet, APAP, ♣Apo-Acetaminophen, Aspirin Free Anacin, Aspirin Free Pain Relief, Children's Pain Reliever, Dapacin, Feverall, Extra Strength Dynafed E.X., Extra Strength Dynafed (Billups, P.J.), Genapap, Genebs, Halenol, Infant's Pain Reliever, Liquiprin, Mapap, Maranox, Meda, Neopap, ♣Novo-Gesic, Oraphen-PD, Panadol, paracetamol, Redutemp, Ridenol, Silapap, Tapanol, Tempra, Tylenol, Uni-Ace

Classification
Therapeutic: antipyretics, nonopioid analgesics

Pregnancy Category B

Indications
Mild pain. Fever.

Action
Inhibits the synthesis of prostaglandins that may serve as mediators of pain and fever, primarily in the CNS. Has no significant anti-inflammatory properties or GI toxicity. **Therapeutic Effects:** Analgesia. Antipyresis.

Pharmacokinetics
Absorption: Well absorbed following oral administration. Rectal absorption is variable.
Distribution: Widely distributed. Crosses the placenta; enters breast milk in low concentrations.
Metabolism and Excretion: 85–95% metabolized by the liver. Metabolites may be toxic in overdose situation. Metabolites excreted by the kidneys.
Half-life: Neonates: 2–5 hr. Adults: 1–3 hr.

TIME/ACTION PROFILE (analgesia and antipyresis)

ROUTE	ONSET	PEAK	DURATION
PO	0.5–1 hr	1–3 hr	3–8 hr†
Rect	0.5–1 hr	1–3 hr	3–4 hr

†Depends on dose

Contraindications/Precautions
Contraindicated in: Previous hypersensitivity; Products containing alcohol, aspartame, saccharin, sugar, or tartrazine (FDC yellow dye #5) should be avoided in patients who have hypersensitivity or intolerance to these compounds.
Use Cautiously in: Hepatic disease/renal disease (lower chronic doses recommended); Chronic alcohol use/abuse; Malnutrition.

Adverse Reactions/Side Effects
GI: HEPATIC FAILURE, HEPATOTOXICITY (overdose).
GU: renal failure (high doses/chronic use). **Hemat:** neutropenia, pancytopenia, leukopenia.
Derm: rash, urticaria.

Interactions
Drug-Drug: Chronic high-dose acetaminophen (>2 g/day) may ↑ risk of bleeding with **warfarin** (PT should be monitored regularly and INR should not exceed 4). Hepatotoxicity is additive with other **hepatotoxic substances**, including **alcohol**. Concurrent use of **sulfinpyrazone**, **isoniazid**, **rifampin**, **rifabutin**, **phenytoin**, **barbiturates**, and **carbamazepine** may ↑ the risk of acetaminophen-induced liver damage (limit self-medication); these agents will also ↓ therapeutic effects of acetaminophen. Concurrent **NSAIDs** ↑ the risk of adverse renal effects (avoid chronic concurrent use). **Propranolol** ↓ metabolism and may ↑ effects. May ↓ effects of **lamotrigine** and **zidovudine**.

Route/Dosage
Children ≤12 yr should not receive >5 doses/24 hr without notifying physician or other health care professional.
PO (Adults and Children >12 yr): 325–650 mg q 4–6 hr or 1 g 3–4 times daily or 1300 mg q 8 hr (not to exceed 4 g or 2.5 g/24 hr in patients with hepatic/renal impairment).
PO (Children 1–12 yr): 10–15 mg/kg/dose q 4–6 hr as needed (not to exceed 5 doses/24 hr).
PO (Infants): 10–15 mg/kg/dose q 4–6 hr as needed (not to exceed 5 doses/24 hr).
PO (Neonates): 10–15 mg/kg/dose q 6–8 hr as needed.
Rect (Adults and Children >12 yr): 325–650 mg q 4–6 hr as needed or 1 g 3–4 times/day (not to exceed 4 g/24 hr).
Rect (Children 1–12 yr): 10–20 mg/kg/dose q 4–6 hr as needed.
Rect (Infants): 10–20 mg/kg/dose q 4–6 hr as needed.
Rect (Neonates): 10–15 mg/kg/dose q 6–8 hr as needed.

acetaminophen 113

Availability (generic available)
Chewable tablets (fruit, bubblegum, or grape flavor): 80 mg^{OTC}, 160 mg^{OTC}. **Tablets:** 160 mg^{OTC}, 325 mg^{OTC}, 500 mg^{OTC}, 650 mg^{OTC}. **Caplets:** 325 mg^{OTC}, 500 mg^{OTC}. **Solution (berry, fruit, and grape flavor):** 100 mg/mL^{OTC}. **Liquid (mint):** 160 mg/5 mL^{OTC}, 500 mg/15 mL^{OTC}. **Elixir (grape and cherry flavor):** 160 mg/5 mL^{OTC}. **Drops:** 100 mg/mL ^{OTC}. **Suspension:** ✣ 100 mg/mL^{OTC}, ✣ 160 mg/5 mL^{OTC}. **Syrup:** 160 mg/5 mL^{OTC}. **Suppositories:** 80 mg^{OTC}, 120 mg^{OTC}, 325 mg^{OTC}, 650 mg^{OTC}. *In combination with:* many other medications. See Appendix B.

NURSING IMPLICATIONS

Assessment
- Assess overall health status and alcohol usage before administering acetaminophen. Patients who are malnourished or chronically abuse alcohol are at higher risk of developing hepatotoxicity with chronic use of usual doses of this drug.
- Assess amount, frequency, and type of drugs taken in patients self-medicating, especially with OTC drugs. Prolonged use of acetaminophen increases the risk of adverse renal effects. For short-term use, combined doses of acetaminophen and salicylates should not exceed the recommended dose of either drug given alone.
- **Pain:** Assess type, location, and intensity prior to and 30–60 min following administration.
- **Fever:** Assess fever; note presence of associated signs (diaphoresis, tachycardia, and malaise).
- *Lab Test Considerations:* Evaluate hepatic, hematologic, and renal function periodically during prolonged, high-dose therapy.
- May alter results of blood glucose monitoring. May cause falsely ↓ values when measured with glucose oxidase/peroxidase method, but probably not with hexokinase/G6PD method. May also cause falsely ↑ values with certain instruments; see manufacturer's instruction manual.
- Increased serum bilirubin, LDH, AST, ALT, and prothrombin time may indicate hepatotoxicity.
- *Toxicity and Overdose:* If overdose occurs, **acetylcysteine** (Acetadote) is the antidote.

Potential Nursing Diagnoses
Acute pain (Indications)
Risk for imbalanced body temperature (Indications)

Implementation
- When combined with opioids do not exceed the maximum recommended daily dose of acetaminophen.
- **PO:** Administer with a full glass of water.
- May be taken with food or on an empty stomach.

Patient/Family Teaching
- Advise patient to take medication exactly as directed and not to take more than the recommended amount. Chronic excessive use of > 4 g/day (2 g in chronic alcoholics) may lead to hepatotoxicity, renal or cardiac damage. Adults should not take acetaminophen longer than 10 days and children not longer than 5 days unless directed by health care professional. Short-term doses of acetaminophen with salicylates or NSAIDs should not exceed the recommended daily dose of either drug alone.
- Advise patient to avoid alcohol (3 or more glasses per day increase the risk of liver damage) if taking more than an occasional 1–2 doses and to avoid taking concurrently with salicylates or NSAIDs for more than a few days, unless directed by health care professional.
- Pedi: Advise parents or caregivers to check concentrations of liquid preparations. Errors have resulted in serious liver damage. Have parents or caregivers determine the correct formulation and dose for their child (based on the child's age/weight), and demonstrate how to measure it using an appropriate measuring device.
- Inform patients with diabetes that acetaminophen may alter results of blood glucose monitoring. Advise patient to notify health care professional if changes are noted.
- Caution patient to check labels on all OTC products. Advise patients to avoid taking more than one product containing acetaminophen at a time to prevent toxicity.
- Advise patient to consult health care professional if discomfort or fever is not relieved by routine doses of this drug or if fever is greater than 39.5°C (103°F) or lasts longer than 3 days.

Evaluation/Desired Outcomes
- Relief of mild pain.
- Reduction of fever.

✣ = Canadian drug name. ▆ = Genetic implication.
*CAPITALS indicates life-threatening; underlines indicate most frequent.

acetaZOLAMIDE
(a-seet-a-**zole**-a-mide)
✤Acetazolam, ✤Apo-Acetazolamide, Diamox, Diamox Sequels

Classification
Therapeutic: anticonvulsants, antiglaucoma agents, diuretics, ocular hypotensive agent
Pharmacologic: carbonic anhydrase inhibitors

Pregnancy Category C

Indications
Lowering of intraocular pressure in the treatment of glaucoma. Management of acute altitude sickness. Edema due to congestive heart failure. Adjunct to the treatment of refractory seizures. **Unlabeled Use:** Reduce cerebrospinal fluid production in hydrocephalus. Prevention of renal calculi composed of uric acid or cystine.

Action
Inhibition of carbonic anhydrase in the eye results in decreased secretion of aqueous humor. Inhibition of renal carbonic anhydrase, resulting in self-limiting urinary excretion of sodium, potassium, bicarbonate, and water. CNS inhibition of carbonic anhydrase and resultant diuresis may ↓ abnormal neuronal firing. Alkaline diuresis prevents precipitation of uric acid or cystine in the urinary tract. **Therapeutic Effects:** Lowering of intraocular pressure. Control of some types of seizures. Prevention and treatment of acute altitude sickness. Diuresis and subsequent mobilization of excess fluid. Prevention of uric acid or cystine renal calculi.

Pharmacokinetics
Absorption: Dose dependent; erratic with doses >10 mg/kg/day.
Distribution: Crosses the placenta and blood-brain barrier; enters breast milk.
Protein Binding: 95%.
Metabolism and Excretion: Excreted mostly unchanged in urine.
Half-life: 2.4–5.8 hr.

TIME/ACTION PROFILE (lowering of intraocular pressure)

ROUTE	ONSET	PEAK	DURATION
PO	1–1.5 hr	2–4 hr	8–12 hr
PO-ER	2 hr	8–18 hr	18–24 hr
IV	2 min	15 min	4–5 hr

Contraindications/Precautions
Contraindicated in: Hypersensitivity or cross-sensitivity with sulfonamides may occur; Hepatic disease or insufficiency; Concurrent use with ophthalmic carbonic anhydrase inhibitors (brinzolamide, dorzolamide) is not recommended; OB: Avoid during first trimester of pregnancy.
Use Cautiously in: Chronic respiratory disease; Electrolyte abnormalities; Gout; Renal disease (dosage reduction necessary for CCr <50 mL/min); Diabetes mellitus; OB:Use with caution during second or third trimester of pregnancy; Lactation:Safety not established.

Adverse Reactions/Side Effects
CNS: depression, tiredness, weakness, drowsiness. **EENT:** transient nearsightedness. **GI:** anorexia, metallic taste, nausea, vomiting, melena. **GU:** crystalluria, renal calculi. **Derm:** STEVENS-JOHNSON SYNDROME, rashes. **Endo:** hyperglycemia. **F and E:** hyperchloremic acidosis, hypokalemia, growth retardation (in children receiving chronic therapy). **Hemat:** APLASTIC ANEMIA, HEMOLYTIC ANEMIA, LEUKOPENIA **Metab:** weight loss, hyperuricemia. **Neuro:** paresthesias. **Misc:** allergic reactions including ANAPHYLAXIS

Interactions
Drug-Drug: Excretion of **barbiturates**, **aspirin**, and **lithium** is ↑ and may lead to ↓ effectiveness. Excretion of **amphetamine**, **quinidine**, **procainamide**, and possibly **tricyclic antidepressants** is ↓ and may lead to toxicity. May ↑ **cyclosporine** levels.

Route/Dosage
PO (Adults): *Glaucoma (open angle)*—250–1000 mg/day in 1–4 divided doses (up to 250 mg q 4 hr) or 500-mg extended-release capsules twice daily. *Epilepsy*—4–16 mg/kg/day in 1–4 divided doses (maximum 30 mg/kg/day or 1 g/day). *Altitude sickness*—250 mg 2–4 times daily started 24–48 hr before ascent, continued for 48 hr or longer to control symptoms. *Antiurolithic*—250 mg at bedtime. *Edema*—250–375 mg/day. *Urine alkalinization*—5 mg/kg/dose repeated 2–3 times over 24 hr.
PO (Children): *Glaucoma*—8–30 mg/kg (300–900 mg/m^2/day) in 3 divided doses (usual range 10–15 mg/kg/day). *Edema*—5 mg/kg/dose once daily. *Epilepsy*—4–16 mg/kg/day in 1–4 divided doses (maximum 30 mg/kg/day or 1 g/day).
PO (Neonates): *Hydrocephalus*—5 mg/kg/dose q 6 hr ↑ by 25 mg/kg/day up to a maximum of 100 mg/kg/day.
IV (Adults): *Glaucoma (closed angle)*—250–500 mg, may repeat in 2–4 hr to a maximum of 1 g/day. *Edema*—250–375 mg/day.

acetaZOLAMIDE 115

IV (Children): *Glaucoma*—5–10 mg/kg q 6 hr, not to exceed 1 g/day. *Edema*—5 mg/kg/dose once daily.

IV (Neonates): *Hydrocephalus*—5 mg/kg/dose q 6 hr ↑ by 25 mg/kg/day up to a maximum of 100 mg/kg/day.

Availability (generic available)
Tablets: 125 mg, 250 mg. **Extended-release capsules:** 500 mg. **Injection:** 500 mg.

NURSING IMPLICATIONS
Assessment
- Observe for signs of hypokalemia (muscle weakness, malaise, fatigue, ECG changes, vomiting).
- Assess for allergy to sulfonamides.
- **Intraocular Pressure:** Assess for eye discomfort or decrease in visual acuity.
- **Seizures:** Monitor neurologic status in patients receiving acetazolamide for seizures. Initiate seizure precautions.
- **Altitude Sickness:** Monitor for decrease in severity of symptoms (headache, nausea, vomiting, fatigue, dizziness, drowsiness, shortness of breath). Notify health care professional immediately if neurologic symptoms worsen or if patient becomes more dyspneic and rales or crackles develop.
- **Edema:** Monitor intake and output ratios and daily weight during therapy.
- ***Lab Test Considerations:*** Serum electrolytes, complete blood counts, and platelet counts should be evaluated initially and periodically throughout prolonged therapy. May cause ↓ potassium, bicarbonate, WBCs, and RBCs. May cause ↑ serum chloride.
- May cause ↑ in serum and urine glucose; monitor serum and urine glucose carefully in diabetic patients.
- May cause false-positive results for urine protein and 17-hydroxysteroid tests.
- May cause ↑ blood ammonia, bilirubin, uric acid, urine urobilinogen, and calcium. May ↓ urine citrate.

Potential Nursing Diagnoses
Disturbed sensory perception (visual) (Indications)

Implementation
- Do not confuse acetazolamide with acetohexamide.
- Encourage fluids to 2000–3000 mL/day, unless contraindicated, to prevent crystalluria and stone formation.
- A potassium supplement without chloride should be administered concurrently with acetazolamide.
- **PO:** Give with food to minimize GI irritation. Tablets may be crushed and mixed with fruit-flavored syrup to minimize bitter taste for patients with difficulty swallowing. Extended-release capsules may be opened and sprinkled on soft food, but do not crush, chew, or swallow contents dry. Extended-release capsules are only indicated for glaucoma and altitude sickness; do not use for epilepsy or diuresis.
- **IM:** Extremely painful; avoid if possible.

IV Administration
- **Direct IV:** ***Diluent:*** Dilute 500 mg of acetazolamide in at least 5 mL of sterile water for injection. Use reconstituted solution within 24 hr. ***Concentration:*** 100 mg/mL. ***Rate:*** Not to exceed 500 mg/min.
- **Intermittent Infusion:** ***Diluent:*** Further dilute in 50–100 mL of D5W, D10W, 0.45% NaCl, 0.9% NaCl, LR, or combinations of dextrose and saline or dextrose and LR solution. ***Concentration:*** 5–10 mg/mL. ***Rate:*** Infuse over 15–30 min.

Patient/Family Teaching
- Instruct patient to take as directed. Take missed doses as soon as possible unless almost time for next dose. Do not double doses. Patients on anticonvulsant therapy may need to gradually withdraw medication.
- Advise patient to report numbness or tingling of extremities, weakness, rash, sore throat, unusual bleeding or bruising, fever, or signs/symptoms of a sulfonamide adverse reaction (Stevens-Johnson syndrome [flu-like symptoms, spreading red rash, or skin/mucous membrane blistering], toxic epidermal necrolysis [widespread peeling/blistering of skin]) to health care professional. If hematopoietic reactions, fever, rash, hepatic, or renal problems occur, acetazolamide should be discontinued.
- May occasionally cause drowsiness. Caution patient to avoid driving and other activities that require alertness until response to the drug is known.
- Caution patient to use sunscreen and wear protective clothing to prevent photosensitivity reactions.

✱ = Canadian drug name. ▮ = Genetic implication.
*CAPITALS indicates life-threatening; underlines indicate most frequent.

- Advise patient to consult health care professional before taking other Rx, OTC, or herbal products.
- **Intraocular Pressure:** Advise patient of the need for periodic ophthalmologic exams; loss of vision may be gradual and painless.

Evaluation/Desired Outcomes
- Decrease in intraocular pressure when used for glaucoma. If therapy is not effective or patient is unable to tolerate one carbonic anhydrase inhibitor, using another may be effective and more tolerable.
- Decrease in the frequency of seizures.
- Reduction of edema.
- Prevention of altitude sickness.
- Prevention of uric acid or cystine stones in the urinary tract.

---

acetylcysteine
(a-se-teel-**sis**-teen)
Acetadote, ✤Mucomyst, ✤Parvolex

Classification
Therapeutic: antidotes (for acetaminophen toxicity), mucolytic

Pregnancy Category B

Indications
PO: Antidote for the management of potentially hepatotoxic overdosage of acetaminophen (administer within 24 hours of ingestion). **IV:** Antidote for the management of potentially hepatotoxic overdosage of acetaminophen (administer within 8–10 hours of ingestion). **Inhaln:** Mucolytic in the management of conditions associated with thick viscid mucous secretions. **Unlabeled Use:** Prevention of radiocontrast-induced renal dysfunction (oral).

Action
PO: Decreases the buildup of a hepatotoxic metabolite in acetaminophen overdosage. **IV:** Decreases the buildup of a hepatotoxic metabolite in acetaminophen overdosage. **Inhaln:** Degrades mucus, allowing easier mobilization and expectoration. **Therapeutic Effects: PO:** Prevention or lessening of liver damage following acetaminophen overdose. **Inhaln:** Lowers the viscosity of mucus.

Pharmacokinetics
Absorption: Absorbed from the GI tract following oral administration. Action is local following inhalation; remainder may be absorbed from pulmonary epithelium.
Distribution: Crosses the placenta; 0.47 L/kg.
Protein Binding: 83% bound to plasma proteins.
Metabolism and Excretion: Partially metabolized by the liver, 22% excreted renally.
Half-life: *Adults*—5.6 hr (↑ in hepatic impairment) *newborns*—11 hr.

TIME/ACTION PROFILE

ROUTE	ONSET	PEAK	DURATION
PO (antidote)	unknown	30–60 min	4 hr
Inhaln (mucolytic)	1 min	5–10 min	short

Contraindications/Precautions
Contraindicated in: Hypersensitivity.
Use Cautiously in: Severe respiratory insufficiency, asthma, or history of bronchospasm; History of GI bleeding (oral only); OB, Lactation: Safety not established.

Adverse Reactions/Side Effects
CNS: drowsiness. **CV:** vasodilation. **EENT:** rhinorrhea. **Resp:** bronchospasm, bronchial/tracheal irritation, chest tightness, increased secretions. **GI:** nausea, vomiting, stomatitis. **Derm:** rash, clamminess, pruritus, urticaria. **Misc:** allergic reactions (primarily with IV), including ANAPHYLAXIS, ANGIOEDEMA, chills, fever.

Interactions
Drug-Drug: Activated charcoal may adsorb orally administered acetylcysteine and decrease its effectiveness as an antidote.

Route/Dosage
Acetaminophen Overdose
PO (Adults and Children): 140 mg/kg initially, followed by 70 mg/kg q 4 hr for 17 additional doses.
IV (Adults and Children): *Loading dose*—150 mg/kg over 15 min initially followed by *First maintenance dose*—50 mg/kg over 4 hr, then *second maintenance dose*—100 mg/kg over 16 hr.

Mucolytic
Inhaln (Adults and Children): *Nebulization via face mask*—3–5 mL of 20% solution or 6–10 mL of the 10% solution 3–4 times daily (range—1–10 mL of 20% solution or 2–20 mL of 10% solution q 2–6 hr); *nebulization via tent or croupette*—volume of 10–20% solution required to maintain heavy mist; *direct instillation*—1–2 mL of 10–20% solution q 1–4 hr; *intratracheal instillation via tracheostomy*—1–2 mL of 10–20% solution q 1–4 hr (up to 2–5 mL of 20% solution via tracheal catheter into

acetylcysteine 117

particular segments of the bronchopulmonary tree).

Prevention of Radiocontrast-Induced Renal Dysfunction
PO (Adults): 600 mg twice daily for 2 days, beginning the day before the procedure.

Availability (generic available)
Solution for inhalation: 10% in 4-, 10-, and 30-mL vials, 20% in 4-, 10-, 30-, and 100−mL vials. **Solution for injection:** 20% in 30−mL vials.

NURSING IMPLICATIONS

Assessment
- **Antidote in Acetaminophen Overdose:** Assess type, amount, and time of acetaminophen ingestion. Assess plasma acetaminophen levels. Initial levels are drawn at least 4 hr after ingestion of acetaminophen. Plasma level determinations may be difficult to interpret following ingestion of extended-release preparations. Do not wait for results to administer dose.
- *IV:* Assess for anaphylactoid reaction. Erythema and flushing are common, usually occurring 30−60 min after initiating infusion, and may resolve with continued administration. If rash, hypotension, wheezing, dyspnea occur, initiate treatment for anaphylaxis (antihistamine and epinephrine). Acetylcysteine infusion should be interrupted until symptoms resolve and carefully restarted. If anaphylactoid reaction recurs, discontinue acetylcysteine and use alternative form of treatment.
- Monitor AST, ALT, and bilirubin levels along with prothrombin time every 24 hr for 96 hr in patients with plasma acetaminophen levels indicating potential hepatotoxicity.
- Monitor cardiac and renal function (creatinine, BUN), serum glucose, and electrolytes. Maintain fluid and electrolyte balance, correct hypoglycemia, and administer vitamin K or fresh frozen plasma or clotting factor concentrate if prothrombin time ratio exceeds 1.5 or 3, respectively.
- Assess patient for nausea, vomiting, and urticaria. Notify health care professional if these occur.
- **Mucolytic:** Assess respiratory function (lung sounds, dyspnea) and color, amount, and consistency of secretions before and immediately following treatment to determine effectiveness of therapy.

Potential Nursing Diagnoses
Risk for self-directed violence (Indications)
Ineffective airway clearance (Indications)
Deficient knowledge, related to medication regimen (Patient/Family Teaching)

Implementation
- After opening, solution for inhalation may turn light purple; does not alter potency. Refrigerate open vials and discard after 96 hr.
- Drug reacts with rubber and metals (iron, nickel, copper); avoid contact with these substances.
- **PO: Acetaminophen Overdose**—First empty stomach contents by inducing emesis or lavage. Dilute 20% solution with cola, water, or juice to a final concentration of 1:3 for patients weighing up to 20 kg or with enough diluent to make a 5% solution for patients weighing more than 20 kg, to increase palatability. May be administered by duodenal tube if patient is unable to swallow. If patient vomits loading dose or maintenance doses within 1 hr of administration, readminister dose.

IV Administration

- **Intermittent Infusion:** Most effective if administered within 8 hr of acetaminophen ingestion. Dilute in D5W. *For loading dose:* Dilute 150 mg/kg in 200 mL. *For 1st Maintenance Dose:* Dilute 50 mg/kg in 500 mL. *For 2nd Maintenance Dose:* Dilute 100 mg/kg in 1000 mL. Adjust fluid volume for patients <40 kg or requiring fluid restriction. Vials are single-use. Discard after using. Reconstituted solution is stable for 24 hr at room temperature. ***Rate:*** Administer *Loading Dose* over 15 min.
- Administer *1st Maintenance Dose* over 4 hr.
- Administer *2nd Maintenance Dose* over 16 hr.
- **Inhaln: Mucolytic**—Encourage adequate fluid intake (2000−3000 mL/day) to decrease viscosity of secretions.
- For nebulization, the 20% solution may be diluted with 0.9% NaCl for injection or inhalation or sterile water for injection or inhalation. May use 10% solution undiluted. May be administered by nebulization, or 1−2 mL may be instilled directly into airway. During administration, when 25% of medication remains in nebulizer, dilute with equal amount of 0.9% NaCl or sterile water.
- An increased volume of liquefied bronchial secretions may occur following administration.

= Canadian drug name. = Genetic implication.
*CAPITALS indicates life-threatening; underlines indicate most frequent.

- Have suction equipment available for patients unable to effectively clear airways.
- If bronchospasm occurs during treatment, discontinue and consult health care professional regarding possible addition of bronchodilator to therapy. Patients with asthma or hyperactive airway disease should be given a bronchodilator prior to acetylcysteine to prevent bronchospasm.
- Rinse patient's mouth and wash face following treatment, as drug leaves a sticky residue.

Patient/Family Teaching
- **Acetaminophen Overdose:** Explain purpose of medication to patient.
- **Inhaln:** Instruct patient to clear airway by coughing deeply before taking aerosol treatment.
- Inform patient that unpleasant odor of this drug becomes less noticeable as treatment progresses and medicine dissipates.

Evaluation/Desired Outcomes
- Decreased acetaminophen levels.
- No further increase in hepatic damage during acetaminophen overdose therapy.
- Decreased dyspnea and clearing of lung sounds when used as a mucolytic.
- Prevention of radiocontrast-induced renal dysfunction.

---

acyclovir (ay-**sye**-kloe-veer)
♣Avirax, Zovirax

Classification
Therapeutic: antivirals
Pharmacologic: purine analogues

Pregnancy Category B (PO, IV), C (topical)

Indications
PO: Recurrent genital herpes infections. Localized cutaneous herpes zoster infections (shingles) and chickenpox (varicella). **IV:** Severe initial episodes of genital herpes in nonimmunosuppressed patients. Mucosal or cutaneous herpes simplex infections or herpes zoster infections (shingles) in immunosuppressed patients. Herpes simplex encephalitis. **Topical:** *Cream*—Recurrent herpes labialis (cold sores). *Ointment*—Treatment of limited non–life-threatening herpes simplex infections in immunocompromised patients (systemic treatment is preferred).

Action
Interferes with viral DNA synthesis. **Therapeutic Effects:** Inhibition of viral replication, decreased viral shedding, and reduced time for healing of lesions.

Pharmacokinetics
Absorption: Despite poor absorption (15–30%), therapeutic blood levels are achieved.
Distribution: Widely distributed. CSF concentrations are 50% of plasma. Crosses placenta; enters breast milk.
Protein Binding: <30%.
Metabolism and Excretion: >90% eliminated unchanged by kidneys; remainder metabolized by liver.
Half-life: Neonates: 4 hr; Children 1–12 yr: 2–3 hr; Adults: 2–3.5 hr (↑ in renal failure).

TIME/ACTION PROFILE (antiviral blood levels)

ROUTE	ONSET	PEAK	DURATION
PO	unknown	1.5–2.5 hr	4 hr
IV	prompt	end of infusion	8 hr

Contraindications/Precautions
Contraindicated in: Hypersensitivity to acyclovir or valacyclovir.
Use Cautiously in: Pre-existing serious neurologic, hepatic, pulmonary, or fluid and electrolyte abnormalities; Renal impairment (dose alteration recommended if CCr <50 mL/min); **Geri:** Due to age related ↓ in renal function; Obese patients (dose should be based on ideal body weight); Patients with hypoxia; **OB, Lactation:** Safety not established.

Adverse Reactions/Side Effects
CNS: SEIZURES, dizziness, headache, hallucinations, trembling. **GI:** diarrhea, nausea, vomiting, elevated liver enzymes, hyperbilirubinemia, abdominal pain, anorexia. **GU:** RENAL FAILURE, crystalluria, hematuria, renal pain. **Derm:** STEVENS-JOHNSON SYNDROME, acne, hives, skin rashes, unusual sweating. **Endo:** changes in menstrual cycle. **Hemat:** THROMBOTIC THROMBOCYTOPENIC PURPURA/HEMOLYTIC UREMIC SYNDROME (high doses in immunosuppressed patients). **Local:** pain, phlebitis, local irritation. **MS:** joint pain. **Misc:** polydipsia.

Interactions
Drug-Drug: **Probenecid** ↑ blood levels of acyclovir. ↑ blood levels and risk of toxicity from **theophylline**; dose adjustment may be necessary. ↓ blood levels and may ↓ effectiveness of **valproic acid** or **hydantoins**. Concurrent use of other **nephrotoxic drugs** ↑ risk of adverse renal effects. **Zidovudine** and IT **methotrexate** may ↑ risk of CNS side effects.

Route/Dosage

Initial Genital Herpes
PO (Adults and Children): 200 mg q 4 hr while awake (5 times/day) for 7–10 days or 400 mg q 8 hr for 7–10 days; maximum dose in children: 80 mg/kg/day in 3–5 divided doses.
IV (Adults and Children): 5 mg/kg q 8 hr or 750 mg/m²/day divided q 8 hr for 5–7 days.

Chronic Suppressive Therapy for Recurrent Genital Herpes
PO (Adults and Children): 400 mg twice daily or 200 mg 3–5 times/day for up to 12 mo. Maximum dose in children: 80 mg/kg/day in 2–5 divided doses.

Intermittent Therapy for Recurrent Genital Herpes
PO (Adults and Children): 200 mg q 4 hr while awake (5 times/day) or 400 mg q 8hr or 800 mg q 12 hr for 5 days, start at first sign of symptoms. Maximum dose in children: 80 mg/kg/day in 2–5 divided doses.

Acute Treatment of Herpes Zoster in Immunosuppressed Patients
PO (Adults): 800 mg q 4 hr while awake (5 times/day) for 7–10 days. *Prophylaxis*—400 mg 5 times/day.
PO (Children): 250–600 mg/m²/dose 4–5 times/day.

Herpes Zoster in Immunocompetent Patients
PO (Adults and Children): 4000 mg/day in 5 divided doses for 5–7 days, maximum dose in children: 80 mg/kg/day in 5 divided doses.

Chickenpox
PO (Adults and Children): 20 mg/kg (not to exceed 800 mg/dose) qid for 5 days. Start within 24 hr of rash onset.

Mucosal and Cutaneous Herpes Simplex Infections in Immunosuppressed Patients
IV (Adults and Children >12 yr): 5 mg/kg q 8 hr for 7 days.
IV (Children <12 yr): 10 mg/kg q 8 hr for 7 days.
Topical (Adults): 0.5 in. ribbon of 5% *ointment* for every 4-square-in. area q 3 hr (6 times/day) for 7 days.

Herpes Simplex Encephalitis
IV (Adults): 10 mg/kg q 8 hr for 14–21 days.
IV (Children 3 mo–12 yr): 10 mg/kg q 8 hr for 14–21 days.
IV (Children birth–3 mo): 20 mg/kg q 8 hr for 14–21 days.
IV (Neonates, premature): 10 mg/kg q 12 hr for 14–21 days.

Varicella Zoster Infections in Immunosuppressed Patients
IV (Adults): 10 mg/kg q 8 hr for 7–10 days.
IV (Children <12 yr): 10 mg/kg q 8 hr for 7–10 days.

Renal Impairment
PO, IV (Adults and Children): *CCr >50 mL/min/1.73 m²*—no dosage adjustment needed; *CCr 25–50 mL/min/1.73 m²*—administer normal dose q 12 hr; *CCr 10–25 mL/min/1.73 m²*—administer normal dose q 24 hr; *CCr 0–10 mL/min/1.73 m²*—50% of dose q 24 hr.
IV (Neonates): *SCr 0.8–1.1 mg/dL:* Administer 20 mg/kg/dose q 12 hr; *SCr 1.2–1.5 mg/dL:* Administer 20 mg/kg/dose q 24 hr; *SCr >1.5 mg/dL:* Administer 10 mg/kg/dose q 24 hr.

Herpes labialis
Topical (Adults and Children >12 yr): Apply 5 times/day for 4 days; start at first symptoms.

Availability (generic available)
Capsules: 200 mg. **Cost:** *Generic*—$12.99/30. **Tablets:** 400 mg, 800 mg. **Cost:** *Generic*—400 mg $14.50/30, 800 mg $24.99/30. **Suspension (banana flavor):** 200 mg/5 mL. **Cost:** $123.97/473 mL. **Powder for injection:** 500 mg/vial, 1000 mg/vial. **Solution for injection:** 25 mg/mL in 20-mL and 40-mL vials, 50 mg/mL in 10-mL and 20-mL vials. **Cream:** 5% in 2-g and 5-g tubes. **Cost:** $51.36/2-g tube, $115.99/5-g tube. *In combination with:* hydrocortisone (Lipsovir). See Appendix B. **Ointment:** 5% in 15-g tubes. **Cost:** $129.99/15-g tube.

NURSING IMPLICATIONS

Assessment
- Assess lesions before and daily during therapy.
- Monitor neurologic status in patients with herpes encephalitis.
- **Lab Test Considerations:** Monitor BUN, serum creatinine, and CCr before and during therapy. ↑ BUN and serum creatinine levels or ↓ CCr may indicate renal failure.

Potential Nursing Diagnoses
Risk for impaired skin integrity (Indications)
Risk for infection (Patient/Family Teaching)

Implementation
- Acyclovir treatment should be started as soon as possible after herpes simplex symptoms appear and within 24 hr of a herpes zoster outbreak.
- **PO:** Acyclovir may be administered with food or on an empty stomach, with a full glass of water.
- Shake oral suspension well before administration.

IV Administration
- **IV:** Maintain adequate hydration (2000–3000 mL/day), especially during first 2 hr after IV infusion, to prevent crystalluria.
- Observe infusion site for phlebitis. Rotate infusion site to prevent phlebitis.
- Acyclovir injectable should not be administered topically, IM, subcut, PO, or in the eye.
- **Intermittent Infusion:** Reconstitute 500-mg or 1-g vial with 10 mL or 20 mL, respectively, of sterile water for injection. Do not reconstitute with bacteriostatic water with benzyl alcohol or parabens. Shake well to dissolve completely. *Diluent:* Dilute in at least 100 mL of D5W, 0.9% NaCl, dextrose/saline combinations or LR. *Concentration:* 7 mg/mL. Patients requiring fluid restriction: 10 mg/mL. *Rate:* Administer via infusion pump over 1 hr to minimize renal tubular damage.
- Use reconstituted solution within 12 hr. Once diluted for infusion, the solution should be used within 24 hr. Refrigeration results in precipitation, which dissolves at room temperature.
- **Y-Site Compatibility:** alfentanil, allopurinol, amikacin, aminophylline, amphotericin B cholesteryl, amphotericin B liposome, ampicillin, anidulafungin, argatroban, atracurium, bivalirudin, bumetanide, buprenorphine, busulfan, butorphanol, calcium chloride, calcium gluconate, carboplatin, cefazolin, cefoperazone, cefotaxime, cefoxitin, ceftazidime, ceftizoxime, ceftriaxone, cefuroxime, chloramphenicol, cimetidine, cisplatin, clindamycin, cyclophosphamide, cyclosporine, cytarabine, dactinomycin, dantrolene, dexamethasone, dexmeditomidine, digoxin, dimenhydrinate, diphenhydramine, docetaxel, doripenem, doxacurium, doxorubicin liposome, doxycycline, enalaprilat, ephedrine, ertapenem, erythromycin lactobionate, etoposide, etoposide phosphate, famotidine, fentanyl, filgrastim, fluconazole, fluorouracil, furosemide, gentamicin, glycopyrrolate, heparin, hetastarch, hydrocortisone, hydromorphone, ifosfamide, imipenem/cilastatin, insulin, isoproterenol, linezolid, lorazepam, magnesium sulfate, mannitol, mechlorethamine, melphalan, methohexital, methotrexate, methylprednisolone, metoprolol, metronidazole, milrinone, mitoxantrone, multivitamin infusion, nafcillin, naloxone, nesiritide, nitroglycerin, octreotide, oxacillin, oxytocin, paclitaxel, pancuronium, pantoprazole, pemetrexed, penicillin G potassium, pentobarbital, perphenazine, phenobarbital, potassium chloride, propofol, propranolol, ranitidine, remifentanil, rituximab, rocuronium, sodium acetate, sodium bicarbonate, succinylcholine, sufentanil, teniposide, theophylline, thiopental, thiotepa, tigecycline, tirofiban, tobramycin, trastuzumab, trimethoprim/sulfamethoxazole, vancomycin, vasopressin, vincristine, voriconazole, zidovudine.
- **Y-Site Incompatibility:** amifostine, amphotericin B colloidal, ampicillin/sulbactam, amsacrine, aztreonam, cefepime, chlorpromazine, ciprofloxacin, codeine, daptomycin, diazepam, dobutamine, dopamine, doxorubicin hydrochloride, epinephrine, epirubicin, eftifibatide, esmolol, fenoldopam, fludarabine, foscarnet, gemcitabine, haloperidol, hydralazine, hydroxyzine, idarubicin, ketorolac, labetalol, levofloxacin, lidocaine, methyldopate, midazolam, nitroprusside, ondansetron, palonosetron, pentamidine, phenylephrine, phenytoin, piperacillin/tazobactam, potassium phosphates, procainamide, prochlorperazine, promethazine, quinupristin/dalfopristin, sargramostim, sodium phosphates, streptozocin, tacrolimus, ticarcillin/clavulanate, vecuronium, verapamil, vinorelbine.
- **Topical:** Apply to skin lesions only; do not use in the eye.

Patient/Family Teaching
- Advise patient to take medication as directed for the full course of therapy. Take missed doses as soon as possible but not just before next dose is due; do not double doses. Acyclovir should not be used more frequently or longer than prescribed.
- Advise patients that the additional use of OTC creams, lotions, and ointments may delay healing and may cause spreading of lesions.
- Inform patient that acyclovir is not a cure. The virus lies dormant in the ganglia, and acyclovir

will not prevent the spread of infection to others.
- Advise patient that condoms should be used during sexual contact and that no sexual contact should be made while lesions are present.
- Patient should consult health care professional if symptoms are not relieved after 7 days of topical therapy or if oral acyclovir does not decrease the frequency and severity of recurrences. Immunocompromised patients may require a longer time, usually 2 weeks, for crusting over of lesions.
- Instruct women with genital herpes to have yearly Papanicolaou smears because they may be more likely to develop cervical cancer.
- **Topical:** Instruct patient to apply ointment in sufficient quantity to cover all lesions every 3 hr, 6 times/day for 7 days. 0.5-in. ribbon of ointment covers approximately 4 square in. Use a finger cot or glove when applying to prevent inoculation of other areas or spread to other people. Keep affected areas clean and dry. Loose-fitting clothing should be worn to prevent irritation.
- Avoid drug contact in or around eyes. Report any unexplained eye symptoms to health care professional immediately; ocular herpetic infection can lead to blindness.

Evaluation/Desired Outcomes
- Crusting over and healing of skin lesions.
- Decrease in frequency and severity of recurrences.
- Acceleration of complete healing and cessation of pain in herpes zoster.
- Decrease in intensity of chickenpox.

adalimumab (a-da-li-mu-mab)
Humira

Classification
Therapeutic: antirheumatics
Pharmacologic: DMARDs, monoclonal antibodies

Pregnancy Category B

Indications
Treatment of moderately to severely active rheumatoid arthritis in patients who have responded inadequately to other DMARDs; may be used with methotrexate or other DMARDs. Psoriatic arthritis. Active ankylosing spondylitis. Crohn's disease. Moderate to severely active polyarticular juvenile (≥ 4 yr) idiopathic arthritis (to be used as monotherapy or with methotrexate). Moderate to severe chronic plaque psoriasis in patients who are candidates for systemic therapy or phototherapy and when other systemic therapies are deemed inappropriate.

Action
Neutralizes and prevents the action of tumor necrosis factor (TNF), resulting in anti-inflammatory and antiproliferative activity. **Therapeutic Effects:** Decreased pain and swelling with decreased rate of joint destruction in patients with rheumatoid arthritis, psoriatic arthritis, juvenile arthritis, and ankylosing spondylitis. Reduced signs and symptoms of Crohn's disease. Reduced severity of plaques.

Pharmacokinetics
Absorption: 64% absorbed after subcut administration.
Distribution: Synovial fluid concentrations are 31–96% of serum.
Metabolism and Excretion: Unknown.
Half-life: 14 days (range 10–20 days).

TIME/ACTION PROFILE (improvement)

ROUTE	ONSET	PEAK	DURATION
Subcut	8–26 wk	131 hr*	2 wk†

*Blood level
†Following discontinuation

Contraindications/Precautions
Contraindicated in: Hypersensitivity; Concurrent use of anakinra; Active infection (including chronic or localized); Lactation: Potential for serious side effects in the infant; discontinue drug or provide formula.
Use Cautiously in: History of recurrent infection or underlying illness/treatment predisposing to infection; Patients residing, or who have resided, where tuberculosis or histoplasmosis is endemic; Pre-existing or recent onset CNS demyelinating disorders; History of lymphoma; Geri: ↑ risk of infection/malignancy; OB: Use only if clearly needed; Pedi: Children <4 yr (safety not established); ↑ risk of lymphoma, leukemia, and other malignancies.

Adverse Reactions/Side Effects
CNS: <u>headache</u>. **CV:** hypertension. **GI:** abdominal pain, nausea. **GU:** hematuria. **Derm:** <u>rash</u>, psoriasis. **Hemat:** LEUKEMIA, neutropenia, thrombocytopenia. **Local:** <u>injection site reactions</u>. **Metab:** hypercholesterolemia, hyperlipidemia. **MS:** back

pain. **Misc:** allergic reactions including ANAPHYLAXIS, INFECTIONS (including reactivation tuberculosis and invasive fungal infections), MALIGNANCY.

Interactions
Drug-Drug: Concurrent use with **anakinra** or other **TNF blocking agents** ↑ risk of serious infections and is contraindicated. **Live vaccinations** should not be given concurrently.

Route/Dosage
Rheumatoid Arthritis, Ankylosing Spondylitis, and Psoriatic Arthritis
Subcut (Adults): 40 mg every other week; patients not receiving concurrent methotrexate may receive additional benefit by increasing dose to 40 mg once weekly.

Crohn's Disease
Subcut (Adults): 160 mg initially on Day 1 (given as four 40-mg injections in one day or as two 40-mg injections given in two consecutive days), followed by 80 mg 2 wk later on Day 15. Two wk later (Day 29), begin maintenance dose of 40 mg every other wk. Aminosalicylates, corticosteroids, and/or immunomodulatory agents may be continued during therapy.

Juvenile Idiopathic Arthritis
Subcut (Children 4–17 yr): *15– <30 kg*—30 mg every other wk; *≥30 kg*—40 mg every other wk.

Plaque Psoriasis
Subcut (Adults): 80 mg initially, then in 1 wk, begin regimen of 40 mg every other wk.

Availability
Solution for subcut injection (prefilled syringes): 20 mg/0.4 mL, 40 mg/0.8 mL. **Pen:** Single use prefilled glass syringe containing 40 mg (0.8 mL).

NURSING IMPLICATIONS

Assessment
- Assess pain and range of motion before and periodically during therapy.
- Assess for signs of infection (fever, dyspnea, flu-like symptoms, frequent or painful urination, redness or swelling at the site of a wound), including tuberculosis, prior to injection. Adalimumab is contraindicated in patients with active infection. New infections should be monitored closely; most common are upper respiratory tract infections, bronchitis, and urinary tract infections. Infections may be fatal, especially in patients taking immunosuppressive therapy.
- Monitor for injection site reactions (redness and/or itching, rash, hemorrhage, bruising, pain, or swelling). Rash will usually disappear within a few days. Application of a towel soaked in cold water may relieve pain or swelling.
- Assess patient for latex allergy. Needle cover of syringe contains latex and should not be handled by persons sensitive to latex.
- Monitor patient for signs of anaphylaxis (urticaria, dyspnea, facial edema) following injection. Medications (antihistamines, corticosteroids, epinephrine) and equipment should be readily available in the event of a severe reaction. Discontinue adalimumab immediately if anaphylaxis or other severe allergic reaction occurs.
- Assess patient for latent tuberculosis with a tuberculin skin test prior to initiation of therapy. Treatment of latent tuberculosis should be started before therapy with adalimumab.
- Assess for signs and symptoms of systemic fungal infections (fever, malaise, weight loss, sweats, cough, dypsnea, pulmonary infiltrates, serious systemic illness with or without concomitant shock). Ascertain if patient lives in or has traveled to areas of endemic mycoses. Consider empiric antifungal treatment for patients at risk of histoplasmosis and other invasive fungal infections until the pathogens are identified. Consult with an infectious diseases specialist. Consider stopping adalimumab until the infection has been diagnosed and adequately treated.
- **Lab Test Considerations:** May cause agranulocytosis, granulocytopenia, leukopenia, pancytopenia, and polycythemia.
- Monitor CBC with differential periodically during therapy. May cause leukopenia, neutropenia, thrombocytopenia, and pancytopenia. Discontinue adalimumab if symptoms of blood dyscrasias (persistent fever) occur.

Potential Nursing Diagnoses
Acute pain (Indications)
Risk for infection (Side Effects)

Implementation
- Administer a tuberculin skin test prior to administration of adalimumab. Patients with active latent TB should be treated for TB prior to therapy.
- Immunizations should be current prior to initiating therapy. Patients on adalimumab may receive concurrent vaccinations, except for live vaccines.
- Administer initial injection under supervision of a health care professional.

- Do not administer solutions that are discolored or contain particulate matter. Discard unused solution.
- Other DMARDs should be continued during adalimumab therapy.
- **Subcut:** Administer at a 45° angle in upper thighs or abdomen, avoiding the 2 inches around the navel. Put pressure on injection site for 10 sec, do not rub. Rotate injection sites; avoid areas that are tender, bruised, hard, or red.

Patient/Family Teaching
- Instruct patient on the correct technique for administering adalimumab. Review patient information sheet, preparation of dose, administration sites and technique, and disposal of equipment into a puncture-resistant container.
- Advise patient to use calendar stickers provided by manufacturer to assist in remembering when dose is due. If a dose is missed, instruct patient to administer as soon as possible, then take next dose according to regular schedule. If more than prescribed dose is taken, caution patient to consult health care professional or the HUMIRA Patient Resource Center at 1-800-4HUMIRA (448-6472).
- Caution patient to notify health care professional immediately if signs of infection, severe rash, swollen face, or difficulty breathing occurs while taking adalimumab.
- Advise patient to consult health care professional before taking other Rx or OTC medications or herbal products.
- Instruct patient to notify health care professional of medication regimen prior to treatment or surgery.
- **Pen:** Clean area for injection with alcohol swab. Hold pen with gray cap pointing up. Check solution through window; if discolored, cloudy, or contains flakes, discard solution. Turn pen over and point cap down to make sure solution reaches fill line; if not, do not use and contact pharmacist. Remove gray cap exposing the needle and the plum cap exposing the button; removing the plum cap activates the pen. Pinch skin and place pen, with window visible, against skin at a 90° angle and press button until a click is heard. Hold pen in place until all solution is injected (10 seconds) and yellow marker is visible in window and has stopped moving. Continue to pinch skin throughout injection. Remove needle and press with a gauze pad or cotton ball for 10 seconds. Do not rub injection site. Dispose of pen into a puncture-resistant container.

Evaluation/Desired Outcomes
- Decreased pain and swelling with decreased rate of joint destruction in patients with rheumatoid arthritis.
- Decreased signs and symptoms, slowed progression of joint destruction, and improved physical function in patients with psoriatic arthritis.
- Reduced signs and symptoms of ankylosing spondylitis.
- Decreased signs and symptoms and maintenance of remission in patients with Crohn's disease.
- Reduced pain and swelling in patients moderate to severe polyarticular juvenile idiopathic arthritis (JIA) in children 4 yr of age and older.
- Reduced severity of plaques in patients with severe chronic plaque psoriasis.

---

adenosine (a-**den**-oh-seen)
Adenocard, Adenoscan

Classification
Therapeutic: antiarrhythmics

Pregnancy Category C

Indications
Conversion of paroxysmal supraventricular tachycardia (PSVT) to normal sinus rhythm when vagal maneuvers are unsuccessful. As a diagnostic agent (with noninvasive techniques) to assess myocardial perfusion defects occurring as a consequence of coronary artery disease.

Action
Restores normal sinus rhythm by interrupting reentrant pathways in the AV node. Slows conduction time through the AV node. Also produces coronary artery vasodilation. **Therapeutic Effects:** Restoration of normal sinus rhythm.

Pharmacokinetics
Absorption: Following IV administration, absorption is complete.
Distribution: Taken up by erythrocytes and vascular endothelium.
Metabolism and Excretion: Rapidly converted to inosine and adenosine monophosphate.
Half-life: <10 sec.

adenosine

TIME/ACTION PROFILE (antiarrhythmic effect)

ROUTE	ONSET	PEAK	DURATION
IV	immediate	unknown	1–2 min

Contraindications/Precautions
Contraindicated in: Hypersensitivity; 2nd- or 3rd-degree AV block or sick sinus syndrome, unless a functional artificial pacemaker is present. **Use Cautiously in:** Patients with a history of asthma (may induce bronchospasm); Unstable angina; OB, Lactation:Safety not established.

Adverse Reactions/Side Effects
CNS: apprehension, dizziness, headache, head pressure, light-headedness. **EENT:** blurred vision, throat tightness. **Resp:** shortness of breath, chest pressure, hyperventilation. **CV:** facial flushing, transient arrhythmias, chest pain, hypotension, palpitations. **GI:** metallic taste, nausea. **Derm:** burning sensation, facial flushing, sweating. **MS:** neck and back pain. **Neuro:** numbness, tingling. **Misc:** heaviness in arms, pressure sensation in groin.

Interactions
Drug-Drug: Carbamazepine may ↑ risk of progressive heart block. **Dipyridamole** ↑ effects of adenosine (dosage reduction of adenosine recommended). Effects of adenosine ↑ by **theophylline** or **caffeine** (larger doses of adenosine may be required). Concurrent use with **digoxin** may ↑ risk of ventricular fibrillation.

Route/Dosage
IV (Adults and Children >50 kg): *Antiarrhythmic*—6 mg by rapid IV bolus; if no results, repeat 1–2 min later as 12-mg rapid bolus. This dose may be repeated (single dose not to exceed 12 mg). *Diagnostic use*—140 mcg/kg/min for 6 min (0.84 mg/kg total).
IV (Children <50 kg): *Antiarrhythmic*—0.05–0.1 mg/kg as a rapid bolus, may repeat in 1–2 min; if response is inadequate, may increase by 0.05–0.1 mg/kg until sinus rhythm is established or maximum dose of 0.3 mg/kg is used.

Availability (generic available)
Injection: 6-mg/2-mL vial (Adenocard), 3 mg/1 mL in 30-mL vial (Adenoscan).

NURSING IMPLICATIONS

Assessment
- Monitor heart rate frequently (every 15–30 sec) and ECG continuously during therapy. A short, transient period of 1st-, 2nd-, or 3rd-degree heart block or asystole may occur following injection; usually resolves quickly due to short duration of adenosine. Once conversion to normal sinus rhythm is achieved, transient arrhythmias (premature ventricular contractions, atrial premature contractions, sinus tachycardia, sinus bradycardia, skipped beats, AV nodal block) may occur, but generally last a few seconds.
- Monitor blood pressure during therapy.
- Assess respiratory status (breath sounds, rate) following administration. Patients with history of asthma may experience bronchospasm.

Potential Nursing Diagnoses
Decreased cardiac output (Indications)

Implementation
- Do not confuse adenosine (Adenocard) with adenosine phosphate.

IV Administration
- **IV:** Crystals may occur if adenosine is refrigerated. Warm to room temperature to dissolve crystals. Solution must be clear before use. Do not administer solutions that are discolored or contain particulate matter. Discard unused portions.
- **Direct IV:** *Diluent:*Administer undiluted. *Concentration:*3 mg/mL. *Rate:*Administer over 1–2 seconds via peripheral IV as proximal as possible to trunk. Slow administration may cause increased heart rate in response to vasodilation. Follow each dose with 20 mL rapid saline flush to ensure injection reaches systemic circulation.
- **Intermittent Infusion (for use in diagnostic testing):** *Diluent:*Administer 30-mL vial undiluted. *Concentration:*3 mg/mL. *Rate:* Administer at a rate of 140 mcg/kg/min over 6 min for a total dose of 0.84 mg/kg. Thallium-201 should be injected as close to the venous access as possible at the midpoint (after 3 min) of the infusion.
- **Y-Site Compatibility:** abciximab, Thallium-201.

Patient/Family Teaching
- Caution patient to change positions slowly to minimize orthostatic hypotension. Doses >12 mg decrease blood pressure by decreasing peripheral vascular resistance.
- Instruct patient to report facial flushing, shortness of breath, or dizziness.

Evaluation/Desired Outcomes
- Conversion of supraventricular tachycardia to normal sinus rhythm.
- Diagnosis of myocardial perfusion defects.

albumin (human)
(al-**byoo**-min)
Albuminar, Albutein, Buminate, normal human serum albumin, Plasbumin

Classification
Therapeutic: volume expanders
Pharmacologic: blood products, colloids

Pregnancy Category C

Indications
Expansion of plasma volume and maintenance of cardiac output in situations associated with fluid volume deficit, including shock, hemorrhage, and burns. Temporary replacement of albumin in diseases associated with low levels of plasma proteins, such as nephrotic syndrome or end-stage liver disease, resulting in relief or reduction of associated edema.

Action
Provides colloidal oncotic pressure, which serves to mobilize fluid from extravascular tissues back into the intravascular space. Requires concurrent administration of appropriate crystalloid. **Therapeutic Effects:** Increase in intravascular fluid volume.

Pharmacokinetics
Absorption: Following IV administration, absorption is essentially complete.
Distribution: Confined to the intravascular space, unless capillary permeability is increased.
Metabolism and Excretion: Probably degraded by the liver.
Half-life: 2–3 wk.

TIME/ACTION PROFILE (oncotic effect)

ROUTE	ONSET	PEAK	DURATION
IV	15–30 min	unknown	24 hr

Contraindications/Precautions
Contraindicated in: Allergic reactions to albumin; Severe anemia; CHF; Normal or increased intravascular volume.
Use Cautiously in: Severe hepatic or renal disease; Dehydration (additional fluids may be required); Patients requiring sodium restriction; Preterm neonates (infuse slowly due to increased risk of intravascular hemorrhage).

Adverse Reactions/Side Effects
CNS: headache. **CV:** PULMONARY EDEMA, fluid overload, hypertension, hypotension, tachycardia. **GI:** increased salivation, nausea, vomiting. **Derm:** rash, urticaria. **MS:** back pain. **Misc:** chills, fever, flushing.

Interactions
Drug-Drug: None significant.

Route/Dosage
Dose is highly individualized and depends on condition being treated.

Hypovolemic shock—5% Albumin
IV (Adults): 25 g (500 mL), may be repeated within 30 min.
IV (Children): 0.5–1 g/kg/dose (10–20 mL/kg/dose) may repeat as needed (maximum 6 g/kg/day).
IV (Infants and Neonates): 0.25–0.5 g/kg/dose (5–10 mL/kg/dose).

Hypoproteinemia—25% Albumin
IV (Adults): 50–75 g.
IV (Children, Infants, and Neonates): 0.5–1 g/kg/dose, may repeat every 1–2 days; doses up to 1.5 g/kg/day have been added to hyperalimentation solutions and given over 24 hr.

Nephrotic Syndrome—25% Albumin
IV (Adults): 12.5–50 g/day in 3–4 divided doses.
IV (Children and Infants): 0.25–1 g/kg/dose.

Availability
Injection: 5% (50 mg/mL), 25% (250 mg/mL).

NURSING IMPLICATIONS

Assessment
- Monitor vital signs, CVP, and intake and output before and frequently throughout therapy. If fever, tachycardia, or hypotension occurs, stop infusion and notify physician immediately. Antihistamines may be required to suppress this hypersensitivity response. Hypotension may also result from infusing too rapidly. May be given without regard to patient's blood group.
- Assess for signs of vascular overload (elevated CVP, rales/crackles, dyspnea, hypertension, jugular venous distention) during and after administration.
- **Surgical Patients:** Assess for increased bleeding after administration caused by increased blood pressure and circulating blood volume. Albumin does not contain clotting factors.
- *Lab Test Considerations:* Serum albumin levels should increase with albumin therapy.

- Monitor serum sodium levels; may cause ↑ concentrations.
- Infusions of normal serum albumin may cause false ↑ of alkaline phosphatase levels.
- Hemorrhage: Monitor hemoglobin and hematocrit levels. These values may ↓ because of hemodilution.

Potential Nursing Diagnoses
Decreased cardiac output (Indications)
Deficient fluid volume (Indications)
Excess fluid volume (Side Effects)

Implementation
- Follow manufacturer's recommendations for administration. Administer through a large-gauge (at least 20-gauge) needle or catheter. Record lot number in patient record.
- Solution should be clear amber; 25% albumin solution is equal to 5 times the osmotic value of plasma. Do not administer solutions that are discolored or contain particulate matter. Each liter of both 5% and 25% albumin contains 130–160 mEq of sodium and is thus no longer labeled "salt-poor" albumin.
- Administration of large quantities of normal serum albumin may need to be supplemented with whole blood to prevent anemia. If more than 1000 mL of 5% normal serum albumin is given or if hemorrhage has occurred, the administration of whole blood or packed RBCs may be needed. Hydration status should be monitored and maintained with additional fluids.

IV Administration
- **Intermittent Infusion:** *Diluent:* Administer 5% normal serum albumin undiluted. Normal serum albumin 25% may be administered undiluted or diluted in 0.9% NaCl, D5W, or sodium lactate injection; do not dilute in sterile water (may result in hypotonic-associated hemolysis which may be fatal). Infusion must be completed within 4 hr. *Concentration:* 5%: 50 mg/mL undiluted. 25%: 250 mg/mL undiluted. *Rate:* Rate of administration is determined by concentration of solution, blood volume, indication, and patient response (usual rate over 30–60 min). In patients with normal blood volume, rate of 5% and 25% solutions should not exceed 2–4 mL/min and 1 mL/min, respectively, for both adults and children.
- **Hypovolemia:** 5% or 25% normal serum albumin may be administered as rapidly as tolerated and repeated in 15–30 min if necessary. **Burns:** Rate after the first 24 hr should be set to maintain a plasma albumin level of 2.5 g/100 mL or a total serum protein level of 5.2 g/100 mL. **Hypoproteinemia:** Normal serum albumin 25% is the preferred solution because of the increased concentration of protein. The rate should not exceed 2–3 mL/min of 25% or 5–10 mL/min of 5% solution to prevent circulatory overload and pulmonary edema. This treatment provides a temporary rise in plasma protein until the hypoproteinemia is corrected.
- **Y-Site Compatibility:** diltiazem, lorazepam.
- **Y-Site Incompatibility:** fat emulsion, midazolam, vancomycin, verapamil.
- **Solution Compatibility:** 0.9% NaCl, D5W, D5/0.9% NaCl, D5/0.45% NaCl, sodium lactate ⅙M, D5/LR, and LR.

Patient/Family Teaching
- Explain the purpose of this solution to the patient.
- Instruct patient to report signs and symptoms of hypersensitivity reaction.

Evaluation/Desired Outcomes
- Increase in blood pressure and blood volume when used to treat shock and burns.
- Increased urinary output reflects the mobilization of fluid from extravascular tissues.
- Elevated serum plasma protein in patients with hypoproteinemia.

---

albuterol (al-byoo-ter-ole)
Accuneb, ♣Apo-Salvent, ♣Gen-Salbutamol, ♣Novo-Salmol, Proair HFA, Proventil HFA, ♣Ventodisk, Ventolin HFA, ♣Ventolin nebules, VoSpire ER

Classification
Therapeutic: bronchodilators
Pharmacologic: adrenergics

Pregnancy Category C

Indications
Used as a bronchodilator to control and prevent reversible airway obstruction caused by asthma or COPD. **Inhaln:** Used as a quick-relief agent for acute bronchospasm and for prevention of exercise-induced bronchospasm. **PO:** Used as a long-term control agent in patients with chronic/persistent bronchospasm.

Action
Binds to beta$_2$-adrenergic receptors in airway smooth muscle, leading to activation of adenyl cyclase and increased levels of cyclic-3′, 5′-adenosine monophosphate (cAMP). Increases in cAMP

albuterol

activate kinases, which inhibit the phosphorylation of myosin and decrease intracellular calcium. Decreased intracellular calcium relaxes smooth muscle airways. Relaxation of airway smooth muscle with subsequent bronchodilation. Relatively selective for beta$_2$ (pulmonary) receptors. **Therapeutic Effects:** Bronchodilation.

Pharmacokinetics
Absorption: Well absorbed after oral administration but rapidly undergoes extensive metabolism.
Distribution: Small amounts appear in breast milk.
Metabolism and Excretion: Extensively metabolized by the liver and other tissues.
Half-life: Oral 2.7–5 hr; Inhalation: 3.8 hr.

TIME/ACTION PROFILE (bronchodilation)

ROUTE	ONSET	PEAK	DURATION
PO	15–30 min	2–3 hr	4–6 hr or more
PO–ER	30 min	2–3 hr	12 hr
Inhaln	5–15 min	60–90 min	3–6 hr

Contraindications/Precautions
Contraindicated in: Hypersensitivity to adrenergic amines.
Use Cautiously in: Cardiac disease; Hypertension; Hyperthyroidism; Diabetes; Glaucoma; Seizure disorders; Excess inhaler use may lead to tolerance and paradoxical bronchospasm; OB, Lactation, Pedi: Safety not established for pregnant women near term, breastfeeding women, and children <2 yr; Geri: ↑ risk of adverse reactions; may require dose ↓.

Adverse Reactions/Side Effects
CNS: nervousness, restlessness, tremor, headache, insomnia (Pedi: occurs more frequently in young children than adults), hyperactivity in children. **Resp:** PARADOXICAL BRONCHOSPASM (excessive use of inhalers). **CV:** chest pain, palpitations, angina, arrhythmias, hypertension. **GI:** nausea, vomiting. **Endo:** hyperglycemia. **F and E:** hypokalemia. **Neuro:** tremor.

Interactions
Drug-Drug: Concurrent use with other **adrenergic agents** will have ↑ adrenergic side effects. Use with **MAO inhibitors** may lead to hypertensive crisis. **Beta blockers** may negate therapeutic effect. May ↓ serum **digoxin** levels. Cardiovascular effects are potentiated in patients receiving **tricyclic antidepressants**. Risk of hypokalemia ↑ concurrent use of **potassium-losing diuretics**. Hypokalemia ↑ the risk of **digoxin** toxicity.
Drug-Natural Products: Use with caffeine-containing herbs (**cola nut**, **guarana**, **tea**, **coffee**) ↑ stimulant effect.

Route/Dosage
PO (Adults and Children ≥12 yr): 2–4 mg 3–4 times daily (not to exceed 32 mg/day) or 4–8 mg of extended-release tablets twice daily.
PO (Geriatric Patients): Initial dose should not exceed 2 mg 3–4 times daily, may be ↑ carefully (up to 32 mg/day).
PO (Children 6–12 yr): 2 mg 3–4 times daily or 0.3–0.6 mg/kg/day as extended-release tablets divided twice daily; may be carefully ↑ as needed (not to exceed 8 mg/day).
PO (Children 2–6 yr): 0.1 mg/kg 3 times daily (not to exceed 2 mg 3 times daily initially); may be carefully ↑ to 0.2 mg/kg 3 times daily (not to exceed 4 mg 3 times daily).
Inhaln (Adults and Children ≥4 yr): *Via metered-dose inhaler*—2 inhalations q 4–6 hr or 2 inhalations 15 min before exercise (90 mcg/spray); some patients may respond to 1 inhalation. *NIH Guidelines for acute asthma exacerbation: Children*—4–8 puffs q 20 min for 3 doses then q 1–4 hr; *Adults*—4–8 puffs q 20 min for up to 4 hr then q 1–4 hr prn.
Inhaln (Adults and Children >12 yr): *NIH Guidelines for acute asthma exacerbation via nebulization or IPPB*—2.5–5 mg q 20 min for 3 doses then 2.5–10 mg q 1–4 hr prn; *Continuous nebulization*—10–15 mg/hr.
Inhaln (Children 2–12 yr): *NIH Guidelines for acute asthma exacerbation via nebulization or IPPB*—0.15 mg/kg/dose (minimum dose 2.5 mg) q 20 min for 3 doses then 0.15–0.3 mg/kg (not to exceed 10 mg) q 1–4 hr prn *or* 1.25 mg 3–4 times daily for children 10–15 kg *or* 2.5 mg 3–4 times daily for children >15 kg; *Continuous nebulization*—0.5–3 mg/kg/hr.

Availability (generic available)
Tablets: 2 mg, 4 mg. **Cost:** *Generic*—2 mg $62.96/270, 4 mg $49.49/270. **Extended-release tablets:** 4 mg, 8 mg. **Cost:** 4 mg $265.43/180, 8 mg $488.93/180. **Oral syrup (strawberry-flavored):** 2 mg/5 mL. **Cost:** *Generic*—$11.42/480 mL. **Metered-dose aerosol:** 90 mcg/inhalation in 6.7-g, 8.5-g, 17-g, and 18-g canisters (200 metered inhalations), ✽ 100 mcg/spray. **Cost:** *Proair HFA*—$35.99/8.5-g canister;

128 alemtuzumab

Proventil HFA—$45.99/6.7-g canister; *Ventolin HFA*—$37.99/18-g canister. **Inhalation solution:** 0.63 mg/3 mL, 1.25 mg/3 mL, 0.83 mg/mL in vials and 3 mL unit dose, ✱1 mg/mL, ✱2 mg/mL, 5 mg/mL. **Cost:** *Generic*—5 mg/mL $15.99/20 mL, 0.63 mg/mL $8.99/3 mL, 0.83 mg/mL $18.99/3 mL (25 vials). **Powder for inhalation (Ventodisk):** ✱200 mcg, ✱400 mcg. *In combination with:* ipratropium (Combivent, DuoNeb). See Appendix B.

NURSING IMPLICATIONS

Assessment
- Assess lung sounds, pulse, and blood pressure before administration and during peak of medication. Note amount, color, and character of sputum produced.
- Monitor pulmonary function tests before initiating therapy and periodically during therapy.
- Observe for paradoxical bronchospasm (wheezing). If condition occurs, withhold medication and notify health care professional immediately.
- *Lab Test Considerations:* May cause transient ↓ in serum potassium concentrations with nebulization or higher-than-recommended doses.

Potential Nursing Diagnoses
Ineffective airway clearance (Indications)

Implementation
- **PO:** Administer oral medication with meals to minimize gastric irritation.
- Extended-release tablets should be swallowed whole; do not break, crush, or chew.
- **Inhaln:** Shake inhaler well, and allow at least 1 min between inhalations of aerosol medication. Prime the inhaler before first use by releasing 4 test sprays into the air away from the face. Pedi: Use spacer for children < 8 yr of age.
- For nebulization or IPPB, the 0.5-, 0.83-, 1-, and 2-mg/mL solutions do not require dilution before administration. The 5 mg/mL (0.5%) solution must be diluted with 1–2.5 mL of 0.9% NaCl for inhalation. Diluted solutions are stable for 24 hr at room temperature or 48 hr if refrigerated.
- For nebulizer, compressed air or oxygen flow should be 6–10 L/min; a single treatment of 3 mL lasts about 10 min.
- IPPB usually lasts 5–20 min.

Patient/Family Teaching
- Instruct patient to take albuterol as directed. If on a scheduled dosing regimen, take missed dose as soon as remembered, spacing remaining doses at regular intervals. Do not double doses or increase the dose or frequency of doses. Caution patient not to exceed recommended dose; may cause adverse effects, paradoxical bronchospasm (more likely with first dose from new cannister), or loss of effectiveness of medication.
- Instruct patient to contact health care professional immediately if shortness of breath is not relieved by medication or is accompanied by diaphoresis, dizziness, palpitations, or chest pain.
- Instruct patient to prime unit with 4 sprays before using and to discard cannister after 200 sprays. Actuators should not be changed among products.
- Inform patient that these products contain hydrofluoralkane (HFA) and the propellant and are described as non-CFC or CFC-free (contain no chlorofluorocarbons).
- Advise patient to consult health care professional before taking any OTC medications, natural/herbal products, or alcohol concurrently with this therapy. Caution patient also to avoid smoking and other respiratory irritants.
- Inform patient that albuterol may cause an unusual or bad taste.
- **Inhaln:** Instruct patient in the proper use of the metered-dose inhaler or nebulizer (see Appendix D).
- Advise patients to use albuterol first if using other inhalation medications and allow 5 min to elapse before administering other inhalant medications unless otherwise directed.
- Advise patient to rinse mouth with water after each inhalation dose to minimize dry mouth.
- Instruct patient to notify health care professional if no response to the usual dose of albuterol or if contents of one canister are used in less than 2 wk.
- Pedi:Caution adolescents and their parents about overuse of inhalers, which can cause heart damage and life-threatening arrhythmias.

Evaluation/Desired Outcomes
- Prevention or relief of bronchospasm.

---

alclometasone, See CORTICOSTEROIDS (TOPICAL/LOCAL).

HIGH ALERT

alemtuzumab
(a-lem-**too**-zoo-mab)
Campath

alemtuzumab

Classification
Therapeutic: antineoplastics
Pharmacologic: monoclonal antibodies

Pregnancy Category C

Indications
Treatment of B-cell chronic lymphocytic leukemia in patients who have been treated with alkylating agents and in which fludarabine therapy has failed.

Action
Binds to the CD52 antigen found on the surface of B- and T-lymphocytes and other white blood cells; resulting in lysis. **Therapeutic Effects:** Lysis of leukemic cells with eventual improvement in hematologic parameters.

Pharmacokinetics
Absorption: IV administration results in complete bioavailability.
Distribution: Binds to CD52 receptors.
Metabolism and Excretion: Unknown.
Half-life: 12 days.

TIME/ACTION PROFILE (hematologic parameters)

ROUTE	ONSET	PEAK	DURATION
IV	unknown	2–4 mos‡	7–11 mos‡‡

‡Median time to response
‡‡Duration of response

Contraindications/Precautions
Contraindicated in: Hypersensitivity; Systemic infections; Underlying immunodeficiency, including HIV infection; Lactation: Discontinue breastfeeding during and for 3 mos following last dose of alemtuzumab.
Use Cautiously in: Patients with ischemic heart disease or in patients on antihypertensive medications; Women and men with reproduction potential should use contraception during treatment and for 6 mos after therapy; OB: Should be administered only if clearly needed.

Adverse Reactions/Side Effects
CNS: depression, dizziness, drowsiness, fatigue, headache, weakness. **Resp:** bronchospasm, cough, dyspnea. **CV:** hypertension, hypotension, tachycardia. **GI:** abdominal pain, anorexia, constipation, stomatitis. **Derm:** rash, sweating. **F and E:** edema. **Hemat:** NEUTROPENIA, PANCYTOPENIA/MARROW HYPOPLASIA, anemia, lymphopenia, thrombocytopenia. **MS:** back pain, skeletal pain. **Misc:** infusion-related events, infection, sepsis.

Interactions
Drug-Drug: Additive bone marrow depression with other **antineoplastics** or **radiation therapy**. May ↓ antibody response to and increase the risk of adverse reactions to **live-virus vaccines**.

Route/Dosage
IV (Adults): 3 mg/day initially, as tolerated increase dose to 10 mg/day and then 30 mg/day given three times weekly for up to 12 weeks; single doses should not exceed 30 mg or more than 90 mg/wk.

Availability
Solution for injection (requires further dilution): 30 mg/3 mL in single-use ampules.

NURSING IMPLICATIONS

Assessment
- Monitor for infusion reactions (hypotension, rigors, fever, shortness of breath, bronchospasm, chills, rash). Premedicate with an oral antihistamine and acetaminophen 30 min prior to initial dose, dose increases, and as clinically indicated. Monitor blood pressure and hypotensive symptoms in patients with ischemic heart disease with extra care. Antihistamines, acetaminophen, antiemetics, meperidine, corticosteroids, and incremental dose escalation have been used to prevent and treat infusion-related reactions. Initiate therapy at lowest dose and increase gradually. If therapy is interrupted for 7 or more days, reinstitute with gradual dose escalation.
- *Lab Test Considerations:* Obtain CBC and platelet counts weekly during therapy and more frequently if worsening anemia, neutropenia, or thrombocytopenia is observed. For first occurrence of ANC <250 cells/mm^3 and/or platelet count <25,000 cells/mm^3, withhold alemtuzumab therapy. When ANC >500 cells/mm^3 and platelet count is >50,000 cells/mm^3, resume at same dose. If delay of 7 days or more occurred initiate therapy at 3 mg and escalate to 10 mg and then to 30 mg as tolerated. For second occurrence of ANC <250 cells/mm^3 and/or platelet count <25,000 cells/mm^3, withhold alemtuzumab. When ANC >500 cells/mm^3 and platelet count >50,000 cells/mm^3, resume therapy at 10 mg. If delay is 7 days or more, initiate therapy at 3 mg and escalate to 10 mg only. For third occurrence of ANC <250 cells/mm^3 and/or platelet count <25,000 cells/

✹ = Canadian drug name. ▮ = Genetic implication.
*CAPITALS indicates life-threatening; underlines indicate most frequent.

mm³, discontinue alemtuzumab therapy permanently. For a decrease of ANC and/or platelet count of 50% of baseline value in patients initiating therapy with a baseline ANC of <500 cells/mm³ and/or a baseline platelet count of 25,000 cells/mm³, withhold therapy. When baseline levels return, resume therapy. If delay is 7 days or more, initiate therapy at 3 mg and escalate to 10 mg and 30 mg as tolerated.
- Assess CD4 counts after treatment until recovery to ≥200 cells cells/mm³.

Potential Nursing Diagnoses
Risk for infection (Side Effects)
Risk for injury (Adverse Reactions)

Implementation
- **High Alert:** Fatalities have occurred with chemotherapeutic agents. Before administering, clarify all ambiguous orders; double check single, daily, and course-of-therapy dose limits; have second practitioner independently double check original order, calculations, and infusion pump settings. Alemtuzumab should only be administered under the supervision of a physician experienced in the use antineoplastic therapy.
- Administer via IV only. Inspect solution for particulate matter or discoloration. Do not administer solutions that contain particulate matter or are discolored.

IV Administration
- Withdraw necessary amount from ampule into syringe. Filter with a sterile low-protein binding, non–fiber-releasing 5 micron filter prior to dilution.
- **Intermittent Infusion:** *Diluent:* Dilute with 100 mL of 0.9% NaCl or D5W. Gently invert bag to mix. Dispose of syringe and unused drug product according to institutional guidelines. Use within 8 hr of dilution. Store at room temperature or in refrigerator. Protect solution from light. *Rate:* Administer over 2 hr.
- **Y-Site Incompatibility:** No data is available regarding mixing with other solutions and medications. Do not add to or infuse simultaneously with other solutions or medications.

Patient/Family Teaching
- Inform patient and family of purpose of alemtuzumab.
- Caution patient to avoid immunizations with a live virus due to immunosuppression.

Evaluation/Desired Outcomes
- Improvement in hematologic parameters in patients with B-cell chronic lymphocytic leukemia.

alendronate (a-len-drone-ate)
Fosamax

Classification
Therapeutic: bone resorption inhibitors
Pharmacologic: biphosphonates

Pregnancy Category C

Indications
Treatment and prevention of postmenopausal osteoporosis. Treatment of osteoporosis in men. Treatment of Paget's disease of the bone. Treatment of corticosteroid-induced osteoporosis in patients (men and women) who are receiving ≥7.5 mg of prednisone/day (or equivalent) with evidence of decreased bone mineral density.

Action
Inhibits resorption of bone by inhibiting osteoclast activity. **Therapeutic Effects:** Reversal of the progression of osteoporosis with decreased fractures. Decreased progression of Paget's disease.

Pharmacokinetics
Absorption: Poorly absorbed (0.6–0.8%) after oral administration.
Distribution: Transiently distributes to soft tissue, then distributes to bone.
Metabolism and Excretion: Excreted in urine.
Half-life: 10 yr (reflects release of drug from skeleton).

TIME/ACTION PROFILE (inhibition of bone resorption)

ROUTE	ONSET	PEAK	DURATION
PO	1 mo	3–6 mo	3 wk–7 mo†

†After discontinuation of alendronate

Contraindications/Precautions
Contraindicated in: Renal insufficiency (CCr <35 mL/min); OB, Lactation:Safety not established.
Use Cautiously in: Patients with active GI pathology (dysphagia, esophageal disease, gastritis, duodenitis, ulcers); Pre-existing hypocalcemia or vitamin D deficiency; Concurrent dental surgery (may ↑ risk of jaw osteonecrosis).

Adverse Reactions/Side Effects
CNS: headache. **EENT:** blurred vision, conjunctivitis, eye pain/inflammation. **CV:** atrial fibrillation. **GI:** abdominal distention, abdominal pain, acid regurgitation, constipation, diarrhea, dyspepsia, dysphagia, esophageal cancer, esophageal ulcer, flatulence, gastritis, nausea, taste perversion, vomiting. **Derm:** erythema, photosensitivity, rash.

alendronate 131

MS: musculoskeletal pain, osteonecrosis (primarily of jaw).

Interactions
Drug-Drug: Calcium supplements, antacids, and **other oral medications** ↓ the absorption of alendronate. Doses >10 mg/day ↑ risk of adverse GI events when used with **NSAIDs**. IV **ranitidine** ↑ blood levels.
Drug-Food: Food significantly ↓ absorption. **Caffeine (coffee, tea, cola), mineral water**, and **orange juice** also ↓ absorption.

Route/Dosage
PO (Adults): *Treatment of osteoporosis*—10 mg once daily or 70 mg once weekly. *Prevention of osteoporosis*—5 mg once daily or 35 mg once weekly. *Paget's disease*—40 mg once daily for 6 mo. Re-treatment may be considered for patients who relapse. *Treatment of corticosteroid-induced osteoporosis in men and premenopausal women*—5 mg once daily. *Treatment of corticosteroid-induced osteoporosis in postmenopausal women not receiving estrogen*—10 mg once daily.

Availability (generic available)
Tablets: 5 mg, 10 mg, 35 mg, 40 mg, 70 mg. **Cost:** 5 mg $248.19/90, 10 mg $240.97/90, 35 mg $235.97/12, 40 mg $177.89/30, 70 mg $239.96/12. **Oral solution (raspberry flavor):** 70 mg/75 mL. **Cost:** $27.99/75 mL. *In combination with:* Cholecalciferol (Fosamax plus D) See Appendix B.

NURSING IMPLICATIONS

Assessment
- **Osteoporosis:** Assess patients for low bone mass before and periodically during therapy.
- **Paget's Disease:** Assess for symptoms of Paget's disease (bone pain, headache, decreased visual and auditory acuity, increased skull size).
- *Lab Test Considerations:* Osteoporosis: Assess serum calcium before and periodically during therapy. Hypocalcemia and vitamin D deficiency should be treated before initiating alendronate therapy. May cause mild, transient elevations of calcium and phosphate.
- **Paget's Disease:** Monitor alkaline phosphatase before and periodically during therapy. Alendronate is indicated for patients with alkaline phosphatase twice the upper limit of normal.

Potential Nursing Diagnoses
Risk for injury (Indications)

Implementation
- Do not confuse Fosamax (alendronate) with Flomax (tamsulosin).
- **PO:** Administer first thing in the morning with 6–8 oz plain water 30 min before other medications, beverages, or food. Swallow tablets whole; do not crush, break, or chew.

Patient/Family Teaching
- Instruct patient on the importance of taking exactly as directed, first thing in the morning, 30 min before other medications, beverages, or food. Waiting longer than 30 min will improve absorption. Alendronate should be taken with 6–8 oz plain water (mineral water, orange juice, coffee, and other beverages decrease absorption). If a dose is missed, skip dose and resume the next morning; do not double doses or take later in the day. If a weekly dose is missed, take the morning after remembered and resume the following week on the chosen day. Do not take 2 tablets on the same day. Do not discontinue without consulting health care professional.
- Caution patient to remain upright for 30 min following dose to facilitate passage to stomach and minimize risk of esophageal irritation. Advise patient to discontinue alendronate and notify health care provider if pain or difficulty swallowing, retrosternal pain, or new/worsening heartburn occur.
- Advise patient to eat a balanced diet and consult health care professional about the need for supplemental calcium and vitamin D.
- Encourage patient to participate in regular exercise and to modify behaviors that increase the risk of osteoporosis (stop smoking, reduce alcohol consumption).
- Advise patient to inform health care professional of alendronate therapy prior to dental surgery.
- Caution patient to use sunscreen and protective clothing to prevent photosensitivity reactions.
- Advise patient to notify health care professional if blurred vision, eye pain, or inflammation occur.
- Advise female patient to notify health care professional if pregnancy is planned or suspected or if she is breastfeeding.

✺ = Canadian drug name.   = Genetic implication.
*CAPITALS indicates life-threatening; underlines indicate most frequent.

Evaluation/Desired Outcomes
- Prevention of or decrease in the progression of osteoporosis in postmenopausal women.
- Treatment of osteoporosis in men.
- Decrease in the progression of Paget's disease.
- Treatment of corticosteroid-induced osteoporosis.

alfuzosin (al-fyoo-zo-sin)
Uroxatral

Classification
Therapeutic: urinary tract antispasmodics
Pharmacologic: peripherally acting antiadrenergics

Pregnancy Category B

Indications
Management of symptomatic benign prostatic hyperplasia (BPH).

Action
Selectively blocks alpha$_1$- adrenergic receptors in the lower urinary tract to relax smooth muscle in the bladder neck and prostate. **Therapeutic Effects:** Increased urine flow and decreased symptoms of BPH.

Pharmacokinetics
Absorption: 49% absorbed following oral administration; food enhances absorption.
Distribution: Unknown.
Metabolism and Excretion: Mostly metabolized by the liver (CYP3A4 enzyme system); 11% excreted unchanged in urine.
Half-life: 10 hr.

TIME/ACTION PROFILE

ROUTE	ONSET	PEAK	DURATION
PO-ER	within hr	8 hr	24 hr

Contraindications/Precautions
Contraindicated in: Hypersensitivity; Moderate to severe hepatic impairment; Potent inhibitors of the CYP3A4 enzyme system; Concurrent use of other alpha-adrenergic blocking agents; Severe renal impairment; Pedi:Children.
Use Cautiously in: Congenital or acquired QTc prolongation or concurrent use of other drugs known to prolong QTc; Mild hepatic impairment; Symptomatic hypotension; Concurrent use of antihypertensive agents or nitrates (↑ risk of postural hypotension); Previous hypotensive episode with other medications; Geri:Consider age-related changes in body mass and cardiac, renal, and hepatic function when prescribing.

Adverse Reactions/Side Effects
CNS: dizziness, fatigue, headache. **EENT:** intraoperative floppy iris syndrome. **Resp:** bronchitis, sinusitis, pharyngitis. **CV:** postural hypotension. **GI:** abdominal pain, constipation, dyspepsia, nausea. **GU:** erectile dysfunction.

Interactions
Drug-Drug: **Ketoconazole**, **itraconazole**, and **ritonavir** ↓ metabolism and significantly ↑ levels and effects (concurrent use contraindicated). Levels are ↑ by **cimetidine**, **atenolol**, and **diltiazem**. Alfuzosin ↑ levels and may ↑ effects of **atenolol** and **diltiazem** (monitor blood pressure and heart rate). ↑ risk of hypotension with **antihypertensives**, **nitrates**, and acute ingestion of **alcohol**.

Route/Dosage
PO (Adults): 10 mg once daily.

Availability
Extended-release tablets: 10 mg. **Cost:** $229.96/90.

NURSING IMPLICATIONS

Assessment
- Assess for symptoms of benign prostatic hyperplasia (urinary hesitancy, feeling of incomplete bladder emptying, interruption of urinary stream, impairment of size and force of urinary stream, terminal urinary dribbling, straining to start flow, dysuria, urgency) before and periodically during therapy.
- Assess patient for orthostatic reaction and syncope. Monitor BP (lying and standing) and pulse frequently during initial dose adjustment and periodically thereafter. May occur within a few hr after initial doses and occasionally thereafter.
- Rule out prostatic carcinoma before therapy; symptoms are similar.

Potential Nursing Diagnoses
Risk for injury (Side Effects)
Noncompliance (Patient/Family Teaching)

Implementation
- **PO:** Administer with food at the same meal each day. Tablets must be swallowed whole; do not crush, break, or chew.

Patient/Family Teaching
- Instruct patient to take medication with the same meal each day. Take missed doses as soon as remembered. If not remembered until next day, omit; do not double doses.
- May cause dizziness or drowsiness. Advise patient to avoid driving or other activities requir-

aliskiren **133**

ing alertness until response to the medication is known.
- Caution patient to avoid sudden changes in position to decrease orthostatic hypotension.
- Advise patient to consult health care professional before taking any cough, cold, or allergy remedies.
- Instruct patient to notify health care professional of medication regimen before any surgery, especially cataract surgery.
- Advise patient to notify health care professional if angina, frequent dizziness, or fainting occurs.
- Emphasize the importance of follow-up exams to evaluate effectiveness of medication.
- Geri: Assess risk for falls; implement fall prevention program and instruct patient and family in preventing falls at home.

Evaluation/Desired Outcomes
- Decreased symptoms of benign prostatic hyperplasia.

---

aliskiren (a-lis-ki-ren)
Tekturna

Classification
Therapeutic: antihypertensives
Pharmacologic: renin inhibitors

Pregnancy Category C

Indications
Treatment of hypertension (alone or with other agents).

Action
Inhibition of renin results in decreased formation of angiotensin II, a powerful vasoconstrictor.
Therapeutic Effects: Decreased blood pressure.

Pharmacokinetics
Absorption: Poorly absorbed (bioavailability 2.5%).
Distribution: Unknown.
Metabolism and Excretion: 2% excreted unchanged in urine, remainder is probably metabolized (CYP3A4 enzyme system).
Half-life: 24 hr.

TIME/ACTION PROFILE (antihypertensive effect)

ROUTE	ONSET	PEAK	DURATION
PO	unknown	2 wk	24 hr

Contraindications/Precautions
Contraindicated in: Hypersensitivity; OB: May cause fetal injury or death; Concurrent use with cyclosporine.
Use Cautiously in: Salt or volume depletion (correct before use); Severe renal impairment; Pedi: Safety not established.

Adverse Reactions/Side Effects
Resp: cough. **GI:** abdominal pain, diarrhea (↑ in females and elderly), dyspepsia, reflux. **Misc:** ANGIOEDEMA.

Interactions
Drug-Drug: Blood levels are ↓ by **irbesartan**. Blood levels are ↑ by **atorvastatin**, **ketoconazole**, and **cyclosporine** (concurrent use with cyclosporine not recommended). May ↓ effects of **furosemide**. Antihypertensive effects may be ↑ by other **antihypertensives**, **diuretics**, and **nitrates**. ↑ risk of hyperkalemia with concurrent use of **ACE inhibitors**, **angiotensin II receptor antagonists**, **potassium supplements**, **potassium-sparing diuretics**, or **potassium-containing salt substitutes**.
Drug-Food: High fat meals significantly ↓ absorption.

Route/Dosage
PO (Adults): 150 mg/day initially; may be ↑ to 300 mg/day.

Availability
Tablets: 150 mg, 300 mg. *In combination with:* hydrochlorothiazide (Tekturna HCT) and valsartan (Valturna); see Appendix B.

NURSING IMPLICATIONS

Assessment
- Monitor blood pressure and pulse frequently during initial dose adjustment and periodically during therapy. Notify health care professional of significant changes. If an excessive fall in BP occurs, place patient in a supine position and administer IV 0.9% NaCl, if necessary. A transient hypotensive response does not contraindicate further therapy.
- Monitor frequency of prescription refills to determine adherence.
- *Lab Test Considerations:* May cause minor ↑ in BUN, serum creatinine, potassium, uric acid, and creatine kinase.
- May cause small ↓ in hemoglobin and hematocrit.

Potential Nursing Diagnoses
Noncompliance (Patient/Family Teaching)

Implementation
- Correct volume or sodium depletion prior to initiating therapy.
- **PO:** Administer at the same time each day without regard to meals.

Patient/Family Teaching
- Instruct patient to take aliskiren as directed at the same time each day, even if feeling better. Take missed doses as soon as remembered, but not if almost time for next dose. Do not double doses. Do not share medication with others, even with same condition; may be harmful.
- May cause dizziness. Caution patient to lie down and notify health care professional. Also, avoid driving and other activities requiring alertness until response to aliskiren is known.
- Advise patient to report signs and symptoms of angioedema (swelling of face, extremities, eyes, lips, tongue, difficulty swallowing, or breathing) to health care professional immediately.
- Instruct patient to notify health care professional prior to taking other Rx, OTC, or herbal products.
- Advise female patients to notify health care professional if pregnancy is planned or suspected or if breastfeeding. If pregnancy is detected, discontinue aliskiren as soon as possible.

Evaluation/Desired Outcomes
- Decrease in blood pressure without appearance of side effects. Antihypertensive effect is 90% attained by 2 wk.

---

allopurinol (al-oh-**pure**-i-nole)
Alloprim, ✤Apo-Allopurinol, Lopurin, ✤Purinol, Zyloprim

Classification
Therapeutic: antigout agents, antihyperuricemics
Pharmacologic: xanthine oxidase inhibitors

Pregnancy Category C

Indications
PO: Prevention of attack of gouty arthritis and nephropathy. **PO, IV:** Treatment of secondary hyperuricemia, which may occur during treatment of tumors or leukemias.

Action
Inhibits the production of uric acid by inhibiting the action of xanthine oxidase. **Therapeutic Effects:** Lowering of serum uric acid levels.

Pharmacokinetics
Absorption: Well absorbed (80%) following oral administration.
Distribution: Widely distributed in tissue and breast milk.
Protein Binding: <1%.
Metabolism and Excretion: Metabolized to oxypurinol, an active compound with a long half-life. 12% excreted unchanged, 76% excreted as oxypurinol.
Half-life: 1–3 hr (oxypurinol 18–30 hr).

TIME/ACTION PROFILE (hypouricemic effect)

ROUTE	ONSET	PEAK	DURATION
PO, IV	1–2 days	1–2 wk	1–3 wk†

†Duration after discontinuation of allopurinol

Contraindications/Precautions
Contraindicated in: Hypersensitivity.
Use Cautiously in: Acute attacks of gout; Renal insufficiency (dose reduction required if CCr <20 mL/min); Dehydration (adequate hydration necessary); OB, Lactation: Rarely used; Geri: Begin at lower end of dosage range.

Adverse Reactions/Side Effects
CV: hypotension, flushing, hypertension, bradycardia, and heart failure (reported with IV administration). **CNS:** drowsiness. **GI:** diarrhea, hepatitis, nausea, vomiting. **GU:** renal failure, hematuria. **Derm:** rash (discontinue drug at first sign of rash), urticaria. **Hemat:** bone marrow depression. **Misc:** hypersensitivity reactions.

Interactions
Drug-Drug: Use with **mercaptopurine** and **azathioprine** ↑ bone marrow depressant properties—doses of these drugs should be ↓. Use with **ampicillin** or **amoxicillin** ↑ risk of rash. Use with **oral hypoglycemic agents** and **warfarin** ↑ effects of these drugs. Use with **thiazide diuretics** or **ACE inhibitors** ↑ risk of hypersensitivity reactions. Large doses of allopurinol may ↑ risk of **theophylline** toxicity. May ↑ **cyclosporine** levels.

Route/Dosage
Management of Gout
PO (Adults and Children >10 yr): *Initially*—100 mg/day; increase at weekly intervals based on serum uric acid (not to exceed 800 mg/day). Doses >300 mg/day should be given in divided

allopurinol **135**

doses; *Maintenance dose*—100–200 mg 2–3 times daily. Doses of ≤300 mg may be given as a single daily dose.

Management of Secondary Hyperuricemia
PO (Adults and Children >10 yr): 600–800 mg/day in 2–3 divided doses starting 1–2 days before chemotherapy or radiation.
PO (Children 6–10 yr): 10 mg/kg/day in 2–3 divided doses (maximum 800 mg/day) or 300 mg daily in 2–3 divided doses.
PO (Children <6 yr): 10 mg/kg/day in 2–3 divided doses (maximum 800 mg/day) or 150 mg daily in 3 divided doses.
IV (Adults and Children >10 yr): 200–400 mg/m^2/day (up to 600 mg/day) as a single daily dose or in divided doses q 8–24 hr.
IV (Children <10 yr): 200 mg/m^2/day initially as a single daily dose or in divided doses q 8–24 hr (maximum dose 600 mg/day).

Renal Impairment
(Adults and Children): *CCr >50 mL/min*—No dosage change; *CCr 10–50 mL/min*—Reduce dosage to 50% of recommended; *CCr <10 mL/min*—Reduce dosage to 30% of recommended.

Availability (generic available)
Tablets: 100 mg, 300 mg. **Cost:** *Generic*—100 mg $12.99/100, 300 mg $22.99/100. **Injection:** 500 mg/vial.

NURSING IMPLICATIONS

Assessment
- Monitor intake and output ratios. Decreased kidney function can cause drug accumulation and toxic effects. Ensure that patient maintains adequate fluid intake (minimum 2500–3000 mL/day) to minimize risk of kidney stone formation.
- Assess patient for rash or more severe hypersensitivity reactions. Discontinue allopurinol immediately if rash occurs. Therapy should be discontinued permanently if reaction is severe. Therapy may be reinstated after a mild reaction has subsided, at a lower dose (50 mg/day with very gradual titration). If skin rash recurs, discontinue permanently.
- **Gout:** Monitor for joint pain and swelling. Addition of colchicine or NSAIDs may be necessary for acute attacks. Prophylactic doses of colchicine or an NSAID should be administered concurrently during the first 3–6 mo of therapy because of an increased frequency of acute attacks of gouty arthritis during early therapy.
- *Lab Test Considerations:* Serum and urine uric acid levels usually begin to ↓ 2–3 days after initiation of oral therapy.
- Monitor blood glucose in patients receiving oral hypoglycemic agents. May cause hypoglycemia.
- Monitor hematologic, renal, and liver function tests before and periodically during therapy, especially during the first few months. May cause ↑ serum alkaline phosphatase, bilirubin, AST, and ALT levels. ↓ CBC and platelets may indicate bone marrow depression. ↑ BUN, serum creatinine, and CCr may indicate nephrotoxicity. These are usually reversed with discontinuation of therapy.

Potential Nursing Diagnoses
Acute pain (Indications)

Implementation
- **PO:** May be administered after milk or meals to minimize gastric irritation; give with plenty of fluid. May be crushed and given with fluid or mixed with food for patients who have difficulty swallowing.

IV Administration
- **Intermittent Infusion:** *Diluent:* Reconstitute each 500 mg vial with 25 mL of sterile water for injection. Solution should be clear and almost colorless with only slight opalescence. Dilute to desired concentration with 0.9% NaCl or D5W. Administer within 10 hr of reconstitution; do not refrigerate. Do not administer solutions that are discolored or contain particulate matter. *Concentration:* Not >6 mg/mL. *Rate:* Infusion should be initiated 24–48 hr before start of chemotherapy known to cause tumor cell lysis. Rate of infusion depends on volume of infusate (100–300 mg doses may be infused over 30 minutes). May be administered as a single infusion or equally divided infusions at 6-, 8-, or 12-hr intervals.
- **Y-Site Compatibility:** acyclovir, aminophylline, aztreonam, bleomycin, bumetanide, buprenorphine, butorphanol, calcium gluconate, carboplatin, cefazolin, cefotetan, ceftazidime, ceftizoxime, ceftriaxone, cefuroxime, cisplatin, cyclophosphamide, dactinomycin, dexamethasone sodium phosphate, doxorubicin liposome, enalaprilat, etoposide, famotidine, filgrastim, fluconazole, fludarabine, fluorouracil,

136 almotriptan

furosemide, ganciclovir, granisetron, heparin, hydrocortisone, hydromorphone, ifosfamide, lorazepam, mannitol, mesna, methotrexate, metronidazole, mitoxandrone, morphine, piperacillin, potassium chloride, ranitidine, teniposide, thiotepa, ticarcillin/clavulanate, trimethoprim/sulfamethoxazole, vancomycin, vinblastine, vincristine, zidovudine.

- **Y-Site Incompatibility:** amikacin, amphotericin B, carmustine, cefotaxime, chlorpromazine, cimetidine, clindamycin, cytarabine, dacarbazine, daunorubicin, diphenhydramine, doxorubicin, doxycycline, droperidol, floxuridine, gentamicin, haloperidol, idarubicin, imipenem/cilastatin, mechlorethamine, meperidine, methylprednisolone sodium succinate, metoclopramide, minocycline, nalbuphine, ondansetron, prochlorperazine, promethazine, sodium bicarbonate, streptozocin, tobramycin, vinorelbine.

Patient/Family Teaching
- Instruct patient to take allopurinol as directed. Take missed doses as soon as remembered. If dosing schedule is once daily, do not take if remembered the next day. If dosing schedule is more than once a day, take up to 300 mg for the next dose.
- Instruct patient to continue taking allopurinol along with an NSAID or colchicine during an acute attack of gout. Allopurinol helps prevent, but does not relieve, acute gout attacks.
- Alkaline diet may be ordered. Urinary acidification with large doses of vitamin C or other acids may increase kidney stone formation (see Appendix M). Advise patient of need for increased fluid intake.
- May occasionally cause drowsiness. Caution patient to avoid driving or other activities requiring alertness until response to drug is known.
- Instruct patient to report skin rash, blood in urine, or influenza symptoms (chills, fever, muscle aches and pains, nausea, or vomiting) to health care professional immediately; skin rash may indicate hypersensitivity.
- Advise patient that large amounts of alcohol increase uric acid concentrations and may decrease the effectiveness of allopurinol.
- Emphasize the importance of follow-up exams to monitor effectiveness and side effects.

Evaluation/Desired Outcomes
- Decreased serum and urinary uric acid levels. May take 2–6 wk to observe clinical improvement in patients treated for gout.

almotriptan (al-moe-trip-tan)
Axert

Classification
Therapeutic: vascular headache suppressants
Pharmacologic: 5-HT$_1$ agonists

Pregnancy Category C

Indications
Acute treatment of migraine headache (for adolescents, migraines should be ≥4 hr in duration).

Action
Acts as an agonist at specific 5-HT$_1$ receptor sites in intracranial blood vessels and sensory trigeminal nerves. **Therapeutic Effects:** Cranial vessel vasoconstriction with associated decrease in release of neuropeptides and resultant decrease in migraine headache.

Pharmacokinetics
Absorption: Well absorbed following oral administration (70%).
Distribution: Unknown.
Metabolism and Excretion: 40% excreted unchanged in urine; 27% metabolized by monoamine oxidase-A (MAO-A); 12% metabolized by cytochrome P450 hepatic enzymes (3A4 and 2D6); 13% excreted in feces as unchanged and metabolized drug.
Half-life: 3–4 hr.

TIME/ACTION PROFILE (Blood levels)

ROUTE	ONSET	PEAK	DURATION
PO	unknown	1–3 hr	unknown

Contraindications/Precautions
Contraindicated in: Hypersensitivity; Ischemic cardiovascular, cerebrovascular, or peripheral vascular syndromes (including ischemic bowel disease); History of significant cardiovascular disease; Uncontrolled hypertension; Should not be used within 24 hr of other 5-HT$_1$ agonists or ergot-type compounds (dihydroergotamine); Basilar or hemiplegic migraine; Concurrent MAO-A inhibitor therapy or within 2 wk of discontinuing MAO-A inhibitor therapy.
Use Cautiously in: Cardiovascular risk factors (hypertension, hypercholesterolemia, cigarette smoking, obesity, diabetes, strong family history, menopausal women or men >40 yr); use only if cardiovascular status has been evaluated and determined to be safe and first dose is administered under supervision; Impaired hepatic or renal function; Hypersensitivity to sulfonamides (cross-

almotriptan

sensitivity may occur); OB, Lactation: Safety not established; Pedi: Safety not established in children <12 yr.

Adverse Reactions/Side Effects
CNS: drowsiness, headache. **CV:** CORONARY ARTERY VASOSPASM, MI, myocardial ischemia, VENTRICULAR FIBRILLATION, VENTRICULAR TACHYCARDIA. **GI:** dry mouth, nausea. **Neuro:** paresthesia.

Interactions
Drug-Drug: Concurrent use with **MAO-A inhibitors** ↑ blood levels and the risk of adverse reactions (concurrent use or use within 2 wk or MAO inhibitor is contraindicated). Concurrent use with other **5-HT$_1$ agonists** or **ergot-type compounds** (**dihydroergotamine**) may result in additive vasoactive properties (avoid use within 24 hr of each other). ↑ serotonin levels and serotonin syndrome may occur when used concurrently with **SSRI and SNRI antidepressants**. Blood levels and effects may be ↑ by **ketoconazole**, **itraconazole**, **ritonavir**, and **erythromycin** (inhibitors of CYP3A4 enzymes).

Route/Dosage
PO (Adults and Children ≥12 yr): 6.25–12.5 mg initially, may repeat in 2 hr; not to exceed 2 doses per 24-hr period.

Hepatic/Renal Impairment
PO (Adults): 6.25 mg initially, may repeat in 2 hr; not to exceed 2 doses per 24-hr period.

Availability
Tablets: 6.25 mg, 12.5 mg.

NURSING IMPLICATIONS

Assessment
- Assess pain location, character, intensity, and duration and associated symptoms (photophobia, phonophobia, nausea, vomiting) during migraine attack.
- Monitor for serotonin syndrome in patients taking SSRIs or SNRIs concurrently with almotriptan.

Potential Nursing Diagnoses
Acute pain (Indications)

Implementation
- **PO:** Tablets should be swallowed whole with liquid.

Patient/Family Teaching
- Inform patient that almotriptan should only be used during a migraine attack. It is meant to be used for relief of migraine attacks but not to prevent or reduce the number of attacks.
- Instruct patient to administer almotriptan as soon as symptoms of a migraine attack appear, but it may be administered any time during an attack. If migraine symptoms return, a second dose may be used. Allow at least 2 hr between doses, and do not use more than 2 doses in any 24-hr period.
- If first dose does not relieve headache, additional almotriptan doses are not likely to be effective; notify health care professional.
- Caution patient not to take almotriptan within 24 hr of another vascular headache suppressant.
- Advise patient that lying down in a darkened room following almotriptan administration may further help relieve headache.
- Caution patient not to use almotriptan if she is pregnant, suspects she is pregnant, plans to become pregnant, or is breastfeeding. Adequate contraception should be used during therapy.
- Advise patient to notify health care professional prior to next dose of almotriptan if pain or tightness in the chest occurs during use. If pain is severe or does not subside, notify health care professional immediately. If feelings of tingling, heat, flushing, heaviness, pressure, drowsiness, dizziness, tiredness, or sickness develop discuss with health care professional at next visit.
- May cause dizziness or drowsiness. Caution patient to avoid driving or other activities requiring alertness until response to medication is known.
- Advise patient to avoid alcohol, which aggravates headaches, during almotriptan use.
- Advise patient to consult health care professional before taking other Rx, OTC, or herbal products concurrently with almotriptan. Patients concurrently taking SSRI or SNRI antidepressants should notify health care professional promptly if signs of serotonin syndrome (mental status changes: agitation, hallucinations, coma; autonomic instability: tachycardia, labile blood pressure, hyperthermia; neuromuscular aberrations: hyperreflexia, incoordination; and/or gastrointestinal symptoms: nausea, vomiting, diarrhea) occur.

Evaluation/Desired Outcomes
- Relief of migraine attack.

alprazolam (al-**pray**-zoe-lam)
✣ Apo-Alpraz, ✣ Novo-Alprazol, Niravam, ✣ Nu-Alpraz, Xanax, Xanax XR

Classification
Therapeutic: antianxiety agents
Pharmacologic: benzodiazepines

Schedule IV

Pregnancy Category D

Indications
Treatment of Generalized Anxiety Disorder (GAD). Panic Disorder. Management of anxiety associated with depression. **Unlabeled Use:** Management of symptoms of premenstrual syndrome (PMS). Insomnia, irritable bowel syndrome (IBS) and other somatic symptoms associated with anxiety. Used as an adjunct with acute mania, acute psychosis.

Action
Acts at many levels in the CNS to produce anxiolytic effect. May produce CNS depression. Effects may be mediated by GABA, an inhibitory neurotransmitter. **Therapeutic Effects:** Relief of anxiety.

Pharmacokinetics
Absorption: Well absorbed (90%) from the GI tract; absorption is slower with extended-release tablets.
Distribution: Widely distributed, crosses blood-brain barrier. Probably crosses the placenta and enters breast milk. Accumulation is minimal.
Metabolism and Excretion: Metabolized by the liver (CYP3A4 enzyme system) to an active compound that is subsequently rapidly metabolized.
Half-life: 12–15 hr.

TIME/ACTION PROFILE (sedation)

ROUTE	ONSET	PEAK	DURATION
PO	1–2 hr	1–2 hr	up to 24 hr

Contraindications/Precautions
Contraindicated in: Hypersensitivity; Cross-sensitivity with other benzodiazepines may exist; Pre-existing CNS depression; Severe uncontrolled pain; Angle-closure glaucoma, obstructive sleep apnea, pulmonary disease; Pregnancy and lactation; Concurrent itraconazole or ketoconazole; OB, Lactation: Use in pregnancy or lactation may cause CNS depression, flaccidity, feeding difficulties, and seizures in infant.
Use Cautiously in: Renal Impairment, Hepatic dysfunction (↓ dose required); Concurrent use with nefazodone, fluvoxamine, cimetidine, fluoxetine, hormonal contraceptives, propoxyphene, diltiazem, isoniazid, erythromycin, clarithromycin, grapefruit juice (↓ dose may be necessary); History of suicide attempt or alcohol/drug dependence, debilitated patients (↓ dose required); Pedi: Safety and efficacy not established. Decreased dosage and frequent monitoring required; Geri: Elderly patients have increased sensitivity to benzodiazepines. Appears on Beers list and is associated with increased risk of falls (↓ dose required) and excessive CNS effects.

Adverse Reactions/Side Effects
CNS: dizziness, drowsiness, lethargy, confusion, hangover, headache, mental depression, paradoxical excitation. **EENT:** blurred vision. **GI:** constipation, diarrhea, nausea, vomiting, weight gain. **Derm:** rashes. **Misc:** physical dependence, psychological dependence, tolerance.

Interactions
Drug-Drug: Alcohol, **antidepressants**, other **benzodiazepines**, **antihistamines**, and **opioid analgesics**—concurrent use results in ↑ CNS depression. **Hormonal contraceptives**, **disulfiram**, **fluoxetine**, **isoniazid**, **metoprolol**, **propoxyphene**, **propranolol**, **valproic acid**, **CYP3A4 inhibitors** (**erythromycin**, **ketoconazole**, **itraconazole**, **fluvoxamine**, **cimetidine**, **nefazodone**) ↓ metabolism of alprazolam, ↑ blood levels and ↑ its actions (dose adjustments may be necessary). May ↓ efficacy of **levodopa**. **CYP3A4 inducers** (**rifampin**, **carbamazepine**, or **barbiturates**) ↑ metabolism and ↓ effects of alprazolam. Sedative effects may be ↓ by **theophylline**. Cigarette smoking ↓ blood levels and effects.
Drug-Natural Products: Kava-kava, valerian, or chamomile can ↑ CNS depression.
Drug-Food: Concurrent ingestion of **grapefruit juice** ↑ blood levels.

Route/Dosage

Anxiety
PO (Adults): 0.25–0.5 mg 2–3 times daily (not >4 mg/day; begin with 0.25 mg 2–3 times daily in geriatric/debilitated patients).

Panic Attacks
PO (Adults): 0.5 mg 3 times daily; may be increased by 1 mg or less every 3–4 days as needed (not >10 mg/day). *Extended–release tablets (Xanax XR)*—0.5–1 mg once daily in the morning, may be increased every 3–4 days by not more than 1 mg/day; up to 10 mg/day (usual range 3–6 mg/day).

Availability (generic available)
Tablets: 0.25 mg, 0.5 mg, 1 mg, 2 mg. **Cost:** 0.25 mg $98.21/100, 0.5 mg $122.35/100, 1 mg $163.25/100, 2 mg $277.56/100. **Extended-release tablets:** 0.5 mg, 1 mg, 2 mg, 3 mg. **Orally disintegrating tablets (orange):** 0.25 mg, 0.5 mg, 1 mg, 2 mg.

NURSING IMPLICATIONS

Assessment
- Assess degree and manifestations of anxiety and mental status (orientation, mood, behavior) prior to and periodically during therapy.
- Assess patient for drowsiness, light-headedness, and dizziness. These symptoms usually disappear as therapy progresses. Dose should be reduced if these symptoms persist.
- Geri: Assess CNS effects and risk of falls. Institute falls prevention strategies.
- Prolonged high-dose therapy may lead to psychological or physical dependence. Risk is greater in patients taking >4 mg/day. Restrict the amount of drug available to patient. Assess regularly for continued need for treatment.
- **Lab Test Considerations:** Monitor CBC and liver and renal function periodically during long-term therapy. May cause ↓ hematocrit and neutropenia.
- ***Toxicity and Overdose:*** Flumazenil is the antidote for alprazolam toxicity or overdose. (Flumazenil may induce seizures in patients with a history of seizures disorder or who are on tricyclic antidepressants.)

Potential Nursing Diagnoses
Anxiety (Indications)
Risk for injury (Side Effects)
Risk for falls (Side Effects)

Implementation
- Do not confuse Xanax (alprazolam) with Zantac (ranitidine).
- If early morning anxiety or anxiety between doses occurs, the same total daily dose should be divided into more frequent intervals.
- **PO:** May be administered with food if GI upset occurs. Administer greatest dose at bedtime to avoid daytime sedation.
- Tablets may be crushed and taken with food or fluids if patient has difficulty swallowing. Do not crush, break, or chew extended-release tablets.
- Taper by 0.5 mg q 3 days to prevent withdrawal. Some patients may require longer tapering period (months).
- For *orally disintegrating tablets:* Remove tablet from bottle with dry hands just prior to taking medication. Place tablet on tongue. Tablet will dissolve with saliva; may also be taken with water. Remove cotton from bottle and reseal tightly to prevent moisture from entering bottle. If only ½ tablet taken, discard unused portion immediately; may not remain stable.

Patient/Family Teaching
- Instruct patient to take medication exactly as directed; do not skip or double up on missed doses. If a dose is missed, take within 1 hr; otherwise, skip the dose and return to regular schedule. If medication is less effective after a few weeks, check with health care professional; do not increase dose. Abrupt withdrawal may cause sweating, vomiting, muscle cramps, tremors, and seizures.
- May cause drowsiness or dizziness. Caution patient to avoid driving and other activities requiring alertness until response to the medication is known. Geri: Instruct patient and family how to reduce falls risk at home.
- Advise patient to avoid drinking grapefruit juice during therapy.
- Advise patient to avoid the use of alcohol or other CNS depressants concurrently with alprazolam. Instruct patient to consult health care professional before taking Rx, OTC, or herbal products concurrently with this medication.
- Inform patient that benzodiazepines are usually prescribed for short-term use and do not cure underlying problems.
- Teach other methods to decrease anxiety (exercise, support group, relaxation techniques).
- Advise patient to not share medication with anyone.

Evaluation/Desired Outcomes
- Decreased sense of anxiety without CNS side effects.
- Decreased frequency and severity of panic attacks.
- Decreased symptoms of premenstrual syndrome.

alteplase, See THROMBOLYTIC AGENTS.

aluminum hydroxide
AlternaGEL, Alu-Cap, ✹ Alugel, Aluminet, Alu-Tab, Amphojel, Basalgel, Dialume

Classification
Therapeutic: antiulcer agents, hypophosphatemics
Pharmacologic: antacids, phosphate binders

Pregnancy Category UK

Indications
Lowering of phosphate levels in patients with chronic renal failure. Adjunctive therapy in the treatment of peptic, duodenal, and gastric ulcers. Hyperacidity, indigestion, reflux esophagitis.

Action
Binds phosphate in the GI tract. Neutralizes gastric acid and inactivates pepsin. **Therapeutic Effects:** Lowering of serum phosphate levels. Healing of ulcers and decreased pain associated with ulcers or gastric hyperacidity. Constipation limits use alone in the treatment of ulcer disease. Frequently found in combination with magnesium-containing compounds.

Pharmacokinetics
Absorption: With chronic use, small amounts of aluminum are systemically absorbed.
Distribution: If absorbed, aluminum distributes widely, crosses the placenta, and enters breast milk. Concentrates in the CNS with chronic use.
Metabolism and Excretion: Mostly excreted in feces. Small amounts absorbed are excreted by the kidneys.
Half-life: Unknown.

TIME/ACTION PROFILE

ROUTE	ONSET	PEAK	DURATION
PO†	hr–days	days–wk	days
PO‡	15–30 min	30 min	30 min–3 hr

†Hypophosphatemic effect
‡Antacid effect

Contraindications/Precautions
Contraindicated in: Severe abdominal pain of unknown cause.
Use Cautiously in: Hypercalcemia; Hypophosphatemia; OB: Generally considered safe; chronic high-dose therapy should be avoided.

Adverse Reactions/Side Effects
GI: constipation. **F and E:** hypophosphatemia.

Interactions
Drug-Drug: Absorption of **tetracyclines, chlorpromazine, iron salts, isoniazid, digoxin,** or **fluoroquinolones** may be decreased. **Salicylate** blood levels may be decreased. **Quinidine, mexiletine,** and **amphetamine** levels may be increased if enough antacid is ingested such that urine pH is increased.

Route/Dosage
Hypophosphatemia
PO (Adults): 1.9–4.8 g (30–40 mL of regular suspension or 15–20 mL of concentrated suspension) 3–4 times daily.
PO (Children): 50–150 mg/kg/24 hr in 4–6 divided doses; titrate to normal serum phosphate levels.

Antacid
PO (Adults): 500–1500 mg (5–30 mL) 3–6 times daily.

Availability (generic available)
Capsules: 475 mg^{OTC}, 500 mg^{OTC}. **Tablets:** 300 mg^{OTC}, 500 mg^{OTC}, 600 mg^{OTC}. **Suspension:** 320 mg/5 mL^{OTC}, 450 mg/5 mL^{OTC}, 600 mg/5 mL^{OTC}, 675 mg/5 mL^{OTC}. **In combination with:** magnesium carbonate, calcium carbonate, simethicone, and mineral oil. See Appendix B.

NURSING IMPLICATIONS
Assessment
- Assess location, duration, character, and precipitating factors of gastric pain.
- *Lab Test Considerations:* Monitor serum phosphate and calcium levels periodically during chronic use of aluminum hydroxide.
- May cause increased serum gastrin and decreased serum phosphate concentrations.
- In treatment of severe ulcer disease, guaiac stools, and emesis, monitor pH of gastric secretions.

Potential Nursing Diagnoses
Acute pain (Indications)
Constipation (Side Effects)

Implementation
- Antacids cause premature dissolution and absorption of enteric-coated tablets and may interfere with absorption of other oral medications. Separate administration of aluminum hydroxide and oral medications by at least 1–2 hr.

- Tablets must be chewed thoroughly before swallowing to prevent their entering small intestine in undissolved form. Follow with a glass of water.
- Shake liquid preparations well before pouring. Follow administration with water to ensure passage into stomach.
- Liquid dosage forms are considered more effective than tablets.
- **Hypophosphatemic:** For phosphate lowering, follow dose with full glass of water or fruit juice.
- **Antacid:** May be given in conjunction with magnesium-containing antacids to minimize constipation, except in patients with renal failure. Administer 1 and 3 hr after meals and at bedtime for maximum antacid effect.
- For treatment of peptic ulcer, aluminum hydroxide may be administered every 1–2 hr while the patient is awake or diluted with 2–3 parts water and administered intragastrically every 30 min for 12 or more hr per day. Physician may order NG tube clamped after administration.
- For reflux esophagitis, administer 15 mL 20–40 min after meals and at bedtime.

Patient/Family Teaching
- Instruct patient to take aluminum hydroxide exactly as directed. If on a regular dosing schedule and a dose is missed, take as soon as remembered if not almost time for next dose; do not double doses.
- Advise patient not to take aluminum hydroxide within 1–2 hr of other medications without consulting health care professional.
- Advise patients to check label for sodium content. Patients with CHF or hypertension, or those on sodium restriction, should use low-sodium preparations.
- Inform patients of potential for constipation from aluminum hydroxide.
- **Hypophosphatemia:** Patients taking aluminum hydroxide for hyperphosphatemia should be taught the importance of a low-phosphate diet.
- **Antacid:** Caution patient to consult health care professional before taking antacids for more than 2 wk if problem is recurring, if taking other medications, if relief is not obtained, or if symptoms of gastric bleeding (black tarry stools, coffee-ground emesis) occur.

Evaluation/Desired Outcomes
- Decrease in serum phosphate levels.
- Decrease in GI pain and irritation.
- Increase in the pH of gastric secretions. In treatment of peptic ulcer, antacid therapy should be continued for at least 4–6 wk after symptoms have disappeared because there is no correlation between disappearance of symptoms and healing of ulcers.

amcinonide, See CORTICOSTEROIDS (TOPICAL/LOCAL).

amifostine (a-mi-fos-teen)
Ethyol

Classification
Therapeutic: cytoprotective agents

Pregnancy Category C

Indications
Reduces renal toxicity from cisplatin. Reduces the incidence of moderate to severe xerostomia from postoperative radiation for head and neck cancer in which the radiation port includes a large portion of the parotid glands.

Action
Converted by alkaline phosphatase in tissue to a free thiol compound that binds and detoxifies damaging metabolites of cisplatin and reactive oxygen species generated by radiation. **Therapeutic Effects:** Decreased renal damage from cisplatin. Decreased severity of xerostomia following radiation for head and neck cancer.

Pharmacokinetics
Absorption: IV administration results in complete bioavailability.
Distribution: Unknown.
Metabolism and Excretion: Rapidly cleared from plasma; converted to cytoprotective compounds by alkaline phosphatase in tissues.
Half-life: 8 min.

TIME/ACTION PROFILE

ROUTE	ONSET	PEAK	DURATION
IV	unknown	unknown	unknown

Contraindications/Precautions
Contraindicated in: Known sensitivity to aminothiol compounds; Hypotension or dehydration;

amifostine

Lactation: Use an alternative to breast milk; Concurrent antineoplastic therapy for other tumors (especially malignancies of germ cell origin).
Use Cautiously in: OB, Pedi: Safety not established; Geri: Geriatric patients or patients with cardiovascular disease have ↑ risk of adverse reactions.

Adverse Reactions/Side Effects
CNS: dizziness, somnolence. **EENT:** sneezing. **CV:** hypotension. **GI:** hiccups, nausea, vomiting. **Derm:** flushing. **F and E:** hypocalcemia. **Misc:** allergic reactions including ANAPHYLAXIS, STEVENS-JOHNSON SYNDROME, TOXIC EPIDERMAL NECROLYSIS, TOXODERMA, ERYTHEMA MULTIFORMA, EXFOLIATIVE DERMATITIS (↑ when used as a radioprotectant), chills.

Interactions
Drug-Drug: Concurrent use of **antihypertensives** ↑ risk of hypotension.

Route/Dosage

Reduction of Renal Damage with Cisplatin
IV (Adults): 910 mg/m^2 once daily, within 30 min before chemotherapy; if full dose is poorly tolerated, subsequent doses should be ↓ to 740 mg/m^2.

Reduction of Xerostomia from Radiation
IV (Adults): 200 mg/m^2 once daily, as a 3-minute infusion starting 15–30 min before standard fraction radiation therapy.

Availability (generic available)
Powder for injection: 500 mg/vial.

NURSING IMPLICATIONS

Assessment
- Monitor blood pressure before and every 5 min during infusion. Discontinue antihypertensives 24 hr prior to treatment. If significant hypotension requiring interruption of therapy occurs, place patient in Trendelenburg position and administer an infusion of 0.9% NaCl using a separate IV line. If blood pressure returns to normal in 5 min and patient is asymptomatic, infusion may be resumed so that full dose may be given.
- Assess fluid status before administration. Correct dehydration before instituting therapy. Nausea and vomiting are frequent and may be severe. Administer prophylactic antiemetics including dexamethasone 20 mg IV and a serotonin-antagonist antiemetic (dolasetron, granisetron, ondansetron, palonosetron) before and during infusion. Monitor fluid status closely.
- Observe patient for signs and symptoms of anaphylaxis (rash, pruritus, laryngeal edema, wheezing). Discontinue the drug and notify physician or other health care professional immediately if these problems occur. Keep epinephrine, an antihistamine, and resuscitation equipment close by in case of an anaphylactic reaction.
- **Xerostomia:** Assess patient for dry mouth and mouth sores periodically during therapy.
- Monitor patient for skin reactions before, during, and after amifostine administration; reactions may be delayed by several weeks after initiation of therapy. Permanently discontinue amifostine in patients who experience serious or severe cutaneous reactions or cutaneous reactions associated with fever or other symptoms of unknown cause. Withhold therapy and obtain dermatologic consultation and biopsy for cutaneous reactions or mucosal lesions of unknown cause appearing outside of injection site or radiation port, and for erythematous, edematous, or bullous lesions on the palms of the hand or soles of the feet.
- ***Lab Test Considerations:*** Monitor serum calcium concentrations before and periodically during therapy. May cause hypocalcemia. Calcium supplements may be necessary.

Potential Nursing Diagnoses
Risk for injury (Indications)

Implementation

IV Administration

- **Intermittent Infusion: *Diluent:*** Reconstitute with 9.7 mL of sterile 0.9% NaCl. Dilute further with 0.9% NaCl. Do not administer solutions that are discolored or contain particulate matter. Solution is stable for 5 hr at room temperature or 24 hr if refrigerated. ***Concentration:*** Adults: dilute dose to a final volume of 50 mL; Children: 5–40 mg/mL. ***Rate:*** *For renal toxicity:* Administer over 15 min within 30 min before chemotherapy administration. Longer infusion times are not as well tolerated. *For xerostomia:* Administer over 3 min starting 15–30 min prior to radiation therapy.
- **Y-Site Compatibility:** amikacin, aminophylline, amphotericin B liposome, ampicillin, ampicillin/sulbactam, aztreonam, bivalirudin, bleomycin, bumetanide, buprenorphine, butorphanol, calcium gluconate, carboplatin, carmustine, caspofungin, cefazolin, cefotaxime, cefotetan, cefoxitin, ceftazidime, ceftizoxime,

aminocaproic acid 143

ceftriaxone, cefuroxime, cimetidine, ciprofloxacin, clindamycin, cyclophosphamide, cytarabine, dacarbazine, dactinomycin, daptomycin, daunorubicin hydrochloride, dexamethasone, dexmedetomidine, diltiazem, diphenhydramine, dobutamine, docetaxel, dopamine, doxorubicin hydrochloride, doxycycline, droperidol, enalaprilat, epirubicin, ertapenem, etoposide, etoposide phosphate, famotidine, fenoldopam, floxuridine, fluconazole, fludarabine, fluorouracil, furosemide, gemcitabine, gentamicin, granisetron, haloperidol, heparin, hydrocortisone, hydromorphone, idarubicin, ifosfamide, imipenem/cilastatin, leucovorin, levofloxacin, linezolid, lorazepam, magnesium sulfate, mannitol, mechlorethamine, meperidine, mesna, methotrexate, methylprednisolone, metoclopramide, metronidazole, milrinone, mitomycin, morphine, nalbuphine, nesiritide, octreotide, ondansetron, oxaliplatin, paclitaxel, palonosetron, pantoprazole, pemetrexed, piperacillin/tazobactam, plicamycin, potassium chloride, promethazine, ranitidine, rituximab, sodium acetate, sodium bicarbonate, streptozocin, tacrolimus, teniposide, thiotepa, ticarcillin/clavulanate, tigecycline, tirofiban, tobramycin, trastuzumab, trimethoprim/sulfamethoxazole, trimetrexate, vancomycin, vasopressin, vecuronium, vinblastine, vincristine, vinorelbine, voriconazole, zidovudine.

- **Y-Site Incompatibility:** acyclovir, amphotericin B colloidal, cefoperazone, cisplatin, ganciclovir, hydroxyzine, minocycline, prochlorperazine, quinupristin/dalfopristin.

- **Additive Incompatibility:** Do not mix with other solutions or medications.

Patient/Family Teaching
- Explain the purpose of amifostine infusion to patient.
- Inform patient that amifostine may cause hypotension, nausea, vomiting, flushing, chills, dizziness, somnolence, hiccups, and sneezing.
- Advise patient to notify health care professional if skin reactions occur.

Evaluation/Desired Outcomes
- Prevention of renal toxicity associated with repeated administration of cisplatin in patients with ovarian cancer.
- Decreased severity of xerostomia from radiation treatment of head and neck cancer.

amikacin, See AMINOGLYCOSIDES.

amiloride, See DIURETICS (POTASSIUM-SPARING).

aminocaproic acid
(a-mee-noe-ka-**pro**-ik)
Amicar, epsilon aminocaproic acid

Classification
Therapeutic: hemostatic agents
Pharmacologic: fibrinolysis inhibitors

Pregnancy Category C

Indications
Management of acute, life-threatening hemorrhage due to systemic hyperfibrinolysis or urinary fibrinolysis. **Unlabeled Use:** Prevention of recurrent subarachnoid hemorrhage. Prevention of bleeding following oral surgery in hemophiliacs. Management of severe hemorrhage caused by thrombolytic agents.

Action
Inhibits activation of plasminogen. **Therapeutic Effects:** Inhibition of fibrinolysis. Stabilization of clot formation.

Pharmacokinetics
Absorption: Rapidly absorbed following oral administration.
Distribution: Widely distributed.
Metabolism and Excretion: Mostly eliminated unchanged by the kidneys.
Half-life: Unknown.

TIME/ACTION PROFILE (peak blood levels)

ROUTE	ONSET	PEAK	DURATION
PO	unknown	2 hr	N/A
IV	unknown	2 hr	N/A

Contraindications/Precautions
Contraindicated in: Active intravascular clotting.
Use Cautiously in: Upper urinary tract bleeding; Cardiac, renal, or liver disease (dosage reduction may be required); Disseminated intravascular coagulation (should be used concurrently with heparin); OB, Lactation: Safety not established; Pedi: Do not use products containing benzyl alcohol with neonates.

✱ = Canadian drug name. ⚕ = Genetic implication.
*CAPITALS indicates life-threatening; underlines indicate most frequent.

Adverse Reactions/Side Effects
CNS: dizziness, malaise. **EENT:** nasal stuffiness, tinnitus. **CV:** arrhythmias, hypotension (IV only). **GI:** anorexia, bloating, cramping, diarrhea, nausea. **GU:** diuresis, renal failure. **MS:** myopathy.

Interactions
Drug-Drug: Concurrent use with **estrogens, conjugated** may result in a hypercoagulable state. Concurrent use with **clotting factors** may ↑ risk of thromboses.

Route/Dosage

Acute Bleeding Syndromes due to Elevated Fibrinolytic Activity
PO (Adults): 5 g 1st hr, followed by 1–1.25 g q hr for 8 hr or until hemorrhage is controlled; or 6 g over 24 hr after prostate surgery (not >30 g/day).
IV (Adults): 4–5 g over 1st hr, followed by 1 g/hr for 8 hr or until hemorrhage is controlled; or 6 g over 24 hr after prostate surgery (not >30 g/day).
PO, IV (Children): 100 mg/kg or 3 g/m^2 over 1st hr, followed by continuous infusion of 33.3 mg/kg/hr; or 1 g/m^2/hr (total dosage not >18 g/m^2/24 hr).

Subarachnoid Hemorrhage
PO (Adults): *To follow IV*—3 g q 2 hr (36 g/day). If no surgery is performed, continue for 21 days after bleeding stops, then decrease to 2 g q 2 hr (24 g/day) for 3 days, then 1 g q 2 hr (12 g/day) for 3 days.
IV (Adults): 36 g/day for 10 days followed by PO.

Prevention of Bleeding Following Oral Surgery in Hemophiliacs
PO (Adults): 75 mg/kg (up to 6 g) immediately after procedure, then q 6 hr for 7–10 days; syrup may also be used as an oral rinse of 1.25 g (5 mL) 4 times a day for 7–10 days.
IV, PO (Children): *Also for epistaxis*—50–100 mg/kg/dose administered IV every 6 hr for 2–3 days starting 4 hr before the procedure. After completion of IV therapy, aminocaproic acid should be given as 50–100 mg/kg/dose orally every 6 hr for 5–7 days.

Availability
Tablets: 500 mg. **Syrup (raspberry flavor):** 1.25 g/5 mL. **Injection:** 250 mg/mL.

NURSING IMPLICATIONS

Assessment
- Monitor blood pressure, pulse, and respiratory status as indicated by severity of bleeding.
- Monitor for overt bleeding every 15–30 min.
- Monitor neurologic status (pupils, level of consciousness, motor activity) in patients with subarachnoid hemorrhage.
- Monitor intake and output ratios frequently; notify physician if significant discrepancies occur.
- Assess for thromboembolic complications (especially in patients with history). Notify physician of positive Homans' sign, leg pain and edema, hemoptysis, dyspnea, or chest pain.
- *Lab Test Considerations:* Monitor platelet count and clotting factors prior to and periodically throughout therapy in patients with systemic fibrinolysis.
- ↑ CPK, AST, and serum aldolase may indicate myopathy.
- May ↑ serum potassium.

Potential Nursing Diagnoses
Ineffective tissue perfusion (Indications)
Risk for injury (Indications, Side Effects)

Implementation
- Do not confuse Amicar (aminocaproic acid) with Amikin (amikacin).
- **PO:** Syrup may be used as an oral rinse, swished for 30 sec 4 times/day for 7–10 days for the control of bleeding during dental and oral surgery in hemophilic patients. Small amounts may be swallowed, except during 1st and 2nd trimesters of pregnancy. Syrup may be applied with an applicator in children or unconscious patients.

IV Administration
- **IV:** Stabilize IV catheter to minimize thrombophlebitis. Monitor site closely.
- **Intermittent Infusion:** *Diluent:* Do not administer undiluted. Dilute initial 4–5 g dose in 250 mL of sterile water for injection, 0.9% NaCl, D5W, or LR. Do not dilute with sterile water in patients with subarachnoid hemorrhage. *Concentration:* 20 mg/mL. *Rate:* Single doses: Administer over 1 hr. Rapid infusion rate may cause hypotension, bradycardia, or other arrhythmias.
- **Continuous Infusion:** Administer IV solution using infusion pump to ensure accurate dose. Administer via slow IV infusion.
- *Rate:* Initial dose may be followed by a continuous infusion of 1–1.25 g/hr in adults or 33.3 mg/kg/hr in children.
- **Additive Incompatibility:** Do not admix with other medications.

Patient/Family Teaching
- Instruct patient to notify the nurse immediately if bleeding recurs or if thromboembolic symptoms develop.
- IV: Caution patient to make position changes slowly to avoid orthostatic hypotension.

Evaluation/Desired Outcomes
- Cessation of bleeding.
- Prevention of rebleeding in subarachnoid hemorrhage without occurrence of undesired clotting.

AMINOGLYCOSIDES

amikacin (am-i-**kay**-sin)

gentamicin† (jen-ta-**mye**-sin)
♣ Cidomycin, Garamycin, G-Mycin, Jenamicin

kanamycin (kan-a-**mye**-sin)

neomycin (neo-oh-**mye**-sin)
Neo-Fradin

streptomycin (strep-toe-**mye**-sin)

tobramycin† (toe-bra-**mye**-sin)
Nebcin, TOBI

Classification
Therapeutic: anti-infectives
Pharmacologic: aminoglycosides

Pregnancy Category C (gentamicin, topical use of others), D (amikacin, kanamycin, neomycin, streptomycin, tobramycin)

†See Appendix C for ophthalmic use

Indications
Amikacin, gentamicin, kanamycin, and tobramycin: Treatment of serious gram-negative bacillary infections and infections caused by staphylococci when penicillins or other less toxic drugs are contraindicated. **Streptomycin:** In combination with other agents in the management of active tuberculosis. **Neomycin:** Used orally to prepare the GI tract for surgery, to decrease the number of ammonia-producing bacteria in the gut as part of the management of hepatic encephalopathy, and to treat diarrhea caused by *Escherichia coli*. **Tobramycin by inhalation:** Management of *Pseudomonas aeruginosa* in cystic fibrosis patients. **Gentamicin, streptomycin:** In combination with other agents in the management of serious enterococcal infections. **Gentamicin IV:** Prevention of infective endocarditis. **Gentamicin (topical):** Treatment of localized infections caused by susceptible organisms. **Unlabeled Use:** Amikacin: In combination with other agents in the management of *Mycobacterium avium* complex infections.

Action
Inhibits protein synthesis in bacteria at level of 30S ribosome. **Therapeutic Effects:** Bactericidal action. **Spectrum:** Most aminoglycosides notable for activity against: *P. aeruginosa, Klebsiella pneumoniae, E.coli, Proteus, Serratia, Acinetobacter, Staphylococcus aureus*. In treatment of enterococcal infections, synergy with a penicillin is required. Streptomycin and amikacin also active against *Mycobacterium*.

Pharmacokinetics
Absorption: Well absorbed after IM administration. IV administration results in complete bioavailability. Some absorption follows administration by other routes. Minimal systemic absorption with neomycin (may accumulate in patients with renal failure).
Distribution: Widely distributed throughout extracellular fluid; cross the placenta; small amounts enter breast milk. Poor penetration into CSF (↑ when meninges are inflamed).
Metabolism and Excretion: Excretion is >90% renal.
Half-life: 2–4 hr (↑ in renal impairment).

TIME/ACTION PROFILE (blood levels*)

ROUTE	ONSET	PEAK	DURATION
PO (neomycin)	rapid	1–4 hr	N/A
IM	rapid	30–90 min	6–24 hr
IV	rapid	15–30 min†	6–24 hr

*All parenterally administered aminoglycosides
†Postdistribution peak occurs 30 min after the end of a 30-min infusion and 15 min after the end of a 1-hr infusion

Contraindications/Precautions
Contraindicated in: Hypersensitivity to aminoglycosides; Most parenteral products contain bisulfites and should be avoided in patients with known intolerance; Pedi: Products containing benzyl alcohol should be avoided in neonates; Intestinal obstruction (neomycin only).
Use Cautiously in: Renal impairment (dose adjustments necessary; blood level monitoring useful in preventing ototoxicity and nephrotoxicity); Hearing impairment; Neuromuscular diseases

such as myasthenia gravis; Obese patients (dose should be based on ideal body weight); **OB:** Tobramycin and streptomycin may cause congenital deafness; Lactation: Safety not established; **Pedi:** Neonates have ↑ risk of neuromuscular blockade; difficulty in assessing auditory and vestibular function and immature renal function; Geri: Difficulty in assessing auditory and vestibular function and age-related renal impairment.

Adverse Reactions/Side Effects
CNS: ataxia, vertigo. **EENT:** ototoxicity (vestibular and cochlear). **GU:** nephrotoxicity. **GI:** *Neomycin*—diarrhea, nausea, vomiting. **F and E:** hypomagnesemia. **MS:** muscle paralysis (high parenteral doses). **Neuro:** ↑ neuromuscular blockade. **Resp:** apnea. **Misc:** hypersensitivity reactions.

Interactions
Drug-Drug: Inactivated by **penicillins** and **cephalosporins** when coadministered to patients with renal insufficiency. Possible respiratory paralysis after **inhalation anesthetics** or **neuromuscular blocking agents**. ↑ incidence of ototoxicity with **loop diuretics**. ↑ incidence of nephrotoxicity with other **nephrotoxic drugs**. Neomycin may ↑ anticoagulant effects of **warfarin**. Neomycin may ↓ absorption of **digoxin** and **methotrexate**.

Route/Dosage

Amikacin
IM, IV (Adults and Children): 5 mg/kg q 8 hr or 7.5 mg/kg q 12 hr (not to exceed 1.5 g/day). *Mycobacterium avium complex*—7.5–15 mg/kg/day divided q 12–24 hr.
IM, IV (Neonates): *Loading dose*—10 mg/kg; *Maintenance dose*—7.5 mg/kg q 12 hr.

Renal Impairment
IM, IV (Adults): *Loading dose*—7.5 mg/kg, further dosing based on blood level monitoring and renal function assessment.

Gentamicin
Many regimens are used; most involve dosing adjusted on the basis of blood level monitoring and assessment of renal function.
IM, IV (Adults): 1–2 mg/kg q 8 hr (up to 6 mg/kg/day in 3 divided doses); *Once-daily dosing (unlabeled)*—4–7 mg/kg q 24 hr.
IM, IV (Children > 5 yr): 2–2.5 mg/kg/dose q 8 hr; *Once daily*—5–7.5 mg/kg/dose q 24 hr; *Cystic fibrosis*—2.5–3.3 mg/kg/dose q 6–8 hr; *Hemodialysis*—1.25–1.75 mg/kg/dose postdialysis.
IM, IV (Children 1 mo-5 yr): 2.5 mg/kg/dose q 8 hr; *Once daily*—5–7.5 mg/kg/dose q 24 hr; *Cystic fibrosis*—2.5–3.3 mg/kg/dose q 6–8 hr; *Hemodialysis*—1.25–1.75 mg/kg/dose postdialysis.
IM, IV (Neonates full term and/or > 1 wk): *Weight <1200 g*—2.5 mg/kg/dose q 18–24 hr; *Weight 1200–2000 g*—2.5 mg/kg/dose q 8–12 hr; *Weight >2000 g*—2.5 mg/kg/dose q 8 hr; *ECMO*—2.5 mg/kg/dose q 18 hr, subsequent doses based on serum concentrations; *Once daily*—3.5–5 mg/kg/dose q 24 hr.
IM, IV (Neonates premature and/or ≤1 wk): *Weight <1000 g*—3.5 mg/kg/dose q 24 hr; *Weight 1000–1200 g*—2.5 mg/kg/dose q 18–24 hr; *Weight >1200 g*—2.5 mg/kg/dose q 12 hr; *Once daily*—3.5–4 mg/kg/dose q 24 hr.
IT (Adults): 4–8 mg/day.
IT (Infants >3 months and Children): 1–2 mg/day.
IT (Neonates): 1 mg/day.
Topical (Adults and Children >1 month): Apply cream or ointment 3–4 times daily.

Renal Impairment
IM, IV (Adults): Initial dose of 2 mg/kg. Subsequent doses/intervals based on blood level monitoring and renal function assessment.

Kanamycin
IM, IV (Adults and Children and Infants): 5 mg/kg q 8 hr *or* 7.5 mg/kg q 12 hr (not to exceed 15 mg/kg/day).
Inhaln (Adults): 250 mg 2–4 times daily.

Renal Impairment
IM, IV (Adults): 7.5 mg/kg; further dosing and intervals determined by blood level monitoring and assessment of renal function.

Neomycin
PO (Adults): *Preoperative intestinal antisepsis*—1 g q hr for 4 doses, then 1 g q 4 hr for 5 doses *or* 1 g at 1 PM, 2 PM, and 11 PM on day before surgery; *Hepatic encephalopathy*—1–3 g q 6 hr for 5–6 days; may be followed by 4 g/day chronically.
PO (Children): *Preoperative intestinal antisepsis*—15 mg/kg q 4 hr for 2 days *or* 25 mg/kg at 1 PM, 2 PM, and 11 PM on day before surgery; *Hepatic encephalopathy*—12.5–25 mg/kg q 6 hr for 5–6 days (maximum dose = 12 g/day).

Streptomycin
IM (Adults): *Tuberculosis*—1 g/day initially, decreased to 1 g 2–3 times weekly; *Other infections*—250 mg–1 g q 6 hr *or* 500 mg–2 g q 12 hr.

AMINOGLYCOSIDES 147

IM (Children): *Tuberculosis*—20 mg/kg/day (not to exceed 1 g/day); *Other infections*—5–10 mg/kg q 6 hr *or* 10–20 mg/kg q 12 hr.

Renal Impairment
IM (Adults): 1 g initially, further dosing determined by blood level monitoring and assessment of renal function.

Tobramycin
IM, IV (Adults): 1–2 mg/kg q 8 hr *or* 4–6.6 mg/kg/day q 24 hr.
IM, IV (Adults): 3–6 mg/kg/day in 3 divided doses, or 4–6.6 mg/kg once daily.
IM, IV (Children > 5 yr): 6–7.5 mg/kg/day divided q 8 hr, up to 13 mg/kg/day divided q 6–8 hr in cystic fibrosis patients (dosing interval may vary from q 6 hr–q 24 hr, depending on clinical situation).
IM, IV (Children 1 mo–5 yr): 7.5 mg/kg/day divided q 8 hr, up to 13 mg/kg/day divided q 6–8 hr in cystic fibrosis.
IM, IV (Neonates): *Preterm <1000 g*—3.5 mg/kg/dose q 24 hr; *0–4 weeks, <1200 g*—2.5 mg/kg/dose q 18 hr; *Postnatal age <7 days*—2.5 mg/kg/dose q 12 hr; *Postnatal age >7 days,1200–2000 g*—2.5 mg/kg/dose q 8–12 hr; *Postnatal age >7 days, >2000 g*—2.5 mg/kg/dose q 8 hr.
Inhaln (Adults and Children): Standard dose: 40–80 mg 2–3 times/day; High dose: 300 mg twice daily for 28 days, then off for 28 days, then repeat cycle.

Renal Impairment
IM, IV (Adults): 1 mg/kg initially, further dosing determined by blood level monitoring and assessment of renal function.

Availability
Amikacin (generic available)
Injection: 50 mg/mL, 250 mg/mL.

Gentamicin (generic available)
Injection: 10 mg/mL, 40 mg/mL. **Premixed injection:** 40 mg/50 mL, 60 mg/50 mL, 60 mg/100 mL, 70 mg/50 mL, 80 mg/50 mL, 80 mg/100 mL, 90 mg/100 mL, 100 mg/50 mL, 100 mg/100 mL, 120 mg/100 mL. **Topical cream:** 0.1%. **Topical ointment:** 0.1%.

Kanamycin (generic available)
Injection: 250 mg/mL, 333.3 mg/mL.

Neomycin (generic available)
Oral solution: 125 mg/5 mL. **Tablets:** 500 mg.
In combination with: other topical antibiotics or anti-inflammatory agents for skin, ear, and eye infections. See Appendix B.

Streptomycin (generic available)
Injection: ✢ 500 mg/mL, 1 g.

Tobramycin (generic available)
Injection: 10 mg/mL, 40 mg/mL, 1.2-g vial. **Nebulizer solution:** 300 mg/5 mL in 5-mL ampules.

NURSING IMPLICATIONS
Assessment
- Assess for infection (vital signs, wound appearance, sputum, urine, stool, WBC) at beginning of and throughout therapy.
- Obtain specimens for culture and sensitivity before initiating therapy. First dose may be given before receiving results.
- Evaluate eighth cranial nerve function by audiometry before and throughout therapy. Hearing loss is usually in the high-frequency range. Prompt recognition and intervention are essential in preventing permanent damage. Also monitor for vestibular dysfunction (vertigo, ataxia, nausea, vomiting). Eighth cranial nerve dysfunction is associated with persistently elevated peak aminoglycoside levels. Discontinue aminoglycosides if tinnitus or subjective hearing loss occurs.
- Monitor intake and output and daily weight to assess hydration status and renal function.
- Assess for signs of superinfection (fever, upper respiratory infection, vaginal itching or discharge, increasing malaise, diarrhea).
- **Hepatic Encephalopathy:** Monitor neurologic status. Before administering oral medication, assess patient's ability to swallow.
- *Lab Test Considerations:* Monitor renal function by urinalysis, specific gravity, BUN, creatinine, and CCr before and during therapy.
- May cause ↑ BUN, AST, ALT, serum alkaline phosphatase, bilirubin, creatinine, and LDH concentrations.
- May cause ↓ serum calcium, magnesium, potassium, and sodium concentrations (streptomycin and tobramycin).
- *Toxicity and Overdose:* Monitor blood levels periodically during therapy. Timing of blood levels is important in interpreting results. Draw blood for peak levels 1 hr after IM injection and 30 min after a 30-min IV infusion is

✢ = Canadian drug name. ⚕ = Genetic implication.
*CAPITALS indicates life-threatening; underlines indicate most frequent.

148 AMINOGLYCOSIDES

completed. Draw trough levels just before next dose. Peak level for **amikacin** and **kanamycin** is 20–30 mcg/mL; trough level should be <10 mcg/mL. Peak level for **gentamicin** and **tobramycin** should not exceed 10 mcg/mL; trough level should not exceed 2 mcg/mL. Peak level for **streptomycin** should not exceed 25 mcg/mL.

Potential Nursing Diagnoses
Risk for infection (Indications)
Disturbed sensory perception (auditory) (Side Effects)

Implementation
Keep patient well hydrated (1500–2000 mL/day) during therapy.

- **Preoperative Bowel Prep:** Neomycin is usually used in conjunction with erythromycin, a low-residue diet, and a cathartic or enema.
- **PO:** Neomycin may be administered without regard to meals.
- **IM:** IM administration should be deep into a well-developed muscle. Alternate injection sites.
- **IV:** If aminoglycosides and penicillins or cephalosporins must be administered concurrently, administer in separate sites, at least 1 hr apart.

Amikacin

IV Administration

- **Intermittent Infusion:** *Diluent:* Dilute with D5W, D10W, 0.9% NaCl, dextrose/saline combinations, or LR. Solution may be pale yellow without decreased potency. Stable for 24 hr at room temperature. *Concentration:* 10 mg/mL. *Rate:* Infuse over 30–60 min for adults and children and over 1–2 hr in infants.
- **Syringe Incompatibility:** heparin.
- **Y-Site Compatibility:** acyclovir, aldesleukin, alfentanil, amifostine, aminophylline, amiodarone, amsacrine, anidulafungin, ascorbic acid, atracurium, atropine, aztreonam, benztropine, bivalirudin, bumetanide, buprenorphine, butorphanol, calcium chloride, calcium gluconate, carboplatin, caspofungin, cefazolin, cefepime, cefonicid, cefotaxime, cefotetan, cefoxitin, ceftazidime, ceftizoxime, ceftriaxone, cefuroxime, chloramphenicol, chlorpromazine, cimetidine, cisatracurium, cisplatin, clindamycin, codeine, cyanocobalamin, cyclophosphamide, cyclosporine, cytarabine, dactinomycin, daptomycin, dexamethasone, dexmedetomidine, digoxin, diltiazem, diphenhydramine, dobutamine, docetaxel, dopamine, doripenem, doxacurium, doxorubicin hydrochloride, doxycycline, eftifibatide, enalaprilat, ephedrine, epinephrine, epirubicin, epoetin alfa, ertapenem, erythromycin, esmolol, etoposide, etoposide phosphate, famotidine, fentanyl, filgrastim, fluconazole, fludarabine, fluorouracil, foscarnet, furosemide, gemcitabine, gentamicin, glycopyrrolate, granisetron, hydrocortisone, hydromorphone, idarubicin, ifosfamide, imipenem/cilastatin, isoproterenol, ketorolac, labetalol, levofloxacin, lidocaine, linezolid, lorazepam, magnesium sulfate, mannitol, mechlorethamine, melphalan, meperidine, metaraminol, methotrexate, methoxamine, methyldopate, methylprednisolone, metoclopramide, metoprolol, metronidazole, midazolam, milrinone, mitoxantrone, morphine, multivitamins, nafcillin, nalbuphine, naloxone, nicardipine, nitroglycerin, nitroprusside, norepinephrine, octreotide, ondansetron, oxaliplatin, oxytocin, paclitaxel, palonosetron, pantoprazole, papaverine, pemetrexed, penicillin G, pentazocine, perphenazine, phenobarbital, phentolamine, phenylephrine, phytonadione, piperacillin/tazobactam, potassium chloride, procainamide, prochlorperazine, promethazine, propranolol, protamine, pyridoxime, quinupristin/dalfopristin, ranitidine, remifentanil, rituximab, rocuronium, sargramostim, sodium acetate, sodium bicarbonate, strepotkinase, succinylcholine, sufentanil, tacrolimus, teniposide, theophylline, thiamine, thiotepa, ticarcillin/clavulanate, tigecycline, tirofiban, tobramycin, tolazoline, trimethaphan, urokinase, vancomycin, vasopressin, vecuronium, verapamil, vincristine, vinorelbine, voriconazole, warfarin, zidovudine.
- **Y-Site Incompatibility:** allopurinol, amophotericin B cholesteryl, amphotericin B colloidal, amphotericin B liposome, azathioprine, azithromycin, cefoperazone, dantrolene, diazepam, diazoxide, folic acid, ganciclovir, heparin, indomethacin, pentamidine, pentobarbital, phenytoin, propofol, trastuzumab, trimethoprim/sulfamethoxazole.
- **Additive Incompatibility:** Manufacturer does not recommend admixing.

Gentamicin

IV Administration

- **Intermittent Infusion:** *Diluent:* Dilute each dose with D5W, 0.9% NaCl, or LR. Do not use solutions that are discolored or that contain a precipitate. *Concentration:* 10 mg/mL. *Rate:* Infuse slowly over 30 min–2 hr.
- **Syringe Incompatibility:** ampicillin, heparin.

AMINOGLYCOSIDES

- **Y-Site Compatibility:** aldesleukin, alfentanil, alprostadil, amifostine, amikacin, aminophylline, amiodarone, amsacrine, anidulafungin, ascorbic acid, atracurium, atropine, aztreonam, benztropine, bivalirudin, bumetanide, buprenorphine, butorphanol, calcium chloride, calcium gluconate, carboplatin, caspofungin, chlorpromazine, cimetidine, ciprofloxacin, cisatracurium, cisplatin, clindamycin, codeine, cyanocobalamin, cyclophosphamide, cyclosporine, cytarabine, dactinomycin, daptomycin, dexmedetomidine, digoxin, diltiazem, diphenhydramine, dobutamine, docetaxel, dopamine, doripenem, doxacurium, doxapram, doxorubicin, doxorubicin liposome, doxycycline, enalaprilat, ephedrine, epinephrine, epirubicin, eftifibatide, epoetin alfa, ertapenem, erythromycin, esmolol, etoposide, etoposide phosphate, famotidine, fenoldopam, fentanyl, fluconazole, fludarabine, fluorouracil, foscarnet, gemcitabine, glycopyrrolate, granisetron, hydromorphone, ifosfamide, imipenem/cilastatin, isoproterenol, ketorolac, labetalol, levofloxacin, linezolid, lorazepam, magnesium sulfate, mannitol, mechlorethamine, melphalan, meperidine, meropenem, midazolam, metaraminol, methoxamine, methyldopate, methylprednisolone, metoclorpamide, metoprolol, metronidazole, midazolam, milrinone, mitoxantrone, morphine, multivitamins, nafcillin, nalbuphine, naloxone, nicardipine, nitroglycerin, nitroprusside, norepinephrine, octreotide, ondansetron, oxaliplatin, oxytocin, paclitaxel, palonosetron, pancuronium, pantoprazole, papaverine, penicillin G, pentazocine, perphenazine, phenobarbital, phentolamine, phenylephrine, phytonadione, potassium chloride, procainamide, prochlorperazine, promethazine, propranolol, protamine, pyridoxime, ranitidine, remifentanil, rituximab, rocuronium, sargramostim, sodium acetate, sodium bicarbonate, streptokinase, succinylcholine, sufentanil, tacrolimus, teniposide, theophylline, thiamine, thiotepa, ticarcillin/clavulanate, tigecycline, tirofiban, tobramycin, tolazoline, trastuzumab, trimetaphan, urokinase, vancomycin, vasopressin, vecuronium, verapamil, vinorelbine, vitamin B complex with C, voriconazole, zidovudine.
- **Y-Site Incompatibility:** allopurinol, amphotericin B chloesteryl, amphotericin B colloidal, amphotericin B liposome, azathioprine, azithromycin, cefoperazone, cefotetan, chloramphenicol, dantrolene, dexamethasone, diazepam, diazoxide, drotrecogin, folic acid, ganciclovir, heparin, idarubicin, indomethacin, methotrexate, pemetrexed, pentamidine, pentobarbital, phenytoin, propofol, trimethoprim/sulfamethoxazole, warfarin.

Kanamycin

IV Administration

- **Intermittent Infusion:** *Diluent:* Dilute each 500 mg in 100–200 mL or each 1 g in 200–400 mL of D5W, D10W, D5/0.9% NaCl, 0.9% NaCl, or LR. Dilute in a proportionately smaller volume for pediatric patients. Darkening of solution does not alter potency. *Concentration:* 2.5–5 mg/mL. *Rate:* Infuse slowly over 30–60 min.
- **Syringe Incompatibility:** heparin.
- **Y-Site Compatibility:** cyclophosphamide, epinephrine, furosemide, heparin, hydrocortisone, hydromorphone, magnesium sulfate, meperidine, morphine, perphenazine, potassium chloride, vitamin B complex with C.
- **Additive Incompatibility:** Manufacturer does not recommend admixing with other antibacterial agents.

Tobramycin

IV Administration

- **Intermittent Infusion:** *Diluent:* Dilute each dose of tobramycin in 50–100 mL of D5W, D10W, D5/0.9% NaCl, 0.9% NaCl, Ringer's or lactated Ringer's solution. *Concentration:* not >10 mg/mL. Pediatric doses may be diluted in proportionately smaller amounts. Stable for 24 hr at room temperature, 96 hr if refrigerated. *Rate:* Infuse slowly over 30–60 min in both adult and pediatric patients.
- **Syringe Incompatibility:** heparin.
- **Y-Site Compatibility:** acyclovir, aldesleukin, alfentanil, alprostadil, amifostine, aminophylline, amiodarone, amsacrine, anidulafungin, ascorbic acid, atracurium, atropine, aztreonam, bivalirudin, bretylium, bumetanide, buprenorphine, butorphanol, calcium chloride, calcium gluconate, carboplatin, caspofungin, chloramphenicol, cimetidine, ciprofloxacin, cisatracurium, cisplatin, clindamycin, cyanocobalamin, cyclophosphamide, cyclosporine, cytarabine, dactinomycin, daptomycin, dexmedetomidine, digoxin, diltiazem, diphenhyrdamine, dobutamine, docetaxel,

✦ = Canadian drug name. ✦ = Genetic implication.
*CAPITALS indicates life-threatening; underlines indicate most frequent.

AMINOGLYCOSIDES

dopamine, doripenem, doxacurium, doxorubicin hydrochloride, doxorubicin liposome, doxycycline, enalaprilat, ephedrine, epinephrine, epirubicin, epoetin alfa, ertapenem, esmolol, etoposide, etoposide phosphate, famotidine, fenoldopam, fentanyl, filgrastim, fluconazole, fludarabine, fluorouracil, foscarnet, furosemide, gemcitabine, gentamicin, glycopyrrolate, granisetron, hydromorphone, ifosfamide, imipenem/cilastatin, isoproterenol, ketorolac, labetalol, levofloxacin, lidocaine, linezolid, lorazepam, magnesium sulfate, mannitol, mechlorethamine, melphalan, meperidine, metaraminol, methcillin, methotrexate, methoxamine, methyldopate, methylprednisolone, metoclopramide, metoprolol, metronidazole, miconazole, midazolam, milrinone, minocycline, mitoxantrone, morphine, moxalactam, multiple vitamins, nafcillin, nalbuphine, naloxone, nicardipine, nitroglycerin, nitroprusside, norepinephrine, octreotide, ondansetron, oxaliplatin, oxytocin, paclitaxel, palonosetron, pantoprazole, papaverine, penicillin G, pentazocine, perphenazine, phenobarbital, phentolamine, phenylephrine, phytonadione, potassium chloride, procainamide, prochlorperazine, promethazine, propranolol, protamine, pyridoxine, quinapristin/dalfopristin, ranitidine, remifentanil, rituximab, rocuronium, sodium acetate, sodium bicarbonate, streptokinase, succinylcholine, sufentanil, tacrolimus, teniposide, theophylline, thiamine, thiotepa, ticarcillin/clavulanate, tigecycline, tirofiban, tolazoline, trastuzumab, trimethaphan, urokinase, vancomycin, vasopressin, vecuronium, verapamil, vincristine, vinorelbine, voriconazole, zidovudine.

- **Y-Site Incompatibility:** allopurinol, amphotericin B cholesteryl, amphotericin B colloidal, amphotericin B liposome, azathioprine, azithromycin, cefazolin, cefoperazone, cefotetan, ceftriaxone, dantrolene, dexamethasone, diazepam, diazoxide, drotrecogin, folic acid, ganciclovir, heparin, hetastarch, indomethacin, oxacillin, pemetrexed, pentamidine, pentobarbital, phenytoin, piperacillin/tazobactam, propofol, sargramostim, trimethoprim/sulfamethoxazole.
- **Additive Incompatibility:** Manufacturer recommends administering separately; do not admix.
- **Topical:** Cleanse skin before application. Wear gloves during application.

Patient/Family Teaching
- Instruct patient to report signs of hypersensitivity, tinnitus, vertigo, hearing loss, rash, dizziness, or difficulty urinating.
- Advise patient of the importance of drinking plenty of liquids.
- Teach patients with a history of rheumatic heart disease or valve replacement the importance of using antimicrobial prophylaxis before invasive medical or dental procedures.
- **PO:** Instruct patient to take neomycin as directed for full course of therapy. Take missed doses as soon as possible if not almost time for next dose; do not take double doses.
- Caution patient that neomycin may cause nausea, vomiting, or diarrhea.
- **Topical:** Instruct patient to wash affected skin gently and pat dry. Apply a thin film of ointment. Apply occlusive dressing only if directed by health care professional. Patient should assess skin and inform health care professional if skin irritation develops or infection worsens.
- **Inhaln:** Instruct patient to take inhalation twice daily as close to 12 hr apart as possible; not < 6 hr apart. Administer over 10–15 min period using a hand-held PARI LC PLUS reusable nebulizer with a *DeVilbiss Pulmo-Aide* compressor. Do not mix with dornase alpha in nebulizer. Instruct patient on multiple therapies to take others first and use tobramycin last. Tobramycin-induced bronchospasm may be reduced if tobramycin is administered after bronchodilators. Instruct patient to sit or stand upright during inhalation and breathe normally through mouthpiece of nebulizer. Nose clips may help patient breath through mouth. Advise patient to disinfect the nebulizer parts (except tubing) by boiling them in water for a full 10 minutes every other treatment day.

Evaluation/Desired Outcomes
- Resolution of the signs and symptoms of infection. If no response is seen within 3–5 days, new cultures should be taken.
- Prevention of infection in intestinal surgery (neomycin).
- Improved neurologic status in hepatic encephalopathy (neomycin).
- Endocarditis prophylaxis (gentamicin).

aminophylline, See **BRONCHODILATORS (XANTHINES).**

amiodarone **151**

HIGH ALERT

amiodarone
(am-ee-**oh**-da-rone)
Cordarone, Nexterone, Pacerone

Classification
Therapeutic: antiarrhythmics (class III)

Pregnancy Category D

Indications
Life-threatening ventricular arrhythmias unresponsive to less toxic agents. **Unlabeled Use:** **PO:** Management of supraventricular tachyarrhythmias. **IV:** As part of the Advanced Cardiac Life Support (ACLS) and Pediatric Advanced Life Support (PALS) guidelines for the management of ventricular fibrillation/pulseless ventricular tachycardia after cardiopulmonary resuscitation and defibrillation have failed; also for other life-threatening tachyarrhythmias.

Action
Prolongs action potential and refractory period. Inhibits adrenergic stimulation. Slows the sinus rate, increases PR and QT intervals, and decreases peripheral vascular resistance (vasodilation). **Therapeutic Effects:** Suppression of arrhythmias.

Pharmacokinetics
Absorption: Slowly and variably absorbed from the GI tract (35–65%). IV administration results in complete bioavailability.
Distribution: Distributed to and accumulates slowly in body tissues. Reaches high levels in fat, muscle, liver, lungs, and spleen. Crosses the placenta and enters breast milk.
Protein Binding: 96% bound to plasma proteins.
Metabolism and Excretion: Metabolized by the liver, excreted into bile. Minimal renal excretion. One metabolite has antiarrhythmic activity.
Half-life: 13–107 days.

TIME/ACTION PROFILE (suppression of ventricular arrhythmias)

ROUTE	ONSET	PEAK	DURATION
PO	2–3 days (up to 2–3 mo)	3–7 hr	wk–mos
IV	2 hr	3–7 hr	unknown

Contraindications/Precautions
Contraindicated in: Patients with cardiogenic shock; Severe sinus node dysfunction; 2nd- and 3rd-degree AV block; Bradycardia (has caused syncope unless a pacemaker is in place); Hypersensitivity to amiodarone or iodine; OB: Can cause fetal hypo- or hyperthyroidism; Lactation: Enters breast milk and can cause harm to the neonate; use an alternative to breast milk; Pedi: Safety not established; products containing benzyl alcohol should not be used in neonates.
Use Cautiously in: History of CHF; Thyroid disorders; Corneal refractive laser surgery; Severe pulmonary or liver disease; Geri: Initiate therapy at the low end of the dosing range due to ↓ hepatic, renal, or cardiac function; comorbid disease; or other drug therapy.

Adverse Reactions/Side Effects
CNS: confusional states, disorientation, hallucinations, dizziness, fatigue, malaise, headache, insomnia. **EENT:** corneal microdeposits, abnormal sense of smell, dry eyes, optic neuritis, optic neuropathy, photophobia. **Resp:** ADULT RESPIRATORY DISTRESS SYNDROME (ARDS), PULMONARY FIBROSIS, PULMONARY TOXICITY. **CV:** CHF, WORSENING OF ARRHYTHMIAS, bradycardia, hypotension. **GI:** anorexia, constipation, nausea, vomiting, abdominal pain, abnormal sense of taste, liver function abnormalities. **GU:** decreased libido, epididymitis. **Derm:** TOXIC EPIDERMAL NECROLYSIS (rare), photosensitivity, blue discoloration. **Endo:** hypothyroidism, hyperthyroidism. **Neuro:** ataxia, involuntary movement, paresthesia, peripheral neuropathy, poor coordination, tremor.

Interactions
Drug-Drug: ↑ risk of QT prolongation with **fluoroquinolones**, **macrolides**, and **azole antifungals** (undertake concurrent use with caution). ↑ levels of **digoxin** (↓ dose of digoxin by 50%). ↑ levels of **class I antiarrhythmics** (**quinidine**, **mexiletine**, **lidocaine**, or **flecainide**— ↓ doses of other drugs by 30–50%). ↑ levels of **cyclosporine**, **dextromethorphan**, **methotrexate**, **phenytoin**, **carvedilol**, and **theophylline**. **Phenytoin** ↓ amiodarone levels. ↑ activity of **warfarin** (↓ dose of warfarin by 33–50%). ↑ risk of bradyarrhythmias, sinus arrest, or AV heart block with **beta blockers** or **calcium channel blockers**. **Cholestyramine** may ↓ amiodarone levels. **Cimetidine** and **ritonavir** ↑ amiodarone levels. Risk of myocardial depression is ↑ by **volatile anesthetics**. ↑ risk of myopathy with **lovastatin** and **simvastatin** (do not exceed 40 mg/day of regular-release

✦ = Canadian drug name. ☰ = Genetic implication.
*CAPITALS indicates life-threatening; underlines indicate most frequent.

amiodarone

lovastatin, 20 mg/day of extended-release lovastatin, or 20 mg/day of simvastatin).

Drug-Natural Products: St. John's wort induces enzymes that metabolize amiodarone; may ↓ levels and effectiveness. Avoid concurrent use.

Drug-Food: Grapefruit juice inhibits enzymes in the GI tract that metabolize amiodarone resulting in ↑ levels and risk of toxicity; avoid concurrent use.

Route/Dosage
Ventricular Arrhythmias
PO (Adults): 800–1600 mg/day in 1–2 doses for 1–3 wk, then 600–800 mg/day in 1–2 doses for 1 mo, then 400 mg/day maintenance dose.

PO (Children): 10 mg/kg/day (800 mg/1.72 m^2/day) for 10 days or until response or adverse reaction occurs, then 5 mg/kg/day (400 mg/1.72 m^2/day) for several weeks, then decreased to 2.5 mg/kg/day (200 mg/1.72 m^2/day) or lowest effective maintenance dose.

IV (Adults): 150 mg over 10 min, followed by 360 mg over the next 6 hr and then 540 mg over the next 18 hr. Continue infusion at 0.5 mg/min until oral therapy is initiated. If arrhythmia recurs, a small loading infusion of 150 mg over 10 min should be given; in addition, the rate of the maintenance infusion may be increased. *Conversion to initial oral therapy*—If duration of IV infusion was <1 wk, oral dose should be 800–1600 mg/day; if IV infusion was 1–3 wk, oral dose should be 600–800 mg/day; if IV infusion was >3 wk, oral dose should be 400 mg/day. *ACLS guidelines for pulseless VFib/VTach*—300 mg IV push, may repeat once after 3–5 min with 150 mg IV push (maximum cumulative dose 2.2 g/24 hr; unlabeled).

IV: Intraosseous (Children and infants): *PALS guidelines for pulseless VFib/VTach*—5 mg/kg as a bolus; *perfusion tachycardia*—5 mg/kg loading dose over 20–60 min (maximum of 15 mg/kg/day; unlabeled).

Supraventricular Tachycardia
PO (Adults): 600–800 mg/day for 1 wk or until desired response occurs or side effects develop, then decrease to 400 mg/day for 3 wk, then maintenance dose of 200–400 mg/day.

PO (Children): 10 mg/kg/day (800 mg/1.72 m^2/day) for 10 days or until response or side effects occur, then 5 mg/kg/day (400 mg/1.72 m^2/day) for several weeks, then decreased to 2.5 mg/kg/day (200 mg/1.72 m^2/day) or lowest effective maintenance dose.

Availability (generic available)
Tablets: 200 mg, 400 mg. **Cost:** 200 mg $235.39/60. **Injection:** 50 mg/mL (Nexterone does not contain polysorbate 80 or benzyl alcohol). **Cost:** 50 mg $1057.13/10 ampules.

NURSING IMPLICATIONS
Assessment
- Monitor ECG continuously during IV therapy or initiation of oral therapy. Monitor heart rate and rhythm throughout therapy; PR prolongation, slight QRS widening, T-wave amplitude reduction with T-wave widening and bifurcation, and U waves may occur. QT prolongation may be associated with worsening of arrhythmias and should be monitored closely during IV therapy. Report bradycardia or increase in arrhythmias promptly; patients receiving IV therapy may require slowing rate, discontinuing infusion, or inserting a temporary pacemaker.
- Assess pacing and defibrillation threshold in patients with pacemakers and implanted defibrillators at beginning and periodically during therapy.
- Assess for signs of pulmonary toxicity (rales/crackles, decreased breath sounds, pleuritic friction rub, fatigue, dyspnea, cough, wheezing, pleuritic pain, fever, hemoptysis, hypoxia). Chest x-ray and pulmonary function tests are recommended before therapy. Monitor chest x-ray every 3–6 months during therapy to detect diffuse interstitial changes or alveolar infiltrates. Bronchoscopy or gallium radionuclide scan may also be used for diagnosis. Usually reversible after withdrawal, but fatalities have occurred.
- **IV:** Assess for signs and symptoms of ARDS throughout therapy. Report dyspnea, tachypnea, or rales/crackles promptly. Bilateral, diffuse pulmonary infiltrates are seen on chest x-ray.
- Monitor blood pressure frequently. Hypotension usually occurs during first several hours of therapy and is related to rate of infusion. If hypotension occurs, slow rate.
- **PO:** Assess for neurotoxicity (ataxia, proximal muscle weakness, tingling or numbness in fingers or toes, uncontrolled movements, tremors); common during initial therapy, but may occur within 1 wk to several months of initiation of therapy and may persist for more than 1 yr after withdrawal. Dose reduction is recommended. Assist patient during ambulation to prevent falls.
- Ophthalmic exams should be performed before and regularly during therapy and whenever vi-

amiodarone

sual changes (photophobia, halos around lights, decreased acuity) occur. May cause permanent loss of vision.
- Assess for signs of thyroid dysfunction, especially during initial therapy. Lethargy; weight gain; edema of the hands, feet, and periorbital region; and cool, pale skin suggest hypothyroidism and may require decrease in dose or discontinuation of therapy and thyroid supplementation. Tachycardia; weight loss; nervousness; sensitivity to heat; insomnia; and warm, flushed, moist skin suggest hyperthyroidism and may require discontinuation of therapy and treatment with antithyroid agents.
- **Lab Test Considerations:** Monitor liver and thyroid functions before and every 6 months during therapy. Drug effects persist long after discontinuation. Thyroid function abnormalities are common, but clinical thyroid dysfunction is uncommon.
- Monitor AST, ALT, and alkaline phosphatase at regular intervals during therapy, especially in patients receiving high maintenance dose. If liver function studies are 3 times normal or double in patients with elevated baseline levels or if hepatomegaly occurs, dose should be reduced.
- May cause asymptomatic elevations in ANA titer concentrations.

Potential Nursing Diagnoses
Decreased cardiac output (Indications)
Impaired gas exchange (Side Effects)

Implementation
- **High Alert:** IV vasoactive medications are inherently dangerous; fatalities have occurred from medication errors involving amiodarone. Before administering, have second practitioner check original order, dose calculations, and infusion pump settings. Patients should be hospitalized and monitored closely during IV therapy and initiation of oral therapy. IV therapy should be administered only by physicians experienced in treating life-threatening arrhythmias.
- Hypokalemia and hypomagnesemia may decrease effectiveness or cause additional arrhythmias; correct before therapy.
- Monitor closely when converting from IV to oral therapy, especially in geriatric patients.
- **PO:** May be administered with meals and in divided doses if GI intolerance occurs or if daily dose exceeds 1000 mg.

IV Administration
- **IV:** Administer via volumetric pump; drop size may be reduced, causing altered dosing with drop counter infusion sets.
- Administer through an in-line filter.
- Infusions exceeding 2 hr must be administered in glass or polyolefin bottles to prevent adsorption. However, polyvinyl chloride (PVC) tubing must be used during administration because concentrations and infusion rate recommendations have been based on PVC tubing.
- **Direct IV: *Diluent:*** Administer undiluted. May also be diluted in 20–30 mL of D5W or 0.9% NaCl. ***Concentration:*** 50 mg/mL. ***Rate:*** Administer IV push.
- **Intermittent Infusion: *Diluent:*** Dilute 150 mg of amiodarone in 100 mL of D5W. Infusion stable for 2 hr in PVC bag. ***Concentration:*** 1.5 mg/mL. ***Rate:*** Infuse over 10 min. Do not administer IV push.
- **Continuous Infusion: *Diluent:*** Dilute 900 mg (18 mL) of amiodarone in 500 mL of D5W. Infusion stable for 24 hr in glass or polyolefin bottle. ***Concentration:*** 1.8 mg/mL. Concentration may range from 1–6 mg/mL (concentrations >2 mg/mL must be administered via central venous catheter). ***Rate:*** Infuse at a rate of 1 mg/min for the first 6 hr, then decrease infusion rate to 0.5 mg/min and continue until oral therapy initiated.
- **Y-Site Compatibility:** amikacin, amphotericin B colloidal, atracurium, atropine, bumetanide, calcium chloride, calcium gluconate, carboplatin, caspofungin, ceftizoxime, ceftriaxone, cefuroxime, ciprofloxacin, cisplatin, clindamycin, cyclophosphamide, dactinomycin, daptomycin, dexmedetomidine, diltiazem, dobutamine, docetaxel, dopamine, doripenem, doxacurium, doxarubicin, doxycycline, epinephrine, eptifibatide, erythromycin lactobionate, esmolol, etoposide, etoposide phosphate, famotidine, fenoldopam, fentanyl, fluconazole, gemcitabine, gentamicin, granisetron, ifosfamide, insulin, isoproterenol, labetalol, lepirudin, lidocaine, linezolid, lorazepam, meperidine, metaraminol, methylprednisolone, metronidazole, midazolam, milrinone, mitoxantrone, morphine, nesiritide, nitroglycerin, norepinephrine, octreotide, oxaliplatin, palonosetron, pemetrexed, penicillin G potassium, phentolamine, phenylephrine, potassium chloride, procainamide, quinupristin/dalfopristin, rifampin, rocuronium, tacrolimus, teniposide,

tirofiban, tobramycin, vancomycin, vasopressin, vecuronium, vincristine, voriconazole.
- **Y-Site Incompatibility:** aminophylline, ampicillin/sulbactam, argatroban, bivalirudin, ceftazidime, cytarabine, digoxin, doxorubicin hydrochloride, drotrecogin, ertapenem, fludarabine, fluorouracil, heparin, imipenem-cilastatin, levofloxacin, mechlorethamine, methotrexate, micafungin, paclitaxel, piperacillin/tazobactam, potassium phosphates, sodium acetate, sodium bicarbonate, sodium phosphates, thiotepa, tigecycline.

Patient/Family Teaching
- Instruct patient to take amiodarone as directed. Patient should read the *Medication Guide* prior to first dose and with each Rx refill. If a dose is missed, do not take at all. Consult health care professional if more than two doses are missed.
- Advise patient to avoid drinking grapefruit juice during therapy.
- Inform patient that side effects may not appear until several days, weeks, or yr after initiation of therapy and may persist for several months after withdrawal.
- Teach patients to monitor pulse daily and report abnormalities.
- Advise patients that photosensitivity reactions may occur through window glass, thin clothing, and sunscreens. Protective clothing and sunblock are recommended during and for 4 months after therapy. If photosensitivity occurs, dosage reduction may be useful.
- Inform patients that bluish discoloration of the face, neck, and arms is a possible side effect of this drug after prolonged use. This is usually reversible and will fade over several months. Notify health care professional if this occurs.
- Instruct male patients to notify health care professional if signs of epididymitis (pain and swelling in scrotum) occur. May require reduction in dose.
- Advise patient to consult health care professional before taking any other Rx, OTC, or herbal product, especially St. John's wort or cough medicine.
- Caution female patients to avoid breastfeeding during therapy.
- Instruct patient to notify health care professional of medication regimen before treatment or surgery.
- Advise patient to notify health care professional if signs and symptoms of thyroid dysfunction occur.
- Emphasize the importance of follow-up exams, including chest x-ray and pulmonary function tests every 3–6 mo and ophthalmic exams after 6 mo of therapy, and then annually.

Evaluation/Desired Outcomes
- Cessation of life-threatening ventricular arrhythmias. Adverse effects may take up to 4 mo to resolve.

---

amitriptyline
(a-mee-**trip**-ti-leen)
✣ Apo-Amitriptyline, ✣ Elavil, ✣ Levate

Classification
Therapeutic: antidepressants
Pharmacologic: tricyclic antidepressants

Pregnancy Category C

Indications
Depression. **Unlabeled Use:** Anxiety, insomnia, treatment-resistant depression. Chronic pain syndromes (i.e., fibromyalgia, neuropathic pain/chronic pain, headache, low back pain).

Action
Potentiates the effect of serotonin and norepinephrine in the CNS. Has significant anticholinergic properties. **Therapeutic Effects:** Antidepressant action.

Pharmacokinetics
Absorption: Well absorbed from the GI tract.
Distribution: Widely distributed.
Protein Binding: 95% bound to plasma proteins.
Metabolism and Excretion: Extensively metabolized by the liver. Some metabolites have antidepressant activity. Undergoes enterohepatic recirculation and secretion into gastric juices. Probably crosses the placenta and enters breast milk.
Half-life: 10–50 hr.

TIME/ACTION PROFILE (antidepressant effect)

ROUTE	ONSET	PEAK	DURATION
PO	2–3 wk (up to 30 days)	2–6 wk	days–wk

Contraindications/Precautions
Contraindicated in: Angle-closure glaucoma; Known history of QTc prolongation, recent MI, heart failure.
Use Cautiously in: May ↑ risk of suicide attempt/ideation especially during dose early treatment or dose adjustment; risk may be greater in children or adolescents; Patients with pre-existing cardiovascular disease; Prostatic hyperplasia (in-

creased risk of urinary retention); History of seizures (threshold may be ↓); OB: Use only if clearly needed and maternal benefits outweigh risk to fetus Lactation: May cause sedation in infant; Pedi: Safety not established in children <12 yr; Geri: Appears on Beers list. ↑ risk of adverse reactions including falls secondary to sedative and anticholinergic effects.

Adverse Reactions/Side Effects
CNS: SUICIDAL THOUGHTS, lethargy, sedation. EENT: blurred vision, dry eyes, dry mouth. CV: ARRHYTHMIAS, hypotension, ECG changes. GI: constipation, hepatitis, paralytic ileus, increased appetite, weight gain. GU: urinary retention, ↓ libido. Derm: photosensitivity. Endo: changes in blood glucose, gynecomastia. Hemat: blood dyscrasias.

Interactions
Drug-Drug: Amitriptyline is metabolized in the liver by the cytochrome P450 2D6 enzyme, and its action may be affected by drugs that compete for metabolism by this enzyme, including other **antidepressants**, **phenothiazines**, **carbamazepine**, **class 1C antiarrhythmics** including **propafenone**, and **flecainide**; when these drugs are used concurrently with amitriptyline, dosage ↓ of one or the other or both may be necessary. Concurrent use of other drugs that inhibit the activity of the enzyme, including **cimetidine**, **quinidine**, **amiodarone**, and **ritonavir**, may result in ↑ effects of amitriptyline. May cause hypotension, tachycardia, and potentially fatal reactions when used with **MAO inhibitors** (avoid concurrent use—discontinue 2 wk before starting amitriptyline). Concurrent use with **SSRI antidepressants** may result in ↑ toxicity and should be avoided (**fluoxetine** should be stopped 5 wk before starting amitriptyline). Concurrent use with **clonidine** may result in hypertensive crisis and should be avoided. Concurrent use with **levodopa** may result in delayed or ↓ absorption of levodopa or hypertension. Blood levels and effects may be ↓ by **rifamycins** (**rifampin**, **rifapentine**, and **rifabutin**). Concurrent use with **moxifloxacin** ↑ risk of adverse cardiovascular reactions. ↑ CNS depression with other **CNS depressants** including **alcohol**, **antihistamines**, **clonidine**, **opioids**, and **sedative/hypnotics**. **Barbiturates** may alter blood levels and effects. Adrenergic and anticholinergic side effects may be ↑ with other agents having **anticholinergic** properties. **Phenothiazines** or **oral contraceptives** ↑ levels and may cause toxicity. **Nicotine** may ↑ metabolism and alter effects.

Drug-Natural Products: St. John's wort may decrease serum concentrations and efficacy. Concomitant use of **kava-kava**, **valerian**, or **chamomile** can increase CNS depression. Increased anticholinergic effects with **jimson weed** and **scopolia**.

Route/Dosage
PO (Adults): 75 mg/day in divided doses; may be increased up to 150 mg/day *or* 50–100 mg at bedtime, may increase by 25–50 mg up to 150 mg (in hospitalized patients, may initiate with 100 mg/day, increasing total daily dose up to 300 mg).
PO (Geriatric Patients and Adolescents): 10 mg tid and 20 mg at bedtime *or* 25 mg at bedtime initially, slowly increased to 100 mg/day as a single bedtime dose or divided doses.

Availability (generic available)
Tablets: 10 mg, 25 mg, 50 mg, 75 mg, 100 mg, 150 mg. **Cost:** *Generic*— 10 mg $13.32/100, 25 mg $12.22/100, 50 mg $14.20/100, 75 mg $12.21/100, 100 mg $12.21/100, 150 mg $24.42/100. **Syrup:** 10 mg/5 mL.

NURSING IMPLICATIONS
Assessment
- Obtain weight and BMI initially and periodically during treatment.
- Assess fasting glucose and cholesterol levels in overweight/obese individuals.
- Monitor blood pressure and pulse before and during initial therapy. Notify health care professional of decreases in blood pressure (10–20 mm Hg) or sudden increase in pulse rate. Patients taking high doses or with a history of cardiovascular disease should have ECG monitored before and periodically during therapy.
- **Depression:** Monitor mental status (orientation, mood behavior) frequently. Assess for suicidal tendencies, especially during early therapy. Restrict amount of drug available to patient.
- Assess for suicidal tendencies, especially during early therapy. Restrict amount of drug available to patient. Risk may be increased in children, adolescents, and adults ≤24 yrs. After starting therapy, children, adolescents, and young adults should be seen by health care professional at least weekly for 4 wk, every 3

wk for next 4 wk, and on advice of health care professional thereafter.
- **Pain:** Assess intensity, quality, and location of pain periodically during therapy. May require several weeks for effects to be seen. Use pain scale to monitor effectiveness of medication. Assess for sexual dysfunction (decreased libido; erectile dysfunction). **Geri:** Geriatric patients started on amitriptyline may be at an increased risk for falls; start with low dose and monitor closely. Assess for anticholinergic effects (weakness and sedation).
- **Lab Test Considerations:** Assess leukocyte and differential blood counts, liver function, and serum glucose before and periodically during therapy. May cause an ↑ serum bilirubin and alkaline phosphatase. May cause bone marrow depression. Serum glucose may be ↑ or ↓.

Potential Nursing Diagnoses
Ineffective coping (Indications)
Chronic pain (Indications)
Risk for injury (Side Effects)

Implementation
- Dose increases should be made at bedtime because of sedation. Dose titration is a slow process; may take weeks to months. May give entire dose at bedtime. Sedative effect may be apparent before antidepressant effect is noted. May require tapering to avoid withdrawal effects.
- **PO:** Administer medication with or immediately after a meal to minimize gastric upset. Tablet may be crushed and given with food or fluids.

Patient/Family Teaching
- Instruct patient to take medication as directed. If a dose is missed, take as soon as possible unless almost time for next dose; if regimen is a single dose at bedtime, do not take in the morning because of side effects. Advise patient that drug effects may not be noticed for at least 2 wk. Abrupt discontinuation may cause nausea, vomiting, diarrhea, headache, trouble sleeping with vivid dreams, and irritability.
- May cause drowsiness and blurred vision. Caution patient to avoid driving and other activities requiring alertness until response to drug is known.
- Orthostatic hypotension, sedation, and confusion are common during early therapy, especially in geriatric patients. Protect patient from falls and advise patient to make position changes slowly. Institute fall precautions. Advise patient to make position changes slowly. Refer as appropriate for nutrition/weight management and medical management.
- Advise patient to avoid alcohol or other CNS depressant drugs during and for 3–7 days after therapy has been discontinued.
- Advise patient, family and caregivers to look for suicidality, especially during early therapy or dose changes. Notify health care professional immediately if thoughts about suicide or dying, attempts to commit suicide, new or worse depression or anxiety, agitation or restlessness, panic attacks, insomnia, new or worse irritability, aggressiveness, acting on dangerous impulses, mania, or other changes in mood or behavior occur.
- Instruct patient to notify health care professional if urinary retention, dry mouth, or constipation persists. Sugarless candy or gum may diminish dry mouth, and an increase in fluid intake or bulk may prevent constipation. If symptoms persist, dose reduction or discontinuation may be necessary. Consult health care professional if dry mouth persists for >2 wk.
- Caution patient to use sunscreen and protective clothing to prevent photosensitivity reactions. Alert patient that medication may turn urine blue-green in color.
- Inform patient of need to monitor dietary intake. Increase in appetite may lead to undesired weight gain.
- Advise patient to notify health care professional if pregnancy is planned or suspected or if breastfeeding.
- Advise patient to notify health care professional of medication regimen before treatment or surgery. Medication should be discontinued as long as possible before surgery.
- Therapy for depression is usually prolonged and should be continued for at least 3 months to prevent relapse. Emphasize the importance of follow-up exams to monitor effectiveness, side effects, and improve coping skills. Advise patient and family that treatment is not a cure and symptoms can recur after discontinuation of medication. Refer patient to local support group.

Evaluation/Desired Outcomes
- Increased sense of well-being.
- Renewed interest in surroundings.
- Increased appetite.
- Improved energy level.
- Improved sleep.
- Decrease in chronic pain symptoms.

amlodipine **157**

- Full therapeutic effects may be seen 2–6 wk after initiating therapy.

amlodipine (am-loe-di-peen)
Norvasc

Classification
Therapeutic: antihypertensives
Pharmacologic: calcium channel blockers

Pregnancy Category C

Indications
Alone or with other agents in the management of hypertension, angina pectoris, and vasospastic (Prinzmetal's) angina.

Action
Inhibits the transport of calcium into myocardial and vascular smooth muscle cells, resulting in inhibition of excitation-contraction coupling and subsequent contraction. **Therapeutic Effects:** Systemic vasodilation resulting in decreased blood pressure. Coronary vasodilation resulting in decreased frequency and severity of attacks of angina.

Pharmacokinetics
Absorption: Well absorbed after oral administration (64–90%).
Distribution: Probably crosses the placenta.
Protein Binding: 95–98%.
Metabolism and Excretion: Mostly metabolized by the liver.
Half-life: 30–50 hr (↑ in geriatric patients and patients with hepatic impairment).

TIME/ACTION PROFILE (cardiovascular effects)

ROUTE	ONSET	PEAK	DURATION
PO	unknown	6–9	24 hr

Contraindications/Precautions
Contraindicated in: Hypersensitivity; Systolic blood pressure <90 mm Hg.
Use Cautiously in: Severe hepatic impairment (dosage reduction recommended); Aortic stenosis; History of CHF; OB, Lactation, Pedi: Safety not established; Geri: Dose reduction recommended; ↑ risk of hypotension.

Adverse Reactions/Side Effects
CNS: <u>headache</u>, dizziness, fatigue. **CV:** <u>peripheral edema</u>, angina, bradycardia, hypotension, palpitations. **GI:** gingival hyperplasia, nausea. **Derm:** flushing.

Interactions
Drug-Drug: Additive hypotension may occur when used concurrently with **fentanyl**, other **antihypertensives**, **nitrates**, acute ingestion of **alcohol**, or **quinidine**. Antihypertensive effects may be ↓ by concurrent use of **nonsteroidal anti-inflammatory agents**. May ↑ risk of neurotoxicity with **lithium**.
Drug-Food: Grapefruit juice ↑ serum levels and effect.

Route/Dosage
PO (Adults): 5–10 mg once daily; *antihypertensive in fragile or small patients or patients already receiving other antihypertensives*—initiate at 2.5 mg/day, ↑ as required/tolerated (up to 10 mg/day) as an antihypertensive therapy with 2.5 mg/day in patients with hepatic insufficiency.

PO (Geriatric Patients): *Antihypertensive*—Initiate therapy at 2.5 mg/day, ↑ as required/tolerated (up to 10 mg/day); *antianginal*—initiate therapy at 5 mg/day, ↑ as required/tolerated (up to 10 mg/day).

Hepatic Impairment
PO (Adults): *Antihypertensive*—Initiate therapy at 2.5 mg/day, ↑ as required/tolerated (up to 10 mg/day); *antianginal*—initiate therapy at 5 mg/day, ↑ as required/tolerated (up to 10 mg/day).

Availability (generic available)
Tablets: 2.5 mg, 5 mg, 10 mg. **Cost:** *Generic*—2.5 mg $99.97/90, 5 mg $105.97/90, 10 mg $135.96/90. *In combination with:* atorvastatin (Caduet), benazepril (Lotrel), olmesartan (Azor), valsartan (Exforge), and valsartan/hydrochlorothiazide (Exforge HCT). See Appendix B.

NURSING IMPLICATIONS

Assessment
- Monitor blood pressure and pulse before therapy, during dose titration, and periodically during therapy. Monitor ECG periodically during prolonged therapy.
- Monitor intake and output ratios and daily weight. Assess for signs of CHF (peripheral edema, rales/crackles, dyspnea, weight gain, jugular venous distention).
- **Angina:** Assess location, duration, intensity, and precipitating factors of patient's anginal pain.

✦ = Canadian drug name. ▌= Genetic implication.
*CAPITALS indicates life-threatening; <u>underlines</u> indicate most frequent.

- **Lab Test Considerations:** Total serum calcium concentrations are not affected by calcium channel blockers.

Potential Nursing Diagnoses
Ineffective tissue perfusion (Indications)
Acute pain (Indications)

Implementation
- **PO:** May be administered without regard to meals.

Patient/Family Teaching
- Advise patient to take medication as directed, even if feeling well. Take missed doses as soon as possible unless almost time for next dose; do not double doses. May need to be discontinued gradually.
- Advise patient to avoid large amounts (6–8 glasses of grapefruit juice/day) during therapy.
- Instruct patient on correct technique for monitoring pulse. Instruct patient to contact health care professional if heart rate is <50 bpm.
- Caution patient to change positions slowly to minimize orthostatic hypotension.
- May cause drowsiness or dizziness. Advise patient to avoid driving or other activities requiring alertness until response to the medication is known.
- Instruct patient on importance of maintaining good dental hygiene and seeing dentist frequently for teeth cleaning to prevent tenderness, bleeding, and gingival hyperplasia (gum enlargement).
- Instruct patient to avoid concurrent use of alcohol or OTC medications, especially cold preparations, without consulting health care professional.
- Advise patient to notify health care professional if irregular heartbeats, dyspnea, swelling of hands and feet, pronounced dizziness, nausea, constipation, or hypotension occurs or if headache is severe or persistent.
- Caution patient to wear protective clothing and use sunscreen to prevent photosensitivity reactions.
- Advise patient to inform health care professional of medication regimen before treatment or surgery.
- **Angina:** Instruct patient on concurrent nitrate or beta-blocker therapy to continue taking both medications as directed and to use SL nitroglycerin as needed for anginal attacks.
- Advise patient to contact health care professional if chest pain does not improve or worsens after therapy, if it occurs with diaphoresis, if shortness of breath occurs, or if severe, persistent headache occurs.
- Caution patient to discuss exercise restrictions with health care professional before exertion.
- **Hypertension:** Encourage patient to comply with other interventions for hypertension (weight reduction, low-sodium diet, smoking cessation, moderation of alcohol consumption, regular exercise, and stress management). Medication controls but does not cure hypertension.
- Instruct patient and family in proper technique for monitoring blood pressure. Advise patient to take blood pressure weekly and to report significant changes to health care professional.

Evaluation/Desired Outcomes
- Decrease in blood pressure.
- Decrease in frequency and severity of anginal attacks.
- Decrease in need for nitrate therapy.
- Increase in activity tolerance and sense of well-being.

---

amoxicillin (a-mox-i-**sil**-in)
Amoxil, ✱ Apo-Amoxi, DisperMox, Moxatag, ✱ Novamoxin, ✱ Nu-Amoxi, Trimox

Classification
Therapeutic: anti-infectives, antiulcer agents
Pharmacologic: aminopenicillins

Pregnancy Category B

Indications
Treatment of: Skin and skin structure infections, Otitis media, Sinusitis, Respiratory infections, Genitourinary infections. Endocarditis prophylaxis. Postexposure inhalational anthrax prophylaxis. Management of ulcer disease due to *Helicobacter pylori*. **Unlabeled Use:** Lyme disease in children <8 yr.

Action
Binds to bacterial cell wall, causing cell death.
Therapeutic Effects: Bactericidal action; spectrum is broader than penicillins. **Spectrum:** Active against: Streptococci, Pneumococci, Enterococci, *Haemophilus influenzae, Escherichia coli, Proteus mirabilis, Neisseria meningitidis, N. gonorrhoeae, Shigella, Chlamydia trachomatis, Salmonella, Borrelia burgdorferi, H. pylori*.

Pharmacokinetics
Absorption: Well absorbed from duodenum (75–90%). More resistant to acid inactivation than other penicillins.

amoxicillin

Distribution: Diffuses readily into most body tissues and fluids. CSF penetration increased when meninges are inflamed. Crosses placenta; enters breast milk in small amounts.
Metabolism and Excretion: 70% excreted unchanged in the urine; 30% metabolized by the liver.
Half-life: Neonates: 3.7 hr; Infants and Children: 1–2 hr; Adults: 0.7–1.4 hr.

TIME/ACTION PROFILE (blood levels)

ROUTE	ONSET	PEAK	DURATION
PO	30 min	1–2 hr	8–12 hr

Contraindications/Precautions
Contraindicated in: Hypersensitivity to penicillins (cross-sensitivity exists to cephalosporins and other beta-lactams); Tablets for oral suspension (DisperMox) contain aspartame; avoid in patients with phenylketonuria.
Use Cautiously in: Severe renal insufficiency (↓ dose if CCr <30 mL/min); Infectious mononucleosis, acute lymphocytic leukemia, or cytomegalovirus infection (↑ risk of rash); OB, Lactation: Has been used safely.

Adverse Reactions/Side Effects
CNS: SEIZURES (high doses). **GI:** PSEUDOMEMBRANOUS COLITIS, diarrhea, nausea, vomiting, ↑ liver enzymes. **Derm:** rashes, urticaria. **Hemat:** blood dyscrasias. **Misc:** allergic reactions including ANAPHYLAXIS, SERUM SICKNESS, superinfection.

Interactions
Drug-Drug: Probenecid ↓ renal excretion and ↑ blood levels of amoxicillin—therapy may be combined for this purpose. May ↑ effect of **warfarin**. May ↓ effectiveness of **oral contraceptives**. **Allopurinol** may ↑ frequency of rash.

Route/Dosage
Most Infections
PO (Adults): 250–500 mg q 8 hr *or* 500–875 mg q 12 hr (not to exceed 2–3 g/day).
PO (Adults and Children ≥12 yr): *Extended-release tablets (for Strep throat)*—775 mg once daily for 10 days.
PO (Children >3 mo): 25–50 mg/kg/day in divided doses q 8 hr *or* 25–50 mg/kg/day individual doses q 12 hr; *Acute otitis media due to highly resistant strains of S. pneumoniae*— 80–90 mg/kg/day divided q 12 hr; *Postexposure inhalational anthrax prophylaxis*—<40 kg: 45 mg/kg/day in divided doses q 8 hr; >40 kg: 500 mg q 8 hr.
PO (Infants ≤3 mo and neonates): 20–30 mg/kg/day in divided doses q 12 hr.

H. Pylori
PO (Adults): *Triple therapy*—1000 mg amoxicillin twice daily with lansoprazole 30 mg twice daily and clarithromycin 500 mg twice daily for 14 days *or* 1000 mg amoxicillin twice daily with omeprazole 20 mg twice daily and clarithromycin 500 mg twice daily for 14 days *or* amoxicillin 1000 mg twice daily with esomeprazole 40 mg daily and clarithromycin 500 mg twice daily for 10 days. *Dual therapy*—1000 mg amoxicillin three times daily with lansoprazole 30 mg three times daily for 14 days.

Endocarditis Prophylaxis
PO (Adults): 2 g 1 hr prior to procedure.
PO (Children): 50 mg/kg 1 hr prior to procedure (not to exceed adult dose).

Gonorrhea
PO (Adults and Children ≥40 kg): single 3 g dose.
PO (Children >2 yr and <40 kg): 50 mg/kg with probenecid 25 mg/kg as a single dose.

Renal Impairment
PO (Adults CCr 10–30 mL/min): 250–500 mg q 12 hr.

Renal Impairment
PO (Adults CCr <10 mL/min): 250–500 mg q 24 hr.

Availability (generic available)
Chewable tablets (cherry, banana, peppermint flavors): 125 mg, 200 mg, 250 mg, 400 mg. **Cost:** *Generic*—125 mg $17.13/30, 200 mg $16.99/20, 250 mg $13.99/30, 400 mg $16.36/30. **Tablets:** 500 mg, 875 mg. **Cost:** *Generic*—500 mg $12.80/21, 875 mg $24.99/30. **Extended-release tablets:** 775 mg. **Capsules:** 250 mg, 500 mg. **Cost:** *Generic*—250 mg $7.99/30, 500 mg $7.99/30. **Suspension (pediatric drops) (bubblegum flavor):** 50 mg/mL. **Cost:** *Generic*—$7.99/30 mL. **Suspension (strawberry [125 mg/5 mL] and bubblegum [200 mg/5 mL, 250 mg/5 mL, 400 mg/5 mL] flavors):** 125 mg/5 mL, 200 mg/5 mL, 250 mg/5 mL, 400 mg/5 mL. **Cost:** *Generic*—125 mg/5 mL $11.25/100 mL, 250 mg/5 mL $16.92/100 mL, 250 mg/5 mL $7.99/150 mL, 400 mg/5 mL $17.47/100 mL. **Tablets for oral suspension**

(strawberry): 200 mg, 400 mg, 600 mg. *In combination with:* clarithromycin and lansoprazole in a compliance package (Prevpac). See Appendix B.

NURSING IMPLICATIONS
Assessment
- Assess for infection (vital signs; appearance of wound, sputum, urine, and stool; WBC) at beginning of and throughout therapy.
- Obtain a history before initiating therapy to determine previous use of and reactions to penicillins or cephalosporins. Persons with a negative history of penicillin sensitivity may still have an allergic response.
- Observe for signs and symptoms of anaphylaxis (rash, pruritus, laryngeal edema, wheezing). Notify health care professional immediately if these occur.
- Obtain specimens for culture and sensitivity prior to therapy. First dose may be given before receiving results.
- Monitor bowel function. Diarrhea, abdominal cramping, fever, and bloody stools should be reported to health care professional promptly as a sign of pseudomembranous colitis. May begin up to several weeks following cessation of therapy.
- **Lab Test Considerations:** May cause ↑ serum alkaline phosphatase, LDH, AST, and ALT concentrations.
- May cause false-positive direct Coombs' test result.

Potential Nursing Diagnoses
Risk for infection (Indications, Side Effects)
Noncompliance (Patient/Family Teaching)

Implementation
- **PO:** Administer around the clock. May be given without regard to meals or with meals to decrease GI side effects. Capsule contents may be emptied and swallowed with liquids. Extended-release tablets should be swallowed whole; do not crush, break, or chew. Chewable tablets should be crushed or chewed before swallowing with liquids.
- Shake oral suspension before administering. Suspension may be given straight or mixed in formula, milk, fruit juice, water, or ginger ale. Administer immediately after mixing. Discard refrigerated reconstituted suspension after 10 days.
- Mix each *tablet for oral suspension (DisperMox)* in 2 tsp of water. Patient should drink entire mixture, rinse container with a small amount of water and drink to make sure entire dose is taken. Do not chew or swallow tablet. Tablets will not dissolve in mouth. Use only water to dissolve tablets, other liquids are not recommended. Store tablets at room temperature.

Patient/Family Teaching
- Instruct patients to take medication around the clock and to finish the drug completely as directed, even if feeling better. Advise patients that sharing of this medication may be dangerous.
- Review use and preparation of *tablets for oral suspension (DisperMox)*.
- Instruct female patients taking oral contraceptives to use an alternate or additional nonhormonal method of contraception during therapy with amoxicillin and until next menstrual period.
- Advise patient to report the signs of superinfection (furry overgrowth on the tongue, vaginal itching or discharge, loose or foul-smelling stools) and allergy.
- Instruct patient to notify health care professional immediately if diarrhea, abdominal cramping, fever, or bloody stools occur and not to treat with antidiarrheals without consulting health care professional.
- Instruct the patient to notify health care professional if symptoms do not improve.
- Teach patients with a history of rheumatic heart disease or valve replacement the importance of using antimicrobial prophylaxis before invasive medical or dental procedures.
- **Pedi:** Teach parents or caregivers to calculate and measure doses accurately. Reinforce importance of using measuring device supplied by pharmacy or with product, not household items.

Evaluation/Desired Outcomes
- Resolution of the signs and symptoms of infection. Length of time for complete resolution depends on the organism and site of infection.
- Endocarditis prophylaxis.
- Eradication of *H. pylori* with resolution of ulcer symptoms.
- Prevention of inhalational anthrax (postexposure).

---

amoxicillin/clavulanate
(a-mox-i-**sill**-in/klav-yoo-**lan**-ate)
Amoclan, Augmentin, Augmentin ES, Augmentin XR, ✤ Clavulin

amoxicillin/clavulanate **161**

Classification
Therapeutic: anti-infectives
Pharmacologic: aminopenicillins/beta lactamase inhibitors

Pregnancy Category B

Indications
Treatment of a variety of infections including: Skin and skin structure infections, Otitis media, Sinusitis, Respiratory tract infections, Genitourinary tract infections.

Action
Binds to bacterial cell wall, causing cell death; spectrum of amoxicillin is broader than penicillin. Clavulanate resists action of beta-lactamase, an enzyme produced by bacteria that is capable of inactivating some penicillins. **Therapeutic Effects:** Bactericidal action against susceptible bacteria. **Spectrum:** Active against: Streptococci, Pneumococci, Enterococci, *Haemophilus influenzae*, *Escherichia coli*, *Proteus mirabilis*, *Neisseria meningitidis*, *N. gonorrhoeae*, *Staphylococcus aureus*, *Klebsiella pneumoniae*, *Shigella*, *Salmonella*, *Moraxella catarrhalis*.

Pharmacokinetics
Absorption: Well absorbed from the duodenum (75–90%). More resistant to acid inactivation than other penicillins.
Distribution: Diffuses readily into most body tissues and fluids. Does not readily enter brain/CSF; CSF penetration is ↑ in the presence of inflamed meninges. Crosses the placenta and enters breast milk in small amounts.
Metabolism and Excretion: 70% excreted unchanged in the urine; 30% metabolized by the liver.
Half-life: 1–1.3 hr.

TIME/ACTION PROFILE (peak blood levels)

ROUTE	ONSET	PEAK	DURATION
PO	30 min	1–2 hr	8–12 hrhr

Contraindications/Precautions
Contraindicated in: Hypersensitivity to penicillins or clavulanate; Suspension and chewable tablets contain aspartame and should be avoided in phenylketonurics; History of amoxicillin/clavulanate-associated cholestatic jaundice.
Use Cautiously in: Severe renal insufficiency (dose ↓ necessary); Infectious mononucleosis (↑ risk of rash); Hepatic impairment (dose cautiously, monitor liver function).

Adverse Reactions/Side Effects
CNS: SEIZURES (high doses). **GI:** PSEUDOMEMBRANOUS COLITIS, diarrhea, hepatic dysfunction, nausea, vomiting. **GU:** vaginal candidiasis. **Derm:** rashes, urticaria. **Hemat:** blood dyscrasias. **Misc:** allergic reactions including ANAPHYLAXIS and SERUM SICKNESS, superinfection.

Interactions
Drug-Drug: **Probenecid** ↓ renal excretion and ↑ blood levels of amoxicillin—therapy may be combined for this purpose. May ↑ the effect of **warfarin**. Concurrent **allopurinol** therapy ↑ risk of rash. May ↓ the effectiveness of **hormonal contraceptives**.
Drug-Food: Clavulanate absorption is ↓ by a **high fat** meal.

Route/Dosage

Most Infections (Dosing based on amoxicillin component)
PO (Adults and Children >40 kg): 250 mg q 8 hr or 500 mg q 12 hr.

Serious Infections and Respiratory Tract Infections
PO (Adults and Children >40 kg): 875 mg q 12 hr *or* 500 mg q 8 hr; *Acute bacterial sinusitis*—2000 mg q 12 hr for 10 days as extended release (XR) product; *Community-acquired pneumonia*—2000 mg every 12 hr for 7–10 days as extended release (XR) product.

Recurrent/persistent acute otitis media due to Multidrug-resistant *Streptococcus pneumonia*, *H. influenzae*, or *M. catarrhalis*
PO (Children <40 kg): 80–90 mg/kg/day in divided doses q 12 hr for 10 days (as ES formulation only).

Renal Impairment
PO (Adults): *CCr 10–30 mL/min*—250–500 mg q 12 hr (do not use 875 mg tablet); *CCr <10 mL/min*—250–500 mg q 24 hr.

Otitis Media, Sinusitis, Lower Respiratory Tract Infections, Serious Infections
PO (Children ≥3 mo): *200 mg/5 mL or 400 mg/5 mL suspension*—45 mg/kg/day divided q 12 hr; *125 mg/5 mL or 250 mg/5 mL suspension*—40 mg/kg/day divided q 8 hr.

Less Serious Infections
PO (Children ≥3 mo): *200 mg/5 mL or 400 mg/5 mL suspension*—25 mg/kg/day divided q

= Canadian drug name. = Genetic implication.
*CAPITALS indicates life-threatening; underlines indicate most frequent.

12 hr *or* 20 mg/kg/day divided q 8 hr (as 125 mg/ 5 mL or 250 mg/5 mL suspension).
PO (Children <3 mo): 15 mg/kg q 12 hr (125 mg/mL suspension recommended).

Availability (generic available)
Tablets: 250 mg amoxicillin with 125 mg clavulanate, 500 mg amoxicillin with 125 mg clavulanate, 875 mg amoxicillin with 125 mg clavulanate. **Cost:** *Generic*— 250 mg $97.19/30, 500 mg $45.99/20, 875 mg $83.99/20. **Chewable tablets (125 mg and 250 mg are lemon-lime flavor; 200 mg and 400 mg are cherry-banana flavor):** 125 mg amoxicillin with 31.25 mg clavulanate, 200 mg amoxicillin with 28.5 mg clavulanate, 250 mg amoxicillin with 62.5 mg clavulanate, 400 mg amoxicillin with 57 mg clavulanate. **Cost:** *Generic*— 125 mg $39.88/30, 200 mg $36.90/20, 250 mg $76.06/30, 400 mg $63.79/20. **Extended-release tablets (scored):** 1000 mg amoxicillin with 62.5 mg clavulanate. **Cost:** 1000 mg $101.53/28. **Powder for oral suspension (125 mg/5 mL is banana flavor; 200 mg/5ml is fruit flavor; 250 mg/5 mL is orange flavor; 400 mg/5 mL is fruit flavor; 600 mg/5 mL is orange or strawberry-creme flavor):** 125 mg amoxicillin with 31.25 mg clavulanate/5 mL, 200 mg amoxicillin with 28.5 mg clavulanate/5 mL, 250 mg amoxicillin with 62.5 mg clavulanate/5 mL, 400 mg amoxicillin with 57 mg clavulanate/5 mL, 600 mg amoxicillin with 42.9 mg clavulanate/5 mL (ES formulation). **Cost:** *Generic*— 125 mg $27.11/100 mL, 200 mg $40.85/100 mL, 250 mg $51.77/100 mL, 400 mg $69.21/100 mL, 600 mg $35.99/75 mL.

NURSING IMPLICATIONS

Assessment
- Assess for infection (vital signs; appearance of wound, sputum, urine, and stool; WBC) at beginning of and throughout therapy.
- Obtain a history before initiating therapy to determine previous use of and reactions to penicillins or cephalosporins. Persons with a negative history of penicillin sensitivity may still have an allergic response.
- Observe for signs and symptoms of anaphylaxis (rash, pruritus, laryngeal edema, wheezing). Notify health care professional immediately if these occur.
- Obtain specimens for culture and sensitivity prior to therapy. First dose may be given before receiving results.
- Monitor bowel function. Diarrhea, abdominal cramping, fever, and bloody stools should be reported to health care professional promptly as a sign of pseudomembranous colitis. May begin up to several weeks following cessation of therapy.
- *Lab Test Considerations:* May cause ↑ serum alkaline phosphatase, LDH, AST, and ALT concentrations. Elderly men and patients receiving prolonged treatment are at ↑ risk for hepatic dysfunction.
- May cause false-positive direct Coombs' test result.

Potential Nursing Diagnoses
Risk for infection (Indications, Side Effects)
Noncompliance (Patient/Family Teaching)

Implementation
- **PO:** Administer around the clock. Administer at the start of a meal to enhance absorption and to decrease GI side effects. Do not administer with high fat meals; clavulanate absorption is decreased. XR tablet is scored and can be broken for ease of administration. Capsule contents may be emptied and swallowed with liquids. Chewable tablets should be crushed or chewed before swallowing with liquids. Shake oral suspension before administering. Refrigerated reconstituted suspension should be discarded after 10 days.
- Two 250-mg tablets are not bioequivalent to one 500-mg tablet; 250-mg tablets and 250-mg chewable tablets are also not interchangeable. Two 500-mg tablets are not interchangeable with one 1000-mg XR tablet; amounts of clavulanic acid and durations of action are different. Augmentin ES 600 (600 mg/5 mL) does not contain the same amount of clavulanic acid as any of the other Augmentin suspensions. Suspensions are not interchangeable.
- Pedi: Do not administer 250-mg chewable tablets to children <40 kg due to clavulanate content. Children <3 months should receive the 125-mg/5 mL oral solution.

Patient/Family Teaching
- Instruct patients to take medication around the clock and to finish the drug completely as directed, even if feeling better. Advise patients that sharing of this medication may be dangerous.
- Instruct female patients taking oral contraceptives to use an alternate or additional method of contraception during therapy and until next menstrual period.
- Advise patient to report the signs of superinfection (furry overgrowth on the tongue, vaginal itching or discharge, loose or foul-smelling stools) and allergy.

- Instruct patient to notify health care professional immediately if diarrhea, abdominal cramping, fever, or bloody stools occur and not to treat with antidiarrheals without consulting health care professionals.
- Instruct the patient to notify health care professional if symptoms do not improve or if nausea or diarrhea persists when drug is administered with food.
- **Pedi:** Teach parents or caregivers to calculate and measure doses accurately. Reinforce importance of using measuring device supplied by pharmacy or with product, not household items.

Evaluation/Desired Outcomes
- Resolution of the signs and symptoms of infection. Length of time for complete resolution depends on the organism and site of infection.

amphetamine mixtures
(am-**fet**-a-meen)
Amphetamine Salt, Adderall, Adderall XR

Classification
Therapeutic: central nervous system stimulants

Schedule II

Pregnancy Category C

Indications
ADHD. Narcolepsy.

Action
Causes release of norepinephrine from nerve endings. Pharmacologic effects are: CNS and respiratory stimulation, Vasoconstriction, Mydriasis (pupillary dilation). **Therapeutic Effects:** Increased motor activity, mental alertness, and decreased fatigue in narcoleptic patients. Increased attention span in ADHD.

Pharmacokinetics
Absorption: Well absorbed after oral administration.
Distribution: Widely distributed in body tissues, with high concentrations in the brain and CSF. Crosses placenta and enters breast milk.
Metabolism and Excretion: Some metabolism by the liver. Urinary excretion is pH-dependent. Alkaline urine promotes reabsorption and prolongs action.

Half-life: Children 6–12 yrs: 9–11 hr; Adults: 10–13 hr (depends on urine pH).

TIME/ACTION PROFILE (CNS stimulation)

ROUTE	ONSET	PEAK	DURATION
PO	tablet: 0.5–1 hr	tablet: 3 hr capsule: 7 hr	4–6 hr

Contraindications/Precautions
Contraindicated in: Hyperexcitable states including hyperthyroidism; Psychotic personalities; Suicidal or homicidal tendencies; Chemical dependence; Glaucoma; Structural cardiac abnormalities (may ↑ the risk of sudden death); OB: Potentially embryotoxic.
Use Cautiously in: Cardiovascular disease (sudden death has occurred in children with structural cardiac abnormalities or other serious heart problems); History of substance abuse (misuse may result in serious cardiovascular events/sudden death); Hypertension; Diabetes mellitus; Tourette's syndrome (may exacerbate tics); Geri: Geriatric or debilitated patients may be more susceptible to side effects.

Adverse Reactions/Side Effects
CNS: hyperactivity, insomnia, restlessness, tremor, behavioral disturbances, dizziness, hallucinations, headache, mania, irritability, thought disorder. **CV:** SUDDEN DEATH, palpitations, tachycardia, cardiomyopathy (increased with prolonged use, high doses), hypertension, hypotension. **GI:** anorexia, constipation, cramps, diarrhea, dry mouth, metallic taste, nausea, vomiting. **GU:** erectile dysfunction, ↑ libido. **Derm:** urticaria. **Endo:** growth inhibition (with long term use in children). **Misc:** psychological dependence.

Interactions
Drug-Drug: Use with **MAO inhibitors** or **meperidine** can result in hypertensive crisis. ↑ adrenergic effects with other **adrenergics** or **thyroid preparations**. Drugs that alkalinize urine (**sodium bicarbonate, acetazolamide**) ↓ excretion, ↑ effects. Drugs that acidify urine (**ammonium chloride**, large doses of **ascorbic acid**) ↑ excretion, ↓ effects. ↑ risk of hypertension and bradycardia with **beta blockers**. ↑ risk of arrhythmias with **digoxin**. **Tricyclic antidepressants** may ↑ effect of amphetamine but may ↑ risk of arrhythmias, hypertension, or hyperpyrexia.

Drug-Natural Products: Use with St. John's wort may ↑ serious side effects (avoid concurrent use).
Drug-Food: Foods that alkalinize the urine (fruit juices) can ↑ effect of amphetamine.

Route/Dosage
Dose is expressed in total amphetamine content (amphetamine + dextroamphetamine).

ADHD
PO (Children ≥6 yr): 5 mg/day 1–2 times daily; ↑ daily dose by 5 mg at weekly intervals. Sustained-release capsules can be given once daily, tablets every 8–12 hr. If starting therapy with extended-release capsules, start with 10 mg once daily and ↑ by 10 mg/day at weekly intervals (up to 40 mg/day).
PO (Adults): 20 mg/day initially (as extended-release product).
PO (Children 3–5 yr): 2.5 mg/day in the morning; ↑ daily dose by 2.5 mg at weekly intervals not to exceed 40 mg/day.

Narcolepsy
PO (Adults and Children ≥ 12 yr): 10–60 mg/day in divided doses; start with 10 mg/day, ↑ by 10 mg/day at weekly intervals. Sustained-release capsules can be given once daily, tablets every 8–12 hr.
PO (Children 6–12 yr): 5 mg once daily; may ↑ by 5 mg/day at weekly intervals to a maximum of 60 mg/day.

Availability (generic available)
Amount is expressed in total amphetamine content (amphetamine + dextroamphetamine).
Tablets: 5 mg, 7.5 mg, 10 mg, 12.5 mg, 15 mg, 20 mg, 30 mg. **Extended-release capsules:** 5 mg, 10 mg, 15 mg, 20 mg, 25 mg, 30 mg.

NURSING IMPLICATIONS

Assessment
- Monitor blood pressure, pulse, and respiration before and periodically during therapy. Obtain a history (including assessment of family history of sudden death or ventricular arrhythmia), physical exam to assess for cardiac disease, and further evaluation (ECG and echocardiogram), if indicated. If exertional chest pain, unexplained syncope, or other cardiac symptoms occur, evaluate promptly.
- May produce a false sense of euphoria and well-being. Provide frequent rest periods and observe patient for rebound depression after the effects of the medication have worn off.
- Monitor closely for behavior change.
- Has high dependence and abuse potential. Tolerance to medication occurs rapidly; do not increase dose.
- **ADHD:** Monitor weight biweekly and inform physician of significant loss. Pedi: Monitor height periodically in children; inform physician of growth inhibition.
- Assess child's attention span, impulse control, and interactions with others. Therapy may be interrupted at intervals to determine whether symptoms are sufficient to continue therapy.
- **Narcolepsy:** Observe and document frequency of narcoleptic episodes.
- *Lab Test Considerations:* May interfere with urinary steroid determinations.
- May cause ↑ plasma corticosteroid concentrations; greatest in evening.

Potential Nursing Diagnoses
Disturbed thought process (Side Effects)

Implementation
- **PO:** Use the lowest effective dose.
- May be taken without regard to food.
- Extended-release capsules may be swallowed whole or opened and sprinkled on applesauce; swallow contents without chewing. Applesauce should be swallowed immediately; do not store. Do not divide contents of capsule; entire contents of capsule should be taken.
- **ADHD:** Pedi: When symptoms are controlled, dose reduction or interruption of therapy may be possible during summer months or may be given on each of the 5 school days, with medication-free weekends and holidays.

Patient/Family Teaching
- Instruct patient to take medication at least 6 hr before bedtime to avoid sleep disturbances. Missed doses should be taken as soon as remembered up to 6 hr before bedtime. With extended release capsule, avoid afternoon doses to prevent insomnia. Do not double doses. Advise patient and parents to read the *Medication Guide* prior to starting therapy and with each Rx refill. Instruct patient not to alter dose without consulting physician. Abrupt cessation of high doses may cause extreme fatigue and mental depression.
- Inform patient that sharing this medication may be dangerous.
- Inform patient that the effects of drug-induced dry mouth can be minimized by rinsing frequently with water or chewing sugarless gum or candies.
- Advise patient to limit caffeine intake.

- May impair judgment. Advise patient to use caution when driving or during other activities requiring alertness.
- Inform patient that periodic holidays from the drug may be used to assess progress and decrease dependence. Pedi: Children should be given a drug-free holiday each year to reassess symptoms and treatment. Doses will change as children age due to pharmacokinetic changes such as slower hepatic metabolism.
- Advise patient and/or parents to notify health care professional of behavioral changes.
- Advise patient to notify health care professional if nervousness, restlessness, insomnia, dizziness, anorexia, or dry mouth becomes severe. Pedi: If reduced appetite and weight loss are a problem, advise parents to provide high calorie meals when drug levels are low (at breakfast and or bedtime).
- Advise patient to notify health care professional if pregnancy is planned or suspected, or if breastfeeding.
- Caution patients to inform health care professional if they have ever abused or been dependent on alcohol or drugs, or if they are now abusing or dependent on alcohol or drugs.
- Emphasize the importance of routine follow-up exams to monitor progress.
- **Home Care Issues:** Advise parents to notify school nurse of medication regimen.

Evaluation/Desired Outcomes
- Improved attention span.
- Decrease in narcoleptic symptoms.

HIGH ALERT

amphotericin B deoxycholate
(am-foe-**ter**-i-sin)
♣ Fungizone

amphotericin B cholesteryl sulfate
Amphotec

amphotericin B lipid complex
Abelcet

amphotericin B liposome
AmBisome

Classification
Therapeutic: antifungals

Pregnancy Category B

amphotericin B

Indications
IV: Treatment of progressive, potentially fatal fungal infections. The cholesteryl sulfate, lipid complex, and liposome formulations should be considered for patients who are intolerant (e.g., renal dysfunction) or refractory to amphotericin B deoxycholate. **Amphotericin B liposome:** Management of suspected fungal infections in febrile neutropenic patients: Treatment of visceral leishmaniasis, Treatment of cryptococcal meningitis in HIV patients.

Action
Binds to fungal cell membrane, allowing leakage of cellular contents. Toxicity (especially acute infusion reactions and nephrotoxicity) is less with lipid formulations. **Therapeutic Effects:** Can be fungistatic or fungicidal (depends on concentration achieved and susceptibility of organism). **Spectrum:** Active against: Aspergillosis, Blastomycosis, Candidiasis, Coccidioidomycosis, Cryptococcosis, Histoplasmosis, Leishmaniasis (liposomal formulation only), Mucormycosis.

Pharmacokinetics
Absorption: IV administration results in complete bioavailability.
Distribution: Extensively distributed to body tissues and fluids. Poor penetration into CSF.
Metabolism and Excretion: Elimination is very prolonged. Detectable in urine up to 7 wk after discontinuation.
Half-life: Biphasic—initial phase, 24–48 hr; terminal phase, 15 days. *Cholesteryl sulfate*—28 hr. *Lipid complex*—174 hr. *Liposomal*—100–153 hr.

TIME/ACTION PROFILE (blood levels)

ROUTE	ONSET	PEAK	DURATION
IV	rapid	end of infusion	24 hr

Contraindications/Precautions
Contraindicated in: Hypersensitivity; Lactation: Potential for distribution into breast milk and toxicity in infant; discontinue nursing.
Use Cautiously in: Renal impairment or electrolyte abnormalities; Patients receiving concurrent leukocyte transfusions (↑ risk of pulmonary toxicity); OB: Has been used safely.

Adverse Reactions/Side Effects
CNS: anxiety, confusion, headache, insomnia. **Resp:** dyspnea, hypoxia, wheezing. **CV:** chest pain, hypotension, tachycardia, edema, hyperten-

♣ = Canadian drug name. 🧬 = Genetic implication.
*CAPITALS indicates life-threatening; underlines indicate most frequent.

sion. **GI:** diarrhea, hyperbilirubinemia, ↑ liver enzymes, nausea, vomiting, abdominal pain. **GU:** nephrotoxicity, hematuria. **F and E:** hyperglycemia, hypocalcemia, hypokalemia, hypomagnesemia. **Hemat:** anemia, leukopenia, thrombocytopenia. **Derm:** pruritus, rashes. **Local:** phlebitis. **MS:** arthralgia, myalgia. **Misc:** HYPERSENSITIVITY REACTIONS, chills, fever, acute infusion reactions.

Interactions
Drug-Drug: ↑ risk of nephrotoxicity, bronchospasm, and hypotension with **antineoplastics**. Concurrent use with **corticosteroids** ↑ risk of hypokalemia. Concurrent use with **zidovudine** may ↑ the risk of myelotoxicity and nephrotoxicity. Concurrent use with **flucytosine** ↑ antifungal activity but may ↑ the risk of toxicity from flucytosine. Combined use with **azole antifungals** may induce fungal resistance. ↑ risk of nephrotoxicity with other **nephrotoxic agents** such as **aminoglycosides**, **cyclosporine**, or **tacrolimus**. Hypokalemia from amphotericin ↑ the risk of **digoxin** toxicity. Hypokalemia may enhance the curariform effects of **neuromuscular blocking agents**.

Route/Dosage
Specific dosage and duration of therapy depend on nature of infection being treated.

Amphotericin Deoxycholate
IV (Adults): Give test dose of 1 mg. If test dose tolerated, initiate therapy with 0.25 mg/kg/day (doses up to 1.5 mg/kg/day may be used, depending on type of infection) (alternate-day dosing may also be used); *Bladder irrigation*—Instill 50 mcg/mL solution into bladder daily for 5–10 days.
IV (Infants and Children): Give test dose of 0.1 mg/kg (maximum dose 1 mg) or may administer initial dose of 0.25–1 mg/kg/day over 6 hr (without test dose) (some infections may require 1.5 mg/kg/day; alternate-day dosing may be used).
IT (Adults): 25–300 mcg q 48–72 hr, ↑ to 500 mcg–1 mg as tolerated (maximum total dose = 15 mg).
IT (Children): 25–100 mcg q 48–72 hr; ↑ to 500 mcg as tolerated.

Amphotericin B Cholesteryl Sulfate (Amphotec)
IV (Adults and Children): 3–4 mg/kg q 24 hr (no test dose needed).

Amphotericin B Lipid Complex (Abelcet)
IV (Adults and Children): 2.5–5 mg/kg q 24 hr (no test dose needed).

Amphotericin B Liposome (AmBisome)
IV (Adults and Children): *Empiric therapy*—3 mg/kg q 24 hr; *Documented infections*—3–5 mg/kg q 24 hr; *Visceral leishmaniasis (immunocompetent patients)*—3 mg/kg q 24 hr on days 1–5, then 3 mg/kg q 24 hr on days 14 and 21; *Visceral leishmaniasis (immunosuppressed patients)*—4 mg/kg q 24 hr on days 1–5, then 4 mg/kg q 24 hr on days 10, 17, 24, 31, and 38; *Cryptococcal meningitis in HIV patients*—6 mg/kg q 24 hr.

Availability (generic available)
Amphotericin Deoxycholate
Powder for injection: 50 mg/vial.

Amphotericin B Cholesteryl Sulfate
Powder for injection: 50 mg/vial, 100 mg/vial.

Amphotericin B Lipid Complex
Suspension for injection: 5 mg/mL.

Amphotericin B Liposome
Powder for injection: 50 mg/vial.

NURSING IMPLICATIONS

Assessment
- Monitor patient closely during test dose and the first 1–2 hr of each dose for fever, chills, headache, anorexia, nausea, or vomiting. Premedicating with antipyretics, corticosteroids, antihistamines, meperidine, and antiemetics may decrease these reactions. Febrile reaction usually subsides within 4 hr after the infusion is completed.
- Assess injection site frequently for thrombophlebitis or leakage. Drug is very irritating to tissues.
- Monitor vital signs every 15 min during test dose and every 30 min for 2–4 hr after administration. Meperidine and dantrolene have been used to prevent and treat rigors. Assess respiratory status (lung sounds, dyspnea) daily. If respiratory distress occurs, discontinue infusion immediately; anaphylaxis may occur. Equipment for cardiopulmonary resuscitation should be readily available.
- Monitor intake and output and weigh daily. Adequate hydration (2000–3000 mL/day) and maintaining sodium balance may minimize nephrotoxicity.
- ***Lab Test Considerations:*** Monitor CBC, BUN and serum creatinine, and potassium and magnesium levels daily. If BUN and serum creatinine ↑ significantly, may need to discontinue or consider switching to cholesteryl sulfate, lipid complex, or liposomal formulation.

amphotericin B

Potential Nursing Diagnoses
Risk for infection (Indications)

Implementation
- Do not confuse amphotericin B cholesteryl sulfate (Amphotec) with amphotericin deoxycholate, amphotericin B lipid complex (Abelcet), or amphotericin B liposome (AmBisome); they are not interchangeable.
- This drug should be administered IV only to hospitalized patients or those under close supervision. Diagnosis should be confirmed before administration.

Amphotericin B Deoxycholate

IV Administration

- **Test dose:** Reconstitute 50-mg vial with 10 mL of sterile water for injection to achieve a concentration of 5 mg/mL. Reconstituted vial stable for 24 hr at room temperature or 1 wk if refrigerated. ***Diluent:*** Further dilute with 500 mL of D5W. May be diluted in 250 mL of D5W if being administered via a central venous catheter. Protect infusion from light. Infusion stable for 24 hr at room temperature or 2 days if refrigerated. To obtain test dose, withdraw 1 mg (10 mL) from 500 mL infusion and further dilute with D5W to a total volume of 20 mL. ***Concentration:*** 0.05 mg/mL. ***Rate:*** Infuse over 10–30 min to determine patient tolerance. Pedi: Infuse over 30–60 min.
- **Intermittent Infusion:** ***Diluent:*** Reconstitute and dilute 50-mg vial as per the directions above. ***Concentration:*** Final concentration of infusion should not exceed 0.1 mg/mL for peripheral infusion or 0.25 mg/mL for central line administration. ***Rate:*** Infuse slowly over 4–6 hr.
- **Y-Site Compatibility:** aldesleukin, amiodarone, dactinomycin, diltiazem, etoposide, hydromorphone, ifosfamide, lorazepam, nesiritide, octreotide, oxaliplatin, tacrolimus, teniposide, thiotepa, zidovudine.
- **Y-Site Incompatibility:** acyclovir, alfentanil, allopurinol, amifostine, amikacin, ampicillin, ampicillin/sulbactam, amsacrine, anidulafungin, atracurium, atropine, aztreonam, benztropine, bivalirudin, bumetanide, butorphanol, calcium chloride, calcium gluconate, carboplatin, caspofungin, cefepime, cefonocid, cefotetan, ceftizoxime, chloramphenicol, cimetidine, cisplatin, clindamycin, codeine, cyanocobalamin, cyclophosphamide, cytarabine, dantrolene, daptomycin, dexamethasone, dexmedetonidine, diazepam, diazoxide, digoxin, diphenhydramine, dobutamine, docetaxel, dopamine, doxacurium, doxorubicin, doxorubicin liposome, doxycycline, ephedrine, epirubicin, epoetin alfa, eptifibatide, ertapenem, erythromycin, esmolol, etoposide phosphate, famotidine, fenoldopam, filgrastim, fluconazole, fludarabine, fluorouracil, foscarnet, ganciclovir, gemcitabine, gentamicin, glycopyrrolate, granisetron, haloperidol, hetastarch, hydralazine, hydrocortisone, hydroxyzine, idarubicin, inamrinone, isoproterenol, ketorolac, labetalol, levofloxacin, lidocaine, linezolid, melphalan, meperidine, merchlorethamine, meropenem, metaraminol, methotrexate, methoxamine, methylprednisolone, metoclopramide, metoprolol, metronidazole, midazolam, milrinone, mitoxantrone, morphine, nafcillin, nalbuphine, nitroprusside, norepinephrine, ondansetron, oxacillin, paclitaxel, palonosetron, pancuronium, pantoprazole, papaverine, pemetrexed, penicillin G, pentamidine, pentazocine, phentolamine, phenylephrine, phenytoin, piperacillin/tazobactam, potassium chloride, prochlorperazine, promethazine, propofol, propranolol, protamine, pyridoxine, quinupristin/dalfopristin, rituximab, rocuronium, sodium acetate, sodium bicarbonate, succinylcholine, sufentanil, thiamine, tigecycline, tirofiban, tobramycin, tolazoline, trastuzumab, trimethoprim/sulfamethoxazole, urokinase, vancomycin, vasopressin, vecuronium, verapamil, vincristine, vinorelbine, voriconazole.
- **Solution Incompatibility:** LR injection, saline solutions.

Amphotericin B Cholesteryl Sulfate

IV Administration

- **Test Dose:** ***Diluent:*** Reconstitute 50-mg vial with 10 mL and 100-mg vial with 20 mL of sterile water for injection to achieve a concentration of 5 mg/mL. Reconstituted vials are stable for 24 hr if refrigerated. Further dilute with D5W to achieve concentration below. Do not use other diluents. Infusion stable for 24 hr if refrigerated. Protect from light. To obtain test dose, withdraw 10 mL from final preparation. ***Concentration:*** Final concentration of infusion should be approximately 0.6 mg/mL (range 0.16–0.83 mg/mL). ***Rate:*** Infuse over 15–30 min.

- **Intermittent Infusion:** *Diluent:* Prepare infusion according to directions above. *Concentration:* Final concentration of infusion should be approximately 0.6 mg/mL (range 0.16–0.83 mg/mL). *Rate:* Infuse at a rate of 1 mg/kg/hr. If patient tolerates infusion without adverse reactions, infusion time may be shortened to a minimum of 2 hr. If reactions occur or patient cannot tolerate volume, infusion time may be extended. Rapid infusions may cause hypotension, hypokalemia, arrhythmias, and shock.
- **Y-Site Compatibility:** acyclovir, aminophylline, cefoxitin, ceftizoxime, clindamycin, dexamethasone, fentanyl, furosemide, ganciclovir, granisetron, hydrocortisone, ifosfamide, lorazepam, mannitol, methotrexate, methylprednisolone, nitroglycerin, sufentanil, trimethoprim/sulfamethoxazole, vinblastine, vincristine, zidovudine.
- **Y-Site Incompatibility:** alfentanil, amikacin, ampicillin, ampicillin/sulbactam, aztreonam, buprenorphine, butorphanol, calcium chloride, calcium gluconate, carboplatin, cefazolin, cefepime, ceftazidime, ceftriaxone, cimetidine, cisatracurium, cisplatin, cyclophosphamide, cyclosporine, cytarabine, diazepam, digoxin, diphenhydramine, dobutamine, dopamine, doxorubicin, doxorubicin liposome, droperidol, enalaprilat, esmolol, famotidine, fluconazole, fluorouracil, gentamicin, haloperidol, heparin, hydromorphone, hydroxyzine, imipenem/cilastatin, labetalol, leucovorin, lidocaine, magnesium sulfate, meperidine, mesna, metoclopramide, metoprolol, metronidazole, midazolam, mitoxantrone, morphine, nalbuphine, naloxone, ondansetron, paclitaxel, pentobarbital, phenobarbital, phenytoin, piperacillin/tazobactam, potassium chloride, prochlorperazine, promethazine, propranolol, ranitidine, remifentanil, sodium bicarbonate, ticarcillin-clavulanate, tobramycin, vancomycin, vecuronium, verapamil, vinorelbine.
- **Solution Incompatibility:** saline solutions.

Amphotericin B Lipid Complex

IV Administration

- **Intermittent Infusion:** *Diluent:* Shake vial gently until yellow sediment at bottom has dissolved. Withdraw dose from required number of vials with 18-gauge needle. Replace needle from syringe filled with amphotericin B lipid complex with 5-micron filter needle. Each filter needle may be used to filter the contents of no more than 4 vials. Insert filter needle of syringe into IV bag of D5W and empty contents of syringe into bag. Protect from light. Infusion is stable for 6 hr at room temperature or 48 hr if refrigerated. *Concentration:* Final concentration of infusion should be 1 mg/mL; a concentration of 2 mg/mL can be used for pediatric patients or patients who cannot tolerate large volumes of fluid. *Rate:* Do not use an in-line filter. Infuse at a rate of 2.5 mg/kg/hr via infusion pump. If infusion exceeds 2 hr, mix contents by shaking infusion bag every 2 hr. If administering through an existing line, flush line with D5W before infusion or use a separate line.
- **Y-Site Compatibility:** anidulafungin, ertapenem, octreotide.
- **Y-Site Incompatibility:** bivalirudin, caspofungin, daptomycin, tirofiban.
- **Solution Incompatibility:** saline solutions.

Amphotericin B Liposome

IV Administration

- **Intermittent Infusion:** *Diluent:* Reconstitute each 50–mg vial with 12 mL of sterile water for injection to achieve concentration of 4 mg/mL. Immediately shake vial vigorously for at least 30 seconds until all particulate matter is completely dispersed. Reconstituted vials are stable for 24 hr if refrigerated. Withdraw appropriate volume for dilution into a syringe. Attach the 5-micron filter to the syringe and inject syringe contents into an appropriate volume of D5W. Infusion should be administered within 6 hr of dilution. *Concentration:* Final concentration of infusion should be 1–2 mg/mL; a lower concentration (0.2–0.5 mg/mL) may be used for infants and small children. *Rate:* Infuse over 2 hr. Infusion time may be shortened to 1 hr if patient tolerates infusion without any adverse reactions. If discomfort occurs during infusion, duration of infusion may be increased. May be administered through an in-line filter with pore diameter of at least 1 micron. If administering through an existing line, flush line with D5W before infusion or use a separate line.
- **Y-Site Compatibility:** acyclovir, amifostine, aminophylline, anidulafungin, atropine, azithromycin, bivalirudin, bumetanide, buprenorphine, busulfan, butorphanol, carboplatin, carmustine, cefazolin, cefoxitin, ceftizoxime, ceftriaxone, cefuroxime, cimetidine, clindamycin, cyclophosphamide, cytarabine, dactinomycin, daptomycin, dexamethasone, dexmedetomidine, diphenhydramine, doxacurium,

enalaprilat, ephedrine, epinephrine, eptifibatide, ertapenem, esmolol, etoposide, famotidine, fenoldopam, fentanyl, fludarabine, fluorouracil, fosphenytoin, furosemide, granisetron, haloperidol, heparin, hydrocortisone, hydromorphone, ifosfamide, isoproterenol, ketorolac, levorphanol, lidocaine, linezolid, mesna, methotrexate, methylprednisolone, metoprolol, milrinone, mitomycin, nesiritide, nitroglycerin, nitroprusside, octreotide, oxaliplatin, oxytocin, palonosetron, pancuronium, pantoprazole, pemetrexed, pentobarbital, phenobarbital, phenylephrine, piperacillin/tazobactam, potassium chloride, procainamide, ranitidine, sufetanil, tacrolimus, theophylline, thiopental, thiotepa, ticarcillin/clavulanate, tigecycline, trimethoprim/sulfamethoxazole, vasopressin, vincristine, voriconazole, zidovudine.

- **Y-Site Incompatibility:** alfentanil, amikacin, ampicillin, ampicillin/sulbactam, aztreonam, bleomycin, calcium chloride, calcium gluconate, caspofungin, cefepime, cefotaxime, ceftazidime, ciprofloxacin, cisplatin, cyclosporine, dacarbazine, daunorubicin, dexrazoxane, diazepam, digoxin, diltiazem, dobutamine, docetaxel, dolasetron, dopamine, doxorubicin, doxycycline, droperidol, epirubicin, erythromycin, etoposide phosphate, gemcitabine, gentamicin, hetastarch, hydroxyzine, idarubicin, imipenem/cilastatin, inamrinone, labetalol, leucovorin, levofloxacin, lorazepam, magnesium sulfate, mannitol, mechlorethamine, meperidine, meropenem, metoclopramide, metronidazole, midazolam, mitoxantrone, morphine, nalbuphine, naloxone, nicardipine, ondansetron, paclitaxel, pentamidine, phenytoin, potassium phosphates, prochlorperazine, promethazine, propranolol, quinupristin/dalfopristin, sodium bicarbonate, sodium phosphates, teniposide, tobramycin, trimethobenzamide, vancomycin, verapamil, vinblastine, vinorelbine.
- **Solution Incompatibility:** Do not dilute or admix with saline solutions, other medications, or solutions containing a bacteriostatic agent.

Patient/Family Teaching
- Explain need for long duration of IV or topical therapy.
- IV: Inform patient of potential side effects and discomfort at IV site. Advise patient to notify health care professional if side effects occur.
- **Home Care Issue:** Instruct family or caregiver on dilution, rate, and administration of drug and proper care of IV equipment.

Evaluation/Desired Outcomes
- Resolution of signs and symptoms of infection. Several weeks to months of therapy may be required to prevent relapse.

---

ampicillin (am-pi-sil-in)
✦Ampicin, ✦Apo-Ampi, Marcillin, ✦Nu-Ampi, ✦Novo-Ampicillin, Omnipen, Penbritin, Principen, Polycillin, Totacillin

Classification
Therapeutic: anti-infectives
Pharmacologic: aminopenicillins

Pregnancy Category B

Indications
Treatment of the following infections: Skin and skin structure infections, Soft-tissue infections, Otitis media, Sinusitis, Respiratory infections, Genitourinary infections, Meningitis, Septicemia. Endocarditis prophylaxis. **Unlabeled Use:** Prevention of infection in certain high-risk patients undergoing cesarean section.

Action
Binds to bacterial cell wall, resulting in cell death. **Therapeutic Effects:** Bactericidal action; spectrum is broader than penicillin. **Spectrum:** Active against: Streptococci, nonpenicillinase-producing staphylococci, *Listeria*, Pneumococci, Enterococci, *Haemophilus influenzae*, *Escherichia coli*, *Enterobacter*, *Klebsiella*, *Proteus mirabilis*, *Neisseria meningitidis*, *N. gonorrhoeae*, *Shigella*, *Salmonella*.

Pharmacokinetics
Absorption: Moderately absorbed from the duodenum (30–50%).
Distribution: Diffuses readily into body tissues and fluids. CSF penetration is increased in the presence of inflamed meninges. Crosses the placenta; enters breast milk in small amounts.
Metabolism and Excretion: Variably metabolized by the liver (12–50%). Renal excretion is variable (25–60% after oral dosing; 50–85% after IM administration).
Half-life: Neonates: 1.7–4 hr; Children and Adults: 1–1.5 hr (increased in renal impairment).

ampicillin

TIME/ACTION PROFILE (blood levels)

ROUTE	ONSET	PEAK	DURATION
PO	rapid	1.5–2 hr	4–6 hr
IM	rapid	1 hr	4–6 hr
IV	rapid	end of infusion	4–6 hr

Contraindications/Precautions
Contraindicated in: Hypersensitivity to penicillins.
Use Cautiously in: Severe renal insufficiency (dosage reduction required if CCr <10 mL/min); Infectious mononucleosis, acute lymphocytic leukemia or cytomegalovirus infection (increased incidence of rash); Patients allergic to cephalosporins; OB: Has been used during pregnancy; Lactation: Is distributed into breast milk. Can cause rash, diarrhea, and sensitization in the infant.

Adverse Reactions/Side Effects
CNS: SEIZURES (high doses). **GI:** PSEUDOMEMBRANOUS COLITIS, diarrhea, nausea, vomiting. **Derm:** rashes, urticaria. **Hemat:** blood dyscrasias. **Misc:** allergic reactions including ANAPHYLAXIS and SERUM SICKNESS, superinfection.

Interactions
Drug-Drug: **Probenecid** decreases renal excretion and increases blood levels of ampicillin—therapy may be combined for this purpose. Large doses may increase the risk of bleeding with **warfarin**. Incidence of rash increases with concurrent **allopurinol** therapy. May decrease the effectiveness of oral **hormonal contraceptives**.

Route/Dosage
Respiratory and Soft-Tissue Infections
PO (Adults and Children ≥20 kg): 250–500 mg q 6 hr.
PO (Children <20 kg): 50–100 mg/kg/day in divided doses q 6–8 hr (not to exceed 2–3 g/day).
IM, IV (Adults and Children ≥40 kg): 500 mg to 3 g q 6 hr (not to exceed 14 g/day).
IM, IV (Children <40 kg): 100–200 mg/kg/day in divided doses q 6–8 hr (not to exceed 12 g/day).

Bacterial Meningitis Caused by *H. influenzae, Streptococcus pneumoniae*, Group B streptococcus or *N. meningitidis* or Septicemia
IM, IV (Adults): 500 mg to 3 g q 6 hr (not to exceed 14 g/day).
IM, IV (Children >1 mo): 200–400 mg/kg/day in divided doses q 6 hr (not to exceed 12 g/day).
IM, IV (Neonates ≤7 days): 200 mg/kg/day divided q 8 hr.
IM, IV (Neonates >7 days): 300 mg/kg/day divided q 6 hr.

GI/GU Infections Other Than *N. gonorrhoeae*
PO (Adults and Children >20 kg): 250–500 mg q 6 hr (larger doses for more serious/chronic infections).
PO (Children ≤20 kg): 50–100 mg/kg/day in divided doses q 6 hr.

N. gonorrhoeae
PO (Adults): 3 g with 1 g probenecid.
IM, IV (Adults and Children ≥40 kg): 500 mg q 6 hr.
IM, IV (Children <40 kg): 100–200 mg/kg/day in divided doses q 6–8 hr.

Urethritis Caused by *N. gonorrhoeae* in Men
IM, IV (Adults and Children ≥40 kg): 500 mg, repeated 8–12 hr later; additional doses may be necessary for more complicated infections (prostatitis, epididymitis).

Prevention of Bacterial Endocarditis
IM, IV (Adults): 2 g 30 min before procedure (gentamicin may be added for high-risk patients); additional 1 g may be given 6 hr later for high-risk patients.
IM, IV (Children): 50 mg/kg (not to exceed 2 g) 30 min before procedure (gentamicin may be added for high-risk patients); additional 25 mg/kg may be given 6 hr later for high-risk patients.

Renal Impairment
(Adults and Children): CCr ≤10 mL/min—Increase dosing interval to q 12 hr.

Availability
Capsules: 250 mg, 500 mg. **Suspension (wild cherry flavor):** 125 mg/5 mL, 250 mg/5 mL. **Powder for injection:** 125 mg, 250 mg, 500 mg, 1 g, 2 g, 10 g.

NURSING IMPLICATIONS

Assessment
- Assess patient for infection (vital signs, wound appearance, sputum, urine, stool, and WBC) at beginning of and throughout therapy.
- Obtain a history before initiating therapy to determine previous use and reactions to penicillins or cephalosporins. Persons with a negative history of penicillin sensitivity may still have an allergic response.

ampicillin

- Obtain specimens for culture and sensitivity before therapy. First dose may be given before receiving results.
- Observe patient for signs and symptoms of anaphylaxis (rash, pruritus, laryngeal edema, wheezing). Discontinue the drug and notify the physician or other health care professional immediately if these occur. Keep epinephrine, an antihistamine, and resuscitation equipment close by in the event of an anaphylactic reaction.
- Assess skin for "ampicillin rash," a nonallergic, dull red, macular or maculopapular, mildly pruritic rash.
- *Lab Test Considerations:* May cause increased AST and ALT.
- May cause transient decreases in estradiol, total conjugated estriol, estriol-glucuronide, or conjugated estrone in pregnant women.
- May cause a false-positive direct Coombs' test result.
- May cause a false-positive urinary glucose.

Potential Nursing Diagnoses
Risk for infection (Indications, Side Effects)
Noncompliance (Patient/Family Teaching)

Implementation
- Do not confuse with omnipen with imipenem.
- Reserve IM or IV route for moderately severe or severe infections or patients unable to take oral medication. Change to PO as soon as possible.
- **PO:** Administer around the clock on an empty stomach at least 1 hr before or 2 hr after meals with a full glass of water. Capsules may be opened and mixed with water. Reconstituted oral suspensions retain potency for 7 days at room temperature and 14 days if refrigerated. Combination with probenecid should be used immediately after reconstitution.
- **IM:** Reconstitute for IM or IV use by adding sterile water for injection 0.9–1.2 mL to the 125-mg vial, 0.9–1.9 mL to the 250-mg vial, 1.2–1.8 mL to the 500-mg vial, 2.4–7.4 mL to the 1-g vial, and 6.8 mL to the 2-g vial.

IV Administration
- **Direct IV:** *Diluent:* Sterile water for injection. *Concentration:* Add 5 mL of sterile water for injection to each 125-, 250-, or 500-mg vial or at least 7.4–10 mL of diluent to each 1- or 2-g vial. Solution should be used within 1 hr of reconstitution. *Rate:* Doses of 125–500 mg may be given over 3–5 min (not to exceed 100 mg/min). Rapid administration may cause seizures.
- **Intermittent Infusion:** *Diluent:* Reconstitute vials as per the directions above. Further dilute in 50 mL or more of 0.9% NaCl, D5W, D5/0.45% NaCl, or LR. Administer within 4 hr (more stable in NaCl). *Concentration:* Final concentration of infusion should not exceed 30 mg/mL. *Rate:* Infuse over 10–15 min.
- **Y-Site Compatibility:** acyclovir, anidulafungin, bivalirudin, daptomycin, filgrastim, granisetron, heparin, levofloxacin, linezolid, milrinone, palonosetron, pantoprazole, propofol, tacrolimus, voriconazole.
- **Y-Site Incompatibility:** If aminoglycosides and penicillins must be administered concurrently, administer in separate sites at least 1 hr apart, aminophylline, amphotericin B, caspofungin, diazepam, diphenhydramine, dobutamine, dopamine, doxycycline, fenoldopam, fluconazole, ganciclovir, haloperidol, hydroxyzine, lansoprazole, lorazepam, midazolam, nafcillin, nicardipine, nitroprusside, ondansetron, penicillin G potassium, phenytoin, prochlorperazine, promethazine, protamine, quinupristin/dalfopristin, sodium bicarbonate, trimethoprim/sulfamethoxazole, verapamil.

Patient/Family Teaching
- Instruct patient to take medication around the clock and to finish the drug completely as directed, even if feeling better. Advise patients that sharing of this medication can be dangerous. Pedi: Instruct parents and caregivers not to save or use this medication for other infections.
- Advise patient to report the signs of superinfection (furry overgrowth on the tongue, vaginal itching or discharge, loose or foul-smelling stools) and allergy.
- Advise patients taking oral contraceptives to use an alternate or additional nonhormonal method of contraception while taking ampicillin and until next menstrual period.
- Caution patient to notify health care professional if fever and diarrhea occur, especially if stool contains blood, pus, or mucus. Advise patient not to treat diarrhea without consulting health care professional. May occur up to several weeks after discontinuation of medication.
- Instruct the patient to notify health care professional if symptoms do not improve.

✽ = Canadian drug name. ✺ = Genetic implication.
*CAPITALS indicates life-threatening; underlines indicate most frequent.

- Patients with a history of rheumatic heart disease or valve replacement need to be taught the importance of using antimicrobial prophylaxis before invasive medical or dental procedures.
- Lactation: Small amounts of ampicillin in breast milk can cause sensitization and alter intestinal flora of the infant. Instruct patient to monitor infant for reactions and discuss with health care provider possible need to temporarily avoid breastfeeding.

Evaluation/Desired Outcomes
- Resolution of the signs and symptoms of infection. Length of time for complete resolution depends on the organism and site of infection.
- Endocarditis prophylaxis.

ampicillin/sulbactam
(am-pi-**sil**-in/sul-**bak**-tam)
Unasyn

Classification
Therapeutic: anti-infectives
Pharmacologic: aminopenicillins/beta lactamase inhibitors

Pregnancy Category B

Indications
Treatment of the following infections: Skin and skin structure infections, soft-tissue infections, Otitis media, Intra-abdominal infections, Sinusitis, Respiratory infections, Genitourinary infections, Meningitis, Septicemia.

Action
Binds to bacterial cell wall, resulting in cell death; spectrum is broader than that of penicillin. Addition of sulbactam increases resistance to beta-lactamases, enzymes produced by bacteria that may inactivate ampicillin. **Therapeutic Effects:** Bactericidal action. **Spectrum:** Active against: Streptococci, Pneumococci, Enterococci, *Haemophilus influenzae*, *Escherichia coli*, *Proteus mirabilis*, *Neisseria meningitidis*, *N. gonorrhoeae*, *Shigella*, *Salmonella*, *Bacteroides fragilis*, *Moraxella catarrhalis*. Use should be reserved for infections caused by beta-lactamase–producing strains.

Pharmacokinetics
Absorption: Well absorbed from IM sites.
Distribution: Ampicillin diffuses readily into bile, blister and tissue fluids. Poor CSF penetration unless meninges are inflamed. Crosses the placenta; enters breast milk in small amounts.

Metabolism and Excretion: Ampicillin is variably metabolized by the liver (12–50%). Renal excretion is also variable. Sulbactam is eliminated unchanged in urine.
Protein Binding: *Ampicillin*—28%; *sulbactam*—38%.
Half-life: *Ampicillin*—1–1.8 hr; *sulbactam*—1–1.3 hr.

TIME/ACTION PROFILE (blood levels)

ROUTE	ONSET	PEAK	DURATION
IM	rapid	1 hr	6–8 hr
IV	immediate	end of infusion	6–8 hr

Contraindications/Precautions
Contraindicated in: Hypersensitivity to penicillins or sulbactam.
Use Cautiously in: Severe renal insufficiency (dosage reduction required if CCr <30 mL/min); Epstein-Barr virus infection, acute lymphocytic leukemia, or cytomegalovirus infection (increased incidence of rash).

Adverse Reactions/Side Effects
CNS: SEIZURES (high doses). **GI:** PSEUDOMEMBRANOUS COLITIS, diarrhea, nausea, vomiting. **Derm:** rashes, urticaria. **Hemat:** blood dyscrasias. **Local:** pain at IM site, pain at IV site. **Misc:** allergic reactions including ANAPHYLAXIS and SERUM SICKNESS, superinfection, elevated liver enzymes.

Interactions
Drug-Drug: Probenecid decreases renal excretion and increases blood levels of ampicillin—therapy may be combined for this purpose. May potentiate the effect of **warfarin**. Concurrent **allopurinol** therapy (increased incidence of rash). May decrease the effectiveness of **hormonal contraceptives**.

Route/Dosage
Dosage based on ampicillin component.
IM, IV (Adults and Children ≥40 kg): 1–2 g ampicillin q 6–8 hr (not to exceed 12 g ampicillin/day).
IM, IV (Children ≥1 yr): 100–200 mg ampicillin/kg/day divided q 6 hr; *Meningitis*—200–400 mg ampicillin/kg/day divided every 6 hr; maximum dose: 8 g ampicillin/day.
IM, IV (Infants >1 month): 100–150 mg ampicillin/kg/day divided q 6 hr.

Renal Impairment
IM, IV (Adults , Children, and Infants): *CCr 15–29 mL/min*—Administer q 12 hr; *CCr 5–14*—Administer q 24 hr.

ampicillin/sulbactam 173

Availability
Powder for injection: 1.5 g (1 g ampicillin with 500 mg sulbactam), 3 g (2 g ampicillin with 1 g sulbactam), 15 g (10 g ampicillin with 5 g sulbactam).

NURSING IMPLICATIONS

Assessment
- Assess patient for infection (vital signs, wound appearance, sputum, urine, stool, and WBCs) at beginning and throughout therapy.
- Obtain a history before initiating therapy to determine previous use of, and reactions to, penicillins or cephalosporins. Persons with a negative history of penicillin sensitivity may still have an allergic response.
- Obtain specimens for culture and sensitivity before therapy. First dose may be given before receiving results.
- Observe patient for signs and symptoms of anaphylaxis (rash, pruritus, laryngeal edema, wheezing). Discontinue the drug and notify the physician or other health care professional immediately if these occur. Keep epinephrine, an antihistamine, and resuscitation equipment close by in the event of an anaphylactic reaction.
- **Lab Test Considerations:** May cause increased AST, ALT, LDH, bilirubin, alkaline phosphatase, BUN, and creatinine.
- May cause decreased hemoglobin, hematocrit, RBC, WBC, neutrophils, and lymphocytes.
- May cause transient decreases in estradiol, total conjugated estriol, estriol-glucuronide, or conjugated estrone in pregnant women.
- May cause a false-positive Coombs' test result.

Potential Nursing Diagnoses
Risk for infection (Indications, Side Effects)

Implementation
- **IM:** Reconstitute for IM use by adding 3.2 mL of sterile water or 0.5% or 2% lidocaine HCl to the 1.5-g vial or 6.4 mL to the 3-g vial. Administer within 1 hr of preparation, deep IM into well-developed muscle.

IV Administration
- **Direct IV:** *Diluent:* Reconstitute 1.5-g vial with 3.2 mL of sterile water for injection and the 3-g vial with 6.4 mL. *Concentration:* 375 mg ampicillin/sulbactam per mL. *Rate:* Administer over at least 10–15 min within 1 hr of reconstitution. More rapid administration may cause seizures.

- **Intermittent Infusion:** *Diluent:* Reconstitute vials as per the directions above. Further dilute in 50–100 mL of 0.9% NaCl, D5W, D5/0.45% NaCl, or LR. Stability of solution varies from 2–8 hr at room temperature or 3–72 hr if refrigerated, depending on concentration and diluent. *Concentration:* Final concentration of infusion should be 3–45 mg of ampicillin/sulbactam per mL. *Rate:* Infuse over 15–30 min.
- **Y-Site Compatibility:** anidulafungin, bivalirudin, daptomycin, fenoldopam, filgrastim, fluconazole, granisetron, hydromorphone, levofloxacin, linezolid, palonosetron, pantoprazole, tacrolimus, tirofiban, voriconazole.
- **Y-Site Incompatibility:** acyclovir, amiodarone, amphotericin B cholesteryl sulfate, caspofungin, cefotaxime, cefoxitin, ciprofloxacin, diazepam, dobutamine, doxycycline, ganciclovir, haloperidol, hydralazine, hydroxyzine, lansoprazole, lorazepam, methylprednisolone sodium succinate, midazolam, nicardipine, ondansetron, phenytoin, prochlorperazine, promethazine, protamine, quinupristin/dalfopristin, trimethoprim/sulfamethoxazole, verapamil. If aminoglycosides and penicillins must be given concurrently, administer in separate sites at least 1 hr apart.

Patient/Family Teaching
- Advise patient to report signs of superinfection (furry overgrowth on the tongue, vaginal itching or discharge, loose or foul-smelling stools) and allergy.
- Advise patients taking oral contraceptives to use an alternative or additional nonhormonal method of contraception while taking ampicillin/sulbactam and until next menstrual period.
- Caution patient to notify health care professional if fever and diarrhea occur, especially if stool contains blood, pus, or mucus. Advise patient not to treat diarrhea without consulting health care professional. May occur up to several weeks after discontinuation of medication.
- Instruct the patient to notify health care professional if symptoms do not improve.

Evaluation/Desired Outcomes
- Resolution of signs and symptoms of infection. Length of time for complete resolution depends on the organism and site of infection.

✦ = Canadian drug name. ⚕ = Genetic implication.
*CAPITALS indicates life-threatening; underlines indicate most frequent.

anakinra (a-na-kin-ra)
Kineret

Classification
Therapeutic: antirheumatics (DMARD)
Pharmacologic: interleukin antagonists

Pregnancy Category B

Indications
Reduction of the signs and symptoms of moderately to severely active rheumatoid arthritis in patients who have failed other DMARDs (may be used in combination with other DMARDs other than tumor necrosis factor [TNF] blocking agents).

Action
Blocks the destructive effects of interleukin-1 on cartilage and bone resorption by inhibiting its binding at specific tissue receptor sites. **Therapeutic Effects:** Slowed progression of rheumatoid arthritis.

Pharmacokinetics
Absorption: Well absorbed (95%) following subcut administration.
Distribution: Unknown.
Metabolism and Excretion: Unknown.
Half-life: 4–6 hr.

TIME/ACTION PROFILE (clinical response)

ROUTE	ONSET	PEAK	DURATION
Subcut	within 12 wk	unknown	unknown

Contraindications/Precautions
Contraindicated in: Active infections; Hypersensitivity; Hypersensitivity to other *Escherichia coli*–derived products.
Use Cautiously in: Other chronic debilitating illness; Underlying immunosuppression; Renal impairment; OB, Lactation, Pedi: Safety not established; Geri: May be more sensitive to toxicity due to age-related decline in renal function; increased incidence of infection in geriatric population.
Exercise Extreme Caution in: Concurrent use of TNF blocking agents such as etanercept (higher risk of serious infections).

Adverse Reactions/Side Effects
CNS: headache. **GI:** diarrhea, nausea. **Hemat:** neutropenia. **Local:** injection site reactions.
Misc: INFECTIONS, hypersensitivity reactions (rare).

Interactions
Drug-Drug: ↑ risk of serious infection with **TNF blocking agents**, such as **etanercept**. May ↓ antibody response to and increase the risk of adverse reactions from **vaccines**; avoid concurrent administration of **live vaccines**.

Route/Dosage
Subcut (Adults ≥18 yr): 100 mg/day.

Availability
Solution for injection: 100 mg/mL in 1-mL prefilled glass syringes.

NURSING IMPLICATIONS

Assessment
- Assess patient's range of motion and degree of swelling and pain in affected joints before and periodically during therapy.
- Assess for signs and symptoms of infection (fever, elevated WBC) prior to and periodically during therapy. Anakinra should not be instituted in patients with active infections and should be discontinued if patient develops a serious infection.
- Observe patient for hypersensitivity reactions (urticaria, dyspnea, hypotension). Discontinue anakinra if severe reaction occurs. Medications (antihistamines, acetaminophen, corticosteroids, epinephrine) and equipment should be readily available in the event of a severe reaction.
- *Lab Test Considerations:* Monitor neutrophil count prior to and during therapy, then monthly for 3 mo and quarterly thereafter for up to 1 yr.

Potential Nursing Diagnoses
Impaired physical mobility (Indications)
Acute pain (Indications)

Implementation
- Administration of higher than recommended doses did not result in higher responses.
- **Subcut:** Administer 1 dose/day. Do not administer solutions that are discolored or contain particulate matter. Provided in single-use 1-mL prefilled glass syringes.

Patient/Family Teaching
- Inform patient of the signs and symptoms of hypersensitivity reactions and other adverse reactions. Advise patient of appropriate actions if reactions occur.
- Advise patients not to receive live vaccines during therapy with anakinra without consulting health care professional.
- **Home Care Issues:** Instruct patient and family on preparation and correct technique for administration of injection and care and disposal of equipment. Caution patients and caregivers not to reuse needles, syringes, or drug product.

Evaluation/Desired Outcomes
- Reduction of signs and symptoms and slowed progression of moderate to severe active rheumatoid arthritis.

anastrozole (a-nass-troe-zole)
Arimidex

Classification
Therapeutic: antineoplastics
Pharmacologic: aromatase inhibitors

Pregnancy Category X

Indications
Adjuvant treatment of postmenopausal hormone receptor-positive early breast cancer. Initial therapy in women with postmenopausal hormone receptor-positive or hormone receptor unknown, locally advanced, or metastatic breast cancer. Advanced postmenopausal breast cancer in women with disease progression despite tamoxifen therapy.

Action
Inhibits the enzyme aromatase, which is partially responsible for conversion of precursors to estrogen. **Therapeutic Effects:** Lowers levels of circulating estrogen, which may halt progression of estrogen-sensitive breast cancer.

Pharmacokinetics
Absorption: 83–85% absorbed following oral administration.
Distribution: Unknown.
Metabolism and Excretion: 85% metabolized by the liver; 11% excreted renally.
Half-life: 50 hr.

TIME/ACTION PROFILE (lowering of serum estradiol)

ROUTE	ONSET	PEAK	DURATION
PO	within 24 hr	14 days	6 days†

†Following cessation of therapy

Contraindications/Precautions
Contraindicated in: OB: Potential harm to fetus or spontaneous abortion.
Use Cautiously in: Women with childbearing potential; Ischemic heart disease; Lactation, Pedi: Safety not established.

Adverse Reactions/Side Effects
CNS: headache, weakness, dizziness. **EENT:** pharyngitis. **Resp:** dyspnea, increased cough. **CV:** MYOCARDIAL INFARCTION, angina, peripheral edema. **GI:** nausea, abdominal pain, anorexia, constipation, diarrhea, dry mouth, vomiting. **GU:** pelvic pain, vaginal bleeding, vaginal dryness. **Derm:** rash, including mucocutaneous disorders, sweating. **Metab:** hypercholesterolemia, weight gain. **MS:** back pain, arthritis, bone pain, carpal tunnel syndrome, fracture. **Neuro:** paresthesia. **Misc:** allergic reactions including ANGIOEDEMA, URTICARIA, and ANAPHYLAXIS, hot flashes, pain.

Interactions
Drug-Drug: None significant.

Route/Dosage
PO (Adults): 1 mg daily.

Availability
Tablets: 1 mg. **Cost:** $795.94/90.

NURSING IMPLICATIONS

Assessment
- Assess patient for pain and other side effects periodically during therapy.
- *Lab Test Considerations:* May cause ↑ GTT, AST, ALT, alkaline phosphatase, total cholesterol, and LDL cholesterol levels.

Potential Nursing Diagnoses
Acute pain (Side Effects)

Implementation
- **PO:** Take medication consistently with regard to food.

Patient/Family Teaching
- Instruct patient to take medication as directed. Take missed doses as soon as remembered unless it is almost time for next dose. Do not double doses. Advise patient to read the *Patient Information* leaflet before starting and with each Rx refill; changes may occur.
- Inform patient of potential for adverse reactions, and advise patient to notify health care professional immediately if allergic reactions (swelling of the face, lips, tongue, and/or throat, difficulty in swallowing and/or breathing), liver problems (general feeling of not being well, yellowing of skin or whites of eyes, pain on the right side of abdomen), skin reactions (lesions, ulcers, or blisters), or chest pain occurs.
- Advise patient that vaginal bleeding may occur during first few weeks after changing over from other hormonal therapy. Continued bleeding should be evaluated.

♦ = Canadian drug name. ⚡ = Genetic implication.
*CAPITALS indicates life-threatening; underlines indicate most frequent.

- Teach patient to report increase in pain so treatment can be initiated.
- Advise patient to notify health care professional immediately if pregnancy is planned or suspected.

Evaluation/Desired Outcomes
- Slowing of disease progression in women with advanced breast cancer.

ANGIOTENSIN-CONVERTING ENZYME (ACE) INHIBITORS

benazepril (ben-**aye**-ze-pril)
Lotensin

captopril (**kap**-toe-pril)
Capoten

enalapril/enalaprilat
(e-**nal**-a-pril/e-**nal**-a-pril-at)
Vasotec, Vasotec IV

fosinopril (foe-**sin**-oh-pril)
Monopril

lisinopril (lyse-**in**-oh-pril)
Prinivil, Zestril

moexipril (moe-**eks**-i-pril)
Univasc

perindopril (pe-**rin**-do-pril)
Aceon, ✣ Coversyl

quinapril (**kwin**-a-pril)
Accupril

ramipril (ra-**mi**-pril)
Altace

trandolapril (tran-**doe**-la-pril)
Mavik

Classification
Therapeutic: antihypertensives
Pharmacologic: ACE inhibitors

Pregnancy Category C (first trimester), D (second and third trimester; all trimesters for perindopril)

Indications
Alone or with other agents in the management of hypertension. **Captopril, enalapril, fosinopril, lisinopril, quinapril, ramipril, trandolapril:** Management of CHF. **Captopril, lisinopril, ramipril, trandolapril:** Reduction of risk of death or development of CHF following MI. **Enalapril:** Slowed progression of left ventricular dysfunction into overt heart failure. **Ramipril:** Reduction of the risk of MI, stroke, and death from cardiovascular disease in patients at risk (>55 yr old with a history of CAD, stroke, peripheral vascular disease, or diabetes with another cardiovascular risk factor). **Captopril:** ↓ progression of diabetic nephropathy. **Perindopril:** Reduction of risk of death from cardiovascular causes or non-fatal MI in patients with stable CAD.

Action
ACE inhibitors block the conversion of angiotensin I to the vasoconstrictor angiotensin II. ACE inhibitors also prevent the degradation of bradykinin and other vasodilatory prostaglandins. ACE inhibitors also ↑ plasma renin levels and ↓ aldosterone levels. Net result is systemic vasodilation. **Therapeutic Effects:** Lowering of blood pressure in hypertensive patients. Improved symptoms in patients with CHF (selected agents only). ↓ development of overt heart failure (enalapril only). Improved survival and ↓ development of overt CHF after MI (selected agents only). ↓ risk of death from cardiovascular causes or MI in patients with stable CAD (perindopril only). ↓ risk of MI, stroke or death from cardiovascular causes in high-risk patients (ramipril only). ↓ progression of diabetic nephropathy (captopril only).

Pharmacokinetics
Absorption: *Benazepril*—37% absorbed after oral administration. *Captopril*—60–75% absorbed after oral administration (↓ by food). *Enalapril*—55–75% absorbed after oral administration. *Enalaprilat*—IV administration results in complete bioavailability. *Fosinopril*—36% absorbed after oral administration. *Lisinopril*—25% absorbed after oral administration (much variability). *Moexipril*—13% bioavailability as moexiprilat after oral administration (↓ by food). *Perindopril*—25% bioavailability as perindoprilat after oral administration. *Quinapril*—60% absorbed after oral administration (high-fat meal may ↓ absorption). *Ramipril*—50–60% absorbed after oral administration. *Trandolapril*—70% bioavailability as trandolapril at after oral administration.

Distribution: All ACE inhibitors cross the placenta. *Benazepril, captopril, enalapril, fosinopril, quinapril* and *trandolapril*—Enter breast milk. *Lisinopril*—Minimal penetration of CNS. *Ramipril*—Probably does not enter breast milk. *Trandolapril*—Enters breast milk.

Protein Binding: *Benazepril*—95%, *Fosinopril*—99.4%, *Moexipril*—90%, *Quinapril*—97%.

ANGIOTENSIN-CONVERTING ENZYME (ACE) INHIBITORS

Metabolism and Excretion: *Benazepril*—Converted by the liver to benazeprilat, the active metabolite. 20% excreted by kidneys; 11–12% nonrenal (biliary elimination). *Captopril*—50% metabolized by the liver to inactive compounds, 50% excreted unchanged by the kidneys. *Enalapril, enalaprilat*—Enalapril is converted by the liver to enalaprilat, the active metabolite; primarily eliminated by the kidneys. *Fosinopril*—Converted by the liver and GI mucosa to fosinoprilat, the active metabolite—50% excreted in urine, 50% in feces. *Lisinopril*—100% eliminated by the kidneys. *Moexipril*—Converted by liver and GI mucosa to moexiprilat, the active metabolite; 13% excreted in urine, 53% in feces. *Perindopril*—Converted by the liver to perindoprilat, the active metabolite; primarily excreted in urine. *Quinapril*—Converted by the liver, GI mucosa, and tissue to quinaprilat, the active metabolite; 96% eliminated by the kidneys. *Ramipril*—Converted by the liver to ramiprilat, the active metabolite; 60% excreted in urine, 40% in feces. *Trandolapril*—Converted by the liver to trandolaprilat, the active metabolite; 33% excreted in urine, 66% in feces.

Half-life: *Benazeprilat*—10–11 hr. *Captopril*—2 hr (↑ in renal impairment). *Enalapril*—2 hr (↑ in renal impairment). *Enalaprilat*—35–38 hr (↑ in renal impairment). *Fosinoprilat*—12 hr. *Lisinopril*—12 hr (↑ in renal impairment). *Moexiprilat*—2–9 hr (↑ in renal impairment). *Perindoprilat*—3–10 hr (↑ in renal impairment). *Quinaprilat*—3 hr (↑ in renal impairment). *Ramiprilat*—13–17 hr (↑ in renal impairment). *Trandolaprilat*—10 hr (↑ in renal impairment).

TIME/ACTION PROFILE (effect on blood pressure—single dose†)

ROUTE	ONSET	PEAK	DURATION
Benazepril	within 1 hr	2–4 hr	24 hr
Captopril	15–60 min	60–90 min	6–12 hr
Enalapril PO	1 hr	4–8 hr	12–24 hr
Enalapril IV	15 min	1–4 hr	4–6 hr
Fosinopril	within 1 hr	2–6 hr	24 hr
Lisinopril	1 hr	6 hr	24 hr
Moexipril	within 1 hr	3–6 hr	up to 24 hr
Perindoprilat	within 1–2 hr	3–7 hr	up to 24 hr
Quinapril	within 1 hr	2–4 hr	up to 24 hr
Ramipril	within 1–2 hr	3–6 hr	24 hr
Trandolapril	within 1–2 hr	4–10 hr	up to 24 hr

†Full effects may not be noted for several weeks

Contraindications/Precautions

Contraindicated in: Hypersensitivity; History of angioedema with previous use of ACE inhibitors; OB: Can cause injury or death of fetus; Lactation: Certain ACE inhibitors appear in breast milk; discontinue drug or use formula.

Use Cautiously in: Renal impairment, hepatic impairment, hypovolemia, hyponatremia, concurrent diuretic therapy; ▓ Black patients with hypertension (monotherapy less effective, may require additional therapy; ↑ risk of angioedema); Women of childbearing potential; Surgery/anesthesia (hypotension may be exaggerated); Pedi: Safety not established for most agents; benazepril, fosinopril, and lisinopril may be used in children ≥6 yr (captopril and enalapril may be used in children of all ages); Geri: Initial dose reduction recommended for most agents due to age-related decline in renal function.

Exercise Extreme Caution in: Family history of angioedema.

Adverse Reactions/Side Effects

CNS: dizziness, drowsiness, fatigue, headache, insomnia, vertigo, weakness. **Resp:** cough, dyspnea. **CV:** hypotension, chest pain, edema, tachycardia. **Endo:** hyperuricemia. **GI:** taste disturbances, abdominal pain, anorexia, constipation, diarrhea, nausea, vomiting. **GU:** erectile dysfunction, proteinuria, renal dysfunction, renal failure. **Derm:** flushing, pruritis, rashes. **F and E:** hyperkalemia. **Hemat:** AGRANULOCYTOSIS, neutropenia (captopril only). **MS:** back pain, muscle cramps, myalgia. **Misc:** ANGIOEDEMA, fever.

Interactions

Drug-Drug: Excessive hypotension may occur with concurrent use of **diuretics** and other **antihypertensives**. ↑ risk of hyperkalemia with concurrent use of **potassium supplements, potassium-sparing diuretics, potassium-containing salt substitutes**, or **angiotensin II receptor antagonists**. Antihypertensive response may be ↓ by **NSAIDs**. Absorption of fosinopril may be ↓ by **antacids** (separate administration by 1–2 hr). ↑ levels and may ↑ risk of **lithium** toxicity. Quinapril may ↓ absorption of **tetracycline, doxycycline**, and **fluoroquinolones** (because of magnesium in tablets). Telmisartan may ↑ **ramipril** levels; concurrent use not recommended.

Drug-Food: Food significantly ↓ absorption of captopril and moexipril (administer drugs 1 hr before meals).

✦ = Canadian drug name. ▓ = Genetic implication.
*CAPITALS indicates life-threatening; underlines indicate most frequent.

Route/Dosage

Benazepril
PO (Adults): 10 mg once daily, ↑ gradually to maintenance dose of 20–40 mg/day in 1–2 divided doses (begin with 5 mg/day in patients receiving diuretics).
PO (Children ≥6 yr): 0.2 mg/kg once daily; may be titrated up to 0.6 mg/kg/day (or 40 mg/day).

Renal Impairment
PO (Adults): *CCr <30 mL/min*—Initiate therapy with 5 mg once daily.

Renal Impairment
PO (Children ≥6 yr): *CCr <30 mL/min*—Contraindicated.

Captopril
PO (Adults): *Hypertension*—12.5–25 mg 2–3 times daily, may be ↑ at 1–2 wk intervals up to 150 mg 3 times daily (begin with 6.25–12.5 mg 2–3 times daily in patients receiving diuretics) (maximum dose = 450 mg/day); *CHF*—25 mg 3 times daily (6.25–12.5 mg 3 times daily in patients who have been vigorously diuresed); titrated up to target dose of 50 mg 3 times daily; *Post-MI*—6.25-mg test dose, followed by 12.5 mg 3 times daily, may be ↑ up to 50 mg 3 times daily; *Diabetic nephropathy*—25 mg 3 times daily.
PO (Children): *CHF*—0.3 mg/kg–0.5 mg/kg/dose 3 times daily, titrate up to a maximum of 6 mg/kg/day in 2–4 divided doses; *Older Children*—6.25–12.5 mg/dose q 12–24 hr, titrate up to a maximum of 6 mg/kg/day in 2–4 divided doses.
PO (Infants): *CHF*—0.15–0.3 mg/kg/dose, titrate up to a maximum of 6 mg/kg/day in 1–4 divided doses.
PO (Neonates): *CHF*—0.05–0.1 mg/kg/dose q 8–24 hr, may ↑ as needed up to 0.5 mg/kg q 6–24 hr; *Premature neonates*—0.01 mg/kg/dose q 8–12 hr.

Renal Impairment
PO (Adults): *CCr 10–50 mL/min*—Administer 75% of dose; *CCr <10 mL/min*—Administer 50% of dose.

Enalapril/Enalaprilat
PO (Adults): *Hypertension*—2.5–5 mg once daily, ↑ as required up to 40 mg/day in 1–2 divided doses (initiate therapy at 2.5 mg once daily in patients receiving diuretics); *CHF*—2.5 mg 1–2 times daily, titrated up to target dose of 10 mg twice daily; begin with 2.5 mg once daily in patients with hyponatremia (serum sodium <130 mEq/L); *Asymptomatic left ventricular dysfunction*—2.5 mg twice daily, titrated up to a target dose of 10 mg twice daily.
PO (Children and Neonates): *Hypertension*—0.1 mg/kg/day q 12–24 hr (once a day in neonates); may be slowly titrated up to a maximum of 0.5 mg/kg/day.
IV (Adults): *Hypertension*—0.625–1.25 mg (0.625 mg if receiving diuretics) q 6 hr; can be titrated up to 5 mg q 6 hr.
IV (Children and Neonates): *Hypertension*—5–10 mcg/kg/dose given q 8–24 hr.

Renal Impairment
PO, IV (Adults): *Hypertension CCr 10–50 mL/min*—Administer 75% of dose; *CCr <10 mL/min*—Administer 50% of dose.

Renal Impairment
PO, IV (Children and Neonates): *CCr <30 mL/min*—Contraindicated.

Fosinopril
PO (Adults): *Hypertension*—10 mg once daily, may be ↑ as required up to 80 mg/day. *CHF*—10 mg once daily (5 mg once daily in patients who have been vigorously diuresed), may be ↑ over several weeks up to 40 mg/day.
PO (Children ≥6 yr and >50 kg): *Hypertension*-5–10 mg once daily.

Lisinopril
PO (Adults): *Hypertension*—10 mg once daily, can be ↑ up to 20–40 mg/day (initiate therapy at 5 mg/day in patients receiving diuretics); *CHF*—5 mg once daily; may be titrated every 2 wk up to 40 mg/day; begin with 2.5 mg once daily in patients with hyponatremia (serum sodium <130 mEq/L); *Post-MI*—5 mg once daily for 2 days, then 10 mg daily.
PO (Children ≥6 yr): *Hypertension*—0.07 mg/kg once daily (up to 5 mg/day), may be titrated every 1–2 wk up to 0.6 mg/kg/day (or 40 mg/day).

Renal Impairment
PO (Adults): *CCr 10–30 mL/min*—Begin with 5 mg once daily; may be slowly titrated up to 40 mg/day; *CCr <10ml/min*—Begin with 2.5 mg once daily; may be slowly titrated up to 40 mg/day.

ANGIOTENSIN-CONVERTING ENZYME (ACE) INHIBITORS

Renal Impairment
(Children ≥6 yr): *CCr <30 mL/min*—Contraindicated.

Moexipril
PO (Adults): 7.5 mg once daily, may be ↑ up to 30 mg/day in 1–2 divided doses (begin with 3.75 mg/day in patients receiving diuretics).

Renal Impairment
PO (Adults): *CCr ≤40 mL/min*—Initiate therapy at 3.75 mg once daily, may be titrated upward carefully to 15 mg/day.

Perindopril
PO (Adults): *Hypertension*—4 mg once daily, may be slowly titrated up to 16 mg/day in 1–2 divided doses (should not exceed 8 mg/day in elderly patients) (begin with 2–4 mg/day in 1–2 divided doses in patients receiving diuretics); *Stable CAD*—4 mg once daily for 2 weeks, may be ↑, if tolerated, to 8 mg once daily; for elderly patients, begin with 2 mg once daily for 1 week (may be ↑, if tolerated, to 4 mg once daily for 1 week, then, ↑ as tolerated to 8 mg once daily).

Renal Impairment
PO (Adults): *CCr 30–60 mL/min*—2 mg/day initially, may be slowly titrated up to 8 mg/day in 1–2 divided doses.

Quinapril
PO (Adults): *Hypertension*—10–20 mg once daily initially, may be titrated q 2 wk up to 80 mg/day in 1–2 divided doses (initiate therapy at 5 mg/day in patients receiving diuretics); *CHF*—5 mg twice daily initially, may be titrated at weekly intervals up to 20 mg twice daily.

Renal Impairment
PO (Adults): *CCr >60 mL/min*—Initiate therapy at 10 mg/day; *CCr 30–60 mL/min*—Initiate therapy at 5 mg/day; *CCr 10–30 mL/min*—Initiate therapy at 2.5 mg/day.

Ramipril
PO (Adults): *Hypertension*—2.5 mg once daily, may be ↑ slowly up to 20 mg/day in 1–2 divided doses (initiate therapy at 1.25 mg/day in patients receiving diuretics). *CHF post-MI*—1.25–2.5 mg twice daily initially, may be ↑ slowly up to 5 mg twice daily. *Reduction in risk of MI, stroke, and death from cardiovascular causes*—2.5 mg once daily for 1 wk, then 5 mg once daily for 3 wk, then ↑ as tolerated to 10 mg once daily (can also be given in 2 divided doses).

Renal Impairment
PO (Adults): *CCr <40 mL/min*—Initiate therapy at 1.25 mg once daily, may be slowly titrated up to 5 mg/day in 1–2 divided doses.

Trandolapril
PO (Adults): *Hypertension*—1 mg once daily (2 mg once daily in black patients); *CHF post-MI*—Initiate therapy at 1 mg once daily, titrate up to 4 mg once daily if possible.

Renal Impairment
PO (Adults): *CCr <30 mL/min*—Initiate therapy at 0.5 mg once daily, may be slowly titrated upward (maximum dose = 4 mg/day).

Hepatic Impairment
PO (Adults): Initiate therapy at 0.5 mg once daily, may be slowly titrated upward (maximum dose = 4 mg/day).

Availability

Benazepril (generic available)
Tablets: 5 mg, 10 mg, 20 mg, 40 mg. *In combination with:* amlodipine (Lotrel) and hydrochlorothiazide (Lotensin HCT). See Appendix B.

Captopril (generic available)
Tablets: 12.5 mg, 25 mg, 50 mg, 100 mg. *In combination with:* hydrochlorothiazide (Capozide). See Appendix B.

Enalapril (generic available)
Tablets: 2.5 mg, 5 mg, 10 mg, 20 mg. *In combination with:* hydrochlorothiazide (Vaseretic). See Appendix B.

Enalaprilat (generic available)
Injection: 1.25 mg/mL.

Fosinopril (generic available)
Tablets: 10 mg, 20 mg, 40 mg. *In combination with:* hydrochlorothiazide. See Appendix B.

Lisinopril (generic available)
Tablets: 2.5 mg, 5 mg, 10 mg, 20 mg, 30 mg, 40 mg. *In combination with:* hydrochlorothiazide (Prinzide, Zestoretic). See Appendix B.

Moexipril (generic available)
Tablets: 7.5 mg, 15 mg. *In combination with:* hydrochlorothiazide (Uniretic).

Perindopril (generic available)
Tablets: 2 mg, 4 mg, 8 mg.

✦ = Canadian drug name. ▮ = Genetic implication.
*CAPITALS indicates life-threatening; underlines indicate most frequent.

Quinapril (generic available)
Tablets: 5 mg, 10 mg, 20 mg, 40 mg. *In combination with:* hydrochlorothiazide (Accuretic, Quinaretic). See Appendix B.

Ramipril (generic available)
Capsules: 1.25 mg, 2.5 mg, 5 mg, 10 mg. **Cost:** 1.25 mg $133.41/90, 2.5 mg $165.97/90, 5 mg $175.98/90, 10 mg $195.97/90.

Trandolapril (generic available)
Tablets: 1 mg, 2 mg, 4 mg. *In combination with:* verapamil (Tarka). See Appendix B.

NURSING IMPLICATIONS
Assessment
- **Hypertension:** Monitor blood pressure and pulse frequently during initial dose adjustment and periodically during therapy. Notify health care professional of significant changes.
- Monitor frequency of prescription refills to determine adherence.
- Assess patient for signs of angioedema (dyspnea, facial swelling).
- **CHF:** Monitor weight and assess patient routinely for resolution of fluid overload (peripheral edema, rales/crackles, dyspnea, weight gain, jugular venous distention).
- *Lab Test Considerations:* Monitor BUN, creatinine, and electrolyte levels periodically. Serum potassium, BUN and creatinine may be ↑, whereas sodium levels may be ↓. If ↑ BUN or serum creatinine concentrations occur, dose reduction or withdrawal may be required.
- Monitor CBC periodically during therapy. Certain drugs may rarely cause slight ↓ in hemoglobin and hematocrit, leukopenia, and eosinophilia.
- May cause ↑ AST, ALT, alkaline phosphatase, serum bilirubin, uric acid, and glucose.
- Assess urine protein prior to and periodically during therapy for up to 1 yr in patients with renal impairment or those receiving >150 mg/day of captopril. If excessive or ↑ proteinuria occurs, re-evaluate ACE inhibitor therapy.
- *Captopril:* May cause positive ANA titer.
- *Captopril:* May cause false-positive test results for urine acetone.
- *Captopril:* Monitor CBC with differential prior to initiation of therapy, every 2 wk for the first 3 mo, and periodically for up to 1 yr in patients at risk for neutropenia (patients with renal impairment or collagen-vascular disease) or at first sign of infection. Discontinue therapy if neutrophil count is <1000/mm³.

Potential Nursing Diagnoses
Decreased cardiac output (Indications, Side Effects)
Noncompliance (Patient/Family Teaching)

Implementation
- Do not confuse Lotensin (benazepril) with Loniten (minoxidil) or lovastatin. Do not confuse enalapril with Eldepryl (seligiline). Do not confuse Monopril (fosinopril) with Accupril (quinapril), minoxidil, or Monoket (isosorbide mononitrate). Do not confuse Prinivil (lisinopril) with Plendil (felodipine) or Prilosec (omeprazole). Do not confuse Accupril (quinapril) with Accutane (isotretinoin). Do not confuse Altace (ramipril) with Artane (trihexyphenidyl).
- Correct volume depletion, if possible, before initiation of therapy.
- **PO:** Precipitous drop in blood pressure during first 1–3 hr after first dose may require volume expansion with normal saline but is not normally considered an indication for stopping therapy. Discontinuing diuretic therapy or cautiously increasing salt intake 2–3 days before initiation may ↓ risk of hypotension. Monitor closely for at least 1 hr after blood pressure has stabilized. Resume diuretics if blood pressure is not controlled.

Benazepril
- **PO:** For patients with difficulty swallowing tablets, pharmacist may compound oral suspension; stable for 30 days if refrigerated. Shake suspension before each use.

Captopril
- **PO:** Administer 1 hr before or 2 hr after meals. May be crushed if patient has difficulty swallowing. Tablets may have a sulfurous odor.
- An oral solution may be prepared by crushing a 25-mg tablet and dissolving it in 25–100 mL of water. Shake for at least 5 min and administer within 30 min.

Enalapril
- **PO:** For patients with difficulty swallowing tablets, pharmacist may compound oral suspension. Shake suspension before each use.

Enalaprilat
IV Administration
- **Direct IV:** *Diluent:* May be administered undiluted. *Concentration:* 1.25 mg/mL. *Rate:* Administer over at least 5 min.
- **Intermittent Infusion:** *Diluent:* Dilute in up to 50 mL of D5W, 0.9% NaCl, D5/0.9% NaCl,

ANGIOTENSIN-CONVERTING ENZYME (ACE) INHIBITORS 181

or D5/LR. Diluted solution is stable for 24 hr.
Rate: Administer as a slow infusion over at least 5 min.

- **Y-Site Compatibility:** acyclovir, alfentanil, allopurinol, amifostine, amikacin, aminophylline, amphotericin B liposome, ascorbic acid, atracurium, atropine, azathioprine, aztreonam, benztropine, bivalirudin, bretylium, bumetanide, buprenorphine, butorphanol, calcium chloride, calcium gluconate, carboplatin, cefazolin, cefonicid, cefoperazone, cefotaxime, cefotetan, cefoxitin, ceftazidime, ceftizoxime, ceftriaxone, cefuroxime, cephalothin, cephapirin, chloramphenicol, cimetidine, cisatracurium, cladribine, clindamycin, cyanocobalamin, cyclophosphamide, cyclosporine, cytarabine, dactinomycin, daptomycin, dexamethasone sodium phosphate, dexmedetomidine, dextran 40, digoxin, diltiazem, diphenhydramine, dobutamine, docetaxel, dopamine, doripenem, doxacurium, doxorubicin hydrochloride, doxorubicin liposome, doxycycline, ephedrine, epinephrine, epirubicin, epoetin, ertapenem, erythromycin lactobionate, esmolol, etoposide, etoposide phosphate, famotidine, fenoldopam, fentanyl, filgrastim, fluconazole, fludarabine, fluorouracil, folic acid, furosemide, ganciclovir, gemcitabine, gentamicin, granisetron, heparin, hetastarch, hydrocortisone sodium succinate, hydromorphone, ifosfamide, imipenem/cilastatin, indomethacin, insulin, isoproterenol, ketorolac, labetalol, levofloxacin, lidocaine, linezolid, lorazepam, magnesium sulfate, mannitol, mechlorethamine, melphalan, meperidine, meropenem, metaraminol, methicillin, methotrexate, methoxamine, methyldopate, methylprednisolone sodium succinate, metoclopramide, metoprolol, metronidazole, mezlocillin, miconazole, midazolam, milrinone, minocycline, mitoxantrone, morphine, moxalactam, multiple vitamin infusion, nafcillin, nalbuphine, naloxone, netilmicin, nicardipine, nitroglycerin, nitroprusside, norepinephrine, octreotide, ondansetron, oxacillin, oxaliplatin, oxytocin, paclitaxel, palonosetron, papaverine, pemetrexed, penicillin G potassium, pentamidine, pentazocine, pentobarbital, phenobarbital, phentolamine, phenylephrine, phytonadione, piperacillin/tazobactam, potassium chloride, potassium phosphate, procainamide, prochlorperazine, promethazine, propofol, propranolol, protamine, pyridoxine, quinupristin/dalfopristin, ranitidine, remifentanil, ritodrine, rituximab, rocuronium, sodium acetate, sodium bicarbonate, streptokinase, succinylcholine, sufentanil, tacrolimus, teniposide, tetracycline, theophylline, thiamine, thiotepa, ticarcillin/clavulanate, tigecycline, tirofiban, tobramycin, tolazoline, trastuzumab, trimethaphan, urokinase, vancomycin, vasopressin, vecuronium, verapamil, vincristine, vinorelbine, voriconazole.
- **Y-Site Incompatibility:** amphotericin B cholesteryl sulfate, caspofungin, cefepime, dantrolene, diazepam, diazoxide, lansoprazole, phenytoin.
- **Additive Compatibility:** dobutamine, dopamine, heparin, meropenem, nitroglycerin, nitroprusside, potassium chloride.

Lisinopril

- **PO:** For patients with difficulty swallowing tablets, pharmacist may compound oral suspension; stable at room temperature for 4 wk. Shake suspension before each use.

Moexipril

- **PO:** Administer moexipril on an empty stomach, 1 hr before a meal.

Ramipril

- **PO:** Capsules may be opened and sprinkled on applesauce, or dissolved in 4 oz water or apple juice for patients with difficulty swallowing. Effectiveness is same as capsule. Prepared mixtures can be stored for up to 24 hr at room temperature or up to 48 hr if refrigerated.

Trandolapril

- **PO:** May be taken with or without food.

Patient/Family Teaching

- Instruct patient to take medication as directed at the same time each day, even if feeling well. Take missed doses as soon as possible but not if almost time for next dose. Do not double doses. Warn patient not to discontinue ACE inhibitor therapy unless directed by health care professional.
- Caution patient to avoid salt substitutes or foods containing high levels of potassium or sodium unless directed by healthcare professional (see Appendix M).
- Caution patient to change positions slowly to minimize hypotension. Use of alcohol, standing for long periods, exercising, and hot weather may ↑ orthostatic hypotension.

= Canadian drug name. = Genetic implication.
*CAPITALS indicates life-threatening; underlines indicate most frequent.

- Advise patient to consult health care professional before taking any Rx, OTC, or herbal products, especially cough, cold, or allergy remedies.
- May cause dizziness. Caution patient to avoid driving and other activities requiring alertness until response to medication is known.
- Advise patient to inform health care professional of medication regimen prior to treatment or surgery.
- Advise patient that medication may cause impairment of taste that generally resolves within 8–12 wk, even with continued therapy.
- Instruct patient to notify health care professional if rash; mouth sores; sore throat; fever; swelling of hands or feet; irregular heart beat; chest pain; dry cough; hoarseness; swelling of face, eyes, lips, or tongue; difficulty swallowing or breathing occur; or if taste impairment or skin rash persists. Persistent dry cough may occur and may not subside until medication is discontinued. Consult health care professional if cough becomes bothersome. Also notify health care professional if nausea, vomiting, or diarrhea occurs and continues.
- Emphasize the importance of follow-up examinations to monitor progress.
- Advise women of childbearing age to use contraception and notify health care professional if pregnancy is planned or suspected. If pregnancy is detected, discontinue medication as soon as possible.
- **Hypertension:** Encourage patient to comply with additional interventions for hypertension (weight reduction, low sodium diet, discontinuation of smoking, moderation of alcohol consumption, regular exercise, and stress management). Medication controls but does not cure hypertension.
- Instruct patient and family on correct technique for monitoring blood pressure. Advise them to check blood pressure at least weekly and to report significant changes to health care professional.

Evaluation/Desired Outcomes
- Decrease in blood pressure without appearance of excessive side effects.
- Decrease in signs and symptoms of CHF (some drugs may also improve survival).
- Decrease in development of overt CHF (enalapril).
- Reduction of risk of death or development of CHF following MI.
- Reduction of risk of death from cardiovascular causes and MI in patients with stable CAD (perindopril).
- Reduction of risk of MI, stroke, or death from cardiovascular causes in patients at high-risk for these events (ramipril).
- Decrease in progression of diabetic nephropathy (captopril).

ANGIOTENSIN II RECEPTOR ANTAGONISTS

candesartan (can-de-**sar**-tan)
Atacand

eprosartan (ep-roe-**sar**-tan)
Teveten

irbesartan (ir-be-**sar**-tan)
Avapro

losartan (loe-**sar**-tan)
Cozaar

olmesartan (ole-me-**sar**-tan)
Benicar

telmisartan (tel-mi-**sar**-tan)
Micardis

valsartan (val-**sar**-tan)
Diovan

Classification
Therapeutic: antihypertensives
Pharmacologic: angiotensin II receptor antagonists

Pregnancy Category C (first trimester), D (second and third trimesters)

Indications
Alone or with other agents in the management of hypertension. Treatment of diabetic nephropathy in patients with type 2 diabetes and hypertension (irbesartan and losartan only). Management of CHF (New York Heart Association class II-IV) in patients who cannot tolerate ACE inhibitors (candesartan and valsartan only) or in combination with an ACE inhibitor and beta-blocker (candesartan only). Prevention of stroke in patients with hypertension and left ventricular hypertrophy (losartan only). Reduction of risk of death from cardiovascular causes in patients with left ventricular systolic dysfunction after MI (valsartan only).

Action
Blocks vasoconstrictor and aldosterone-producing effects of angiotensin II at receptor sites, including vascular smooth muscle and the adrenal

ANGIOTENSIN II RECEPTOR ANTAGONISTS 183

glands. **Therapeutic Effects:** Lowering of blood pressure. Slowed progression of diabetic nephropathy (irbesartan and losartan only). Reduced cardiovascular death and hospitalizations due to CHF in patients with CHF (candesartan and valsartan only). Decreased risk of cardiovascular death in patients with left ventricular systolic dysfunction who are post-MI (valsartan only). Decreased risk of stroke in patients with hypertension and left ventricular hypertrophy (effect may be less in black patients) (losartan only).

TIME/ACTION PROFILE (antihypertensive effect with chronic dosing)

ROUTE	ONSET	PEAK	DURATION
Candesartan	2–4 hr	4 wk	24 hr
Eprosartan	1–2 hr	2–3 wk	12–24 hr
Irbesartan	within 2 hr	2 wk	24 hr
Losartan	6 hr	3–6 wk	24 hr
Olmesartan	within 1 wk	2 wk	24 hr
Telmisartan	within 3 hr	4 wk	24 hr
Valsartan	within 2 hr	4 wk	24 hr

Pharmacokinetics
Absorption: *Candesartan*—Candesartan cilexetil is converted to candesartan, the active component; 15% bioavailability of candesartan; *Eprosartan*—13% absorbed after oral administration; *Irbesartan*—60–80% absorbed after oral administration; *Losartan*—well absorbed, with extensive first-pass hepatic metabolism, resulting in 33% bioavailability; *Olmesartan*—Olmesartan medoxomil is converted to olmesartan, the active component; 26% bioavailability of olmesartan; *Telmisartan*—42–58% absorbed following oral administration (bioavailability ↑ in patients with hepatic impairment); *Valsartan*—10–35% absorbed following oral administration.
Distribution: All angiotensin receptor blockers (ARBs) cross the placenta; *Candesartan*—enters breast milk.
Protein Binding: All ARBs are >90% protein-bound.
Metabolism and Excretion: *Candesartan*—Minor metabolism by the liver; 33% excreted in urine, 67% in feces (via bile); *Eprosartan*—Excreted primarily unchanged in feces via biliary excretion; *Irbesartan*—Some hepatic metabolism; 20% excreted in urine, 80% in feces; *Losartan*—Undergoes extensive first-pass hepatic metabolism; 14% is converted to an active metabolite. 4% excreted unchanged in urine; 6% excreted in urine as active metabolite; some biliary elimination; *Olmesartan*—30–50% excreted unchanged in urine, remainder eliminated in feces via bile; *Telmisartan*—Excreted mostly unchanged in feces via biliary excretion; *Valsartan*—Minor metabolism by the liver; 13% excreted in urine, 83% in feces.
Half-life: *Candesartan*—9 hr; *Eprosartan*—20 hr; *Irbesartan*—11–15 hr; *Losartan*—2 hr (6–9 hr for metabolite); *Olmesartan*—13 hr; *Telmisartan*—24 hr; *Valsartan*—6 hr.

Contraindications/Precautions
Contraindicated in: Hypersensitivity; OB: Can cause injury or death of fetus; Lactation: Discontinue drug or provide formula.
Use Cautiously in: CHF (may result in azotemia, oliguria, acute renal failure and/or death); Volume- or salt-depleted patients or patients receiving high doses of diuretics (correct deficits before initiating therapy or initiate at lower doses); Black patients (may not be effective); Impaired renal function due to primary renal disease or CHF (may worsen renal function); Obstructive biliary disorders (telmisartan) or hepatic impairment (candesartan, losartan, or telmisartan); Women of childbearing potential; Pedi: Safety not established in children <18 yr (< 6 yr for losartan).

Adverse Reactions/Side Effects
CNS: <u>dizziness</u>, anxiety, depression, fatigue, headache, insomnia, weakness. **CV:** <u>hypotension</u>, chest pain, edema, tachycardia. **Derm:** rashes. **EENT:** nasal congestion, pharyngitis, rhinitis, sinusitis. **GI:** abdominal pain, diarrhea, drug-induced hepatitis, dyspepsia, nausea, vomiting. **GU:** impaired renal function. **F and E:** hyperkalemia. **MS:** arthralgia, back pain, myalgia. **Misc:** ANGIOEDEMA.

Interactions
Drug-Drug: Antihypertensive effect may be blunted by **NSAIDs**. ↑ antihypertensive effects with other **antihypertensives** and **diuretics**. Telmisartan may ↑ serum **digoxin** levels. Concurrent use of **potassium-sparing diuretics**, **potassium-containing salt substitutes**, **angiotensin-converting enzyme inhibitors**, or **potassium supplements** may ↑ risk of hyperkalemia. Candesartan may ↑ serum **lithium** levels. Irbesartan and losartan may ↑ effects of **amiodarone**, **fluoxetine**, **glimepiride**, **glipizide**, **phenytoin**, **rosiglitazone**, and **warfarin**. **Rifampin** may ↓ effects of losartan.

✱ = Canadian drug name. = Genetic implication.
*CAPITALS indicates life-threatening; <u>underlines</u> indicate most frequent.

Route/Dosage

Candesartan
PO (Adults): *Hypertension*—16 mg once daily; may be ↑ up to 32 mg/day in 1–2 divided doses (begin therapy at a lower dose in patients who are receiving diuretics or are volume depleted). *CHF*—4 mg once daily initially, dose may be doubled at 2 wk intervals up to target dose of 32 mg once daily.

Hepatic Impairment
PO (Adults): *Moderate hepatic impairment*—Initiate at a lower dose.

Eprosartan
PO (Adults): 600 mg once daily; may be ↑ to 800 mg/day (in 1–2 divided doses) (usual range 400–800 mg/day).

Renal Impairment
PO (Adults): *CCr <60 mL/min*—Do not exceed 600 mg/day.

Irbesartan
PO (Adults): *Hypertension*—150 mg once daily; may be ↑ to 300 mg once daily. Initiate therapy at 75 mg once daily in patients who are receiving diuretics or are volume depleted. *Type 2 diabetic nephropathy*—300 mg once daily.

Losartan
PO (Adults): *Hypertension*—50 mg once daily initially (range 25–100 mg/day as a single daily dose or 2 divided doses) (initiate therapy at 25 mg once daily in patients who are receiving diuretics or are volume depleted). *Prevention of stroke in patients with hypertension and left ventricular hypertrophy*—50 mg once daily initially; hydrochlorothiazide 12.5 mg once daily should be added and/or dose of losartan ↑ to 100 mg once daily followed by an ↑ in hydrochlorothiazide to 25 mg once daily based on blood pressure response. *Type 2 diabetic nephropathy*—50 mg once daily, may ↑ to 100 mg once daily depending on blood pressure response.

Hepatic Impairment
PO (Adults): 25 mg once daily initially; may be ↑ as tolerated.
PO (Children > 6 yr): *Hypertension*—0.7 mg/kg once daily (up to 50 mg/day), may be titrated up to 1.4 mg/kg/day (or 100 mg/day).

Renal Impairment
PO (Children > 6 yr): *CCr <30 mL/min*—Contraindicated.

Olmesartan
PO (Adults): 20 mg once daily; may be ↑ up to 40 mg once daily (patients who are receiving diuretics or are volume-depleted should be started on lower doses).

Telmisartan
PO (Adults): 40 mg once daily (volume-depleted patients should start with 20 mg once daily); may be titrated up to 80 mg/day.

Valsartan
PO (Adults): *Hypertension*—80 mg or 160 mg once daily initially in patients who are not volume-depleted; may be ↑ to 320 mg once daily; *CHF*—40 mg twice daily, may be titrated up to target dose of 160 mg twice daily as tolerated; *Post-MI*—20 mg twice daily (may be initiated ≥ 12 hr after MI); dose may be titrated up to target dose of 160 mg twice daily, as tolerated.

Availability

Candesartan
Tablets: 4 mg, 8 mg, 16 mg, 32 mg. **Cost:** 4 mg $154.54/90, 8 mg $155.97/90, 16 mg $155.97/90, 32 mg $215.96/90. *In combination with:* hydrochlorothiazide (Atacand HCT; see Appendix B).

Eprosartan
Tablets: 400 mg, 600 mg. *In combination with:* hydrochlorothiazide (Teveten HCT; see Appendix B).

Irbesartan
Tablets: 75 mg, 150 mg, 300 mg. **Cost:** 75 mg $149.97/90, 150 mg $165.97/90, 300 mg $199.97/90. *In combination with:* hydrochlorothiazide (Avalide; see Appendix B).

Losartan
Tablets: 25 mg, 50 mg, 100 mg. **Cost:** 25 mg $157.96/90, 50 mg $162.98/90, 100 mg $219.97/90. *In combination with:* hydrochlorothiazide (Hyzaar; see Appendix B).

Olmesartan
Tablets: 5 mg, 20 mg, 40 mg. **Cost:** 5 mg $149.97/90, 20 mg $153.50/90, 40 mg $179.96/90. *In combination with:* hydrochlorothiazide (Benicar HCT; amlodipine (Azor); see Appendix B).

Telmisartan
Tablets: 20 mg, 40 mg, 80 mg. **Cost:** 20 mg $50.32/28, 40 mg $58.99/30, 80 mg $65.99/30. *In combination with:* hydrochlorothiazide (Micardis HCT; see Appendix B).

ANGIOTENSIN II RECEPTOR ANTAGONISTS

Valsartan
Tablets: 40 mg, 80 mg, 160 mg, 320 mg. **Cost:** 40 mg $151.97/90, 80 mg $179.97/90, 160 mg $179.97/90, 320 mg $261.95/90. *In combination with:* aliskiren (Valturna); amlodipine (Exforge); hydrochlorothiazide (Diovan HCT); amlodipine and hydrochlorothiazide (Exforge HCT; See Appendix B).

NURSING IMPLICATIONS

Assessment
- Assess blood pressure (lying, sitting, standing) and pulse periodically during therapy. Notify health care professional of significant changes.
- Monitor frequency of prescription refills to determine adherence.
- Assess patient for signs of angioedema (dyspnea, facial swelling). May rarely cause angioedema.
- **CHF:** Monitor daily weight and assess patient routinely for resolution of fluid overload (peripheral edema, rales/crackles, dyspnea, weight gain, jugular venous distention).
- *Lab Test Considerations:* Monitor renal function and electrolyte levels periodically. Serum potassium, BUN, and serum creatinine may be ↑.
- May cause ↑ AST, ALT, and serum bilirubin (candesartan and olmesartan only).
- May cause ↑ uric acid, slight ↓ in hemoglobin and hematocrit, neutropenia, and thrombocytopenia.

Potential Nursing Diagnoses
Risk for injury (Adverse Reactions)
Noncompliance (Patient/Family Teaching)

Implementation
- Do not confuse valsartan with losartan.
- Correct volume depletion, if possible, prior to initiation of therapy.
- **PO:** May be administered without regard to meals.

Losartan
- **PO:** For patients with difficulty swallowing tablets, pharmacist can compound oral suspension; stable for 4 wk if refrigerated. Shake suspension before each use.

Patient/Family Teaching
- Emphasize the importance of continuing to take as directed, even if feeling well. Take missed doses as soon as remembered if not almost time for next dose; do not double doses. Instruct patient to take medication at the same time each day. Warn patient not to discontinue therapy unless directed by health care professional.
- Caution patient to avoid salt substitutes containing potassium or food containing high levels of potassium or sodium unless directed by health care professional. See Appendix M.
- Caution patient to avoid sudden changes in position to decrease orthostatic hypotension. Use of alcohol, standing for long periods, exercising, and hot weather may increase orthostatic hypotension.
- Advise women of childbearing age to use contraception and notify health care professional if pregnancy is suspected or planned. If pregnancy is detected, discontinue medication as soon as possible.
- May cause dizziness. Caution patient to avoid driving or other activities requiring alertness until response to medication is known.
- Advise patient to consult health care professional before taking any OTC or herbal cough, cold, or allergy remedies or other medications.
- Instruct patient to notify health care professional of medication regimen prior to treatment or surgery.
- Instruct patient to notify health care professional if swelling of face, eyes, lips, or tongue occurs, or if difficulty swallowing or breathing occurs.
- Emphasize the importance of follow-up exams to evaluate effectiveness of medication.
- **Hypertension:** Encourage patient to comply with additional interventions for hypertension (weight reduction, low-sodium diet, discontinuation of smoking, moderation of alcohol consumption, regular exercise, stress management). Medication controls but dose not cure hypertension.
- Instruct patient and family on proper technique for monitoring blood pressure. Advise them to check blood pressure at least weekly and to report significant changes.

Evaluation/Desired Outcomes
- Decrease in blood pressure without appearance of excessive side effects.
- Slowed progression of diabetic nephropathy (irbesartan, losartan).
- Decreased cardiovascular death and CHF-related hospitalizations in patients with CHF (candesartan).

- Decreased hospitalizations in patients with CHF (valsartan).
- Decreased risk of cardiovascular death in patients with left ventricular systolic dysfunction after MI (valsartan).
- Reduced risk of stroke in patients with hypertension and left ventricular hypertrophy (losartan).

anidulafungin
(a-**ni**-du-la-fun-gin)
Eraxis

Classification
Therapeutic: antifungals
Pharmacologic: echinocandins

Pregnancy Category C

Indications
Candidemia and other serious candidal infections including intra-abdominal abscess, peritonitis. Esophageal candidiasis.

Action
Inhibits the synthesis of fungal cell wall. **Therapeutic Effects:** Death of susceptible fungi. **Spectrum:** Active against *Candida albicans*, *C. glabrata*, *C. parapsilosis*, and *C. tropicalis*.

Pharmacokinetics
Absorption: IV administration results in complete bioavailability.
Distribution: Crosses the placenta.
Metabolism and Excretion: Undergoes chemical degradation without hepatic metabolism; <1% excreted in urine.
Half-life: 40–50 hr.

TIME/ACTION PROFILE (blood levels)

ROUTE	ONSET	PEAK	DURATION
IV	rapid	end of infusion	24 hr

Contraindications/Precautions
Contraindicated in: Hypersensitivity.
Use Cautiously in: Underlying liver disease (may worsen); OB, Lactation: Pregnancy or lactation; Pedi: Safe use in children not established.

Adverse Reactions/Side Effects
Resp: dyspnea. **CV:** hypotension. **GI:** diarrhea, ↑ liver enzymes. **Derm:** flushing, rash, urticaria. **F and E:** hypokalemia.

Interactions
Drug-Drug: None noted.

Route/Dosage
IV (Adults): *Esophageal candidiasis*—100 mg loading dose on day 1, then 50 mg daily. *Candidemia and other candidal infections*—200 mg loading dose on day 1, then 100 mg daily.

Availability
Lyophilized powder for IV use (requires reconsitution): 50 mg/vial.

NURSING IMPLICATIONS
Assessment
- Assess infected area and monitor cultures before and periodically during therapy.
- Specimens for culture should be taken before instituting therapy. Therapy may be started before results are obtained.
- **Lab Test Considerations:** May cause ↑ ALT, AST, alkaline phosphatase, and hepatic enzymes.
- May cause hypokalemia.
- May cause neutropenia and leukopenia.

Potential Nursing Diagnoses
Risk for infection (Indications)

Implementation

IV Administration

- **Intermittent Infusion:** Reconstitute each 50 mg vial with 15 mL of companion diluent (20% Dehydrated Alcohol in Water for injection) for a concentration of 3.33 mg/mL. **Diluent:** Further dilute within 24 hr by transferring contents of reconstituted vial into IV bag of D5W or 0.9% NaCl. For the 50 mg dose, dilute with 85 mL for an infusion volume of 100 mL. For the 100 mg dose, dilute with 170 mL for an infusion volume of 200 mL. For the 200 mg dose, dilute with 340 mL for a total infusion volume of 400 mL. **Concentration:** Final concentration should not exceed 0.5 mg/mL. Do not administer solutions that are discolored or contain particulate matter. Store reconstituted solution at room temperature; do not freeze. **Rate:** Administer at a rate not to exceed 1.1 mg/min.
- **Y-Site Compatibility:** acyclovir, amikacin, aminophylline, amphotericin B lipid complex, amphotericin B liposome, ampicillin, ampicillin/sulbactam, bivalirudin, carboplatin, cefazolin, cefepime, cefoxitin, ceftazidime, ceftizoxime, ceftriaxone, cefuroxime, cimetidine, ciprofloxacin, cisplatin, clindamycin, cyclophosphamide, cyclosporine, cytarabine, daunorubicin hydrochloride, dexamethasone, digoxin, dobutamine, docetaxel, dopamine,

ANTIFUNGALS (TOPICAL) 187

doripenem, doxorubicin hydrochloride, epinephrine, erythromycin, etoposide phosphate, famotidine, fentanyl, fluconazole, fluorouracil, furosemide, ganciclovir, gemcitabine, gentamicin, heparin, hydrocortisone, hydromorphone, ifosfamide, imipenem/cilastatin, leucovorin, levofloxacin, linezolid, meperidine, meropenem, methylprednisolone, metronidazole, midazolam, morphine, mycophenolate, norepinephrine, octreotide, oxytocin, paclitaxel, pantoprazole, phenylephrine, piperacillin/tazobactam, potassium chloride, quinupristin/dalfopristin, ranitidine, tacrolimus, ticarcillin/clavulanate, tirofiban, tobramycin, trimethoprim/sulfamethoxazole, vancomycin, vincristine, voriconazole, zidovudine.

- **Y-Site Incompatibility:** amphotericin B colloidal, ertapenem, sodium bicarbonate.

Patient/Family Teaching
- Explain purpose of medication to patient.
- Instruct patient to notify health care professional if diarrhea becomes pronounced.

Evaluation/Desired Outcomes
- Resolution of clinical and laboratory indications of fungal infections. Duration of therapy should be based on the patients clinical response. Therapy should be continued for at least 14 days after the last positive culture. For esophageal candidiasis, treatment should continue for at least 7 days following resolution of symptoms.

ANTIFUNGALS (TOPICAL)

butenafine (byoo-**ten**-a-feen)
Lotrimin Ultra, Mentax

ciclopirox (sye-kloe-**peer**-ox)
Loprox, Penlac, ✦ Stieprox

clotrimazole (kloe-**trye**-ma-zole)
✦ Canesten, ✦ Clotrimaderm, Cruex, Lotrimin AF, ✦ Lotriderm, Mycelex

econazole (ee-**kon**-a-zole)

ketoconazole (kee-toe-**kon**-a-zole)
Extina, Kuric, Nizoral, Nizoral A-D, Xolegel

miconazole (mye-**kon**-a-zole)
Fungoid, Lotrimin AF, Micatin, ✦ Micozole, Zeasorb-AF

naftifine (**naff**-ti-feen)
Naftin

nystatin (nye-**stat**-in)
Mycostatin, ✦ Nadostine, ✦ Nyaderm, Nystop

oxiconazole (ox-i-**kon**-a-zole)
Oxistat

sulconazole (sul-**kon**-a-zole)
Exelderm

terbinafine (ter-**bin**-a-feen)
Lamisil AT

tolnaftate (tol-**naff**-tate)
✦ Pitrex, Podactin, Tinactin, Ting

Classification
Therapeutic: antifungals (topical)

Pregnancy Category B (butenafine, ciclopirox, clotrimazole, naftifine, oxiconazole, terbinafine), C (econazole, ketoconazole, miconazole, sulconazole, tolnaftate), UK (nystatin)

Indications
Treatment of a variety of cutaneous fungal infections, including cutaneous candidiasis, tinea pedis (athlete's foot), tinea cruris (jock itch), tinea corporis (ringworm), tinea versicolor, seborrheic dermatitis, dandruff, and onychomycosis of fingernails and toes.

Action
Butenafine, nystatin, clotrimazole, econazole, ketoconazole, miconazole, naftifine, oxiconazole, sulconazole, and terbinafine affect the synthesis of the fungal cell wall, allowing leakage of cellular contents. Tolnaftate distorts the hyphae and stunts mycelial growth in fungi. Ciclopirox inhibits the transport of essential elements in the fungal cell, disrupting the synthesis of DNA, RNA, and protein.
Therapeutic Effects: Decrease in symptoms of fungal infection.

Pharmacokinetics
Absorption: Absorption through intact skin is minimal.
Distribution: Distribution after topical administration is primarily local.
Metabolism and Excretion: Metabolism and excretion not known following local application.
Half-life: *Butenafine*—35 hr; *Ciclopirox*—5.5 hr (gel); *Terbinafine*—21 hr.

✦ = Canadian drug name. ❢ = Genetic implication.
*CAPITALS indicates life-threatening; underlines indicate most frequent.

ANTIFUNGALS (TOPICAL)

TIME/ACTION PROFILE (resolution of symptoms/lesions†)

ROUTE	ONSET	PEAK	DURATION
Butenafine	unknown	up to 4 wk	unknown
Tolnaftate	24–72 hr	unknown	unknown

† Only the drugs with known information included in this table

Contraindications/Precautions
Contraindicated in: Hypersensitivity to active ingredients, additives, preservatives, or bases; Some products contain alcohol or bisulfites and should be avoided in patients with known intolerance.
Use Cautiously in: Nail and scalp infections (may require additional systemic therapy); OB, Lactation: Safety not established.

Adverse Reactions/Side Effects
Local: burning, itching, local hypersensitivity reactions, redness, stinging.

Interactions
Drug-Drug: Either not known or insignificant.

Route/Dosage

Butenafine
Topical (Adults and Children >12 yr): Apply once daily for 2 wk for tinea corporis, tinea cruris, or tinea versicolor. Apply once daily for 4 wk or once daily for 7 days for tinea pedis.

Ciclopirox
Topical (Adults and Children >10 yr): *Cream/lotion*—Apply twice daily for 2–4 wk; *Topical solution (nail lacquer)*—Apply to nails at bedtime or 8 hr prior to bathing for up to 48 wk. Each daily application should be made over the previous coat and then removed with alcohol every 7 days; *Gel*—Apply twice daily for 4 wk; *Shampoo*—5–10 mL applied to scalp, lather and leave on for 3 min, rinse; repeat twice weekly for 4 wk (at least 3 days between applications).

Clotrimazole
Topical (Adults and Children >3 yr): Apply twice daily for 1–4 wk.

Econazole
Topical (Adults and Children): Apply once daily for tinea pedis (for 4 wk), tinea cruris (for 2 wk), tinea corporis (for 2 wk), or tinea versicolor (for 2 wk). Apply twice daily for cutaneous candidiasis (for 2 wk).

Ketoconazole
Topical (Adults): Apply cream once daily for cutaneous candidiasis (for 2 wk), tinea corporis (for 2 wk), tinea cruris (for 2 wk), tinea pedis (for 6 wk), or tinea versicolor (for 2 wk). Apply cream twice daily for seborrheic dermatitis (for 4 wk). For dandruff, use shampoo twice weekly (wait 3–4 days between treatments) for 4 wk, then intermittently.

Miconazole
Topical (Adults and Children >2 yr): Apply twice daily. Treat tinea cruris for 2 wk and tinea pedis or tinea corporis for 4 wk.

Naftifine
Topical (Adults): Apply cream once daily for up to 4 wk. Apply gel twice daily for up to 4 wk.

Nystatin
Topical (Adults and Children): Apply 2–3 times daily until healing is complete.

Oxiconazole
Topical (Adults and Children): Apply cream or lotion 1–2 times daily for tinea pedis (for 4 wk), tinea corporis (for 2 wk), or tinea cruris (for 2 wk). Apply cream once daily for tinea versicolor (for 2 wk).

Sulconazole
Topical (Adults): Apply 1–2 times daily (twice daily for tinea pedis). Treat tinea corporis, tinea cruris, or tinea versicolor for 3 wk, and tinea pedis for 4 wk.

Terbinafine
Topical (Adults): Apply twice daily for tinea pedis (for 1 wk) or daily for tinea cruris or tinea corporis for 1 wk.

Tolnaftate
Topical (Adults): Apply twice daily for tinea cruris (for 2 wk), tinea pedis (for 4 wk), or tinea corporis (for 4 wk).

Availability

Butenafine
Cream: 1%[Rx, OTC].

Ciclopirox (generic available)
Cream: 0.77%. **Lotion:** 0.77%. **Nail lacquer:** 8%. **Shampoo:** 1%.

Clotrimazole (generic available)
Cream: 1%[OTC]. **Solution:** 1%[OTC]. *In combination with:* betamethasone (Lotrisone). See Appendix B.

Econazole (generic available)
Cream: 1%.

ANTIFUNGALS (TOPICAL)

Ketoconazole (generic available)
Cream: 2%. **Shampoo:** 1%^OTC, 2%. **Foam:** 2%. **Gel:** 2%.

Miconazole (generic available)
Cream: 2%^Rx, OTC. **Lotion powder:** 2%^OTC. **Ointment:** 2%^OTC. **Powder:** 2%^OTC. **Spray powder:** 2%^OTC. **Spray liquid:** 2%^OTC. **Solution:** 2%^OTC. **Tincture:** 2%^OTC. *In combination with:* zinc oxide (Vusion). See Appendix B.

Naftifine
Cream: 1%^Rx, OTC. **Gel:** 1%^OTC.

Nystatin (generic available)
Cream: 100,000 units/g^Rx, OTC. **Ointment:** 100,000 units/g^Rx, OTC. **Powder:** 100,000 units/g^Rx, OTC. *In combination with:* triamcinolone. See Appendix B.

Oxiconazole
Cream: 1%. **Lotion:** 1%.

Sulconazole
Cream: 1%. **Solution:** 1%.

Terbinafine (generic available)
Cream: 1%^OTC. **Spray liquid:** 1%^OTC.

Tolnaftate (generic available)
Cream: 1%^OTC. **Solution:** 1%^OTC. **Powder:** 1%^OTC. **Spray powder:** 1%^OTC. **Spray liquid:** 1%^OTC.

NURSING IMPLICATIONS

Assessment
- Inspect involved areas of skin and mucous membranes before and frequently during therapy. Increased skin irritation may indicate need to discontinue medication.

Potential Nursing Diagnoses
Risk for impaired skin integrity (Indications)
Risk for infection (Indications)

Implementation
- Do not confuse Lotrimin (clotrimazole) with Lotrisone (betamethasone/clotrimazole). Do not confuse Kuric (ketoconazole) with Carac (fluorouracil).
- Consult health care professional for proper cleansing technique before applying medication.
- Choice of vehicle is based on use. Ointments, creams, and liquids are used as primary therapy. Lotion is usually preferred in intertriginous areas; if cream is used, apply sparingly to avoid maceration. Powders are usually used as adjunctive therapy but may be used as primary therapy for mild conditions (especially for moist lesions).
- **Topical:** Apply small amount to cover affected area completely. Avoid the use of occlusive wrappings or dressings unless directed by health care professional.
- **Nail lacquer:** Avoid contact with skin other than skin immediately surrounding treated nail. Avoid contact with eyes or mucous membranes. Removal of unattached, infected nail, as frequently as monthly, by health care professional is needed with use of this medication. Up to 48 wk of daily application and professional removal may be required to achieve clear or almost clear nail. Six months of treatment may be required before results are noticed.
- **Ciclopirox or Ketoconazole shampoo:** Moisten hair and scalp thoroughly with water. Apply sufficient shampoo to produce enough lather to wash scalp and hair and gently massage it over the entire scalp area for approximately 1 min. Rinse hair thoroughly with warm water. Repeat process, leaving shampoo on hair for an additional 3 min. After the 2nd shampoo, rinse and dry hair with towel or warm air flow. Shampoo twice a week for 4 wk with at least 3 days between each shampooing and then intermittently as needed to maintain control.
- **Ketoconazole foam:** Hold container upright and dispense foam into cap of can or other smooth surface; dispensing directly on to hand is not recommended as the foam begins to melt immediately on contact with warm skin. Pick up small amounts with fingertips and gently massage into affected areas until absorbed. Move hair to allow direct application to skin.

Patient/Family Teaching
- Instruct patient to apply medication as directed for full course of therapy, even if feeling better. Emphasize the importance of avoiding the eyes.
- Caution patient that some products may stain fabric, skin, or hair. Check label information. Fabrics stained from cream or lotion can usually be cleaned by handwashing with soap and warm water; stains from ointments can usually be removed with standard cleaning fluids.
- Patients with athlete's foot should be taught to wear well-fitting, ventilated shoes, to wash affected areas thoroughly, and to change shoes and socks at least once a day.

ANTIFUNGALS (VAGINAL)

- Advise patient to report increased skin irritation or lack of response to therapy to health care professional.
- **Nail lacquer:** File away loose nail and trim nails every 7 days after solution is removed with alcohol. Do not use nail polish on treated nails. Inform health care professional if patient has diabetes mellitus before using.

Evaluation/Desired Outcomes
- Decrease in skin irritation and resolution of infection. Early relief of symptoms may be seen in 2–3 days. For *Candida,* tinea cruris, and tinea corporis, 2 wk are needed, and for tinea pedis, therapeutic response may take 3–4 wk. Recurrent fungal infections may be a sign of systemic illness.

ANTIFUNGALS (VAGINAL)

butoconazole
(byoo-toe-**kon**-a-zole)
Gynezole-1, Mycelex-3

clotrimazole (kloe-**trye**-ma-zole)
✤Canesten, ✤Clotrimaderm, Gyne-Lotrimin-3, Mycelex-7, ✤Trivagizole-3

miconazole (mye-**kon**-a-zole)
Monistat-1, Monistat-3, Monistat-7, Vagistat-3

nystatin (nye-**stat**-in)
Mycostatin

terconazole (ter-**kon**-a-zole)
Terazol-3, Terazol-7

tioconazole (tye-oh-**kon**-a-zole)
1–Day, Monistat-1Day, Vagistat-1

Classification
Therapeutic: antifungals (vaginal)

Pregnancy Category A (nystatin), B (clotrimazole), C (butoconazole, miconazole, terconazole, tioconazole)

Indications
Treatment of vulvovaginal candidiasis.

Action
Affects the permeability of the fungal cell wall, allowing leakage of cellular contents. Not active against bacteria. **Therapeutic Effects:** Inhibited growth and death of susceptible *Candida,* with decrease in accompanying symptoms of vulvovaginitis (vaginal burning, itching, discharge).

Pharmacokinetics
Absorption: Absorption through intact skin is minimal.
Distribution: Unknown. Action is primarily local.
Metabolism and Excretion: Negligible with local application.
Half-life: Not applicable.

TIME/ACTION PROFILE

ROUTE	ONSET	PEAK	DURATION
All agents	rapid	unknown	24 hr

Contraindications/Precautions
Contraindicated in: Hypersensitivity to active ingredients, additives, or preservatives; OB: Safety not established; Lactation: Safety not established.
Use Cautiously in: None noted.

Adverse Reactions/Side Effects
GU: itching, pelvic pain, vulvovaginal burning.

Interactions
Drug-Drug: Concurrent use of vaginal miconazole with **warfarin** ↑ risk of bleeding/bruising (appropriate monitoring recommended).

Route/Dosage
Butoconazole
Vag (Adults and Children ≥12 yr): 1 applicatorful (5 g) at bedtime for 3 days (Mycelex-3) *or* one applicatorful single dose (Gynezole-1).

Clotrimazole
Vag (Adults and Children >12 yr): *Vaginal tablets*—100 mg at bedtime for 7 nights (preferred regimen for pregnancy) *or* 200 mg at bedtime for 3 nights. *Vaginal cream*—1 applicatorful (5 g) of 1% cream at bedtime for 7 days *or* 1 applicatorful (5 g) of 2% cream at bedtime for 3 days.

Miconazole
Vag (Adults and Children ≥12 yr): *Vaginal suppositories*—one 100-mg suppository at bedtime for 7 days *or* one 200-mg suppository at bedtime for 3 days *or* one 1200-mg suppository as a single dose. *Vaginal cream*—1 applicatorful of 2% cream at bedtime for 7 days *or* 1 applicatorful of 4% cream at bedtime for 3 days. *Combination packages*—contain a cream or suppositories as well as an external vaginal cream (may be used twice daily for up to 7 days, as needed, for symptomatic management of itching).

Nystatin
Vag (Adults): 100,000 units (1 tablet) daily for 2 wk.

Terconazole
Vag (Adults): *Vaginal cream*—1 applicatorful (5 g) of 0.4% cream at bedtime for 7 days *or* 1 applicatorful (5 g) of 0.8% cream at bedtime for 3 days. *Vaginal suppositories*—1 suppository (80 mg) at bedtime for 3 days.

Tioconazole
Vag (Adults and Children ≥12 yr): 1 applicatorful (4.6 g) at bedtime as a single dose.

Availability
Butoconazole
Vaginal cream: 2%[Rx, OTC].

Clotrimazole (generic available)
Vaginal tablets: 100 mg[OTC], 200 mg[OTC]. **Vaginal cream:** 1%[OTC], 2%[OTC].

Miconazole (generic available)
Vaginal cream: 2%[OTC], 4%[OTC]. **Vaginal suppositories:** 100 mg[OTC], 200 mg[Rx, OTC]. ***In combination with:*** combination package of 3 200-mg suppositories and 2% external cream[OTC]; one 1200-mg suppository and 2% external cream[OTC]; 4% vaginal cream and 2% external cream[OTC]; 7 100-mg suppositories and 2% external cream[OTC]; 2% vaginal cream and 2% external cream[OTC].

Nystatin (generic available)
Vaginal tablets: 100,000 units.

Terconazole (generic available)
Vaginal cream: 0.4%, 0.8%. **Vaginal suppositories:** 80 mg.

Tioconazole
Vaginal ointment: 6.5%[OTC].

NURSING IMPLICATIONS

Assessment
- Inspect involved areas of skin and mucous membranes before and frequently during therapy. Increased skin irritation may indicate need to discontinue medication.

Potential Nursing Diagnoses
Risk for infection (Indications)
Risk for impaired skin integrity (Indications)

Implementation
- Consult physician or other health care professional for proper cleansing technique before applying medication.
- Nystatin vaginal tablets should be refrigerated.
- **Vag:** Applicators are supplied for vaginal administration.

Patient/Family Teaching
- Instruct patient to apply medication as directed for full course of therapy, even if feeling better. Therapy should be continued during menstrual period.
- Instruct patient on proper use of vaginal applicator. Medication should be inserted high into the vagina at bedtime. Instruct patient to remain recumbent for at least 30 min after insertion. Advise use of sanitary napkins to prevent staining of clothing or bedding.
- Advise patient to avoid using tampons while using this product.
- Advise patient to consult health care professional regarding intercourse during therapy. Vaginal medication may cause minor skin irritation in sexual partner. Advise patient to refrain from sexual contact during therapy or have male partner wear a condom. Some products may weaken latex contraceptive devices. Another method of contraception should be used during treatment.
- Advise patient to report to health care professional increased skin irritation or lack of response to therapy. A second course may be necessary if symptoms persist.
- Advise patient to dispose of applicator after each use (except for terconazole).

Evaluation/Desired Outcomes
- Decrease in skin irritation and vaginal discomfort. Therapeutic response is usually seen after 1 wk. Diagnosis should be reconfirmed with smears or cultures before a second course of therapy to rule out other pathogens associated with vulvovaginitis. Recurrent vaginal infections may be a sign of systemic illness.

---

aprepitant (a-prep-i-tant)
Emend

Classification
Therapeutic: antiemetics
Pharmacologic: neurokinin antagonists

Pregnancy Category B

Indications
Prevention of acute and delayed nausea and vomiting caused by initial/repeat treatment with highly emetogenic chemotherapy (with other antiemetics). Prevention of postoperative nausea and vomiting.

aprepitant

Action
Acts as a selective antagonist at substance P/neurokinin 1 (NK_1) receptors in the brain. **Therapeutic Effects:** Decreased nausea and vomiting associated with chemotherapy. Augments the antiemetic effects of dexamethasone and 5-HT_3 antagonists (ondansetron).

Pharmacokinetics
Absorption: 60–65% absorbed following oral administration.
Distribution: Crosses the blood brain barrier; remainder of distribution unknown.
Metabolism and Excretion: Mostly metabolized by the liver (CYP3A4 enzyme system); not renally excreted.
Half-life: 9–13 hr.

TIME/ACTION PROFILE (antiemetic effect)

ROUTE	ONSET	PEAK	DURATION
PO	1 hr	4 hr*	24 hr

*Blood level

Contraindications/Precautions
Contraindicated in: Hypersensitivity; Concurrent use with pimozide (risk of life-threatening adverse cardiovascular reactions); Lactation: May cause unwanted effects in nursing infants.
Use Cautiously in: Concurrent use with any agents metabolized by CYP3A4 (see Drug-Drug Interactions); OB: Use only if clearly needed; Pedi: Safety not established.

Adverse Reactions/Side Effects
CV: dizziness, fatigue, weakness. **GI:** diarrhea. **Misc:** hiccups.

Interactions
Drug-Drug: Aprepitant inhibits, induces, and is metabolized by the CYP3A4 enzyme system; it also induces the CYP2C9 system. Concurrent use with other medications that are metabolized by CYP3A4 may result in increased toxicity from these agents including **docetaxel**, **paclitaxel**, **etoposide**, **irinotecan**, **ifosfamide**, **imatinib**, **vinorelbine**, **vinblastine**, **vincristine**, **midazolam**, **triazolam**, and **alprazolam**; concurrent use should be undertaken with caution. Concurrent use with **drugs that significantly inhibit the CYP3A4 enzyme system** including (**ketoconazole**, **itraconazole**, **nefazodone**, **clarithromycin**, **ritonavir**, **nelfinavir**, and **diltiazem**) may ↑ blood levels and effects of aprepitant. Concurrent use with **drugs that induce the CYP3A4 enzyme system** including **rifampin**, **carbamazepine**, and **phenytoin** may ↓ blood levels and effects of aprepitant. ↑ blood levels and effects of **dexamethasone** (regimen reflects a 50% dose reduction); a similar effect occurs with **methylprednisolone** (↓ IV dose by 25%, ↓ PO dose by 50% when used concurrently). May ↓ the effects of **warfarin** (careful monitoring for 2 wk recommended), **oral contraceptives** (use alternate method), **tolbutamide**, and **phenytoin**.

Route/Dosage
PO (Adults): *Chemotherapy*—125 mg 1 hr prior to chemotherapy, then 80 mg once daily for 2 days (with dexamethasone 12 mg PO 30 min prior to chemotherapy, then 8 mg once daily for 3 days and ondansetron 32 mg IV 30 min prior to chemotherapy); *Postoperative*—40 mg given within 3 hr prior to induction of anesthesia.

Availability
Capsules: 40 mg, 80 mg, 125 mg.

NURSING IMPLICATIONS

Assessment
- Assess nausea, vomiting, appetite, bowel sounds, and abdominal pain prior to and following administration.
- Monitor hydration, nutritional status, and intake and output. Patients with severe nausea and vomiting may require IV fluids in addition to antiemetics.
- ***Lab Test Considerations:*** Monitor clotting status closely during the 2 wk period, especially at 7–10 days, following aprepitant therapy in patients on chronic warfarin therapy.
- May cause mild, transient ↑ in alkaline phosphatase, AST, ALT, and BUN.
- May cause proteinuria, erythrocyturia, leukocyturia, hyperglycemia, hyponatremia, and ↑ leukocytes.
- May cause ↓ hemoglobin and WBC.

Potential Nursing Diagnoses
Risk for deficient fluid volume (Indications)
Imbalanced nutrition: less than body requirements (Indications)

Implementation
- For chemotherapy, aprepitant is given as part of a regimen that includes a corticosteroid and a 5-HT_3 antagonist (see Route/Dosage).
- **PO:** Administer daily for 3 days. *Day 1*—administer 125 mg 1 hr prior to chemotherapy. *Days 2 and 3*—administer 80 mg once in the morning. May be administered without regard to food.

Patient/Family Teaching
- Instruct patient to take aprepitant as directed. Direct patient to read the patient package insert

before starting therapy and to reread it each time the prescription is renewed.
- Instruct patient to notify health care professional if nausea and vomiting occur prior to administration.
- Advise patient to notify health care professional prior to taking any other Rx, OTC, or herbal products.
- Caution patient that aprepitant may decrease the effectiveness of oral contraceptives. Advise patient to use alternate nonhormonal methods of contraception. Advise patient to notify health care professional if pregnancy is planned or suspected or if breastfeeding.
- Advise patient and family to use general measures to decrease nausea (begin with sips of liquids and small, nongreasy meals; provide oral hygiene; remove noxious stimuli from environment).
- Advise patient to notify health care professional promptly if symptoms of allergic reactions (hives, rash, itching, difficulty breathing, or swallowing) occur.

Evaluation/Desired Outcomes
- Decreased nausea and vomiting associated with chemotherapy.
- Prevention of postoperative nausea and vomiting.

HIGH ALERT

argatroban (ar-gat-tro-ban)
Argatroban

Classification
Therapeutic: anticoagulants
Pharmacologic: thrombin inhibitors

Pregnancy Category B

Indications
Prophylaxis or treatment of thrombosis in patients with heparin-induced thrombocytopenia. As an anticoagulant in patients with or at risk for heparin-induced thrombocytopenia who are undergoing percutaneous coronary intervention (PCI).

Action
Inhibits thrombin by binding to its receptor sites. Inhibition of thrombin prevents activation of factors V, VIII, and XII; the conversion of fibrinogen to fibrin; platelet adhesion and aggregation.
Therapeutic Effects: Decreased thrombus formation and extension with decreased sequelae of thrombosis (emboli, postphlebitic syndromes).

Pharmacokinetics
Absorption: IV administration results in complete bioavailability.
Distribution: Unknown.
Metabolism and Excretion: Mostly metabolized by the liver; excreted primarily in feces via biliary excretion. 16% excreted unchanged in urine, 14% excreted unchanged in feces.
Half-life: 39–51 min (↑ in hepatic impairment).

TIME/ACTION PROFILE (anticoagulant effect)

ROUTE	ONSET	PEAK	DURATION
IV	immediate	1–3 hr	2–4 hr

Contraindications/Precautions
Contraindicated in: Major bleeding; Hypersensitivity; Lactation: Lactation.
Use Cautiously in: Hepatic impairment (↓ initial infusion rate recommended); OB: Use only if clearly needed; Pedi: Safety not established.

Adverse Reactions/Side Effects
CV: hypotension. **GI:** diarrhea, nausea, vomiting. **Hemat:** BLEEDING. **Misc:** allergic reactions including ANAPHYLAXIS, fever.

Interactions
Drug-Drug: Risk of bleeding may be ↑ by concurrent use of **antiplatelet agents, thrombolytic agents,** or **other anticoagulants**.
Drug-Natural Products: ↑ bleeding risk with **anise, arnica, chamomile, clove, feverfew, garlic, ginger, ginkgo, Panax ginseng,** and others.

Route/Dosage
IV (Adults): 2 mcg/kg/min as a continuous infusion; adjust infusion rate on the basis of activated partial thromboplastin time (aPTT). *Patients undergoing PCI*—350 mcg/kg bolus followed by infusion at 25 mcg/kg/min, activated clotting time (ACT) should be assessed 5–10 min later. If ACT is 300–450 sec, procedure may be started. If ACT < 300 sec, give additional bolus of 150 mcg/kg and ↑ infusion rate to 30 mcg/kg/min. If ACT is >450 sec infusion rate should be ↓ to 15 mcg/kg/min and ACT rechecked after 5–10 min. If thrombotic complications occur or ACT drops to < 300 sec, an additional bolus of 150 mcg/kg may be given and the infusion rate ↑ to 40 mcg/kg/min followed by ACT monitoring. If anticoagulation is required after surgery, lower infusion rates should be used.

Hepatic Impairment
IV (Adults): 0.5 mcg/kg/min as a continuous infusion; adjust infusion rate on the basis of aPTT.

Availability
Solution for injection: 100 mg/mL.

NURSING IMPLICATIONS

Assessment
- Monitor vital signs periodically during therapy. Unexplained decreases in blood pressure may indicate hemorrhage. Assess patient for bleeding. Arterial and venous punctures, IM injections, and use of urinary catheters, nasotracheal intubation, and nasogastric tubes should be minimized. Noncompressible sites for IV access should be avoided. Monitor for blood in urine, lower back pain, pain or burning on urination. If bleeding cannot be controlled with pressure, decrease dose or discontinue argatroban immediately.
- Monitor for signs of anaphylaxis (rash, coughing, dyspnea) throughout therapy.
- *Lab Test Considerations:* Monitor aPTT prior to initiation of continuous infusion, 2 hours after initiation of therapy, and periodically during therapy to confirm aPTT is within desired therapeutic range.
- For patients undergoing PCI, monitor ACT as described in Route and Dose section.
- Assess hemoglobin, hematocrit, and platelet count prior to, and periodically during, argatroban therapy. May cause ↓ hemoglobin and hematocrit. Unexplained ↓ hematocrit may indicate hemorrhage.
- Use of argatroban concurrently with multiple doses of warfarin will result in more prolonged prothrombin time and international normalized ratio (INR) (although there is not an ↑ in vitamin K-dependent factor X_a activity) than when warfarin is used alone. Monitor INR daily during concomitant therapy. Repeat INR 4–6 hr after argatroban is discontinued. If the repeat value is below the desired therapeutic value for warfarin alone, restart argatroban therapy and continue until the desired therapeutic range for warfarin alone is reached. To obtain the INR for warfarin alone when the dose of argatroban is >2 mcg/kg/min the argatroban dose should be temporarily reduced to 2 mcg/kg/min; the INR for combined therapy may then be obtained 4–6 hr after argatroban dose was reduced.
- *Toxicity and Overdose:* There is no specific antidote for argatroban. If overdose occurs, discontinue argatroban. Anticoagulation parameters usually return to baseline within 2–4 hr after discontinuation.

Potential Nursing Diagnoses
Ineffective tissue perfusion (Indications)

Implementation
- All parenteral anticoagulants should be discontinued before argatroban therapy is initiated. Oral anticoagulation may be initiated with maintenance dose of warfarin; do not administer loading dose. Discontinue argatroban therapy when INR for combined therapy is >4.

IV Administration
- **IV:** Solution is slightly viscous, clear, and colorless to pale yellow. Do not administer solutions that are cloudy or contain particulate matter. Discard unused portion.
- **Direct IV:** *Diluent:* Bolus dose of 350 mcg/kg should be given prior to continuous infusion in patients undergoing PCI. For Diluent information, see Continuous Infusion section below. *Rate:* Administer bolus over 3–5 min.
- **Continuous Infusion:** *Diluent:* Dilute each 100 mg/mL in 0.9% NaCl, D5W, or LR. Mix by repeated inversion for 1 min. Solution may show a slight haziness that disappears upon mixing. *Concentration:* 1 mg/mL. *Rate:* Based on patient's weight (See Route/Dosage section). Dose adjustment may be made 2 hr after starting infusion or changing dose until steady-state aPTT is 1.5–3 times the initial baseline value (not to exceed 100 sec).
- **Y-Site Compatibility:** acyclovir, anidulafungin, atropine, bivalirudin, daptomycin, diltiazem, diphenhydramine, dobutamine, dopamine, eptifibatide, ertapenem, fenoldopam, fentanyl, furosemide, hydrocortisone, hydromorphone, lidocaine, lorazepam, metoprolol, midazolam, milrinone, morphine, nesiritide, nitroglycerin, nitroprusside, norepinephrine, octreotide, ondansetron, oxytocin, pancuronium, phenylephrine, teniposide, tigecycline, tirofiban, vasopressin, vecuronium, verapamil.
- **Y-Site Incompatibility:** amiodarone.

Patient/Family Teaching
- Inform patient of the purpose of argatroban.
- Instruct patient to notify health care professional immediately if any bleeding is noted.

Evaluation/Desired Outcomes
- Decreased thrombus formation and extension.
- Decreased sequelae of thrombosis (emboli, post-phlebitic syndromes).

aripiprazole (a-ri-pip-ra-zole)
Abilify

Classification
Therapeutic: antipsychotics, mood stabilizers
Pharmacologic: dihydrocarbostyril

Pregnancy Category C

Indications
Schizophrenia. Acute and maintenance therapy of manic and mixed episodes associated with bipolar disorder (as monotherapy or with lithium or valproate). Adjunct treatment of depression in adults. Agitation associated with schizophrenia or bipolar disorder.

Action
Psychotropic activity may be due to agonist activity at dopamine D_2 and serotonin $5-HT_{1A}$ receptors and antagonist activity at the $5-HT_{2A}$ receptor. Also has $alpha_1$ adrenergic blocking activity. **Therapeutic Effects:** Decreased manifestations of schizophrenia. Decreased mania in bipolar patients. Decreased symptoms of depression. Decreased agitation associated with schizophrenia or bipolar disorder.

Pharmacokinetics
Absorption: Well absorbed (87%) following oral administration; 100% following IM injection.
Distribution: Extensive extravascular distribution.
Protein Binding: *aripiprazole and dehydro-aripiprazole*—>99%.
Metabolism and Excretion: Mostly metabolized by the liver (CYP3A4 and CYP2D6 isoenzymes); the CYP2D6 enzyme system exhibits genetic polymorphism; ~7% of population may be poor metabolizers and may have significantly ↑ aripiprazole concentrations and an ↑ risk of adverse effects (may need smaller doses); one metabolite (dehydro-aripiprazole) has antipsychotic activity. 18% excreted unchanged in feces; <1% excreted unchanged in urine.
Half-life: *Aripiprazole*—75 hr; *dehydro-aripiprazole*—94 hr.

TIME/ACTION PROFILE (antipsychotic effect)

ROUTE	ONSET	PEAK	DURATION
PO	unknown	2 wk	unknown
IM	unknown	1–3 hr	unknown

Contraindications/Precautions
Contraindicated in: Hypersensitivity; Lactation: Presumed to be excreted in breast milk; discontinue drug or bottle feed.
Use Cautiously in: Known cardiovascular or cerebrovascular disease; Conditions which cause hypotension (dehydration, treatment with antihypertensives or diuretics); Diabetes (may ↑ risk of hyperglycemia); Seizure disorders; Patients at risk for aspiration pneumonia; Concurrent ketoconazole or other potential CYP3A4 inhibitors (↓ aripiprazole dose by 50%); Concurrent quinidine, fluoxetine, paroxetine, or other potential CYP2D6 inhibitors; Concurrent carbamazepine or other potential CYP3A4 inducers; OB: Use only if benefit outweighs risk to fetus; Pedi: May ↑ risk of suicide attempt/ideation especially during dose early treatment or dose adjustment; risk may be greater in children, adolescents, and young adults taking antidepressants (safe use in children/adolescents not established); Geri: ↑ risk of mortality in elderly patients treated for dementia-related psychosis.

Adverse Reactions/Side Effects
CNS: SUICIDAL THOUGHTS, drowsiness, extrapyramidal reactions, akathisia, confusion, depression, fatigue, hostility, insomnia, lightheadedness, manic reactions, impaired cognitive function, nervousness, restlessness, seizures, tardive dyskinesia. **Resp:** dyspnea. **CV:** bradycardia, chest pain, edema, hypertension, orthostatic hypotension, tachycardia. **EENT:** blurred vision, conjunctivitis, ear pain. **GI:** constipation, anorexia, ↑ salivation, nausea, vomiting, weight loss. **GU:** urinary incontinence. **Hemat:** AGRANULOCYTOSIS, anemia, leukopenia, neutropenia. **Derm:** dry skin, ecchymosis, skin ulcer, sweating. **MS:** muscle cramps, neck pain. **Metab:** hyperglycemia. **Neuro:** abnormal gait, tremor. **Misc:** NEUROLEPTIC MALIGNANT SYNDROME, ↓ heat regulation.

Interactions
Drug-Drug: Ketoconazole or **other potential CYP3A4 inhibitors** ↓ metabolism and ↑ effects (↓ aripiprazole dose by 50%). **Quinidine, fluoxetine, paroxetine,** or **other potential CYP2D6 inhibitors** ↓ metabolism and ↑ effects (↓ aripiprazole dose by at least 50%). Concurrent **carbamazepine** or **other potential CYP3A4 inducers** ↑ metabolism and ↓ effects (double aripiprazole dose; then ↓ to 10–15 mg/day when interfering drug is withdrawn).

Route/Dosage

Schizophrenia
PO (Adults): 10 or 15 mg daily; doses up to 30 mg/day have been used; increments in dosing should not be made before 2 wk at a given dose.
PO (Children 13–17 yr): 2 mg daily; ↑ to 5 mg daily after 2 days, and then to target dose of 10 mg daily after another 2 days; may further ↑ dose in 5-mg increments if needed (max: 30 mg/day).

Bipolar mania
PO (Adults): 15 mg daily as monotherapy or with lithium or valproate; may ↑ to 30 mg daily, based on response.
PO (Children 10–17 yr): 2 mg daily; ↑ to 5 mg daily after 2 days, and then to target dose of 10 mg daily after another 2 days; may further ↑ dose in 5-mg increments if needed (max: 30 mg/day).

Depression
PO (Adults): 2–5 mg daily, may titrate upward at 1-wk intervals to 5–10 mg daily; not to exceed 15 mg/day.

Agitation Associated with Schizophrenia or Bipolar Disorder
IM (Adults): 9.75 mg/day, may use a dose of 5.25 mg based on clinical situation. May give additional doses up to a cumulative dose of 30 mg/day, if needed.

Availability
Tablets: 2 mg, 5 mg, 10 mg, 15 mg, 20 mg, 30 mg. **Cost:** 2 mg $999.90/90, 5 mg $999.90/90, 10 mg $1,035.88/90, 15 mg $999.88/90, 20 mg $1,375.83/90, 30 mg $1,375.83/90. **Tablets, orally disintegrating:** 10 mg, 15 mg. **Oral solution (orange cream):** 1 mg/mL. **Injection:** 9.75 mg/1.3 mL single-dose vials.

NURSING IMPLICATIONS

Assessment
- Assess mental status (orientation, mood, behavior) before and periodically during therapy. Assess for suicidal tendencies, especially during early therapy for depression. Restrict amount of drug available to patient. Risk may be increased in children, adolescents, and adults ≤24 yrs.
- Assess weight and BMI initially and throughout therapy.
- Obtain fasting blood glucose and cholesterol levels initially and periodically during therapy.
- Monitor blood pressure (sitting, standing, lying), pulse, and respiratory rate before and periodically during therapy.
- Observe patient carefully when administering medication to ensure that medication is actually taken and not hoarded or cheeked.
- Monitor patient for onset of akathisia (restlessness or desire to keep moving) and extrapyramidal side effects (*parkinsonian*—difficulty speaking or swallowing, loss of balance control, pill rolling of hands, masklike face, shuffling gait, rigidity, tremors; and *dystonic*—muscle spasms, twisting motions, twitching, inability to move eyes, weakness of arms or legs) periodically throughout therapy. Report these symptoms.
- Monitor for tardive dyskinesia (uncontrolled rhythmic movement of mouth, face, and extremities; lip smacking or puckering; puffing of cheeks; uncontrolled chewing; rapid or worm-like movements of tongue). Notify health care professional immediately if these symptoms occur, as these side effects may be irreversible.
- Monitor for development of neuroleptic malignant syndrome (fever, muscle rigidity, altered mental status, respiratory distress, tachycardia, seizures, diaphoresis, hypertension or hypotension, pallor, tiredness, loss of bladder control). Notify health care professional immediately if these symptoms occur.
- *Lab Test Considerations:* May cause ↑ creatinine phosphokinase.
- Monitor CBC frequently during initial months of therapy in patients with pre-existing or history of low WBC. May cause leukopenia, neutropenia, or agranulocytosis. Discontinue therapy if this occurs.

Potential Nursing Diagnoses
Disturbed thought process (Indications)
Imbalanced nutrition: risk for more than body requirements (Side Effects)

Implementation
- **PO:** Administer once daily without regard to meals.
- Do not open the blister until ready to administer. For single tablet removal, open the package and peel back the foil on the blister to expose the tablet. Do not push the tablet through the foil; may damage tablet. Immediately upon opening the blister, using dry hands, remove the tablet and place the entire orally disintegrating tablet on the tongue. Tablet disintegration occurs rapidly in saliva. Take tablet without liquid; but if needed, it can be taken with liquid. Do not attempt to split the tablet.

asenapine

asenapine (a-sen-a-peen)
Saphris

Classification
Therapeutic: antipsychotics, mood stabilizers
Pharmacologic: dibenzo-oxepino pyrroles

Pregnancy Category C

Indications
Acute treatment of schizophrenia. Acute treatment of manic/mixed episodes associated with bipolar I disorder.

Action
May act through combined antagonism of dopaminergic (D_2) and $5-HT_{2A}$ receptors. **Therapeutic Effects:** Decreased symptoms of acute schizophrenia and mania/mixed episodes of bipolar I disorder.

Pharmacokinetics
Absorption: 35% absorbed following sublingual administration.
Distribution: Rapidly distributed throughout the body. Vd is approximately 20–25 L/kg: 95% bound to plasma proteins.
Metabolism and Excretion: Highly metabolized; primarily by CYP1A2 and UGTA14 enzyme systems 50% excreted in urine, 40% in feces, primarily as metabolites.
Half-life: 24 hr.

TIME/ACTION PROFILE (anitpsychotic effect))

ROUTE	ONSET	PEAK	DURATION
SL	unknown	0.5–1.5 hr†	12–24 hr

† Blood levels.

Contraindications/Precautions
Contraindicated in: Dementia-related psychoses; Severe hepatic impairment; Lactation: Avoid use during lactation.
Use Cautiously in: History of cardiac arrhythmias, congenital QT prolongation, electrolyte abnormalities (especially hypomagnesemia or hypokalemia; correct prior to use) or concurrent use of medications known to prolong the QTc interval; may ↑ risk of life-threatening arrhythmias; History of seizures or conditions/medications known to ↓ seizure threshold; History of leukopenia/neutropenia; Strenuous exercise, exposure to extreme heat, concurrent medications with anticholinergic activity, or risk of dehydration; Geri: ↑

- **IM:** IM route should be used for agitation. Convert to oral dose as soon as possible. Administer IM; for dose of 5.25 mg use 0.7 mL, 9.75 mg use 1.3 mL, and 15 mg use 2 mL of aripiprazole solution. Solution should be clear and colorless; do not administer solutions that are discolored or contain a precipitate.

Patient/Family Teaching
- Advise patient to take medication as directed and not to skip doses or double up on missed doses. Take missed doses as soon as remembered unless almost time for the next dose.
- Inform patient of possibility of extrapyramidal symptoms and tardive dyskinesia. Instruct patient to report these symptoms immediately.
- Advise patient to make position changes slowly to minimize orthostatic hypotension.
- Medication may cause drowsiness and lightheadedness. Caution patient to avoid driving or other activities requiring alertness until response to medication is known.
- Advise patient and family to notify health care professional if thoughts about suicide or dying, attempts to commit suicide; new or worse depression; new or worse anxiety; feeling very agitated or restless; panic attacks; trouble sleeping; new or worse irritability; acting aggressive; being angry or violent; acting on dangerous impulses; an extreme increase in activity and talking; other unusual changes in behavior or mood occur.
- Caution patient to avoid taking alcohol or other CNS depressants concurrently with this medication.
- Advise patient that extremes in temperature should be avoided, because this drug impairs body temperature regulation.
- Advise patient to notify health care professional of medication regimen prior to treatment or surgery.
- Emphasize the importance of routine follow-up exams and continued participation in psychotherapy as indicated.

Evaluation/Desired Outcomes
- Decrease in excitable, paranoic, or withdrawn behavior.
- Decrease incidence of mood swings in patients with bipolar disorders.
- Increased sense of well-being in patients with depression.
- Decreased agitation associated with schizophrenia or bipolar disorder.

♣ = Canadian drug name. ☰ = Genetic implication.
CAPITALS indicates life-threatening; underlines indicate most frequent.

risk of adverse reactions; consider age-related ↓ in hepatic function, cardiovascular status, and concurrent medications; History of suicide attempt; Geri: ↑ risk of mortality in elderly patients treated for dementia-related psychosis; OB: Use only when potential benefit justifies the potential risk; Pedi: safe and effective use has not been established.

Adverse Reactions/Side Effects
CNS: NEUROLEPTIC MALIGNANT SYNDROME, SEIZURES, SUICIDAL THOUGHTS, akathisia, dizziness, drowsiness, extrapyramidal symptoms, anxiety, fatigue, syncope, tardive dyskinesia. **CV:** bradycardia, orthostatic hypotension, QTc prolongation, tachycardia. **GI:** oral hypoesthesia, dry mouth, dyspepsia. **Endo:** hyperglycemia, hyperprolactinemia. **Metab:** weight gain, ↑ appetite.

Interactions
Drug-Drug: Concurrent use of **drugs known to prolong QTc** including **Class 1A antiarrhythmics** such as **quinidine** and **procainamide** or **Class 3 antiarrhythmics** including **amiodarone** and **sotalol** or other **antipsychotics** including **ziprasidone**, **chlorpromazine** or **thioridazine** or certain **antibiotics** such as **gatifloxacin** or **moxifloxacin**; may ↑ risk of torsade de pointes and/or sudden death. Concurrent use should be avoided. **Fluvoxamine**, a strong inhibitor of CYP1A2, ↑ levels and risk of toxicity; use cautiously. Similar effects may occur with **paroxetine**, a CYP2D6 substrate and inhibitor. Drugs having similar properties (**substrates/inhibitors of CYP2D6**) should also be used cautiously with asenapine. ↑ risk of CNS depression with other **CNS depressants** including **antihistamines**, some **antidepressants**, **sedative/hypnotics**, and **alcohol**.

Route/Dosage
SL (Adults): *Schizophrenia*—5 mg twice daily; *Bipolar Disorder*—10 mg twice daily, may be decreased to 5 mg twice daily if tolerated poorly.

Availability
Sublingual tablets: 5 mg, 10 mg.

NURSING IMPLICATIONS

Assessment
- Assess mental status (orientation, mood, behavior) before and periodically during therapy. Assess for suicidal tendencies. Restrict amount of drug available to patient. Risk may be increased in children, adolescents, and adults ≤24 yrs.
- Assess weight and BMI initially and throughout therapy.
- Monitor blood pressure (sitting, standing, lying) and pulse before and periodically during therapy.
- Observe patient carefully when administering medication to ensure that medication is actually taken and not hoarded or cheeked.
- Monitor patient for onset of akathisia (restlessness or desire to keep moving) and extrapyramidal side effects (*parkinsonian*—difficulty speaking or swallowing, loss of balance control, pill rolling of hands, masklike face, shuffling gait, rigidity, tremors; and *dystonic*—muscle spasms, twisting motions, twitching, inability to move eyes, weakness of arms or legs) periodically throughout therapy. Report these symptoms.
- Monitor for tardive dyskinesia (uncontrolled rhythmic movement of mouth, face, and extremities; lip smacking or puckering; puffing of cheeks; uncontrolled chewing; rapid or worm-like movements of tongue). Notify health care professional immediately if these symptoms occur, as these side effects may be irreversible.
- Monitor for development of neuroleptic malignant syndrome (fever, muscle rigidity, altered mental status, respiratory distress, tachycardia, seizures, diaphoresis, hypertension or hypotension, pallor, tiredness, loss of bladder control). Discontinue asenapine and notify health care professional immediately if these symptoms occur.
- Monitor for symptoms related to hyperprolactinemia (menstrual abnormalities, galactorrhea, sexual dysfunction).
- *Lab Test Considerations:* Obtain fasting blood glucose and cholesterol levels initially and periodically during therapy.
- Monitor CBC frequently during initial months of therapy in patients with pre-existing or history of low WBC. May cause leukopenia, neutropenia, or agranulocytosis. Monitor patients with neutropenia for fever or other symptoms of infection and treat promptly. Discontinue therapy if ANC <1000/mm^3 occurs.
- May cause transient ↑ in serum ALT.

Potential Nursing Diagnoses
Disturbed thought process (Indications)

Implementation
- **SL:** Open packet immediately before use by firmly pressing thumb button and pulling out tablet pack. Do not push tablet through or cut or tear tablet pack. Peel back colored tab and gently remove tablet. Place tablet under tongue and allow to dissolve completely; dissolves in saliva within seconds. Avoid eating or drinking

for 10 min after administration. Slide tablet pack back into case until it clicks.

Patient/Family Teaching
- Advise patient to take medication as directed and not to skip doses or double up on missed doses. Take missed doses as soon as remembered unless almost time for the next dose.
- Inform patient of possibility of extrapyramidal symptoms and tardive dyskinesia. Instruct patient to report these symptoms immediately.
- Advise patient to make position changes slowly to minimize orthostatic hypotension.
- Medication may cause drowsiness and dizziness. Caution patient to avoid driving or other activities requiring alertness until response to medication is known.
- Advise patient and family to notify health care professional if thoughts about suicide or dying, attempts to commit suicide; new or worse depression; new or worse anxiety; feeling very agitated or restless; panic attacks; trouble sleeping; new or worse irritability; acting aggressive; being angry or violent; acting on dangerous impulses; an extreme increase in activity and talking; other unusual changes in behavior or mood occur.
- Caution patient to notify health care professional before taking other Rx, OTC, or herbal products and to avoid taking alcohol or other CNS depressants concurrently with this medication.
- Advise patient that extremes in temperature should be avoided, because this drug impairs body temperature regulation.
- Advise patient to notify health care professional of medication regimen prior to treatment or surgery.
- Advise female patients to notify health care professional if pregnancy is planned or suspected and to avoid breastfeeding during therapy.
- Emphasize the importance of routine follow-up exams and continued participation in psychotherapy as indicated.

Evaluation/Desired Outcomes
- Decrease in excitable, paranoic, or withdrawn behavior.
- Decrease incidence of mood swings in patients with bipolar disorders.
- Decreased agitation associated with schizophrenia or bipolar disorder.

---

asparaginase 199

HIGH ALERT

asparaginase
(a-spare-a-ji-nase)
Elspar, ✳ Kidrolase

Classification
Therapeutic: antineoplastics
Pharmacologic: enzymes

Pregnancy Category C

Indications
Part of combination chemotherapy in the treatment of acute lymphocytic leukemia (ALL).

Action
Catalyst in the conversion of asparagine (an amino acid) to aspartic acid and ammonia. Depletes asparagine in leukemic cells. **Therapeutic Effects:** Death of leukemic cells.

Pharmacokinetics
Absorption: Is absorbed from IM sites.
Distribution: Remains in the intravascular space. Poor penetration into the CSF.
Metabolism and Excretion: Slowly sequestered in the reticuloendothelial system.
Half-life: IV: 8–30 hr; IM: 39–49 hr.

TIME/ACTION PROFILE (depletion of asparagine)

ROUTE	ONSET	PEAK†	DURATION
IM	immediate	14–24 hr	23–33 days
IV	immediate	unknown	23–33 days

†Plasma levels of asparaginase

Contraindications/Precautions
Contraindicated in: Previous hypersensitivity; Lactation: May cause unwanted effects in the nursing infant.
Use Cautiously in: History of hypersensitivity reactions; Severe liver disease; Renal or pancreatic disease; CNS depression; Clotting abnormalities; Chronic debilitating illnesses; OB: Use only if the potential benefit justifies the potential risk to the fetus.

Adverse Reactions/Side Effects
CNS: SEIZURES, agitation, coma, confusion, depression, dizziness, fatigue, hallucinations, headache, irritability, somnolence. **GI:** nausea, vomiting, anorexia, cramps, hepatotoxicity, pancreatitis, weight loss. **Derm:** rashes, urticaria. **Endo:** hyperglycemia. **Hemat:** coagulation abnormalities, transient bone marrow depression.

✳ = Canadian drug name. 🧬 = Genetic implication.
*CAPITALS indicates life-threatening; underlines indicate most frequent.

Metab: hyperammonemia, hyperuricemia. **Misc:** hypersensitivity reactions including ANAPHYLAXIS.

Interactions
Drug-Drug: May negate the antineoplastic activity of **methotrexate**. May enhance the hepatotoxicity of other **hepatotoxic drugs**. Concurrent IV use with or immediately preceding **vincristine** and **prednisone** may result in ↑ neurotoxicity and hyperglycemia. May alter the response to **live vaccines** (↓ antibody response, ↑ risk of adverse reactions).

Route/Dosage
Various other regimens may be used.

Multiple-Agent Induction Regimen (in Combination with Vincristine and Prednisone)
IV (Children): 1000 IU/kg/day for 10 successive days beginning on day 22 of regimen.
IM (Children): 6000 IU/m^2 on days 4, 7, 10, 13, 16, 19, 22, 25, 28.

Single-Agent Therapy for Acute Lymphocytic Leukemia
IV (Adults and Children): 200 IU/kg daily for 28 days.

Desensitization Regimen
IV (Adults and Children): Administer 1 IU, then double dose every 10 min until total dose for that day has been given or reaction occurs.

Test Dose
Intradermal (Adults and Children): 2 IU.

Availability
Injection: 10,000-IU vial (with mannitol).

NURSING IMPLICATIONS

Assessment
- Monitor vital signs before and frequently during therapy. Inform physician if fever or chills occur.
- Monitor intake and output. Notify physician of significant discrepancies. Encourage patient to drink 2000–3000 mL/day to promote excretion of uric acid. Allopurinol and alkalinization of the urine may be used to prevent urate stone formation.
- Monitor for hypersensitivity reaction (urticaria, diaphoresis, facial swelling, joint pain, hypotension, bronchospasm). Epinephrine and resuscitation equipment should be readily available. Reaction may occur up to 2 hr after administration. If patient requires continued therapy, pegaspargase is an alternative.
- Assess nausea, vomiting, and appetite. Weigh weekly. An antiemetic may be given before administration.
- Monitor effect and neurologic status. Notify physician if depression, drowsiness, or hallucinations occur. Symptoms usually resolve 2–3 days after drug is discontinued.
- *Lab Test Considerations:* Monitor CBC before and periodically throughout therapy. May alter coagulation studies. Platelets, PT, PTT, and thrombin time may be ↑. May cause ↑ BUN.
- Hepatotoxicity may be manifested by ↑ AST, ALT, alkaline phosphatase, bilirubin, or cholesterol. Liver function test results usually return to normal after therapy. May cause pancreatitis; monitor frequently for ↑ amylase or glucose.
- Monitor blood glucose during therapy. May cause hyperglycemia treatable with fluids and insulin. May be fatal.
- May cause ↑ serum and urine uric acid concentrations.
- May interfere with thyroid function tests.

Potential Nursing Diagnoses
Risk for injury (Side Effects)
Risk for infection (Side Effects)

Implementation
- *High Alert:* Fatalities have occurred with chemotherapeutic agents. Before administering, clarify all ambiguous orders; double-check single, daily, and course-of-therapy dose limits; have second practitioner independently double check original order and dose calculations. Do not confuse asparaginase with pegaspargase.
- Solution should be prepared in a biologic cabinet. Wear gloves, gown, and mask while handling medication. Discard equipment in specially designated containers. See Appendix L.
- If coagulopathy develops, apply pressure to venipuncture sites; avoid IM injections.
- **Test Dose:** Intradermal test dose must be performed before initial dose; doses must be separated by more than 1 wk. Reconstitute vial with 5 mL of sterile water for injection or 0.9% NaCl for injection (without preservatives). Add 0.1 mL of this 2000-IU/mL solution to 9.9 mL additional diluent to yield a 20-IU/mL solution. Inject 0.1 mL (2 IU) intradermally. Observe site for 1 hr for formation of wheal. Wheal is indicative of a positive reaction.
- **Desensitization Therapy:** Begin by administering 1 IU intravenously. Double dose every 10 min if hypersensitivity does not occur until full daily dose is administered.

- **IM:** Prepare for IM dose by adding 2 mL of 0.9% NaCl for injection (without preservatives) to the 10,000-IU vial. Shake vial gently. Administer no more than 2 mL per injection site.

IV Administration

- **Direct IV:** *Diluent:* Prepare *Elspar* IV dose by diluting 10,000-IU vial with 5 mL of sterile water for injection or 0.9% NaCl (without preservatives). If gelatinous fibers are present, administration through a 5-micron filter will not alter potency. Administration through a 0.2-micron filter may cause loss of potency. Solution should be clear after reconstitution. Discard if cloudy. Stable for 8 hr if refrigerated. Prepare *Kidrolase* for IM or IV administration by adding 4 mL sterile water to 10,000 IU vial and rotate gently to dissolve. Unused reconstituted solution is stable for 14 days if refrigerated. May be further diluted with 0.9% NaCl or D5W. *Concentration:* Dilute doses in 50–250 mL of diluent. *Rate:* Administer through Y-site of rapidly flowing IV of D5W or 0.9% NaCl over 30–60 min. Maintain IV infusion for 2 hr after dose.
- **Y-Site Compatibility:** methotrexate, sodium bicarbonate.
- **Additive Incompatibility:** Information unavailable. Do not admix with other drugs.

Patient/Family Teaching

- Instruct patient to notify health care professional if abdominal pain, severe nausea and vomiting, jaundice, fever, chills, sore throat, bleeding or bruising, excess thirst or urination, or mouth sores occur. Caution patient to avoid crowds and persons with known infections. Instruct patient to use soft toothbrush and electric razor, and to be especially careful to avoid falls. Patients should also be cautioned not to drink alcoholic beverages or take medication containing aspirin or NSAIDs because these may precipitate gastric bleeding.
- Advise both men and women not to conceive a child while taking asparaginase. Barrier methods of contraception are recommended.
- Instruct patient not to receive any vaccinations without advice of health care professional. Advise parents that this may alter immunization schedule.
- Emphasize need for periodic lab tests to monitor for side effects.

Evaluation/Desired Outcomes

- Improvement of hematologic status in patients with leukemia.

---

aspirin, See SALICYLATES.

---

atazanavir (a-ta-zan-a-veer)
Reyataz

Classification
Therapeutic: antiretrovirals
Pharmacologic: protease inhibitors

Pregnancy Category B

Indications
HIV infection (with other antiretrovirals).

Action
Inhibits the action of HIV protease, preventing maturation of virions. **Therapeutic Effects:** ↑ CD4 cell counts and ↓ viral load with subsequent slowed progression of HIV and its sequelae.

Pharmacokinetics
Absorption: Rapidly absorbed (↑ by food).
Distribution: Enters cerebrospinal fluid and semen.
Metabolism and Excretion: 80% metabolized (CYP3A); 13% excreted unchanged in urine.
Half-life: 7 hr.

TIME/ACTION PROFILE (blood levels)

ROUTE	ONSET	PEAK	DURATION
PO	rapid	2.5 hr	24 hr

Contraindications/Precautions
Contraindicated in: Hypersensitivity; Severe hepatic impairment; Concurrent use of ergotamine, ergonovine, dihydroergotamine, methylergonovine, midazolam, pimozide, triazolam, rifampin, irinotecan, lovastatin, simvastatin, indinavir, proton-pump inhibitors (for treatment-experienced patients), efavirenz (for treatment-experienced patients), or St. John's wort; Pedi: ↑ risk of kernicterus in infants <3 mo.
Use Cautiously in: Mild to moderate hepatic impairment; Pre-existing conduction system disease (marked first-degree AV block or second- or third-degree AV block) or concurrent use of other drugs that increase the PR interval (especially those metabolized by CYP3A4, including verapamil or diltiazem); Diabetes mellitus; Hemo-

---

♣ = Canadian drug name. 🧬 = Genetic implication.
*CAPITALS indicates life-threatening; underlines indicate most frequent.

philia (↑ risk of bleeding); **Pedi:** Children <6 yr (safety not established); **OB:** Use only if clearly needed; Breastfeeding is not recommended if HIV-infected.

Adverse Reactions/Side Effects
When used in combination with other antiretrovirals.
CNS: headache, depression, dizziness, insomnia. **CV:** ↑ PR interval, heart block. **GI:** nausea, abdominal pain, ↑ bilirubin, cholelithiasis, diarrhea, jaundice, vomiting, ↑ transaminases. **Derm:** rash. **Endo:** hyperglycemia. **Metab:** fat redistribution. **MS:** myalgia. **Misc:** fever.

Interactions
Drug-Drug: Atazanavir is an inhibitor of CYP3A and UGT1A1 enzyme systems. It is also a substrate of CYP3A. ↑ levels of **ergotamine, ergonovine, dihydroergotamine, methylergonovine, midazolam, pimozide, triazolam, lovastatin, simvastatin,** and **irinotecan**; concurrent use may result in life-threatening CNS, cardiovascular, hematologic, or musculoskeletal toxicity and is contraindicated. Combination therapy with **tenofovir** may lead to ↓ virologic response and possible resistance (100 mg **ritonavir** should be added to boost blood levels and dose of atazanavir ↓ to 300 mg/day). Levels are significantly ↓ by **rifampin** and **St. John's wort**; may promote viral resistance, avoid concurrent use. Levels are significantly ↓ by **omeprazole**; do not exceed omeprazole dose of 20 mg/day when used with atazanavir and ritonavir in treatment-naive patients (should be taken at least 12 hr before atazanavir and ritonavir); should not be used in treatment-experienced patients. Concurrent use with **indinavir** may ↑ risk of hyperbilirubinemia and should be avoided. Concurrent use with **didanosine** buffered tablets will ↓ absorption and levels; give atazanavir with food 2 hr before or 1 hr after **didanosine**. **Efavirenz** ↓ levels and may promote viral resistance; 600 mg efavirenz should be given with atazanavir 400 mg/day and ritonavir 100 mg/day to counteract this effect in treatment-naive patients (should not be used with atazanavir in treatment-experienced patients). ↑ **saquinavir** levels. Levels are ↑ by **ritonavir**; ↓ atazanavir dose to 300 mg/day. **Nevirapine** may ↓ levels and atazanavir may ↑ **nevirapine** levels; avoid concurrent use. **Antacids** or **buffered medications** will ↓ absorption; atazanavir should be given 2 hr before or 1 hr after. ↑ levels of **lidocaine, amiodarone,** or **quinidine**; blood level monitoring is recommended. ↑ risk of bleeding with **warfarin**. ↑ of **tricyclic antidepressants**; blood level monitoring is recommended. ↑ levels of **rifabutin**; ↓ rifabutin dose by 75% (150 mg every other day or 3 times weekly). ↑ levels of **diltiazem** and its active metabolite; ↓ diltiazem dose by 50% and ECG monitoring recommended. Similar precautions may be needed with **felodipine, nifedipine, nicardipine,** and **verapamil**. ↑ levels of **fluticasone**; consider alternative therapy; should not be used when atazanavir used with ritonavir. ↓ levels of **voriconazole** when atazanavir is used with ritonavir; avoid concurrent use. **Voriconazole** may also ↑ levels of atazanavir (when used without ritonavir). ↑ levels of **ketoconazole** or **itraconazole** when atazanavir is used with ritonavir. ↑ levels of **trazodone**; ↓ dose of trazodone. ↑ levels of **sildenafil, vardenafil,** and **tadalafil**; ↓ **sildenafil** dose to 25 mg every 48 hr; ↓ **vardenafil** dose to 2.5 mg every 72 hr; ↓ **tadalafil** dose to 10 mg every 72 hr. Exercise caution and monitor for hypertension, visual changes, and priapism. ↑ levels and risk of myopathy from **atorvastatin** or **rosuvastatin** (use lowest dose of these agents or consider fluvastatin or pravastatin). Levels may be ↓ by **histamine H$_2$ antagonists**, promoting viral resistance; separate doses by at least 10 hr. ↑ levels of **cyclosporine, sirolimus,** and **tacrolimus**; monitor immunosuppressant blood levels. ↑ levels of **clarithromycin**; ↓ clarithromycin dose by 50% or consider alternative therapy. May ↓ levels of some **estrogens** found in **hormonal contraceptives**; use alternative nonhormonal method of contraception. Concurrent use of other **drugs known to** ↑ **PR interval** may ↑ risk of heart block.

Route/Dosage
PO (Adults): *Therapy-naive*— 400 mg once daily *or* 300 mg once daily with ritonavir 100 mg once daily; should be used at a dose of 300 mg once daily with ritonavir 100 mg once daily if used concomitantly with tenofovir, H2 receptor antagonist, or proton pump inhibitor; should be used at a dose of 400 mg once daily with ritonavir 100 mg once daily if used concomitantly with efavirenz. *Therapy-experienced*— 300 mg once daily with ritonavir 100 mg once daily; should be used at dose of 400 mg once daily with ritonavir 100 mg once daily if used with tenofovir and a H2 receptor antagonist.

PO (Children ≥6 yr and Therapy-Naive): *15–24 kg*— 150 mg once daily with ritonavir 80 mg once daily; *25–31 kg*— 200 mg once daily with ritonavir 100 mg once daily; *32–38 kg*— 250 mg once daily with ritonavir 100 mg once daily; *6–12 yr and ≥39 kg*— 300 mg once daily with ritonavir

100 mg once daily; ≥*13 yr and* ≥*39 kg*— 400 mg once daily.
PO (Children ≥6 yr and Therapy-Experienced): *25–31 kg*— 200 mg once daily with ritonavir 100 mg once daily; *32–38 kg*— 250 mg once daily with ritonavir 100 mg once daily; ≥*39 kg*— 300 mg once daily with ritonavir 100 mg once daily.

Renal Impairment
PO (Adults): *Therapy-Naive and HD*— 300 mg once daily with ritonavir 100 mg once daily; *Therapy-Experienced and HD*— contraindicated.

Hepatic Impairment
PO (Adults): *Moderate hepatic impairment*— 300 mg once daily (do not use with ritonavir).

Availability
Capsules: 100 mg, 150 mg, 200 mg, 300 mg.

NURSING IMPLICATIONS

Assessment
- Assess for change in severity of HIV symptoms and for symptoms of opportunistic infections throughout therapy.
- Assess for rash which can occur within initial 8 wk of therapy. Usually resolves within 2 weeks without altering therapy. Discontinue therapy if rash becomes severe.
- **Lab Test Considerations:** Monitor viral load and CD4 cell count regularly during therapy.
- May cause ↑ serum amylase, lipase and hyperglycemia.
- May ↑ liver enzymes.
- May ↑ creatine kinase.
- May cause ↓ hemoglobin, neutrophils, and platelets.
- May cause ↑ in unconjugated bilirubin; reversible on discontinuation.

Potential Nursing Diagnoses
Risk for infection (Indications)
Noncompliance (Patient/Family Teaching)

Implementation
- **PO:** Administer daily with food to enhance absorption. Capsules should be swallowed whole; do not open.

Patient/Family Teaching
- Emphasize the importance of taking atazanavir with food as directed. Advise patient to read the *Patient Information* before taking and with each Rx refill; may be updated. Atazanavir must always be used in combination with other antiretroviral drugs. Do not take more than prescribed amount and do not stop taking without consulting health care professional. Take missed doses as soon as remembered, then return to regular dose schedule. If within 6 hr of next dose, omit dose and take next dose at regular time. Do not double doses.
- Instruct patient that atazanavir should not be shared with others.
- Inform patient that atazanavir does not cure HIV or prevent associated or opportunistic infections. Atazanavir does not reduce the risk of transmission of HIV to others through sexual contact or blood contamination. Caution patient to use a condom and to avoid sharing needles or donating blood to prevent spreading the HIV virus to others. Advise patient that atazanavir may cause lipodystrophy (redistribution or accumulation of body fat) and the long-term effects of atazanavir are unknown at this time.
- Instruct patient to consult health care professional before taking other Rx, OTC, or herbal products, especially St. John's wort; interactions may be fatal.
- May cause dizziness. Caution patient to notify health care professional if this occurs and to avoid driving and other activities requiring alertness until response to medication is known.
- Notify health care professional immediately if yellowing of eyes, change in heart rhythm, or high blood sugar occur.
- Emphasize the importance of regular follow-up exams and blood counts to determine progress and monitor for side effects.
- Inform patient that redistribution and accumulation of body fat may occur, causing central obesity, dorsocervical fat enlargement (buffalo hump), peripheral wasting, breast enlargement, and cushingoid appearance. The cause and long-term effects are not known.
- Instruct females using hormonal contraceptives to use an alternative nonhormonal method of contraception. Advise patient to notify health care professional if pregnancy is planned or suspected or if breastfeeding. If pregnant patient is exposed to atazanavir, register patient in *Antiretroviral Pregnancy Registry* by calling 1-800-258-4263.

Evaluation/Desired Outcomes
- Delayed progression of HIV and decreased opportunistic infections in patients with HIV.

- Decrease in viral load and increase in CD4 cell counts.

atenolol (a-ten-oh-lole)
♣ Apo-Atenolol, ♣ Novo-Atenolol, Tenormin

Classification
Therapeutic: antianginals, antihypertensives
Pharmacologic: beta blockers

Pregnancy Category D

Indications
Management of hypertension. Management of angina pectoris. Prevention of MI.

Action
Blocks stimulation of beta$_1$(myocardial)-adrenergic receptors. Does not usually affect beta$_2$(pulmonary, vascular, uterine)-receptor sites. **Therapeutic Effects:** Decreased blood pressure and heart rate. Decreased frequency of attacks of angina pectoris. Prevention of MI.

Pharmacokinetics
Absorption: 50–60% absorbed after oral administration.
Distribution: Minimal penetration of CNS. Crosses the placenta and enters breast milk.
Metabolism and Excretion: 40–50% excreted unchanged by the kidneys; remainder excreted in feces as unabsorbed drug.
Half-life: 6–9 hr.

TIME/ACTION PROFILE (cardiovascular effects)

ROUTE	ONSET	PEAK	DURATION
PO	1 hr	2–4 hr	24 hr

Contraindications/Precautions
Contraindicated in: Uncompensated CHF; Pulmonary edema; Cardiogenic shock; Bradycardia or heart block.
Use Cautiously in: Renal impairment (dosage reduction recommended if CCr ≤35 mL/min); Hepatic impairment; Geriatric patients (increased sensitivity to beta blockers; initial dosage reduction recommended); Pulmonary disease (including asthma; beta selectivity may be lost at higher doses); Diabetes mellitus (may mask signs of hypoglycemia); Thyrotoxicosis (may mask symptoms); Patients with a history of severe allergic reactions (intensity of reactions may be increased); OB: Crosses the placenta and may cause fetal/neonatal bradycardia, hypotension, hypoglycemia, or respiratory depression; Lactation, Pedi: Safety not established.

Adverse Reactions/Side Effects
CNS: fatigue, weakness, anxiety, depression, dizziness, drowsiness, insomnia, memory loss, mental status changes, nervousness, nightmares. **EENT:** blurred vision, stuffy nose. **Resp:** bronchospasm, wheezing. **CV:** BRADYCARDIA, CHF, PULMONARY EDEMA, hypotension, peripheral vasoconstriction. **GI:** constipation, diarrhea, liver function abnormalities, nausea, vomiting. **GU:** erectile dysfunction, decreased libido, urinary frequency. **Derm:** rashes. **Endo:** hyperglycemia, hypoglycemia. **MS:** arthralgia, back pain, joint pain. **Misc:** drug-induced lupus syndrome.

Interactions
Drug-Drug: General anesthesia, IV **phenytoin**, and **verapamil** may cause additive myocardial depression. Additive bradycardia may occur with **digoxin**. Additive hypotension may occur with other **antihypertensives**, acute ingestion of **alcohol**, or **nitrates**. Concurrent use with **amphetamine**, **cocaine**, **ephedrine**, **epinephrine**, **norepinephrine**, **phenylephrine**, or **pseudoephedrine** may result in unopposed alpha-adrenergic stimulation (excessive hypertension, bradycardia). Concurrent **thyroid** administration may decrease effectiveness. May alter the effectiveness of **insulins** or **oral hypoglycemic agents** (dosage adjustments may be necessary). May decrease the effectiveness of **theophylline**. May decrease the beneficial beta$_1$-cardiovascular effects of **dopamine** or **dobutamine**. Use cautiously within 14 days of **MAO inhibitor** therapy (may result in hypertension).

Route/Dosage
PO (Adults): *Antianginal*—50 mg once daily; may be increased after 1 wk to 100 mg/day (up to 200 mg/day). *Antihypertensive*—25–50 mg once daily; may be increased after 2 wk to 50–100 mg once daily. *MI*—50 mg, then 50 mg 12 hr later, then 100 mg/day as a single dose or in 2 divided doses for 6–9 days or until hospital discharge.

Renal Impairment
PO (Adults): *CCr 15–35 mL/min*—dosage should not exceed 50 mg/day; *CCr <15 mL/min*—dosage should not exceed 50 mg every other day.

Availability (generic available)
Tablets: 25 mg, 50 mg, 100 mg. *Cost:* Generic—25 mg $11.99/90, 50 mg $12.99/90, 100 mg $15.89/90. *In combination with:* chlorthalidone (Tenoretic). See Appendix B.

NURSING IMPLICATIONS

Assessment
- Monitor blood pressure, ECG, and pulse frequently during dosage adjustment period and periodically throughout therapy.
- Monitor intake and output ratios and daily weights. Assess routinely for CHF (dyspnea, rales/crackles, weight gain, peripheral edema, jugular venous distention).
- Monitor frequency of prescription refills to determine adherence.
- **Angina:** Assess frequency and characteristics of angina periodically throughout therapy.
- ***Lab Test Considerations:*** May cause ↑ BUN, serum lipoprotein, potassium, triglyceride, and uric acid levels.
- May cause ↑ ANA titers.
- May cause ↑ in blood glucose levels.
- ***Toxicity and Overdose:*** Monitor patients receiving beta blockers for signs of overdose (bradycardia, severe dizziness or fainting, severe drowsiness, dyspnea, bluish fingernails or palms, seizures). Notify physician immediately if these signs occur.

Potential Nursing Diagnoses
Decreased cardiac output (Side Effects)
Noncompliance (Patient/Family Teaching)

Implementation
- **PO:** Take apical pulse before administering drug. If <50 bpm or if arrhythmia occurs, withhold medication and notify physician or other health care professional.

Patient/Family Teaching
- Instruct patient to take atenolol as directed at the same time each day, even if feeling well; do not skip or double up on missed doses. Take missed doses as soon as possible up to 8 hr before next dose. Abrupt withdrawal may cause life-threatening arrhythmias, hypertension, or myocardial ischemia.
- Advise patient to make sure enough medication is available for weekends, holidays, and vacations. A written prescription may be kept in wallet in case of emergency.
- Teach patient and family how to check pulse and blood pressure. Instruct them to check pulse daily and blood pressure biweekly and to report significant changes.
- May cause drowsiness or dizziness. Caution patients to avoid driving or other activities that require alertness until response to the drug is known.
- Advise patients to change positions slowly to minimize orthostatic hypotension.
- Caution patient that atenolol may increase sensitivity to cold.
- Instruct patient to consult health care professional before taking any OTC medications, especially cold preparations, concurrently with this medication.
- Patients with diabetes should closely monitor blood glucose, especially if weakness, malaise, irritability, or fatigue occurs. Medication does not block sweating as a sign of hypoglycemia.
- Advise patient to notify health care professional if slow pulse, difficulty breathing, wheezing, cold hands and feet, dizziness, light-headedness, confusion, depression, rash, fever, sore throat, unusual bleeding, or bruising occurs.
- Instruct patient to inform health care professional of medication regimen before treatment or surgery.
- Advise patient to carry identification describing disease process and medication regimen at all times.
- **Hypertension:** Reinforce the need to continue additional therapies for hypertension (weight loss, sodium restriction, stress reduction, regular exercise, moderation of alcohol consumption, and smoking cessation). Medication controls but does not cure hypertension.

Evaluation/Desired Outcomes
- Decrease in blood pressure.
- Reduction in frequency of angina.
- Increase in activity tolerance.
- Prevention of MI.

---

atomoxetine
(a-to-**mox**-e-teen)
Strattera

Classification
Therapeutic: agents for attention deficit disorder
Pharmacologic: selective norepinephrine reuptake inhibitors

Pregnancy Category C

Indications
Attention-Deficit/Hyperactivity Disorder (ADHD).

atomoxetine

Action
Selectively inhibits the presynaptic transporter of norepinephrine. **Therapeutic Effects:** Increased attention span.

Pharmacokinetics
Absorption: Well absorbed following oral administration.
Distribution: Unknown.
Protein Binding: 98%.
Metabolism and Excretion: Mostly metabolized by the liver (CYP2D6 enzyme pathway). ▓ A small percentage of the population are poor metabolizers and will have higher blood levels with ↑ effects.
Half-life: 5 hr.

TIME/ACTION PROFILE

ROUTE	ONSET	PEAK	DURATION
PO	unknown	1–2 hr	12–24 hr

Contraindications/Precautions
Contraindicated in: Concurrent or within 2 wk therapy with MAO inhibitors; Angle-closure glaucoma.
Use Cautiously in: Hypertension, tachycardia, cardiovascular or cerebrovascular disease; Pre-existing psychiatric illness; May ↑ risk of suicide attempt/ideation especially during dose early treatment or dose adjustment; risk may be greater in children or adolescents; Concurrent albuterol or vasopressors (↑ risk of adverse cardiovascular reactions); OB: Use only if benefits outweigh risks to fetus; Lactation, Pedi: Safety not established.

Adverse Reactions/Side Effects
CNS: SUICIDAL THOUGHTS, dizziness, fatigue, mood swings, behavioral disturbances, hallucinations, mania, thought disorder; *Adults*, insomnia. **CV:** hypertension, orthostatic hypotension, syncope, tachycardia. **GI:** dyspepsia, severe liver injury (rare), nausea, vomiting; *Adults*, dry mouth, constipation. **Derm:** rash, urticaria. **GU:** *Adults*—dysmenorrhea, ejaculatory problems, ↓ libido, erectile dysfunction, urinary hesitation, urinary retention. **Metab:** ↓ appetite, weight/growth loss. **Misc:** allergic reactions including ANGIONEUROTIC EDEMA.

Interactions
Drug-Drug: Concurrent use with **MAO inhibitors** may result in serious, potentially fatal reactions (do not use within 2 wk of each other). ↑ risk of cardiovascular effects with **albuterol** or **vasopressors** (use cautiously). **Drugs which inhibit the CYP2D6 enzyme pathway** (**quinidine**, **fluoxetine**, **paroxetine**) will increase blood levels and effects, dose ↓ recommended.

Route/Dosage
PO (Children and adolescents <70 kg): 0.5 mg/kg/day initially, may be ↑ every 3 days to a daily target dose of 1.2 mg/kg, given as a single dose in the morning or evenly divided doses in the morning and late afternoon/early evening (not to exceed 1.4 mg/kg/day or 100 mg/day whichever is less). *If taking concurrent CYP2D6 inhibitor (quinidine, fluoxetine, paroxetine)*—0.5 mg/kg/day initially, may ↑ if needed to 1.2 mg/kg/day after 4 wk.
PO (Adults, adolescents, and children >70 kg): 40 mg/day initially, may be ↑ every 3 days to a daily target dose of 80 mg/day given as a single dose in the morning or evenly divided doses in the morning and late afternoon/early evening; may be further ↑ after 2–4 wk up to 100 mg/day. *If taking concurrent CYP2D6 inhibitor (quinidine, fluoxetine, paroxetine)*—40 mg/day initially, may ↑ if needed to 80 mg/day after 4 wk.

Hepatic Impairment
PO (Adults and Children): *Moderate hepatic impairment (Child-Pugh Class B)*— ↓ initial and target dose by 50%; *Severe hepatic impairment (Child-Pugh Class C)*— ↓ initial and target dose to 25% of normal.

Availability
Capsules: 10 mg, 18 mg, 25 mg, 40 mg, 60 mg, 80 mg, 100 mg. **Cost:** 10 mg $368.58/90, 18 mg $433.13/90, 25 mg $369.98/90, 40 mg $389.95/90, 60 mg $389.95/90, 80 mg $435.93/90, 100 mg $439.96/90.

NURSING IMPLICATIONS

Assessment
- Assess attention span, impulse control, and interactions with others.
- Monitor blood pressure and pulse periodically during therapy. Obtain a history (including assessment of family history of sudden death or ventricular arrhythmia), physical exam to assess for cardiac disease, and further evaluation (ECG and echocardiogram), if indicated. If exertional chest pain, unexplained syncope, or other cardiac symptoms occur, evaluate promptly.
- Monitor growth, body height, and weight in children.
- Assess for signs of liver injury (pruritus, dark urine, jaundice, right upper quadrant tenderness, unexplained "flu-like" symptoms) during

therapy. Monitor liver function tests at first sign of liver injury. Discontinue and do not restart atomoxetine in patients with jaundice or laboratory evidence of liver injury.
- Monitor closely for notable changes in behavior that could indicate the emergence or worsening of suicidal thoughts or behavior or depression.

Potential Nursing Diagnoses
Disturbed thought process (Indications)
Impaired social interaction (Indications)

Implementation
- **PO:** Administer without regard to food. Capsules should be swallowed whole; do not open, crush, or chew. Doses may be discontinued without tapering.

Patient/Family Teaching
- Instruct patient to take medication as directed. Take missed doses as soon as possible, but should not take more than the total daily amount in any 24-hr period. Advise patient and parents to read the *Medication Guide* prior to starting therapy and with each Rx refill.
- Inform patient that sharing this medication may be dangerous.
- Advise patient to notify health care professional immediately if signs of liver injury occur.
- Advise patient and family to notify health care professional if thoughts about suicide or dying, attempts to commit suicide; new or worse depression; new or worse anxiety; feeling very agitated or restless; panic attacks; trouble sleeping; new or worse irritability; acting aggressive; being angry or violent; acting on dangerous impulses; an extreme increase in activity and talking; other unusual changes in behavior or mood occur.
- Caution patient to consult health care professional prior to taking other Rx, OTC, dietary supplements, or herbal products.
- May cause dizziness. Caution patient to avoid driving or other activities requiring alertness until response to medication is known.
- Advise female patients to notify health care professional if pregnancy is planned or suspected or if they are breastfeeding.
- Pedi: Advise parents to notify school nurse of medication regimen.

Evaluation/Desired Outcomes
- Improved attention span and social interactions in ADHD.

---

atorvastatin, See HMG-CoA REDUCTASE INHIBITORS (statins).

atovaquone (a-toe-va-kwone)
Mepron

Classification
Therapeutic: anti-infectives

Pregnancy Category C

Indications
Treatment of mild to moderate *Pneumocystis jirovecii* pneumonia (PCP) in patients who are unable to tolerate trimethoprim/sulfamethoxazole. Prophylaxis of *PCP*.

Action
Inhibits the action of enzymes necessary to nucleic acid and ATP synthesis. **Therapeutic Effects:** Active against *P. jirovecii*.

Pharmacokinetics
Absorption: Absorption is poor but is increased by food, particularly fat.
Distribution: Enters CSF in very low concentrations (<1% of plasma levels).
Protein Binding: >99.9%.
Metabolism and Excretion: Undergoes enterohepatic recycling; elimination occurs in feces.
Half-life: 2.2–2.9 days.

TIME/ACTION PROFILE (blood levels)

ROUTE	ONSET	PEAK	DURATION
PO	unknown	1–8 hr; 24–96 hr†	12 hr

†Two peaks are due to enterohepatic recycling.

Contraindications/Precautions
Contraindicated in: Hypersensitivity; Lactation: May appear in breast milk.
Use Cautiously in: ↓ hepatic, renal, or cardiac function (dose modification may be necessary); GI disorders (absorption may be limited); OB: Safety not established; Pedi: Safety not established.

Adverse Reactions/Side Effects
CNS: headache, insomnia. **Resp:** cough. **GI:** diarrhea, nausea, vomiting. **Derm:** rash. **Misc:** fever.

Interactions
Drug-Drug: May interact with **drugs that are highly bound to plasma proteins** (does not appear to interact with phenytoin).

Drug-Food: Food ↑ absorption.

Route/Dosage
Treatment
PO (Adults): 750 mg twice daily for 21 days.
PO (Children): 40 mg/kg/day (unlabeled).

Prevention
PO (Adults and Adolescents 13–16 yr): 1500 mg once daily.

Availability
Suspension: 750 mg/5 mL.

NURSING IMPLICATIONS

Assessment
- Assess patient for signs of infection (vital signs, lung sounds, sputum, WBCs) at beginning of and throughout therapy.
- Obtain specimens prior to initiating therapy. First dose may be given before receiving results.
- *Lab Test Considerations:* Monitor hematologic and hepatic functions. May cause mild, transient anemia and neutropenia. May also cause ↑ serum amylase, AST, ALT, and alkaline phosphatase.
- Monitor electrolytes. May cause hyponatremia.

Potential Nursing Diagnoses
Risk for infection (Indications, Side Effects)
Deficient knowledge, related to medication regimen (Patient/Family Teaching)

Implementation
- **PO:** Administer with food twice daily for 21 days for treatment and once daily for prevention.

Patient/Family Teaching
- Instruct patient to take atovaquone exactly as directed around the clock for the full course of therapy, even if feeling better. Emphasize the importance of taking atovaquone with food, especially foods high in fat; taking without food may decrease plasma concentrations and effectiveness.
- Advise patient to notify health care professional if rash occurs.

Evaluation/Desired Outcomes
- Resolution of the signs and symptoms of infection.

---

atropine† (at-ro-peen)
Atro-Pen

Classification
Therapeutic: antiarrhythmics
Pharmacologic: anticholinergics, antimuscarinics

Pregnancy Category C
†See Appendix C for ophthalmic use

Indications
IM: Given preoperatively to decrease oral and respiratory secretions. **IV:** Treatment of sinus bradycardia and heart block. **PO:** Adjunctive therapy in the management of peptic ulcer and irritable bowel syndrome. **IV:** Reversal of adverse muscarinic effects of anticholinesterase agents (neostigmine, physostigmine, or pyridostigmine). **IM, IV:** Treatment of anticholinesterase (organophosphate pesticide) poisoning. **Inhaln:** Treatment of exercise-induced bronchospasm.

Action
Inhibits the action of acetylcholine at postganglionic sites located in: Smooth muscle, Secretory glands, CNS (antimuscarinic activity). Low doses decrease: Sweating, Salivation, Respiratory secretions. Intermediate doses result in: Mydriasis (pupillary dilation), Cycloplegia (loss of visual accommodation), Increased heart rate. GI and GU tract motility are decreased at larger doses. **Therapeutic Effects:** Increased heart rate. Decreased GI and respiratory secretions. Reversal of muscarinic effects. May have a spasmolytic action on the biliary and genitourinary tracts.

Pharmacokinetics
Absorption: Well absorbed following oral, subcut, or IM administration.
Distribution: Readily crosses the blood-brain barrier. Crosses the placenta and enters breast milk.
Metabolism and Excretion: Mostly metabolized by the liver; 30–50% excreted unchanged by the kidneys.
Half-life: Children <2 yr: 4–10 hr; Children >2 yr: 1.5–3.5 hr; Adults: 4–5 hr.

TIME/ACTION PROFILE (inhibition of salivation)

ROUTE	ONSET	PEAK	DURATION
PO	30 min	30–60 min	4–6 hr
IM, subcut	rapid	15–50 min	4–6 hr
IV	immediate	2–4 min	4–6 hr

Contraindications/Precautions
Contraindicated in: Hypersensitivity; Angle-closure glaucoma; Acute hemorrhage; Tachycardia secondary to cardiac insufficiency or thyrotoxicosis; Obstructive disease of the GI tract.

atropine

Use Cautiously in: Intra-abdominal infections; Prostatic hyperplasia; Chronic renal, hepatic, pulmonary, or cardiac disease; OB, Lactation: Safety not established; IV administration may produce fetal tachycardia; Pedi: Infants with Down syndrome have increased sensitivity to cardiac effects and mydriasis. Children may have increased susceptibility to adverse reactions. Exercise care when prescribing to children with spastic paralysis or brain damage; Geri: Increased susceptibility to adverse reactions.

Adverse Reactions/Side Effects
CNS: drowsiness, confusion, hyperpyrexia. **EENT:** blurred vision, cycloplegia, photophobia, dry eyes, mydriasis. **CV:** tachycardia, palpitations, arrhythmias. **GI:** dry mouth, constipation, impaired GI motility. **GU:** urinary hesitancy, retention, impotency. **Resp:** tachypnea, pulmonary edema. **Misc:** flushing, decreased sweating.

Interactions
Drug-Drug: ↑ anticholinergic effects with other **anticholinergics**, including **antihistamines**, **tricyclic antidepressants**, **quinidine**, and **disopyramide**. Anticholinergics may alter the absorption of other **orally administered drugs** by slowing motility of the GI tract. **Antacids** ↓ absorption of **anticholinergics**. May ↑ GI mucosal lesions in patients taking oral **potassium chloride** tablets. May alter response to **beta-blockers**.

Route/Dosage

Preanesthesia (To Decrease Salivation/Secretions)
IM, IV, Subcut, PO (Adults): 0.4–0.6 mg 30–60 min pre-op.
IM, IV, Subcut, PO (Children > 5 kg): 0.01–0.02 mg/kg/dose 30–60 min preop to a maximum of 0.4 mg/dose; minimum: 0.1 mg/dose.
IM, IV, Subcut, PO (Children < 5 kg): 0.02 mg/kg/dose 30–60 min preop then q 4–6 hr as needed.

Bradycardia
IV (Adults): 0.5–1 mg; may repeat as needed q 5 min, not to exceed a total of 2 mg (q 3–5 min in Advanced Cardiac Life Support guidelines) or 0.04 mg/kg (total vagolytic dose).
IV (Children): 0.02 mg/kg (maximum single dose is 0.5 mg in children and 1 mg in adolescents); may repeat q 5 min up to a total dose of 1 mg in children (2 mg in adolescents).

Endotracheal (Children): use the IV dose and dilute before administration.

Reversal of Adverse Muscarinic Effects of Anticholinesterases
IV (Adults): 0.6–12 mg for each 0.5–2.5 mg of neostigmine methylsulfate or 10–20 mg of pyridostigmine bromide concurrently with anticholinesterase.

Organophosphate Poisoning
IM (Adults): 2 mg initially, then 2 mg q 10 min as needed up to 3 times total.
IV (Adults): 1–2 mg/dose q 10–20 min until atropinic effects observed then q 1–4 hr for 24 hr; up to 50 mg in first 24 hr and 2 g over several days may be given in severe intoxication.
IM (Children >10 yr >90 lbs): 2 mg.
IM (Children 4–10 yr 40–90 lbs): 1 mg.
IM (Children 6 mo–4 yr 15–40 lbs): 0.5 mg.
IV (Children): 0.02–0.05 mg/kg q 10–20 min until atropinic effects observed then q 1–4 hr for 24 hr.

Bronchospasm
Inhaln (Adults): 0.025–0.05 mg/kg/dose q 4–6 hr as needed; maximum 2.5 mg/dose.
Inhaln (Children): 0.03–0.05 mg/kg/dose 3–4 times/day; maximum 2.5 mg/dose.

Availability (generic available)
Tablets: 0.4 mg. *In combination with:* phenobarbital oral solution (Antrocol). See Appendix B. **Injection:** 0.05 mg/mL, 0.1 mg/mL, 0.4 mg/mL, 1 mg/mL, 0.5 mg/0.7 mL Auto-injector, 1 mg/0.7 mL Auto-injector, 2 mg/0.7 mL Auto-injector.

NURSING IMPLICATIONS

Assessment
- Assess vital signs and ECG tracings frequently during IV drug therapy. Report any significant changes in heart rate or blood pressure, or increased ventricular ectopy or angina to physician promptly.
- Monitor intake and output ratios in elderly or surgical patients because atropine may cause urinary retention.
- Assess patients routinely for abdominal distention and auscultate for bowel sounds. If constipation becomes a problem, increasing fluids and adding bulk to the diet may help alleviate constipation.
- ***Toxicity and Overdose:*** If overdose occurs, physostigmine is the antidote.

Potential Nursing Diagnoses
Decreased cardiac output (Indications)
Impaired oral mucous membrane (Side Effects)
Constipation (Side Effects)

Implementation
- **PO:** Oral doses of atropine may be given without regard to food.
- **IM:** Intense flushing of the face and trunk may occur 15–20 min following IM administration. In children, this response is called "atropine flush" and is not harmful.

IV Administration
- **Direct IV:** *Diluent:* Administer undiluted. **Rate:** Administer over 1 min; more rapid administration may be used during cardiac resuscitation (follow with 20 mL saline flush). Slow administration (over >1 min) may cause a paradoxical bradycardia (usually resolved in approximately 2 min).
- **Y-Site Compatibility:** abciximab, amikacin, aminophylline, amiodarone, argatroban, buprenorphine, butorphanol, etomidate, famotidine, fenoldopam, fentanyl, heparin, hydrocortisone sodium succinate, hydromorphone, inamrinone, meropenem, methadone, morphine, nafcillin, potassium chloride, sufentanil, tirofiban, vitamin B complex with C.
- **Y-Site Incompatibility:** thiopental.
- **Endotracheal:** Dilute with 5–10 mL of 0.9% NaCl.
- **Rate:** Inject directly into the endotracheal tube followed by several positive pressure ventilations.

Patient/Family Teaching
- Instruct patient to take as directed. Take missed doses as soon as remembered unless almost time for next dose. Do not double doses.
- May cause drowsiness. Caution patients to avoid driving or other activities requiring alertness until response to medication is known.
- Instruct patient that oral rinses, sugarless gum or candy, and frequent oral hygiene may help relieve dry mouth.
- Caution patients that atropine impairs heat regulation. Strenuous activity in a hot environment may cause heat stroke.
- Instruct patient to consult health care professional before taking any OTC medications or herbal products concurrently with atropine.
- **Pedi:** Instruct parents or caregivers that medication may cause fever and to notify health care professional before administering to a febrile child.
- **Geri:** Inform male patients with benign prostatic hyperplasia that atropine may cause urinary hesitancy and retention. Changes in urinary stream should be reported to health care professional.

Evaluation/Desired Outcomes
- Increase in heart rate.
- Dryness of mouth.
- Reversal of muscarinic effects.

---

azacitidine (a-za-**sye**-ti-deen)
Vidaza

Classification
Therapeutic: antineoplastics
Pharmacologic: nucleoside analogues

Pregnancy Category D

Indications
Myelodysplastic syndromes including: some refractory anemias, chronic myelomonocytic leukemia.

Action
Inhibits DNS synthesis. **Therapeutic Effects:** Death of rapidly replicating cells, particularly malignant ones.

Pharmacokinetics
Absorption: Rapidly absorbed following subcutaneous administration; 89% bioavailable.
Distribution: Unknown.
Metabolism and Excretion: 85% excreted in urine; some hepatic metabolism may occur. Less than 1% fecal elimination.
Half-life: 4 hr.

TIME/ACTION PROFILE (effects on bone marrow)

ROUTE	ONSET	PEAK	DURATION
Subcut	unknown	unknown	unknown

Contraindications/Precautions
Contraindicated in: Hypersensitivity; Advanced malignant hepatic tumors; OB: Potential for congenital anomalies; Lactation: Potential for serious side effects in infants.
Use Cautiously in: Renal impairment; Liver disease; OB: Patients with child-bearing potential (male and female) due to potential fetal harm; Pedi: Safety not established.

Adverse Reactions/Side Effects
CNS: fatigue. **GI:** HEPATOTOXICITY, constipation, diarrhea, nausea, vomiting. **GU:** nephrotoxicity, renal tubular acidosis. **Derm:** ecchymosis. **F and**

azacitidine 211

E: hypokalemia. **Hemat:** anemia, neutropenia, thrombocytopenia. **Local:** injection site erythema. **Misc:** allergic reactions including ANAPHYLAXIS, fever.

Interactions
Drug-Drug: Additional bone marrow depression may occur with other **antineoplastics**.

Route/Dosage
Subcut, IV (Adults): 75 mg/m²/day for 7 days every 4 wk; may be increased to 100 mg/m²/day for 7 days every 4 wk if no beneficial effect occurs after 2 cycles. Continue for as long as patient benefits.

Availability
Suspension for injection (requires reconstitution): 100 mg/vial.

NURSING IMPLICATIONS

Assessment
- Monitor for bone marrow depression. Assess for bleeding (bleeding gums, bruising, petechiae, stools, urine, and emesis) and avoid IM injections and taking rectal temperatures if platelet count is low. Apply pressure to venipuncture sites for 10 min. Assess for signs of infection during neutropenia. Anemia may occur. Monitor for increased fatigue, dyspnea, and orthostatic hypotension.
- Assess patient for nausea and vomiting during therapy. Premedicate patient before each dose.
- Monitor for signs of anaphylaxis (facial edema, wheezing, dizziness, fainting, tachycardia, hypotension). Discontinue medication immediately and report symptoms. Epinephrine and resuscitation equipment should be readily available.
- *Lab Test Considerations:* Monitor CBC with differential and platelet count prior to each dosing cycle. If baseline WBC is more than 3×10^9/L, ANC is more than 1.5×10^9/L, and platelets are more than 75×10^9/L, then dose is adjusted based on nadir counts for each cycle. If ANC is less than 0.5×10^9 and platelets are less than 25×10^9 then decrease dose by 50%. If ANC is $0.5 – 1.5 \times 10^9$ and platelets are $25 – 50 \times 10^9$ then decrease dose to 67% in next course. If ANC is greater than 1.5×10^9 and platelets are greater than 50, then 100% of dose can be given in subsequent cycle.
- Obtain liver chemistries and serum creatinine prior to initiation of therapy.
- Monitor renal function during therapy. If serum bicarbonate is less than 20 mEq/L, reduce dose by 50% in next course. If unexplained ↑ in BUN or serum creatinine occur, delay next cycle until values return to normal or baseline and decrease dose by 50% in next course.
- May cause hypokalemia.

Potential Nursing Diagnoses
Risk for infection (Adverse Reactions)
Risk for injury (Adverse Reactions)

Implementation
- Solution should be prepared in a biologic cabinet. Wear gloves, gown, and mask while handling medication. If powder or solution comes in contact with skin or mucosa, wash thoroughly with soap and water. Discard equipment in specially designated containers (see Appendix L).
- **Subcut:** Reconstitute by adding 4 mL of sterile water for injection slowly into the azacitadine vial for a concentration of 25 mg/mL. Invert vial 2–3 times and rotate gently until suspension is uniform. Suspension will be cloudy. Stable for up to 1 hr at room temperature; must be administered within 1 hr of reconstitution. Suspension may also be refrigerated for up to 8 hr; may be allowed to equilibrate to room temperature for up to 30 min. Invert syringe 2–3 times and roll syringe gently between palms immediately prior to administration to mix suspension.
- Divide doses greater than 4 mL equally into 2 syringes and administer into separate sites. Rotate sites (thigh, abdomen, upper arm) with new injections at least one inch from old site. Do not use site that is bruised, tender, red, or hard.

IV Administration
- **Intermittent Infusion:** *Diluent:* Reconstitute each vial with 10 mL sterile water for injection. Shake vigorously or roll vial until all solids are dissolved. Solution should be clear; do not administer solutions that are not clear or contain particulate matter. *Concentration:* 10 mg/mL. Withdraw solution from required number of vials and inject into 50–100 mL of 0.9% NaCl or LR. Solution is stable for 1 hr at room temperature. *Rate:* Infuse over 10–40 min. Infusion must be completed within 1 hr of reconstitution.
- **Solution Incompatibility:** 5% dextrose, hespan, solutions containing bicarbonate.

Patient/Family Teaching
- Instruct patient to notify health care professional promptly if fever; chills; cough; hoarseness; sore throat; signs of infection; lower back or side pain; painful or difficult urination; bleeding gums; bruising; petechiae; blood in stools, urine, or emesis; increased fatigue; dyspnea; or orthostatic hypotension occurs. Caution patient to avoid crowds and persons with known infections. Instruct patient to use soft toothbrush and electric razor and to avoid falls. Caution patient not to drink alcoholic beverages or take medication containing aspirin or NSAIDs; may precipitate gastric bleeding.
- May cause dizziness. Caution patient to avoid driving or other activities requiring alertness until response to medication is known.
- Advise patient to notify health care professional if they have underlying liver or renal disease.
- OB: Advise both male and female patients of the need for contraception during therapy.

Evaluation/Desired Outcomes
- Improved bone marrow and blood counts.

---

azathioprine
(ay-za-**thye**-oh-preen)
Azasan, Imuran

Classification
Therapeutic: immunosuppressants
Pharmacologic: purine antagonists

Pregnancy Category D

Indications
Prevention of renal transplant rejection (with corticosteroids, local radiation, or other cytotoxic agents). Treatment of severe, active, erosive rheumatoid arthritis unresponsive to more conventional therapy. **Unlabeled Use:** Management of Crohn's disease.

Action
Antagonizes purine metabolism with subsequent inhibition of DNA and RNA synthesis. **Therapeutic Effects:** Suppression of cell-mediated immunity and altered antibody formation.

Pharmacokinetics
Absorption: Readily absorbed after oral administration.
Distribution: Crosses the placenta. Enters breast milk in low concentrations.
Metabolism and Excretion: Metabolized to mercaptopurine, which is further metabolized (one route is by thiopurine methyltransferase [TPMT] to form an inactive metabolite). Minimal renal excretion of unchanged drug.
Half-life: 3 hr.

TIME/ACTION PROFILE

ROUTE	ONSET	PEAK	DURATION
PO (anti-inflammatory)	6–8 wk	12 wk	unknown
IV (immunosuppression)	days–wk	unknown	days–wk

Contraindications/Precautions
Contraindicated in: Hypersensitivity; Concurrent use of mycophenolate; OB: Has been shown to cause fetal harm; Lactation: Appears in breast milk.
Use Cautiously in: Infections; Malignancies; ↓ bone marrow reserve; Previous or concurrent radiation therapy; Other chronic debilitating illnesses; Severe renal impairment/oliguria (↑ sensitivity); Patients with TPMT enzyme deficiency (substantial dosage ↓ are required to avoid hematologic adverse events); OB: Patients with childbearing potential.

Adverse Reactions/Side Effects
EENT: retinopathy. **Resp:** pulmonary edema. **GI:** anorexia, hepatotoxicity, nausea, vomiting, diarrhea, mucositis, pancreatitis. **Derm:** alopecia, rash. **Hemat:** anemia, leukopenia, pancytopenia, thrombocytopenia. **MS:** arthralgia. **Misc:** SERUM SICKNESS, chills, fever, Raynaud's phenomenon, retinopathy.

Interactions
Drug-Drug: Additive myelosuppression with **antineoplastics**, **cyclosporine**, and **myelosuppressive agents**. **Allopurinol** inhibits the metabolism of azathioprine, increasing toxicity. Dose of azathioprine should be ↓ by 25–33% with concurrent allopurinol. May ↓ antibody response to **live-virus vaccines** and ↑ the risk of adverse reactions.
Drug-Natural Products: Concomitant use with **echinacea** and **melatonin** may interfere with immunosuppression.

Route/Dosage

Renal Allograft Rejection Prevention
PO, IV (Adults and Children): 3–5 mg/kg/day initially; maintenance dose 1–3 mg/kg/day.

Rheumatoid Arthritis
PO (Adults and Children): 1 mg/kg/day for 6–8 wk, ↑ by 0.5 mg/kg/day q 4 wk until response

azathioprine

or up to 2.5 mg/kg/day, then ↓ by 0.5 mg/kg/day q 4–8 wk to minimal effective dose.

Availability (generic available)
Tablets: 50 mg, 75 mg, 100 mg. **Injection:** 100 mg/vial.

NURSING IMPLICATIONS

Assessment
- Assess for infection (vital signs, sputum, urine, stool, WBC) during therapy.
- Monitor intake and output and daily weight. Decreased urine output may lead to toxicity with this medication.
- **Rheumatoid Arthritis:** Assess range of motion; degree of swelling, pain, and strength in affected joints; and ability to perform activities of daily living before and periodically during therapy.
- *Lab Test Considerations:* Monitor renal, hepatic, and hematologic functions before beginning therapy, weekly during the 1st mo, bimonthly for the next 2–3 mo, and monthly thereafter.
- Leukocyte count of <3000 or platelet count of <100,000/mm³ may necessitate a reduction in dose or temporary discontinuation.
- A ↓ in hemoglobin may indicate bone marrow suppression.
- Hepatotoxicity may be manifested by ↑ alkaline phosphatase, bilirubin, AST, ALT, and amylase concentrations. Usually occurs within 6 mo of transplant, rarely with rheumatoid arthritis, and is reversible on discontinuation of azathioprine.
- May ↓ serum and urine uric acid and plasma albumin.

Potential Nursing Diagnoses
Risk for infection (Indications)

Implementation
- Do not confuse Imuran (azathioprine) with IMDUR (isosorbide mononitrate). Do not confuse azaTHIOprine with azaCITIDine.
- Protect transplant patients from staff members and visitors who may carry infection. Maintain protective isolation as indicated.
- **PO:** May be administered with or after meals or in divided doses to minimize nausea.

IV Administration
- **IV:** Reconstitute 100 mg with 10 mL of sterile water for injection. Swirl vial gently until completely dissolved. Reconstituted solution may be administered up to 24 hr after preparation.
- Prepare solution in a biologic cabinet. Wear gloves, gown, and mask while handling medication. Discard equipment in specially designated containers (see Appendix L).
- **Direct IV:** *Diluent:* 0.9% NaCl, 0.45%NaCl, or D5W. *Concentration:* 10 mg/mL. *Rate:* Give over 5 min.
- **Intermittent Infusion:** *Diluent:* Solution may be further diluted in 50 mL with 0.9% NaCl, 0.45% NaCl, or D5W. Do not admix. *Rate:* Usually infused over 30–60 min; may range 5 min–8 hr.
- **Y-Site Compatibility:** alfentanil, atracurium, atropine, benztropine, calcium gluconate, cyanocobalamin, cyclosporine, enalaprilat, epoetin alfa, erythromycin, fentanyl, fluconazole, folic acid, furosemide, glycopyrrolate, heparin, insulin, mannitol, mechlorethamine, metoprolol, naloxone, nitroglycerin, oxytocin, penicillin G, potassium chloride, propranolol, protamine, sufentanil, trimetaphan, vasopressin.
- **Y-Site Incompatibility:** amikacin, ampicillin/sulbactam, ascorbic acid, aztreonam, bumetanide, buprenorphine, butorphanol, calcium chloride, cefazolin, cefoperazone, cefotaxime, cefotetan, cefoxitin, ceftazidime, ceftriaxone, cefuroxime, chloramphenicol, chlorpromazine, cimetidine, clindamycin, dantrolene, diazepam, diazoxide, diphenhydramine, dobutamine, doxycycline, ephedrine, epinephrine, esmolol, famotidine, ganciclovir, gentamicin, haloperidol, hydralazine, hydrocortisone, hydroxyzine, imipenem/cilastatin, inamrinone, isoproterenol, ketorolac, labetalol, lidocaine, magnesium sulfate, meperidine, metaraminol, methoxamine, methyldopate, miconazole, midazolam, morphine, multivitamins, nafcillin, nalbuphine, nitroprusside, norepinephrine, ondansetron, papaverine, pentamidine, pentazocine, phenylephrine, phenytoin, procainamide, prochlorperazine, promethazine, pyridoxime, rocuronium, sodium bicarbonate, streptokinase, succinylcholine, tacrolimus, theophylline, thiamine, tobramycin, tolazoline, trimethoprim/sulfamethoxazole, vancomycin, verapamil.

Patient/Family Teaching
- Instruct patient to take azathioprine as directed. If a dose is missed on a once-daily regimen, omit dose; if on several-times-a-day dosing, take as soon as possible or double next

dose. Consult health care professional if more than 1 dose is missed or if vomiting occurs shortly after dose is taken. Do not discontinue without consulting health care professional.
- Advise patient to report unusual tiredness or weakness; cough or hoarseness; fever or chills; lower back or side pain; painful or difficult urination; severe diarrhea; black, tarry stools; blood in urine; or transplant rejection to health care professional immediately.
- Reinforce the need for lifelong therapy to prevent transplant rejection.
- Instruct the patient to consult health care professional before taking any Rx, OTC, or herbal products, or receiving any vaccinations while taking this medication.
- Advise patient to avoid contact with persons with contagious diseases and persons who have recently taken oral poliovirus vaccine or other live viruses.
- This drug may have teratogenic properties. Advise patient to use contraception during and for at least 4 mo after therapy is completed.
- Emphasize the importance of follow-up exams and lab tests.
- **Rheumatoid Arthritis:** Concurrent therapy with salicylates, NSAIDs, or corticosteroids may be necessary. Patient should continue physical therapy and adequate rest. Explain that joint damage will not be reversed; goal is to slow or stop disease process.

Evaluation/Desired Outcomes
- Prevention of transplant rejection.
- Decreased stiffness, pain, and swelling in affected joints in 6–8 wk in rheumatoid arthritis. Therapy is discontinued if no improvement in 12 wk.

---

azithromycin
(aye-zith-roe-mye-sin)
Zithromax, Zmax

Classification
Therapeutic: agents for atypical mycobacterium, anti-infectives
Pharmacologic: macrolides

Pregnancy Category B

Indications
Treatment of the following infections due to susceptible organisms: Upper respiratory tract infections, including streptococcal pharyngitis, acute bacterial exacerbations of chronic bronchitis and tonsillitis; Lower respiratory tract infections, including bronchitis and pneumonia; Acute otitis media; Skin and skin structure infections; Nongonococcal urethritis, cervicitis, gonorrhea, and chancroid. Prevention of disseminated *Mycobacterium avium* complex (MAC) infection in patients with advanced HIV infection. *Extended-release suspension (ZMax)* Acute bacterial sinusitis and community-acquired pneumonia in adults. **Unlabeled Use:** Prevention of bacterial endocarditis. Treatment of cystic fibrosis lung disease.

Action
Inhibits protein synthesis at the level of the 50S bacterial ribosome. **Therapeutic Effects:** Bacteriostatic action against susceptible bacteria.
Spectrum: Active against the following gram-positive aerobic bacteria: *Staphylococcus aureus*, *Streptococcus pneumoniae*, *S. pyogenes* (group A strep). Active against these gram-negative aerobic bacteria: *Haemophilus influenzae*, *Moraxella catarrhalis*, *Neisseria gonorrhoeae*. Also active against: *Mycoplasma*, *Legionella*, *Chlamydia pneumoniae*, *Ureaplasma urealyticum*, *Borrelia burgdorferi*, *M. avium*. Not active against methicillin-resistant *S. aureus*.

Pharmacokinetics
Absorption: Rapidly absorbed (40%) after oral administration. IV administration results in complete bioavailability.
Distribution: Widely distributed to body tissues and fluids. Intracellular and tissue levels exceed those in serum; low CSF levels.
Metabolism and Excretion: Mostly excreted unchanged in bile; 4.5% excreted unchanged in urine.
Half-life: 11–14 hr after single dose; 2–4 days after several doses; 59 hr after extended release suspension.

TIME/ACTION PROFILE (serum)

ROUTE	ONSET	PEAK	DURATION
PO	rapid	2.5–3.2 hr	24 hr
IV	rapid	end of infusion	24 hr

Contraindications/Precautions
Contraindicated in: Hypersensitivity to azithromycin, erythromycin, or other macrolide anti-infectives.
Use Cautiously in: Severe liver impairment (dose adjustment may be required); Severe renal impairment (CCr <10 mL/min); Myasthenia gravis (may worsen symptoms); OB, Lactation: Safety not established; Pedi: Safety not established in children <5 yr.

azithromycin 215

Adverse Reactions/Side Effects
CNS: dizziness, seizures, drowsiness, fatigue, headache. **CV:** chest pain, hypotension, palpitations, QT prolongation (rare). **GI:** PSEUDOMEMBRANOUS COLITIS, abdominal pain, diarrhea, nausea, cholestatic jaundice, elevated liver enzymes, dyspepsia, flatulence, melena, oral candidiasis. **GU:** nephritis, vaginitis. **Hemat:** anemia, leukopenia, thrombocytopenia. **Derm:** STEVENS-JOHNSON SYNDROME, TOXIC EPIDERMAL NECROLYSIS, photosensitivity, rashes. **EENT:** ototoxicity. **F and E:** hyperkalemia. **Misc:** ANGIOEDEMA.

Interactions
Drug-Drug: **Aluminum-** and **magnesium-containing antacids** ↓ peak levels. **Nelfinavir** ↑ levels (monitor carefully); azithromycin also ↓ nelfinavir levels. **Efavirenz** ↑ levels. May ↑ the effects and risk of toxicity of **warfarin** and **zidovudine**. Other macrolide anti-infectives have been known to ↑ levels and effects of **digoxin**, **theophylline**, **ergotamine**, **dihydroergotamine**, **triazolam**, **carbamazepine**, **cyclosporine**, **tacrolimus**, and **phenytoin**; careful monitoring of concurrent use is recommended.

Route/Dosage
Most Respiratory and Skin Infections
PO (Adults): 500 mg on 1st day, then 250 mg/day for 4 more days (total dose of 1.5 g); *Acute bacterial sinusitis*—500 mg once daily for 3 days or single 2-g dose of extended-release suspension (Zmax).
PO (Children ≥ 6 months): 10 mg/kg (not >500 mg/dose) on 1st day, then 5 mg/kg (not >250 mg/dose) for 4 more days. *Pharyngitis/tonsilitis*—12 mg/kg once daily for 5 days (not >500 mg/dose); *Acute bacterial sinusitis*—10 mg/kg/day for three days.

Otitis media
PO (Children ≥6 mo): 30 mg/kg single dose (not >1500 mg/dose) *or* 10 mg/kg/day as a single dose (not >500 mg/dose) for 3 days *or* 10 mg/kg as a single dose (not >500 mg/dose) on 1st day, then 5 mg/kg as a single dose (not >250 mg/dose) daily for 4 more days.

Acute bacterial exacerbations of chronic bronchitis
PO (Adults): 500 mg on 1st day, then 250 mg/day for 4 more days (total dose of 1.5 g) *or* 500 mg daily for 3 days.

Community-Acquired Pneumonia
IV, PO (Adults): *More severe*—500 mg IV q 24 hr for at least 2 doses, then 500 mg PO q 24 hr for a total of 7–10 days; *less severe*—500 mg PO, then 250 mg/day PO for 4 more days or 2 g single dose as extended-release suspension (Zmax).
PO (Children >6 mo): 10 mg/kg on 1st day, then 5 mg/kg for 4 more days.

Pelvic Inflammatory Disease
IV, PO (Adults): 500 mg IV q 24 hr for 1–2 days, then 250 mg PO q 24 hr for a total of 7 days.

Endocarditis Prophylaxis
PO (Adults): 500 mg 1 hr before procedure.
PO (Children): 15 mg/kg 1 hr before procedure.

Nongonococcal Urethritis, Cervicitis, Chancroid, Chlamydia
PO (Adults): Single 1-g dose.
PO (Children): *Chancroid:* Single 20-mg/kg dose (not >1000 mg/dose). *Urethritis or cervicitis:* Single 10-mg/kg dose (not >1000 mg/dose).

Gonorrhea
PO (Adults): Single 2-g dose.

Prevention of Disseminated MAC Infection
PO (Adults): 1.2 g once weekly (alone or with rifabutin).
PO (Children): 5 mg/kg once daily (not >250 mg/dose) or 20 mg/kg (not >1200 mg/dose) once weekly (alone or with rifabutin).

Cystic Fibrosis
PO (Children ≥6 yrs, weight ≥25 kg to <40 kg): 250 mg q MWF. ≥40 kg: 500 mg q MWF.

Availability (generic available)
Tablets: 250 mg, 500 mg, 600 mg. **Cost:** *Generic*—250 mg $15.99/6, 500 mg $44.32/3, 600 mg $399.99/30. **Powder for oral suspension (cherry, creme de vanilla, and banana flavor):** 1 g/pkt. **Cost:** $93.99/3 packets. **Powder for oral suspension (cherry, creme de vanilla, and banana flavor):** 100 mg/5 mL in 15-mL bottles, 200 mg/5 mL in 15-mL, 22.5-mL, and 30-mL bottles. **Cost:** *Zithromax*—100 mg/5 mL $44.99/15 mL, 200 mg/5 mL $43.99/22.5 mL, 200 mg/5 mL $43.99/30 mL; *Generic*—200 mg/5 mL $32.27/15 mL. **Extended-release oral suspension (ZMax) (cherry-banana):** 2-g

single-dose bottle. **Powder for injection:** 500 mg/vial.

NURSING IMPLICATIONS
Assessment
- Assess patient for infection (vital signs; appearance of wound, sputum, urine, and stool; WBC) at beginning of and throughout therapy.
- Obtain specimens for culture and sensitivity before initiating therapy. First dose may be given before receiving results.
- Observe for signs and symptoms of anaphylaxis (rash, pruritus, laryngeal edema, wheezing). Notify health care professional immediately if these occur.
- Assess patient for skin rash frequently during therapy. Discontinue azithromycin at first sign of rash; may be life-threatening. Stevens-Johnson syndrome or toxic epidermal necrolysis may develop. Treat symptomatically; may recur once treatment is stopped.
- *Lab Test Considerations:* May cause ↑ serum bilirubin, AST, ALT, LDH, and alkaline phosphatase concentrations.
- May cause ↑ creatine phosphokinase, potassium, prothrombin time, BUN, serum creatinine, and blood glucose concentrations.
- May occasionally cause ↓ WBC and platelet count.

Potential Nursing Diagnoses
Risk for infection (Indications, Side Effects)
Noncompliance (Patient/Family Teaching)

Implementation
- Do not confuse azithromycin with erythromycin.
- *Zmax extended release oral suspension* is not bioequivalent or interchangeable with azithromycin oral suspension.
- **PO:** Administer 1 hr before or 2 hr after meals.
- For administration of single 1-g packet, thoroughly mix entire contents of packet with 2 oz (60 mL) of water. Drink entire contents immediately; add an additional 2 oz of water, mix and drink to assure complete consumption of dose. Do not use the single packet to administer doses other than 1000 mg of azithromycin. Pedi: 1-g packet is not for pediatric use.
- For *Zmax,* shake suspension well and drink entire contents of bottle. Use within 12 hr of reconstitution. If patient vomits within 1 hr of administration, contact prescriber for instructions. *Zmax* may be taken without regard to antacids containing magnesium or aluminum hydroxide.

IV Administration
- **Intermittent Infusion:** *Diluent:* Reconstitute each 500-mg vial with 4.8 mL of sterile water for injection to achieve a concentration of 100 mg/mL. Reconstituted solution is stable for 24 hr at room temperature. Further dilute the 500-mg dose in 250 mL or 500 mL of 0.9% NaCl, 0.45% NaCl, D5W, LR, D5/0.45% NaCl, or D5/LR. Infusion is stable for 24 hr at room temperature or for 7 days if refrigerated. *Concentration:* Final concentration of infusion is 1–2 mg/mL. *Rate:* Administer the 1-mg/mL solution over 3 hr or the 2-mg/mL solution over 1 hr. Do not administer as a bolus.
- **Y-Site Compatibility:** amphotericin B liposome, bivalirudin, carboplatin, cisplatin, daptomycin, dexmedetomidine, diphenhydramine, docetaxel, dolasetron, doripenem, droperidol, ertapenem, fenoldopam, fluorouracil, hetastarch, mechlorethamine, meperidine, nesiritide, octreotide, ondansetron, oxaliplatin, oxytocin, palonosetron, pantoprazole, pemetrexed, rocuronium, sodium acetate, thiotepa, tigecycline, tirofiban, vasopressin, vincristine, voriconazole.
- **Y-Site Incompatibility:** amikacin, aztreonam, cefotaxime, ceftazidime, ceftriaxone, cefuroxime, ciprofloxacin, clindamycin, epirubicin, famotidine, fentanyl, furosemide, gentamicin, imipenem-cilastatin, ketorolac, mitoxantrone, morphine, piperacillin-tazobactam, potassium chloride, quinupristin/dalfopristin, ticarcillin-clavulanate, tobramycin.

Patient/Family Teaching
- Instruct patients to take medication as directed and to finish the drug completely, even if they are feeling better. Take missed doses as soon as possible unless almost time for next dose; do not double doses. Advise patients that sharing of this medication may be dangerous.
- Instruct patient not to take azithromycin with food or antacids.
- May cause drowsiness and dizziness. Caution patient to avoid driving or other activities requiring alertness until response to medication is known.
- Advise patient to use sunscreen and protective clothing to prevent photosensitivity reactions.
- Advise patient to report symptoms of chest pain, palpitations, yellowing of skin or eyes, or signs of superinfection (black, furry overgrowth on the tongue; vaginal itching or discharge; loose or foul-smelling stools) or rash.
- Instruct patient to notify health care professional if fever and diarrhea develop, especially

azithromycin 217

if stool contains blood, pus, or mucus. Advise patient not to treat diarrhea without advice of health care professional.
- Advise patients being treated for nongonococcal urethritis or cervicitis that sexual partners should also be treated.
- Instruct parents, caregivers, or patient to notify health care professional if symptoms do not improve.
- Pedi: Tell parents or caregivers that medication is generally well tolerated in children. Most common side effects in children are mild diarrhea and rash. Tell parents to notify health care practitioner if these occur.

Evaluation/Desired Outcomes
- Resolution of the signs and symptoms of infection. Length of time for complete resolution depends on the organism and site of infection.

baclofen (bak-loe-fen)
Kemstro, Lioresal

Classification
Therapeutic: antispasticity agents, skeletal muscle relaxants (centrally acting)

Pregnancy Category C

Indications
PO: Treatment of reversible spasticity due to multiple sclerosis or spinal cord lesions. **IT:** Treatment of severe spasticity originating in the spinal cord. **Unlabeled Use:** Management of pain in trigeminal neuralgia.

Action
Inhibits reflexes at the spinal level. **Therapeutic Effects:** Decreased muscle spasticity; bowel and bladder function may also be improved.

Pharmacokinetics
Absorption: Well absorbed after oral administration.
Distribution: Widely distributed; crosses the placenta.
Metabolism and Excretion: 70–80% eliminated unchanged by the kidneys.
Half-life: 2.5–4 hr.

TIME/ACTION PROFILE (effects on spasticity)

ROUTE	ONSET	PEAK	DURATION
PO	hr–wk	unknown	unknown
IT	0.5–1 hr	4 hr	4–8 hr

Contraindications/Precautions
Contraindicated in: Hypersensitivity; Orally-disintegrating tablets contain aspartame and should not be used in patients with phenylketonuria.
Use Cautiously in: Patients in whom spasticity maintains posture and balance; Patients with epilepsy (may ↓ seizure threshold); Renal impairment (↓ dose may be required); OB, Lactation, Pedi: Safety not established; Geri: Geriatric patients are at ↑ risk of CNS side effects.

Adverse Reactions/Side Effects
CNS: SEIZURES (IT), dizziness, drowsiness, fatigue, weakness, confusion, depression, headache, insomnia. **EENT:** nasal congestion, tinnitus. **CV:** edema, hypotension. **GI:** nausea, constipation. **GU:** frequency. **Derm:** pruritus, rash. **Metab:** hyperglycemia, weight gain. **Neuro:** ataxia. **Misc:** hypersensitivity reactions, sweating.

Interactions
Drug-Drug: ↑ CNS depression with other **CNS depressants** including **alcohol, antihistamines, opioid analgesics,** and **sedative/hypnotics.** Use with **MAO inhibitors** may lead to ↑ CNS depression or hypotension.
Drug-Natural Products: Concomitant use of **kava-kava, valerian,** or **chamomile** can ↑ CNS depression.

Route/Dosage
PO (Adults): 5 mg 3 times daily. May increase q 3 days by 5 mg/dose up to 80 mg/day (some patients may have a better response to 4 divided doses).
IT (Adults): 100–800 mcg/day infusion; dose is determined by response during screening phase.
IT (Children): 25–1200 mcg/day infusion (average 275 mcg/day); dose is determined by response during screening phase.

Availability (generic available)
Tablets: 10 mg, 20 mg. *Cost: Generic*—10 mg $78.16/270, 20 mg $137.92/270. **Orally-disintegrating tablets (Kemstro) (orange):** 10 mg, 20 mg. **Intrathecal injection:** 50 mcg/mL, 500 mcg/mL, 2000 mcg/mL.

NURSING IMPLICATIONS

Assessment
- Assess muscle spasticity before and periodically during therapy.
- Observe patient for drowsiness, dizziness, or ataxia. May be alleviated by a change in dose.
- **IT:** Monitor patient closely during test dose and titration. Resuscitative equipment should be immediately available for life-threatening or intolerable side effects.
- *Lab Test Considerations:* May cause ↑ in serum glucose, alkaline phosphatase, AST, and ALT levels.

Potential Nursing Diagnoses
Impaired wheelchair mobility (Indications)
Risk for injury (Adverse Reactions)

Implementation
- **PO:** Administer with milk or food to minimize gastric irritation.
- For *orally disintegrating tablets,* just prior to administration place tablet on tongue with dry hands. Tablet will disintegrate, then swallow with saliva or water. Administration with liquid is not necessary.

♦ = Canadian drug name. ᴴ = Genetic implication.
*CAPITALS indicates life-threatening; underlines indicate most frequent.

- **IT:** For *screening phase,* dilute for a concentration of 50 mcg/mL with sterile preservative-free NaCl for injection. Test dose should be administered over at least 1 min. Observe patient for a significant decrease in muscle tone or frequency or severity of spasm. If response is inadequate, 2 additional test doses, each 24 hr apart, 75 mcg/1.5 mL and 100 mcg/2 mL respectively, may be administered. Patients with an inadequate response should not receive chronic IT therapy.
- Dose titration for implantable IT pumps is based on patient response. If no substantive response after dose increase, check pump function and catheter patency.

Patient/Family Teaching
- Instruct patient to take baclofen as directed. Take a missed dose within 1 hr; do not double doses. Caution patient to avoid abrupt withdrawal of this medication because it may precipitate an acute withdrawal reaction (hallucinations, increased spasticity, seizures, mental changes, restlessness). Discontinue baclofen gradually over 2 wk or more.
- May cause dizziness and drowsiness. Advise patient to avoid driving or other activities requiring alertness until response to drug is known.
- Instruct patient to change positions slowly to minimize orthostatic hypotension.
- Advise patient to avoid concurrent use of alcohol or other CNS depressants while taking this medication.
- Instruct patient to notify health care professional if frequent urge to urinate or painful urination, constipation, nausea, headache, insomnia, tinnitus, depression, or confusion persists. Geri: Geriatric patients are at greater risk for these side effects.
- Advise patient to report signs and symptoms of hypersensitivity (rash, itching) promptly.
- **IT:** Caution patient and caregiver not to discontinue IT therapy abruptly. May result in fever, mental status changes, exaggerated rebound spasticity, and muscle rigidity. Advise patient not to miss scheduled refill appointments and to notify health care professional promptly if signs of withdrawal occur.

Evaluation/Desired Outcomes
- Decrease in muscle spasticity and associated musculoskeletal pain with an increased ability to perform activities of daily living.
- Decreased pain in patients with trigeminal neuralgia. May take weeks to obtain optimal effect.

---

basiliximab (ba-sil-**ix**-i-mab)
Simulect

Classification
Therapeutic: immunosuppressants
Pharmacologic: monoclonal antibodies

Pregnancy Category B

Indications
Prevention of acute organ rejection in patients undergoing renal transplantation; used with corticosteroids and cyclosporine.

Action
Binds to and blocks specific interleukin-2 (IL-2) receptor sites on activated T lymphocytes. **Therapeutic Effects:** Prevention of acute organ rejection following renal transplantation.

Pharmacokinetics
Absorption: IV administration results in complete bioavailability.
Distribution: Unknown.
Metabolism and Excretion: Unknown.
Half-life: 7.2 days.

TIME/ACTION PROFILE (effect on immune function)

ROUTE	ONSET	PEAK	DURATION
IV	2 hr	unknown	36 days

Contraindications/Precautions
Contraindicated in: Hypersensitivity; OB: May affect fetal developing immune system; Lactation: May enter breast milk.
Use Cautiously in: Women with childbearing potential; Geri: Due to greater incidence of infection.

Adverse Reactions/Side Effects
Noted for patients receiving corticosteroids and cyclosporine in addition to basiliximab.
CNS: dizziness, headache, insomnia, weakness. **EENT:** abnormal vision, cataracts. **Resp:** coughing. **CV:** HEART FAILURE, edema, hypertension, angina, arrhythmias, hypotension. **GI:** abdominal pain, constipation, diarrhea, dyspepsia, moniliasis, nausea, vomiting, GI bleeding, gingival hyperplasia, stomatitis. **Derm:** acne, wound complications, hypertrichosis, pruritus. **Endo:** hyperglycemia, hypoglycemia. **F and E:** acidosis, hypercholesterolemia, hyperkalemia, hyperuricemia, hypocalcemia, hypokalemia, hypophosphatemia. **Hemat:** bleeding, coagulation abnormalities. **MS:** back pain, leg pain. **Neuro:** tremor, neuropathy, paresthesia. **Misc:** hypersensitivity

basiliximab

reactions including ANAPHYLAXIS, <u>infection</u>, <u>weight gain</u>, chills.

Interactions
Drug-Drug: Immunosuppression may be ↑ with other **immunosuppressants**.
Drug-Natural Products: Concomitant use with **echinacea** and **melatonin** may interfere with immunosuppression.

Route/Dosage
IV (Adults and Children ≥35 kg): 20 mg given 2 hr before transplantation; repeated 4 days after transplantation. Second dose should be withheld if complications or graft loss occurs.
IV (Children <35 kg): 10 mg given 2 hr before transplantation; repeated 4 days after transplantation. Second dose should be withheld if complications or graft loss occurs.

Availability
Powder for reconstitution: 20 mg/vial, 10 mg/vial.

NURSING IMPLICATIONS

Assessment
- Monitor for signs of anaphylactic or hypersensitivity reactions (hypotension, tachycardia, cardiac failure, dyspnea, wheezing, bronchospasm, pulmonary edema, respiratory failure, urticaria, rash, pruritus, sneezing) at each dose. Onset of symptoms is usually within 24 hr. Resuscitation equipment and medications for treatment of severe hypersensitivity should be readily available. If a severe hypersensitivity reaction occurs, basiliximab therapy should be permanently discontinued. Patients who have previously received basiliximab should only receive subsequent therapy with extreme caution.
- Monitor for infection (fever, chills, rash, sore throat, purulent discharge, dysuria). Notify physician immediately if these symptoms occur; may necessitate discontinuation of therapy.
- ***Lab Test Considerations:*** May cause ↑ or ↓ hemoglobin, hematocrit, serum glucose, potassium, and calcium concentrations.
- May cause ↑ serum cholesterol levels.
- May cause ↑ BUN, serum creatinine, and uric acid concentrations.
- May cause ↓ serum magnesium, phosphate, and platelet levels.

Potential Nursing Diagnoses
Risk for infection (Side Effects)

Implementation

IV Administration
- Basiliximab is usually administered concurrently with cyclosporine and corticosteroids.
- Reconstitute with 2.5 mL or 5 mL of sterile water for injection for the 10 mg or 20 mg vial, respectively. Shake gently to dissolve powder.
- **Direct IV:** ***Diluent:*** May be administered undiluted. Bolus administration may be associated with nausea, vomiting, and local reactions (pain). ***Concentration:*** 4 mg/mL. ***Rate:*** Administer over 20–30 min via peripheral or central line.
- **Intermittent Infusion:** ***Diluent:*** Dilute further with 25–50 mL of 0.9% NaCl or D5W. Gently invert bag to mix; do not shake, to avoid foaming. Solution is clear to opalescent and colorless; do not administer solutions that are discolored or contain particulate matter. Discard unused portion. Administer within 4 hr or may be refrigerated for up to 24 hr. Discard after 24 hr. ***Concentration:*** 0.08–0.16 mg/mL. ***Rate:*** Administer over 20–30 min via peripheral or central line.
- **Additive Incompatibility:** Do not admix; do not administer in IV line containing other medications.

Patient/Family Teaching
- Explain purpose of medication to patient. Explain that patient will need to resume lifelong therapy with other immunosuppressive drugs after completion of basiliximab course.
- May cause dizziness. Caution patient to avoid driving or other activities requiring alertness until response is known.
- Instruct patient to continue to avoid crowds and persons with known infections, because basiliximab also suppresses the immune system.

Evaluation/Desired Outcomes
- Prevention of acute organ rejection in patients receiving renal transplantation.

becaplermin (be-kap-lerm-in)
Regranex

Classification
Therapeutic: wound/ulcer/decubiti healing agent
Pharmacologic: platelet-derived growth factors

Pregnancy Category C

Indications
Treatment of lower extremity diabetic neuropathic ulcers extending to subcut tissue or beyond and having adequate blood supply.

Action
Promotes chemotaxis of cells involved in wound repair and enhances formation of granulation tissue. **Therapeutic Effects:** Improved healing.

Pharmacokinetics
Absorption: Minimal absorption (<3%).
Distribution: Action is primarily local.
Metabolism and Excretion: Unknown.
Half-life: Unknown.

TIME/ACTION PROFILE (improvement in ulcer healing)

ROUTE	ONSET	PEAK	DURATION
Topical	within 10 wk	unknown	unknown

Contraindications/Precautions
Contraindicated in: Known hypersensitivity to becaplermin or parabens; Known neoplasm at site of application; Wounds that close by primary intention.
Use Cautiously in: Known malignancy; OB, Lactation, Pedi: Safety not established.

Adverse Reactions/Side Effects
Derm: erythematous rash at application site.
Misc: MALIGNANCY (MAY LEAD TO ↑ MORTALITY, ESPECIALLY WITH USE OF ≥3 TUBES).

Interactions
Drug-Drug: None known.

Route/Dosage
Topical (Adults): Length of gel *in inches* from 15- or 7.5-g tube = length × width of ulcer area × 0.6; from the 2-g tube = length × width of ulcer area × 1.3. Length of gel *in centimeters* from 15- or 7.5-g tube = length × width of ulcer area ÷ 4; from the 2-g tube = length × width of ulcer area ÷ 2; for 12 hr each day.

Availability
Gel: 100 mcg/g (0.01%) in 2-, 7.5-, and 15-g tubes.

NURSING IMPLICATIONS

Assessment
- Assess size, color, drainage, and skin surrounding wound at weekly or biweekly intervals. Amount of gel to be applied is recalculated based on wound size.

Potential Nursing Diagnoses
Impaired tissue integrity (Indications)
Deficient knowledge, related to medication regimen (Patient/Family Teaching)

Implementation
- **Topical:** Calculated amount is applied as a thin layer (1/16-in. thick) and covered with a moist saline dressing for 12 hr; dressing is removed, ulcer rinsed and redressed with moist dressing without becaplermin for rest of day. Process is repeated daily.
- Store gel in refrigerator; do not freeze. Do not use beyond expiration date on crimped end of tube.

Patient/Family Teaching
- Instruct patient on proper technique for application. Wash hands before applying gel and use cotton swab or tongue depressor to aid in application. Tip of tube should not come in contact with ulcer or any other surface; recap tightly after each use. Squeeze calculated amount of gel onto a clean, firm, nonabsorbable surface (wax paper). Spread gel with swab or tongue depressor over the ulcer surface in an even layer to the thickness of a dime. Cover with a saline-moistened gauze dressing.
- Do not apply more than calculated amount; has not been shown to be beneficial. If a dose is missed, apply as soon as remembered. If not remembered until next day, skip dose and return to regular dosing schedule. Do not double doses.
- After 12 hr, rinse ulcer gently with saline or water to remove residual gel and cover with saline-moistened gauze.
- Emphasize the importance of strict wound care and non–weight-bearing program.

Evaluation/Desired Outcomes
- Improved healing of ulcers. If the ulcer does not decrease in size by 30% within 10 wk or if complete healing has not occurred within 20 wk, continuation of therapy should be reassessed.

beclomethasone, See CORTICOSTEROIDS (INHALATION).

beclomethasone, See CORTICOSTEROIDS (NASAL).

benazepril, See ANGIOTENSIN-CONVERTING ENZYME (ACE) INHIBITORS.

bendamustine
(ben-da-**muss**-teen)
Treanda

Classification
Therapeutic: antineoplastics
Pharmacologic: benzimidazoles

Pregnancy Category D

Indications
Chronic lymphocytic leukemia. Indolent B-cell non-Hodgkin's lymphoma that has progressed during or within 6 months of receiving rituximab or a rituximab-containing regimen.

Action
Damages DNA resulting in death of rapidly replicating cells. **Therapeutic Effects:** Decreased proliferation of leukemic cells. Death of lymphoma cells.

Pharmacokinetics
Absorption: IV administration results in complete bioavailability.
Distribution: Distributes freely into red blood cells.
Protein Binding: 94–96%.
Metabolism and Excretion: Mostly metabolized (partially by the CYP1A2 enzyme system; 90% excreted in feces; some renal elimination. Although metabolites have antineoplastic activity, levels are extremely low.
Half-life: 40 min.

TIME/ACTION PROFILE (blood levels)

ROUTE	ONSET	PEAK	DURATION
IV	rapid	end of infusion	unknown

Contraindications/Precautions
Contraindicated in: Hypersensitivity to bendamustine or mannitol; CCr <40 mL/min. Use with caution in lesser degrees of renal impairment; Moderate or severe hepatic impairment; OB: Pregnancy or lactation.
Use Cautiously in: Patients at risk for tumor lysis syndrome (concurrent allopurinol recommended); Mild hepatic impairment; Mild to moderate renal impairment; Patients with child-bearing potential; Geri: Elderly patients may be more susceptible to adverse reactions; Pedi: Safety not established.

Adverse Reactions/Side Effects
CNS: fatigue, weakness. **Resp:** cough. **GI:** nausea, vomiting, diarrhea. **Derm:** TOXIC EPIDERMAL NECROLYSIS, STEVENS-JOHNSON SYNDROME, skin reactions. **Hemat:** anemia, LEUKOPENIA, NEUTROPENIA, THROMBOCYTOPENIA. **Metab:** hyperuricemia. **Misc:** MALIGNANCY, TUMOR LYSIS SYNDROME, allergic reactions including ANAPHYLAXIS, fever, infusion reactions.

Interactions
Drug-Drug: Concurrent use of **CYP1A2 inducers/inhibitors** can alter levels of bendamustine. **Inhibitors of CYP1A2** including **fluvoxamine** and **ciprofloxacin** may ↑ levels of bendamustine and ↓ levels of active metabolites. **Inducers of CYP1A2** including **omeprazole** and **smoking** may ↓ levels of bendamustine and ↑ levels of its active metabolites. Consider alternative treatments.

Route/Dosage
Chronic Lymphocytic Leukemia
IV (Adults): 100 mg/m^2 on days 1 and 2 of a 28-day cycle, up to 6 cycles; dose modification required for toxicity.

Non-Hodgkin's Lymphoma
IV (Adults): 120 mg/m^2 on days 1 and 2 of a 21-day cycle, up to 8 cycles; dose modification required for toxicity.

Availability
Lyophilized powder for injection (requires reconstitution): 100 mg vial.

NURSING IMPLICATIONS

Assessment
- Monitor for bone marrow depression. Assess for bleeding (bleeding gums, bruising, petechiae, guaiac stools, urine, and emesis) and

avoid IM injections and taking rectal temperatures if platelet count is low. Apply pressure to venipuncture sites for 10 min. Assess for signs of infection during neutropenia; anemia may occur; monitor for increased fatigue, dyspnea, and orthostatic hypotension.
- Monitor for symptoms of infusion reactions (fever, chills, pruritus, rash). May rarely cause severe allergic and anaphylactic reactions, especially in second and subsequent cycles. Discontinue therapy if severe reactions occur. Ask patient about symptoms suggestive of infusion reactions after first cycle of therapy. Consider using antihistamines, antipyretics, and corticosteroids in patients who previously experienced Grade 1 or 2 reactions. Consider discontinuation of therapy in patients with Grade 3 or 4 reactions.
- Assess for tumor lysis syndrome. Usually occurs during first cycle of bendamustine. May lead to acute renal failure and death. Maintain adequate volume status, close monitoring of blood chemistry, especially potassium and uric acid levels, and use allopurinol during first 1–2 wk of therapy in high risk patients.
- Assess for skin reactions (rash, toxic skin reactions, bullous exanthema). Withhold or discontinue therapy if reactions are progressive or severe. If non-hematologic toxicity is ≥ Grade 3, reduce dose to 50 mg/m^2 on Days 1 and 2 of each cycle.
- Monitor intake and output, appetite, and nutritional intake. Assess for nausea and vomiting. Administration of an antiemetic before and during therapy and adjusting diet as tolerated may help maintain fluid and electrolyte balance and nutritional status.
- **Lab Test Considerations:** Monitor CBC with differential and platelet count before and during therapy. The hematologic nadirs occur wk 3. Recovery usually occurs in 28 days. Withhold dose and notify physician if ANC is ≥1 × 10^9/L and platelet count is ≥75,000 × 10^9/L. *For patients treated for chronic lymphocytic leukemia:* If hemotologic toxicity ≥Grade 3, reduce dose to 50 mg/m^2 on Days 1 and 2. If Grade 3 or greater toxicity recurs, reduce dose to 25 mg/m^2 on Days 1 and 2. *For patients treated for non-Hodgkin's lymphoma:* If hematologic toxicity ≥Grade 4, reduce dose to 90 mg/m^2 on Days 1 and 2. If Grade 4 or greater toxicity recurs, reduce dose to 60 mg/m^2 on Days 1 and 2.
- Monitor blood chemistry, especially serum potassium and uric acid before and periodically during therapy. Allopurinol may be used during first wk of therapy to prevent tumor lysis syndrome.

Potential Nursing Diagnoses
Risk for infection (Side Effects)

Implementation
- **High Alert:** Fatalities have occurred with chemotherapeutic agents. Before administering, clarify all ambiguous orders; double check single, daily, and course-of-therapy dose limits; have second practitioner independently double-check original order, calculations, and infusion pump settings.

IV Administration
- Prepare solution in a biologic cabinet. Wear gloves and safety glasses while handling medication. Discard equipment in designated containers.
- **Intermittent Infusion:** Reconstitute each 100-mg vial with 20 mL of Sterile Water for Injection. Solution should be clear, colorless to pale yellow. Do not administer solutions that are discolored or contain a precipitate. ***Concentration:*** 5 mg/mL. ***Diluent:*** Withdraw volume needed and transfer to 500 mL of 0.9% NaCl or 2.5% dextrose/0.45% NaCl within 30 min of reconstitution. Mix thoroughly.
- Diluted solution is stable for 24 hr when refrigerated or 3 hr at room temperature; administration must be completed within this period. Solution contains no preservatives; discard unused solution. ***Rate:*** Chronic Lymphocytic Leukemia—Administer 100 mg/m^2 over 30 min. *Non-Hodgkin's lymphoma*—Administer 120 mg/m^2 over 60 min.
- **Additive Incompatibility:** Do not admix or dilute with other solutions or medication.

Patient/Family Teaching
- Instruct patient to notify health care professional if fever; chills; sore throat; signs of infection; lower back or side pain; difficult or painful urination; shortness of breath; fatigue; bleeding gums; bruising; petechiae; or blood in urine, stool, or emesis occurs.
  Caution patient to avoid crowds and persons with known infections. Instruct patient to use soft toothbrush and electric razor. Caution patients to avoid alcoholic beverages and products containing aspirin or NSAIDs; may precipitate gastric bleeding.
- Instruct patient to notify health care professional immediately if symptoms of allergic reactions (rash, facial swelling, or difficulty breathing) or nausea, vomiting or diarrhea occur.

- May cause tiredness. Caution patient to avoid driving and other activities requiring alertness until response to medication is known.
- Advise patient this medication may have teratogenic effects. Contraception should be used by both men and women during and for at least 3 months following completion of therapy. Advise women not to breastfeed during therapy.
- Instruct patient not to receive any vaccinations without advice of health care professional.
- Emphasize need for periodic lab tests to monitor for side effects.

Evaluation/Desired Outcomes
- Improvement in hematologic parameters.

---

benzathine penicillin G, See PENICILLINS.

---

benztropine (benz-troe-peen)
♣ Apo-Benztropine, Cogentin

Classification
Therapeutic: antiparkinson agents
Pharmacologic: anticholinergics

Pregnancy Category C

Indications
Adjunctive treatment of all forms of Parkinson's disease, including drug-induced extrapyramidal effects and acute dystonic reactions.

Action
Blocks cholinergic activity in the CNS, which is partially responsible for the symptoms of Parkinson's disease. Restores the natural balance of neurotransmitters in the CNS. **Therapeutic Effects:** Reduction of rigidity and tremors.

Pharmacokinetics
Absorption: Well absorbed following PO and IM administration.
Distribution: Unknown.
Metabolism and Excretion: Unknown.
Half-life: Unknown.

TIME/ACTION PROFILE (antidyskinetic activity)

ROUTE	ONSET	PEAK	DURATION
PO	1–2 hr	several days	24 hr
IM, IV	within min	unknown	24 hr

Contraindications/Precautions
Contraindicated in: Hypersensitivity; Children <3 yr; Angle-closure glaucoma; Tardive dyskinesia.
Use Cautiously in: Prostatic hyperplasia; Seizure disorders; Cardiac arrhythmias; OB, Lactation: Safety not established; Geri: ↑ risk of adverse reactions.

Adverse Reactions/Side Effects
CNS: confusion, depression, dizziness, hallucinations, headache, sedation, weakness. **EENT:** blurred vision, dry eyes, mydriasis. **CV:** arrhythmias, hypotension, palpitations, tachycardia. **GI:** constipation, dry mouth, ileus, nausea. **GU:** hesitancy, urinary retention. **Misc:** decreased sweating.

Interactions
Drug-Drug: Additive anticholinergic effects with **drugs sharing anticholinergic properties**, such as **antihistamines**, **phenothiazines**, **quinidine**, **disopyramide**, and **tricyclic antidepressants**. Counteracts the cholinergic effects of **bethanechol**. **Antacids** and **antidiarrheals** may ↓ absorption.
Drug-Natural Products: ↑ anticholinergic effect with **angel's trumpet**, **jimson weed**, and **scopolia**.

Route/Dosage
Parkinsonism
PO (Adults): 1–2 mg/day in 1–2 divided doses (range 0.5–6 mg/day).

Acute Dystonic Reactions
IM, IV (Adults): 1–2 mg, then 1–2 mg PO twice daily.

Drug-Induced Extrapyramidal Reactions
PO, IM, IV (Adults): 1–4 mg given once or twice daily (1–2 mg 2–3 times daily may also be used PO).

Availability (generic available)
Tablets: 0.5 mg, 1 mg, 2 mg. Injection: 1 mg/mL.

NURSING IMPLICATIONS

Assessment
- Assess parkinsonian and extrapyramidal symptoms (restlessness or desire to keep moving, rigidity, tremors, pill rolling, masklike face, shuffling gait, muscle spasms, twisting motions, difficulty speaking or swallowing, loss of balance control) before and throughout therapy.

♣ = Canadian drug name. ᛋ = Genetic implication.
*CAPITALS indicates life-threatening; underlines indicate most frequent.

- Assess bowel function daily. Monitor for constipation, abdominal pain, distention, or absence of bowel sounds.
- Monitor intake and output ratios and assess patient for urinary retention (dysuria, distended abdomen, infrequent voiding of small amounts, overflow incontinence).
- Patients with mental illness are at risk of developing exaggerated symptoms of their disorder during early therapy with benztropine. Withhold drug and notify physician or other health care professional if significant behavioral changes occur.
- **IM/IV:** Monitor pulse and blood pressure closely and maintain bedrest for 1 hr after administration. Advise patients to change positions slowly to minimize orthostatic hypotension.

Potential Nursing Diagnoses
Impaired physical mobility (Indications)
Risk for injury (Indications)

Implementation
- **PO:** Administer with food or immediately after meals to minimize gastric irritation. May be crushed and administered with food if patient has difficulty swallowing.
- **IM:** Parenteral route is used only for dystonic reactions.

IV Administration
- **Direct IV:** IV route is rarely used because onset is same as with IM route. *Rate:* Administer at a rate of 1 mg over 1 min.
- **Syringe Compatibility:** metoclopramide, perphenazine.
- **Y-Site Compatibility:** fluconazole, tacrolimus.

Patient/Family Teaching
- Encourage patient to take benztropine as directed. Take missed doses as soon as possible, up to 2 hr before the next dose. Taper gradually when discontinuing or a withdrawal reaction may occur (anxiety, tachycardia, insomnia, return of parkinsonian or extrapyramidal symptoms).
- May cause drowsiness or dizziness. Advise patient to avoid driving or other activities that require alertness until response to the drug is known.
- Instruct patient that frequent rinsing of mouth, good oral hygiene, and sugarless gum or candy may decrease dry mouth. Patient should notify health care professional if dryness persists (saliva substitutes may be used). Also, notify the dentist if dryness interferes with use of dentures.
- Caution patient to change positions slowly to minimize orthostatic hypotension.
- Instruct patient to notify health care professional if difficulty with urination, constipation, abdominal discomfort, rapid or pounding heartbeat, confusion, eye pain, or rash occurs.
- Advise patient to confer with health care professional before taking OTC medications, especially cold remedies, or drinking alcoholic beverages.
- Caution patient that this medication decreases perspiration. Overheating may occur during hot weather. Patient should notify health care professional if unable to remain indoors in an air-conditioned environment during hot weather.
- Advise patient to avoid taking antacids or antidiarrheals within 1–2 hr of this medication.
- Emphasize the importance of routine follow-up exams.

Evaluation/Desired Outcomes
- Decrease in tremors and rigidity and an improvement in gait and balance. Therapeutic effects are usually seen 2–3 days after the initiation of therapy.

---

betamethasone, See
CORTICOSTEROIDS (SYSTEMIC).

---

betamethasone, See
CORTICOSTEROIDS (TOPICAL/LOCAL).

---

bevacizumab
(be-va-**kiz**-oo-mab)
Avastin

Classification
Therapeutic: antineoplastics
Pharmacologic: monoclonal antibodies

Pregnancy Category C

Indications
Metastatic colon or rectal carcinoma (with IV 5-fluorouracil). First line treatment of patients with unresectable, locally advanced, recurrent or metastatic non-squamous, non-small cell lung cancer with carboplatin and paclitaxel. Patients who have not received chemotherapy for metastatic HER2 negative breast cancer (with paclitaxel). Patients with progressive glioblastoma fol-

lowing prior therapy. Metastatic renal cell carcinoma (with interferon alfa).

Action
A monoclonal antibody that binds to vascular endothelial growth factor (VEGF), preventing its attachment to binding sites on vascular endothelium, thereby inhibiting growth of new blood vessels (angiogenesis). **Therapeutic Effects:** Decreased metastatic disease progression and microvascular growth.

Pharmacokinetics
Absorption: IV administration results in complete bioavailability.
Distribution: Unknown.
Metabolism and Excretion: Unknown.
Half-life: 20 days (range 11–50 days).

TIME/ACTION PROFILE

ROUTE	ONSET	PEAK	DURATION
IV	rapid	end of infusion	14 days

Contraindications/Precautions
Contraindicated in: Hypersensitivity; Recent hemoptysis or other serious recent bleeding episode; First 28 days after major surgery; OB: Angiogenesis is critical to the developing fetus. Contraindicated unless benefit to mother outweighs potential fetal harm. Lactation: Discontinue nursing during treatment and, due to long half-life, for several weeks following treatment.
Use Cautiously in: Cardiovascular disease; Pedi: Safety not established; Geri: ↑ risk of serious adverse reactions including arterial thromboembolic events.

Adverse Reactions/Side Effects
CNS: reversible posterior leukoencephalopathy syndrome (RPLS). **CV:** CHF, THROMBOEMBOLIC EVENTS, hypertension, hypotension. **Resp:** HEMOPTYSIS, non-gastrointestinal fistulas, nasal septum perforation. **GI:** GI PERFORATION. **GU:** nephrotic syndrome, proteinuria. **Hemat:** BLEEDING. **Misc:** WOUND DEHISCENCE, impaired wound healing, infusion reactions.

Interactions
Drug-Drug: ↑ blood levels of SN 38 (the active metabolite of **irinotecan**); significance is not known. ↑ risk of microangiopathic hemolytic anemia when used with **sunitinib**; concurrent use should be avoided.

Route/Dosage
Colon Cancer
IV (Adults): 5 mg/kg infusion every 14 days.
Lung Cancer
IV (Adults): 15 mg/kg infusion every 3 wk.
Breast Cancer
IV (Adults): 10 mg/kg infusion q 14 days.
Glioblastoma
IV (Adults): 10 mg/kg infusion q 14 days.
Renal Cell Carcinoma
IV (Adults): 10 mg/kg infusion q 14 days.

Availability
Solution for injection (requires dilution): 100 mg/4 mL vial, 400 mg/16 mL vial.

NURSING IMPLICATIONS
Assessment
- Assess for signs of GI perforation (abdominal pain associated with constipation and vomiting), fistula formation, and wound dehiscence during therapy; therapy should be discontinued.
- Assess for signs of hemorrhage (epistaxis, hemoptysis, bleeding) and thromboembolic events (stroke, MI, deep vein thrombosis, pulmonary embolus) during therapy; may require discontinuation.
- Monitor BP every 2–3 wk during therapy. Temporarily suspend therapy during severe hypertension not controlled with medical management; permanently discontinue if hypertensive crisis occurs.
- Assess for infusion reactions (stridor, wheezing) during therapy.
- Assess for signs of CHF (dyspnea, peripheral edema, rales/crackles, jugular venous distension) during therapy.
- Monitor for signs of RPLS (headache, seizure, lethargy, confusion, blindness). Hypertension may or may not be present. May occur within 16 hr to 1 yr of initiation of therapy. Treat hypertension if present and discontinue bevacizumab therapy. Symptoms usually resolve within days.
- ***Lab Test Considerations:*** Monitor serial urinalysis for proteinuria during therapy. Patients with a 2+ or greater urine dipstick require further testing with a 24–hr urine collec-

tion. Suspend therapy for ≥2 grams of proteinuria/24 hours and resume when proteinuria is <2 gm/24 hours. Discontinue therapy in patients with nephrotic syndrome.
- May cause leukopenia, thrombocytopenia, hypokalemia, and bilirubinemia.

Potential Nursing Diagnoses
Ineffective tissue perfusion (Adverse Reactions)

Implementation
- Avoid administration for at least 28 days following major surgery; surgical incision should be fully healed due to potential for impaired wound healing.

IV Administration
- **Intermittent Infusion: *Diluent:*** Dilute prescribed dose in 100 mL of 0.9% NaCl. Do not shake. Discard unused portions. Do not administer solution that is discolored or contains particulate matter. Stable if refrigerated for up to 8 hr. ***Rate:*** Administer initial dose over 90 min. If well tolerated, second infusion may be administered over 60 min. If well tolerated, all subsequent infusions may be administered over 30 min. **Do not administer as an IV push or bolus.**
- **Additive Incompatibility:** Do not mix or administer with dextrose solutions.

Patient/Family Teaching
- Inform patient of purpose of medication.
- Advise patient to report any signs of bleeding immediately to health care professional.

Evaluation/Desired Outcomes
- Decreased metastatic disease progression and microvascular growth.

---

bicalutamide
(bye-ka-**loot**-a-mide)
Casodex

Classification
Therapeutic: antineoplastics
Pharmacologic: antiandrogens

Pregnancy Category X

Indications
Treatment of metastatic prostate carcinoma in conjunction with luteinizing hormone–releasing hormone (LHRH) analogs (goserelin, leuprolide).

Action
Antagonizes the effects of androgen at the cellular level. **Therapeutic Effects:** Decreased spread of prostate carcinoma.

Pharmacokinetics
Absorption: Well absorbed after oral administration.
Distribution: Unknown.
Protein Binding: 96%.
Metabolism and Excretion: Mostly metabolized by the liver.
Half-life: 5.8 days.

TIME/ACTION PROFILE (blood levels)

ROUTE	ONSET	PEAK	DURATION
PO	unknown	31.3 hr	unknown

Contraindications/Precautions
Contraindicated in: Hypersensitivity; Women.
Use Cautiously in: Moderate to severe liver impairment; Pedi: Safety not established.

Adverse Reactions/Side Effects
CNS: weakness, dizziness, headache, insomnia. **Resp:** dyspnea. **CV:** chest pain, hypertension, peripheral edema. **GI:** constipation, diarrhea, nausea, abdominal pain, ↑ liver enzymes, vomiting. **GU:** hematuria, erectile dysfunction, incontinence, nocturia, urinary tract infections. **Derm:** alopecia, rashes, sweating. **Endo:** breast pain, gynecomastia. **Hemat:** anemia. **Metab:** hyperglycemia, weight loss. **MS:** back pain, pelvic pain, bone pain. **Neuro:** paresthesia. **Misc:** generalized pain, hot flashes, flu-like syndrome, infection.

Interactions
Drug-Drug: May ↑ the effect of **warfarin**. ↑ risk of hyperglycemia with **LHRH analogs**.

Route/Dosage
PO (Adults): 50 mg once daily (must be given concurrently with LHRH analog or following surgical castration).

Availability (generic available)
Tablets: 50 mg.

NURSING IMPLICATIONS

Assessment
- Assess patient for adverse GI effects. Diarrhea is the most common cause of discontinuation of therapy.
- ***Lab Test Considerations:*** Monitor serum prostate-specific antigen (PSA) periodically to determine response to therapy. If levels rise, assess patient for disease progression. May require periodic LHRH analogue administration without bicalutamide.
- Monitor liver function tests before and periodically during therapy. May cause ↑ serum alkaline phosphatase, AST, ALT, and bilirubin con-

bimatoprost (lash, ophthalmic) 229

centrations. If transaminases ↑ >2 times normal, bicalutamide should be discontinued; levels usually return to normal after discontinuation.
- May cause ↑ BUN and serum creatinine, and ↓ hemoglobin and WBCs.

Potential Nursing Diagnoses
Diarrhea (Adverse Reactions)

Implementation
- Start treatment with bicalutamide at the same time as LHRH analogue.
- **PO:** May be administered in the morning or evening, without regard to food.

Patient/Family Teaching
- Instruct patient to take bicalutamide as directed at the same time each day. Do not discontinue without consulting health care professional.
- Advise patient not to take other medications without consulting health care professional.
- Instruct patient to report severe or persistent diarrhea.
- Discuss with patient the possibility of hair loss. Explore methods of coping.
- Emphasize the importance of regular follow-up exams and blood tests to determine progress; monitor for side effects.

Evaluation/Desired Outcomes
- Decreased spread of prostate carcinoma.

---

bimatoprost (lash, ophthalmic) (bi-mat-o-prost)
Latisse

Classification
Therapeutic: hair regrowth stimulants
Pharmacologic: prostaglandins

Pregnancy Category C

Indications
Treatment of eyelash hypotrichosis.

Action
Increases the percent of hair in eyelashes and prolongs the duration of growth phase. **Therapeutic Effects:** Increases eyelash growth, improving length, thickness, and darkness.

Pharmacokinetics
Absorption: Minimal systemic absorption.
Distribution: Small amounts absorbed are widely distributed.
Metabolism and Excretion: Highly metabolized; 67% excreted in urine, 25% in feces mostly as metabolites.
Half-life: 45 min.

TIME/ACTION PROFILE (improvement in eyelash growth)

ROUTE	ONSET	PEAK	DURATION
Topical	2 mos	4 mos	4 wk or more*

*Following discontinuation.

Contraindications/Precautions
Contraindicated in: Hypersensitivity.
Use Cautiously in: Active intraocular inflammation; Patients with aphakia, pseudophakia with a torn posterior lens capsule, or know risk factors for macular edema; OB: Use in pregnancy only if potential benefit justifies potential risk to the fetus; Lactation: Use cautiously during lactation; Pedi: Safe and effective use in children has not been established.

Adverse Reactions/Side Effects
EENT: conjunctival hyperemia, eye pruritus, hyperpigmentation of eyelids, macular edema, permanent pigmentation of the iris.

Interactions
Drug-Drug: May ↓ the intraocular pressure lowering effect of **prostaglandin analogs**.

Route/Dosage
Topical (Adults): Apply to upper eyelid margin nightly.

Availability
Ophthalmic solution: 0.3 mg/mL provided as 3 mL in a 5-mL bottle.

NURSING IMPLICATIONS

Assessment
- Monitor intraocular pressure in patients with a history of increased intraocular pressure or who are using prostaglandin analogs for intraocular pressure reduction concurrently.

Potential Nursing Diagnoses
Disturbed body image (Indications)

Implementation
- **Topical:** Apply once each night using the accompanying sterile applicators. Additional applications will not increase the growth of eyelashes.

Patient/Family Teaching
- Instruct patient on correct application of bimatoprost. If a dose is missed, omit and apply next

evening; do not double dose. Patient should wash face and remove all makeup and contact lenses prior to application. Contact lenses may be reinserted 15 min following administration. Place one drop of medication on the disposable sterile applicator and brush cautiously along the skin of the upper eyelid margin at the base of the eyelashes. Use only the applicator supplied with the product. Use each applicator for one eye then discard; reuse may result in contamination and infection. If solution gets into the eye, it is not harmful and does not need to be rinsed. Do not apply to lower lash line. Blot any excess solution outside upper eyelid margin with a tissue or other absorbent material. Do not allow tip of bottle or applicator to come in contact with surrounding structures, fingers, or any other unintended surface to avoid contamination. Instruct patient to read the *Patient Information* guide prior to use and with each Rx refill, in case of new information.

- Inform patient that eyelid skin may darken with use of bimatoprost; may be reversible with discontinuation of medication. Instillation directly into eye may result in increased brown iris pigmentation; usually permanent.
- Inform patient of potential for hair growth occurring outside target treatment area if medication repeatedly touched same area of skin.
- Advise patient to notify health care professional immediately if eye trauma or infection, sudden decrease in visual acuity, conjunctivitis, or eyelid reactions occur or if having ocular surgery.
- Instruct patient to notify health care professional of bimatoprost use prior to intraocular pressure examinations.
- Advise female patients to notify health care professional if pregnancy is planned or suspected or if breastfeeding.

Evaluation/Desired Outcomes

- Increased length, thickness, and darkness of eyelashes. Onset is gradual and may not be noticed for 2 mos. Length, thickness, number of eyelashes, and/or direction of eyelash growth may vary between eyes. Upon discontinuation, eyelashes usually return to pretreatment level within 4 wk to mos.

---

bisacodyl (bis-a-**koe**-dill)
Bisac-Evac, ✦Bisaco-Lax, ✦Bisacolax, Caroid, Carter's Little Pills, Dacodyl, Deficol, Dulcagen, Dulcolax, Feen-a-Mint, Fleet Laxative, ✦Laxit,

Modane, Reliable Gentle Laxative, Theralax, Women's Gentle Laxative

Classification
Therapeutic: laxatives
Pharmacologic: stimulant laxatives

Pregnancy Category UK

Indications
Treatment of constipation. Evacuation of the bowel before radiologic studies or surgery. Part of a bowel regimen in spinal cord injury patients.

Action
Stimulates peristalsis. Alters fluid and electrolyte transport, producing fluid accumulation in the colon. **Therapeutic Effects:** Evacuation of the colon.

Pharmacokinetics
Absorption: Variable absorption follows oral administration; rectal absorption is minimal; action is local in the colon.
Distribution: Small amounts of metabolites excreted in breast milk.
Metabolism and Excretion: Small amounts absorbed are metabolized by the liver.
Half-life: Unknown.

TIME/ACTION PROFILE (evacuation of bowel)

ROUTE	ONSET	PEAK	DURATION
PO	6–12 hr	unknown	unknown
Rectal	15–60 min	unknown	unknown

Contraindications/Precautions
Contraindicated in: Hypersensitivity; Abdominal pain; Obstruction; Nausea or vomiting (especially with fever or other signs of an acute abdomen).
Use Cautiously in: Severe cardiovascular disease; Anal or rectal fissures; Excess or prolonged use (may result in dependence); OB, Lactation: May be used during pregnancy and lactation.

Adverse Reactions/Side Effects
GI: abdominal cramps, nausea, diarrhea, rectal burning. **F and E:** hypokalemia (with chronic use). **MS:** muscle weakness (with chronic use). **Misc:** protein-losing enteropathy, tetany (with chronic use).

Interactions
Drug-Drug: Antacids, histamine H_2-receptor antagonists, and **gastric acid–pump inhibitors** may remove enteric coating of tablets resulting in gastric irritation/dyspepsia. May ↓ the absorption of other **orally administered drugs** because of ↑ motility and ↓ transit time.

Drug-Food: Milk may remove enteric coating of tablets, resulting in gastric irritation/dyspepsia.

Route/Dosage
PO (Adults and Children ≥12 yr): 5–15 mg (up to 30 mg/day) as a single dose.
PO (Children 3–11 yr): 5–10 mg (0.3 mg/kg) as a single dose.
Rect (Adults and Children ≥12 yr): 10 mg single dose.
Rect (Children 2–11 yr): 5–10 mg single dose.
Rect (Children <2 yr): 5 mg single dose.

Availability (generic available)
Enteric-coated tablets: 5 mg^OTC. Enteric coated and delayed release: 5 mg^OTC. Suppositories: 5 mg^OTC, 10 mg^OTC. Rectal suspension: 10 mg/30 mL^OTC. *In combination with:* In Bowel Preparation kits with Magnesium citrate (Evac-Q-Kwik^OTC, EZ-EM Prep Kit^OTC, LiquiPrep Bowel Evacuant^OTC, Tridate Bowel Cleansing Kit^OTC), Phosphate/biphosphate (Fleet Prep Kit. No. 1^OTC, Fleet Prep Kit No.2^OTC, Fleet Prep Kit No.3^OTC), sennosides (X-Prep Bowel Evacuant Kit #1^OTC), sennosides, magnesium citrate, magnesium sulfate (X-Prep Bowel Evacuant Kit #2^OTC). See Appendix B.

NURSING IMPLICATIONS

Assessment
- Assess patient for abdominal distention, presence of bowel sounds, and usual pattern of bowel function.
- Assess color, consistency, and amount of stool produced.

Potential Nursing Diagnoses
Constipation (Indications)

Implementation
- May be administered at bedtime for morning results.
- **PO:** Taking on an empty stomach will produce more rapid results.
- Do not crush or chew enteric-coated tablets. Take with a full glass of water or juice.
- Do not administer oral doses within 1 hr of milk or antacids; this may lead to premature dissolution of tablet and gastric or duodenal irritation.
- **Rect:** Suppository or enema can be given at the time a bowel movement is desired. Lubricate suppositories with water or water-soluble lubricant before insertion. Encourage patient to retain the suppository or enema 15–30 min before expelling.

Patient/Family Teaching
- Advise patients, other than those with spinal cord injuries, that laxatives should be used only for short-term therapy. Prolonged therapy may cause electrolyte imbalance and dependence.
- Advise patient to increase fluid intake to at least 1500–2000 mL/day during therapy to prevent dehydration.
- Encourage patients to use other forms of bowel regulation (increasing bulk in the diet, increasing fluid intake, or increasing mobility). Normal bowel habits may vary from 3 times/day to 3 times/wk.
- Instruct patients with cardiac disease to avoid straining during bowel movements (Valsalva maneuver).
- Advise patient that bisacodyl should not be used when constipation is accompanied by abdominal pain, fever, nausea, or vomiting.

Evaluation/Desired Outcomes
- Soft, formed bowel movement when used for constipation.
- Evacuation of colon before surgery or radiologic studies, or for patients with spinal cord injuries.

---

bismuth subsalicylate
(biz-muth sub-sa-lis-i-late)
Bismatrol, Kaopectate, Kao-Tin, Kapectolin, Peptic Relief, Pepto-Bismol

Classification
Therapeutic: antidiarrheals, antiulcer agents
Pharmacologic: adsorbents

Pregnancy Category C

Indications
Mild to moderate diarrhea. Nausea, abdominal cramping, heartburn, and indigestion that may accompany diarrheal illnesses. Treatment of ulcer disease associated with *Helicobacter pylori* (with anti-infectives). Treatment/prevention of traveler's (enterotoxigenic *Escherichia coli*) diarrhea. **Unlabeled Use:** Chronic infantile diarrhea.

Action
Promotes intestinal adsorption of fluids and electrolytes. Decreases synthesis of intestinal prostaglandins. **Therapeutic Effects:** Relief of diar-

rhea. Eradication of *H. pylori* with decreased recurrence of ulcer disease (with other agents).

Pharmacokinetics
Absorption: Bismuth is not absorbed; salicylate split from parent compound is >90% absorbed from the small intestine. Salicylate is highly bound to albumin.
Distribution: Salicylate crosses the placenta and enters breast milk.
Metabolism and Excretion: Bismuth is excreted unchanged in the feces. Salicylate undergoes extensive hepatic metabolism.
Half-life: Salicylate—2–3 hr for low doses; 15–30 hr with larger doses.

TIME/ACTION PROFILE (relief of diarrhea and other GI symptoms)

ROUTE	ONSET	PEAK	DURATION
PO	within 24 hr	unknown	unknown

Contraindications/Precautions
Contraindicated in: Aspirin hypersensitivity; cross-sensitivity with NSAIDs or oil of wintergreen may occur. Pedi: During or after recovery from chickenpox or flu-like illness (contains salicylate, which can cause Reye's syndrome). Geri: Geriatric patients who may have fecal impaction.
Use Cautiously in: Patients undergoing radiologic examination of the GI tract (bismuth is radiopaque); Diabetes mellitus; Gout; OB, Lactation: Safety not established; avoid chronic use of large doses; Pedi, Geri: Potential for impaction.

Adverse Reactions/Side Effects
GI: constipation, gray-black stools, impaction (infants, debilitated patients).

Interactions
Drug-Drug: If taken with **aspirin**, may ↑ the risk of salicylate toxicity. May ↓ absorption of **tetracycline** or **fluoroquinolones** (separate administration by 2–4 hr). May ↓ effectiveness of **probenecid** (large doses).

Route/Dosage
PO (Adults): *Antidiarrheal*—2 tablets or 30 mL (15 mL of extra/maximum strength) q 30 min *or* 2 tablets q 60 min as needed (not to exceed 4.2 g/24 hr). *Antiulcer*—524 mg 4 times daily (as 2 tablets, 30 mL of regular strength suspension or 15 mL of extra/maximum strength).
PO (Children 9–12 yr): 1 tablet or 15 mL (7.5 mL of extra/maximum strength) q 30–60 min (not to exceed 2.1 g/24 hr).
PO (Children 6–9 yr): 10 mL (5 mL of extra/maximum strength) q 30–60 min (not to exceed 1.4 g/24 hr).
PO (Children 3–6 yr): 5 mL (2.5 mL of extra/maximum strength) q 30–60 min (not to exceed 704 mg/24 hr).

Availability (generic available)
Tablets: 262 mg^{OTC}. **Chewable tablets (cherry and other flavors):** 262 mg^{OTC}, ✦300 mg^{OTC}. **Liquid (cherry, caramel, peppermint, and other flavors):** 262 mg/15 mL^{OTC}, ✦264 mg/15 mL^{OTC}, 525 mg/15 mL^{OTC}. *In combination with:* metronidazole and tetracycline (Helidac—convenience package) (Pylera—combination capsule). See Appendix B.

NURSING IMPLICATIONS
Assessment
- **Diarrhea:** Assess the frequency and consistency of stools, presence of nausea and indigestion, and bowel sounds before and during therapy.
- Assess fluid and electrolyte balance and skin turgor for dehydration if diarrhea is prolonged.
- **Ulcers:** Assess for epigastric or abdominal pain and frank or occult blood in the stool, emesis, or gastric aspirate.
- *Lab Test Considerations:* Chronic high doses may cause falsely ↑ uric acid levels with colorimetric assay.
- May interfere with radiologic examination of the GI tract.
- May cause abnormal results with alkaline phosphatase, AST, and ALT tests.
- May cause ↓ potassium levels and serum T_3 and T_4 concentrations.
- Large doses of salicylates may also cause prolonged prothrombin time (PT).
- For additional lab test considerations related to salicylate content, see salicylates monograph.

Potential Nursing Diagnoses
Diarrhea (Indications)
Constipation (Side Effects)

Implementation
- **PO:** Shake liquid before using. Chewable tablets may be chewed or allowed to dissolve before swallowing.

Patient/Family Teaching
- Instruct patient to take medication exactly as directed.
- Inform patient that medication may temporarily cause stools and tongue to appear gray-black.
- Instruct patient that this medication contains aspirin. Advise patient taking concurrent aspirin products to discontinue bismuth subsalicylate if tinnitus, ringing in the ears, occurs.

- **Diarrhea:** Instruct patient to notify health care professional if diarrhea persists for more than 2 days or if accompanied by a high fever.
- U.S. Centers for Disease Control and Prevention warn against giving salicylates to children or adolescents with varicella (chickenpox) or influenza-like or viral illnesses because of a possible association with Reye's syndrome.
- **Ulcers:** Advise patient to consult health care professional before taking other OTC ulcer remedies concurrently with bismuth subsalicylate.

Evaluation/Desired Outcomes
- Decrease in diarrhea.
- Decrease in symptoms of indigestion.
- Prevention of traveler's diarrhea.
- Treatment of ulcers.

---

bisoprolol (bis-oh-proe-lol)
Monocor, Zebeta

Classification
Therapeutic: antihypertensives
Pharmacologic: beta blockers

Pregnancy Category C

Indications
Management of hypertension.

Action
Blocks stimulation of beta$_1$(myocardial)-adrenergic receptors. Does not usually affect beta$_2$(pulmonary, vascular, uterine)-receptor sites. **Therapeutic Effects:** Decreased blood pressure and heart rate.

Pharmacokinetics
Absorption: Well absorbed after oral administration, but 20% undergoes first-pass hepatic metabolism.
Distribution: Unknown.
Metabolism and Excretion: 50% excreted unchanged by the kidneys; remainder renally excreted as metabolites; 2% excreted in feces.
Half-life: 9–12 hr.

TIME/ACTION PROFILE (antihypertensive effect)

ROUTE	ONSET	PEAK	DURATION
PO	unknown	1–4 hr	24 hr

Contraindications/Precautions
Contraindicated in: Uncompensated CHF; Pulmonary edema; Cardiogenic shock; Bradycardia or heart block.
Use Cautiously in: Renal impairment (dosage reduction recommended); Hepatic impairment (dosage reduction recommended); Pulmonary disease (including asthma; beta$_1$ selectivity may be lost at higher doses); avoid use if possible; Diabetes mellitus (may mask signs of hypoglycemia); Thyrotoxicosis (may mask symptoms); Patients with a history of severe allergic reactions (intensity of reactions may be increased); OB, Lactation, Pedi: Safety not established; crosses the placenta and may cause fetal/neonatal bradycardia, hypotension, hypoglycemia, or respiratory depression; Geri: Increased sensitivity to beta blockers; initial dosage reduction recommended.

Adverse Reactions/Side Effects
CNS: fatigue, weakness, anxiety, depression, dizziness, drowsiness, insomnia, memory loss, mental status changes, nervousness, nightmares. **EENT:** blurred vision, stuffy nose. **Resp:** bronchospasm, wheezing. **CV:** BRADYCARDIA, CHF, PULMONARY EDEMA, hypotension, peripheral vasoconstriction. **GI:** constipation, diarrhea, liver function abnormalities, nausea, vomiting. **GU:** erectile dysfunction, decreased libido, urinary frequency. **Derm:** rashes. **Endo:** hyperglycemia, hypoglycemia. **MS:** arthralgia, back pain, joint pain. **Misc:** drug-induced lupus syndrome.

Interactions
Drug-Drug: General anesthetics, **IV phenytoin**, and **verapamil** may cause additive myocardial depression. Additive bradycardia may occur with **digoxin**. Additive hypotension may occur with other **antihypertensives**, acute ingestion of **alcohol**, or **nitrates**. Concurrent use with **amphetamine**, **cocaine**, **ephedrine**, **epinephrine**, **norepinephrine**, **phenylephrine**, or **pseudoephedrine** may result in unopposed alpha-adrenergic stimulation (excessive hypertension, bradycardia). Concurrent thyroid preparation administration may decrease effectiveness. May alter the effectiveness of **insulins** or **oral hypoglycemic agents** (dosage adjustments may be necessary). May decrease the effectiveness of **theophylline**. May decrease the beneficial beta$_1$-cardiovascular effects of **dopamine** or **dobutamine**. Use cautiously within 14 days of **MAO inhibitor** therapy (may result in hypertension).

✷ = Canadian drug name. ◨ = Genetic implication.
*CAPITALS indicates life-threatening; underlines indicate most frequent.

Route/Dosage
PO (Adults): 5 mg once daily, may be increased to 10 mg once daily (range 2.5–20 mg/day).

Renal Impairment
Hepatic Impairment
PO (Adults): *CCr <40 mL/min*—Initiate therapy with 2.5 mg/day, titrate cautiously.

Availability (generic available)
Tablets: 5 mg, 10 mg. **Cost:** 5-mg and 10-mg tablets $35.75/30 tablets. ***In combination with:*** hydrochlorothiazide (Ziac). See Appendix B.

NURSING IMPLICATIONS
Assessment
- Monitor blood pressure, ECG, and pulse frequently during dosage adjustment period and periodically throughout therapy.
- Monitor intake and output ratios and daily weights. Assess routinely for signs and symptoms of CHF (dyspnea, rales/crackles, weight gain, peripheral edema, jugular venous distention).
- Monitor frequency of prescription refills to determine adherence.
- ***Lab Test Considerations:*** May cause increased BUN, serum lipoprotein, potassium, triglyceride, and uric acid levels.
- May cause increased ANA titers.
- May cause increase in blood glucose levels.

Potential Nursing Diagnoses
Decreased cardiac output (Side Effects)
Noncompliance (Patient/Family Teaching)

Implementation
- **PO:** Take apical pulse before administering. If <50 bpm or if arrhythmia occurs, withhold medication and notify physician or other health care professional.
- May be administered without regard to meals.

Patient/Family Teaching
- Instruct patient to take medication exactly as directed, at the same time each day, even if feeling well; do not skip or double up on missed doses. If a dose is missed, it should be taken as soon as possible up to 4 hr before next dose. Abrupt withdrawal may precipitate life-threatening arrhythmias, hypertension, or myocardial ischemia.
- Teach patient and family how to check pulse and blood pressure. Instruct them to check pulse daily and blood pressure biweekly and to report significant changes to health care professional.
- May cause drowsiness. Caution patients to avoid driving or other activities that require alertness until response to the drug is known.
- Advise patients to change positions slowly to minimize orthostatic hypotension.
- Caution patient that this medication may increase sensitivity to cold.
- Instruct patient to consult health care professional before taking any OTC medications, especially cold preparations, concurrently with this medication. Patients on antihypertensive therapy should also avoid excessive amounts of coffee, tea, and cola.
- Diabetics should closely monitor blood glucose, especially if weakness, malaise, irritability, or fatigue occurs. Medication does not block dizziness or sweating as signs of hypoglycemia.
- Advise patient to notify health care professional if slow pulse, difficulty breathing, wheezing, cold hands and feet, dizziness, light-headedness, confusion, depression, rash, fever, sore throat, unusual bleeding, or bruising occurs.
- Instruct patient to inform health care professional of medication regimen before treatment or surgery.
- Advise patient to carry identification describing disease process and medication regimen at all times.
- **Hypertension:** Reinforce the need to continue additional therapies for hypertension (weight loss, sodium restriction, stress reduction, regular exercise, moderation of alcohol consumption, and smoking cessation). Medication controls but does not cure hypertension.

Evaluation/Desired Outcomes
- Decrease in blood pressure.

HIGH ALERT

bivalirudin (bi-val-i-**roo**-din)
Angiomax

Classification
Therapeutic: anticoagulants
Pharmacologic: thrombin inhibitors

Pregnancy Category B

Indications
Used in conjunction with aspirin to reduce the risk of acute ischemic complications in patients with unstable angina who are undergoing percutaneous transluminal angioplasty (PCTA) or percutaneous coronary intervention (PCI). Patients with or at risk of heparin-induced thrombocyto-

bivalirudin

penia (HIT) and thrombosis syndrome (HITTS) who are undergoing PCI.

Action
Specifically and reversibly inhibits thrombin by binding to its receptor sites. Inhibition of thrombin prevents activation of factors V, VIII, and XII; the conversion of fibrinogen to fibrin; platelet adhesion and aggregation. **Therapeutic Effects:** Decreased acute ischemic complications in patients with unstable angina (death, MI, or the urgent need for revascularization procedures).

Pharmacokinetics
Absorption: IV administration results in complete bioavailability.
Distribution: Unknown.
Metabolism and Excretion: Cleared from plasma by a combination of renal mechanisms and proteolytic breakdown.
Half-life: 25 min (↑ in renal impairment).

TIME/ACTION PROFILE (anticoagulant effect)

ROUTE	ONSET	PEAK	DURATION
IV	immediate	unknown	1–2 hr

Contraindications/Precautions
Contraindicated in: Active major bleeding; Hypersensitivity.
Use Cautiously in: Any disease state associated with an ↑ risk of bleeding; Heparin-induced thrombocytopenia or heparin-induced thrombocytopenia-thrombosis syndrome; Patients with unstable angina not undergoing PTCA; Patients with other acute coronary syndromes; Concurrent use with other platelet aggregation inhibitors (safety not established); Renal impairment (↓ infusion rate if GFR <30 mL/min); Lactation, Pedi: Safety not established; OB: Use only if clearly needed.

Adverse Reactions/Side Effects
CNS: headache, anxiety, insomnia, nervousness. **CV:** hypotension, bradycardia, hypertension. **GI:** nausea, abdominal pain, dyspepsia, vomiting. **Hemat:** BLEEDING. **Local:** injection site pain. **MS:** back pain. **Misc:** pain, fever, pelvic pain.

Interactions
Drug-Drug: Risk of bleeding may be ↑ by concurrent use of **abciximab, heparin, low molecular weight heparins, clopidogrel, thrombolytics**, or any other **drugs that inhibit coagulation**.
Drug-Natural Products: ↑ risk of bleeding with **arnica, chamomile, clove, dong quai, feverfew, garlic, ginger, gingko, Panax ginseng**, and others.

Route/Dosage
IV (Adults): 0.75 mg/kg as a bolus injection, followed by an infusion at a rate of 1.75 mg/kg/hr for the duration of the PCI procedure. An activated clotting time (ACT) should be performed 5 min after bolus dose and an additional bolus dose of 0.3 mg/kg may be administered if needed. Continuation of the infusion (at a rate of 1.75 mg/kg/hr) for up to 4 hr post-procedure is optional. If needed, the infusion may be continued beyond this initial 4 hr at a rate of 0.2 mg/kg/hr for up to 20 hr. Therapy should be initiated prior to the procedure and given in conjunction with aspirin.

Renal Impairment
IV (Adults): No ↓ in the bolus dose is needed in any patient with renal impairment. *GFR 10–29 mL/min*— ↓ infusion rate to 1 mg/kg/hr; *Dialysis-dependent patients (off dialysis)*— ↓ infusion rate to 0.25 mg/kg/hr. ACT should be monitored in all patients with renal impairment.

Availability
Powder for injection: 250 mg/vial.

NURSING IMPLICATIONS

Assessment
- Assess for bleeding. Most common is oozing from the arterial access site for cardiac catheterization. Arterial and venous punctures, IM injections, and use of urinary catheters, nasotracheal intubation, and nasogastric tubes should be minimized. Noncompressible sites for IV access should be avoided. If bleeding cannot be controlled with pressure, discontinue bivalirudin immediately.
- Monitor vital signs. May cause bradycardia, hypertension, or hypotension. An unexplained decrease in blood pressure may indicate hemorrhage.
- *Lab Test Considerations:* Assess hemoglobin, hematocrit, and platelet count prior to bivalirudin therapy and periodically during therapy. May cause ↓ hemoglobin and hematocrit. An unexplained ↓ in hematocrit may indicate hemorrhage.
- Monitor ACT periodically in patients with renal dysfunction.

Potential Nursing Diagnoses
Ineffective tissue perfusion (Indications)

Implementation
- Administer IV just prior to PTCA, in conjunction with aspirin 300 mg to 325 mg/day. Do not administer IM.

IV Administration
- **Direct IV:** (for bolus dose) Reconstitute each 250-mg vial with 5 mL of sterile water for injection. Reconstituted vials are stable for 24 hr if refrigerated. *Diluent:* Further dilute in 50 mL of D5W or 0.9% NaCl. Withdraw bolus dose out of bag. Infusion is stable for 24 hr at room temperature. *Concentration:* Final concentration of infusion is 5 mg/mL. *Rate:* Administer as a bolus injection.
- **Intermittent Infusion:** Reconstitute each 250-mg vial as per the above directions. *Diluent:* Further dilute in 50 mL of D5W or 0.9% NaCl. If infusion is to be continued after 4 hr (at a rate of 0.2 mg/kg/hr), reconstituted vial should be diluted in 500 mL of D5W or 0.9% NaCl. Infusion is stable for 24 hr at room temperature. *Concentration:* 5 mg/mL (for infusion rate of 1.75 mg/kg/hr); 0.5 mg/mL (for infusion rate of 0.2 mg/kg/hr). *Rate:* Based on patient's weight (see Route/Dosage section).
- **Y-Site Compatibility:** acyclovir, allopurinol, amifostine, amikacin, aminocaproic acid, aminophylline, amphotericin B liposome, ampicillin, ampicillin-sulbactam, anidulafungin, argatroban, arsenic trioxide, atracurium, atropine, azithromycin, aztreonam, bleomycin, bumetanide, buprenorphine, busulfan, butorphanol, calcium chloride, calcium gluconate, carboplatin, carmustine, cefazolin, cefepime, cefoperazone, cefotaxime, cefoxitin, ceftazidime, ceftozoxime, ceftriaxone, cefuroxime, chloramphenicol, cimetidine, ciprofloxacin, cisatracurium, cisplatin, clindamycin, cyclophosphamide, cyclosporine, cytarabine, dacarbazine, dactinomycin, daptomycin, daunorubicin, dexamethasone, dexmedetomidine, dexrazoxane, digoxin, diltiazem, diphenhydramine, docetaxel, dolasetron, dopamine, doxorubicin, doxorubicin liposome, doxycycline, droperidol, enaprilat, ephedrine, epinephrine, epirubicin, epoprostenol, eptifibatide, ertapenem, erythromycin, esmolol, etoposide, etoposide phosphate, famotidine, fenoldopam, fentanyl, fluconazole, fludarabine, fluorouracil, foscarnet, fosphenytoin, furosemide, ganciclovir, gemcitabine, gentamicin, glycopyrrolate, granisetron, haloperidol, heparin, hydralazine, hydrocortisone, hydromorphone, idarubicin, ifosfamide, imipenem/cilastatin, inamrinone, insulin, irinotecan, isoproterenol, ketorolac, labetalol, leucovorin, levofloxacin, lidocaine, linezolid, lorazepam, magnesium sulfate, mannitol, mechlorethamine, melaphalan, meperidine, meropenem, mesna, methohexital, methotrexate, methyldopate, methylprednisolone, metoclopramide, metoprolol, metronidazole, midazolam, milrinone, mitomycin, mitoxantrone, morphine, mycophenolate, nafcillin, nalbuphine, naloxone, nesiritide, nicardipine, nitroglycerin, nitroprusside, norepinephrine, octreotide, ondansetron, oxaliplatin, oxytocin, paclitaxel, palonosetron, pamidronate, pancuronium, pemetrexed, pentobarbital, phenobarbital, phenylephrine, piperacillin-tazobactam, potassium acetate, potassium chloride, potassium phosphate, procainamide, promethazine, ranitidine, remifentanil, rocuronium, sodium acetate, sodium bicarbonate, sodium phosphates, streptozocin, succinylcholine, sufentanil, tacrolimus, teniposide, theophylline, thiopental, thiotepa, ticarcillin-clavulanate, tigecycline, tirofiban, tobramycin, topotecan, trimethoprim/sulfamethoxazole, vasopressin, vecuronium, verapamil, vinblastine, vincristine, vinorelbine, voriconazole, warfarin, zidovudine, zolendronic acid.
- **Y-Site Incompatibility:** alteplase, amiodarone, amphotericin B, amphotericin B lipid complex, caspofungin, chlorpromazine, dantrolene, diazepam, pentamidine, pentazocine, phenytoin, prochlorperazine, quinupristin/dalfopristin, reteplase, streptokinase, vancomycin.

Patient/Family Teaching
- Inform patient of the purpose of bivalirudin.
- Instruct patient to notify health care professional immediately if any bleeding is noted.

Evaluation/Desired Outcomes
- Decreased acute ischemic complications in patients with unstable angina (death, MI or the urgent need for revascularization procedures).

HIGH ALERT

bleomycin (blee-oh-**mye**-sin)
Blenoxane

Classification
Therapeutic: antineoplastics
Pharmacologic: antitumor antibiotics

Pregnancy Category D

Indications
Treatment of: Lymphomas, Squamous cell carcinoma, Testicular embryonal cell carcinoma, Choriocarcinoma, Teratocarcinoma. Intrapleural ad-

bleomycin 237

ministration to prevent the reaccumulation of malignant effusions.

Action
Inhibits DNA and RNA synthesis. **Therapeutic Effects:** Death of rapidly replicating cells, particularly malignant ones.

Pharmacokinetics
Absorption: Well absorbed from IM and subcut sites. Absorption follows intrapleural and intraperitoneal administration.
Distribution: Widely distributed, concentrates in skin, lungs, peritoneum, kidneys, and lymphatics.
Metabolism and Excretion: 60–70% excreted unchanged by the kidneys.
Half-life: 2 hr (↑ in renal impairment).

TIME/ACTION PROFILE (tumor response)

ROUTE	ONSET	PEAK	DURATION
IV, IM, Subcut	2–3 wk	unknown	unknown

Contraindications/Precautions
Contraindicated in: Hypersensitivity; OB, Lactation: Potential for fetal, infant harm.
Use Cautiously in: Renal impairment (dose ↓ required if CCr <35 mL/min); Pulmonary impairment; Nonmalignant chronic debilitating illness; Patients with childbearing potential; Geri: ↑ risk of pulmonary toxicity and reduction in renal function.

Adverse Reactions/Side Effects
CNS: aggressive behavior, disorientation, weakness. **Resp:** PULMONARY FIBROSIS, pneumonitis. **CV:** hypotension, peripheral vasoconstriction. **GI:** anorexia, nausea, stomatitis, vomiting. **Derm:** hyperpigmentation, mucocutaneous toxicity, alopecia, erythema, rashes, urticaria, vesiculation. **Hemat:** anemia, leukopenia, thrombocytopenia. **Local:** pain at tumor site, phlebitis at IV site. **Metab:** weight loss. **Misc:** ANAPHYLACTOID REACTIONS, chills, fever.

Interactions
Drug-Drug: Hematologic toxicity ↑ with concurrent use of **radiation therapy** and other **antineoplastics**. Concurrent use with **cisplatin** ↓ elimination of bleomycin and may ↑ toxicity. ↑ risk of pulmonary toxicity with other **antineoplastics** or thoracic **radiation therapy**. **General anesthesia** ↑ the risk of pulmonary toxicity. ↑ risk of Raynaud's phenomenon when used with **vinblastine**.

Route/Dosage
Lymphoma patients should receive initial test doses of 2 units or less for the first 2 doses.
IV, IM, Subcut (Adults and Children): 0.25–0.5 unit/kg (10–20 units/m^2) weekly or twice weekly initially. If favorable response, lower maintenance doses given (1 unit/day or 5 units/wk IM or IV). May also be given as continuous IV infusion at 0.25 unit/kg or 15 units/m^2/day for 4–5 days.
Intrapleural (Adults): 15–20 units instilled for 4 hr, then removed.

Availability (generic available)
Injection: 15 units/vial, 30 units/vial.

NURSING IMPLICATIONS
Assessment
- Monitor vital signs before and frequently during therapy.
- Assess for fever and chills. May occur 3–6 hr after administration and last 4–12 hr.
- Monitor for anaphylactic (fever, chills, hypotension, wheezing) and idiosyncratic (confusion, hypotension, fever, chills, wheezing) reactions. Keep resuscitation equipment and medications on hand. Lymphoma patients are at particular risk for idiosyncratic reactions that may occur immediately or several hours after therapy, usually after the first or second dose.
- Assess respiratory status for dyspnea and rales/crackles. Monitor chest x-ray before and periodically during therapy. Pulmonary toxicity occurs primarily in geriatric patients (age 70 or older) who have received 400 or more units or at lower doses in patients who received other antineoplastics or thoracic radiation. May occur 4–10 wk after therapy. Discontinue and do not resume bleomycin if pulmonary toxicity occurs.
- Assess nausea, vomiting, and appetite. Weigh weekly. Modify diet as tolerated. Antiemetics may be given before administration.
- *Lab Test Considerations:* Monitor CBC before and periodically during therapy. May cause thrombocytopenia and leukopenia (nadir occurs in 12 days and usually returns to pretreatment levels by day 17).
- Monitor baseline and periodic renal and hepatic function.

✦ = Canadian drug name.　█ = Genetic implication.
*CAPITALS indicates life-threatening; underlines indicate most frequent.

Potential Nursing Diagnoses
Risk for injury (Side Effects)
Disturbed body image (Side Effects)

Implementation
- **High Alert:** Fatalities have occurred with chemotherapeutic agents. Before administering, clarify all ambiguous orders; double-check single, daily, and course-of-therapy dose limits; have second practitioner independently double-check original order and dose calculations.
- Prepare solution in a biologic cabinet. Wear gloves, gown, and mask while handling medication. Discard equipment in specially designated containers.
- Lymphoma patients should receive a 1- or 2-unit test dose 2–4 hr before initiation of therapy. Monitor closely for anaphylactic reaction. May not detect reactors.
- Premedication with acetaminophen, corticosteroids, and diphenhydramine may reduce drug fever and risk of anaphylaxis.
- Reconstituted solution is stable for 24 hr at room temperature and for 14 days if refrigerated.
- **IM, Subcut:** Reconstitute vial with 1–5 mL of sterile water for injection, 0.9% NaCl, or bacteriostatic water for injection. Do not reconstitute with diluents containing benzyl alcohol when used for neonates.

IV Administration
- **Intermittent Infusion:** Prepare IV doses by diluting 15-unit vial with at least 5 mL of 0.9% NaCl. **Diluent:** Further dilute dose in 50 to 1000 mL of D5W or 0.9% NaCl. **Rate:** Administer slowly over 10 min.
- **Y-Site Compatibility:** allopurinol, amifostine, aminocaproic acid, aminophylline, amiodarone, anidulafungin, atracurium, aztreonam, bivalirudin, bumetanide, busulfan, calcium chloride, calcium gluconate, carboplatin, carmustine, caspofungin, cefepime, chlorpromazine, cimetidine, cisatracurium, cisplatin, codeine, cyclophosphamide, cyclosporine, cytarabine, dacarbazine, dactinomycin, daptomycin, daunorubicin, dexamethasone, dexmedetomidine, dexrazoxane, digoxin, diltiazem, diphenhydramine, dobutamine, docetaxel, dopamine, doxacurium, doxorubicin, doxorubicin liposome, droperidol, enalaprilat, epinephrine, epirubicin, ertapenem, esmolol, etoposide, etoposide phosphate, famotidine, fenoldopam, filgrastim, fludarabine, fluorouracil, fospehnytoin, furosemide, gemcitabine, glycopyrrolate, granisetron, haloperidol, heparin, hetastarch, hydralazine, hydrocortisone, idarubicin, ifosfamide, inamrinone, insulin, isoproterenol, ketorolac, labetalol, leucovorin calcium, levofloxacin, lidocaine, magnesium sulfate, mannitol, mechlorethamine, melphalan, meperidine, mesna, metaraminol, methotrexate, methyldopate, methylprednisolone, metoclopramide, metoprolol, milrinone, mitomycin, mitoxantrone, naloxone, nesiritide, nicardipine, nitroglycerin, norepinephrine, octreotide, ondansetron, oxaliplatin, paclitaxel, palonosetron, pancuronium, pantoprazole, pemetrexed, phentolamine, phenylephrine, piperacillin/tazobactam, potassium chloride, potassium phosphates, procainamide, quinupristin/dalfopristin, rituximab, sargramostim, sodium acetate, teniposide, thiotepa, tirofiban, trastuzumab, vinblastine, vincristine, vinorelbine, voriconazole.
- **Y-Site Incompatibility:** amphotericin B liposome, dantrolene, phenytoin, tigecycline.
- **Intrapleural:** Dissolve 60 units in 50–100 mL of 0.9% NaCl.
- May be administered through thoracotomy tube. Position patient as directed.

Patient/Family Teaching
- Instruct patient to notify health care professional if fever, chills, wheezing, faintness, diaphoresis, shortness of breath, prolonged nausea and vomiting, or mouth sores occur.
- Encourage patient not to smoke because this may worsen pulmonary toxicity.
- Explain to the patient that skin toxicity may manifest itself as skin sensitivity, hyperpigmentation (especially at skin folds and points of skin irritation), and skin rashes and thickening.
- Instruct patient to inspect oral mucosa for erythema and ulceration. If ulceration occurs, advise patient to use sponge brush and rinse mouth with water after eating and drinking. Opioid analgesics may be required if pain interferes with eating.
- Discuss with patient the possibility of hair loss. Explore coping strategies.
- Advise patient of the need for contraception during therapy.
- Instruct patient not to receive any vaccinations without advice of health care professional.
- Emphasize need for periodic lab tests to monitor for side effects.

Evaluation/Desired Outcomes
- Decrease in tumor size without evidence of hypersensitivity or pulmonary toxicity.

bortezomib (bor-tez-o-mib)
Velcade

Classification
Therapeutic: antineoplastics
Pharmacologic: proteasome inhibitors

Pregnancy Category D

Indications
Multiple myeloma (as initial therapy or after progression); with melphalan and prednisone). Mantle cell lymphoma after at least one other therapy.

Action
Inhibits proteasome, a regulator of intracellular protein catabolism, resulting in disruption of various intracellular processes. Cytotoxic to a variety of cancerous cells. **Therapeutic Effects:** Death of rapidly replicating cells, particularly malignant ones.

Pharmacokinetics
Absorption: IV administration results in complete bioavailability.
Distribution: Unknown.
Metabolism and Excretion: Mostly metabolized by the liver (P450 enzymes); excretion is unknown.
Half-life: 9–15 hr.

TIME/ACTION PROFILE

ROUTE	ONSET	PEAK	DURATION
IV	unknown	38 days*	unknown

*Median time to response based on clinical parameters

Contraindications/Precautions
Contraindicated in: Hypersensitivity to bortezomib, boron, or mannitol; OB: Potential fetal harm.; Lactation: Potential for serious adverse reaction in nursing infants.
Use Cautiously in: OB: Women with childbearing potential; Hepatic impairment (may ↑ levels, risk of toxicity); History of or risk factors for CHF; Pedi: Safety not established.

Adverse Reactions/Side Effects
CNS: fatigue, malaise, weakness, dizziness, syncope. **EENT:** blurred vision, diplopia. **CV:** hypotension, CHF. **Resp:** pneumonia. **GI:** anorexia, constipation, diarrhea, nausea, vomiting. **Hemat:** BLEEDING, anemia, neutropenia, thrombocytopenia. **Neuro:** peripheral neuropathy. **Misc:** fever, tumor lysis syndrome.

Interactions
Drug-Drug: Concurrent neurotoxic medications including **amiodarone**, some **antivirals**, **nitrofuratoin**, **isoniazid**, or **HMG-CoA reductase inhibitors** may ↑ risk of peripheral neuropathy.

Route/Dosage
IV (Adults): 1.3 mg/m^2 twice weekly for 2 wk (days 1, 4, 8, and 11) followed by a 10-day rest; further cycles/doses depend on response and toxicity.

Availability
Lyophilized powder for injection (requires reconstitution): 3.5 mg/vial.

NURSING IMPLICATIONS

Assessment
- Monitor vital signs frequently during therapy. May cause fever and orthostatic hypotension requiring adjustment of antihypertensives, hydration, or administration of mineralocorticoids.
- Monitor for GI adverse effects. May require antidiarrheals, antiemetics, and fluid and electrolyte replacement to prevent dehydration. Weigh weekly; modify diet as tolerated.
- Monitor for signs and symptoms of tumor lysis syndrome (tachypnea, tachycardia, hypotension, pulmonary edema). Patients with high tumor burden prior to treatment are at increased risk.
- **Lab Test Considerations:** Monitor CBC and platelet count frequently during therapy. The nadir of thrombocytopenia is day 11 and recovery is usually by next cycle. Occurs more commonly in cycles 1 and 2, but may occur throughout therapy. May require discontinuation of therapy.
- Monitor blood glucose levels closely in patients taking oral hypoglycemic agents; may require adjustment of antidiabetic agent dose.

Potential Nursing Diagnoses
Risk for injury (Adverse Reactions)

Implementation
- Should be administered under the supervision of a physician experienced in the use of antineoplastic therapy.
- Prepare solution in a biologic cabinet. Wear gloves, gown, and mask, while handling medication. Discard equipment in specially designated containers.

BRONCHODILATORS (XANTHINES)

IV Administration

- **Direct IV:** Reconstitute each vial with 3.5 mL of 0.9% NaCl. Solution should be clear and colorless; do not administer solutions that are discolored or contain particulate matter. Administer reconstituted solution within 8 hr at room temperature; 3 of the 8 hr may be stored in a syringe. *Rate:* Administer as a bolus injection twice weekly for 2 wk followed by a 10-day rest period. At least 72 hr should elapse between consecutive doses.
- If peripheral neuropathy is Grade 1 (paresthesia or loss of reflexes without pain or loss of function) continue prescribed dose. If paresthesia is Grade 1 with pain or Grade 2 (interfering with function but not with daily activities) reduce dose to 1.0 mg/m². If peripheral neuropathy is Grade 2 with pain or Grade 3 (interfering with activities of daily living) withhold dose until toxicity resolves, then re-initiate with a reduced dose of 0.7 mg/m² and decrease frequency to once/wk. If peripheral neuropathy is Grade 4 (permanent sensory loss that interferes with daily function) discontinue bortezomib.

Patient/Family Teaching

- Caution the patient that dehydration may occur with vomiting or diarrhea. Advise patient to maintain fluid intake and to notify health care professional if dizziness or fainting occurs.
- Instruct patient to contact health care professional if they experience new or worsening signs of peripheral neuropathy.
- May cause dizziness and blurred vision. Caution patient to avoid driving or other activities requiring alertness until response to medication is known.
- Advise patient to consult health care professional before taking Rx, OTC, or herbal products.
- Advise patient of the need for contraception and to avoid breastfeeding during therapy.

Evaluation/Desired Outcomes

- Decrease in serum and urine myeloma protein.
- Decrease in size and spread of malignancy.

BRONCHODILATORS (XANTHINES)

aminophylline (am-in-**off**-i-lin)
♣ Phyllocontin, Truphylline

theophylline (thee-**off**-i-lin)
♣ Apo-Theo LA, ♣ Novo-Theophyl SR, ♣ PMS-Theophylline, ♣ Pulmophylline, Quibron-T, Theochron, Theo-24, Uniphyl

Classification
Therapeutic: bronchodilators
Pharmacologic: xanthines

Pregnancy Category C

Indications
Long-term control of reversible airway obstruction caused by asthma or COPD. Increases diaphragmatic contractility (aminophylline). **Unlabeled Use:** Respiratory and myocardial stimulant in premature infant apnea (apnea of prematurity) (aminophylline).

Action
Inhibit phosphodiesterase, producing increased tissue concentrations of cyclic adenosine monophosphate (cAMP). Increased levels of cAMP result in: Bronchodilation, CNS stimulation, Positive inotropic and chronotropic effects, Diuresis, Gastric acid secretion. **Therapeutic Effects:** Bronchodilation.

Pharmacokinetics
Absorption: Aminophylline releases theophylline after administration. Well absorbed from oral dosage forms; absorption from extended-release dosage forms is slow but complete.
Distribution: Widely distributed; crosses the placenta; breast milk concentrations are 70% of plasma levels; not distributed into adipose tissue.
Metabolism and Excretion: Aminophylline is converted to theophylline; theophylline is 90% metabolized by the liver to several metabolites (including the active metabolites, caffeine and 3–methylxanthine) which may accumulate in neonates; metabolites are renally excreted; 10% excreted unchanged by the kidneys.
Half-life: *Theophylline*—Premature infants: 20–30 hr; Term infants: 11–25 hr; Children 1–4 yr: 3.4 hr; Children 6–17 yr: 3.7 hr; Adults: 9–10 hr (increased in patients >60 yr, patients with CHF or liver disease; decreased in cigarette smokers).

TIME/ACTION PROFILE (bronchodilation)

ROUTE	ONSET†	PEAK	DURATION
Aminophylline PO	15–60 min	1–2 hr	6–8 hr
Aminophylline PO–ER	unknown	4–7 hr	8–12 hr
Aminophylline IV	rapid	end of infusion	6–8 hr
Theophylline PO	rapid	1–2 hr	6 hr

BRONCHODILATORS (XANTHINES) 241

| Theophylline delayed PO–ER | 4–8 hr | 8–24 hr |
| Theophylline rapid IV | end of infusion | 6–8 hr |

†Provided that a loading dose has been given and steady-state blood levels exist

Contraindications/Precautions
Contraindicated in: Hypersensitivity to aminophylline or theophylline.
Use Cautiously in: CHF, liver disease, or hypothyroidism (dosage reduction required); Cardiac arrhythmias; Peptic ulcer disease; Seizure disorder; OB: Has been used safely; Lactation: Safety not established; Pedi: Dosage reduction required in children <1 yr; Geri, OB: Dosage reduction required due to enhanced potential for adverse reaction.

Adverse Reactions/Side Effects
CNS: SEIZURES, anxiety, headache, insomnia, irritability. **CV:** ARRHYTHMIAS, tachycardia, angina, palpitations. **GI:** nausea, vomiting, anorexia. **Neuro:** tremor. **Derm:** rashes.

Interactions
Drug-Drug: Additive CV and CNS side effects with **adrenergics (sympathomimetic)**. May ↓ the therapeutic effect of **lithium** and **phenytoin**. **Nicotine** (cigarettes, gum, transdermal patches), **barbiturates, phenytoin, nevirapine**, and **rifampin** may ↑ metabolism and may ↓ effectiveness. **Erythromycin, beta blockers, clarithromycin, calcium channel blockers, cimetidine, doxycycline, estrogens, hormonal contraceptives, disulfiram, fluvoxamine, isoniazid, ketoconazole, mexiletine, nefazodone, protease inhibitors, quinidine**, some **fluoroquinolones**, and large doses of **allopurinol** ↓ metabolism and may lead to toxicity.
Drug-Natural Products: Caffeine-containing herbs (**cola nut, guarana, maté, tea, coffee**) may ↑ serum levels and risk of CNS and cardiovascular side effects. ↓ serum levels and effectiveness with **St. John's wort**.
Drug-Food: Excessive regular intake of **charcoal-broiled foods** may ↓ effectiveness.

Route/Dosage
Dose should be determined by theophylline serum level monitoring. Loading dose should be decreased or eliminated if theophylline preparation has been used in preceding 24 hr. Aminophylline is 80% theophylline (100 mg aminophylline = 80 mg theophylline). Extended-release (controlled-release, sustained-release) products may be given q 8–24 hr, depending upon the formulation.

Aminophylline

PO (Adults and Children): See theophylline for oral doses.

IV (Adults): *Loading dose*—6 mg/kg (4.7 mg/kg of theophylline) given over 20–30 min, followed by 0.7 mg/kg/hr (0.56 mg/kg/hr of theophylline) via continuous infusion (non-smokers); an infusion rate of 0.9 mg/kg/hr (0.72 mg/kg/hr of theophylline) should be used for smokers.

IV (Geriatric Patients and Adult Patients with Cor Pulmonale): *Loading dose*—6 mg/kg (4.7 mg/kg of theophylline) given over 20–30 min, followed by 0.6 mg/kg/hr (0.47 mg/kg/hr of theophylline) via continuous infusion.

IV (Adults with CHF or Liver Failure): *Loading dose*—6 mg/kg (4.7 mg/kg of theophylline) given over 20–30 min, followed by 0.5 mg/kg/hr (0.39 mg/kg/hr of theophylline) via continuous infusion.

IV (Children 12–16 yr): *Loading dose:* 6 mg/kg (4.7 mg/kg of theophylline) given over 20–30 min, followed by 0.7 mg/kg/hr (0.56 mg/kg/hr of theophylline) via continuous infusion.

IV (Children 9–12 yr): *Loading dose:* 6 mg/kg (4.7 mg/kg of theophylline) given over 20–30 min, followed by 0.9 mg/kg/hr (0.72 mg/kg/hr of theophylline) via continuous infusion.

IV (Children 1–9 yr): *Loading dose:* 6 mg/kg (4.7 mg/kg of theophylline) given over 20–30 min, followed by 1–1.2 mg/kg/hr (0.8–0.96 mg/kg/hr of theophyllne) via continuous infusion.

IV (Children 6 mo–1 yr): *Loading dose:* 6 mg/kg (4.7 mg/kg of theophylline) given over 20–30 min, followed by 0.6–0.7 mg/kg/hr (0.48–0.56 mg/kg/hr of theophylline) via continuous infusion.

IV (Infants 6 wk–6 mo): *Loading dose*—6 mg/kg (4.7 mg/kg of theophylline) given over 20–30 min, followed by 0.5 mg/kg/hr (0.4 mg/kg/hr of theophylline) via continuous infusion.

Theophylline

PO (Adults Healthy, Non-smoking): *Loading dose*—5 mg/kg, followed by 10 mg/kg/day divided q 8–12 hr (not to exceed 900 mg/day).

PO (Adults with CHF, Cor Pulmonale, or Liver Dysfunction): *Loading dose*—5 mg/kg, followed by 5 mg/kg/day divided q 8–12 hr (not to exceed 400 mg/day).

✹ = Canadian drug name. ⬛ = Genetic implication.
*CAPITALS indicates life-threatening; underlines indicate most frequent.

242 BRONCHODILATORS (XANTHINES)

PO (Children 12–16 yr, Non-smoking): *Loading dose*—5 mg/kg, followed by 13 mg/kg/day divided q 8–12 hr.
PO (Children 9–12 yr, adolescent and adult smokers < 50 yr): *Loading dose*—5 mg/kg, followed by 16 mg/kg/day divided q 8–12 hr.
PO (Children 1–9 yr): *Loading dose*—5 mg/kg, followed by 20–24 mg/kg/day divided q 8–12 hr.
PO (Infants 6 mo–1 yr): *Loading dose*—5 mg/kg, followed by 12–18 mg/kg/day divided q 6–8 hr.
PO (Infants 6 wk–6 mo): *Loading dose*—5 mg/kg, followed by 10 mg/kg/day divided q 6–8 hr.
PO (Neonates up to 6 wk): *Loading dose*—4 mg/kg, followed by 4 mg/kg/day divided q 12 hr.
IV (Adults and Children): See aminophylline for IV doses.

Availability

Aminophylline (generic available)
Tablets: 100 mg, 200 mg. **Extended-release tablets:** ♣ 225 mg, ♣ 350 mg. **Oral solution:** 105 mg/5 mL. **Suppositories:** 250 mg, 500 mg. **Injection:** 25 mg/mL.

Theophylline (generic available)
Sustained-release tablets (8–12 hr): 300 mg. **Extended-release tablets (12–24 hr):** 100 mg, 200 mg, 300 mg, 450 mg. **Controlled-release tablets (24 hr):** 400 mg, 600 mg. **Extended-release capsules (12 hr):** 125 mg, 200 mg, 300 mg. **Extended-release capsules (24 hr):** 100 mg, 200 mg, 300 mg, 400 mg. **Elixir (orange/raspberry, mixed fruit, and other flavors):** 80 mg/15 mL. **Injection (with dextrose):** 0.8 mg/mL, 1.6 mg/mL, 2 mg/mL, 3.2 mg/mL, 4 mg/mL.

NURSING IMPLICATIONS

Assessment
- Assess blood pressure, pulse, respiratory status (rate, lung sounds, use of accessory muscles, number and severity of apnea spells in infants) before and throughout therapy. Ensure that oxygen therapy is correctly instituted during acute asthma attacks.
- Monitor intake and output ratios for an increase in diuresis or fluid overload.
- Patients with a history of cardiovascular problems should be monitored for chest pain and ECG changes (PACs, supraventricular tachycardia, PVCs, ventricular tachycardia). Resuscitative equipment should be readily available.
- Monitor pulmonary function tests before and periodically during therapy to determine therapeutic efficacy in patients with chronic bronchitis or emphysema.
- *Lab Test Considerations:* Monitor ABGs, acid-base, and fluid and electrolyte balance in patients receiving parenteral therapy or whenever required by patient's condition.
- ***Toxicity and Overdose:*** Monitor drug levels routinely, especially in patients requiring high doses or during prolonged intensive therapy. Serum sample should be obtained at time of peak absorption. Peak levels should be evaluated 30 min after a 30 min IV loading dose, 12–24 hr after initiation of a continuous infusion and 1–2 hr after rapid-acting oral forms, and 4–12 hr after extended-release oral forms. Therapeutic plasma levels range from 10–15 mcg/mL for asthma and 6–14 mcg/mL for apnea of prematurity. Drug levels in excess of 20 mcg/mL are associated with toxicity. Caffeine ingestion may falsely elevate drug concentration levels.
- Observe patient for symptoms of drug toxicity (anorexia, nausea, vomiting, stomach cramps, diarrhea, confusion, headache, restlessness, flushing, increased urination, insomnia, tachycardia, arrhythmias, seizures). Notify physician or other health care professional immediately if these occur. Tachycardia, ventricular arrhythmias, or seizures may be the first sign of toxicity. Geri: Patients over 60 yr have increased risk of toxicity and sensitivity to toxic effects due to age-related pharmacodynamic and pharmacokinetic changes. Theophylline doses should not exceed 400 mg/d. Assess frequently.

Potential Nursing Diagnoses
Ineffective airway clearance (Indications)
Activity intolerance (Indications)

Implementation
- Administer around the clock to maintain therapeutic plasma levels. Once-a-day doses should be administered in the morning.
- Do not refrigerate elixirs; crystals may form. Crystals should dissolve when liquid is warmed to room temperature.
- Wait at least 4–6 hr after stopping IV therapy to begin immediate-release oral dosage; for extended-release oral dosage form, give first oral dose at time of IV discontinuation.
- **PO:** Administer oral preparations with food or a full glass of water to minimize GI irritation. Food slows but does not reduce the extent of absorption. May be administered 1 hr before or 2 hr after meals for more rapid absorption.

BRONCHODILATORS (XANTHINES) 243

Swallow tablets whole; do not crush, break, or chew enteric-coated or extended-release tablets (extended-release tablets may be broken if scored). Pedi: Use calibrated measuring device to ensure accurate dose of liquid preparations.

Aminophylline

IV Administration

- **IV:** *Diluent:* May be diluted in D5W, D10W, D20W, 0.9% NaCl, 0.45% NaCl, D5/0.9% NaCl, D5/0.45% NaCl, D5/0.25% NaCl, or LR. *Concentration:* 1 mg/mL (maximum 25 mg/mL). Mixture is stable for 24 hr if refrigerated.
- Do not administer discolored or precipitated solution. Flush main IV line before administration.
- If extravasation occurs, local injection of 1% procaine and application of heat may relieve pain and promote vasodilation.
- **Loading Dose:** Administer over 20–30 min.
- **Rate:** Do not exceed 20–25 mg/min in adults or 0.36 mg/kg/min in children. Administer via infusion pump to ensure accurate dosage. Rapid administration may cause chest pain, dizziness, hypotension, tachypnea, flushing, arrhythmias, or a reaction to the solution or administration technique (chills; fever; redness, pain, or swelling at injection site).
- **Continuous Infusion:** Usually given as a loading dose in a small volume followed by continuous infusion in larger volume.
- **Rate:** See Route and Dosage section for rates.
- **Syringe Compatibility:** heparin, metoclopramide.
- **Syringe Incompatibility:** doxapram.
- **Y-Site Compatibility:** allopurinol, amifostine, amphotericin B cholesteryl sulfate complex, ceftazidime, cimetidine, cladribine, docetaxel, doxorubicin liposome, enalaprilat, esmolol, etoposide, famotidine, filgrastim, fluconazole, fludarabine, foscarnet, gemcitabine, granisetron, inamrinone, labetalol, melphalan, meropenem, morphine, paclitaxel, pancuronium, piperacillin/tazobactam, potassium chloride, propofol, ranitidine, remifentanil, sargramostim, tacrolimus, teniposide, thiotepa, tolazoline, vecuronium, vitamin B complex with vitamin C.
- **Y-Site Incompatibility:** amiodarone, ciprofloxacin, dobutamine, hydralazine, ondansetron, vinorelbine, warfarin.
- **Additive Incompatibility:** Admixing is not recommended because of dose titration and incompatibilities.

Theophylline

IV Administration

- **Continuous Infusion:** Premixed IV theophylline and 5% dextrose are packed in a moisture-barrier overwrap. Remove immediately before administration and squeeze bag to check for leaks. Discard if solution is not clear.
- **Loading Dose:** Administer over 20–30 min. If patient has had another form of theophylline before loading dose, serum theophylline level should be obtained and loading dose proportionately reduced.
- **Rate:** Do not exceed 20–25 mg/min. Rapid administration may cause chest pain, dizziness, hypotension, tachypnea, flushing, arrhythmias, or a reaction to the solution or administration technique (chills; fever; redness, pain, or swelling at injection site). Infusion rate may be increased after 12 hr. Administer via infusion pump to ensure accurate dosage. Monitor ECG continuously; tachyarrhythmias may occur.
- **Y-Site Compatibility:** acyclovir, ampicillin, ampicillin/sulbactam, aztreonam, cefazolin, cefotetan, ceftazidime, ceftriaxone, cimetidine, cisatracurium, clindamycin, diltiazem, dobutamine, dopamine, doxycycline, erythromycin lactobionate, famotidine, fluconazole, gentamicin, haloperidol, heparin, hydrocortisone sodium succinate, lidocaine, methyldopate, methylprednisolone sodium succinate, metronidazole, midazolam, milrinone, nafcillin, nitroglycerin, nitroprusside, penicillin G potassium, piperacillin, potassium chloride, ranitidine, remifentanil, ticarcillin, ticarcillin/clavulanate, tobramycin, vancomycin.
- **Y-Site Incompatibility:** hetastarch, phenytoin.
- **Additive Incompatibility:** Admixing is not recommended because of dose titration and incompatibilities.

Patient/Family Teaching

- Emphasize the importance of taking only the prescribed dose at the prescribed time intervals. Missed doses should be taken as soon as possible or omitted if close to next dose.
- Encourage the patient to drink adequate liquids (2000 mL/day minimum) to decrease the viscosity of the airway secretions.

✦ = Canadian drug name. = Genetic implication.
*CAPITALS indicates life-threatening; underlines indicate most frequent.

- Advise patient to avoid OTC cough, cold, or breathing preparations without consulting health care professional. These medications may increase side effects and cause arrhythmias.
- Encourage patients not to smoke. A change in smoking habits may necessitate a change in dosage.
- Advise patient to minimize intake of xanthine-containing foods or beverages (colas, coffee, chocolate) and not to eat charcoal-broiled foods daily.
- Instruct patient not to change brands without consulting health care professional.
- Advise patient to contact health care professional promptly if the usual dose of medication fails to produce the desired results, symptoms worsen after treatment, or toxic effects occur.
- Emphasize the importance of having serum levels routinely tested every 6–12 mo.

Evaluation/Desired Outcomes
- Increased ease in breathing.
- Clearing of lung fields on auscultation.
- Respiratory and myocardial stimulation in apnea of infancy (aminophylline).

---

budesonide, See CORTICOSTEROIDS (INHALATION).

---

budesonide, See CORTICOSTEROIDS (NASAL).

---

budesonide, See CORTICOSTEROIDS (SYSTEMIC).

---

bumetanide (byoo-met-a-nide)
Bumex, ✣Burinex

Classification
Therapeutic: diuretics
Pharmacologic: loop diuretics

Pregnancy Category C

Indications
Edema due to heart failure, hepatic disease, or renal impairment.

Action
Inhibits the reabsorption of sodium and chloride from the loop of Henle and distal renal tubule. Increases renal excretion of water, sodium chloride, magnesium, potassium, and calcium. Effectiveness persists in impaired renal function.
Therapeutic Effects: Diuresis and subsequent mobilization of excess fluid (edema, pleural effusions).

Pharmacokinetics
Absorption: Well absorbed after oral or IM administration.
Distribution: Widely distributed.
Protein Binding: 72–96%.
Metabolism and Excretion: Partially metabolized by liver; 50% eliminated unchanged by kidneys and 20% excreted in feces.
Half-life: 60–90 min (6 hr in neonates).

TIME/ACTION PROFILE (diuretic effect)

ROUTE	ONSET	PEAK	DURATION
PO	30–60 min	1–2 hr	4–6 hr
IM	30–60 min	1–2 hr	4–6 hr
IV	2–3 min	15–45 min	2–3 hr

Contraindications/Precautions
Contraindicated in: Hypersensitivity; Cross-sensitivity with thiazides and sulfonamides may occur; Hepatic coma or anuria.
Use Cautiously in: Severe liver disease (may precipitate hepatic coma; concurrent use with potassium-sparing diuretics may be necessary); Electrolyte depletion; Diabetes mellitus; Increasing azotemia; Lactation, Pedi: Safety not established; bumetanide is a potent displacer of bilirubin and should be used cautiously in critically ill or jaundiced neonates because of risk of kernicterus. Injection contains benzyl alcohol, which may cause gasping syndrome in neonates; Geri: May have increased risk of side effects, especially hypotension and electrolyte imbalance, at usual doses.

Adverse Reactions/Side Effects
CNS: dizziness, encephalopathy, headache. **EENT:** hearing loss, tinnitus. **CV:** hypotension. **GI:** diarrhea, dry mouth, nausea, vomiting. **GU:** excessive urination. **Derm:** photosensitivity, pruritis, rash. **Endo:** hyperglycemia, hyperuricemia. **F and E:** dehydration, hypocalcemia, hypochloremia, hypokalemia, hypomagnesemia, hyponatremia, hypovolemia, metabolic alkalosis. **MS:** arthralgia, muscle cramps, myalgia. **Misc:** increased BUN.

Interactions
Drug-Drug: ↑ hypotension with **antihypertensives**, **nitrates**, or acute ingestion of **alcohol**. ↑ risk of hypokalemia with other **diuretics**, **amphotericin B**, **stimulant laxatives**, and **corticosteroids**. Hypokalemia may ↑ risk of **digoxin** toxicity and ↑ risk of arrhythmia in

bumetanide

patients taking drugs that prolong the QT interval. ↓ **lithium** excretion, may cause **lithium** toxicity. ↑ risk of ototoxicity with **aminoglycosides**. **NSAIDS** ↓ effects of bumetanide.

Route/Dosage
PO (Adults): 0.5–2 mg/day given in 1–2 doses; titrate to desired response (maximum daily dose = 10 mg/day).
IM, IV (Adults): 0.5–1 mg/dose, may repeat q 2–3 hr as needed (up to 10 mg/day).

Availability (generic available)
Tablets: 0.5 mg, 1 mg, 2 mg, ✦ 5 mg. **Cost:** *Generic*—0.5 mg $37.32/100, 1 mg $31.31/100, 2 mg $49.97/100. **Injection:** 0.25 mg/mL.

NURSING IMPLICATIONS

Assessment
- Assess fluid status during therapy. Monitor daily weight, intake and output ratios, amount and location of edema, lung sounds, skin turgor, and mucous membranes. Notify physician or other health care professional if thirst, dry mouth, lethargy, weakness, hypotension, or oliguria occurs.
- Monitor blood pressure and pulse before and during administration. Monitor frequency of prescription refills to determine compliance.
- Assess patients receiving digoxin for anorexia, nausea, vomiting, muscle cramps, paresthesia, and confusion; ↑ risk of digoxin toxicity due to potassium-depleting effect of diuretic. Potassium supplements or potassium-sparing diuretics may be used concurrently to prevent hypokalemia.
- Assess patient for tinnitus and hearing loss. Audiometry is recommended for patients receiving prolonged high-dose IV therapy. Hearing loss is most common after rapid or high-dose IV administration in patients with decreased renal function or those taking other ototoxic drugs.
- Assess for allergy to sulfonamides.
- Geri: Diuretic use is associated with increased risk for falls in older adults. Assess falls risk and implement fall prevention strategies.
- ● *Lab Test Considerations:* Monitor electrolytes, renal and hepatic function, serum glucose, and uric acid levels before and periodically during therapy. May cause ↓ serum sodium, potassium, calcium, and magnesium concentrations. May also cause ↑ BUN, serum glucose, creatinine, and uric acid levels.

Potential Nursing Diagnoses
Excess fluid volume (Indications)
Risk for deficient fluid volume (Side Effects)

Implementation
- Do not confuse Bumex (bumetanide) with Buprenex (buprenorphine).
- If administering twice daily, give last dose no later than 5pm to minimize disruption of sleep cycle.
- IV is preferred over IM for parenteral administration.
- **PO:** May be taken with food to minimize gastric irritation.

IV Administration
- **Direct IV:** *Diluent:* Administer undiluted. *Concentration:* 0.25 mg/mL. *Rate:* Administer slowly over 1–2 min.
- **Continuous Infusion:** *Diluent:* May dilute in D5W or 0.9% NaCl. May also administer as undiluted drug. Protect from light. *Concentration:* Not to exceed 0.25 mg/mL. *Rate:* Infuse over 5 min. May be administered over 12 hr for patients with renal impairment.
- **Y-Site Compatibility:** acyclovir, amikacin, aminophylline, amiodarone, atropine, aztreonam, bivalirudin, calcium chloride, calcium gluconate, caspofungin, cefazolin, cefepime, cefotaxime, cefoxitin, ceftazidime, ceftizoxime, ceftriaxone, cefuroxime, chloramphenicol, cimetidine, cisatracurium, clindamycin, cyclosporine, daptomycin, dexamethasone, dexmedetomidate, digoxin, diltiazem, diphenhydramine, dobutamine, dopamine, doxycycline, enalaprilat, epinephrine, ertapenem, erythromycin, esmolol, famotidine, fentanyl, filgrastim, fluconazole, gentamicin, granisetron, heparin, hydrocortisone sodium succinate, hydromorphone, imipenem, insulin, isoproterenol, ketorolac, labetalol, levofloxacin, lidocaine, linezolid, lorazepam, magnesium sulfate, meperidine, methylprednisolone sodium succinate, metoclopramide, metoprolol, metronidazole, micafungin, milrinone, morphine, nafcillin, nitroglycerin, nitroprusside, norepinephrine, ondansetron, palonosetron, pantoprazole, penicillin G potassium, phenylephrine, phytonadione, piperacillin/tazobactam, potassium chloride, procainamide, promethazine, propofol, propranolol, protamine, ranitidine, rifampin, sodium bicarbonate, tacrolimus, ticarcillin/clavulanate, tirofi-

✦ = Canadian drug name. ▌= Genetic implication.
*CAPITALS indicates life-threatening; underlines indicate most frequent.

ban, tobramycin, vancomycin, vasopressin, verapamil, voriconazole.
- **Y-Site Incompatibility:** diazepam, fenoldopam, ganciclovir, haloperidol, nesiritide, phenytoin, quinupristin/dalfopristin, sulfamethoxazole/trimethoprim.

Patient/Family Teaching
- Instruct patient to take bumetanide as directed. Take missed doses as soon as possible; do not double doses.
- Caution patient to change positions slowly to minimize orthostatic hypotension. Caution patient that drinking alcohol, exercising during hot weather, or standing for long periods may enhance orthostatic hypotension.
- Instruct patient to consult health care professional regarding a diet high in potassium. See Appendix M.
- Advise patient to contact health care professional of gain more than 3 lbs in one day.
- Advise patient to consult health care professional before taking Rx, OTC, or herbal products concurrently with therapy.
- Instruct patient to notify health care professional of medication regimen before treatment or surgery.
- Caution patient to use sunscreen and protective clothing to prevent photosensitivity reactions.
- Advise patient to contact health care professional immediately if muscle weakness, cramps, nausea, dizziness, numbness, or tingling of extremities occurs.
- Advise patients with diabetes to monitor blood glucose closely; may cause increased levels.
- Emphasize the importance of routine follow-up examinations.
- Geri: Caution older patients or their caregivers about increased risk for falls. Suggest strategies for fall prevention.

Evaluation/Desired Outcomes
- Decrease in edema.
- Decrease in abdominal girth and weight.
- Increase in urinary output.

---

bupivacaine, See EPIDURAL LOCAL ANESTHETICS.

HIGH ALERT

buprenorphine
(byoo-pre-**nor**-feen)
Buprenex, Subutex

Classification
Therapeutic: opioid analgesics
Pharmacologic: opioid agonists/antagonists

Schedule III

Pregnancy Category C

Indications
IM, IV: Management of moderate to severe acute pain. **SL:** Treatment of opioid dependence; suppresses withdrawal symptoms in opioid detoxification.

Action
Binds to opiate receptors in the CNS. Alters the perception of and response to painful stimuli while producing generalized CNS depression. Has partial antagonist properties that may result in opioid withdrawal in physically dependent patients when used as an analgesic. **Therapeutic Effects: IM, IV:** Decreased severity of pain. **SL:** Suppression of withdrawal symptoms during detoxification and maintenance from heroin or other opioids. Produces a relatively mild withdrawal compared to other agents.

Pharmacokinetics
Absorption: Well absorbed after IM and SL use; IV administration results in complete bioavailability.
Distribution: Crosses the placenta; enters breast milk. CNS concentration is 15–25% of plasma.
Protein Binding: 96%.
Metabolism and Excretion: Mostly metabolized by the liver mostly via the CYP3A4 enzyme system; one metabolite is active.
Half-life: 2–3 hr (parenteral).

TIME/ACTION PROFILE (analgesia)

ROUTE	ONSET	PEAK	DURATION
IM	15 min	60 min	6 hr†
IV	rapid	less than 60 min	6 hr†

†4–5 hr in children

Contraindications/Precautions
Contraindicated in: Hypersensitivity; Lactation: Enters breast milk; avoid use or discontinue nursing.
Use Cautiously in: Increased intracranial pressure; Severe renal, hepatic, or pulmonary disease; Hypothyroidism; Adrenal insufficiency; Alcoholism; Debilitated patients (dose reduction required); Undiagnosed abdominal pain; Prostatic hyperplasia; OB: Safety not established; neonatal withdrawal may occur in infants born to patients receiving SL buprenorphine during pregnancy; Geri: Dose reduction required.

Adverse Reactions/Side Effects
CNS: <u>confusion</u>, <u>dysphoria</u>, <u>hallucinations</u>, <u>sedation</u>, dizziness, euphoria, floating feeling, headache, unusual dreams. **EENT:** blurred vision, diplopia, miosis (high doses). **Resp:** respiratory depression. **CV:** hypertension, hypotension, palpitations. **GI:** <u>nausea</u>, constipation, dry mouth, ileus, vomiting. **GU:** urinary retention. **Derm:** <u>sweating</u>, clammy feeling. **Misc:** physical dependence, psychological dependence, tolerance.

Interactions
Drug-Drug: Use with extreme caution in patients receiving **MAO inhibitors** (↑ CNS and respiratory depression and hypotension— ↓ buprenorphine dose by 50%; may need to ↓ **MAO inhibitor** dose). ↑ CNS depression with **alcohol**, **antihistamines**, **antidepressants**, and **sedative/hypnotics**. May ↓ effectiveness of other **opioid analgesics**. Inhibitors of the CYP3A4 enzyme system including **azole antifungals (itraconazole, ketoconazole)**, **erythromycin**, **protease inhibitor antiretrovirals (ritonavir, indinavir, saquinavir)** ↑ blood levels and effects; dose reduction may be necessary during concurrent use. Inducers of the CYP3A4 enzyme system including **carbamazepine**, **rifampin**, or **phenytoin** ↓ blood levels and effects; dose modification may be necessary during concurrent use. Concurrent abuse of IV buprenorphine and **benzodiazepines** may result in coma and death.
Drug-Natural Products: Concomitant use of **kava-kava**, **valerian**, **chamomile**, or **hops** can ↑ CNS depression.

Route/Dosage
Analgesia
IM, IV (Adults): 0.3 mg q 4–6 hr as needed. May repeat initial dose after 30 min (up to 0.3 mg q 4 hr or 0.6 mg q 6 hr); 0.6-mg doses should be given only IM.
IM, IV (Children 2–12 yr): 2–6 mcg (0.002–0.006 mg)/kg q 4–6 hr.

Treatment of opioid dependence
SL (Adults): 12–16 mg/day as a single dose.

Availability (generic available)
Sublingual tablets: 2 mg, 8 mg. *In combination with:* naloxone (Suboxone). See Appendix B. **Injection:** 300 mcg (0.3 mg)/mL.

NURSING IMPLICATIONS
Assessment
- **Pain:** Assess type, location, and intensity of pain before and 1 hr after IM and 5 min (peak) after IV administration. When titrating opioid doses, increases of 25–50% should be administered until there is either a 50% reduction in the patient's pain rating on a numerical or visual analogue scale or the patient reports satisfactory pain relief. A repeat dose can be safely administered at the time of the peak if previous dose is ineffective and side effects are minimal. Single doses of 600 mcg (0.6 mg) should be administered IM. Patients requiring doses higher than 600 mcg (0.6 mg) should be converted to an opioid agonist. Buprenorphine is not recommended for prolonged use or as first-line therapy for acute or cancer pain.
- An equianalgesic chart (see Appendix K) should be used when changing routes or when changing from one opioid to another.
- Assess level of consciousness, blood pressure, pulse, and respirations before and periodically during administration. If respiratory rate is <10/min, assess level of sedation. Dose may need to be decreased by 25–50%. Buprenorphine 0.3–0.4 mg has approximately equal analgesic and respiratory depressant effects to morphine 10 mg.
- Assess previous analgesic history. Antagonistic properties may induce withdrawal symptoms (vomiting, restlessness, abdominal cramps, increased blood pressure and temperature) in patients who are physically dependent on opioid agonists. Symptoms may occur up to 15 days after discontinuation and persist for 1–2 wk.
- Buprenorphine has a lower potential for dependence than other opioids; however, prolonged use may lead to physical and psychological dependence and tolerance. This should not prevent patient from receiving adequate analgesia. Most patients receiving buprenorphine for pain do not develop psychological dependence. If tolerance develops, changing to an opioid agonist may be required to relieve pain.
- **Opioid Dependence:** Assess patient for signs and symptoms of opioid withdrawal before and during therapy.
- *Lab Test Considerations:* May cause ↑ serum amylase and lipase levels.
- Monitor liver function tests prior to and periodically during therapy for opioid dependence.

buprenorphine

- *Toxicity and Overdose:* If an opioid antagonist is required to reverse respiratory depression or coma, naloxone (Narcan) is the antidote. Dilute the 0.4-mg ampule of naloxone in 10 mL of 0.9% NaCl and administer 0.5 mL (0.02 mg) by direct IV push every 2 min. For children and patients weighing <40 kg, dilute 0.1 mg of naloxone in 10 mL of 0.9% NaCl for a concentration of 10 mcg/mL and administer 0.5 mcg/kg every 1–2 min. Titrate dose to avoid withdrawal, seizures, and severe pain. Naloxone may not completely reverse respiratory depressant effects of buprenorphine; may require mechanical ventilation, oxygen, IV fluids, and vasopressors.

Potential Nursing Diagnoses
Acute pain (Indications)
Risk for injury (Side Effects)
Ineffective coping (Indications)

Implementation
- *High Alert:* Accidental overdose of opioid analgesics has resulted in fatalities. Before administering, clarify all ambiguous orders; have second practitioner independently check original order, dose calculations, route of administration, and infusion pump programming. Do not confuse Buprenex (buprenorphine) with Bumex (bumetanide).
- **Pain:** Explain therapeutic value of medication before administration to enhance the analgesic effect.
- Regularly administered doses may be more effective than prn administration. Analgesic is more effective if given before pain becomes severe.
- Coadministration with nonopioid analgesics has additive effects and may permit lower opioid doses.
- **SL:** Administer sublingually. Usually takes 2–10 min for tablets to dissolve. If more than one tablet is prescribed, place multiple tablets under the tongue or 2 at a time until all tablets are dissolved. Do not chew or swallow; decreases amount of medication absorbed.
- **IM:** Administer IM injections deep into well-developed muscle. Rotate sites of injections.

IV Administration
- **Direct IV:** May give IV undiluted. *High Alert:* Administer slowly. Rapid administration may cause respiratory depression, hypotension, and cardiac arrest. *Rate:* Give over at least 2 minutes.
- **Syringe Compatibility:** glycopyrrolate, heparin, midazolam.
- **Y-Site Compatibility:** allopurinol, amifostine, aztreonam, cefipime, cisatracurium, cladribine, docetaxel, etoposide phosphate, filgrastim, gemcitabine, granisetron, linezolid, melphalan, oxaliplatin, pemetrexed, piperacillin/tazobactam, propofol, remifentanil, teniposide, thiotepa, vinorelbine.
- **Y-Site Incompatibility:** amphotericin B cholesteryl sulfate, doxorubicin liposome.
- **Solution Compatibility:** 0.9% NaCl, D5W, D5/0.9% NaCl, lactated Ringer's injection, Ringer's injection.
- **Opioid Dependence:** Must be prescribed by health care professional with special training. Induction is usually started with buprenorphine (Subutex) over 3–4 days. Initial dose should be administered at least 4 hr after last opioid dose and preferably when early signs of opioid whitdrawal appear. Once patient is on a stable dose, maintenance therapy with buprenorphine/naloxone (Suboxone) is preferred for continued, unsupervised treatment.

Patient/Family Teaching
- Medication may cause drowsiness or dizziness. Advise patient to call for assistance when ambulating and to avoid driving or other activities requiring alertness until response to medication is known.
- Advise patient to avoid concurrent use of alcohol or other CNS depressants.
- Advise patient to notify health care professional before taking other Rx or OTC medication or herbal products.
- **Pain:** Instruct patient on how and when to ask for pain medication.
- Encourage patients on bedrest to turn, cough, and deep-breathe every 2 hr to prevent atelectasis.
- Instruct patient to change positions slowly to minimize orthostatic hypotension.
- Advise patient that good oral hygiene, frequent mouth rinses, and sugarless gum or candy may decrease dry mouth.
- **Opioid Dependence:** Instruct patient in the correct use of medication; directions for use must be followed exactly. Medication must be used regularly, not occasionally. Take missed doses as soon as remembered; if almost time for next dose, skip missed dose and return to regular dosing schedule. Do not take 2 doses at once unless directed by health care professional. Do not discontinue use without consulting health care professional; abrupt discontinuation may cause withdrawal symptoms. If

buPROPion **249**

medication is discontinued, flush unused tablets down the toilet.
- Caution patient that buprenorphine may be a target for people who abuse drugs; store medications in a safe place to protect them from theft. Selling or giving this medication to others is against the law.
- Caution patient that injection of *Suboxone* can lead to bad withdrawal symptoms.
- Advise patient if admitted to the emergency room to inform treating physician and emergency room staff of physical dependence on opioids and of treatment regimen.
- Advise patient to notify health care professional promptly if faintness, dizziness, confusion, slowed breathing, skin or whites of eyes turn yellow, urine turns dark, light-colored stools, decreased appetite, nausea, or abdominal pain occur.

Evaluation/Desired Outcomes
- Decrease in severity of pain without a significant alteration in level of consciousness or respiratory status.
- Suppression of withdrawal symptoms during detoxification and maintenance from heroin or other opioids.

---

buPROPion (byoo-proe-pee-on)
Aplenzin, Budeprion SR, Budeprion XL, Wellbutrin, Wellbutrin SR, Wellbutrin XL, Zyban

Classification
Therapeutic: antidepressants, smoking deterrents
Pharmacologic: aminoketones

Pregnancy Category B

Indications
Treatment of depression (with psychotherapy). Depression in patients with seasonal affective disorder (XL only). Smoking cessation (Zyban only). **Unlabeled Use:** Treatment of ADHD in adults (SR only). To increase sexual desire in women.

Action
Decreases neuronal reuptake of dopamine in the CNS. Diminished neuronal uptake of serotonin and norepinephrine (less than tricyclic antidepressants). **Therapeutic Effects:** Diminished depression. Decreased craving for cigarettes.

Pharmacokinetics
Absorption: Although well absorbed, rapidly and extensively metabolized by the liver.
Distribution: Unknown.
Metabolism and Excretion: Extensively metabolized by the liver. Some conversion to active metabolites.
Half-life: 14 hr (active metabolites may have longer half-lives).

TIME/ACTION PROFILE (antidepressant effect)

ROUTE	ONSET	PEAK	DURATION
PO	1–3 wk	unknown	unknown

Contraindications/Precautions
Contraindicated in: Hypersensitivity; History of bulimia, and anorexia nervosa; Concurrent MAO inhibitor or ritonavir therapy; Lactation: Potential for serious adverse reactions in nursing infants.
Use Cautiously in: Renal/hepatic impairment (↓ dose recommended); Recent history of MI; History of suicide attempt; Unstable cardiovascular status; May ↑ risk of suicide attempt/ideation especially during early treatment or dose adjustment; this risk appears to be greater in adolescents or children; OB: Use only if benefit to patient outweighs potential risk to fetus; Geri: ↑ risk of drug accumulation; ↑ sensitivity to effects.
Exercise Extreme Caution in: History of seizures, head trauma or concurrent medications that ↓ seizure threshold (theophylline, antipsychotics, antidepressants, systemic corticosteroids); Severe hepatic cirrhosis (↓ dose required); Pedi: ↑ risk of suicidal thinking and behavior. Observe carefully, especially at initiation of therapy and during ↑ or ↓ in dose.

Adverse Reactions/Side Effects
CNS: SEIZURES, SUICIDAL THOUGHTS/BEHAVIOR, agitation, headache, depression, hostility, insomnia, mania, psychoses. **GI:** dry mouth, nausea, vomiting, change in appetite, weight gain, weight loss. **Derm:** photosensitivity. **Endo:** hyperglycemia, hypoglycemia, syndrome of inappropriate ADH secretion. **Neuro:** tremor.

Interactions
Drug-Drug: ↑ risk of adverse reactions when used with **amantadine**, **levodopa**, or **MAO inhibitors** (concurrent use of MAO inhibitors is contraindicated). ↑ risk of seizures with **phenothiazines**, **antidepressants**, **theophylline**, **corticosteroids**, **OTC stimulants/anorectics**,

---
✦ = Canadian drug name. ☤ = Genetic implication.
*CAPITALS indicates life-threatening; underlines indicate most frequent.

buPROPion

or cessation of **alcohol** or **benzodiazepines** (avoid or minimize alcohol use). Blood levels ↑ by **ritonavir** (avoid concurrent use). **Carbamazepine** may ↓ blood levels and effectiveness. Concurrent use with **nicotine** replacement may cause hypertension. ↑ risk of bleeding with **warfarin**. Bupropion and one of its metabolites inhibit the CYP2D6 enzyme system and may ↑ levels and risk of toxicity from **antidepressants** (SSRIs and tricyclic), some **beta blockers**, **antiarrhythmics**, and **antipsychotics**.

Route/Dosage
Depression
PO (Adults): *Immediate-release*—100 mg twice daily initially; after 3 days may ↑ to 100 mg 3 times daily; after at least 4 wk of therapy, may ↑ up to 450 mg/day in divided doses (not to exceed 150 mg/dose; wait at least 6 hr between doses at the 300 mg/day dose or at least 4 hr between doses at the 450-mg/day dose). *Sustained-release*—150 mg once daily in the morning; after 3 days, may ↑ to 150 mg twice daily with at least 8 hr between doses; after at least 4 wk of therapy, may ↑ to a maximum daily dose of 400 mg given as 200 mg twice daily. *Extended-release (Wellbutrin XL)*—150 mg once daily in the morning, may be ↑ after 4 days to 300 mg once daily; some patients may require up to 450 mg/day as a single daily dose. *Extended-release (Aplenzin)*—174 mg once daily in the morning, may be ↑ after 4 days to 348 mg once daily; some patients may require up to 522 mg/day as a single daily dose.

Seasonal Affective Disorder
PO (Adults): 150 mg/day in the morning; if dose is well tolerated, ↑ to 300 mg/day in one wk. Doses should be tapered to 150 mg/day for 2 wk before discontinuing.

Smoking cessation
PO (Adults): *Zyban*—150 mg once daily for 3 days, then 150 mg twice daily for 7–12 wk (doses should be at least 8 hr apart).

Availability (generic available)
Tablets: 75 mg, 100 mg. **Cost:** *Generic*—75 mg $54.99/90, 100 mg $66.99/90. **Sustained-release tablets:** 100 mg, 150 mg, 200 mg. **Cost:** *Generic*—100 mg $189.97/180, 150 mg $163.93/180, 200 mg $334.96/180. **Extended-release tablets (Wellbutrin XL):** 150 mg, 300 mg. **Cost:** *Generic*—150 mg $367.97/90, 300 mg $365.96/90. **Extended-release tablets (Aplenzin):** 174 mg, 348 mg, 522 mg.

NURSING IMPLICATIONS
Assessment
- Monitor mood changes. Inform health care professional if patient demonstrates significant increase in anxiety, nervousness, or insomnia.
- Assess mental status and mood changes, especially during initial few months of therapy and during dose changes. Risk may be increased in children, adolescents, and adults ≤24 yrs. Inform health care professional if patient demonstrates significant increase in signs of depression (depressed mood, loss of interest in usual activities, significant change in weight and/or appetite, insomnia or hypersomnia, psychomotor agitation or retardation, increased fatigue, feelings of guilt or worthlessness, slowed thinking or impaired concentration, suicide attempt or suicidal ideation). Restrict amount of drug available to patient.
- *Lab Test Considerations:* Monitor hepatic and renal function closely in patients with kidney or liver impairment to prevent ↑ serum and tissue bupropion concentrations.

Potential Nursing Diagnoses
Ineffective coping (Indications)

Implementation
- Do not confuse bupropion with buspirone. Do not administer bupropion (Wellbutrin) with Zyban, which contain the same ingredients.
- Administer doses in equally spaced time increments during the day to minimize the risk of seizures. Risk of seizures increases four fold in doses greater than 450 mg per day.
- May be initially administered concurrently with sedatives to minimize agitation. This is not usually required after the 1st wk of therapy.
- Insomnia may be decreased by avoiding bedtime doses. May require treatment during 1st wk of therapy.
- May be administered with food to lessen GI irritation.
- Nicotine patches, gum, inhalers, and spray may be used concurrently with bupropion.
- When converting from other brands of bupropion to *Aplenzin*, 348 mg/day *Aplenzin* is equivalent to 300 mg/day bupropion HCl and 174 mg/day *Aplenzin* is equivalent to 150 mg/day bupropion HCl.
- **PO:** Sustained-release or extended-release tablets should be swallowed whole; do not break, crush, or chew.
- **Seasonal Affective Disorder:** Begin administration in autumn prior to the onset of depressive symptoms. Continue therapy through win-

ter and begin to taper and discontinue in early spring.

Patient/Family Teaching
- Instruct patient to take bupropion as directed. Take missed doses as soon as possible and space day's remaining doses evenly at not less than 4-hr intervals. Missed doses for smoking cessation should be omitted. Do not double doses or take more than prescribed. May require 4 wk or longer for full effects. Do not discontinue without consulting health care professional. May require gradual reduction before discontinuation.
- May impair judgment or motor and cognitive skills. Caution patient to avoid driving and other activities requiring alertness until response to medication is known.
- Advise patient, family, and caregivers to look for suicidality, especially during early therapy or dose changes. Notify health care professional immediately if thoughts about suicide or dying, attempts to commit suicide, new or worse depression or anxiety, agitation or restlessness, panic attacks, insomnia, new or worse irritability, aggressiveness, acting on dangerous impulses, mania, or other changes in mood or behavior occur.
- Advise patient to avoid alcohol during therapy and to consult with health care professional before taking other medications with bupropion, such as Zyban.
- Inform patient that frequent mouth rinses, good oral hygiene, and sugarless gum or candy may minimize dry mouth. If dry mouth persists for more than 2 wk, consult health care professional regarding use of saliva substitute.
- Advise patient to notify health care professional if rash or other troublesome side effects occur.
- Inform patient that unused shell of XL tablets may appear in stool; this is normal.
- Advise patient to use sunscreen and protective clothing to prevent photosensitivity reactions.
- Instruct female patients to inform health care professional if pregnancy is planned or suspected.
- Advise patient to notify health care professional of medication regimen before treatment or surgery.
- Emphasize the importance of follow-up exams to monitor progress. Encourage patient participation in psychotherapy.
- **Smoking Cessation:** Smoking should be stopped during the 2nd week of therapy to allow for the onset of bupropion and to maximize the chances of quitting.
- Advise patient to stop taking bupropion and contact a health care professional immediately if agitation, depressed mood, and any changes in behavior that are not typical of nicotine withdrawal, or if suicidal thoughts or behavior occur.

Evaluation/Desired Outcomes
- Increased sense of well-being.
- Renewed interest in surroundings. Acute episodes of depression may require several months of treatment.
- Cessation of smoking.

---

busPIRone (byoo-**spye**-rone)
BuSpar

Classification
Therapeutic: antianxiety agents

Pregnancy Category B

Indications
Management of anxiety.

Action
Binds to serotonin and dopamine receptors in the brain. Increases norepinephrine metabolism in the brain. **Therapeutic Effects:** Relief of anxiety.

Pharmacokinetics
Absorption: Rapidly absorbed.
Distribution: Unknown.
Protein Binding: 95% bound to plasma proteins.
Metabolism and Excretion: Extensively metabolized by the liver (CYP3A4 enzyme system); 20–40% excreted in feces.
Half-life: 2–3 hr.

TIME/ACTION PROFILE (relief of anxiety)

ROUTE	ONSET	PEAK	DURATION
PO	7–10 days	3–4 wk	unknown

Contraindications/Precautions
Contraindicated in: Hypersensitivity; Severe hepatic or renal impairment; Concurrent use of MAO inhibitors; Ingestion of large amounts of grapefruit juice.
Use Cautiously in: Patients receiving other antianxiety agents (other agents should be slowly withdrawn to prevent withdrawal or rebound phenomenon); Patients receiving other psychotropics; Lactation, OB, Pedi: Safety not established.

Adverse Reactions/Side Effects
CNS: dizziness, drowsiness, excitement, fatigue, headache, insomnia, nervousness, weakness, personality changes. **EENT:** blurred vision, nasal congestion, sore throat, tinnitus, altered taste or smell, conjunctivitis. **Resp:** chest congestion, hyperventilation, shortness of breath. **CV:** chest pain, palpitations, tachycardia, hypertension, hypotension, syncope. **GI:** nausea, abdominal pain, constipation, diarrhea, dry mouth, vomiting. **GU:** changes in libido, dysuria, urinary frequency, urinary hesitancy. **Derm:** rashes, alopecia, blisters, dry skin, easy bruising, edema, flushing, pruritus. **Endo:** irregular menses. **MS:** myalgia. **Neuro:** incoordination, numbness, paresthesia, tremor. **Misc:** clamminess, sweating, fever.

Interactions
Drug-Drug: Use with **MAO inhibitors** may result in hypertension and is not recommended. **Erythromycin**, **nefazodone**, **ketoconazole**, **itraconazole**, **ritonavir**, and other **inhibitors of CYP3A4** ↑ blood levels and effects of buspirone; dose reduction is recommended (decrease to 2.5 mg twice daily with erythromycin, decrease to 2.5 mg once daily with nefazodone). **Rifampin**, **dexamethasone**, **phenytoin**, **phenobarbital**, **carbamazepine**, and other **inducers of CYP3A4** ↓ blood levels and effects of buspirone; dose adjustment may be necessary. Avoid concurrent use with **alcohol**.
Drug-Natural Products: Concomitant use of **kava-kava**, **valerian**, or **chamomile** can ↑ CNS depression.
Drug-Food: Grapefruit juice ↑ serum levels and effect; ingestion of large amounts of grapefruit juice is not recommended.

Route/Dosage
PO (Adults): 7.5 mg twice daily; increase by 5 mg/day q 2–4 days as needed (not to exceed 60 mg/day). Usual dose is 20–30 mg/day (in 2 divided doses).

Availability (generic available)
Tablets: 5 mg, 7.5 mg, 10 mg, 15 mg, 30 mg. **Cost:** *Generic* — 5 mg $79.97/180, 7.5 mg $110.97/180, 10 mg $128.99/180, 15 mg $129.40/180, 30 mg $267.93/180.

NURSING IMPLICATIONS
Assessment
- Assess degree and manifestations of anxiety before and periodically during therapy.
- Buspirone does not appear to cause physical or psychological dependence or tolerance. However, patients with a history of drug abuse should be assessed for tolerance or dependence. Restrict amount of drug available to these patients.

Potential Nursing Diagnoses
Anxiety (Indications)
Risk for injury (Side Effects)

Implementation
- Do not confuse buspirone with bupropion.
- Patients changing from other antianxiety agents should receive gradually decreasing doses. Buspirone will not prevent withdrawal symptoms.
- PO: May be administered with food to minimize gastric irritation. Food slows but does not alter extent of absorption.

Patient/Family Teaching
- Instruct patient to take buspirone exactly as directed. Take missed doses as soon as possible if not just before next dose; do not double doses. Do not take more than amount prescribed.
- May cause dizziness or drowsiness. Caution patient to avoid driving or other activities requiring alertness until response to the medication is known.
- Advise patient to avoid concurrent use of alcohol or other CNS depressants.
- Advise patient to consult health care professional before taking OTC medications or herbal products with this drug.
- Instruct patient to notify health care professional if any chronic abnormal movements occur (dystonia, motor restlessness, involuntary movements of facial or cervical muscles) or if pregnancy is suspected.
- Emphasize the importance of follow-up exams to determine effectiveness of medication.

Evaluation/Desired Outcomes
- Increase in sense of well-being.
- Decrease in subjective feelings of anxiety. Some improvement may be seen in 7–10 days. Optimal results take 3–4 wk of therapy. Buspirone is usually used for short-term therapy (3–4 wk). If prescribed for long-term therapy, efficacy should be periodically assessed.

HIGH ALERT

busulfan (byoo-sul-fan)
Busulfex, Myleran

Classification
Therapeutic: antineoplastics
Pharmacologic: alkylating agents

Pregnancy Category D

busulfan 253

Indications
PO: Treatment of chronic myelogenous leukemia (CML) and bone marrow disorders. **IV:** With cyclophosphamide as a conditioning regimen before allogenic hematopoietic progenitor cell transplantation for CML.

Action
Disrupts nucleic acid function and protein synthesis (cell-cycle phase–nonspecific). **Therapeutic Effects:** Death of rapidly growing cells, especially malignant ones.

Pharmacokinetics
Absorption: Rapidly absorbed from the GI tract.
Distribution: Unknown.
Metabolism and Excretion: Extensively metabolized by the liver.
Half-life: 2.5 hr.

TIME/ACTION PROFILE (effects on blood counts)

ROUTE	ONSET	PEAK	DURATION
PO	1–2 wk	weeks	up to 1 mo†
IV	unknown	unknown	13 days‡

†Complete recovery may take up to 20 mo
‡After administration of last dose

Contraindications/Precautions
Contraindicated in: Hypersensitivity; Failure to respond to previous courses; OB, Lactation: Potential for serious side effects in fetus or infant. **Use Cautiously in:** Active infections; ↓ bone marrow reserve; Obese patients (base dose on ideal body weight); Other chronic debilitating diseases; Patients with childbearing potential; Geri: Begin therapy at lower end of dose range due to ↑ frequency of impaired cardiac, hepatic, or renal function.

Adverse Reactions/Side Effects
Incidence and severity of adverse reactions and side effects are increased with IV use.
CNS: *IV*—SEIZURES, CEREBRAL HEMORRHAGE/COMA, anxiety, confusion, depression, dizziness, headache, encephalopathy, mental status changes, weakness. **EENT:** *PO*—cataracts; *IV*, epistaxis, pharyngitis, ear disorders. **CV:** hepatic veno-oclusive disease (↑ allogenic transplantation). **Resp:** *PO*—PULMONARY FIBROSIS; *IV*, alveolar hemorrhage, asthma, atelectasis, cough, hemoptysis, hypoxia, pleural effusion, pneumonia, rhinitis, sinusitis. **CV:** *PO*—CARDIAC TAMPONADE (WITH HIGH-DOSE CYCLOPHOSPHAMIDE); *IV*, chest pain, hypotension, tachycardia, thrombosis, arrhythmias, atrial fibrillation, cardiomegaly, ECG changes, edema, heart block, hypertension, left-sided heart failure, pericardial effusion, ventricular extrasystoles. **GI:** *PO*—drug-induced hepatitis, nausea, vomiting; *IV*, abdominal enlargement, anorexia, constipation, diarrhea, dry mouth, hematemesis, nausea, rectal discomfort, vomiting, abdominal pain, dyspepsia, hepatomegaly, pancreatitis, stomatitis. **GU:** oliguria, dysuria, hematuria. **Derm:** *PO*—itching, rashes, acne, alopecia, erythema nodosum, exfoliative dermatitis, hyperpigmentation. **Endo:** *PO*—sterility, gynecomastia. **F and E:** hypokalemia, hypomagnesemia, hypophosphatemia. **Hemat:** BONE MARROW DEPRESSION. **Local:** inflammation/pain at injection site. **Metab:** *PO and IV*—hyperuricemia; *IV*, hyperglycemia. **MS:** arthralgia, myalgia, back pain. **Misc:** allergic reactions, chills, fever, infection.

Interactions
Drug-Drug: Concurrent or previous (within 72 hr) use of **acetaminophen** may ↓ elimination and ↑ toxicity. Concurrent use with high-dose **cyclophosphamide** in patients with thalassemia may result in cardiac tamponade. Concurrent use with **itraconazole** or **phenytoin** ↓ blood level effectiveness. Long-term continuous therapy with **thioguanine** may ↑ risk of hepatic toxicity. ↑ bone marrow suppression with other **antineoplastics** or **radiation therapy**. May ↓ the antibody response to and ↑ risk of adverse reactions from **live-virus vaccines**.

Route/Dosage
Many other regimens are used. See current protocols for up-to-date dosage.
PO (Adults): *Induction*—1.8 mg/m^2/day or 60 mcg (0.06 mg)/kg/day until WBCs <15,000/mm^3. Usual dose is 4–8 mg/day (range 1–12 mg/day). *Maintenance*—1–3 mg/day.
PO (Children): 0.06–0.12 mg/kg/day or 1.8–4.6 mg/m^2/day initially. Titrate dose to maintain WBC of approximately 20,000/mm^3.
IV (Adults): 0.8 mg/kg q 6 hr (dose based on ideal body weight or actual weight, whichever is less; in obese patients, dosage should be based on adjusted ideal body weight) for 4 days (total of 16 doses); given in combination with cyclophosphamide.

Availability
Tablets: 2 mg. **Solution for injection:** 6 mg/mL.

NURSING IMPLICATIONS
Assessment
- **High Alert:** Monitor for bone marrow depression. Assess for bleeding (bleeding gums, bruising, petechiae, guaiac stools, urine, emesis) and avoid IM injections and taking rectal temperatures. Apply pressure to venipuncture sites for at least 10 min. Assess for signs of infection (fever, chills, sore throat, cough, hoarseness, lower back or side pain, difficult or painful urination) during neutropenia. Anemia may occur. Monitor for increased fatigue, dyspnea, and orthostatic hypotension. Notify health care professional if these symptoms occur.
- Monitor intake and output ratios and daily weights. Report significant changes in totals.
- Monitor for symptoms of gout (increased uric acid, joint pain, lower back or side pain, swelling of feet or lower legs). Encourage patient to drink at least 2 L of fluid each day. Allopurinol may be given to decrease uric acid levels. Alkalinization of urine may be ordered to increase excretion of uric acid.
- Assess for pulmonary fibrosis (fever, cough, shortness of breath) periodically during and after therapy. Discontinue therapy at the first sign of pulmonary fibrosis. Usually occurs 8 mo–10 yr (average 4 yr) after initiation of therapy.
- **IV:** Premedicate patient with phenytoin before IV administration to minimize the risk of seizures.
- Administer antiemetics before IV administration and on a fixed schedule throughout IV administration.
- **Lab Test Considerations:** Monitor CBC with differential and platelet count before and weekly during therapy. The nadir of leukopenia occurs within 10–15 days and the nadir of WBC at 11–30 days. Recovery usually occurs within 12–20 wk. Notify physician if WBC is <15,000/mm³ or if a precipitous drop occurs. Institute thrombocytopenia precautions if platelet count is <150,000/mm³. Bone marrow depression may be severe and progressive, with recovery taking 1 mo–2 yr after discontinuation of therapy.
- Monitor serum ALT, bilirubin, alkaline phosphatase, and uric acid before and periodically during therapy. May cause ↑ uric acid levels.
- May cause false-positive cytology results of breast, bladder, cervix, and lung tissues.

Potential Nursing Diagnoses
Disturbed body image (Side Effects)
Risk for injury (Side Effects)
Risk for infection (Side Effects)

Implementation
- **High Alert:** Fatalities have occurred with chemotherapeutic agents. Before administering, clarify all ambiguous orders; double check single, daily, and course-of-therapy dose limits; have second practitioner independently double check original order, calculations, and infusion pump settings.
- **PO:** Administer at the same time each day. Administer on an empty stomach to decrease nausea and vomiting.

IV Administration
- **IV:** Prepare solution in a biologic cabinet. Wear gloves, gown, and mask while handling IV medication. Discard IV equipment in specially designated containers.
- **Intermittent Infusion:** *Diluent:* Dilute with 10 times the volume of busulfan using 0.9% NaCl or D5W. *Concentration:* ≥0.5 mg/mL. When drawing busulfan from vial, use needle with 5-micron nylon filter provided, remove calculated volume from vial, remove needle and filter, replace needle and inject busulfan into diluent. Do not use polycarbonate syringes with busulfan. Only use filters provided with busulfan. Always add busulfan to diluent, not diluent to busulfan. Solution diluted with 0.9% NaCl or D5W is stable for 8 hr at room temperature and solution diluted with 0.9% NaCl is stable for 12 hr if refrigerated. Administration must be completed during this time. Solution is clear and colorless; do not administer solutions that are discolored or contain a precipitate. *Rate:* Administer via central venous catheter over 2 hr every 6 hr for 4 days for a total of 16 doses. Use infusion pump to administer entire dose over 2 hr.
- **Y-Site Compatibility:** acyclovir, amphotericin B liposome, anidulafungin, bivalirudin, bleomycin, caspofungin, codeine, daptomycin, dexmedetomidine, diltiazem, docetaxel, ertapenem, fenoldopam, granisetron, hetastarch, hydromorphone, levofloxacin, linezolid, lorazepam, meperidine, metronidazole, milrinone, nesiritide, octreotide, ondansetron, paclitaxel, palonosetron, pancuronium, piperacillin/tazobactam, quinupristin/dalfopristin, rituximab, sodium acetate, tacrolimus, tigecycline, tirofiban, trastuzumab, vasopressin.

BUTALBITAL COMPOUND

(byoo-**tal**-bi-tal)

butalbital, acetaminophen†
Axocet, Bucet, Bupap, Butex Forte, Dolgic, Marten-Tab, Phrenilin, Phrenilin Forte, Repap CF, Sedapap, Tencon, Triaprin

butalbital, acetaminophen, caffeine†
Endolor, Esgic, Esgic-Plus, Fioricet, Margesic, Medigesic, Repan, Triad

butalbital, aspirin, caffeine‡
Fiorinal, Fiortal, ✲Tecnal

Classification
Therapeutic: nonopioid analgesics (combination with barbiturate)
Pharmacologic: barbiturates

Schedule III (products with aspirin only)

Pregnancy Category D

†For information on acetaminophen component in formulation, see acetaminophen monograph

‡For information on aspirin component in formulation, see salicylates monograph

Indications
Management of mild to moderate pain.

Action
Contain an analgesic (aspirin or acetaminophen) for relief of pain, a barbiturate (butalbital) for its sedative effect, and some contain caffeine, which may be of benefit in vascular headaches. **Therapeutic Effects:** Decreased severity of pain with some sedation.

Pharmacokinetics
Absorption: Well absorbed.
Distribution: Widely distributed; cross the placenta and enter breast milk.
Metabolism and Excretion: Mostly metabolized by the liver.
Half-life: 35 hr.

TIME/ACTION PROFILE

ROUTE	ONSET	PEAK	DURATION
PO	15–30 min	1–2 hr	2–6 hr

Contraindications/Precautions
Contraindicated in: Hypersensitivity to individual components; Cross-sensitivity may occur; Co-

- **Y-Site Incompatibility:** idarubicin, thiotepa, vecuronium, voriconazole.

Patient/Family Teaching
- Instruct patient to take medication as directed, at the same time each day, even if nausea and vomiting are a problem. Consult health care professional if vomiting occurs shortly after dose is taken. If a dose is missed, do not take at all; do not double doses.
- Advise patient to notify health care professional if fever; sore throat; signs of infection; lower back or side pain; difficult or painful urination; sores in the mouth or on the lips; chills; dyspnea; persistent cough; bleeding gums; bruising; petechiae; or blood in urine, stool, or emesis occurs. Instruct patient to use soft toothbrush and electric razor. Caution patient not to drink alcoholic beverages or take products containing aspirin or NSAIDs.
- Caution patient to avoid crowds and persons with known infections. Health care professional should be informed immediately if symptoms of infection occur.
- Discuss with patient the possibility of hair loss. Explore methods of coping.
- Review with patient the need for contraception during therapy. Women need to use contraception even if amenorrhea occurs.
- Instruct patient not to receive any vaccinations without advice of health care professional.
- Advise patient to notify health care professional if unusual bleeding; bruising; or flank, stomach, or joint pain occurs. Advise patients on long-term therapy to notify health care professional immediately if cough, shortness of breath, and fever occur or if darkening of skin, diarrhea, dizziness, fatigue, anorexia, confusion, or nausea and vomiting become pronounced.
- Inform patient of increased risk of a second malignancy with busulfan.

Evaluation/Desired Outcomes
- Decrease in leukocyte count to within normal limits.
- Decreased night sweats.
- Increase in appetite.
- Increased sense of well-being. Therapy is resumed when leukocyte count reaches 50,000/mm^3.

BUTALBITAL COMPOUND

matose patients or those with pre-existing CNS depression; Uncontrolled severe pain; Aspirin should be avoided in patients with bleeding disorders or thrombocytopenia; Acetaminophen should be avoided in patients with severe hepatic or renal disease; Caffeine should be avoided in patients with severe cardiovascular disease; Pregnancy or lactation; Porphyria.

Use Cautiously in: History of suicide attempt or drug addiction; Chronic alcohol use/abuse (for aspirin and acetaminophen content); Geri: Appears on Beers list. Geriatric patients are at increased risk for side effects (dosage reduction recommended); Use should be short-term only; Children (safety not established).

Adverse Reactions/Side Effects
CNS: *caffeine*—drowsiness, hangover, delirium, depression, excitation, headache (with chronic use), insomnia, irritability, lethargy, nervousness, vertigo. **Resp:** respiratory depression. **CV:** *caffeine*—palpitations, tachycardia. **GI:** *caffeine*—constipation, diarrhea, epigastric distress, heartburn, nausea, vomiting. **Derm:** dermatitis, rash. **Misc:** hypersensitivity reactions including ANGIOEDEMA and SERUM SICKNESS, physical dependence, psychological dependence, tolerance.

Interactions
Drug-Drug: Additive CNS depression with other **CNS depressants**, including **alcohol**, **antihistamines**, **antidepressants**, **opioid analgesics**, and **sedative/hypnotics**. May increase the liver metabolism and decrease the effectiveness of other drugs including **hormonal contraceptives**, **chloramphenicol**, **acebutolol**, **propranolol**, **metoprolol**, **timolol**, **doxycycline**, **corticosteroids**, **tricyclic antidepressants**, **phenothiazines**, **phenylbutazone**, and **quinidine**. **MAO inhibitors**, **primidone**, and **valproic acid** may prevent metabolism and increase the effectiveness of butalbital. May enhance the hematologic toxicity of **cyclophosphamide**.
Drug-Natural Products: **St. John's wort** may decrease barbiturate effect. Concurrent use of **kava-kava**, **valerian**, **skullcap**, **chamomile**, or **hops** can increase CNS depression.

Route/Dosage
PO (Adults): 1–2 capsules or tablets (50–100 mg butalbital) every 4 hr as needed for pain (not to exceed 4 g acetaminophen or aspirin/24 hr).

Availability (generic available)
Tablets and capsules: 50 mg. *In combination with:* aspirin, acetaminophen, caffeine, and codeine Rx. See Appendix B.

NURSING IMPLICATIONS
Assessment
- Assess type, location, and intensity of pain before and 60 min following administration.
- Prolonged use may lead to physical and psychological dependence and tolerance. This should not prevent patient from receiving adequate analgesia. Most patients who receive butalbital compound for pain do not develop psychological dependence.
- Assess frequency of use. Frequent, chronic use may lead to daily headaches in headache-prone individuals because of physical dependence on caffeine and other components. Chronic headaches from overmedication are difficult to treat and may require hospitalization for treatment and prophylaxis.

Potential Nursing Diagnoses
Acute pain (Indications)
Risk for injury (Side Effects)

Implementation
- Do not confuse Fiorinal with Fioricet.
- Explain therapeutic value of medication before administration to enhance the analgesic effect.
- Regularly administered doses may be more effective than prn administration. Analgesic is more effective if given before pain becomes severe.
- Medication should be discontinued gradually after long-term use to prevent withdrawal symptoms.
- **PO:** Oral doses should be administered with food, milk, or a full glass of water to minimize GI irritation.

Patient/Family Teaching
- Instruct patient to take medication exactly as directed. Do not increase dose because of the habit-forming potential of butalbital. If medication appears less effective after a few weeks, consult health care professional. Doses of acetaminophen or aspirin should not exceed the maximum recommended daily dose. Chronic excessive use of >4 g/day (2 g in chronic alcoholism) may lead to hepatotoxicity, renal or cardiac damage.
- Advise patients with vascular headaches to take medication at first sign of headache. Lying down in a quiet, dark room may also be helpful. Medications taken for prophylaxis should be continued.
- May cause drowsiness or dizziness. Advise patient to avoid driving and other activities requiring alertness until response to medication is known.

- Caution patient to avoid concurrent use of alcohol or other CNS depressants.
- Advise patient to use an additional nonhormonal method of contraception while taking butalbital compound.

Evaluation/Desired Outcomes
- Decrease in severity of pain without a significant alteration in level of consciousness.

butenafine, See ANTIFUNGALS (TOPICAL).

butoconazole, See ANTIFUNGALS (VAGINAL).

HIGH ALERT

butorphanol (byoo-**tor**-fa-nole)
Stadol, Stadol NS

Classification
Therapeutic: opioid analgesics
Pharmacologic: opioid agonists/antagonists

Schedule IV

Pregnancy Category C

Indications
Management of moderate to severe pain. Analgesia during labor. Sedation before surgery. Supplement in balanced anesthesia.

Action
Binds to opiate receptors in the CNS. Alters the perception of and response to painful stimuli while producing generalized CNS depression. Has partial antagonist properties that may result in opioid withdrawal in physically dependent patients. **Therapeutic Effects:** Decreased severity of pain.

Pharmacokinetics
Absorption: Well absorbed from IM sites and nasal mucosa.
Distribution: Crosses the placenta and enters breast milk.
Metabolism and Excretion: Mostly metabolized by the liver; 11–14% excreted in the feces. Minimal renal excretion.
Half-life: 3–4 hr.

TIME/ACTION PROFILE (analgesia)

ROUTE	ONSET	PEAK	DURATION
IM	within 15 min	30–60 min	3–4 hr
IV	within mins	4–5 min	2–4 hr
Intranasal	within 15 min	1–2 hr	4–5 hr

Contraindications/Precautions
Contraindicated in: Hypersensitivity; Patients physically dependent on opioids (may precipitate withdrawal).
Use Cautiously in: Head trauma; Increased intracranial pressure; Severe renal, hepatic, or pulmonary disease (increase interval to q 6–8 hr initially in hepatic/renal impairment); Hypothyroidism; Adrenal insufficiency; Alcoholism; Undiagnosed abdominal pain; Prostatic hyperplasia; OB, Lactation, Pedi: Safety not established but has been used during labor (may cause respiratory depression in the newborn); Geri: Decrease usual dose by 50%; give at twice the usual interval initially.

Adverse Reactions/Side Effects
CNS: confusion, dysphoria, hallucinations, sedation, euphoria, floating feeling, headache, unusual dreams. **EENT:** blurred vision, diplopia, miosis (high doses). **Resp:** respiratory depression. **CV:** hypertension, hypotension, palpitations. **GI:** nausea, constipation, dry mouth, ileus, vomiting. **GU:** urinary retention. **Derm:** sweating, clammy feeling. **Misc:** physical dependence, psychological dependence, tolerance.

Interactions
Drug-Drug: Use with extreme caution in patients receiving **MAO inhibitors** (may produce severe, potentially fatal reactions—reduce initial dose of butorphanol to 25% of usual dose). Additive CNS depression with **alcohol, antidepressants, antihistamines**, and **sedative/hypnotics**. May precipitate withdrawal in patients who are physically dependent on **opioids** and have not been detoxified. May ↓ effects of concurrently administered **opioids**.
Drug-Natural Products: Concomitant use of **kava-kava**, **valerian**, **chamomile**, or **hops** can ↑ CNS depression.

Route/Dosage
IM (Adults): 2 mg q 3–4 hr as needed (range 1–4 mg).
IV (Adults): 1 mg q 3–4 hr as needed (range 0.5–2 mg).
IM, IV (Geriatric Patients): 1 mg q 4–6 hr, increased as necessary.

Intranasal (Adults): 1 mg (1 spray in 1 nostril) initially. An additional dose may be given 60–90 min later. This sequence may be repeated in 3–4 hr. If pain is severe, an initial dose of 2 mg (1 spray in each nostril) may be given. May be repeated in 3–4 hr.
Intranasal (Geriatric Patients): 1 mg (1 spray in 1 nostril) initially. An additional dose may be given 90–120 min later. This sequence may be repeated in 3–4 hr.

Availability (generic available)
Injection: 1 mg/mL, 2 mg/mL. **Intranasal solution:** 10 mg/mL, in 2.5-mL metered-dose spray pump (14–15 doses; 1 mg/spray).

NURSING IMPLICATIONS
Assessment
- Assess type, location, and intensity of pain before and 30–60 min after IM, 5 min after IV, and 60–90 min after intranasal administration. When titrating opioid doses, increases of 25–50% should be administered until there is either a 50% reduction in the patient's pain rating on a numerical or visual analogue scale or the patient reports satisfactory pain relief. A repeat dose can be safely administered at the time of the peak if previous dose is ineffective and side effects are minimal. Patients requiring doses higher than 4 mg should be converted to an opioid agonist. Butorphanol is not recommended for prolonged use or as first-line therapy for acute or cancer pain.
- An equianalgesic chart (see Appendix K) should be used when changing routes or when changing from one opioid to another.
- Assess blood pressure, pulse, and respirations before and periodically during administration. If respiratory rate is <10/min, assess level of sedation. Dose may need to be decreased by 25–50%. Respiratory depression does not increase in severity, only in duration, with increased dosage.
- Assess previous analgesic history. Antagonistic properties may induce withdrawal symptoms (vomiting, restlessness, abdominal cramps, increased blood pressure and temperature) in patients who are physically dependent on opioid agonists.
- Butorphanol has a lower potential for dependence than other opioids; however, prolonged use may lead to physical and psychological dependence and tolerance. This should not prevent the patient from receiving adequate analgesia. Most patients receiving butorphanol for pain do not develop psychological dependence.

If tolerance develops, changing to an opioid agonist may be required to relieve pain.
- ***Lab Test Considerations:*** May cause ↑ serum amylase and lipase levels.
- ***Toxicity and Overdose:*** If an opioid antagonist is required to reverse respiratory depression or coma, naloxone (Narcan) is the antidote. Dilute the 0.4-mg ampule of naloxone in 10 mL of 0.9% NaCl and administer 0.5 mL (0.02 mg) by direct IV push every 2 min. For children and patients weighing <40 kg, dilute 0.1 mg of naloxone in 10 mL of 0.9% NaCl for a concentration of 10 mcg/mL and administer 0.5 mcg/kg every 1–2 min. Titrate dose to avoid withdrawal, seizures, and severe pain.

Potential Nursing Diagnoses
Acute pain (Indications)
Risk for injury (Side Effects)
Disturbed sensory perception (visual, auditory) (Side Effects)

Implementation
- ***High Alert:*** Accidental overdosage of opioid analgesics has resulted in fatalities. Before administering, clarify all ambiguous orders; have second practitioner independently check original order, dose calculations, route of administration, and infusion pump programming. Do not confuse Stadol with Haldol.
- Explain therapeutic value of medication before administration to enhance the analgesic effect.
- Regularly administered doses may be more effective than prn administration. Analgesic is more effective if given before pain becomes severe.
- Coadministration with nonopioid analgesics may have additive analgesic effects and permit lower opioid doses.
- **IM:** Administer IM injections deep into well-developed muscle. Rotate sites of injections.

IV Administration
- **Direct IV:** ***Diluent:*** May give IV undiluted. ***Concentration:*** 1–2 mg/mL. ***Rate:*** Administer over 3–5 min. ***High Alert:*** Rapid administration may cause respiratory depression, hypotension, and cardiac arrest.
- **Syringe Compatibility:** atropine, chlorpromazine, cimetidine, diphenhydramine, droperidol, fentanyl, hydroxyzine, meperidine, metoclopramide, midazolam, morphine, pentazocine, perphenazine, prochlorperazine, promethazine, scopolamine, thiethylperazine.
- **Syringe Incompatibility:** dimenhydrinate, pentobarbital.
- **Y-Site Compatibility:** allopurinol sodium, amifostine, aztreonam, bivalirudin, cefepime,

cisatracurium, cladribine, dexmedetomidine, docetaxel, doxorubicin liposome, enalaprilat, esmolol, etoposide phosphate, fenoldopam, filgrastim, fludarabine, gemcitabine, granisetron, labetalol, linezolid, melphalan, nicardipine, oxaliplatin, paclitaxel, pemetrexed, piperacillin/tazobactam, propofol, remifentanil, sargramostim, teniposide, thiotepa, vinorelbine.

- **Y-Site Incompatibility:** amphotericin B cholesteryl sulfate complex, lansoprazole, midazolam.
- **Intranasal:** Administer 1 spray in 1 nostril.

Patient/Family Teaching

- Instruct patient on how and when to ask for pain medication.
- Medication may cause drowsiness or dizziness. Advise patient to call for assistance when ambulating and to avoid driving or other activities requiring alertness until response to the medication is known.
- Encourage patients on bedrest to turn, cough, and deep-breathe every 2 hr to prevent atelectasis.
- Instruct patient to change positions slowly to minimize orthostatic hypotension.
- Caution patient to avoid concurrent use of alcohol or other CNS depressants with this medication.
- Advise patient that good oral hygiene, frequent mouth rinses, and sugarless gum or candy may decrease dry mouth.
- **Intranasal:** Instruct patient on proper use of nasal spray. See package insert for detailed instructions. Instruct patient to replace protective clip and clear cover after use and to store the unit in the child resistant container. Caution patient that medication should not be used by anyone other than the person for whom it was prescribed. Excess medication should be disposed of as soon as it is no longer needed. To dispose of, unscrew cap, rinse bottle and pump with water, and dispose of in waste can.
- If 2-mg dose is prescribed, administer additional spray in other nostril. May cause dizziness and dysphoria. Patient should remain recumbent after administration of 2-mg dose until response to medication is known.

Evaluation/Desired Outcomes

- Decrease in severity of pain without a significant alteration in level of consciousness or respiratory status.

cabergoline (ka-ber-goe-leen)

Classification
Therapeutic: antihyperprolactinemic
Pharmacologic: dopamine agonists

Pregnancy Category B

Indications
Treatment of hyperprolactinemia (idiopathic or pituitary in origin). **Unlabeled Use:** Adjunctive treatment of Parkinson's disease.

Action
Inhibits secretion of prolactin by acting as a dopamine agonist. In Parkinson's, dopamine agonists directly stimulate neural dopamine receptors.
Therapeutic Effects: Decreased secretion of prolactin in hyperprolactinemia. Reduced involuntary movements associated with Parkinson's disease.

Pharmacokinetics
Absorption: Well absorbed but undergoes extensive first-pass hepatic metabolism.
Distribution: Widely distributed; concentrates in pituitary.
Metabolism and Excretion: Extensively metabolized by the liver; <4% excreted unchanged in urine.
Protein Binding: 40–42%.
Half-life: 63–69 hr.

TIME/ACTION PROFILE (effect on serum prolactin levels)

ROUTE	ONSET	PEAK	DURATION
PO	unknown	2–3 hr	unknown

Contraindications/Precautions
Contraindicated in: Hypersensitivity to cabergoline or ergot alkaloids; Uncontrolled hypertension; History of pulmonary, pericardial, valvular, or retroperitoneal fibrotic disorders; Lactation: Has been associated with hypertension, stroke, and seizures. Not to be used for suppression of physiologic lactation.
Use Cautiously in: Hepatic impairment; OB: Use in pregnancy only if clearly needed; Pedi: Safety not established.

Adverse Reactions/Side Effects
CNS: dizziness, headache, depression, drowsiness, fatigue, nervousness, vertigo, weakness.
Resp: PULMONARY FIBROSIS, pleural effusion.
EENT: abnormal vision. **CV:** VALVULAR DISORDERS, postural hypotension, hot flashes. **GI:** constipation, nausea, abdominal pain, dyspepsia, vomiting. **GU:** dysmenorrhea. **Endo:** breast pain. **Neuro:** paresthesia.

Interactions
Drug-Drug: ↑ risk of hypotension with **antihypertensives**. May ↑ the effects of **sibutramine**, **SSRIs**, and other **serotonin agonists** (induces serotonin syndrome). Effectiveness may be ↓ by **phenothiazines**, **butyrophenones** (**haloperidol**), **thioxanthenes**, or **metoclopramide** (avoid concurrent use).

Route/Dosage
PO (Adults): 0.25 mg twice weekly; may be ↑ at 4-wk intervals up to 1 mg twice weekly.

Availability (generic available)
Tablets: 0.5 mg.

NURSING IMPLICATIONS

Assessment
- Monitor blood pressure before and frequently during initial therapy. Initial doses >1 mg may cause orthostatic hypotension. Use with caution when administering concurrently with other medications that lower blood pressure. Supervise ambulation and transfer during initial dosing to prevent injury from hypotension.
- Evaluate the cardiac status and consider echocardiography periodically in patients receiving long-term treatment. Monitor for signs or symptoms of valvular disorders (dyspnea, edema, CHF, new cardiac murmur). Use lowest dose and reassess need for therapy periodically.
- **Parkinson's Disease:** Assess symptoms (restlessness or desire to keep moving, rigidity, tremors, pill rolling, masklike face, shuffling gait, muscle spasms, twisting motions, difficulty speaking or swallowing, loss of balance control) before and during therapy.
- *Lab Test Considerations:* Monitor serum prolactin concentrations monthly until normalized (<20 mcg/liter in women and <15 mcg/liter in men).

Potential Nursing Diagnoses
Risk for injury (Side Effects)
Impaired physical mobility (Indications)

Implementation
- **PO:** May be taken without regard to food.

Patient/Family Teaching
- Instruct patient to take medication exactly as directed. Take missed doses as soon as possible within 1 or 2 days. If not remembered until time of next dose, double dose. If nausea occurs, discuss with health care professional.
- May cause drowsiness and dizziness. Caution patient to avoid driving and other activities requiring alertness until response to medication is known.
- Advise patient to change positions slowly to minimize orthostatic hypotension.
- Caution patient to avoid concurrent use of alcohol during therapy.
- Advise women to consult with health care professional regarding a nonhormonal method of birth control. Women should contact health care professional promptly if pregnancy is planned or suspected.
- Instruct patients taking cabergoline for pituitary tumors to inform health care professional immediately if signs of tumor enlargement occur (blurred vision, sudden headache, severe nausea, and vomiting).
- Advise patient to notify health care professional if signs of valvular disorders (shortness of breath, swelling in extremities) occurs.
- Emphasize the importance of regular follow-up exams to determine effectiveness and monitor side effects.

Evaluation/Desired Outcomes
- Decrease in galactorrhea in patients with hyperprolactinemia.
- After a normal serum prolactin level has been maintained for more than 6 mo, cabergoline may be discontinued. Serum prolactin levels should be monitored periodically to determine necessity of reinstituting cabergoline.
- Decrease in tremor, rigidity, and bradykinesia.
- Improvement in balance and gait in patients with Parkinson's disease.

---

caffeine citrate
(ka-**feen** si-trate)
Cafcit

Classification
Therapeutic: central nervous system stimulants
Pharmacologic: respiratory stimulants

Pregnancy Category C

Indications
Short-term treatment of idiopathic apnea of prematurity in infants between 28 and <33 wk gestational age.

Action
Increases levels of cyclic AMP by inhibiting phosphodiesterase. Acts as a bronchial smooth muscle relaxant. Suggested mechanisms of action include: Stimulation of the respiratory center, Increased minute ventilation, Decreased threshold to hypercapnea, Increased response to hypercapnea, Increased skeletal muscle tone, Decreased diaphragmatic fatigue, Increased metabolic rate, Increased oxygen consumption. **Therapeutic Effects:** Decrease in periods of apnea.

Pharmacokinetics
Absorption: IV administration results in complete bioavailability; also absorbed after oral administration.
Distribution: Rapidly distributes to the brain; CSF levels in neonates are similar to plasma levels.
Metabolism and Excretion: Mostly metabolized by the liver (cytochrome P450 1A2) enzymes; 3–8% converted to theophylline.
Half-life: Infants >9 months, Children, and Adults: 5 hr; *Neonates*—3–4 days.

TIME/ACTION PROFILE

ROUTE	ONSET	PEAK	DURATION
IV	rapid	end of infusion	24 hr
PO	rapid	30 min–2 hr	24 hr

Contraindications/Precautions
Contraindicated in: Hypersensitivity.
Use Cautiously in: History of seizure disorders; History of cardiovascular disease; Pedi: Increased risk of toxicity in neonates with impaired hepatic or renal function.

Adverse Reactions/Side Effects
CNS: insomnia, irritability, jitteriness, restlessness. **CV:** tachycardia. **GI:** NECROTIZING ENTEROCOLITIS, feeding intolerance, gastritis, GI bleeding. **GU:** increased urine output. **Derm:** dry skin, rash, skin breakdown. **Endo:** hypoglycemia, hyperglycemia. **MS:** muscle tremors, twitches.

Interactions
Drug-Drug: Cimetidine, fluconazole, and ketoconazole ↓ metabolism (dose reduction of caffeine may be necessary). **Phenobarbital** and **phenytoin** may ↑ caffeine metabolism (↑ doses of caffeine may be necessary). Because caffeine is a significant metabolite of **theophylline**, concurrent administration is not recommended.

Route/Dosage
IV (Neonates): *Loading dose* — 20 mg/kg caffeine citrate (10 mg/kg caffeine base).
IV, PO (Neonates): *Maintenance dose* — starting 24 hr after loading dose 5 mg/kg caffeine citrate (2.5 mg/kg caffeine base) q 24 hr.

Availability (generic available)
Solution for injection: 20 mg/mL caffeine citrate (10 mg/mL caffeine base) in 3-mL vials. **Oral solution:** 20 mg/mL caffeine citrate (10 mg/mL caffeine base) in 3-mL vials.

NURSING IMPLICATIONS

Assessment
- Assess respiratory status frequently throughout therapy.
- Monitor patient for signs of necrotizing enterocolitis (abdominal distension, vomiting, bloody stools, lethargy). May be fatal.
- **Lab Test Considerations:** Monitor serum caffeine levels before and periodically during therapy in infants previously treated with theophylline or in infants whose mothers consumed caffeine before delivery.
- Monitor serum glucose levels. May cause hypoglycemia or hyperglycemia.
- **Lab Test Considerations:** Therapeutic range: 8–20 mcg/mL.
- ***Toxicity and Overdose:*** Serum caffeine levels of >50 mcg/mL have been associated with serious toxicity. Monitor serum levels and adjust dose in neonates with impaired hepatic or renal function to avoid toxicity.

Potential Nursing Diagnoses
Ineffective breathing pattern (Indications)

Implementation
- **PO:** Maintenance doses may also be administered orally.

IV Administration
- **Intermittent Infusion:** Solution should be clear, without particulate matter. ***Rate:*** Initial *loading dose* should be administered over 30 min. *Maintenance doses* may be administered over 10 min every 24 hr beginning 24 hr after loading dose. Syringe pump should be used to ensure accurate delivery.
- **Syringe Compatibility:** alprostadil, amikacin, aminophylline, calcium gluconate, cefotaxime, cimetidine, clindamycin, dexamethasone, dobutamine, dopamine, epinephrine, fentanyl, gentamicin, heparin, isoproterenol, lidocaine, metoclopramide, morphine, nitroprusside, pancuronium, penicillin G, phenobarbital, phenylephrine, sodium bicarbonate, vancomycin.
- **Syringe Incompatibility:** acyclovir, furosemide, lorazepam, nitroglycerin, oxacillin, pantoprazole.
- **Y-Site Compatibility:** doxapram, levofloxacin.
- **Additive Compatibility:** amino acids, calcium gluconate, D5W, D50W, dopamine, fat emulsion, heparin, fentanyl.

Patient/Family Teaching
- Instruct parent on correct technique for administration. Measure oral dose accurately with a 1-mL syringe. If apnea events continue, consult health care professional; do not increase dose.
- Advise parent to consult health care professional immediately if signs of necrotizing enterocolitis occur.

Evaluation/Desired Outcomes
- Decrease in apneic episodes in premature infant.

CALCITONIN

calcitonin (salmon)
(kal-si-**toe**-nin)
Miacalcin

calcitonin (rDNA)
Fortical

Classification
Therapeutic: hypocalcemics
Pharmacologic: hormones

Pregnancy Category C

Indications
IM, Subcut: Treatment of Paget's disease of bone. Adjunctive therapy for hypercalcemia. **IM, Subcut, Intranasal:** Management of postmenopausal osteoporosis.

Action
Inhibits osteoclastic bone resorption and promotes renal excretion of calcium. **Therapeutic Effects:** Decreased rate of bone turnover. Lowering of serum calcium.

Pharmacokinetics
Absorption: Completely absorbed from IM and subcut sites. Rapidly absorbed from nasal mu-

cosa; absorption is 3% compared with parenteral administration.
Distribution: Unknown.
Metabolism and Excretion: Rapidly metabolized in kidneys, blood, and tissues.
Half-life: 40–90 min.

TIME/ACTION PROFILE

ROUTE	ONSET	PEAK	DURATION
IM, subcut†	Unknown	2 hr	6–8 hr
Intranasal‡	rapid	31–39 min	Unknown

†Effects on serum calcium; effects on serum alkaline phosphates and urinary hydroxyproline in Paget's disease may require 6–24 months of continuous treatment
‡Serum levels of administered calcitonin

Contraindications/Precautions
Contraindicated in: Hypersensitivity to calcitonin, salmon protein or gelatin diluent (in some products); OB, Lactation: Use is not recommended.
Use Cautiously in: Pedi: Safety not established.

Adverse Reactions/Side Effects
CNS: *nasal only*—headaches. **EENT:** *nasal only*—rhinitis, epistaxis, nasal irritation. **GI:** *IM, subcut*—nausea, vomiting. **GU:** *IM, subcut*—urinary frequency. **Derm:** rashes. **Local:** injection site reactions. **MS:** *nasal*—arthralgia, back pain. **Misc:** allergic reactions including ANAPHYLAXIS, facial flushing, swelling.

Interactions
Drug-Drug: Previous bisphosphonate therapy, including **alendronate**, **risedronate**, **etidronate**, **ibandronate** or **pamidronate**, may ↓ response to calcitonin.

Route/Dosage
Postmenopausal osteoporosis
IM, Subcut (Adults): 100 IU every other day.
Intranasal (Adults): 1 spray (200 IU)/day in alternating nostrils.

Paget's disease
IM, Subcut (Adults): 100 IU/day initially, after titration, maintenance dose is usually 50 IU/day or every other day.

Hypercalcemia
IM, Subcut (Adults): 4 IU/kg q 12 hr; if adequate response not achieved, may increase dose after 1–2 days to 8 IU/kg q 12 hr, and if necessary after 2 more days may be increased to 8 IU/kg q 6 hr.

Availability (generic available)
Injection : 200 IU/mL in 2-mL vials. **Cost:** $50.89/vial. **Nasal spray:** 200 IU/actuation in 3.7-mL bottles. **Cost:** *Miacalcin*—$112.22/bottle.

NURSING IMPLICATIONS
Assessment
- Observe patient for signs of hypersensitivity (skin rash, fever, hives, anaphylaxis, serum sickness). Keep epinephrine, antihistamines, and oxygen nearby in the event of a reaction.
- Assess patient for signs of hypocalcemic tetany (nervousness, irritability, paresthesia, muscle twitching, tetanic spasms, seizures) during the first several doses of calcitonin. Parenteral calcium, such as calcium gluconate, should be available in case of this event.
- **Intranasal:** Assess nasal mucosa, septum, turbinates, and mucosal blood vessels periodically during therapy. If severe ulceration occurs, drug should be discontinued.
- *Lab Test Considerations:* Monitor serum calcium and alkaline phosphatase periodically during therapy. Levels should normalize within a few months of initiation of therapy.
- Urine hydroxyproline (24 hr) may be monitored periodically in patients with Paget's disease.

Potential Nursing Diagnoses
Acute pain (Indications)
Risk for injury (Indications, Side Effects)

Implementation
- In patients with suspected sensitivity to calcitonin, skin test should be considered before starting therapy. Test dose is prepared in a dilution of 10 IU/mL by withdrawing 0.05 mL in a tuberculin syringe and filling to 1 mL with 0.9% NaCl for injection. Mix well and discard 0.9 mL. Administer 0.1 mL intradermally on inner aspect on forearm and observe site for 15 min. More than mild erythema or wheal constitutes positive response.
- Store injection and unopened nasal spray bottle in refrigerator. Nasal spray bottle in use can be stored at room temperature.
- **IM, Subcut:** Inspect injection site for the appearance of redness, swelling, or pain. Rotate injection sites. Subcut is the preferred route. Use IM route if dose exceeds 2 mL in volume. Use multiple sites to minimize inflammatory reaction.

Patient/Family Teaching
- Advise patient to take calcitonin as directed. If dose is missed and medication is scheduled for twice a day, take only if possible within 2 hr of correct time. If scheduled for daily dose, take

only if remembered that day. If scheduled for every other day, take when remembered and restart alternate day schedule. If taking 1 dose 3 times weekly (Mon, Wed, Fri), take missed dose the next day and set each injection back 1 day; resume regular schedule the following week. Do not double doses.
- Instruct patient in the proper method of self-injection and care and disposal of equipment.
- Advise patient to report signs of hypercalcemic relapse (deep bone or flank pain, renal calculi, anorexia, nausea, vomiting, thirst, lethargy) or allergic response promptly.
- Reassure patient that flushing and warmth following injection are transient and usually last about 1 hr.
- Explain that nausea following injection tends to decrease even with continued therapy.
- Instruct patient to follow low-calcium diet if recommended by health care professional (see Appendix M). Women with postmenopausal osteoporosis should adhere to a diet high in calcium and vitamin D.
- **Osteoporosis:** Advise patients receiving calcitonin for the treatment of osteoporosis that exercise has been found to arrest and reverse bone loss. The patient should discuss any exercise limitations with health care professional before beginning program.
- **Intranasal:** Instruct patient on correct use of nasal spray. Demonstrate procedure for use. Before first use, activate pump by holding upright and depressing white side arms down toward bottle 5 times until a full spray is emitted. Following activation, place nozzle firmly in nostril with head in an upright position and depress the pump toward the bottle. The pump should NOT be primed before each daily use. Discard bottle 30 days after first use.
- Advise patient to notify health care professional if significant nasal irritation occurs.

Evaluation/Desired Outcomes
- Lowered serum calcium levels.
- Decreased bone pain.
- Slowed progression of postmenopausal osteoporosis. Significant increases in bone marrow density may be seen as early as 6 months after initiation of therapy.

---

calcitriol, See VITAMIN D COMPOUNDS.

CALCIUM SALTS

calcium acetate (25% Ca or 12.6 mEq/g)
(**kal**-see-um **ass**-e-tate)
PhosLo

calcium carbonate (40% Ca or 20 mEq/g)
(**kal**-see-um **kar**-bo-nate)
Alka-Mints, Amitone, ✤Apo-Cal, BioCal, Calcarb, Calci-Chew, Calciday, Calcilac, Calci-Mix, ✤Calcite, ✤Calglycine, Cal-Plus, ✤Calsan, Caltrate, Chooz, Dicarbosil, Equilet, Gencalc, Liqui-Cal, Liquid Cal-600, Maalox Antacid Caplets, Mallamint, ✤Mylanta Lozenges, Nephro-Calci, ✤Nu-Cal, Os-Cal, Oysco, Oyst-Cal, Oystercal, Rolaids Calcium Rich, Surpass, Surpass Extra Strength, Titralac, Tums, Tums E-X

calcium chloride (27% Ca or 13.6 mEq/g)
(**kal**-see-um **kloh**-ride)

calcium citrate (21% Ca or 12 mEq/g) (**kal**-see-um **si**-trate)
Cal-Citrate 250, Citrical, Citrical Liquitab

calcium gluconate (9% Ca or 4.5 mEq/g)
(**kal**-see-um **gloo**-koh-nate)
Kalcinate

calcium lactate (13% Ca or 6.5 mEq/g) (**kal**-see-um **lak**-tate)
Cal-Lac

tricalcium phosphate (39% Ca or 19.5 mEq/g)
(tri-**kal**-see-um **foss**-fate)
Posture

Classification
Therapeutic: mineral and electrolyte replacements/supplements

Pregnancy Category C (calcium acetate, calcium chloride, calcium gluconate injections), UK (calcium carbonate, calcium citrate, calcium lactate, tricalcium phosphate)

Indications
PO, IV: Treatment and prevention of hypocalcemia. **PO:** Adjunct in the prevention of postmenopausal osteoporosis. **IV:** Emergency treatment of hyperkalemia and hypermagnesemia and adjunct in cardiac arrest or calcium channel blocking agent toxicity (calcium chloride, calcium gluconate). **Calcium carbonate:** May be used as an antacid. **Calcium acetate:** Control of hyperphosphatemia in end-stage renal disease.

Action
Essential for nervous, muscular, and skeletal systems. Maintain cell membrane and capillary permeability. Act as an activator in the transmission of nerve impulses and contraction of cardiac, skeletal, and smooth muscle. Essential for bone formation and blood coagulation. **Therapeutic Effects:** Replacement of calcium in deficiency states. Control of hyperphosphatemia in end-stage renal disease without promoting aluminum absorption (calcium acetate).

Pharmacokinetics
Absorption: Absorption from the GI tract requires vitamin D. IV administration results in complete bioavailability.
Distribution: Readily enters extracellular fluid. Crosses the placenta and enters breast milk.
Metabolism and Excretion: Excreted mostly in the feces; 20% eliminated by the kidneys.
Half-life: Unknown.

TIME/ACTION PROFILE (effects on serum calcium)

ROUTE	ONSET	PEAK	DURATION
PO	unknown	unknown	unknown
IV	immediate	immediate	0.5–2 hr

Contraindications/Precautions
Contraindicated in: Hypercalcemia; Renal calculi; Ventricular fibrillation.
Use Cautiously in: Patients receiving digitalis glycosides; Severe respiratory insufficiency; Renal disease; Cardiac disease.

Adverse Reactions/Side Effects
CNS: syncope (IV only), tingling. **CV:** CARDIAC ARREST (IV only), arrhythmias, bradycardia. **GI:** constipation, nausea, vomiting. **GU:** calculi, hypercalciuria. **Local:** phlebitis (IV only).

Interactions
Drug-Drug: Hypercalcemia ↑ the risk of **digoxin** toxicity. Chronic use with **antacids** in renal insufficiency may lead to milk-alkali syndrome. Ingestion by mouth ↓ the absorption of orally administered **tetracyclines**, **fluoroquinolones**, **phenytoin**, and **iron salts**. Excessive amounts may ↓ the effects of **calcium channel blockers**. ↓ absorption of **etidronate** and **risedronate** (do not take within 2 hr of calcium supplements). Concurrent use with **diuretics (thiazide)** may result in hypercalcemia. May ↓ the ability of **sodium polystyrene sulfonate** to decrease serum potassium.
Drug-Food: Cereals, spinach, or rhubarb may ↓ the absorption of calcium supplements. Calcium acetate should not be given concurrently with other calcium supplements.

Route/Dosage
Doses are expressed in mg, g, or mEq of calcium.
PO (Adults): *Prevention of hypocalcemia, treatment of depletion, osteoporosis*—1–2 g/day. *Antacid*—0.5–1.5 g as needed (calcium carbonate only). *Hyperphosphatemia in end-stage renal disease (calcium acetate only)*—Amount necessary to control serum phosphate and calcium.

PO (Children): *Supplementation*—45–65 mg/kg/day.

PO (Infants): *Neonatal hypocalcemia*—50–150 mg/kg (not to exceed 1 g).

IV (Adults): *Emergency treatment of hypocalcemia, cardiac standstill*—7–14 mEq. *Hypocalcemic tetany*—4.5–16 mEq; repeat until symptoms are controlled. *Hyperkalemia with cardiac toxicity*—2.25–14 mEq; may repeat in 1–2 min. *Hypermagnesemia*—7 mEq.

IV (Children): *Emergency treatment of hypocalcemia*—1–7 mEq. *Hypocalcemic tetany*—0.5–0.7 mEq/kg 3–4 times daily.

IV (Infants): *Emergency treatment of hypocalcemia*—<1 mEq. *Hypocalcemic tetany*—2.4 mEq/kg/day in divided doses.

Availability (generic available)
Calcium Acetate
Tablets: 250 mg (65 mg Ca)^OTC, 667 mg (169 mg Ca)^OTC, 668 mg (169 mg Ca)^OTC, 1 g (250 mg Ca)^OTC. **Capsules:** 500 mg (125 mg Ca)^OTC.

Calcium Carbonate
Tablets: 500 mg (200 mg Ca)^OTC, 600 mg (240 mg Ca)^OTC, 650 mg (260 mg Ca)^OTC, 667 mg (266.8 mg Ca)^OTC, 1 g (400 mg Ca)^OTC, 1.25 g (500 mg Ca)^OTC, 1.5 g (600 mg Ca)^OTC. **Chewable tablets:** 350 mg (300 mg Ca)^OTC, 420 mg (168 mg Ca)^OTC, 450 mg ^OTC, 500 mg (200 mg Ca)^OTC, 750 mg (300 mg Ca)^OTC, 1 g (400 mg Ca)^OTC, 1.25 g (500 mg Ca)^OTC. **Gum tablets:** 300 mg ^OTC, 450 mg ^OTC, 500 mg (200 mg Ca)^OTC. **Capsules:** 1.25 g (500 mg Ca)^OTC. **Lozenges:** 600 mg (240 mg

CALCIUM SALTS

Ca)^{OTC}. **Oral suspension:** 1.25 g (500 mg Ca)/5 mL^{OTC}. **Powder:** 6.5 g (2400 mg Ca)/packet^{OTC}.

Calcium Chloride
Injection: 10% (1.36 mEq/mL).

Calcium Citrate
Tablets: 250 mg^{OTC}.

Calcium Gluconate
Tablets: 500 mg (45 mg Ca)^{OTC}, 650 mg (58.5 mg Ca)^{OTC}, 975 mg (87.75 mg Ca)^{OTC}, 1 g (90 mg Ca)^{OTC}. **Injection:** 10% (0.45 mEq/mL).

Calcium Lactate
Tablets: 325 mg (42.45 mg Ca)^{OTC}, 500 mg ^{OTC}, 650 mg (84.5 mg Ca)^{OTC}.

Tricalcium Phosphate
Tablets: 600 mg (234 mg Ca)^{OTC}.

NURSING IMPLICATIONS

Assessment
- **Calcium Supplement/Replacement:** Observe patient closely for symptoms of hypocalcemia (paresthesia, muscle twitching, laryngospasm, colic, cardiac arrhythmias, Chvostek's or Trousseau's sign). Notify health care professional if these occur. Protect symptomatic patients by elevating and padding siderails and keeping bed in low position.
- Monitor blood pressure, pulse, and ECG frequently throughout parenteral therapy. May cause vasodilation with resulting hypotension, bradycardia, arrhythmias, and cardiac arrest. Transient increases in blood pressure may occur during IV administration, especially in geriatric patients or in patients with hypertension.
- Assess IV site for patency. Extravasation may cause cellulitis, necrosis, and sloughing.
- Monitor patient on digoxin for signs of toxicity.
- **Antacid:** When used as an antacid, assess for heartburn, indigestion, and abdominal pain. Inspect abdomen; auscultate bowel sounds.
- *Lab Test Considerations:* Monitor serum calcium or ionized calcium, chloride, sodium, potassium, magnesium, albumin, and parathyroid hormone (PTH) concentrations before and periodically during therapy for treatment of hypocalcemia.
- May cause ↓ serum phosphate concentrations with excessive and prolonged use. When used to treat hyperphosphatemia in renal failure patients, monitor phosphate levels.
- *Toxicity and Overdose:* Assess patient for nausea, vomiting, anorexia, thirst, severe constipation, paralytic ileus, and bradycardia. Contact health care professional immediately if these signs of hypercalcemia occur.

Potential Nursing Diagnoses
Imbalanced nutrition: less than body requirements (Indications)
Risk for injury, related to osteoporosis or electrolyte imbalance (Indications)

Implementation
- *High Alert:* Errors with IV calcium gluconate and chloride have occurred secondary to confusion over which salt is ordered. Clarify incomplete orders. Confusion has occurred with milligram doses of calcium chloride and calcium gluconate, which are not equal. Chloride and gluconate forms are routinely available on most hospital crash carts; specify form of calcium desired. Doses should be expressed in mEq.
- Do not confuse Os-Cal (calcium carbonate) with Asacol (mesalamine).
- In arrest situations, the use of calcium chloride is now limited to patients with hyperkalemia, hypocalcemia, and calcium channel blocker toxicity.
- **PO:** Administer calcium carbonate or phosphate 1–1.5 hr after meals and at bedtime. Chewable tablets should be well chewed before swallowing. Dissolve effervescent tablets in glass of water. Follow oral doses with a full glass of water, except when using calcium carbonate as a phosphate binder in renal dialysis. Administer on an empty stomach before meals to optimize effectiveness in patients with hyperphosphatemia.
- **IM:** IM administration of calcium salts can cause severe necrosis and tissue sloughing. Do not administer IM.

IV Administration
- **IV:** IV solution should be warmed to body temperature and given through a small-bore needle in a large vein to minimize phlebitis. Do not administer through a scalp vein. May cause cutaneous burning sensation, peripheral vasodilation, and drop in blood pressure. Patient should remain recumbent for 30–60 min after IV administration.
- If infiltration occurs, discontinue IV. May be treated with application of heat, elevation, and local infiltration of normal saline, 1% procaine HCl, or hyaluronidase.

= Canadian drug name. = Genetic implication.
*CAPITALS indicates life-threatening; underlines indicate most frequent.

- **High Alert:** Administer slowly. High concentrations may cause cardiac arrest. Rapid administration may cause tingling, sensation of warmth, and a metallic taste. Halt infusion if these symptoms occur, and resume infusion at a slower rate when they subside.
- Do not administer solutions that are not clear or that contain a precipitate.

Calcium Chloride

IV Administration

- **Direct IV:** May be administered undiluted by IV push.
- **Intermittent/Continuous Infusion:** May be diluted with D5W, D10W, 0.9% NaCl, D5/0.25% NaCl, D5/0.45% NaCl, D5/0.9% NaCl, or D5/LR.
- **Rate:** Maximum rate for adults is 0.7–1.4 mEq/min (0.5–1 mL of 10% solution); for children, 0.5 mL/min.
- **Y-Site Compatibility:** acyclovir, alfentanil, amikacin, aminophylline, amiodarone, anidulafungin, ascorbic acid, atracurium, atropine, aztreonam, benztropine, bivalirudin, bleomycin, bumetanide, buprenorphine, butorphanol, calcium gluconate, carboplatin, caspofungin, cefonocid, cefotaxime, cefotetan, cefoxitin, ceftizoxime, chloramphenicol, chlorpromazine, cimetidine, clindamycin, cyanocobalamin, cyclophosphamide, cyclosporine, cytarabine, dactinomycin, daptomycin, dexmedetomidine, digoxin, diltiazem, diphenhydramine, dobutamine, docetaxel, dopamine, doxacurium, doxapram, doxorubicin, doxycycline, enalaprilat, ephedrine, epinephrine, epirubicin, epoetin alfa, eptifibatide, ertapenem, erythromycin, esmolol, etoposide, etoposide phosphate, famotidine, fenoldopam, fentanyl, fluconazole, fludarabine, furosemide, gemcitabine, gentamicin, glycopyrrolate, granisetron, heparin, hetastarch, hydromorphone, idarubicin, ifosfamide, inamrinone, insulin, isoproterenol, labetalol, lidocaine, linezolid, lorazepam, mannitol, mechlorethamine, meperidine, metaraminol, methotrexate, methoxamine, methyldopate, metoclopramide, metoprolol, metronidazole, micafungin, midazolam, milrinone, mitoxantrone, morphine, multivitamin, nafcillin, nalbuphine, naloxone, nesiritide, nitroglycerin, nitroprusside, norepinephrine, octreotide, ondansetron, oxaliplatin, oxytocin, paclitaxel, palonosetron, pancuronium, papaverine, penicillin G, pentazocine, pentobarbital, phenobarbital, phentolamine, phenylephrine, phytonadione, piperacillin/tazobactam, potassium chloride, procainamide, promethazine, propranolol, protamine, pyridoxime, ranitidine, rocuronium, streptokinase, succinylcholine, sufentanil, tacrolimus, teniposide, theophylline, thiamine, thiotepa, ticarcillin/clavulanate, tigecycline, tirofiban, tobramycin, tolazoline, trimetaphan, urokinase, vancomycin, vasopressin, vencuronium, verapamil, vincristine, vinorelbine, voriconazole.
- **Y-Site Incompatibility:** amphotericin B cholesteryl, amphotericin B colloidal, amphotericin B liposome, azathioprine, cefazolin, cefoperazone, ceftazidime, ceftriaxone, cefuroxime, dantrolene, dexamethasone, diazepam, diazoxide, fluorouracil, folic acid, haloperidol, hydrocortisone, indomethacin, ketorolac, magnesium sulfate, methylprednisolone, oxacillin, pantoprazole, pemetrexed, phenytoin, prochlorperazine, propofol, quinupristin/dalfopristin, sodium bicarbonate, trimethoprim/sulfamethoxazole.

Calcium Gluconate

IV Administration

- **Direct IV:** Administer slowly by direct IV push. **Rate:** Maximum administration rate for adults is 1.5–2 mL/min.
- **Continuous Infusion:** May be further diluted in 1000 mL of D5W, D10W, D20W, D5/0.9% NaCl, 0.9% NaCl, D5/LR, or LR.
- **Rate:** Administer at a rate not to exceed 200 mg/min over 12–24 hr.
- **Y-Site Compatibility:** acyclovir, aldesleukin, alfentanil, allopurinol, amifostine, amikacin, aminophylline, amiodarone, anidulafungin, ascorbic acid, atracurium, atropine, azathioprine, aztreonam, benztropine, bivalirudin, bleomycin, bumetanide, buprenorphine, butorphanol, calcium chloride, carboplatin, caspofungin, cefazolin, cefepime, cefonocid, cefoperazone, cefotaxime, cefotetan, cefoxitin, ceftazidime, ceftizoxime, cefuroxime, chloramphenicol, chlorpromazine, cimetidine, ciprofloxacin, cisatracurium, cisplatin, cladribine, clindamycin, codeine, cyanocobalamin, cyclophosphamide, cyclosporine, cytarabine, dactinomycin, daptomycin, dexmedetomidine, digoxin, diltiazem, diphenhydramine, dobutamine, docetaxel, dopamine, doripenem, doxacurium, doxapram, doxorubicin, doxorubicin liposome, doxycycline, enalaprilat, ephedrine, epinephrine, epirubicin, epoetin alfa, eptifibatide, ertapenem, erythromycin, esmolol, etoposide, etoposide phosphate, famotidine, fenoldopam, fentanykl, filgrastim, fludar-

abine, fluorouracil, folic acid, furosemide, ganciclovir, gemcitabine, gentamicin, glycopyrrolate, granisetron, heparin, hetastarch, hydromorphone, idarubicin, ifosfamide, insulin, isoproterenol, labetalol, levofloxacin, lidocaine, linezolid, lorazepam, magnesium sulfate, mannitol, mechlorethamine, melphalan, meperidine, metaraminol, methotrexate, methoxamine, methyldopate, metoclopramide, metoprolol, metronidazole, micafungin, midazolam, milrinone, mitoxantrone, morphine, multivitamins, nafcillin, nalbuphine, naloxone, nesiritide, nicardipine, nitroglycerin, nitroprusside, norepinephrine, octreotide, ondansetron, oxaliplatin, oxytocin, paclitaxel, palonosetron, pancuronium, pantoprazole, papaverine, penicillin G, pentamidine, pentaziocine, pentobarbital, phenobarbital, phentolamine, phenylephrine, phytonadione, piperacillin/tazobactam, potassium chloride, procainamide, promethazine, propofol, propranolol, protamine, pyridoxime, ranitidine, remifentanil, rituximab, rocuronium, sargramostim, sodium acetate, streptokinase, succinylcholine, sufentanil, tacrolimus, teniposide, theophylline, thiamine, thiotepa, ticarcillin/clavulanate, tigecycline, tirofiban, tobramycin, tolazoline, trastuzumab, trimetaphan, urokinase, vancomycin, vasopressin, vecuronium, verapamil, vincristine, vinorelbine, vitamin B complex with C, voriconazole.

- **Y-Site Incompatibility:** amphotericin B cholesteryl, amphotericin B colloidal, amphotericin B liposome, ceftriaxone, dantrolene, dexamethazone, diazepam, diazoxide, inamrinone, indomethacin, methylprednisolone, oxacillin, pemetrexed, phenytoin, quinupristin/dalfopristin, sodium bicarbonate, sodium phosphates, trimethoprim/sulfamethoxazole.

Patient/Family Teaching
- Instruct patient not to take enteric-coated tablets within 1 hr of calcium carbonate; this will result in premature dissolution of the tablets.
- Do not administer concurrently with foods containing large amounts of oxalic acid (spinach, rhubarb), phytic acid (brans, cereals), or phosphorus (milk or dairy products). Administration with milk products may lead to milk-alkali syndrome (nausea, vomiting, confusion, headache). Do not take within 1–2 hr of other medications if possible.
- Instruct patients on a regular schedule to take missed doses as soon as possible, then go back to regular schedule.
- Advise patient that calcium carbonate may cause constipation. Review methods of preventing constipation (increasing bulk in diet, increasing fluid intake, increasing mobility) and using laxatives. Severe constipation may indicate toxicity.
- Advise patient to avoid excessive use of tobacco or beverages containing alcohol or caffeine.
- **Calcium Supplement:** Encourage patients to maintain a diet adequate in vitamin D (see Appendix M).
- **Osteoporosis:** Advise patients that exercise has been found to arrest and reverse bone loss. Patient should discuss any exercise limitations with health care professional before beginning program.

Evaluation/Desired Outcomes
- Increase in serum calcium levels.
- Decrease in the signs and symptoms of hypocalcemia.
- Resolution of indigestion.
- Control of hyperphosphatemia in patients with renal failure (calcium acetate only).

---

candesartan, See ANGIOTENSIN II RECEPTOR ANTAGONISTS.

HIGH ALERT

capecitabine
(kap-pe-**site**-a-been)
Xeloda

Classification
Therapeutic: antineoplastics
Pharmacologic: antimetabolites

Pregnancy Category D

Indications
Metastatic colorectal cancer. Adjuvant treatment for Dukes' C colon cancer following primary resection. Metastatic breast cancer that has worsened despite prior therapy with anthracycline (daunorubicin, doxorubicin, idarubicin) (to be used in combination with docetaxel). Metastatic breast cancer that is resistant to both paclitaxel and an anthracycline (daunorubicin, doxorubicin, idarubicin) or is resistant to paclitaxel and further anthracycline therapy is contraindicated.

Action

⚠ Converted in tissue to 5-fluorouracil (5-FU), which inhibits DNA and RNA synthesis by preventing thymidine production. The enzyme responsible for the final step in the conversion to 5-FU may be found in higher concentrations in some tumors. **Therapeutic Effects:** Death of rapidly replicating cells, particularly malignant ones.

Pharmacokinetics

Absorption: Well absorbed after oral administration.
Distribution: Unknown.
Metabolism and Excretion: ⚠ Metabolized mostly in tissue and by the liver to 5-FU; 5-FU is metabolized by dihydropyrimidine dehydrogenase to a less toxic compound; inactive metabolites are excreted primarily in urine.
Half-life: 45 min.

TIME/ACTION PROFILE (blood levels)

ROUTE	ONSET	PEAK	DURATION
PO	unknown†	1.5 hr (2 hr for 5-FU)‡	unknown

†Onset of antineoplastic effect is 6 wk
‡Peak 5-FU levels occur at 2 hr

Contraindications/Precautions

Contraindicated in: Hypersensitivity to capecitabine or 5-FU; Dihydropyrimidine dehydrogenase deficiency ⚠ (patients at ↑ risk of 5-FU toxicity); Severe renal impairment (CCr <30 mL/min); OB: Potential for fetal harm or death; Lactation: Potential for serious adverse effects in nursing infants.
Use Cautiously in: Mild-moderate renal impairment (↓ starting dose to 75% in patients with CCr 30–50 mL/min); Hepatic dysfunction; Coronary artery disease; Pedi: Safety not established; Geri: ↑ risk of severe diarrhea in patients ≥80 yr.

Adverse Reactions/Side Effects

CNS: fatigue, headache, dizziness, insomnia. **EENT:** eye irritation, epistaxis, rhinorrhea. **CV:** edema, chest pain. **GI:** DIARRHEA, NECROTIZING ENTEROCOLITIS, abdominal pain, anorexia, constipation, dysgeusia, hyperbilirubinemia, nausea, stomatitis, vomiting, dyspepsia, xerostomia. **Derm:** dermatitis, hand-and-foot syndrome, nail disorder, alopecia, erythema, rashes. **F and E:** dehydration. **Hemat:** anemia, leukopenia, thrombocytopenia. **MS:** arthralgia, myalgia. **Neuro:** peripheral neuropathy. **Resp:** cough, dyspnea. **Misc:** fever.

Interactions

Drug-Drug: May ↑ risk of bleeding with **warfarin** (frequent monitoring of PT/INR recommended). Toxicity ↑ by concurrent **leucovorin**. **Antacids** may ↑ absorption. May ↑ blood levels and risk of toxicity from **phenytoin** (may need to ↓ phenytoin dose).
Drug-Food: Food ↑ absorption, although capecitabine should be given within 30 min after a meal.

Route/Dosage

PO (Adults): 1250 mg/m^2 twice daily for 14 days, followed by 7-day rest period; given in 3-wk cycles.

Renal Impairment

PO (Adults CCr 30-50 mL/min): ↓ initial dose to 75% of usual.

Availability

Tablets: 150 mg, 500 mg.

NURSING IMPLICATIONS

Assessment

- Assess mucous membranes, number and consistency of stools, and frequency of vomiting. Assess for signs of infection (fever, chills, sore throat, cough, hoarseness, pain in lower back or side, difficult or painful urination). Assess for bleeding (bleeding gums; bruising; petechiae; and guaiac-test stools, urine, and emesis). Avoid IM injections and taking rectal temperatures. Apply pressure to venipuncture sites for 10 min. Anemia may occur. Monitor for increased fatigue, dyspnea, and orthostatic hypotension.
- Notify health care professional if symptoms of toxicity (stomatitis, uncontrollable vomiting, diarrhea, fever) occur; drug may need to be discontinued or dose decreased. Patients with severe diarrhea should be monitored carefully and given fluid and electrolyte replacement if they become dehydrated.
- Assess patient for hand-and-foot syndrome. Symptoms include numbness, dysesthesia or paresthesia, tingling, painless or painful swelling, erythema, desquamation, blistering, and severe pain.
- *Lab Test Considerations:* Monitor hepatic (serum alkaline phosphatase, AST, ALT, and bilirubin), renal, and hematologic (hematocrit, hemoglobin, leukocyte, platelet count) function before and periodically during therapy. May cause leukopenia, anemia, and thrombocytopenia. Leukopenia may require discontinuation of therapy. Therapy should be interrupted

if serum bilirubin ↑ to 1.5 times normal or greater; may be reinstituted after bilirubin returns to normal.
- **Lab Test Considerations:** Monitor PT or INR frequently in patients receiving warfarin and capecitabine to adjust warfarin dose. May cause ↑ bleeding within a few days of initiation of therapy to 1 mo following discontinuation of therapy. Risk is greater in patients over 60 yr.

Potential Nursing Diagnoses
Risk for infection (Side Effects)
Imbalanced nutrition: less than body requirements (Side Effects)

Implementation
- **High Alert:** Fatalities have occurred with chemotherapeutic agents. Before administering, clarify all ambiguous orders; double-check single, daily, and course-of-therapy dose limits; have second practitioner independently double-check original order and dose calculations. Do not confuse capecitabine (Xeloda) with orlistat (Xenical).
- Dose modifications are based on degree of toxicity encountered. Once a dose has been reduced because of toxicity, it should not be increased at a later time. See manufacturer's recommendations.
- **PO:** Administer every 12 hr for 2 wk, followed by a 1-wk rest period. Tablets should be taken with water within 30 min after a meal.

Patient/Family Teaching
- Instruct patient to take medication every 12 hr with water within 30 min after a meal. Missed doses should be omitted; continue regular schedule. Do not double dose.
- Inform patient of the most common side effects. Instruct patient to notify health care provider immediately if any of the following occur: diarrhea (>4 bowel movements in a day or any diarrhea at night), vomiting (more than once in 24 hr), nausea (loss of appetite and significant decrease in daily food intake), stomatitis (pain, redness, swelling, or sore in mouth), hand-and-foot syndrome (pain, swelling, or redness of hands and/or feet), fever or infection (temperature of ≥100.5° F or other signs of infection).
- Instruct patient to notify health care professional if he or she is taking folic acid.
- Instruct patient to notify health care professional if fever; chills; sore throat; signs of infection; yellowing of skin or eyes; abdominal pain; joint or flank pain; swelling of feet or legs; bleeding gums; bruising; petechiae; or blood in urine, stool, or emesis occurs. Caution patient to avoid crowds and persons with known infections. Instruct patient to use soft toothbrush and electric razor. Patients should be cautioned not to drink alcoholic beverages or take products containing aspirin or NSAIDs.
- Advise patient to rinse mouth with clear water after eating and drinking and to avoid flossing to minimize stomatitis. Viscous lidocaine may be used if mouth pain interferes with eating. Stomatitis pain may require treatment with opioid analgesics.
- Review with patient the need for contraception during therapy.
- Emphasize the importance of routine follow-up lab tests to monitor progress and to check for side effects.

Evaluation/Desired Outcomes
- Tumor regression.

---

capsaicin (kap-**say**-sin)
✤Axsam, Capsin, Capzasin-P, Dolorac, No Pain-HP, Pain Doctor, Pain-X, R-Gel, Rid • a • Pain • HP, Zostrix, Zostrix-HP

Classification
Therapeutic: nonopioid analgesics (topical)

Pregnancy Category UK

Indications
Temporary management of pain due to rheumatoid arthritis and osteoarthritis. Treatment of pain associated with postherpetic neuralgia or diabetic neuropathy. **Unlabeled Use:** Treatment of postmastectomy pain syndrome. Treatment of complex regional pain syndrome.

Action
May deplete and prevent the reaccumulation of a chemical (substance P) responsible for transmitting painful impulses from peripheral sites to the CNS. **Therapeutic Effects:** Relief of discomfort associated with painful peripheral syndromes.

Pharmacokinetics
Absorption: Unknown.
Distribution: Unknown.
Metabolism and Excretion: Unknown.
Half-life: Unknown.

✤ = Canadian drug name. ❄ = Genetic implication.
*CAPITALS indicates life-threatening; underlines indicate most frequent.

TIME/ACTION PROFILE

ROUTE	ONSET	PEAK	DURATION
topical	1–2 wk	2–4 wk†	unknown

†May take up to 6 wk for head and neck neuralgias

Contraindications/Precautions
Contraindicated in: Hypersensitivity to capsaicin or hot peppers; Not for use near eyes or on open or broken skin.
Use Cautiously in: OB, Lactation, Pedi: Safety not established for pregnant women, breastfeeding infants, or children <2 yr.

Adverse Reactions/Side Effects
Resp: cough. **Derm:** transient burning.

Interactions
Drug-Drug: None significant.

Route/Dosage
Topical (Adults and Children ≥2 yr): Apply to affected areas 3–4 times daily.

Availability
Cream: 0.025%^OTC, 0.075%^OTC. **Gel:** 0.05%^OTC. **Lotion:** 0.025%^OTC. **Roll-on:** 0.075%^OTC. *In combination with:* methylsalicylate (Ziks^OTC). See Appendix B.

NURSING IMPLICATIONS

Assessment
- Assess pain intensity and location before and periodically throughout therapy.

Potential Nursing Diagnoses
Chronic pain (Indications)
Noncompliance (Patient/Family Teaching)

Implementation
- **Topical:** Apply to affected area not more than 3–4 times daily. Avoid getting medication into eyes or on broken or irritated skin. Do not bandage tightly.
- Topical lidocaine may be applied during the first 1–2 wk of treatment to reduce initial discomfort.

Patient/Family Teaching
- Instruct patient on the correct method for application of capsaicin. Rub cream into affected area well so that little or no cream is left on the surface. Gloves should be worn during application or hands should be washed immediately after application. If application is to hands for arthritis, do not wash hands for at least 30 min after application.
- Advise patient to apply missed doses as soon as possible unless almost time for next dose. Pain relief lasts only as long as capsaicin is used regularly.
- Advise patient that transient burning may occur with application, especially if applied fewer than 3–4 times daily. Burning usually disappears after the first few days but may continue for 2–4 wk or longer. Burning is increased by heat, sweating, bathing in warm water, humidity, and clothing. Burning usually decreases in frequency and intensity the longer capsaicin is used. Decreasing number of daily doses will not lessen burning but may decrease amount of pain relief and may prolong period of burning.
- Caution patient to flush area with water if capsaicin gets into eyes and to wash with warm, but not hot, soapy water if capsaicin gets on other sensitive areas of the body.
- Instruct patient with herpes zoster (shingles) not to apply capsaicin cream until lesions have healed completely.
- Advise patient to discontinue use and notify health care professional if pain persists longer than 1 month, worsens, or if signs of infection are present.

Evaluation/Desired Outcomes
- Decrease in discomfort associated with:
- Postherpetic neuropathy.
- Diabetic neuropathy.
- Rheumatoid arthritis.
- Osteoarthritis. Pain relief usually begins within 1–2 wk with arthritis, 2–4 wk with neuralgias, and 4–6 wk with neuralgias of the head and neck.

---

captopril, See ANGIOTENSIN-CONVERTING ENZYME (ACE) INHIBITORS.

---

carbamazepine
(kar-ba-**maz**-e-peen)
✦Apo-Carbamazepine, Carbatrol, Epitol, Equetro, ✦Novo-Carbamaz, Tegretol, ✦Tegretol CR, Tegretol-XR, Teril

Classification
Therapeutic: anticonvulsants, mood stabilizers

Pregnancy Category D

Indications
Treatment of tonic-clonic, mixed, and complex-partial seizures. Management of pain in trigeminal neuralgia or diabetic neuropathy. **Equetro only:**

carbamazepine

Acute mania and mixed mania. **Unlabeled Use:** Other forms of neurogenic pain.

Action
Decreases synaptic transmission in the CNS by affecting sodium channels in neurons. **Therapeutic Effects:** Prevention of seizures. Relief of pain in trigeminal neuralgia. Decreased mania.

Pharmacokinetics
Absorption: Absorption is slow but complete. Suspension produces earlier, higher peak, and lower trough levels.
Distribution: Widely distributed. Crosses the blood-brain barrier. Crosses the placenta rapidly and enters breast milk in high concentrations.
Protein Binding: *Carbamazepine*—75–90%; *epoxide*—50%.
Metabolism and Excretion: Extensively metabolized in the liver by cytochrome P450 3A4 to active epoxide metabolite; epoxide metabolite has anticonvulsant and antineuralgic activity.
Half-life: *Carbamazepine*—single dose—25–65 hr, chronic dosing—*Children*—8–14 hr; *Adults*—12–17 hr; *epoxide*—34±9 hr.

TIME/ACTION PROFILE (anticonvulsant activity)

ROUTE	ONSET	PEAK	DURATION
PO	up to one month†	4–5 hr‡	6–12 hr
PO-ER	up to one month†	2–3–12 hr‡	12 hr

†Onset of antineuralgic activity is 8–72 hr
‡Listed for tablets; peak level occurs 1.5 hr after a chronic dose of suspension

Contraindications/Precautions
Contraindicated in: Hypersensitivity; Bone marrow suppression; Concomitant use or use within 14 days of MAO inhibitors; OB: Use only during pregnancy if potential benefits outweigh risks to the fetus; additional vitamin K during last weeks of pregnancy has been recommended; Lactation: Discontinue drug or bottle feed.
Use Cautiously in: All patients (may ↑ risk of suicidal thoughts/behaviors); Cardiac or hepatic disease; Renal failure (dosing adjustment required for ClCr < 10 mL/min; ↑ intraocular pressure; Geri: Older men with prostatic hyperplasia may be at ↑ risk for acute urinary retention or difficulty initiating stream.
Exercise Extreme Caution in: ⚕ Patients positive for HLA-B*1502 allele (unless benefits clearly outweigh the risks).

Adverse Reactions/Side Effects
CNS: SUICIDAL THOUGHTS, ataxia, drowsiness, fatigue, psychosis, sedation, vertigo. **EENT:** blurred vision, nystagmus, corneal opacities. **Resp:** pneumonitis. **CV:** CHF, edema, hypertension, hypotension, syncope. **GI:** hepatitis, pancreatitis, weight gain. **GU:** hesitancy, urinary retention. **Derm:** photosensitivity, rashes, STEVENS-JOHNSON SYNDROME, TOXIC EPIDERMAL NECROLYSIS, urticaria. **Endo:** syndrome of inappropriate antidiuretic hormone (SIADH), hyponatremia. **Hemat:** AGRANULOCYTOSIS, APLASTIC ANEMIA, THROMBOCYTOPENIA, eosinophilia, leukopenia. **Misc:** chills, fever, lymphadenopathy, ↑ liver enzymes, multiorgan hypersensitivity reactions, hepatic failure (rare).

Interactions
Drug-Drug: May ↑ metabolism of and therefore ↓ levels/ effectiveness of **corticosteroids**, **doxycycline**, **felbamate**, **quinidine**, **warfarin**, **estrogen-containing contraceptives**, **barbiturates**, **cyclosporine**, **benzodiazepines**, **theophylline**, **lamotrigine**, **phenytoin**, **topiramate**, **valproic acid**, **bupropion**, and **haloperidol**. **Danazol** ↑ blood levels (avoid concurrent use if possible). Concurrent use (within 2 wk) of **MAO inhibitors** may result in hyperpyrexia, hypertension, seizures, and death. **Verapamil**, **diltiazem**, **propoxyphene**, **itraconazole**, **ketoconazole**, **erythromycin**, **clarithromycin**, **SSRIs**, **antidepressants**, or **cimetidine** may inhibit the hepatic metabolism of carbamazepine and ↑ levels; may cause toxicity. Enzyme inducers such as **rifampin**, **phenobarbital**, **phenytoin**, **primidone**, and **methosuximide** may ↓ serum concentration of carbamazepine. May ↑ risk of hepatotoxicity from **isoniazid**. **Felbamate** ↓ carbamazepine levels but ↑ levels of active metabolite. May ↓ effectiveness and ↑ risk of toxicity from **acetaminophen**. May ↑ risk of CNS toxicity from **lithium**. May ↓ duration of action of **nondepolarizing neuromuscular blocking agents**.
Drug-Food: Grapefruit juice ↑ serum levels and oral bioavailability by 40% and therefore may ↑ effects.

Route/Dosage
PO (Adults): *Anticonvulsant*—200 mg twice daily (tablets) or 100 mg 4 times daily (suspension); increase by 200 mg/day q 7 days until therapeutic levels are achieved (range is 600–1200 mg/day in divided doses q 6–8 hr; not to exceed

---
✚ = Canadian drug name. ⚕ = Genetic implication.
*CAPITALS indicates life-threatening; underlines indicate most frequent.

1 g/day in 12–15-yr-olds. Extended-release products are given twice daily (XR, CR). *Antineuralgic*— 100 mg twice daily or 50 mg 4 times daily (suspension); increase by up to 200 mg/day until pain is relieved, then maintenance dose of 200–1200 mg/day in divided doses (usual range, 400–800 mg/day).

PO (Children 6–12 yr): 100 mg twice daily (tablets) or 50 mg 4 times daily (suspension). ↑ by 100 mg weekly until therapeutic levels are obtained (usual range 400–800 mg/day; not to exceed 1 g/day). Extended-release products (XR, CR) are given twice daily.

PO (Children <6 yr): 10–20 mg/kg/day in 2–3 divided doses; may be ↑ at weekly intervals until optimal response and therapeutic levels are achieved. Usual maintenance dose is 250–350 mg/day (not to exceed 35 mg/kg/day).

Availability (generic available)
Tablets: 200 mg. **Cost:** *Generic*— $25.97/180. **Chewable tablets:** 100 mg, ❀ 200 mg. **Cost:** *Generic*— 100 mg $21.98/180. **Extended-release capsules:** 100 mg, 200 mg, 300 mg. **Cost:** 100 mg $235.66/180, 200 mg $226.49/180, 300 mg $216.88/180. **Extended-release tablets:** 100 mg, 200 mg, 400 mg. **Cost:** 100 mg $83.93/180, 200 mg $143.93/180, 400 mg $279.94/180. **Oral suspension (citrus/vanilla flavor):** 100 mg/5 mL. **Cost:** *Generic*— $28.26/450 mL.

NURSING IMPLICATIONS

Assessment
- Monitor closely for notable changes in behavior that could indicate the emergence or worsening of suicidal thoughts or behavior or depression.
- ❚ Monitor for changes in skin condition in early therapy. Stevens-Johnson syndrome and toxic epidermal necrolysis are significantly more common in patients with a particular human leukocyte antigen (HLA) allele, HLA-B*1502 (occurs almost exclusively in patients with Asian ancestry, including South Asian Indians). Screen patients of Asian ancestry for the HLA-B*1502 allele before starting treatment with carbamazepine. If positive, carbamazepine should not be started unless the expected benefit outweighs increased risk of serious skin reactions. Patients who have been taking carbamazepine for more than a few months without developing skin reactions are at low risk of these events ever developing.
- **Seizures:** Assess frequency, location, duration, and characteristics of seizure activity.
- **Trigeminal Neuralgia:** Assess for facial pain (location, intensity, duration). Ask patient to identify stimuli that may precipitate facial pain (hot or cold foods, bedclothes, touching face).
- **Bipolar Disorder:** Assess mental status (mood, orientation, behavior) and cognitive abilities before and periodically during therapy.
- *Lab Test Considerations:* Monitor CBC, including platelet count, reticulocyte count, and serum iron, weekly during the first 2 mo and yearly thereafter for evidence of potentially fatal blood cell abnormalities. Medication should be discontinued if bone marrow depression occurs.
- ❚ Perform genetic testing for the HLA-B*1502 allele in patients of Asian ancestry prior to beginning therapy.
- Liver function tests, urinalysis, and BUN should be routinely performed. May cause ↑ AST, ALT, serum alkaline phosphatase, bilirubin, BUN, urine protein, and urine glucose levels.
- Monitor serum ionized calcium levels every 6 mo or if seizure frequency increases. Thyroid function tests and ionized serum calcium concentrations may be ↓; hypocalcemia ↓ seizure threshold.
- Monitor ECG and serum electrolytes before and periodically during therapy. May cause hyponatremia.
- May occasionally cause ↑ serum cholesterol, high-density lipoprotein, and triglyceride concentrations.
- May cause false-negative pregnancy test results with tests that determine human chorionic gonadotropin.
- *Toxicity and Overdose:* Serum blood levels should be routinely monitored during therapy. Therapeutic levels range from 4–12 mcg/mL.

Potential Nursing Diagnoses
Risk for injury (Indications, Side Effects)
Chronic pain (Indications)
Disturbed thought process (Indications)

Implementation
- Implement seizure precautions as indicated.
- **PO:** Administer medication with food to minimize gastric irritation. May take at bedtime to reduce daytime sedation. Tablets may be crushed if patient has difficulty swallowing. Do not crush or chew extended-release tablets. Extended-release capsules may be opened and the contents sprinkled on applesauce or other similar foods.

- Do not administer suspension simultaneously with other liquid medications or diluents; mixture produces an orange rubbery mass.

Patient/Family Teaching
- Instruct patient to take carbamazepine around the clock, as directed. Take missed doses as soon as possible but not just before next dose; do not double doses. Notify health care professional if more than one dose is missed. Medication should be gradually discontinued to prevent seizures. Instruct patient to read the *Medication Guide* before starting and with each Rx refill; changes may occur.
- May cause dizziness or drowsiness. Advise patients to avoid driving or other activities requiring alertness until response to medication is known.
- Instruct patients that behavioral changes, skin rash, fever, sore throat, mouth ulcers, easy bruising, petechiae, unusual bleeding, abdominal pain, chills, rash, pale stools, dark urine, or jaundice should be reported to health care professional immediately. Advise patient and family to notify health care professional if thoughts about suicide or dying, attempts to commit suicide; new or worse depression; new or worse anxiety; feeling very agitated or restless; panic attacks; trouble sleeping; new or worse irritability; acting aggressive; being angry or violent; acting on dangerous impulses; an extreme increase in activity and talking, other unusual changes in behavior or mood occur.
- Inform patient that coating of *Tegretol XR* is not absorbed, but is excreted in feces and may be visible in stool.
- Advise patient not to take alcohol or other CNS depressants concurrently with this medication.
- Caution patients to use sunscreen and protective clothing to prevent photosensitivity reactions.
- Inform patient that frequent mouth rinses, good oral hygiene, and sugarless gum or candy may help reduce dry mouth. Saliva substitute may be used. Consult dentist if dry mouth persists >2 wk.
- Advise female patients to use a nonhormonal form of contraception while taking carbamazepine.
- Instruct patient to notify health care professional of medication regimen before treatment or surgery.
- Emphasize the importance of follow-up lab tests and eye exams to monitor for side effects.

- Inform patient and family that the Manic-Depressive and Depressive Association can offer support for mania.
- **Seizures:** Advise patients to carry identification describing disease and medication regimen at all times.

Evaluation/Desired Outcomes
- Absence or reduction of seizure activity.
- Decrease in trigeminal neuralgia pain. Patients with trigeminal neuralgia who are pain-free should be re-evaluated every 3 mo to determine minimum effective dose.
- Decreased mania and depressive symptoms in Bipolar I disorder.

---

carbidopa/levodopa
(kar-bi-doe-pa/lee-voe-doe-pa)
Parcopa, Sinemet, Sinemet CR

Classification
Therapeutic: antiparkinson agents
Pharmacologic: dopamine agonists

Pregnancy Category C (carbidopa/levodopa)

Indications
Parkinson's disease. Not useful for drug-induced extrapyramidal reactions.

Action
Levodopa is converted to dopamine in the CNS, where it serves as a neurotransmitter. Carbidopa, a decarboxylase inhibitor, prevents peripheral destruction of levodopa. **Therapeutic Effects:** Relief of tremor and rigidity in Parkinson's syndrome.

Pharmacokinetics
Absorption: Well absorbed following oral administration.
Distribution: Widely distributed. *Levodopa*—enters the CNS in small concentrations. *Carbidopa*—does not cross the blood-brain barrier but does cross the placenta. Both enter breast milk.
Metabolism and Excretion: *Levodopa*—mostly metabolized by the GI tract and liver. *Carbidopa*—30% excreted unchanged by the kidneys.
Half-life: *Levodopa*—1 hr; *carbidopa*—1–2 hr.

✦ = Canadian drug name.   ❦ = Genetic implication.
*CAPITALS indicates life-threatening; underlines indicate most frequent.

carbidopa/levodopa

TIME/ACTION PROFILE (antiparkinson effects)

ROUTE	ONSET	PEAK	DURATION
Carbidopa	unknown	unknown	5–24 hr
Levodopa	10–15 min	unknown	5–24 hr or more
Carbidopa/levodopa sustained release	unknown	2 hr	12 hr

Contraindications/Precautions

Contraindicated in: Hypersensitivity; Angle-closure glaucoma; MAO inhibitor therapy; Malignant melanoma; Undiagnosed skin lesions; Some products contain tartrazine, phenylalanine, or aspartame and should be avoided in patients with known hypersensitivity.
Use Cautiously in: History of cardiac, psychiatric, or ulcer disease; OB, Pedi: Safety not established; Lactation: May ↓ serum prolactin.

Adverse Reactions/Side Effects

CNS: involuntary movements, anxiety, dizziness, hallucinations, memory loss, psychiatric problems, urges (gambling, sexual). **EENT:** blurred vision, mydriasis. **GI:** nausea, vomiting, anorexia, dry mouth, hepatotoxicity. **Derm:** melanoma. **Hemat:** hemolytic anemia, leukopenia. **Misc:** darkening of urine or sweat.

Interactions

Drug-Drug: Use with **MAO inhibitors** may result in hypertensive reactions. ↑ risk of arrhythmias with **inhalation hydrocarbon anesthetics** (especially **halothane**; if possible discontinue 6–8 hr before anesthesia). **Phenothiazines, haloperidol, papaverine, phenytoin,** and **reserpine** may ↓ effect of levodopa. Large doses of **pyridoxine** may ↓ beneficial effects of levodopa. Concurrent use with **methyldopa** may alter the effectiveness of levodopa and ↑ risk of CNS side effects. ↑ hypotension may result with concurrent **antihypertensives**. **Anticholinergics** may ↓ absorption of levodopa. ↑ risk of adverse reactions with **selegilene** or **cocaine**.
Drug-Natural Products: Kava-kava may ↓ levodopa effectiveness.
Drug-Food: Ingestion of foods containing large amounts of **pyridoxine** may ↓ effect of levodopa.

Route/Dosage

Carbidopa/Levodopa

PO (Adults): 25 mg carbidopa/100 mg levodopa 3 times daily; may be ↑ every 1–2 days until desired effect is achieved (max = 8 tablets of 25 mg carbidopa/100 mg levodopa/day).

Carbidopa/Levodopa Extended-Release

PO (Adults): *Patients not currently receiving levodopa*— 50 mg carbidopa/200 mg levodopa twice daily (minimum of 6 hr apart) initially. *Conversion from standard carbidopa/levodopa*— initiate therapy with at least 10% more levodopa content/day (may need up to 30% more) given at 4–8 hr intervals while awake. Allow 3 days between dosage changes; some patients may require larger doses and shorter dosing intervals.

Availability

Carbidopa/Levodopa (generic available)
Tablets: 10 mg carbidopa/100 mg levodopa, 25 mg carbidopa/100 mg levodopa, 25 mg carbidopa/250 mg levodopa. **Orally-disintegrating tablets (mint):** 10 mg carbidopa/100 mg levodopa, 25 mg carbidopa/100 mg levodopa, 25 mg carbidopa/250 mg levodopa. **Extended-release tablets:** 25 mg carbidopa/100 mg levodopa, 50 mg carbidopa/200 mg levodopa. *In combination with:* entacapone (Stalevo); see Appendix B.

NURSING IMPLICATIONS

Assessment

- Assess parkinsonian symptoms (akinesia, rigidity, tremors, pill rolling, shuffling gait, mask-like face, twisting motions, and drooling) during therapy. "On-off phenomenon" may cause symptoms to appear or improve suddenly.
- Assess blood pressure and pulse frequently during period of dose adjustment.
- *Lab Test Considerations:* May cause false-positive test results in Coombs' test.
- May cause ↑ serum glucose. Dipstick for urine ketones may reveal false-positive results.
- Monitor hepatic and renal function and CBC periodically in patients on long-term therapy. May cause ↑ AST, ALT, bilirubin, alkaline phosphatase, LDH, and serum protein-bound iodine concentrations. May cause ↓ BUN, creatinine, and uric acid.
- May cause ↓ hemoglobin, ↓ hematocrit, agranulocytosis, hemolytic and nonhemolytic anemia, thrombocytopenia, leukopenia, and ↑ WBC.
- *Toxicity and Overdose:* Assess for signs of toxicity (involuntary muscle twitching, facial grimacing, spasmodic eye winking, exaggerated protrusion of tongue, behavioral changes). Consult health care professional if symptoms occur.

Potential Nursing Diagnoses
Impaired physical mobility (Indications)
Risk for injury (Indications)

Implementation
- In the carbidopa/levodopa combination, the number following the drug name represents the milligrams of each respective drug.
- In preoperative patients or patients who are NPO, confer with health care professional about continuing medication administration.
- **PO:** Administer on a regular schedule.
- Controlled-release tablets may be administered as whole or half tablets, but they should not be crushed or chewed.
- For *orally disintegrating tablets,* just prior to administration remove tablet from bottle with dry hands. Immediately place tablet on top of tongue. Tablet will dissolve in seconds, then swallow with saliva. Administration with liquid is not necessary.

Patient/Family Teaching
- Instruct patient to take this medication at regular intervals as directed. Do not change dose regimen or take additional antiparkinson drugs, including more carbidopa/levodopa, without consulting health care professional. Take missed doses as soon as remembered, unless next scheduled dose is within 2 hr; do not double doses.
- Explain that gastric irritation may be decreased by eating food shortly after taking medications but that high-protein meals may impair levodopa's effects. Dividing the daily protein intake among all the meals may help ensure adequate protein intake and drug effectiveness. Do not drastically alter diet during carbidopa/levodopa therapy without consulting health care professional.
- May cause sudden onset of sleep, drowsiness, or dizziness. Advise patient to avoid driving and other activities that require alertness until response to drug is known.
- Caution patient to change positions slowly to minimize orthostatic hypotension. Health care professional should be notified if orthostatic hypotension occurs.
- Instruct patient that frequent rinsing of mouth, good oral hygiene, and sugarless gum or candy may decrease dry mouth.
- Caution patient to monitor skin lesions for any changes. Health care professional should be notified promptly because carbidopa/levodopa may activate malignant melanoma.
- Advise patient to confer with health care professional before taking OTC medications, especially cold remedies. Large amounts of vitamin B_6 (pyridoxine) and iron may interfere with the action of levodopa.
- Inform patient that harmless darkening of saliva, urine, or sweat may occur.
- Advise patient to notify health care professional if palpitations, urinary retention, involuntary movements, behavioral changes, severe nausea and vomiting, new skin lesions, or new or increased gambling, sexual, or other intense urges occur. Dose reduction may be required.
- Inform patient that sometimes a "wearing-off" effect may occur at end of dosing interval. Notify health care professional if this poses a problem to lifestyle.

Evaluation/Desired Outcomes
- Resolution of parkinsonian signs and symptoms. Therapeutic effects usually become evident after 2–3 wk of therapy but may require up to 6 mo. Patients who take this medication for several yr may experience a decrease in the effectiveness of this drug. Effectiveness may sometimes be restored after a "drug holiday."

---

carbonyl iron, See IRON SUPPLEMENTS.

HIGH ALERT

carboplatin (kar-boe-**pla**-tin)
Paraplatin, ✦Paraplatin-AQ

Classification
Therapeutic: antineoplastics
Pharmacologic: alkylating agents

Pregnancy Category D

Indications
Advanced ovarian carcinoma (with other agents). Palliative treatment of ovarian carcinoma unresponsive to other modalities.

Action
Inhibits DNA synthesis by producing cross-linking of parent DNA strands (cell-cycle phase–nonspecific). **Therapeutic Effects:** Death of rapidly replicating cells, particularly malignant ones.

carboplatin

Pharmacokinetics
Absorption: IV administration results in complete bioavailability.
Distribution: Unknown.
Protein Binding: Platinum is irreversibly bound to plasma proteins.
Metabolism and Excretion: Excreted mostly by the kidneys.
Half-life: *Carboplatin*—2.6–5.9 hr (increased in renal impairment); *platinum*—5 days.

TIME/ACTION PROFILE (effects on blood counts)

ROUTE	ONSET	PEAK	DURATION
IV	unknown	21 days	28 days

Contraindications/Precautions
Contraindicated in: Hypersensitivity to carboplatin, cisplatin, or mannitol; OB: Pregnancy or lactation.
Use Cautiously in: Hearing loss; Electrolyte abnormalities; Renal impairment (dose reduction recommended if creatinine <60 mL/min); Active infections; Diminished bone marrow reserve (dose reduction recommended); Other chronic debilitating illnesses; Geri: ↑ risk of thrombocytopenia, consider renal function in dose determination; Patients with childbearing potential; Pedi: Safe use in children not established.

Adverse Reactions/Side Effects
CNS: weakness. **EENT:** ototoxicity. **GI:** abdominal pain, nausea, vomiting, constipation, diarrhea, hepatitis, stomatitis. **GU:** gonadal suppression, nephrotoxicity. **Derm:** alopecia, rash. **F and E:** hypocalcemia, hypokalemia, hypomagnesemia, hyponatremia. **Hemat:** ANEMIA, LEUKOPENIA, THROMBOCYTOPENIA. **Metab:** hyperuricemia. **Neuro:** peripheral neuropathy. **Misc:** hypersensitivity reactions including ANAPHYLACTIC-LIKE REACTIONS.

Interactions
Drug-Drug: ↑ nephrotoxicity and ototoxicity with other **nephrotoxic** and **ototoxic drugs (aminoglycosides, loop diuretics)**. ↑ bone marrow depression with other **bone marrow–depressing drugs** or **radiation therapy**. May ↓ antibody response to **live-virus vaccines** and ↑ risk of adverse reactions.

Route/Dosage
Other dosing formulas are used.
IV (Adults): *Initial treatment*—300 mg/m^2 with cyclophosphamide at 4-wk intervals. *Treatment of refractory tumors*—360 mg/m^2 as a single dose; may be repeated at 4-wk intervals, depending on response.

Renal Impairment
IV (Adults): *CCr 41–59 mL/min*—initial dose 250 mg/m^2; *CCr 16–40 mL/min*—initial dose 200 mg/m^2.

Availability (generic available)
Lyophilized powder for injection: 50-mg vials, 150-mg vials, 450-mg vials. **Aqueous solution for injection:** 50-mg/5-ml vial, 150-mg/15-mL vial, 450-mg/45-mL vial, 600-mg/60-mL vial.

NURSING IMPLICATIONS

Assessment
- Assess for nausea and vomiting; often occur 6–12 hr after therapy (1–4 hr for aqueous solution) and may persist for 24 hr. Prophylactic antiemetics may be used. Adjust diet as tolerated to maintain fluid and electrolyte balance and ensure adequate nutritional intake. May require discontinuation of therapy.
- Assess patients receiving *Paraplatin-AQ* for neurotoxicity (paresthesias in a stocking—glove distribution, areflexia, loss of proprioception and vibratory sensations). Discontinue therapy when symptoms are first observed. May progress further even after stopping therapy. May be irreversible.
- Monitor for bone marrow depression. Assess for bleeding (bleeding gums, bruising, petechiae, guaiac stools, urine, and emesis) and avoid IM injections and rectal temperatures if platelet count is low. Apply pressure to venipuncture sites for 10 min. Assess for signs of infection during neutropenia. Anemia may occur and may be cumulative; transfusions are frequently required. Monitor for increased fatigue, dyspnea, and orthostatic hypotension.
- Monitor for signs of anaphylaxis (rash, urticaria, pruritus, facial swelling, wheezing, tachycardia, hypotension). Discontinue medication immediately and notify physician if these occur. Epinephrine and resuscitation equipment should be readily available.
- Audiometry is recommended before initiation of therapy and subsequent doses. Ototoxicity manifests as tinnitus and unilateral or bilateral hearing loss in high frequencies and becomes more frequent and severe with repeated doses. Ototoxicity is more pronounced in children.
- *Lab Test Considerations:* Monitor CBC, differential, and clotting studies before and weekly during therapy. For *Paraplatin:* The nadirs of thrombocytopenia and leukopenia occur after 21 days and recover by 30 days after a dose. Nadir of granulocyte counts usually occurs after 21–28 days and recovers by day 35.

Withhold subsequent doses until neutrophil count is >2000/mm^3 and platelet count is > 100,000/mm^3. For *Paraplatin-AQ:* The nadirs of thrombocytopenia and leukopenia occur between days 18 and 23 and recover by day 39. Anemia also occurs with the same frequency and timing as thrombocytopenia and leukopenia.
- Monitor renal function and serum electrolytes before initiation of therapy and before each course of carboplatin. Nephrotoxicity with *Paraplatin-AQ* is cumulative and is potentiated by aminoglycoside antibiotics. Monitor serum creatinine, BUN, creatinine clearance, and magnesium, sodium, potassium, and calcium levels prior to initiating therapy and before each subsequent dose. May cause ↑ BUN and serum creatinine concentrations and ↓ CCr. May cause ↓ serum potassium, calcium, magnesium, and sodium concentrations. Renal function must return to normal before each dose of *Paraplatin-AQ* is given.
- Monitor hepatic function before and periodically during therapy. May cause ↑ serum bilirubin, alkaline phosphatase, and AST concentrations.
- *Paraplatin-AQ* may cause hyperuricemia, usually occurring 3–5 days after therapy. Allopurinol may be used to ↓ uric acid levels.
- *Paraplatin-AQ* may cause ↑ serum amylase levels.

Potential Nursing Diagnoses
Risk for infection (Adverse Reactions)
Risk for injury (Side Effects)

Implementation
- **High Alert:** Fatalities have occurred with chemotherapeutic agents. Before administering, clarify all ambiguous orders; double-check single, daily, and course-of-therapy dose limits; have second practitioner independently double-check original order, calculations, and infusion pump settings.
- **High Alert:** Do not confuse carboplatin with cisplatin. Do not confuse Paraplatin (carboplatin) with Platinol (cisplatin).
- **High Alert:** Carboplatin should be administered in a monitored setting under the supervision of a physician experienced in cancer chemotherapy.

IV Administration
- Solution should be prepared in a biologic cabinet. Wear gloves, gown, and mask while handling medication. Discard equipment in specially designated containers.
- Do not use aluminum needles or equipment during preparation or administration; aluminum reacts with the drug.

Paraplatin
- **Intermittent Infusion:** Reconstitute to a concentration of 10 mg/mL with sterile water for injection, D5W, or 0.9% NaCl for injection. *Diluent:*May be further diluted in D5W or 0.9% NaCl. *Concentration:*0.5 mg/mL. Stable for 8 hr at room temperature.
- May also be administered over 24 hr or by dividing total dose into 5 consecutive pulse doses; may decrease nausea and vomiting but does not decrease nephrotoxicity or ototoxicity. *Rate:*Administer over 15–60 min.
- **Y-Site Compatibility:** allopurinol, amifostine, anidlafungin, aztreonam, cefepime, cladribine, doxorubicin liposome, etoposide phosphate, filgrastim, fludarabine, gemcitabine, granisetron, linezolid, melphalan, ondansetron, oxaliplatin, paclitaxel, palonosetron, pemetrexed, piperacillin/tazobactam, propofol, sargramostim, teniposide, thiotepa, topotecan, vinorelbine.
- **Y-Site Incompatibility:** amphotericin B cholesteryl sulfate complex, lansoprazole.

Paraplatin-AQ
- Hydrate patient with 1–2 liters of fluid infused over 8–12 hr prior to therapy.
- Adequate hydration and urinary output must be maintained for 24 hr following infusion.
- **Intermittent Infusion:** *Diluent:*Dilute Paraplatin-AQ with 2 liters of D5/0.45% NaCl containing 37.5 g of mannitol. Do not dilute with D5W. If diluted solution is not to be used within 6 hr, protect solution from light. Do not refrigerate.

Patient/Family Teaching
- Instruct patient to notify health care professional promptly if fever; chills; sore throat; signs of infection; lower back or side pain; difficult or painful urination; bleeding gums; bruising; pinpoint red spots on skin; blood in stools, urine, or emesis; increased fatigue, dyspnea, or orthostatic hypotension occurs.
- Caution patient to avoid crowds and persons with known infections. Instruct patient to use soft toothbrush and electric razor and to avoid falls. Caution patients not to drink alcoholic

beverages or take medication containing aspirin or NSAIDs because they may precipitate gastric bleeding.
- Instruct patient to promptly report any numbness or tingling in extremities or face, decreased coordination, difficulty with hearing or ringing in the ears, unusual swelling, or weight gain to health care professional.
- Instruct patient not to receive any vaccinations without advice of health care professional and to avoid contact with persons who have received oral polio vaccine within the past several months.
- Advise patient of the need for contraception (if patient is not infertile as a result of surgical or radiation therapy).
- Instruct patient to inspect oral mucosa for erythema and ulceration. If ulceration occurs, advise patient to notify health care professional, rinse mouth with water after eating, and use sponge brush. Mouth pain may require treatment with opioids.
- Discuss with patient the possibility of hair loss. Explore methods of coping.
- Emphasize the need for periodic lab tests to monitor for side effects.

Evaluation/Desired Outcomes
- Decrease in size or spread of ovarian carcinoma.

---

carisoprodol
(kar-i-**sop**-roe-dole)
Soma, Vanadom

Classification
Therapeutic: skeletal muscle relaxants (centrally acting)

Pregnancy Category UK

Indications
Adjunct to rest and physical therapy in the treatment of muscle spasm associated with acute painful musculoskeletal conditions.

Action
Skeletal muscle relaxation, probably due to CNS depression. **Therapeutic Effects:** Skeletal muscle relaxation.

Pharmacokinetics
Absorption: Well absorbed after oral administration.
Distribution: Crosses the placenta; high concentrations in breast milk.
Metabolism and Excretion: Mostly metabolized by the liver.

Half-life: 8 hr.

TIME/ACTION PROFILE (skeletal muscle relaxation)

ROUTE	ONSET	PEAK	DURATION
PO	30 min	unknown	4–6 hr

Contraindications/Precautions
Contraindicated in: Hypersensitivity to carisoprodol or to meprobamate; Porphyria or suspected porphyria.
Use Cautiously in: Severe liver or kidney disease; OB, Lactation, Pedi: Safety not established for pregnant women, breastfeeding infants, or children <16 yr; Geri: Poorly tolerated due to anticholinergic effects. Appears on Beers list.

Adverse Reactions/Side Effects
CNS: dizziness, drowsiness, agitation, ataxia, depression, headache, insomnia, irritability, syncope. **Resp:** asthma attacks. **CV:** hypotension, tachycardia. **GI:** epigastric distress, hiccups, nausea, vomiting. **Derm:** flushing, rashes. **Hemat:** eosinophilia, leukopenia. **Misc:** ANAPHYLACTIC SHOCK, fever, psychological dependence, severe idiosyncratic reaction.

Interactions
Drug-Drug: Additive CNS depression with other **CNS depressants** including **alcohol**, **antihistamines**, **opioid analgesics**, and **sedative/hypnotics**.
Drug-Natural Products: Concomitant use of **kava-kava**, **valerian**, **skullcap**, **chamomile**, or **hops** can increase CNS depression.

Route/Dosage
PO (Adults ≥16 yrs): 250–350 mg 4 times daily for no > 2–3 wk.

Availability (generic available)
Tablets: 250 mg, 350 mg. *In combination with:* aspirin (Soma compound) and codeine. See Appendix B.

NURSING IMPLICATIONS
Assessment
- Assess patient for pain, muscle stiffness, and range of motion before and periodically throughout therapy.
- Observe patient for idiosyncratic symptoms that may appear within minutes or hours of administration during the first dose. Symptoms include extreme weakness, quadriplegia, dizziness, ataxia, dysarthria, visual disturbances, agitation, euphoria, confusion, and disorientation. Usually subsides over several hours.

carmustine **281**

- Geri:Assess geriatric patients for anticholinergic effects (sedation and weakness).

Potential Nursing Diagnoses
Acute pain (Indications)
Impaired bed mobility (Indications)
Risk for injury (Side Effects)

Implementation
- Do not confuse Soma with Soma Compound.
- Provide safety measures as indicated. Supervise ambulation and transfer of patients.
- **PO:** Administer with food to minimize GI irritation. Give dose at bedtime.

Patient/Family Teaching
- Instruct patient to take medication as directed. Missed doses should be taken within 1 hr; if not, omit and return to regular dosing schedule. Do not double doses.
- Encourage patient to comply with additional therapies prescribed for muscle spasm (rest, physical therapy, heat, etc.).
- May cause dizziness or drowsiness. Advise patient to avoid driving or other activities requiring alertness until response to drug is known.
- Instruct patient to change positions slowly to minimize orthostatic hypotension.
- Advise patient to avoid concurrent use of alcohol and other CNS depressants while taking this medication.
- Instruct patient to notify health care professional if signs of allergy (rash, hives, swelling of tongue or lips, dyspnea) or idiosyncratic reaction occur.

Evaluation/Desired Outcomes
- Decreased musculoskeletal pain and muscle spasticity.
- Increased range of motion.

HIGH ALERT

carmustine (kar-mus-teen)
BCNU, BiCNU, Gliadel

Classification
Therapeutic: antineoplastics
Pharmacologic: alkylating agents

Pregnancy Category D

Indications
Alone or with other treatments (surgery, radiation) in the management of: Brain tumors, Multiple myeloma, Hodgkin's disease, Other lymphomas.

Action
Inhibits DNA and RNA synthesis (cell-cycle phase–nonspecific). **Therapeutic Effects:** Death of rapidly replicating cells, especially malignant ones.

Pharmacokinetics
Absorption: Following IV administration, absorption is complete. Following implantation, action is primarily local.
Distribution: Highly lipid soluble; readily penetrates CSF. Enters breast milk.
Metabolism and Excretion: Rapidly metabolized. Some metabolites have antineoplastic activity.
Half-life: *Biologic*—15–30 min; *chemical*—5 min.

TIME/ACTION PROFILE (effect on platelet counts)

ROUTE	ONSET	PEAK	DURATION
IV	days	4–5 wk	6 wk

Contraindications/Precautions
Contraindicated in: Hypersensitivity; Pregnancy or lactation.
Use Cautiously in: Infections; Depressed bone marrow reserve; Geriatric patients (consider age related decrease in body mass, renal/hepatic/cardiovascular function, concurrent medications and chronic illnesses); Impaired pulmonary, hepatic, or renal function; Other chronic debilitating illnesses; Patients with childbearing potential.

Adverse Reactions/Side Effects
Resp: PULMONARY FIBROSIS, pulmonary infiltrates. **GI:** hepatotoxicity, nausea, vomiting, anorexia, diarrhea, esophagitis. **GU:** renal failure. **Derm:** alopecia. **Hemat:** LEUKOPENIA, THROMBOCYTOPENIA, anemia. **Local:** pain at IV site.

Interactions
Drug-Drug: ↑ bone marrow depression with other **antineoplastics** or **radiation therapy**. **Smoking** ↑ risk of pulmonary toxicity. May ↓ antibody response to **live-virus vaccines** and ↑ risk of adverse reactions. Myelosuppression may be ↑ by **cimetidine**.

Route/Dosage
IV (Adults and Children): 150–200 mg/m² single dose every 6–8 wk *or* 75–100 mg/m²/day for 2 days q 6 wk *or* 40 mg/m²/day for 5 days q 6 wk.

carmustine

Intracavitary (Adults): Up to 61.6 mg (8 implants) placed in cavity created during surgical resection of brain tumor.

Availability
Injection: 100-mg vial. **Intracavitary wafer:** 7.7 mg in packages of 8.

NURSING IMPLICATIONS
Assessment
- Monitor vital signs before and frequently during therapy.
- Monitor for bone marrow depression. Assess for bleeding (bleeding gums, bruising, petechiae, guaiac stools, urine, and emesis) and avoid IM injections and taking rectal temperatures if platelet count is low. Apply pressure to venipuncture sites for 10 min. Assess for signs of infection during neutropenia. Anemia may occur; monitor for increased fatigue, dyspnea, and orthostatic hypotension.
- Assess respiratory status for dyspnea or cough. Pulmonary toxicity usually occurs after high cumulative doses or several courses of therapy but may also occur following 1–2 courses of low doses. Symptoms may be rapid or gradual in onset; damage may be reversible or irreversible. Delayed pulmonary fibrosis may occur yr after therapy. Notify physician promptly if symptoms occur.
- Monitor IV site closely. Carmustine is an irritant. Instruct patient to notify nurse immediately if discomfort occurs at IV site. Discontinue IV immediately if infiltration occurs. Ice may be applied to site. May cause hyperpigmentation of skin along vein.
- Monitor intake and output, appetite, and nutritional intake. Assess for nausea and vomiting, which occur within 2 hr of administration and persist for 4–6 hr. Administration of an antiemetic before and during therapy and adjusting diet as tolerated may help maintain fluid and electrolyte balance and nutritional status.
- **Lab Test Considerations:** Monitor CBC with differential and platelet count before and throughout therapy. The nadir of thrombocytopenia occurs in 4–5 wk; the nadir of leukopenia in 5–6 wk. Recovery usually occurs in 6–7 wk but may take 10–12 wk after prolonged therapy. Withhold dose and notify physician if platelet count is <100,000/mm^3 or leukocyte count is <4000/mm^3. Anemia is usually mild.
- Monitor serum bilirubin, AST, ALT, and LDH before and periodically during therapy. May cause mild, reversible ↑ in AST, alkaline phosphatase, and bilirubin.
- Monitor BUN, serum creatinine, and uric acid before and periodically during therapy. Notify physician if BUN is elevated.

Potential Nursing Diagnoses
Risk for injury (Side Effects)
Disturbed body image (Side Effects)

Implementation
- **High Alert:** Fatalities have occurred with chemotherapeutic agents. Before administering, clarify all ambiguous orders; double-check single, daily, and course-of-therapy dose limits; have second practitioner independently double-check original order, calculations, and infusion pump settings.

IV Administration
- Solution should be prepared in a biologic cabinet. Wear gloves, gown, and mask while handling medication. Discard equipment in designated containers. Contact with skin may cause transient hyperpigmentation.
- **Intermittent Infusion:** Dilute contents of each 100-mg vial with 3 mL of absolute ethyl alcohol provided as a diluent. Dilute this solution with 27 mL of sterile water for injection. **Concentration:** 3.3 mg/mL. **Diluent:** May be further diluted with 500 mL of D5W or 0.9% NaCl in a glass container.
- Solution is clear and colorless. Do not use vials that contain an oily film, which indicates decomposition. Reconstituted solution is stable for 24 hr when refrigerated and protected from light. Solution contains no preservatives; do not use as a multidose vial.
- IV lines may be flushed with 5–10 mL of 0.9% NaCl before and after carmustine infusion to minimize irritation at the injection site. **Rate:** Administer dose over 1–2 hr at rate of <3 mg/mL/min. Rapid infusion rate may cause local pain, burning at site, and flushing. Facial flushing occurs within 2 hr and may persist for 4 hr.
- **Y-Site Compatibility:** amifostine, aztreonam, cefepime, etoposide, filgrastim, fludarabine, gemcitabine, granisetron, melphalan, ondansetron, piperacillin/tazobactam, sargramostim, teniposide, thiotepa, vinorelbine.
- **Additive Incompatibility:** allopurinol, sodium bicarbonate.

Patient/Family Teaching
- Instruct patient to notify health care professional if fever; chills; sore throat; signs of infection; lower back or side pain; difficult or painful urination; bleeding gums; bruising;

petechiae; or blood in urine, stool, or emesis occurs.Caution patient to avoid crowds and persons with known infections. Instruct patient to use soft toothbrush and electric razor. Patients should be cautioned not to drink alcoholic beverages or to take products containing aspirin or NSAIDs.

- Instruct patient to notify health care professional if shortness of breath or increased cough occurs. Encourage patient not to smoke, because smokers are at greater risk for pulmonary toxicity.
- Instruct patient to inspect oral mucosa for redness and ulceration. If mouth sores occur, advise patient to use sponge brush and rinse mouth with water after eating and drinking. Stomatitis may require treatment with opioid analgesics.
- Discuss with patient the possibility of hair loss. Explore coping strategies.
- Advise patient of the need for contraception.
- Instruct patient not to receive any vaccinations without advice of health care professional.
- Emphasize need for periodic lab tests to monitor for side effects.

Evaluation/Desired Outcomes
- Decrease in size and spread of tumor.
- Improvement in hematologic parameters in nonsolid cancers.

carvedilol (kar-**ve**-dil-ole)
Coreg, Coreg CR

Classification
Therapeutic: antihypertensives
Pharmacologic: beta blockers

Pregnancy Category C

Indications
Hypertension. CHF (ischemic or cardiomyopathic) with digoxin, diuretics, and ACE inhibitors. Left ventricular dysfunction after myocardial infarction.

Action
Blocks stimulation of beta$_1$ (myocardial) and beta$_2$ (pulmonary, vascular, and uterine)-adrenergic receptor sites. Also has alpha$_1$ blocking activity, which may result in orthostatic hypotension.
Therapeutic Effects: Decreased heart rate and blood pressure. Improved cardiac output, slowing of the progression of CHF and decreased risk of death.

Pharmacokinetics
Absorption: Well absorbed but rapidly undergoes extensive first-pass hepatic metabolism, resulting in 25–35% bioavailability. Food slows absorption.
Distribution: Unknown.
Protein Binding: 98%.
Metabolism and Excretion: Extensively metabolized (primarily by CYP2D6 and CYP2C9; the CYP2D6 enzyme system exhibits genetic polymorphism); ~7% of population may be poor metabolizers and may have significantly ↑ carvedilol concentrations and an ↑ risk of adverse effects); excreted in feces via bile, <2% excreted unchanged in urine.
Half-life: 7–10 hr.

TIME/ACTION PROFILE (cardiovascular effects)

ROUTE	ONSET	PEAK	DURATION
PO	within 1 hr	1–2 hr	12 hr
PO-CR	unknown	5 hr	24 hr

Contraindications/Precautions
Contraindicated in: History of serious hypersensitivity reaction (Stevens-Johnson syndrome, angioedema, anaphylaxis); Pulmonary edema; Cardiogenic shock; Bradycardia, heart block or sick sinus syndrome (unless a pacemaker is in place); Uncompensated CHF requiring IV inotropic agents (wean before starting carvedilol); Severe hepatic impairment; Asthma or other bronchospastic disorders.
Use Cautiously in: CHF (condition may deteriorate during initial therapy); Renal impairment; Hepatic impairment; Diabetes mellitus (may mask signs of hypoglycemia); Thyrotoxicosis (may mask symptoms); Peripheral vascular disease; History of severe allergic reactions (intensity of reactions may be increased); OB:Crosses placenta and may cause fetal/neonatal bradycardia, hypotension, hypoglycemia, or respiratory depression); Lactation, Pedi:Safety not established; Geri: ↑ sensitivity to beta blockers; initial dose reduction recommended.

Adverse Reactions/Side Effects
CNS: dizziness, fatigue, weakness, anxiety, depression, drowsiness, insomnia, memory loss, mental status changes, nervousness, nightmares. **EENT:** blurred vision, dry eyes, nasal stuffiness. **Resp:** bronchospasm, wheezing. **CV:** BRADYCARDIA, CHF, PULMONARY EDEMA **GI:** diarrhea, constipation, nausea. **GU:** erectile dysfunction, ↓ li-

---

✦= Canadian drug name.   = Genetic implication.
*CAPITALS indicates life-threatening; underlines indicate most frequent.

bido. **Derm:** STEVENS-JOHNSON SYNDROME, TOXIC EPIDERMAL NECROLYSIS, itching, rashes, urticaria. **Endo:** hyperglycemia, hypoglycemia. **MS:** arthralgia, back pain, muscle cramps. **Neuro:** paresthesia. **Misc:** ANAPHYLAXIS, ANGIOEDEMA, drug-induced lupus syndrome.

Interactions
Drug-Drug: General anesthetics, IV phenytoin, diltiazem, and verapamil may cause ↑ myocardial depression. ↑ risk of bradycardia with digoxin. Amiodarone or fluconazole may ↑ levels. ↑ hypotension may occur with other antihypertensives, acute ingestion of alcohol, or nitrates. Concurrent use with clonidine ↑ hypotension and bradycardia. May ↑ withdrawal phenomenon from clonidine (discontinue carvedilol first). Concurrent administration of thyroid preparations may ↓ effectiveness. May alter the effectiveness of insulins or oral hypoglycemic agents (dose adjustments may be necessary). May ↓ effectiveness of theophylline. May ↓ beneficial beta$_1$-cardiovascular effects of dopamine or dobutamine. Use cautiously within 14 days of MAO inhibitor therapy (may result in hypotension/bradycardia). Cimetidine may ↑ toxicity from carvedilol. Concurrent NSAIDs may ↓ antihypertensive action. Effectiveness may be ↓ by rifampin. May ↑ serum digoxin levels. May ↑ blood levels of cyclosporine (monitor blood levels).

Route/Dosage
PO (Adults): *Hypertension*—6.25 mg twice daily, may be ↑ q 7–14 days up to 25 mg twice daily *or extended-release*—20 mg once daily, dose may be doubled every 7–14 days up to 80 mg once daily; *CHF*—3.125 mg twice daily for 2 wk; may be ↑ to 6.25 mg twice daily. Dose may be doubled q 2 wk as tolerated (not to exceed 25 mg twice daily in patients <85 kg or 50 mg twice daily in patients >85 kg) *or extended-release*—10 mg once daily, dose may be doubled every 2 wk as tolerated up to 80 mg once daily; *Left ventricular dysfunction after MI*—6.25 mg twice daily, ↑ after 3–10 days to 12.5 twice daily then to target dose of 25 mg twice daily; some patients may require lower initial doses and slower titration *or extended-release*—20 mg once daily, dose may be doubled every 3–10 days up to 80 mg once daily.

Availability (generic available)
Tablets: 3.125 mg, 6.25 mg, 12.5 mg, 25 mg. **Cost:** *Generic*—3.125 mg $89.95/180, 6.25 mg $79.94/180, 12.5 mg $79.94/180, 25 mg $89.93/180. **Extended-release capsules:** 10 mg, 20 mg, 40 mg, 80 mg. **Cost:** all strengths $333.97/90.

NURSING IMPLICATIONS
Assessment
- Monitor blood pressure and pulse frequently during dose adjustment period and periodically during therapy. Assess for orthostatic hypotension when assisting patient up from supine position.
- Monitor intake and output ratios and daily weight. Assess patient routinely for evidence of fluid overload (peripheral edema, dyspnea, rales/crackles, fatigue, weight gain, jugular venous distention). Patients may experience worsening of symptoms during initiation of therapy for CHF.
- **Hypertension:** Check frequency of refills to determine adherence.
- *Lab Test Considerations:* May cause ↑ BUN, serum lipoprotein, potassium, triglyceride, and uric acid levels.
- May cause ↑ ANA titers.
- May cause ↑ in blood glucose levels.
- *Toxicity and Overdose:* Monitor patients receiving beta blockers for signs of overdose (bradycardia, severe dizziness or fainting, severe drowsiness, dyspnea, bluish fingernails or palms, seizures). Notify health care professional immediately if these signs occur.

Potential Nursing Diagnoses
Decreased cardiac output (Side Effects)
Noncompliance (Patient/Family Teaching)

Implementation
- Do not confuse carvedilol with captopril or carteolol.
- Discontinuation of concurrent clonidine should be gradual, with carvedilol discontinued first over 1-2 wk with limitation of physical activity; then, after several days, discontinue clonidine.
- **PO:** Take apical pulse before administering. If <50 bpm or if arrhythmia occurs, withhold medication and notify health care professional.
- Administer with food to minimize orthostatic hypotension.
- Extended-release capsules should be taken in the morning and swallowed whole; do not crush, break, or chew. Extended-release capsules may be opened and sprinkled on cold applesauce and taken immediately; do not store mixture.
- To convert from immediate-release to extended-release product, doses of 3.125 mg

twice daily can be converted to 10 mg daily; doses of 6.25 mg twice daily can be converted to 20 mg daily; doses of 12.5 mg twice daily can be converted to 40 mg daily; and doses of 25 mg twice daily can be converted to 80 mg daily.

Patient/Family Teaching
- Instruct patient to take medication as directed, at the same time each day, even if feeling well. Do not skip or double up on missed doses. Take missed doses as soon as possible up to 4 hr before next dose. Abrupt withdrawal may precipitate life-threatening arrhythmias, hypertension, or myocardial ischemia.
- Advise patient to make sure enough medication is available for weekends, holidays, and vacations. A written prescription may be kept in wallet in case of emergency.
- Teach patient and family how to check pulse and blood pressure. Instruct them to check pulse daily and blood pressure biweekly. Advise patient to hold dose and contact health care professional if pulse is <50 bpm or blood pressure changes significantly.
- May cause drowsiness or dizziness. Caution patients to avoid driving or other activities that require alertness until response to the drug is known.
- Advise patient to change positions slowly to minimize orthostatic hypotension, especially during initiation of therapy or when dose is increased.
- Caution patient that this medication may increase sensitivity to cold.
- Instruct patient to consult health care professional before taking any Rx, OTC, or herbal products, especially cold preparations, concurrently with this medication.
- Patients with diabetes should closely monitor blood glucose, especially if weakness, malaise, irritability, or fatigue occurs. Medication may mask some signs of hypoglycemia, but dizziness and sweating may still occur.
- Advise patient to notify health care professional if slow pulse, difficulty breathing, wheezing, cold hands and feet, dizziness, confusion, depression, rash, fever, sore throat, unusual bleeding, or bruising occurs.
- Instruct patient to inform health care professional of medication regimen before treatment or surgery.
- Advise patient to carry identification describing disease process and medication regimen at all times.
- **Hypertension:** Reinforce the need to continue additional therapies for hypertension (weight loss, sodium restriction, stress reduction, regular exercise, moderation of alcohol consumption, and smoking cessation). Medication controls but does not cure hypertension.

Evaluation/Desired Outcomes
- Decrease in blood pressure without appearance of detrimental side effects.
- Decrease in severity of CHF.

---

caspofungin (kas-po-fun-gin)
Cancidas

Classification
Therapeutic: antifungals (systemic)
Pharmacologic: echinocandins

Pregnancy Category C

Indications
Invasive aspergillosis refractory to, or intolerant of, other therapies. Candidemia and associated serious infections (intra-abdominal abscesses, peritonitis, pleural space infections). Esophageal candidiasis. Suspected fungal infections in febrile neutropenic patients.

Action
Inhibits the synthesis of β (1, 3)-D-glucan, a necessary component of the fungal cell wall. **Therapeutic Effects:** Death of susceptible fungi.

Pharmacokinetics
Absorption: IV administration results in complete bioavailability.
Distribution: Widely distributed to tissues.
Protein Binding: 97%.
Metabolism and Excretion: Slowly and extensively metabolized; <1.5% excreted unchanged in urine.
Half-life: Polyphasic: β phase—9–11 hr; γ phase—40–50 hr.

TIME/ACTION PROFILE

ROUTE	ONSET	PEAK	DURATION
IV	unknown	end of infusion	24 hr

Contraindications/Precautions
Contraindicated in: Hypersensitivity; Concurrent use with cyclosporine.

caspofungin

Use Cautiously in: Moderate hepatic impairment (decreased maintenance dose recommended); Pedi: Children <3 mo (safety not established).

Adverse Reactions/Side Effects
CNS: headache. **GI:** diarrhea, nausea, vomiting. **Derm:** flushing. **Local:** venous irritation at injection site. **Misc:** allergic reactions including ANAPHYLAXIS, fever.

Interactions
Drug-Drug: Concurrent use with **cyclosporine** is not recommended due to ↑ risk of hepatic toxicity. May ↓ blood levels and effects of **tacrolimus**. Blood levels and effectiveness may be ↓ by **rifampin**; maintenance dose should be ↑ to 70 mg (in patients with normal liver function). Blood levels and effectiveness also may be ↓ by **efavirenz, nelfinavir, nevirapine, phenytoin, dexamethasone,** or **carbamazepine**; an ↑ in the maintenance dose to 70 mg should be considered in patients who are not clinically responding.

Route/Dosage
IV (Adults): 70 mg initially followed by 50 mg daily, duration determined by clinical situation and response; *Esophageal candidiasis*—50 mg daily, duration determined by clinical situation and response.

IV (Children ≥3 mo): 70 mg/m^2 (max: 70 mg) initially followed by 50 mg/m^2 daily (max: 70 mg/day), duration determined by clinical situation and response.

Moderate Hepatic Impairment (Child-Pugh Score 5–6)
IV (Adults): 70 mg initially followed by 35 mg daily, duration determined by clinical situation and response.

Availability
Powder for injection: 50 mg/vial, 70 mg/vial.

NURSING IMPLICATIONS

Assessment
- Assess patient for signs and symptoms of fungal infections prior to and periodically during therapy.
- Monitor patient for signs of anaphylaxis (rash, dyspnea, stridor) during therapy.
- *Lab Test Considerations:* May cause ↑ serum alkaline phosphatase, AST, ALT, eosinophils, and urine protein and RBCs. May also cause ↓ serum potassium, hemoglobin, hematocrit, and WBCs.

Potential Nursing Diagnoses
Risk for infection (Indications)

Implementation
IV Administration

- **Intermittent Infusion:** *Diluent:* Allow refrigerated vial to reach room temperature. *For 70-mg or 50-mg dose*—Reconstitute vials with 10.8 mL of 0.9% NaCl, sterile water for injection, Bacteriostatic Water for Injection with methylparaben and propylparaben, or Bacteriostatic Water for Injection with 0.9% benzyl alcohol. Do not dilute with dextrose solutions. Reconstituted solution is stable for 1 hr at room temperature. Withdraw 10 mL from vial and add to 250 mL of 0.9% NaCl, 0.45% NaCl, 0.225% NaCl, or LR. The 50-mg dose also can be diluted in 100 mL when volume restriction is necessary. Infusion is stable for 24 hr at room temperature or 48 hr if refrigerated. *For 35-mg dose*—Reconstitute a 50-mg or 70-mg vial as per the directions above. Remove the volume of drug equal to the calculated loading dose or calculated maintenance dose based on a concentration of 7 mg/mL (if reconstituted from the 70-mg vial) or a concentration of 5 mg/mL (if reconstituted from the 50-mg vial). White cake should dissolve completely. Mix gently until a clear solution is obtained. Do not use a solution that is cloudy, discolored, or contains precipitates. *Concentration:* 0.14–0.47 mg/mL. *Rate:* Infuse over 1 hr.

- **Y-Site Compatibility:** acyclovir, amikacin, aminophylline, amiodarone, aztreonam, bumetanide, calcium chloride, calcium gluconate, ceftizoxime, cimetidine, ciprofloxacin, cisatracurium, cyclosporine, daptomycin, diltiazem, diphenhydramine, dobutamine, dolasetron, dopamine, doxycycline, droperidol, epinephrine, erythromycin, esmolol, famotidine, fenoldopam, fentanyl, fluconazole, ganciclovir, gentamicin, granisetron, haloperidol, hydrocortisone sodium succinate, hydromorphone, imipenem/cilastatin, insulin, isoproterenol, labetalol, levofloxacin, linezolid, magnesium sulfate, meperidine, meropenem, metoclopramide, metoprolol, midazolam, milrinone, morphine, moxifloxacin, nicardipine, nitroglycerin, norepinephrine, ondansetron, palonosetron, phenylephrine, procainamide, prochlorperazine, promethazine, propranolol, quinupristin/dalfopristin, tacrolimus, tirofiban, tobramycin, vancomycin, vasopressin, vecuronium, verapamil.

- **Y-Site Incompatibility:** amphotericin B, ampicillin, ampicillin/sulbactam, azithromycin,

cefazolin, cefepime, cefotaxime, cefoxitin, ceftazidime, ceftriaxone, cefuroxime, chloramphenicol, clindamycin, dexamethasone sodium phosphate, diazepam, digoxin, enalaprilat, ertapenem, furosemide, heparin, hydralazine, ketorolac, lidocaine, lorazepam, methylprednisolone sodium succinate, metronidazole, nafcillin, nitroprusside, pamidronate, pancuronium, pantoprazole, phenytoin, piperacillin/tazobactam, potassium chloride, potassium phosphate, ranitidine, sodium bicarbonate, ticarcillin/clavulanate, trimethoprim/sulfamethoxazole.
- **Solution Incompatibility:** Solutions containing dextrose.

Patient/Family Teaching
- Explain the purpose of caspofungin to patient and family.

Evaluation/Desired Outcomes
- Decrease in signs and symptoms of fungal infections. Duration of therapy is determined based on severity of underlying disease, recovery from immunosuppression, and clinical response.

---

cefaclor, See CEPHALOSPORINS—SECOND GENERATION.

---

cefadroxil, See CEPHALOSPORINS—FIRST GENERATION.

---

cefazolin, See CEPHALOSPORINS—FIRST GENERATION.

---

cefdinir, See CEPHALOSPORINS—THIRD GENERATION.

---

cefditoren, See CEPHALOSPORINS—THIRD GENERATION.

---

cefepime (seff-e-peem)
Maxipime

Classification
Therapeutic: anti-infectives
Pharmacologic: fourth-generation cephalosporins

Pregnancy Category B

Indications
Treatment of the following infections caused by susceptible organisms: Uncomplicated skin and skin structure infections, Bone and joint infections, Uncomplicated and complicated urinary tract infections, Respiratory tract infections, Complicated intra-abdominal infections (with metronidazole), Septicemia. Empiric treatment of febrile neutropenic patients.

Action
Binds to the bacterial cell wall membrane, causing cell death. **Therapeutic Effects:** Bactericidal action against susceptible bacteria. **Spectrum:** Similar to that of second- and third-generation cephalosporins, but activity against staphylococci is less, whereas activity against gram-negative pathogens is greater, even for organisms resistant to first-, second-, and third-generation agents. Notable is increased action against: *Enterobacter*, *Haemophilus influenzae* (including β-lactamase-producing strains), *Escherichia coli*, *Klebsiella pneumoniae*, *Neisseria*, *Proteus*, *Providencia*, *Pseudomonas aeruginosa*, *Serratia*, *Moraxella catarrhalis* (including β-lactamase-producing strains). Not active against methicillin-resistant staphylococci or enterococci.

Pharmacokinetics
Absorption: Well absorbed after IM administration; IV administration results in complete bioavailability.
Distribution: Widely distributed. Crosses the placenta; enters breast milk in low concentrations. Some CSF penetration.
Metabolism and Excretion: 85% excreted unchanged in urine.
Half-life: 2 hr (increased in renal impairment).

TIME/ACTION PROFILE

ROUTE	ONSET	PEAK	DURATION
IM	rapid	1–2 hr	12 hr
IV	rapid	end of infusion	12 hr

Contraindications/Precautions
Contraindicated in: Hypersensitivity to cephalosporins; Serious hypersensitivity to penicillins.

cefepime

Use Cautiously in: Renal impairment (↓ dosing/ ↑ dosing interval recommended if CCr ≤60 mL/min); History of GI disease, especially colitis; Patients with hepatic dysfunction or poor nutritional status (may be at increased risk of bleeding); Geriatric patients (dose adjustment due to age-related decrease in renal function may be necessary); OB, Lactation, Pedi: Pregnancy, lactation, and children <2 mo (safety not established).

Adverse Reactions/Side Effects
CNS: SEIZURES (high doses in patients with renal impairment), encephalopathy, headache. **GI:** PSEUDOMEMBRANOUS COLITIS, diarrhea, nausea, vomiting. **Derm:** rashes, pruritus, urticaria. **Hemat:** bleeding, eosinophilia, hemolytic anemia, neutropenia, thrombocytopenia. **Local:** pain at IM site, phlebitis at IV site. **Misc:** allergic reactions including ANAPHYLAXIS, superinfection, fever.

Interactions
Drug-Drug: Probenecid ↓ excretion and ↑ blood levels. Concurrent use of **loop diuretics** or **aminoglycosides** may ↑ risk of nephrotoxicity.

Route/Dosage
IM (Adults): *Mild-to-moderate uncomplicated or complicated urinary tract infections due to Escherichia coli*—0.5–1 g every 12 hr.
IV (Adults): *Moderate-to-severe pneumonia*—1–2 g every 12 hr. *Mild-to-moderate uncomplicated or complicated urinary tract infections* 0.5–1 g every 12 hr. *Severe uncomplicated or complicated urinary tract infections, moderate-to-severe uncomplicated skin and skin structure infections, complicated intra-abdominal infections*—2 g every 12 hr. *Empiric treatment of febrile neutropenia*—2 g every 8 hr.
IV (Children 2 mo–16 yr): *Uncomplicated and complicated urinary tract infections, uncomplicated skin and skin structure infections, pneumonia*—50 mg/kg every 12 hr (not to exceed 2 g/dose). *Febrile neutropenia*—50 mg/kg every 8 hr (not to exceed 2 g/dose).

Renal Impairment
IM, IV (Adults): (See Manufacturer's specific recommendations) *CCr 30–60 mL/min*—0.5–1 g every 24 hr or 2 g every 12–24 hr; *CCr 11–29 mL/min*—0.5–2 g every 24 hr; *CCr <11 mL/min*—250 mg–1 g every 24 hr.

Availability (generic available)
Powder for injection: 500 mg, 1 g, 2 g.

NURSING IMPLICATIONS
Assessment
- Assess patient for infection (vital signs; appearance of wound, sputum, urine, and stool; WBC) at beginning of and throughout therapy.
- Before initiating therapy, obtain a history to determine previous use of and reactions to penicillins or cephalosporins. Persons with a negative history of penicillin sensitivity may still have an allergic response.
- Obtain specimens for culture and sensitivity before initiating therapy. First dose may be given before receiving results.
- Observe patient for signs and symptoms of anaphylaxis (rash, pruritus, laryngeal edema, wheezing). Discontinue the drug and notify health care professional immediately if these symptoms occur. Keep epinephrine, an antihistamine, and resuscitation equipment close by in the event of an anaphylactic reaction.
- Monitor bowel function. Diarrhea, abdominal cramping, fever, and bloody stools should be reported to health care professional promptly as a sign of pseudomembranous colitis. May begin up to several weeks following cessation of therapy.
- *Lab Test Considerations:* May cause positive results for Coombs' test in patients receiving high doses or in neonates whose mothers were given cephalosporins before delivery.
- May cause ↑ serum AST, ALT, bilirubin, BUN, and creatinine.
- May rarely cause leukopenia, neutropenia, thrombocytopenia, and eosinophilia.

Potential Nursing Diagnoses
Risk for infection (Indications, Side Effects)
Diarrhea (Adverse Reactions)
Deficient knowledge, related to medication regimen (Patient/Family Teaching)

Implementation
- **IM:** Reconstitute IM doses with sterile or bacteriostatic water for injection, 0.9% NaCl, or D5W. May be diluted with lidocaine to minimize injection discomfort.
- Inject deep into a well-developed muscle mass; massage well.
- IM route should only be used for treatment of mild-to-moderate uncomplicated or complicated urinary tract infections due to *Escherichia coli*.

IV Administration
- **IV:** Monitor injection site frequently for phlebitis (pain, redness, swelling). Change sites every 48–72 hr to prevent phlebitis.

- If aminoglycosides are administered concurrently, administer in separate sites, if possible, at least 1 hr apart. If second site is unavailable, flush lines between medications.
- **Intermittent Infusion:** Reconstitute with 5 mL sterile water, 0.9% NaCl, or D5W for the 500-mg vial, or 10 mL for the 1-g or 2-g vials. ***Diluent:***Dilute further in 50–100 mL of D5W, 0.9% NaCl, D10W, D5/0.9% NaCl, or D5/LR. ***Concentration:***Maximum 18 mg/mL.
- Solution is stable for 24 hr at room temperature and 7 days if refrigerated. ***Rate:***Administer over 30 min.
- **Y-Site Compatibility:** ampicillin-sulbactam, anidulafungin, aztreonam, bivalirudin, bleomycin, bumetanide, buprenorphine, butorphanol, calcium gluconate, carboplatin, carmustine, cyclophosphamide, cytarabine, dactinomycin, dexamethasone sodium phosphate, dexmedetomidine, docetaxel, doxacurium, doxorubicin liposome, fenoldopam, fluconazole, fludarabine, fluorouracil, furosemide, granisetron, hetastarch, hydrocortisone sodium phosphate, hydrocortisone sodium succinate, hydromorphone, imipenem-cilastatin, insulin, ketamine, leukovorin, levofloxacin, linezolid, lorazepam, melphalan, mesna, methotrexate, methylprednisolone sodium succinate, metronidazole, milrinone, mycophenolate, octreotide, oxytocin, paclitaxel, palonosetron, piperacillin-tazobactam, ranitidine, remifentanil, rocuronium, sargramostim, sodium acetate, sodium bicarbonate, sufentanil, thiotepa, ticarcillin-clavulanate, tigecycline, tirofiban, trimethoprim/sulfamethoxazole, vasopressin, zidovudine.
- **Y-Site Incompatibility:** acyclovir, amphotericin B cholesteryl, amphotericin B colloidal, amphotericin B liposome, caspofungin, chlorpromazine, cimetidine, ciprofloxacin, cisplatin, dacarbazine, daunorubicin, diazepam, diltiazem, diphenhydramine, doxorubicin hydrochloride, droperidol, enalaprilat, epirubicin, erythromycin, etoposide, etoposide phosphate, famotidine, filgrastim, floxuridine, ganciclovir, gemcitabine, haloperidol, hydroxyzine, idarubicin, ifosfamide, magnesium sulfate, mannitol, mechlorethamine, meperidine, metoclopramide, midazolam, mitomycin, mitoxantrone, nalbuphine, nesiritide, nicardipine, ondansetron, oxaliplatin, pantoprazole, pemetrexed, phenytoin, plicamycin, prochlorperazine, promethazine, quinupristin/dalfopristin, streptozocin, tacrolimus, theophylline, vecuronium, vinblastine, vincristine, vinorelbine, voriconazole.

Patient/Family Teaching
- Advise patient to report signs of superinfection (furry overgrowth on the tongue, vaginal itching or discharge, loose or foul-smelling stools) and allergy.
- Instruct patient to notify health care professional if fever and diarrhea develop, especially if stool contains blood, pus, or mucus. Advise patient not to treat diarrhea without consulting health care professional.

Evaluation/Desired Outcomes
- Resolution of the signs and symptoms of infection. Length of time for complete resolution depends on the organism and site of infection.

---

cefixime, See CEPHALOSPORINS—THIRD GENERATION.

---

cefoperazone, See CEPHALOSPORINS—THIRD GENERATION.

---

cefotaxime, See CEPHALOSPORINS—THIRD GENERATION.

---

cefotetan, See CEPHALOSPORINS—SECOND GENERATION.

---

cefoxitin, See CEPHALOSPORINS—SECOND GENERATION.

---

cefpodoxime, See CEPHALOSPORINS—THIRD GENERATION.

---

cefprozil, See CEPHALOSPORINS—SECOND GENERATION.

---

ceftazidime, See CEPHALOSPORINS—THIRD GENERATION.

✣ = Canadian drug name.   ⚡ = Genetic implication.
*CAPITALS indicates life-threatening; underlines indicate most frequent.

ceftibuten, See CEPHALOSPORINS—THIRD GENERATION.

ceftizoxime, See CEPHALOSPORINS—THIRD GENERATION.

ceftriaxone, See CEPHALOSPORINS—THIRD GENERATION.

cefuroxime, See CEPHALOSPORINS—SECOND GENERATION.

celecoxib (sel-e-**kox**-ib)
Celebrex

Classification
Therapeutic: antirheumatics, nonsteroidal anti-inflammatory agents
Pharmacologic: COX-2 inhibitors

Pregnancy Category C

Indications
Relief of signs and symptoms of osteoarthritis, rheumatoid arthritis, ankylosing spondylitis and juvenile rheumatoid arthritis. Reduction of the number of adenomatous colorectal polyps in familial adenomatous polyposis (FAP), as an adjunct to usual care (endoscopic surveillance, surgery). Management of acute pain including primary dysmenorrhea.

Action
Inhibits the enzyme COX-2. This enzyme is required for the synthesis of prostaglandins. Has analgesic, anti-inflammatory, and antipyretic properties. **Therapeutic Effects:** Decreased pain and inflammation caused by arthritis or spondylitis. Decreased number of colorectal polyps. Decreased pain.

Pharmacokinetics
Absorption: Bioavailability unknown.
Distribution: 97% bound to plasma proteins; extensive tissue distribution.
Metabolism and Excretion: Mostly metabolized by the hepatic CYP2C9 isoenzyme; the CYP2C9 enzyme system exhibits genetic polymorphism; poor metabolizers may have significantly ↑ celecoxib concentrations and an ↑ risk of adverse effects; <3% excreted unchanged in urine and feces.
Half-life: 11 hr.

TIME/ACTION PROFILE (pain reduction)

ROUTE	ONSET	PEAK	DURATION
PO	24–48 hr	unknown	12–24 hr†

†After discontinuation.

Contraindications/Precautions
Contraindicated in: Hypersensitivity; Cross-sensitivity may exist with other NSAIDs, including aspirin; History of allergic-type reactions to sulfonamides; History of asthma, urticaria, or allergic-type reactions to aspirin or other NSAIDs, including the aspirin triad (asthma, nasal polyps, and severe hypersensitivity reactions to aspirin); Advanced renal disease; Severe hepatic dysfunction; Peri-operative pain from coronary artery bypass graft (CABG) surgery; OB: Should not be used in late pregnancy (may cause premature closure of the ductus arteriosus).
Use Cautiously in: Cardiovascular disease or risk factors for cardiovascular disease (may ↑ risk of serious cardiovascular thrombotic events, myocardial infarction, and stroke, especially with prolonged use); Pre-existing renal disease, heart failure, liver dysfunction, concurrent diuretic or ACE inhibitor therapy (↑ risk of renal impairment); Hypertension or fluid retention; Renal insufficiency (may precipitate acute renal failure); Serious dehydration (correct deficits before administering); Patients who are known or suspected to be poor CYP2C9 metabolizers (↓ initial dose by 50%); Pre-existing asthma; Pedi: Safety not established in children <2 yrs or for longer than 6 mo; Geri: Concurrent therapy with corticosteroids or anticoagulants, long duration of NSAID therapy, history of smoking, alcoholism, geriatric patients, or poor general health status (↑ risk of GI bleeding); Lactation: Lactation.
Exercise Extreme Caution in: History of ulcer disease or GI bleeding.

Adverse Reactions/Side Effects
CNS: dizziness, headache, insomnia. **CV:** MYOCARDIAL INFARCTION, STROKE, THROMBOSIS, edema. **GI:** GI BLEEDING, abdominal pain, diarrhea, dyspepsia, flatulence, nausea. **Derm:** EXFOLIATIVE DERMATITIS, STEVENS-JOHNSON SYNDROME, TOXIC EPIDERMAL NECROLYSIS, rash.

Interactions
Drug-Drug: CYP2C9 inhibitors may ↑ levels. May ↓ effectiveness of **ACE inhibitors**, **thiazide diuretics**, and **furosemide**. **Fluconazole** ↑ levels (use lowest recommended dosage). May ↑ risk of bleeding with **warfarin** and **aspirin**. May ↑ serum **lithium** levels. Does not inhibit the cardioprotective effect of low-dose **aspirin**.

Route/Dosage
PO (Adults): *Osteoarthritis*—200 mg once daily *or* 100 mg twice daily. *Rheumatoid arthritis*—100–200 mg twice daily. *Ankylosing spondylitis*—200 mg once daily *or* 100 mg twice daily; dose may be ↑ after 6 wk to 400 mg daily. *Familial adenomatous polyposis*—400 mg twice daily. *Acute pain, including dysmenorrhea*—400 mg initially, then a 200-mg dose if needed on the first day; then 200 mg twice daily as needed.

Hepatic Impairment
PO (Adults): *Moderate hepatic impairment (Child-Pugh Class B)*— ↓ dose by 50%.
PO (Children ≥2 yrs, ≥10 kg–≤25 kg): *Juvenile rheumatoid arthritis*—50 mg twice daily.
PO (Children ≥2 yrs, ≥25 kg): *Juvenile rheumatoid arthritis*—100 mg twice daily.

Availability
Capsules: 50 mg, 100 mg, 200 mg, 400 mg.
Cost: 100 mg $213.29/100, 200 mg $362.17/100, 400 mg $524.26/100.

NURSING IMPLICATIONS

Assessment
- Assess range of motion, degree of swelling, and pain in affected joints before and periodically throughout therapy.
- Assess patient for allergy to sulfonamides, aspirin, or NSAIDs. Patients with these allergies should not receive celecoxib.
- Monitor patient for signs of Stevens-Johnson syndrome and toxic epidermal necrolysis. Discontinue celecoxib at first sign of rash.
- ***Lab Test Considerations:*** May cause ↑ AST and ALT levels.
- May cause hypophosphatemia and ↑ BUN.

Potential Nursing Diagnoses
Impaired physical mobility (Indications)
Acute pain (Indications)

Implementation
- Do not confuse with Celexa (citalopram) or Cerebyx (fosphenytoin).
- **PO:** May be administered without regard to meals. Capsules may be opened and sprinkled on applesauce and ingested immediately with water. Mixture may be stored in the refrigerator for up to 6 hr.

Patient/Family Teaching
- Instruct patient to take celecoxib exactly as directed. Do not take more than prescribed dose. Increasing doses does not appear to increase effectiveness. Use lowest effective dose for shortest period of time.
- Advise patient to notify health care professional promptly if sign or symptom of GI toxicity (abdominal pain, black stools), skin rash, unexplained weight gain, edema, or chest pain occurs. Patients should discontinue celecoxib and notify health care professional if signs and symptoms of hepatotoxicity (nausea, fatigue, lethargy, pruritus, jaundice, upper right quadrant tenderness, flu-like symptoms) occur.
- Advise patient to notify health care professional if pregnancy is planned or suspected.
- Advise patients with FAP to continue routine surveillance procedures.

Evaluation/Desired Outcomes
- Reduction in joint pain in patients with osteoarthritis.
- Reduction in joint tenderness, pain, and joint swelling in patients with rheumatoid arthritis and juvenile rheumatoid arthritis.
- Decreased number of colonic polyps in patients with FAP.

---

cephalexin, See CEPHALOSPORINS—FIRST GENERATION.

CEPHALOSPORINS—FIRST GENERATION

cefadroxil (sef-a-**drox**-ill)
Duricef

cefazolin (sef-**a**-zoe-lin)
Ancef

cephalexin (sef-a-**lex**-in)
✤Apo-Cephalex, ✤DOM-Cephalexin, Keflex, ✤Nu-Cephalex, Panixine, ✤PMS-Cephalexin

Classification
Therapeutic: anti-infectives
Pharmacologic: first-generation cephalosporins

Pregnancy Category B

Indications
Treatment of the following infections caused by susceptible organisms: Skin and skin structure infections (including burn wounds), Pneumonia,

---

✤ = Canadian drug name. ≡ = Genetic implication.
*CAPITALS indicates life-threatening; underlines indicate most frequent.

CEPHALOSPORINS—FIRST GENERATION

Urinary tract infections, Bone and joint infections, Septicemia. Not suitable for the treatment of meningitis. **Cefadroxil:** Pharyngitis and/or tonsillitis. **Cefazolin:** Perioperative prophylaxis, biliary tract infections, genital infections, bacterial endocarditis prophylaxis for dental and upper respiratory tract procedures. **Cephalexin:** Otitis media.

Action
Bind to bacterial cell wall membrane, causing cell death. **Therapeutic Effects:** Bactericidal action against susceptible bacteria. **Spectrum:** Active against many gram-positive cocci including: *Streptococcus pneumoniae*, Group A beta-hemolytic streptococci, Penicillinase-producing staphylococci. Not active against: Methicillin-resistant staphylococci, *Bacteroides fragilis*, *Enterococcus*. Active against some gram-negative rods including: *Klebsiella pneumoniae*, *Proteus mirabilis*, *Escherichia coli*.

Pharmacokinetics
Absorption: *Cefadroxil* and *cephalexin* are well absorbed following oral administration. *Cefazolin* is well absorbed following IM administration. **Distribution:** Widely distributed. Cefazolin penetrates bone and synovial fluid well. All cross the placenta and enter breast milk in low concentrations. Minimal CSF penetration.
Metabolism and Excretion: Excreted almost entirely unchanged by the kidneys.
Half-life: *Cefadroxil*—60–120 min; *cefazolin*—90–150 min; *cephalexin*—50–80 min; (all are ↑ in renal impairment).

TIME/ACTION PROFILE (blood levels)

ROUTE	ONSET	PEAK	DURATION
Cefadroxil PO	rapid	1.5–2 hr	12–24 hr
Cefazolin IM	rapid	0.5–2 hr	6–12 hr
Cefazolin IV	rapid	5 min	6–12 hr
Cephalexin PO	rapid	1 hr	6–12 hr

Contraindications/Precautions
Contraindicated in: Hypersensitivity to cephalosporins; Serious hypersensitivity to penicillins.
Use Cautiously in: Renal impairment (dosage ↓ and/or ↑ dosing interval recommended for: *cefadroxil and cephalexin*, if CCr ≤50 mL/min, and *cefazolin*, if CCr <30 mL/min; History of GI disease, especially colitis; Geri: Dosage adjustment due to age-related ↓ in renal function may be necessary; OB, Lactation: Half-life is shorter and blood levels lower during pregnancy; have been used safely.

Adverse Reactions/Side Effects
CNS: SEIZURES (high doses). **GI:** PSEUDOMEMBRANOUS COLITIS, diarrhea, nausea, vomiting, cramps. **Derm:** STEVENS-JOHNSON SYNDROME, rashes, pruritis, urticaria. **Hemat:** agranulocytosis, eosinophilia, hemolytic anemia, neutropenia, thrombocytopenia. **Local:** pain at IM site, phlebitis at IV site. **Misc:** allergic reactions including ANAPHYLAXIS and SERUM SICKNESS, superinfection.

Interactions
Drug-Drug: Probenecid ↓ excretion and ↑ blood levels of renally excreted cephalosporins. Concurrent use of **loop diuretics** or **aminoglycosides** may ↑ risk of renal toxicity.

Route/Dosage
Cefadroxil
PO (Adults): *Pharyngitis and tonsillitis*—500 mg q 12 hr or 1 g q 24 hr for 10 days. *Skin and soft-tissue infections*—500 mg q 12 hr or 1 g q 24 hr. *Urinary tract infections*—500 mg–1 g q 12 hr or 1–2 g q 24 hr.
PO (Children): *Pharyngitis, tonsillitis, or impetigo*—15 mg/kg q 12 hr or 30 mg/kg q 24 hr for 10 days. *Skin and soft-tissue infections*—15 mg/kg q 12 hr. *Urinary tract infections*—15 mg/kg q 12 hr.

Renal Impairment
PO (Adults): *CCr 25–50 mL/min*—500 mg q 12 hr; *CCr 10–25 mL/min*—500 mg q 24 hr; *CCr <10 mL/min*—500 mg q 36 hr.

Cefazolin
IM, IV (Adults): *Moderate to severe infections*—500 mg–2 g q 6–8 hr (maximum 12 g/day). *Mild infections with gram-positive cocci*—250–500 mg q 8 hr. *Uncomplicated urinary tract infections*—1 g q 12 hr. *Pneumococcal pneumonia*—500 mg q 12 hr. *Infective endocarditis or septicemia*—1–1.5 g q 6 hr. *Perioperative prophylaxis*—1 g given 30–60 min prior to incision. Additional 500 mg–1 g should be given for surgeries ≥2 hr. 500 mg–1 g should then be given for all surgeries q 6–8 hr for 24 hr postoperatively.
IM, IV (Children and Infants >1 mo): 16.7–33.3 mg/kg q 8 hr (maximum 6 g/day); *Bacterial endocarditis prophylaxis in penicillin-allergic patients:* -25 mg/kg 30 minutes prior to procedure (maximum dose = 1 g).
IM, IV (Neonates ≤7 days): 40 mg/kg/day divided q 12 hr.
IM, IV (Neonates >7 days and ≤2 kg): 40 mg/kg/day divided q 12 hr.

CEPHALOSPORINS—FIRST GENERATION

IM, IV (Neonates >7 days and >2 kg): 60 mg/kg/day divided q 8 hr.

Renal Impairment
IM, IV (Adults): *CCr 10–30 mL/min*—Administer q 12 hr; *CCr ≤10 mL/min*—Administer q 24 hr.

Cephalexin
PO (Adults): *Most infections*—250–500 mg q 6 hr. *Uncomplicated cystitis, skin and soft-tissue infections, streptococcal pharyngitis*—500 mg q 12 hr.
PO (Children): *Most infections*—25–50 mg/kg/day divided q 6–8 hr (can be administered q 12 hr in skin/skin structure infections or streptococcal pharyngitis). *Otitis media*—18.75–25 mg/kg q 6 hr (maximum = 4 g/day).

Renal Impairment
PO (Adults): *CCr 10–50 mL/min*—500 mg q 8–12 hr; *CCr <10 mL/min*—250–500 mg q 12–24 hr.

Availability

Cefadroxil (generic available)
Capsules: 500 mg. **Tablets:** 1 g. **Oral suspension (orange-pineapple flavor):** 250 mg/5 mL, 500 mg/5 mL.

Cefazolin (generic available)
Powder for injection: 500 mg, 1 g, 10 g, 20 g.
Premixed containers: 500 mg/50 mL D5W, 1 g/50 mL D5W.

Cephalexin (generic available)
Capsules: 250 mg, 333 mg, 500 mg, 750 mg. **Tablets:** 250 mg, 500 mg. **Oral suspension:** 100 mg/mL, 125 mg/5 mL, 250 mg/5 mL.

NURSING IMPLICATIONS

Assessment
- Assess for infection (vital signs; appearance of wound, sputum, urine, and stool; WBC) at beginning and during therapy.
- Before initiating therapy, obtain a history to determine previous use of and reactions to penicillins or cephalosporins. Persons with a negative history of penicillin sensitivity may still have an allergic response.
- Obtain specimens for culture and sensitivity before initiating therapy. First dose may be given before receiving results.
- Observe patient for signs and symptoms of anaphylaxis (rash, pruritus, laryngeal edema, wheezing). Discontinue drug and notify health care professional immediately if these problems occur. Keep epinephrine, an antihistamine, and resuscitation equipment close by in case of an anaphylactic reaction.
- Monitor bowel function. Diarrhea, abdominal cramping, fever, and bloody stools should be reported to health care professional promptly as a sign of pseudomembranous colitis. May begin up to several weeks following cessation of therapy.
- ***Lab Test Considerations:*** May cause positive results for Coombs' test in patients receiving high doses or in neonates whose mothers were given cephalosporins before delivery.
- May cause ↑ serum AST, ALT, alkaline phosphatase, bilirubin, LDH, BUN, creatinine.
- May rarely cause leukopenia, neutropenia, agranulocytosis, thrombocytopenia, or eosinophilia.

Potential Nursing Diagnoses
Risk for infection (Indications, Side Effects)
Diarrhea (Adverse Reactions)

Implementation
- **PO:** Administer around the clock. May be administered on full or empty stomach. Administration with food may minimize GI irritation. Shake oral suspension well before administering. Refrigerate oral suspensions.

Cefazolin
- **IM:** Reconstitute IM doses with 2 mL or 2.5 mL of sterile water for injection to achieve a final concentration of 225–330 mg/mL.
- Inject deep into a well-developed muscle mass; massage well.

IV Administration
- **IV:** Monitor site frequently for thrombophlebitis (pain, redness, swelling). Change sites every 48–72 hr to prevent phlebitis.
- Do not use solutions that are cloudy or contain a precipitate.
- If aminoglycosides are administered concurrently, administer in separate sites, if possible, at least 1 hr apart. If second site is unavailable, flush line between medications.
- **Direct IV:** ***Diluent:***0.9% NaCl, D5W, D10W, dextrose/saline combinations, D5/LR. ***Concentration:***100 mg/mL. May use up to 138 mg/mL in fluid-restricted patients. ***Rate:***May administer over 3–5 min.

CEPHALOSPORINS—SECOND GENERATION

- **Intermittent Infusion:** ***Diluent:*** Reconstituted 500-mg or 1-g solution may be diluted in 50–100 mL of 0.9% NaCl, D5W, D10W, dextrose/saline combinations, D5/LR. Solution is stable for 24 hr at room temperature and 10 days if refrigerated. ***Concentration:*** 20 mg/mL. ***Rate:*** Administer over 10–60 min.
- **Syringe Compatibility:** heparin.
- **Y-Site Compatibility:** acyclovir, alfentanil, allopurinol, alprostadil, amifostine, aminophylline, amphotericin B liposome, anidulafungin, ascorbic acid, atracurium, atropine, aztreonam, bivalirudin, bumetanide, buprenorphine, butorphanol, calcium gluconate, carboplatin, cefonicid, cefoperazone, cefotetan, cefoxitin, ceftazidime, ceftizoxime, ceftriaxone, cefuroxime, chloramphenicol, cimetidine, cisplatin, clindamycin, cyanocobalamin, cyclophosphamide, cyclosporine, cytarabine, dactinomycin, daptomycin, dexamethasone, dexmedetomidine, digoxin, diltiazem, docetaxel, doxacurium, doxapram, doxorubicin liposome, enalaprilat, ephedrine, epinephrine, epirubicin, epoetin alfa, esmolol, etoposide, etoposide phosphate, fenoldopam, fentanyl, filgrastim, fluconazole, fludarabine, fluorouracil, folic acid, foscarnet, gemcitabine, glycopyrrolate, granisetron, heparin, hydrocortisone, ifosfamide, imipenem/cilastatin, indomethacin, insulin, isoproterenol, ketorolac, lidocaine, linezolid, lorazepam, mannitol, mechlorethamine, melphalan, meperidine, metaraminol, methotrexate, methoxamine, methyldopate, methylprednisolone, metoclopramide, metoprolol, metronidazole, midazolam, milrinone, morphine, multivitamins, nafcillin, nalbuphine, naloxone, nesiritide, nicardipine, nitroglycerin, nitroprusside, norepinephrine, octreotide, ondansetron, oxacillin, oxaliplatin, oxytocin, paclitaxel, palonosetron, pancuronium, pantoprazole, penicillin G, perphenazine, phenobarbital, phenylephrine, phytonadione, potassium chloride, procainamide, propofol, propranolol, ranitidine, remifentanil, rituximab, sargramostim, sodium acetate, sodium bicarbonate, streptokinase, succinylcholine, sufentanil, tacrolimus, teniposide, theophylline, thiamine, thiotepa, ticarcillin/clavulanate, tigecycline, tirofiban, tolazoline, trastuzumab, trimetaphan, urokinase, vasopressin, vecuronium, verapamil, vincristine, vitamin B complex with C, voriconazole, warfarin.
- **Y-Site Incompatibility:** amphotericin B cholesteryl, azathioprine, calcium chloride, caspofungin, cefotaxime, chlorpromazine, dantrolene, diazepam, diazoxide, diphenhydramine, dobutamine, dopamine, doxorubicin hydrochloride, doxycycline, erythromycin, ganciclovir, haloperidol, hydralazine, hydroxyzine, idarubicin, levofloxacin, mitoxantrone, papaverine, pemetrexed, pentamidine, pentazocine, pentobarbital, phentolamine, phenytoin, prochlorperazine, promethazine, quinupristin/dalfopristin, sodium citrate, tobramycin, trimethoprim/sulfamethoxazole, vinorelbine.

Patient/Family Teaching
- Instruct patient to take medication around the clock at evenly spaced times and to finish the medication completely as directed, even if feeling better. Take missed doses as soon as possible unless almost time for next dose; do not double doses. Advise patient that sharing this medication may be dangerous.
- **Pedi:** Instruct parents or caregivers to use calibrated measuring device with liquid preparations.
- Advise patient to report signs of superinfection (furry overgrowth on the tongue, vaginal itching or discharge, loose or foul-smelling stools) and allergy.
- Instruct patient to notify health care professional if fever and diarrhea develop, especially if diarrhea contains blood, mucus, or pus. Advise patient not to treat diarrhea without consulting health care professional.

Evaluation/Desired Outcomes
- Resolution of signs and symptoms of infection. Length of time for complete resolution depends on the organism and site of infection.
- Decreased incidence of infection when used for prophylaxis.

CEPHALOSPORINS—SECOND GENERATION

cefaclor (**sef**-a-klor)
♣Ceclor, Raniclor

cefotetan (sef-oh-**tee**-tan)

cefoxitin (se-**fox**-i-tin)
Mefoxin

cefprozil (sef-**proe**-zil)
Cefzil

cefuroxime (se-fyoor-**ox**-eem)
Ceftin, Zinacef

CEPHALOSPORINS—SECOND GENERATION

Classification
Therapeutic: anti-infectives
Pharmacologic: second-generation cephalosporins

Pregnancy Category B

Indications
Treatment of the following infections caused by susceptible organisms: Respiratory tract infections, Skin and skin structure infections, Bone and joint infections (not cefaclor or cefprozil), Urinary tract infections (not cefprozil). **Cefotetan and cefoxitin:** Intra-abdominal and gynecologic infections. **Cefuroxime:** Meningitis, gynecologic infections, and Lyme disease. **Cefaclor, cefprozil, cefuroxime:** Otitis media. **Cefoxitin and cefuroxime:** Septicemia. **Cefotetan, cefoxitin, cefuroxime:** Perioperative prophylaxis.

Action
Bind to bacterial cell wall membrane, causing cell death. **Therapeutic Effects:** Bactericidal action against susceptible bacteria. **Spectrum:** Similar to that of first-generation cephalosporins but have ↑ activity against several other gram-negative pathogens including: *Haemophilus influenzae, Escherichia coli, Klebsiella pneumoniae, Morganella morganii, Neisseria gonorrhoeae* (including penicillinase-producing strains), *Proteus, Providencia, Serratia marcescens, Moraxella catarrhalis.* Not active against methicillin-resistant staphylococci or enterococci. **Cefuroxime:** Active against *Borrelia burgdorferi.* **Cefotetan and cefoxitin:** Active against *Bacteroides fragilis.*

Pharmacokinetics
Absorption: *Cefotetan, cefoxitin,* and *cefuroxime*—well absorbed following IM administration. *Cefaclor, cefprozil,* and *cefuroxime*—well absorbed following oral administration.
Distribution: Widely distributed. Penetration into CSF is poor, but adequate for cefuroxime (IV) to be used in treating meningitis. All cross the placenta and enter breast milk in low concentrations.
Metabolism and Excretion: Excreted primarily unchanged by the kidneys.
Half-life: *Cefaclor*—30–60 min; *cefotetan*—3–4.6 hr; *cefoxitin*—40–60 min; *cefprozil*—90 min; *cefuroxime*—60–120 min; (all are ↑ in renal impairment).

TIME/ACTION PROFILE

ROUTE	ONSET	PEAK	DURATION
Cefaclor PO	rapid	30–60 min	6–12 hr
Cefaclor PO-CD	unknown	unknown	12 hr
Cefotetan IM	rapid	1–3 hr	12 hr
Cefotetan IV	rapid	end of infusion	12 hr
Cefoxitin IM	rapid	30 min	4–8 hr
Cefoxitin IV	rapid	end of infusion	4–8 hr
Cefprozil PO	unknown	1–2 hr	12–24 hr
Cefuroxime PO	unknown	2–3 hr	8–12 hr
Cefuroxime IM	rapid	15–60 min	6–12 hr
Cefuroxime IV	rapid	end of infusion	6–12 hr

Contraindications/Precautions
Contraindicated in: Hypersensitivity to cephalosporins; Serious hypersensitivity to penicillins.
Use Cautiously in: Renal impairment (↓ dose/ ↑ dosing interval recommended for: *cefotetan* if CCr ≤30 mL/min, *cefoxitin* if CCr ≤50 mL/min, *cefprozil* if CCr <30 mL/min, *cefuroxime* if CCr ≤20 mL/min); **Cefotetan and cefoxitin:** Patients with hepatic dysfunction, poor nutritional state, or cancer may be at ↑ risk for bleeding; History of GI disease, especially colitis; *Cefprozil (oral suspension)* contains aspartame and should be avoided in patients with phenylketonuria; Geri:Dose adjustment due to age-related ↓ in renal function may be necessary; may also be at ↑ risk for bleeding with *cefotetan* or *cefoxitin*; OB, Lactation:Have been used safely.

Adverse Reactions/Side Effects
CNS: SEIZURES(high doses). **GI:** PSEUDOMEMBRANOUS COLITIS, <u>diarrhea</u>, cramps, nausea, vomiting. **Derm:** <u>rashes</u>, urticaria. **Hemat:** agranulocytosis, bleeding (↑ with cefotetan and cefoxitin), eosinophilia, hemolytic anemia, neutropenia, thrombocytopenia. **Local:** <u>pain</u> at IM site, <u>phlebitis</u> at IV site. **Misc:** allergic reactions including ANAPHYLAXISand SERUM SICKNESS, superinfection.

Interactions
Drug-Drug: Probenecid ↓ excretion and ↑ blood levels. If **alcohol** is ingested within 48–72 hr of cefotetan, a disulfiram-like reaction may occur. Cefotetan may ↑ risk of bleeding with **anticoagulants**, **antiplatelet agents**, **thrombolytics**, and **NSAIDs**. **Antacids** ↓ absorption of

✽= Canadian drug name.   = Genetic implication.
*CAPITALS indicates life-threatening; underlines indicate most frequent.

cefaclor. Concurrent use of **aminoglycosides** or **loop diuretics** may ↑ risk of nephrotoxicity.

Route/Dosage

Cefaclor
PO (Adults): 250–500 mg q 8 hr or 375–500 mg q 12 hr as extended-release tablets.
PO (Children >1 mo): 6.7–13.4 mg/kg q 8 hr or 10–20 mg/kg q 12 hr (up to 1 g/day).

Cefotetan
IM, IV (Adults): *Most infections*—1–2 g q 12 hr. *Severe/life-threatening infections*—2–3 g q 12 hr. *Urinary tract infections*—500 mg–2 g q 12 hr *or* 1–2 g q 24 hr. *Perioperative prophylaxis*-1–2 g 30–60 min before initial incision (one-time dose).

Renal Impairment
IM, IV (Adults): *CCr 10–30 mL/min*—Usual adult dose q 24 hr or ½ usual adult dose q 12 hr; *<CCr 10 mL/min*—Usual adult dose q 48 hr or ¼ usual adult dose q 12 hr.

Cefoxitin
IM, IV (Adults): *Most infections*—1 g q 6–8 hr. *Severe infections*—1 g q 4 hr or 2 g q 6–8 hr. *Life-threatening infections*—2 g q 4 hr or 3 g q 6 hr. *Perioperative prophylaxis*—2 g 30–60 min before initial incision, then 2 g q 6 hr for up to 24 hr.
IM, IV (Children and Infants >3 mo): *Most infections*—13.3–26.7 mg/kg q 4 hr *or* 20–40 mg/kg q 6 hr. *Perioperative prophylaxis*—30–40 mg/kg within 60 min of initial incision, then 30–40 mg/kg q 6 hr for up to 24 hr.

Renal Impairment
IM, IV (Adults): *CCr 30–50 mL/min*—1–2 g q 8–12 hr; *CCr 10–29 mL/min*—1–2 g q 12–24 hr; *CCr 5–9 mL/min*—0.5–1 g q 12–24 hr; *CCr <5 mL/min*—0.5–1 g q 24–48 hr.

Cefprozil
PO (Adults): *Most infections*—250–500 mg q 12 hr *or* 500 mg q 24 hr.
PO (Children 6 mo–12 yr): *Otitis media*—15 mg/kg q 12 hr. *Acute sinusitis*—7.5–15 mg/kg q 12 hr (higher dose should be used for moderate-to-severe infections).
PO (Children 2–12 yr): *Pharyngitis/tonsillitis*—7.5 mg/kg q 12 hr. *Skin/skin structure infections*—20 mg/kg q 24 hr.

Renal Impairment
PO (Adults and Children ≥6 mo): *CCr <30 mL/min*—½ of usual dose at normal dosing interval.

Cefuroxime
Cefuroxime oral tablets and oral suspension are not bioequivalent and are not substitutable on a mg-to-mg basis.
PO (Adults and Children >12 yr): *Pharyngitis/tonsillitis, maxillary sinusitis, uncomplicated UTIs*—250 mg q 12 hr. *Bronchitis, uncomplicated skin/skin structure infections*—250–500 mg q 12 hr. *Gonorrhea*—1 g (single dose). *Lyme disease*—500 mg q 12 hr for 20 days.
PO (Children 3 mo–12 yr): *Otitis media, acute bacterial maxillary sinusitis, impetigo*—15 mg/kg q 12 hr as oral suspension (not to exceed 1 g/day) *or* 250 mg q 12 hr as tablets. *Pharyngitis/tonsillitis*—10 mg/kg q 12 hr as oral suspension (not to exceed 500 mg/day).
IM, IV (Adults): *Uncomplicated urinary tract infections, skin/skin structure infections, disseminated gonococcal infections, uncomplicated pneumonia*—750 mg every 8 hr. *Bone/joint infections, severe or complicated infections*—1.5 g every 8 hr. *Life-threatening infections*—1.5 g every 6 hr. *Meningitis*—3 g every 8 hr. *Perioperative prophylaxis*—1.5 g IV 30–60 min before initial incision; 750 mg IM/IV every 8 hr can be given when procedure prolonged. *Prophylaxis during open-heart surgery*—1.5 g IV at induction of anesthesia and then every 12 hr for 3 additional doses. *Gonorrhea*—1.5 g IM (750 mg in two sites) with 1 g probenecid PO.
IM, IV (Children and Infants >3 mo): *Most infections*—12.5–25 mg/kg q 6 hr *or* 16.7–33.3 mg/kg q 8 hr (maximum dose = 6 g/day). *Bone and joint infections*—50 mg/kg q 8 hr (maximum dose = 6 g/day). *Bacterial meningitis*—50–60 mg/kg q 6 hr *or* 66.7–80 mg/kg q 8 hr.

Renal Impairment
IM, IV (Adults): *CCr 10–20 mL/min*—750 mg q 12 hr; *CCr <10 mL/min*—750 mg q 24 hr.

Availability

Cefaclor (generic available)
Capsules: 250 mg, 500 mg. **Chewable tablets (fruity):** 125 mg, 187 mg, 250 mg, 375 mg. **Extended-release tablets (CD):** 375 mg, 500 mg. **Oral suspension (strawberry):** 125 mg/5 mL, 187 mg/5 mL, 250 mg/5 mL, 375 mg/5 mL.

Cefotetan (generic available)
Powder for injection: 1 g, 2 g, 10 g. **Premixed containers:** 1 g/50 mL, 2 g/50 mL.

Cefoxitin (generic available)
Powder for injection: 1 g, 2 g, 10 g. **Premixed containers:** 1 g/50 mL D5W, 2 g/50 mL D5W.

CEPHALOSPORINS—SECOND GENERATION

Cefprozil (generic available)
Tablets: 250 mg, 500 mg. **Oral suspension (bubblegum flavor):** 125 mg/5 mL, 250 mg/5 mL.

Cefuroxime (generic available)
Tablets: 250 mg, 500 mg. **Oral suspension (tutti-frutti flavor):** 125 mg/5 mL, 250 mg/5 mL. **Powder for injection:** 750 mg, 1.5 g, 7.5 g. **Premixed containers:** 750 mg/50 mL, 1.5 g/50 mL.

NURSING IMPLICATIONS

Assessment
- Assess for infection (vital signs; appearance of wound, sputum, urine, and stool; WBC) at beginning and during therapy.
- Before initiating therapy, obtain a history to determine previous use of and reactions to penicillins or cephalosporins. Persons with a negative history of penicillin sensitivity may still have an allergic response.
- Obtain specimens for culture and sensitivity before initiating therapy. First dose may be given before receiving results.
- Observe patient for signs and symptoms of anaphylaxis (rash, pruritus, laryngeal edema, wheezing). Discontinue the drug immediately if these symptoms occur. Keep epinephrine, an antihistamine, and resuscitation equipment close by in the event of an anaphylactic reaction.
- Monitor bowel function. Diarrhea, abdominal cramping, fever, and bloody stools should be reported to health care professional promptly as a sign of pseudomembranous colitis. May begin up to several weeks following cessation of therapy.
- *Lab Test Considerations:* May cause positive results for Coombs' test in patients receiving high doses or in neonates whose mothers were given cephalosporins before delivery.
- *Cefotetan*—monitor prothrombin time and assess patient for bleeding (guaiac stools; check for hematuria, bleeding gums, ecchymosis) daily in high-risk patients; may cause hypoprothrombinemia.
- May cause ↑ serum AST, ALT, alkaline phosphatase, bilirubin, LDH, BUN, and creatinine.
- *Cefoxitin* may cause falsely ↑ test results for serum and urine creatinine; do not obtain serum samples within 2 hr of administration.
- May rarely cause leukopenia, neutropenia, agranulocytosis, thrombocytopenia, and eosinophilia.

Potential Nursing Diagnoses
Risk for infection (Indications, Side Effects)
Diarrhea (Adverse Reactions)
Deficient knowledge, related to medication regimen (Patient/Family Teaching)

Implementation
- Do not confuse Cefotan (cefotetan) with Ceftin (cefuroxime).
- Do not confuse Ceftin (cefuroxime) with Cefzil (cefprozil).
- Do not confuse cefuroxime with cefotaxime.
- **PO:** Administer around the clock. May be administered on full or empty stomach. Administration with food may minimize GI irritation. Shake oral suspension well before administering.
- Administer cefaclor extended-release tablets with food; do not crush, break, or chew.
- Do not administer *cefaclor* within 1 hr of antacids.
- *Cefuroxime* tablets should be swallowed whole, not crushed; crushed tablets have a strong, persistent bitter taste. Tablets may be taken without regard to meals. Suspension must be taken with food. Shake well each time before using. Tablets and suspension are not interchangeable.
- **IM:** Reconstitute IM doses with sterile or bacteriostatic water for injection or 0.9% NaCl for injection. May be diluted with lidocaine to minimize injection discomfort.
- Inject deep into a well-developed muscle mass; massage well.

IV Administration
- **IV:** Change sites every 48–72 hr to prevent phlebitis. Monitor site frequently for thrombophlebitis (pain, redness, swelling).
- If aminoglycosides are administered concurrently, administer in separate sites if possible, at least 1 hr apart. If second site is unavailable, flush line between medications.
- **Direct IV:** Dilute each cephalosporin in at least 1 g/10 mL. Do not use preparations containing benzyl alcohol for neonates. *Rate:* Administer slowly over 3–5 min.

Cefotetan
- **Intermittent Infusion:** *Diluent:* Reconstituted solution may be further diluted in 50–

CEPHALOSPORINS—SECOND GENERATION

100 mL of D5W or 0.9% NaCl. Solution may be colorless or yellow. Solution is stable for 24 hr at room temperature or 96 hr if refrigerated. ***Concentration:*** 10–40 mg/mL. ***Rate:*** Administer over 20–30 min.

- **Y-Site Compatibility:** acyclovir, alfentanil, allopurinol, amifostine, aminophylline, ascorbic acid, atropine, aztreonam, bivalirudin, bumetanide, buprenorphine, butorphanol, calcium chloride, cafazolin, calcium gluconate, carboplatin, cefonicid, cefoperazone, cefotaxime, cefoxitin, ceftizoxime, ceftriaxone, cefuroxime chloramphenicol, cimetidine, cisplatin, clindamycin, cyanocobalamin, cyclophosphamide, cyclosporine, cytarabine, dactinomycin, daptomycin, dexamethasone, dexmedetomidate, digoxin, diltiazem, docetaxel, dopamine, doxacurium, enalaprilat, ephedrine, epinephrine, epoetin alfa, etoposide, etoposide phosphate, fenoldopam, fentanyl, filgrastim, fluconazole, fludarabine, fluorouracil, folic acid, furosemide, gemcitabine, glycopyrrolate, granisetron, heparin, hetastarch, hydrocortisone, hydromorphone, ifosfamide, imipenem/cilastatin, isoproterenol, ketorolac, levofloxacin, lidocaine, linezolid, lorazepam, magnesium sulfate, mannitol, mechlorethamine, melphalan, metaraminol, methotrexate, methoxamine, methyldopate, methylprednisolone, metoclopramide, metoprolol, metronidazole, milrinone, mitoxantrone, morphine, multivitamins, nafcillin, nalbuphine, naloxone, nesiritide, nitroglycerin, nitroprusside, norepinephrine, octreotide, oxacillin, oxaliplatin, oxytocin, paclitaxel, palonosetron, penicillin G, phenylephrine, phytonadione, potassium chloride, procainamide, propofol, propranolol, pyridoxime, ranitidine, remifentanil, rituximab, rocuronium, sargramostim, sodium acetate, streptokinase, succinylcholine, sufentanil, tacrolimus, teniposide, theophylline, thiamine, thiotepa, ticarcillin/clavulanate, tigecycline, tirofiban, trimetaphan, urokinase, vasopressin, vecuronium, verapamil, vincristine, voriconazole.
- **Y-Site Incompatibility:** amphotericin B colloidal, amphotericin B liposome, azathioprine, caspofungin, chlorpromazine, dantrolene, diazepam, diazoxide, diphenhydramine, dobutamine, doxorubicin hydrochloride, doxycycline, epirubicin, erythromycin, esmolol, ganciclovir, gentamicin, haloperidol, hydralazine, hydroxyzine, inamrinone, indomethacin, labetalol, pantoprazole, papaverine, pemetrexed, pentamidine, pentazocine, pentobarbital, phenobarbital, phentolamine, phenytoin, prochlorperazine, promethazine, protamine, quinupristin/dalfopristin, sodium bicarbonate, tobramycin, trastuzumab, trimethoprim/sulfamethoxazole, vinorelbine.

Cefoxitin

- **Intermittent Infusion:** ***Diluent:*** Reconstituted solution may be further diluted in 50–100 mL of D5W, D10W, 0.9% NaCl, dextrose/saline combinations, D5/LR, Ringer's or LR. Stable for 24 hr at room temperature and 1 wk if refrigerated. Darkening of powder does not alter potency. ***Concentration:*** 40 mg/mL. ***Rate:*** Administer over 30–60 min.
- **Continuous Infusion:** May be diluted in 500–1000 mL for continuous infusion.
- **Syringe Compatibility:** heparin.
- **Y-Site Compatibility:** acyclovir, alfentanil, amifostine, aminophylline, amphotericin B cholesteryl, amphotericin B liposome, anidulafungin, ascorbic acid, atracurium, atropine, aztreonam, bivalirudin, bumetanide, buprenorphine, butorphanol, calcium chloride, calcium gluconate, carboplatin, cefazolin, cefonicid, cefoperazone, cefotaxime, cefotetan, ceftazidime, ceftriaxone, cefuroxime, chloramphenicol, cimetidine, cisplatin, clindamycin, cyanocobalamin, cyclophosphamide, cyclosporine, cytarabine, dactinomycin, daptomycin, dexamethasone, dexmedetomidine, digoxin, diltiazem, docetaxel, dopamine, doxacurium, doxorubicin liposome, enalaprilat, ephedrine, epinephrine, epoetin alfa, esmolol, etoposide, etoposide phosphate, fentanyl, fluconazole, fludarabine, fluorouracil, folic acid, foscarnet, furosemide, gemcitabine, glycopyrrolate, granisetron, heparin, hydrocortisone, hydromorphone, ifosfamide, imipenem/cilastatin, indomethacin, isoproterenol, ketorolac, lidocaine, linezolid, lorazepam, magnesium sulfate, mannitol, mechlorethamine, meperidine, metaraminol, methotrexate, methoxamine, methyldopate, metoclopramide, metoprolol, metronidazole, midazolam, milrinone, morphine, multivitamins, nafcillin, nalbuphine, naloxone, nesiritide, nitroglycerin, nitroprusside, norepinephrine, octreotide, ondansetron, oxacillin, oxaliplatin, oxytocin, paclitaxel, palonosetron, pantoprazole, penicillin G, perphenazine, phenylephrine, phytonadione, potassium chloride, procainamide, propofol, propranolol, pyridoxime, ranitidine, remifentanil, rituximab, rocuronium, sodium acetate, streptokinase, succinylcholine, sufentanil, tacrolimus, teniposide, theophylline, thiamine, thiotepa, ticarcillin/clavulanate, tigecycline, tirofiban, tolazoline, trimetaphan, urokinase,

CEPHALOSPORINS—SECOND GENERATION

vasopressin, vecuronium, verapamil, vincristine, voriconazole.

- **Y-Site Incompatibility:** ampicillin/sulbactam, azathioprine, caspofungin, ceftizoxime, chlorpromazine, dantrolene, diazepam, diazoxide, diphenhydramine, dobutamine, doxorubiucin hydrochloride, doxycycline, epirubicin, erythromycin, fenoldopam, fligrastim, ganciclovir, haloperidol, hydralazine, hydroxyzine, inamrinone, insulin, labetalol, levofloxacin, methylprednisolone, mitoxantrone, papaverine, pemetrexed, pentamidine, pentazocine, pentobarbital, phenobarbital, phentolamine, phenytoin, prochlorperazine, promethazine, protamine, quinupristin/dalfopristin, sodium bicarbonate, trastuzumab, trimethoprim/sulfamethoxazole, vinorelbine.

Cefuroxime

- **Intermittent Infusion:** *Diluent:*Solution may be further diluted in 50–100 mL of 0.9% NaCl, D5W, D10W, or dextrose/saline combinations. Stable for 24 hr at room temperature and 48 hr if refrigerated. *Concentration:* 10–40 mg/mL. *Rate:*Administer over 15–60 min.
- **Continuous Infusion:** May also be diluted in 500–1000 mL for continuous infusion.
- **Y-Site Compatibility:** acyclovir, alfentanil, allopurinol, amifostine, aminophylline, amiodarone, amphotericin B liposome, anidulafungin, ascorbic acid, atracurium, atropine, aztreonam, bivalirudin, bumetanide, buprenorphine, butorphanol, calcium gluconate, carboplatin, cefazolin, cefonicid, cefoperazone, cefotaxime, cefotetan, cefoxitin, ceftazidime, ceftizoxime, ceftriaxone, chloramphenicol, cimetidine, cisplatin, clindamycin, cyclophosphamide, cyanocobalamin, cyclosporine, cytarabine, dactinomycin, daptomycin, dexmedetomidine, digoxin, diltiazem, docetaxel, dopamine, doxacurium, enalaprilat, ephedrine, epinephrine, epoetin alfa, erythromycin, esmolol, etoposide, etoposide phosphate, famotidine, fenoldopam, fentanyl, fludarabine, fluorouracil, folic acid, foscarnet, furosemide, gemcitabine, glycopyrrolate, granisetron, heparin, hetastarch, hydrocortisone, hydromorphone, ifosfamide, imipenem/cilastatin, indomethacin, insulin, isoproterenol, ketorolac, levofloxacin, lidocaine, linezolid, lorazepam, mannitol, mechlorethamine, melphalan, meperidine, metaraminol, methotrexate, methoxamine, methyldopate, methylprednisolone, metoclopramide, metoprolol, metronidazole, milrinone, morphine, multivitamins, nafcillin, nalbuphine, naloxone, nesiritide, nitroglycerin, nitroprusside, norepinephrine, octreotide, ondansetron, oxacillin, oxaliplatin, oxytocin, paclitaxel, palonosetron, pancuronium, pantoprazole, pemetrexed, penicillin G, perphenazine, phenylephrine, phytonadione, potassium chloride, procainamide, propofol, propranolol, pyridoxine, ranitidine, remifentanil, rituximab, rocuronium, sargramostim, sodium acetate, streptokinase, succinylcholine, sufentanil, tacrolimus, teniposide, theophylline, thiamine, thiotepa, ticarcillin/clavulanate, tigecycline, tirofiban, tolazoline, trastuzumab, trimetaphan, urokinase, vasopressin, vecuronium, verapamil, vincristine, voriconazole.
- **Y-Site Incompatibility:** azathioprine, azithromycin, calcium chloride, caspofungin, chlorpromazine, dantrolene, dexamethasone, diazepam, diazoxide, diphenhydramine, dobutamine, doxorubicin hydrochloride, doxycycline, epirubicin, filgrastim, ganciclovir, haloperidol, hydralazine, hydroxyzine, inamrinone, labetalol, magnesium sulfate, midazolam, mitoxantrone, papaverine, pentamidine, penatzocine, pentobarbital, phenobarbital, phentolamine, phenytoin, prochlorperazine, promethazine, protamine, quinupristin/dalfopristin, sodium bicarbonate, trimethoprim/sulfamethoxazole, vinorelbine.

Patient/Family Teaching

- Instruct patient to take medication around the clock at evenly spaced times and to finish the medication completely, even if feeling better. Take missed doses as soon as possible unless almost time for next dose; do not double doses. Advise patient that sharing of this medication may be dangerous.
- Pedi:Instruct parents or caregivers to use calibrated measuring device with liquid preparations.
- Advise patient to report signs of superinfection (furry overgrowth on the tongue, vaginal itching or discharge, loose or foul-smelling stools) and allergy.
- Caution patients that concurrent use of alcohol with *cefotetan* may cause a disulfiram-like reaction (abdominal cramps, nausea, vomiting, headache, hypotension, palpitations, dyspnea, tachycardia, sweating, flushing). Alcohol and

alcohol-containing medications should be avoided during and for several days after therapy.
- Instruct patient to notify health care professional if fever and diarrhea develop, especially if stool contains blood, pus, or mucus. Advise patient not to treat diarrhea without consulting health care professional.

Evaluation/Desired Outcomes
- Resolution of signs and symptoms of infection. Length of time for complete resolution depends on the organism and site of infection.
- Decreased incidence of infection when used for prophylaxis.

CEPHALOSPORINS—THIRD GENERATION

cefdinir (sef-di-nir)
Omnicef

cefditoren (sef-dye-tor-en)
Spectracef

cefixime (sef-ik-seem)
Suprax

cefoperazone (sef-oh-per-a-zone)

cefotaxime (sef-oh-taks-eem)
Claforan

cefpodoxime (sef-poe-dox-eem)
Vantin

ceftazidime (sef-tay-zi-deem)
Fortaz, Tazicef

ceftibuten (sef-tye-byoo-ten)
Cedax

ceftizoxime (sef-ti-zox-eem)
Cefizox

ceftriaxone (sef-try-ax-one)
Rocephin

Classification
Therapeutic: anti-infectives
Pharmacologic: third-generation cephalosporins

Pregnancy Category B

Indications
Treatment of the following infections caused by susceptible organisms: Skin and skin structure infections (not cefixime), Urinary and gynecologic infections (not cefdinir, cefditoren, or ceftibuten), Respiratory tract infections (not cefdinir, cefditoren, or ceftibuten). **Cefotaxime, ceftazidime, ceftizoxime, ceftriaxone:** Meningitis and bone/joint infections. **Cefoperazone, cefotaxime, ceftazidime, ceftizoxime, ceftriaxone:** Intra-abdominal infections and septicemia. **Cefdinir, cefixime, cefpodoxime, ceftibuten, ceftriaxone:** Otitis media. **Cefotaxime, ceftriaxone:** Perioperative prophylaxis. **Ceftazidime:** Febrile neutropenia. **Cefotaxime, ceftriaxone:** Lyme disease.

Action
Bind to the bacterial cell wall membrane, causing cell death. **Therapeutic Effects:** Bactericidal action against susceptible bacteria. **Spectrum:** Similar to that of second-generation cephalosporins, but activity against staphylococci is less, whereas activity against gram-negative pathogens is greater, even for organisms resistant to first- and second-generation agents. Notable is increased action against: *Enterobacter, Haemophilus influenzae, Escherichia coli, Klebsiella pneumoniae, Neisseria gonorrhoeae, Citrobacter, Morganella, Proteus, Providencia, Serratia, Moraxella catarrhalis, Borrelia burgdorferi.* Some agents have activity against *N. meningitidis* (cefotaxime, ceftazidime, ceftizoxime, ceftriaxone). Some agents have enhanced activity against *Pseudomonas aeruginosa* (ceftazidime, cefoperazone). Not active against methicillin-resistance staphylococci or enterococci. Some agents have activity against anaerobes, including *Bacteroides fragilis* (cefoperazone, cefotaxime, ceftizoxime, ceftriaxone).

Pharmacokinetics
Absorption: *Cefoperazone, cefotaxime, ceftazidime, ceftizoxime,* and *ceftriaxone* are well absorbed after IM administration. *Ceftibuten* is well absorbed after oral administration; *cefixime* 40–50% absorbed after oral administration (oral suspension); *cefdinir* 16–25% absorbed after oral administration. *Cefditoren pivoxil* and *cefpodoxime proxetil* are prodrugs that are converted to their active components in GI tract during absorption (*cefditoren*—14% absorbed [↑ by high-fat meal]; *cefpodoxime*—50% absorbed).
Distribution: Widely distributed. Cross the placenta; enter breast milk in low concentrations. CSF penetration better than with first- and second-generation agents.
Protein Binding: *Cefoperazone* and *ceftriaxone* ≥90%.
Metabolism and Excretion: *Cefdinir, ceftazidime, cefditoren,* and *ceftizoxime*—>85% excreted in urine. *Cefpodoxime*—30% excreted in

CEPHALOSPORINS—THIRD GENERATION

urine. *Cefoperazone*—excreted in the bile. *Ceftibuten, ceftriaxone,* and *cefotaxime*—partly metabolized and partly excreted in the urine. *Cefixime*—50% excreted unchanged in urine, ≥10% in bile.

Half-life: *Cefdinir*—1.7 hr; *cefditoren*—1.6 hr; *cefixime*—3–4 hr; *cefoperazone*—2 hr; *cefotaxime*—1–1.5 hr; *cefpodoxime*—2–3 hr; *ceftazidime*—2 hr; *ceftibuten*—2 hr; *ceftizoxime*—1.4–1.9 hr; *ceftriaxone*—6–9 hr (all except *cefoperazone* and *ceftriaxone* are ↑ in renal impairment).

TIME/ACTION PROFILE

ROUTE	ONSET	PEAK	DURATION
Cefdinir PO	rapid	2–4 hr	12–24 hr
Cefditoren PO	rapid	1.5–3 hr	12 hr
Cefixime PO	rapid	2–6 hr	24 hr
Cefoperazone IM	rapid	1–2 hr	12 hr
Cefoperazone IV	rapid	end of infusion	12 hr
Cefotaxime IM	rapid	0.5 hr	4–12 hr
Cefotaxime IV	rapid	end of infusion	4–12 hr
Cefpodoxime PO	unknown	2–3 hr	12 hr
Ceftazidime IM	rapid	1 hr	6–12 hr
Ceftazidime IV	rapid	end of infusion	6–12 hr
Ceftibuten PO	rapid	3 hr	24 hr
Ceftizoxime IM	rapid	0.5–1.5 hr	6–12 hr
Ceftizoxime IV	rapid	end of infusion	6–12 hr
Ceftriaxone IM	rapid	1–2 hr	12–24 hr
Ceftriaxone IV	rapid	end of infusion	12–24 hr

Contraindications/Precautions

Contraindicated in: Hypersensitivity to cephalosporins; Serious hypersensitivity to penicillins; Pedi:Hyperbilirubinemic neonates (ceftriaxone only; may lead to kernicterus); Pedi:Neonates ≤28 days requiring calcium-containing IV solutions (↑ risk of precipitation formation); Carnitine deficiency or inborn errors of metabolism (cefditoren only); Hypersensitivity to milk protein (ceftidoren only; contains sodium caseinate).

Use Cautiously in: Renal impairment (↓ dosing/ ↑ dosing interval recommended for: *cefdinir* if CCr <30 mL/min, *cefixime* if CCr ≤60 mL/min, *cefotaxime* if CCr <20 mL/min, *cefpodoxime* if CCr <30 mL/min, *ceftazidime* if CCr ≤50 mL/min, *ceftibuten* and *cefditoren* if CCr <50 mL/min, *ceftizoxime* if CCr ≤80 mL/min); Hepatic/biliary impairment or combined hepatic/biliary/renal impairment (dose reduction/ ↑ dosing interval recommended for *cefoperazone*); Combined severe hepatic and renal impairment (dose reduction/ ↑ dosing interval recommended for *ceftriaxone*); Diabetes (*ceftibuten* and *cefdinir* suspension contain sucrose); History of GI disease, especially colitis; Patients with poor nutritional status, malabsorption states, or alcoholism may be at ↑ risk for bleeding with *cefoperazone*; Geri:Dose adjustment due to age-related ↓ in renal function may be necessary; OB, Lactation:Have been used safely.

Adverse Reactions/Side Effects

CNS: SEIZURES(high doses), headache. **GI:** PSEUDOMEMBRANOUS COLITIS, diarrhea, nausea, vomiting, cholelithiasis (ceftriaxone), cramps. **Derm:** STEVENS-JOHNSON SYNDROME, rashes, urticaria. **Hemat:** agranulocytosis, bleeding (↑ with cefoperazone), eosinophilia, hemolytic anemia, lymphocytosis, neutropenia, thrombocytopenia, thrombocytosis. **GU:** hematuria, vaginal moniliasis. **Local:** pain at IM site, phlebitis at IV site. **Misc:** allergic reactions including ANAPHYLAXIS and SERUM SICKNESS, superinfection.

Interactions

Drug-Drug: **Probenecid** ↓ excretion and ↑ serum levels (cefdinir, cefditoren, cefixime, cefotaxime, cefpodoxime, ceftizoxime, ceftriaxone). Ingestion of **alcohol** within 48–72 hr of cefoperazone may result in a disulfiram-like reaction. Cefoperazone may ↑ risk of bleeding with **anticoagulants**, **antiplatelet agents**, **thrombolytic agents**, and **NSAIDS**. Concurrent use of **loop diuretics** or **nephrotoxic agents** including **aminoglycosides** may ↑ risk of nephrotoxicity. **Antacids** ↓ absorption of cefdinir, cefditoren, and cefpodoxime. **Iron supplements** ↓ absorption of cefdinir. **H₂-receptor antagonists** ↓ absorption of cefditoren and cefpodoxime. Cefixime may ↑ **carbamazepine** levels. Ceftriaxone should not be administered concomitantly with any calcium-containing solutions.

Route/Dosage

Cefdinir

PO (Adults ≥13 yr): 300 mg q 12 hr *or* 600 mg q 24 hr (use q 12 hr dosing only for community-acquired pneumonia or skin and skin structure infections).

PO (Children 6 mo–12 yr): 7 mg/kg q 12 hr (use only for skin/skin structure infections) *or* 14 mg/kg q 24 hr; dose should not exceed 600 mg/day.

Renal Impairment
PO (Adults and Children ≥13 yr): *CCr <30 mL/min*—300 mg q 24 hr.

Renal Impairment
PO (Children 6 mo–12 yr): *CCr <30 mL/min*—7 mg/kg q 24 hr.

Cefditoren
PO (Adults and Children ≥12 yr): *Pharyngitis/tonsillitis, skin/skin structure infections*—200 mg twice daily; *Acute bacterial exacerbation of chronic bronchitis or community acquired pneumonia*—400 mg twice daily.

Renal Impairment
PO (Adults): *CCr 30–49 mL/min*—dose should not exceed 200 mg twice daily; *CCr <30 mL/min*—dose should not exceed 200 mg once daily.

Cefixime
PO (Adults and Children >12 yr or >50 kg): *Most infections*—400 mg once daily; *Gonorrhea*—400 mg single dose.
PO (Children): 8 mg/kg once daily *or* 4 mg/kg q 12h.

Renal Impairment
PO (Adults): *CCr 21–60 mL/min*—75% of standard dose once daily; *CCr ≤20 mL/min*—50% of standard dose once daily.

Cefoperazone
IM, IV (Adults): *Mild to moderate infections*—1–2 g q 12 hr. *Severe infections*—2–4 g q 8 hr *or* 1.5–3 g q 6 hr.

Hepatic/Renal Impairment
IM, IV (Adults): *Impaired hepatic function/biliary obstruction*—daily dose should not exceed 4 g; *combined hepatic and renal impairment*—daily dose should not exceed 1–2 g.

Cefotaxime
IM, IV (Adults and Children >12 yr): *Most uncomplicated infections*—1 g q 12 hr. *Moderate or severe infections*—1–2 g q 6–8 hr. *Life-threatening infections*—2 g q 4 hr (maximum dose = 12 g/day). *Gonococcal urethritis/cervicitis or rectal gonorrhea in females*—500 mg IM (single dose). *Rectal gonorrhea in males*—1 g IM (single dose). *Perioperative prophylaxis*—1 g 30–90 min before initial incision (one-time dose).

IM, IV (Children 1 mo–12 yr): *<50 kg*—100–200 mg/kg/day divided q 6–8 hr. *Meningitis*—200 mg/kg/day divided q 6 hr. *Invasive pneumococcal meningitis*—225–300 mg/kg/day divided q 6–8 hr. *≥50 kg*—see adult dosing.
IV (Neonates 1–4 wk): 50 mg/kg q 6–8 hr.
IV (Neonates ≤1 wk): 50 mg/kg q 8–12 hr.

Renal Impairment
(Adults): *CCr <20 mL/min*— ↓ dose by 50%.

Cefpodoxime
PO (Adults): *Most infections*—200 mg q 12 hr. *Skin and skin structure infections*—400 mg q 12 hr. *Urinary tract infections/pharyngitis*—100 mg q 12 hr. *Gonorrhea*—200 mg single dose.
PO (Children 2 mo–12 yr): *Pharyngitis/tonsillitis/otitis media/acute maxillary sinusitis*—5 mg/kg q 12 hr (not to exceed 200 mg/dose).

Renal Impairment
PO (Adults): *CCr <30 mL/min*— ↑ dosing interval to q 24 hr.

Ceftazidime
IM, IV (Adults and Children ≥12 yr): *Pneumonia and skin/skin structure infections*—500 mg–1 g q 8 hr. *Bone and joint infections*—2 g q 12 hr. *Severe and life-threatening infections*—2 g q 8 hr. *Complicated urinary tract infections*—500 mg q 8–12 hr. *Uncomplicated urinary tract infections*—250 mg q 12 hr. *Cystic fibrosis lung infection caused by P. aeruginosa*—30–50 mg/kg q 8 hr (maximum dose = 6 g/day).
IM, IV (Children 1 mo–12 yr): 33.3–50 mg/kg q 8 hr (maximum dose = 6 g/day).
IM, IV (Neonates ≤4 wk): 50 mg/kg q 8–12 hr.

Renal Impairment
IM, IV (Adults): *CCr 31–50 mL/min*—1 g q 12 hr; *CCr 16–30 mL/min*—1 g q 24 hr; *CCr 6–15 mL/min*—500 mg q 24 hr; *CCr <5 mL/min*—500 mg q 48 hr.

Ceftibuten
PO (Adults and Children ≥12 yr): 400 mg q 24 hr for 10 days.
PO (Children 6 mo–12 yr): 9 mg/kg q 24 hr for 10 days (maximum dose = 400 mg/day).

Renal Impairment
PO (Adults): *CCr 30–49 mL/min*—200 mg q 24 hr as capsules *or* 4.5 mg/kg q 24 hr as suspension; *CCr 5–29 mL/min*—100 mg q 24 hr as capsules *or* 2.25 mg/kg q 24 hr as suspension.

CEPHALOSPORINS—THIRD GENERATION 303

Ceftizoxime
IM, IV (Adults): *Severe infections*—1–2 g q 8–12 hr. *Life-threatening infections*—3–4 g q 8 hr. *Uncomplicated urinary tract infections*—500 mg q 12 hr. *Gonococcal urethritis/cervicitis*—1 g IM (single dose).
IM, IV (Children >6 mo): 50 mg/kg q 6–8 hr (not to exceed 200 mg/kg/day).

Renal Impairment
IM, IV (Adults): *CCr 50–79 mL/min*—500 mg–1.5 g q 8 hr; *CCr 5–49 mL/min*—250 mg–1 g q 12 hr; *CCr 0–4 mL/min*—500 mg–1 g q 48 hr or 250–500 mg q 24 hr.

Ceftriaxone
IM, IV (Adults): *Most infections*—1–2 g q 12–24 hr. *Gonorrhea*—250 mg IM (single dose). *Meningitis*—2 g q 12 hr. *Perioperative prophylaxis*—1 g 30–120 min before initial incision (single dose).
IM, IV (Children): *Most infections*—25–37.5 mg/kg q 12 hr or 50–75 mg/kg q 24 hr; dose should not exceed 2 g/day. *Meningitis*—100 mg/kg q 24 hr or 50 mg/kg q 12 hr; dose should not exceed 4 g/day. *Acute otitis media*—50 mg/kg IM single dose; dose should not exceed 1 g. *Uncomplicated gonorrhea*—125 mg IM (single dose).

Availability

Cefdinir (generic available)
Oral suspension (strawberry): 125 mg/5 mL, 250 mg/5 mL. **Cost:** *Generic*—125 mg/5 mL $73.40/100 mL, 250 mg/5 mL $83.87/60 mL. **Capsules:** 300 mg. **Cost:** $104.99/20.

Cefditoren
Tablets: 200 mg.

Cefixime
Oral suspension (strawberry): 100 mg/5 mL. **Tablets:** 400 mg.

Cefoperazone (generic available)
Powder for injection: 1 g, 2 g, 10 g. **Premixed containers:** 1 g/50 mL, 2 g/50 mL.

Cefotaxime (generic available)
Powder for injection: 500 mg, 1 g, 2 g, 10 g, 20 g. **Premixed containers:** 1 g/50 mL, 2 g/50 mL.

Cefpodoxime (generic available)
Tablets: 100 mg, 200 mg. **Oral suspension (lemon creme):** 50 mg/5 mL, 100 mg/5 mL.

Ceftazidime (generic available)
Powder for injection: 500 mg, 1 g, 2 g, 6 g. **Premixed containers:** 1 g/50 mL, 2 g/50 mL.

Ceftibuten
Capsules: 400 mg. **Oral suspension (cherry):** 90 mg/5 mL.

Ceftizoxime
Powder for injection: 1 g, 2 g, 10 g. **Premixed containers:** 1 g/50 mL, 2 g/50 mL.

Ceftriaxone (generic available)
Powder for injection: 250 mg, 500 mg, 1 g, 2 g, 10 g. **Premixed containers:** 1 g/50 mL, 2 g/50 mL.

NURSING IMPLICATIONS

Assessment
- Assess for infection (vital signs; appearance of wound, sputum, urine, and stool; WBC) at beginning of and throughout therapy.
- Before initiating therapy, obtain a history to determine previous use of and reactions to penicillins or cephalosporins. Persons with a negative history of penicillin sensitivity may still have an allergic response.
- Obtain specimens for culture and sensitivity before initiating therapy. First dose may be given before receiving results.
- Observe for signs and symptoms of anaphylaxis (rash, pruritus, laryngeal edema, wheezing). Discontinue drug and notify health care professional immediately if these symptoms occur. Keep epinephrine, an antihistamine, and resuscitation equipment close by in the event of an anaphylactic reaction.
- Monitor bowel function. Diarrhea, abdominal cramping, fever, and bloody stools should be reported to health care professional promptly as a sign of pseudomembranous colitis. May begin up to several weeks following cessation of therapy.
- Pedi: Assess newborns for jaundice and hyperbilirubinemia before making decision to use ceftriaxone (should not be used in jaundiced or hyperbilirubinemic neonates).
- *Lab Test Considerations:* May cause positive results for Coombs' test in patients receiving high doses or in neonates whose mothers were given cephalosporins before delivery.
- Monitor prothrombin time and assess patient for bleeding (guaiac stools; check for hematuria, bleeding gums, ecchymosis) daily in pa-

tients receiving *cefoperazone* or *cefditoren*, as this agent may cause hypoprothrombinemia.
- May cause ↑ serum AST, ALT, alkaline phosphatase, bilirubin, LDH, BUN, and creatinine.
- May rarely cause leukopenia, neutropenia, agranulocytosis, thrombocytopenia, eosinophilia, lymphocytosis, and thrombocytosis.

Potential Nursing Diagnoses
Risk for infection (Indications, Side Effects)
Diarrhea (Adverse Reactions)
Deficient knowledge, related to medication regimen (Patient/Family Teaching)

Implementation
- Cefditoren is not recommended for prolonged use since other piralate-containing compounds have caused clinical manifestations of carnitine deficiency when used over a period of months.
- **PO:** Administer around the clock. May be administered on full or empty stomach. Administration with food may minimize GI irritation. Shake oral suspension well before administering. Administer *cefditoren* with meals to enhance absorption. Administer *cefpodoxime tablets* with meals to enhance absorption (the suspension may be administered without regard to meals. Administer *ceftibuten* at least 1 hr before or 2 hr after meals.
- *Cefixime oral suspension* should be used to treat otitis media (results in higher peak concentrations than tablets).
- Do not administer *cefdinir* or *cefpodoxime* within 2 hr before or after an antacid. Do not administer *cefpodoxime* within 2 hr before or after an H₂ receptor antagonist. Do not administer *cefdinir* within 2 hr before or after iron supplements. Do not administer *cefditoren* concomitantly with antacids.
- **IM:** Reconstitute IM doses with sterile or bacteriostatic water for injection or 0.9% NaCl for injection. May be diluted with lidocaine to minimize injection discomfort.
- Inject deep into a well-developed muscle mass; massage well.

IV Administration

- **IV:** Monitor injection site frequently for phlebitis (pain, redness, swelling). Change sites every 48–72 hr to prevent phlebitis.
- If aminoglycosides are administered concurrently, administer in separate sites, if possible, at least 1 hr apart. If second site is unavailable, flush lines between medications.
- **Direct IV:** Dilute cephalosporins in at least 1 g/10 mL. Avoid direct IV administration of *cefoperazone* and *ceftriaxone*. Do not use preparations containing benzyl alcohol for neonates. *Rate:*Administer slowly over 3–5 min.

Cefoperazone
- **Intermittent Infusion:** Reconstitute each gram with at least 5 mL of sterile or bacteriostatic water for injection or 0.9% NaCl. Shake vigorously and allow to stand for visualization and clarity. Solution may be colorless to straw colored. *Diluent:*Dilute each gram in solution in 50–100 mL of 0.9% NaCl, D5W, D10W, dextrose/saline combinations, D5/LR, or LR. *Concentration:*2–50 mg/mL Solution is stable for 24 hr at room temperature and 5 days if refrigerated. *Rate:*Administer over 15–30 min.
- **Continuous Infusion:** For continuous infusion, concentration should be 2–25 mg/mL.
- **Syringe Compatibility:** heparin.
- **Y-Site Compatibility:** acyclovir, alfentanil, allopurinol, aminophylline, ascorbic acid, atropine, aztreonam, bivalirudin, bumetanide, buprenorphine, butorphanol, calcium gluconate, carboplatin, cefazolin, cefonicid, cefotaxime, cefotetan, cefoxitin, ceftazidime, ceftizoxime, ceftriaxone, cefuroxime, chloramphenicol, cisplatin, clindamycin, cyanocobalamin, cyclophosphamide, cyclosporine, cytarabine, dactinomycin, dexamethasone, dexmedetomidine, digoxin, docetaxel, enalaprilat, epinephrine, epoetin alfa, eftifibatide, etoposide, etoposide phosphate, fenoldopam, fentanyl, fluconazole, fludarabine, fluorouracil, folic acid, foscarnet, furosemide, glycopyrrolate, granisetron, heparin, hydrocortisone, hydromorphone, ifosfamide, imipenem/cilastatin, isoproterenol, ketorolac, lidocaine, linezolid, mannitol, mechlorethamine, melphalan, methotrexate, methylprednisolone, metoclopramide, metoprolol, metronidazole, multivitamins, nafcillin, naloxone, nitroglycerin, nitroprusside, norepinephrine, oxacillin, oxytocin, paclitaxel, penicillin G, pentobarbital, phenobarbital, phenylephrine, phytonadione, potassium chloride, procainamide, propofol, propranolol, ranitidine, rituximab, sodium acetate, sodium bicarbonate, streptokinase, succinylcholine, sufentanil, tacrolimus, teniposide, theophylline, thiotepa, ticarcillin/clavulanate, urokinase, vasopressin, vincristine.
- **Y-Site Incompatibility:** amifostine, amikacin, amphotericin B cholesteryl, amphotericin B liposome, atracurium, azathioprine, benztropine, calcium chloride, caspofungin, chlorpromazine, cimetidine, cisatracurium, codeine, dantrolene, diazepam, diazoxide, di-

CEPHALOSPORINS—THIRD GENERATION

phenhydramine, dobutamine, dopamine, doxacurium, doxorubicin, doxorubicin liposome, doxycycline, epirubicin, filgrastim, ganciclovir, gemcitabine, gentamicin, haloperidol, hydralazine, hydroxyzine, idarubicin, inamrinone, indomethacin, insulin, labetalol, levofloxacin, meperidine, metaraminol, methoxamine, methyldopate, midazolam, mitoxantrone, nalbuphine, nesiritide, nicardipine, ondansetron, oxaliplatin, pantoprazole, papaverine, pentamidine, pentazocine, perphenazine, phentolamine, phenytoin, prochlorperazine, promethazine, protamine, pyridoxime, quinupristin/dalfopristin, rocuronium, sargramostim, thiamine, tobramycin, tolazoline, trastuzumab, trimetaphan, trimethoprim/sulfamethoxazole, vancomycin, verapamil, vinorelbine.

Cefotaxime

- **Intermittent Infusion:** *Diluent:* Reconstituted solution may be further diluted in 50–100 mL of D5W, D10W, LR, dextrose/saline combinations, or 0.9% NaCl. Solution may appear light yellow to amber. Solution is stable for 24 hr at room temperature and 5 days if refrigerated. *Concentration:* 20–60 mg/mL. *Rate:* Administer over 20–30 min.
- **Syringe Compatibility:** heparin.
- **Y-Site Compatibility:** acyclovir, alfentanil, alprostadin, amifostine, aminophylline, ascorbic acid, atracurium, atropine, aztreonam, benztropine, bivalirudin, bumetanide, buprenorphine, butorphanol, calcium chloride, calcium gluconate, carboplatin, cefonocid, cefoperazone, cefotetan, cefoxitin, ceftriaxone, cefuroxime, cimetidine, cisplain, clindamycin, cyanocobalamin, cyclophosphamide, cyclosporine, cytarabine, dactinomycin, daptomycin, dexamethasone, dexmedetomidine, digoxin, diltiazem, docetaxel, dopamine, doxacurium, doxycyline, enalaprilat, ephedrine, epinephrine, epirubicin, epoetin, erythromycin, esmolol, etoposide, etoposide phosphate, famotidine, fenoldopam, fentanyl, fludarabine, fluorouracil, folic acid, furosemide, glycopyrrolate, granisetron, heparin, hydrocortisone, hydromorphone, ifosfamide, imipenem/cilastatin, insulin, isoproterenol, ketorolac, lidocaine, linezolid, lorazepam, magnesium sulfate, mannitol, mechlorethamine, melphalan, meperidine, metaraminol, methotrexate, methoxamine, methyldopate, metoclopramide, metoprolol, metronidazole, miconazole, midazolam, milrinone, morphine, multivitamins, nafcillin, nalbuphine, naloxone, nesiritide, nitroglycerin, nitroprusside, norepinephrine, octreotide, ondansetron, oxacillin, oxaliplatin, oxytocin, paclitaxel, palonosetron, penicillin G, perphenazine, phenylephrine, phytonadione, potassium chloride, procainamide, propofol, propranolol, pyridoxime, ranitidine, remifentanil, ritodrine, rituximab, rocuronium, sargramostim, sodium acetate, streptokinase, succinylcholine, sufentanil, tacrolimus, teniposide, theophylline, thiamine, thiotepa, ticarcillin/clavulanate, tigecycline, tirofiban, tolazoline, trimethaphan, urokinase, vasopressin, verapamil, vinorelbine, voriconazole.
- **Y-Site Incompatibility:** allopurinol, amphotericin B liposome, ampicillin/sulbactam, azathioprine, azithromycin, caspofungin, cefazolin, ceftazidime, ceftizoxime, chloramphenicol, chlorpromazine, dantrolene, diazepam, diazoxide, diphenhydramine, doxorubicin hydrochloride, filgrastim, ganciclovir, gemcitabine, haloperidol, hydralazine, hydroxyzine, inamrinone, labetalol, methylprednisolone, mitoxantrone, pantoprazole, papaverine, pemetrexed, pentamidine, pentazocine, pentobarbital, phenobarbital, phenytoin, prochlorperazine, promethazine, quinupristin/dalfopristin, sodium bicarbonate, trastuzumab, trimethoprim/sulfamethoxazole, vecuronium.

Ceftazidime

- **Intermittent Infusion:** *Diluent:* Reconstituted solution may be further diluted in at least 1 g/10 mL of 0.9% NaCl, D5W, D10W, dextrose/saline combinations, or LR. Dilution causes CO_2 to form inside vial, resulting in positive pressure; vial may require venting after dissolution to preserve sterility of vial. Not required with L-arginine formulation (Ceptaz). Solution may appear yellow to amber; darkening does not alter potency. Solution is stable for 18 hr at room temperature and 7 days if refrigerated. *Concentration:* 40 mg/mL. *Rate:* Administer over 15–30 min.
- **Y-Site Compatibility:** acyclovir, alfentanil, allopurinol, amifostine, aminophylline, anidulafungin, atropine, aztreonam, bivalirudin, bumetanide, buprenorphine, butorphanol, calcium gluconate, carboplatin, cefazolin, cefonicid, ceforperazone, cefotetan, cefoxitin, ceftizoxime, ceftriaxone, cefuroxime, cimetidine, ciprofloxacin, cisplatin, clindamycin, cya-

nocobalamin, cyclophosphamide, cyclosporine, cytarabine, dactinomycin, daptomycin, dexamethasone, dexmedetomidine, digoxin, diltiazem, docetaxel, dopamine, doxacurium, doxapram, enalaprilat, ephedrine, epinephrine, epoetin alfa, esmolol, etoposide, etoposide phosphate, famotidine, fenoldopam, fentanyl, filgrastim, fludarabine, fluorouracil, folic acid, foscarnet, furosemide, gemcitabine, glycopyrrolate, granisetron, heparin, hetastarch, hydrocortisone, hydromorphone, ifosfamide, imipenem/cilastatin, indomethacin, insulin, isoproterenol, ketamine, ketorolac, labetalol, levofloxacin, lidocaine, linezolid, lorazepam, magnesium sulfate, mannitol, mechlorethamine, melphalan, meperidine, metaraminol, methotrexate, methoxamine, methyldopate, methylprednisolone, metoclopramide, metoprolol, metronidazole, milrinone, morphine, multivitamins, nafcillin, nalbuphine, naloxone, nesiritide, nitroglycerin, norepinephrine, octreotide, oxacillin, oxaliplatin, oxytocin, paclitaxel, palonosetron, pantoprazole, penicillin G, phenobarbital, phentolamine, phenylephrine, phytonadione, potassium chloride, procainamide, propranolol, pyridoxime, ranitidine, remifentanil, rituximab, rocuronium, sodium acetate, sodium bicarbonate, sodium citrate, streptokinase, succinylcholine, sufentanil, tacrolimus, teniposide, thiotepa, ticarcillin/clavulanate, tigecycline, tirofiban, tolazoline, trastuzumab, trimethaphan, urokinase, vasopressin, vecuronium, vincristine, vinorelbine, voriconazole, zidovudine.

- **Y-Site Incompatibility:** amiodarone, amphotericin B cholesteryl, amphotericin B liposome, amsacrine, ascorbic acid, atracurium, azathioprine, azithromycin, calcium chloride, caspofungin, cefotaxime, chloramphenicol, chlorpromazine, diazepam, diazoxide, diphenhydramine, doxorubicin hydrochloride, doxorubicin liposome, doxycycline, epirubicin, ganciclovir, haloperidol, hydralazine, hydroxyzine, idarubicin, inamrinone, midazolam, mitoxantrone, nitroprusside, papaverine, pemetrexed, pentamidine, pentazocine, phenytoin, prochlorperazine, promethazine, protamine, quinupristin/dalfopristin, thiamine, trimethoprim/sulfamethoxazole, verapamil, warfarin.

Ceftizoxime

- **Intermittent Infusion:** *Diluent:*Reconstituted solution may be further diluted in 50–100 mL of D5W, D10W, 0.9% NaCl, dextrose/saline combinations, or LR. Solution is stable for 8 hr at room temperature and 48 hr if refrigerated. *Concentration:*20 mg/mL. *Rate:* Administer over 15–30 min.

- **Y-Site Compatibility:** acyclovir, alfentanil, allopurinol, amifostine, aminophylline, amiodarone, amphotericin B cholesteryl, amphotericin B liposome, anidulafungin, ascorbic acid, atracurium, atropine, aztreonam, benztropine, bivalirudin, bumetanide, buprenorphine, butorphanol, calcium chloride, calcium gluconate, carboplatin, caspofungin, cefazolin, cefoperazone, cefotetan, ceftazidime, ceftriaxone, cefuroxime, cimetidine, cisplatin, clindamycin, cyanocobalamin, cyclophosphamide, cyclosporine, cytarabine, dactinomycin, dactomycin, dexamethasone, dexmedetomidine, digoxin, diltiazem, diphenhyrdamine, docetaxel, dopamine, doxacurium, doxorubicin hydrochloride, doxorubicin liposome, enalaprilat, ephedrine, ephinephrine, epirubicin, epoetin, esmolol, etoposide, etoposide phosphate, fenoldopam, fentanyl, fluconazole, fludarabine, fluorouracil, folic acid, foscarnet, furosemide, gemcitabine, glycopyrrolate, granisetron, heparin, hetastarch, hydrocortisone, hydromorphone, ifosfamide, imipenem/cilastatin, insulin, isoproterenol, ketorolac, labetalol, levofloxaxin, lidocaine, linezolid, lorazepam, magnesium chloride, mannitol, mechlorethamine, melphalan, meperidine, methotrexate, methoxamine, methyldopate, metoclopramide, metoprolol, metronidazole, midazolam, milrinone, mitoxantrone, morphine, multivitamins, nafcillin, naloxone, nesiritide, nicardipine, nitroglycerin, nitroprusside, norepinephrine, octreotide, ondansetron, oxaliplatin, oxytocin, paclitaxel, palonosetron, pantoprazole, pemetrexed, penicillin G, phenobarbital, phenylephrine, phytonadione, potassium chloride, propofol, propranolol, ranitidine, remifentanil, ritodrine, rituximab, rocuronium, sargramostim, sodium acetate, sodium bicarbonate, streptokinase, succinylcholine, sufentanil, tacrolimus, teniposide, theophylline, thiotepa, ticarcillin/clavulanate, tigecycline, tirofiban, trastuzumab, trimethaphan, vasopressin, verapamil, vincristine, vinorelbine, voriconazole.

- **Y-Site Incompatibility:** amphotericin B colloidal, cefotaxime, cefoxitin, chloramphenicool, chlorpromazine, dantrolene, diazepam, diazoxide, doxycycline, ethromycin, filgrastim, ganciclovir, haloperidol, hydralazine, hydroxyzine, inamrinone, nalbuphine, papaverine, pentamadine, pentazocine, phenytoin, procainamide, prochlorperazine, promethazine, protamine, pyridoxime, quinupristin/dalfopristin, thiamine, trimethoprim/sulfamethoxazole.

Ceftriaxone

- **Intermittent Infusion:** Reconstitute each 250-mg vial with 2.4 mL, each 500-mg vial with 4.8 mL, each 1-g vial with 9.6 mL, and each 2-g vial with 19.2 mL of sterile water for injection, 0.9% NaCl, or D5W for a concentration of 100 mg/mL. *Diluent:* Solution may be further diluted in 50–100 mL of 0.9% NaCl, D5W, D10W, D5/0.45% NaCl, or LR. Solution may appear light yellow to amber. Solution is stable for 3 days at room temperature. *Concentration:* 40 mg/mL. *Rate:* Administer over 10–30 min.

- **Y-Site Compatibility:** acyclovir, alfentanil, allopurinol, amifostine, aminophylline, amiodarone, amphotericin B liposome, anidulafungin, atracurium, atropine, aztreonam, bivalirudin, bumetanide, buprenorphine, butorphanol, carboplatin, cefazolin, cefonocid, cefoperazone, cefotaxime, cefotetan, cefoxitin, ceftazidime, ceftizoxime, cefuroxime, cimetidine, cisatracurium, cisplatin, cyanocobalamin, cyclophosphamide, cyclosporine, cytarabine, dactinomycin, daptomycin, dexamethasone, dexmedetomidine, digoxin, diltiazem, docetaxel, dopamine, doxacurium, doxorubicin liposome, doxycycline, drotrecogin, enalaprilat, ephedrine, epinephrine, epoetin alfa, epitifibitide, erythromycin, esmolol, etoposide, etoposide phosphate, fenoldopam, fentanyl, fludarabine, fluorouracil, folic acid, foscarnet, furosemide, gemcitabine, glycopyrrolate, granisetron, heparin, hetastarch, hydrocortisone, hydromorphone, ifosfamide, indomethacin, insulin, isoproterenol, ketorolac, levofloxacin, lidocaine, linezolid, lorazepam, mannitol, mechlorethamine, melphalan, meperidine, metaraminol, methotrexate, methoxamine, methyldopate, methylprednisolone, metoclopramide, metoprolol, metronidazole, midazolam, milrinone, morphine, multivitamins, nafcillin, nalbuphine, naloxone, nesiritide, nitroglycerin, nitroprusside, norepinephrine, octreotide, oxacillin, oxaliplatin, oxytocin, paclitaxel, palonosetron, pantoprazole, pemetrexed, penicillin G, phenobarbital, phentolamine, phenylephrine, phytonadione, potassium chloride, procainamide, propofol, propranolol, pyridoxime, ranitidine, remifentanil, rituximab, rocuronium, sargramostim, sodium acetate, sodium bicarbonate, streptokinase, succinylcholine, sufentanil, tacrolimus, teniposide, theophylline, thiamine, thiotepa, ticarcillin/clavulanate, tigecycline, tirofiban, tolazoline, trastuzumab, trimethaphan, urokinase, vasopressin, vecuronium, verapamil, vincristine, voriconazole, warfarin, zidovudine.

- **Y-Site Incompatibility:** amphotericin B cholesteryl, amsacrine, ascorbic acid, azathioprine, azithromycin, calcium chloride, calcium gluconate, caspofungin, chloramphenicol, chlorpromazine, clindamycin, dantrolene, diazepam, diazoxide, diphenhydramine, dobutamine, doxorubicin hydrochloride, epirubicin, filgrastim, ganciclovir, haloperidol, hetastarch, hydralazine, hydroxyzine, idarubicin, imipenem/cilastatin, inamrinone, labetalol, lactated ringers, magnesium sulfate, mitoxantrone, pentamidine, pentazocine, pentobarbital, phenytoin, prochlorperazine, promethazine, protamine, quinupristin/dalfopristin, Ringer's injection, trimethoprim/sulfamethoxazole, tobramycin, vinorelbine. Calcium-containing solutions, including parenteral nutrition, should not be mixed or co-administered, even via different infusion lines at different sites in patients <28 days old. In older patients, flush line thoroughly between infusions.

Patient/Family Teaching

- Instruct patient to take medication around the clock and to finish the medication completely, even if feeling better. Take missed doses as soon as possible unless almost time for next dose; do not double doses. Advise patient that sharing of this medication may be dangerous.
- Pedi: Instruct parents or caregivers to use calibrated measuring device with liquid preparations.
- Advise patient to report signs of superinfection (furry overgrowth on the tongue, vaginal itching or discharge, loose or foul-smelling stools) and allergy.
- Caution patients that concurrent use of alcohol with *cefoperazone* may cause a disulfiram-like reaction (abdominal cramps, nausea, vomiting, headache, hypotension, palpitations, dyspnea, tachycardia, sweating, flushing). Alcohol and alcohol-containing medications should be avoided during and for several days after therapy.
- Instruct patient to notify health care professional if fever and diarrhea develop, especially if stool contains blood, pus, or mucus. Advise patient not to treat diarrhea without consulting health care professional.

Evaluation/Desired Outcomes
- Resolution of the signs and symptoms of infection. Length of time for complete resolution depends on the organism and site of infection.
- Decreased incidence of infection when used for prophylaxis.

certolizumab pegol
(ser-toe-**liz**-u-mab)
Cimzia

Classification
Therapeutic: gastrointestinal anti-inflammatories, antirheumatics
Pharmacologic: tumor necrosis factor blockers, DMARDs, monoclonal antibodies

Pregnancy Category B

Indications
Moderately-to-severely active Crohn's disease when response to conventional therapy has been inadequate. Moderately-to-severely active rheumatoid arthritis.

Action
Neutralizes tumor necrosis factor (TNF), a prime mediator of inflammation; pegolation provides a long duration of action. **Therapeutic Effects:** Decreased signs/symptoms of Crohn's disease. Decreased pain and swelling, decreased rate of joint destruction and improved physical function in rheumatoid arthritis.

Pharmacokinetics
Absorption: 80% absorbed following SC administration.
Distribution: Unknown.
Metabolism and Excretion: Unknown.
Half-life: 14 days.

TIME/ACTION PROFILE (blood levels)

ROUTE	ONSET	PEAK	DURATION
Subcut	unknown	50–120 hr	2–4 wk

Contraindications/Precautions
Contraindicated in: Active untreated infection; Hepatitis B reactivation; Concurrent use of anakinra.
Use Cautiously in: History of recurrent infections, concurrent immunosupressants, medical conditions associated with increased risk of infection, current residence in areas where tuberculosis or histoplasmosis is endemic, history of hepatitis B infection (may reactivate); History of demyelinating disorders (may exacerbate); History of heart failure; Geri:May ↑ risk of infections; OB:Use in pregnancy only if clearly needed; avoid breastfeeding; Pedi:Safety not established; ↑ risk of lymphoma, leukemia, and other malignancies.

Adverse Reactions/Side Effects
Derm: psoriasis, skin reactions (rarely severe).
Hemat: LEUKEMIA, hematologic reactions. **MS:** arthralgia. **Misc:** allergic reactions including ANAPHYLAXIS, INFECTIONS (including reactivation tuberculosis and invasive fungal infections), MALIGNANCY, lupus-like syndrome.

Interactions
Drug-Drug: Concurrent use with **anakinra** ↑ risk of serious infections (contraindicated). May ↓ antibody response to or ↑ risk of adverse reactions to **live vaccines** (contraindicated).

Route/Dosage
Crohn's Disease
Subcut (Adults): 400 mg initially, repeat 2 and 4 wk later; may be followed by maintenance dose of 400 mg every 4 wk.

Rheumatoid Arthritis
Subcut (Adults): 400 mg initially, repeat 2 and 4 wk later; then maintenance dose of 200 mg every 2 wk (400 mg every 4 wk may be used alternatively).

Availability
Lyophilized powder for subcutaneous injection (requires reconstitution): 200 mg/vial.
Prefilled syringe: 200 mg/mL.

NURSING IMPLICATIONS

Assessment
- **Crohn's Disease:** Assess abdominal pain and frequency, quantity, and consistency of stools at beginning and during therapy.
- **Arthritis:** Assess pain and range of motion before and periodically during therapy.
- Assess for signs of infection (fever, sore throat, dyspnea, WBC) prior to and during therapy. Monitor all patients for active TB during therapy, even if initial test was negative. Do not begin certolizumab during an active infection, including chronic or localized infections. If infection develops, monitor closely and discontinue certolizumab if infection becomes serious.
- Evaluate patients at risk for hepatitis B virus (HBV) infection for prior evidence of HBV infection before initiating therapy. Monitor carriers of HBV closely for clinical and lab signs of active HBV infection during and for several

months following discontinuation of therapy. If HBV reactivation occurs, discontinue certolizumab and initiate antiviral therapy.
- Monitor for signs of hypersensitivity reactions (angioedema, dyspnea, hypotension, rash, serum sickness, urticaria). If reactions occur, discontinue certolizumab and treat symptomatically.
- Assess for signs and symptoms of systemic fungal infections (fever, malaise, weight loss, sweats, cough, dypsnea, pulmonary infiltrates, serious systemic illness with or without concomitant shock). Ascertain if patient lives in or has traveled to areas of endemic mycoses. Consider empiric antifungal treatment for patients at risk of histoplasmosis and other invasive fungal infections until the pathogens are identified. Consult with an infectious diseases specialist. Consider stopping certolizumab until the infection has been diagnosed and adequately treated.
- *Lab Test Considerations:* May cause anemia, leukopenia, pancytopenia, and thrombocytopenia.
- Monitor CBC with differential periodically during therapy. May cause leukopenia, neutropenia, thrombocytopenia, and pancytopenia. Discontinue certolizumab if symptoms of blood dyscrasias (persistent fever) occur.
- May cause ↑ liver enzymes.
- May cause erroneously ↑ aPTT.

Potential Nursing Diagnoses
Risk for infection (Side Effects)

Implementation
- Perform test for latent TB. If positive, begin treatment for TB prior to starting certolizumab therapy.
- Bring medication to room temperature prior to reconstituting. Reconstitute 2 vials for each dose by adding 1 mL of Sterile Water for injection to each vial, using a 20-gauge needle, for a concentration of 200 mg/mL. Gently swirl so all powder comes into contact with sterile water; do not shake. Leave vials undisturbed for as long as 30 min to fully reconstitute. Solution is clear and colorless to pale yellow; do not administer solutions that are discolored or contain particulate matter. Do not leave reconstituted solution at room temperature for >2 hr prior to injection. May be refrigerated for up to 24 hr prior to injection; do not freeze.
- **Subcut:** Bring solution to room temperature prior to injection. Using a new 20-gauge needle for each vial, withdraw reconstituted solution into 2 separate syringes each containing 1 mL (200 mg/mL) of certolizumab. Switch each 20-gauge needle to a 23-gauge needle and inject the full contents of each syringe subcut into separate sides of the abdomen or thigh.

Patient/Family Teaching
- Advise patient of potential benefits and risks of certolizumab. Advise patient to read the *Medication Guide* prior to starting therapy.
- Inform patient of risk of infection. Advise patient to notify health care professional if symptoms of infection (fever, cough, flu-like symptoms, or open cuts or sores), including TB or reactivation of HBV infection, occur.
- Counsel patient about possible risk of lymphoma and other malignancies while receiving certolizumab.
- Advise patient to notify health care professional if signs of hypersensitivity reactions (rash, swollen face, difficulty breathing), or new or worsening medical conditions such as heart or neurological disease or autoimmune disorders occur and to report signs of bone marrow depression (bruising, bleeding, or persistent failure.
- Instruct patient to consult health care professional prior to taking any Rx, OTC, vitamins, or herbal products.
- Advise patient to notify health care professional if pregnancy is planned or suspected or if breastfeeding.

Evaluation/Desired Outcomes
- Decrease in signs and symptoms of Crohn's disease.
- Decreased pain and swelling with decreased rate of joint destruction in patients with rheumatoid arthritis.

---

cetirizine (se-ti-ra-zeen)
Zyrtec

Classification
Therapeutic: allergy, cold, and cough remedies, antihistamines
Pharmacologic: piperazines (peripherally selective)

Pregnancy Category B

cetirizine

Indications
Relief of allergic symptoms caused by histamine release including: Seasonal and perennial allergic rhinitis, Chronic urticaria.

Action
Antagonizes the effects of histamine at H_1-receptor sites; does not bind to or inactivate histamine. Anticholinergic effects are minimal and sedation is dose related. **Therapeutic Effects:** Decreased symptoms of histamine excess (sneezing, rhinorrhea, ocular tearing and redness, pruritus).

Pharmacokinetics
Absorption: Well absorbed following oral administration.
Distribution: Unknown.
Protein Binding: 93%.
Metabolism and Excretion: Excreted primarily unchanged by the kidneys.
Half-life: 7.4–9 hr (decreased in children to 6.2 hr, increased in renal impairment up to 19–21 hr).

TIME/ACTION PROFILE (antihistaminic effects)

ROUTE	ONSET	PEAK	DURATION
PO	30 min	4–8 hr	24 hr

Contraindications/Precautions
Contraindicated in: Hypersensitivity to cetirizine, hydroxyzine or any component; Lactation: Excreted in breast milk; not recommended for use.
Use Cautiously in: Patients with hepatic or renal impairment (dosage reduction recommended if $CCr \leq 31$ mL/min or hepatic function is impaired); OB, Pedi:Safety not established for pregnant women or children <6 mo; Geri:Initiate at lower doses.

Adverse Reactions/Side Effects
CNS: dizziness, drowsiness (significant with doses >10 mg/day), fatigue. **EENT:** pharyngitis. **GI:** dry mouth.

Interactions
Drug-Drug: Additive CNS depression may occur with **alcohol**, **opioid analgesics**, or **sedative/hypnotics**. **Theophylline** may decrease clearance and increase toxicity.

Route/Dosage
PO (Adults and children >6 yr): 5–10 mg given once or divided twice daily.
PO (Children 2–5 yr): 2.5 mg once daily initially, may be increased to 5 mg once daily or 2.5 mg every 12 hr.
PO (Children 1–2 yr): 2.5 mg once daily; may be increased to 2.5 mg every 12 hr.
PO (Children 6–12 mo): 2.5 once daily.

Hepatic/Renal Impairment
PO (Adults and Children >12 yr): *CCr $\leq$31 mL/min, hepatic impairment or hemodialysis*— 5 mg once daily.
PO (Children 6–11 yr): start therapy at <2.5 mg/day.
PO (Children <6 yr): use not recommended.

Availability (generic available)
Tablets: 5 mg[OTC], 10 mg[OTC]. **Cost:** 5 mg $76.99/30, 10 mg $75.99/30. **Chewable tablets (grape):** 5 mg[OTC], 10 mg[OTC]. **Cost:** 5 mg $75.99/30, 10 mg $75.99/30. **Syrup (banana-grape and bubblegum flavors):** 1 mg/mL in 120-mL and 480-mL bottles[OTC]. **Cost:** $41.99/120 mL, $145.97/480 mL. ***In combination with:*** pseudoephedrine (Zyrtec-D 12 Hour) (See Appendix B).

NURSING IMPLICATIONS

Assessment
- Assess allergy symptoms (rhinitis, conjunctivitis, hives) before and periodically during therapy.
- Assess lung sounds and character of bronchial secretions. Maintain fluid intake of 1500–2000 mL/day to decrease viscosity of secretions.
- *Lab Test Considerations:* May cause false-negative result in allergy skin testing.

Potential Nursing Diagnoses
Ineffective airway clearance (Indications)
Risk for injury (Adverse Reactions)

Implementation
- Do not confuse Zyrtec (cetirizine) with Zantac (ranitidine) or Zyprexa (olanzapine).
- **PO:** Administer once daily without regard to food.

Patient/Family Teaching
- Instruct patient to take medication as directed.
- May cause dizziness and drowsiness. Caution patient to avoid driving or other activities requiring alertness until response to medication is known.
- Advise patient to avoid taking alcohol or other CNS depressants concurrently with this drug.
- Advise patient that good oral hygiene, frequent rinsing of mouth with water, and sugarless gum or candy may minimize dry mouth. Patient should notify dentist if dry mouth persists >2 wk.

- Instruct patient to contact health care professional if dizziness occurs or if symptoms persist.

Evaluation/Desired Outcomes
- Decrease in allergic symptoms.

♦ cetuximab (se-**tux**-i-mab)
Erbitux

Classification
Therapeutic: antineoplastics
Pharmacologic: monoclonal antibodies

Pregnancy Category C

Indications
Locally or regionally advanced squamous cell carcinoma of the head and neck with radiation. Recurrent or metastatic squamous cell carcinoma of the head and neck progressing after platinum-based therapy. Epidermal growth factor receptor (EGFR) expressing metastatic colorectal cancer in patients who have not responded to irinotecan and oxaliplatin. Metastatic colorectal cancer (with irinotecan) when tumors express the EGFR and have not responded or are intolerant to irinotecan alone.

Action
♦ Binds specifically to EGFR, thereby preventing the binding of endogenous epidermal growth factor (EGF). This prevents cell growth and differentiation processes. Combination with irinotecan enhances antitumor effects of irinotecan. **Therapeutic Effects:** Decreased tumor growth and spread.

Pharmacokinetics
Absorption: IV administration results in complete bioavailability.
Distribution: Unknown.
Metabolism and Excretion: Unknown.
Half-life: 97–114 hr.

TIME/ACTION PROFILE

ROUTE	ONSET	PEAK	DURATION
IV	unknown	unknown	unknown

Contraindications/Precautions
Contraindicated in: Hypersensitivity to cetuximab or murine (mouse) proteins; ♦ Patients whose tumors have KRAS mutations in codon 12 or 13 (not effective); OB, Lactation: Pregnancy or lactation.

Use Cautiously in: Exposure to sunlight (may exacerbate dermatologic toxicity); Pedi: Safety not established.

Adverse Reactions/Side Effects
Most adverse reactions reflect combination therapy with irinotecan.
CNS: malaise, depression, headache, insomnia. **EENT:** conjunctivitis. **Resp:** dyspnea, ↑ cough, interstitial lung disease. **CV:** PULMONARY EMBOLISM. **GI:** abdominal pain, constipation, diarrhea, nausea, vomiting, anorexia, stomatitis. **GU:** renal failure. **Derm:** acneform dermatitis, hypertrichosis, nail disorder, pruritus, skin desquamation, skin infection. **F and E:** dehydration, hypomagnesemia, peripheral edema. **Hemat:** anemia, leukopenia. **MS:** back pain. **Metab:** weight loss. **Misc:** INFUSION REACTIONS, fever, desquamation of mucosal epithelium.

Interactions
Drug-Drug: None noted.

Route/Dosage

Head & Neck Cancer with Radiation
IV (Adults): 400 mg/m^2 administered 1 wk prior to initiation of radiation therapy, followed by weekly maintenance doses of 250 mg/m^2 for the duration of radiation therapy. Complete infusion 1 hr prior to radiation therapy; dose modification recommended for dermatologic toxicity.

Head and Neck Cancer Monotherapy
IV (Adults): 400 mg/m^2 initial loading dose, followed by weekly maintenance doses of 250 mg/m^2 until disease progression or unacceptable toxicity; dose modification recommended for dermatologic toxicity.

Colorectal Cancer
IV (Adults): 400 mg/m^2 initial loading dose, followed by weekly maintenance doses of 250 mg/m^2; dose modification recommended for dermatologic toxicity.

Availability
Solution for injection: 2 mg/mL.

NURSING IMPLICATIONS

Assessment
- Assess for infusion reaction (rapid onset of airway obstruction [bronchospasm, stridor, hoarseness], urticaria, hypotension, loss of consciousness, myocardial infarction, cardiopulmonary arrest) for at least 1 hr following in-

fusion. Longer observation periods may be required for those who experience infusion reactions. Most reactions occur during first dose, but may also occur in later doses. For severe reactions, immediately stop infusion and discontinue cetuximab permanently. Epinephrine, corticosteroids, IV antihistamines, bronchodilators, and oxygen should be available for reactions.Mild to moderate reactions (chills, fever, dyspnea) may be managed by slowing rate of infusion and administration of antihistamines.
- Assess for onset or worsening of pulmonary symptoms. Interrupt therapy to determine nature of symptoms. If interstitial lung disease is confirmed, discontinue cetuximab and treat appropriately.
- Assess for dermatologic toxicities (acneform rash, skin drying and fissuring, inflammatory and infectious sequelae [blepharitis, cheilitis, cellulitis, cyst]). Treat symptomatically. Acneform rash usually occurs within initial 2 wk of therapy and resolves following cessation, but may continue up to 28 days following therapy.
- **Lab Test Considerations:** May cause anemia and leukopenia.
- Monitor serum electrolytes periodically during and for at least 8 wk following infusion. May cause hypomagnesemia, hypocalcemia, and hypokalemia; may occur from days to months after initiation of therapy. May require electrolyte replacement.

Potential Nursing Diagnoses
Ineffective breathing pattern (Adverse Reactions)
Impaired skin integrity (Adverse Reactions)

Implementation
- Premedicate with histamine₁ antagonist (diphenhydramine 50 mg) 30–60 min prior to first dose; base subsequent administration on presence and severity of infusion reactions.
- Administer through a low protein binding 0.22-micrometer in-line filter placed as proximal to patient as possible. Solution should be clear and colorless and may contain a small amount of white amorphous cetuximab particles. Do not shake or dilute.
- Can be administered via infusion pump or syringe pump. Cetuximab should be piggybacked to the patient's infusion line.
- Observe patient for 1 hr following infusion.

IV Administration
- **Intermittent Infusion:** *For administration via infusion pump:* Draw up volume of a vial using vented spike needle or other transfer device. Transfer to a sterile evacuated container or bag. Repeat with new needle for each vial until calculated volume is in container. Affix infusion line and prime with cetuximab before starting infusion.
- *For administration via syringe pump:* Draw up volume of a vial using sterile syringe attached to an appropriate vented spike needle. Place syringe into syringe driver of a syringe pump and set rate. Connect infusion line and prime with cetuximab. Use a new needle and filter for each vial. **Diluent:**Do not dilute. **Concentration:**2 mg/mL. **Rate:**Administer over 2 hr at a rate not to exceed 10 mg/min. Use 0.9% NaCl to flush line at end of infusion.

Patient/Family Teaching
- Explain purpose of cetuximab and potential side effects to patient.
- Advise patient to report dermatologic changes and signs and symptoms of infusion reactions (fever, chills, or breathing problems) promptly.
- Caution patient to wear sunscreen and hats and limit sun exposure during therapy during and for 2 mo following last dose of cetuximab.
- Advise both female and male patients to use adequate contraception during and for 6 mo following therapy and to avoid breastfeeding during and for 2 mo following therapy.

Evaluation/Desired Outcomes
- Decreased tumor growth and spread.

HIGH ALERT

chloral hydrate
(klor-al hye-drate)
Aquachloral, ✣Novo-Chlorhydrate, ✣PMS-Chloral Hydrate

Classification
Therapeutic: sedative/hypnotics

Schedule IV

Pregnancy Category C

Indications
Short-term sedative and hypnotic (effectiveness decreases after 2 wk of use). Sedation or reduction of anxiety preoperatively (anesthetic adjunct) or prior to diagnostic procedures.

Action
Converted to trichloroethanol, which is the active drug. Has generalized CNS depressant properties.
Therapeutic Effects: Sedation or induction of sleep.

chloral hydrate

Pharmacokinetics
Absorption: Well absorbed following oral or rectal administration.
Distribution: Widely distributed. Crosses the placenta and enters breast milk in low concentrations.
Metabolism and Excretion: Converted by liver to trichloroethanol, which is active. Trichloroethanol is, in turn, metabolized by the liver and kidneys to inactive compounds.
Half-life: *Chloral hydrate*—Infants: 1 hr. *Trichloroethanol*—Neonates: 8.5–66 hr; Children: 10 hr; Adults: 8–11 hr.

TIME/ACTION PROFILE (sedation)

ROUTE	ONSET	PEAK	DURATION
PO	30 min	1 hr	4–8 hr
Rectal	0.5–1 hr	1 hr	4–8 hr

Contraindications/Precautions
Contraindicated in: Hypersensitivity; Severe cardiac disease; Severe renal impairment (ClCr <50 mL/min); Coma or pre-existing CNS depression; Uncontrolled severe pain; OB: Crosses placenta; chronic use during pregnancy may cause withdrawal symptoms in the neonate; Lactation: Excreted in human milk, use by nursing mothers may cause sedation in the infant; Esophagitis, gastritis, or ulcer disease; Proctitis (rectal use); Tartrazine hypersensitivity (some rectal products); Impaired respiratory function; Sleep apnea.
Use Cautiously in: Hepatic dysfunction; History of suicide attempt or substance abuse; Obstructive sleep apnea; Pedi: May cause direct hyperbilirubinemia in neonates; Geri, Pedi: Dosage reduction recommended.

Adverse Reactions/Side Effects
CNS: excess sedation, disorientation, dizziness, hangover, headache, incoordination, irritability, paradoxical excitation (children). **Resp:** respiratory depression. **GI:** diarrhea, nausea, vomiting, flatulence. **Derm:** rashes. **Misc:** tolerance, physical dependence, psychological dependence.

Interactions
Drug-Drug: Additive CNS depression with other **CNS depressants**, including **alcohol**, **antihistamines**, **antidepressants**, **sedative/hypnotics**, and **opioid analgesics**. May potentiate **warfarin**. When given within 24 hr of IV **furosemide**, may cause diaphoresis, changes in blood pressure, and flushing. May increase metabolism and decrease effects of **phenytoin**. May increase toxicity of **ifosfamide** and **cyclophosphamide**.
Drug-Natural Products: Concomitant use of **kava-kava**, **valerian**, **skullcap**, **chamomile**, or **hops** can increase CNS depression.

Route/Dosage
PO (Adults): *Hypnotic*—500–1000 mg 15–30 min before bedtime. *Preoperative sedation*—500 mg–1000 mg 30 min before surgery. *Daytime sedation*—250 mg 3 times daily. Single dose/daily dose should not >2 g.
PO (Geriatric Patients): *Hypnotic*—250 mg 15–30 min before bedtime.
Rect (Adults): *Sedation*—325 mg 3 times daily. *Hypnotic*—500–1000 mg. Single dose/daily dose should not >2 g.
PO, Rect (Children >1 month): *Pre-electroencephalogram sedation*—20–25 mg/kg 30–60 min prior. *Sedation prior to dental/medical procedures*—50–75 mg/kg 30–60 min prior; may repeat within 30 min if needed; single dose should not exceed 1 g total for infants or 2 g total for children. *Hypnotic*—50 mg/kg; maximum 2 g/day. *Sedation/anxiety:* 25–50 mg/kg/day divided q 6–8 hr; maximum 500 mg/dose.
PO, Rect (Neonates): 25 mg/kg/dose prior to a procedure.

Availability (generic available)
Capsules: 500 mg. **Syrup:** 500 mg/5 mL. **Suppositories:** 325 mg, 500 mg.

NURSING IMPLICATIONS

Assessment
- Assess mental status (orientation, mood, behavior) and potential for abuse prior to administering this medication. Prolonged use may lead to physical and psychological dependence. Limit amount of drug available to the patient.
- Assess sleep pattern before and periodically throughout therapy.
- Geri: Assess CNS effects and risk for falls. Institute fall prevention strategies.
- Assess level of consciousness at time of peak effect. Notify physician or other health care professional if desired sedation does not occur or if paradoxical reaction occurs.
- *Lab Test Considerations:* Interferes with tests for urinary 17-hydroxycorticosteroids and urinary catecholamines.

Potential Nursing Diagnoses
Insomnia (Indications)
Anxiety (Indications)

Risk for injury (Side Effects)
Ineffective coping (Indications)
Sleep deprivation (Indications)
Risk for falls (Side Effects)
Acute confusion (Side Effects)

Implementation

- **_High Alert:_** Pedi:Chloral hydrate overdosage has resulted in fatalities in children. Only accept orders written in milligrams, not volume (teaspoons) or concentration. Chloral hydrate should be administered to children only by trained staff in the health care setting. When administered to children for sedation before outpatient procedures, administer at the facility where procedure is to be performed. Repeated doses should be used with great caution in neonates, as drug and metabolites accumulate and may lead to toxicity. Continue monitoring until level of consciousness is safe for discharge.
- Before administering, reduce external stimuli and provide comfort measures to increase effectiveness of medication.
- Refer for psychotherapy if ineffective coping is basis for sleep pattern disturbance.
- Protect patient from injury. Place bed-side rails up. Assist with ambulation. Remove cigarettes from patients receiving hypnotic dose.
- **PO:** Capsules should be swallowed whole with a full glass of water or juice to minimize gastric irritation; do not chew.Dilute syrup in a half glass of water, juice, ginger ale, or formula to mask taste.
- **Rect:** If suppository is too soft for insertion, chill in refrigerator for 30 min or run under cold water before removing foil wrapper.

Patient/Family Teaching

- Instruct patient to take chloral hydrate exactly as directed. Missed doses should be omitted; do not double doses. If used for 2 wk or longer, abrupt withdrawal may result in CNS excitement, tremor, anxiety, hallucinations, and delirium.
- Chloral hydrate causes drowsiness and dizziness. Caution patient to avoid driving or other activities requiring alertness until response to medication is known.
- Caution patient that concurrent alcohol use may create an additive effect that results in tachycardia, vasodilation, flushing, headache, hypotension, and pronounced CNS depression. Alcohol and other CNS depressants should be avoided while taking chloral hydrate.
- Advise patient to discontinue use and notify health care professional if skin rash, dizziness, irritability, impaired thought processes, headache, or motor incoordination occurs.
- Teach sleep hygiene techniques (dark room, quiet, bedtime ritual, limit daytime napping, avoid nicotine and caffeine).

Evaluation/Desired Outcomes

- Sedation.
- Improvement in sleep pattern.

---

chlordiazepoxide
(klor-dye-az-e-**pox**-ide)
✦Apo-Chlordiazepoxide, Libritabs, Librium, ✦Mitran, ✦Novopoxide, ✦Poxi

Classification
Therapeutic: antianxiety agents, sedative/hypnotics
Pharmacologic: benzodiazepines

Schedule IV

Pregnancy Category D

Indications
Adjunct management of anxiety. Treatment of alcohol withdrawal. Adjunct management of anxiety associated with acute myocardial infarction.

Action
Acts at many levels of the CNS to produce anxiolytic effect. Depresses the CNS, probably by potentiating GABA, an inhibitory neurotransmitter.
Therapeutic Effects: Sedation. Relief of anxiety.

Pharmacokinetics
Absorption: Well absorbed from the GI tract. IM absorption may be slow and unpredictable.
Distribution: Widely distributed. Crosses the blood-brain barrier. Crosses the placenta; enters breast milk. Recommend to discontinue drug or bottle feed.
Metabolism and Excretion: Highly metabolized by the liver. Some products of metabolism are active as CNS depressants.
Half-life: 5–30 hr.

TIME/ACTION PROFILE (sedation)

ROUTE	ONSET	PEAK	DURATION
PO	1–2 hr	0.5–4 hr	up to 24 hr
IM	15–30 min	unknown	unknown
IV	1–5 min	unknown	0.25–1 hr

Contraindications/Precautions
Contraindicated in: Hypersensitivity; Some products contain tartrazine and should be avoided in patients with known intolerance;

chlordiazepoxide 315

Cross-sensitivity with other benzodiazepines may occur; Comatose patients or those with pre-existing CNS depression; Uncontrolled severe pain; Pulmonary disease; Angle-closure glaucoma; Porphyria; OB, Lactation: May cause CNS depression, flaccidity, feeding difficulties, and weight loss in infants; Pedi: Not for use in children ≤6 yr.
Use Cautiously in: Hepatic dysfunction; Severe renal impairment; History of suicide attempt or substance abuse; Geri: Long-acting benzodiazepines cause prolonged sedation in the elderly. Appears on Beers list and is associated with increased risk of falls (↓ dose required or consider short-acting benzodiazepine); Debilitated patients (initial dose reduction required).

Adverse Reactions/Side Effects
CNS: dizziness, drowsiness, hangover, headache, mental depression, paradoxical excitation, sedation. **EENT:** blurred vision. **GI:** constipation, diarrhea, nausea, vomiting, weight gain. **Derm:** rashes. **Local:** pain at IM site. **Misc:** physical dependence, psychological dependence, tolerance.

Interactions
Drug-Drug: **Alcohol**, **antidepressants**, **antihistamines**, and **opioid analgesics**—concurrent use results in additive CNS depression. **Cimetidine**, **oral contraceptives**, **disulfiram**, **fluoxetine**, **isoniazid**, **ketoconazole**, **metoprolol**, **propoxyphene**, **propranolol**, or **valproic acid** may enhance effects. May ↓ efficacy of **levodopa**. **Rifampin** or **barbiturates** may ↓ effectiveness of chlordiazepoxide. Sedative effects may be ↓ by **theophylline**.
Drug-Natural Products: Concomitant use of **kava-kava**, **valerian**, **chamomile**, or **hops** can ↑ CNS depression.

Route/Dosage
PO (Adults): *Alcohol withdrawal*—50–100 mg, repeated until agitation is controlled (up to 400 mg/day). *Anxiety*—5–25 mg 3–4 times daily.
PO (Geriatric Patients or Debilitated Patients): *Anxiety*—5 mg 2–4 times daily initially, increased as needed.
PO (Children >6 yr): *Anxiety*—5 mg 2–4 times daily, up to 10 mg 2–3 times daily.
IM, IV (Adults): *Alcohol withdrawal*—50–100 mg initially; may be repeated in 2–4 hr. *Anxiety*—50–100 mg initially, then 25–50 mg 3–4 times daily as required (25–50 mg initially in geriatric patients). *Preoperative sedation*—50–100 mg 1 hr preop.
IM, IV (Geriatric Patients or Debilitated Patients): *Anxiety/sedation*—25–50 mg/dose.
IM, IV (Children >12 yr): *Anxiety/sedation*—25–50 mg/dose.

Availability (generic available)
Capsules: 5 mg, 10 mg, 25 mg. **Tablets:** 5 mg, 10 mg, 25 mg. **Injection:** 100-mg ampule. *In combination with:* amitriptyline (Limbitrol DS), clidinium (Librax). See Appendix B.

NURSING IMPLICATIONS
Assessment
- Assess for anxiety and level of sedation (ataxia, dizziness, slurred speech) periodically during therapy.
- Assess degree and manifestations of anxiety and mental status (orientation, mood, behavior) prior to and periodically during therapy.
- Monitor blood pressure, heart rate, and respiratory rate frequently when administering parenterally. Report significant changes immediately.
- Prolonged high-dose therapy may lead to psychological or physical dependence. Restrict the amount of drug available to patient.
- Geri: Assess risk of falls and institute fall prevention strategies.
- **Alcohol Withdrawal:** Assess for tremors, agitation, delirium, and hallucinations. Protect patient from injury. Institute seizure precautions.
- Geri: Assess risk of falls and institute fall prevention strategies.
- *Lab Test Considerations:* Patients on prolonged therapy should have CBC and liver function tests evaluated periodically. May cause ↑ in serum bilirubin, AST, and ALT.
- May alter results of urine 17-ketosteroids and 17-ketogenic steroids. May cause ↓ response on metyrapone tests and decreased thyroidal uptake of ^{123}I and ^{131}I.
- *Toxicity and Overdose:* Flumazenil reverses sedation caused by chlordiazepoxide toxicity or overdose. (Flumazenil may induce seizures in patients with a history of seizure disorder or who are on tricyclic antidepressants.)

Potential Nursing Diagnoses
Anxiety (Indications)
Risk for injury (Side Effects)
Ineffective coping
Dysfunctional family processes: alcoholism

chlorpheniramine

Implementation
- Do not confuse Librium with Librax.
- IV administration is usually the preferred route for parenteral administration because of the slow, erratic absorption after IM administration.
- After parenteral administration, have patient remain recumbent and observe for 3–8 hr or longer, depending on patient's response.
- Equipment to maintain a patent airway should be immediately available when chlordiazepoxide is administered intravenously.
- Use parenteral solution immediately after reconstitution and discard any unused portion.
- **PO:** Administer after meals or with milk to minimize GI irritation. Tablets may be crushed and taken with food or fluids if patient has difficulty swallowing. Administer greater dose at bedtime to avoid daytime sedation. Do not discontinue abruptly; taper by 10 mg every 3 days to reduce chance of withdrawal effects. Some patients may require longer taper period (months). Monitor patients closely with seizure disorder as abrupt withdrawal may precipitate seizures.
- **IM:** Reconstitute only with 2 mL of diluent provided by manufacturer. Do not use solution if opalescent or hazy. Agitate gently to minimize bubbling. Administer slowly, deep into a well-developed muscle mass to minimize pain at injection site. Solution reconstituted with IM diluent should not be given IV.

IV Administration
- **Direct IV: *Diluent:*** Reconstitute 100 mg in 5 mL of 0.9% NaCl or sterile water for injection. Do not use IM diluent. ***Concentration:*** 20 mg/mL. ***Rate:*** Administer prescribed dose slowly over at least 1 min. Rapid administration may cause apnea, hypotension, bradycardia, or cardiac arrest.
- **Y-Site Compatibility:** heparin, hydrocortisone sodium succinate, potassium chloride, vitamin B complex with C.

Patient/Family Teaching
- Instruct patient to take chlordiazepoxide as directed. If medication is less effective after a few weeks, check with health care professional; do not increase dose. Medication should be tapered at the completion of long-term therapy. Sudden cessation of medication may lead to withdrawal (insomnia, irritability, nervousness, tremors).
- May cause drowsiness or dizziness. Caution patient to avoid driving or other activities requiring alertness until response to medication is known. Geri:Instruct patient and family how to reduce falls risk at home.
- Advise patient to avoid the use of alcohol and other CNS depressants concurrently with this medication.
- Instruct patient to consult health care professional before taking OTC medications.
- Instruct patient to notify health care professional if pregnancy is planned or suspected.
- Advise patient that benzodiazepines do not cure underlying problems. Psychotherapy is beneficial in addressing source of anxiety and improving coping skills.
- Teach other methods to decrease anxiety, such as exercise, use of support group (e.g., Alcoholics Anonymous), or relaxation techniques.
- Teach patient not to share medication with anyone.

Evaluation/Desired Outcomes
- Decreased sense of anxiety.
- Increased ability to cope.
- Decreased delirium tremens and more rational ideation when used for alcohol withdrawal.

---

chlorothiazide, See DIURETICS (THIAZIDE).

---

chlorpheniramine
(klor-fen-**ir**-a-meen)
Aller-Chlor, Allergy, Chlo-Amine, Chlorate, Chlor-Trimeton, Chlor-Trimeton Allergy 4 Hour, Chlor-Trimeton Allergy 8 Hour, Chlor-Trimeton Allergy 12 Hour, ✤Chlor-Tripolon, ✤Novo-Pheniram, PediaCare Allergy Formula, Phenetron, Telechlor, Teldrin

Classification
Therapeutic: allergy, cold, and cough remedies, antihistamines

Pregnancy Category B

Indications
Relief of allergic symptoms caused by histamine release, including: Nasal allergies, Allergic dermatoses. Management of severe allergic or hypersensitivity reactions, including anaphylaxis and transfusion reactions.

Action
Antagonizes the effects of histamine at H_2-receptor sites; does not bind to or inactivate histamine.

chlorpheniramine

Therapeutic Effects: Decreased symptoms of histamine excess (sneezing, rhinorrhea, nasal and ocular pruritus, ocular tearing, and redness).

Pharmacokinetics
Absorption: Well absorbed following oral and parenteral administration.
Distribution: Widely distributed. Minimal amounts excreted in breast milk. Crosses the blood-brain barrier.
Metabolism and Excretion: Extensively metabolized by the liver.
Half-life: 12–15 hr.

TIME/ACTION PROFILE (antihistaminic effects)

ROUTE	ONSET	PEAK	DURATION
PO	15–30 min	6 hr	4–12 hr
PO–ER	unknown	unknown	8–24 hr
Subcut	unknown	unknown	4–12 hr
IM	unknown	unknown	4–12 hr
IV	rapid	unknown	4–12 hr

Contraindications/Precautions
Contraindicated in: Hypersensitivity; Acute attacks of asthma; Lactation: Avoid use or use alternative feeding method; Known alcohol intolerance (some liquid forms); Pedi: Children <4 yr (OTC cough and cold products containing this medication should be avoided).
Use Cautiously in: Angle-closure glaucoma; Liver disease; Geri: Appears on Beers list. Geriatric patients are more susceptible to adverse reactions due to anticholinergic effects; OB: Safety not established.

Adverse Reactions/Side Effects
CNS: drowsiness, dizziness, excitation (in children). **EENT:** blurred vision. **CV:** hypertension, arrhythmias, hypotension, palpitations. **GI:** dry mouth, constipation, obstruction. **GU:** retention, urinary hesitancy.

Interactions
Drug-Drug: ↑ CNS depression with other **CNS depressants**, including **alcohol**, **opioid analgesics**, and **sedative/hypnotics**. **MAO inhibitors** intensify and prolong anticholinergic effects of antihistamines. ↑ anticholinergic effects with other **drugs possessing anticholinergic properties**, including **antidepressants**, **atropine**, **haloperidol**, **phenothiazines**, **quinidine**, and **disopyramide**.

Route/Dosage
PO (Adults): 4 mg q 4–6 hr *or* 8–12 mg of extended-release formulation q 8–12 hr (not to exceed 24 mg/day).
PO (Geriatric Patients): 4 mg twice daily *or* 8 mg of extended-release formulation at bedtime.
PO (Children 6–12 yr): 2 mg 3–4 times daily (not to exceed 12 mg/day).

Injectable formulation is available only in Canada
Subcut, IM, IV (Adults): 5–40-mg single dose (not to exceed 40 mg/day).
Subcut (Children): 87.5 mcg (0.0875 mg)/kg or 2.5 mg/m^2 q 6 hr as needed.

Availability (generic available)
Tablets: 4 mg$^{Rx, OTC}$, 8 mg$^{Rx, OTC}$, 12 mg$^{Rx, OTC}$. **Chewable tablets (orange flavor):** 2 mg$^{Rx, OTC}$. **Timed-release tablets:** 8 mg$^{Rx, OTC}$, 12 mg$^{Rx, OTC}$. **Timed-release capsules:** 8 mg$^{Rx, OTC}$, 12 mg$^{Rx, OTC}$. **Syrup:** 1 mg/5 mL$^{Rx, OTC}$, 2 mg/5 mL$^{Rx, OTC}$, ✦2.5 mg/5 mL$^{Rx, OTC}$. **Injection:** 10 mg/mL, 100 mg/mL. *In combination with:* Codeine (Codeprex), pseudoephedrine (Advil), and decongestants$^{Rx, OTC}$. See Appendix B.

NURSING IMPLICATIONS

Assessment
- Assess allergy symptoms (rhinitis, conjunctivitis, hives) prior to and periodically during therapy.
- Monitor pulse and blood pressure before initiating and throughout IV therapy.
- Caution parents to avoid OTC cough and cold products while breastfeeding or to children <4 yrs.
- Geri: Assess for adverse anticholinergic effects (delirium, acute confusion, dizziness, dry mouth, blurred vision, urinary retention, constipation, tachycardia).
- Assess lung sounds and character of bronchial secretions. Maintain fluid intake of 1500–2000 mL/day to decrease viscosity of secretions.
- *Lab Test Considerations:* May cause false-negative reactions on allergy skin tests; discontinue 4 days prior to testing.

Potential Nursing Diagnoses
Ineffective airway clearance (Indications)
Risk for injury (Adverse Reactions)

✦ = Canadian drug name. ▨ = Genetic implication.
*CAPITALS indicates life-threatening; underlines indicate most frequent.

Implementation
- **PO:** Administer oral doses with food or milk to decrease GI irritation. Extended-release tablets and capsules should be swallowed whole; do not crush, break, or chew.Chewable tablets should not be swallowed whole; chew well before swallowing.
- **Subcut, IM:** The 100-mg/mL solution is recommended for IM or subcut routes only. The 10-mg/mL solution may be used for IM, subcut, or IV.

IV Administration
- **Direct IV:** *Diluent:*May be given undiluted. Use only the 10 mg/mL strength for IV administration. *Concentration:*10 mg/mL. *Rate:* Administer each 10-mg dose over at least 1 min.

Patient/Family Teaching
- Instruct patient to take chlorpheniramine as directed.
- Geri:Teach patient and family about anticholinergic effects and to contact health care professional if effects persist.
- May cause drowsiness. Caution patient to avoid driving or other activities requiring alertness until response to drug is known.
- Caution patient to avoid using alcohol or other CNS depressants concurrently with this drug.
- Advise patient that good oral hygiene, frequent rinsing of mouth with water, and sugarless gum or candy may help relieve dryness of mouth.
- Instruct patient to contact health care professional if symptoms persist.

Evaluation/Desired Outcomes
- Decrease in allergic symptoms.

---

chlorproMAZINE
(klor-**proe**-ma-zeen)
✱Chlorpromanyl, ✱Largactil, ✱Novo-Chlorpromazine

Classification
Therapeutic: antiemetics, antipsychotics
Pharmacologic: phenothiazines

Pregnancy Category C

Indications
Second-line treatment for schizophrenia and psychoses after failure with atypical antipsychotics. Hyperexcitable, combative behavior in children. Nausea and vomiting. Intractable hiccups. Preoperative sedation. Acute intermittent porphyria.
Unlabeled Use: Vascular headache. Bipolar disorder.

Action
Alters the effects of dopamine in the CNS. Has significant anticholinergic/alpha-adrenergic blocking activity. **Therapeutic Effects:** Diminished signs/symptoms of psychosis. Relief of nausea/vomiting/intractable hiccups. Decreased symptoms of porphyria.

Pharmacokinetics
Absorption: Variable absorption from tablets. Well absorbed following IM administration.
Distribution: Widely distributed; high CNS concentrations. Crosses the placenta; enters breast milk.
Protein Binding: ≥90%.
Metabolism and Excretion: Highly metabolized by the liver and GI mucosa. Some metabolites are active.
Half-life: 30 hr.

TIME/ACTION PROFILE (antipsychotic activity, antiemetic activity, sedation)

ROUTE	ONSET	PEAK	DURATION
PO	30–60 min	unknown	4–6 hr
IM	unknown	unknown	4–8 hr
IV	rapid	unknown	unknown

Contraindications/Precautions
Contraindicated in: Hypersensitivity; Hypersensitivity to sulfites (injectable); Cross-sensitivity with other phenothiazines may occur; Angle-closure glaucoma; Bone marrow depression; Severe liver/cardiovascular disease; Concurrent pimozide use.

Use Cautiously in: Diabetes; Respiratory disease; Prostatic hyperplasia; CNS tumors; Epilepsy; Intestinal obstruction; OB, Lactation:Safety not established. Discontinue drug or bottle feed; Pedi: Children with acute illnesses, infections, gastroenteritis, or dehydration (↑ risk of extrapyramidal reactions); Geri: ↑ risk of mortality in elderly patients treated for dementia-related psychosis; Geri:Geriatric/debilitated patients (↓ initial dose).

Adverse Reactions/Side Effects
CNS: NEUROLEPTIC MALIGNANT SYNDROME, sedation, extrapyramidal reactions, tardive dyskinesia. **EENT:** blurred vision, dry eyes, lens opacities. **CV:** hypotension (↑ with IM, IV), tachycardia. **GI:** constipation, dry mouth, anorexia, hepatitis, ileus, priapism. **GU:** urinary retention. **Derm:** photosensitivity, pigment changes, rashes. **Endo:** galactorrhea, amenorrhea. **Hemat:** AGRANULOCYTOSIS, leukopenia. **Metab:** hyperthermia. **Misc:** allergic reactions.

chlorproMAZINE 319

Interactions
Drug-Drug: Concurrent use with **pimozide** ↑ the risk of potentially serious cardiovascular reactions. May alter serum **phenytoin** levels. ↓ pressor effect of **norepinephrine** and eliminates bradycardia. Antagonizes peripheral vasoconstriction from **epinephrine** and may reverse some of its actions. May ↓ elimination and ↑ effects of **valproic acid**. May ↓ the pharmacologic effects of **amphetamine** and **related compounds**. May ↓ the effectiveness of **bromocriptine**. May ↑ blood levels and effects of **tricyclic antidepressants**. **Antacids** or **adsorbent antidiarrheals** may ↓ adsorption; administer 1 hr before or 2 hr after chlorpromazine. ↑ risk of anticholinergic effects with **antihistamines**, **tricyclic antidepressants**, **quinidine**, or **disopyramide**. Premedication with chlorpromazine ↑ the risk of neuromuscular excitation and hypotension when followed by **barbiturate** anesthesia. **Barbiturates** may ↑ metabolism and ↓ effectiveness. Chlorpromazine may ↓ **barbiturate** levels. Additive hypotension with **antihypertensives**. Additive CNS depression with **alcohol**, **antidepressants**, **antihistamines**, **MAO inhibitors**, **opioid analgesics**, **sedative/hypnotics**, or **general anesthetics**. Concurrent use with **lithium** may produce disorientation, unconsciousness, or extrapyramidal symptoms. Concurrent use with **meperidine** may produce excessive sedation and hypotension. Concurrent use with **propranolol** ↑ blood levels of both drugs.
Drug-Natural Products: Concomitant use of **kava-kava**, **valerian**, **chamomile**, or **hops** can ↑ CNS depression. ↑ anticholinergic effects with **angel's trumpet**, **jimson weed**, and **scopolia**.

Route/Dosage
PO (Adults): *Psychoses*—10–25 mg 2–4 times daily; may ↑ every 3–4 days (usual dose is 200 mg/day; up to 1 g/day). *Nausea and vomiting*—10–25 mg q 4 hr as needed. *Preoperative sedation*—25–50 mg 2–3 hr before surgery. *Hiccups/porphyria*—25–50 mg 3–4 times daily.
PO (Children): *Psychoses/nausea and vomiting*—0.55 mg/kg (15 mg/m²) q 4–6 hr as needed. *Preoperative sedation*—0.55 mg/kg (15 mg/m²) 2–3 hr before surgery.
IM (Adults): *Severe psychoses*—25–50 mg initially, may be repeated in 1 hr; ↑ to maximum of 400 mg q 3–12 hr if needed (up to 1 g/day). *Nausea/vomiting*—25 mg initially, may repeat with 25–50 mg q 3–4 hr as needed. *Nausea/vomiting during surgery*—12.5 mg, may be repeated in 30 min as needed. *Preoperative sedation*—12.5–25 mg 1–2 hr prior to surgery. *Hiccups/tetanus*—25–50 mg 3–4 times daily. *Porphyria*—25 mg q 6–8 hr until patient can take PO.
IM (Children 6 mo): *Psychoses/nausea and vomiting*—0.55 mg/kg (15 mg/m²) q 6–8 hr (not to exceed 40 mg/day in children 6 mo–5 yr, or 75 mg/day in children 5–12 yr). *Nausea/vomiting during surgery*—0.275 mg/kg, may repeat in 30 min as needed. *Preoperative sedation*—0.55 mg/kg 1–2 hr prior to surgery. *Tetanus*—0.55 mg/kg q 6–8 hr.
IV (Adults): *Nausea/vomiting during surgery*—up to 25 mg. *Hiccups/tetanus*—25–50 mg. *Porphyria*—25 mg q 8 hr.
IV (Children): *Nausea/vomiting during surgery*—0.275 mg/kg. *Tetanus*—0.55 mg/kg.

Availability (generic available)
Tablets: 10 mg, 25 mg, 50 mg, 100 mg, 200 mg.
Injection: 25 mg/mL.

NURSING IMPLICATIONS
Assessment
- Assess mental status (orientation, mood, behavior) prior to and periodically during therapy.
- Assess weight and BMI initially and throughout therapy.
- Assess fasting blood glucose and cholesterol levels initially and periodically throughout therapy. Refer as appropriate for nutritional/weight and medical management.
- Assess positive (hallucinations, delusions, agitation) and negative (social withdrawal) symptoms of schizophrenia.
- Monitor blood pressure (sitting, standing, lying), pulse, and respiratory rate prior to and frequently during the period of dose adjustment.
- Observe patient carefully when administering medication to ensure medication is actually taken and not hoarded.
- Assess fluid intake and bowel function. Increased bulk and fluids in the diet may help minimize constipation.
- Monitor patient for onset of akathisia (restlessness or desire to keep moving) and ex-trapyr-amidal side effects (*parkinsonian*—difficulty speaking or swallowing, loss of balance con-

✦ = Canadian drug name. ᴳ = Genetic implication.
*CAPITALS indicates life-threatening; underlines indicate most frequent.

trol, pill rolling of hands, mask-like face, shuffling gait, rigidity, tremors; and *dystonic*—muscle spasms, twisting motions, twitching, inability to move eyes, weakness of arms or legs) every 2 mo during therapy and 8–12 wk after therapy has been discontinued. Notify health care professional if these symptoms occur; reduction in dose or discontinuation may be necessary. Trihexyphenidyl, diphenhydramine, or benzotropine may be used to control these symptoms. Benzodiazepines may alleviate symptoms of akathisia.
- Monitor for tardive dyskinesia (uncontrolled rhythmic movement of mouth, face, and extremities; lip smacking or puckering; puffing of cheeks; uncontrolled chewing; rapid or worm-like movements of tongue, excessive eye blinking). Report these symptoms immediately; may be irreversible.
- Monitor for development of neuroleptic malignant syndrome (fever, respiratory distress, tachycardia, convulsions, diaphoresis, hypertension or hypotension, pallor, tiredness, severe muscle stiffness, loss of bladder control). Report these symptoms immediately.
- **Preoperative Sedation:** Assess level of anxiety prior to and following administration.
- **Vascular Headache:** Assess type, location, intensity, and duration of pain and accompanying symptoms.
- *Lab Test Considerations:* Monitor CBC, liver function tests, and ocular exams periodically throughout therapy. May cause ↓ hematocrit, hemoglobin, leukocytes, granulocytes, platelets. May cause ↑ bilirubin, AST, ALT, and alkaline phosphatase. Agranulocytosis occurs 4–10 wk after initiation of therapy, with recovery 1–2 wk following discontinuation. May recur if medication is restarted.Liver function abnormalities may require discontinuation of therapy. May cause false-positive or false-negative pregnancy tests and false-positive urine bilirubin test results.

Potential Nursing Diagnoses
Disturbed thought process (Indications)
Imbalanced nutrition: risk for more than body requirements (Side Effects)

Implementation
- Do not confuse chlorpromazine with chlorpropamide or prochlorperazine.
- Keep patient recumbent for at least 30 min following parenteral administration to minimize hypotensive effects.
- Phenothiazines should be discontinued 48 hr before and not resumed for 24 hr following metrizamide myelography, because they lower the seizure threshold.
- **Hiccups:** Initial treatment is with oral doses. If hiccups persist 2–3 days, IM injection may be used, followed by IV infusion.
- **PO:** Administer oral doses with food, milk, or a full glass of water to minimize gastric irritation. Tablets may be crushed.
- **IM:** Do not inject subcut. Inject slowly into deep, well-developed muscle. May be diluted with 0.9% NaCl or 2% procaine. Lemon-yellow color does not alter potency of solution. Do not administer solution that is markedly discolored or contains a precipitate.

IV Administration

- **Direct IV:** *Diluent:*Dilute with 0.9% NaCl. *Concentration:*Do not exceed 1 mg/mL. *Rate:*Inject slowly at a rate of at least 1 mg/min for adults and 0.5 mg/min for children.
- **Continuous Infusion:** *Diluent:*May further dilute 25–50 mg in 500–1000 mL of D5W, D10W, 0.45% NaCl, 0.9% NaCl, Ringer's or lactated Ringer's injection, dextrose/Ringer's or dextrose/lactated Ringer's combinations.
- **Syringe Compatibility:** atropine , benztropine, butorphanol, diphenhydramine, doxapram, droperidol, fentanyl, glycopyrrolate, hydromorphone, hydroxyzine, meperidine, metoclopramide, midazolam, morphine, pentazocine, scopolamine.
- **Syringe Incompatibility:** cimetidine, heparin, pantoprazole, pentobarbital, thiopental.
- **Y-Site Compatibility:** alfentanyl, amikacin, amsacrine, anidulafungin, ascorbic acid, atracurium, atropine, benztropine, bleomycin, buprenorphine, butorphanol, calcium chloride, calcium gluconate, caspofungin, cimetidine, cisatracurium, cisplatin, cladribine, cyclophosphamide, cyclosporine, cytarabine, dactinomycin, daptomycin, dexmedetomidine, digoxin, diltiazem, diphenhydramine, dobutamine, docetaxel, dopamine, doxacurium, doxorubicin, doxorubicin liposome, doxycycline, enalaprilat, ephedrine, epinephrine, epirubicin, erythromycin, esmolol, etoposide, famotidine, fenoldopam, filgrastim, fluconazole, gemcitabine, gentamicin, glycopyrrolate, granisetron, heparin, hetastarch, hydrocortisone, hydromorphone, idarubicin, ifosfamide, isoproterenol, labetalol, levofloxacin, lidocaine, lorazepam, magnesium sulfate, mannitol, mechlorethamine, meperidine, methoxamine, methyldopate, methylprednisolone, metoclopramide, metoprolol, metronidazole, midazolam, milrinone, mitoxantrone, morphine, multivitamins,

nafcillin, nalbuphine, naloxone, nitroglycerin, norepinephrine, octreotide, ondansetron, oxacillin, oxaliplatin, palonosetron, pancuronium, papaverine, pentamidine, pentazocine, phentolamine, phytonadione, potassium chloride, procainamide, prochlorperazine, propofol, propranolol, protamine, pyridoxime, quinupristin/dalfopristin, ranitidine, rituximab, rocuronium, sodium acetate, succinylcholine, sufentanil, tacrolimus, teniposide, theophylline, thiamine, thiotepa, tirofiban, tolazoline, trimetaphan, vancomycin, vasopressin, vecuronium, verapamil, vincristine, vinorelbine, vitamin B complex with C, voriconazole.

- **Y-Site Incompatibility:** acyclovir, allopurinol, aminophylline, amphotericin B cholesteryl, amphotericin B colloidal, amphotericin B liposome, ampicillin, ampicillin/sulbactam, azathioprine, aztreonam, bivalirudin, bumetanide, carboplatin, cefazolin, cefepime, cefonocid, cefoperazone, cefotaxime, cefotetan, cefoxitin, ceftizoxime, ceftriaxone, cefuroxime, chloramphenicol, clindamycin, dantrolene, dexamethasone, diazepam, diazoxide, eftifibatide, epoetin alfa, ertapenem, etoposide phosphate, fludarabine, fluorouracil, folic acid, furosemide, gancilovir, hydralazine, imipenem/cilastatin, inamrinone, indomethacin, insulin, ketorolac, linezolid, melphalan, methotrexate, nitroprusside, paclitaxel, pantoprazole, pemetrexed, pentobarbital, phenobarbital, phytonadione, piperacillin/tazobactam, sargramostim, sodium bicarbonate, streptokinase, ticarcillin/clavulante, tigecycline, trastuzumab, trimethoprim/sulfamethoxazole.

Patient/Family Teaching
- Advise patient to take medication as directed and not to skip doses or double up on missed doses. If a dose is missed, take within 1 hr or omit dose and return to regular schedule. Abrupt withdrawal may lead to gastritis, nausea, vomiting, dizziness, headache, tachycardia, and insomnia.
- Inform patient of possibility of extrapyramidal symptoms and tardive dyskinesia. Instruct patient to report these symptoms immediately to health care professional.
- Advise patient to change positions slowly to minimize orthostatic hypotension.
- Medication may cause drowsiness. Caution patient to avoid driving or other activities requiring alertness until response to the medication is known.
- Caution patient to avoid taking alcohol or other CNS depressants concurrently with this medication.
- Advise patient to use sunscreen and protective clothing when exposed to the sun. Exposed surfaces may develop a temporary pigment change (ranging from yellow-brown to grayish purple). Extremes of temperature (exercise, hot weather, hot baths or showers) should also be avoided, because this drug impairs body temperature regulation.
- Instruct patient to use frequent mouth rinses, good oral hygiene, and sugarless gum or candy to minimize dry mouth. Consult health care professional if dry mouth continues for 2 wk.
- Advise patient not to take chlorpromazine within 2 hr of antacids or antidiarrheal medication.
- Inform patient that this medication may turn urine a pink-to-reddish-brown color.
- Advise patient to notify health care professional of medication regimen prior to treatment or surgery.
- Instruct patient to notify health care professional promptly if sore throat, fever, unusual bleeding or bruising, rash, weakness, tremors, visual disturbances, dark-colored urine, or clay-colored stools occur.
- Emphasize the importance of routine follow-up exams to monitor response to medication and detect side effects. Encourage continued participation in psychotherapy as indicated.
- Treatment is not a cure since symptoms can recur after discontinuation of medication.

Evaluation/Desired Outcomes
- Decrease in excitable, manic behavior. Therapeutic effects may not be seen for 7–8 wk.
- Relief of nausea and vomiting.
- Relief of hiccups.
- Preoperative sedation.
- Management of porphyria.
- Relief of vascular headache.
- Decrease in positive (hallucinations, delusions, agitation) symptoms of schizophrenia.

chlorthalidone (thiazide–like), See DIURETICS (THIAZIDE).

chlorzoxazone
(klor-**zox**-a-zohn)
Parafon Forte DSC

Classification
Therapeutic: skeletal muscle relaxants (centrally acting)

Pregnancy Category C

Indications
Adjunct to rest and physical therapy in the treatment of muscle spasm associated with acute painful musculoskeletal conditions.

Action
Skeletal muscle relaxation, probably due to CNS depression. **Therapeutic Effects:** Skeletal muscle relaxation with decreased discomfort.

Pharmacokinetics
Absorption: Readily absorbed after oral administration.
Distribution: Unknown.
Metabolism and Excretion: Mostly metabolized by the liver; <1% excreted unchanged in urine.
Half-life: 1.1 hr.

TIME/ACTION PROFILE (skeletal muscle effects)

ROUTE	ONSET	PEAK	DURATION
PO	within 1 hr	1–2 hr	3–4 hr

Contraindications/Precautions
Contraindicated in: Hypersensitivity; Porphyria.
Use Cautiously in: Underlying cardiovascular disease; Impaired renal or hepatic function; OB, Lactation, Pedi:Safety not established; Geri:Appears on Beers list. Poorly tolerated due to anticholinergic effects.

Adverse Reactions/Side Effects
CNS: dizziness, drowsiness. **GI:** GI BLEEDING constipation, diarrhea, heartburn, nausea, vomiting. **Derm:** allergic dermatitis. **Hemat:** AGRANULOCYTOSIS anemia. **Misc:** allergic reactions including ANGIOEDEMA

Interactions
Drug-Drug: ↑ risk of CNS depression with other **CNS depressants**, including **alcohol, antihistamines, antidepressants, sedative/hypnotics,** or **opioid analgesics**.
Drug-Natural Products: Concomitant use of **kava-kava, valerian, skullcap, chamomile,** or **hops** can ↑ CNS depression.

Route/Dosage
PO (Adults): 250–750 mg 3–4 times daily.
PO (Children): 20 mg/kg or 600 mg/m²/day in 3–4 divided doses.

Availability (generic available)
Tablets: 250 mg, 500 mg. **Cost:** *250 mg generic*—$29.86/100; *500 mg Parafon Forte DSC*—$126.84/100; *generic*—$102.96/100

NURSING IMPLICATIONS

Assessment
- Assess patient for pain, muscle stiffness, and range of motion before and periodically during therapy.
- Geri:Assess geriatric patients for anticholinergic effects (sedation and weakness).

Potential Nursing Diagnoses
Acute pain (Indications)
Impaired physical mobility (Indications)
Risk for injury (Side Effects)

Implementation
- **PO:** May be administered with meals to minimize gastric irritation. Tablets may be crushed and mixed with food or liquid for ease of administration.

Patient/Family Teaching
- Instruct patient to take medication as directed; do not take more than the prescribed amount. Missed doses should be taken within 1 hr of time ordered; otherwise, omit and return to normal dosage schedule. Do not double doses.
- Medication may cause drowsiness and dizziness. Caution patient to avoid driving or other activities requiring alertness until response to drug is known.
- Advise patient to avoid concurrent use of alcohol or other CNS depressants with this medication.
- If constipation becomes a problem, advise patient that increasing fluid intake and bulk in diet and stool softeners may alleviate this condition.

Evaluation/Desired Outcomes
- Relief of muscular spasm in acute skeletal muscle conditions.

---

cholecalciferol, See VITAMIN D COMPOUNDS.

---

cholestyramine
(koe-less-**tear**-a-meen)
LoCHOLEST, LoCHOLEST Light, Prevalite, Questran, Questran Light

cholestyramine

Classification
Therapeutic: lipid-lowering agents
Pharmacologic: bile acid sequestrants

Pregnancy Category C

Indications
Management of primary hypercholesterolemia. Pruritus associated with elevated levels of bile acids. **Unlabeled Use:** Diarrhea associated with excess bile acids.

Action
Bind bile acids in the GI tract, forming an insoluble complex. Result is increased clearance of cholesterol. **Therapeutic Effects:** Decreased plasma cholesterol and low-density lipoproteins (LDLs). Decreased pruritus.

Pharmacokinetics
Absorption: Action takes place in the GI tract. No absorption occurs.
Distribution: No distribution.
Metabolism and Excretion: After binding bile acids, insoluble complex is eliminated in the feces.
Half-life: Unknown.

TIME/ACTION PROFILE (hypocholesterolemic effects)

ROUTE	ONSET	PEAK	DURATION
PO	24–48 hr	1–3 wk	2–4 wk

Contraindications/Precautions
Contraindicated in: Hypersensitivity; Complete biliary obstruction; Some products contain aspartame and should be avoided in patients with phenylketonuria.
Use Cautiously in: History of constipation.
Exercise Extreme Caution in: Children (may cause intestinal obstruction; deaths have occurred).

Adverse Reactions/Side Effects
EENT: irritation of the tongue. **GI:** abdominal discomfort, constipation, nausea, fecal impaction, flatulence, hemorrhoids, perianal irritation, steatorrhea, vomiting. **Derm:** irritation, rashes. **F and E:** hyperchloremic acidosis. **Metab:** vitamin A, D, and K deficiency.

Interactions
Drug-Drug: May decrease absorption/effects of orally administered **acetaminophen, amiodarone, clindamycin, clofibrate, digoxin, diuretics, gemfibrozil, glipizide, corticosteroids, imipramine, mycophenolate, methotrexate, methyldopa, niacin, NSAIDs, penicillin, phenytoin, phosphates, propranolol, tetracyclines, tolbutamide, thyroid preparations, ursodiol, warfarin,** and **fat-soluble vitamins (A, D, E,** and **K)**. May decrease absorption of other **orally administered medications**.

Route/Dosage
PO (Adults): 4 g 1–2 times daily (initially, may be increased as needed/tolerated up to 24 g/day in 6 divided doses).
PO (Children): 240 mg/kg/day in 2–3 divided doses (not >8 g/day).

Availability (generic available)
Powder for suspension with aspartame (strawberry flavor [LoCHOLEST], unflavored [Prevalite, Questran Light]): 4 g cholestyramine/packet or scoop. **Powder for suspension (strawberry flavor [LoCHOLEST], unflavored [Questran, generic]):** 4 g cholestyramine/packet or scoop.

NURSING IMPLICATIONS

Assessment
- **Hypercholesterolemia:** Obtain a diet history, especially in regard to fat consumption.
- **Pruritus:** Assess severity of itching and skin integrity. Dose may be decreased when relief of pruritus occurs.
- **Diarrhea:** Assess frequency, amount, and consistency of stools.
- *Lab Test Considerations:* Serum cholesterol and triglyceride levels should be evaluated before initiating, frequently during first few months and periodically throughout therapy. Discontinue medication if paradoxical increase in cholesterol level occurs.
- May cause an increase in AST, ALT, phosphorus, chloride, and alkaline phosphatase and a decrease in serum calcium, sodium, and potassium levels.
- May also cause prolonged prothrombin times.

Potential Nursing Diagnoses
Constipation (Side Effects)
Noncompliance (Patient/Family Teaching)

Implementation
- Parenteral or water-miscible forms of fat-soluble vitamins (A, D, and K) and folic acid may be ordered for patients on chronic therapy.
- **PO:** Administer before meals.

- Scoops for powdered preparations may not be exchangable between products.
- Administer other medications 1 hr before or 4–6 hr after the administration of this medication.

Patient/Family Teaching
- Instruct patient to take medication exactly as directed; do not skip doses or double up on missed doses.
- Instruct patient to take medication before meals. Mix cholestyramine with 4–6 oz water, milk, fruit juice, or other noncarbonated beverages. Shake vigorously. Slowly stir in a large glass. Rinse glass with small amount of additional beverage to ensure all medication is taken. May also mix with highly fluid soups, cereals, or pulpy fruits (applesauce, crushed pineapple). Allow powder to sit on fluid and hydrate for 1–2 min before mixing. Do not take dry. Variations in the color of cholestyramine do not alter stability.
- Advise patient that this medication should be used in conjunction with dietary restrictions (fat, cholesterol, carbohydrates, alcohol), exercise, and cessation of smoking.
- Explain that constipation may occur. Increase in fluids and bulk in diet, exercise, stool softeners, and laxatives may be required to minimize the constipating effects. Instruct patient to notify health care professional if constipation, nausea, flatulence, and heartburn persist or if stools become frothy and foul smelling.
- Advise patient to notify health care professional if unusual bleeding or bruising; petechiae; or black, tarry stools occur. Treatment with vitamin K may be necessary.

Evaluation/Desired Outcomes
- Decrease in serum low-density lipoprotein cholesterol levels. Therapy is usually discontinued if the clinical response remains poor after 3 mo of therapy.
- Decrease in severity of pruritus. Relief usually occurs 1–3 wk after therapy is initiated.
- Decrease in frequency and severity of diarrhea.

---

choline and magnesium salicylates, See SALICYLATES.

---

choline salicylate, See SALICYLATES.

---

ciclesonide, See CORTICOSTEROIDS (NASAL).

---

ciclopirox, See ANTIFUNGALS (TOPICAL).

---

cidofovir (sye-doe-foe-veer)
Vistide

Classification
Therapeutic: antivirals

Pregnancy Category C

Indications
Management of cytomegalovirus (CMV) retinitis in HIV-infected patients (with probenecid).

Action
Suppresses replication of CMV by inhibiting viral DNA synthesis. **Therapeutic Effects:** Slows progression of CMV retinitis; may not be curative.

Pharmacokinetics
Absorption: IV administration results in complete bioavailability.
Distribution: Unknown.
Metabolism and Excretion: Excreted mostly unchanged by the kidneys.
Half-life: Unknown.

TIME/ACTION PROFILE

ROUTE	ONSET	PEAK	DURATION
IV	rapid	end of infusion	unknown

Contraindications/Precautions
Contraindicated in: Hypersensitivity to cidofovir, probenecid, or sulfonamides; Serum Cr >1.5 mg/dL, CCr ≤55 mL/min, or urine protein ≥100 mg/dL (≥2+ proteinuria); Concurrent use of foscarnet, amphotericin B, aminoglycoside anti-infectives, NSAIDs, or IV pentamidine.
Use Cautiously in: Pregnancy or children (safety not established); breastfeeding is not recommended in HIV-positive patients.
Exercise Extreme Caution in: Any condition or medication that increases the risk of dehydration.

Adverse Reactions/Side Effects
CNS: headache, weakness. **EENT:** decreased intraocular pressure, hearing loss, iritis, ocular hypotony, uveitis. **Resp:** dyspnea, pneumonia. **GI:** HEPATIC DYSFUNCTION, PANCREATITIS, abdominal pain, nausea, vomiting, anorexia, diarrhea. **GU:** RENAL FAILURE, proteinuria. **Derm:** alopecia, rash. **F and E:** decreased serum bicarbonate. **Hemat:** neutropenia, anemia. **Metab:** METABOLIC ACIDOSIS. **Misc:** chills, fever, infection.

Interactions
Drug-Drug: ↑ risk of nephrotoxicity with **aminoglycosides**, **amphotericin B**, **foscarnet**, and **pentamidine** and should be avoided; wait 7 days after giving other nephrotoxic agents. **Probenecid**, which is required concurrently, may interact with **acetaminophen**, **acyclovir**, **ACE inhibitors**, **barbiturates**, **benzodiazepines**, **bumetanide**, **methotrexate**, **famotidine**, **furosemide**, **NSAIDs**, **theophylline**, and **zidovudine**.

Route/Dosage
IV (Adults): 5 mg/kg once weekly for 2 wk, followed by 5 mg/kg every 2 wk (must be given with probenecid).

Renal Impairment
IV (Adults): *Increase in serum creatinine of 0.3–0.4 mg/dL*—decrease dose to 3 mg/kg; discontinue if serum creatinine increases ≥0.5 mg/dL over baseline.

Availability
Solution for injection: 75 mg/mL in 5-mL ampules.

NURSING IMPLICATIONS

Assessment
- Monitor vision for progression of CMV retinitis. Monitor ocular symptoms, intraocular pressure, and visual acuity periodically.
- Antiemetics and administration after a meal may minimize nausea and vomiting associated with probenecid. If allergic reactions occur in association with probenecid, pretreatment with antihistamines or acetaminophen should be considered.
- Monitor vital signs periodically. May cause fever, hypotension, and tachycardia. Monitor patients for early signs and symptoms of infection.
- ***Lab Test Considerations:*** Renal function, measured by serum Cr and urine protein, must be monitored within 48 hr before each dose and throughout cidofovir therapy. In patients with proteinuria, administer IV hydration and repeat urine protein test. If renal function deteriorates, dose modification or temporary discontinuation should be considered.
- Monitor WBC before each dose. Granulocytopenia may occur.
- May cause hyperglycemia, hyperlipemia, hypocalcemia, hypokalemia, and elevated alkaline phosphatase, AST, and ALT.

Potential Nursing Diagnoses
Risk for infection (Indications)

Implementation
- Probenecid and saline prehydration must be given with cidofovir to minimize renal toxicity. *Probenecid* must be administered 2 g orally given 3 hr before, then 1 g given 2 hr and 8 hr after completion of cidofovir infusion. *Saline prehydration* with 1 L of 0.9% NaCl must be given over 1–2 hr before cidofovir. A second liter over 1–3 hr is recommended concurrently with or after cidofovir.
- Patients receiving foscarnet, amphotericin B, aminoglycoside, NSAIDs, or IV pentamidine should wait at least 7 days after these agents to begin cidofovir.

IV Administration
- **Intermittent Infusion:** *Diluent:* Dilute in 100 mL of 0.9% NaCl. Solution is stable for 24 hr if refrigerated. Allow refrigerated solution to return to room temperature before administration. *Rate:* Administer over 1 hr.
- **Additive Incompatibility:** Information unavailable. Do not admix with other solutions or medications.

Patient/Family Teaching
- Inform patient that cidofovir is not a cure for CMV retinitis and that retinitis may continue to progress during and after therapy.
- Inform patient that concurrent antiretroviral therapy may be continued. However, zidovudine therapy should be temporarily discontinued or decreased by 50% on the days of cidofovir therapy because of the effects of probenecid on zidovudine.
- Advise patient of the possibility of renal toxicity from cidofovir. Emphasize the importance of routine lab tests to monitor renal function.
- Inform patient that cidofovir may have teratogenic effects. Women should use contraception during and for 1 mo after therapy. Men should use barrier contraception during and for 3 mo after therapy.
- Discuss with patient the possibility of hair loss. Explore coping strategies.
- Advise patients to have routine ophthalmologic exams after cidofovir therapy.

Evaluation/Desired Outcomes
- Decrease in symptoms and arrest of progression of CMV retinitis in HIV-infected patients.

cilostazol (sil-os-tah-zol)
Pletal

Classification
Therapeutic: antiplatelet agents
Pharmacologic: platelet aggregation inhibitors

Pregnancy Category C

Indications
Reduction of the symptoms of intermittent claudication as measured by increased walking distance.

Action
Inhibits the enzyme cyclic adenosine monophosphate (cAMP) phosphodiesterase III (PDE III), which results in increased cAMP in platelets and blood vessels, producing inhibition of platelet aggregation and vasodilation. **Therapeutic Effects:** Reduced symptoms of intermittent claudication with improved walking distance.

Pharmacokinetics
Absorption: Slowly absorbed after oral administration.
Distribution: Unknown.
Protein Binding: 95–98% bound to plasma proteins; one active metabolite is 97.4% bound, the other is 66% bound.
Metabolism and Excretion: Extensively metabolized by the liver, two metabolites have platelet aggregation inhibitory activity; metabolites are mostly excreted by the kidneys.
Half-life: *Cilostazol and its active metabolites*—11–13 hr.

TIME/ACTION PROFILE (symptom reduction)

ROUTE	ONSET	PEAK	DURATION
PO	2–4 wk	up to 12 wk	unknown

Contraindications/Precautions
Contraindicated in: Hypersensitivity; CHF; OB: Potential for congenital defects, stillbirth, and low birth weight; Lactation:Potential risk to nursing infants; discontinue or bottle feed.
Use Cautiously in: Pedi:Safety not established.

Adverse Reactions/Side Effects
CNS: headache, dizziness. **CV:** palpitations, tachycardia. **GI:** diarrhea.

Interactions
Drug-Drug: Concurrent administration of **ketoconazole**, **itraconazole**, **erythromycin**, **diltiazem**, **fluconazole**, **miconazole**, **fluvoxamine**, **fluoxetine**, **nefazodone**, **sertraline**, or **omeprazole** decreases metabolism and increases levels and activity of cilostazol (use lower doses). Concurrent use with **aspirin** has additive effects on platelet function.
Drug-Food: Grapefruit juice inhibits metabolism and increases effects; concurrent use should be avoided.

Route/Dosage
PO (Adults): 100 mg twice daily (50 mg twice daily if receiving inhibitors of cilostazol metabolism).

Availability (generic available)
Tablets: 50 mg, 100 mg.

NURSING IMPLICATIONS

Assessment
- Assess patient for intermittent claudication before and periodically during therapy.
- *Lab Test Considerations:* May occasionally cause anemia, hyperlipemia, hyperuricemia, and albuminuria. May prolong bleeding time.

Potential Nursing Diagnoses
Activity intolerance (Indications)

Implementation
- **PO:** Administer on an empty stomach, 1 hr before or 2 hr after meals.
- Do not administer with grapefruit juice. May increase cilostazol levels.

Patient/Family Teaching
- Instruct patient to take cilostazol on an empty stomach, exactly as directed.
- May cause dizziness. Caution patient to avoid driving or other activities requiring alertness until response to medication is known.
- Advise patient to avoid smoking; nicotine constricts blood vessels.

Evaluation/Desired Outcomes
- Relief from cramping in calf muscles, buttocks, thighs, and feet during exercise.
- Improvement in walking endurance. Therapeutic effects may be seen in 2–4 wk.

---

cimetidine, See HISTAMINE H_2 ANTAGONISTS.

---

cinacalcet (sin-a-kal-set)
Sensipar

cinacalcet

Classification
Therapeutic: hypocalcemics
Pharmacologic: calcimimetic agents

Pregnancy Category C

Indications
Secondary hyperparathyroidism in patients who are being hemodialyzed. Hypercalcemia caused by parathyroid carcinoma.

Action
Increases sensitivity of calcium-sensing receptors located on the surface of chief cells of parathyroid gland to levels of extracellular calcium. This decreases parathyroid hormone production with resultant decrease in serum calcium. **Therapeutic Effects:** Decreased bone turnover and fibrosis. Decreased serum calcium.

Pharmacokinetics
Absorption: Well absorbed following oral administration, absorption is enhanced by food and further enhanced by a high fat meal.
Distribution: Unknown.
Protein Binding: 93–97%.
Metabolism and Excretion: Highly metabolized by CYP3A4, CYP2D6, and CYP1A2 enzyme systems; 80% excreted in urine as metabolites, 15% in feces.
Half-life: 30–40 hr.

TIME/ACTION PROFILE (effect on PTH levels)

ROUTE	ONSET	PEAK	DURATION
PO	rapid	2–6 hr	6–12 hr

Contraindications/Precautions
Contraindicated in: Hypersensitivity; Serum calcium <8.4 mg/dL; Lactation: Discontinue drug or bottle-feed.

Use Cautiously in: History of seizure disorder; Chronic kidney disease patients who are not being dialyzed (↑ risk of hypocalcemia); Parathyroid hormone level <150 pg/mL (dose reduction or discontinuation may be warranted); Moderate to severe hepatic impairment; OB: Use only if benefits justify risks to fetus; Pedi: Safety not established.

Adverse Reactions/Side Effects
GI: nausea, vomiting. **F and E:** hypocalcemia.
Metab: adynamic bone disease.

Interactions
Drug-Drug: Inhibits CYP2D6 and may ↑ levels of **flecainide**, **vinblastine**, **thioridazine**, **metoprolol**, **carvedilol**, and most **tricyclic antidepressants**; dose adjustments may be necessary. Blood levels are ↑ by **strong CYP3A4 inhibitors** including **ketoconazole**, **itraconazole**, and **erythromycin**; monitoring and dose adjustment may be necessary.

Route/Dosage
PO (Adults): 30 mg twice daily, titrate every 2–4 wk up to 90 mg 3–4 times daily in response to serum calcium monitoring.

Availability
Tablets: 30 mg, 60 mg, 90 mg.

NURSING IMPLICATIONS

Assessment
- Monitor for signs and symptoms of hypocalcemia (paresthesias, myalgias, cramping, tetany, convulsions) during therapy. If calcium levels decrease to below normal, serum calcium may be increased by adjusting dose (see Lab Test Considerations) and providing supplemental serum calcium, initiating or increasing dose of calcium-based phosphate binder or vitamin D.
- *Lab Test Considerations:* Monitor serum calcium and phosphorous levels within 1 wk after initiation of therapy or dose adjustment and monthly for patients with hyperparathyroidism or every 2 mo for patients with parathyroid carcinoma once maintenance dose has been established, especially in patients with a history of seizure disorder. Therapy should not be initiated in patients with serum calcium less than the lower limit of normal (8.4 mg/dL).
- If serum calcium ↓ below 8.4 mg/dL but remains above 7.5 mg/dL, or if symptoms of hypocalcemia occur, use calcium-containing phosphate binders and/or vitamin D sterols to ↑ serum calcium. If serum calcium ↓ below 7.5 mg/dL, or if symptoms of hypocalcemia persist and the dose of vitamin D cannot be ↑, withhold administration of cinacalcet until serum calcium levels reach 8.0 mg/dL, and/or symptoms of hypocalcemia resolve. Re-initiate therapy using next lowest dose of cinacalcet.
- Monitor serum parathyroid hormone (iPTH) levels 1 to 4 wk after initiation of therapy or dose adjustment, and every 1 to 3 mo after maintenance dose has been established. If iPTH levels ↓ below 150–300 pg/mL, reduce dose or discontinue cinacalcet.

- Monitor liver function tests in patients with moderate to severe hepatic impairment during therapy.

Potential Nursing Diagnoses
Deficient knowledge, related to medication regimen (Patient/Family Teaching)

Implementation
- Cinacalcet may be used alone or in combination with vitamin D and/or phosphate binders.
- **PO:** Administer with food or shortly after a meal. Take tablets whole, do not divide.

Patient/Family Teaching
- Instruct patient to take cinacalcet as directed.
- Advise patient to report signs and symptoms of hypocalcemia to health care professional promptly.

Evaluation/Desired Outcomes
- Decreased serum calcium levels.

HIGH ALERT

cisplatin (sis-pla-tin)
✦Platinol, Platinol-AQ

Classification
Therapeutic: antineoplastics
Pharmacologic: alkylating agents

Pregnancy Category D

Indications
Metastatic testicular and ovarian carcinoma. Advanced bladder cancer. Head and neck cancer. Cervical cancer. Lung cancer. Other tumors.

Action
Inhibits DNA synthesis by producing cross-linking of parent DNA strands (cell-cycle phase–nonspecific). **Therapeutic Effects:** Death of rapidly replicating cells, particularly malignant ones.

Pharmacokinetics
Absorption: IV administration results in complete bioavailability.
Distribution: Widely distributed; accumulates for months; enters breast milk.
Metabolism and Excretion: Excreted mainly by the kidneys.
Half-life: 30–100 hr.

TIME/ACTION PROFILE (effects on blood counts)

ROUTE	ONSET	PEAK	DURATION
IV	unknown	18–23 days	39 days

Contraindications/Precautions
Contraindicated in: Hypersensitivity; Pregnancy or lactation.
Use Cautiously in: Hearing loss; Renal impairment (dosage ↓ recommended); CHF; Electrolyte abnormalities; Active infections; Bone marrow depression; Geriatric patients (↑ risk of nephrotoxicity, peripheral neuropathy); Chronic debilitating illnesses; Patients with childbearing potential.

Adverse Reactions/Side Effects
CNS: SEIZURES, malaise, weakness. **EENT:** ototoxicity, tinnitus. **GI:** severe nausea, vomiting, diarrhea, hepatotoxicity. **GU:** nephrotoxicity, sterility. **Derm:** alopecia. **F and E:** hypocalcemia, hypokalemia, hypomagnesemia. **Hemat:** LEUKOPENIA, THROMBOCYTOPENIA, anemia. **Local:** phlebitis at IV site. **Metab:** hyperuricemia. **Neuro:** peripheral neuropathy. **Misc:** anaphylactoid reactions.

Interactions
Drug-Drug: ↑ nephrotoxicity and ototoxicity with other **nephrotoxic** and **ototoxic drugs** (**aminoglycosides, loop diuretics**). ↑ risk of hypokalemia and hypomagnesemia with **loop diuretics** and **amphotericin B**. May ↓ **phenytoin** levels. ↑ bone marrow depression with other **antineoplastics** or **radiation therapy**. May ↓ antibody response to **live-virus vaccines** and ↑ adverse reactions.

Route/Dosage
Other regimens are used.
IV (Adults): *Metastatic testicular tumors*—20 mg/m^2 daily for 5 days repeated q 3–4 wk. *Metastatic ovarian cancer*—75–100 mg/m^2, repeat q 4 wk in combination with cyclophosphamide *or* 100 mg/m^2 q 3 wk if used as a single agent. *Advanced bladder cancer*—50–70 mg/m^2 q 3–4 wk as a single agent.

Availability (generic available)
Powder for injection: 10-mg, 50-mg vials. **Injection:** 1 mg/mL in 50- and 100-mg vials.

NURSING IMPLICATIONS

Assessment
- Monitor vital signs frequently during administration. Report significant changes.
- Monitor intake and output and specific gravity frequently during therapy. Report discrepancies immediately. To reduce the risk of nephrotoxicity, maintain a urinary output of at least 100 mL/hr for 4 hr before initiating and for at least 24 hr after administration.
- Encourage patient to drink 2000–3000 mL/day to promote excretion of uric acid. Allopuri-

nol and alkalinization of the urine may be used to help prevent uric acid nephropathy.
- Assess patency of IV site frequently during therapy. Cisplatin may cause severe irritation and necrosis of tissue if extravasation occurs. If a large amount of highly concentrated cisplatin solution extravasates, mix 4 mL of 10% sodium thiosulfate with 6 mL of sterile water or 1.6 mL of 25% sodium thiosulfate with 8.4 mL of sterile water and inject 1–4 mL (1 mL for each mL extravasated) through existing line or cannula. Inject subcut if needle has been removed. Sodium thiosulfate inactivates cisplatin.
- Severe and protracted nausea and vomiting usually occur 1–4 hr after a dose; vomiting may last for 24 hr. Administer parenteral antiemetic agents 30–45 min before therapy and routinely around the clock for the next 24 hr. Monitor amount of emesis and notify health care professional if emesis exceeds guidelines to prevent dehydration. Nausea and anorexia may persist for up to 1 wk.
- Monitor for bone marrow depression. Assess for bleeding (bleeding gums, bruising, petechiae, stools, urine, and emesis) and avoid IM injections and taking rectal temperatures if platelet count is low. Apply pressure to venipuncture sites for 10 min. Assess for signs of infection during neutropenia. Anemia may occur. Monitor for increased fatigue, dyspnea, and orthostatic hypotension.
- Monitor for signs of anaphylaxis (facial edema, wheezing, dizziness, fainting, tachycardia, hypotension). Discontinue medication immediately and report symptoms. Epinephrine and resuscitation equipment should be readily available.
- Medication may cause ototoxicity and neurotoxicity. Assess patient frequently for dizziness, tinnitus, hearing loss, loss of coordination, loss of taste, or numbness and tingling of extremities; may be irreversible. Notify health care professional promptly if these occur. Audiometry should be performed before initiation of therapy and before subsequent doses. Hearing loss is more frequent with children and usually occurs first with high frequencies and may be unilateral or bilateral.
- Monitor for inadvertent cisplatin overdose. Doses >100 mg/m^2/cycle once every 3–4 wk are rarely used. Differentiate daily doses from total dose/cycle. Symptoms of high cumulative doses include muscle cramps (localized, painful involuntary skeletal muscle contractions of sudden onset and short duration) and are usually associated with advanced stages of peripheral neuropathy.
- **Lab Test Considerations:** Monitor CBC with differential and platelet count before and routinely throughout therapy. The nadir of leukopenia, thrombocytopenia, and anemia occurs within 18–23 days and recovery 39 days after a dose. Withhold further doses until WBC is >4000/mm^3 and platelet count is >100,000/mm^3.
- Monitor BUN, serum creatinine, and CCr before initiation of therapy and before each course of cisplatin to detect nephrotoxicity. May cause ↑ BUN and creatinine and ↓ calcium, magnesium, phosphate, sodium, and potassium levels that usually occur the 2nd wk after a dose. Do not administer additional doses until BUN is <25 mg/100 mL and serum creatinine is <1.5 mg/100 mL. May cause ↑ uric acid level, which usually peaks 3–5 days after a dose.
- May cause transiently ↑ serum bilirubin and AST concentrations.
- May cause positive Coombs' test result.

Potential Nursing Diagnoses
Risk for infection (Adverse Reactions)
Risk for injury (Side Effects)

Implementation
- *High Alert:* Fatalities have occurred with chemotherapeutic agents. Before administering, clarify all ambiguous orders; double-check single, daily, and course-of-therapy dose limits; have second practitioner independently double-check original order, calculations, and infusion pump settings. Do not confuse with carboplatin. To prevent confusion, orders should include generic and brand names. Administer under the supervision of a physician experienced in the use of cancer chemotherapeutic agents.
- Solution should be prepared in a biologic cabinet. Wear gloves, gown, and mask while handling medication. If powder or solution comes in contact with skin or mucosa, wash thoroughly with soap and water. Discard equipment in specially designated containers (see Appendix L).
- Hydrate patient with at least 1–2 L of IV fluid 8–12 hr before initiating therapy with cispla-

tin. Amifostine may be administered to minimize nephrotoxicity.
- Do not use aluminum needles or equipment during preparation or administration. Aluminum reacts with this drug, forms a black or brown precipitate, and renders the drug ineffective.
- Unopened vials of powder and constituted solution must not be refrigerated.

IV Administration

- **Intermittent Infusion:** Reconstitute 10-mg vials with 10 mL of sterile water for injection and 50-mg vial with 50 mL. Stable for 20 hr if reconstituted with sterile water, for 72 hr with bacteriostatic water. Do not refrigerate, because crystals will form. Solution should be clear and colorless; discard if turbid or if it contains precipitates.
- *Diluent:* Dilution in 2 L of 5% dextrose in 0.3% or 0.45% NaCl containing 37.5 g of mannitol is recommended. *Concentration:* Keep under 0.5 mg/mL to prevent tissue necrosis. *Rate:* Variable. Maximum rate 1 mg/min.
- **Continuous Infusion:** Has been administered as continuous infusion over 24 hr to 5 days with resultant decrease in nausea and vomiting. *High Alert:* Clarify dose to ensure cumulative dosage is not confused with daily dose; errors may be fatal.
- **Syringe Compatibility:** bleomycin, cyclophosphamide, doxapram, doxorubicin, droperidol, fluorouracil, furosemide, heparin, leucovorin calcium, methotrexate, metoclopramide, mitomycin, vinblastine, vincristine.
- **Y-Site Compatibility:** allopurinol, aztreonam, bleomycin, chlorpromazine, cimetidine, cladribine, cyclophosphamide, dexamethasone, diphenhydramine, doxorubicin, doxorubicin liposome, droperidol, etoposide, famotidine, filgrastim, fludarabine, fluorouracil, furosemide, ganciclovir, gemcitabine, granisetron, heparin, hydromorphone, leucovorin calcium, linezolid, lorazepam, melphalan, methotrexate, methylprednisolone, metoclopramide, mitomycin, morphine, ondansetron, paclitaxel, palonosetron, pemetrexed, prochlorperazine edisylate, promethazine, propofol, ranitidine, sargramostim, teniposide, topotecan, vinblastine, vincristine, vinorelbine.
- **Y-Site Incompatibility:** amifostine, amphotericin B cholesteryl sulfate, cefepime, lansoprazole, piperacillin/tazobactam, thiotepa.
- **Additive Compatibility:** etoposide, floxuridine, ifosfamide, leucovorin calcium, magnesium sulfate, mannitol, ondansetron, 0.9% NaCl, D5/0.9% NaCl.
- **Additive Incompatibility:** fluorouracil, mesna, thiotepa.

Patient/Family Teaching

- Instruct patient to report pain at injection site immediately.
- Instruct patient to notify health care professional promptly if fever; chills; cough; hoarseness; sore throat; signs of infection; lower back or side pain; painful or difficult urination; bleeding gums; bruising; petechiae; blood in stools, urine, or emesis; increased fatigue; dyspnea; or orthostatic hypotension occurs. Caution patient to avoid crowds and persons with known infections. Instruct patient to use soft toothbrush and electric razor and to avoid falls. Caution patient not to drink alcoholic beverages or take medication containing aspirin or NSAIDs; may precipitate gastric bleeding.
- Instruct patient to report promptly any numbness or tingling in extremities or face, difficulty with hearing or tinnitus, unusual swelling, or joint pain.
- Instruct patient not to receive any vaccinations without advice of health care professional.
- Advise patient of the need for contraception, although cisplatin may cause infertility.
- Emphasize the need for periodic lab tests to monitor for side effects.

Evaluation/Desired Outcomes

- Decrease in size or spread of malignancies. Therapy should not be administered more frequently than every 3–4 wk, and only if lab values are within acceptable parameters and patient is not exhibiting signs of ototoxicity or other serious adverse effects.

---

citalopram (si-tal-oh-pram)
Celexa

Classification
Therapeutic: antidepressants
Pharmacologic: selective serotonin reuptake inhibitors (SSRIs)

Pregnancy Category C

Indications
Depression. **Unlabeled Use:** Premenstrual dysphoric disorder (PMDD). Obsessive-compulsive discorder (OCD). Panic disorder. Generalized anxiety disorder (GAD). Post-traumatic stress disorder (PTSD). Social anxiety disorder (social phobia).

citalopram **331**

Action
Selectively inhibits the reuptake of serotonin in the CNS. **Therapeutic Effects:** Antidepressant action.

Pharmacokinetics
Absorption: 80% absorbed after oral administration.
Distribution: Enters breast milk.
Metabolism and Excretion: Mostly metabolized by the liver (10% by CYP3A4 and 2C19 enzymes); excreted unchanged in urine.
Half-life: 35 hr.

TIME/ACTION PROFILE (antidepressant effect)

ROUTE	ONSET	PEAK	DURATION
PO	1–4 wk	unknown	unknown

Contraindications/Precautions
Contraindicated in: Hypersensitivity; Concurrent MAO inhibitor or pimozide therapy.
Use Cautiously in: History of mania; History of suicide attempt/ideation (↑ risk during early therapy and during dose adjustment); History of seizure disorder; Illnesses or conditions that are likely to result in altered metabolism or hemodynamic responses; Severe renal or hepatic impairment; OB: Use during third trimester may result in neonatal serotonin syndrome requiring prolonged hospitalization, respiratory and nutritional support; Lactation: Present in breast milk and may result in lethargy with ↓ feeding in infants; weigh risk/benefits; Pedi: May ↑ risk of suicide attempt/ideation especially during early treatment or dose adjustment in children/adolescents (unlabeled for pediatric use); Geri: ↓ doses recommended.

Adverse Reactions/Side Effects
CNS: NEUROLEPTIC MALIGNANT SYNDROME, SUICIDAL THOUGHTS, apathy, confusion, drowsiness, insomnia, weakness, agitation, amnesia, anxiety, ↓ libido, dizziness, fatigue, impaired concentration, ↑ depression, migraine headache. **EENT:** abnormal accommodation. **Resp:** cough. **CV:** postural hypotension, tachycardia. **GI:** abdominal pain, anorexia, diarrhea, dry mouth, dyspepsia, flatulence, ↑ saliva, nausea, altered taste, ↑ appetite, vomiting. **GU:** amenorrhea, dysmenorrhea, ejaculatory delay, erectile dysfunction, polyuria. **Derm:** sweating, photosensitivity, pruritus, rash. **Metab:** weight loss, weight gain. **F and E:** hyponatremia. **MS:** arthralgia, myalgia. **Neuro:** tremor, paresthesia. **Misc:** SEROTONIN SYNDROME, fever, yawning.

Interactions
Drug-Drug: May cause serious, potentially fatal reactions when used with **MAO inhibitors**; allow at least 14 days between citalopram and **MAO inhibitors**. Concurrent use with **pimozide** may result in prolongation of the QTc interval and is contraindicated. Drugs that affect serotonergic neurotransmitter systems, including **linezolid**, **tramadol**, and **triptans** ↑ risk of serotonin syndrome. Use cautiously with other **centrally acting drugs** (including **alcohol**, **antihistamines**, **opioid analgesics**, and **sedative/hypnotics**; concurrent use with **alcohol** is not recommended). **Cimetidine** may ↑ levels. Serotonergic effects may be ↑ by **lithium** (concurrent use should be carefully monitored). **Ketoconazole**, **itraconazole**, **erythromycin**, and **omeprazole** may ↑ levels. **Carbamazepine** may ↓ blood levels. May ↑ levels of **metoprolol**. Use cautiously with **tricyclic antidepressants** due to unpredictable effects on serotonin and norepinephrine reuptake. ↑ risk of bleeding with **aspirin**, **NSAIDs**, **clopidogrel**, or **warfarin**.
Drug-Natural Products: ↑ risk of serotonergic side effects including serotonin syndrome with **St. John's wort** and **SAMe**.

Route/Dosage
PO (Adults): 20 mg once daily initially, may be ↑ by 20 mg/day at weekly intervals, up to 60 mg/day (usual dose is 40 mg/day).
PO (Geriatric Patients): 20 mg once daily initially, may be ↑ to 40 mg/day only in nonresponding patients.

Hepatic Impairment
PO (Adults): 20 mg once daily initially, may be ↑ to 40 mg/day only in nonresponding patients.

Availability (generic available)
Tablets: 10 mg, 20 mg, 40 mg. **Cost:** *Generic*— 10 mg $89.97/90, 20 mg $89.97/90, 40 mg $89.97/90. **Oral solution (peppermint flavor):** 10 mg/5 mL. **Cost:** *Generic*— 10 mg/5 mL $114.00/240 mL.

NURSING IMPLICATIONS

Assessment
- Monitor mood changes during therapy.
- Assess for suicidal tendencies, especially during early therapy and dose changes. Restrict amount of drug available to patient. Risk may be increased in children, adolescents, and

adults ≤24 yr. After starting therapy, children, adolescents, and young adults should be seen by health care professional at least weekly for 4 wk, every 3 wk for the next 4 wk, and on advice of health care professional thereafter.
- Assess for sexual dysfunction (erectile dysfunction; decreased libido).
- Assess for serotonin syndrome (mental changes [agitation, hallucinations, coma], autonomic instability [tachycardia, labile blood pressure, hyperthermia], neuromuscular aberrations [hyperreflexia, incoordination], and/or GI symptoms [nausea, vomiting, diarrhea]), especially in patients taking other serotonergic drugs (SSRIs, SNRIs, triptans).

Potential Nursing Diagnoses
Ineffective coping (Indications)
Risk for injury (Side Effects)
Sexual dysfunction (Side Effects)

Implementation
- Do not confuse with Celebrex (celecoxib), Cerebyx (fosphenytoin), Zyprexa (olanzapine), or Lexapro (escitalopram).
- **PO:** Administer as a single dose in the morning or evening without regard to food.

Patient/Family Teaching
- Instruct patient to take citalopram as directed.
- May cause drowsiness, dizziness, impaired concentration, and blurred vision. Caution patient to avoid driving and other activities requiring alertness until response to the drug is known.
- Advise patient to avoid alcohol or other CNS depressant drugs during therapy and to consult health care professional before taking other Rx, OTC, or herbal products.
- Caution patient to change positions slowly to minimize dizziness.
- Advise patient, family, and caregivers to look for suicidality, especially during early therapy or dose changes. Notify health care professional immediately if thoughts about suicide or dying, attempts to commit suicide, new or worse depression or anxiety, agitation or restlessness, panic attacks, insomnia, new or worse irritability, aggressiveness, acting on dangerous impulses, mania, or other changes in mood or behavior or if symptoms of serotonin syndrome occur.
- Advise patient to use sunscreen and wear protective clothing to prevent photosensitivity reactions.
- Inform patient that frequent mouth rinses, good oral hygiene, and sugarless gum or candy may minimize dry mouth. If dry mouth persists for more than 2 wk, consult health care professional regarding use of saliva substitute.
- Instruct female patients to inform health care professional if pregnancy is planned or suspected, or if they plan to breastfeed. If used during pregnancy should be tapered during third trimester to avoid neonatal serotinin syndrome.
- Caution patients that citalopram should not be used for at least 14 days after discontinuing MAO inhibitors, and at least 14 days should be allowed after stopping citalopram before starting an MAO inhibitor.
- Emphasize the importance of follow-up exams to monitor progress.

Evaluation/Desired Outcomes
- Increased sense of well-being.
- Renewed interest in surroundings. May require 1–4 wk of therapy to obtain antidepressant effects.

HIGH ALERT

cladribine (klad-ri-been)
Leustatin

Classification
Therapeutic: antineoplastics
Pharmacologic: antimetabolites

Pregnancy Category D

Indications
Management of active hairy cell leukemia manifested as anemia, leukopenia, thrombocytopenia, or clinical symptoms. **Unlabeled Use:** chronic lymphocytic leukemia, chronic myelogenous leukemia, non-Hodgkin's lymphomas, progressive multiple sclerosis.

Action
Inhibits DNA synthesis. **Therapeutic Effects:** Death of rapidly replicating cells, particularly malignant ones.

Pharmacokinetics
Absorption: IV administration results in complete bioavailability.
Distribution: Extensively distributed to body tissues; penetrates into cerebrospinal fluid.
Metabolism and Excretion: Unknown.
Half-life: 3–22 hr.

cladribine **333**

TIME/ACTION PROFILE (noted as effect on peripheral counts)

ROUTE	ONSET	PEAK	DURATION†
Platelets	unknown	unknown	12 days
Absolute neutrophil count	unknown	unknown	5 wk
Hemoglobin	unknown	unknown	8 wk

†Time to normalization of counts

Contraindications/Precautions
Contraindicated in: Hypersensitivity; Diluent contains benzyl alcohol and should be avoided in patients with known intolerance; OB, Lactation: Pregnant or lactating patients.
Use Cautiously in: Patients with active infections; Patients taking medications that cause immunosuppression or bone marrow depression; Impaired hepatic or renal function (↑ risk of toxicity); Patients with childbearing potential; Pedi: Children (safety not established).

Adverse Reactions/Side Effects
CNS: fatigue, headache, dizziness, insomnia, malaise, weakness. **EENT:** epistaxis. **Resp:** abnormal breath sounds, cough, dyspnea. **CV:** edema, tachycardia. **GI:** anorexia, diarrhea, nausea, vomiting, abdominal pain, constipation. **Derm:** rash, erythema, petechiae, pruritus, sweating. **Hemat:** NEUTROPENIA, anemia, thrombocytopenia. **Local:** injection site reactions, phlebitis, thrombosis. **MS:** arthralgia, myalgia. **Misc:** chills, fever, infection, trunk pain.

Interactions
Drug-Drug: Additive bone marrow depression may occur with other **antineoplastics** or **radiation therapy**.

Route/Dosage
IV (Adults): *Hairy cell leukemia*– 0.09 mg/kg/day for 7 days.

Availability
Injection: 1 mg/mL.

NURSING IMPLICATIONS
Assessment
- Monitor for bone marrow depression. Assess for fever, chills, sore throat, and signs of infection. Monitor platelet count throughout therapy. Assess for bleeding (bleeding gums, bruising, petechiae; test stool, urine, and emesis for blood). Avoid administering IM injections and taking rectal temperatures. Apply pressure to venipuncture site for 10 min. Anemia may occur. Monitor for increased fatigue and dyspnea.
- Monitor IV site for phlebitis.
- Monitor intake and output. Development of uric acid nephropathy in patients with leukemia and lymphoma may be prevented with adequate oral hydration and allopurinol, if needed.
- *Lab Test Considerations:* Monitor CD4 T-lymphocyte count and CD8 T-lymphocyte count before initiation of therapy and periodically during and after therapy. Cladribine causes prolonged depression of CD4 and CD8 lymphocyte subset counts, with recovery taking at least 6–12 mo.
- Monitor hemoglobin, hematocrit, leukocyte, and platelet counts before and periodically throughout therapy, especially during the first 4–8 wk after treatment. During the first 2 wk after therapy, platelet counts, absolute neutrophil count (ANC), and hemoglobin decrease. Transfusions of platelets and red blood cells may be required. Platelet count, ANC, and hemoglobin usually return to normal levels by day 12, week 5, and week 8, respectively.
- Monitor renal and hepatic function before and periodically during therapy. May cause nephrotoxicity, resulting in elevated serum creatinine, anuria, and acidosis.
- Monitor serum uric acid concentrations before and periodically during therapy, especially in patients with high tumor burden. May cause elevated serum and uric acid concentrations. May require alkalinization of the urine.
- *Toxicity and Overdose:* May cause irreversible neurologic toxicity, resulting in motor weakness progressing to paraparesis or quadriparesis with high doses. If symptoms occur, discontinue cladribine. There is no known antidote.

Potential Nursing Diagnoses
Risk for infection (Indications)
Risk for injury (Adverse Reactions)

Implementation
- *High Alert:* Fatalities have occurred with chemotherapeutic agents. Before administering, clarify all ambiguous orders; double-check single, daily, and course-of-therapy dose limits; have second practitioner independently double-check original order, calculations, and infusion pump settings.

✤ = Canadian drug name.   = Genetic implication.
*CAPITALS indicates life-threatening; underlines indicate most frequent.

clarithromycin

- Prepare solution in a biologic cabinet. Wear gloves, gown, and mask while handling IV medication. Discard IV equipment in specially designated containers (see Appendix L).

IV Administration

- **Continuous Infusion:** *Diluent:* Add the daily dose to 500 mL of 0.9% NaCl for injection. Solution is stable for 24 hr at room temperature or 8 days if refrigerated.
- May also be prepared as a 7-day solution with bacteriostatic 0.9% NaCl for infusion via *Pharmacia Deltec* medication cassettes. *Rate:* Administer as a continuous infusion over 24 hr.
- **Y-Site Compatibility:** aminophylline, bumetanide, buprenorphine, butorphanol, calcium gluconate, carboplatin, chlorproamzine, cimetidine, cisplatin, cyclophosphamide, cytarabine, dexamethasone, diphenhydramine, dobutamine, dopamine, doxorubicin hydrochloride, droperidol, enalaprilat, etoposide, famotidine, furosemide, granisetron, haloperidol, heparin, hydrocortisone, hydromorphone, idarubicin, leucovorin, lorazepam, mannitol, meperidine, mesna, methylprednisolone, metoclopramide, mitoxantrone, morphine, nalbuphine, ondansetron, paclitaxel, potassium chloride, prochlorperazine, promethazine, ranitidine, sodium bicarbonate, teniposide, vincristine.
- **Additive Incompatiblity:** D5W. Do not admix with other medications or solutions.

Patient/Family Teaching

- Instruct patient to notify health care professional promptly in the event of fever; sore throat; signs of infection; bleeding gums; bruising; petechiae; blood in urine, stool, or emesis; unusual swelling; joint pain; shortness of breath; or confusion. Caution patient to avoid crowds and persons with known infections. Instruct patient to use soft toothbrush and electric razor and to be especially careful to avoid falls. Patients should also be cautioned not to drink alcoholic beverages or to take products containing aspirin or NSAIDs because these may precipitate GI hemorrhage.
- Advise patient to use nonhormonal contraceptive measures during and for at least 4 mo after completion of therapy.
- Instruct patient not to receive any vaccinations without advice of health care professional.

Evaluation/Desired Outcomes

- Improvement in hematologic status in patients with leukemia.

clarithromycin
(kla-**rith**-roe-mye-sin)
Biaxin, Biaxin XL

Classification
Therapeutic: agents for atypical mycobacterium, anti-infectives, antiulcer agents
Pharmacologic: macrolides

Pregnancy Category C

Indications
Respiratory tract infections including streptococcal pharyngitis, sinusitis, bronchitis and pneumonia. Treatment (with ethambutol) and prevention of disseminated *Mycobacterium avium* complex (MAC). Treatment of following pediatric infections: Otitis media, Sinusitis, Pharyngitis, Skin/skin structure infections. Part of a combination regimen for ulcer disease due to *Helicobacter pylori*. Endocarditis prophylaxis.

Action
Inhibits protein synthesis at the level of the 50S bacterial ribosome. **Therapeutic Effects:** Bacteriostatic action. **Spectrum:** Active against these gram-positive aerobic bacteria: *Staphylococcus aureus*, *Staphylococcus pneumoniae*, *S. pyogenes* (group A strep). Active against these gram-negative aerobic bacteria: *Haemophilus influenzae*, *Moraxella catarrhalis*. Also active against: *Mycoplasma*, *Legionella*, *H. pylori*, *M. avium*.

Pharmacokinetics
Absorption: Rapidly absorbed (50%) after oral administration.
Distribution: Widely distributed; tissue levels may exceed those in serum.
Protein Binding: 65–70%.
Metabolism and Excretion: 10–15% converted by the liver to 14-hydroxyclarithromycin, which has anti-infective activity; 20–30% excreted unchanged in urine. Metabolized by and also inhibits the CYP3A enzyme system.
Half-life: Dose-dependent and prolonged with renal dysfunction *250-mg dose*—3–4 hr; *500-mg dose*—5–7 hr.

TIME/ACTION PROFILE (serum levels)

ROUTE	ONSET	PEAK	DURATION
PO	unknown	2 hr	12 hr
PO-XL	unknown	4 hr	24 hr

Contraindications/Precautions
Contraindicated in: Hypersensitivity to clarithromycin, erythromycin, or other macrolide anti-

clarithromycin

infectives; Concurrent use of pimozide; OB: Avoid use during pregnancy unless no alternatives are available; Lactation: Not recommend for breast-feeding women.

Use Cautiously in: Severe liver or renal impairment (dose adjustment required if CCr <30 mL/min); Myasthenia gravis.

Adverse Reactions/Side Effects

CNS: headache. **Derm:** pruritus, rash, Stevens-Johnson syndrome. **GI:** PSEUDOMEMBRANOUS COLITIS, abdominal pain/discomfort, abnormal taste, diarrhea, dyspepsia, nausea.

Interactions

Drug-Drug: Clarithromycin is an inhibitor of the CYP3A enzyme system. Concurrent use with other agents metabolized by this system can ↑ levels and risk of toxicity. May prolong the QT interval and ↑ risk of arrhythmias with **pimozide**; concurrent use is contraindicated. Similar effects may occur with antiarrhythmics; ECG should be monitored for QTc prolongation and serum levels monitored. May ↑ serum levels and the risk of toxicity from **carbamazepine**, some **benzodiazepines (midazolam, triazolam, alprazolam), cyclosporine, buspirone, disopyramide, ergot alkaloids, felodipine, omeprazole, tacrolimus, digoxin,** or **theophylline**. **Ritonavir** ↑ blood levels (↓ clarithromycin dose in patients with CC <60 mL/min). ↑ levels of **HMG-CoA reductase inhibitors** and may ↑ risk of rhabdomyolysis. May ↑ effect of **warfarin** and **sildenafil** (dose reduction may be warranted). May ↑ or ↓ effects of **zidovudine**. Blood levels are ↑ by **delavirdine** and **fluconazole**. Blood levels may be ↓ by **rifampin** and **rifabutin**. ↑ risk of colchicine toxicty when administered with **colchicine**, especially in the elderly.

Route/Dosage

PO (Adults): *Pharyngitis/tonsillitis*—250 mg q 12 hr for 10 days; *Acute maxillary sinusitis*—500 mg q 12 hr for 14 days or 1000 mg once daily for 14 days as XL tablets; *Acute exacerbation of chronic bronchitis*—250–500 mg q 12 hr for 7–14 days or 1000 mg once daily for 7 days as XL tablets; *Community-Acquired pneumonia*—250 mg q 12 hr for 7–14 days or 1000 mg once daily for 7 days as XL tablets; *skin/skin structure infections*—250 mg q 12 hr for 7–14 days; *H. pylori*—500 mg 2–3 times daily with a proton pump inhibitor (lansoprazole or omeprazole) or ranitidine with or without amoxicillin for 10–14 days; *Endocarditis prophylaxis*—500 mg 1 hr before procedure; *MAC prophylaxis/treatment*—500 mg twice daily, for active infection another antimycobacterial is required.

PO (Children): *Most infections*—15 mg/kg/day divided q 12 hr for 7–14 days (up to 500 mg/dose for MAC). *Endocarditis prophylaxis*—15 mg/kg 1 hr before procedure.

Renal Impairment

PO (Adults): *CCr <30 mL/min*—250 mg 1-2 times daily, a 500-mg initial dose may be used.
PO (Children): *CCr <30 mL/min*—decrease dose by 50% or double dosing interval.

Availability (generic available)

Tablets: 250 mg, 500 mg. **Cost:** *Generic*—250 mg $73.32/20, 500 mg $73.32/20. **Extended-release tablets:** 500 mg. **Cost:** $109.99/20. **Oral suspension (fruit punch and vanilla flavors):** 125 mg/5 mL, 250 mg/5 mL. **Cost:** *Generic*—125 mg/5 mL $39.98/100 mL, 250 mg/5 mL $71.38/100 mL. *In combination with:* amoxicillin and lansoprazole as part of a compliance package (Prevpac); See Appendix B.

NURSING IMPLICATIONS

Assessment

- Assess patient for infection (vital signs; appearance of wound, sputum, urine, and stool; WBC) at beginning of and during therapy.
- Obtain specimens for culture and sensitivity before initiating therapy. First dose may be given before receiving results.
- **Ulcers:** Assess patient for epigastric or abdominal pain and frank or occult blood in the stool, emesis, or gastric aspirate.
- *Lab Test Considerations:* May rarely cause ↑ serum AST, ALT, and alkaline phosphatase concentrations.
- May occasionally cause ↑ BUN.

Potential Nursing Diagnoses

Risk for infection (Indications, Side Effects)
Noncompliance (Patient/Family Teaching)

Implementation

- **PO:** Administer around the clock, without regard to meals. Food slows but does not decrease the extent of absorption.
- Administer XL tablets with food or milk; do not crush, break or chew.

- Shake suspension well before administration. Store suspension at room temperature; do not refrigerate.
- Do not administer within 4 hr of zidovudine.

Patient/Family Teaching
- Instruct patient to take medication around the clock and to finish the drug completely as directed, even if feeling better. Take missed doses as soon as possible, unless almost time for next dose. Do not double doses. Advise patient that sharing of this medication may be dangerous.
- Advise patient to report the signs of superinfection (black, furry overgrowth on the tongue; vaginal itching or discharge; loose or foul-smelling stools).
- Instruct patient to notify health care professional if fever and diarrhea develop, especially if stool contains blood, pus, or mucus. Advise patient not to treat diarrhea without consulting health care professional.
- Caution patients taking zidovudine that clarithromycin and zidovudine must be taken at least 4 hr apart.
- Advise patient to notify health care professional if pregnancy is planned or suspected.
- Instruct the patient to notify health care professional if symptoms do not improve within a few days.

Evaluation/Desired Outcomes
- Resolution of the signs and symptoms of infection. Length of time for complete resolution depends on the organism and site of infection.
- Treatment of ulcers.
- Endocarditis prophylaxis.

---

clevidipine (kle-vi-di-peen)
Cleviprex

Classification
Therapeutic: antihypertensives
Pharmacologic: calcium channel blockers (dihydropyridine)

Indications
Reduction of blood pressure when oral therapy is not feasible/desirable.

Action
Inhibits calcium transport into vascular smooth muscle, resulting in inhibition of excitation-contraction coupling and subsequent contraction. Decreases systemic vascular resistance; does not reduce cardiac filling pressure (pre-load). Has no effect on venous capacitance vessels. **Therapeutic Effects:** Decreases blood pressure.

Pharmacokinetics
Absorption: IV administration results in complete bioavailibility.
Distribution: Unknown.
Protein Binding: >99.5%.
Metabolism and Excretion: Rapidly metabolized by esterases in plasma and tissue to inactive metabolites; metabolites are excreted in urine (63–74%) and feces (7–22%).
Half-life: *Initial phase*—1 min; *terminal phase*—15 min.

TIME/ACTION PROFILE

ROUTE	ONSET	PEAK	DURATION
IV	2–4 min	30 min*	end of infusion

*Time to target blood pressure.

Contraindications/Precautions
Contraindicated in: Hypersensitivity; Allergy to soybeans, eggs/egg products, defective lipid metabolism including pathologic hyperlipidemia, lipoid nephrosis or acute pancreatitis; severe aortic stenosis.
Use Cautiously in: Geri: Titrate dose cautiously, initiate therapy at low end of dose range; consider age-related decrease in hepatic, renal or cardiac function, concomitant diseases, or other drug therapy; OB: Use only if maternal benefit outweighs potential risk to fetus; Lactation: Consider possible infant exposure; Pedi: Safety not established for patients <18 yr.

Adverse Reactions/Side Effects
CNS: headache. **CV:** CHF, hypotension, rebound hypertension, reflex tachycardia. **GI:** nausea, vomiting. **MS:** arthralgia.

Interactions
Drug-Drug: ↑ risk of excess hypotension with other **antihypertensives**. Does not protect against effects of abrupt **beta blocker** withdrawal.

Route/Dosage
IV (Adults): *Initial dose:* 1–2 mg/hr; *Dose titration:* Double dose every 90 sec initially; as blood pressure approaches goal, increase dose by less than doubling and lengthen the time between dose adjustments to every 5–10 min. Usual dose required is 4–6 mg/hour. Severe hypertensive patients may require higher doses with a maximum of 16 mg/hr or less. Doses up to 32 mg/hr have been used, but generally should not exceed 21 mg/hr in a 24 hr period due to lipid load.

Availability
Emulsion for injection 0.5 mg/mL: 50 mL vial, 100 mL vial. **Cost:** wholesale cost $145/50-mL vial, $290/100-mL vial.

NURSING IMPLICATIONS
Assessment
- Monitor blood pressure and heart rate during infusion, and until vital signs stabilize. Hypotension and reflex tachycardia may occur with rapid upward titration. Monitor patients receiving prolonged clevidipine infusions and who have not been transitioned to other antihypertensive therapies for the possibility of rebound hypertension for at least 8 hr after infusion is stopped; additional adjustments may be needed.

Potential Nursing Diagnoses
Ineffective tissue perfusion (Indications)

Implementation
- Discontinue clevidipine or titrate downward during initiation of oral therapy; consider time to onset of the oral agent's effect. Continue blood pressure monitoring until desired effect is achieved.

IV Administration
- **Intermittent Infusion:** *Diluent:* Do not dilute. Invert vial gently several times before use to ensure emulsion uniformity prior to administration. Solution is milky white; inspect for particulate matter and discoloration. Commercially available standard plastic cannulae may be used to administer the infusion. Administer via central line or peripheral line. Solution is in single-use vials; discard unused portion 4 hr after stopper puncture. Store in refrigerator; once emulsion reaches room temperature, stable for 2 mo, do not re-refrigerate. *Rate:* Initiate intravenous infusion at 1-2 mg/hr. Administer using an infusion device allowing calibrated infusion rates.
- **Y-Site Compatibility:** Water for Injection, USP, 0.9% NaCl, D5W, D5/0.9% NaCl, D5/LR, LR, 10% amino acid.
- **Y-Site Incompatibility:** Do not administer in the same line as other medications.

Patient/Family Teaching
- Inform patient of the rationale for use of clevidipine.
- Advise patients to contact a health care professional immediately if signs of a new hypertensive emergency (neurological symptoms, visual changes, evidence of CHF) occur.
- Advise female patients to notify health care professional if pregnancy is planned or suspected or if breastfeeding.
- Encourage patients with underlying hypertension to continue follow-up care and to continue taking their oral antihypertensive medication(s) as directed.

Evaluation/Desired Outcomes
- Decrease in blood pressure.

---

clindamycin (klin-da-mye-sin)
Cleocin, Cleocin T, Clinda-Derm, Clindagel, Clindesse, ClindaMax, Clindets, C/T/S, ✤ Dalacin C, ✤ Dalacin T, Evoclin

Classification
Therapeutic: anti-infectives

Pregnancy Category B

Indications
PO, IM, IV: Treatment of: Skin and skin structure infections, Respiratory tract infections, Septicemia, Intra-abdominal infections, Gynecologic infections, Osteomyelitis, Endocarditis prophylaxis. **Topical:** Severe acne. **Vag:** Bacterial vaginosis. **Unlabeled Use: PO, IM, IV:** Treatment of *Pneumocystis carinii* pneumonia, CNS toxoplasmosis, and babesiosis.

Action
Inhibits protein synthesis in susceptible bacteria at the level of the 50S ribosome. **Therapeutic Effects:** Bactericidal or bacteriostatic, depending on susceptibility and concentration. **Spectrum:** Active against most gram-positive aerobic cocci, including: Staphylococci, *Streptococcus pneumoniae*, other streptococci, but not enterococci. Has good activity against those anaerobic bacteria that cause bacterial vaginosis, including *Bacteroides fragilis*, *Gardnerella vaginalis*, *Mobiluncus* spp, *Mycoplasma hominis*, and *Corynebacterium*. Also active against *P. jirovecii* and *Toxoplasma gondii*.

Pharmacokinetics
Absorption: Well absorbed following PO/IM administration. Minimal absorption following topical/vaginal use.
Distribution: Widely distributed. Does not significantly cross blood-brain barrier. Crosses the placenta; enters breast milk.
Protein Binding: 94%.
Metabolism and Excretion: Mostly metabolized by the liver.

✤ = Canadian drug name. ▓ = Genetic implication.
*CAPITALS indicates life-threatening; underlines indicate most frequent.

clindamycin

Half-life: Neonates: 3.6–8.7 hr; Infants up to 1 yr: 3 hr; Children and adults: 2–3 hr.

TIME/ACTION PROFILE (blood levels)

ROUTE	ONSET	PEAK	DURATION
PO	rapid	60 min	6–8 hr
IM	rapid	1–3 hr	6–8 hr
IV	rapid	end of infusion	6–8 hr

Contraindications/Precautions
Contraindicated in: Hypersensitivity; Previous pseudomembranous colitis; Severe liver impairment; Diarrhea; Known alcohol intolerance (topical solution, suspension).
Use Cautiously in: OB: Safety not established for systemic and topical; approved for vaginal use in 3rd trimester of pregnancy; Lactation: Has been used safely but appears in breast milk and exposes infant to drug and its side effects.

Adverse Reactions/Side Effects
CNS: dizziness, headache, vertigo. **CV:** arrhythmias, hypotension. **GI:** PSEUDOMEMBRANOUS COLITIS, diarrhea, bitter taste (IV only), nausea, vomiting. **Derm:** rashes. **Local:** phlebitis at IV site.

Interactions
Drug-Drug: Kaolin/pectin may ↓ GI absorption. May enhance the neuromuscular blocking action of other **neuromuscular blocking agents**. **Topical:** Concurrent use with **irritants**, **abrasives**, or **desquamating agents** may result in additive irritation.

Route/Dosage
PO (Adults): *Most infections*—150–450 mg q 6 hr. *P. carinii pneumonia*—1200–1800 mg/day in divided doses with 15–30 mg Primaquine/day (unlabeled). *CNS toxoplasmosis*—1200–2400 mg/day in divided doses with pyrimethamine 50–100 mg/day (unlabeled); *Bacterial endocarditis prophylaxis*—600 mg 1 hr before procedure.
PO (Children >1 mo): 10–30 mg/kg/day divided q 6–8 hr; maximum dose 1.8 g/day. *Bacterial endocarditis prophylaxis*—20 mg/kg 1 hr before procedure.
IM, IV (Adults): *Most infections*—300–600 mg q 6–8 hr *or* 900 mg q 8 hr (up to 4.8 g/day IV has been used); single IM doses of >600 mg are not recommended). *P. carinii pneumonia*—2400–2700 mg/day in divided doses with Primaquine (unlabeled). *Toxoplasmosis*—1200–4800 mg/day in divided doses with pyrimethamine. *Bacterial endocarditis prophylaxis*—600 mg 30 min before procedure.
IM, IV (Children >1 mo): 25–40 mg/kg/day divided q 6–8 hr; maximum dose: 4.8 g/day. *Bacterial endocarditis prophylaxis*—20 mg/kg 30 min before procedure; maximum dose: 600 mg.
IM, IV (Infants <1 mo and <2 kg): 5 mg/kg q 8–12 hr ≥*2 kg*—20–30 mg/kg/day divided q 6–8 hr.
Vag (Adults and Adolescents): *Cleocin, Clindamax*—1 applicatorful (5 g) at bedtime for 3 or 7 days (7 days in pregnant patients); *Clindesse*—one applicatorful (5 g) single dose; *or* 1 suppository (100 mg) at bedtime for 3 nights.
Topical (Adults and Adolescents): *Solution*—1% solution/suspension applied twice daily (range 1–4 times daily). *Foam, gel*—1% foam or gel applied once daily.

Availability (generic available)
Capsules: 75 mg, 150 mg, 300 mg. **Oral suspension:** 75 mg/5 mL. **Injection:** 150 mg/mL. **Premixed infusion:** 300 mg/50 mL, 600 mg/50 mL, 900 mg/50 mL. **Topical:** 1% lotion, gel, foam, solution, suspension, single-use applicators. *In combination with:* benzoyl peroxide (Acanya, BenzaClin, Duac); (see Appendix B).
Vaginal cream: 2%. **Vaginal suppositories (ovules):** 100 mg. *In combination with:* tretinoin (Ziana); (see Appendix B).

NURSING IMPLICATIONS

Assessment
- Assess for infection (vital signs; appearance of wound, sputum, urine, and stool; WBC) at beginning of and during therapy.
- Obtain specimens for culture and sensitivity prior to initiating therapy. First dose may be given before receiving results.
- Monitor bowel elimination. Diarrhea, abdominal cramping, fever, and bloody stools should be reported to health care professional promptly as a sign of pseudomembranous colitis. This may begin up to several weeks following the cessation of therapy.
- Assess patient for hypersensitivity (skin rash, urticaria).
- *Lab Test Considerations:* Monitor CBC; may cause transient ↓ in leukocytes, eosinophils, and platelets.
- May cause ↑ alkaline phosphatase, bilirubin, CPK, AST, and ALT concentrations.

Potential Nursing Diagnoses
Risk for infection (Indications, Side Effects)
Diarrhea (Side Effects)

Implementation
- **PO:** Administer with a full glass of water. May be given with or without meals. Shake liquid

preparations well. Do not refrigerate. Stable for 14 days at room temperature.
- **IM:** Do not administer >600 mg in a single IM injection.

IV Administration
- **Intermittent Infusion:** *Diluent:* Vials must be diluted before use. Dilute a dose of 300 mg or 600 mg in 50 mL and a dose of 900 mg or 1200 mg in 100 mL. Compatible diluents include D5W, 0.9% NaCl, D5/0.9% NaCl, D5/0.45% NaCl, or LR. Admixed solution stable for 16 days at room temperature. Premixed infusion is already diluted and ready to use. *Concentration:* Not to exceed 18 mg/mL. *Rate:* Not exceed 30 mg/min. Hypotension and cardiopulmonary arrest have been reported following rapid IV administration.
- **Y-Site Compatibility:** acyclovir, alfentanil, amifostine, amikacin, aminophylline, amiodarone, amphotericin B cholesteryl, amphotericin B liposome, amsacrine, anakinra, anidulafungin, ascorbic acid, atropine, aztreonam, bivalirudin, bumetanide, buprenorphine, butorphanol, calcium chloride, calcium gluconate, carboplatin, cefazolin, cefoperazone, cefotaxime, cefotetan, cefoxitin, ceftazidime, ceftizoxime, cefuroxime, chloramphenicol, cimetidine, cisatracurium, cisplatin, cyanocobalamin, cyclophosphamide, cyclosporine, cytarabine, dactinomycin, daptomycin, dexamethasone sodium phosphate, dexmedetomidine, digoxin, diltiazem, diphenhydramine, docetaxel, dopamine, doxorubicin hydrochloride, doxorubicin liposome, doxycycline, enalaprilat, ephedrine, epinephrine, epirubicin, epoetin alpha, esmolol, etoposide, etoposide phosphate, famotidine, fenoldopam, fentanyl, fludarabine, fluorouracil, folic acid, foscarnet, furosemide, gemcitabine, gentamicin, glycopyrrolate, granisetron, heparin, hydrocortisone sodium succinate, hydromorphone, ifosfamide, imipenem/cilastatin, indomethacin, insulin, isoproterenol, ketorolac, labetalol, levofloxacin, lidocaine, linezolid, lorazepam, magnesium sulfate, mannitol, mechlorethamine, melphalan, meperidine, metaraminol, methotrexate, methoxamine, methyldopa, methylprednisolone sodium succinate, metoclopramide, metoprolol, metronidazole, midazolam, milrinone, morphine, multivitamins, nafcillin, nalbuphine, naloxone, nesiritide, netilmicin, nicardipine, nitroglycerin, nitroprusside, norepinephrine, octreotide, ondansetron, oxacillin, oxaliplatin, oxytocin, paclitaxel, palonosetron, pantoprazole, pemetrexed, penicillin G, perphenazine, phenobarbital, phenylephrine, phytonadione, piperacillin/tazobactam, potassium chloride, procainamide, propofol, propranolol, protamine, pyridoxine, ranitidine, remifentanil, rocuronium, sargramostim, sodium acetate, sodium bicarbonate, streptokinase, succinylcholine, sufentanil, tacrolimus, teniposide, theophylline, thiamine, thiotepa, ticarcillin/clavulanate, tigecycline, tirofiban, tobramycin, tolazoline, urokinase, vancomycin, vasopressin, vecuronium, verapamil, vincristine, vinorelbine, vitamin B complex with C, voriconazole, zidovudine.
- **Y-Site Incompatibility:** allopurinol, amphotericin B colloidal, azathioprine, azithromycin, caspofungin, ceftriaxone, chlorpromazine, dantrolene, diazepam, filgrastim, ganciclovir, haloperidol, hydroxyzine, idarubicin, inamrinone, minocycline, mitoxantrone, pentamidine, phenytoin, prochlorperazine, promethazine, quinupristin/dalfopristin, trimethoprim/sulfamethoxazole, trastuzumab.
- **Vag:** Applicators are supplied for vaginal administration. When treating bacterial vaginosis, concurrent treatment of male partner is not usually necessary.
- **Topical:** Contact with eyes, mucous membranes, and open cuts should be avoided during topical application. If accidental contact occurs, rinse with copious amounts of cool water.
- Wash affected areas with warm water and soap, rinse, and pat dry prior to application. Apply to entire affected area.

Patient/Family Teaching
- Instruct patient to take medication around the clock at evenly spaced times and to finish the drug completely as directed, even if feeling better. Take missed doses as soon as possible unless almost time for next dose. Do not double doses. Advise patient that sharing of this medication may be dangerous.
- Instruct patient to notify health care professional immediately if diarrhea, abdominal cramping, fever, or bloody stools occur and not to treat with antidiarrheals without consulting health care professional.
- Advise patient to report signs of superinfection (furry overgrowth on the tongue, vaginal or anal itching or discharge).

- Notify health care professional if no improvement within a few days.
- Patients with a history of rheumatic heart disease or valve replacement need to be taught the importance of antimicrobial prophylaxis before invasive medical or dental procedures.
- **IV:** Inform patient that bitter taste occurring with IV administration is not clinically significant.
- **Vag:** Instruct patient on proper use of vaginal applicator. Insert high into vagina at bedtime. Instruct patient to remain recumbent for at least 30 min following insertion. Advise patient to use sanitary napkin to prevent staining of clothing or bedding. Continue therapy during menstrual period.
- Advise patient to refrain from vaginal sexual intercourse during treatment.
- Caution patient that mineral oil in clindamycin cream may weaken latex or rubber contraceptive devices. Such products should not be used within 72 hr of vaginal cream.
- **Topical:** Caution patient applying topical clindamycin that solution is flammable (vehicle is isopropyl alcohol). Avoid application while smoking or near heat or flame.
- Advise patient to notify health care professional if excessive drying of skin occurs.
- Advise patient to wait 30 min after washing or shaving area before applying.

Evaluation/Desired Outcomes
- Resolution of the signs and symptoms of infection. Length of time for complete resolution depends on the organism and site of infection.
- Endocarditis prophylaxis.
- Improvement in acne vulgaris lesions. Improvement should be seen in 6 wk but may take 8–12 wk for maximum benefit.

---

clobetasol, See CORTICOSTEROIDS (TOPICAL/LOCAL).

---

clocortolone, See CORTICOSTEROIDS (TOPICAL/LOCAL).

---

clofarabine (klo-**far**-a-been)
Clolar

Classification
Therapeutic: antineoplastics
Pharmacologic: antimetabolites

Pregnancy Category D

Indications
Refractory/relapsed acute lymphoblastic leukemia in children 1–21 yr.

Action
Converted intracellularly to the active 5'-triphosphate metabolite which acts as a purine nucleoside antimetabolite; net result is inhibition of DNA synthesis. Produces a rapid reduction of peripheral leukemia cells. **Therapeutic Effects:** Death of rapidly replicating cells, particularly malignant ones.

Pharmacokinetics
Absorption: IV administration results in complete bioavailability.
Distribution: unknown.
Metabolism and Excretion: 46–60% excreted unchanged in urine.
Half-life: 5.2 hr.

TIME/ACTION PROFILE (effect on WBCs)

ROUTE	ONSET	PEAK	DURATION
IV	rapid	unknown	2–6 wk

Contraindications/Precautions
Contraindicated in: None; OB, Lactation: Pregnancy or lactation.
Use Cautiously in: Hepatic or renal impairment; Concurrent use of nephrotoxic or hepatotoxic drugs.

Adverse Reactions/Side Effects
CNS: fatigue. **Resp:** pharyngitis. **CV:** pericardial effusion, tachycardia, edema. **GI:** diarrhea, hepatic toxicity, nausea, abdominal pain, constipation, mucositis, vomiting. **F and E:** dehydration. **Hemat:** NEUTROPENIA, anemia, thrombocytopenia. **Local:** injection site pain. **Misc:** SYSTEMIC INFLAMMATORY RESPONSE SYNDROME, TUMOR LYSIS SYNDROME, infections, fever, chills.

Interactions
Drug-Drug: Concurrent use of **hepato- or nephrotoxoc drugs** ↑ risk of hepato- and nephrotoxicity and should be avoided for the 5-day treatment period.

Route/Dosage
IV (Children 1–21 yr): 52 mg/m^2 daily for 5 days; cycle may be repeated every 2–6 wk.

Availability
Solution for IV administration: 20 mg/mL vials.

NURSING IMPLICATIONS

Assessment
- Monitor respiratory status and blood pressure during clofabarine infusion.

clonazepam 341

- Monitor for bone marrow depression. Assess for bleeding (bleeding gums, bruising, petechiae, guaiac stools, urine, and emesis) and avoid IM injections and rectal temperatures if platelet count is low. Apply pressure to venipuncture sites for 10 min. Assess for signs of infection during neutropenia. Anemia may occur. Monitor for increased fatigue, dyspnea, and orthostatic hypotension.
- Monitor for signs and symptoms of tumor lysis syndrome and cytokine release (tachypnea, tachycardia, hypotension, pulmonary edema) that could develop into systemic inflammatory response syndrome (SIRS), capillary leak syndrome (pleural and pericardial effusions) and organ dysfunction. Administer continuous IV fluids throughout the 5 days of therapy to reduce effects of tumor lysis syndrome and other adverse drug reactions. Administer prophylactic corticosteroids (hydrocortisone 100 mg/m^2 of Days 1 and 3) and allopurinol if hyperuricemia is expected. If significant signs or symptoms of SIRS or capillary leak syndrome occur, discontinue clofarabine immediately; diuretics and albumin may be used; may be fatal. Clofarabine may be reinstituted, usually at a lower dose, when the patient is stable.
- Assess for nausea and diarrhea. Prevent dehydration. Discontinue clofarabine administration if hypotension occurs during 5 days of therapy. If hypotension resolves without pharmacological intervention, clofarabine may be reinstituted, usually at a lower dose.
- **Lab Test Considerations:** Monitor CBC and platelet counts at regular intervals during therapy and more frequently if levels are abnormal. May cause anemia, leukopenia, thrombocytopenia, neutropenia, febrile neutropenia, and infection.
- Monitor hepatic and renal function frequently during therapy. May cause ↑ AST, ALT, and bilirubin; usually occur within 1 wk of administration and return to baseline within several days. May cause ↑ serum creatinine.

Potential Nursing Diagnoses
Risk for infection (Adverse Reactions)

Implementation
- Administer under the supervision of a physician experienced in the use of cancer chemotherapeutic agents.

IV Administration
- **Intermittent Infusion:** *Diluent:* Dilute with 50 mL of 5% D5W or 0.9% NaCl and filter through a sterile 0.2 micron syringe filter. Solution is clear and practically colorless. *Concentration:* 0.4 mg/mL Store at room temperature; use within 24 hr of preparation. *Rate:* Administer over 2 hr daily for 5 consecutive days.
- **Y-Site Incompatibility:** Do not administer other medications through same IV line.

Patient/Family Teaching
- Advise patient to consult health care professional if dizziness, fainting spells, or decreased urine output occur during therapy.
- Advise patient to consult health care professional prior to taking Rx, OTC, or herbal product during clofarabine therapy.

Evaluation/Desired Outcomes
- Rapid reduction in peripheral leukemia cells.

---

clonazepam (kloe-na-ze-pam)
Klonopin, ♣ Rivotril, ♣ Syn-Clonazepam

Classification
Therapeutic: anticonvulsants
Pharmacologic: benzodiazepines

Schedule IV

Pregnancy Category C

Indications
Prophylaxis of: Petit mal, Petit mal variant, Akinetic, Myoclonic seizures. Panic disorder with or without agoraphobia. **Unlabeled Use:** Uncontrolled leg movements during sleep. Neuralgias. Sedation. Adjunct management of acute mania, acute psychosis, or insomnia.

Action
Anticonvulsant effects may be due to presynaptic inhibition. Produces sedative effects in the CNS, probably by stimulating inhibitory GABA receptors. **Therapeutic Effects:** Prevention of seizures. Decreased manifestations of panic disorder.

Pharmacokinetics
Absorption: Well absorbed from the GI tract.
Distribution: Probably crosses the blood-brain barrier and the placenta.

Metabolism and Excretion: Mostly metabolized by the liver.
Half-life: 18–50 hr.

TIME/ACTION PROFILE (anticonvulsant activity)

ROUTE	ONSET	PEAK	DURATION
PO	20–60 min	1–2 hr	6–12 hr

Contraindications/Precautions
Contraindicated in: Hypersensitivity to clonazepam or other benzodiazepines; Severe liver disease.
Use Cautiously in: All patients (may ↑ risk of suicidal thoughts/behaviors); Angle-closure glaucoma; Obstructive sleep apnea; Chronic respiratory disease; History of porphyria; Do not discontinue abruptly; OB: Safety not established; chronic use during pregnancy may result in withdrawal in the neonate; Lactation: May enter breast milk; discontinue drug or bottle feed; Pedi: Safety not established; Geri: May experience excessive sedation at usual doses; decreased dosage recommended.

Adverse Reactions/Side Effects
CNS: SUICIDAL THOUGHTS, behavioral changes, drowsiness, fatigue, slurred speech, ataxia, sedation, abnormal eye movements, diplopia, nystagmus. **Resp:** increased secretions. **CV:** palpitations. **GI:** constipation, diarrhea, hepatitis, weight gain. **GU:** dysuria, nocturia, urinary retention. **Hemat:** anemia, eosinophilia, leukopenia, thrombocytopenia. **Neuro:** ataxia, hypotonia. **Misc:** fever, physical dependence, psychological dependence, tolerance.

Interactions
Drug-Drug: Alcohol, antidepressants, antihistamines, other benzodiazepines, and opioid analgesics—concurrent use results in ↑ CNS depression. Cimetidine, hormonal contraceptives, disulfiram, fluoxetine, isoniazid, ketoconazole, metoprolol, propoxyphene, propranolol, or valproic acid may ↓ metabolism of clonazepam, ↑ its actions. May ↓ efficacy of levodopa. Rifampin or barbiturates may ↑ metabolism and ↓ effectiveness of clonazepam. Sedative effects may be ↓ by theophylline. May ↑ serum phenytoin levels. Phenytoin may ↓ serum clonazepam levels.
Drug-Natural Products: Concomitant use of kava-kava, valerian, or chamomile can ↑ CNS depression.

Route/Dosage
PO (Adults): 0.5 mg 3 times daily; may ↑ by 0.5–1 mg q 3 days. Total daily maintenance dose not to exceed 20 mg. *Panic disorder*—0.125 mg twice daily; ↑ after 3 days toward target dose of 1 mg/day (some patients may require up to 4 mg/day).
PO (Children <10 yr or 30 kg): Initial daily dose 0.01–0.03 mg/kg/day (not to exceed 0.05 mg/kg/day) given in 2–3 equally divided doses; ↑ by no more than 0.25–0.5 mg q 3 days until therapeutic blood levels are reached (not to exceed 0.2 mg/kg/day).

Availability (generic available)
Tablets: 0.5 mg, 1 mg, 2 mg. **Cost:** *Generic*—0.5 mg $29.99/100, 1 mg $29.99/100, 2 mg $26.66/100. **Orally-disintegrating tablets:** 0.125 mg, 0.25 mg, 0.5 mg, 1 mg, 2 mg. **Cost:** *Generic*—0.125 mg $69.99/60, 0.25 mg $72.99/60, 0.5 mg $70.99/60, 2 mg $100.00/60.

NURSING IMPLICATIONS
Assessment
- Observe and record intensity, duration, and location of seizure activity.
- Assess degree and manifestations of anxiety and mental status (orientation, mood, behavior) prior to and periodically during therapy.
- Assess need for continued treatment regularly.
- Assess patient for drowsiness, unsteadiness, and clumsiness. These symptoms are dose related and most severe during initial therapy; may decrease in severity or disappear with continued or long-term therapy.
- Monitor closely for notable changes in behavior that could indicate the emergence or worsening of suicidal thoughts or behavior or depression.
- *Lab Test Considerations:* Patients on prolonged therapy should have CBC and liver function test results evaluated periodically. May cause an ↑ in serum bilirubin, AST, and ALT.
- May cause ↓ thyroidal uptake of sodium iodide, ^{123}I, and ^{131}I.
- *Toxicity and Overdose:* Therapeutic serum concentrations are 20–80 mg/mL. Flumazenil antagonizes clonazepam toxicity or overdose (may induce seizures in patients with history of seizure disorder or who are on tricyclic antidepressants).

Potential Nursing Diagnoses
Risk for injury (Indications, Side Effects)

Implementation
- Do not confuse clonazepam with clonidine or clorazepate.
- Institute seizure precautions for patients on initial therapy or undergoing dose manipulations.

- **PO:** Administer with food to minimize gastric irritation. Tablets may be crushed if patient has difficulty swallowing. Administer largest dose at bedtime to avoid daytime sedation. Taper by 0.25 mg every 3 days to decrease signs and symptoms of withdrawal. Some patients may require longer taper period (months).

Patient/Family Teaching
- Instruct patient to take medication exactly as directed. Take missed doses within 1 hr or omit; do not double doses. Abrupt withdrawal of clonazepam may cause status epilepticus, tremors, nausea, vomiting, and abdominal and muscle cramps. Instruct patient to read the *Medication Guide* before starting and with each Rx refill, changes may occur.
- Advise patient to not share medication with others.
- Medication may cause drowsiness or dizziness. Advise patient to avoid driving or other activities requiring alertness until response to drug is known.
- Caution patient to avoid taking alcohol or other CNS depressants concurrently with this medication.
- Advise patient to notify health care professional of medication regimen prior to treatment or surgery.
- Instruct patient and family to notify health care professional of unusual tiredness, bleeding, sore throat, fever, clay-colored stools, yellowing of skin, or behavioral changes. Advise patient and family to notify health care professional if thoughts about suicide or dying, attempts to commit suicide; new or worse depression; new or worse anxiety; feeling very agitated or restless; panic attacks; trouble sleeping; new or worse irritability; acting aggressive; being angry or violent; acting on dangerous impulses; an extreme increase in activity and talking, other unusual changes in behavior or mood occur.
- Patient on anticonvulsant therapy should carry identification at all times describing disease process and medication regimen.
- Emphasize the importance of follow-up exams to determine effectiveness of the medication.
- Advise patient that clonazepam is usually prescribed for short-term use and does not cure underlying problems.

Evaluation/Desired Outcomes
- Decrease or cessation of seizure activity without undue sedation. Dose adjustments may be required after several months of therapy.
- Decrease in frequency and severity of panic attacks.
- Relief of leg movements during sleep.
- Decrease in pain from neuralgia.

clonidine (klon-i-deen)
Catapres, Catapres-TTS, ✽Dixarit, Duraclon

Classification
Therapeutic: antihypertensives
Pharmacologic: adrenergics (centrally acting)

Pregnancy Category C

Indications
PO, Transdermal: Management of mild to moderate hypertension. **Epidural:** Management of cancer pain unresponsive to opioids alone. **Unlabeled Use:** Management of opioid withdrawal. Treatment of attention-deficit hyperactivity disorder (ADHD). Adjunctive treatment of neuropathic pain.

Action
Stimulates alpha-adrenergic receptors in the CNS, which results in decreased sympathetic outflow inhibiting cardioacceleration and vasoconstriction centers. Prevents pain signal transmission to the CNS by stimulating alpha-adrenergic receptors in the spinal cord. **Therapeutic Effects:** Decreased blood pressure. Decreased pain.

Pharmacokinetics
Absorption: Well absorbed from the GI tract and skin. Enters systemic circulation following epidural use. Some absorption follows sublingual administration.
Distribution: Widely distributed; enters CNS. Crosses the placenta readily; enters breast milk in high concentrations.
Metabolism and Excretion: Mostly metabolized by the liver; 40–50% eliminated unchanged in urine.
Half-life: *Neonates*—44–72 hr; *Children*—8–12 hr; *Adults: Plasma*—12–22 hr; *CNS*—1.3 hr.

TIME/ACTION PROFILE (PO, TD = antihypertensive effect; epidural = analgesia)

ROUTE	ONSET	PEAK	DURATION
PO	30–60 min	2–4 hr	8–12 hr
Transdermal	2–3 days	unknown	7 days†
Epidural	unknown	unknown	unknown

†8 hr following removal of patch

Contraindications/Precautions
Contraindicated in: Hypersensitivity; *Epidural*—injection site infection, anticoagulant therapy, or bleeding problems.
Use Cautiously in: Serious cardiac or cerebrovascular disease; Renal insufficiency; Pedi: Evaluation for cardiac disease should precede initiation of therapy for ADHD in children; Geri: Appear on Beers list due to increased risk of orthostatic hypotension and adverse CNS effects in geriatric patients (↓ dose recommended); OB, Lactation: Safety not established.

Adverse Reactions/Side Effects
CNS: drowsiness, depression, dizziness, nervousness, nightmares. **CV:** bradycardia, hypotension (↑ with epidural), palpitations. **GI:** dry mouth, constipation, nausea, vomiting. **GU:** erectile dysfunction. **Derm:** rash, sweating. **F and E:** sodium retention. **Metab:** weight gain. **Misc:** withdrawal phenomenon.

Interactions
Drug-Drug: Additive sedation with **CNS depressants**, including **alcohol**, **antihistamines**, **opioid analgesics**, and **sedative/hypnotics**. Additive hypotension with other **antihypertensives** and **nitrates**. Additive bradycardia with **beta blockers**, **diltiazem**, **verapamil**, or **digoxin**. **MAO inhibitors**, **amphetamines**, or **tricyclic antidepressants** may ↓ antihypertensive effect. Withdrawal phenomenon may be ↑ by discontinuation of **beta blockers**. Epidural clonidine prolongs the effects of epidurally administered **local anesthetics**. May ↓ effectiveness of **levodopa**.

Route/Dosage
PO (Adults and Adolescents ≥12 yrs): 100 mcg (0.1 mg) bid, ↑ by 100–200 mcg (0.1–0.2 mg)/day q 2–4 days. *Usual maintenance dose* is 200–600 mcg (0.2–0.6 mg)/day in 2–3 divided doses (up to 2.4 mg/day). *Urgent treatment*—200 mcg (0.2 mg) loading dose, then 100 mcg (0.1 mg) q hr until blood pressure is controlled or 800 mcg (0.8 mg) total has been administered; follow with maintenance dosing. *Opioid withdrawal*—300 mcg (0.3 mg)–1.2 mg/day, may be ↓ by 50%/day for 3 days, then discontinued or ↓ by 100–200 mcg (0.1–0.2 mg)/day.
PO (Geriatric Patients): 100 mcg (0.1 mg) at bedtime initially, ↑ as needed.
PO (Children): *Hypertension*—Initial 5–10 mcg/kg/day divided BID-TID, then increase gradually to 5–25 mcg/kg/day in divided doses q 6 hr; maximum dose: 0.9 mg/day. *ADHD*—0.05 mg/day, then increase q 3–7 days by 0.05 mg/day to 3–5 mcg/kg/day divided TID-QID; maximum dose: 0.5 mg/day. *Neuropathic pain*—2 mcg/kg/dose q 4–6 hr then increase gradually over days up to 4 mcg/kg/dose q 4–6 hr.
Transdermal (Adults): *Hypertension*—Transdermal system delivering 100–300 mcg (0.1–0.3 mg)/24 hr applied every 7 days. Initiate with 100 mcg (0.1 mg)/24 hr system; dosage increments may be made q 1–2 wk when system is changed.
Transdermal (Children): Once stable oral dose is reached, children may be switched to a transdermal system equivalent closest to the total daily oral dose.
Epidural (Adults): 30 mcg/hr initially; titrated according to need.
Epidural (Children): 0.5 mcg/kg/hr initially; titrated according to need up to 2 mcg/kg/hr.

Availability (generic available)
Tablets: ✱ 25 mcg (0.025 mg), 100 mcg (0.1 mg), 200 mcg (0.2 mg), 300 mcg (0.3 mg). **Cost:** *Generic*—0.1 mg $21.65/100, 0.2 mg $12.21/100, 0.3 mg $26.65/100. **Transdermal systems:** Catapres-TTS 1, releases 0.1 mg/24 hr, Catapres-TTS 2, releases 0.2 mg/24 hr, Catapres-TTS 3, releases 0.3 mg/24 hr. **Cost:** Catapres-TTS 1 $85.99/4 patches, Catapres-TTS 2 $139.97/4 patches, Catapres-TTS 3 $194.97/4 patches. **Solution for epidural injection:** 100 mcg/mL, 500 mcg/mL. *In combination with:* chlorthalidone (Clorpres). See Appendix B.

NURSING IMPLICATIONS
Assessment
- Monitor intake and output ratios and daily weight, and assess for edema daily, especially at beginning of therapy.
- Monitor blood pressure and pulse frequently during initial dose adjustment and periodically throughout therapy. Report significant changes.
- **Pain:** Assess location, character, and intensity of pain prior to, frequently during first few days, and routinely throughout administration.
- Monitor for fever as potential sign of catheter infection.

clonidine

- **Opioid Withdrawal:** Monitor patient for signs and symptoms of opioid withdrawal (tachycardia, fever, runny nose, diarrhea, sweating, nausea, vomiting, irritability, stomach cramps, shivering, unusually large pupils, weakness, difficulty sleeping, gooseflesh).
- *Lab Test Considerations:* May cause transient ↑ in blood glucose levels.
- May cause ↓ urinary catecholamine and vanillylmandelic acid (VMA) concentrations; these may ↑ on abrupt withdrawal.
- May cause weakly positive Coombs' test result.

Potential Nursing Diagnoses
Chronic pain (Indications)
Risk for injury (Side Effects)

Implementation

- Do not confuse Catapres (clonidine) with Cataflam (diclofenac).
- Do not confuse clonidine with clonazepam (Klonopin).
- In the perioperative setting, continue clonidine up to 4 hr prior to surgery and resume as soon as possible thereafter. Do not interrupt *transdermal clonidine* during surgery. Monitor blood pressure carefully.
- **PO:** Administer last dose of the day at bedtime.
- A 0.1 mg/mL oral suspension may be compounded for pediatric patients.
- **Transdermal:** Transdermal system should be applied once every 7 days. May be applied to any hairless site; avoid cuts or calluses. Absorption is greater when placed on chest or upper arm and decreased when placed on thigh. Rotate sites. Wash area with soap and water; dry thoroughly before application. Apply firm pressure over patch to ensure contact with skin, especially around edges. Remove old system and discard. System includes a protective adhesive overlay to be applied over medication patch to ensure adhesion, should medication patch loosen.
- **Epidural:** Dilute 500 mcg/mL with 0.9% NaCl for a concentration of 100 mcg/mL. Do not administer solutions that are discolored or contain a precipitate. Discard unused portion.

Patient/Family Teaching

- Instruct patient to take clonidine at the same time each day, even if feeling well. Take missed dosed as soon as remembered. If more than 1 oral dose in a row is missed or if transdermal system is late in being changed by 3 or more days, consult health care professional. All routes of clonidine should be gradually discontinued over 2–4 days to prevent rebound hypertension.
- Advise patient to make sure enough medication is available for weekends, holidays, and vacations. A written prescription may be kept in wallet in case of emergency.
- Clonidine may cause drowsiness, which usually diminishes with continued use. Advise patient to avoid driving or other activities requiring alertness until response to medication is known.
- Caution patient to avoid sudden changes in position to decrease orthostatic hypotension. Use of alcohol, standing for long periods, exercising, and hot weather may increase orthostatic hypotension.
- If dry mouth occurs, frequent mouth rinses, good oral hygiene, and sugarless gum or candy may decrease effect. If dry mouth continues for more than 2 wk, consult health care professional.
- Caution patient to avoid concurrent use of alcohol or other CNS depressants with this medication.
- Advise patient to consult health care professional before taking other Rx, OTC, or herbal products, especially cough, cold, or allergy remedies.
- Advise patient to notify health care professional of medication regimen prior to treatment or surgery.
- Advise patient to notify health care professional if itching or redness of skin (with transdermal patch), mental depression, swelling of feet and lower legs, paleness or cold feeling in fingertips or toes, or vivid dreams or nightmares occur. May require discontinuation of therapy, especially with depression.
- **Hypertension:** Encourage patient to comply with additional interventions for hypertension (weight reduction, low-sodium diet, discontinuation of smoking, moderation of alcohol consumption, regular exercise, and stress management). Medication helps control but does not cure hypertension.
- Instruct patient and family on proper technique for blood pressure monitoring. Advise them to check blood pressure at least weekly and report significant changes.
- **Transdermal:** Instruct patient on proper application of transdermal system. Do not cut or trim unit. Transdermal system can remain in place during bathing or swimming.

= Canadian drug name. ᚷ = Genetic implication.
*CAPITALS indicates life-threatening; underlines indicate most frequent.

- Advise patient referred for MRI test to discuss patch with referring health care professional and MRI facility to determine if removal of patch is necessary prior to test and for directions for replacing patch.

Evaluation/Desired Outcomes
- Decrease in blood pressure.
- Decrease in severity of pain.
- Decrease in the signs and symptoms of opioid withdrawal.

---

clopidogrel (kloh-**pid**-oh-grel)
Plavix

Classification
Therapeutic: antiplatelet agents
Pharmacologic: platelet aggregation inhibitors

Pregnancy Category B

Indications
Reduction of atherosclerotic events (MI, stroke, vascular death) in patients at risk for such events including recent MI, acute coronary syndrome (unstable angina/non–Q-wave MI), stroke, or peripheral vascular disease.

Action
Inhibits platelet aggregation by irreversibly inhibiting the binding of ATP to platelet receptors.
Therapeutic Effects: Decreased occurrence of atherosclerotic events in patients at risk.

Pharmacokinetics
Absorption: Well absorbed following oral administration; rapidly metabolized to an active antiplatelet compound. Parent drug has no antiplatelet activity.
Distribution: Unknown.
Protein Binding: *Clopidogrel*—98%; *active metabolite*—94%.
Metabolism and Excretion: Rapidly and extensively converted by the liver (CYP2C19) to its active metabolite, which is then eliminated 50% in urine and 45% in feces; 2% of Whites, 4% of Blacks, and 14% of Asians have CYP2C19 genotype that results in reduced metabolism of clopidogrel (poor metabolizers) into its active metabolite (may result in ↓ antiplatelet effects).
Half-life: 8 hr (active metabolite).

TIME/ACTION PROFILE (effects on platelet function)

ROUTE	ONSET	PEAK	DURATION
PO	within 24 hr	3–7 days	5 days†

†Following discontinuation

Contraindications/Precautions
Contraindicated in: Hypersensitivity; Pathologic bleeding (peptic ulcer, intracranial hemorrhage); Lactation.
Use Cautiously in: Patients at risk for bleeding (trauma, surgery, or other pathologic conditions); History of GI bleeding/ulcer disease; Concurrent use of strong CYP2C19 inhibitors; Severe hepatic impairment; OB, Lactation, Pedi: Safety not established; use in pregnancy only if clearly indicated.

Adverse Reactions/Side Effects
Incidence of adverse reactions similar to that of aspirin.
CNS: depression, dizziness, fatigue, headache. **EENT:** epistaxis. **Resp:** cough, dyspnea. **CV:** chest pain, edema, hypertension. **GI:** GI BLEEDING, abdominal pain, diarrhea, dyspepsia, gastritis. **Derm:** pruritus, purpura, rash. **Hemat:** BLEEDING, NEUTROPENIA, THROMBOTIC THROMBOCYTOPENIC PURPURA. **Metab:** hypercholesterolemia. **MS:** arthralgia, back pain. **Misc:** fever, hypersensitivity reactions.

Interactions
Drug-Drug: Concurrent **abciximab**, **eptifibatide**, **tirofiban**, **aspirin**, **NSAIDs**, **heparin**, **LMWHs**, **thrombolytic agents**, **ticlopidine**, or **warfarin** may ↑ risk of bleeding. May ↓ metabolism and ↑ effects of **phenytoin**, **tolbutamide**, **tamoxifen**, **torsemide**, **fluvastatin**, and many **NSAIDs**. Concurrent use of strong CYP2C19 inhibitors (e.g. **omeprazole**, **esomeprazole**, **cimetidine**, **fluconazole**, **ketoconazole**, **voriconazole**, **etravirine**, **felbamate**, **fluoxetine**, or **fluvoxamine**) may ↓ antiplatelet effects (concurrent use not recommended).
Drug-Natural Products: ↑ bleeding risk with **anise**, **arnica**, **chamomile**, **clove**, **fenugreek**, **feverfew**, **garlic**, **ginger**, **ginkgo**, **Panax ginseng**, and others.

Route/Dosage

Recent MI, Stroke, or Peripheral Vascular Disease
PO (Adults): 75 mg once daily.

Acute Coronary Syndrome
PO (Adults): 300 mg initially, then 75 mg once daily; aspirin 75–325 mg once daily should be given concurrently.

Availability
Tablets: 75 mg, 300 mg. **Cost:** $389.68/90.

clorazepate (klor-az-e-pate)
✦ Apo-Clorazepate, Gen-XENE, ✦ Novo-Clopate, Tranxene, Tranxene-SD

Classification
Therapeutic: anticonvulsants, sedative/hypnotics
Pharmacologic: benzodiazepines

Schedule IV

Pregnancy Category UK

NURSING IMPLICATIONS

Assessment
- Assess patient for symptoms of stroke, peripheral vascular disease, or MI periodically during therapy.
- Monitor patient for signs of thrombotic thrombocytic purpura (thrombocytopenia, microangiopathic hemolytic anemia, neurologic findings, renal dysfunction, fever). May rarely occur, even after short exposure (<2 wk). Requires prompt treatment.
- **Lab Test Considerations:** Monitor bleeding time during therapy. Prolonged bleeding time, which is time- and dose-dependent, is expected.
- Monitor CBC with differential and platelet count periodically during therapy. Neutropenia and thrombocytopenia may rarely occur.
- May cause ↑ serum bilirubin, hepatic enzymes, total cholesterol, nonprotein nitrogen (NPN), and uric acid concentrations.

Potential Nursing Diagnoses
Risk for injury (Indications, Side Effects)

Implementation
- Discontinue clopidogrel 5–7 days before planned surgical procedures.
- **PO:** Administer once daily without regard to food.

Patient/Family Teaching
- Instruct patient to take medication exactly as directed. Take missed doses as soon as possible unless almost time for next dose; do not double doses.
- Advise patient to notify health care professional promptly if fever, chills, sore throat, or unusual bleeding or bruising occurs.
- Advise patient to notify health care professional of medication regimen prior to treatment or surgery.
- Advise patient to consult health care professional before taking any Rx, OTC, or herbal products, especially those containing aspirin or NSAIDs or proton pump inhibitors.

Evaluation/Desired Outcomes
- Prevention of stroke, MI, and vascular death in patients at risk.

Indications
Management of simple partial seizures. Anxiety disorder, symptoms of anxiety. Acute alcohol withdrawl. **Unlabeled Use:** Anxiety associated with acute myocardial infarction.

Action
Acts at many levels in the CNS to produce anxiolytic effect and CNS depression (by stimulating inhibitory GABA receptors). Produces skeletal muscle relaxation (by inhibiting spinal polysynaptic afferent pathways). Also has anticonvulsant effect (enhances presynaptic inhibition). **Therapeutic Effects:** Relief of anxiety. Sedation. Prevention of seizures.

Pharmacokinetics
Absorption: Well absorbed from the GI tract as desmethyldiazepam.
Distribution: Widely distributed. Crosses the placenta; enters breast milk.
Metabolism and Excretion: Metabolized by the liver; some conversion to active compounds.
Half-life: 48 hr.

TIME/ACTION PROFILE (sedation)

ROUTE	ONSET	PEAK	DURATION
PO	1–2 hr	1–2 hr	up to 24 hr†

†May last longer in geriatric patients

Contraindications/Precautions
Contraindicated in: Hypersensitivity; Cross-sensitivity with other benzodiazepines may occur; Pre-existing CNS depression; Severe uncontrolled pain; Angle-closure glaucoma; OB, Lactation: May cause CNS depression, flaccidity, feeding difficulties, and seizures in infant. In lactation discontinue drug or bottle-feed.
Use Cautiously in: All patients (may ↑ risk of suicidal thoughts/behaviors); Pre-existing hepatic dysfunction; Patients who may be suicidal or have

---

✦ = Canadian drug name. ⚡ = Genetic implication.
*CAPITALS indicates life-threatening; underlines indicate most frequent.

been addicted to drugs in the past; Debilitated patients (dosage reduction required); Severe pulmonary disease; Geri: Long-acting benzodiazepines cause prolonged sedation in the elderly. Appears on Beers list and is associated with increased risk of falls (↓ dose required or consider short-acting benzodiazepine).

Adverse Reactions/Side Effects
CNS: SUICIDAL THOUGHTS, dizziness, drowsiness, lethargy, hangover, headache, mental depression, slurred speech, ataxia, paradoxical excitation. **EENT:** blurred vision. **Resp:** respiratory depression. **GI:** constipation, diarrhea, nausea, vomiting, weight gain (unusual). **Derm:** rashes. **Misc:** physical dependence, psychological dependence, tolerance.

Interactions
Drug-Drug: **Alcohol**, **antidepressants**, **antihistamines**, and **opioid analgesics**—concurrent use results in ↑ CNS depression. **Cimetidine**, **hormonal contraceptives**, **disulfiram**, **fluoxetine**, **isoniazid**, **ketoconazole**, **metoprolol**, **propoxyphene**, **propranolol**, or **valproic acid** may ↓ metabolism of clorazepate, ↑ its actions. May ↓ efficacy of **levodopa**. **Rifampin** or **barbiturates** may ↓ metabolism and ↓ effectiveness of clorazepate. Sedative effects may be ↓ by **theophylline**.
Drug-Natural Products: Concomitant use of **kava-kava**, **valerian**, or **chamomile** ↑ CNS depression.

Route/Dosage
Prescribe largest dose at bedtime to avoid daytime sedation. Can be used on prn basis for anxiety.
PO (Adults): *Anxiety*—7.5–15 mg 2–4 times daily *or* 15 mg at bedtime initially. May also be given in a single dose of 11.25–22.5 mg at bedtime. *Alcohol withdrawal*—30 mg initially, then 15 mg 2–4 times daily on 1st day, then gradually ↓ over subsequent days. *Anticonvulsant*—7.5 mg 3 times daily; can ↑ by no more than 7.5 mg/day at weekly intervals (daily dose not to exceed 90 mg).
PO (Geriatric Patients or Debilitated Patients): *Anxiety*—3.75–15 mg/day, may be ↑.
PO (Children 9–12 yr): *Anticonvulsant*—7.5 mg twice daily initially, may ↑ by 7.5 mg/wk (not to exceed 60 mg/day).

Availability (generic available)
Tablets: 3.75 mg, 7.5 mg, 11.25 mg, 15 mg, 22.5 mg.

NURSING IMPLICATIONS
Assessment
- Assess for drowsiness, unsteadiness, and clumsiness. Symptoms are dose related and most severe during initial therapy; may decrease in severity or disappear with continued or long-term therapy.
- Prolonged high-dose therapy may lead to psychological or physical dependence. Restrict amount of drug available to patient.
- Conduct regular assessment for continued need for treatment.
- Monitor closely for notable changes in behavior that could indicate the emergence or worsening of suicidal thoughts or behavior or depression.
- **Anxiety:** Assess degree and manifestations of anxiety and mental status (orientation, mood, behavior) prior to and periodically during therapy.
- **Alcohol Withdrawal:** Assess patient experiencing alcohol withdrawal for tremors, agitation, delirium, and hallucinations. Protect from injury. Institute seizure precautions.
- **Seizures:** Observe and record intensity, duration, and location of seizure activity.
- Geri: Assess risk of falls and institute fall prevention strategies.
- *Lab Test Considerations:* Patients on prolonged therapy should have CBC and liver function tests evaluated periodically. May cause an ↑ in serum bilirubin, AST, and ALT.
- May cause ↓ thyroidal uptake of sodium iodide ^{123}I and ^{131}I.
- *Toxicity and Overdose:* Flumazenil is the antidote for clorazepate toxicity or overdose (flumazenil may induce seizures in patients with a history of seizures disorder or who are on tricyclic antidepressants).

Potential Nursing Diagnoses
Anxiety (Indications)
Risk for injury (Indications, Side Effects)
Risk for falls (Side Effects)

Implementation
- Do not confuse clorazepate with clonazepam.
- **PO:** If gastric irritation is a problem, may be administered with food or fluids. Capsule should be swallowed whole; do not open.
- Avoid administration of antacids within 1 hr of medication, because absorption of clorazepate may be delayed.
- Use lowest effective dose for shortest period of time. Taper by 0.5 mg q 3 days to prevent with-

clozapine **349**

drawal. Some patients may require longer tapering period (months).

Patient/Family Teaching
- Instruct patient to take medication as directed, not to skip or double up on missed doses. Abrupt withdrawal may cause status epilepticus, tremors, nausea, vomiting, and abdominal and muscle cramps. Instruct patient to read the *Medication Guide* before starting and with each Rx refill, changes may occur.
- May cause drowsiness or dizziness. Advise patient to avoid driving or other activities requiring alertness until response to drug is known. Geri: Instruct patient and family how to reduce falls risk at home.
- Caution patient to avoid alcohol or other CNS depressants concurrently with this medication.
- Instruct patient and family to notify health care professional of unusual tiredness, bleeding, sore throat, fever, clay-colored stools, yellowing of skin, or behavioral changes. Advise patient and family to notify health care professional if thoughts about suicide or dying, attempts to commit suicide; new or worse depression; new or worse anxiety; feeling very agitated or restless; panic attacks; trouble sleeping; new or worse irritability; acting aggressive; being angry or violent; acting on dangerous impulses; an extreme increase in activity and talking, other unusual changes in behavior or mood occur.
- Instruct patient to contact health care professional immediately if pregnancy is planned or suspected.
- Advise patient to notify health care professional of medication regimen prior to treatment or surgery.
- Emphasize the importance of follow-up exams to determine effectiveness of the medication.
- **Seizures:** Patients on anticonvulsant therapy should carry identification describing disease process and medication regimen at all times.

Evaluation/Desired Outcomes
- Increase in sense of well-being.
- Decrease in subjective feelings of anxiety.
- Control of acute alcohol withdrawal.
- Decrease or cessation of seizure activity without undue sedation.

clotrimazole, See ANTIFUNGALS (TOPICAL).

clotrimazole, See ANTIFUNGALS (VAGINAL).

clozapine (kloe-za-peen)
Clozaril, FazaClo

Classification
Therapeutic: antipsychotics

Pregnancy Category B

Indications
Schizoprenia unresponsive to or intolerant of standard therapy with other antipsychotics (treatment refractory). To reduce recurrent suicidal behavior in schizophrenic patients.

Action
Binds to dopamine receptors in the CNS. Also has anticholinergic and alpha-adrenergic blocking activity. Produces fewer extrapyramidal reactions and less tardive dyskinesia than standard antipsychotics but carries high risk of hematologic abnormalities. **Therapeutic Effects:** Diminished schizophrenic behavior. Diminished suicidal behavior.

Pharmacokinetics
Absorption: Well absorbed after oral administration.
Distribution: Rapid and extensive distribution; crosses blood-brain barrier and placenta.
Protein Binding: 95%.
Metabolism and Excretion: Mostly metabolized on first pass through the liver (by CYP1A2, CYP2D6, and CYP3A4 isoenzymes); (the CYP2D6 enzyme system exhibits genetic polymorphism; ~7% of population may be poor metabolizers and may have significantly ↑ clozapine concentrations and an ↑ risk of adverse effects).
Half-life: 8–12 hr.

TIME/ACTION PROFILE (antipsychotic effect)

ROUTE	ONSET	PEAK	DURATION
PO	unknown	wk	4–12 hr

Contraindications/Precautions
Contraindicated in: Hypersensitivity; Bone marrow depression; Severe CNS depression/coma; Uncontrolled epilepsy; Granulocytopenia; Lactation: Discontinue drug or bottle-feed.
Use Cautiously in: Prostatic enlargement; Angle-closure glaucoma; Malnourished patients or

= Canadian drug name. = Genetic implication.
*CAPITALS indicates life-threatening; underlines indicate most frequent.

patients with cardiovascular, hepatic, or renal disease (use lower initial dose, titrate more slowly); Diabetes; Seizure disorder; Pedi: Children <16 yr (safety not established); Geri: ↑ risk of mortality in elderly patients treated for dementia-related psychosis.

Adverse Reactions/Side Effects
CNS: NEUROLEPTIC MALIGNANT SYNDROME, SEIZURES, dizziness, sedation. **EENT:** visual disturbances. **CV:** MYOCARDITIS, hypotension, tachycardia, ECG changes, hypertension. **GI:** constipation, abdominal discomfort, dry mouth, ↑ salivation, nausea, vomiting, weight gain. **Derm:** rash, sweating. **Endo:** hyperglycemia. **Hemat:** AGRANULOCYTOSIS, LEUKOPENIA. **Neuro:** extrapyramidal reactions. **Misc:** fever.

Interactions
Drug-Drug: ↑ anticholinergic effects with other **agents having anticholinergic properties,** including **antihistamines**, **quinidine**, **disopyramide**, and **antidepressants**. Concurrent use with **SSRI antidepressants** (especially **fluvoxamine**), **cimetidine**, **ciprofloxacin**, and **erythromycin** ↑ blood levels and risk of toxicity. ↑ CNS depression with **alcohol**, **antidepressants**, **antihistamines**, **opioid analgesics**, or **sedative/hypnotics**. ↑ hypotension with **nitrates**, acute ingestion of **alcohol**, or **antihypertensives**. ↑ risk of bone marrow suppression with **antihypertensives** or **radiation therapy**. Use with **lithium** ↑ risk of adverse CNS reactions, including seizures. **Phenytoin**, **nicotine**, and **rifampin** may ↓ levels and lead to ↓ efficacy.
Drug-Natural Products: Caffeine-containing herbs (**cola nut**, **tea**, **coffee**) may ↑ serum levels and side effects. **St. John's wort** may ↓ blood levels and efficacy.

Route/Dosage
PO (Adults): 25 mg 1–2 times daily initially; ↑ by 25–50 mg/day over a period of 2 wk up to target dose of 300–450 mg/day. May ↑ by up to 100 mg/day once or twice further (not to exceed 900 mg/day). Treatment should be continued for at least 2 yr in patients with suicidal behavior.

Availability (generic available)
Tablets: 25 mg, 100 mg. **Orally-disintegrating tablets (mint):** 25 mg, 100 mg.

NURSING IMPLICATIONS

Assessment
- Monitor patient's mental status (orientation, mood, behavior) before and periodically during therapy.
- Monitor blood pressure (sitting, standing, lying) and pulse rate before and frequently during initial dose titration.
- Assess weight and BMI initially and throughout therapy.
- Assess fasting blood glucose and cholesterol levels initially and throughout therapy. Refer as appropriate for nutritional/weight management and medical management.
- Observe patient carefully when administering medication to ensure that medication is actually taken and not hoarded or cheeked.
- Monitor for signs of myocarditis (unexplained fatigue, dyspnea, tachypnea, fever, chest pain, palpitations, other signs and symptoms of heart failure, ECG changes, such as ST-T wave abnormalities, arrhythmias, or tachycardia during first month of therapy). If these occur, clozapine should be discontinued and not restarted.
- Monitor patient for onset of akathisia (restlessness or desire to keep moving) and extrapyramidal side effects (*parkinsonian*—difficulty speaking or swallowing, loss of balance control, pill-rolling motion of hands, mask-like face, shuffling gait, rigidity, tremors and dystonic muscle spasms, twisting motions, twitching, inability to move eyes, weakness of arms or legs) every 2 mo during therapy and 8–12 wk after therapy has been discontinued. Notify health care professional if these symptoms occur; reduction in dose or discontinuation of medication may be necessary. Trihexyphenidyl or benzotropine may be used to control these symptoms.
- Although not yet reported for clozapine, monitor for possible tardive dyskinesia (uncontrolled rhythmic movement of mouth, face, and extremities, lip smacking or puckering, puffing of cheeks, uncontrolled chewing, rapid or worm-like movements of tongue). Report these symptoms immediately; may be irreversible.
- Monitor frequency and consistency of bowel movements. Increasing bulk and fluids in the diet may help to minimize constipation.
- Clozapine lowers the seizure threshold. Institute seizure precautions for patients with history of seizure disorder.
- Transient fevers may occur, especially during first 3 wk of therapy. Fever is usually self-limiting but may require discontinuation of medication. Also, monitor for development of neuroleptic malignant syndrome (fever, respiratory distress, tachycardia, seizures, diaphoresis, hypertension or hypotension, pallor, tiredness). Notify health care professional immediately if these symptoms occur.

- **Lab Test Considerations:** Monitor WBC, absolute neutrophil count (ANC), and differential count before initiation of therapy and WBC and ANC weekly for the first 6 months, then biweekly during therapy and weekly for 4 wk after discontinuation of clozapine. Because of the risk of agranulocytosis, clozapine is available only in a 1-wk supply through the **Clozaril Patient Management System,** which combines WBC testing, patient monitoring, and controlled distribution through participating pharmacies. If WBC is <3000 mm^3 or granulocyte count is <1500 mm^3, withhold clozapine, increase frequency of WBC monitoring according to management system guidelines, and monitor patient for signs and symptoms of infection. If acceptable WBC and ANC levels were maintained during first 6 months of continuous therapy, monitoring may decrease to every 2 wk. If levels are maintained for second 6 months, WBC and ANC may be monitored every 4 wk thereafter.
- **Toxicity and Overdose:** Overdose is treated with activated charcoal and supportive therapy. Monitor patient for several days because of risk of delayed effects.
- Avoid use of epinephrine and its derivatives when treating hypotension, and avoid quinidine and procainamide when treating arrhythmias.

Potential Nursing Diagnoses
Risk for other-directed violence (Indications)
Disturbed thought process (Indications)
Risk for injury (Side Effects)

Implementation
- **PO:** Administer capsules with food or milk to decrease gastric irritation.
- Leave oral disintegrating tablet in blister until time of use. Do not push tablet through foil. Just before use, peel foil and gently remove disintegrating tablet. Immediately place tablet in mouth and allow to disintegrate and swallow with saliva. If ½ tablet dose used, destroy other half of tablet.

Patient/Family Teaching
- Instruct patient to take medication as directed. Patients on long-term therapy may need to discontinue gradually over 1–2 wk.
- Explain purpose and procedures for *Clozaril Patient Management System* to patient.
- Inform patient of possibility of extrapyramidal symptoms. Instruct patient to report these symptoms immediately.
- Inform patient that cigarette smoking can decrease clozapine levels. Risk for relapse increases if patient begins or increases smoking.
- Advise patient to change positions slowly to minimize orthostatic hypotension.
- May cause seizures and drowsiness. Caution patient to avoid driving or other activities requiring alertness while taking clozapine.
- Caution patient to avoid concurrent use of alcohol, other CNS depressants, and Rx, OTC, and herbal products without consulting health care professional.
- Instruct patient to use frequent mouth rinses, good oral hygiene, and sugarless gum or candy to minimize dry mouth.
- Advise patient to notify health care professional of medication regimen before treatment or surgery.
- Instruct patient to notify health care professional promptly if unexplained fatigue, dyspnea, tachypnea, chest pain, palpitations, sore throat, fever, lethargy, weakness, malaise, or flu-like symptoms occur or if pregnancy is planned or suspected.
- Advise female patients to notify health care professional if pregnancy is planned or suspected, or if breast-feeding or planning to breast-feed.
- Advise patient of need for continued medical follow-up for psychotherapy, eye exams, and laboratory tests.

Evaluation/Desired Outcomes
- Decreased positive symptoms (delusions, hallucinations) of schizophrenia.
- Decrease in negative symptoms (social withdrawal, flat, blunt affect) of schizophrenia.

HIGH ALERT

codeine (koe-deen)
✦ Paveral

Classification
Therapeutic: allergy, cold, and cough remedies, antitussives, opioid analgesics
Pharmacologic: opioid agonists

Schedule II, III, IV, V (depends on content)

Pregnancy Category C

Indications
Management of mild to moderate pain. Antitussive (in smaller doses). **Unlabeled Use:** Management of diarrhea.

Action
Binds to opiate receptors in the CNS. Alters the perception of and response to painful stimuli while producing generalized CNS depression. Decreases cough reflex. Decreases GI motility.
Therapeutic Effects: Decreased severity of pain. Suppression of the cough reflex. Relief of diarrhea.

Pharmacokinetics
Absorption: 50% absorbed from the GI tract. Completely absorbed from IM sites. Oral and parenteral doses are not equal.
Distribution: Widely distributed. Crosses the placenta; enters breast milk.
Metabolism and Excretion: Mostly metabolized by the liver (primarily via CYP2D6); 10% converted to morphine; the CYP2D6 enzyme system exhibits genetic polymorphism (some patients [1–10% Whites, 3% African Americans, 16–28% North Africans/Ethiopians/Arabs] may be ultra-rapid metabolizers and may have ↑ morphine concentrations and an ↑ risk of adverse effects); 5–15% excreted unchanged in urine.
Half-life: 2.5–4 hr.

TIME/ACTION PROFILE (analgesia)

ROUTE	ONSET	PEAK	DURATION
PO	30–45 min	60–120 min	4 hr
IM	10–30 min	30–60 min	4 hr
Subcut	10–30 min	unknown	4 hr

Contraindications/Precautions
Contraindicated in: Hypersensitivity.
Use Cautiously in: Head trauma; Increased intracranial pressure; Severe renal, hepatic, or pulmonary disease; Hypothyroidism; Adrenal insufficiency; Alcoholism; Geri: Geriatric or debilitated patients (dose reduction required; more susceptible to CNS depression, constipation); Undiagnosed abdominal pain; Geri: Prostatic hyperplasia; OB: Has been used during labor; respiratory depression may occur in the newborn; OB, Lactation: Avoid chronic use.

Adverse Reactions/Side Effects
CNS: confusion, sedation, dysphoria, euphoria, floating feeling, hallucinations, headache, unusual dreams. **EENT:** blurred vision, diplopia, miosis. **Resp:** respiratory depression. **CV:** hypotension, bradycardia. **GI:** constipation, nausea, vomiting. **GU:** urinary retention. **Derm:** flushing, sweating. **Misc:** physical dependence, psychological dependence, tolerance.

Interactions
Drug-Drug: Use with extreme caution in patients receiving **MAO inhibitors** (↓ initial dose to 25% of usual dose). Additive CNS depression with **alcohol**, **antidepressants**, **antihistamines**, and **sedative/hypnotics**. Administration of **partial antagonists** (**buprenorphine**, **butorphanol**, **nalbuphine**, or **pentazocine**) may precipitate opioid withdrawal in physically dependent patients. **Nalbuphine** or **pentazocine** may ↓ analgesia.
Drug-Natural Products: Concomitant use of **kava-kava**, **valerian**, **skullcap**, **chamomile**, or **hops** can ↑ CNS depression.

Route/Dosage
PO (Adults): *Analgesic*—15–60 mg q 3–6 hr as needed. *Antitussive*—10–20 mg q 4–6 hr as needed (not to exceed 120 mg/day). *Antidiarrheal*—30 mg up to 4 times daily.
PO (Children 6–12 yr): *Analgesic*—0.5 mg/kg (15 mg/m^2) q 4–6 hr (up to 4 times daily) as needed. *Antitussive*—5–10 mg q 4–6 hr as needed (not to exceed 60 mg/day). *Antidiarrheal*—0.5 mg/kg up to 4 times daily.
PO (Children 2–5 yr): *Analgesic*—0.5 mg/kg (15 mg/m^2) q 4–6 hr (up to 4 times daily) as needed. *Antitussive*—0.25 mg/kg up to 4 times daily. *Antidiarrheal*—0.5 mg/kg up to 4 times daily.
IM, IV, Subcut (Adults): *Analgesic*—15–60 mg q 4–6 hr as needed.
IM, IV, Subcut (Infants and Children): *Analgesic*—0.5 mg/kg (15 mg/m^2) q 4–6 hr as needed.

Availability (generic available)
Tablets: 15 mg, 30 mg, 60 mg. **Oral solution:** ✤ 10 mg/5 mL. **Injection:** 30 mg/mL, 60 mg/mL. *In combination with:* antihistamines, decongestants, antipyretics, caffeine, butalbital, and nonopioid analgesics. See Appendix B.

NURSING IMPLICATIONS
Assessment
- Assess blood pressure, pulse, and respirations before and periodically during administration. If respiratory rate is <10/min, assess level of sedation. Physical stimulation may be sufficient to prevent significant hypoventilation. Dose may need to be decreased by 25–50%. Initial drowsiness will diminish with continued use.
- Assess bowel function routinely. Prevention of constipation should be instituted with increased intake of fluids, bulk, and laxatives to minimize constipating effects. Stimulant laxa-

tives should be administered routinely if opioid use exceeds 2–3 days, unless contraindicated.
- **Pain:** Assess type, location, and intensity of pain before and 1 hr (peak) after administration. When titrating opioid doses, increases of 25–50% should be administered until there is either a 50% reduction in the patient's pain rating on a numerical or visual analogue scale or the patient reports satisfactory pain relief. A repeat dose can be safely administered at the time of the peak if previous dose is ineffective and side effects are minimal.
- An equianalgesic chart (see Appendix K) should be used when changing routes or when changing from one opioid to another.
- Prolonged use may lead to physical and psychological dependence and tolerance. This should not prevent patient from receiving adequate analgesia. Most patients who receive codeine for pain do not develop psychological dependence. If progressively higher doses are required, consider conversion to a stronger opioid.
- **Cough:** Assess cough and lung sounds during antitussive use.
- *Lab Test Considerations:* May cause ↑ plasma amylase and lipase concentrations.
- *Toxicity and Overdose:* If an opioid antagonist is required to reverse respiratory depression or coma, naloxone (Narcan) is the antidote. Dilute the 0.4-mg ampule of naloxone in 10 mL of 0.9% NaCl and administer 0.5 mL (0.02 mg) by direct IV push every 2 min. For children and patients weighing <40 kg, dilute 0.1 mg of naloxone in 10 mL of 0.9% NaCl for a concentration of 10 mcg/mL and administer 0.5 mcg/kg every 2 min. Titrate dose to avoid withdrawal, seizures, and severe pain.

Potential Nursing Diagnoses
Acute pain (Indications)
Disturbed sensory perception (visual, auditory) (Side Effects)
Risk for injury (Side Effects)

Implementation
- *High Alert:* Accidental overdosage of opioid analgesics has resulted in fatalities. Before administering, clarify all ambiguous orders; have second practitioner independently check dose calculations and route of administration.
- *High Alert:* Do not confuse codeine with Cardene (nicardipine) or Lodine (etodolac).
- Explain therapeutic value of medication before administration to enhance the analgesic effect.
- Regularly administered doses may be more effective than prn administration. Analgesic is more effective if given before pain becomes severe.
- Coadministration with nonopioid analgesics may have additive analgesic effects and permit lower doses.
- Medications should be discontinued gradually after long-term use to prevent withdrawal symptoms.
- When combined with nonopioid analgesics (aspirin, acetaminophen) #2 = 15 mg, #3 = 30 mg, #4 = 60 mg codeine. Codeine as an individual drug is a Schedule II substance. In combination with other drugs, tablet form is Schedule III, and elixir or cough suppressant is Schedule V (see Appendix J).
- **PO:** Oral doses may be administered with food or milk to minimize GI irritation.
- **IM, Subcut:** Do not administer solution that is more than slightly discolored or contains a precipitate.

IV Administration
- **Direct IV:** Codeine is usually administered IM or subcut, but slow IV injection has been used.
- **Syringe Compatibility:** dimenhydrinate, glycopyrrolate, hydroxyzine.
- **Y-Site Compatibility:** amifostine, amikacin, aminophylline, ammonium chloride, ampicillin/sulbactam, aztreonam, bleomycin, bumetanide, busulfan, calcium gluconate, carboplatin, carmustine, cefazolin, cefotaxime, cefotetan, cefoxitin, ceftazidime, ceftizoxime, ceftriaxone, cefuroxime, chlorpormazine, cimetidine, ciprofloxacin, cisplatin, clindamycin, cyclophosphamide, cyclosporine, cytarabine, dactinomycin, daunorubicin, dexamethasone, dexrazoxane, digoxin, diphenhydramine, dobutamine, docetaxel, dopamine, doxorubicin, doxycycline, droperidol, enalaprilat, etoposide, etoposide phosphate, famotidine, floxuridine, fluconazole, fludarabine, fluorouracil, gemcitabine, gentanicin, haloperidol, heparin, hydrocortisone, idarubicin, ifosfamide, imipenem/cilastatin, leucovorin, magnesium sulfate, mesna, metoclopramide, metronidazole, mitomycin, mitoxantrone, ondansetron, paclitaxel, plicamycin, potassium chloride, prochlorperazine, promethazine, ranitidine, sodium bicarbonate, streptozocin, teniposide, theophylline, thi-

354 colchicine

otepa, tobramycin, topotecan, trimethobenzamide, vancomycin, vinblastine, vincristine, vinorelbine, zidovudine.
- **Y-Site Incompatibility:** acyclovir, amobarbital, amphotericin B colloidal, ampicillin, cefoperazone, chlorothiazide, furosemide, ganciclovir, lorazepam, mannitol, methotrexate, methylprednisolone, pentobarbital, phenobarbital, phenytoin, piperacillin/tazobactam, thiopental, trimethoprim/sulfamethoxazole.

Patient/Family Teaching
- Instruct patient on how and when to ask for and take pain medication.
- Codeine may cause drowsiness or dizziness. Advise patient to call for assistance when ambulating or smoking. Caution ambulatory patient to avoid driving or other activities requiring alertness until response to medication is known.
- Advise patient to change positions slowly to minimize orthostatic hypotension.
- Caution patient to avoid concurrent use of alcohol or other CNS depressants with this medication.
- Encourage patient to turn, cough, and breathe deeply every 2 hr to prevent atelectasis.
- Advise patient that good oral hygiene, frequent mouth rinses, and sugarless gum or candy may decrease dry mouth.

Evaluation/Desired Outcomes
- Decrease in severity of pain without a significant alteration in level of consciousness or respiratory status.
- Suppression of cough.
- Control of diarrhea.

HIGH ALERT

colchicine (kol-chi-seen)
Colcrys

Classification
Therapeutic: antigout agents

Pregnancy Category D

Indications
Acute attacks of gouty arthritis. Familial Mediterranean fever. **Unlabeled Use:** Treatment of hepatic cirrhosis and prevention of recurrences of gout.

Action
Interferes with the functions of WBCs in initiating and perpetuating the inflammatory response to monosodium urate crystals. **Therapeutic Effects:** Decreased pain and inflammation in acute attacks of gout. Reduced number of attacks of familial Mediterranean fever.

Pharmacokinetics
Absorption: Absorbed from the GI tract, then re-enters GI tract from biliary secretions, when more absorption may occur; bioavailability = 45%.
Distribution: Concentrates in WBCs.
Metabolism and Excretion: Partially metabolized by the liver by CYP3A4; also a substrate for P-glycoprotein. Secreted in bile back into GI tract; eliminated in the feces. 40–65% excreted in the urine as unchanged drug.
Half-life: 27–31 hr.

TIME/ACTION PROFILE (anti-inflammatory activity)

ROUTE	ONSET	PEAK	DURATION
PO	12 hr	24–72 hr	unknown

Contraindications/Precautions
Contraindicated in: Hypersensitivity; Use of P-glycoprotein inhibitors or strong CYP3A4 inhibitors in patients with renal or hepatic impairment.
Use Cautiously in: Geri: Elderly or debilitated patients (toxicity may be cumulative); Renal impairment (dose ↓ suggested if CCr <80 mL/min); OB, Lactation, Pedi: Safety not established.

Adverse Reactions/Side Effects
GI: diarrhea, nausea, vomiting, abdominal pain. **Derm:** alopecia. **Hemat:** AGRANULOCYTOSIS, APLASTIC ANEMIA, leukopenia, thrombocytopenia. **Neuro:** peripheral neuritis.

Interactions
Drug-Drug: Additive bone marrow depression may occur with **bone marrow depressants** or **radiation therapy**. Strong **CYP3A4 inhibitors** (e.g., **atazanavir, clarithromycin, indinavir, itraconazole, ketoconazole, nefazodone, nelfinavir, ritonavir, saquinavir,** or **telithromycin**) moderate **CYP3A4 inhibitors** (e.g., **aprepitant, diltiazem, erythromycin, fluconazole, fosamprenavir,** or **verapamil**) and **P-glycoprotein inhibitors** (e.g., **cyclosporine** or **ranolazine**) may ↑ levels and risk of toxicity (↓ colchicine dose). ↑ risk of rhabdomyolysis with **HMG-CoA reductase inhibitors**, **gemfibrozil**, or **fenofibrate**. Additive adverse GI effects with **NSAIDs**. May cause reversible malabsorption of **vitamin B$_{12}$**.
Drug-Food: Grapefruit juice may ↑ levels and risk of toxicity (↓ colchicine dose).

colchicine   **355**

Route/Dosage
Acute Gout Attacks
PO (Adults): 1.2 mg initially, then 0.6 mg 1 hr later (maximum dose of 1.8 mg in 1 hr); *Concomitant use of strong CYP3A4 inhibitors*— 0.6 mg initially, then 0.3 mg 1 hr later (do not repeat treatment course for ≥3 days); *Concomitant use of moderate CYP3A4 inhibitors*—1.2 mg × 1 dose (do not repeat for ≥3 days); *Concomitant use of P-glycoprotein inhibitors*— 0.6 mg × 1 dose (do not repeat for ≥3 days).

Renal Impairment
PO (Adults): *CCr <30 mL/min*—1.2 mg initially, then 0.6 mg 1 hr later; do not repeat treatment course for ≥2 wk; *Dialysis*—0.6 mg × 1 dose; do not repeat treatment course for ≥2 wk.

Prevention of Recurrent Gout Attacks (unlabeled use)
PO (Adults): 0.6 mg daily (may be used up to 3 times daily or as little as 1–4 times weekly).

Familial Mediterranean Fever
PO (Adults and Children >12 yr): 1.2–2.4 mg daily (in 1–2 divided doses); may ↑ or ↓ dose in 0.3 mg/day increments based on safety and efficacy; *Concomitant use of strong CYP3A4 inhibitors or P-glycoprotein inhibitors*—Do not exceed 0.6 mg/day (may be given as 0.3 mg twice daily); *Concomitant use of moderate CYP3A4 inhibitors*—Do not exceed 1.2 mg/day (may be given as 0.6 mg twice daily).
PO (Children 6–12 yr): 0.9–1.8 mg daily (in 1–2 divided doses).
PO (Children 4–6 yr): 0.3–1.8 mg daily (in 1–2 divided doses).

Renal Impairment
PO (Adults): *CCr 30–80 mL/min*—dose reduction may be necessary; *CCr <30 mL/min or dialysis*—0.3 mg/day.

Availability (generic available)
Tablets: 0.6 mg, ✽1 mg. **Cost:** *Generic*— $18.12/90.

NURSING IMPLICATIONS

Assessment
- ***High Alert:*** Assess patient for toxicity (weakness, abdominal discomfort, nausea, vomiting, diarrhea, delirium, seizures, sense of suffocation, dilated pupils, difficulty swallowing, ascending paralysis, oliguria), withhold drug and report symptoms immediately.
- Monitor intake and output ratios. Fluids should be encouraged to promote a urinary output of at least 2000 mL/day.
- **Gout:** Assess involved joints for pain, mobility, and edema throughout therapy. During initiation of therapy, monitor for drug response every 1–2 hr.
- **Familial Mediterranean fever:** Assess for signs and symptoms of familial Mediterranean fever (abdominal pain, chest pain, fever, chills, recurrent joint pain, red and swollen skin lesions) periodically during therapy.
- ***Lab Test Considerations:*** In patients receiving prolonged therapy, monitor baseline and periodic CBC; report significant ↓ in values. May cause ↓ platelet count, leukopenia, aplastic anemia, and agranulocytosis.
- May cause ↑ in AST and alkaline phosphatase.
- May cause false-positive results for urine hemoglobin.
- May interfere with results of urinary 17-hydroxycorticosteroid concentrations.
- ***Toxicity and Overdose:*** Assess patient for toxicity (weakness, abdominal discomfort, nausea, vomiting, diarrhea). If these symptoms occur, discontinue medication and notify physician or other health care professional. Opioids may be needed to treat diarrhea.

Potential Nursing Diagnoses
Acute pain (Indications)
Impaired walking (Indications)

Implementation
- ***High Alert:*** Colchicine overdose can be fatal. Cumulative dose should not exceed 4 mg. Cumulative dose should not exceed 2 mg in geriatric and renal patients. After dosing limit has been reached, do not administer any additional colchicine by any route for 21 days.
- Intermittent therapy with 3 days between courses may be used to decrease risk of toxicity.
- **PO:** Administer oral doses with food to minimize gastric irritation.

Patient/Family Teaching
- Review medication administration schedule. Take missed doses as soon as remembered unless almost time for next dose. Do not double doses.
- Instruct patients taking prophylactic doses not to increase to therapeutic doses during an acute attack to prevent toxicity. An NSAID or

✽ = Canadian drug name.   ▦ = Genetic implication.
*CAPITALS indicates life-threatening; underlines indicate most frequent.

corticosteroid, preferably via intrasynovial injection, should be used to treat acute attacks.
- Advise patient to avoid grapefruit and grapefruit juice during therapy; may increase risk of toxicity.
- Advise patient to follow recommendations of health care professional regarding weight loss, diet, and alcohol consumption.
- Instruct patient to report nausea, vomiting, abdominal pain, diarrhea, unusual bleeding, bruising, sore throat, fatigue, malaise, or rash promptly. Medication should be withheld if gastric symptoms indicative of toxicity occur.
- Advise patient to notify health care professional before taking any other Rx, OTC, or herbal products.
- Surgery may precipitate an acute attack of gout. Advise patient to confer with health care professional regarding dose 3 days before surgical or dental procedures.

Evaluation/Desired Outcomes
- Decrease in pain and swelling in affected joints within 12 hr.
- Relief of symptoms within 24–48 hr.
- Prevention of acute gout attacks.
- Reduced number of attacks of familial Mediterranean fever.

colesevelam (koe-le-**sev**-e-lam)
Welchol

Classification
Therapeutic: lipid-lowering agents
Pharmacologic: bile acid sequestrants

Pregnancy Category B

Indications
Adjunctive therapy to diet and exercise for the reduction of LDL cholesterol in patients with primary hypercholesterolemia; may be used alone or in combination with hepatic hydroxymethylglutaryl coenzyme A (HMG-CoA) reductase inhibitor. Adjunctive therapy to diet and exercise to improve glycemic control in patients with type 2 diabetes.

Action
Binds bile acids in the GI tract. Result in increased clearance of cholesterol. Mechanism for lowering blood glucose unknown. **Therapeutic Effects:** Decreased cholesterol and blood glucose.

Pharmacokinetics
Absorption: Not absorbed; action is primarily local in the GI tract.
Distribution: Unknown.
Metabolism and Excretion: Unknown.
Half-life: Unknown.

TIME/ACTION PROFILE (cholesterol-lowering effect)

ROUTE	ONSET	PEAK	DURATION
PO	24–48 hr	2 wk	unknown

Contraindications/Precautions
Contraindicated in: Hypersensitivity; Bowel obstruction; Triglycerides >500 mg/dL; History of pancreatitis due to hypertriglyceridemia.
Use Cautiously in: Triglycerides >300 mg/dL; Dysphagia, swallowing disorders, severe GI motility disorders, or major GI tract surgery; Pregnancy, lactation, or children (safety not established).

Adverse Reactions/Side Effects
GI: constipation, dyspepsia.

Interactions
Drug-Drug: May ↓ absorption of **glyburide**, **levothyroxine**, **phenytoin**, **estrogen-containing oral contraceptives** (give ≥4 hr before colesevelam).

Route/Dosage
PO (Adults): 3 tablets twice daily or 6 tablets once daily.

Availability
Tablets: 625 mg.

NURSING IMPLICATIONS

Assessment
- Obtain a diet history, especially in regard to fat consumption.
- ***Lab Test Considerations:*** Monitor serum total cholesterol, LDL, and triglyceride levels before initiating, and periodically during therapy.

Potential Nursing Diagnoses
Constipation (Side Effects)
Noncompliance (Patient/Family Teaching)

Implementation
- **PO:** Administer once or twice daily with meals. Colesevelam should be taken with a liquid.

Patient/Family Teaching
- Instruct patient to take medication as directed; do not skip doses or double up on missed doses.
- Advise patient that this medication should be used in conjunction with diet restrictions (fat, cholesterol, carbohydrates, alcohol), exercise, and cessation of smoking.

Evaluation/Desired Outcomes
- Decrease in serum total choesterol, LDL cholesterol, apolipoprotein, and blood glucose levels.

colestipol (koe-**les**-ti-pole)
Colestid

Classification
Therapeutic: lipid-lowering agents
Pharmacologic: bile acid sequestrants

Pregnancy Category UK

Indications
Management of primary hypercholesterolemia. Pruritus associated with elevated levels of bile acids. **Unlabeled Use:** Diarrhea associated with excess bile acids.

Action
Binds bile acids in the GI tract, forming an insoluble complex. Result is increased clearance of cholesterol. **Therapeutic Effects:** Decreased plasma cholesterol and LDL. Decreased pruritus.

Pharmacokinetics
Absorption: Action takes place in the GI tract. No absorption occurs.
Distribution: No distribution.
Metabolism and Excretion: After binding bile acids, insoluble complex is eliminated in the feces.
Half-life: Unknown.

TIME/ACTION PROFILE (hypocholesterolemic effects)

ROUTE	ONSET	PEAK	DURATION
PO	24–48 hr	1 mo	1 mo

Contraindications/Precautions
Contraindicated in: Hypersensitivity; Complete biliary obstruction; Some products contain aspartame and should be avoided in patients with phenylketonuria.
Use Cautiously in: History of constipation.
Exercise Extreme Caution in: Pedi: May cause potentially fatal intestinal obstruction in children.

Adverse Reactions/Side Effects
EENT: irritation of the tongue. **GI:** abdominal discomfort, constipation, nausea, fecal impaction, flatulence, hemorrhoids, perianal irritation, steatorrhea, vomiting. **Derm:** irritation, rashes. **F and E:** hyperchloremic acidosis. **Metab:** vitamin A, D, and K deficiency.

Interactions
Drug-Drug: May decrease absorption/effects of orally administered **acetaminophen**, **amiodarone**, **clindamycin**, **clofibrate**, **digoxin**, **diuretics**, **gemfibrozil**, **glipizide**, **corticosteroids**, **imipramine**, **mycophenolate**, **methotrexate**, **methyldopa**, **niacin**, **NSAIDs**, **penicillin**, **phenytoin**, **phosphates**, **propranolol**, **tetracyclines**, **tolbutamide**, **thyroid preparations**, **ursodiol**, **warfarin**, and **fat-soluble vitamins (A, D, E,** and **K)**. May decrease absorption of other **orally administered medications**.

Route/Dosage
PO (Adults): *Granules*—5 g 1–2 times daily, may be increased q 1–2 mo up to 30 g/day in 1–2 doses. *Tablets*—2 g 1–2 times daily, may be increased q 1–2 mo up to 16 g/day in 1–2 doses.

Availability
Granules for suspension (unflavored): 5 g/packet or scoop. **Flavored granules for suspension with aspartame (orange flavor):** 5 g/packet or scoop. **Tablets:** 1 g.

NURSING IMPLICATIONS

Assessment
- **Hypercholesterolemia:** Obtain a diet history, especially in regard to fat consumption.
- **Pruritus:** Assess severity of itching and skin integrity. Dose may be decreased when relief of pruritus occurs.
- **Diarrhea:** Assess frequency, amount, and consistency of stools.
- *Lab Test Considerations:* Serum cholesterol and triglyceride levels should be evaluated before initiating, frequently during first few months and periodically throughout therapy. Discontinue medication if paradoxical increase in cholesterol level occurs.
- May cause an increase in AST, ALT, phosphorus, chloride, and alkaline phosphatase and a decrease in serum calcium, sodium, and potassium levels.
- May also cause prolonged PT.

Potential Nursing Diagnoses
Constipation (Side Effects)
Noncompliance (Patient/Family Teaching)

Implementation
- Parenteral or water-miscible forms of fat-soluble vitamins (A, D, K) and folic acid may be ordered for patients on chronic therapy.

- **PO:** Administer before meals.
- Scoops for powdered preparations may not be exchangable between products.
- Administer other medications 1 hr before or 4–6 hr after the administration of this medication.
- Colestipol tablets should be swallowed whole; do not crush, break, or chew.

Patient/Family Teaching
- Instruct patient to take medication exactly as directed; do not skip doses or double up on missed doses.
- Instruct patient to take medication before meals. Colestipol can be mixed with water, juice, or carbonated beverages. Slowly stir in a large glass. Rinse glass with small amount of additional beverage to ensure all medication is taken. May also mix with highly fluid soups, cereals, or pulpy fruits (applesauce, crushed pineapple). Allow powder to sit on fluid and hydrate for 1–2 min before mixing. Do not take dry.
- Advise patient that this medication should be used in conjunction with diet restrictions (fat, cholesterol, carbohydrates, alcohol), exercise, and cessation of smoking.
- Explain that constipation may occur. Increase in fluids and bulk in diet, exercise, stool softeners, and laxatives may be required to minimize the constipating effects. Instruct patient to notify health care professional if constipation, nausea, flatulence, and heartburn persist or if stools become frothy and foul smelling.
- Advise patient to notify health care professional if unusual bleeding or bruising; petechiae; or black, tarry stools occur. Treatment with vitamin K may be necessary.

Evaluation/Desired Outcomes
- Decrease in serum LDL cholesterol levels. Therapy is usually discontinued if the clinical response remains poor after 3 mo of therapy.
- Decrease in severity of pruritus. Relief usually occurs 1–3 wk after therapy is initiated.
- Decrease in frequency and severity of diarrhea.

CONTRACEPTIVES, HORMONAL MONOPHASIC ORAL CONTRACEPTIVES

ethinyl estradiol/desogestrel
(**eth**-in-il es-tra-**dye**-ole/dess-oh-**jess**-trel)
Apri 28, Desogen, Ortho-Cept, Reclipsen, Solia

ethinyl estradiol/drospirenone
(**eth**-in-il es-tra-**dye**-ole/droe-**spy**-re-nown)
Ocella, Yasmin, Yaz

ethinyl estradiol/ethynodiol
(**eth**-in-il es-tra-**dye**-ole/e-thye-noe-**dye**-ole)
Kelnor 1/35, Zovia 1/35, Zovia 1/50

ethinyl estradiol/levonorgestrel
(**eth**-in-il es-tra-**dye**-ole/lee-voe-nor-**jess**-trel)
Aviane-28, Lessina-28, Levlen-28, Levora-28, Lutera, Nordette-28, Portia-28, Sronyx

ethinyl estradiol/norethindrone
(**eth**-in-il es-tra-**dye**-ole/nor-eth-**in**-drone)
Balziva-28, Brevicon-28, Femcon Fe, Junel 21 1/20, Junel 21 1.5/20, Junel Fe 1/20, Junel Fe 1.5/30, Loestrin 21 1/20, Loestrin 21 1.5/30, Loestrin Fe 1/20, Loestrin Fe 1.5/30, Microgestin, Microgestin Fe 1/20, Modicon, Necon 0.5/35, Necon 1/35, Norethin 1/35E, Norinyl 1+35, Nortrel 0.5/35, Nortrel 1/35, Ortho-Novum 1/35, Ovcon 35, Ovcon 50, Zenchant

ethinyl estradiol/norgestimate
(**eth**-in-il es-tra-**dye**-ole/nor-**jes**-ti-mate)
MonoNessa, Ortho-Cyclen, Previfem, Sprintec

ethinyl estradiol/norgestrel
(**eth**-in-il es-tra-**dye**-ole/nor-**jess**-trel)
Cryselle, Lo/Ovral 28, Low-Ogestrel 28, Ogestrel 28

mestranol/norethindrone
(**mes**-tre-nole/nor-eth-**in**-drone)
Necon 1/50, Norinyl 1+50

BIPHASIC ORAL CONTRACEPTIVES

ethinyl estradiol/desogestrel
(**eth**-in-il es-tra-**dye**-ole/dess-oh-**jess**-trel)
Kariva, Mircette

ethinyl estradiol/norethindrone
(**eth**-in-il es-tra-**dye**-ole/nor-eth-**in**-drone)

CONTRACEPTIVES, HORMONAL

Necon 10/11, Ortho-Novum 10/11

TRIPHASIC ORAL CONTRACEPTIVES

ethinyl estradiol/desogestrel
(eth-in-il es-tra-dye-ole/dess-oh-jess-trel)
Cesia, Cyclessa, Velivet

ethinyl estradiol/levonorgestrel
(eth-in-il ess-tra-dye-ole/lee-voe-nor-jess-trel)
Enpresse, Tri-Levlen, Trivora 28

ethinyl estradiol/norethindrone
(eth-in-il es-tra-dye-ole/nor-eth-in-drone)
Aranelle, Leena, Necon 7/7/7, Nortrel 7/7/7, Ortho-Novum 7/7/7, Tilia Fe, Tri-Legest Fe, Tri-Norinyl

ethinyl estradiol/norgestimate
(eth-in-il es-tra-dye-ole/nor-jess-ti-mate)
Ortho Tri-Cyclen, Ortho Tri-Cyclen Lo, Tri-Lo-Sprintec, Tri-Nessa, Tri-Previfem, Tri-Sprintec

EXTENDED-CYCLE ORAL CONTRACEPTIVE

ethinyl estradiol/levonorgestrel
(eth-in-il ess-tra-dye-ole/lee-voe-nor-jess-trel)
Jolessa, LoSeasonique, Lybrel, Quasense, Seasonale, Seasonique

PROGESTIN-ONLY ORAL CONTRACEPTIVES

norethindrone (nor-eth-in-drone)
Errin, Camila, Jolivette, Micronor, Nor-QD

PROGRESSIVE ESTROGEN ORAL CONTRACEPTIVES

norethindrone/ethinyl acetate
(nor-eth-in-drone/eth-in-il a-se-tate)
Estrostep, Estrostep Fe

CONTRACEPTIVE IMPLANT

etonorgestrel (e-toe-nor-jess-trel)
Implanon

EMERGENCY CONTRACEPTIVE

levonorgestrel
(lee-voe-nor-jess-trel)
Plan B

INJECTABLE CONTRACEPTIVE

medroxyprogesterone
(me-drox-ee-proe-jess-te-rone)
Depo-Provera, Depo-subQ Provera 104

INTRAUTERINE CONTRACEPTIVE

levonorgestrel
(lee-voe-nor-jess-trel)
Mirena

VAGINAL RING CONTRACEPTIVE

ethinyl estradiol/etonogestrel
(eth-in-il ess-tra-dye-ole/e-toe-noe-jess-trel)
NuvaRing

TRANSDERMAL CONTRACEPTIVE

ethinyl estradiol/norelgestromin
(eth-in-il ess-tra-dye-ole/nor-el-jess-troe-min)
Ortho Evra

Classification
Therapeutic: contraceptive hormones

Pregnancy Category X

Indications
Prevention of pregnancy. Regulation of menstrual cycle. Emergency contraception (some products). Treatment of heavy menstrual bleeding in women who choose to use intrauterine contraception as their method of contraception (Mirena). Treatment of premenstrual dysphoric disorder (Yaz, Yasmin). Management of acne in women >14 yr who desire contraception, have no health problems, and have failed topical treatment.

Action
Monophasic Oral Contraceptives: Provide a fixed dosage of estrogen/progestin over a 21-day cycle. Ovulation is inhibited by suppression of follicle-stimulating hormone (FSH) and luteinizing

---
♣ = Canadian drug name. ♦ = Genetic implication.
*CAPITALS indicates life-threatening; underlines indicate most frequent.

hormone (LH). May alter cervical mucus and the endometrial environment, preventing penetration by sperm and implantation of the egg. **Biphasic Oral Contraceptives:** Ovulation is inhibited by suppression of FSH and LH. May alter cervical mucus and the endometrial environment, preventing penetration by sperm and implantation of the egg. In addition, smaller dose of progestin in phase 1 allows for proliferation of endometrium. Larger amount in phase 2 allows for adequate secretory development. **Triphasic Oral Contraceptives:** Ovulation is inhibited by suppression of FSH and LH. May alter cervical mucus and the endometrial environment, preventing penetration by sperm and implantation of the egg. Varying doses of estrogen/progestin may more closely mimic natural hormonal fluctuations. **Extended-cycle:** Provides continuous estrogen/progestin for 84 days (365 days for Lybrel), then off for 7 days (low-dose estrogen-only tablet taken during these 7 days with LoSeasonique and Seasonique), resulting in 4 menstrual periods/year (no periods/year for Lybrel). **Progressive Estrogen:** Contains constant amount of progestin with 3 progressive doses of estrogen. **Progestin-Only Contraceptives/Contraceptive Implant/Intrauterine Levonorgestrel/Medroxyprogesterone Injection:** Mechanism not clearly known. May alter cervical mucus and the endometrial environment, preventing penetration by sperm and implantation of the egg. Ovulation may also be suppressed. **Emergency Contraceptive Pills (ECPs):** Inhibit ovulation/fertilization; may also alter tubal transport of sperm/egg and prevent implantation. **Vaginal Ring, Transdermal Patch:** inhibits ovulation, decreases sperm entry into uterus, and decreases likelihood of implantation. **Anti-acne effect:** Combination of estrogen/progestin may increase sex hormone binding globulin (SHBG) resulting in decreased unbound testosterone, which may be a cause of acne.
Therapeutic Effects: Prevention of pregnancy. Decreased severity of acne. Decrease in menstrual blood loss. Decrease in premenstrual dysphoric disorder.

Pharmacokinetics
Absorption: *Ethinyl estradiol*—rapidly absorbed; *norethindrone*—65% absorbed; *Desogesrtrel and levonorgestrel*—100% absorbed. Others are well absorbed after oral administration. Slowly absorbed from implant, subcutaneous or IM injection. Some absorption follows intrauterine implantation.
Distribution: Unknown.

Protein Binding: *Ethinyl estradiol*—97–98%. *Drospirenone*—97%.
Metabolism and Excretion: *Ethinyl estradiol and norethindrone*—undergo extensive first-pass hepatic metabolism. *Mestranol*—is rapidly converted to ethinyl estradol. *Desogestrel*—is rapidly metabolized to 3-keto-desogestgrel, the active metabolite. Most agents are metabolized by the liver.
Half-life: *Ethinyl estradiol*—6–20 hr; *Levonorgestrel*—45 hr; *Norethindrone*—5–14 hr; *Desogestrel (metabolite)*—38 ± 20 hr; *Drospirenone*—30 hr; *Norgestimate (metabolite)*—12–20 hr; *others*—unknown.

TIME/ACTION PROFILE (prevention of pregnancy)

ROUTE	ONSET	PEAK	DURATION
PO	1 mo	1 mo	1 mo†
Implant	1 mo	1 mo	5 yr
Intrauterine system	1 mo	1 mo	3 yr
IM	1 mo	1 mo	3 mo
Subcut	unknown	1 wk	3 mo

†Only during month of taking contraceptive

Contraindications/Precautions
Contraindicated in: OB: Pregnancy; History of thromboembolic disease (e.g., DVT, PE, MI, stroke); Valvular heart disease; Major surgery with extended periods of immobility; Diabetes with vascular involvement; Headache with focal neurological symptoms; Uncontrolled hypertension; History of breast, endometrial, or estrogen-dependent cancer; Abnormal genital bleeding; Liver disease; Hypersensitivity to parabens (injectable only); *Intrauterine levonorgestrel only*— Intrauterine anomaly, postpartum endometriosis, multiple sexual partners, pelvic inflammatory disease, liver disease, genital actinomycosis, immunosuppression, IV drug abuse, untreated genitourinary infection, history of ectopic pregnancy; Some products contain tartrazine and should be avoided in patients with known hypersensitivity intolerance; Lactation: Avoid use.
Use Cautiously in: History of cigarette smoking or age >30–35 yr (↑ risk of cardiovascular or thromboembolic phenomenon); Presence of other cardiovascular risk factors (obesity, hyperglycemia, elevated lipids, hypertension); History of diabetes mellitus, bleeding disorders, concurrent anticoagulant therapy or headaches; Pedi: Avoid use before menarche.

Adverse Reactions/Side Effects
CNS: depression, migraine headache. **EENT:** contact lens intolerance, optic neuritis, retinal

CONTRACEPTIVES, HORMONAL

thrombosis. **CV:** CEREBRAL HEMORRHAGE, CEREBRAL THROMBOSIS, CORONARY THROMBOSIS, PULMONARY EMBOLISM, edema, hypertension, Raynaud's phenomenon, thromboembolic phenomena, thrombophlebitis. **GI:** abdominal cramps, bloating, cholestatic jaundice, gallbladder disease, liver tumors, nausea, vomiting. **GU:** amenorrhea, breakthrough bleeding, dysmenorrhea, spotting. *Intrauterine levonorgestrel only*—uterine imbedment/uterine rupture. **Derm:** melasma, rash. **Endo:** hyperglycemia. **MS:** *Injectable medroxyprogesterone only*—bone loss. **Misc:** weight change.

Interactions
Drug-Drug: Oral contraceptive efficacy may be ↓ by **penicillins**, **chloramphenicol**, **barbiturates**, chronic **alcohol** use, **carbamazepine**, **oxcarbazepine**, **felbamate**, systemic **corticosteroids**, **phenytoin**, **topiramate**, **primidone**, **modafinil**, **rifampin**, **rifabutin**, some **protease inhibitor antiretrovirals** (including **ritonavir**), or **tetracyclines**. May ↑ effects/risk of toxicity of some **benzodiazepines**, **beta blockers**, **corticosteroids**, **cyclosporine**, and **theophylline**. ↑ risk of hepatic toxicity with **dantrolene** (estrogen only). **Indinavir**, **itraconazole**, **ketoconazole**, **fluconazole**, and **atorvastatin** may ↑ effects/risk of toxicity. Smoking ↑ risk of thromboembolic phenomena (estrogen only). May ↓ levels of **acetaminophen**, **temazepam**, **lamotrigine**, **lorazepam**, **oxazepam**, or **morphine**. *Drosperinone-containing products only*—concurrent use with **NSAIDs**, **potassium-sparing diuretics**, **potasssium supplements**, **ACE inhibitors**, or **angiotensin II receptor antagonists** may result in hyperkalemia.
Drug-Natural Products: Concomitant use with **St. John's wort** may ↓ contraceptive efficacy and cause breakthrough bleeding and irregular menses.

Route/Dosage
Monophasic Oral Contraceptives
PO (Adults): On 21-day regimen, take first tablet on first Sunday after menses begins (take on Sunday if menses begins on Sunday) for 21 days, then skip 7 days and begin again. Regimen may also be started on first day of menses, continue for 21 days, then skip 7 days and begin again. Some regimens contain 7 placebo tablets, so that 1 tablet is taken every day for 28 days.

Biphasic Oral Contraceptives
PO (Adults): Given in 2 phases. First phase is 10 days of smaller amount of progestin. Second phase is larger amount of progestin. Amount of estrogen remains constant for same length of time (total of 21 days), then skip 7 days and begin again. Some regimens contain 7 placebo tablets for 28-day regimen.

Triphasic Oral Contraceptives
PO (Adults): Progestin amount varies throughout 21-day cycle. Estrogen component stays the same or may vary. Some regimens contain 7 placebo tablets for 28-day regimen.

Extended-Cycle Contraceptive
PO (Adults): *LoSeasonique, Seasonale and Seasonique*. Start taking first active pill on first Sunday after menses begins (if first day is Sunday, begin then), continue for 84 days of active pill, followed by 7 days of placebo tablets (low-dose estrogen tablets for LoSeasonique and Seasonique), then resume 84/7 cycle again. For *Lybrel*, begin taking the first pill during the first day of the menstrual cycle and start the next pack the day after the previous pack ends.

Progestin-Only Oral Contraceptives
PO (Adults): Start on first day of menses. Taken daily and continuously.

Progressive Estrogen Oral Contraceptives
PO (Adults): Estrogen amount increases q 7 days throughout 21-day cycle. Progestin component stays the same. Some regimens contain 7 placebo tablets for 28-day regimen.

Emergency Contraceptive
PO (Adults and Adolescents): *Plan B*—1 tablet within 72 hr of unprotected intercourse followed by 1 more tablet 12 hr later; *Lo/Ovral*—4 white tablets within 72 hr of unprotected intercourse followed by 4 more white tablets 12 hr later; *Levlen, Nordette*—4 light orange tablets within 72 hr of unprotected intercourse followed by 4 more light orange tablets 12 hr later; *Triphasil, Tri-Levlen*—4 yellow tablets within 72 hr of unprotected intercourse followed by 4 more yellow tablets 12 hr later.

Injectable Contraceptive
medroxyprogesterone (Depo-Provera)
IM (Adults): 150 mg within first 5 days of menses or within 5 days postpartum, if not breastfeed-

CONTRACEPTIVES, HORMONAL

ing. If breastfeeding, give 6 wk postpartum; repeat q 3 mo.

medroxyprogesterone (Depo-Sub Q Provera 104)
Subcut (Adults): 104 mg within first 5 days of menses or within 5 days postpartum, if not breastfeeding. If breastfeeding, give 6 wk postpartum; repeat q 12–14 wk.

Intrauterine Contraceptive
Intrauterine (Adults): Insert one device into uterine cavity within 7 days of menses or immediately after 1st trimester abortion; releases 20 mcg levonorgestrel/day over 5 yr.

Vaginal Ring Contraceptive
Vag (Adults): One ring inserted on or prior to day 5 of menstrual cycle. Ring is left in place for 3 wk, then removed for 1 wk, then a new ring is inserted.

Transdermal Patch
Transdermal (Adults): Patch is applied on day 1 of menstrual cycle (or convenient day in first week), changed weekly thereafter for 3 weeks. Week 4 is patch-free. Cycle is then repeated.

Acne
PO (Adults): Ortho Tri-Cyclen only, taken daily for 21 days, off for 7 days.

Availability

Combination Estrogen/Progestin Oral Contraceptives (generic available)
Oral contraceptive tablets: Usually in monthly packs with enough (21) active tablets to complete a 28-day cycle. Some contain 7 inert tablets to complete the cycle with or without supplemental iron. **Cost:** *Apri*—$179.93/6 cycles; *Estrostep Fe*—$354.26/6 cycles; *Femcon Fe*—$338.97/6 cycles; *Kariva*—$239.94/6 cycles; *Levora*—$151.94/6 cycles; *Low-Ogestrel*—$151.94/6 cycles; *Necon 0.5/35*—$125.95/6 cycles; *Ovcon 35*—$322.44/6 cycles; *Sprintec*—$143.10/6 cycles; *Tri-Nessa*—$137.94/6 cycles; *Trivora-28*—$139.94/6 cycles; *Yasmin*—$299.90/6 cycles; *Yaz*—$307.96/6 cycles.

Extended-Cycle Contraceptive
Tablets: LoSeasonique—active tablets containing 0.02 mg ethinyl estradiol, 0.1 mg levonorgestrel, and 7 tablets containing 0.01 mg ethinyl estradiol; Seasonale—84 active tablets containing 0.03 mg ethinyl estradiol and 0.15 mg levonorgestrel and 7 inactive tablets; Seasonique—active tablets containing 0.03 mg ethinyl estradiol, 0.15 mg levonorgestrel, and 7 tablets containing 0.01 mg ethinyl estradiol; Lybrel—28 active tablets containing 0.09 mg levonorgestrel and 0.02 mg ethinyl estradiol. **Cost:** *Lybrel*—$49.99/28 tablets; *Seasonale*—$181.98/91 tablets; *Seasonique*—$165.98/91 tablets.

Levonorgestrel (generic available)
Emergency contraceptives: 2 tablets containing 0.75 mg levonorgestrel (Plan B). **Implant:** Rod contains 68 mg etonogestrel. **Intrauterine system:** contains 52 mg levonorgestrel (releases 20 mcg/day).

Medroxyprogesterone (generic available)
Injectable IM: 150 mg/mL. **Injectable Subcutaneous:** 104 mg/0.65 mL (in pre-filled syringes).

Vaginal Ring Contraceptive
Ring: delivers 0.015 mg ethinyl estradiol and 0.120 mg etonogestrel/day. **Cost:** $289.95/6 rings.

Transdermal Patch
Patch: contains 0.75 mg ethinyl estradiol and 6 mg of norelgestromin; releases 20 mg ethinyl estradiol/150 mg norelgestromin per 24 hr. **Cost:** $299.95/18 patches.

NURSING IMPLICATIONS

Assessment
- Assess blood pressure before and periodically during therapy.
- **Acne:** Assess skin lesion before and periodically during therapy.
- *Lab Test Considerations:* Monitor hepatic function periodically during therapy.
- *Estrogens only*—May cause ↑ serum glucose, sodium, triglyceride, VHDL, total cholesterol, prothrombin, and factors VII, VIII, IX, and X levels. May cause ↓ LDL and antithrombin III levels.
- May cause false interpretations of thyroid function tests.
- *Progestins only*—May cause ↑ LDL concentrations. May cause ↓ serum alkaline phosphatase and HDL concentrations.

Potential Nursing Diagnoses
Noncompliance (Patient/Family Teaching)

Implementation
- **PO:** Oral doses may be administered with or immediately after food to reduce nausea. Chewable tablets may be swallowed whole or chewed; if chewed follow with 8 ounces of liquid.
- For extended-cycle tablets, *Jolessa, Quasense, Seasonale, Seasonique,* or *LoSeasonique*—

take active tablets for 84 days and followed by the placebo tablets for 7 days; for *Lybrel*—Take 1 pill each day for 28 days, then start the next set of pills daily for the next 28 days.
- For *Emergency Contraception*—Tablets are taken as soon as possible and within 72 hr after unprotected intercourse. Two doses are taken 12 hr apart. Emergency contraception products are available without a prescription to women 17 or older and by prescription for women under 17 yr.
- **Subcut:** Shake vigorously before use to form a uniform suspension. Inject slowly (over 5–7 seconds) at a 45° angle into fatty area of anterior thigh or abdomen every 12 to 14 wk. If more than 14 wk elapse between injections, rule out pregnancy prior to administration. Do not rub area after injection.
- When switching from other hormonal contraceptives, administer within dosing period (7 days after taking last active pill, removing patch or ring, or within the dosing period for IM injection).
- **IM:** Shake vial vigorously just before use to ensure uniform suspension. Administer deep IM into gluteal or deltoid muscle. If period between injections is >14 wk, determine that patient is not pregnant before administering the drug.
- Injectable medroxyprogesterone may lead to bone loss, especially in women younger than 21 yr. Injectable medroxyprogesterone should be used for >2 yr only if other methods of contraception are inadequate. If used long term, women should use supplemental calcium and vitamin D, and monitor bone mineral density.
- **Intrauterine system:** Should be inserted by a trained health care provider. Health care providers are advised to become thoroughly familiar with the insertion instructions before attempting insertion. Following insertion counsel patient on what to expect following insertion. Give patient *Follow-up Reminder Card* provided with product. Discuss expected bleeding patterns during the first months of use. Prescribe analgesics, if indicated. Patients should be reexamined and evaluated 4 to 12 weeks after insertion and once a year thereafter, or more frequently if clinically indicated.

Patient/Family Teaching

- Instruct patient to take oral medication as directed at the same time each day. Pills should be taken in proper sequence and kept in the original container. Advise patient not to skip pills even if not having sex very often.
- *If single daily dose is missed:* Take as soon as remembered; if not until next day, take 2 tablets and continue on regular dosing schedule. *If 2 days in a row are missed:* Take 2 tablets a day for the next 2 days and continue on regular dosing schedule, using a second method of birth control for the remaining cycle. *If 3 days in a row are missed:* Discontinue medication and use another form of birth control until period begins or pregnancy is ruled out; then begin a new cycle of tablets. *For 28-day dosing schedule:* If schedule is followed for first 21 days and 1 dose is missed of the last 7 tablets, it is important to take the 1st tablet of next month's cycle on the regularly scheduled day.
- Advise patient taking *Jolessa, Quasense, Seasonale, Sesonique,* or *LoSeasonique extended-cycle tablets* that withdrawal bleeding should occur during the 7 days following discontinuation of the active tablets. If withdrawal bleeding does not occur, notify health care professional. Advise patient taking *Lybrel* that no withdrawal bleeding should occur.
- For initial use of *Jolessa, Quasense, Seasonale, Sesonique,* or *LoSeasonique extended cycle tablets,* caution patient to use a nonhormonal method of contraception until she has taken the first 7 days of active tablets. Each 91-day cycle should start on the same day of the week. If started later than the proper day or 2 or more days are missed, a second nonhormonal method of contraception should be used until she has taken the pink tablet for 7 days. Transient spotting or bleeding may occur. If bleeding is persistent or prolonged, notify health care professional.
- Advise patient taking extended cycle tablets that spotting or light bleeding may occur, especially during first 3 months. Continue medication; notify health care professional if bleeding lasts >7 days.
- Advise patient of the need to use another form of contraception for the first 3 wk when beginning to use *oral contraceptives*.
- Advise patient that a second method of birth control should also be used during each cycle in which any of the following are used: *Oral contraceptives*—ampicillin, corticosteroids, antiretroviral protease inhibitors, barbiturates, carbamazepine, chloramphenicol, dihydroergotamine, corticosteroids (systemic), mineral

CONTRACEPTIVES, HORMONAL

oil, oral neomycin, oxcarbazepine, penicillin V, phenylbutazone, primidone, rifampin, sulfonamides, tetracyclines, topiramate, or valproic acid.
- Explain dose schedule and maintenance routine. Discontinuing medication suddenly may cause withdrawal bleeding.
- If nausea becomes a problem, advise patient that eating solid food often provides relief. If nausea persists or vomiting or diarrhea occur, use a nonhormonal method of contraception and notify health care professional.
- Advise patient to report signs and symptoms of fluid retention (swelling of ankles and feet, weight gain), thromboembolic disorders (pain, swelling, tenderness in extremities, headache, chest pain, blurred vision), mental depression, hepatic dysfunction (yellowed skin or eyes, pruritus, dark urine, light-colored stools), or abnormal vaginal bleeding. Women with a strong family history of breast cancer, fibrocystic breast disease, abnormal mammograms, or cervical dysplasia should be monitored for breast cancer at least yearly.
- Instruct patient to stop taking medication and notify health care professional if pregnancy is suspected.
- Caution patient that cigarette smoking during estrogen therapy may increase risk of serious side effects, especially for women over age 35.
- Caution patients to use sunscreen and protective clothing to prevent increased pigmentation.
- Caution patient that hormonal contraceptives do not protect against HIV or other sexually transmitted diseases.
- Advise patient to notify health care professional of medication regimen before treatment or surgery.
- Emphasize the importance of routine follow-up physical exams including blood pressure; breast, abdomen, and pelvic examinations; and Papanicolaou smears every 6–12 mo.
- **IM, Subcut:** Advise patient to maintain adequate amounts of dietary calcium and vitamin D to help prevent bone loss.
- **Transdermal:** Instruct patient on application of patch. First patch should be applied within 24 hr of menstrual period. If applied after Day 1 of menstrual period, a nonhormonal method of contraception should be used for the next 7 days. Day of application becomes *Patch Change Day*. Patches are worn for 1 wk and changed on the same day of each wk for 3 wk. Week 4 is patch-free. Withdrawal bleeding is expected during this time.
- Apply patch to clean, dry, intact, healthy skin on buttock, abdomen, upper outer arm, or upper torso in a place where it won't be rubbed by tight clothing. Do not place on skin that is red, irritated, or cut, and do not place on breasts. Do not apply make-up, creams, lotions, powders, or other topical products to area of patch application.
- To apply patch open foil pouch by tearing along edge using fingers. Peel pouch apart and open flat. Grasp a corner of the patch firmly and remove gently from foil pouch. Use fingernail to lift one corner of the patch and peel patch **and** the plastic liner off the foil liner. Do not remove clear liner as patch is removed. Peel away half of the clear liner without touching sticky surface. Apply the sticky surface and remove the rest of the liner. Press down firmly with palm of hand for 10 seconds; make sure the edges stick well.
- On *Patch Change Day* remove patch and apply new one immediately. Used patch still contains some active hormones; fold in half so it sticks to itself and throw away. Apply new patches to a new spot to prevent skin irritation; may be applied in same anatomic area.
- Following patch-free week, apply a new patch on *Patch Change Day*, the day after Day 28, no matter when the menstrual cycle begins.
- If patch becomes partially or completely detached for less than 1 day, reapply patch or apply new patch. If patch is detached for more than 1 day, apply a new patch immediately and use a nonhormonal form of contraception for the next 7 days. Cycle will now start over with a new *Patch Change Day*. If patch is no longer sticky, apply a new patch; do not use tape or wraps to keep patch in place.
- If patch is not changed on *Patch Change Day* in the first week of the cycle, apply new patch immediately upon remembering and use a nonhormonal method of contraception for next 7 days. If patch change is missed in for 1 or 2 days during Week 2 or 3, apply new patch immediately and apply next patch on usual *Patch Change Day*. No backup contraception is needed. If patch change is missed for more than 2 days during Week 2 or 3, stop the cycle and start a new 4-wk contraceptive cycle by applying new patch immediately and using a nonhormonal method of contraception for the next 7 days. If patch is not removed on *Patch Change Day* in Week 4, remove as soon as remembered and start next cycle on usual *Patch Change Day*. No additional contraception is needed.

- Advise patient referred for MRI test to discuss patch with referring health care professional and MRI facility to determine if removal of patch is necessary prior to test and for directions for replacing patch.
- **NuvaRing:** *If a hormonal contraceptive was not used in the past month,* insert *NuvaRing* between Days 1 and 5 of the menstrual cycle (Day 1 = first day of menstrual period), even if bleeding has not finished. Use a nonhormonal method of birth control other than a diaphragm during the first 7 days of ring use. *If switching from a combination estrogen/progesterone oral contraceptive,* insert *NuvaRing* any time during first 7 days after last tablet and no later than the day a new pill cycle would have started. No extra birth control is needed. *If switching from a mini-pill,* start using *NuvaRing* on any day of the month; do not skip days between last pill and first day of *NuvaRing* use. *If switching from an implant,* start using *NuvaRing* on same day implant is removed. *If switching from an injectable contraceptive,* start using *NuvaRing* on the day when next injection is due. *If switching from a progestin-containing IUD,* start using *NuvaRing* on the same day as IUD is removed. A nonhormonal method of contraception, other than the diaphragm, should be used for the first 7 days of *NuvaRing* use when switching from the mini-pill, implant, injectable contraceptive, or IUD.
- *NuvaRing* comes in a reclosable foil pouch. Instruct patient to wash hands, then remove *NuvaRing* from pouch; keep pouch for ring disposal. Using a position of comfort (lying down, squatting, or standing with one leg up), hold *NuvaRing* between thumb and index finger and press opposite sides of the ring together. Gently push folded ring into vagina. Exact position is not important for function of *NuvaRing*. Most women do not feel *NuvaRing* once it is in place. If discomfort is felt, *NuvaRing* may not be inserted far enough into vagina; use finger to push further into vagina. *There is no danger of NuvaRing being pushed in too far or getting lost.* Once inserted, leave *NuvaRing* in place for 3 wk.
- Remove ring 3 wk after insertion on same day and time of insertion. Remove by hooking finger under forward rim or by holding ring between index and middle finger and pulling out. Place ring in foil pouch and dispose; do not throw in toilet. Menstrual period will usually start 2–3 days after ring is removed and may not have finished before next ring is inserted. To continue contraceptive protection, new ring must be inserted 1 wk after last one was removed, even if menstrual period has not stopped.
- If *NuvaRing* slips out of vagina and has been out less than 3 hr, contraceptive protection is still in place. *NuvaRing* can be rinsed in cool to tepid water and should be reinserted as soon as possible. If ring is lost, insert a new ring and continue same schedule as lost ring. If *NuvaRing* has been out of vagina for more than 3 hr, a nonhormonal method of contraception, other than a diaphragm, should be used for the next 7 days.
- *If NuvaRing has been left in for an extra wk or less (4 wk total or less),* remove and insert a new ring after a 1-wk ring-free break. If *NuvaRing* has been left in place for more than 4 wk, woman should check to be sure she is not pregnant. A nonhormonal method of contraception, other than a diaphragm, must be used for the next 7 days.
- **Intrauterine system:** Advise patient to notify health care professional if pelvic pain or pain during sex, unusual vaginal discharge or genital sores, unexplained fever, exposure to sexually transmitted infections, very severe or migraine headaches, yellowing of skin or whites of the eyes, very severe vaginal bleeding or bleeding that lasts a long time occurs, if a menstrual period is missed, or if *Mirena's* threads cannot be felt.

Evaluation/Desired Outcomes
- Prevention of pregnancy.
- Regulation of the menstrual cycle.
- Decrease in menstrual blood loss.
- Decrease in acne.
- Decrease in symptoms of premenstrual dysphoric disorder.

CORTICOSTEROIDS (INHALATION)

beclomethasone
(be-kloe-**meth**-a-sone)
QVAR

budesonide (byoo-**dess**-oh-nide)
Pulmicort Respules, Pulmicort Flexhaler

flunisolide (floo-**niss**-oh-lide)
AeroBid, AeroBid-M, Aerospan

fluticasone (floo-**ti**-ka-sone)
Flovent Diskus, Flovent HFA

mometasone (mo-**met**-a-sone)
Asmanex

Classification
Therapeutic: antiasthmatics, anti-inflammatories (steroidal)
Pharmacologic: corticosteroids (inhalation)

Pregnancy Category B (budesonide), C (all others)

Indications
Maintenance treatment of asthma as prophylactic therapy. May decrease the need for or eliminate use of systemic corticosteroids in patients with asthma.

Action
Potent, locally acting anti-inflammatory and immune modifier. **Therapeutic Effects:** Decreased frequency and severity of asthma attacks. Improves asthma symptoms.

Pharmacokinetics
Absorption: *Beclomethasone*—20%; *budesonide*—6–13% (Flexhaler), 6% (Respules); *flunisolide*—40%; *fluticasone*—<7% (aerosol), 18% (powder); *mometasone*—<1%. Action is primarily local after inhalation.
Distribution: 10–25% is deposited in airways if a spacer device is not used. All cross the placenta and enter breast milk in small amounts.
Metabolism and Excretion: *Beclomethasone*—after inhalation, beclomethasone dipropionate is converted to beclomethasone monopropionate, an active metabolite that adds to its potency, primarily excreted in feces (<10% excreted in urine; *Budenoside, flunisolide, fluticasone, mometasone*—metabolized by the liver after absorption from lungs; *Budenoside*—60% excreted in urine, 40% in feces; *flunisolide*—50% excreted in urine, 50% in feces; *fluticasone*—primarily excreted in feces (<5% excreted in urine); *mometasone*—75% excreted in feces.
Half-life: *Beclomethasone*—2.8 hr; *budesonide*—2–3.6 hr; *flunisolide*—1.8 hr; *fluticasone*—7.8 hr; *mometasone*—5 hr.

TIME/ACTION PROFILE (improvement in symptoms)

ROUTE	ONSET	PEAK	DURATION
Inhalation	within 24 hr‡	1–4 wk†	unknown

†Improvement in pulmonary function; decreased airway responsiveness may take longer.
‡2–8 days for budesonide respule.

Contraindications/Precautions
Contraindicated in: Some products contain alcohol or lactose and should be avoided in patients with known hypersensitivity or intolerance; Acute attack of asthma/status asthmaticus.
Use Cautiously in: Active untreated infections; Diabetes or glaucoma; Underlying immunosuppression (due to disease or concurrent therapy); Systemic corticosteroid therapy (should not be abruptly discontinued when inhalation therapy is started; additional corticosteroids needed in stress or trauma); Hepatic dysfunction (fluticasone); OB, Lactation: Safety not established; Pedi: Prolonged or high-dose therapy may lead to complications.

Adverse Reactions/Side Effects
CNS: headache, agitation, depression, dizziness, fatigue, insomnia, restlessness. **EENT:** dysphonia, hoarseness, cataracts, nasal congestion, pharyngitis, sinusitis. **Resp:** bronchospasm, cough, wheezing. **GI:** diarrhea, dry mouth, dyspepsia, esophageal candidiasis, taste disturbances, nausea. **Endo:** adrenal suppression (↑ dose, long-term therapy only), decreased growth (children), ↓ bone mineral density (fluticasone). **MS:** back pain. **Misc:** CHURG-STRAUSS SYNDROME.

Interactions
Drug-Drug: Ketoconazole ↑ levels of budesonide, fluticasone, and mometasone. **Ritonavir** ↑ levels of budesonide and fluticasone; avoid using with fluticasone. **Itraconazole, clarithromycin,** and **erythromycin** ↑ levels of budesonide.

Route/Dosage
Beclomethasone
Inhaln (Adults and Children ≥12 yr): *Previously on bronchodilators alone*—40–80 mcg twice daily (not to exceed 320 mcg twice daily); *Previously on inhaled corticosteroids*—40–160 mcg twice daily (not to exceed 320 mcg twice daily).
Inhaln (Children 5–11 yr): *Previously on bronchodilators alone*—40 mcg twice daily (not to exceed 80 mcg twice daily); *Previously on inhaled corticosteroids*—40 mcg twice daily (not to exceed 80 mcg twice daily).

CORTICOSTEROIDS (INHALATION) 367

Budesonide (Pulmicort Flexhaler)
Inhaln (Adults): 180–360 mcg twice daily (not to exceed 720 mcg twice daily).
Inhaln (Children ≥6 yr): 180–360 mcg twice daily (not to exceed 360 mcg twice daily).

Budesonide (Pulmicort Respules)
Inhaln (Children 1–8 yr): *Previously on bronchodilators alone*—0.5 mg once daily or 0.25 mg twice daily (not to exceed 0.5 mg/day); *Previously on other inhaled corticosteroids*—0.5 mg once daily or 0.25 mg twice daily (not to exceed 1 mg/day); *Previously on oral corticosteroids*—1 mg once daily or 0.5 mg twice daily (not to exceed 1 mg/day).

Flunisolide
Aerobid and Aerospan inhalers are not interchangeable; the dosage changes when switching from one product to another
Inhaln (Adults and Children >15 yr [Aerobid/Aerobid-M Inhaler]): 500 mcg (2 inhalations) twice daily (not to exceed 4 inhalations twice daily).
Inhaln (Adults and Children ≥12 yr [Aerospan Inhaler]): 160 mcg (2 inhalations) twice daily (not to exceed 4 inhalations twice daily).
Inhaln (Children 6–15 yr [Aerobid/Aerobid-M Inhaler]): 500 mcg (2 inhalations) twice daily (not to exceed 2 inhalations twice daily).
Inhaln (Children 6–11 yr [Aerospan Inhaler]): 80 mcg (1 inhalation) twice daily (not to exceed 2 inhalations twice daily).

Fluticasone (Aerosol Inhaler)
Inhaln (Adults and Children ≥12 yr): *Previously on bronchodilators alone*—88 mcg twice daily initially, may be ↑ up to 440 mcg twice daily; *Previously on other inhaled corticosteroids*—88–220 mcg twice daily initially, may be ↑ up to 440 mcg twice daily; *Previously on oral corticosteroids*—440 mcg twice daily initially, may be ↑ up to 880 mcg twice daily.
Inhaln (Children 4–11 yr): 88 mcg twice daily (not to exceed 88 mcg twice daily).

Fluticasone (Dry Powder Inhaler)
Inhaln (Adults and Children ≥12 yr): *Previously on bronchodilators alone*—100 mcg twice daily initially, may be ↑ up to 500 mcg twice daily; *Previously on other inhaled corticosteroids*—100–250 mcg twice daily initially, may be ↑ up to 500 mcg twice daily; *Previously on oral corticosteroids*—500–1000 mcg twice daily.
Inhaln (Children 4–11 yr): *Previously on bronchodilators alone*—50 mcg twice daily initially, may be ↑ up to 100 mcg twice daily; *Previously on other inhaled corticosteroids*—50 mcg twice daily, may be ↑ up to 100 mcg twice daily.

Mometasone
Inhaln (Adults and Children >12 yr): *Previously on bronchodilators or other inhaled corticosteroids*—220 mcg (1 inhalation) once daily, up to 440 mcg/day as a single dose or 2 divided doses; *Previously on oral corticosteroids*—440 mcg (2 inhalations) twice daily (not to exceed 880 mcg/day).

Availability

Beclomethasone
Inhalation aerosol: 40 mcg/metered inhalation in 7.3-g canister (delivers 100 metered inhalations), 80 mcg/metered inhalation in 7.3-g canister (delivers 100 metered inhalations). **Cost:** 40 mcg/metered inhalation $41.32/7.3–g canister; 80 mcg metered inhalation $52.04/7.3-g canister.

Budesonide
Inhalation powder (Flexhaler): 90 mcg/metered inhalation (delivers 60 metered inhalations), 180 mcg/metered inhalation (delivers 120 metered inhalations). **Inhalation suspension (Respules):** 0.25 mg/2 mL in single-dose ampules (5 ampules/envelope), 0.5 mg/2 mL in single-dose ampules (5 ampules/envelope), 1 mg/2 mL in single-dose ampules (5 ampules/envelope). **Cost:** 0.25 mg/2 mL $158.99/20 ampules, 0.5 mg/2 mL $187.00/30 ampules. *In combination with:* formoterol (Symbicort). See Appendix B.

Flunisolide
Inhalation aerosol (Aerobid): 250 mcg/metered inhalation in 7-g canisters (delivers 100 metered inhalations). **Inhalation aerosol-menthol (Aerobid-M):** 250 mcg/metered inhalation in 7-g canisters (delivers 100 metered inhalations). **Inhalation aerosol (Aerospan):** 80 mcg/metered inhalation in 5.1-g canisters (delivers 60 metered inhalations) or 8.9-g canisters (delivers 120 metered inhalations).

Fluticasone
Inhalation aerosol (Flovent-HFA): 44 mcg/metered inhalation in 10.6-g canisters (delivers

CORTICOSTEROIDS (INHALATION)

120 metered inhalations), 110 mcg/metered inhalation in 12-g canisters (delivers 120 metered inhalations), 220 mcg/metered inhalation in 12-g canisters (delivers 120 metered inhalations). **Cost:** 44 mcg/inhalation $90.00/inhaler, 110 mcg/inhalation $118.99/inhaler, 220 mcg/inhalation $193.52/inhaler. **Powder for inhalation (Flovent Diskus):** 50 mcg, 100 mcg, 250 mcg. *In combination with:* salmeterol (Advair). See Appendix B.

Mometasone
Powder for inhalation (Twisthaler): 110 mcg (delivers 100 mcg/metered inhalation; in packages of 7 and 30 inhalation units), 220 mcg (delivers 200 mcg/metered inhalation; in packages of 14, 30, 60, and 120 inhalation units).

NURSING IMPLICATIONS
Assessment
- Monitor respiratory status and lung sounds. Assess pulmonary function tests periodically during and for several months after a transfer from systemic to inhalation corticosteroids.
- Assess patients changing from systemic corticosteroids to inhalation corticosteroids for signs of adrenal insufficiency (anorexia, nausea, weakness, fatigue, hypotension, hypoglycemia) during initial therapy and periods of stress. If these signs appear, notify health care professional immediately; condition may be life-threatening.
- Monitor for withdrawal symptoms (joint or muscular pain, lassitude, depression) during withdrawal from oral corticosteroids.
- Monitor growth rate in children receiving chronic therapy; use lowest possible dose.
- May cause decreased bone mineral density during prolonged therapy. Monitor patients with increased risk (prolonged immobilization, family history of osteoporosis, post-menopausal status, tobacco use, advanced age, poor nutrition, chronic use of drugs that can reduce bone mass [anticonvulsants, oral corticosteroids]) for fractures.
- *Lab Test Considerations:* Periodic adrenal function tests may be ordered to assess degree of hypothalamic-pituitary-adrenal (HPA) axis suppression in chronic therapy. Children and patients using higher than recommended doses are at highest risk for HPA suppression.
- May cause ↑ serum and urine glucose concentrations if significant absorption occurs.

Potential Nursing Diagnoses
Ineffective airway clearance (Indications)
Risk for infection (Side Effects)
Deficient knowledge, related to medication regimen (Patient/Family Teaching)

Implementation
- After the desired clinical effect has been obtained, attempts should be made to decrease dose to lowest amount required to control symptoms. Gradually decrease dose every 2–4 wk as long as desired effect is maintained. If symptoms return, dose may briefly return to starting dose.
- **Inhaln:** Allow at least 1 min between inhalations.

Patient/Family Teaching
- Advise patient to take medication as directed. Take missed doses as soon as remembered unless almost time for next dose. Instruct patient to read the *Patient Information and Instructions for Use* before using and with each Rx refill, in case of new information. Advise patient not to discontinue medication without consulting health care professional; gradual decrease is required.
- Advise patients using inhalation corticosteroids and bronchodilator to use bronchodilator first and to allow 5 min to elapse before administering the corticosteroid, unless otherwise directed by health care professional.
- Advise patient that inhalation corticosteroids should not be used to treat an acute asthma attack but should be continued even if other inhalation agents are used.
- Patients using inhalation corticosteroids to control asthma may require systemic corticosteroids for acute attacks. Advise patient to use regular peak flow monitoring to determine respiratory status.
- Caution patient to avoid smoking, known allergens, and other respiratory irritants.
- Advise patient to notify physician if sore throat or sore mouth occurs.
- Advise female patients to notify health care professional if pregnancy is planned or suspected or if breastfeeding.
- Instruct patient whose systemic corticosteroids have been recently reduced or withdrawn to carry a warning card indicating the need for supplemental systemic corticosteroids in the event of stress or severe asthma attack unresponsive to bronchodilators.
- **Metered-Dose Inhaler:** Instruct patient in the proper use of the metered-dose inhaler. Most inhalers require priming before first use. Shake inhaler well. Exhale completely, and then close lips firmly around mouthpiece. While breathing in deeply and slowly, press

down on canister. Hold breath for as long as possible to ensure deep instillation of medication. Remove inhaler from mouth and breathe out gently. Allow 1–2 min between inhalations. Rinse mouth with water or mouthwash after each use to minimize fungal infections, dry mouth, and hoarseness. Clean the mouthpiece weekly with clean, dry tissue or cloth. Do not place in water (see Appendix D).

- **Pulmicort Flexhaler:** Advise patient to follow instructions supplied. Before first-time use, prime unit by turning cover and lifting off; hold upright with mouthpiece up and twist brown grip fully to right, then fully to left until it clicks. To administer dose, hold upright, twist brown grip fully to right, then fully to left until it clicks. Turn head away from inhaler and exhale (do not blow into inhaler). Do not shake inhaler. Place mouthpiece between lips and inhale deeply and forcefully. Remove inhaler from mouth and exhale (do not exhale into mouthpiece). Repeat procedure if 2nd dose required. Replace cover; rinse mouth with water (do not swallow).

- **Pulmicort Respules:** Administer with a jet nebulizer connected to adequate air flow, equipped with a mouthpiece or face mask. Adjust face mask to avoid exposing eyes to nebulized medication. Wash face after use of face mask. Ultrasonic nebulizers are not adequate for administration and not recommended. Store respules upright, away from heat and protected from light. Do not refrigerate or freeze. Respules are stable for 2 wk at room temperature after opening aluminum foil envelope. Open respules must be used promptly. Unused respules should be returned to aluminum foil envelope.

- **Flovent Diskus:** Do not use with a spacer. Exhale completely and then close lips firmly around mouthpiece. While breathing in deeply and slowly, press down on canister. Hold breath for as long as possible to ensure deep instillation of medication. Remove inhaler from mouth and breathe out gently. Allow 1–2 min between inhalations. After inhalation, rinse mouth with water and spit out (see Appendix D). Never wash the mouthpiece or any part of the Diskus inhaler. Discard Diskus inhaler device 6 wk (50-mcg strength) or 2 mo (100-mcg and 250-mcg strengths) after removal from protective foil overwrap pouch or after all blisters have been used (whichever comes first).

- **Asmanex Twisthaler:** Advise patient to remove cap while device is in upright position. To administer dose, exhale fully, then place mouthpiece between lips and inhale deeply and forcefully. Remove device from mouth and hold breath for 10 sec before exhaling (do not exhale into mouthpiece). Wipe the mouthpiece dry, if necessary, and replace the cap on the device. Rinse mouth with water. Advise patient to discard twisthaler 45 days from opening or when dose counter reads "00", whichever comes first.

Evaluation/Desired Outcomes

- Management of the symptoms of chronic asthma.
- Improvement in symptoms of asthma.

CORTICOSTEROIDS (NASAL)

beclomethasone (be-kloe-**meth**-a-sone)
Beconase AQ, ✦Rivanase AQ

budesonide (byoo-**dess**-oh-nide)
Rhinocort Aqua

ciclesonide (sye-**kles**-oh-nide)
Omnaris

flunisolide (floo-**niss**-oh-lide)
Nasarel, ✦Rhinalar

fluticasone (floo-**ti**-ka-sone)
Flonase, Veramyst

mometasone (moe-**met**-a-sone)
Nasonex

triamcinolone (trye-am-**sin**-oh-lone)
AllerNaze, Nasacort AQ

Classification
Therapeutic: anti-inflammatories (steroidal)
Pharmacologic: corticosteroids (nasal)

Pregnancy Category B (budesonide), C (all others)

Indications
Seasonal or perennial allergic rhinitis. Nonallergic rhinitis (fluticasone). Treatment of nasal polyps.

✦ = Canadian drug name. ❚ = Genetic implication.
*CAPITALS indicates life-threatening; <u>underlines</u> indicate most frequent.

CORTICOSTEROIDS (NASAL)

Action
Potent, locally acting anti-inflammatory and immune modifier. **Therapeutic Effects:** ↓ in symptoms of allergic or nonallergic rhinitis. ↓ in symptoms of nasal polyps.

Pharmacokinetics
Absorption: *Beclomethasone*—44% absorbed; *budesonide*—34% absorbed; *flunisolide*—50% absorbed; *ciclesonide, fluticasone, mometasone*—negligible absorption. Action of all agents is primarily local following nasal use.
Distribution: All agents cross the placenta and enter breast milk in small amounts.
Metabolism and Excretion: Following absorption from nasal mucosa, corticosteroids are rapidly and extensively metabolized by the liver.
Half-life: *Beclomethasone*—2.7 hr; *budesonide*—2–3 hr; *ciclesonide*—unknown; *flunisolide*—1–2 hr; *fluticasone*—7.8 hr; *mometasone*—5.8 hr; *triamcinolone*—3–5.4 hr.

TIME/ACTION PROFILE (improvement in symptoms)

ROUTE	ONSET	PEAK	DURATION
Beclomethasone	1–3 days	up to 2 wk	unknown
Budesonide	1–2 days	2 wk	unknown
Ciclesonide	1–2 days	2–5 wk	unknown
Flunisolide	few days	up to 3 wk	unknown
Fluticasone	few days	unknown	unknown
Mometasone	within 2 days	1–2 wk	unknown
Triamcinolone	few days	3–4 days	unknown

Contraindications/Precautions
Contraindicated in: Some products contain alcohol, propylene, or polyethylene glycol and should be avoided in patients with known hypersensitivity or intolerance.
Use Cautiously in: Active untreated infections; Diabetes or glaucoma; Underlying immunosuppression (due to disease or concurrent therapy); Systemic corticosteroid therapy (should not be abruptly discontinued when intranasal therapy is started); Recent nasal trauma, septal ulcers, or surgery (wound healing may be impaired by nasal corticosteroids; OB, Lactation, Pedi: Pregnancy, lactation, or children <12 yr (triamcinolone [AllerNaze]) or <6 yr (beclomethasone, budesonide, ciclesonide, flunisolide) or <4 yr (fluticasone [Flonase]) or <2 yr (fluticasone [Veramyst], mometasone, triamcinolone [Nasacort AQ]) (safety not established; prolonged or high-dose therapy may lead to complications).

Adverse Reactions/Side Effects
CNS: dizziness, headache. **EENT:** epistaxis, nasal burning, nasal irritation, nasal congestion, pharyngitis, rhinorrhea, sneezing, tearing eyes. **GI:** dry mouth, esophageal candidiasis, nausea, vomiting. **Derm:** rash (fluticasone), urticaria (fluticasone). **Endo:** adrenal suppression (high-dose, long-term therapy only), growth suppression (children). **Resp:** bronchospasm, cough. **Misc:** ANAPHYLAXIS, ANGIOEDEMA.

Interactions
Drug-Drug: Ketoconazole ↑ effects of budesonide, ciclesonide, and fluticasone. **Ritonavir** ↑ effects of fluticasone (avoid concurrent use).

Route/Dosage

Beclomethasone
Intranasal (Adults and Children ≥12 yr): 1–2 sprays in each nostril twice daily (not to exceed 2 sprays in each nostril twice daily).
Intranasal (Children 6–12 yr): 1–2 sprays in each nostril twice daily; once adequate control achieved, ↓ dose to 1 spray in each nostril twice daily.

Budesonide
Intranasal (Adults and Children ≥12 yr): 1 spray in each nostril once daily (not to exceed 4 sprays in each nostril once daily).
Intranasal (Children 6–11 yr): 1 spray in each nostril once daily (not to exceed 2 sprays in each nostril once daily).

Ciclesonide
Intranasal (Adults and Children ≥6 yr): 2 sprays in each nostril once daily (not to exceed 2 sprays in each nostril/day).

Flunisolide
Intranasal (Adults and Children >14 yr): 2 sprays in each nostril twice daily, may be ↑ to 2 sprays in each nostril 3 times daily if greater effect needed after 4–7 days (not to exceed 8 sprays in each nostril/day).
Intranasal (Children 6–14 yr): 1 spray in each nostril 3 times daily or 2 sprays in each nostril twice daily (not to exceed 4 sprays in each nostril/day).

Fluticasone
Intranasal (Adults and Children ≥12 yrs): *Flonase*—2 sprays in each nostril once daily or 1 spray in each nostril twice daily; after several days, attempt to ↓ dose to 1 spray in each nostril once daily. Patients ≥12 yr with seasonal allergic rhinitis may also use 2 sprays in each nostril once

CORTICOSTEROIDS (NASAL)

daily on an as-needed basis; *Veramyst*—2 sprays in each nostril once daily or 1 spray in each nostril twice daily; after several days, attempt to ↓ dose to 1 spray in each nostril once daily.
Intranasal (Children >4 yr): *Flonase*—1 spray in each nostril once daily (not to exceed 2 sprays in each nostril/day).
Intranasal (Children 2–11 yrs): *Veramyst*—1 spray in each nostril daily; may ↑ to 2 sprays if no response. Once symptoms are controlled, attempt to ↓ dose to 1 spray/day.

Mometasone
Intranasal (Adults and Children >12 yr): *Treatment of seasonal and perennial allergic rhinitis*—2 sprays in each nostril once daily (not to exceed 2 sprays in each nostril once daily).
Intranasal (Adults): *Nasal polyps*—2 sprays in each nostril twice daily (not to exceed 2 sprays in each nostril twice daily).
Intranasal (Children 2–11 yr): *Treatment of seasonal and perennial allergic rhinitis*—1 spray in each nostril once daily.

Triamcinolone
Intranasal (Adults and Children >12 yr): *AllerNaze or Nasacort AQ*—2 sprays in each nostril once daily.
Intranasal (Children 6–11 yr): *Nasacort AQ*—1 spray in each nostril once daily (not to exceed 2 sprays in each nostril/day).
Intranasal (Children 2–5 yr): *Nasacort AQ*—1 spray in each nostril once daily.

Availability

Beclomethasone
Nasal spray: 42 mcg/metered spray in 25-g bottles (delivers 180 metered sprays), ✽ 50 mcg/metered spray in 25-g bottles (delivers 200 metered sprays).

Budesonide
Nasal spray: 32 mcg/metered spray in 8.6-g canister (delivers 120 metered sprays). **Cost:** $92.99/bottle.

Ciclesonide
Nasal spray: 50 mcg/metered spray in 12.5-g bottle (delivers 120 metered sprays).

Flunisolide (generic available)
Nasal solution: 25 mcg/metered spray in 25-mL bottle (delivers 200 metered sprays), 29 mcg/metered spray in 25-mL bottle (delivers 200 metered sprays).

Fluticasone (generic available)
Nasal spray (Flonase): 50 mcg/metered spray in 16-g bottle (delivers 120 metered sprays). **Cost:** *Generic*—$59.99/bottle. **Nasal spray (Veramyst):** 27.5 mcg/spray in a 10-g bottle (delivers 120 sprays).

Mometasone
Nasal spray (scent-free): 50 mcg/metered spray in 17-g bottle (delivers 120 metered sprays). **Cost:** $89.24/bottle.

Triamcinolone
Nasal spray (AllerNaze): 50 mcg/metered spray in 15-mL bottle (120 metered sprays). **Nasal spray (Nasacort AQ):** 55 mcg/metered spray in 16.5-g bottle (120 metered sprays). **Cost:** $89.99/16.5-g bottle.

NURSING IMPLICATIONS

Assessment
- Monitor degree of nasal stuffiness, amount and color of nasal discharge, and frequency of sneezing.
- Patients on long-term therapy should have periodic otolaryngologic examinations to monitor nasal mucosa and passages for infection or ulceration.
- Monitor growth rate in children receiving chronic therapy; use lowest possible dose.
- *Lab Test Considerations:* Periodic adrenal function tests may be ordered to assess degree of hypothalamic-pituitary-adrenal (HPA) axis suppression in chronic therapy. Children and patients using higher than recommended doses are at highest risk for HPA suppression.

Potential Nursing Diagnoses
Ineffective airway clearance (Indications)
Risk for infection (Side Effects)
Deficient knowledge, related to medication regimen (Patient/Family Teaching)

Implementation
- After desired clinical effect has been obtained, attempt to decrease dose to lowest amount. Gradually decrease dose every 2–4 wk as long as desired effect is maintained. If symptoms return, dose may briefly return to starting dose.
- **Intranasal:** Patients also using a nasal decongestant should be given decongestant 5–15 min before corticosteroid nasal spray. If patient

✽ = Canadian drug name. ▮ = Genetic implication.
*CAPITALS indicates life-threatening; underlines indicate most frequent.

is unable to breathe freely through nasal passages, instruct patient to blow nose gently in advance of medication administration.

Patient/Family Teaching
- Advise patient to take medication as directed. Take missed doses as soon as remembered unless almost time for next dose.
- Caution patient not to exceed maximal daily dose of nasal spray.
- Instruct patient in correct technique for administering nasal spray (see Appendix D). Most nasal sprays include directions with pictures. Instruct patient to read patient information sheet prior to use. Shake well before use. Warn patient that temporary nasal stinging may occur.
- Instruct patient to gently blow nose to clear nostrils prior to administering dose.
- Instruct patient to stop medication and notify health care professional immediately if signs of anaphylaxis (rash, hives, difficulty breathing, swollen lips or throat) occur.
- Advise patient to consult health care professional before taking other Rx, OTC, or herbal products with fluticasone.
- Advise female patients to notify health care professional if pregnancy is planned or suspected or if breastfeeding.
- Instruct patient to notify health care professional if symptoms do not improve within 1 month, if symptoms worsen, or if sneezing or nasal irritation occurs.

Evaluation/Desired Outcomes
- Resolution of nasal stuffiness, discharge, and sneezing in seasonal or perennial allergic rhinitis or nonallergic rhinitis.
- Reduction in symptoms of nasal polyps.

CORTICOSTEROIDS (SYSTEMIC)
short-acting corticosteroids

cortisone (**kor**-ti-sone)
✤ Cortone

hydrocortisone
(hye-droe-**kor**-ti-sone)
Cortef, Cortenema, Solu-Cortef

intermediate-acting corticosteroids

methylPREDNISolone
(meth-ill-pred-**niss**-oh-lone)
A-Methapred, Depo-Medrol, Medrol, Solu-Medrol

predniSOLONE
(pred-**niss**-oh-lone)
Orapred, Orapred ODT, Pediapred, Prelone

predniSONE (**pred**-ni-sone)
Sterapred

triamcinolone
(trye-am-**sin**-oh-lone)
Aristospan, Kenalog, Trivaris

long-acting corticosteroids

betamethasone
(bay-ta-**meth**-a-sone)
✤ Betnelan, ✤ Betnesol, Celestone, ✤ Selestoject

budesonide (byoo-**des**-oh-nide)
Entocort EC

dexamethasone
(dex-a-**meth**-a-sone)
DexPak

Classification
Therapeutic: antiasthmatics, corticosteroids
Pharmacologic: corticosteroids (systemic)

Pregnancy Category B (prednisone), C (betamethasone, budesonide, dexamethasone, hydrocortisone, methylprednisolone, prednisolone, triamcinolone), D (cortisone)

Indications
Cortisone, hydrocortisone: Management of adrenocortical insufficiency. **Betamethasone, dexamethasone, hydrocortisone, prednisolone, prednisone, methylprednisolone, triamcinolone:** Used systemically and locally in a wide variety of chronic diseases including: Inflammatory, Allergic, Hematologic, Neoplastic, Autoimmune disorders. **Methylprednisolone, prednisone:** With other immunosuppressants in the prevention of organ rejection in transplantation surgery. Asthma. **Dexamethasone:** Management of cerebral edema: Diagnostic agent in adrenal disorders. **Budesonide:** Treatment of mild to moderate Crohn's disease. **Unlabeled Use:** Short-term administration to high-risk mothers before delivery to prevent respiratory distress syndrome in the newborn (betamethasone, dexamethasone). Adjunctive therapy of hypercalcemia (prednisone, prednisolone, methylprednisolone). Management of acute spinal cord injury (methylprednisolone). Adjunctive management of nausea and vomiting from chemotherapy (dexamethasone, prednisone, prednisolone, methylpredniso-

CORTICOSTEROIDS (SYSTEMIC)

lone). Management of croup (dexamethasone). Treatment of airway edema prior to extubation (dexamethasone). Facilitation of ventilator weaning in neonates with bronchopulmonary dysplasia (dexamethasone).

Action
In pharmacologic doses, all agents suppress inflammation and the normal immune response. All agents have numerous intense metabolic effects (see Adverse Reactions/Side Effects). Suppress adrenal function at chronic doses of *betamethasone*—0.6 mg/day; *cortisone, hydrocortisone*—20 mg/day; *dexamethasone*—0.75 mg/day; *methylprednisolone, triamcinolone*—4 mg/day; *prednisone/prednisolone*—5 mg/day. **Cortisone, hydrocortisone:** Replace endogenous cortisol in deficiency states. **Cortisone, hydrocortisone:** Have potent mineralocorticoid (sodium-retaining) activity. **Prednisolone, prednisone:** Have minimal mineralocorticoid activity. **Betamethasone, dexamethasone, methylprednisolone, triamcinolone:** Have negligible mineralocorticoid activity. **Budesonide:** Local anti-inflammatory activity in the lumen of the GI tract. **Therapeutic Effects:** Suppression of inflammation and modification of the normal immune response. Replacement therapy in adrenal insufficiency. **Budesonide:** Improvement in symptoms/sequelae of Crohn's disease.

Pharmacokinetics
Absorption: Well absorbed after oral administration (except budesonide). Sodium phosphate and sodium succinate salts are rapidly absorbed after IM administration. Acetate and acetonide salts are slowly but completely absorbed after IM administration. Absorption from local sites (intraarticular, intralesional) is slow but complete. Bioavailability of budesonide is 9–21%.
Distribution: All are widely distributed, cross the placenta, and probably enter breast milk.
Metabolism and Excretion: All are metabolized mostly by the liver to inactive metabolites. *Cortisone* is converted by the liver to hydrocortisone. *Prednisone* is converted by the liver to prednisolone, which is then metabolized by the liver.
Half-life: *Betamethasone*—3–5 hr (plasma), 36–54 hr (tissue). *Budesonide*—2.0–3.6 hr. *Cortisone*—0.5 hr (plasma), 8–12 hr (tissue). *Dexamethasone*—3–4.5 hr (plasma), 36–54 hr (tissue). *Hydrocortisone*—1.5–2 hr (plasma), 8–12 hr (tissue). *Methylprednisolone*—>3.5 hr (plasma), 18–36 hr (tissue). *Prednisolone*—2.1–3.5 hr (plasma), 18–36 hr (tissue). *Prednisone*—3.4–3.8 hr (plasma), 18–36 hr (tissue). *Triamcinolone*—2–5 hr (plasma), 18–36 hr (tissue).

TIME/ACTION PROFILE (anti-inflammatory activity)

ROUTE	ONSET	PEAK	DURATION
Betamethasone PO	unknown	1–2 hr	3.25 days
Betamethasone IM (acetate/sodium phosphate)	1–3 hr	unknown	1 wk
Budesonide PO	unknown	unknown	unknown
Cortisone PO	rapid	2 hr	1.25–1.5 days
Dexamethasone PO	unknown	1–3 hr	2.75 days
Dexamethasone IM, IV (sodium phosphate)	rapid	unknown	2.75 days
Hydrocortisone PO	unknown	1–2 hr	1.25–1.5 days
Hydrocortisone IM (sodium succinate)	rapid	1 hr	variable
Hydrocortisone IV (sodium succinate)	rapid	unknown	unknown
Methylprednisolone PO	unknown	1–2 hr	1.25–1.5 days
Methylprednisolone IM (acetate)	6–48 hr	4–8 days	1–4 wk
Methylprednisolone IM, IV (sodium succinate)	rapid	unknown	unknown
Prednisolone PO	unknown	1–2 hr	1.25–1.5 days
Prednisone PO	unknown	1–2 hr	1.25–1.5 days
Triamcinolone IM (acetonide)	24–48 hr	unknown	1–6 wk
Triamcinolone Intralesional (hexacetonide)	slow	unknown	4 days–4 wk

Contraindications/Precautions
Contraindicated in: Active untreated infections (may be used in patients being treated for some forms of meningitis); Lactation: Avoid chronic use; Known alcohol, bisulfite, or tartrazine hypersensitivity or intolerance (some products contain these and should be avoided in susceptible patients); Administration of live virus vaccines.
Use Cautiously in: Chronic treatment (will lead to adrenal suppression; use lowest possible dose for shortest period of time); Hypothyroidism; Cirrhosis; Pedi: Children (chronic use will result in ↓ growth; use lowest possible dose for shortest period of time); Stress (surgery, infections); supplemental doses may be needed; Potential infections may mask signs (fever, inflammation); OB: Safety not established; Pedi: Neonates (avoid use of benzyl alcohol containing injectable preparations; use preservative-free formulations).

Adverse Reactions/Side Effects
Adverse reactions/side effects are much more common with high-dose/long-term therapy. **CNS:** depression, euphoria, headache, ↑ intracranial pressure (children only), personality changes, psychoses, restlessness. **EENT:** cataracts, ↑ intraocular pressure. **CV:** hypertension. **GI:** PEPTIC ULCERATION, anorexia, nausea, vomiting. **Derm:** acne, ↓ wound healing, ecchymoses, fragility, hirsutism, petechiae. **Endo:** adrenal suppression, hyperglycemia. **F and E:** fluid retention (long-term high doses), hypokalemia, hypokalemic alkalosis. **Hemat:** THROMBOEMBOLISM, thrombophlebitis. **Metab:** weight gain. **MS:** muscle wasting, osteoporosis, avascular necrosis of joints, muscle pain. **Misc:** cushingoid appearance (moon face, buffalo hump), ↑ susceptibility to infection.

Interactions
Drug-Drug: ↑ risk of hypokalemia with **thiazide** and **loop diuretics**, or **amphotericin B**. Hypokalemia may ↑ risk of **digoxin** toxicity. May increase requirement for **insulin** or **oral hypoglycemic agents**. **Phenytoin**, **phenobarbital**, and **rifampin** ↑ metabolism; may ↓ effectiveness. **Hormonal contraceptives** may ↓ metabolism. ↑ risk of adverse GI effects with **NSAIDs** (including aspirin). At chronic doses that suppress adrenal function, may ↓ antibody response to and ↑ risk of adverse reactions from **live-virus vaccines**. May increase serum concentrations of **cyclosporine** and **tacrolimus**. May ↑ risk of tendon rupture from **fluoroquinolones**. **Antacids** ↓ absorption of prednisone and dexamethasone. Known inhibitors of the CYP3A4 enzyme including **ketoconazole**, **itraconazole**, **ritonavir**, **indinavir**, **saquinavir**, and **erythromycin** may ↑ blood levels and effects of budesonide (↓ dose may be necessary). May ↓ **isoniazid** levels and effectiveness. May antagonize the effects of **anticholinergic agents** in myasthenia gravis.
Drug-Food: Grapefruit juice ↑ serum levels and effects of budesonide (avoid concurrent use).

Route/Dosage
Betamethasone
PO (Adults): 0.6–7.2 mg/day as single daily dose or in divided doses.
PO (Children): *Adrenocortical insufficiency*—17.5 mcg/kg/day (500 mcg/m^2/day) in 3 divided doses. *Other uses*—62.5–250 mcg/kg/day (1.875–7.5 mg/m^2/day) in 3 divided doses.
IM (Adults): 0.5–9 mg as betamethasone sodium phosphate/acetate suspension. *Prevention of respiratory distress syndrome in newborn*—12 mg daily for 2–3 days before delivery (unlabeled).
IM (Children): *Adrenocortical insufficiency*—17.5 mcg/kg/day (500 mcg/m^2/day) in 3 divided doses every 3rd day or 5.8–8.75 mcg/kg (166–250 mcg/m^2)/day as a single dose.

Budesonide
PO (Adults): *Active Crohn's disease*—9 mg once daily in the morning for ≤8 weeks, may repeat 8 wk course for recurring episodes. *Maintenance of remission*—6 mg once daily for up to 3 months; once symptoms are controlled, taper to complete cessation.

Cortisone
PO (Adults): 25–300 mg/day in divided doses q 12–24 hr.
PO (Children): *Adrenocortical insufficiency*—0.7 mg/kg/day (20–25 mg/m^2/day) in divided doses q 8 hr. *Other uses*—2.5–10 mg/kg/day (75–300 mg/m^2/day) in divided doses q 6–8 hr.

Dexamethasone
PO, IM, IV (Adults): *Anti-inflammatory*—0.75–9 mg daily in divided doses q 6–12 hr. *Airway edema or extubation*—0.5–2 mg/kg/day divided q 6 hr; begin 24 hr prior to extubation and continue for 24 hr post-extubation. *Cerebral edema*—10 mg IV, then 4 mg IM or IV q 6 hr until maximal response achieved, then switch to PO regimen and taper over 5–7 days.
PO, IM, IV (Children): *Airway edema or extubation*—0.5–2 mg/kg/day divided q 6 hr; begin

24 hr prior to extubation and continue for 24 hr post-extubation. *Anti-inflammatory*—0.08–0.3 mg/kg/day or 2.5–10 mg/m²/day divided q 6–12 hr. *Physiologic replacement*—0.03–0.15 mg/kg/day or 0.6–0.75 mg/m²/day divided q 6–12 hr.

PO (Adults): *Suppression test*—1 mg at 11PM or 0.5 mg q 6 hr for 48 hr.

IV (Children): *Chemotherapy-induced emesis*—5–20 mg given 15–30 min before treatment; *Cerebral edema*—Loading dose 1–2 mg/kg followed by 1–1.5 mg/kg/day divided q 4–6 hr for 5 days (not to exceed 16 mg/day); then taper over 1–6 wk; *Bacterial meningitis*—0.6 mg/kg/day divided q 6 hr × 4 days (start at time of first antibiotic dose).

IV, PO (Adults): *Chemotherapy-induced emesis*—10–20 mg given 15–30 min before each treatment or 10 mg q 12 hr on each treatment day; *Delayed nausea/vomiting*—4–10 mg PO 1–2 times/day for 2–4 days *or* 8 mg PO q 12 hr for 2 days, then 4 mg PO q 12 hr for 2 days *or* 20 mg PO 1 hr before chemotherapy, then 10 mg PO q 12 hr after chemotherapy, then 8 mg PO q 12 hr for 2 days, then 4 mg PO q 12 hr for 2 days.

IS (Adults): 0.4–6 mg/day.

Hydrocortisone

PO (Adults): 20–240 mg/day in 1–4 divided doses.

PO (Children): *Adrenocortical insufficiency*—0.56 mg/kg/day (15–20 mg/m²/day) as a single dose or in divided doses. *Other uses*—2–8 mg/kg/day (60–240 mg/m²/day) as a single dose or in divided doses.

IM, IV (Adults): 100–500 mg q 2–6 hr (range 100–8000 mg/day).

IM, IV (Children): *Adrenocortical insufficiency*—0.186–0.28 mg/kg/day (10–12 mg/m²/day) in 3 divided doses. *Other uses*—0.666–4 mg/kg (20–120 mg/m²) q 12–24 hr.

Rect (Adults): *Retention enema*—100 mg nightly for 21 days or until remission occurs.

Methylprednisolone

PO (Adults): *Multiple sclerosis*—160 mg/day for 7 days, then 64 mg every other day for 1 mo. *Other uses*—2–60 mg/day as a single dose or in 2–4 divided doses. *Asthma exacerbations*—120–180 mg/day in divided doses 3–4 times/day for 48 hr, then 60–80 mg/day in 2 divided doses.

PO (Children): *Anti-inflammatory/Immunosuppressive*—0.5–1.7 mg/kg/day (5–25 mg/m²/day) in divided doses q 6–12 hr. *Asthma exacerbations*—1 mg/kg q 6 hr for 48 hr, then 1–2 mg/kg/day (maximum: 60 mg/day) divided twice daily.

IM, IV (Adults): *Most uses: methylprednisolone sodium succinate*—40–250 mg q 4–6 hr. *High-dose "pulse" therapy: methylprednisolone sodium succinate*—30 mg/kg IV q 4–6 hr for up to 72 hr. *Status asthmaticus: methylprednisolone sodium succinate*—2 mg/kg IV, then 0.5–1 mg/kg IV q 6 hr for up to 5 days. *Multiple sclerosis: methylprednisolone sodium succinate*—160 mg/day for 7 days, then 64 mg every other day for 1 mo. *Adjunctive therapy of* Pneumocystis jirovecii *pneumonia in AIDS patients: methylprednisolone sodium succinate*—30 mg twice daily for 5 days, then 30 mg once daily for 5 days, then 15 mg once daily for 10 days. *Acute spinal cord injury: methylprednisolone sodium succinate*—30 mg/kg IV over 15 min initially, followed in 45 min with a continuous infusion of 5.4 mg/kg/hr for 23 hr (unlabeled).

IM, IV (Children): *Anti-inflammatory/Immunosuppressive*—0.5–1.7 mg/kg/day (5–25 mg/m²/day) in divided doses q 6–12 hr. *Acute spinal cord injury: methylprednisolone sodium succinate*—30 mg/kg IV over 15 min initially, followed in 45 min with a continuous infusion of 5.4 mg/kg/hr for 23 hr (unlabeled). *Status asthmaticus*—2 mg/kg IV, then 0.5–1 mg/kg IV q 6 hr. *Lupus nephritis*—30 mg/kg IV every other day for 6 doses.

IM (Adults): *Methylprednisolone acetate*—40–120 mg daily, weekly, or every 2 wk.

Prednisolone

PO (Adults): *Most uses*—5–60 mg/day as a single dose or in divided doses. *Multiple sclerosis*—200 mg/day for 7 days, then 80 mg every other day for 1 mo. *Asthma exacerbations*—120–180 mg/day in divided doses 3–4 times/day for 48 hr, then 60–80 mg/day in 2 divided doses.

PO (Children): *Anti-inflammatory/Immunosuppressive*—0.1–2 mg/kg/day in 1–4 divided doses; *Nephrotic syndrome*—2 mg/kg/day (60 mg/m²/day) in 1–3 divided doses daily (maximum dose: 80 mg/day) until urine is protein-free for 4–6 weeks, followed by 2 mg/kg/dose (40 mg/m²/dose) every other day in the morning; gradually taper off over 4–6 weeks; *Asthma exacerbations*—1 mg/kg q 6 hr for 48 hr, then 1–2 mg/kg/day (maximum: 60 mg/day) divided twice daily.

Prednisone

PO (Adults): *Most uses*—5–60 mg/day as a single dose or in divided doses. *Multiple sclerosis*—200 mg/day for 1 wk, then 80 mg every other day for 1 mo. *Adjunctive therapy of* P. jirovecii *pneumonia in AIDS patients*—40 mg twice daily for 5 days, then 40 mg once daily for 5 days, then 20 mg once daily for 10 days.
PO (Children): *Nephrotic syndrome*—2 mg/kg/day initially given in 1–3 divided doses (maximum 80 mg/day) until urine is protein free for 4–6 weeks. Maintenance dose of 2 mg/kg/day every other day in the morning, gradually taper off after 4–6 weeks. *Asthma exacerbation*—1 mg/kg q 6 hr for 48 hr, then 1–2 mg/kg/day (maximum 60 mg/day) in divided doses twice daily.

Triamcinolone

IM (Adults): *Triamcinolone acetonide*—40–80 mg q 4 wk.
Intra-articular (Adults): *Triamcinolone hexacetonide*—2–20 mg q 3–4 wk (dose depends on size of joint to be injected, amount of inflammation, and amount of fluid present).
IM (Children): *Triamcinolone acetonide*—40 mg q 4 wk or 30–200 mcg/kg (1–6.25 mg/m²) q 1–7 days.

Availability

Betamethasone
Tablets: ✱ 0.5 mg. **Oral solution (cherry-or-ange flavor):** 0.6 mg/5 mL. **Effervescent tablets:** ✱ 0.5 mg. **Extended-release tablets:** ✱ 1 mg. **Suspension for injection (sodium phosphate and acetate):** 6 mg (total)/mL.

Budesonide
Capsules (enteric-coated): 3 mg.

Cortisone (generic available)
Tablets: 25 mg.

Dexamethasone (generic available)
Tablets: 0.5 mg, 0.75 mg, 1 mg, 1.5 mg, 2 mg, 4 mg, 6 mg. **Elixir (raspberry flavor):** 0.5 mg/5 mL. **Oral solution (cherry flavor):** 0.5 mg/5 mL, 1 mg/mL. **Solution for injection (sodium phosphate):** 4 mg/mL, 10 mg/mL.

Hydrocortisone (generic available)
Tablets: 5 mg, 10 mg, 20 mg. **Enema:** 100 mg/60 mL. **Powder for injection (sodium succinate):** 100 mg, 250 mg, 500 mg, 1 g.

Methylprednisolone (generic available)
Tablets: 2 mg, 4 mg, 8 mg, 16 mg, 32 mg. **Powder for injection (sodium succinate):** 40 mg, 125 mg, 500 mg, 1 g, 2 g. **Suspension for injection (acetate):** 20 mg/mL, 40 mg/mL, 80 mg/mL.

Prednisolone (generic available)
Tablets: 5 mg. **Orally disintegrating tablets (grape flavor):** 10 mg, 15 mg, 30 mg. **Oral solution:** 5 mg/5 mL, 10 mg/5 mL, 15 mg/5 mL, 20 mg/5 mL.

Prednisone (generic available)
Tablets: 1 mg, 2.5 mg, 5 mg, 10 mg, 20 mg, 50 mg. **Oral solution:** 1 mg/mL, 5 mg/mL.

Triamcinolone (generic available)
Suspension for injection (acetonide): 10 mg/mL, 40 mg/mL, 80 mg/mL. **Suspension for injection (hexacetonide):** 5 mg/mL, 20 mg/mL.

NURSING IMPLICATIONS

Assessment
- These drugs are indicated for many conditions. Assess involved systems before and periodically during therapy.
- Assess for signs of adrenal insufficiency (hypotension, weight loss, weakness, nausea, vomiting, anorexia, lethargy, confusion, restlessness) before and periodically during therapy.
- Monitor intake and output ratios and daily weights. Observe patient for peripheral edema, steady weight gain, rales/crackles, or dyspnea. Notify health care professional if these occur.
- Children should have periodic evaluations of growth.
- **Cerebral Edema:** Assess for changes in level of consciousness and headache during therapy.
- **Budesonide:** Assess signs of Crohn's disease (diarrhea, crampy abdominal pain, fever, bleeding from rectum) during therapy.
- **Rect:** Assess symptoms of ulcerative colitis (diarrhea, bleeding, weight loss, anorexia, fever, leukocytosis) periodically during therapy.
- *Lab Test Considerations:* Monitor serum electrolytes and glucose. May cause hyperglycemia, especially in persons with diabetes. May cause hypokalemia. Patients on prolonged therapy should routinely have CBC, serum electrolytes, and serum and urine glucose evaluated. May ↓ WBCs. May ↓ serum potassium and calcium and ↑ serum sodium concentrations.
- Guaiac-test stools. Promptly report presence of guaiac-positive stools.
- May ↑ serum cholesterol and lipid values. May ↓ uptake of thyroid ^{123}I or [131]I.
- Suppress reactions to allergy skin tests.
- Periodic adrenal function tests may be ordered to assess degree of hypothalamic-pituitary-ad-

CORTICOSTEROIDS (SYSTEMIC)

renal axis suppression in systemic and chronic topical therapy.
- **Dexamethasone Suppression Test:** : To diagnose Cushing's syndrome: Obtain baseline cortisol level; administer dexamethasone at 11 PM and obtain cortisol levels at 8 AM the next day. Normal response is a ↓ cortisol level.
- Alternative method: Obtain baseline 24-hr urine for 17-hydroxycorticosteroid (OHCS) concentrations, then begin 48-hr administration of dexamethasone. Second 24-hr urine for 17-OHCS is obtained after 24 hr of dexamethasone.

Potential Nursing Diagnoses
Risk for infection (Side Effects)
Disturbed body image (Side Effects)

Implementation
- Do not confuse prednisone with prednisolone, methylprednisolone, or primidone. Do not confuse hydrocortisone with hydrocodone.
- If dose is ordered daily or every other day, administer in the morning to coincide with the body's normal secretion of cortisol.
- Periods of stress, such as surgery, may require supplemental systemic corticosteroids.
- Patients with mild to moderate Crohn's disease may be switched from oral prednisolone without adrenal insufficiency by gradually decreasing prednisolone doses and adding budesonide.
- **PO:** Administer with meals to minimize GI irritation.
- Tablets may be crushed and administered with food or fluids for patients with difficulty swallowing. Capsules should be swallowed whole; do not crush, break, or chew.
- Use calibrated measuring device to ensure accurate dose of liquid forms.
- For orally disintegrating tablets (ODT), remove tablet from blister just prior to dosing. Peel blister pack open, and place tablet on tongue; may be swallowed whole or allowed to dissolve in mouth, with or without water. Tablets are friable; do not cut, split, or break.
- Avoid consumption of grapefruit juice during therapy with budesonide or methylprednisolone.
- **IM, Subcut:** Shake suspension well before drawing up. IM doses should not be administered when rapid effect is desirable. Do not dilute with other solution or admix. Do not administer suspensions IV.

Dexamethasone

IV Administration

- **Direct IV:** *Diluent:* May be given undiluted. *Concentration:* 4–10 mg/mL. *Rate:* Administer over 1–4 min if dose is <10 mg.
- **Intermittent Infusion:** *Diluent:* High-dose therapy should be added to D5W or 0.9% NaCl solution. Solution should be clear and colorless to light yellow; use diluted solution within 24 hr. *Concentration:* Up to 10 mg/mL. *Rate:* Administer infusions over 15–30 min.
- **Syringe Compatibility:** caffeine citrate, dimenhydrate, furosemide, granisetron, ketamine, metoclopramide, octreotide, palonosetron, ranitidine, sufentanil.
- **Syringe Incompatibility:** doxapram, glycopyrrolate, haloperidol, pantoprazole.
- **Y-Site Compatibility:** acyclovir, alfentanil, allopurinol, amifostine, amikacin, aminophylline, amphotericin B cholesteryl, amphotericin B liposome, amsacrine, anidulafungin, ascorbic acid, atracurium, atropine, aztreonam, bivalirudin, bumetanide, buprenorphine, butorphanol, carboplatin, cefazolin, cefepime, cefonocid, cefoperazone, cefotaxime, cefotetan, cefoxitin, ceftazidime, ceftizoxime, ceftriaxone, chloramphenicol, cimetidine, cisatracurium, cisplatin, cladribine, clindamycin, cyanocobalamin, cyclophosphamide, cyclosporine, cytarabine, dactinomycin, daptomycin, dexmedetomidine, digoxin, docetaxel, dopamine, doripenem, doxacurium, doxorubicin, doxorubicin liposome, enalaprilat, ephedrine, epinephrine, epoetin alfa, ertapenem, etoposide, etoposide phosphate, famotidine, fentanyl, filgrastim, fluconazole, fludarabine, fluorouracil, foscarnet, furosemide, ganciclovir, gemcitabine, glycopyrrolate, granisetron, heparin, hydromorphone, ifosfamide, imipenem/cilastatin, indomethacin, insulin, isoproterenol, ketorolac, levofloxacin, lidocaine, linezolid, lorazepam, mannitol, mechlorethamine, melphalan, meropenem, metaraminol, methadone, methoxamine, methyldopa, metoclopramide, metoprolol, metronidazole, milrinone, morphine, multivitamin, nafcillin, nalbuphine, naloxone, nitroglycerin, nitroprusside, norepinephrine, octreotide, ondansetron, oxaliplatin,

---

✦ = Canadian drug name.   ❖ = Genetic implication.
*CAPITALS indicates life-threatening; underlines indicate most frequent.

oxytocin, paclitaxel, palonosetron, pemetrexed, penicillin G, pentobarbital, phenobarbital, phenylephrine, phytonadione, piperacillin/tazobactam, potassium chloride, procainamide, propofol, propranolol, pyridoxime, ranitidine, remifentanil, rituximab, rocuronium, sargramostim, sodium acetate, sodium bicarbonate, streptokinase, succinylcholine, sufentanil, tacrolimus, teniposide, theophylline, thiamine, thiotepa, ticarcillin/clavulanate, tigecycline, tirofiban, tolazoline, trastuzumab, trimethaphan, urokinase, vancomycin, vasopressin, vecuronium, verapamil, vincristine, vinorelbine, vitamin B complex with C, voriconazole, zidovudine.

- **Y-Site Incompatibility:** amphotericin B colloidal, calcium chloride, calcium gluconate, caspofungin, cefuroxime, chlorpormazine, ciprofloxacin, dantrolene, diazepam, diazoxide, diphenhydramine, dobutamine, doxycycline, epirubicin, erythromycin, esmolol, fenoldopam, gentamicin, haloperidol, hydroxyzine, idarubicin, inamrinone, labetalol, magnesium sulfate, midazolam, mitoxantrone, pantoprazole, papaverine, pentamidine, pentazocine, phentolamine, phenytoin, prochlorperazine, promethazine, protamine, quinapristin/dalfopristin, tobramycin, topotecan, trimethoprim/sulfamethoxazole.

Hydrocortisone

IV Administration

- **Direct IV:** *Diluent:* Reconstitute with provided solution (i.e., Act-O-Vials) or 2 mL of bacteriostatic water or saline for injection. *Concentration:* 50 mg/mL. *Rate:* Administer each 100 mg over at least 30 sec. Doses 500 mg and larger should be infused over at least 10 min.
- **Intermittent/Continuous Infusion:** *Diluent:* May be added to 50–1000 mL of D5W, 0.9% NaCl, or D5/0.9% NaCl. Diluted solutions should be used within 24 hr. *Concentration:* 1–5 mg/mL. Concentrations of up to 60 mg/mL have been used in fluid restricted adults. *Rate:* Administer over 20–30 min or at prescribed rate.
- **Hydrocortisone sodium succinate Y-Site Compatibility:** acyclovir, alfentanil, allopurinol, amifostine, amikacin, aminophylline, amphotericin B cholesteryl, amphotericin B liposome, amsacrine, anidulafungin, argatroban, ascorbic acid, atracurium, atropine, aztreonam, bivalirudin, bumetanide, buprenorphine, butorphanol, carboplatin, caspofungin, cefazolin, cefepime, cefonocid, cefoperazone, cefotaxime, cefotetan, cefoxitin, ceftazidime, ceftizoxime, ceftriaxone, cefuroxime, chloramphenicol, chlorpromazine, cimetidine, cisatracurium, cisplatin, cladribine, clindamycin, cyanocobalamin, cyclophosphamide, cyclosporine, cytarabine, dactinomycin, daptomycin, dexmedetomidine, digoxin, docetaxel, dopamine, doripenem, doxacurium, doxorubicin hydrochloride, doxorubicin liposome, droperidol, edrophonium, enalaprilat, ephedrine, epinephrine, epirubicin, epoetin alfa, ertapenem, erythromycin, conjugated estrogens, ethacrynate, etoposide, famotidine, fenoldopam, fentanyl, filgrastim, fluconazole, fludarabine, fluorouracil, folic acid, foscarnet, furosemide, gallium nitrate, gemcitabine, glycopyrrolate, granisetron, heparin, hydromorphone, ifosfamide, imiepnem/cilastatin, indomethacin, insulin, isoproterenol, kanamycin, ketorolac, levofloxacin, lidocaine, linezolid, lorazepam, mannitol, mechlorethamine, melphalan, metaraminol, methotrexate, methoxamine, methyldopate, methylergonovine, metoclopramide, metoprolol, metronidazole, milrinone, mitoxantrone, morphine, multivitamins, nafcillin, naloxone, neostigmine, nesiritide, nicardipine, nitroglycerin, nitroprusside, norepinephrine, octreotide, ondansetron, oxacillin, oxaliplatin, oxytocin, paclitaxel, palonosetron, pancuronium, pantoprazole, pemetrexed, penicillin G potassium, pentobarbital, phenobarbital, phentolamine, phenylephrine, phytonadione, piperacillin/tazobactam, potassium chloride, procainamide, prochlorperazine, propofol, propranolol, pyridostigmine, ranitidine, remifentanil, rituximab, scopolamine, sodium acetate, sodium bicarbonate, succinylcholine, sufentanil, tacrolimus, teniposide, theophylline, thiotepa, ticarcillin/clavulanate, tigecycline, tirofiban, trastuzumab, trimethaphan, trimethobenzamide, urokinase, vasopressin, vecuronium, verapamil, vincristine, vinorelbine, voriconazole.

- **Y-Site Incompatibility:** amphotericin B colloidal, azathioprine, calcium chloride, ciprofloxacin, dantrolene, diazepam, diazoxide, dobutamine, doxycycline, ganciclovir, haloperidol, idarubicin, labetalol, lansoprazole, nalbuphine, pentamidine, phenytoin, protamine, pyridoxime, quinapristin/dalfopristin, rocuronium, sargramostim, thiamine, trimethoprim/sulfamethoxazole.

Methylprednisolone

IV Administration

- **Direct IV:** *Diluent:* Reconstitute with provided solution (Act-O-Vials, Univials) or 2 mL of bacteriostatic water (with benzyl alcohol) for injection. Use preservative-free diluent for use in neonates. Acetate injection is not for IV use. *Concentration:* Maximum concentration 125 mg/mL. *Rate:* Low dose (<1.8 mg/kg or <125 mg/dose): May be administered direct IV push over 1 to several minutes. Moderate dose (2 mg/kg or 250 mg/dose): give over 15–30 min. High dose (15 mg/kg or 500 mg/dose): give over 30 min. Doses 15 mg/kg or 1 g give over 1 hour.
- **Intermittent/Continuous Infusion:** *Diluent:* May be diluted further in D5W, 0.9% NaCl, or D5/0.9% NaCl and administered as intermittent or continuous infusion at the prescribed rate. *Concentration:* Maximum 2.5 mg/mL. Solution may form a haze upon dilution.
- **Syringe Compatibility:** granisetron, metoclopramide.
- **Syringe Incompatibility:** pantoprazole.
- **Y-Site Compatibility:** acyclovir, alfentanil, alprostadil, amifostine, amikacin, aminophylline, amiodarone, amphotericin B cholesteryl, amphotericin B liposome, anidulafungin, ascorbic acid, atracurium, atropine, aztreonam, bivalirudin, bumetanide, buprenorphine, butorphanol, carboplatin, cefazolin, cefepime, cefoperazone, cefotetan, ceftazidime, ceftriaxone, cefuroxime, chloramphenicol, chlorpromazine, cimetidine, cisplatin, cladribine, clindamycin, cyanocobalamin, cyclophosphamide, cyclosproine, cytarabine, dactinomycin, daptomycin, dexmedetomidine, digoxin, dobutamine, dopamine, doxacurium, doxorubicin liposome, enalaprilat, ephedrine, epinephrine, epoetin alfa, ertapenem, erythromycin, etoposide, famotidine, fentanyl, fludarabine, fluorouracil, folic acid, furosemide, gentamicin, glycopyrrolate, granisetron, hydromorphone, ifosphamide, imiepnem/cilastatin, insulin, isoproterenol, ketorolac, labetalol, levofloxacin, linezolid, lorazepam, mannitol, mechlorethamine, melphalan, metaraminol, methotrexate, methoxamine, methyldopate, metronidazole, metoprolol, metronidazole, milrinone, morphine, multivitamin, nafcillin, naloxone, nesiritide, nicardipine, nitroglycerin, nitroprusside, norepinephrine, octreotide, oxaliplatin, oxytocin, pemetrexed, penicillin G, pentobarbital, phenobarbital, phenylephrine, piperacillin/tazobactam, procainamide, prochlorperazine, propranolol, ranitidine, remifentanil, rituximab, sodium acetate, sodium bicarbonate, streptokinase, succinylcholine, sufentanil, tacrolimus, teniposide, theophylline, thiotepa, ticarcillin/clavulanate, tirofiban, tobramycin, tolazoline, topotecan, trastuzumab, vancomycin, vasopressin, verapamil, vincristine, voriconazole.
- **Y-Site Incompatibility:** allopurinol, amphotericin B colloidal, amphotericin B liposome, ampicillin/sulbactam, amsacrine, calcium chloride, calcium gluconate, caspofungin, cefotaxime, cefoxitin, ciprofloxacin, dantrolene, diazepam, diazoxide, diphenhydramine, docetaxel, doxycycline, epirubicin, etoposide phosphate, fenoldopam, filgrastim, ganciclovir, gemcitabine, haloperidol, hydralazine, ketamine, lansoprazole, magnesium sulfate, mitoxantrone, nalbuphine, paclitaxel, palonosetron, pantoprazole, papaverine, pentamidine, pentazocine, phenytoin, promethazine, propofol, protamine, pyridoxime, quinapristin/dalfopristin, rocuronium, sargramostim, thiamine, trimethoprim/sulfamethoxazole, vecuronium, vinorelbine.
- **Rect:** Position patient on left side and administer nightly for 21 days. Enema should be retained for at least 1 hr and preferably all night. May use sedatives and antidiarrheals to facilitate retention.

Patient/Family Teaching

- Instruct patient on correct technique of medication administration. Advise patient to take medication as directed. Take missed doses as soon as remembered unless almost time for next dose. Do not double doses. Stopping the medication suddenly may result in adrenal insufficiency (anorexia, nausea, weakness, fatigue, dyspnea, hypotension, hypoglycemia). If these signs appear, notify health care professional immediately. This can be life threatening.
- Corticosteroids cause immunosuppression and may mask symptoms of infection. Instruct patient to avoid people with known contagious illnesses and to report possible infections immediately.

- *Prelone* syrup should not be refrigerated, *Pediapred* solution may be refrigerated, *Orapred* solution should be refrigerated.
- Caution patient to avoid vaccinations without first consulting health care professional.
- Review side effects with patient. Instruct patient to inform health care professional promptly if severe abdominal pain or tarry stools occur. Patient should also report unusual swelling, weight gain, tiredness, bone pain, bruising, nonhealing sores, visual disturbances, or behavior changes.
- Advise patient to notify health care professional of medication regimen before treatment or surgery.
- Discuss possible effects on body image. Explore coping mechanisms.
- Instruct patient to inform health care professional if symptoms of underlying disease return or worsen.
- Advise patient to carry identification describing disease process and medication regimen in the event of emergency in which patient cannot relate medical history.
- Explain need for continued medical follow-up to assess effectiveness and possible side effects of medication. Periodic lab tests and eye exams may be needed.
- **Long-term Therapy:** Encourage patient to eat a diet high in protein, calcium, and potassium, and low in sodium and carbohydrates (see Appendix M). Alcohol should be avoided during therapy; may ↑ risk of GI irritation.
- If rectal dose used 21 days, decrease to every other night for 2–3 weeks to decrease gradually.

Evaluation/Desired Outcomes
- Decrease in presenting symptoms with minimal systemic side effects.
- Suppression of the inflammatory and immune responses in autoimmune disorders, allergic reactions, and neoplasms.
- Management of symptoms in adrenal insufficiency.
- Improvement of symptoms/sequelae of Crohn's disease (decreased frequency of liquid stools, decreased abdominal complaints, improved sense of well being).
- Improvement in symptoms of ulcerative colitis. Clinical symptoms usually improve in 3–5 days. Mucosal appearance may require 2–3 months to improve.

CORTICOSTEROIDS (TOPICAL/LOCAL)

alclometasone (al-kloe-**met**-a-sone)
Aclovate

amcinonide (am-**sin**-oh-nide)
✢Cyclocort

betamethasone (bay-ta-**meth**-a-sone)
✢Betacort, ✢Betaderm, Beta-Val, ✢Betnovate, ✢Celestoderm, Dermabet, Diprolene, Diprolene AF, ✢Ectosone, Luxiq, ✢Metaderm, ✢Novobetamet, ✢Prevex, ✢Topilene, ✢Topisone, Valnac

clobetasol (kloe-**bay**-ta-sol)
Clobex, Cormax, ✢Dermovate, Embeline, Embeline E, Olux, Olux-E, Temovate, Temovate E

clocortolone (kloe-**kor**-toe-lone)
Cloderm

desonide (**des**-oh-nide)
Desonate, DesOwen, Verdeso

desoximetasone (dess-ox-i-**met**-a-sone)
Topicort, Topicort-LP

diflorasone (dye-**flor**-a-sone)
Psorcon

fluocinolone (floo-oh-**sin**-oh-lone)
Capex, Derma-Smoothe/FS, ✢Fluoderm, ✢Fluolar, ✢Fluonide, Synalar, ✢Synamol

fluocinonide (floo-oh-**sin**-oh-nide)
✢Lidemol, Lidex, Lidex-E, ✢Lyderm, ✢Topsyn, Vanos

flurandrenolide (flure-an-**dren**-oh-lide)
Cordran, Cordran-SP, ✢Drenison

fluticasone (floo-**tik**-a-sone)
Cutivate

halcinonide (hal-**sin**-oh-nide)
Halog

halobetasol (hal-oh-**bay**-ta-sol)
Ultravate

CORTICOSTEROIDS (TOPICAL/LOCAL)

hydrocortisone
(hye-droe-**kor**-ti-sone)
Acticort, Aeroseb-HC, Ala-Cort, Ala-Scalp, Alphaderm, Anusol HC, Bactine, ✸ Barriere-HC, CaldeCORT Anti-Itch, Carmol HC, Cetacort, ✸ Cortacet, Cortaid, ✸ Cortate, Cort-Dome, ✸ Cortef Feminine Itch, Corticaine, ✸ Corticreme, Cortifair, Cortifoam, Cortizone, Dermacort, DermiCort, Dermtex HC, ✸ Emo-Cort, FoilleCort, Gynecort, Hemril-HC, Hi-Cor, Hycort, ✸ Hyderm, Hydro-Tex, Hytone, Lacti-Care-HC, Lanacort 9-1-1, Lemoderm, Locoid, ✸ Novohydrocort, Nutracort, Orabase-HCA, Pandel, Penecort, Pharma-Cort, Prevex HC, Proctocort, Rhulicort, Synacort, Texacort, ✸ Unicort, Westcort

mometasone (moe-**met**-a-sone)
✸ Elocom, Elocon

prednicarbate (pred-ni-**kar**-bate)
Dermatop

triamcinolone
(trye-am-**sin**-oh-lone)
Kenalog, ✸ Triaderm, ✸ Trianide, Triderm

Classification
Therapeutic: anti-inflammatories (steroidal)
Pharmacologic: corticosteroids (topical)

Pregnancy Category C

Indications
Management of inflammation and pruritis associated with various allergic/immunologic skin problems.

Action
Suppress normal immune response and inflammation. **Therapeutic Effects:** Suppression of dermatologic inflammation and immune processes.

Pharmacokinetics
Absorption: Minimal. Prolonged use on large surface areas, application of large amounts, or use of occlusive dressings may ↑ systemic absorption.
Distribution: Remain primarily at site of action.
Metabolism and Excretion: Usually metabolized in skin; some have been modified to resist local metabolism and have a prolonged local effect.
Half-life: *Betamethasone*—3–5 hr (plasma), 36–54 hr (tissue). *Dexamethasone*—3–4.5 hr (plasma), 36–54 hr (tissue). *Hydrocortisone*—1.5–2 hr (plasma), 8–12 hr (tissue). *Triamcinolone*—2–>5 hr (plasma), 18–36 hr (tissue).

TIME/ACTION PROFILE (response depends on condition being treated)

ROUTE	ONSET	PEAK	DURATION
Topical	min–hr	hr–days	hr–days

Contraindications/Precautions
Contraindicated in: Hypersensitivity or known intolerance to corticosteroids or components of vehicles (ointment or cream base, preservative, alcohol); Untreated bacterial or viral infections.
Use Cautiously in: Hepatic dysfunction; Diabetes mellitus, cataracts, glaucoma, or tuberculosis (use of large amounts of high-potency agents may worsen condition); Patients with pre-existing skin atrophy; OB, Lactation: Chronic use at high dosages may result in adrenal suppression in mother and growth suppression in children; Pedi: Children may be more susceptible to adrenal and growth suppression. Clobetasol not recommended for children <12 yr; desoximetasone not recommended for children <10 yr.

Adverse Reactions/Side Effects
Derm: allergic contact dermatitis, atrophy, burning, dryness, edema, folliculitis, hypersensitivity reactions, hypertrichosis, hypopigmentation, irritation, maceration, miliaria, perioral dermatitis, secondary infection, striae. **Misc:** adrenal suppression (↑ dose, long-term therapy).

Interactions
Drug-Drug: None significant.

Route/Dosage
Topical (Adults and Children): 1–4 times daily (depends on product, preparation, and condition being treated).
Rect (Adults): hydrocortisone *Aerosol foam*—90 mg 1–2 times/day for 2–3 wk; then adjusted.

Availability

Alclometasone (generic available)
Cream: 0.05%. **Ointment:** 0.05%.

CORTICOSTEROIDS (TOPICAL/LOCAL)

Amcinonide (generic available)
Cream: 0.1%. Lotion: 0.1%. Ointment: 0.1%.

Betamethasone (generic available)
Cream: 0.05%, 0.1%. Gel: 0.05%. Lotion: 0.05%, 0.1%. Ointment: 0.05%, 0.1%. Aerosol Foam: 0.12%. *In combination with:* clotrimazole (Lotrisone), calcipotriene (Taclonex); see Appendix B.

Clobetasol (generic available)
Cream: 0.05%. Emollient cream: 0.05%. Foam: 0.05%. Gel: 0.05%. Ointment: 0.05%. Foam: 0.05%. Lotion: 0.05%. Scalp solution: 0.05%. Shampoo: 0.05%. Spray: 0.05%.

Clocortolone
Cream: 0.1%.

Desonide (generic available)
Cream: 0.05%. Foam: 0.05%. Gel: 0.05%. Ointment: 0.05%. Lotion: 0.05%.

Desoximetasone (generic available)
Cream: 0.05%, 0.25%. Gel: 0.05%. Ointment: 0.25%.

Diflorasone (generic available)
Cream: 0.05%. Ointment: 0.05%.

Fluocinolone (generic available)
Cream: 0.01%, 0.025%. Ointment: 0.025%. Solution: 0.01%. Shampoo: 0.01%. Oil: 0.01%.

Fluocinonide (generic available)
Cream: 0.05%, 0.1%. Gel: 0.05%. Ointment: 0.05%. Solution: 0.05%.

Flurandrenolide
Cream: 0.025%, 0.05%. Ointment: 0.025%, 0.05%. Lotion: 0.05%. Tape: 4 mcg/m^2.

Fluticasone (generic available)
Cream: 0.05%. Lotion: 0.05%. Ointment: 0.005%.

Halcinonide
Cream: 0.1%. Ointment: 0.1%. Solution: 0.1%.

Halobetasol (generic available)
Cream: 0.05%. Ointment: 0.05%.

Hydrocortisone (generic available)
Cream: 0.1%, 0.2%, 0.5%[Rx, OTC], 1%[Rx, OTC], 2.5%. Gel: 1%[Rx, OTC]. Ointment: 0.1%, 0.2%, 0.5%[Rx, OTC], 1%[Rx, OTC], 2.5%. Lotion: 1%[Rx, OTC], 2.5%. Solution: 1%, 2.5%. Spray: 0.5%[Rx, OTC], 1%[Rx, OTC]. Rectal cream: 1%. Rectal aerosol: 10%. *In combination with:* acetic acid, antifungals, anti-infectives, antihistamines, urea, and benzoyl peroxide in various otic and topical preparations; acyclovir (Lipsovir cream). See Appendix B.

Mometasone (generic available)
Cream: 0.1%. Ointment: 0.1%. Lotion: 0.1%.

Prednicarbate (generic available)
Cream: 0.1%.

Triamcinolone (generic available)
Cream: 0.025%, 0.1%, 05%. Ointment: 0.025%, 0.1%, 0.5%. Lotion: 0.025%, 0.1%. Spray: 0.2 mg/2-sec spray. *In combination with:* acetic acid, antifungals, anti-infectives, antihistamines, urea, and benzoyl peroxide in various otic and topical preparations. See Appendix B.

NURSING IMPLICATIONS

Assessment
- Assess affected skin before and daily during therapy. Note degree of inflammation and pruritus. Notify health care professional if symptoms of infection (increased pain, erythema, purulent exudate) develop.
- ***Lab Test Considerations:*** Adrenal function tests may be ordered to assess degree of hypothalamic-pituitary-adrenal (HPA) axis suppression in long-term topical therapy. Children and patients with dose applied to a large area, using an occlusive dressing, or using high-potency products are at highest risk for HPA suppression.
- May cause ↑ serum and urine glucose concentrations if significant absorption occurs.

Potential Nursing Diagnoses
Risk for impaired skin integrity (Indications)
Risk for infection (Side Effects)

Implementation
- Choice of vehicle depends on site and type of lesion. Ointments are more occlusive and preferred for dry, scaly lesions. Creams should be used on oozing or intertriginous areas, where the occlusive action of ointments might cause folliculitis or maceration. Creams may be preferred for esthetic reasons even though they may dry skin more than ointments. Gels, aerosols, lotions, and solutions are useful in hairy areas.
- **Topical:** Apply *ointments, creams,* or *gels* sparingly as a thin film to clean, slightly moist skin. Wear gloves. Apply occlusive dressing only if specified by health care professional.

- Apply *lotion, solution,* or *gel* to hair by parting hair and applying a small amount to affected area. Rub in gently. Protect area from washing, clothing, or rubbing until medication has dried. Hair may be washed as usual but not right after applying medication.
- Use *aerosols* by shaking well and spraying on affected area, holding container 3–6 in. away. Spray for about 2 seconds to cover an area the size of a hand. Do not inhale. If spraying near face, cover eyes.

Patient/Family Teaching
- Instruct patient on correct technique of medication administration. Emphasize importance of avoiding the eyes. Apply missed doses as soon as remembered unless almost time for the next dose.
- Caution patient to use only as directed. Avoid using cosmetics, bandages, dressings, or other skin products over the treated area unless directed by health care professional.
- Advise parents of pediatric patients not to apply tight-fitting diapers or plastic pants on a child treated in the diaper area; these garments work as an occlusive dressing and may cause more of the drug to be absorbed.
- Caution women that medication should not be used extensively, in large amounts, or for protracted periods if they are pregnant or planning to become pregnant.
- Advise patient to consult health care professional before using medicine for condition other than indicated.
- Instruct patient to inform health care professional if symptoms of underlying disease return or worsen or if symptoms of infection develop.

Evaluation/Desired Outcomes
- Resolution of skin inflammation, pruritus, or other dermatologic conditions.

---

cortisone, See CORTICOSTEROIDS (SYSTEMIC).

---

cyanocobalamin, See VITAMIN B$_{12}$ PREPARATIONS.

---

cyclobenzaprine
(sye-kloe-**ben**-za-preen)
Amrix, Flexeril

Classification
Therapeutic: skeletal muscle relaxants (centrally acting)

Pregnancy Category B

Indications
Management of acute painful musculoskeletal conditions associated with muscle spasm. **Unlabeled Use:** Management of fibromyalgia.

Action
Reduces tonic somatic muscle activity at the level of the brainstem. Structurally similar to tricyclic antidepressants. **Therapeutic Effects:** Reduction in muscle spasm and hyperactivity without loss of function.

Pharmacokinetics
Absorption: Well absorbed from the GI tract.
Distribution: Unknown.
Protein Binding: 93%.
Metabolism and Excretion: Mostly metabolized by the liver.
Half-life: 1–3 days.

TIME/ACTION PROFILE (skeletal muscle relaxation)

ROUTE	ONSET	PEAK†	DURATION
PO	within 1 hr	3–8 hr	12–24 hr
Extended release	unk	unk	24 hr

†Full effects may not occur for 1–2 wk

Contraindications/Precautions
Contraindicated in: Hypersensitivity; Should not be used within 14 days of MAO inhibitor therapy; Immediate period after MI; Severe or symptomatic cardiovascular disease; Cardiac conduction disturbances; Hyperthyroidism.
Use Cautiously in: Cardiovascular disease; Geri: Appears on Beers list. Poorly tolerated due to anticholinergic effects; OB, Lactation, Pedi: Pregnancy, lactation, and children <15 yr (safety not established).

Adverse Reactions/Side Effects
CNS: dizziness, drowsiness, confusion, fatigue, headache, nervousness. **EENT:** dry mouth,

blurred vision. **CV:** arrhythmias. **GI:** constipation, dyspepsia, nausea, unpleasant taste. **GU:** urinary retention.

Interactions
Drug-Drug: Additive CNS depression with other **CNS depressants**, including **alcohol**, **antihistamines**, **opioid analgesics**, and **sedative/hypnotics**. Additive anticholinergic effects with **drugs possessing anticholinergic properties**, including **antihistamines**, **antidepressants**, **atropine**, **disopyramide**, **haloperidol**, and **phenothiazines**. Avoid use within 14 days of **MAO inhibitors** (hyperpyretic crisis, seizures, and death may occur).
Drug-Natural Products: Concomitant use of **kava-kava**, **valerian**, **chamomile**, or **hops** can ↑ CNS depression.

Route/Dosage
PO (Adults): *Acute painful musculoskeletal conditions*— 10 mg 3 times daily (range 20–40 mg/day in 2–4 divided doses; not to exceed 60 mg/day) *or* extended-release, 15–30 mg once daily. *Fibromyalgia*— 5–40 mg at bedtime (unlabeled).

Availability (generic available)
Tablets : 5 mg, 10 mg. **Cost:** *Generic*— 5 mg $18.85/100, 10 mg $18.86/100. **Extended-release capsules (Amrix):** 15 mg, 30 mg. **Cost:** 15 mg $773.97/90.

NURSING IMPLICATIONS

Assessment
- Assess patient for pain, muscle stiffness, and range of motion before and periodically throughout therapy.
- **Geri:** Assess geriatric patients for anticholinergic effects (sedation and weakness).

Potential Nursing Diagnoses
Acute pain (Indications)
Impaired physical mobility (Indications)
Risk for injury (Side Effects)

Implementation
- Do not confuse cyclobenzaprine with cyproheptadine.
- **PO:** May be administered with meals to minimize gastric irritation.
- Swallow extended-release capsules whole; do not open, crush, or chew.

Patient/Family Teaching
- Instruct patient to take medication as directed; do not take more than the prescribed amount. Taken missed doses within 1 hr of time ordered; otherwise, return to normal dose schedule. Do not double doses.
- Medication may cause drowsiness, dizziness, and blurred vision. Caution patient to avoid driving or other activities requiring alertness until response to drug is known.
- Advise patient to avoid concurrent use of alcohol or other CNS depressants with this medication.
- If constipation becomes a problem, advise patient that increasing fluid intake and bulk in diet and stool softeners may alleviate this condition.
- Advise patient to notify health care professional if symptoms of urinary retention (distended abdomen, feeling of fullness, overflow incontinence, voiding small amounts) occur.
- Inform patient that good oral hygiene, frequent mouth rinses, and sugarless gum or candy may help relieve dry mouth.

Evaluation/Desired Outcomes
- Relief of muscular spasm in acute skeletal muscle conditions. Maximum effects may not be evident for 1–2 wk. Use is usually limited to 2–3 wk; however, has been effective for at least 12 wk in the management of fibromyalgia.

HIGH ALERT

cyclophosphamide
(sye-kloe-**fos**-fa-mide)
✦ Procytox

Classification
Therapeutic: antineoplastics, immunosuppressants
Pharmacologic: alkylating agents

Pregnancy Category D

Indications
Alone or with other modalities in the management of: Hodgkin's disease, Malignant lymphomas, Multiple myeloma, Leukemias, Mycosis fungoides, Neuroblastoma, Ovarian carcinoma, Breast carcinoma, and a variety of other tumors. Minimal change nephrotic syndrome in children. **Unlabeled Use:** Severe active rheumatoid arthritis or Wegener's granulomatosis.

Action
Interferes with DNA replication and RNA transcription, ultimately disrupting protein synthesis

(cell-cycle phase–nonspecific). **Therapeutic Effects:** Death of rapidly replicating cells, particularly malignant ones. Also has immunosuppressant action in smaller doses.

Pharmacokinetics
Absorption: Inactive parent drug is well absorbed from the GI tract. Converted to active drug by the liver.
Distribution: Widely distributed. Limited penetration of the blood-brain barrier. Crosses the placenta; enters breast milk.
Metabolism and Excretion: Converted to active drug by the liver; 30% eliminated unchanged by the kidneys.
Half-life: 4–6.5 hr.

TIME/ACTION PROFILE (effects on blood counts)

ROUTE	ONSET	PEAK	DURATION
PO, IV	7 days	7–15 days	21 days

Contraindications/Precautions
Contraindicated in: Hypersensitivity; OB, Lactation: Pregnancy or lactation.
Use Cautiously in: Active infections; Bone marrow depression; Other chronic debilitating illnesses; OB: Patients with childbearing potential.

Adverse Reactions/Side Effects
Resp: PULMONARY FIBROSIS. **CV:** MYOCARDIAL FIBROSIS, hypotension. **GI:** anorexia, nausea, vomiting. **GU:** HEMORRHAGIC CYSTITIS, hematuria. **Derm:** alopecia. **Endo:** gonadal suppression, syndrome of inappropriate antidiuretic hormone (SIADH). **Hemat:** LEUKOPENIA, thrombocytopenia, anemia. **Metab:** hyperuricemia. **Misc:** secondary neoplasms.

Interactions
Drug-Drug: Phenobarbital or **rifampin** may ↑ toxicity of cyclophosphamide. Concurrent **allopurinol** or **thiazide diuretics** may exaggerate bone marrow depression. May prolong neuromuscular blockade from **succinylcholine**. Cardiotoxicity may be additive with other **cardiotoxic agents** (e.g., **cytarabine, daunorubicin, doxorubicin**). May ↓ serum **digoxin** levels. Additive bone marrow depression with other **antineoplastics** or **radiation therapy**. May potentiate the effects of **warfarin**. May ↓ antibody response to **live-virus vaccines** and ↑ risk of adverse reactions. Prolongs the effects of **cocaine**.

Route/Dosage
Many regimens are used.
PO (Adults): 1–5 mg/kg/day.
PO (Children): *Induction*—2–8 mg/kg/day (60–250 mg/m²/day) in divided doses for 6 days or longer. *Maintenance*—2–5 mg/kg (50–150 mg/m²/day) twice weekly.
IV (Adults): 40–50 mg/kg in divided doses over 2–5 days *or* 10–15 mg/kg q 7–10 days *or* 3–5 mg/kg twice weekly *or* 1.5–3 mg/kg/day. Other regimens may use larger doses.
IV (Children): *Induction*—2–8 mg/kg/day (60–250 mg/m²/day) in divided doses for 6 days or longer. Total dose for 7 days may be given as a single weekly dose. *Maintenance*—10–15 mg/kg every 7–10 days or 30 mg/kg q 3–4 wk.

Availability (generic available)
Tablets: 25 mg, 50 mg. **Injection:** 500 mg, ✤ 750 mg, 1 g, 2 g.

NURSING IMPLICATIONS
Assessment
- Monitor blood pressure, pulse, respiratory rate, and temperature frequently during administration. Report significant changes.
- Monitor urinary output frequently during therapy. To reduce the risk of hemorrhagic cystitis, fluid intake should be at least 3000 mL/day for adults and 1000–2000 mL/day for children. May be administered with mesna.
- Monitor for bone marrow depression. Assess for bleeding (bleeding gums, bruising, petechiae, guaiac stools, urine, and emesis) and avoid IM injections and taking rectal temperatures if platelet count is low. Apply pressure to venipuncture sites for 10 min. Assess for signs of infection during neutropenia. Anemia may occur. Monitor for increased fatigue, dyspnea, and orthostatic hypotension.
- Assess nausea, vomiting, and appetite. Weigh weekly. Antiemetics may be given 30 min before administration of medication to minimize GI effects. Anorexia and weight loss can be minimized by feeding frequent light meals.
- Encourage patient to drink 2000–3000 mL/day to promote excretion of uric acid. Alkalinization of the urine may be used to help prevent uric acid nephropathy.
- Assess cardiac and respiratory status for dyspnea, rales/crackles, weight gain, edema. Pulmonary toxicity may occur after prolonged therapy. Cardiotoxicity may occur early in therapy and is characterized by symptoms of CHF.

- **Lab Test Considerations:** Monitor CBC with differential and platelet count before and periodically during therapy. The nadir of leukopenia occurs in 7–12 days (recovery in 17–21 days). Leukocytes should be maintained at 2500–4000/mm³. May also cause thrombocytopenia (nadir 10–15 days), and rarely causes anemia.
- Monitor BUN, creatinine, and uric acid before and frequently during therapy to detect nephrotoxicity.
- Monitor ALT, AST, LDH, and serum bilirubin before and frequently during therapy to detect hepatotoxicity.
- Urinalysis should be evaluated before initiating therapy and frequently during therapy to detect hematuria or change in specific gravity indicative of SIADH.
- May suppress positive reactions to skin tests for *Candida*, mumps, *Trichophyton*, and tuberculin purified-protein derivative (PPD). May also produce false-positive results in Papanicolaou smears.

Potential Nursing Diagnoses
Risk for infection (Side Effects)
Disturbed body image (Side Effects)

Implementation
- **High Alert:** Fatalities have occurred with chemotherapeutic agents. Before administering, clarify all ambiguous orders; double-check single, daily, and course-of-therapy dose limits; have second practitioner independently double-check original order, calculations, and infusion pump settings. Do not confuse cyclophosphamide with cyclosporine. Do not confuse Cytoxan (cyclophosphamide) with Cytozar (cytarabine) or Cytotec (misoprostol).
- **PO:** Administer medication on an empty stomach. If severe gastric irritation develops, medication may be given with food.
- Oral solution can be formed by diluting powder for injection in aromatic elixir to a concentration of 1–5 mg of cyclophosphamide/mL. Reconstituted preparations should be refrigerated and used within 2 wk.
- **IV:** Prepare solution for IV administration in a biologic cabinet. Wear gloves, gown, and mask while handling IV medication. Discard IV equipment in specially designated containers.
- Prepare IV solution by diluting each 100 mg with 5 mL of sterile water or bacteriostatic water for injection containing parabens. Shake solution gently and allow to stand until clear. Use solution without bacteriostatic water within 6 hr. Solution prepared with bacteriostatic water is stable for 24 hr at room temperature, 6 days if refrigerated.

IV Administration
- **Direct IV:** Administer reconstituted solution undiluted. ***Concentration:*** 20 mg/mL. ***Rate:*** Administer at a rate of 100 mg/min.
- **Intermittent Infusion:** ***Diluent:*** May be further diluted in up to 250 mL of D5W, 0.9% NaCl, 0.45% NaCl, dextrose/saline combinations, LR, or dextrose/Ringer's solution. ***Concentration:*** 20–25 mg/mL. ***Rate:*** Administer over 30–60 min..
- **Syringe Compatibility:** bleomycin, cisplatin, doxapram, doxorubicin, droperidol, fluorouracil, furosemide, heparin, leucovorin calcium, methotrexate, metoclopramide, mitomycin, vinblastine, vincristine.
- **Y-Site Compatibility:** acyclovir, alfentanil, allopurinol, amifostine, amikacin, aminocaproic acid, aminophylline, amiodarone, amphotericin B liposome, ampicillin, ampicillin/sulbactam, anidulafungin, atracurium, aztreonam, bivalirudin, bleomycin, bumetanide, buprenorphine, butorphanol, calcium chloride, calcium gluconate, carboplatin, caspofungin, cefazolin, cefepime, cefoperazone, cefotaxime, cefoxitin, ceftazidime, ceftizoxime, ceftriaxone, cefuroxime, chloramphenicol, chlorpromazine, cimetidine, ciprofloxacin, cisatracurium, cisplatin, cladribine, clindamycin, codeine, cyclosporine, cytarabine, dactinomycin, dapotomycin, daunorubicin, dexamethasone, dexmedetomidine, dexrazoxane, digoxin, diltiazem, diphenhydramine, dobutamine, docetaxel, dolasetron, dopamine, doripenem, doxacurium, doxorubicin, doxorubicin liposome, doxycycline, droperidol, enalaprilat, ephedrine, epinephrine, epirubicin, ertapenem, erythromycin, esmolol, etoposide, etoposide phosphate, famotidine, fenoldopam, fentanyl, filgrastim, fluconazole, fludarabine, fluorouracil, foscarnet, fosphenytoin, furosemide, ganciclovir, gemcitabine, gentamicin, granisetron, haloperidol, heparin, hetastarch, hydrocortisone, hydromorphone, idarubicin, imipenem/cilastatin, inamrinone, insulin, isoproterenol, kanamycin, ketorolac, labetalol, leucovorin calcium, levofloxacin, levorphanol, lidocaine, linezolid, lorazepam, magnesium sulfate, mannitol, melphalan, meperidine, meropenem, mesna, methohexital, methotrexate, methylprednisolone, metoclopramide, metoprolol, metronidazole, midazolam, milrinone, mitomycin, mitoxantrone, morphine, nafcillin, nalbuphine, naloxone, nesiritide, nitroglycerin, nitroprus-

side, norepinephrine, octreotide, ondansetron, oxacillin, oxaliplatin, paclitaxel, palonosetron, pancuronium, pantoprazole, pemetrexed, penicillin G potassium, pentamidine, pentobarbital, phenobarbital, phenylephrine, piperacillin/tazobactam, potassium chloride, potassium phosphates, procainamide, prochlorperazine, promethazine, propofol, propranolol, quinupristin/dalfopristin, ranitidine, remifentanil, rituximab, rocuronium, sargramostim, sodium acetate, sodium bicarbonate, sodium phosphates, succinylcholine, sufentanil, tacrolimus, teniposide, theophylline, thiopental, thiotepa, ticarcillin/clavulanate, tigecycline, tirofiban, tobramycin, topotecan, trastuzumjab, trimethoprim/sulfamethoxazole, vancomycin, vasopressin, vecuronium, verapamil, vinblastine, vincristine, vinorelbine, voriconazole, zidovudine.
- **Y-Site Incompatibility:** amphotericin B cholesteryl, amphotericin B colloidal, diazepam, phenytoin.

Patient/Family Teaching
- Instruct patient to take dose in early morning. Emphasize need for adequate fluid intake for 72 hr after therapy. Patient should void frequently to decrease bladder irritation from metabolites excreted by the kidneys. Report hematuria immediately. If a dose is missed, contact health care professional.
- Instruct patient to notify health care professional promptly if fever; sore throat; signs of infection; lower back or side pain; difficult or painful urination; sores in the mouth or on the lips; yellow discoloration of skin or eyes; bleeding gums; bruising; petechiae; blood in urine, stool, or emesis; unusual swelling; joint pain; shortness of breath; or confusion occurs. Caution patient to avoid crowds and persons with known infections. Instruct patient to use soft toothbrush and electric razor and to avoid falls. Patient should also be cautioned not to drink alcoholic beverages or to take products containing aspirin or NSAIDs; may precipitate GI hemorrhage.
- Advise patient that this medication may cause sterility and menstrual irregularities or cessation of menses. This drug is also teratogenic, and contraceptive measures should continue for at least 4 mo after completion of therapy.
- Discuss with patient the possibility of hair loss. Explore methods of coping. May also cause darkening of skin and fingernails.
- Instruct patient not to receive any vaccinations without advice of health care professional.

Evaluation/Desired Outcomes
- Decrease in size or spread of malignant tumors.
- Improvement of hematologic status in patients with leukemia. Maintenance therapy is instituted if leukocyte count remains between 2500 and 4000/mm^3 and if patient does not demonstrate serious side effects.
- Management of minimal change nephrotic syndrome in children.

---

cycloSPORINE†
(**sye**-kloe-spor-een)
Neoral, Sandimmune, Gengraf

Classification
Therapeutic: immunosuppressants, antirheumatics (DMARD)
Pharmacologic: polypeptides (cyclic)

Pregnancy Category C
†See Appendix C for ophthalmic use

Indications
PO, IV: Prevention and treatment of rejection in renal, cardiac, and hepatic transplantation (with corticosteroids). **PO:** Treatment of severe active rheumatoid arthritis (Neoral only). Treatment of severe recalcitrant psoriasis in adult nonimmunocompromised patients (Neoral only). **Unlabeled Use:** Management of recalcitrant ulcerative colitis. Treatment of steroid resistant nephrotic syndrome. Treatment of severe steroid resistant autoimmune disease. Prevention and treatment of graft vs. host disease in bone marrow transplant patients.

Action
Inhibits normal immune responses (cellular and humoral) by inhibiting interleukin-2, a factor necessary for initiation of T-cell activity. **Therapeutic Effects:** Prevention of rejection reactions. Slowed progression of rheumatoid arthritis or psoriasis.

Pharmacokinetics
Absorption: Erratically absorbed (range 10–60%) after oral administration, with significant

first-pass metabolism by the liver. Microemulsion (Neoral) has better bioavailability.
Distribution: Widely distributed, mainly into extracellular fluid and blood cells. Crosses the placenta; enters breast milk.
Protein Binding: 90–98%.
Metabolism and Excretion: Extensively metabolized by the liver (first pass); excreted in bile, small amounts excreted unchanged in urine.
Half-life: Children—7 hr; adults—19 hr.

TIME/ACTION PROFILE (blood levels)

ROUTE	ONSET	PEAK	DURATION
PO	unknown†	2–6 hr	unknown
IV	unknown	end of infusion	unknown

†Onset of action in rheumatoid arthritis is 4–8 wk and may last 4 wk after discontinuation; for psoriasis, onset is 2–6 wk and lasts 6 wk following discontinuation

Contraindications/Precautions
Contraindicated in: Hypersensitivity to cyclosporine or polyoxyethylated castor oil (vehicle for IV form); OB, Lactation: Should not be given unless benefits outweigh risks; Disulfiram therapy or known alcohol intolerance (IV and oral liquid dose forms contain alcohol); Psoriasis patients receiving immunosuppressants or radiation; Uncontrolled hypertension.
Use Cautiously in: Severe hepatic impairment (dose ↓ recommended); Renal impairment (frequent dose changes may be necessary); Active infection; Pedi: Larger or more frequent doses may be required.

Adverse Reactions/Side Effects
CNS: SEIZURES, tremor, confusion, flushing, headache, psychiatric problems. **CV:** hypertension. **GI:** diarrhea, hepatotoxicity, nausea, vomiting, abdominal discomfort, anorexia, pancreatitis. **GU:** nephrotoxicity. **Derm:** hirsutism, acne. **F and E:** hyperkalemia, hypomagnesemia. **Hemat:** anemia, leukopenia, thrombocytopenia. **Metab:** hyperlipidemia, hyperuricemia. **Neuro:** hyperesthesia, paresthesia. **Misc:** gingival hyperplasia, hypersensitivity reactions, infections (including activation of latent viral infections such as BK virus-associated nephropathy).

Interactions
Drug-Drug: ↑ blood levels and/or risk of toxicity with **azithromycin, clarithomycin, amphotericin B, aminoglycosides, amiodarone,** anabolic steroids, some **calcium channel blockers, cimetidine, colchicine, danazol, erythromycin, fluconazole, fluoroquinolones, ketoconazole, itraconazole, metoclopramide, methotrexate, miconazole, nefazodone NSAIDs, melphalan, protease inhibitors quinupristin/dalfopristin,** or **hormonal contraceptives**. ↑ nephrotoxicity with **acyclovir, amphotericin B, aminoglycosides, NSAIDs, trimethoprim, ciprofloxacin,** and **vancomycin**. ↑ immunosuppression with other **immunosuppressants** (cyclophosphamide, azathioprine, corticosteroids). **Barbiturates, phenytoin, rifampin, rifabutin, carbamazepine, oxcarbamazepine** or **sulfonamides** may ↓ effect of cyclosporine. ↑ risk of hyperkalemia with **potassium-sparing diuretics, potassium supplements,** or **ACE inhibitors**. ↑ serum levels/risk of toxicity from **digoxin** (↓ digoxin dose by 50%). Prolongs the action of **neuromuscular blocking agents**. ↑ risk of seizures with **imipenem/cilastatin**. May ↓ antibody response to **live-virus vaccines** and ↑ risk of adverse reactions. ↑ risk of rhabdomyolysis with **HMG-CoA reductase inhibitors**. May ↑ levels and risk of toxicity from **etoposide**. Concurrent use with **tacrolimus** should be avoided. **Orlistat** ↓ absorption; avoid concurrent use. May ↑ levels and the risk of hypoglycemia from **repaglinide**.
Drug-Natural Products: Concomitant use with **echinacea** and **melatonin** may interfere with immunosuppression. Use with **St. John's wort** may cause ↓ serum levels and organ rejection for transplant patients.
Drug-Food: Concurrent ingestion of **grapefruit or grapefruit juice** ↑ absorption and should be avoided. **Food** ↓ absorption of microemulsion products (Neoral).

Route/Dosage
Doses are adjusted on the basis of serum level monitoring.

Prevention of Transplant Rejection (Sandimmune)
PO (Adults and Children): 14–18 mg/kg/dose 4–12 hr before transplant then 5–15 mg/kg/day divided q 12–24 hr postoperatively, taper by 5% weekly to maintenance dose of 3–10 mg/kg/day.
IV (Adults and Children): 5–6 mg/kg/dose 4–12 hr before transplant, then 2–10 mg/kg/day in divided doses q 8–24 hr; change to PO as soon as possible.

Prevention of Transplant Rejection (Neoral)
PO (Adults and Children): 4–12 mg/kg/day divided q 12 hr (dose varies depending on organ transplanted).

cycloSPORINE **389**

Rheumatoid Arthritis (Neoral only)
PO (Adults and Children): 2.5 mg/kg/day given in 2 divided doses; may ↑ by 0.5–0.75 mg/kg/day after 8 and 12 weeks, up to 4 mg/kg/day. ↓ dose by 25–50% if adverse reactions occur.

Severe Psoriasis (Neoral only)
PO (Adults): 2.5 mg/kg/day given in 2 divided doses, for at least 4 wk; then may ↑ by 0.5 mg/kg/day q 2 wk, up to 4 mg/kg/day. ↓ dose by 25–50% if adverse reactions occur.

Autoimmune Diseases (Neoral only)
PO (Adults and Children): 1–3 mg/kg/day.

Availability (generic available)
Microemulsion soft gelatin capsules (Gengraf, Neoral): 25 mg, 100 mg. **Cost:** *Gengraf*—25 mg $227.97/180, 100 mg $949.52/180; *Neoral*—25 mg $239.96/180, 100 mg $956.36/180. **Microemulsion oral solution (Gengraf, Neoral):** 100 mg/mL. **Cost:** *Neoral*—$301.71/50 mL. **Soft gelatin capsules (Sandimmune):** 25 mg, 100 mg. **Cost:** 25 mg $337.25/180, 100 mg $1,280.00/180. **Oral solution (Sandimmune):** 100 mg/mL. **Cost:** *Neoral*—$363.18/50 mL. **Injection (Sandimmune):** 50 mg/mL in 5-mL ampules.

NURSING IMPLICATIONS

Assessment
- Monitor serum creatinine level, intake and output ratios, daily weight, and blood pressure during therapy. Report significant changes.
- **Prevention of Transplant Rejection:** Assess for symptoms of organ rejection throughout therapy.
- **IV:** Monitor patient for signs and symptoms of hypersensitivity (wheezing, dyspnea, flushing of face or neck) continuously during at least the first 30 min of each treatment and frequently thereafter. Oxygen, epinephrine, and equipment for treatment of anaphylaxis should be available with each IV dose.
- **Arthritis:** Assess pain and limitation of movement prior to and during administration.
- Prior to initiating therapy, perform a physical exam including blood pressure on 2 occasions to determine baseline. Monitor blood pressure every 2 wk during initial 3 mo, then monthly if stable. If hypertension occurs, dose should be reduced.
- **Psoriasis:** Assess skin lesions prior to and during therapy.

- *Lab Test Considerations:* Measure serum creatinine, BUN, CBC, magnesium, potassium, uric acid, and lipids at baseline, every 2 wk during initial therapy, and then monthly if stable. Nephrotoxicity may occur; report significant increases.
- May cause hepatotoxicity; monitor for ↑ AST, ALT, alkaline phosphatase, amylase, and bilirubin.
- May cause ↑ serum potassium and uric acid levels and ↓ serum magnesium levels.
- Serum lipid levels may be ↑.
- *Toxicity and Overdose:* Evaluate serum cyclosporine levels periodically during therapy. Dose may be adjusted daily, in response to levels, during initiation of therapy. Guidelines for desired serum levels will vary among institutions.

Potential Nursing Diagnoses
Chronic pain (Indications)
Risk for infection (Side Effects)

Implementation
- Do not confuse cyclosporine with cyclophosphamide or cycloserine.
- Given with other immunosuppressive agents. Protect transplant patients from staff and visitors who may carry infection. Maintain protective isolation as indicated.
- Microemulsion products (Neoral) and other products (Sandimmune) are not interchangeable.
- **PO:** Draw up oral solution in the pipette provided with the medication. Mix oral solution with milk, chocolate milk, apple juice or orange juice, preferably at room temperature. Stir well and drink at once. Use a glass container and rinse with more diluent to ensure that total dose is taken. Administer oral doses with meals. Wipe pipette dry; do not wash after use.

IV Administration
- **Intermittent Infusion:** *Diluent:* Dilute each 1 mL (50 mg) of IV concentrate immediately before use with 20–100 mL of D5W or 0.9% NaCl for injection. Solution is stable for 24 hr in D5W. In 0.9% NaCl, it is stable for 6 hr in a polyvinylchloride container and 12 hr in a glass container at room temperature. *Concentration:* 2.5 mg/mL. *Rate:* Infuse slowly over 2–6 hr via infusion pump.
- **Continuous Infusion:** May be administered over 24 hr.

= Canadian drug name. = Genetic implication.
*CAPITALS indicates life-threatening; underlines indicate most frequent.

- **Y-Site Compatibility:** acyclovir, alfentanil, amikacin, aminophylline, anidulafungin, ascorbic acid, atracurium, atropine, azathioprine, azotreonam, bivalirudin, bumetanide, buprenorphine, butorphanol, calcium chloride, calcium gluconate, carboplatin, caspofungin, cefazolin, cefonicid, cefoperazone, cefotaxime, cefotetan, cefoxitin, ceftazidime, ceftizoxime, ceftriaxone, cefuroxime, chloramphenicol, chlorpromazine, cimetidine, cisplatin, clindamycin, cyclophosphamide, cytarabine, dactinomycin, daptomycin, dexamethasone, dexmedetomidine, digoxin, diltiazem, diphenhydramine, dobutamine, docetaxel, dopamine, doripenem, doxacurium, doxarubicin hydrochloride, doxycycline, enalaprilat, ephedrine, epinephrine, epirubicin, epoetin alfa, ertapenem, erythromycin, esmolol, etoposide, etoposide phosphate, famotidine, fenoldopam, fentanyl, fluconazole, fludarabine, fluorouracil, folic acid, furosemide, ganciclovir, gemcitabine, gentamicin, glycopyrrolate, granisetron, heparin, hetastarch, hydrocortisone, hydromorphone, ifosfamide, imipenem/cilastatin, indomethacin, isoproterenol, ketorolac, labetalol, levofloxacin, lidocaine, linezolid, lorazepam, mannitol, mechlorethamine, meperidine, methotrexate, methoxamine, methyldopate, methylprednisolone, metoclopramide, metoprolol, metronidazole, micafungin, midazolam, milrinone, mitoxantrone, morphine, multivitamins, nafcillin, naloxone, nesiritide, nitroglycerin, nitroprusside, norepinephrine, octreotide, ondansetron, oxacillin, oxaliplatin, oxytocin, paclitaxel, palonosetron, pantoprazole, papaverine, pemetrexed, penicillin G, pentamidine, pentazocine, phentolamine, phenylephrine, phytonadione, piperacillin/tazobactam, potassium chloride, prochlorperazine, promethazine, propofol, propranolol, protamine, pyridoxime, quinupristin/dalfopristin, ranitidine, sargramostim, sodium acetate, sodium bicarbonate, streptokinase, succinylcholine, sufentanil, tacrolimus, teniposide, theophylline, thimine, thiotepa, ticarcillin/clavulanate, tigecycline, tirofiban, tobramycin, trimetaphan, urokinase, vancomycin, vasopressin, vecuronium, verapamil, vincristine, vinorelbine.
- **Y-Site Incompatibility:** amphotericin B cholesteryl, amphotericin B liposome, cyanocobalamin, dantrolene, diazepam, diazoxide, drotrecogin, pentobarbital, phenobarbital, phenytoin, rituximab, trastuzumab, trimethoprim/sulfamethoxazole, voriconazole.

Patient/Family Teaching
- Instruct patient to take medication at the same time each day and with regard to food, as directed. Do not skip doses or double up on missed doses. Take missed doses as soon as remembered within 12 hr. Do not discontinue medication without advice of health care professional.
- Reinforce the need for lifelong therapy to prevent transplant rejection. Review symptoms of rejection for transplanted organ, and stress need to notify health care professional immediately if they occur.
- Instruct patients and/or parents to notify health care professional if diarrhea develops; decreases absorption of cyclosporine and can result in rejection.
- Instruct patient to avoid grapefruit and grapefruit juice to prevent interaction with cyclosporine.
- Advise patient of common side effects (nephrotoxicity, increased blood pressure, hand tremors, increased facial and body hair, gingival hyperplasia). Advise patients that if hair growth is excessive, depilatories, or waxing, can be used.
- Teach patient the correct method for monitoring blood pressure. Instruct patient to notify health care professional of significant changes in blood pressure or if hematuria, increased frequency, cloudy urine, decreased urine output, fever, sore throat, tiredness, or unusual bruising occurs.
- Instruct patient on proper oral hygiene. Meticulous oral hygiene and dental examinations for teeth cleaning and plaque control every 3 mo will help decrease gingival inflammation and hyperplasia.
- Instruct patient to consult health care professional before taking any OTC medications or receiving any vaccinations while taking this medication.
- Advise patient to notify health care professional if pregnancy is planned or suspected.
- Emphasize the importance of follow-up exams and lab tests.

Evaluation/Desired Outcomes
- Prevention of rejection of transplanted tissues.
- Decrease in severity of pain.
- Increased ease of joint movement.
- Decrease in progression of psoriasis.

cyproheptadine
(si-proe-**hep**-ta-deen)
Periactin, PMS-Cyproheptadine

cyproheptadine

Classification
Therapeutic: allergy, cold, and cough remedies, antihistamines

Pregnancy Category B

Indications
Relief of allergic symptoms caused by histamine release including: Seasonal and perennial allergic rhinitis, Chronic urticaria, Cold urticaria. **Unlabeled Use:** Stimulation of appetite.

Action
Antagonizes the effects of histamine at H-receptor sites; does not bind to or inactivate histamine. Also blocks the effects of serotonin, which may result in increased appetite. **Therapeutic Effects:** Decreased symptoms of histamine excess (sneezing, rhinorrhea, nasal and ocular pruritus, ocular tearing and redness). Decreased cold urticaria.

Pharmacokinetics
Absorption: Apparently well absorbed after oral dosing.
Distribution: Unknown.
Metabolism and Excretion: Mostly metabolized by the liver.
Half-life: Unknown.

TIME/ACTION PROFILE (antihistaminic effects)

ROUTE	ONSET	PEAK	DURATION
PO	15–60 min	1–2 hr	8 hr

Contraindications/Precautions
Contraindicated in: Hypersensitivity; Acute attacks of asthma; Lactation; Known alcohol intolerance (syrup only).
Use Cautiously in: Geri: Appears on Beers list. Geriatric patients are sensitive to anticholinergic effects and have increased risk for side effects; Angle-closure glaucoma; Liver disease; Pregnancy (safety not established).

Adverse Reactions/Side Effects
CNS: drowsiness, excitation (increased in children). **EENT:** blurred vision. **CV:** arrhythmias, hypotension, palpitations. **GI:** dry mouth, constipation. **GU:** hesitancy, retention. **Derm:** photosensitivity, rashes. **Misc:** weight gain.

Interactions
Drug-Drug: Additive CNS depression with other **CNS depressants**, including **alcohol**, **opioid analgesics**, and **sedative/hypnotics**. MAO inhibitors may intensify and prolong the anticholinergic effects of **antihistamines**.

Route/Dosage
PO (Adults): 4 mg q 8 hr (range 4–20 mg/day in 3 divided doses; up to 0.5 mg/kg/day).
PO (Children 6–14 yr): 2–4 mg q 8–12 hr (not to exceed 16 mg/day).
PO (Children 2–6 yr): 2 mg q 8–12 hr (not to exceed 12 mg/day).

Availability (generic available)
Tablets: 4 mg, ❋ 4 mg^OTC. Syrup: 2 mg/5 mL, ❋ 2 mg/5 mL^OTC.

NURSING IMPLICATIONS

Assessment
- Geri: Assess for adverse anticholinergic effects (delirium, acute confusion, dizziness, dry mouth, blurred vision, urinary retention, constipation, tachycardia).
- **Allergy:** Assess symptoms (rhinitis, conjunctivitis, hives) prior to and periodically throughout therapy.
- Assess lung sounds and respiratory function prior to and periodically throughout therapy. May cause thickening of bronchial secretions. Maintain fluid intake of 1500–2000 mL/day to decrease viscosity of secretions.
- **Appetite Stimulant:** Monitor food intake and weight routinely.
- *Lab Test Considerations:* May cause false-negative reactions on allergy skin tests; discontinue 72 hr prior to testing.
- Increased serum amylase and prolactin concentrations may occur when cyproheptadine is administered with a thyrotropin-releasing hormone.

Potential Nursing Diagnoses
Ineffective airway clearance (Indications)
Risk for injury (Side Effects)

Implementation
- Do not confuse cyproheptadine with cyclobenzaprine.
- **PO:** Administer with food, water, or milk to minimize gastric irritation.

Patient/Family Teaching
- Instruct patient to take cyproheptadine exactly as directed. Missed dose should be taken as soon as remembered. Do not double doses. Syrup should be accurately measured using calibrated medication cup or measuring device.

- Medication may cause drowsiness. Advise patient to avoid driving or other activities requiring alertness until response to the drug is known.
- Advise patient to use sunscreen and protective clothing to prevent a photosensitivity reaction.
- Caution patient to avoid concurrent use of alcohol and other CNS depressants.
- Advise patient that frequent mouth rinses, good oral hygiene, and sugarless gum or candy may decrease dry mouth. Patient should notify dentist if dry mouth persists for >2 wk.
- Geri: Teach patient and family about anticholinergic effects and to contact a health care provider if such effects persist.

Evaluation/Desired Outcomes
- Alleviation of allergic symptoms.
- Alleviation of cold urticaria.
- Improvement of appetite.

HIGH ALERT

cytarabine (sye-tare-a-been)
Ara-C, cytosine arabinoside,
✦Cytosar, Cytosar-U, DepoCyt

Classification
Therapeutic: antineoplastics
Pharmacologic: antimetabolites

Pregnancy Category D

Indications
IV: Used mainly in combination chemotherapeutic regimens for the treatment of leukemias and non-Hodgkin's lymphomas. **IT:** Treatment of lymphomatous meningitis.

Action
Inhibits DNA synthesis by inhibiting DNA polymerase (cell-cycle S-phase–specific). **Therapeutic Effects:** Death of rapidly replicating cells, particularly malignant ones.

Pharmacokinetics
Absorption: Absorption occurs from subcut sites, but blood levels are lower than with IV administration; IT administration results in negligible systemic exposure.
Distribution: Widely distributed; IV- and subcut-administered cytarabine crosses the blood-brain barrier but not in sufficient quantities. Crosses the placenta.
Metabolism and Excretion: Metabolized mostly by the liver; <10% excreted unchanged by the kidneys. Metabolism to inactive drug in the CSF is negligible because the enzyme that metabolizes it is present in very low concentrations in the CSF.
Half-life: *IV, subcut* — 1–3 hr; *IT* — 100–236 hr.

TIME/ACTION PROFILE (IV, subcut — effects on WBCs; IT — levels in CSF)

ROUTE	ONSET	PEAK	DURATION
Subcut, IV (1st phase)	24 hr	7–9 days	12 days
Subcut, IV (2nd phase)	15–24 days	15–24 days	25–34 days
IT	rapid	5 hr	14–28 days

Contraindications/Precautions
Contraindicated in: Hypersensitivity; OB: Pregnancy or lactation; Active meningeal infection (IT only).
Use Cautiously in: Active infections; Decreased bone marrow reserve; Renal/hepatic disease; Other chronic debilitating illnesses; OB: Patients with childbearing potential.

Adverse Reactions/Side Effects
CNS: CNS dysfunction (high dose), confusion, drowsiness, headache. **EENT:** corneal toxicity (high dose), hemorrhagic conjunctivitis (high dose). **Resp:** PULMONARY EDEMA (high dose). **CV:** edema. **GI:** nausea, vomiting, hepatitis, hepatotoxicity, severe GI ulceration (high dose), stomatitis. **GU:** urinary incontinence. **Derm:** alopecia, rash. **Endo:** sterility. **Hemat:** *(less with IT use)* — anemia, leukopenia, thrombocytopenia. **Metab:** hyperuricemia. **Neuro:** *Intrathecal only* — CHEMICAL ARACHNOIDITIS, abnormal gait. **Misc:** cytarabine syndrome, fever.

Interactions
Drug-Drug: ↑ bone marrow depression with other **antineoplastics** or **radiation therapy**. ↑ risk of cardiomyopathy when used in high-dose regimens with **cyclophosphamide**. May ↓ antibody response to **live-virus vaccines** and ↑ risk of adverse reactions. May ↓ absorption of **digoxin** tablets. May ↓ the efficacy of **gentamicin** when used to treat *Klebsiella pneumoniae* infections. Recent treatment with **asparaginase** may ↑ risk of pancreatitis. ↑ neurotoxicity with concurrently administered IT antineoplastics (IT only).

Route/Dosage
Dose regimens vary widely.
IV (Adults): *Induction dose* — 200 mg/m^2/day for 5 days q 2 wk as a single agent *or* 2–6 mg/kg/day (100–200 mg/m^2/day) as a single daily dose

cytarabine **393**

or in 2–3 divided doses for 5–10 days or until remission occurs as part of combination chemotherapy. *Maintenance*—70–200 mg/m²/day for 2–5 days monthly. *Refractory leukemias/lymphomas*—3 g/m² q 12 hr for up to 12 doses. **Subcut, IM (Adults):** *Maintenance*—1–1.5 mg/kg q 1–4 wk.
IT (Adults): *Depo Cyt Induction*—50 mg (intraventricular or lumbar puncture) every 14 days for 2 doses (weeks 1 and 3); *consolidation*—50 mg (intraventricular or lumbar puncture) every 14 days for 3 doses (weeks 5, 7, and 9), followed by one additional dose at week 13; *maintenance*—50 mg (intraventricular or lumbar puncture) every 28 days for 4 doses (weeks 17, 21, 25, and 29). If drug-related neurotoxicity occurs, dose should be reduced to 25 mg or discontinued (dexamethasone 4 mg PO/IV twice daily for 5 days should be started concurrently with IT cytarabine).

Availability (generic available)
Powder for injection: 100 mg, 500 mg, 1 g, 2 g. **Sustained-release liposome injection for IT use:** 50 mL/5-mL vial.

NURSING IMPLICATIONS
Assessment
- Monitor for bone marrow depression. Assess for bleeding (bleeding gums, bruising, petechiae, guaiac stools, urine, and emesis) and avoid IM injections and taking rectal temperatures if platelet count is low. Apply pressure to venipuncture sites for 10 min. Assess for signs of infection during neutropenia. Anemia may occur. Monitor for increased fatigue, dyspnea, and orthostatic hypotension.
- Monitor intake and output ratios and daily weights. Report significant changes in totals.
- Monitor for symptoms of gout (increased uric acid, joint pain, edema). Encourage patient to drink at least 2 L of fluid each day. Allopurinol may decrease uric acid levels. Alkalinization of urine may increase excretion of uric acid.
- Assess nutritional status. Nausea and vomiting may occur within 1 hr of administration, especially if IV dose is administered rapidly, less severe if medication is infused slowly. Administering an antiemetic prior to and periodically throughout therapy and adjusting diet as tolerated may help maintain fluid and electrolyte balance and nutritional status.
- Monitor patient for development of *cytarabine* or *ara-C syndrome* (fever, myalgia, bone pain, chest pain, maculopapular rash, conjunctivitis, malaise), which usually occurs 6–12 hr following administration. Corticosteroids may be used for treatment or prevention. If patient responds to corticosteroids, continue cytarabine and corticosteroids.
- Assess patient for respiratory distress and pulmonary edema. Occurs with high doses rarely; may be fatal.
- Monitor patient for signs of anaphylaxis (rash, dyspnea, swelling). Epinephrine, corticosteroids, and resuscitation equipment should be readily available.
- **IT:** Chemical arachnoiditis (nausea, vomiting, headache, fever, back pain, CSF pleocytosis and neck rigidity, neck pain, or meningism) is an expected side effect of IT cytarabine. Incidence and severity of symptoms may be decreased with coadministration of dexamethasone.
- Monitor patients receiving IT therapy continuously for the development of neurotoxicity (myelopathy, personality changes, dysarthria, ataxia, confusion, somnolence, coma). If neurotoxicity develops, decrease amount of subsequent doses and discontinue if neurotoxicity persists. Risk may be increased if cytarabine is administered intrathecally and IV within a few days.
- *Lab Test Considerations:* Monitor CBC with differential and platelet count prior to and frequently during therapy. Leukocyte counts begin to drop within 24 hr of administration. The initial nadir occurs in 7–9 days. After a small ↑ in the count, the second, deeper nadir occurs 15–24 days after administration. Platelet counts begin to ↓ 5 days after a dose, with a nadir at 12–15 days. Leukocyte and thrombocyte counts usually begin to ↑ 10 days after the nadirs. Therapy is usually withdrawn if leukocyte count is <1000/mm³ or platelet count is <50,000/mm³. Bone marrow aspirations are recommended every 2 wk until remission occurs.
- Monitor renal (BUN and creatinine) and hepatic function (AST, ALT, bilirubin, alkaline phosphatase, and LDH) prior to and routinely during therapy.
- May cause ↑ uric acid concentrations.

Potential Nursing Diagnoses
Risk for infection (Adverse Reactions)
Risk for injury (Side Effects)

Implementation

- **_High Alert:_** Fatalities have occurred with chemotherapeutic agents. Before administering, clarify all ambiguous orders; double-check single, daily, and course-of-therapy dose limits; have second practitioner independently double-check original order, calculations, and infusion pump settings.
- **_High Alert:_** Do not confuse cytarabine with Cytoxan (cyclophosphamide). Do not confuse Cytosar (cytarabine) with Cytovene (ganciclovir) or Cytoxan. Do not confuse high-dose and regular therapy. Fatalities have occurred with high-dose therapy.
- Solution should be prepared in a biologic cabinet. Wear gloves, gown, and mask while handling IV medication. Discard IV equipment in specially designated containers (see Appendix L).
- May be given subcut, direct IV, intermittent IV, continuous IV, or IT.
- **IV, Subcut:** Reconstitute 100-mg vials with 5 mL of bacteriostatic water for injection with benzyl alcohol 0.9% for a concentration of 20 mg/mL. Reconstitute 500-mg vials with 10 mL for a concentration of 50 mg/mL, 1-g vials with 10 mL, and 2-g vials with 20 mL for a concentration of 100 mg/mL. Reconstituted solution is stable for 48 hr. Do not administer a cloudy or hazy solution.

IV Administration

- **Direct IV:** _Diluent:_ Administer undiluted. _Concentration:_ 100 mg/mL. _Rate:_ Administer each 100 mg over 1–3 min.
- **Intermittent Infusion:** _Diluent:_ May be further diluted in 0.9% NaCl, D5W, D10W, D5/0.9% NaCl, Ringer's solution, LR, or D5/LR. _Concentration:_ Dilute doses in 100 mL of diluent. _Rate:_ Infuse over 15–30 min.
- **Continuous Infusion:** Rate and concentration for IV infusion are ordered individually.
- **Syringe Compatibility:** metoclopramide.
- **Y-Site Compatibility:** amifostine, amsacrine, aztreonam, cefepime, chlorpromazine, cimetidine, cladribine, dexamethasone phosphate, diphenhydramine, doxorubicin liposome, droperidol, etoposide phosphate, famotidine, filgrastim, fludarabine, furosemide, gemcitabine, gentamicin, granisetron, heparin, hydrocortisone, hydromorphone, idarubicin, linezolid, lorazepam, melphalan, methotrexate, methylprednisolone, metoclopramide, morphine, ondansetron, paclitaxel, pemetrexed, piperacillin/tazobactam, prochlorperazine, promethazine, propofol, ranitidine, sargramostim, sodium bicarbonate, teniposide, thiotepa, vinorelbine.
- **Y-Site Incompatibility:** allopurinol, amphotericin B cholesteryl sulfate complex, ganciclovir, lansoprazole.
- **Additive Compatibility:** methotrexate, mitoxantrone, ondansetron, potassium chloride, sodium bicarbonate, vincristine.
- **Additive Incompatibility:** fluorouracil, heparin, regular insulin, nafcillin, oxacillin, penicillin G sodium.
- **IT:** Patients receiving _liposomal cytarabine_ should be started on dexamethasone 4 mg twice daily PO or IV for 5 days beginning on the day of liposomal cytarabine injection.
- Allow vial to warm to room temperature. Gently agitate or invert vial to resuspend particles immediately before withdrawal from vial. No further reconstitution or dilution is required with _liposomal cytarabine_. Reconstitute _conventional cytarabine_ with preservative-free 0.9% NaCl or autologous spinal fluid. Use immediately to prevent bacterial contamination.
- Liposomal cytarabine must be used within 4 hr of withdrawal from the vial. Discard unused portions. Inject directly into CSF via intraventricular reservoir or by direct injection into lumbar sac. Do not use in-line filters.
- Instruct patient to lie flat for 1 hr following IT injection. Monitor for immediate toxic reactions.

Patient/Family Teaching

- Caution patient to avoid crowds and persons with known infections. Report symptoms of infection (fever, chills, cough, hoarseness, sore throat, lower back or side pain, painful or difficult urination) immediately.
- Instruct patient to report unusual bleeding. Advise patient of thrombocytopenia precautions (use soft toothbrush and electric razor, avoid falls, do not drink alcoholic beverages or take medication containing aspirin or NSAIDs; may precipitate gastric bleeding).
- Instruct patient to inspect oral mucosa for redness and ulceration. If mouth sores occur, advise patient to use sponge brush and rinse mouth with water after eating and drinking. Stomatitis may require treatment with opioid analgesics.
- Advise patient that this medication may have teratogenic effects. Contraception should be used during therapy and for at least 4 mo after therapy is concluded.
- Instruct patient not to receive any vaccinations without advice of health care professional.

- Emphasize the need for periodic lab tests to monitor for side effects.
- **IT:** Inform patient about the expected side effects (headache, nausea, vomiting, fever) and about early signs of neurotoxicity. Instruct patient to notify health care professional if these signs occur.
- Emphasize the importance of taking dexamethasone with lyposomal cytarabine.

Evaluation/Desired Outcomes
- Improvement of hematopoietic values in leukemias.
- Decrease in size and spread of the tumor in non-Hodgkin's lymphomas. Therapy is continued every 2 wk until patient is in complete remission or thrombocyte count or leukocyte count falls below acceptable levels.
- Treatment of lymphomatous meningitis.

HIGH ALERT
dacarbazine (da-**kar**-ba-zeen)
✤ DTIC, DTIC-Dome

Classification
Therapeutic: antineoplastics
Pharmacologic: alkylating agents

Pregnancy Category C

Indications
Treatment of metastatic malignant melanoma (single agent). Treatment of Hodgkin's disease as second-line therapy (with other agents).

Action
Disrupts DNA and RNA synthesis (cell-cycle phase–nonspecific). **Therapeutic Effects:** Death of rapidly growing tissue cells, especially malignant ones.

Pharmacokinetics
Absorption: IV administration results in complete bioavailability.
Distribution: Large volume of distribution; probably concentrates in liver; some CNS penetration.
Metabolism and Excretion: 50% metabolized by the liver, 50% excreted unchanged by the kidneys.
Half-life: 5 hr (↑ in renal and hepatic dysfunction).

TIME/ACTION PROFILE (effects on blood counts)

ROUTE	ONSET	PEAK	DURATION
IV (WBCs)	16–20 days	21–25 days	3–5 days
IV (platelets)	unknown	16 days	3–5 days

Contraindications/Precautions
Contraindicated in: Hypersensitivity; OB, Lactation: Pregnancy or lactation.
Use Cautiously in: Active infections; Bone marrow depression; Pedi: Children (safety not established); Renal dysfunction; Hepatic dysfunction.

Adverse Reactions/Side Effects
GI: HEPATIC NECROSIS, anorexia, nausea, vomiting, diarrhea, hepatic vein thrombosis. **Derm:** alopecia, facial flushing, photosensitivity, rash. **Endo:** gonadal suppression. **Hemat:** anemia, leukopenia, thrombocytopenia. **Local:** pain at IV site, phlebitis at IV site, tissue necrosis. **MS:** myalgia. **Neuro:** facial paresthesia. **Misc:** ANAPHYLAXIS, fever, flu-like syndrome, malaise.

Interactions
Drug-Drug: Additive bone marrow depression with other **antineoplastics**. **Carbamazepine, phenobarbital, rifampin,** and **aminoglutethimide** may ↑ metabolism and decrease effectiveness. Blood levels may be ↑ with **amiodarone, ciprofloxacin, fluvoxamine, ketoconazole, norfloxacin, ofloxacin, isoniazid,** or **miconazole.** May ↓ antibody response to **live-virus vaccines** and ↑ risk of adverse reactions.

Route/Dosage
Other regimens are used.
IV (Adults): *Malignant melanoma*—2–4.5 mg/kg/day for 10 days administered every 4 wk *or* 250 mg/m^2/day for 5 days administered every 3 wk. *Hodgkin's disease*—150 mg/m^2/day for 5 days (in combination with other agents) administered every 4 wk *or* 375 mg/m^2 (in combination with other agents) administered every 15 days.

Availability
Powder for injection: 200 mg.

NURSING IMPLICATIONS
Assessment
- Monitor vital signs prior to and frequently during therapy.
- Monitor for bone marrow depression. Assess for bleeding (bleeding gums, bruising, petechiae, guaiac stools, urine, and emesis) and avoid IM injections and rectal temperatures if platelet count is low. Apply pressure to venipuncture sites for 10 min. Assess for signs of infection during neutropenia. Anemia may occur. Monitor for increased fatigue, dyspnea, and orthostatic hypotension.
- Monitor IV site closely. Dacarbazine is an irritant. Instruct patient to notify health care professional immediately if discomfort at IV site occurs. Discontinue IV immediately if infiltration occurs. Applications of hot packs may relieve pain, burning sensation, and irritation at injection site.
- Monitor intake and output, appetite, and nutritional intake. Assess for nausea and vomiting, which may be severe and last 1–12 hr. Administration of an antiemetic prior to and periodically during therapy, restricting oral intake for 4–6 hr prior to administration, and adjusting diet as tolerated may help maintain fluid and electrolyte balance and nutritional status. Nausea usually decreases on subsequent doses.

✤ = Canadian drug name. ⚡ = Genetic implication.
*CAPITALS indicates life-threatening; underlines indicate most frequent.

- **Lab Test Considerations:** Monitor CBC and differential prior to and periodically throughout therapy. The nadir of thrombocytopenia occurs in 16 days. The nadir of leukopenia occurs in 3–4 wk. Recovery begins in 5 days. Withhold dose and notify physician if platelet count is <100,000/mm³ or leukocyte count is <4000/mm³.
- Monitor for increased AST, ALT, BUN, and serum creatinine. May cause hepatic necrosis.

Potential Nursing Diagnoses
Risk for infection (Side Effects)
Risk for injury (Side Effects)

Implementation
- **High Alert:** Fatalities have occurred with chemotherapeutic agents. Before administering, clarify all ambiguous orders; double-check single, daily, and course-of-therapy dose limits; have second practitioner independently double-check original order, calculations, and infusion pump settings.

IV Administration
- Prepare solution in a biologic cabinet. Wear gloves, gown, and mask while handling medication. Discard equipment in designated containers (see Appendix L).
- Reconstitute each 200-mg vial with 19.7 mL of sterile water for injection. Solution is colorless or clear yellow. Do not use solution that has turned pink. **Concentration:** 10 mg/mL solution is stable for 8 hr at room temperature and for 72 hr if refrigerated.
- **Intermittent Infusion: *Diluent:*** Further dilute with up to 250 mL of D5W or 0.9% NaCl. Stable for 24 hr if refrigerated or 8 hr at room temperature. ***Rate:*** Administer over 30–60 min.
- **Y-Site Compatibility:** amifostine, aztreonam, bivalirudin, caspofungin, daptomycin, dexmedetomidine, docetaxel, doxorubicin liposome, ertapenem, etoposide phosphate, fenoldopam, filgrastim, fludarabine, granisetron, hetastarch, levofloxacin, mechlorethamine, melphalan, nesiritide, octreotide, ondansetron, oxaliplatin, paclitaxel, palonosetron, quinupristin/dalfopristin, sargramostim, teniposide, thiotepa, tigecycline, tirofiban, vinorelbine, voriconazole.
- **Y-Site Incompatibility:** allopurinol, amphotericin B liposome, cefepime, pantoprazole, pemetrexed, piperacillin/tazobactam.

Patient/Family Teaching
- Instruct patient to notify health care professional if fever; chills; sore throat; signs of infection; bleeding gums; bruising; petechiae; abdominal pain; yellowing of eyes; or blood in urine, stool, or emesis occurs. Caution patient to avoid crowds and persons with known infections. Instruct patient to use soft toothbrush and electric razor. Patients should be cautioned not to drink alcoholic beverages or take products containing aspirin or NSAIDs; may increase GI irritation.
- May cause photosensitivity. Instruct patient to avoid sunlight or wear protective clothing and use sunscreen for 2 days after therapy.
- Instruct patient to inform health care professional if flu-like syndrome occurs. Symptoms include fever, myalgia, and general malaise. May occur after several courses of therapy. Usually occurs 1 wk after administration. May persist for 1–3 wk. Acetaminophen may be used for relief of symptoms.
- Discuss with patient the possibility of hair loss. Explore coping strategies.
- Advise patient of the need for a nonhormonal method of contraception.
- Instruct patient not to receive any vaccinations without advice of health care professional.

Evaluation/Desired Outcomes
- Decrease in size and spread of malignant melanoma or Hodgkin's lymphoma.

---

dalteparin, See HEPARINS (LOW MOLECULAR WEIGHT).

---

dantrolene (dan-troe-leen)
Dantrium

Classification
Therapeutic: skeletal muscle relaxants (direct acting)

Pregnancy Category C

Indications
PO: Treatment of spasticity associated with: Spinal cord injury, Stroke, Cerebral palsy, Multiple sclerosis. Prophylaxis of malignant hyperthermia. **IV:** Emergency treatment of malignant hyperthermia. **Unlabeled Use:** Management of neuroleptic malignant syndrome.

Action
Acts directly on skeletal muscle, causing relaxation by decreasing calcium release from sarcoplasmic reticulum in muscle cells. Prevents intense catabolic process associated with malignant hyperthermia. **Therapeutic Effects:** Reduction

dantrolene

of muscle spasticity. Prevention of malignant hyperthermia.

Pharmacokinetics
Absorption: 35% absorbed after oral administration.
Distribution: Unknown.
Metabolism and Excretion: Almost entirely metabolized by the liver.
Half-life: 8.7 hr.

TIME/ACTION PROFILE (effects on spasticity)

ROUTE	ONSET	PEAK	DURATION
PO	1 wk	unknown	6–12 hr
IV	rapid	rapid	unknown

Contraindications/Precautions
Contraindicated in: No contraindications to IV form in treatment of hyperthermia; OB, Lactation: Pregnancy and lactation; Situations in which spasticity is used to maintain posture or balance.
Use Cautiously in: Cardiac, pulmonary, or previous liver disease; Women, patients >35 yr (↑ risk of hepatotoxicity).

Adverse Reactions/Side Effects
CNS: drowsiness, muscle weakness, confusion, dizziness, headache, insomnia, malaise, nervousness. **EENT:** excessive lacrimation, visual disturbances. **Resp:** pleural effusions. **CV:** changes in BP, tachycardia. **GI:** HEPATOTOXICITY, diarrhea, anorexia, cramps, dysphagia, GI bleeding, vomiting. **GU:** crystalluria, dysuria, frequency, erectile dysfunction, incontinence, nocturia. **Derm:** pruritus, sweating, urticaria. **Hemat:** eosinophilia. **Local:** irritation at IV site, phlebitis. **MS:** myalgia. **Misc:** chills, drooling, fever.

Interactions
Drug-Drug: Additive CNS depression with **CNS depressants**, including **alcohol**, **antihistamines**, **opioid analgesics**, **sedative/hypnotics**, and parenteral **magnesium sulfate**. ↑ risk of hepatotoxicity with other **hepatotoxic agents** or **estrogens**. ↑ risk of arrhythmias with **verapamil**. ↑ neuromuscular blocking effects of **vecuronium**.
Drug-Natural Products: Concomitant use of **kava-kava**, **valerian**, **chamomile**, or **hops** can increase CNS depression.

Route/Dosage
PO (Adults): *Spasticity*—25 mg/day initially; ↑ by 25 mg/day q 4–7 days until desired response or total of 100 mg 4 times daily is reached. *Prevention of malignant hyperthermia*—4–8 mg/kg/day in 3–4 divided doses for 1–2 days before procedure, last dose 3–4 hr preop. *Post-hyperthermic crisis follow-up*—4–8 mg/kg/day in 3–4 divided doses for 1–3 days after IV treatment.

PO (Children >5 yr): *Spasticity*—0.5 mg/kg twice daily; ↑ by 0.5 mg/kg/day q 4–7 days until desired response is obtained or dosage of 3 mg/kg 4 times daily is reached (not to exceed 400 mg/day). *Prevention of malignant hyperthermia*—4–8 mg/kg/day in 3–4 divided doses for 1–2 days before procedure, last dose 3–4 hr preop. *Post-hyperthermic crisis follow-up*—4–8 mg/kg/day in 3–4 divided doses for 1–3 days after IV treatment.

IV (Adults and Children): *Treatment of malignant hyperthermia*—at least 1 mg/kg (up to 3 mg/kg), continued until symptoms decrease or a cumulative dose of 10 mg/kg has been given. If symptoms reappear, dose may be repeated. *Prevention of malignant hyperthermia*—2.5 mg/kg before anesthesia.

Availability (generic available)
Capsules: 25 mg, 50 mg, 100 mg. **Powder for injection:** 20 mg/vial.

NURSING IMPLICATIONS

Assessment
- Assess bowel function periodically. Persistent diarrhea may warrant discontinuation of therapy.
- **Muscle Spasticity:** Assess neuromuscular status and muscle spasticity before initiating therapy and periodically during its course to determine response to therapy.
- **Malignant Hyperthermia:** Assess previous anesthesia history of all surgical patients. Also assess for family history of reactions to anesthesia (malignant hyperthermia or perioperative death).
- Monitor ECG, vital signs, electrolytes, and urine output continuously when administering IV for malignant hyperthermia.
- Monitor patient for difficulty swallowing and choking during meals on the day of administration.
- *Lab Test Considerations:* Monitor liver function frequently during therapy. Liver function abnormalities (↑ AST, ALT, alkaline phosphatase, bilirubin, GGTP) may require discontinuation of therapy.

- Evaluate renal function and CBC before and periodically during therapy in patients receiving prolonged therapy.

Potential Nursing Diagnoses
Impaired physical mobility (Indications)
Acute pain (Indications)
Risk for injury (Side Effects)

Implementation
- Do not confuse Dantrium (dantrolene) with danazol.
- **PO:** If gastric irritation becomes a problem, may be administered with food. Oral suspensions may be made by opening capsules and adding them to fruit juices or other liquid. Drink immediately after mixing.
- Oral dose for spasticity should be divided into 4 doses/day.

IV Administration
- **Direct IV:** *Diluent:* Reconstitute each 20 mg with 60 mL of sterile water for injection (without a bacteriostatic agent). Shake until solution is clear. Solution must be used within 6 hr. Administer without further dilution. Protect diluted solution from direct light. ***Concentration:*** 0.333 mg/mL. *Rate:* Administer each single dose by rapid continuous IV push through Y-tubing or 3-way stopcock. Follow immediately with subsequent doses as indicated. Medication is very irritating to tissues; observe infusion site frequently to avoid extravasation.
- **Intermittent Infusion:** Prophylactic dose has been administered as an infusion. *Rate:* Administer over 1 hr before anesthesia.
- **Y-Site Compatibility:** acyclovir, paclitaxel, palonosetron.
- **Y-Site Incompatibility:** alfentanil, amikacin, aminophylline, amphotericin B colloidal, ampicillin, ampicillin/sulbactam, ascorbic acid, atracurium, atropine, azathioprine, aztreonam, bivalirudin, bumetanide, buprenorphine, butorphanol, caclium chloride, calcium gluconate, caspofungin, cefazolin, cefonocid, cefoperazone, cefotaxime, cefotetan, cefoxitin, ceftazidime, ceftizoxime, ceftriaxone, cefuroxime, chloramphenicol, chlorpromazine, cimetidine, cisplatin, clindamycin, cyanocobalamin, cyclosporine, dactinomycin, daptomycin, dexamethasone, diazepam, diazoxide, digoxin, diltiazem, diphenhydramine, dobutamine, docetaxel, dopamine, doxycycline, enalaprilat, ephedrine, epinephrine, epoetin alfa, ertapenem, erythromycin, esmolol, etoposide, etoposide phosphate, famotidine, fenoldopam, fentanyl, fluconazole, fludarabine, folic acid, furosemide, ganciclovir, gemcitabine, gentamicin, glycopyrrolate, granisetron, haloperidol, heparin, hetastarch, hydralazine, hydrocortisone, hydromorphone, hydroxyzine, imipenem/cilastatin, inamrinone, indomethacin, insulin, isoproterenol, ketorolac, labetalol, lidocaine, linezolid, lorazepam, magnesium sulfate, mannitol, mechlorethamine, meperidine, metaraminol, methoxamine, methyldopate, methylprednisolone, metoclopramide, metoprolol, metronidazole, midazolam, milrinone, mitoxantrone, morphine, multivitamins, nafcillin, nalbuphine, naloxone, nesiritide, nitroglycerin, nitroprusside, norepinephrine, octreotide, ondansetron, oxacillin, oxaliplatin, oxytocin, pantoprazole, papaverine, pemetrexed, penicillin G, pentamidine, pentazocine, pentobarbital, phenobarbital, phentolamine, phenylephrine, phenytoin, phytonadione, piperacillin/tazobactam, potassium chloride, procainamide, prochlorperazine, proimethazine, propranolol, protamine, pyridoxime, ranitidine, sodium acetate, sodium bicarbonate, streptokinase, succinylcholine, sufentanil, tacrolimus, teniposide, theophylline, thiamine, thiotepa, ticarcillin/clavulanate, tigecycline, tirofiban, tobramycin, tolazoline, trimethoprim/sulfamethoxazole, urokinase, vancomycin, vasopressin, vecuronium, verapamil, vinorelbine, voriconazole.

Patient/Family Teaching
- Advise patient not to take more medication than the amount prescribed to minimize risk of hepatotoxicity and other side effects. If a dose is missed, do not take unless remembered within 1 hr. Do not double doses.
- May cause dizziness, drowsiness, visual disturbances, and muscle weakness. Advise patient to avoid driving and other activities requiring alertness until response to drug is known. After IV dose for surgery, patients may experience decreased grip strength, leg weakness, lightheadedness, and difficulty swallowing for up to 48 hr. Caution patients to avoid activities requiring alertness and to use caution when walking down stairs and eating during this period.
- Advise patient to avoid taking alcohol or other CNS depressants concurrently with this medication.
- Instruct patient to notify health care professional if rash; itching; yellow eyes or skin; dark urine; or clay-colored, bloody, or black, tarry stools occur or if nausea, weakness, malaise,

fatigue, or diarrhea persists. May require discontinuation of therapy.
- Advise patient to wear sunscreen and protective clothing to prevent photosensitivity reactions.
- Emphasize the importance of follow-up exams to check progress in long-term therapy and blood tests to monitor for side effects.
- **Malignant Hyperthermia:** Patients with malignant hyperthemia should carry identification describing disease process at all times.

Evaluation/Desired Outcomes
- Relief of muscle spasm in musculoskeletal conditions. One wk or more may be required to see improvement; if there is no observed improvement in 45 days, the medication is usually discontinued.
- Prevention of or decrease in temperature and skeletal rigidity in malignant hyperthermia.

---

daptomycin (dap-to-**mye**-sin)
Cubicin

Classification
Therapeutic: anti-infectives
Pharmacologic: cyclic lipopeptide antibacterial agents

Pregnancy Category B

Indications
Complicated skin and skin structure infections caused by aerobic Gram-positive bacteria.

Action
Causes rapid depolarization of membrane potential following binding to bacterial membrane; this results in inhibition of protein, DNA, and RNA synthesis. **Therapeutic Effects:** Death of bacteria with resolution of infection. **Spectrum:** Active against *Staphylococcus aureus* (including methicillin-resistant strains), *Streptococcus pyogenes*, *S. pyogenes agalactiae*, some *S. dysgalactiae*, and *Enterococcus faecalis* (vancomycin-susceptible strains).

Pharmacokinetics
Absorption: IV administration results in complete bioavailability.
Distribution: Unknown.
Protein Binding: 92%.
Metabolism and Excretion: Metabolism not known; mostly excreted by kidneys.
Half-life: 8.1 hr.

TIME/ACTION PROFILE

ROUTE	ONSET	PEAK	DURATION
IV	rapid	end of infusion	24 hr

Contraindications/Precautions
Contraindicated in: Hypersensitivity.
Use Cautiously in: CCr <30 mL/min (dose reduction required); Geri: May have ↓ clinical response with ↑ risk of adverse reactions; OB: Use only if clearly needed; Lactation: Lactation; Pedi: Safety not established.

Adverse Reactions/Side Effects
CNS: dizziness. **Resp:** dyspnea. **CV:** hypertension, hypotension. **GI:** PSEUDOMEMBRANOUS COLITIS, constipation, diarrhea, nausea, vomiting, ↑ liver function tests. **GU:** renal failure. **Derm:** pruritus, rash. **Hemat:** anemia. **Local:** injection site reactions. **MS:** ↑ CPK. **Misc:** fever.

Interactions
Drug-Drug: Tobramycin ↑ blood levels. Concurrent **HMG-CoA reductase inhibitors** may ↑ the risk of myopathy.

Route/Dosage
IV (Adults): 4 mg/kg every 24 hr.

Renal Impairment
IV (Adults): *CCr <30 mL/min*—4 mg/kg every 48 hr.

Availability
Powder for injection: 500 mg/vial.

NURSING IMPLICATIONS
Assessment
- Assess patient for infection (vital signs; appearance of wound, sputum, urine, and stool; WBC) at beginning of and throughout therapy.
- Monitor bowel function. Diarrhea, abdominal cramping, fever, and bloody stools should be reported to health care professional promptly as a sign of pseudomembranous colitis. May begin up to several weeks following cessation of therapy.
- Monitor patient for development of muscle pain or weakness, particularly of distal extremities. Discontinue daptomycin in patients with unexplained signs and symptoms of myopathy in conjunction with CPK elevation >1000 U/L, or in patients without reported symptoms who have marked elevations in CPK >2000 U/L. Consider temporarily suspending agents asso-

ciated with rhabdomyolysis, (HMG-CoA reductase inhibitors) in patients receiving daptomycin.
- **Lab Test Considerations:** Monitor CPK weekly, more frequently in patients with unexplained ↑. Discontinue daptomycin if CPK >1000 units/L and signs and symptoms of myopathy occur. In patients with renal insufficiency, monitor both renal function and CPK more frequently.
- May cause false prolongation of PT and ↑ INR.

Potential Nursing Diagnoses
Risk for infection (Indications, Side Effects)

Implementation
IV Administration
- **Intermittent Infusion:** *Diluent:* Reconstitute 500-mg vial with 10 mL of 0.9% NaCl inserted toward wall of vial. Rotate vial gently to wet powder. Allow to stand for 10 min undisturbed. Swirl vial gently to completely reconstitute solution. Reconstituted vials are stable for 12 hr at room temperature or 48 hr if refrigerated. Dilute further in 50 mL of 0.9% NaCl. Solution is stable for 12 hr at room temperature or 48 hr if refrigerated. Do not administer solutions that are cloudy or contain a precipitate. *Rate:* Infuse over 30 min. Do not infuse daptomycin with ReadyMED® elastomeric infusion pumps due to incompatibility.
- **Y-Site Compatibility:** alfentanil, amifostine, amikacin, aminocaproic acid, aminophylline, amiodarone, amphotericin B liposome, ampicillin, ampicillin/sulbactam, argatroban, atenolol, azithromycin, aztreonam, bivalirudin, bumetanide, buprenorphine, busulfan, butorphanol, calcium chloride, calcium gluconate, carboplatin, carmustine, caspofungin, cefazolin, cefepime, cefotaxime, cefotetan, cefoxitin, ceftazidime, ceftizoxime, ceftriaxone, cefuroxime, chloramphenicol, cimetidine, ciprofloxacin, cisatracurium, cisplatin, clindamycin, cyclophosphamide, cyclosporine, dacarbazine, dactinomycin, daunorubicin hydrochloride, dexamethasone sodium phosphate, dexmedetomidine, dexrazoxane, diazepam, digoxin, diltiazem, diphenhydramine, dobutamine, docetaxel, dolasetron, dopamine, doripenem, doxorubicin hydrochloride, doxorubicin liposome, doxycycline, droperidol, enalaprilat, epinephrine, epirubicin, eptifibatide, ertapenem, erythromycin, esmolol, etoposide, etoposide phosphate, famotidine, fenoldopam, fentanyl, fluconazole, fludarabine, fluorouracil, foscarnet, fosphenytoin, furosemide, ganciclovir, gentamicin, glycopyrrolate, granisetron, haloperidol, heparin, hydralazine, hydrocortisone sodium succinate, hydromorphone, idarubicin, ifosfamide, insulin, irinotecan, isoproterenol, ketorolac, labetalol, leucovorin, levofloxacin, lidocaine, linezolid, lorazepam, magnesium sulfate, mannitol, mechlorethamine, melphalan, meperidine, meropenem, mesna, metaraminol, methyldopa, methylprednisolone sodium succinate, metoclopramide, metoprolol, midazolam, milrinone, mitoxantrone, morphine, moxifloxacin, mycophenolate mofetil, nafcillin, nalbuphine, naloxone, nicardipine, nitroprusside, norepinephrine, octreotide, ondansetron, oxaliplatin, oxytocin, paclitaxel, palonosetron, pamidronate, pancuronium, pemetrexed, pentamidine, phentolamine, phenylephrine, phenyobarbital, piperacillin/tazobactam, potassium acetate, potassium chloride, potassium phosphate, procainamide, prochlorperazine, promethazine, propranolol, quinupristin/dalfopristin, ranitidine, rocuronium, sodium acetate, sodium bicarbonate, sodium phosphate, succinylcholine, tacrolimus, teniposide, theophylline, thiotepa, ticarcillin/clavulanate, tigecycline, tirofiban, tobramycin, topotecan, trimethobenzamide, trimethoprim/sulfamethoxazole, vasopressin, vecuronium, verapamil, vinblastine, vincristine, vinorelbine, voriconazole, zidovudine, zoledronic acid.
- **Y-Site Incompatibility:** acyclovir, allopurinol, amphotericin B colloidal, amphotericin B lipid complex, cytarabine, dantrolene, gemcitabine, imipenem/cilastatin, methotrexate, metronidazole, minocycline, mitomycin, nesiritide, nitroglycerin, pantoprazole, pentazocine, pentobarbital, phenytoin, remifentanil, streptozocin, sufentanil, thiopental, vancomycin.
- **Solution Incompatibility:** D5W.

Patient/Family Teaching
- Inform patient of purpose of medication.
- Instruct patient to notify health care professional if fever and diarrhea develop, especially if stool contains blood, pus, or mucus. Advise patient not to treat diarrhea without consulting health care professional.
- May cause dizziness. Caution patient to avoid driving or other activities requiring alertness until response to medication is known.

Evaluation/Desired Outcomes
- Resolution of the signs and symptoms of infection. Length of time for complete resolution depends on the organism and site of infection.

darbepoetin (dar-be-**poh**-e-tin)
Aranesp

Classification
Therapeutic: antianemics
Pharmacologic: hormones (rDNA)

Pregnancy Category C

Indications
Anemia associated with chronic renal failure. Chemotherapy-induced anemia in patients with non-myeloid malignancies.

Action
Stimulates erythropoiesis (production of red blood cells). **Therapeutic Effects:** Maintains and may elevate red blood cell counts, decreasing the need for transfusions.

Pharmacokinetics
Absorption: 30–50% following subcut administration; IV administration results in complete bioavailability.
Distribution: Confined to the intravascular space.
Metabolism and Excretion: Unknown.
Half-life: *Subcut*—49 hr; *IV*—21 hr.

TIME/ACTION PROFILE (increase in RBCs)

ROUTE	ONSET	PEAK	DURATION
IV, subcut	2–6 wk	unknown	unknown

Contraindications/Precautions
Contraindicated in: Hypersensitivity; Uncontrolled hypertension; Patients receiving chemotherapy when anticipated outcome is cure.
Use Cautiously in: History of hypertension; Underlying hematologic diseases, including hemolytic anemia, sickle-cell anemia, thalassemia and porphyria (safety not established); OB, Lactation, Pedi: Safety not established.

Adverse Reactions/Side Effects
CNS: SEIZURES, dizziness, fatigue, headache, weakness. **Resp:** cough, dyspnea, bronchitis. **CV:** CHF, MI, STROKE, THROMBOTIC EVENTS (especially with hemoglobin >12 g/dL), edema, hypertension, hypotension, chest pain. **GI:** abdominal pain, nausea, diarrhea, vomiting, constipation. **Derm:** pruritus. **Hemat:** pure red cell aplasia. **MS:** myalgia, arthralgia, back pain, limb pain. **Misc:** fever, allergic reactions, flu-like syndrome, sepsis, ↑ mortality and ↑ tumor growth (with hemoglobin ≥12 g/dL).

Interactions
Drug-Drug: None reported.

Route/Dosage

Anemia due to Chronic Renal Failure
(Use lowest dose that will gradually increase hemoglobin level and avoid RBC transfusion).
IV, Subcut (Adults): *Starting treatment with darbepoetin (no previous epoetin)*—0.45 mcg/kg once weekly (may start with 0.75 mcg/kg q 2 wk in patients not on dialysis); adjust dose to attain target Hgb of 10–12 g/dL; if Hgb ↑ by >1.0 g/dL in 2 wk or if the Hgb is ↑ and nearing 12 g/dL, ↓ dose by 25%; if Hgb ↑ by <1.0 g/dL after 4 wk of therapy (with adequate iron stores), ↑ dose by 25%; do not ↑ dose more frequently than q 4 wk. *Conversion from epoetin to darbepoetin*—weekly epoetin dose <2500 units = 6.25 mcg/week darbepoetin, weekly epoetin dose 2500–4999 units = 12.5 mcg/week darbepoetin, weekly epoetin dose 5000–10,999 units = 25 mcg/week darbepoetin, weekly epoetin dose 11,000–17,999 units = 40 mcg/week darbepoetin, weekly epoetin dose 18,000–33,999 units = 60 mcg/week darbepoetin, weekly epoetin dose 34,000–89,999 units = 100 mcg/week darbepoetin, weekly epoetin dose >90,000 units = 200 mcg/week darbepoetin.

Anemia due to Chemotherapy
(Use only for chemotherapy-related anemia and discontinue when chemotherapy course is completed; do not initiate if hemoglobin ≥10 g/dL.)
Subcut (Adults): 2.25 mcg/kg weekly or 500 mcg q 3 wk; target Hgb should not exceed 12 g/dL. If Hgb ↑ by >1.0 g/dL in 2 wk or if the Hgb >12 g/dL or Hgb reaches level to avoid transfusion, ↓ dose by 40%; if Hgb ↑ by <1.0 g/dL after 6 wk of therapy, ↑ dose to 4.5 mcg/kg .

Availability
Albumin solution for injection: 25 mcg/mL 1-mL vial, 40 mcg/mL 1-mL vial, 60 mcg/mL 1-mL vial, 100 mcg/mL 1-mL vial, 150 mcg/mL 0.75-mL vial, 200 mcg/mL 1-mL vial, 300 mcg/mL 1-mL vial, 500 mcg/mL 1-mL vial. **Pre-filled syringes:** 60 mcg/0.3 mL, 100 mcg/0.5 mL, 200 mcg/0.4 mL.

NURSING IMPLICATIONS

Assessment
• Monitor blood pressure before and during therapy. Inform health care professional if severe hypertension is present or if blood pres-

sure begins to increase. Additional antihypertensive therapy may be required during initiation of therapy.
- Monitor response for symptoms of anemia (fatigue, dyspnea, pallor).
- Monitor dialysis shunts (thrill and bruit) and status of artificial kidney during hemodialysis. May need to increase heparin dose to prevent clotting. Monitor patients with underlying vascular disease for impaired circulation.
- Monitor for allergic reactions (rash, utricaria). Discontinue darbepoetin if signs of anaphylaxis (dyspnea, laryngeal swelling) occur.
- **Lab Test Considerations:** May cause ↑ in WBCs and platelets. May ↓ bleeding times.
- Monitor serum ferritin, transferrin, and iron levels prior to and during therapy to assess need for concurrent iron therapy. Transferrin saturation should be at least 20% and ferritin should be at least 100 ng/mL.
- Monitor hemoglobin before and weekly during initial therapy, for 4 wk after a change in dose, and regularly after target range has been reached and maintenance dose is determined. Monitor other hematopoietic parameters (CBC with differential and platelet count) before and periodically during therapy. Hemoglobin increases of more than 1.0 g/dL in any 2-week period or hemoglobin >12 g/dL increases the likelihood of life-threatening cardiovascular complications, cardiac arrest, neurologic events (seizures, stroke), hypertensive reactions, CHF, vascular thrombosis/ischemia/infarction, acute MI, and fluid overload/edema.
- If increase in hemoglobin is less than 1 g/dL over 4 wk and iron stores are adequate, dose may be increased by 25% of previous dose.
- Monitor renal function studies and electrolytes closely; resulting increased sense of well-being may lead to decreased compliance with other therapies for renal failure.

Potential Nursing Diagnoses
Activity intolerance (Indications)

Implementation
- Transfusions are still required for severe symptomatic anemia. Supplemental iron should be initiated with darbepoetin and continued during therapy. Correct deficiencies of folic acid or vitamin B_{12} prior to therapy.
- Institute seizure precautions in patients who experience greater than a 1.0 g/dL increase in hemoglobin in a 2-wk period or exhibit any change in neurologic status.
- *For conversion from epoetin alfa to darbepoetin,* if epoetin was administered 2–3 times/wk administer darbepoetin once a week. If patient was receiving epoetin once/wk, darbepoetin may be administered once every 2 wk. Route of administration should remain consistent.
- Dose adjustments should not be more frequent than once/month.
- Do not shake vial; inactivation of medication may occur. Do not administer vials containing solution that is discolored or contains particulate matter. Discard vial immediately after withdrawing dose. Do not pool unused portions.
- **Subcut:** This route is often used for patients not requiring dialysis.

IV Administration
- **Direct IV:** Administer undiluted. *Rate:* May be administered as direct injection or bolus over 1–3 min into IV tubing or via venous line at end of dialysis session.
- **Y-Site Incompatibility:** Do not administer in conjunction with other drugs or solutions.

Patient/Family Teaching
- Explain rationale for concurrent iron therapy (increased red blood cell production requires iron).
- Discuss possible return of menses and fertility in women of childbearing age. Patient should discuss contraceptive options with health care professional.
- Discuss ways of preventing self-injury in patients at risk for seizures. Driving and activities requiring continuous alertness should be avoided.
- Inform patient that use of darbepoetin may result in shortened overall survival and/or ↓ time to tumor progression.
- **Anemia of Chronic Renal Failure**: Stress importance of compliance with dietary restrictions, medications, and dialysis. Foods high in iron and low in potassium include liver, pork, veal, beef, mustard and turnip greens, peas, eggs, broccoli, kale, blackberries, strawberries, apple juice, watermelon, oatmeal, and enriched bread. Darbepoetin will result in increased sense of well-being, but it does not cure underlying disease.
- **Home Care Issues:** Home dialysis patients determined to be able to safely and effectively administer darbepoetin should be taught proper dosage, administration technique with syringe, auto-injector or IV use, and disposal of equipment. *Information for Patients and Caregivers* should be provided to patient along with medication.

Evaluation/Desired Outcomes
- Increase in hemoglobin not to exceed 12 g/dL with improvement in symptoms of anemia in patients with chronic renal failure or with chemotherapy-induced anemia.

⚇ darifenacin (dar-i-fen-a-sin)
Enablex

Classification
Therapeutic: urinary tract antispasmodics
Pharmacologic: anticholinergics

Pregnancy Category C

Indications
Overactive bladder with symptoms (urge incontinence, urgency, frequency).

Action
Acts as a muscarinic (cholinergic) receptor antagonist; antagonizes bladder smooth muscle contraction. **Therapeutic Effects:** Decreased symptoms of overactive bladder.

Pharmacokinetics
Absorption: 15–19% absorbed.
Distribution: Unknown.
Protein Binding: 98%.
Metabolism and Excretion: Extensively metabolized by the CYP2D6 enzyme system in most individuals; ⚇ poor metabolizers (7% of Caucasians, 2% of African Americans) have less CYP2D6 activity with less metabolism occurring. Some metabolism via CYP3A4 enzyme system. 60% excreted renally as metabolites, 40% in feces as metabolites.
Half-life: 13–19 hr.

TIME/ACTION PROFILE

ROUTE	ONSET	PEAK	DURATION
PO	unknown	7 hr	24 hr

Contraindications/Precautions
Contraindicated in: Hypersensitivity; Urinary retention; Gastric retention; Uncontrolled angle-closure glaucoma; Severe hepatic impairment.
Use Cautiously in: Concurrent use of CYP3A4 inhibitors (use lower dose/clinical monitoring may be necessary); Moderate hepatic impairment (lower dose recommended); Bladder outflow obstruction; GI obstructive disorders, ↓ GI motility, severe constipation or ulcerative colitis; Myasthenia gravis; Angle-closure glaucoma; Lactation, Pedi: Safety not established; OB: Use only if maternal benefit outweighs fetal risk.

Adverse Reactions/Side Effects
CNS: dizziness. **EENT:** blurred vision. **GI:** constipation, dry mouth, dyspepsia, nausea. **Metab:** heat intolerance. **Misc:** ANGIOEDEMA.

Interactions
Drug-Drug: Blood levels and risk of toxicity are ↑ by concurrent use of strong CYP3A4 inhibitors including **ketoconazole**, **itraconazole**, **ritonavir**, **nelfinavir**, **clarithromycin**, and **nefazodone**; daily dose should not exceed 7.5 mg. Concurrent use of moderate inhibitors of CYP3A4, especially those with narrow therapeutic indices, including **flecainide**, **thioridazine**, and **tricyclic antidepressants**, should be undertaken with caution.

Route/Dosage
PO (Adults): 7.5 mg once daily, may be ↑ after 2 wk to 15 mg once daily.

Availability
Extended-release tablets: 7.5 mg, 15 mg.

NURSING IMPLICATIONS

Assessment
- Monitor voiding pattern and assess symptoms of overactive bladder (urinary urgency, urinary incontinence, urinary frequency) to and periodically during therapy.

Potential Nursing Diagnoses
Impaired urinary elimination (Indications)

Implementation
- **PO:** Administer once daily without regard to food. Extended-release tablets must be swallowed whole; do not break, crush, or chew.

Patient/Family Teaching
- Instruct patient to take darifenacin as directed. Advise patient to read the *Patient Information* before starting therapy and with each prescription refill. If a dose is missed, skip dose and take next day; do not take 2 doses in same day.
- Do not share darifenacin with others; may be dangerous.
- Inform patient of potential anticholinergic side effects (constipation, urinary retention, blurred vision, heat prostration in a hot environment).
- May cause dizziness and blurred vision. Caution patient to avoid driving and other activities that require alertness until response to medication is known.
- Advise patient to consult health care professional prior to taking Rx, OTC, or herbal products with darifenacin.

♣ = Canadian drug name. ⚇ = Genetic implication.
*CAPITALS indicates life-threatening; underlines indicate most frequent.

Evaluation/Desired Outcomes
- Decrease in symptoms of overactive bladder (urge urinary incontinence, urgency, frequency).

---

darunavir (da-ru-na-veer)
Prezista

Classification
Therapeutic: antiretrovirals
Pharmacologic: protease inhibitors

Pregnancy Category C

Indications
HIV infection (must be used with ritonavir and with other antiretrovirals).

Action
Inhibits HIV-1 protease, selectively inhibiting the cleavage of HIV-encoded specific polyproteins in infected cells. This prevents the formation of mature virus particles. **Therapeutic Effects:** Increased CD4 cell counts and decreased viral load with subsequent slowed progression of HIV infection and its sequelae.

Pharmacokinetics
Absorption: *Without ritonavir*—37% absorbed following oral administration; *with ritonavir*—82%. Food ↑ absorption by 30%.
Distribution: Unknown.
Protein Binding: 95% bound to plasma proteins.
Metabolism and Excretion: Extensively metabolized by CYP3A enzyme system. 41% eliminated unchanged in feces, 8% in urine.
Half-life: 15 hr.

TIME/ACTION PROFILE

ROUTE	ONSET	PEAK	DURATION
PO	unknown	2.5–4 hr	12 hr

Contraindications/Precautions
Contraindicated in: Concurrent dihydroergotamine, ergonovine, ergotamine, methylergonovine, midazolam, pimozide, triazolam, lovastatin, simvastatin, rifampin, or St. John's wort; Lactation: HIV may be transmitted in human milk; **Pedi:** Children <3 yr.
Use Cautiously in: Hepatic impairment; Sulfa allergy; **Geri:** Consider age-related impairment in hepatic function, concurrent chronic disease states and drug therapy; **OB:** Use in pregnancy only if maternal benefit outweighs fetal risk; **Pedi:** Children 3–6 yr (safety not established).

Adverse Reactions/Side Effects
Based on concurrent use with ritonavir.
GI: HEPATOTOXICITY, constipation, diarrhea, nausea, vomiting. **Endo:** hyperglycemia. **Metab:** body fat redistribution. **Derm:** rash.

Interactions
Drug-Drug: Darunavir and ritonavir are both inhibitors of CYP3A and are metabolized by CYP3A. Multiple drug-drug interactions can be expected with drugs that share, inhibit, or induce these pathways. Consult product information for more specific details. **Rifampin** ↑ metabolism and may ↓ antiretroviral effectiveness, concurrent use is contraindicated. ↓ metabolism of and may ↑ risk of ergot toxicity with **dihydroergotamine, ergonovine, ergotamine,** or **methylergonovine**; concurrent use is contraindicated. ↓ metabolism of and may ↑ risk of myopathy with **lovastatin** and **simvastatin**; concurrent use is contraindicated. ↑ levels and risk of cardiotoxicity with **pimozide**; concurrent use is contraindicated. ↑ levels and risk of excess CNS depression with **midazolam** or **triazolam**; concurrent use is contraindicated. Concurrent use with **indinavir** may ↑ darunavir and indinavir levels. ↑ levels and risk of myopathy from **atorvastatin, rosuvastatin,** or **pravastatin** (use lowest dose of these agents or consider fluvastatin). Concurrent use with **efavirenz** results in ↓ darunavir levels and ↑ efavirenz levels; use combination cautiously. **Lopivavir/ritonavir** may ↓ levels; although concurrent use is not recommended, additional ritonavir may be required. **Saquinavir** may ↓ levels; concurrent use is not recommended. ↑ levels of **lidocaine, quinidine, propafenone, flecainide,** and **amiodarone**; use cautiously and with available blood level monitoring. ↑ **digoxin** levels; blood level monitoring recommended. May ↑ **carbamazepine** levels; blood level monitoring recommended. May ↓ **phenytoin** or **phenobarbital** levels; blood level monitoring recommended. ↓ levels of **warfarin**; monitor INR. ↑ levels of **trazodone** and **desipramine**; use cautiously and ↓ dose if necessary. ↑ levels of **clarithromycin**; ↓ dose of clarithromycin if CCr ≤60 mL/min. **Ketoconazole** and **itraconazole** may levels. ↑ levels of **ketoconazole** and **itraconazole**; daily dose of itraconazole or ketoconazole should not be >200 mg. ↓ levels of **voriconazole**; concurrent use not recommended. Concurrent use with **rifabutin** ↑ rifabutin levels and ↓ darunavir levels; (may be due to ritonavir); ↓ rifabutin dose to 150 mg every other day. ↑ levels of **beta-blockers**; may need to ↓ dose. ↑ levels of **felodi-**

pine, **nifedipine**, or **nicardipine**; monitor clinical response carefully. **Dexamethasone** ↓ levels. May ↑ levels of **inhaled fluticasone**; choose alternative inhaled corticosteroid. ↑ levels of **cyclosporine**, **tacrolimus**, or **sirolimus**; blood level monitoring recommended. ↓ levels of **methadone**. ↑ **risperidone** and **thioridazine** levels; may need to ↓ dose. May ↑ levels of **sildenafil**, **vardenafil** or **tadalafil**; may result in hypotension, syncope, visual changes, and prolonged erection (↓ dose of sildenafil to 25 mg q 48 hr, vardenafil to 2.5 mg q 72 hr, and tadalafil to 10 mg q 72 hr recommended). ↓ levels of **sertraline** and **paroxetine**; adjust dose by clinical response. May ↓ levels and contraceptive efficacy of some estrogen-based **hormonal contraceptives** including **ethinyl estradiol** (alternative or additional methods of contraception recommended).

Drug-Natural Products: St. John's wort ↑ metabolism and may ↓ antiretroviral effectiveness; concurrent use is contraindicated.

Route/Dosage
PO (Adults): *Therapy-naive*—800 mg (two 400-mg tablets) with ritonavir 100 mg once daily; *Therapy-experienced*—600 mg (one 600-mg tablet or two 300-mg tablets) with ritonavir 100 mg twice daily.

PO (Children ≥6 yr): *20–29 kg*—375 mg with ritonavir 50 mg twice daily; *30–39 kg*—450 mg with ritonavir 60 mg twice daily; *≥40 kg*—600 mg with ritonavir 100 mg twice daily.

Availability
Tablets: 75 mg, 150 mg, 300 mg, 400 mg, 600 mg.

NURSING IMPLICATIONS

Assessment
- Assess patient for change in severity of HIV symptoms and for symptoms of opportunistic infections during therapy.
- Assess for allergy to sulfonamides.
- Monitor patient for development of rash; usually maculopapular and self-limited. Discontinue therapy if severe.
- **Lab Test Considerations:** Monitor viral load and CD4 counts regularly during therapy.
- May cause ↑ serum AST, ALT, GGT, total bilirubin, alkaline phosphatase, pancreatic amylase, pancreatic lipase, triglycerides, total cholesterol, and uric acid concentrations. Monitor hepatic function prior to and periodically during therapy. Hepatotoxicity may require interruption or discontinuation of therapy.

Potential Nursing Diagnoses
Risk for infection (Indications)
Noncompliance (Patient/Family Teaching)

Implementation
- **PO:** Must be administered with a meal or light snack along with ritonavir 100 mg to be effective. The type of food is not important. Tablets should be swallowed whole with water or milk; do not chew.

Patient/Family Teaching
- Emphasize the importance of taking darunavir with ritonavir exactly as directed, at evenly spaced times throughout day. Do not take more than prescribed amount and do not stop taking without consulting health care professional. If a dose of darunavir or ritonavir is missed by more than 6 hr, wait and take next dose at regularly scheduled time. If missed by less than 6 hr, take darunavir and ritonavir immediately and then take next dose at regularly scheduled time. If a dose is skipped, do not double doses. Advise patient to read the *Patient Information* sheet before starting therapy and with each Rx renewal in case changes have been made.
- Instruct patient that darunavir should not be shared with others.
- Advise patient to avoid taking other Rx, OTC, or herbal products without consulting health care professional. These medications interact with many other drugs.
- Inform patient that darunavir does not cure AIDS or prevent associated or opportunistic infections. Darunavir does not reduce the risk of transmission of HIV to others through sexual contact or blood contamination. Caution patient to use a condom during sexual contact and to avoid sharing needles or donating blood to prevent spreading the AIDS virus to others. Advise patient that the long-term effects of darunavir are unknown at this time.
- Inform patient that darunavir may cause hyperglycemia and hepatotoxicity. Advise patient to notify health care professional if signs of hyperglycemia (increased thirst or hunger; unexplained weight loss; increased urination; fatigue; or dry, itchy skin) or hepatotoxicity (unexplained fatigue, anorexia, nausea, jaundice, abdominal pain or dark urine) occur.
- Advise patients taking oral contraceptives to use a nonhormonal method of birth control

during darunavir therapy. Advise female patients to avoid breastfeeding during therapy with darunavir.
- Inform patient that redistribution and accumulation of body fat may occur, causing central obesity, dorsocervical fat enlargement (buffalo hump), peripheral wasting, breast enlargement, and cushingoid appearance. The cause and long-term effects are not known.
- Emphasize the importance of regular follow-up exams and blood counts to determine progress and monitor for side effects.

Evaluation/Desired Outcomes
- Delayed progression of AIDS and decreased opportunistic infections in patients with HIV.
- Decrease in viral load and improvement in CD4 cell counts.

HIGH ALERT

DAUNOrubicin hydrochloride
(daw-noe-**roo**-bi-sin **hye**-dro-**klor**-ide)
Cerubidine

Classification
Therapeutic: antineoplastics
Pharmacologic: anthracyclines

Pregnancy Category D

Indications
In combination with other antineoplastics in the treatment of leukemias.

Action
Forms a complex with DNA, which subsequently inhibits DNA and RNA synthesis (cell-cycle phase-nonspecific). **Therapeutic Effects:** Death of rapidly replicating cells, particularly malignant ones. Also has immunosuppressive properties.

Pharmacokinetics
Absorption: Administered IV only, resulting in complete bioavailability.
Distribution: Widely distributed. Crosses the placenta.
Metabolism and Excretion: Extensively metabolized by the liver. Converted partially to a compound that also has antineoplastic activity (daunorubicinol); 40% eliminated by biliary excretion.
Half-life: *Daunorubicin* — 18.5 hr. *Daunorubicinol* — 26.7 hr.

TIME/ACTION PROFILE (effects on blood counts)

ROUTE	ONSET	PEAK	DURATION
IV	7–10 days	10–14 days	21 days

Contraindications/Precautions
Contraindicated in: Hypersensitivity to daunorubicin or any other components in the formulation; Symptomatic CHF/arrhythmias; Pregnant or lactating women.
Use Cautiously in: Active infections or decreased bone marrow reserve; Geriatric patients or patients with other chronic debilitating illnesses (dosage reduction recommended for patients ≥60 yr); May reactivate skin lesions produced by previous radiation therapy; Hepatic or renal impairment (dosage reduction recommended if serum creatinine >3 mg/dL or serum bilirubin >1.2 mg/dL); Patients who have received previous anthracycline therapy or who have underlying cardiovascular disease (increased risk of cardiotoxicity); Patients with childbearing potential.

Adverse Reactions/Side Effects
EENT: rhinitis, abnormal vision, sinusitis. **CV:** CARDIOTOXICITY, arrhythmias. **GI:** nausea, vomiting, esophagitis, hepatotoxicity, stomatitis. **GU:** red urine, gonadal suppression. **Derm:** alopecia. **Hemat:** anemia, leukopenia, thrombocytopenia. **Local:** phlebitis at IV site. **Metab:** hyperuricemia. **Misc:** chills, fever.

Interactions
Drug-Drug: Additive myelosuppression with other **antineoplastics**. May decrease antibody response to **live-virus vaccines** and increase risk of adverse reactions. **Cyclophosphamide** increases the risk of cardiotoxicity. Increased risk of hepatic toxicity with other **hepatotoxic agents**.

Route/Dosage
Other dose regimens are used. In adults, cumulative dose should not exceed 550 mg/m^2 (450 mg/m^2 if previous chest radiation).
IV (Adults <60 yr): 45 mg/m^2/day for 3 days in first course, then for 2 days of second course (as part of combination regimen).
IV (Adults ≥60 yr): 30 mg/m^2/day for 3 days in first course, then for 2 days of second course (as part of combination regimen).
IV (Children >2 yr): 25 mg/m^2 once weekly (as part of combination regimen). In children <2 yr or BSA <0.5 m^2, dosage should be determined on a mg/kg basis.

DAUNOrubicin hydrochloride

Availability (generic available)
Powder for injection: 20 mg/vial. **Solution for injection:** 5 mg/mL in 4-mL vials (20 mg).

NURSING IMPLICATIONS
Assessment
- Monitor vital signs before and frequently during therapy.
- Monitor for bone marrow depression. Assess for bleeding (bleeding gums; bruising; petechiae; guaiac stools, urine, and emesis) and avoid IM injections and taking rectal temperatures if platelet count is low. Apply pressure to venipuncture sites for 10 min. Assess for signs of infection during neutropenia. Anemia may occur. Monitor for increased fatigue, dyspnea, and orthostatic hypotension.
- Assess IV site frequently for inflammation or infiltration. Instruct patient to notify nurse immediately if pain or irritation at injection site occurs. If extravasation occurs, infusion must be stopped and restarted in another vein to avoid damage to subcut tissue. Notify physician immediately. Daunorubicin is a vesicant. Standard treatments include local injections of steroids and application of ice compresses.
- Monitor intake and output, appetite, and nutritional intake. Assess for nausea and vomiting, which, although mild, may persist for 24–48 hr. Administration of an antiemetic before and periodically during therapy and adjusting diet as tolerated may help maintain fluid and electrolyte balance and nutritional status. Encourage fluid intake of 2000–3000 mL/day. Allopurinol and alkalinization of the urine may be used to help prevent urate stone formation.
- Assess patient for evidence of cardiotoxicity, which manifests as CHF (peripheral edema, dyspnea, rales/crackles, weight gain, jugular venous distention) and usually occurs 1–6 mo after initiation of therapy. Chest x-ray, echocardiography, ECGs, and radionuclide angiography determination of ejection fraction may be ordered before and periodically throughout therapy. A 30% decrease in QRS voltage and decrease in systolic ejection fraction are early signs of cardiotoxicity. Patients who receive total cumulative doses >550/mm^2, who have a history of cardiac disease, or who have received mediastinal radiation are at greater risk of developing cardiotoxicity. May be irreversible and fatal, but usually responds to early treatment.
- *Lab Test Considerations:* Monitor uric acid levels.
- *Daunorubicin hydrochloride:* Monitor CBC and differential before and periodically throughout therapy. The leukocyte count nadir occurs 10–14 days after administration. Recovery usually occurs within 21 days after administration of daunorubicin.
- Monitor AST, ALT, LDH, and serum bilirubin. May cause transiently ↑ serum alkaline phosphatase, bilirubin, and AST concentrations.

Potential Nursing Diagnoses
Risk for infection (Adverse Reactions)
Decreased cardiac output (Side Effects)

Implementation
- *High Alert:* Fatalities have occurred with chemotherapeutic agents. Before administering, clarify all ambiguous orders; double-check single, daily, and course-of-therapy dose limits; have second practitioner independently double-check original order, calculations, and infusion pump settings. Do not confuse daunorubicin hydrochloride (Cerubidine) with daunorubicin citrate liposome (DaunoXome) or with doxorubicin (Adriamycin, Rubex) or doxorubicin hydrochloride liposome (Doxil). To prevent confusion, orders should include generic and brand name.
- Solution should be prepared in a biologic cabinet. Wear gloves, gown, and mask while handling IV medication. Discard IV equipment in specially designated containers.
- **IV:** Reconstitute each 20 mg with 4 mL of sterile water for injection for a concentration of 5 mg/mL. Shake gently to dissolve. Reconstituted medication is stable for 24 hr at room temperature, 48 hr if refrigerated. Protect from sunlight.
- Do not use aluminum needles when reconstituting or injecting daunorubicin, as aluminum darkens the solution.

IV Administration
- **Direct IV:** *Diluent:* Dilute further in 10–15 mL of 0.9% NaCl. Administer direct IV push through Y-site into free-flowing infusion of 0.9% NaCl or D5W. *Rate:* Administer over at least 2–3 min. Rapid administration rate may cause facial flushing or erythema along the vein.
- **Intermittent Infusion:** *Diluent:* May also be diluted in 50–100 mL of 0.9% NaCl. *Rate:*

✦ = Canadian drug name. ✱ = Genetic implication.
*CAPITALS indicates life-threatening; underlines indicate most frequent.

Administer 50 mL over 10–15 min or 100 mL over 30–45 min.
- **Y-Site Compatibility:** amifostine, etoposide, filgrastim, gemcitabine, granisetron, melphalan, methotrexate, ondansetron, sodium bicarbonate, teniposide, thiotepa, vinorelbine.
- **Y-Site Incompatibility:** allopurinol, aztreonam, cefepime, fludarabine, lansoprazole, piperacillin/tazobactam.
- **Additive Incompatibility:** Manufacturer does not recommend admixing daunorubicin hydrochloride.

Patient/Family Teaching
- Instruct patient to notify health care professional if fever; chills; sore throat; signs of infection; bleeding gums; bruising; petechiae; or blood in urine, stool, or emesis occurs. Caution patient to avoid crowds and persons with known infections. Instruct patient to use soft toothbrush and electric razor. Patient should be cautioned not to drink alcoholic beverages or take products containing aspirin or NSAIDs.
- Instruct patient to inspect oral mucosa for erythema and ulceration. If ulceration occurs, advise patient to use sponge brush and rinse mouth with water after eating and drinking. Stomatitis pain may require management with opioid analgesics. Period of highest risk is 3–7 days after administration of dose.
- Instruct patient to notify health care professional immediately if irregular heartbeat, shortness of breath, or swelling of lower extremities occurs.
- Discuss with patient possibility of hair loss. Explore methods of coping. Regrowth of hair usually begins within 5 wk after discontinuing therapy.
- Inform patient that medication may turn urine reddish color for 1–2 days after administration.
- Inform patient that this medication may cause irreversible gonadal suppression. Advise patient that this medication may have teratogenic effects. Contraception should be used during therapy and for at least 4 mo after therapy is concluded.
- Instruct patient not to receive any vaccinations without advice of health care professional.
- Emphasize the need for periodic lab tests to monitor for side effects.

Evaluation/Desired Outcomes
- Improvement of hematologic status in patients with leukemia.

HIGH ALERT

decitabine (de-sit-a-been)
Dacogen

Classification
Therapeutic: antineoplastics

Pregnancy Category D

Indications
Treatment of various myelodysplastic syndromes (MDS).

Action
Inhibits DNA methyltransferase, causing apoptosis. Has more effect on rapidly replicating cells.
Therapeutic Effects: Improved hematologic and clinical manifestations of MDS.

Pharmacokinetics
Absorption: IV administration results in complete bioavailability.
Distribution: Unknown.
Metabolism and Excretion: Mostly metabolized by the liver.
Half-life: 0.5 hr.

TIME/ACTION PROFILE (blood levels)

ROUTE	ONSET	PEAK	DURATION
IV	rapid	end of infusion	unknown

Contraindications/Precautions
Contraindicated in: Hypersensitivity; OB: Pregnancy or lactation.
Use Cautiously in: Patients with child-bearing potential (males and females); Impaired hepatic/renal function; Geri: Elderly patients may be more sensitive to effects; Pedi: Safety in children not established.

Adverse Reactions/Side Effects
CNS: confusion, fatigue, insomnia, depression, lethargy. **EENT:** blurred vision. **Resp:** cough. **CV:** atrial fibrillation, pulmonary edema, tachycardia. **GI:** abdominal pain, constipation, diarrhea, stomatitis, vomiting, abnormal liver function tests. **Derm:** petechiae, rash. **F and E:** edema, hypokalemia, hypomagnesemia, ascites. **Hemat:** BLEEDING, anemia, neutropenia, thrombocytopenia. **Local:** injection site irritation. **Metab:** hyperglycemia. **MS:** arthralgia, myalgia. **Misc:** INFECTION, fever, lymphadenopathy.

Interactions
Drug-Drug: ↑ risk of myelosuppression with other **antineoplastics**, **immunosuppressants**, or **radiation therapy**. May ↓ antibody re-

sponse to and ↑ risk of adverse reactions from **live virus vaccines**.

Route/Dosage
IV (Adults): *First treatment cycle*—15 mg/m^2 as a continuous infusion over 3 hours repeated every 8 hours for 3 days. *Subsequent cycles*—cycle should be repeated every 6 wk for a minimum of 4 cycles; treatment may be continued as long as the patient continues to benefit. Dose adjustment/delay may be required for hematologic toxicity, renal or hepatic impairment, or infection.

Availability
Lyophilized powder for injection (requires reconstitution): 50 mg/vial.

NURSING IMPLICATIONS
Assessment
- Monitor for bone marrow depression. Assess for bleeding (bleeding gums, bruising, petechiae, guaiac stools, urine, and emesis) and avoid IM injections and taking rectal temperatures if platelet count is low. Apply pressure to venipuncture sites for 10 min. Assess for signs of infection during neutropenia. Anemia may occur. Monitor for increased fatigue, dyspnea, and orthostatic hypotension.
- *Lab Test Considerations:* Monitor CBC prior to each dosing cycle and periodically as needed. May cause neutropenia, thrombocytopenia, and anemia; occur more frequently in 1st or 2nd cycle. Use early institution of growth factors and antimicrobial agents to prevent infections.
- Obtain liver chemistries and serum creatinine prior to initiation of treatment. May cause hyperbilirubinemia and hypoalbuminemia.
- May cause hyperglycemia, hypomagnesemia, hyponatremia, hypokalemia, and hyperkalemia.

Potential Nursing Diagnoses
Risk for infection (Adverse Reactions)

Implementation
- *High Alert:* Fatalities have occurred with chemotherapeutic agents. Before administering, clarify all ambiguous orders; double-check single, daily, and course-of-therapy dose limits; have second practitioner independently double-check original order, calculations, and infusion pump settings.
- Solution should be prepared in a biologic cabinet. Wear gloves, gown, and mask while handling IV medication. Discard IV equipment in specially designated containers (see Appendix L).
- Pre-medicate patient with standard anti-emetic therapy.
- If hematologic recovery (ANC ≥1,000 cells/mm^3 and platelets ≥50,000 cells/mm^3) from previous treatment cycle requires more than 6, but less than 8 wk—delay dosing for up to 2 wk and temporarily reduce dose to 11 mg/m^2 (33 mg/m^2/day, 99 mg/m^2/cycle) upon restarting therapy.
- If hematologic recovery requires more than 8, but less than 10 wk—Patient should be assessed for disease progression (by bone marrow aspirates); in the absence of progression, delay dose for up to 2 more wk and reduce dose as above upon restarting, then maintain or increase in subsequent cycles as clinically indicated.
- **Intermittent Infusion:** Reconstitute with 10 mL of Sterile Water for injection for a concentration of 5 mg/mL. Immediately after reconstitution, dilute further with 0.9% NaCl, D5W, or LR for a final concentration of 0.1–1.0 mg/mL. Unless used within 15 min of reconstitution, dilute solution must be prepared using cold infusion fluids and refrigerated until administration (maximum of 7 hr). *Rate:* Administer over 3 hr.

Patient/Family Teaching
- Caution patient to avoid crowds and persons with known infections. Report symptoms of infection (fever, chills, cough, hoarseness, sore throat, lower back or side pain, painful or difficult urination) immediately.
- Instruct patient to report unusual bleeding. Advise patient of thrombocytopenia precautions (use soft toothbrush and electric razor, avoid falls, do not drink alcoholic beverages or take medication containing aspirin or NSAIDs; may precipitate gastric bleeding).
- Inform patient that this medication may have teratogenic effects. Advise women to avoid becoming pregnant during treatment and advise men not to father a child during or for 2 months after treatment.

Evaluation/Desired Outcomes
- Improved hematologic and clinical manifestations of MDS.

deferoxamine
(de-fer-**ox**-a-meen)
Desferal

Classification
Therapeutic: antidotes
Pharmacologic: heavy metal antagonists

Pregnancy Category C

Indications
Acute toxic iron ingestion. Secondary iron overload syndromes associated with multiple transfusion therapy.

Action
Chelates unbound iron, forming a water-soluble complex (ferrioxamine) in plasma that is easily excreted by the kidneys. **Therapeutic Effects:** Removal of excess iron. Also chelates aluminum.

Pharmacokinetics
Absorption: Poorly absorbed after oral administration. Well absorbed after IM administration and subcut administration.
Distribution: Appears to be widely distributed.
Metabolism and Excretion: Metabolized by tissues and plasma enzymes. Unchanged drug and chelated form excreted by the kidneys; 33% of iron removed is eliminated in the feces via biliary excretion.
Half-life: 1 hr.

TIME/ACTION PROFILE (effects on hematologic parameters)

ROUTE	ONSET	PEAK	DURATION
IV	rapid	unknown	unknown
IM	unknown	unknown	unknown
Subcut	unknown	unknown	unknown

Contraindications/Precautions
Contraindicated in: Severe renal disease; Anuria; OB: Early pregnancy or childbearing potential (however, may be used safely in pregnant patients with moderate-to-severe acute iron intoxication).
Use Cautiously in: Pedi: Children <3 yr (safety not established).

Adverse Reactions/Side Effects
EENT: blurred vision, cataracts, ototoxicity. **CV:** hypotension, tachycardia. **GI:** abdominal pain, diarrhea. **GU:** red urine. **Derm:** erythema, flushing, urticaria. **Local:** induration at injection site, pain at injection site. **MS:** leg cramps. **Misc:** allergic reactions, fever, shock after rapid IV administration.

Interactions
Drug-Drug: Ascorbic acid may ↑ effectiveness of deferoxamine but may also ↑ cardiac iron toxicity.

Route/Dosage
Acute Iron Ingestion
IM, IV (Adults and Children ≥3 yr): 1 g, then 500 mg q 4 hr for 2 doses. Additional doses of 500 mg q 4–12 hr may be needed (not to exceed 6 g/24 hr).

Chronic Iron Overload
IM, IV (Adults and Children ≥3 yr): 500 mg–1 g daily IM; additional doses of 2 g should be given IV for each unit of blood transfused (not to exceed 1 g/day in absence of transfusions; 6 g/day if patient receives transfusions).
Subcut (Adults and Children ≥3 yr): 1–2 g/day (20–40 mg/kg/day) infused over 8–24 hr.

Availability (generic available)
Powder for injection: 500 mg/vial, 2 g/vial.

NURSING IMPLICATIONS
Assessment
- In acute poisoning, assess time, amount, and type of iron preparation ingested.
- Monitor signs of iron toxicity: early acute (abdominal pain, bloody diarrhea, emesis), late acute (decreased level of consciousness, shock, metabolic acidosis).
- Monitor vital signs closely, especially during IV administration. Report hypotension, erythema, urticaria, or signs of allergic reaction. Keep epinephrine, an antihistamine, and resuscitation equipment close by in the event of an anaphylactic reaction.
- May cause oculotoxicity or ototoxicity. Report decreased visual acuity or hearing loss. Audiovisual exams should be performed every 3 mo in patients with chronic iron overload.
- Monitor intake and output and urine color. Inform health care professional if patient is anuric. Chelated iron is excreted primarily by the kidneys; urine may turn red.
- *Lab Test Considerations:* Monitor serum iron, total iron binding capacity (TIBC), ferritin levels, and urinary iron excretion before and periodically during therapy.
- Monitor liver function studies to assess damage from iron poisoning.

Potential Nursing Diagnoses
Risk for injury poisoning (Indications)

Implementation

- IM route is preferred in acute iron intoxication unless patient is in shock.
- Reconstitute 500-mg vial with 2 mL and 2-g vial with 8 mL of sterile water for injection for a concentration of 213 mg/mL. Dissolve powder completely before administration. Solution is yellow and is stable for 1 wk after reconstitution if protected from light. Discard unused portion.
- Used in conjunction with induction of emesis or gastric aspiration and lavage with sodium bicarbonate, and supportive measures for shock and metabolic acidosis in acute poisoning.
- **IM:** Administer deep IM and massage well. Rotate sites. IM administration may cause transient severe pain.
- **Subcut:** Reconstitute 500-mg vial with 5 mL and 2-g vial with 20 mL of sterile water for injection. *Concentration:* 95 mg/mL. Subcut route used to treat chronically elevated iron therapy is administered into abdominal subcut tissue via infusion pump for 8–24 hr per treatment.
- **IV:** Reconstitute 500-mg vial with 5 mL and 2-g vial with 20 mL of sterile water for injection. *Concentration:* 95 mg/mL. *Diluent:* D5W, 0.9% NaCl, 0.45% NaCl, or LR. Dissolve powder completely before administration. Solution is clear and colorless to slightly yellow. Administer within 3 hr of reconstitution; 24 hr if prepared under laminar flow hood. Discard unused portion. *Rate:* Maximum infusion rate is 15 mg/kg/hr for first 1000 mg. May be followed by 500 mg infused over 4 hr at a slower rate not to exceed 125 mg/hr. Rapid infusion rate may cause hypotension, erythema, urticaria, wheezing, convulsions, tachycardia, or shock.
- May be administered at the same time as blood transfusion in persons with chronically elevated serum iron levels. Use separate site for administration.

Patient/Family Teaching

- Reinforce need to keep iron preparations, all medications, and hazardous substances out of the reach of children.
- Reassure patient that red coloration of urine is expected and reflects excretion of excess iron.
- May cause dizziness or impairment of vision or hearing. Caution patient to avoid driving or other activities requiring alertness until response from medication is known.
- Advise patient not to take vitamin C preparations without consulting health care professional, because tissue toxicity may increase.
- Encourage patients requiring chronic therapy to keep follow-up appointments for lab tests. Eye and hearing exams may be monitored every 3 mo.

Evaluation/Desired Outcomes

- Return of serum iron concentrations to a normal level (50–150 mcg/100 mL).

---

desipramine (dess-**ip**-ra-meen)
Norpramin, ✣ Pertofrane

Classification
Therapeutic: antidepressants
Pharmacologic: tricyclic antidepressants

Pregnancy Category C

Indications

Depression. **Unlabeled Use:** Chronic pain syndromes. Anxiety. Insomnia.

Action

Potentiates the effect of serotonin and norepinephrine in the CNS. Has significant anticholinergic properties. **Therapeutic Effects:** Antidepressant action (may develop only over several weeks).

Pharmacokinetics

Absorption: Well absorbed from the GI tract.
Distribution: Widely distributed.
Protein Binding: 90–92%.
Metabolism and Excretion: Extensively metabolized by the liver. One metabolite is pharmacologically active (2-hydroxydesipramine). Undergoes enterohepatic recirculation and secretion into gastric juices. Small amounts enter breast milk.
Half-life: 12–27 hr.

TIME/ACTION PROFILE (antidepressant effect)

ROUTE	ONSET	PEAK	DURATION
PO	2–3 wk	2–6 wk	days–wk

Contraindications/Precautions

Contraindicated in: Angle-closure glaucoma; Recent MI, heart failure, known history of QTc prolongation.
Use Cautiously in: Patients with pre-existing cardiovascular disease; Prostatic hyperplasia (↑ susceptibility to urinary retention); History of sei-

zures (threshold may be ↓); May ↑ risk of suicide attempt/ideation especially during early treatment or dose adjustment; risk may be greater in children or adolescents; OB: Use during pregnancy only if maternal benefit outweighs risks to fetus; use during lactation may result in neonatal sedation; Pedi: Safety not established in children <12 yr; Geri: ↑ sensitivity to effects.

Adverse Reactions/Side Effects
CNS: drowsiness, fatigue. **EENT:** blurred vision, dry eyes, dry mouth. **CV:** ARRHYTHMIAS, hypotension, ECG changes. **GI:** constipation, drug-induced hepatitis, paralytic ileus, increased appetite, weight gain. **GU:** urinary retention, decreased libido. **Derm:** photosensitivity. **Endo:** changes in blood glucose, gynecomastia. **Hemat:** blood dyscrasias.

Interactions
Drug-Drug: Desipramine is metabolized in the liver by the cytochrome P450 2D6 enzyme and its action may be affected by drugs which compete for metabolism by or alter the activity of this enzyme including other **antidepressants**, **phenothiazines**, **carbamazepine**, **class 1C antiarrthythmics** (**propafenone**, **flecainide**, **encainide**); when used concurrently dose reduction of one or the other or both may be necessary. Concurrent use of other drugs that inhibit the activity of the enzyme, including **cimetidine**, **quinidine**, **amiodarone**, and **ritonavir**, may result in ↑ effects. May cause hypotension, tachycardia, and potentially fatal reactions when used with **MAO inhibitors** (avoid concurrent use—discontinue 2 wk prior to). Concurrent use with **SSRI antidepressants** may result in ↑ toxicity and should be avoided (fluoxetine should be stopped 5 wk before). Concurrent use with **clonidine** may result in hypertensive crisis and should be avoided. **Phenytoin** may ↓ levels and effectiveness; ↑ doses of desipramine may be required to treat depression. Concurrent use with **levodopa** may result in delayed/↓ absorption of levodopa or hypertension. Blood levels and effects may be ↓ by **rifamycins**, **carbamazepine**, and **barbiturates**. Concurrent use with **moxifloxacin** ↑ risk of adverse cardiovascular reactions. ↑ CNS depression with other **CNS depressants** including **alcohol**, **antihistamines**, **clonidine**, **opioid analgesics**, and **sedative/hypnotics**. **Barbiturates** may alter blood levels and effects. **Adrenergic** and **anticholinergic** side effects may be ↑ with other **agents having these properties**. **Hormonal contraceptives** ↑ levels and may cause toxicity. **Cigarette smoking** may ↑ metabolism and alter effects.

Drug-Natural Products: Concomitant use of **kava-kava**, **valerian**, or **chamomile** can ↑ CNS depression. ↑ anticholinergic effects with **jimson weed** and **scopolia**.

Route/Dosage
PO (Adults): 100–200 mg/day as a single dose or in divided doses (up to 300 mg/day).
PO (Geriatric Patients): 25–50 mg/day in divided doses (up to 150 mg/day).
PO (Children >12 yr): 25–50 mg/day in divided doses, increased as needed up to 100 mg/day.
PO (Children 6–12 yr): 10–30 mg/day (1–5 mg/kg/day) in divided doses.

Availability (generic available)
Tablets: 10 mg, 25 mg, 50 mg, 75 mg, 100 mg, 150 mg.

NURSING IMPLICATIONS

Assessment
- Obtain weight and BMI initially and periodically throughout therapy.
- Assess FBS and cholesterol levels for overweight/obese individuals.
- Refer as appropriate for nutrition/weight management and medical management.
- Monitor blood pressure and pulse prior to and during initial therapy. Notify physician or other health care professional of decreases in blood pressure (10–20 mm Hg) or sudden increase in pulse rate. Patients taking high doses or with a history of cardiovascular disease should have ECG monitored prior to and periodically during therapy.
- **Depression:** Monitor mental status (orientation, mood, behavior) frequently. Assess for suicidal tendencies, especially during early therapy. Restrict amount of drug available to patient.
- **Pain:** Assess intensity, quality, and location of pain periodically throughout therapy. Use pain scale to monitor effectiveness of medication.
- *Lab Test Considerations:* Assess leukocyte and differential blood counts, liver function, and serum glucose periodically. May cause an ↑ serum bilirubin and alkaline phosphatase. May cause bone marrow depression. Serum glucose may be ↑ or ↓.
- *Lab Test Considerations:* Serum levels may be monitored in patients who fail to respond to usual therapeutic dose.

Potential Nursing Diagnoses
Ineffective coping (Indications)
Risk for injury (Side Effects)

Impaired oral mucous membrane (Side Effects)
Impaired urinary elimination (Side Effects)
Chronic pain (Indications)
Risk for constipation (Side Effects)
Sexual dysfunction (Side Effects)

Implementation

- Do not confuse desipramine with clomipramine, imipramine, or nortriptyline.
- Dose increases should be made at bedtime because of sedation. Dose titration is a slow process; may take weeks to months. May give entire dose at bedtime.
- Taper to avoid withdrawal effects. Reduce dose by half for 3 days then reduce again by half for 3 days, then discontinue.
- **PO:** Administer medication with or immediately after a meal to minimize gastric upset. Tablet may be crushed and given with food or fluids.

Patient/Family Teaching

- Instruct patient to take medication as directed. Take missed doses as soon as possible unless almost time for next dose; if regimen is a single dose at bedtime, do not take in the morning because of side effects. Advise patient that drug effects may not be noticed for at least 2 wk. Abrupt discontinuation may cause nausea; vomiting; diarrhea; headache; trouble sleeping, with vivid dreams; and irritability.
- May cause drowsiness and blurred vision. Caution patient to avoid driving and other activities requiring alertness until response to drug is known.
- Orthostatic hypotension, sedation, and confusion are common during early therapy, especially in the elderly. Protect patient from falls. Institute fall precautions. Advise patient to make position changes slowly.
- Advise patient to avoid alcohol or other CNS depressant drugs during and for 3–7 days after therapy has been discontinued.
- Instruct patient to notify health care professional if urinary retention, dry mouth, or constipation persists. Sugarless candy or gum may diminish dry mouth, and an increase in fluids or bulk may prevent constipation. If symptoms persist, dose reduction or discontinuation may be necessary. Consult health care professional if dry mouth persists for more than 2 wk.
- Caution patient to use sunscreen and protective clothing to prevent photosensitivity reactions.
- Inform patient of need to monitor dietary intake. Increase in appetite may lead to undesired weight gain.
- Alert patient that medication may turn urine blue-green in color.
- Advise patient to notify health care professional of medication regimen prior to treatment or surgery.
- Therapy for depression is usually prolonged. Emphasize the importance of follow-up exams to monitor effectiveness and side effects and to improve coping skills.
- Refer to local support group.

Evaluation/Desired Outcomes

- Increased sense of well-being.
- Renewed interest in surroundings.
- Increased appetite.
- Improved energy level.
- Improved sleep.
- Decrease in chronic pain symptoms.
- Full therapeutic effects may be seen 2–6 wk after initiating therapy.

---

desirudin (des-i-**rude**-in)
Iprivask

Classification
Therapeutic: anticoagulants
Pharmacologic: thrombin inhibitors

Pregnancy Category C

Indications

Prevention of deep-vein thrombosis (DVT) after hip-replacement surgery.

Action

Selectively inhibits free and clot-bound thrombin. Inhibition of thrombin prevents activation of factors V, VIII, and XII; conversion of fibrinogen to fibrin; platelet adhesion and aggregation. **Therapeutic Effects:** Decreased incidence of DVT and subsequent pulmonary embolism after hip-replacement surgery.

Pharmacokinetics

Absorption: Completely absorbed following subcutaneous administration.
Distribution: Binds specifically and directly to thrombin.
Metabolism and Excretion: 40–50% excreted unchanged by kidneys; some metabolism in kidneys and pancreas.
Half-life: 2 hr.

✦ = Canadian drug name.   ✶ = Genetic implication.
*CAPITALS indicates life-threatening; <u>underlines</u> indicate most frequent.

desirudin

TIME/ACTION PROFILE (effect on aPTT)

ROUTE	ONSET	PEAK	DURATION
Subcut	rapid	1–3 hr	12 hr

Contraindications/Precautions
Contraindicated in: Hypersensitivity to natural or recombinant hirudins; Active bleeding; Coagulation disorders.
Use Cautiously in: Renal impairment (dosage change recommended if CCr ≤60 mL/min); Geriatric patients (due to age-related renal impairment); Hepatic impairment; Pregnancy (use only if benefits to mother outweigh fetal risk); Lactation, children (safety not established).
Exercise Extreme Caution in: Spinal/epidural anesthesia (increased risk of spinal/epidural hematomas and their sequelae, especially when used with NSAIDs, platelet inhibitors, or other anticoagulants).

Adverse Reactions/Side Effects
GI: nausea. **Hemat:** BLEEDING, anemia. **Local:** injection site reactions, wound secretion.

Interactions
Drug-Drug: Dextran 40, **systemic corticosteroids**, **thrombolytics**, and other **anticoagulants** ↑ risk of bleeding (discontinue if possible; if not, monitor laboratory and clinical status closely). Agents altering platelet function including **salicylates**, **NSAIDs**, **clopidogrel**, **ticlopidine**, **dipyridamole**, and **glycoprotein IIb/IIIa antagonists** also ↑ risk of bleeding.

Route/Dosage
Subcut (Adults): 15 mg every 12 hr, start 5–15 min prior to surgery, but after regional block (if used), for up to 12 days.

Renal Impairment
Subcut (Adults): *CCr 31–60 mL/min*—start with 5 mg every 12 hr; further doses determined by daily aPTT; *CCr <31 mL/min*—start with 1.7 mg every 12 hr; further doses determined by daily aPTT.

Availability
Lyophilized powder for injection (requires reconstitution with specific diluent): 15.75 mg/vial with 0.6 mL ampule of diluent (contains mannitol, delivers 15 mg dose).

NURSING IMPLICATIONS

Assessment
- Assess for signs of bleeding (bleeding gums, nosebleed, unusual bruising; black, tarry stools; hematuria; fall in hematocrit or blood pressure; guaiac-positive stools; bleeding from surgical site). Notify physician if these occur.
- Assess patient for evidence of thrombosis. Symptoms depend on area of involvement. Notify physician immediately; may require urgent treatment.
- Monitor patients with epidural catheters frequently for signs of neurological impairment (midline back pain, numbness or weakness in lower limbs, bowel and/or bladder dysfunction). Notify physician immediately if these occur.
- Observe injection sites for hematomas, ecchymosis, or inflammation.
- ***Lab Test Considerations:*** Monitor activated partial thromboplastin time (aPTT) daily in patients with increased risk of bleeding and/or renal impairment. Monitor serum creatinine daily in patients with renal impairment. Peak aPTT should not exceed two times control. Reduce dose or discontinue desirudin until aPTT is <2 times control; resume at a lower dose.
- If a patient is switched from oral anticoagulants to desirudin or from desirudin to oral anticoagulants, measure anticoagulant activity closely.
- Thrombin time is not suitable for monitoring desirudin.
- Monitor CBC. If hematocrit ↓ unexpectedly, assess patient for potential bleeding sites.

Potential Nursing Diagnoses
Ineffective tissue perfusion (Indications)
Risk for injury (Adverse Reactions)

Implementation
- Reconstitute each vial with 0.5 mL of diluent provided for a concentration of 15.75 mg of desirudin/0.5 mL. Shake vial gently until fully reconstituted to a clear colorless solution. Do not administer solutions that are discolored, cloudy, or contain a particulate matter. Reconstituted solution should be used immediately, but is stable for 24 hr at room temperature and protected from light. Discard unused solution.
- **Subcut:** Withdraw all reconstituted solution into syringe with a 26- or 27-gauge, 1/2-inch length needle. Inject entire contents subcutaneously which will deliver 15 mg. Patient should be sitting or lying down during administration. Rotate sites between left and right anterolateral and left and right posterolateral thigh or abdominal wall. Inject entire length of needle while pinching skin between thumb and forefinger; continue to pinch skin throughout injection. Do not rub injection site following injection to prevent bruising.

- **Syringe Incompatibility:** Do not mix with other diluents or medications.

Patient/Family Teaching
- Advise patient to report symptoms of unusual bleeding or bruising to health care professional immediately.
- Instruct patient not to take aspirin, NSAIDs, or herbal products during therapy without consulting health care professional.

Evaluation/Desired Outcomes
- Decreased incidence of DVT and subsequent pulmonary embolism after hip-replacement surgery.

---

desloratadine
(dess-lor-**a**-ta-deen)
Clarinex

Classification
Therapeutic: allergy, cold, and cough remedies, antihistamines
Pharmacologic: piperidines

Pregnancy Category C

Indications
Symptoms of allergic rhinitis (seasonal and perennial). Chronic idiopathic urticaria.

Action
Blocks peripheral effects of histamine released during allergic reactions. **Therapeutic Effects:** Decreased symptoms of allergic reactions (nasal stuffiness, red swollen eyes). Decreased pruritus, reduction in number and size of hives in chronic idiopathic urticaria.

Pharmacokinetics
Absorption: Well absorbed; absorption for orally-disintegrating tablets and oral tablets is identical.
Distribution: Enters breast milk.
Metabolism and Excretion: Extensively metabolized to 3-hydroxydesloratadine, an active metabolite; small percentage of patients may be slow metabolizers.
Half-life: 27 hr.

TIME/ACTION PROFILE (antihistaminic effects)

ROUTE	ONSET	PEAK	DURATION
PO	unknown	3 hr	24 hr

Contraindications/Precautions
Contraindicated in: Hypersensitivity; OB: Lactation.

Use Cautiously in: Patients with hepatic or renal impairment (↓ dose to 5 mg every other day); Geri: Dosing for the elderly should consider ↓ hepatic, renal, or cardiac function, concomitant diseases, other drug therapy and ↑ risk of adverse reactions; Pedi: Children <6 mo (safety not established).

Adverse Reactions/Side Effects
CNS: drowsiness (rare). **EENT:** pharyngitis. **GI:** dry mouth. **Misc:** allergic reactions including AN-APHYLAXIS.

Interactions
Drug-Drug: The following interactions may occur, but are less likely to occur with desloratidine than with more sedating antihistamines. **MAO inhibitors** may ↑ and prolong effects of antihistamines. ↑ CNS depression may occur with other **CNS depressants** including **alcohol**, **antidepressants**, **opioids**, and **sedative/hypnotics**.

Route/Dosage
PO (Adults and Children ≥12 yr): 5 mg once daily.

Hepatic Impairment
Renal Impairment
PO (Adults and Children ≥12 yr): 5 mg every other day.
PO (Children 6–11 yr): 2.5 mg once daily.
PO (Children 12 mo–5 yr): 1.25 mg once daily.
PO (Children 6–12 mo): 1 mg once daily.

Availability
Tablets: 5 mg. **Cost:** $292.91/90. **Orally-disintegrating tablets (RediTabs) (tutti frutti):** 2.5 mg, 5 mg. **Cost:** 2.5 mg $319.29/90, 5 mg $307.89/90. **Syrup (bubblegum):** 0.5 mg/mL. **Cost:** $168.58/473 mL. *In combination with:* pseudoephedrine (Clarinex-D 12 Hour, Clarinex-D 24 Hour; see Appendix B).

NURSING IMPLICATIONS

Assessment
- Assess allergy symptoms (rhinitis, conjunctivitis, hives) before and periodically during therapy.
- Assess lung sounds and character of bronchial secretions. Maintain fluid intake of 1500–

desmopressin

2000 mL/day to decrease viscosity of secretions.
- **Lab Test Considerations:** May cause false-negative result on allergy skin testing.

Potential Nursing Diagnoses
Ineffective airway clearance (Indications)
Risk for injury (Adverse Reactions)

Implementation
- **PO:** May be administered without regard to meals.
- **Pedi:** Use calibrated measuring device to ensure accurate dose of syrup for children.
- *For rapidly disintegrating tablets (Reditabs):* Place on tongue. Tablet disintegrates rapidly. May be taken with or without water. Administer immediately after opening the blister.

Patient/Family Teaching
- Instruct patients to take desloratidine as directed. Do not increase dose or frequency; does not increase effectiveness and may increase side effects.
- May rarely cause drowsiness. Caution patient to avoid driving or other activities requiring alertness until response to medication is known.
- Advise patient to avoid taking alcohol or other CNS depressants concurrently with this drug.
- Advise patient that good oral hygiene, frequent rinsing of mouth with water, and sugarless gum or candy may minimize dry mouth. Patient should notify dentist if dry mouth persists >2 wk.

Evaluation/Desired Outcomes
- Decrease in allergic symptoms.

---

desmopressin
(des-moe-**press**-in)
DDAVP, DDAVP Rhinal Tube, DDAVP Rhinyle Drops, Stimate

Classification
Therapeutic: hormones
Pharmacologic: antidiuretic hormones

Pregnancy Category B

Indications
PO, Subcut, IV, Intranasal: Treatment of central diabetes insipidus caused by a deficiency of vasopressin. **IV, Intranasal:** Controls bleeding in certain types of hemophilia and von Willebrand's disease. **PO:** Primary nocturnal enuresis.

Action
An analogue of naturally occurring vasopressin (antidiuretic hormone). Primary action is enhanced reabsorption of water in the kidneys.
Therapeutic Effects: Prevention of nocturnal enuresis. Maintenance of appropriate body water content in diabetes insipidus. Control of bleeding in certain types of hemophilia or von Willebrand's disease.

Pharmacokinetics
Absorption: 5% absorbed following oral administration; some 10–20% absorbed from nasal mucosa.
Distribution: Distribution not fully known. Enters breast milk.
Metabolism and Excretion: Unknown.
Half-life: 75 min.

TIME/ACTION PROFILE (PO, intranasal = antidiuretic effect; IV = effect on factor VIII activity)

ROUTE	ONSET	PEAK	DURATION
PO	1 hr	4–7 hr	unknown
Intranasal	1 hr	1–5 hr	8–20 hr
IV	within min	15–30 min	3 hr†

†4–24 hr in mild hemophilia A

Contraindications/Precautions
Contraindicated in: Hypersensitivity; Hypersensitivity to chlorobutanol; Patients with type IIB or platelet-type (pseudo) von Willebrand's disease; Hyponatremia.
Use Cautiously in: Angina pectoris; Hypertension; Patients at risk for hyponatremia; OB, Lactation: Safety not established.

Adverse Reactions/Side Effects
CNS: SEIZURES, drowsiness, headache, listlessness. **EENT:** *intranasal*—nasal congestion, rhinitis. **Resp:** dyspnea. **CV:** hypertension, hypotension, tachycardia (large IV doses only). **GI:** mild abdominal cramps, nausea. **GU:** vulval pain. **Derm:** flushing. **F and E:** water intoxication/hyponatremia. **Local:** phlebitis at IV site.

Interactions
Drug-Drug: **Chlorpropamide**, **clofibrate**, or **carbamazepine** may enhance the antidiuretic response to desmopressin. **Demeclocycline**, **lithium**, or **norepinephrine** may diminish the antidiuretic response to desmopressin. Large doses may enhance the effects of **vasopressors**.

Route/Dosage

Primary Nocturnal Enuresis
PO (Adults and Children ≥6 yr): 0.2 mg at bedtime; may be titrated up to 0.6 mg at bedtime to achieve desired response.

Diabetes Insipidus

PO (Adults and Children): 0.05 mg twice daily; adjusted as needed (usual range: 0.1–1.2 mg/day in 2–3 divided doses).
Intranasal (Adults): *DDAVP*–0.1–0.4 mL/day in 1–3 divided doses.
Intranasal (Children 3 mo–12 yr): *DDAVP*–0.05–0.3 mL/day in 1–2 divided doses.
Subcut, IV (Adults): 2–4 mcg/day in 2 divided doses.

Hemophilia A/von Willebrand's disease
Intranasal (Adults and Children ≥50 kg): *Stimate*—1 spray (150 mcg) in each nostril.
Intranasal (Adults and Children <50 kg): *Stimate*—1 spray (150 mcg) in one nostril.
IV (Adults and Children >3 mo): 0.3 mcg/kg, repeated as needed.

Availability (generic available)
Tablets: 0.1 mg, 0.2 mg. **Nasal spray (DDAVP):** 10 mcg/spray—5-mL bottle (0.1 mg/mL) contains 50 doses). **Nasal spray (Stimate):** 150 mcg/spray. **Rhinal tube delivery system-nasal solution:** 2.5-mL vials with applicator tubes (0.1 mg/mL). **Injection:** 4 mcg/mL.

NURSING IMPLICATIONS

Assessment
- Chronic intranasal use may cause tolerance or if administered more frequently than every 24–48 hr IV tachyphylaxis (short-term tolerance) may develop.
- **Nocturnal Enuresis:** Monitor frequency of enuresis throughout therapy. Use cautiously in patients at risk for water intoxication with hyponatremia.
- **Diabetes Insipidus:** Monitor urine and plasma osmolality and urine volume frequently. Assess patient for symptoms of dehydration (excessive thirst, dry skin and mucous membranes, tachycardia, poor skin turgor). Weigh patient daily and assess for edema.
- **Hemophilia:** Monitor plasma factor VIII coagulant, factor VIII antigen, and ristocetin cofactor. May also assess activated partial thromboplastin time (aPTT) for hemophilia A and skin bleeding time for von Willebrand's disease. Assess patient for signs of bleeding.
- Monitor blood pressure and pulse during IV infusion.
- Monitor intake and output and adjust fluid intake (especially in children and elderly) to avoid overhydration in patients receiving desmopressin for hemophilia.
- ***Toxicity and Overdose:*** Signs and symptoms of water intoxication include confusion, drowsiness, headache, weight gain, difficulty urinating, seizures, and coma.
- Treatment of overdose includes decreasing dose and, if symptoms are severe, administration of furosemide.

Potential Nursing Diagnoses
Deficient fluid volume (Indications)
Excess fluid volume (Adverse Reactions)

Implementation
- IV desmopressin has 10 times the antidiuretic effect of intranasal desmopressin.
- **PO:** Begin oral doses 12 hr after last intranasal dose. Monitor response closely.
- **Diabetes Insipidus:** Parenteral dose for antidiuretic effect is administered direct IV or subcut.
- **Hemophilia:** Parenteral dose for control of bleeding is administered via IV infusion. If used preoperatively, administer 30 min prior to procedure.

IV Administration

- **Direct IV:** (for diabetes insipidus) ***Diluent:*** Administer undiluted. ***Concentration:*** 4 mcg/mL. ***Rate:*** Administer over 1 min.
- **Intermittent Infusion (for hemophilia and von Willebrand's disease):** ***Diluent:*** Dilute each dose in 50 mL of 0.9% NaCl for adults and children >10 kg and in 10 mL in children weighing <10 kg. ***Rate:*** Infuse slowly over 15–30 min.
- **Y-Site Compatibility:** No information available.
- **Intranasal:** If intranasal dose is used preoperatively, administer 2 hr before procedure.

Patient/Family Teaching
- Advise patient to notify health care professional if bleeding is not controlled or if headache, dyspnea, heartburn, nausea, abdominal cramps, vulval pain, or severe nasal congestion or irritation occurs.
- Caution patient to avoid concurrent use of alcohol with this medication.
- **Diabetes Insipidus:** Instruct patient on intranasal administration. Medication is supplied with a flexible calibrated catheter (rhinyle). Draw solution into rhinyle. Insert one end of tube into nostril, blow on the other end to de-

posit solution deep into nasal cavity. An air-filled syringe may be attached to the plastic catheter for children, infants, or obtunded patients. Tube should be rinsed under water after each use.
- If nasal spray is used, prime pump prior to first use by pressing down 4 times. Caution patient that nasal spray should not be used beyond the labeled number of sprays; subsequent sprays may not deliver accurate dose. Do not attempt to transfer remaining solution to another bottle.
- Instruct patient to take missed doses as soon as remembered but not if it is almost time for the next dose. Do not double doses.
- Advise patient that rhinitis or upper respiratory infection may decrease effectiveness of this therapy. If increased urine output occurs, patient should contact health care professional for dosage adjustment.
- Patients with diabetes insipidus should carry identification at all times describing disease process and medication regimen.

Evaluation/Desired Outcomes
- Decreased frequency of nocturnal enuresis.
- Decrease in urine volume.
- Relief of polydipsia.
- Increased urine osmolality.
- Control of bleeding in hemophilia.

---

desonide, See CORTICOSTEROIDS (TOPICAL/LOCAL).

---

desoximetasone, See CORTICOSTEROIDS (TOPICAL/LOCAL).

---

desvenlafaxine
(des-ven-la-fax-een)
Pristiq

Classification
Therapeutic: antidepressants
Pharmacologic: selective serotonin/norepinephrine reuptake inhibitors

Pregnancy Category C

Indications
Major depressive disorder.

Action
Inhibits serotonin and norepinephrine reuptake in the CNS. **Therapeutic Effects:** Decrease in depressive symptomatology, with fewer relapses/recurrences.

Pharmacokinetics
Absorption: 80% absorbed following oral administration.
Distribution: Enters breast milk.
Metabolism and Excretion: 55% metabolized by the liver, 45% excreted unchanged in urine.
Half-life: 10 hr.

TIME/ACTION PROFILE (blood levels)

ROUTE	ONSET	PEAK	DURATION
PO	unknown	7.5 hr	24 hr

Contraindications/Precautions
Contraindicated in: Hypersensitivity to venlafaxine or desvenlafaxine; Concurrent MAO inhibitors or within 14 days of stopping an MAO inhibitor; after desvenlafaxine is stopped wait 7 days until starting an MAO inhibitor; Should not be used concurrently with venlafaxine.
Use Cautiously in: Untreated cerebrovascular or cardiovascular disease, including untreated hypertension (control blood pressure before initiating therapy); Bipolar disorder (may activate mania/hypomania); History of ↑ intraocular pressure/angle-closure glaucoma; Renal impairment (consider modifications, dose should not exceed 50 mg/day, especially in moderate to severe renal impairment); History of seizures or neurologic impairment; Hepatic impairment (dose should not exceed 100 mg/day); Geri: Consider age-related decrease in renal function, decreased body mass, concurrent disease states, and medications; OB, Lactation: Use in pregnancy or lactation only if maternal benefit outweighs fetal/infant risk; Pedi: ↑ risk of suicidal thinking and behavior (suicidality) in children and adolescents with major depressive disorder and other psychiatric disorders. Observe closely for suicidality and behavior changes.

Adverse Reactions/Side Effects
CNS: NEUROLEPTIC MALIGNANT SYNDROME, SEIZURES, SUICIDAL THOUGHTS, anxiety, dizziness, drowsiness, insomnia, headache. **EENT:** ↑ intraocular pressure, mydriasis. **Resp:** eosinophilic pneumonia, interstitial lung disease. **CV:** hypertension. **GI:** ↓ appetite, constipation, nausea. **GU:** male sexual dysfunction. **Derm:** sweating. **F and E:** hyponatremia. **Hemat:** ↑ risk of bleeding. **Metab:** hypercholesterolema, hyperlipidemia. **Misc:** SEROTONIN SYNDROME.

desvenlafaxine **421**

Interactions
Drug-Drug: Concurrent use with **MAO inhibitors** may result in serious, potentially fatal reactions (wait at least 2 wk after stopping MAO inhibitor before initiating desvenlafaxine; wait at least 1 wk after stopping desvenlafaxine before starting an MAO inhibitor). ↑ risk of bleeding with other **drugs that ↑ bleeding risk** including **anticoagulants**, **antithrombotics**, **platelet aggregation inhibitors**, and **NSAIDs**. Use cautiously with other **CNS-active drugs**, including **alcohol** or **sedative/hypnotics**; effects of combination are unknown. Drugs that affect serotonergic neurotransmitter systems, including **linezolid**, **tramadol**, and **triptans** ↑ risk of serotonin syndrome. **Ketoconazole** may ↑ the effects of desvenlafaxine.

Route/Dosage
PO (Adults): 50 mg once daily.

Renal Impairment
PO (Adults): *CCr 30–50 mL/min*—50 mg/day; *CCr <30 mL/min*—50 mg every other day.

Availability
Extended-release tablets: 50 mg, 100 mg.

NURSING IMPLICATIONS

Assessment
- Assess mental status and mood changes, especially during initial few months of therapy and during dose changes. Inform health care professional if patient demonstrates significant increase in signs of depression (depressed mood, loss of interest in usual activities, significant change in weight and/or appetite, insomnia or hypersomnia, psychomotor agitation or retardation, increased fatigue, feelings or guilt or worthlessness, slowed thinking or impaired concentration, suicide attempt or suicidal ideation).
- Assess suicidal tendencies, especially in early therapy. Restrict amount of drug available to patient. Risk may be increased in children, adolescents, and adults ≤24 yr.
- Monitor blood pressure before and periodically during therapy. Sustained hypertension may be dose related; decrease dose or discontinue therapy if this occurs.
- Monitor appetite and nutritional intake; weigh weekly. Report continued weight loss. Adjust diet as tolerated to support nutritional status.
- Assess for serotonin syndrome (mental changes [agitation, hallucinations, coma], autonomic instability [tachycardia, labile blood pressure, hyperthermia], neuromuscular aberations [hyper reflexia, incoordination], and/or GI symptoms [nausea, vomiting, diarrhea]), especially in patients taking other serotonergic drugs (SSRIs, SNRIs, triptans).
- *Lab Test Considerations:* May cause ↑ fasting serum total cholesterol, LDL, cholesterol, and triglycerides.
- May cause transient proteinuria, not usually associated with ↑ BUN or creatinine.
- May cause hyponatremia.

Potential Nursing Diagnoses
Ineffective coping (Indications)
Risk for injury (Side Effects)

Implementation
- **PO:** Administer at the same time each day, with or without food. Tablets should be swallowed whole; do not crush, break, chew, or dissolve.

Patient/Family Teaching
- Instruct patient to take medication exactly as directed at the same time each day. Take missed doses as soon as possible unless almost time for next dose. Do not double doses or discontinue abruptly; gradually decrease before discontinuation.
- Advise patient, family and caregivers to look for suicidality, especially during early therapy or dose changes. Notify health care professional immediately if thoughts about suicide or dying, attempts to commit suicide, new or worse depression or anxiety, agitation or restlessness, panic attacks, insomnia, new or worse irritability, aggressiveness, acting on dangerous impulses, mania, or other changes in mood or behavior or if symptoms of serotonin syndrome occur.
- May cause drowsiness or dizziness. Caution patient to avoid driving or other activities requiring alertness until response to the drug is known.
- Caution patient to avoid taking alcohol or other CNS-depressant drugs during therapy and not to take other Rx, OTC, or herbal products without consulting health care professional.
- Instruct female patients to inform health care professional if pregnancy is planned or suspected or if breastfeeding.
- Instruct patient to notify health care professional if signs of allergy (rash, hives, swelling, difficulty breathing) occur.

✱ = Canadian drug name. ▦ = Genetic implication.
*CAPITALS indicates life-threatening; underlines indicate most frequent.

- Emphasize the importance of follow-up exams to monitor progress. Encourage patient participation in psychotherapy.

Evaluation/Desired Outcomes
- Increased sense of well-being.
- Renewed interest in surroundings. Need for therapy should be periodically reassessed. Therapy is usually continued for several mo.

---

dexamethasone, See CORTICOSTEROIDS (SYSTEMIC).

---

dexlansoprazole
(dex-lan-**soe**-pra-zole)
Dexilant

Classification
Therapeutic: antiulcer agents
Pharmacologic: proton-pump inhibitors

Pregnancy Category B

Indications
Healing/maintenance of healing of erosive esophagitis (EE). Tretment of heartburn from non-erosive gastroesophageal reflux disease (GERD).

Action
Binds to an enzyme in the presence of acidic gastric pH, preventing the final transport of hydrogen ions into the gastric lumen. **Therapeutic Effects:** Diminished accumulation of acid in the gastric lumen, with lessened acid reflux.

Pharmacokinetics
Absorption: Well absorbed following oral administration.
Distribution: Unknown.
Protein Binding: 96–99%.
Metabolism and Excretion: Extensively metabolized by the liver (CYP2C19 and CYP3A4 enzyme systems are involved); patients who are poor metabolizers may have higher blood levels; no active metabolites. No renal elimination.
Half-life: 1–2 hr.

TIME/ACTION PROFILE (blood levels)

ROUTE	ONSET	PEAK*	DURATION
PO	unknown	1–2 hr (1st); 4–5 hr (2nd)	24 hr

*Reflects effects of delayed release capsule.

Contraindications/Precautions
Contraindicated in: Hypersensitivity; Severe hepatic impairment; Lactation: Lactation.

Use Cautiously in: Moderate hepatic impairment (daily dose should not exceed 30 mg); Pedi: Safety not established.

Adverse Reactions/Side Effects
GI: abdominal pain, diarrhea, flatulence, nausea, vomiting.

Interactions
Drug-Drug: ↓ levels of **atazanavir**; do not administer concurrently. May ↓ absorption of drugs requiring acid pH for absorption, including **amipcillin**, **iron salts**, and **ketoconazole**. May increase effect of **warfarin**. May ↓ the antiplatelet effects of **clopidogrel**.

Route/Dosage
PO (Adults): Healing of EE—60 mg once daily for up to 8 wk; maintenance of healing of EE—30 mg once daily for up to 6 mo; GERD—30 mg once daily for 4 wk.

Hepatic Impairment
PO (Adults): Moderate hepatic impairment—daily dose should not exceed 30 mg.

Availability
Delayed release capsules: 30 mg, 60 mg.

NURSING IMPLICATIONS

Assessment
- Assess patient routinely for epigastric or abdominal pain and for frank or occult blood in stool, emesis, or gastric aspirate.
- **Lab Test Considerations:** May cause abnormal liver function tests, including ↑ AST, ALT, and ↑ or ↓ serum bilirubin.
- May cause ↑ serum creatinine and BUN, ↑ blood glucose, and ↑ serum potassium levels.
- May cause ↓ platelet levels.
- May also cause ↑ gastrin and total protein levels.
- Monitor INR and prothrombin time in patients taking warfarin.

Potential Nursing Diagnoses
Acute pain (Indications)

Implementation
- **PO:** May be administered without regard to food. Swallow capsules whole or may be opened and sprinkled on 1 tbsp of applesauce and swallowed immediately for patients with difficulty swallowing.

Patient/Family Teaching
- Instruct patient to take medication as directed for the full course of therapy, even if feeling better. Take missed doses as soon as remembered. Brand name was formerly Kapidex.

dexmedetomidine **423**

- Advise patient to avoid alcohol, products containing aspirin or NSAIDs, and foods that may cause an increase in GI irritation.
- Advise patient to report onset of black, tarry stools; diarrhea; or abdominal pain to health care professional promptly.
- Advise female patients to notify health care professional if pregnancy is planned or suspected or if breastfeeding.
- Instruct patient to consult health care professional prior to taking other Rx, OTC, or herbal products.

Evaluation/Desired Outcomes
- Decrease in abdominal pain heartburn, gastric irritation and bleeding in patients with GERD; may require up to 4 wk of therapy.
- Healing in patients with erosive esophagitis; may require up to 8 wk of therapy for healing and 6 mo of therapy for maintenance.

---

dexmedetomidine
(dex-me-de-**to**-mi-deen)
Precedex

Classification
Therapeutic: sedative/hypnotics

Pregnancy Category C

Indications
Sedation of initially intubated and mechanically ventilated patients during treatment in an intensive care setting; should not be used for >24 hr. Sedation of non-intubated patients before and/or during surgical and other procedures.

Action
Acts as a relatively selective alpha-adrenergic agonist with sedative properties. **Therapeutic Effects:** Sedation.

Pharmacokinetics
Absorption: IV administration results in complete bioavailability.
Distribution: Unknown.
Protein Binding: 94%.
Metabolism and Excretion: Mostly metabolized by the liver, some metabolism by P450 enzyme system. Metabolites are mostly excreted in urine.
Half-life: 2 hr.

TIME/ACTION PROFILE (sedation)

ROUTE	ONSET	PEAK	DURATION
IV	rapid	unknown	unknown

Contraindications/Precautions
Contraindicated in: Hypersensitivity.
Use Cautiously in: Hepatic impairment (lower doses may be required); Advanced heart block; Geri: ↑ risk of bradycardia and hypotension; OB, Lactation, Pedi: Safety not established.

Adverse Reactions/Side Effects
Resp: hypoxia. **CV:** BRADYCARDIA, SINUS ARREST, hypotension, transient hypertension. **GI:** nausea, vomiting. **Hemat:** anemia. **Misc:** fever.

Interactions
Drug-Drug: Sedation is enhanced by **anesthetics**, other **sedative/hypnotics**, and **opioid analgesics**.
Drug-Natural Products: Concomitant use of **kava-kava, valerian, skullcap, chamomile,** or **hops** can ↑ CNS depression.

Route/Dosage
ICU Sedation
IV (Adults): *Loading infusion*—1 mcg/kg over 10 min followed by *maintenance infusion* of 0.2–0.7 mcg/kg/hr for maximum of 24 hr; rate is adjusted to achieve desired level of sedation.

Procedural Sedation
IV (Adults): *Loading infusion*—1 mcg/kg (0.5 mcg/kg for ophthalmic surgery or patients >65 yr) over 10 min followed by *maintenance infusion* of 0.6 mcg/kg/hr; rate is adjusted to achieve desired level of sedation (usual range 0.2–1 mcg/kg/hr) (maintenance infusion of 0.7 mcg/kg/hr recommended for fiberoptic intubation until endotracheal tube secured).

Availability
Injection: 100 mcg/mL in 2-mL ampules and vials.

NURSING IMPLICATIONS
Assessment
- Assess level of sedation throughout therapy. Dose is adjusted based on level of sedation.
- Monitor ECG and blood pressure continuously throughout therapy. May cause hypotension, bradycardia, and sinus arrest.
- ***Toxicity and Overdose:*** Atropine IV may be used to modify the vagal tone.

✶ = Canadian drug name.   = Genetic implication.
*CAPITALS indicates life-threatening; underlines indicate most frequent.

Potential Nursing Diagnoses
Anxiety (Indications)

Implementation
- Dexmedetomidine should be administered only in intensive care settings with continuous monitoring.

IV Administration
- **Continuous Infusion:** *Diluent:* To prepare infusion, withdraw 2 mL of dexmedetomidine and add to 48 mL of 0.9 NaCl for a total of 50 mL. *Concentration:* 4 mcg/mL. Shake gently. Solution should be clear; do not administer solutions that are discolored or contain particulate matter. Ampules and vials are for single use only. *Rate:* Administer *loading infusion* over 10 minutes, followed by *maintenance infusion* of 0.2–0.7 mcg/kg/hr for ICU sedation and 0.2–1.0 mcg/kg/hr for procedural sedation. Adjust dose to achieve desired level of sedation. Administer via infusion pump to ensure accurate rate.
- **Y-Site Compatibility:** 0.9% NaCl, 20% mannitol, acyclovir, alfentanil, allopurinol, amifostine, amikacin, aminocaproic acid, aminophylline, amiodarone, amphotericin B liposome, ampicillin, ampicillin/sulbactam, atropine, azithromycin, aztreonam, bivalirudin, bleomycin, bumetanide, buprenorphine, busulfan, butorphanol, calcium chloride, calcium gluconate, carboplatin, carmustine, caspofungin, cefazolin, cefepime, cefoperazone, cefotaxime, cefotetan, cefoxitin, ceftazidime, ceftizoxime, ceftriaxone, cefuroxime, chlorpromazine, cimetidine, ciprofloxacin, cisatracurium, cisplatin, clindamycin, cyclophosphamide, cyclosporine, cytarabine, dacarbazine, dactinomycin, daptomycin, daunorubicin hydrochloride, D5W, dexamethasone, dexrazoxane, digoxin, diltiazem, diphenhydramine, dobutamine, docetaxel, dolasetron, dopamine, doxacurium, doxorubicin hydrochloride, doxycycline, droperidol, enalaprilat, epinephrine, ertapenem, erythromycin, esmolol, etomidate, etoposide, etoposide phosphate, famotidine, fenoldopam, fentanyl, fluconazole, fludarabine, fluorouracil, foscarnet, fosphenytoin, furosemide, gancyclovir, gemcitabine, gentamicin, glycopyrrolate, granisetron, haloperidol, heparin, hydrocortisone, hydromorphone, idarubicin, ifosfamide, imipenem/cilastatin, insulin, isoproterenol, ketorolac, labetalol, leucovorin, levofloxacin, lidocaine, linezolid, lorazepam, magnesium sulfate, mannitol, mechlorethamine, meperidine, meropenem, mesna, methohexital, methotrexate, methylprednisolone, metoclopramide, metoprolol, metronidazole, midazolam, milrinone, minocycline, mitomycin, mitoxantrone, morphine, nalbuphine, naloxone, nesiritide, nicardipine, nitroglycerin, nitroprusside, norepinephrine, octreotide, ondansetron, oxaliplatin, oxytocin, paclitaxel, palonosetron, pancuronium, pemetrexed, pentamidine, pentobarbital, phenobarbital, phenylephrine, piperacillin/tazobactam, plasma substitute, potassium chloride, potassium phosphate, procainamide, prochlorperazine, promethazine, propofol, propranolol, quinapristin/dalfopristin, ranitidine, remifentanil, rocuronium, sodium acetate, sodium bicarbonate, sodium phosphate, succinylcholine, sufentanil, tacrolimus, teniposide, theophylline, thiopental, thiotepa, ticarcillin/clavulanate, tigecycline, tirofiban, tobramycin, topotecan, vancomycin, vasopressin, vecuronium, verapamil, vinblastine, vincristine, vinorelbine, voriconazole, zidovudine.
- **Y-Site Incompatibility:** amphotericin B colloidal, diazepam, pantoprazole, phenytoin.

Patient/Family Teaching
- Explain to patient and family the purpose of the medication.

Evaluation/Desired Outcomes
- Sedation for up to 24 hr.

---

dexmethylphenidate
(dex-meth-ill-**fen**-i-date)
Focalin, Focalin XR

Classification
Therapeutic: central nervous system stimulants

Schedule II

Pregnancy Category C

Indications
Adjunctive treatment of ADHD.

Action
Produces CNS and respiratory stimulation with weak sympathomimetic activity. **Therapeutic Effects:** Increased attention span in ADHD.

Pharmacokinetics
Absorption: Readily absorbed following oral administration.
Distribution: Unknown.

dexmethylphenidate

Metabolism and Excretion: Mostly metabolized by the liver; inactive metabolites are renally excreted.
Half-life: 2.2 hr.

TIME/ACTION PROFILE (improvement in symptoms)

ROUTE	ONSET	PEAK	DURATION
PO	7 days	1 mo	unknown

Contraindications/Precautions

Contraindicated in: Hypersensitivity; Hyperexcitable states (marked anxiety, agitation, or tension); Hyperthyroidism; Psychotic personalities, suicidal or homicidal tendencies; Glaucoma; Motor tics, family history or diagnosis of Tourette's syndrome; Concurrent use of MAO inhibitors; Should not be used to treat depression or prevent/treat normal fatigue; Psychoses (may exacerbate symptoms).

Use Cautiously in: Cardiovascular disease (sudden death has occurred in children with structural cardiac abnormalities or other serious heart problems); Hyperthyroidism; Hypertension; Diabetes mellitus; Geri: Geriatric/debilitated patients; Continual use (may result in psychological or physical dependence); Seizure disorders (may lower seizure threshold); OB, Lactation, Pedi: Pregnancy, lactation, or children <6 yr (safety not established; use in pregnancy only if clearly needed).

Adverse Reactions/Side Effects

CNS: behavioral disturbances, hallucinations, insomnia, mania, nervousness, thought disorder. **EENT:** visual disturbances. **CV:** SUDDEN DEATH, tachycardia. **GI:** abdominal pain, anorexia, nausea. **Metab:** growth suppression, weight loss (may occur with prolonged use). **Neuro:** twitching. **Misc:** fever.

Interactions

Drug-Drug: Concurrent use with or use within 14 days following discontinuation of **MAO inhibitors** may result in hypertensive crisis and is contraindicated. May ↓ effects of **antihypertensives**. May ↑ effects of **vasopressors**. May cause serious adverse reactions with **clonidine**. May ↑ effects of **warfarin, phenobarbital, phenytoin**, some **antidepressants**; dose adjustments may be necessary.

Route/Dosage

Tablets

PO (Adults and Children ≥6 yr): *Patients not previously taking methylphenidate*—2.5 mg twice daily, may be ↑ weekly as needed up to 10 mg twice daily; *Patients currently taking methylphenidate*—starting dose is 1/2 of the methylphenidate dose, up to 10 mg twice daily.

Extended-release capsules

PO (Adults): *Patients not previously taking methylphenidate*—10 mg once daily, may be ↑ by 10 mg after 1 wk to 20 mg/day; *Patients currently taking methylphenidate*—starting dose is 1/2 of the methylphenidate dose, up to 20 mg/day given as a single daily dose; *Patients currently taking dexmethylphenidate*—give same daily dose as a single dose.

PO (Children ≥6 yr): *Patients not previously taking methylphenidate*—5 mg once daily, may be ↑ by 5 mg weekly up to 20 mg/day; *Patients currently taking methylphenidate*—starting dose is 1/2 of the methylphenidate dose, up to 20 mg/day, given as a single daily dose; *Patients currently taking dexmethylphenidate*—give same daily dose as a single dose.

Availability (generic available)

Tablets: 2.5 mg, 5 mg, 10 mg. Cost: *Generic*—2.5 mg $69.90/100, 5 mg $89.90/100, 10 mg $129.90/100. **Extended-release capsules:** 5 mg, 10 mg, 15 mg, 20 mg.

NURSING IMPLICATIONS

Assessment

- Assess child's attention span, impulse control, and interactions with others. Therapy may be interrupted at intervals to determine whether symptoms are sufficient to continue therapy.
- Monitor blood pressure, pulse, and respiration before administering and periodically during therapy. Obtain a history (including assessment of family history of sudden death or ventricular arrhythmia), physical exam to assess for cardiac disease, and further evaluation (ECG and echocardiogram), if indicated. If exertional chest pain, unexplained syncope, or other cardiac symptoms occur, evaluate promptly.
- Monitor weight biweekly and inform health care professional of significant loss. Pedi: Monitor height periodically in children; report growth inhibition.
- Monitor closely for behavior change.

✤ = Canadian drug name. 🧬 = Genetic implication.
*CAPITALS indicates life-threatening; underlines indicate most frequent.

- Dexmethylphenidate has the potential for dependence and abuse. Prolonged use may result in tolerance.
- **Lab Test Considerations:** Monitor CBC, differential, and platelet count periodically in patients receiving prolonged therapy.

Potential Nursing Diagnoses
Disturbed thought process (Side Effects)

Implementation
- **PO:** Administer twice daily at least 4 hr apart without regard to meals.
- Administer XR tablets once daily in the morning. Capsules should be swallowed whole. For patients with difficulty swallowing, capsules can be opened and sprinkled on a spoonful of applesauce. Mixture should be consumed immediately; do not store for future use.

Patient/Family Teaching
- Instruct patient to take medication as directed. If more than prescribed amount is taken, notify health care professional immediately. If a dose is missed, take the remaining doses for that day at regularly spaced intervals; do not double doses. Take the last dose before 6PM to minimize the risk of insomnia. Instruct patient not to alter dose without consulting health care professional. Abrupt cessation with high doses may cause extreme fatigue and mental depression. Advise patient and parents to read the *Medication Guide* prior to starting therapy and with each Rx refill.
- Inform patient that sharing this medication may be dangerous.
- Advise patient to check weight 2–3 times weekly and report weight loss to health care professional.
- Advise patient to consult with health care professional prior to taking other prescription, OTC, or herbal products concurrently with dexmethylphenidate.
- May rarely cause dizziness or drowsiness. Caution patient to avoid driving or activities requiring alertness until response to medication is known.
- Advise patient to notify health care professional if nervousness, restlessness, insomnia, dizziness, anorexia, or dry mouth becomes severe. Pedi: If reduced appetite and weight loss are a problem, advise parents to provide high calorie meals when drug levels are low (at breakfast and or bedtime).
- Advise patient and/or parents to notify health care professional of behavioral changes.
- Inform patient that health care professional may order periodic holidays from the drug to assess progress and to decrease dependence.
- Advise patient to notify health care professional if pregnancy is planned or suspected, or if breastfeeding.
- Caution patients to inform health care professional if they have ever abused or been dependent on alcohol or drugs, or if they are now abusing or dependent on alcohol or drugs.
- Emphasize the importance of routine follow-up exams to monitor progress.
- **Home Care Issues:** Advise parents to notify school nurse of medication regimen.

Evaluation/Desired Outcomes
- Improved attention span, decreased impulsiveness and hyperactivity in ADHD. If improvement is not seen within 1 month, discontinue dexmethylphenidate.

---

dexrazoxane (dex-ra-zox-ane)
Totect, Zinecard

Classification
Therapeutic: cardioprotective agents

Pregnancy Category C

Indications
Reducing incidence and severity of cardiomyopathy from doxorubicin in women with metastatic breast cancer who have already received a cumulative dose of doxorubicin >300 mg/m². Treatment of extravasation resulting from IV anthracycline chemotherapy.

Action
Acts as an intracellular chelating agent. **Therapeutic Effects:** Diminishes the cardiotoxic effects of doxorubicin. Decreased damage from extravasation of anthracyclines.

Pharmacokinetics
Absorption: IV administration results in complete bioavailability.
Distribution: Unknown.
Metabolism and Excretion: Some metabolism occurs; 42% eliminated in urine.
Half-life: 2.1–2.5 hr.

TIME/ACTION PROFILE (cardioprotective effect)

ROUTE	ONSET	PEAK	DURATION
IV	rapid	unknown	unknown

dexrazoxane **427**

Contraindications/Precautions
Contraindicated in: Any other type of chemotherapy except other anthracyclines (doxorubicin-like agents).
Use Cautiously in: CCr <40 mL/min (dose reduction required); OB: Pregnancy, lactation, or children (safety not established).

Adverse Reactions/Side Effects
Hemat: myelosuppression. **Local:** pain at injection site.

Interactions
Drug-Drug: Myelosuppression may be ↑ by **antineoplastics** or **radiation therapy**. Antitumor effects of concurrent combination chemotherapy with **fluorouracil** and **cyclophosphamide** may be ↓ by dexrazoxane.

Route/Dosage
Cardioprotective
IV (Adults): 10 mg of dexrazoxane/1 mg doxorubicin.
Renal Impairment
IV (Adults): decrease dose by 50%.
Extravasation protection
IV (Adults): 1000 mg/m^2 (maximum 2000 mg) given on days 1 and 2, and followed by a dose of 500 mg/m^2 (maximum 1000 mg) on day 3.
Renal Impairment
IV (Adults CCr <40 mL/min): decrease dose by 50%.

Availability (generic available)
Injection (Zinecard): 250-mg vial, 500-mg vial.
Injection (Totect): 500-mg vial.

NURSING IMPLICATIONS

Assessment
- **Cardioprotective:** Assess extent of cardiomyopathy (cardiomegaly on x-ray, basilar rales, S gallop, dyspnea, decline in left ventricular ejection fraction) prior to and periodically during therapy.
- **Extravasation protection:** Assess site of extravasation for pain, burning, swelling, and redness.
- ***Lab Test Considerations:*** Monitor CBC and platelet count frequently during therapy. Thrombocytopenia, leukopenia, neutropenia, and granulocytopenia from chemotherapy may be more severe at nadir with dexrazoxane therapy.
- Monitor liver function tests periodically during therapy. May cause reversible ↑ of liver enzymes.

Potential Nursing Diagnoses
Decreased cardiac output (Indications)
Risk for impaired skin integrity (Indications)

Implementation
- Solution should be prepared in a biologic cabinet. Wear gloves, gown, and mask while handling IV medication. Discard IV equipment in specially designated containers (see Appendix L).
- Do not administer solutions that are discolored or contain particulate matter. Reconstituted solution and diluted solution are stable in an IV bag for 6 hr at room temperature or if refrigerated. Discard unused solutions.

IV Administration
- **Cardioprotective:** Doxorubicin should be administered within 30 min following dexrazoxane administration.
- **Direct IV: *Diluent:*** Reconstitute dexrazoxane with 0.167 molar (M/6) sodium lactate injection. ***Concentration:*** 10 mg/mL. ***Rate:*** Administer via slow IV push.
- **Intermittent Infusion: *Diluent:*** Reconstituted solution may also be diluted with 0.9% NaCl or D5W. Solution is stable for 6 hr at room temperature or refrigerated. ***Concentration:*** 1.3–5 mg/mL. ***Rate:*** May also be administered via rapid IV infusion over 15–30 min.
- **Additive Incompatibility:** Do not mix with other medications.
- **Extravasation Protection:** Administer as soon as possible within 6 hr of extravasation. Remove cooling procedures, such as ice packs, at least 15 min before administration to allow sufficient blood flow to area of extravasation.
- **Intermittent Infusion: *Diluent:*** Dilute each vial in 50 mL of diluent provided by manufacturer. Add contents of all vials into 1000 mL of 0.9% NaCl for further dilution. Solution is slightly yellow. Use diluted solutions within 2 hr of dilution. Store at room temperature. ***Rate:*** Administer over 1–2 hr.

Patient/Family Teaching
- Explain the purpose of the medication to the patient.
- Emphasize the need for continued monitoring of cardiac function.

- Advise patient to notify health care professional if pregnancy is suspected or planned. Dexrazoxane may be teratogenic.

Evaluation/Desired Outcomes
- Reduction of incidence and severity of cardiomyopathy associated with doxorubicin administration in women with metastatic breast cancer.
- Decrease in late sequalae (site pain, fibrosis, atrophy, and local sensory disturbance) following extravasation of anthracycline chemotherapeutic agents.

dextroamphetamine
(dex-troe-am-**fet**-a-meen)
Dexedrine

Classification
Therapeutic: central nervous system stimulants
Pharmacologic: amphetamines

Schedule II

Pregnancy Category C

Indications
Adjunct management of ADHD. Narcolepsy. **Unlabeled Use:** Exogenous obesity.

Action
Produces CNS stimulation by releasing norepinephrine from nerve endings. Pharmacologic effects: CNS and respiratory stimulation, Vasoconstriction, Mydriasis (pupillary dilation), Contraction of the urinary bladder sphincter.
Therapeutic Effects: Increased motor activity and mental alertness and decreased fatigue in narcoleptic patients. Increased attention span in ADHD.

Pharmacokinetics
Absorption: Well absorbed.
Distribution: Widely distributed; high concentrations in brain and CSF. Crosses the placenta; enters breast milk; potentially embryotoxic.
Metabolism and Excretion: Some metabolism by the liver. Urinary excretion is pH-dependent. Alkaline urine promotes reabsorption and prolongs action.
Half-life: 10–12 hr (6.8 hr in children).

TIME/ACTION PROFILE (CNS stimulation)

ROUTE	ONSET	PEAK	DURATION
PO	1–2 hr	3 hr	2–10 hr
PO-ER	unknown	unknown	up to 24 hr

Contraindications/Precautions
Contraindicated in: OB, Lactation: Pregnancy or lactation; Hyperexcitable states, including hyperthyroidism; Psychotic personalities; Suicidal or homicidal tendencies; Glaucoma; Some products contain tartrazine; avoid in patients with known hypersensitivity.
Use Cautiously in: Cardiovascular disease (sudden death has occurred in children with structural cardiac abnormalities or other serious heart problems); Hypertension; Diabetes mellitus; History of substance abuse; Debilitated patients; Continual use (may produce psychological dependence or physical addiction); Geri: Appears on Beers list. Elderly are at ↑ risk for cardiovascular side effects.

Adverse Reactions/Side Effects
CNS: hyperactivity, insomnia, restlessness, tremor, behavioral disturbances, depression, dizziness, hallucinations, headache, irritability, mania, thought disorder. **CV:** SUDDEN DEATH, palpitations, tachycardia, arrhythmias, hypertension. **GI:** anorexia, constipation, cramps, diarrhea, dry mouth, metallic taste, nausea, vomiting. **GU:** erectile dysfunction, ↑ libido. **Derm:** urticaria. **Misc:** physical dependence, psychological dependence.

Interactions
Drug-Drug: ↑ adrenergic effects with other **adrenergics**. Use with **MAO inhibitors** can result in hypertensive crisis. Alkalinizing the urine (**sodium bicarbonate**, **acetazolamide**) prolongs effect. Acidification of urine (**ammonium chloride**, large doses of **ascorbic acid**) ↓ effect. **Phenothiazines** may ↓ effect of dextroamphetamine. May antagonize the response to **antihypertensives**. ↑ risk of cardiovascular side effects with **beta blockers** or **tricyclic antidepressants**.
Drug-Natural Products: St. John's wort may ↑ serious side effects, concurrent use is not recommended. Use with caffeine-containing herbs (**guarana**, **tea**, **coffee**) ↑ stimulant effect. St. John's wort may ↑ serious side effects, concurrent use is not recommended.

Route/Dosage

Attention-Deficit Hyperactivity Disorder
PO (Adults): 5–40 mg/day in divided doses. Sustained-release capsules should not be used as initial therapy.
PO (Children ≥ 6 yr): 5 mg 1–2 times daily, ↑ by 5 mg daily at weekly intervals (maximum: 40 mg/day). Sustained-release capsules should not be used as initial therapy.

PO (Children 3–5 yr): 2.5 mg/day, ↑ by 2.5 mg daily at weekly intervals (maximum: 40 mg/day).

Narcolepsy
PO (Adults): 5–60 mg/day single dose or in divided doses. Sustained-release capsules should not be used as initial therapy.
PO (Children ≥12 yr): 10 mg/day, ↑ by 10 mg/day at weekly intervals until response is obtained or 60 mg is reached.
PO (Children 6–12 yr): 5 mg/day, ↑ by 5 mg/day at weekly intervals until response is obtained or 60 mg is reached.

Exogenous obesity
PO (Adults and Children >12 yr): 5–30 mg/day in divided doses of 5–10 mg given 30–60 min before meals.

Availability (generic available)
Tablets: 5 mg, 10 mg. **Sustained-release capsules:** 5 mg, 10 mg, 15 mg.

NURSING IMPLICATIONS

Assessment
- Monitor blood pressure, pulse, and respiration before administering and periodically during therapy. Obtain a history (including assessment of family history of sudden death or ventricular arrhythmia), physical exam to assess for cardiac disease, and further evaluation (ECG and echocardiogram), if indicated. If exertional chest pain, unexplained syncope, or other cardiac symptoms occur, evaluate promptly.
- Has high dependence and abuse potential. Tolerance to medication occurs rapidly; do not increase dose.
- Monitor closely for behavior change.
- Geri: Not recommended for use in elderly secondary to risk for hypertension, angina, and MI.
- **ADHD:** Monitor weight biweekly and inform health care professional of significant loss. Pedi: Monitor height periodically in children; report growth inhibition.
- Assess child's attention span, impulse control, and interactions with others. Therapy may be interrupted at intervals to determine whether symptoms are sufficient to continue therapy.
- **Narcolepsy:** Observe and document frequency of narcoleptic episodes.
- May produce a false sense of euphoria and well-being. Provide frequent rest periods and observe patient for rebound depression after the effects of the medication have worn off.
- **Lab Test Considerations:** May interfere with urinary steroid determinations.
- May cause ↑ plasma corticosteroid concentrations; greatest in evening.

Potential Nursing Diagnoses
Disturbed thought process (Side Effects)

Implementation
- Do not confuse Adderall (dextroamphetamine/amphetamine) with Inderal (propranolol).
- Therapy should utilize the lowest effective dose.
- **PO:** Sustained-release capsules should be swallowed whole; do not break, crush, or chew.
- **ADHD:** Pedi: When symptoms are controlled, dose reduction or interruption of therapy may be possible during summer months or may be given on each of the 5 school days with medication-free weekends and holidays.

Patient/Family Teaching
- Instruct patient to take medication at least 6 hr before bedtime to avoid sleep disturbances. Take missed doses as soon as remembered up to 6 hr before bedtime. Do not double doses. Advise patient and parents to read the *Medication Guide* prior to starting therapy and with each Rx refill. Instruct patient not to alter dose without consulting health care professional. Abrupt cessation of high doses may cause extreme fatigue and mental depression.
- Inform patient that sharing this medication may be dangerous.
- Inform patient that the effects of drug-induced dry mouth can be minimized by rinsing frequently with water or chewing sugarless gum or candies.
- Advise patient to avoid the intake of large amounts of caffeine.
- Medication may impair judgment. Advise patients to use caution when driving or during other activities requiring alertness.
- Advise patient to notify health care professional if nervousness, restlessness, insomnia, dizziness, anorexia, or dry mouth becomes severe. Pedi: If reduced appetite and weight loss are a problem, advise parents to provide high calorie meals when drug levels are low (at breakfast and/or bedtime).
- Advise patient and/or parents to notify health care professional of behavioral changes.

�֍ = Canadian drug name. ≋ = Genetic implication.
*CAPITALS indicates life-threatening; underlines indicate most frequent.

- Inform patient that periodic holiday from the drug may be ordered to assess progress and decrease dependence.
- Advise patient to notify health care professional if pregnancy is planned or suspected, or if breastfeeding.
- Caution patients to inform health care professional if they have ever abused or been dependent on alcohol or drugs, or if they are now abusing or dependent on alcohol or drugs.
- Emphasize the importance of routine follow-up exams to monitor progress.
- **Home Care Issues:** Advise parents to notify school nurse of medication regimen.

Evaluation/Desired Outcomes
- Improved attention span. Therapy should be interrupted and reassessed periodically.
- Decrease in narcoleptic symptoms.

---

dextromethorphan
(dex-troe-meth-**or**-fan)
✤ Balminil DM, Benylin Adult, Benylin Pediatric, ✤ Broncho-Grippol-DM, ✤ Calmylin #1, Children's Hold, Creo-Terpin, Delsym, DexAlone, ✤ DM Syrup, Drixoral Liquid Cough Caps, ElixSure Children's Cough Syrup, Hold, ✤ Koffex, Little Colds Cough Formula Drops, Mediquell, ✤ Neo-DM, ✤ Ornex • DM, PediCare Infant's Long Acting Cough Drops, Pertussin Cough Suppressant, Pertussin CS, Pertussin ES, ✤ Robidex, Robitussin Cough Calmers, Robitussine CoughGels, Robitussin Maximum Strength Cough Suppressant, Robitussin Pediatric, ✤ Sedatuss, Simply Cough, Sucrets Cough Control Formula, TheraFlu Thin Strips Long Acting Cough, Triaminic Thin Strips Long Acting Cough, Vicks 44 Cough Relief, Vicks Formula 44 Pediatric Formula

Classification
Therapeutic: allergy, cold, and cough remedies, antitussives

Pregnancy Category C

Indications
Symptomatic relief of coughs caused by minor viral upper respiratory tract infections or inhaled irritants. Most effective for chronic nonproductive cough. A common ingredient in nonprescription cough and cold preparations.

Action
Suppresses the cough reflex by a direct effect on the cough center in the medulla. Related to opioids structurally but has no analgesic properties. **Therapeutic Effects:** Relief of irritating nonproductive cough.

Pharmacokinetics
Absorption: Rapidly absorbed from the GI tract. Extended-release product is slowly absorbed.
Distribution: Unknown. Probably crosses the placenta and enters breast milk.
Metabolism and Excretion: Metabolized to dextrorphan, an active metabolite. Dextromethorphan and dextrorphan are renally excreted.
Half-life: Unknown.

TIME/ACTION PROFILE (cough suppression)

ROUTE	ONSET	PEAK	DURATION
PO	15–30 min	unknown	3–6 hr†
PO-ER	unknown	unknown	9–12 hr

†Up to 8 hr for gelcaps

Contraindications/Precautions
Contraindicated in: Hypersensitivity; Patients taking MAO inhibitors or SSRIs; Should not be used for chronic productive coughs; Some products contain alcohol and should be avoided in patients with known intolerance.
Use Cautiously in: Cough that lasts more than 1 wk or is accompanied by fever, rash, or headache—health care professional should be consulted; History of drug abuse or drug-seeking behavior (capsules have been abused resulting in deaths); Diabetes (some products contain sucrose); OB: Pregnancy (has been used safely); Lactation: Lactation; Pedi: Children <4 yr (OTC cough and cold products containing this medication should be avoided).

Adverse Reactions/Side Effects
CNS: *high dose*—dizziness, sedation. **GI:** nausea.

Interactions
Drug-Drug: Use with **MAO inhibitors** may result in serotonin syndrome (nausea, confusion, changes in blood pressure); concurrent use should be avoided. ↑ CNS depression with **antihistamines**, **alcohol**, **antidepressants**, **sedative/hypnotics**, or **opioids**. **Amiodarone**, **fluoxetine**, or **quinidine** may ↑ blood levels and adverse reactions from dextromethorphan.

Route/Dosage
PO (Adults and Children >12 yr): 10–20 mg q 4 hr *or* 30 mg q 6–8 hr *or* 60 mg of extended-release preparation bid (not to exceed 120 mg/day).

PO (Children 6–12 yr): 5–10 mg q 4 hr *or* 15 mg q 6–8 hr *or* 30 mg of extended-release preparation q 12 hr (not to exceed 60 mg/day).
PO (Children 4–6 yr): 2.5–5 mg q 4 hr *or* 7.5 mg q 6–8 hr *or* 15 mg of extended-release preparation q 12 hr (not to exceed 30 mg/day).

Availability
Gelcaps: 30 mg^OTC. **Lozenges (cherry):** 2.5 mg^OTC, 5 mg^OTC. **Liquid (cherry, grape):** 3.5 mg/5 mL^OTC, 5 mg/5 mL, 7.5 mg/5 mL^OTC, 15 mg/5 mL^OTC, 30 mg/5 mL^OTC. **Syrup (cherry, cherry bubblegum):** 7.5 mg/5 mL^OTC, 15 mg/15 mL^OTC, 10 mg/5 mL^OTC. **Extended-release suspension (orange):** 30 mg/5 mL^OTC. **Drops (Grape):** 7.5 mg/0.8 mL^OTC, 7.5 mg/1 mL^OTC. **Orally-disintegrating strips (cherry, grape):** 7.5 mg^OTC, 15 mg^OTC. *In combination with:* antihistamines, decongestants, and expectorants in cough and cold preparations^OTC. See Appendix B.

NURSING IMPLICATIONS

Assessment
- Assess frequency and nature of cough, lung sounds, and amount and type of sputum produced. Unless contraindicated, maintain fluid intake of 1500–2000 mL to decrease viscosity of bronchial secretions.

Potential Nursing Diagnoses
Ineffective airway clearance (Indications)

Implementation
- Dextromethorphan 15–30 mg is equivalent in cough suppression to codeine 8–15 mg.
- **PO:** Do not give fluids immediately after administering to prevent dilution of vehicle. Shake oral suspension well before administration.

Patient/Family Teaching
- Instruct patient to cough effectively: Sit upright and take several deep breaths before attempting to cough.
- Advise patient to minimize cough by avoiding irritants, such as cigarette smoke, fumes, and dust. Humidification of environmental air, frequent sips of water, and sugarless hard candy may also decrease the frequency of dry, irritating cough.
- Caution patient to avoid taking more than the recommended dose or taking alcohol or other CNS depressants concurrently with this medication; fatalities have occurred. Caution parents to avoid OTC cough and cold products while breastfeeding or to children <4 yrs.
- May occasionally cause dizziness. Caution patient to avoid driving or other activities requiring alertness until response to the medication is known.
- Advise patient that any cough lasting over 1 wk or accompanied by fever, chest pain, persistent headache, or skin rash warrants medical attention.

Evaluation/Desired Outcomes
- Decrease in frequency and intensity of cough without eliminating patient's cough reflex.

---

diazepam (dye-az-e-pam)
✦Apo-Diazepam, Diastat, ✦Diazemuls, ✦Novodipam, ✦ PMS-Diazepam, Valium, ✦Vivol

Classification
Therapeutic: antianxiety agents, anticonvulsants, sedative/hypnotics, skeletal muscle relaxants (centrally acting)
Pharmacologic: benzodiazepines

Schedule IV

Pregnancy Category D

Indications
Adjunct in the management of: Anxiety Disorder, Athetosis, Anxiety relief prior to cardioversion (injection), Stiffman Syndrome, Preoperative sedation, Conscious sedation (provides light anesthesia and anterograde amnesia). Treatment of status epilepticus/uncontrolled seizures (injection). Skeletal muscle relaxant. Management of the symptoms of alcohol withdrawal. **Unlabeled Use:** Anxiety associated with acute myocardial infarction, insomnia.

Action
Depresses the CNS, probably by potentiating GABA, an inhibitory neurotransmitter. Produces skeletal muscle relaxation by inhibiting spinal polysynaptic afferent pathways. Has anticonvulsant properties due to enhanced presynaptic inhibition. **Therapeutic Effects:** Relief of anxiety. Sedation. Amnesia. Skeletal muscle relaxation. Decreased seizure activity.

Pharmacokinetics
Absorption: Rapidly absorbed from the GI tract. Absorption from IM sites may be slow and unpredictable. Well absorbed (90%) from rectal mucosa.

Distribution: Widely distributed. Crosses the blood-brain barrier. Crosses the placenta; enters breast milk.

Metabolism and Excretion: Highly metabolized by the hepatic P450 enzymes (CYP2C19 and CYP3A4); the CYP2C19 enzyme system exhibits genetic polymorphism; 15–20% of Asian patients and 3–5% of Caucasian and Black patients may be poor metabolizers and may have significantly ↑ diazepam concentrations and an ↑ risk of adverse effects. Some products of metabolism are active as CNS depressants.

Half-life: Neonates: 50–95 hr; Infants 1 month–2 yr: 40–50 hr; Children 2–12 yr: 15–21 hr; Children 12–16 yr: 18–20 hr; Adults: 20–50 hr (up to 100 hr for metabolites).

TIME/ACTION PROFILE (sedation)

ROUTE	ONSET	PEAK	DURATION
PO	30–60 min	1–2 hr	up to 24 hr
IM	within 20 min	0.5–1.5 hr	unknown
IV	1–5 min	15–30 min	15–60 min†
Rectal	2–10 min	1–2 hr	4–12 hr

†In status epilepticus, anticonvulsant duration is 15–20 min

Contraindications/Precautions

Contraindicated in: Hypersensitivity; Cross-sensitivity with other benzodiazepines may occur; Comatose patients; Myasthenia gravis; Severe pulmonary impairment; Sleep apnea; Severe hepatic dysfunction; Pre-existing CNS depression; Uncontrolled severe pain; Angle-closure glaucoma; Some products contain alcohol, propylene glycol, or tartrazine and should be avoided in patients with known hypersensitivity or intolerance; OB: ↑ risk of congenital malformations; Pedi: Children <6 mo (for oral; safety not established); Lactation: Recommend to discontinue drug or bottle-feed.

Use Cautiously in: Severe renal impairment; History of suicide attempt or drug dependence; Debilitated patients (dose reduction required); Patients with low albumin; Pedi: Metabolites can accumulate in neonates. Injection contains benzyl alcohol which can cause potentially fatal gasping syndrome in neonates; Geri: Long-acting benzodiazepines cause prolonged sedation in the elderly. Appears on *Beers list* and is associated with ↑ risk of falls (↓ dose required or consider short-acting benzodiazepine).

Adverse Reactions/Side Effects

CNS: dizziness, drowsiness, lethargy, depression, hangover, ataxia, slurred speech, headache, paradoxical excitation. **EENT:** blurred vision. **Resp:** respiratory depression. **CV:** hypotension (IV only). **GI:** constipation, diarrhea (may be caused by propylene glycol content in oral solution), nausea, vomiting, weight gain. **Derm:** rashes. **Local:** pain (IM), phlebitis (IV), venous thrombosis. **Misc:** physical dependence, psychological dependence, tolerance.

Interactions

Drug-Drug: Alcohol, **antidepressants**, **antihistamines**, and **opioid analgesics**—concurrent use results in additive CNS depression. **Cimetidine**, **hormonal contraceptives**, **disulfiram**, **fluoxetine**, **isoniazid**, **ketoconazole**, **metoprolol**, **propoxyphene**, **propranolol**, or **valproic acid** may ↓ the metabolism of diazepam, enhancing its actions. May ↓ the efficacy of **levodopa**. **Rifampin** or **barbiturates** may ↑ the metabolism and ↓ effectiveness of diazepam. Sedative effects may be ↓ by **theophylline**. Concurrent use of **ritonavir** is not recommended.

Drug-Natural Products: Concomitant use of **kava-kava**, **valerian**, or **chamomile** can ↑ CNS depression.

Route/Dosage

Antianxiety

PO (Adults): 2–10 mg 2–4 times daily.
IM, IV (Adults): 2–10 mg, may repeat in 3–4 hr as needed.
PO (Children >6 mo): 1–2.5 mg 3–4 times daily.
IM, IV (Children >1 mo): 0.04–0.3 mg/kg/dose q 2–4 hr to a maximum of 0.6 mg/kg within an 8 hr period if necessary.

Precardioversion

IV (Adults): 5–15 mg 5–10 min precardioversion.

Pre-endoscopy

IV (Adults): 2.5–20 mg.
IM (Adults): 5–10 mg 30 min pre-endoscopy.

Pediatric Conscious Sedation for Procedures

PO (Children >6 mo): 0.2–0.3 mg/kg (not to exceed 10 mg/dose) 45–60 min prior to procedure.

Status Epilepticus/Acute Seizure Activity

IV (Adults): 5–10 mg, may repeat q 10–15 min to a total of 30 mg, may repeat regimen again in 2–4 hr (IM route may be used if IV route unavailable); larger doses may be required.
IM, IV (Children ≥5 yr): 0.05–0.3 mg/kg/dose given over 3–5 min q 15–30 min to a total dose of 10 mg, repeat q 2–4 hr.

diazepam

IM, IV (Children 1 mo–5 yr): 0.05–0.3 mg/kg/dose given over 3–5 min q 15–30 min to maximum dose of 5 mg, repeat in 2–4 hr if needed.
IV (Neonates): 0.1–0.3 mg/kg/dose given over 3–5 min q 15–30 min to maximum dose of 2 mg.
Rect (Adults and Children >12 yr): 0.2 mg/kg; may repeat 4–12 hr later.
Rect (Children 6–11 yr): 0.3 mg/kg; may repeat 4–12 hr later.
Rect (Children 2–5 yr): 0.5 mg/kg; may repeat 4–12 hr later.

Febrile Seizure Prophylaxis
PO (Children >1 mo): 1 mg/kg/day divided q 8 hr at first sign of fever and continue for 24 hr after fever is gone.

Skeletal Muscle Relaxation
PO (Adults): 2–10 mg 3–4 times daily.
PO (Geriatric Patients or Debilitated Patients): 2–2.5 mg 1–2 times daily initially.
PO (Children >6 mo): 1–2.5 mg 3–4 times daily.
IM, IV (Adults): 5–10 mg; may repeat in 2–4 hr (larger doses may be required for tetanus).
IM, IV (Geriatric Patients or Debilitated Patients): 2–5 mg; may repeat in 2–4 hr (larger doses may be required for tetanus).
IM, IV (Children ≥5 yr): *Tetanus*—5–10 mg q 3–4 hr.
IM, IV (Children >1 mo): *Tetanus*—1–2 mg q 3–4 hr.

Alcohol Withdrawal
PO (Adults): 10 mg 3–4 times in first 24 hr, decrease to 5 mg 3–4 times daily.
IM, IV (Adults): 10 mg initially, then 5–10 mg in 3–4 hr as needed; larger or more frequent doses have been used.

Psychoneurotic Reactions
IM, IV (Adults): 2–10 mg, may be repeated in 3–4 hr.

Availability (generic available)
Tablets: 2 mg, 5 mg, 10 mg. **Cost:** *Generic*—2 mg $7.99/30, 5 mg $7.99/30, 10 mg $7.99/30.
Oral solution: 1 mg/mL, 5 mg/mL (Intensol).
Solution for injection: 5 mg/mL (contains 10% alcohol and 40% propylene glycol). **Rectal gel delivery system:** 2.5 mg, 10 mg, 20 mg.

NURSING IMPLICATIONS

Assessment
- Monitor blood pressure, pulse, and respiratory rate prior to and periodically throughout therapy and frequently during IV therapy.
- Assess IV site frequently during administration; diazepam may cause phlebitis and venous thrombosis.
- Prolonged high-dose therapy may lead to psychological or physical dependence. Restrict amount of drug available to patient. Observe depressed patients closely for suicidal tendencies.
- Conduct regular assessment of continued need for treatment.
- Geri: Assess risk of falls and institute fall prevention strategies.
- **Anxiety:** Assess mental status (orientation, mood, behavior) and degree of anxiety.
- Assess level of sedation (ataxia, dizziness, slurred speech) prior to and periodically throughout therapy.
- **Seizures:** Observe and record intensity, duration, and location of seizure activity. The initial dose of diazepam offers seizure control for 15–20 min after administration. Institute seizure precautions.
- **Muscle Spasms:** Assess muscle spasm, associated pain, and limitation of movement prior to and during therapy.
- **Alcohol Withdrawal:** Assess patient experiencing alcohol withdrawal for tremors, agitation, delirium, and hallucinations. Protect patient from injury.
- *Lab Test Considerations:* Evaluate hepatic and renal function and CBC periodically during prolonged therapy.
- ***Toxicity and Overdose:*** Flumazenil is an adjunct in the management of toxicity or overdose. (Flumazenil may induce seizures in patients with a history of seizures disorder or who are on tricyclic antidepressants.)

Potential Nursing Diagnoses
Anxiety (Indications)
Impaired physical mobility (Indications)
Risk for injury (Side Effects)

Implementation
- Do not confuse diazepam with lorazepam or ditropan.
- Patient should be kept on bedrest and observed for at least 3 hr following parenteral administration.

- If opioid analgesics are used concurrently with parenteral diazepam, decrease opioid dose by ⅓ and titrate dose to effect.
- Use lowest effective dose. Taper by 2 mg every 3 days to decrease withdrawal symptoms. Some patients may require longer taper periods (mos).
- **PO:** Tablets may be crushed and taken with food or water if patient has difficulty swallowing.
- Mix Intensol preparation with liquid or semisolid food such as water, juices, soda, applesauce, or pudding. Administer entire amount immediately. Do not store.
- **IM:** IM injections are painful and erratically absorbed. If IM route is used, inject deeply into deltoid muscle for maximum absorption.

IV Administration

- **IV:** Resuscitation equipment should be available when diazepam is administered IV.
- **Direct IV:** *Diluent:* For IV administration do not dilute or mix with any other drug. If direct IV push is not feasible, administer IV push into tubing as close to insertion site as possible. Continuous infusion is not recommended due to precipitation in IV fluids and absorption of diazepam into infusion bags and tubing. Injection may cause burning and venous irritation; avoid small veins. *Concentration:* 5 mg/mL. *Rate:* Administer slowly at a rate of 5 mg/min in adults. Infants and children should receive 1–2 mg/min. Rapid injection may cause apnea, hypotension, bradycardia, or cardiac arrest.
- **Y-Site Compatibility:** daptomycin, docetaxel, fentanyl, methadone, piperacillin/tazobactam, teniposide.
- **Y-Site Incompatibility:** acyclovir, alfentanil, amikacin, aminophylline, amphotericin B cholesteryl sulfate, amphotericin B colloidal, amphotericin B liposome, ampicillin, ampicillin/sulbactam, anidulafungin, ascorbic acid, atracurium, atropine, azathioprine, aztreonam, bivalirudin, bumetanide, buprenorphine, butorphanol, calcium chloride, calcium gluconate, carboplatin, caspofungin, cefazolin, cefepime, cefonocid, cefoperazone, cefotaxime, cefotetan, cefoxitin, ceftazidime, ceftizoxime, ceftriaxone, cefuroxime, chloramphenicol, chlorpromazine, cimetidine, cisplatin, clindamycin, cyanocobalamin, cyclophosphamide, cyclosporine, cytarabine, dactinomycin, dantrolene, dexamethasone, dexmedetomidine, diazoxide, digoxin, diltiazem, diphenhydramine, dopamine, doripenem, doxacurium, doxorubicin, doxycycline, eftifibatide, enalaprilat, ephedrine, epinephrine, epirubicin, epoetin alfa, erythromycin, esmolol, etoposide, etoposide phosphate, famotidine, fenoldopam, fluconazole, fludarabine, fluorouracil, folic acid, foscarnet, furosemide, ganciclovir, gemcitabine, gentamicin, glycopyrrolate, granisetron, haloperidol, heparin, hetastarch, hydralazine, hydrocortisone, hydroxyzine, idarubicin, ifosfamide, imipenem/cilastatin, inamrinone, indomethacin, insulin, isoproterenol, ketorolac, labetalol, levofloxacin, lidocaine, linezolid, magnesium chloride, mannitol, mechlorethamine, meperidine, meropenem, metaraminol, methotrexate, methoxamine, methyldopate, methylprednisolone, metoclopramide, metoprolol, metronidazole, midazolam, milrinone, mitoxantrone, multivitamin, nalbuphine, naloxone, nesiritide, nitroglycerin, nitroprusside, norepinephrine, octreotide, oxacillin, oxaliplatin, oxytocin, paclitaxel, palonosetron, pancuronium, pantoprazole, papaverine, pemetrexed, penicillin G, pentamidine, pentazocine, pentobarbital, phenobarbital, phentolamine, phenylephrine, phenytoin, phytonadione, potassium chloride, procainamide, prochlorperazine, promethazine, propofol, propranolol, protamine, pyridoxine, quinupristin/dalfopristin, ranitidine, rocuronium, sodium acetate, sodium bicarbonate, streptokinase, succinylcholine, tacrolimus, theophylline, thiamine, thiotepa, ticarcillin/clavulanate, tigecycline, tirofiban, tobramycin, tolazoline, trimetaphan, trimethoprim/sulfamethoxazole, urokinase, vancomycin, vasopressin, vecuronium, verapamil, vincristine, vinorelbine, vitamin B complex with C, voriconazole.
- **Rect:** Do not repeat *Diastat* rectal dose more than 5 times/mo or 1 episode every 5 days. Round dose up to next available dose unit.
- Diazepam injection has been used for rectal administration. Instill via catheter or cannula fitted to the syringe or directly from a 1-mL syringe inserted 4–5 cm into the rectum. A dilution of diazepam injection with propylene glycol containing 1 mg/mL has also been used.
- Do not dilute with other solutions, IV fluids, or medications.

Patient/Family Teaching

- Instruct patient to take medication as directed and not to take more than prescribed or increase dose if less effective after a few weeks without checking with health care professional. Review package insert for Diastat rectal gel with patient/caregiver prior to administration.

Abrupt withdrawal of diazepam may cause insomnia, unusual irritability or nervousness, and seizures. Advise patient that sharing of this medication may be dangerous.
- Medication may cause drowsiness, clumsiness, or unsteadiness. Advise patient to avoid driving or other activities requiring alertness until response to medication is known. *Geri:* Advise geriatric patients of increased risk for CNS effects and potential for falls.
- Caution patient to avoid taking alcohol or other CNS depressants concurrently with this medication.
- Advise patient to notify health care professional if pregnancy is planned or suspected.
- Emphasize the importance of follow-up examinations to determine effectiveness of the medication.
- **Seizures:** Patients on anticonvulsant therapy should carry identification describing disease process and medication regimen at all times.

Evaluation/Desired Outcomes
- Decrease in anxiety level. Full therapeutic antianxiety effects occur after 1–2 wk of therapy.
- Decreased recall of surgical or diagnostic procedures.
- Control of seizures.
- Decrease in muscle spasms.
- Decreased tremulousness and more rational ideation when used for alcohol withdrawal.

DICLOFENAC† (dye-kloe-fen-ak)
diclofenac potassium (oral)
Cambia, Cataflam, Zipsor
diclofenac sodium (oral)
✤ Apo-Diclo, Voltaren, Voltaren XR
diclofenac sodium (topical gel)
Solaraze, Voltaren Gel
diclofenac epolamine (topical patch)
Flector

Classification
Therapeutic: nonopioid analgesics, nonsteroidal anti-inflammatory agents

Pregnancy Category B (3% gel), C (oral, 1% gel, patch)

†For ophthalmic use see Appendix C

Indications
PO: Management of inflammatory disorders including: Rheumatoid arthritis, Osteoarthritis, Ankylosing spondylitis. Primary dysmenorrhea. Relief of mild to moderate pain. Acute treatment of migraines (powder for oral solution). **Topical:** Management of: Actinic keratoses (Solaraze), Osteoarthritis (Voltaren Gel). **Transdermal:** Acute pain due to minor strains, sprains, and contusions.

Action
Inhibits prostaglandin synthesis. **Therapeutic Effects:** Suppression of pain and inflammation. Relief of acute migraine attacks. **Topical**: Clearance of actinic keratosis lesions.

Pharmacokinetics
Absorption: Undergoes first-pass metabolism by liver which results in 50% bioavailability. Oral diclofenac sodium is a delayed-release dose form. Diclofenac potassium is an immediate-release dose form. 6–10% of topical gel is systemically absorbed.
Distribution: Crosses the placenta.
Protein Binding: >99%.
Metabolism and Excretion: Metabolized by the liver to several metabolites; 65% excreted in urine, 35% in bile.
Half-life: 2 hr.

TIME/ACTION PROFILE

ROUTE	ONSET	PEAK	DURATION
PO (inflammation)	few days-1 wk	≥2 wk	unknown
PO (pain)	30 min	unknown	up to 8 hr
Top (gel and patch)	unknown	10–20 hr	unknown

Contraindications/Precautions
Contraindicated in: Hypersensitivity to diclofenac or other components of formulation; Cross-sensitivity may occur with other NSAIDs including aspirin; Active GI bleeding/ulcer disease; Patients undergoing coronary artery bypass graft surgery.
Use Cautiously in: Severe renal/hepatic disease; Cardiovascular disease or risk factors for cardiovascular disease (may ↑ risk of serious cardiovascular thrombotic events, myocardial infarction, and stroke, especially with prolonged use); Heart failure; History of porphyria; History of peptic ulcer disease and/or GI bleeding; Geri: Dose reduction recommended; more susceptible to adverse reactions, including GI bleeding; Bleeding tendency or concurrent anticoagulant therapy;

436 DICLOFENAC

OB, Lactation: Not recommended for use during second half of pregnancy; Pedi: Safety not established.

Adverse Reactions/Side Effects
For oral diclofenac unless noted.
CNS: dizziness, headache. **CV:** hypertension. **EENT:** tinnitus. **GI:** GI BLEEDING, abdominal pain, constipation, diarrhea, dyspepsia, flatulence, heartburn, ↑ liver enzymes, nausea, vomiting. **GU:** acute renal failure, hematuria. **Derm:** EXFOLIATIVE DERMATITIS, STEVENS-JOHNSON SYNDROME, TOXIC EPIDERMAL NECROLYSIS, pruritis, rashes, eczema, photosensitivity. **F and E:** edema. **Hemat:** anemia, prolonged bleeding time. **Local:** *Topical only*—contact dermatitis, dry skin, exfoliation. **Misc:** allergic reactions including ANAPHYLAXIS.

Interactions
Primarily noted for oral administration.
Drug-Drug: ↑ adverse GI effects with **aspirin**, other **NSAIDs**, or **corticosteroids**. May ↓ effectiveness of **diuretics** or **antihypertensives**. May ↑ levels/risk of toxicity from **cyclosporine**, **lithium**, or **methotrexate**. ↑ risk of bleeding with some **cephalosporins**, **thrombolytic agents**, **antiplatelet agents**, or **warfarin**. Concurrent use of oral **NSAIDs** during topical diclofenac therapy should be minimized.
Drug-Natural Products: ↑ bleeding risk with **arnica**, **chamomile**, **clove**, **dong quai**, **feverfew**, **garlic**, **ginger**, **ginkgo**, **Panax ginseng**, and others.

Route/Dosage
Different formulations of oral diclofenac (diclofenac sodium enteric-coated tablets, diclofenac sodium extended-release tablets, and diclofenac potassium immediate-release tablets) are not bioequivalent and should not be substituted on a mg-to-mg basis.

Diclofenac Potassium
PO (Adults): *Analgesic/antidysmenorrheal (Cataflam)*—100 mg initially, then 50 mg 3 times daily as needed; *Analgesic (Zipsor)*—25 mg 4 times daily; *Rheumatoid arthritis (Cataflam)*—50 mg 3–4 times daily; *Osteoarthritis (Cataflam)*—50 mg 2–3 times daily; *Osteoarthritis (Cambria)*—one packet (50 mg) given as a single dose.

Diclofenac Sodium
PO (Adults): *Rheumatoid arthritis (delayed-release [enteric-coated] tablets)*—50 mg 3–4 times daily *or* 75 mg twice daily (usual maintenance dose 25 mg 3 times daily). *Rheumatoid arthritis (extended-release tablets)*—100 mg once daily; if unsatisfactory response, dose may be ↑ to 100 mg twice daily. *Osteoarthritis (delayed-release [enteric-coated] tablets)*—50 mg 2–3 times daily *or* 75 mg twice daily. *Osteoarthritis (extended-release tablets)*—100 mg once daily. *Ankylosing spondylitis (delayed-release [enteric-coated] tablets)*—25 mg 4 times daily, with an additional 25 mg given at bedtime, if necessary.
Topical (Adults): *Solaraze*—Apply to lesions twice daily for 60–90 days; *Voltaren gel*—Lower extremities (knees, ankles, feet): Apply 4 g to affected area 4 times daily (maximum of 16 g per joint/day); Upper extremities (elbows, wrists, hands): Apply 2 g to affected area 4 times daily (maximum of 8 g per joint/day); Maximum total body dose should not exceed 32 g/day.

Diclofenac Epolamine
Topical (Adults): *Flector*—Apply 1 patch to most painful area twice daily.

Availability (generic available)
Diclofenac potassium immediate-release tablets (Cataflam): 50 mg. **Cost:** Generic—$59.98/100. **Diclofenac potassium liquid-filled capsules (Zipsor):** 50 mg. **Diclofenac potassium powder for oral solution (Cambria):** 50 mg/packet. **Diclofenac sodium delayed-release (enteric-coated) tablets (Voltaren):** ✹ 25 mg, 50 mg, 75 mg. **Cost:** Generic—50 mg $37.08/100, 75 mg $44.98/100. **Diclofenac sodium extended-release tablets (Voltaren XR):** ✹ 75 mg, 100 mg. **Cost:** Generic—100 mg $208.78/90. **Diclofenac sodium gel:** 1% (Voltaren gel), 3% (Solaraze). **Diclofenac epolamine topical patch:** 180 mg/patch. *In combination with:* 200 mcg misoprostol (Arthrotec). See Appendix B.

NURSING IMPLICATIONS

Assessment
- Patients who have asthma, aspirin-induced allergy, and nasal polyps are at ↑ risk for developing hypersensitivity reactions.
- Monitor blood pressure closely during initiation of treatment and periodically during therapy in patients with hypertension.
- **Pain:** Assess pain and limitation of movement; note type, location, and intensity before and 30–60 min after administration.
- **Arthritis:** Assess arthritic pain (note type, location, intensity) and limitation of movement before and periodically during therapy.
- **Actinic Keratosis:** Assess lesions prior to and periodically during therapy.

DICLOFENAC 437

- **Lab Test Considerations:** Diclofenac has minimal effect on bleeding time and platelet aggregation.
- May cause ↓ in hemoglobin and hematocrit.
- Monitor CBC and liver function tests within 8 wk of initiating diclofenac therapy and periodically during therapy. May cause ↑ serum alkaline phosphatase, LDH, AST, and ALT concentrations.
- Monitor BUN and serum creatinine periodically during therapy. May cause ↑ BUN and serum creatinine.

Potential Nursing Diagnoses
Acute pain (Indications)
Impaired physical mobility (Indications)

Implementation
- Do not confuse Cataflam (diclofenac) with Catapres (clonidine).
- Administration in higher than recommended doses does not provide increased effectiveness but may cause increased side effects. Use lowest effective dose for shortest period of time.
- **PO:** Take with food or milk to minimize gastric irritation. May take first 1–2 doses on an empty stomach for more rapid onset. Do not crush or chew enteric-coated or extended-release tablets.
- **Dysmenorrhea:** Administer as soon as possible after the onset of menses. Prophylactic treatment has not been shown to be effective.
- **Topical:** Gel should be applied to intact skin; do not use on open wounds. An adequate amount of gel should be applied to cover the entire lesion.
- **Transdermal:** Apply patch to the most painful area twice a day. Do not apply to non-intact or damaged skin resulting from any etiology (exudative dermatitis, eczema, infected lesion, burns, wounds). Avoid contact with eyes; wash hands after applying, handling, or removing patch.

Patient/Family Teaching
- Caution patient to avoid concurrent use of alcohol, aspirin, acetaminophen, other NSAIDs, or other OTC medications without consulting health care professional.
- Instruct patient to notify health care professional of medication regimen before treatment or surgery.
- Instruct female patients to inform health care professional if they plan or suspect pregnancy. Caution female patient to avoid use of diclofenac in last trimester of pregnancy and to notify health care professional if breastfeeding.
- May cause serious side effects: CV (MI or stroke), GI (ulcers, bleeding), skin (exfoliative dermatitis, Stevens-Johnson Syndrome, toxic epidermal necrolysis) and hypersensitivity (anaphylaxis). May occur without warning symptoms. Advise patient to stop medication and notify health care professional immediately if symptoms of CV side effects (chest pain, shortness of breath, weakness, slurring of speech), GI side effects (epigastric pain, dyspepsia, melana, hematemesis), skin side effects (skin rash, blisters, fever, itching) or hypersensitivity reactions (difficulty breathing or swelling of face or throat) occur. Inform patient that risk for heart attack or stroke that can lead to death increases with longer use of NSAID medications and in people who have heart disease and that risk of ulcer increases with concurrent use of corticosteroids and anticoagulants, longer use, smoking, drinking alcohol, older age, and having poor health.
- Advise patient to notify health care professional promptly if unexplained weight gain, swelling of arms and legs or hands and feet, nausea, fatigue, lethargy, pruritus, yellowing of skin or eyes, itching, stomach pain, vomiting blood, bloody or tarry stools, or flu-like symptoms occur.
- **PO:** Instruct patient to take diclofenac with a full glass of water and to remain in an upright position for 15–30 min after administration. Take missed doses as soon as possible within 1–2 hr if taking once or twice a day or unless almost time for next dose if taking more than twice a day. Do not double doses.
- May cause drowsiness or dizziness. Caution patient to avoid driving or other activities requiring alertness until response to medication is known.
- Caution patient to wear sunscreen and protective clothing to prevent photosensitivity reactions.
- **Topical:** Advise patient to minimize use of concurrent NSAIDs during topical therapy.
- Instruct patient to avoid covering lesion with occlusive dressing and to avoid applying sunscreen or cosmetics to the affected area.
- Advise patient that it may take up to 1 mo for complete healing of the lesion to occur.
- **Transdermal:** Instruct patient on correct application procedure for patch. Apply patch to

most painful area. Change patch every 12 hr. Remove patch if irritation occurs. Fold used patches so adhesive sticks to itself and discard where children and pets cannot get them. Encourage patient to read the *NSAID Medication Guide* that accompanies the prescription.
- Instruct patients if patch begins to peel off to tape the edges. Do not wear patch during bathing or showering. Bathing should take place between scheduled patch removal and application.
- Advise patient referred for MRI test to discuss patch with referring health care professional and MRI facility to determine if removal of patch is necessary prior to test and for directions for replacing patch.

Evaluation/Desired Outcomes
- Decrease in severity of mild-to-moderate pain.
- Increased ease of joint movement. Patients who do not respond to one NSAID may respond to another. May require 2 wk or more for maximum effects.
- Decrease in or healing of lesions in actinic keratosis. Optimal effect may not be seen until 30 days after discontinuation of therapy. Lesions that do not heal should be re-evaluated.

---

dicloxacillin, See PENICILLINS, PENICILLINASE RESISTANT.

---

dicyclomine
(dye-**sye**-kloe-meen)
Bentyl, ✦ Bentylol, ✦ Formulex, ✦ Spasmoban

Classification
Therapeutic: antispasmodics
Pharmacologic: anticholinergics

Pregnancy Category UK

Indications
Management of irritable bowel syndrome in patients who do not respond to usual interventions (sedation/change in diet).

Action
May have a direct and local effect on GI smooth muscle, reducing motility and tone. **Therapeutic Effects:** Decreased GI motility.

Pharmacokinetics
Absorption: Well absorbed after oral and IM administration.
Distribution: Unknown.
Metabolism and Excretion: 80% eliminated in urine, 10% in feces.
Half-life: 1.8 hr (initial phase), 9–10 hr (terminal phase).

TIME/ACTION PROFILE (antispasmodic effect)

ROUTE	ONSET	PEAK	DURATION
PO, IM	unknown	unknown	unknown

Contraindications/Precautions
Contraindicated in: Hypersensitivity; Obstruction of the GI or GU tract; Reflux esophagitis; Severe ulcerative colitis (risk of paralytic ileus); Unstable cardiovascular status; Glaucoma; Myasthenia gravis; Infants <6 mo; Lactation.
Use Cautiously in: High environmental temperatures (risk of heat prostration); Hepatic/renal impairment; Autonomic neuropathy; Cardiovascular disease; Prostatic hyperplasia; Geri: Appears on Beers list. Geriatric patients have increased sensitivity to anticholinergics; Pregnancy (safety not established).

Adverse Reactions/Side Effects
CNS: confusion (increased in geriatric patients), drowsiness, light-headedness (IM only). **EENT:** blurred vision, increased intraocular pressure. **CV:** palpitations, tachycardia. **GI:** PARALYTIC ILEUS, constipation, heartburn, decreased salivation, dry mouth, nausea, vomiting. **GU:** erectile dysfunction, urinary hesitancy, urinary retention. **Derm:** decreased sweating. **Endo:** decreased lactation. **Local:** pain/redness at IM site. **Misc:** allergic reactions including ANAPHYLAXIS.

Interactions
Drug-Drug: Additive anticholinergic effects with other **anticholinergics**, including **antihistamines**, **quinidine**, and **disopyramide**. May alter the absorption of **other orally administered drugs** by slowing motility of the GI tract. **Antacids** or **adsorbent antidiarrheals** decrease the absorption of anticholinergics. May increase GI mucosal lesions in patients taking oral **potassium chloride** tablets. Increased risk of adverse cardiovascular reactions with **cyclopropane** anesthesia.

Route/Dosage
PO (Adults): 10–20 mg 3–4 times daily (up to 160 mg/day).
PO (Children ≥2 yr): 10 mg 3–4 times daily, adjusted as tolerated.
PO (Children 6 mo–2 yr): 5–10 mg 3–4 times daily, adjusted as tolerated.
IM (Adults): 20 mg q 4–6 hr, adjusted as tolerated.

Availability
Tablets: ✤ 10 mg, 20 mg. **Capsules:** 10 mg, 20 mg. **Syrup:** 10 mg/5 mL. **Solution for injection:** 10 mg/mL.

NURSING IMPLICATIONS
Assessment
- Assess patient for symptoms of irritable bowel syndrome (abdominal cramping, alternating constipation and diarrhea, mucus in stools) before and periodically during therapy.
- Assess patient routinely for abdominal distention and auscultate for bowel sounds. If constipation becomes a problem, increasing fluids and adding bulk to the diet may help alleviate the constipating effects of the drug.
- Monitor intake and output ratios; may cause urinary retention.
- *Lab Test Considerations:* Antagonizes effects of pentagastrin and histamine during the gastric acid secretion test. Avoid administration for 24 hr preceding the test.
- *Toxicity and Overdose:* Severe anticholinergic symptoms may be reversed with physostigmine or neostigmine.

Potential Nursing Diagnoses
Acute pain (Indications)
Diarrhea (Indications)

Implementation
- **PO:** Administer dicyclomine 30 min–1 hr before meals.
- **IM:** Monitor patient after administration; may cause light-headedness and irritation at injection site.

Patient/Family Teaching
- Instruct patient to take dicyclomine exactly as directed and not to take more than the prescribed amount. Missed doses should be taken as soon as remembered if not just before next dose.
- Medication may cause drowsiness and blurred vision. Caution patient to avoid driving or other activities requiring alertness until response to the medication is known.
- Inform patient that frequent oral rinses, sugarless gum or candy, and good oral hygiene may help relieve dry mouth. Consult health care professional regarding use of saliva substitute if dry mouth persists for more than 2 wk.
- Advise patient receiving dicyclomine to make position changes slowly to minimize the effects of drug-induced orthostatic hypotension.
- Caution patient to avoid extremes of temperature. This medication decreases the ability to sweat and may increase the risk of heat stroke.
- Advise patient to consult health care professional before taking any OTC medications concurrently with this therapy.
- Advise patient to notify health care professional immediately if eye pain or increased sensitivity to light occurs. Emphasize the importance of routine eye exams throughout therapy.

Evaluation/Desired Outcomes
- A decrease in the symptoms of irritable bowel syndrome.

---

diflorasone, See CORTICOSTEROIDS (TOPICAL/LOCAL).

HIGH ALERT

digoxin (di-jox-in)
Lanoxicaps, Lanoxin

Classification
Therapeutic: antiarrhythmics, inotropics
Pharmacologic: digitalis glycosides

Pregnancy Category C

Indications
Heart failure. Atrial fibrillation and atrial flutter (slows ventricular rate). Paroxysmal atrial tachycardia.

Action
Increases the force of myocardial contraction. Prolongs refractory period of the AV node. Decreases conduction through the SA and AV nodes. **Therapeutic Effects:** Increased cardiac output (positive inotropic effect) and slowing of the heart rate (negative chronotropic effect).

Pharmacokinetics
Absorption: 60–80% absorbed after oral administration of tablets; 70-85% absorbed after administration of elixir. Absorption from liquid-filled capsules is 90–100%; 80% absorbed from IM sites (IM route not recommended due to pain/irritation).
Distribution: Widely distributed; crosses placenta and enters breast milk.
Metabolism and Excretion: Excreted almost entirely unchanged by the kidneys.
Half-life: 36–48 hr (increased in renal impairment).

✤ = Canadian drug name. ⚡ = Genetic implication.
*CAPITALS indicates life-threatening; underlines indicate most frequent.

440 digoxin

TIME/ACTION PROFILE (antiarrhythmic or inotropic effects, provided that a loading dose has been given)

ROUTE	ONSET	PEAK	DURATION
Digoxin–PO	30–120 min	2–8 hr	2–4 days†
Digoxin–IM	30 min	4–6 hr	2–4 days†
Digoxin–IV	5–30 min	1–4 hr	2–4 days†

†Duration listed is that for normal renal function; in impaired renal function, duration will be longer

Contraindications/Precautions
Contraindicated in: Hypersensitivity; Uncontrolled ventricular arrhythmias; AV block (in absence of pacemaker); Idiopathic hypertrophic subaortic stenosis; Constrictive pericarditis; Known alcohol intolerance (elixir only).
Use Cautiously in: Hypokalemia (greatly ↑ risk of digoxin toxicity); Hypercalcemia (↑ risk of toxicity, especially with mild hypokalemia); Hypomagnesemia (may ↑ risk of digoxin toxicity); Diuretic use (may cause electrolyte abnormalities including hypokalemia and hypomagnesemia); Hypothyroidism; Geri: Very sensitive to toxic effects; dose adjustments required for age-related ↓ in renal function and body weight; Myocardial infarction; Renal impairment (dose ↓ required); Obesity (dose should be based on ideal body weight); OB: Although safety has not been established, has been used during pregnancy without adverse effects on the fetus; Lactation: Similar concentrations in serum and breast milk result in subtherapeutic levels in infant, use with caution.

Adverse Reactions/Side Effects
CNS: fatigue, headache, weakness. **EENT:** blurred vision, yellow or green vision. **CV:** ARRHYTHMIAS, bradycardia, ECG changes, AV block, SA block. **GI:** anorexia, nausea, vomiting, diarrhea. **Hemat:** thrombocytopenia. **Metab:** electrolyte imbalances with acute digoxin toxicity.

Interactions
Drug-Drug: **Thiazide** and **loop diuretics**, **piperacillin**, **ticarcillin**, **amphotericin B**, **corticosteroids**, and excessive use of **laxatives** may cause hypokalemia which may ↑ risk of toxicity. **Amiodarone**, some **benzodiazepines**, **cyclosporine**, **diphenoxylate**, **indomethacin**, **itraconazole**, **propafenone**, **quinidine**, **quinine**, **spironolactone**, and **verapamil** may ↑ levels and lead to toxicity (serum level monitoring/dose reduction may be required). Levels may be ↓ by some **antineoplastics** (**bleomycin**, **carmustine**, **cyclophosphamide**, **cytarabine**, **doxorubicin**, **methotrexate**, **procarbazine**, **vincristine**), **activated charcoal**, **cholestyramine**, **colestipol**, **kaolin/pectin**, **metoclopramide**, **penicillamine**, **rifampin**, or **sulfasalazine**. In a small percentage (10%) of patients gut bacteria metabolize digoxin to inactive compounds; **macrolide anti-infectives** (**erythromycin**, **azithromycin**, **clarithromycin**) and **tetracyclines**, by killing these bacteria, will cause ↑ levels and toxicity; dose may need to be ↓ for up to 9 weeks. Additive bradycardia may occur with **beta blockers**, **diltiazem**, **verapamil**, **clonidine**, and other **antiarrhythmics** (**quinidine**, **disopyramide**). Concurrent use of **sympathomimetics** may ↑ risk of arrthythmias. **Thyroid hormones** may ↓ therapeutic effects.
Drug-Natural Products: **Licorice** and stimulant natural products (**aloe**) may ↑ risk of potassium depletion. **St. John's wort** may ↓ levels and effect.
Drug-Food: Concurrent ingestion of a **high-fiber meal** may ↓ absorption. Administer digoxin 1 hour before or 2 hours after such a meal.

Route/Dosage
For rapid effect, a larger initial loading/digitalizing dose should be given in several divided doses over 12–24 hr. Maintenance doses are determined for digoxin by renal function. All dosing must be evaluated by individual response. In general, doses required for atrial arrhythmias are higher than those for inotropic effect. When determining dose, consider that bioavailability of gelatin capsules (Lanoxicaps) is greater than that of tablets.

IV (Adults): *Digitalizing dose*—0.5–1 mg given as 50% of the dose initially and one quarter of the initial dose in each of 2 subsequent doses at 6-12 hr intervals.
IV (Children >10 yr): *Digitalizing dose*—8–12 mcg/kg given as 50% of the dose initially and one quarter of the initial dose in each of 2 subsequent doses at 6-12 hr intervals.
IV (Children 5–10 yr): *Digitalizing dose*—15–30 mcg/kg given as 50% of the dose initially and one quarter of the initial dose in each of 2 subsequent doses at 6-12 hr intervals.
IV (Children 2–5 yr): *Digitalizing dose*—25–35 mcg/kg given as 50% of the dose initially and one quarter of the initial dose in each of 2 subsequent doses at 6-12 hr intervals.
IV (Children 1–24 mo): *Digitalizing dose*—30–50 mcg/kg given as 50% of the dose initially and one quarter of the initial dose in each of 2 subsequent doses at 6-12 hr intervals.
IV (Infants–full term): 20–30 mcg/kg given as 50% of the dose initially and one quarter of the

digoxin

initial dose in each of 2 subsequent doses at 6-12 hr intervals.
IV (Infants–premature): *Digitalizing dose*—15–25 mcg/kg given as 50% of the dose initially and one quarter of the initial dose in each of 2 subsequent doses at 6-12 hr intervals.
PO (Adults): *Digitalizing dose*—0.75–1.5 mg given as 50% of the dose initially and one quarter of the initial dose in each of 2 subsequent doses at 6–12 hr intervals. *Maintenance dose*—0.125–0.5 mg/day as tablets or 0.350–0.5 mg/day as gelatin capsules, depending on patient's lean body weight, renal function, and serum level.
PO (Geriatric Patients): Initial daily dosage should not exceed 0.125 mg.
PO (Children >10 yr): *Digitalizing dose*—10–15 mcg/kg given as 50% of the dose initially and one quarter of the initial dose in each of 2 subsequent doses at 6-12 hr intervals. *Maintenance dose*—2.5–5 mcg/kg given daily as a single dose.
PO (Children 5–10 yr): *Digitalizing dose*—20–35 mcg/kg given as 50% of the dose initially and one quarter of the initial dose in each of 2 subsequent doses at 6-12 hr intervals. *Maintenance dose*—5–10 mcg/kg given daily in 2 divided doses.
PO (Children 2–5 yr): *Digitalizing dose*—30–40 mcg/kg given as 50% of the dose initially and one quarter of the initial dose in each of 2 subsequent doses at 6-12 hr intervals. *Maintenance dose*—7.5–10 mcg/kg given daily in 2 divided doses.
PO (Children 1–24 mo): *Digitalizing dose*—35–60 mcg/kg given as 50% of the dose initially and one quarter of the initial dose in each of 2 subsequent doses at 6-12 hr intervals. *Maintenance dose*—10–15 mcg/kg given daily in 2 divided doses.
PO (Infants–full term): *Digitalizing dose*—25–35 mcg/kg given as 50% of the dose initially and one quarter of the initial dose in each of 2 subsequent doses at 6-12 hr intervals. *Maintenance dose*—6–10 mcg/kg given daily in 2 divided doses.
PO (Infants–premature): *Digitalizing dose*—20–30 mcg/kg given as 50% of the dose initially and one quarter of the initial dose in each of 2 subsequent doses at 6-12 hr intervals. *Maintenance dose*—5–7.5 mcg/kg given daily in 2 divided doses.

Availability (generic available)
Tablets: 0.125 mg, 0.25 mg. **Cost:** *Lanoxin*—0.125 mg $24.97/90, 0.25 mg $29.97/90; *Generic*—0.125 mg $21.97/90, 0.25 mg $21.97/90. **Capsules:** 0.05 mg, 0.1 mg, 0.2 mg. **Cost:** 0.05 mg $25.99/100, 0.1 mg $33.56/100, 0.2 mg $39.57/100. **Elixir (lime flavor):** 0.05 mg/mL. **Injection:** 0.25 mg/mL. **Pediatric injection:** 0.1 mg/mL.

NURSING IMPLICATIONS

Assessment
- Monitor apical pulse for 1 full min before administering. Withhold dose and notify physician if pulse rate is <60 bpm in an adult, <70 bpm in a child, or <90 bpm in an infant. Also notify health care professional promptly of any significant changes in rate, rhythm, or quality of pulse.
- Pedi: Heart rate varies in children depending on age, ask physician to specify at what heart rates digoxin should be withheld.
- Monitor blood pressure periodically in patients receiving IV digoxin.
- Monitor ECG throughout IV administration and 6 hr after each dose. Notify health care professional if bradycardia or new arrhythmias occur.
- Observe IV site for redness or infiltration; extravasation can lead to tissue irritation and sloughing.
- Monitor intake and output ratios and daily weights. Assess for peripheral edema, and auscultate lungs for rales/crackles throughout therapy.
- Before administering initial loading dose, determine whether patient has taken any digitalis preparations in the preceding 2–3 wk.
- Geri: Digoxin has been associated with an increased risk of falls in the elderly. Assess for falls risk and implement prevention strategies per facility protocol.
- **Lab Test Considerations:** Evaluate serum electrolyte levels (especially potassium, magnesium, and calcium) and renal and hepatic functions periodically during therapy. Notify health care professional before giving dose if patient is hypokalemic. Hypokalemia, hypomagnesemia, or hypercalcemia may make the patient more susceptible to digitalis toxicity. Pedi: Neonates may have falsely elevated serum digoxin concentrations due to a naturally occurring substance chemically similar to di-

442 digoxin

goxin. Geri: Older adults may be toxic even when serum concentrations are within normal range; assess for clinical symptoms of toxicity even when serum levels are normal.

- ***Toxicity and Overdose:*** Therapeutic serum digoxin levels range from 0.5–2 ng/mL. Serum levels may be drawn 6–8 hr after a dose is administered, although they are usually drawn immediately before the next dose. Bacteria in the GI tract can metabolize a substantial amount of digoxin before it is absorbed. Patients receiving erythromycin or tetracycline, which kill gut bacteria, can develop toxicity on their usual doses of digoxin. Geri: Older adults are at increased risk for toxic effects of digoxin (appears on Beers list) due to age-related decreased renal clearance, which can exist even when serum creatinine levels are normal. Digoxin requirements in the older adult may change and a formerly therapeutic dose can become toxic.
- Observe for signs and symptoms of toxicity. In adults and older children, the first signs of toxicity usually include abdominal pain, anorexia, nausea, vomiting, visual disturbances, bradycardia, and other arrhythmias. In infants and small children, the first symptoms of overdose are usually cardiac arrhythmias. If these appear, withhold drug and notify health care professional immediately.
- If signs of toxicity occur and are not severe, discontinuation of digitalis glycoside may be all that is required.
- If hypokalemia is present and renal function is adequate, potassium salts may be administered. Do not administer if hyperkalemia or heart block exists. **Correct any other electrolyte abnormalities.**
- Correction of arrhythmias resulting from digitalis toxicity may be attempted with lidocaine, procainamide, quinidine, propranolol, or phenytoin. Temporary ventricular pacing may be useful in advanced heart block.
- Treatment of life-threatening arrhythmias may include administration of digoxin immune Fab *(Digibind)*, which binds to the digitalis glycoside molecule in the blood and is excreted by the kidneys.

Potential Nursing Diagnoses
Decreased cardiac output (Indications)

Implementation
- **High Alert:** Digoxin has a narrow therapeutic range. Medication errors associated with digoxin include miscalculation of pediatric doses and insufficient monitoring of digoxin levels.

Have second practitioner independently check original order and dose calculations. Monitor therapeutic drug levels.
- For rapid digitalization, the initial dose is higher than the maintenance dose; 50% of the total digitalizing dose is given initially. The remainder of the dose will be administered in 25% increments at 4–8 hr intervals.
- When changing from parenteral to oral dose forms, dose adjustments may be necessary because of pharmacokinetic variations in percentage of digoxin absorbed: 100 mcg (0.1 mg) digoxin injection or 100 mcg (0.1 mg) liquid-filled capsule = 125 mcg (0.125 mg) tablet or 125 mcg (0.125 mg) of elixir.
- **PO:** Administer oral preparations consistently with regard to meals. Tablets can be crushed and administered with food or fluids if patient has difficulty swallowing. Use calibrated measuring device for liquid preparations; calibrated dropper is not accurate for doses of less than 0.2 mL or 10 mcg. Do not alternate between dose forms; bioavailability of capsules is greater than that of tablets or elixir.
- **IM:** Administer deep into gluteal muscle and massage well to reduce painful local reactions. Do not administer more than 2 mL of digoxin in each IM site. IM administration is not generally recommended.

IV Administration
- **Direct IV:** ***Diluent:*** May be administered undiluted. May also dilute 1 mL of digoxin in 4 mL of sterile water for injection, D5W, or 0.9% NaCl. Less diluent will cause precipitation. Use diluted solution immediately. ***Rate:*** Administer over at least 5 min.
- **Y-Site Compatibility:** acyclovir, alfentanil, amikacin, aminophylline, anidulafungin, ascorbic acid, atracurium, atropine, aztreonam, benztropine, bivalirudin, bleomycin, bumetanide, buprenorphine, butorphanol, calcium chloride, calcium gluconate, carboplatin, cefazolin, cefonocid, cefoperazone, cefotaxime, cefotetan, cefoxitin, ceftazidime, ceftizoxime, ceftriaxone, cefuroxime, chloramphenicol, chlorpromazine, cimetidine, ciprofloxacin, cisatracurium, cisplatin, clindamycin, codeine, cyanocobalamin, cyclophosphamide, cyclosporine, cytarabine, dactinomycin, daptomycin, dexamethasone, dexmedetomidine, diltiazem, diphenhydramine, dobutamine, docetaxel, dopamine, doripenem, doxacurium, doxycycline, enalaprilat, ephedrine, epinephrine, epirubicin, epoetin alfa, eptifibatide, ertapenem, erythromycin, esmolol, etoposide, eto-

poside phosphate, famotidine, fenoldopam, fentanyl, fludarabine, fluorouracil, folic acid, furosemide, ganciclovir, gemcitabine, gentamicin, glycopyrrolate, granisetron, heparin, hetastarch, hydrocortisone, hydromorphone, ifosfamide, imipenem/cilastatin, indomethacin, isoproterenol, ketorolac, labetalol, levofloxacin, lidocaine, linezolid, lorazepam, magnesium sulfate, mannitol, mechlorethamine, meperidine, meropenem, metaraminol, methotrexate, methoxamine, methyldopate, methylprednisolone, metoclopramide, metoprolol, metronidazole, midazolam, milrinone, morphine, multivitamins, nafcillin, nalbuphine, naloxone, nesiritide, nitroglycerin, nitroprusside, norepinephrine, octreotide, ondansetron, oxacillin, oxaliplatin, oxytocin, palonosetron, pancuronium, pantoprazole, papaverine, pemetrexed, penicillin G, pentazocine, pentobarbital, phenobarbital, phentolamine, phenylephrine, phytonadione, piperacillin/tazobactam, potassium chloride, procainamide, prochlorperazine, promethazine, propranolol, protamine, pyridoxime, ranitidine, remifentanil, rituximab, rocuronium, sodium acetate, sodium bicarbonate, streptokinase, succinylcholine, sufentanil, tacrolimus, teniposide, theophylline, thiamine, thiotepa, ticarcillin/clavulanate, tigecycline, tirofiban, tobramycin, tolazoline, trastuzumab, trimetaphan, urokinase, vancomycin, vasopressin, vecuronium, verapamil, vincristine, vinorelbine, vitamin B complex with C, voriconazole.
- **Y-Site Incompatibility:** amiodarone, amphotericin B cholesteryl, amphotericin B colloidal, amphotericin B liposome, caspofungin, dantrolene, diazepam, diazoxide, doxorubicin, foscarnet, idarubicin, mitoxantrone, paclitaxel, pentamidine, phenytoin, propofol, quinupristin/dalfopristin, trimethoprim/sulfamethoxazole.

Patient/Family Teaching
- Instruct patient to take medication as directed, at the same time each day. Teach parents or caregivers of infants and children how to accurately measure medication. Take missed doses within 12 hr of scheduled dose or omit. Do not double doses. Consult health care professional if doses for 2 or more days are missed. Do not discontinue medication without consulting health care professional.
- Teach patient to take pulse and to contact health care professional before taking medication if pulse rate is <60 or >100.
- Pedi: Teach parents or caregivers that changes in heart rate, especially bradycardia, are among the first signs of digoxin toxicity in infants and children. Instruct parents or caregivers in apical heart rate assessment and ask them to notify a health care professional if heart rate is outside of range set by health care professional before administering the next scheduled dose.
- Review signs and symptoms of digitalis toxicity with patient and family. Advise patient to notify health care professional immediately if these or symptoms of CHF occur. Inform patient that these symptoms may be mistaken for those of colds or flu.
- Instruct patient to keep digoxin tablets in their original container and not to mix in pill boxes with other medications; they may look similar to and may be mistaken for other medications.
- Advise patient that sharing of this medication can be dangerous.
- Caution patient to avoid concurrent use of other Rx, OTC, and herbal products without consulting health care professional. Advise patient to avoid taking antacids or antidiarrheals within 2 hr of digoxin.
- Advise patient to notify health care professional of this medication regimen before treatment.
- Patients taking digoxin should carry identification describing disease process and medication regimen at all times.
- Geri: Review fall prevention strategies with older adults and their families.
- Emphasize the importance of routine follow-up exams to determine effectiveness and to monitor for toxicity.

Evaluation/Desired Outcomes
- Decrease in severity of CHF.
- Increase in cardiac output.
- Decrease in ventricular response in atrial tachyarrhythmias.
- Termination of paroxysmal atrial tachycardia.

digoxin immune Fab
(di-**jox**-in im-**myoon** fab)
Digibind, DigiFab

digoxin immune Fab

Classification
Therapeutic: antidotes
Pharmacologic: antibody fragments

Pregnancy Category C

Indications
Serious life-threatening overdosage with digoxin.

Action
An antibody produced in sheep that binds antigenically to unbound digoxin in serum. **Therapeutic Effects:** Binding and subsequent removal of digoxin, preventing toxic effects in overdose.

Pharmacokinetics
Absorption: Administered IV only, resulting in complete bioavailability.
Distribution: Widely distributed throughout extracellular space.
Metabolism and Excretion: Excreted by the kidneys as the bound complex (digoxin immune Fab plus digoxin).
Half-life: 14–20 hr.

TIME/ACTION PROFILE (reversal of arrhythmias and hyperkalemia; reversal of inotropic effect may take several hr)

ROUTE	ONSET	PEAK	DURATION
IV	30 min (variable)	unknown	2–6 hr

Contraindications/Precautions
Contraindicated in: No known contraindications.
Use Cautiously in: Known hypersensitivity to sheep proteins or products; Children, pregnancy, or lactation (safety not established).

Adverse Reactions/Side Effects
CV: re-emergence of atrial fibrillation, re-emergence of CHF. **F and E:** HYPOKALEMIA.

Interactions
Drug-Drug: Prevents therapeutic response to **digoxin**.

Route/Dosage
Digibind—38 mg of digoxin immune Fab will bind 0.5 mg of digoxin. Each vial contains 38 mg of digoxin immune Fab; *DigiFab*—40 mg of digoxin immune Fab will bind 0.5 mg of digoxin. Each vial contains 40 mg of digoxin immune Fab.

Known Amount of Digoxin Ingested (Administered)
IV (Adults and Children): *For digitalis glycoside toxicity due to digoxin tablets, oral solution, or IM digoxin*—dose of digoxin ingested (mg) × 0.8/1000 × 38. *For digitalis glycoside toxicity due to digoxin capsules, IV digoxin*—dose of digoxin ingested (mg)/0.5 × 38.

Known Serum Digoxin Concentrations (SDCs)
IV (Adults and Children): *Digibind*—Dose (mg) = SDC (nanograms/mL) × body weight (kg)/100 × 38; *DigiFab*—SDC (nanograms/mL) × body weight (kg)/100 × 40.

Unknown Amount Ingested/SDCs Unavailable
IV (Adults and Children): *Digibind*—760 mg (20 vials); *DigiFab*—800 mg (20 vials).

Toxicity during chronic digoxin therapy
IV (Adults and Children): *Digibind*—228 mg (6 vials); *DigiFab*—240 mg (6 vials).

Availability
Powder for injection, lyophilized (Digibind): 38 mg/vial. **Powder for injection, lyophilized (DigiFab):** 40 mg/vial.

NURSING IMPLICATIONS

Assessment
- Monitor ECG, pulse, blood pressure, and body temperature before and during treatment. Patients with atrial fibrillation may develop a rapid ventricular response as a result of decreased digoxin levels.
- Assess patient for increase in signs of CHF (peripheral edema, dyspnea, rales/crackles, weight gain).
- *Lab Test Considerations:* Monitor serum digoxin levels before administration.
- Monitor serum potassium levels frequently during treatment. Before treatment, hyperkalemia usually coexists with toxicity. Levels may decrease rapidly; hypokalemia should be treated promptly.
- Free serum digoxin levels fall rapidly after administration. Total serum concentrations rise suddenly after administration but are bound to the Fab molecule and are inactive. Total serum concentrations will decrease to undetectable levels within several days. Serum digoxin levels are not valid for 5–7 days after administration.

Potential Nursing Diagnoses
Deficient knowledge, related to medication regimen (Patient/Family Teaching)

Implementation
- Cardiopulmonary resuscitation equipment and medications should be available during administration.

- Delay redigitalization for several days until the elimination of digoxin immune Fab from the body is complete.

IV Administration

- **Intermittent Infusion:** *Diluent:* Reconstitute each vial in 4 mL of sterile water for injection and mix gently. Solution will contain a concentration of 9.5 mg/mL (*Digibind*) or 10 mg/mL (*DigiFab*). May be further diluted with 0.9% NaCl to achieve the concentration below. Reconstituted solution should be used immediately but is stable for 4 hr if refrigerated. For small doses in infants and children, a reconstituted 38-mg vial can be diluted with 34 mL of 0.9% NaCl (*Digibind*) or 36 mL of 0.9% NaCl (*DigiFab*) for a concentration of 1 mg/mL. *Concentration:* 1 mg/mL. *Rate:* Infuse over 30 min through a 0.22-micron membrane filter. If cardiac arrest is imminent, rapid direct IV injection may be used. Do not use rapid direct injection in other patients because of increased risk of adverse reactions. Small doses in infants and children may be administered with a tuberculin syringe.
- **Incompatibility:** Information unavailable. Do not mix with other drugs or solutions.

Patient/Family Teaching

- Explain the procedure and purpose of the treatment to the patient.
- Instruct patient to notify health care provider immediately if signs of delayed allergic reaction (rash, pruritus, urticaria) occur after hospital discharge.

Evaluation/Desired Outcomes

- Resolution of signs and symptoms of digoxin toxicity.
- Decreased digoxin or level without major side effects.

---

dihydroergotamine, See ergotamine.

---

diltiazem (dil-**tye**-a-zem)
♣ Apo-Diltiaz, Cardizem, Cardizem CD, Cardizem LA, Cardizem SR, Cartia XT, Dilacor XR, Diltia XT,
♣ Novo-Diltiazem, Nu-Diltiaz,
♣ Ratio-Diltiazem CD, ♣ Syn-Diltiazem, Taztia XT, Tiazac

diltiazem 445

Classification
Therapeutic: antianginals, antiarrhythmics (class IV), antihypertensives
Pharmacologic: calcium channel blockers

Pregnancy Category C

Indications
Hypertension. Angina pectoris and vasospastic (Prinzmetal's) angina. Supraventricular tachyarrhythmias and rapid ventricular rates in atrial flutter or fibrillation.

Action
Inhibits transport of calcium into myocardial and vascular smooth muscle cells, resulting in inhibition of excitation-contraction coupling and subsequent contraction. **Therapeutic Effects:** Systemic vasodilation resulting in decreased blood pressure. Coronary vasodilation resulting in decreased frequency and severity of attacks of angina. Reduction of ventricular rate in atrial fibrillation or flutter.

Pharmacokinetics
Absorption: Well absorbed, but rapidly metabolized after oral administration.
Distribution: Unknown.
Protein Binding: 70–80%.
Metabolism and Excretion: Mostly metabolized by the liver (CYP3A4 enzyme system).
Half-life: 3.5–9 hr.

TIME/ACTION PROFILE

ROUTE	ONSET	PEAK	DURATION
PO	30 min	2–3 hr	6–8 hr
PO–SR	unknown	unknown	12 hr
PO–CD, XR, LA	unknown	14 days†	up to 24 hr
IV	2–5 min	2–4 hr	unknown

†Maximum antihypertensive effect with chronic therapy

Contraindications/Precautions
Contraindicated in: Hypersensitivity; Sick sinus syndrome; 2nd- or 3rd-degree AV block (unless an artificial pacemaker is in place); Systolic blood pressure <90 mm Hg; Recent MI or pulmonary congestion; Concurrent use of rifampin.
Use Cautiously in: Severe hepatic impairment (↓ dose recommended); Geri: ↓ dose; slower IV infusion rate recommended; ↑ risk of hypotension; consider age-related decrease in body mass, ↓ hepatic/renal/cardiac function, concurrent drug therapy and other disease states); Severe renal impairment; Serious ventricular ar-

rhythmias or CHF; OB, Lactation, Pedi: Safety not established.

Adverse Reactions/Side Effects
CNS: abnormal dreams, anxiety, confusion, dizziness, drowsiness, headache, nervousness, psychiatric disturbances, weakness. **EENT:** blurred vision, disturbed equilibrium, epistaxis, tinnitus. **Resp:** cough, dyspnea. **CV:** ARRHYTHMIAS, CHF, peripheral edema, bradycardia, chest pain, hypotension, palpitations, syncope, tachycardia. **GI:** ↑ liver enzymes, anorexia, constipation, diarrhea, dry mouth, dysgeusia, dyspepsia, nausea, vomiting. **GU:** dysuria, nocturia, polyuria, sexual dysfunction, urinary frequency. **Derm:** dermatitis, erythema multiforme, flushing, sweating, photosensitivity, pruritus/urticaria, rash. **Endo:** gynecomastia, hyperglycemia. **Hemat:** anemia, leukopenia, thrombocytopenia. **Metab:** weight gain. **MS:** joint stiffness, muscle cramps. **Neuro:** paresthesia, tremor. **Misc:** STEVENS-JOHNSON SYNDROME, gingival hyperplasia.

Interactions
Drug-Drug: ↑ hypotension may occur when used with **fentanyl**, other **antihypertensives**, **nitrates**, acute ingestion of **alcohol**, or **quinidine**. Antihypertensive effects may be ↓ by **NSAIDs**. May ↑ **digoxin** levels. Concurrent use with **beta blockers**, **digoxin**, **disopyramide**, or **phenytoin** may result in bradycardia, conduction defects, or CHF. **Phenobarbital** and **phenytoin** may ↑ metabolism and ↓ effectiveness. May ↓ metabolism of and ↑ risk of toxicity from **cyclosporine**, **quinidine**, or **carbamazepine**. **Cimetidine** and **ranitidine** ↑ levels and effects. May ↑ or ↓ the effects of **lithium** or **theophylline**.
Drug-Food: **Grapefruit juice** ↑ levels and effect.

Route/Dosage
PO (Adults): 30–120 mg 3–4 times daily or 60–120 mg twice daily as SR capsules or 180–240 mg once daily as CD or XR capsules or LA tablets (up to 360 mg/day).
IV (Adults): 0.25 mg/kg; may repeat in 15 min with a dose of 0.35 mg/kg. May follow with continuous infusion at 10 mg/hr (range 5–15 mg/hr) for up to 24 hr.

Availability (generic available)
Tablets: 30 mg, 60 mg, 90 mg, 120 mg. **Cost:** *Generic*— 30 mg $12.99/90, 60 mg $14.99/90, 90 mg $15.99/90, 120 mg $19.99/90. **Sustained-release capsules:** 60 mg, 90 mg, 120 mg. **Cost:** *Generic*— 60 mg $80.30/180, 90 mg $124.76/180, 120 mg $199.13/180. **Extended-release capsules (Cardizem CD, Dilacor XR, Tiazac, Cartia XT, Taztia XT):** 120 mg, 180 mg, 240 mg, 300 mg, 360 mg, 420 mg. **Cost:** *Generic*— 120 mg $69.98/90, 180 mg $79.97/90, 240 mg $106.97/90, 300 mg $126.97/90, 360 mg $128.97/90, 420 mg $120.99/90. **Extended-release tablets (Cardizem LA):** 120 mg, 180 mg, 240 mg, 300 mg, 360 mg, 420 mg. **Cost:** 120 mg $183.90/90, 180 mg $189.97/90, 240 mg $225.98/90, 300 mg $330.86/90, 360 mg $339.98/90, 420 mg $363.18/90. **Injection:** 5 mg/mL.

NURSING IMPLICATIONS
Assessment
- Monitor blood pressure and pulse prior to therapy, during dose titration, and periodically during therapy. Monitor ECG periodically during prolonged therapy. May cause prolonged PR interval.
- Monitor intake and output ratios and daily weight. Assess for signs of CHF (peripheral edema, rales/crackles, dyspnea, weight gain, jugular venous distention).
- Monitor frequency of prescription refills to determine adherence.
- Patients receiving digoxin concurrently with calcium channel blockers should have routine serum digoxin levels checked and be monitored for signs and symptoms of digoxin toxicity.
- **Angina:** Assess location, duration, intensity, and precipitating factors of patient's anginal pain.
- **Arrhythmias:** Monitor ECG continuously during administration. Report bradycardia or prolonged hypotension promptly. Emergency equipment and medication should be available. Monitor blood pressure and pulse before and frequently during administration.
- ***Lab Test Considerations:*** Total serum calcium concentrations are not affected by calcium channel blockers.
- Monitor serum potassium periodically. Hypokalemia ↑ the risk of arrhythmias and should be corrected.
- Monitor renal and hepatic functions periodically during long-term therapy. May cause ↑ in hepatic enzymes after several days of therapy, which return to normal on discontinuation of therapy.

Potential Nursing Diagnoses
Acute pain (Indications)
Decreased cardiac output (Adverse Reactions)

Implementation

- Do not confuse Cardizem (diltiazem) with Cardene (nicardipine). Do not confuse Cardizem LA with Cardene SR. Do not confuse Tiazac (diltiazem) with Ziac (bisprolol/hydrochlorothiazide).
- **PO:** May be administered without regard to meals. May be administered with meals if GI irritation becomes a problem.
- Do not open, crush, break, or chew sustained-release capsules or tablets. Empty tablets that appear in stool are not significant. Crush and mix diltiazem with food or fluids for patients having difficulty swallowing.

IV Administration

- **Direct IV:** *Diluent:* Administer bolus dose undiluted. *Concentration:* 5 mg/mL. *Rate:* Administer over 2 min.
- **Continuous Infusion:** *Diluent:* Dilute 125 mg in 100 mL, 250 mg in 250 mL, or 250 mg in 500 mL of 0.9% NaCl, D5W, or D5/0.45% NaCl. Infusion is stable for 24 hr at room temperature or if refrigerated. *Concentration:* 125 mg/125 mL (1 mg/mL), 250 mg/300 mL (0.83 mg/mL), 250 mg/550 mL (0.45 mg/mL). *Rate:* See Route/Dosage section. Titrate to patient's heart rate and blood pressure response.
- **Y-Site Compatibility:** albumin, alfentanil, amifostine, amikacin, amiodarone, amphotericin B colloidal, argatroban, atracurium, aztreonam, bivalirudin, bumetanide, buprenorphine, busulfan, butorphanol, calcium chloride, calcium gluconate, carboplatin, caspofungin, cefazolin, cefotaxime, cefotetan, cefoxitin, ceftazidime, ceftizoxime, ceftriaxone, cefuroxime, chlorpromazine, cimetidine, ciprofloxacin, cisatracurium, cisplatin, clindamycin, cyclophosphamide, cyclosporine, cytarabine, dactinomycin, daptomycin, dexamethasone, dexmedetomidine, digoxin, diphenhydramine, dobutamine, docetaxel, dopamine, doripenem, doxacurium, doxorubicin hydrochloride, doxycycline, droperidol, enalaprilat, ephedrine, epinephrine, epirubicin, ertapenem, erythromycin lactobionate, esmolol, etoposide, etoposide phosphate, famotidine, fenoldopam, fentanyl, fluconazole, fludarabine, foscarnet, fosphenytoin, gemcitabine, gentamicin, glycopyrrolate, granisetron, haloperidol, hetastarch, hydralazine, hydromorphone, ifosfamide, imipenem/cilastatin, inamrinone, isoproterenol, labetalol, levofloxacin, lidocaine, linezolid, lorazepam, magnesium sulfate, mannitol, mechlorethamine, melphalan, meperidine, meropenem, metaraminol, methyldopate, metoclopramide, metoprolol, metronidazole, midazolam, milrinone, mitoxantrone, morphine, multivitamins, nalbuphine, naloxone, nesiritide, nicardipine, nitroglycerin, nitroprusside, norepinephrine, octreotide, ondansetron, oxacillin, oxaliplatin, oxytocin, paclitaxel, palonosetron, pancuronium, pemetrexed, penicillin G potassium, pentamidine, phentolamine, phenylephrine, potassium chloride, potassium phosphates, prochlorperazine, promethazine, propranolol, quinupriostin/dalfopristin, ranitidine, remifentanil, rocuronium, sodium acetate, streptozocin, sufentanil, tacrolimus, teniposide, theophylline, thiotepa, ticarcillin/clavulanate, tigecycline, tirofiban, tobramycin, trimethobenzamide, trimethoprim/sulfamethoxazole, vancomycin, vasopressin, vecuronium, verapamil, vincristine, vinorelbine, voriconazole, zidovudine.
- **Y-Site Incompatibility:** allopurinol, amphotericin B liposome, cefepime, chloramphenicol, dantrolene, diazepam, fluorouracil, furosemide, ganciclovir, ketorolac, methotrexate, micafungin, pantroprazole, pentobarbital, phenobarbital, phenytoin, piperacillin/tazobactam, rifampin, thiopental.

Patient/Family Teaching

- Advise patient to take medication as directed at the same time each day, even if feeling well. Take missed doses as soon as possible unless almost time for next dose; do not double doses. May need to be discontinued gradually.
- Advise patient to avoid large amounts (6–8 glasses of grapefruit juice/day) during therapy.
- Instruct patient on correct technique for monitoring pulse. Instruct patient to contact health care professional if heart rate is <50 bpm.
- Caution patient to change positions slowly to minimize orthostatic hypotension.
- May cause drowsiness or dizziness. Advise patient to avoid driving or other activities requiring alertness until response to the medication is known.
- Instruct patient on importance of maintaining good dental hygiene and seeing dentist frequently for teeth cleaning to prevent tenderness, bleeding, and gingival hyperplasia (gum enlargement).

- Instruct patient to avoid concurrent use of alcohol or OTC medications, especially cough and cold preparations, without consulting health care professional.
- Advise patient to notify health care professional if irregular heartbeats, dyspnea, swelling of hands and feet, pronounced dizziness, nausea, constipation, or hypotension occurs or if headache is severe or persistent.
- Caution patient to wear protective clothing and use sunscreen to prevent photosensitivity reactions.
- **Angina:** Instruct patient on concurrent nitrate or beta-blocker therapy to continue taking both medications as directed and to use SL nitroglycerin as needed for anginal attacks.
- Advise patient to contact health care professional if chest pain does not improve, worsens after therapy, or occurs with diaphoresis; if shortness of breath occurs; or if severe, persistent headache occurs.
- Caution patient to discuss exercise restrictions with health care professional before exertion.
- **Hypertension:** Encourage patient to comply with other interventions for hypertension (weight reduction, low-sodium diet, smoking cessation, moderation of alcohol consumption, regular exercise, and stress management). Medication controls but does not cure hypertension.
- Instruct patient and family in proper technique for monitoring blood pressure. Advise patient to take blood pressure weekly and to report significant changes to health care professional.

Evaluation/Desired Outcomes
- Decrease in blood pressure.
- Decrease in frequency and severity of anginal attacks.
- Decrease in need for nitrate therapy.
- Increase in activity tolerance and sense of well-being.
- Suppression and prevention of tachyarrhythmias.

---

dinoprostone
(dye-noe-**prost**-one)
Cervidil Vaginal Insert, Prepidil Endocervical Gel, Prostin E Vaginal Suppository

Classification
Therapeutic: cervical ripening agent
Pharmacologic: oxytocics, prostaglandins

Pregnancy Category C

Indications
Endocervical Gel, Vaginal Insert: Used to "ripen" the cervix in pregnancy at or near term when induction of labor is indicated. Vaginal Suppository: Induction of midtrimester abortion, Management of missed abortion up to 28 wk, Management of nonmetastatic gestational trophoblastic disease (benign hydatidiform mole).

Action
Produces contractions similar to those occurring during labor at term by stimulating the myometrium (oxytocic effect). Initiates softening, effacement, and dilation of the cervix ("ripening"). Also stimulates GI smooth muscle. **Therapeutic Effects:** Initiation of labor. Expulsion of fetus.

Pharmacokinetics
Absorption: Rapidly absorbed.
Distribution: Unknown. Action is mostly local.
Metabolism and Excretion: Metabolized by enzymes in lung, kidneys, spleen, and liver tissue.
Half-life: Unknown.

TIME/ACTION PROFILE

ROUTE	ONSET	PEAK	DURATION
Cervical ripening (gel)	rapid	30–45 min	unknown
Cervical ripening (insert)	rapid	unknown	12 hr
Abortion time (suppository)	10 min	12–24 hr	2–3 hr

Contraindications/Precautions
Contraindicated in: Hypersensitivity to prostaglandins or additives in the gel or suppository; The gel/insert should be avoided in situations in which prolonged uterine contractions should be avoided, including: Previous cesarean section or uterine surgery, Cephalopelvic disproportion, Traumatic delivery or difficult labor, Multiparity (≥6 term pregnancies), Hyperactive or hypertonic uterus, Fetal distress (if delivery is not imminent), Unexplained vaginal bleeding, Placenta previa, Vasa previa, Active herpes genitalis, Obstetric emergency requiring surgical intervention, Situations in which vaginal delivery is contraindicated; Presence of acute pelvic inflammatory disease or ruptured membranes; Concurrent oxytocic therapy (wait for 30 min after removing insert before using oxytocin).

Use Cautiously in: Uterine scarring; Asthma; Hypotension; Cardiac disease; Adrenal disorders; Anemia; Jaundice; Diabetes mellitus; Epilepsy; Glaucoma; Pulmonary, renal, or hepatic disease; Multiparity (up to 5 previous term pregnancies).

Adverse Reactions/Side Effects
Endocervical Gel, Vaginal Insert.
GU: uterine contractile abnormalities, warm feeling in vagina. **MS:** back pain. **Misc:** fever.

Suppository
CNS: headache, drowsiness, syncope. **Resp:** coughing, dyspnea, wheezing. **CV:** hypotension, hypertension. **GI:** diarrhea, nausea, vomiting. **GU:** UTERINE RUPTURE, urinary tract infection, uterine hyperstimulation, vaginal/uterine pain. **Misc:** allergic reactions including ANAPHYLAXIS, chills, fever.

Interactions
Drug-Drug: Augments the effects of other **oxytocics**.

Route/Dosage
Cervical Ripening
Vag (Adults, Cervical): *Endocervical gel*—0.5 mg; if response is unfavorable, may repeat in 6 hr (not to exceed 1.5 mg/24 hr). *Vaginal insert*—one 10-mg insert.

Abortifacient
Vag (Adults): One 20-mg suppository, repeat q 3–5 hr (not to exceed 240 mg total or longer than 48 hr).

Availability
Endocervical gel (Prepidil): 0.5 mg dinoprostone in 3 g of gel vehicle in a prefilled syringe with catheters. **Vaginal insert (Cervidil):** 10 mg. **Vaginal suppository (Prostin E Vaginal):** 20 mg.

NURSING IMPLICATIONS

Assessment
- **Abortifacient:** Monitor frequency, duration, and force of contractions and uterine resting tone. Opioid analgesics may be administered for uterine pain.
- Monitor temperature, pulse, and blood pressure periodically throughout therapy. Dinoprostone-induced fever (elevation >1.1°C or 2°F) usually occurs within 15–45 min after insertion of suppository. This returns to normal 2–6 hr after discontinuation or removal of suppository from vagina.
- Auscultate breath sounds. Wheezing and sensation of chest tightness may indicate hypersensitivity reaction.
- Assess for nausea, vomiting, and diarrhea in patients receiving suppository. Vomiting and diarrhea occur frequently. Patient should be premedicated with antiemetic and antidiarrheal.
- Monitor amount and type of vaginal discharge. Notify physician or other health care professional immediately if symptoms of hemorrhage (increased bleeding, hypotension, pallor, tachycardia) occur.
- **Cervical Ripening:** Monitor uterine activity, fetal status, and dilation and effacement of cervix continuously throughout therapy. Assess for hypertonus, sustained uterine contractility, and fetal distress. Insert should be removed at the onset of active labor.

Potential Nursing Diagnoses
Deficient knowledge, related to medication regimen (Patient/Family Teaching)

Implementation
- **Abortifacient:** Warm the suppository to room temperature just before use.
- Wear gloves when handling unwrapped suppository to prevent absorption through skin.
- Patient should remain supine for 10 min after insertion of suppository; then she may be ambulatory.
- **Vaginal Insert:** Place vaginal insert transversely in the posterior vaginal fornix immediately after removing from foil package. Warming of insert and sterile conditions are not required. Use vaginal insert only with a retrieval system. Use minimal amount of water-soluble lubricant during insertion; avoid excess because it may hamper release of dinoprostone from insert. Patient should remain supine for 2 hr after insertion, then may ambulate.
- Vaginal insert delivers dinoprostone 0.3 mg/hr over 12 hr. Remove insert at the onset of active labor, before amniotomy, or after 12 hr.
- Oxytocin should not be used during or less than 30 min after removal of insert.
- **Endocervical Gel:** Determine degree of effacement before insertion of the endocervical catheter. Do not administer above the level of the internal os. Use a 20-mm endocervical catheter if no effacement is present and a 10-mm catheter if the cervix is 50% effaced.
- Use caution to prevent contact of dinoprostone gel with skin. Wash hands thoroughly with soap and water after administration.
- Bring gel to room temperature just before administration. Do not force warming with external sources (water bath, microwave). Remove

peel-off seal from end of syringe; then remove the protective end cap and insert end cap into plunger stopper assembly in barrel of syringe. Aseptically remove catheter from package. Firmly attach catheter hub to syringe tip; click is evidence of attachment. Fill catheter with sterile gel by pushing plunger to expel air from catheter before administration to patient. Gel is stable for 24 mo if refrigerated.
- Patient should be in dorsal position with cervix visualized using a speculum. Introduce gel with catheter into cervical canal using sterile technique. Administer gel by gentle expulsion from syringe and then remove catheter. Do not attempt to administer small amount of gel remaining in syringe. Use syringe for only 1 patient; discard syringe, catheter, and unused package contents after using.
- Patient should remain supine for 15–30 min after administration to minimize leakage from cervical canal.
- Oxytocin may be administered 6–12 hr after desired response from dinoprostone gel. If no cervical/uterine response to initial dose of dinoprostone is obtained, repeat dose may be administered in 6 hr.

Patient/Family Teaching
- Explain purpose of medication and vaginal exams.
- **Abortifacient:** Instruct patient to notify health care professional immediately if fever and chills, foul-smelling vaginal discharge, lower abdominal pain, or increased bleeding occurs.
- Provide emotional support throughout therapy.
- **Cervical Ripening:** Inform patient that she may experience a warm feeling in her vagina during administration.
- Advise patient to notify health care professional if contractions become prolonged.

Evaluation/Desired Outcomes
- Complete abortion. Continuous administration for more than 2 days is not usually recommended.
- Cervical ripening and induction of labor.

---

diphenhydrAMINE (oral, parenteral)
(dye-fen-**hye**-dra-meen)
✦ Allerdryl, Allergy Medication, AllerMax, Banophen, Benadryl Dye-Free Alergy, Benadryl Allergy, Benadryl, Compoz, Compoz Nighttime Sleep Aid, Diphen AF, Diphen Cough, Diphenhist, Dormin, Genahist, 40 Winks, Hyrexin-50, ✦ Insomnal, Maximum Strength Nytol, Maximum Strength Sleepinal, Midol PM, Miles Nervine, Nighttime Sleep Aid, Nytol, Scot-Tussin Allergy DM, Siladril, Silphen, Sleep-Eze 3, Sleepwell 2-night, Sominex, Snooze Fast, Sominex, Tusstat, Twilite, Unisom Nighttime Sleep-Aid

Classification
Therapeutic: allergy, cold, and cough remedies, antihistamines, antitussives

Pregnancy Category B

Indications
Relief of allergic symptoms caused by histamine release including: Anaphylaxis, Seasonal and perennial allergic rhinitis, Allergic dermatoses. Parkinson's disease and dystonic reactions from medications. Mild nighttime sedation. Prevention of motion sickness. Antitussive (syrup only).

Action
Antagonizes the effects of histamine at H_1-receptor sites; does not bind to or inactivate histamine. Significant CNS depressant and anticholinergic properties. **Therapeutic Effects:** Decreased symptoms of histamine excess (sneezing, rhinorrhea, nasal and ocular pruritus, ocular tearing and redness, urticaria). Relief of acute dystonic reactions. Prevention of motion sickness. Suppression of cough.

Pharmacokinetics
Absorption: Well absorbed after oral or IM administration but 40–60% of an oral dose reaches systemic circulation due to first-pass metabolism.
Distribution: Widely distributed. Crosses the placenta; enters breast milk.
Metabolism and Excretion: 95% metabolized by the liver.
Half-life: 2.4–7 hr.

TIME/ACTION PROFILE (antihistaminic effects)

ROUTE	ONSET	PEAK	DURATION
PO	15–60 min	2–4 hr	4–8 hr
IM	20–30 min	2–4 hr	4–8 hr
IV	rapid	unknown	4–8 hr

Contraindications/Precautions
Contraindicated in: Hypersensitivity; Acute attacks of asthma; Lactation: Lactation; Known alcohol intolerance (some liquid products).
Use Cautiously in: Severe liver disease; Angle-closure glaucoma; Seizure disorders; Prostatic hyperplasia; Peptic ulcer; May cause paradoxical ex-

diphenhydrAMINE 451

citation in young children; Hyperthyroidism; OB: Safety not established; Geri: Appears on *Beers list*. Geriatric patients are more susceptible to adverse drug reactions and anticholinergic effects (delirium, acute confusion, dizziness, dry mouth, blurred vision, urinary retention, constipation, tachycardia); dose reduction or non-anticholinergic antihistamine recommended.

Adverse Reactions/Side Effects
CNS: drowsiness, dizziness, headache, paradoxical excitation (increased in children). **EENT:** blurred vision, tinnitus. **CV:** hypotension, palpitations. **GI:** anorexia, dry mouth, constipation, nausea. **GU:** dysuria, frequency, urinary retention. **Derm:** photosensitivity. **Resp:** chest tightness, thickened bronchial secretions, wheezing. **Local:** pain at IM site.

Interactions
Drug-Drug: ↑ risk of CNS depression with other **antihistamines**, **alcohol**, **opioid analgesics**, and **sedative/hypnotics**. ↑ anticholinergic effects with **tricyclic antidepressants**, **quinidine**, or **disopyramide**. **MAO inhibitors** intensify and prolong the anticholinergic effects of antihistamines.
Drug-Natural Products: Concomitant use of **kava-kava**, **valerian**, or **chamomile** can ↑ CNS depression.

Route/Dosage
PO (Adults and Children >12 yr): *Antihistaminic/antiemetic/antivertiginic*—25–50 mg q 4–6 hr, not to exceed 300 mg/day. *Antitussive*—25 mg q 4 hr as needed, not to exceed 150 mg/day. *Antidyskinetic*—25–50 mg q 4 hr (not to exceed 400 mg/day). *Sedative/hypnotic*—50 mg 20–30 min before bedtime.
PO (Children 6–12 yr): *Antihistaminic/antiemetic/antivertiginic*—12.5–25 mg q 4–6 hr (not to exceed 150 mg/day). *Antidyskinetic*—1–1.5 mg/kg q 6–8 hr as needed (not to exceed 300 mg/day). *Antitussive*—12.5 mg q 4 hr (not to exceed 75 mg/day). *Sedative/hypnotic*—1 mg/kg/dose 20–30 min before bedtime (not to exceed 50 mg).
PO (Children 2–6 yr): *Antihistaminic/antiemetic/antivertiginic*—6.25–12.5 mg q 4–6 hr (not to exceed 37.5 mg/day). *Antidyskinetic*—1–1.5 mg/kg q 4–6 hr as needed (not to exceed 300 mg/day). *Antitussive*—6.25 mg q 4 hr (not to exceed 37.5 mg/24 hr). *Sedative/hypnotic*—1 mg/kg/dose 20–30 min before bedtime (not to exceed 50 mg).

IM, IV (Adults): 25–50 mg q 4 hr as needed (may need up to 100-mg dose, not to exceed 400 mg/day).
IM, IV (Children): 1.25 mg/kg (37.5 mg/m^2) 4 times daily (not to exceed 300 mg/day).

Availability (generic available)
Capsules: 25 mg$^{Rx, OTC}$, 50 mg$^{Rx, OTC}$. **Tablets:** 25 mg$^{Rx, OTC}$, 50 mg$^{Rx, OTC}$. **Chewable tablets (grape flavor):** 25 mg$^{Rx, OTC}$. **Elixir (cherry and other flavors):** 12.5 mg/5 mL$^{Rx, OTC}$. **Syrup (cherry and raspberry flavor):** 12.5 mg/5 mL$^{Rx, OTC}$. **Injection:** 10 mg/mL, 50 mg/mL. ***In combination with:*** analgesics, decongestants, and expectorants, in OTC pain, sleep, cough, and cold preparations. See Appendix B.

NURSING IMPLICATIONS

Assessment
- Diphenhydramine has multiple uses. Determine why the medication was ordered and assess symptoms that apply to the individual patient. Geri: Appears in the *Beers list*. May cause sedation and confusion due to increased sensitivity to anticholinergic effects. Monitor carefully, assess for confusion, delirium, other anticholinergic side effects and fall risk. Institute measures to prevent falls.
- **Prevention and Treatment of Anaphylaxis:** Assess for urticaria and for patency of airway.
- **Allergic Rhinitis:** Assess degree of nasal stuffiness, rhinorrhea, and sneezing.
- **Parkinsonism and Extrapyramidal Reactions:** Assess movement disorder before and after administration.
- **Insomnia:** Assess sleep patterns.
- **Motion Sickness:** Assess nausea, vomiting, bowel sounds, and abdominal pain.
- **Cough Suppressant:** Assess frequency and nature of cough, lung sounds, and amount and type of sputum produced. Unless contraindicated, maintain fluid intake of 1500–2000 mL daily to decrease viscosity of bronchial secretions.
- **Pruritus:** Assess degree of itching, skin rash, and inflammation.
- ***Lab Test Considerations:*** May ↓ skin response to allergy tests. Discontinue 4 days before skin testing.

Potential Nursing Diagnoses
Insomnia (Indications)
Risk for deficient fluid volume (Indications)
Risk for injury (Side Effects)

Implementation

- Do not confuse Benadryl (diphenhydramine) with Benylin (dextromethorphan), desipramine (Norpramin), or with dimenhydrinate (Dramamine).
- When used for insomnia, administer 20 min before bedtime and schedule activities to minimize interruption of sleep.
- When used for prophylaxis of motion sickness, administer at least 30 min and preferably 1–2 hr before exposure to conditions that may precipitate motion sickness.
- **PO:** Administer with meals or milk to minimize GI irritation. Capsule may be emptied and contents taken with water or food.
- **IM:** Administer 50 mg/mL into well-developed muscle. Avoid subcut injections.

IV Administration

- **Direct IV:** *Diluent:* May be further diluted in 0.9% NaCl, 0.45% NaCl, D5W, D10W, dextrose/saline combinations, Ringer's solution, LR, and dextrose/Ringer's combinations. *Concentration:* 25 mg/mL. *Rate:* Infuse at a rate not to exceed 25 mg/min.
- **Syringe Compatibility:** atropine, butorphanol, chlorpromazine, cimetidine, droperidol, fentanyl, fluphenazine, glycopyrrolate, hydromorphone, hydroxyzine, meperidine, metoclopramide, midazolam, morphine, nalbuphine, pentazocine, perphenazine, prochlorperazine, promethazine, ranitidine, scopolamine, sufentanil.
- **Syringe Incompatibility:** haloperidol, pantoprazole, pentobarbital, phenobarbital, phenytoin, thiopental.
- **Y-Site Compatibility:** abciximab, acyclovir, aldesleukin, alfentanil, amifostine, amikacin, amphotericin B liposome, amsacrine, argatroban, ascorbic acid, atropine, azithromycin, benztropine, bivalirudin, bumetanide, buprenorphine, butorphanol, calcium chloride, calcium gluconate, carboplatin, caspofungin, ceftizoxime, chlorpromazine, cimetidine, ciprofloxacin, cisatracurium, cisplatin, cladribine, clindamycin, cyanocobalamin, cyclophosphamide, cytarabine, dactinomycin, daptomycin, dexmedetomidine, digoxin, diltiazem, dobutamine, docetaxel, dopamine, doripenem, doxorubicin, doxorubicin liposome, doxycycline, enalaprilat, epinephrine, epirubicin, epoetin alfa, ertapenem, erythromycin, esmolol, etoposide phosphate, famotidine, fenoldopam, fentanyl, filgrastim, fluconazole, fludarabine, folic acid, gemcitabine, gentamicin, glycopyrrolate, granisetron, hydromorphone, idarubicin, ifosfamide, imipenem/cilastatin, isoproterenol, labetalol, levofloxacin, lidocaine, linezolid, lorazepam, magnesium sulfate, mannitol, mechlorethamine, melphalan, meperidine, meropenem, methadone, methicillin, methotrexate, methoxamine, methyldopate, metoclopramide, metoprolol, metronidazole, midazolam, minocycline, mitomycin, morphine, multiple vitamins, nalbuphine, naloxone, nesiritide, nitroglycerin, norepinephrine, octreotide, ondansetron, oxaliplatin, oxytocin, paclitaxel, palonosetron, pemetrexed, penicillin G, pentamidine, pentazocine, phentolamine, phenylephrine, phytonadione, piperacillin/tazobactam, potassium chloride, procainamide, prochlorperazine, promethazine, propofol, propranolol, protamine, pyridoxine, quinipristin/dalfopristin, ranitidine, remifentanil, rituximab, rocuronium, sargramostim, sodium acetate, streptokinase, succinylcholine, sufentanil, tacrolimus, teniposide, theophylline, thiamine, thiotepa, ticarcillin/clavulanate, tigecycline, tirofiban, tobramycin, tolazoline, trastuzumab, trimethophan, urokinase, vancomycin, vasopressin, vecuronium, verapamil, vincristine, vinorelbine, vitamin B complex with C, voriconazole.
- **Y-Site Incompatibility:** allopurinol, aminophylline, amphotericin B cholesteryl, amphotericin B colloidal, ampicillin, azathioprine, cefazolin, cefepime, cefoperazone, cefotaxime, cefotetan, cefoxitin, ceftazidime, ceftriaxone, cefuroxime, chloramphenicol, dantrolene, dexamethasone, diazepam, diazoxide, fluorouracil, foscarnet, furosemide, ganciclovir, indomethacin, insulin, ketorolac, methylprednisolone, milrinone, nitroprusside, pantoprazole, pentobarbital, phenobarbital, phenytoin, sodium bicarbonate, trimethoprim/sulfamethoxazole.

Patient/Family Teaching

- Instruct patient to take medication as directed; do not exceed recommended amount. Caution patient not to use oral OTC diphenhydramine products with any other product containing diphenhydramine, including products used topically.
- May cause drowsiness. Caution patient to avoid driving or other activities requiring alertness until response to drug is known.
- May cause dry mouth. Inform patient that frequent oral rinses, good oral hygiene, and sugarless gum or candy may minimize this effect. Notify health care professional if dry mouth persists for more than 2 wk.

- Teach sleep hygiene techniques (dark room, quiet, bedtime ritual, limit daytime napping, avoidance of nicotine and caffeine) to patients taking diphenhydramine to aid sleep.
- Advise patient to use sunscreen and protective clothing to prevent photosensitivity reactions.
- Caution patient to avoid use of alcohol and other CNS depressants concurrently with this medication.
- Pedi: Can cause excitation in children. Caution parents or caregivers about proper dose calculation; overdosage, especially in infants and children, can cause hallucinations, seizures, or death. Caution parents to avoid OTC cough and cold products while breastfeeding or to children <4 yr.
- Geri: Instruct older adults to avoid OTC products that contain diphenhydramine due to increased sensitivity to anticholinergic effects and potential for adverse reactions related to these effects.
- Advise patients taking diphenhydramine in OTC preparations to notify health care professional if symptoms worsen or persist for more than 7 days.

Evaluation/Desired Outcomes
- Prevention of, or decreased urticaria in, anaphylaxis or other allergic reactions.
- Decreased dyskinesia in parkinsonism and extrapyramidal reactions.
- Sedation when used as a sedative/hypnotic.
- Prevention of or decrease in nausea and vomiting caused by motion sickness.
- Decrease in frequency and intensity of cough without eliminating cough reflex.

---

diphenoxylate/atropine
(dye-fen-**ox**-i-late/**a**-troe-peen)
Logen, Lomanate, Lomotil, Lonox

difenoxin/atropine
(dye-fen-**ox**-in/**a**-troe-peen)
Motofen

Classification
Therapeutic: antidiarrheals
Pharmacologic: anticholinergics

Schedule V (diphenoxylate/atropine), IV (difenoxin/atropine)

Pregnancy Category C

Indications
Adjunctive therapy in the treatment of diarrhea.

Action
Inhibits excess GI motility. Structurally related to opioid analgesics but has no analgesic properties. Atropine added to discourage abuse. **Therapeutic Effects:** Decreased GI motility with subsequent decrease in diarrhea.

Pharmacokinetics
Absorption: Well absorbed from the GI tract.
Distribution: Enters breast milk.
Metabolism and Excretion: *Diphenoxylate*—mostly metabolized by the liver with some conversion to an active antidiarrheal compound (difenoxin). *Difenoxin*—metabolized by the liver. Minimal excretion in urine.
Half-life: *Diphenoxylate*—2.5 hr; *difenoxin*—4.5 hr.

TIME/ACTION PROFILE (antidiarrheal action)

ROUTE	ONSET	PEAK	DURATION
Difenoxin–PO	45–60 min	2 hr	3–4 hr
Diphenoxylate–PO	45–60 min	2 hr	3–4 hr

Contraindications/Precautions
Contraindicated in: Hypersensitivity; Severe liver disease; Infectious diarrhea (due to *Escherichia coli*, *Salmonella*, or *Shigella*); Diarrhea associated with pseudomembranous colitis; Dehydrated patients; Angle-closure glaucoma; Children <2 yr; Known alcohol intolerance (some liquid diphenoxylate/atropine products only).
Use Cautiously in: Patients physically dependent on opioids; Inflammatory bowel disease; Geriatric patients (more sensitive to effects); Children (more sensitive to effects, especially Down syndrome patients); Prostatic hyperplasia; Pregnancy, lactation, or children <12 yr (safety not established for difenoxin/atropine in children <12 yr; diphenoxylate/atropine should not be used in children <2 yr).

Adverse Reactions/Side Effects
CNS: dizziness, confusion, drowsiness, headache, insomnia, nervousness. **EENT:** blurred vision, dry eyes. **CV:** tachycardia. **GI:** constipation, dry mouth, epigastric distress, ileus, nausea, vomiting. **GU:** urinary retention. **Derm:** flushing.

Interactions
Drug-Drug: Additive CNS depression with other **CNS depressants** including **alcohol**, **antihista-**

454 dipyridamole

mines, **opioid analgesics**, and **sedative/hypnotics**. Additive anticholinergic properties with other **drugs having anticholinergic properties**, including **tricyclic antidepressants** and **disopyramide**. Use with **MAO inhibitors** may result in hypertensive crisis.
Drug-Natural Products: Increased anticholinergic effects with **angel's trumpet**, **jimson weed**, and **scopolia**.

Route/Dosage
Difenoxin/Atropine
Doses given are in terms of difenoxin—each tablet contains 1 mg difenoxin with 0.025 mg of atropine.
PO (Adults): 2 tablets initially, then 1 tablet after each loose stool or every 3–4 hr as needed (not to exceed 8 tablets/day).

Diphenoxylate/Atropine
Adult doses given are in terms of diphenoxylate—each tablet contains 2.5 mg diphenoxylate with 0.025 mg of atropine; pediatric doses are given in mg of diphenoxylate and in mL of diphenoxylate/atropine liquid; each 5 mL of liquid contains 2.5 mg diphenoxylate with 0.025 mg of atropine.
PO (Adults): 5 mg 3–4 times daily initially, then 5 mg once daily as needed (not to exceed 20 mg/day).
PO (Children): *use liquid only*—0.3–0.4 mg/kg/day in 4 divided doses.

Availability
Difenoxin/Atropine
Tablets: 1 mg difenoxin/0.025 mg atropine.

Diphenoxylate/Atropine (generic available)
Tablets: 2.5 mg diphenoxylate/0.025 mg atropine. **Liquid (cherry flavor):** 2.5 mg diphenoxylate/0.025 mg atropine per 5 mL.

NURSING IMPLICATIONS
Assessment
- Assess the frequency and consistency of stools and bowel sounds prior to and throughout therapy.
- Assess patient's fluid and electrolyte balance and skin turgor for dehydration.
- *Lab Test Considerations:* Liver function tests should be evaluated periodically during prolonged therapy.
- Diphenoxylate/atropine may cause increased serum amylase concentrations.

Potential Nursing Diagnoses
Diarrhea (Indications)
Constipation (Side Effects)

Implementation
- Do not confuse Lomotil with Lamictal (lamontrigine) or Lamisil (terbinafine).
- Risk of dependence increases with high-dose, long-term use. Atropine has been added to discourage abuse.
- **PO:** Diphenoxylate/atropine tablets may be administered with food if GI irritation occurs. Tablets may be crushed and administered with patient's fluid of choice. Use calibrated measuring device for liquid preparations.

Patient/Family Teaching
- Instruct patient to take medication exactly as directed. Do not take more than the prescribed amount because of the habit-forming potential and risk of overdose in children. If on a scheduled dosing regimen, missed doses should be taken as soon as possible unless almost time for next dose. Do not double doses.
- Medication may cause drowsiness. Advise patient to avoid driving or other activities requiring alertness until response to drug is known.
- Advise patient that frequent mouth rinses, good oral hygiene, and sugarless gum or candy may relieve dry mouth.
- Caution patient to avoid alcohol and other CNS depressants concurrently with this medication.
- Advise patient to inform health care professional of medication regimen prior to treatment or surgery.
- Instruct patient to notify health care professional if diarrhea persists or if fever, abdominal pain, or palpitations occur.

Evaluation/Desired Outcomes
- Decrease in diarrhea. Treatment of acute diarrhea should be continued for 24–36 hr before it is considered ineffective.

---

dipyridamole
(dye-peer-**id**-a-mole)
✤ Apo-Dipyridamole, Dipridacot,
✤ Novodipiradol, Persantine, Persantine IV

Classification
Therapeutic: antiplatelet agents, diagnostic agents (coronary vasodilators)
Pharmacologic: platelet adhesion inhibitors

Pregnancy Category B

Indications
PO: Prevention of thromboembolism in patients with prosthetic heart valves (with warfarin). Maintains patency after surgical grafting proce-

dures, including coronary artery bypass (with aspirin). **IV:** As an alternative to exercise in myocardial perfusion scintigraphy (cardiac stress testing with radiotracer imaging).

Action
PO: Decreases platelet aggregation by inhibiting the enzyme phosphodiesterase. **IV:** Produces coronary vasodilation by inhibiting adenosine uptake.
Therapeutic Effects: PO: Inhibition of platelet aggregation and subsequent thromboembolic events. **IV:** In diagnostic thallium imaging, dipyridamole dilates normal coronary arteries, reducing flow to vessels that are narrowed and causing abnormal thallium distribution.

Pharmacokinetics
Absorption: Moderately absorbed (30–60%) after oral administration.
Distribution: Widely distributed. Crosses the placenta; enters breast milk.
Metabolism and Excretion: Metabolized by the liver; excreted in the bile.
Half-life: 10 hr.

TIME/ACTION PROFILE (PO = antiplatelet activity, IV = coronary vasodilation)

ROUTE	ONSET	PEAK	DURATION
PO	unknown	unknown	unknown
IV	unknown	6.5 min†	30 min

†From start of infusion

Contraindications/Precautions
Contraindicated in: Hypersensitivity.
Use Cautiously in: Hypotensive patients; Geri: Appears on Beers list. Geriatric patients may be more susceptible to orthostatic hypotension; Patients with platelet defects; Pregnancy (although safety not established, has been used without harm during pregnancy); Lactation or children <12 yr (safety not established).

Adverse Reactions/Side Effects
CNS: dizziness, headache, syncope; *IV only*, transient cerebral ischemia, weakness. **Resp:** *IV only*—bronchospasm. **CV:** *IV only*—MI, hypotension, arrhythmias, flushing. **GI:** nausea, diarrhea, GI upset, vomiting. **Derm:** rash.

Interactions
Drug-Drug: Additive effects with **aspirin** on platelet aggregation. Risk of bleeding may be ↑ when used with **anticoagulants**, **thrombolytic agents**, **NSAIDs**, **cefoperazone**, **cefotetan**, **valproic acid**, or **sulfinpyrazone**. ↑ risk of hypotension with **alcohol**. **Theophylline** may negate the effects of dipyridamole during diagnostic thallium imaging.

Route/Dosage
PO (Adults): 225–400 mg/day in 3–4 divided doses.
IV (Adults): 570 mcg/kg; maximum dose 60 mg.

Availability (generic available)
Tablets: 25 mg, 50 mg, 75 mg, ✦ 100 mg. **Injection:** 5 mg/mL in 2-mL and 10-ml vials. *In combination with:* aspirin (Aggrenox). See Appendix B.

NURSING IMPLICATIONS

Assessment
- **PO:** Monitor blood pressure and pulse before instituting therapy and regularly during period of dosage adjustment. Geri: Assess geriatric patients for orthostatic hypotension.
- **IV:** Monitor vital signs during and for 10–15 min after infusion. Obtain ECG in at least 1 lead. If severe chest pain or bronchospasm occurs, administer IV aminophylline 50–250 mg at a rate of 50–100 mg over 30–60 sec. If hypotension is severe, place patient in a supine position with head tilting down. If chest pain is unrelieved with aminophylline 250 mg, administer nitroglycerin SL. If chest pain is still unrelieved, treat as myocardial infarction.
- *Lab Test Considerations:* Bleeding time should be monitored periodically throughout therapy.

Potential Nursing Diagnoses
Decreased cardiac output (Indications)
Acute pain (Indications)

Implementation
- **PO:** Administer with a full glass of water at least 1 hr before or 2 hr after meals for faster absorption. If GI irritation occurs, may be administered with or immediately after meals. Tablets may be crushed and mixed with food if patient has difficulty swallowing. Pharmacist may make a suspension.

IV Administration
- **Intermittent Infusion:** *Diluent:* Dilute in at least a 1:2 ratio of 0.45% NaCl, 0.9% NaCl, or D5W for a total volume of 20–50 mL. Undiluted dipyridamole may cause venous irritation. *Rate:* Infuse over 4 min.
- **Y-Site Compatibility:** No information available.

Patient/Family Teaching

- **PO:** Instruct patient to take medication at evenly spaced intervals as directed. Take missed doses as soon as remembered unless the next scheduled dose is within 4 hr. Do not double doses. Benefit of medication may not be apparent to patient; encourage patient to continue taking medication as directed.
- Caution patient to change positions slowly to minimize orthostatic hypotension.
- Advise patient to avoid the use of alcohol, as it may potentiate the hypotensive effects. Tobacco products should also be avoided because nicotine causes vasoconstriction.
- Advise patient to consult health care professional before taking OTC medications concurrently with this medication. Aspirin should be taken only if directed and only in dose prescribed. Advise patient to discuss alternatives for pain relief or fever.
- Instruct patient to notify health care professional if unusual bleeding or bruising occurs. Concurrent use of aspirin or warfarin may increase risk of bleeding but is commonly used with specific indications.
- Advise patient to notify health care professional of medication regimen and whether using concurrent aspirin or warfarin therapy.
- **IV:** Instruct patient to notify health care professional immediately if dyspnea or chest pain occurs.

Evaluation/Desired Outcomes

- Prevention of postoperative thromboembolic complications associated with prosthetic heart valves.
- Maintenance of patency after surgical graft procedures.
- Coronary vasodilation in thallium myocardial perfusion imaging.

DIURETICS (POTASSIUM-SPARING)

amiloride (a-**mill**-oh-ride)
✤ Apo-Amiloride, ✤ Midamor

spironolactone
(speer-oh-no-**lak**-tone)
Aldactone, ✤ Novospiroton

triamterene (trye-**am**-ter-een)
Dyrenium

Classification
Therapeutic: diuretics
Pharmacologic: potassium-sparing diuretics

Pregnancy Category B (amiloride), C (spironolactone, triamterene)

Indications
Counteract potassium loss caused by other diuretics. Used with other agents (thiazides) to treat edema or hypertension. Primary hyperaldosteronism (spironolactone only). **Unlabeled Use:** Spironolactone: Management of CHF (low doses).

Action
Inhibition of sodium reabsorption in the kidney while saving potassium and hydrogen ions (spironolactone achieves this effect by antagonizing aldosterone receptors). **Therapeutic Effects:** Weak diuretic and antihypertensive response when compared with other diuretics. Conservation of potassium.

Pharmacokinetics
Absorption: *Amiloride*—30–90% absorbed; *spironolactone*—>90% absorbed; *triamterene*—30–70% absorbed.
Distribution: *Amiloride* and *triamterene*—widely distributed; all cross the placenta and enter breast milk.
Protein Binding: *Spironolactone* >90%.
Metabolism and Excretion: *Amiloride*—50% eliminated unchanged in urine, 40% excreted in the feces; *spironolactone*—converted by the liver to its active diuretic compound (canrenone); *triamterene*—80% metabolized by the liver, some excretion of unchanged drug.
Half-life: *Amiloride*—6–9 hr; *spironolactone*—78–84 min (spironolactone); 13–24 hr (canrenone); *triamterene*—1.7–2.5 hr.

TIME/ACTION PROFILE (diuretic effect)

ROUTE	ONSET	PEAK	DURATION
Amiloride	2 hr†	6–10 hr†	24 hr†
Spironolactone	unknown	2–3 days‡	2–3 days‡
Triamterene	2–4 hr†	1–several days‡	7–9 hr†

†Single dose
‡Multiple doses

Contraindications/Precautions
Contraindicated in: Hypersensitivity; Hyperkalemia; Anuria; Acute renal insufficiency; Significant renal dysfunction (CCr ≤30 mL/min or SCr >2.5 mg/dL).

DIURETICS (POTASSIUM-SPARING)

Use Cautiously in: Hepatic dysfunction; Geri: Presence of age-related renal dysfunction may lead to ↑ risk of hyperkalemia; Diabetes (↑ risk of hyperkalemia); History of gout or kidney stones (triamterene only); Concurrent use of potassium supplements or potassium-containing salt substitutes; OB, Lactation, Pedi: Safety not established.

Adverse Reactions/Side Effects
CNS: dizziness; *spironolactone only*, clumsiness, headache. **CV:** arrhythmias. **GI:** *amiloride*—constipation, nausea, vomiting. **GU:** *spironolactone*—erectile dysfunction; *triamterene*—nephrolithiasis. **Derm:** *triamterene*—photosensitivity. **Endo:** *spironolactone*—breast tenderness, gynecomastia, irregular menses, voice deepening. **F and E:** hyperkalemia, hyponatremia. **Hemat:** *spironolactone*—agranulocytosis; *triamterene*—hemolytic anemia, thrombocytopenia. **MS:** muscle cramps. **Misc:** allergic reactions.

Interactions
Drug-Drug: ↑ hypotension with acute ingestion of **alcohol**, other **antihypertensives**, or **nitrates**. Use with **ACE inhibitors**, **angiotensin II receptor antagonists**, **NSAIDS**, **potassium supplements**, **cyclosporine**, or **tacrolimus** ↑ risk of hyperkalemia. May ↑ levels/risk of toxicity from **lithium**. Effectiveness may be ↓ by **NSAIDs**. Spironolactone may ↑ effects of **digoxin**.

Route/Dosage
Amiloride
PO (Adults): *HTN*—5–10 mg/day (up to 20 mg).
PO (Children 1–17 yr): 0.4–0.625 mg/kg/day (maximum = 20 mg/day) (unlabeled use).

Spironolactone
PO (Adults): *Edema*—25–200 mg/day in 1–2 divided doses. *HTN*—50–100 mg/day in 1–2 divided doses. *Diuretic-induced hypokalemia*—25–100 mg/day in 1–2 divided doses. *Diagnosis of primary hyperaldosteronism*—100–400 mg/day in 1–2 divided doses. *CHF*—12.5–25 mg/day (unlabeled use).
PO (Children 1–17 yr): *Diuretic, HTN*—1 mg/kg/day in 1–2 divided doses (should not exceed 3.3 mg/kg/day or 100 mg/day) (unlabeled use). *Diagnosis of primary hyperaldosteronism*—125–375 mg/m^2/day in 1–2 divided doses (unlabeled use).

PO (Neonates): 1–3 mg/kg/day in 1–2 divided doses.

Triamterene
PO (Adults): *HTN*—100 mg twice daily (not to exceed 300 mg/day; lower doses in combination products).
PO (Children): *HTN*—1–2 mg/kg/day in 2 divided doses; should not exceed 4 mg/kg/day or 300 mg/day.

Availability
Amiloride (generic available)
Tablets: 5 mg. *In combination with:* hydrochlorothiazide ({Moduret}). See Appendix B.

Spironolactone (generic available)
Tablets: 25 mg, 50 mg, 100 mg. *In combination with:* hydrochlorothiazide (Aldactazide, {Apo-Spirozide}). See Appendix B.

Triamterene
Capsules: 50 mg, 100 mg. *In combination with:* hydrochlorothiazide ({Apo-Triazide}, Dyazide, Maxzide, {Novo-Triamzide}, {Nu-Triazide}, {Pro-Triazide}, {Riva-Zide}). See Appendix B.

NURSING IMPLICATIONS

Assessment
- Monitor intake and output ratios and daily weight during therapy.
- If medication is given as an adjunct to antihypertensive therapy, monitor blood pressure before administering.
- Monitor response of signs and symptoms of hypokalemia (weakness, fatigue, U wave on ECG, arrhythmias, polyuria, polydipsia). Assess patient frequently for development of hyperkalemia (fatigue, muscle weakness, paresthesia, confusion, dyspnea, ECG changes, cardiac arrhythmias). Patients who have diabetes mellitus or kidney disease and geriatric patients are at increased risk of developing these symptoms.
- Periodic ECGs are recommended in patients receiving prolonged therapy.
- **Lab Test Considerations:** Serum potassium levels should be evaluated before and routinely during therapy. Withhold drug and notify physician or other health care professional if patient becomes hyperkalemic.
- Monitor BUN, serum creatinine, and electrolytes before and periodically during therapy. May cause ↑ serum magnesium, BUN, creati-

nine, potassium, and urinary calcium excretion levels. May also cause ↓ sodium levels.
- Discontinue potassium-sparing diuretics 3 days before a glucose tolerance test because of risk of severe hyperkalemia.
- *Spironolactone* may cause false ↑ of plasma cortisol concentrations. Spironolactone should be withdrawn 4–7 days before test.
- Monitor platelet count and total and differential leukocyte count periodically during therapy in patients taking *triamterene*.

Potential Nursing Diagnoses
Excess fluid volume (Indications)

Implementation
- **PO:** Administer in AM to avoid interrupting sleep pattern.
- Administer with food or milk to minimize gastric irritation and to increase bioavailability.
- *Triamterene* capsules may be opened and contents mixed with food or fluids for patients with difficulty swallowing.

Patient/Family Teaching
- Emphasize the importance of continuing to take this medication, even if feeling well. Instruct patient to take medication at the same time each day. Take missed doses as soon as remembered unless almost time for next dose. Do not double doses.
- Caution patient to avoid salt substitutes and foods that contain high levels of potassium or sodium unless prescribed by health care professional.
- May cause dizziness. Caution patient to avoid driving or other activities requiring alertness until response to medication is known.
- Advise patient to consult with health care professional before taking any OTC decongestants, cough or cold preparations, or appetite suppressants concurrently with this medication because of potential for increased blood pressure.
- Advise patients taking *triamterene* to use sunscreen and protective clothing to prevent photosensitivity reactions.
- Instruct patient to notify health care professional of medication regimen before treatment or surgery.
- Advise patient to notify health care professional if muscle weakness or cramps; fatigue; or severe nausea, vomiting, or diarrhea occurs.
- Emphasize the need for follow-up exams to monitor progress.
- **Hypertension:** Reinforce need to continue additional therapies for hypertension (weight loss, restricted sodium intake, stress reduction, moderation of alcohol intake, regular exercise, and cessation of smoking). Medication helps control but does not cure hypertension.
- Teach patient and family the correct technique for checking blood pressure weekly.

Evaluation/Desired Outcomes
- Increase in diuresis and decrease in edema while maintaining serum potassium level in an acceptable range.
- Decrease in blood pressure.
- Prevention of hypokalemia in patients taking diuretics.
- Treatment of hyperaldosteronism.

DIURETICS (THIAZIDE)

chlorothiazide
(klor-oh-**thye**-a-zide)
Diuril, Sodium Diuril

chlorthalidone (thiazide–like)
(klor-**thal**-i-doan)
✦ Apo-Chlorthalidone, Thalitone

hydrochlorothiazide
(hye-droe-klor-oh-**thye**-a-zide)
✦ Apo-Hydro,
✦ Bio-Hydrochlorothiazide,
✦ DOM-Hydrochlorothiazide, Esedrix, Microzide, ✦ Novo-Hydrazide,
✦ Nu-Hydro, Oretic,
✦ PHL-Hydrochlorothiazide,
✦ PMS-Hydrochlorothiazide,
✦ Urozide

Classification
Therapeutic: antihypertensives, diuretics
Pharmacologic: thiazide diuretics

Pregnancy Category B (chlorthalidone, hydrochlorothiazide), C (chlorothiazide)

Indications
Management of mild to moderate hypertension. Treatment of edema associated with: CHF, Renal dysfunction, Cirrhosis, Glucocorticoid therapy, Estrogen therapy.

Action
Increases excretion of sodium and water by inhibiting sodium reabsorption in the distal tubule. Promotes excretion of chloride, potassium, magnesium, and bicarbonate. May produce arteriolar dilation. **Therapeutic Effects:** Lowering of blood pressure in hypertensive patients and diuresis with mobilization of edema.

DIURETICS (THIAZIDE) 459

Pharmacokinetics
Absorption: All are rapidly absorbed after oral administration.
Distribution: All cross the placenta and enter breast milk.
Metabolism and Excretion: All are excreted mainly unchanged by the kidneys.
Half-life: *Chlorothiazide*—1–2 hr; *chlorthalidone*—35–50 hr; *hydrochlorothiazide*—6–15 hr.

TIME/ACTION PROFILE (diuretic effect)

ROUTE	ONSET	PEAK	DURATION
Chlorothiazide PO	2 hr	4 hr	6–12 hr
Chlorothiazide IV	15 min	30 min	2 hr
Chlorthalidone	2 hr	2 hr	48–72 hr
Hydrochlorothiazide†	2 hr	3–6 hr	6–12 hr

†Onset of antihypertensive effect is 3–4 days and does not become maximal for 7–14 days of dosing

Contraindications/Precautions
Contraindicated in: Hypersensitivity (cross-sensitivity with other thiazides or sulfonamides may exist); Some products contain tartrazine and should be avoided in patients with known intolerance; Anuria; Lactation.
Use Cautiously in: Renal or hepatic impairment; OB: Pregnancy (jaundice or thrombocytopenia may be seen in the newborn); Pedi: Avoid use of hydrochlorothiazide oral solution in neonates (contains sodium benzoate, a metabolite of benzyl alcohol, which causes fetal gasping syndrome).

Adverse Reactions/Side Effects
CNS: dizziness, drowsiness, lethargy, weakness. **CV:** hypotension. **GI:** anorexia, cramping, hepatitis, nausea, pancreatitis, vomiting. **Derm:** photosensitivity, rashes. **Endo:** hyperglycemia. **F and E:** <u>hypokalemia</u>, dehydration, hypercalcemia, hypochloremic alkalosis, hypomagnesemia, hyponatremia, hypophosphatemia, hypovolemia. **Hemat:** thrombocytopenia. **Metab:** hypercholesterolemia, hyperuricemia. **MS:** muscle cramps.

Interactions
Drug-Drug: Additive hypotension with other **antihypertensives**, acute ingestion of **alcohol**, or **nitrates**. Additive hypokalemia with **corticosteroids**, **amphotericin B**, **piperacillin**, or **ticarcillin**. ↓ excretion of **lithium**. **Cholestyramine** or **colestipol** ↓ absorption. Hypokalemia ↑ risk of **digoxin** toxicity. **NSAIDs** may ↓ effectiveness.

Route/Dosage
When used as a diuretic in adults, generally given daily, but may be given every other day or 2–3 days/week.

Chlorothiazide
PO (Adults): 125 mg–2 g/day in 1–2 divided doses.
PO (Children >6 mos): 20 mg/kg/day in 1–2 divided doses (maximum dose = 1 g/day).
PO (Neonates ≤6 mo): 10–20 mg/kg q 12 hr (maximum dose = 375 mg/day).
IV (Adults): 500 mg–1 g/day in 1–2 divided doses.
IV (Children >6 mos): 4 mg/kg/day in 1–2 divided doses (maximum dose = 20 mg/kg/day) (unlabeled use).
IV (Neonates ≤6 mo): 1–4 mg/kg q 12 hr (maximum dose = 20 mg/kg/day) (unlabeled use).

Chlorthalidone
PO (Adults): 12.5–100 mg once daily (daily doses above 25 mg are associated with greater likelihood of electrolyte abnormalities).

Hydrochlorothiazide
PO (Adults): 12.5–100 mg/day in 1–2 divided doses (up to 200 mg/day); not to exceed 50 mg/day for hypertension; daily doses above 25 mg are associated with greater likelihood of electrolyte abnormalities.
PO (Children >6 mo): 1–3 mg/kg/day in 2 divided doses (not to exceed 37.5 mg/day).
PO (Children <6 mo): 1–3 mg/kg/day in 2 divided doses.

Availability

Chlorothiazide (generic available)
Tablets: 250 mg, 500 mg. **Oral suspension:** 250 mg/5 mL. **Powder for injection:** 500 mg.

Chlorthalidone (generic available)
Tablets: 25 mg, 50 mg, 100 mg. *In combination with:* atenolol (Tenoretic), clonidine (Clorpres). See Appendix B.

Hydrochlorothiazide (generic available)
Tablets: 25 mg, 50 mg. **Capsules:** 12.5 mg. **Oral solution:** 10 mg/mL, 100 mg/mL

460 DIURETICS (THIAZIDE)

In combination with: numerous antihypertensive agents. See Appendix B.

NURSING IMPLICATIONS
Assessment
- Monitor blood pressure, intake, output, and daily weight and assess feet, legs, and sacral area for edema daily.
- Assess patient, especially if taking digoxin, for anorexia, nausea, vomiting, muscle cramps, paresthesia, and confusion. Notify health care professional if these signs of electrolyte imbalance occur. Patients taking digoxin are at risk of digoxin toxicity because of the potassium-depleting effect of the diuretic.
- If hypokalemia occurs, consideration may be given to potassium supplements or ↓ dose of diuretic.
- Assess patient for allergy to sulfonamides.
- **Hypertension:** Monitor blood pressure before and periodically during therapy.
- Monitor frequency of prescription refills to determine compliance.
- *Lab Test Considerations:* Monitor electrolytes (especially potassium), blood glucose, BUN, serum creatinine, and uric acid levels before and periodically throughout therapy.
- May cause ↑ in serum and urine glucose in diabetic patients.
- May cause ↑ in serum bilirubin, calcium, creatinine, and uric acid, and ↓ in serum magnesium, potassium, sodium, and urinary calcium concentrations.
- May cause ↑ serum cholesterol, low-density lipoprotein, and triglyceride concentrations.

Potential Nursing Diagnoses
Excess fluid volume (Indications)
Risk for deficient fluid volume (Side Effects)
Deficient knowledge, related to medication regimen (Patient/Family Teaching)

Implementation
- Administer in the morning to prevent disruption of sleep cycle.
- Intermittent dose schedule may be used for continued control of edema.
- **PO:** May give with food or milk to minimize GI irritation. Tablets may be crushed and mixed with fluid to facilitate swallowing.

IV Administration
- **Intermittent Infusion: *Diluent:*** Reconstitute chlorothiazide with at least 18 mL of sterile water for injection. Shake to dissolve. Stable for 24 hr at room temperature. May be given undiluted or may be diluted further with D5W or 0.9% NaCl. *Concentration:* Up to 28 mg/mL. *Rate:* If administered undiluted may give by direct IV over 3–5 min. If diluted, may run over 30 min.

Patient/Family Teaching
- Instruct patient to take this medication at the same time each day. If a dose is missed, take as soon as remembered but not just before next dose is due. Do not double doses.
- Instruct patient on use of calibrated dropper for measuring hydrochlorothiazide concentrated oral solution.
- Instruct patient to monitor weight biweekly and notify health care professional of significant changes.
- Caution patient to change positions slowly to minimize orthostatic hypotension. This may be potentiated by alcohol.
- Advise patient to use sunscreen and protective clothing to prevent photosensitivity reactions.
- Instruct patient to discuss dietary potassium requirements with health care professional (see Appendix M).
- Instruct patient to notify health care professional of medication regimen before treatment or surgery.
- Advise patient to report muscle weakness, cramps, nausea, vomiting, diarrhea, or dizziness to health care professional.
- Emphasize the importance of routine follow-up exams.
- **Hypertension:** Advise patients to continue taking the medication even if feeling better. Medication controls but does not cure hypertension.
- Encourage patient to comply with additional interventions for hypertension (weight reduction, low-sodium diet, regular exercise, smoking cessation, moderation of alcohol consumption, and stress management).
- Instruct patient and family in correct technique for monitoring weekly blood pressure.
- Advise patient to consult health care professional before taking OTC medication, especially cough or cold preparations, concurrently with this therapy.

Evaluation/Desired Outcomes
- Decrease in blood pressure.
- Increase in urine output.
- Decrease in edema.

---

divalproex sodium, See VALPROATES.

DOBUTamine

HIGH ALERT

DOBUTamine
(doe-**byoo**-ta-meen)
Dobutrex

Classification
Therapeutic: inotropics
Pharmacologic: adrenergics

Pregnancy Category B

Indications
Short-term (<48 hr) management of heart failure caused by depressed contractility from organic heart disease or surgical procedures.

Action
Stimulates beta$_1$ (myocardial)-adrenergic receptors with relatively minor effect on heart rate or peripheral blood vessels. **Therapeutic Effects:** Increased cardiac output without significantly increased heart rate.

Pharmacokinetics
Absorption: Administered by IV infusion only, resulting in complete bioavailability.
Distribution: Unknown.
Metabolism and Excretion: Metabolized by the liver and other tissues.
Half-life: 2 min.

TIME/ACTION PROFILE (inotropic effects)

ROUTE	ONSET	PEAK	DURATION
IV	1–2 min	10 min	brief (min)

Contraindications/Precautions
Contraindicated in: Hypersensitivity to dobutamine or bisulfites; Idiopathic hypertrophic subaortic stenosis.
Use Cautiously in: History of hypertension (increased risk of exaggerated pressor response); MI; Atrial fibrillation (pretreatment with digitalis glycosides recommended); History of ventricular atopic activity (may be exacerbated); Hypovolemia (correct before administration); Pregnancy or lactation (safety not established).

Adverse Reactions/Side Effects
CNS: headache. **Resp:** shortness of breath. **CV:** hypertension, increased heart rate, premature ventricular contractions, angina pectoris, arrhythmias, hypotension, palpitations. **GI:** nausea, vomiting. **Local:** phlebitis. **Misc:** hypersensitivity reactions including skin rash, fever, bronchospasm or eosinophilia, nonanginal chest pain.

Interactions
Drug-Drug: Use with **nitroprusside** may have a synergistic effect on ↑ cardiac output. **Beta blockers** may negate the effect of dobutamine.
↑ risk of arrhythmias or hypertension with some **anesthetics** (**cyclopropane, halothane**), **MAO inhibitors, oxytocics**, or **tricyclic antidepressants**.

Route/Dosage
IV (Adults and Children): 2.5–15 mcg/kg/min titrate to response (up to 40 mcg/kg/min).
IV (Neonates): 2–15 mcg/kg/min.

Availability
Injection: 12.5 mg/mL in 20-, 40-, and 100-mL vials. **Premixed infusion:** 250 mg/250 mL, 500 mg/500 mL, 500 mg/250 mL, 1000 mg/250 mL.

NURSING IMPLICATIONS

Assessment
- Monitor blood pressure, heart rate, ECG, pulmonary capillary wedge pressure (PCWP), cardiac output, CVP, and urinary output continuously during the administration. Report significant changes in vital signs or arrhythmias. Consult physician for parameters for pulse, blood pressure, or ECG changes for adjusting dose or discontinuing medication.
- Palpate peripheral pulses and assess appearance of extremities routinely throughout dobutamine administration. Notify physician if quality of pulse deteriorates or if extremities become cold or mottled.
- *Lab Test Considerations:* Monitor potassium concentrations during therapy; may cause hypokalemia.
- Monitor electrolytes, BUN, creatinine, and prothrombin time weekly during prolonged therapy.
- *Toxicity and Overdose:* If overdose occurs, reduction or discontinuation of therapy is the only treatment necessary because of the short duration of dobutamine.

Potential Nursing Diagnoses
Decreased cardiac output (Indications)
Ineffective tissue perfusion (Indications)

Implementation
- *High Alert:* IV vasoactive medications are potentially dangerous. Have second practitioner independently check original order, dosage calculations, and infusion pump settings. Do not

---
✦ = Canadian drug name. ☤ = Genetic implication.
*CAPITALS indicates life-threatening; underlines indicate most frequent.

confuse dobutamine with dopamine. If available as floor stock, store in separate areas.
- Correct hypovolemia with volume expanders before initiating dobutamine therapy.
- Administer into a large vein and assess administration site frequently. Extravasation may cause pain and inflammation.

IV Administration

- **Continuous Infusion: *Diluent:*** Vials must be diluted before use. Dilute 250–1000 mg in 250–500 mL of D5W, 0.9% NaCl, 0.45% NaCl, D5/0.45% NaCl, D5/0.9% NaCl, or LR. Admixed infusions stable for 48 hr at room temperature and 7 days if refrigerated. Premixed infusions are already diluted and ready to use. ***Concentration:*** 0.25–5 mg/mL. ***Rate:*** Based on patient's weight (see Route/Dosage section). Administer via infusion pump to ensure precise amount delivered. Titrate to patient response (heart rate, presence of ectopic activity, blood pressure, urine output, CVP, PCWP, cardiac index). Dose should be titrated so heart rate does not increase by >10% of baseline.
- **Y-Site Compatibility:** amifostine, amikacin, amiodarone, anidulafungin, argatroban, atracurium, atropine, aztreonam, bivalirudin, bumetanide, calcium chloride, calcium gluconate, caspofungin, cimetidine, ciprofloxacin, cisatracurium, cyclosporine, cladribine, dexmeditomidine, diazepam, digoxin, diltiazem, diphenhydramine, docetaxel, dopamine, doxorubicin liposome, doxycycline, enalaprilat, epinephrine, eptifibatide, erythromycin, esmolol, etoposide phosphate, famotidine, fenoldopam, fentanyl, fluconazole, gemcitabine, gentamicin, granisetron, haloperidol, hydromorphone, inamrinone, insulin, isoproterenol, labetalol, levofloxacin, lidocaine, linezolid, lorazepam, magnesium sulfate, meperidine, methylprednisolone sodium succinate, metoclopramide, metoprolol, milrinone, morphine, nafcillin, nicardipine, nitroglycerin, norepinephrine, ondansetron, oxaliplatin, palonosetron, pancuronium, phenylephrine, potassium chloride, procainamide, prochlorperazine, promethazine, propofol, propranolol, protamine, ranitidine, remifentanil, streptokinase, tacrolimus, theophylline, thiotepa, tigecycline, tirofiban, tobramycin, tolazoline, vancomycin, vasopressin, vecuronium, verapamil, voriconazole, zidovudine.
- **Y-Site Incompatibility:** acyclovir, alteplase, aminophylline, amphotericin B cholesteryl sulfate, ampicillin, ampicillin/sulbactam, amphotericin B, cefazolin, cefoxitin, ceftriaxone, cefuroxime, chloramphenicol, ertapenem, foscarnet, ganciclovir, hydrocortisone sodium succinate, indomethacin, ketorolac, lansoprazole, micafungin, pantoprazole, pemetrexed, penicillin G potassium, phenytoin, phytonadione, piperacillin/tazobactam, sodium bicarbonate, thiopental, ticarcillin/clavulanate, trimethoprim/sulfamethoxazole, warfarin.

Patient/Family Teaching
- Explain to patient the rationale for instituting this medication and the need for frequent monitoring.
- Advise patient to inform nurse immediately if chest pain; dyspnea; or numbness, tingling, or burning of extremities occurs.
- Instruct patient to notify nurse immediately of pain or discomfort at the site of administration.
- **Home Care Issues:** Instruct caregiver on proper care of IV equipment.
- Instruct caregiver to report signs of worsening CHF (shortness of breath, orthopnea, decreased exercise tolerance), abdominal pain, and nausea or vomiting to health care professional promptly.

Evaluation/Desired Outcomes
- Increase in cardiac output.
- Improved hemodynamic parameters.
- Increased urine output.

HIGH ALERT

docetaxel (doe-se-**tax**-el)
Taxotere

Classification
Therapeutic: antineoplastics
Pharmacologic: taxoids

Pregnancy Category D

Indications
Breast cancer (locally advanced/metastatic breast cancer or with doxorubicin and cyclophosphamide as adjuvant treatment of node-positive disease). Non–small-cell lung cancer (locally advanced/ metastatic) after failure on platinum regimen or with platinum as initial therapy). Advanced metastatic hormone-refractory prostate cancer (with prednisone). Squamous cell carcinoma of the head and neck (inoperable, locally advanced) with cisplatin and fluorouracil.

Action
Interferes with normal cellular microtubule function required for interphase and mitosis. **Therapeutic Effects:** Death of rapidly replicating cells, particularly malignant ones.

Pharmacokinetics
Absorption: IV administration results in complete bioavailability.
Distribution: Unknown.
Metabolism and Excretion: Extensively metabolized by the liver; metabolites undergo fecal elimination.
Half-life: 11.1 hr.

TIME/ACTION PROFILE (effect on blood counts)

ROUTE	ONSET	PEAK	DURATION
IV	rapid	5–9 days	7 days

Contraindications/Precautions
Contraindicated in: Hypersensitivity; Hypersensitivity to polysorbate 80; Known alcohol intolerance; Neutrophil count <1500/mm³; Liver impairment (serum bilirubin > upper limit of normal, ALT and/or AST >1.5 times upper limit of normal, with alkaline phosphatase >2.5 times upper limit of normal); OB: Pregnancy or lactation.
Use Cautiously in: OB: Patients with childbearing potential.

Adverse Reactions/Side Effects
CNS: fatigue, weakness. **Resp:** bronchospasm. **CV:** ASCITES, CARDIAC TAMPONADE, PERICARDIAL EFFUSION, PULMONARY EDEMA, peripheral edema. **GI:** diarrhea, nausea, stomatitis, vomiting. **Derm:** alopecia, rashes, dermatitis, desquamation, edema, erythema, nail disorders. **Hemat:** anemia, thrombocytopenia, leukopenia. **Local:** injection site reactions. **MS:** myalgia, arthralgia. **Neuro:** neurosensory deficits, peripheral neuropathy. **Misc:** hypersensitivity reactions, including ANAPHYLAXIS.

Interactions
Drug-Drug: ↑ bone marrow depression may occur with other **antineoplastics** or **radiation therapy**. **Cyclosporine**, **ketoconazole**, **erythromycin**, or **troleandomycin** may significantly alter the effects of docetaxel.

Route/Dosage
IV (Adults): *Breast cancer*—60–100 mg/m² every 3 wk; *Breast cancer adjuvant therapy*—75 mg/m² every 3 wk for 6 cycles (with doxorubicin and cyclophosphamide); *Non–small-cell lung cancer*—75 mg/m² every 3 wk (alone or with platinum); *Prostate cancer*—75 mg/m² every 3 wk (with oral prednisone); *Squamous cell cancer*—75 mg/m² every 3 wk for 4 cycles (with cisplatin and fluorouracil).

Availability
Injection concentrate: 20 mg/0.5 mL polysorbate 80 with diluent (13% ethanol), 80 mg/2 mL polysorbate 80 with diluent (13% ethanol).

NURSING IMPLICATIONS
Assessment
- Monitor vital signs before and after administration.
- Assess infusion site for patency. Docetaxel is not a vesicant. If extravasation occurs, discontinue docetaxel immediately and aspirate the IV needle. Apply cold compresses to the site for 24 hr.
- Monitor for hypersensitivity reactions continuously during infusion. These are most common after the first and second doses of docetaxel. Reactions may consist of bronchospasm, hypotension, and/or erythema. Mild to moderate reactions may be treated symptomatically and infusion slowed or stopped until reaction subsides. Severe reactions require discontinuation of therapy and symptomatic treatment. Do not readminister docetaxel to patients with previous severe reactions. Severe edema may also occur. Weigh patients before each treatment. Fluid accumulation may result in edema, ascites, and pleural or pericardial effusions. Pretreatment with corticosteroids (such as dexamethasone 8 mg PO twice daily for 5 days, starting 1 day before docetaxel) is recommended to minimize edema and hypersensitivity reactions. PO furosemide may be used to treat edema.
- Monitor for bone marrow depression. Assess for bleeding (bleeding gums, bruising, petechiae; guaiac stools, urine, and emesis) and avoid IM injections and taking rectal temperatures if platelet count is low. Apply pressure to venipuncture sites for 10 min. Assess for signs of infection during neutropenia. Anemia may occur. Monitor for increased fatigue, dyspnea, and orthostatic hypotension.
- Assess patient for rash. May occur on feet or hands but may also occur on arms, face, or thorax, usually with pruritus. Rash usually occurs within 1 wk after infusion and resolves before next infusion.
- Assess for development of neurosensory deficit (paresthesia, dysesthesia, pain, burning). May also cause weakness. Pyridoxine may be used to minimize symptoms. Severe symptoms may require dose reduction or discontinuation.

- Assess patient for arthralgia and myalgia, which are usually relieved by nonopioid analgesics but may be severe enough to require treatment with opioid analgesics.
- **Lab Test Considerations:** Monitor CBC and differential before each treatment. Frequently causes neutropenia (<2000 neutrophils/mm^3); may require dose adjustment. If the neutrophil count is less than 1500/mm^3, dose should be held. Neutropenia is reversible and not cumulative. The nadir is 8 days, with a duration of 7 days. May also cause thrombocytopenia and anemia.
- Monitor liver function studies (AST, ALT, alkaline phosphatase, bilirubin) before each cycle. Doses are usually held if levels are elevated.

Potential Nursing Diagnoses
Risk for infection (Adverse Reactions)
Risk for injury (Adverse Reactions)

Implementation
- **High Alert:** Fatalities have occurred with chemotherapeutic agents. Before administering, clarify all ambiguous orders; double-check single, daily, and course-of-therapy dose limits; have second practitioner independently double-check original order, calculations, and infusion pump settings. Do not confuse Taxotere (docetaxel) with Taxol (paclitaxel).
- Solution should be prepared in a biologic cabinet. Wear gloves, gown, and mask while handling medication. Discard IV equipment in specially designated containers.

IV Administration
- **Continuous Infusion:** *Diluent:* Before dilution, allow vials to stand at room temperature for 5 min. Withdraw entire contents of diluent vial and transfer to vial of docetaxel. Rotate vial gently for 15 sec to mix. Do not shake. Solution should be clear but may contain foam at top. Allow to stand for a few minutes to allow foam to dissipate. All foam need not dissipate before continuing preparation. *Concentration:* To prepare the solution for infusion, withdraw the required amount of 10 mg/mL solution into syringe and inject into 250 mL of 0.9% NaCl or D5W for a concentration of 0.3–0.9 mg/mL. Rotate infusion container to mix infusion thoroughly. Do not administer solutions that are cloudy or contain a precipitate. Solution does not require an in-line filter. Dilute solutions are stable for 8 hr if refrigerated or at room temperature. *Rate:* Administer over 1 hr.
- **Y-Site Compatibility:** acyclovir, amifostine, amikacin, aminophylline, ampicillin, ampicillin/sulbactam, aztreonam, bumetanide, buprenorphine, butorphanol, calcium gluconate, cefazolin, cefepime, cefotaxime, cefotetan, cefoxitin, ceftazidime, ceftizoxime, ceftriaxone, cefuroxime, chlorpromazine, cimetidine, ciprofloxacin, clindamycin, dexamethasone sodium phosphate, diphenhyrdamine, dobutamine, dopamine, doxycycline, droperidol, enalaprilat, famotidine, fluconazole, furosemide, ganciclovir, gemcitabine, gentamicin, granisetron, haloperidol, heparin, hydrocortisone, hydromorphone, imipenem/cilastatin, leucovorin, lorazepam, LR, magnesium sulfate, mannitol, meperidine, meropenem, mesna, metoclopramide, metronidazole, minocycline, morphine, ondansetron, oxaliplatin, palonosetron, pemetrexed, piperacillin, piperacillin/tazobactam, potassium chloride, prochlorperazine, promethazine, ranitidine, sodium bicarbonate, ticarcillin/clavulanate, tobramycin, trimethoprim/sulfamethoxazole, vancomycin, zidovudine.
- **Y-Site Incompatibility:** amphotericin B, doxorubicin liposome, methylprednisolone, nalbuphine.
- **Additive Incompatibility:** Information unavailable. Do not admix with other drugs or solutions.

Patient/Family Teaching
- Advise patient to notify health care professional if fever >101°F; chills; sore throat; signs of infection; bleeding gums; bruising; petechiae; or blood in urine, stool, or emesis occur. Caution patient to avoid crowds and persons with known infections. Instruct patient to use soft toothbrush and electric razor.
- Patient should be cautioned not to drink alcoholic beverages or take products containing aspirin or NSAIDs.
- Fatigue is a frequent side effect of docetaxel. Advise patient that frequent rest periods and pacing of activities may minimize fatigue.
- Instruct patient to notify health care professional if abdominal pain, yellow skin, weakness, paresthesia, gait disturbances, swelling of the feet, or joint or muscle aches occur.
- Instruct patient to inspect oral mucosa for redness and ulceration. If mouth sores occur, advise patient to use sponge brush and rinse mouth with water after eating and drinking.
- Discuss with patient the possibility of hair loss. Complete hair loss usually begins after 1 or 2 treatments and is reversible after discontinuation of therapy. Explore coping strategies.

- Instruct patient not to receive any vaccinations without advice of health care professional.
- Emphasize the need for periodic lab tests to monitor for side effects.

Evaluation/Desired Outcomes
- Decrease in size or spread of malignancy in women with advanced breast cancer.
- Decrease in size or spread of malignancy in locally advanced or metastatic non–small-cell lung cancer.
- Decreased size or spread of advanced metastatic hormone-refractory prostate cancer.

---

docosanol (doe-koe-sa-nole)
Abreva

Classification
Therapeutic: antivirals (topical)

Pregnancy Category B

Indications
Treatment of recurrent oral-facial herpes simplex (cold sores, fever blisters).

Action
Prevents herpes simplex virus from entering cells by preventing viral particles from fusing with cell membranes. **Therapeutic Effects:** Reduced healing time. Decreased duration of symptoms (pain, burning, itching, tingling).

Pharmacokinetics
Absorption: Unknown.
Distribution: Unknown.
Metabolism and Excretion: Unknown.
Half-life: Unknown.

TIME/ACTION PROFILE

ROUTE	ONSET	PEAK	DURATION
Topical	unknown	unknown	unknown

Contraindications/Precautions
Contraindicated in: Hypersensitivity to docosanol or any other components of the formulation (benzyl alcohol, mineral oil, propylene glycol, or sucrose).
Use Cautiously in: Children <12 yr (safety not established); Pregnancy (use only if clearly needed).

Adverse Reactions/Side Effects
All local reactions occured at site of application.
Local: acne, skin, itching, rash.

Interactions
Drug-Drug: None significant.

Route/Dosage
Topical (Adults and Children ≥12 yr): Apply small amount 5 times daily to sores on lips or face until healed.

Availability
Cream: 10% cream in 2 g tubes[OTC].

NURSING IMPLICATIONS

Assessment
- Assess skin lesions prior to and periodically throughout therapy.

Potential Nursing Diagnoses
Impaired skin integrity, impaired (Indications)
Risk for infection, high risk for (Indications)
Deficient knowledge, related to disease process and medication regimen (Patient/Family Teaching)

Implementation
- **Topical:** Cream should be applied to lesions 5 times daily starting at the first sign of a sore or blister.

Patient/Family Teaching
- Instruct patient on correct technique for application of docosanol. Cream should only be applied to lips and face. Avoid application in or near eyes. Emphasize handwashing following application, or touching lesions to prevent spread to others or to other areas of the body.
- Advise patient to begin application of docosanol at the first sign of a sore or blister, even during prodromal stage (feeling of burning, itching, tingling, or numbness).
- Inform patient that docosanol reduces duration of herpes simplex virus episodes but does not cure virus. Viral reactivation may be triggered by ultraviolet radiation or sun exposure, stress, fatigue, chilling, and windburn. Other possible triggers include fever, injury, menstruation, dental work, and infectious diseases (cold, flu).
- Advise patient to notify health care professional if lesions do not heal in 14 days or if fever, rash, or swollen lymph nodes occur.

Evaluation/Desired Outcomes
- Reduction in duration of symptoms (pain, burning, itching, tingling) of herpes simplex virus episodes.

DOCUSATE (dok-yoo-sate)

docusate calcium
DC Softgels, Dioctocal, Pro-Cal-Sof, Sulfolax, Surfak

docusate sodium
Colace, Correctol Stool Softener Soft Gels, Diocto, Docu, Docusoft S, DOK, DOS Softgels, DOS, DOSS, DSS, Dulcolax Stool Softener, Ex-Lax Stool Softener, Fleet Sof-Lax, Modane Soft, Philliips Liqui-Gels, Regulax-SS, ❋Regulex, Silace, Soflax, Stool Softener, Therevac SB

Classification
Therapeutic: laxatives
Pharmacologic: stool softeners

Pregnancy Category C

Indications
PO: Prevention of constipation (in patients who should avoid straining, such as after MI or rectal surgery). **Rect:** Used as enema to soften fecal impaction.

Action
Promotes incorporation of water into stool, resulting in softer fecal mass. May also promote electrolyte and water secretion into the colon. **Therapeutic Effects:** Softening and passage of stool.

Pharmacokinetics
Absorption: Small amounts may be absorbed from the small intestine after oral administration. Absorption from the rectum is not known.
Distribution: Unknown.
Metabolism and Excretion: Amounts absorbed after oral administration are eliminated in bile.
Half-life: Unknown.

TIME/ACTION PROFILE (softening of stool)

ROUTE	ONSET	PEAK	DURATION
PO	24–48 hr (up to 3–5 days)	unknown	unknown
Rectal	2–15 min	unknown	unknown

Contraindications/Precautions
Contraindicated in: Hypersensitivity; Abdominal pain, nausea, or vomiting, especially when associated with fever or other signs of an acute abdomen.

Use Cautiously in: Excessive or prolonged use may lead to dependence; Should not be used if prompt results are desired; OB, Lactation: Has been used safely.

Adverse Reactions/Side Effects
EENT: throat irritation. **GI:** mild cramps. **Derm:** rashes.

Interactions
Drug-Drug: None significant.

Route/Dosage

Docusate Calcium
PO (Adults): 240 mg once daily.

Docusate Sodium
PO (Adults and Children >12 yr): 50–400 mg in 1–4 divided doses.
PO (Children 6–12 yr): 40–150 mg in 1–4 divided doses.
PO (Children 3–6 yr): 20–60 mg in 1–4 divided doses.
PO (Children <3 yr): 10–40 mg in 1–4 divided doses.
Rect (Adults): 50–100 mg or 1 unit containing 283 mg docusate sodium, soft soap, and glycerin.

Availability (generic available)

Docusate Calcium
Capsules: 240 mg[OTC].

Docusate Sodium (generic available)
Tablets: 100 mg[OTC]. **Capsules:** 50 mg[OTC], 100 mg[OTC], 120 mg[OTC], 240 mg[OTC], 250 mg[OTC]. **Syrup:** 20 mg/5 mL[OTC]. **Liquid:** 150 mg/15 mL[OTC]. **Enema:** 283 mg/5 mL[OTC]. *In combination with:* stimulant laxatives[OTC]. See Appendix B.

NURSING IMPLICATIONS

Assessment
- Assess for abdominal distention, presence of bowel sounds, and usual pattern of bowel function.
- Assess color, consistency, and amount of stool produced.

Potential Nursing Diagnoses
Constipation (Indications)

Implementation
- This medication does not stimulate intestinal peristalsis.
- **PO:** Administer with a full glass of water or juice. May be administered on an empty stomach for more rapid results.
- Oral solution may be diluted in milk or fruit juice to decrease bitter taste.
- Do not administer within 2 hr of other laxatives, especially mineral oil. May cause increased absorption.

Patient/Family Teaching
- Advise patients that laxatives should be used only for short-term therapy. Long-term therapy may cause electrolyte imbalance and dependence.
- Encourage patients to use other forms of bowel regulation, such as increasing bulk in the diet, increasing fluid intake (6–8 full glasses/day), and increasing mobility. Normal bowel habits are variable and may vary from 3 times/day to 3 times/wk.
- Instruct patients with cardiac disease to avoid straining during bowel movements (Valsalva maneuver).
- Advise patient not to use laxatives when abdominal pain, nausea, vomiting, or fever is present.
- Advise patient not to take docusate within 2 hr of other laxatives.

Evaluation/Desired Outcomes
- A soft, formed bowel movement, usually within 24–48 hr. Therapy may take 3–5 days for results. Rectal dose forms produce results within 2–15 min.

---

dofetilide (doe-fet-il-ide)
Tikosyn

Classification
Therapeutic: antiarrhythmics (class III)

Pregnancy Category C

Indications
Maintenance of normal sinus rhythm (delay in time to recurrence of atrial fibrillation/atrial flutter [AF/AFl]) in patients with AF/AFl lasting more than one week, and who have been converted to normal sinus rhythm. For the conversion of atrial fibrillation and atrial flutter to normal sinus rhythm.

Action
Blocks cardiac ion channels responsible for transport of potassium. Increases monophasic action potential duration. Increases effective refractory period. **Therapeutic Effects:** Prevention of recurrent AF/AFl. Conversion of AF/AFl to normal sinus rhythm.

Pharmacokinetics
Absorption: Well absorbed (>90%) following oral administration.
Distribution: Unknown.

Metabolism and Excretion: 80% excreted by kidneys via cationic renal secretion, mostly as unchanged drug; 20% excreted as inactive metabolites; some metabolism in the liver via cytochrome P450 system (CYP3A4 isoenzyme).
Half-life: 10 hr.

TIME/ACTION PROFILE (blood levels)

ROUTE	ONSET	PEAK	DURATION
PO	within hours	2-3 hr†	12-24 hr

†Steady state levels are achieved after 2–3 days

Contraindications/Precautions
Contraindicated in: Hypersensitivity; Congenital or acquired prolonged QT syndromes; Baseline QT interval or QTc of >440 msec (500 msec in patients with ventricular conduction abnormalities); Creatinine clearance (CCr) <20 mL/min; Concurrent use of verapamil or agents which inhibit the renal cation transport system including cimetidine, ketoconazole, trimethoprim, megestrol or prochlorperazine; Concurrent use of hydrochlorothiazide; OB: Lactation (use should be avoided).

Use Cautiously in: Underlying electrolyte abnormalities (increased risk of serious arrhythmias; correct prior to administration); CCr 20–60 mL/min (dosage reduction recommended); Severe hepatic impairment; OB: Pregnancy (use only when benefit to patient outweighs potential risk to fetus); Pedi: Children <18 yr (safety not established).

Adverse Reactions/Side Effects
CNS: dizziness, headache. **CV:** VENTRICULAR ARRHYTHMIAS, chest pain, QT interval prolongation.

Interactions
Drug-Drug: Hydrochlorothiazide ↑ dofetilide levels and the risk of QT prolongation with arrhythmias; concurrent use is contraindicated. Concurrent use of renal cation transport inhibitors including **cimetidine**, **trimethoprim**, and **ketoconazole** increases blood levels and the risk of serious arrhythmias and is contraindicated. **Amiloride**, **metformin**, **megestrol**, **prochlorperazine**, and **triamterene** may have similar effects. **Phenothiazines**, **tricyclic antidepressants**, some **macrolides** (including **erythromcyin** and **telithromycin**, and **fluoroquinolones** may prolong QT interval and ↑ risk of arrhythmias; concurrent use is not recommended. Blood levels and risk of arrhythmias is also ↑ by **verapamil**; concurrent use is contra-

indicated and a 2-day washout period is recommended). Inhibitors of the cytochrome P450 system (CY P450 3A4 isoenzyme) including **macrolide anti-infectives**, **azole antifungals**, **protease inhibitor antiretrovirals**, **SSRI antidepressants**, **amiodarone**, **cannabinoids**, **diltiazem**, **nefazodone**, **quinine**, and **zafirlukast** may also ↑ blood levels and the risk of arrhythmias and concurrent use should be undertaken with caution. Should not be used concurrently with other **class I or III antiarrhythmics** due to increased risk of arrhythmias. **Phenothiazines** and **tricyclic antidepressants** also prolong QT interval and should not be used concurrently with dofetilide. Hypokalemia or hypomagnesemia from **potassium-depleting diuretics** increases the risk of arrhythmias; correct abnormalities prior to administration. Concurrent use of **digoxin** may also increase the risk of arrhythmias.
Drug-Food: Grapefruit juice may ↑ levels; avoid concurrent use.

Route/Dosage
Dosing should be adjusted according to renal function and assessment of QT interval.
PO (Adults): *Starting dose*—500 mcg twice daily; *maintenance dose*—250 mcg twice daily (not to exceed 500 mcg twice daily).

Renal Impairment
PO (Adults): *CCr 40–60 mL/min Starting dose*—250 mcg twice daily; *maintenance dose*—125 mcg twice daily; *CCr 20– 40 mL/min Starting dose*—125 mcg twice daily; *maintenance dose*—125 mcg once daily.

Availability
Capsules: 125 mcg, 250 mcg, 500 mcg.

NURSING IMPLICATIONS

Assessment
- Monitor ECG, pulse, and blood pressure continuously during initiation of therapy and for at least 3 days, then periodically during therapy. Evaluate QTc prior to initiation of therapy and every 3 months during therapy. If QTc exceeds 440 msec (500 msec in patients with ventricular conduction abnormalities), discontinue dofetilide and monitor patient until QTc returns to baseline.
- Assess the patient's medication history including OTC, Rx, and natural/herbal products, with emphasis on those that interact with dofetilide (see Interactions).
- ***Lab Test Considerations:*** Creatinine clearance must be calculated for all patients prior to administration and every 3 months during therapy.

Potential Nursing Diagnoses
Decreased cardiac output (Indications)

Implementation
- Dolfetilide must be initiated or reinitiated in a setting that provides continuous ECG monitoring and has personnel trained in the management of serious ventricular arrhythmias. Due to the potential for life-threatening ventricular arrhythmias, dofetilide is usually used for patients with highly symptomatic AF/AFl.
- Patients with AF should be anticoagulated according to usual protocol prior to electrical or pharmacological cardioversion.
- Make sure patient has an adequate supply of dofetilide prior to discharge to prevent interruption of therapy.
- Patients should not be discharged from the hospital within 12 hr of electrical or pharmacological conversion to normal sinus rhythm.
- **PO:** Administer at the same time each day without regard to food.

Patient/Family Teaching
- Instruct patient to take medication as directed, even if feeling well. If a dose is missed, do not double next dose. Take next dose at usual time.
- Patient should read the patient package insert prior to initiation of therapy and reread it each time therapy is renewed. Emphasize the need for compliance with therapy, the potential for drug interactions, and the need for periodic monitoring to minimize the risk of serious arrhythmias.
- Instruct patient or family member on how to take pulse. Advise patient to report changes in pulse rate or rhythm to health care professional.
- May cause dizziness. Caution patient to avoid driving or other activities requiring alertness until response to medication is known.
- Advise patient to inform health care professional of medication regimen prior to treatment or surgery.
- Instruct patient not to take OTC medications with dofetilide without consulting health care professional.
- Advise patient to consult health care professional immediately if they faint, become dizzy, or have fast heartbeats. If health care professional is unavailable instruct patient to go to nearest hospital emergency department, take remaining dofetilide capsules, and show them to the doctor or nurse. If symptoms associated

with altered electrolyte balance such as excessive or prolonged diarrhea, sweating, or vomiting or loss of appetite or thirst occur health care professional should also be notified immediately.
- Emphasize the importance of routine follow-up exams to monitor progress.

Evaluation/Desired Outcomes
- Prevention of recurrent AF/AFl.
- Conversion of AF/AFl to normal sinus rhythm.
- If patients do not convert to normal sinus rhythm within 24 hr of initiation of therapy, electrical conversion should be considered.

---

dolasetron (dol-a-se-tron)
Anzemet

Classification
Therapeutic: antiemetics
Pharmacologic: 5-HT$_3$ antagonists

Pregnancy Category B

Indications
Prevention of nausea and vomiting associated with emetogenic chemotherapy. Prevention and treatment of postoperative nausea/vomiting.

Action
Blocks the effects of serotonin at receptor sites (selective antagonist) located in vagal nerve terminals and in the chemoreceptor trigger zone in the CNS. **Therapeutic Effects:** Decreased incidence and severity of nausea/vomiting associated with emetogenic chemotherapy or surgery.

Pharmacokinetics
Absorption: Well absorbed but rapidly metabolized to hydrodolasetron, the active metabolite.
Distribution: Unknown.
Metabolism and Excretion: 61% of hydrodolasetron is excreted unchanged by the kidneys.
Half-life: *Hydrodolasetron*—8.1 hr (shorter in children).

TIME/ACTION PROFILE (antiemetic effect)

ROUTE	ONSET	PEAK	DURATION
PO	unknown	1–2 hr	up to 24 hr
IV	unknown	15–30 min	up to 24 hr

Contraindications/Precautions
Contraindicated in: Hypersensitivity.
Use Cautiously in: Patients with risk factors for prolongation of cardiac conduction intervals (hypokalemia, hypomagnesemia, concurrent diuretic or antiarrhythmic therapy, congenital QT syndrome, cumulative high-dose anthracycline therapy); Pregnancy or lactation (safety not established).

Adverse Reactions/Side Effects
CNS: headache (increased in cancer patients), dizziness, fatigue, syncope. **CV:** bradycardia, ECG changes, hypertension, hypotension, tachycardia. **GI:** diarrhea, dyspepsia. **GU:** oliguria. **Derm:** pruritus. **Misc:** chills, fever, pain.

Interactions
Drug-Drug: Concurrent **diuretic** or **antiarrhythmic** therapy or cumulative **high-dose anthracycline therapy** may ↑ risk of conduction abnormalities. Blood levels and effects of hydrodolasteron are ↑ by **atenolol** and **cimetidine**. Blood levels and effects of hydrodolasetron are ↓ by **rifampin**.

Route/Dosage

Prevention of Chemotherapy-Induced Nausea/Vomiting
PO (Adults): 100 mg given within 1 hr before chemotherapy.
PO (Children 2–16 yr): 1.8 mg/kg given within 1 hr before chemotherapy (not to exceed 100 mg).
IV (Adults and Children ≥2 yr): 1.8 mg/kg given 30 min before chemotherapy (usual dose in adults is 100 mg; not to exceed 100 mg in children).

Prevention/Treatment of Postoperative Nausea/Vomiting
PO (Adults): 100 mg given within 2 hr before surgery.
PO (Children 2–16 yr): 1.2 mg/kg (up to 100 mg/dose) given within 2 hr before surgery.
IV (Adults): 12.5 mg given 15 min before cessation of anesthesia (prevention) or as soon as nausea or vomiting begins (treatment).
IV (Children 2–16 yr): 0.35 mg/kg (up to 12.5 mg) given 15 min before cessation of anesthesia (prevention) or as soon as nausea or vomiting begins (treatment).

Availability
Tablets: 50 mg, 100 mg. **Injection:** 12.5 mg/0.625 mL ampules, 20 mg/mL in 5-mL vials.

✦ = Canadian drug name. 🧬 = Genetic implication.
*CAPITALS indicates life-threatening; underlines indicate most frequent.

NURSING IMPLICATIONS
Assessment
- Assess patient for nausea, vomiting, abdominal distention, and bowel sounds before and after administration.
- Monitor vital signs after administration. IV administration may be followed by severe hypotension, bradycardia, and syncope.

Potential Nursing Diagnoses
Imbalanced nutrition: less than body requirements (Indications)

Implementation
- **PO:** Administer within 1 hr before chemotherapy or 2 hr before surgery.
- Injectable dolasetron may be mixed in apple or apple-grape juice for oral dosing for pediatric patients. May be stored at room temperature for 2 hr before use.

IV Administration
- **IV:** Administer 30 min before chemotherapy, 15 min before cessation of anesthesia, or postoperatively if nausea and vomiting occur shortly after surgery.
- **Direct IV:** *Diluent:* May be administered undiluted. *Concentration:* 20 mg/mL. *Rate:* Administer over at least 30 sec.
- **Intermittent Infusion:** *Diluent:* May be diluted in 0.9% NaCl, D5W, dextrose/saline combinations, D5/LR, LR, or 10% mannitol solution. Solution is clear and colorless. Stable for 24 hr at room temperature or 48 hr if refrigerated after dilution. *Concentration:* Dilute doses in 50 mL diluent. *Rate:* Administer each dose as an IV infusion over up to 15 min.
- **Y-Site Compatibility:** azithromycin, dexmedetomidine, fenoldopam, oxaliplatin.
- **Y-Site Incompatibility:** Manufacturer recommends not admixing with other medications.

Patient/Family Teaching
- Advise patient to notify health care professional if nausea or vomiting occurs.

Evaluation/Desired Outcomes
- Prevention of nausea and vomiting associated with emetogenic cancer chemotherapy.
- Prevention and treatment of postoperative nausea and vomiting.

---

donepezil (doe-nep-i-zill)
Aricept, Aricept ODT

Classification
Therapeutic: anti-Alzheimer's agents
Pharmacologic: cholinergics (cholinesterase inhibitors)

Pregnancy Category C

Indications
Mild to moderate dementia associated with Alzheimer's disease.

Action
Inhibits acetylcholinesterase thus improving cholinergic function by making more acetylcholine available. **Therapeutic Effects:** May temporarily lessen some of the dementia associated with Alzheimer's disease. Enhances cognition. Does not cure the disease.

Pharmacokinetics
Absorption: Well absorbed after oral administration.
Distribution: Unknown.
Protein Binding: 96%.
Metabolism and Excretion: Partially metabolized by the liver (CYP2D6 and CYP3A4 enzymes) and partially excreted by kidneys (17% unchanged). Two metabolites are pharmacologically active.
Half-life: 70 hr.

TIME/ACTION PROFILE (improvement in symptoms)

ROUTE	ONSET	PEAK	DURATION
PO	unknown	several wk	6 wk†

†Return to baseline after discontinuation

Contraindications/Precautions
Contraindicated in: Hypersensitivity to donepezil or piperidine derivatives.
Use Cautiously in: Patients with underlying cardiac disease, especially sick sinus syndrome or supraventricular conduction defects; Patients with a history of ulcer disease or those currently taking NSAIDs; Patients with a history of seizures; Patients with a history of asthma or obstructive pulmonary disease; OB, Lactation, Pedi: Safety not established; assumed to be secreted in breast milk. Discontinue drug or bottle-feed.

Adverse Reactions/Side Effects
CNS: headache, abnormal dreams, depression, dizziness, drowsiness, fatigue, insomnia, syncope, sedation (unusual). **CV:** atrial fibrillation, hypertension, hypotension, vasodilation. **GI:** diarrhea, nausea, anorexia, vomiting, weight gain (unusual). **GU:** frequent urination. **Derm:** ecchymoses. **Metab:** hot flashes, weight loss. **MS:** arthritis, muscle cramps.

Interactions
Drug-Drug: Exaggerates muscle relaxation from **succinylcholine.** Interferes with the action of **anticholinergics.** ↑ cholinergic effects of **bethanechol.** May ↑ risk of GI bleeding from **NSAIDs. Quinidine** and **ketoconazole** ↓ metabolism of donepezil. **Rifampin, carbamazepine, dexamethasone, phenobarbital,** and **phenytoin** induce the enzymes that metabolize donepezil and may ↓ its effects.
Drug-Natural Products: Jimson weed and **scopolia** may antagonize cholinergic effects.

Route/Dosage
Mild to Moderate Alzheimer's Disease
PO (Adults): 5 mg once daily; after 4–6 wk may increase to 10 mg once daily (dose should not exceed 5 mg/day in frail, elderly females).

Severe Alzheimer's Disease
PO (Adults): 10 mg once daily (dose should not exceed 10 mg/day).

Availability
Tablets: 5 mg, 10 mg. **Cost:** 5 mg $464.97/90, 10 mg $455.97/90. **Orally-disintegrating tablets:** 5 mg, 10 mg. **Cost:** 5 mg $174.65/30, 10 mg $166.85/30.

NURSING IMPLICATIONS

Assessment
- Assess cognitive function (memory, attention, reasoning, language, ability to perform simple tasks) periodically during therapy.
- Administer Mini-Mental Status Exam (MMSE) initially and periodically as a screening tool to rate cognitive functioning.
- Administer Clock Drawing Test initially and periodically as a screening tool to measure severity of dementia.
- Monitor heart rate periodically during therapy. May cause bradycardia.

Potential Nursing Diagnoses
Disturbed thought process (Indications)
Impaired environmental interpretation syndrome (Indications)
Risk for injury (Indications)

Implementation
- **PO:** Administer in the evening just before going to bed. May be taken without regard to food.
- *Oral disintegrating tablets* should be allowed to dissolve on tongue; follow with water.

Patient/Family Teaching
- Emphasize the importance of taking donepezil daily, as directed. Missed doses should be skipped and regular schedule returned to the following day. Do not take more than prescribed; higher doses do not increase effects but may increase side effects.
- Inform patient/family that it may take weeks before improvement in baseline behavior is observed.
- Caution patient and caregiver that donepezil may cause dizziness.
- Advise patient and caregiver to notify health care professional if nausea, vomiting, diarrhea, or changes in color of stool occur or if new symptoms occur or previously noted symptoms increase in severity.
- Advise patient and caregiver to notify health care professional of medication regimen before treatment or surgery.
- Emphasize the importance of follow-up exams to monitor progress; atypical antipsychotics may be used as an adjunct to improve behavior.

Evaluation/Desired Outcomes
- Improvement in cognitive function (memory, attention, reasoning, language, ability to perform simple tasks) in patients with Alzheimer's disease.

HIGH ALERT

DOPamine (dope-a-meen)
Intropin, ✦Revimine

Classification
Therapeutic: inotropics, vasopressors
Pharmacologic: adrenergics

Pregnancy Category C

Indications
Adjunct to standard measures to improve: Blood pressure, Cardiac output, Urine output in treatment of shock unresponsive to fluid replacement. Increase renal perfusion (low doses).

Action
Small doses (0.5–3 mcg/kg/min) stimulate dopaminergic receptors, producing renal vasodilation. Larger doses (2–10 mcg/kg/min) stimulate dopaminergic and beta$_1$-adrenergic receptors, producing cardiac stimulation and renal vasodilation. Doses greater than 10 mcg/kg/min stimulate al-

DOPamine

pha-adrenergic receptors and may cause renal vasoconstriction. **Therapeutic Effects:** Increased cardiac output, increased blood pressure, and improved renal blood flow.

Pharmacokinetics
Absorption: Administered IV only, resulting in complete bioavailability.
Distribution: Widely distributed but does not cross the blood-brain barrier.
Metabolism and Excretion: Metabolized in liver, kidneys, and plasma.
Half-life: 2 min.

TIME/ACTION PROFILE (hemodynamic effects)

ROUTE	ONSET	PEAK	DURATION
IV	1–2 min	up to 10 min	<10 min

Contraindications/Precautions
Contraindicated in: Tachyarrhythmias; Pheochromocytoma; Hypersensitivity to bisulfites (some products).
Use Cautiously in: Hypovolemia; Myocardial infarction; Occlusive vascular diseases; Geri: Older patients may be more susceptible to adverse effects; OB: Pregnancy and lactation (safety not established).

Adverse Reactions/Side Effects
CNS: headache. **EENT:** mydriasis (high dose). **Resp:** dyspnea. **CV:** arrhythmias, hypotension, angina, ECG change, palpitations, vasoconstriction. **GI:** nausea, vomiting. **Derm:** piloerection. **Local:** irritation at IV site.

Interactions
Drug-Drug: Use with **MAO inhibitors**, **ergot alkaloids** (**ergotamine**), **doxapram**, **guanadrel**, or some **antidepressants** results in severe hypertension. Use with IV **phenytoin** may cause hypotension and bradycardia. Use with **general anesthetics** may result in arrhythmias. **Beta blockers** may antagonize cardiac effects.

Route/Dosage
IV (Adults): *Dopaminergic (renal vasodilation) effects*—1–5 mcg/kg/min. *Beta-adrenergic (cardiac stimulation) effects*—5–15 mcg/kg/min. *Alpha-adrenergic (increased peripheral vascular resistance) effects*—>15 mcg/kg/min; infusion rate may be increased as needed.
IV (Children and Infants): 1–20 mcg/kg/min, depending on desired response (1–5 mcg/kg/min has been used to improve renal blood flow).
IV (Neonates): 1–20 mcg/kg/min.

Availability (generic available)
Injection for dilution: 40 mg/mL, 80 mg/mL, 160 mg/mL. **Premixed injection:** 200 mg/250 mL, 400 mg/250 mL, 800 mg/250 mL, 800 mg/500 mL.

NURSING IMPLICATIONS
Assessment
- Monitor blood pressure, heart rate, pulse pressure, ECG, pulmonary capillary wedge pressure (PCWP), cardiac output, CVP, and urinary output continuously during administration. Report significant changes in vital signs or arrhythmias. Consult physician for parameters for pulse, blood pressure, or ECG changes for adjusting dose or discontinuing medication.
- Monitor urine output frequently throughout administration. Report decreases in urine output promptly.
- Palpate peripheral pulses and assess appearance of extremities routinely during dopamine administration. Notify physician if quality of pulse deteriorates or if extremities become cold or mottled.
- If hypotension occurs, administration rate should be increased. If hypotension continues, more potent vasoconstrictors (norepinephrine) may be administered.
- ***Toxicity and Overdose:*** If excessive hypertension occurs, rate of infusion should be decreased or temporarily discontinued until blood pressure is decreased. Although additional measures are usually not necessary because of short duration of dopamine, phentolamine may be administered if hypertension continues.

Potential Nursing Diagnoses
Decreased cardiac output (Indications)
Ineffective tissue perfusion (Indications)

Implementation
- **High Alert:** IV vasoactive medications are potentially dangerous. Have second practitioner independently check original order, dose calculations, and infusion pump settings. Do not confuse dopamine with dobutamine. If both are available as floor stock, store in separate areas.
- Correct hypovolemia with volume expanders before initiating dopamine therapy.
- Extravasation may cause severe irritation, necrosis, and sloughing of tissue. Administer into a large vein and assess administration site frequently. If extravasation occurs, affected area should be infiltrated liberally with 10–15 mL

of 0.9% NaCl containing 5–10 mg of phentolamine. For pediatric patients, use 1 mL of phentolamine dilution to infiltrate (do not exceed 5 mg total). Infiltration within 12 hr of extravasation produces immediate hyperemic changes.

IV Administration

- **Continuous Infusion: *Diluent:*** Dopamine vials must be diluted before use. Dilute 200–800 mg of dopamine in 250–500 mL of 0.9% NaCl, D5W, D5/LR, D5/0.45% NaCl, D5/0.9% NaCl, or LR. Admixed solution is stable for 24 hr. Discard solutions that are cloudy, discolored, or contain a precipitate. Premixed infusions are already diluted and ready to use. ***Concentration:*** 0.8–3.2 mg/mL. ***Rate:*** Based on patient's weight (see Route/Dosage section). Infusion must be administered via infusion pump to ensure precise amount delivered. Titrate to response (blood pressure, heart rate, urine output, peripheral perfusion, presence of ectopic activity, cardiac index). Decrease rate gradually when discontinuing to prevent marked decreases in blood pressure.
- **Y-Site Compatibility:** amifostine, amikacin, aminophylline, amiodarone, anidulafungin, argatroban, atracurium, atropine, aztreonam, bivalirudin, bumetanide, calcium chloride, calcium gluconate, caspofungin, cefotaxime, cefoxitin, ceftazidime, ceftizoxime, ceftriaxone, cefuroxime, cimetidine, ciprofloxacin, cisatracurium, cladribine, clindamycin, cyclosporine, daptomycin, dexamethasone sodium phosphate, dexmedetomidine, digoxin, diltiazem, diphenhydramine, dobutamine, docetaxel, doxorubicin liposome, doxycycline, droperidol, enalaprilat, epinephrine, ertapenem, erythromycin, esmolol, etoposide phosphate, famotidine, fenoldopam, fentanyl, fluconazole, foscarnet, gemcitabine, gentamicin, granisetron, haloperidol, heparin, hydrocortisone sodium succinate, hydromorphone, imipenem/cilastatin, inamrinone, isoproterenol, ketorolac, labetalol, levofloxacin, lidocaine, linezolid, lorazepam, magnesium sulfate, meperidine, methylprednisolone sodium succinate, metoclopramide, metoprolol, metronidazole, micafungin, midazolam, milrinone, morphine, nafcillin, nicardipine, nitroglycerin, nitroprusside, norepinephrine, ondansetron, oxaliplatin, palonosetron, pancuronium, pantoprazole, pemetrexed, penicillin G potassium, phenylephrine, phytonadione, piperacillin/tazobactam, potassium chloride, procainamide, prochlorperazine, promethazine, propofol, propranolol, protamine, ranitidine, remifentanil, sargramostim, streptokinase, tacrolimus, theophylline, thiotepa, ticarcillin/clavulanate, tigecycline, tirofiban, tobramycin, tolazoline, vancomycin, vasopressin, vecuronium, verapamil, vitamin B complex with C, voriconazole, warfarin, zidovudine.
- **Y-Site Incompatibility:** acyclovir, alteplase, amphotericin B cholesteryl sulfate, ampicillin, cefazolin, chloramphenicol, diazepam, ganciclovir, indomethacin, insulin, lansoprazole, phenytoin, thiopental, trimethoprim/sulfamethoxazole.

Patient/Family Teaching
- Explain to patient the rationale for instituting this medication and the need for frequent monitoring.
- Advise patient to inform nurse immediately if chest pain; dyspnea; numbness, tingling, or burning of extremities occurs.
- Instruct patient to inform nurse immediately of pain or discomfort at the site of administration.

Evaluation/Desired Outcomes
- Increase in blood pressure.
- Increase in peripheral circulation.
- Increase in urine output.

---

doripenem (do-ri-pen-em)
Doribax

Classification
Therapeutic: anti-infectives
Pharmacologic: carbapenems

Pregnancy Category B

Indications
Infections caused by susceptible organisms including: complicated intra-abdominal infections, complicated urinary tract infections, including pyelonephritis.

Action
Inhibits bacterial cell wall formation. **Therapeutic Effects:** Bactericidal action against susceptible bacteria. **Spectrum:** Active against the following gram-negative organisms: *Acinetobacter baumanii, Escherichia coli, Klebsiella pneumoniae, Proteus mirabilis,* and *Pseudomonas aeruginosa.* Also active against the following gram-

474 doripenem

positive organisms: *Streptococcus constellatus* and *S. intermedius*. Anaerobic spectrum includes *Bacteroides caccae*, *B. fragilis*, *B. thetaiotaomicron*, *B.uniformis*, *B. vulgatus*, and *Peptostreptococcus micros*.

Pharmacokinetics
Absorption: IV administration results in complete bioavailability.
Distribution: Penetrates renal and peritoneal and retroperitoneal tissues and fluids.
Metabolism and Excretion: Mostly excreted unchanged in urine; minimal metabolism.
Half-life: 1 hr.

TIME/ACTION PROFILE (blood levels)

ROUTE	ONSET	PEAK	DURATION
IV	unknown	end of infusion	8 hr*

*Normal renal function

Contraindications/Precautions
Contraindicated in: Hypersensitivity to doripenem, other carbapenems, or beta-lactams.
Use Cautiously in: Geri: Consider age-related decrease in renal function when choosing dose; Lactation: Use cautiously during lactation; Pedi: Safe use in children has not been established.

Adverse Reactions/Side Effects
CV: headache. **GI:** PSEUDOMEMBRANOUS COLITIS, diarrhea, nausea, ↑ liver enzymes. **Hemat:** anemia. **Local:** phlebitis. **Misc:** allergic reactions including ANAPHYLAXIS, infection with resistant organisms, superinfection.

Interactions
Drug-Drug: May ↓ serum **valproate** levels (↑ risk of seizures).
Drug-Natural Products: May ↓ blood levels of **valproic acid**; this may result in loss of seizure control. **Probenecid** ↓ renal clearance and ↑ blood levels.

Route/Dosage
IV (Adults): 500 mg every 8 hr.

Renal Impairment
IV (Adults): *CCr 30–50 mL/min*—250 mg every 8 hr; *CCr >10–<30 mL/min*—250 mg every 12 hr.

Availability
Powder for injection (requires reconstitution): 500 mg/vial.

NURSING IMPLICATIONS
Assessment
- Assess patient for infection (vital signs; appearance of wound, sputum, urine, and stool; WBC) at beginning of and during therapy.
- Obtain a history before initiating therapy to determine previous use of and reactions to penicillins, cephalosporins, or carbapenems. Persons with a negative history of penicillin sensitivity may still have an allergic response.
- Obtain specimens for culture and sensitivity before initiating therapy. First dose may be given before receiving results.
- Observe patient for signs and symptoms of anaphylaxis (rash, pruritus, laryngeal edema, wheezing). Discontinue the drug and notify the physician immediately if these occur. Have epinephrine, an antihistamine, and resuscitative equipment close by in the event of an anaphylactic reaction.
- *Lab Test Considerations:* May cause ↑ AST, ALT, serum alkaline phosphatase levels.
- May cause anemia.

Potential Nursing Diagnoses
Risk for infection (Indications, Side Effects)

Implementation
- May switch to appropriate oral therapy after at least 3 days of parenteral therapy, once clinical improvement has been demonstrated.

IV Administration
- **Intermittent Infusion:** Reconstitute 500-mg vial with 10 mL of sterile injection or 0.9% NaCl and shake gently to form a suspension of 50 mg/mL. *Diluent:* Withdraw the resulting solution using a 21-gauge needle and add it to 100 mL of 0.9% NaCl or D5W; gently shake until clear. *For moderate or severe renal impairment, withdraw 55 mL of this solution from the bag and discard.* Solution should be clear and colorless to slightly yellow. *Concentration:* Final concentration is 4.5 mg/mL. Suspension is stable for 1 hr prior to dilution in infusion bag. Administer within 8 hr of reconstitution with 0.9% NaCl or 4 hr of reconstitution with D5W at room temperature or 24 hr if refrigerated; do not freeze. *Rate:* Administer over 1 hr. Do not administer direct IV.
- **Y-Site Compatibility:** acyclovir, amikacin, aminophylline, amiodarone, anidulafungin, atropine, azithromycin, bumetanide, calcium gluconate, carboplatin, caspofungin, cimetidine, ciprofloxacin, cisplatin, cyclophosphamide, cyclosporine, daptomycin, dexametha-

sone, digoxin, diltiazem, diphenhydramine, dobutamine, docetaxel, dopamine, doxorubicin, enalaprilat, esmolol, esomeprazole, etoposide phosphate, famotidine, fentanyl, fluconazole, fluorouracil, foscarnet, fucosemide, gemcitabine, gentamicin, granisetron, heparin, hydrocortisone sodium succinate, hydromorphone, ifosfamide, insulin, labetalol, levofloxacin, linezolid, lorazepam, magnesium sulfate, mannitol, meperidine, methotrexate, methylprednisolone, metoclopramide, metronidazole, micafungin, midazolam, milrinone, morphine, moxifloxacin, norepinephrine, ondansetron, paclitaxel, pantoprazole, phenobarbital, phenylephrine, potassium chloride, ranitidine, sodium bicarbonate, sodium phosphate, tacrolimus, tigecycline, tobramycin, vancomycin, voriconazole, zidovudine.

- **Y-Site Incompatibility:** Do not mix with or physically add to solutions containing other medications, diazepam, potassium phosphate, propofol.

Patient/Family Teaching
- Advise patient to report the signs of superinfection (black, furry overgrowth on the tongue; vaginal itching or discharge; loose or foul-smelling stools) and allergy. Consult health care professional before treating with antidiarrheals.
- Caution patient to notify health care professional if fever and diarrhea occur, especially if stool contains blood, pus, or mucus. Advise patient not to treat diarrhea without consulting health care professional. May occur up to several weeks after discontinuation of medication.

Evaluation/Desired Outcomes
- Resolution of the signs and symptoms of infection. Length of time for complete resolution depends on the organism and site of infection. Duration may be extended up to 14 days for patients with concurrent bacteremia.

---

doxazosin (dox-ay-zoe-sin)
Cardura, Cardura XL

Classification
Therapeutic: antihypertensives
Pharmacologic: peripherally acting antiadrenergics

Pregnancy Category C

Indications
Hypertension (alone or with other agents) (immediate-release only). Symptomatic benign prostatic hyperplasia (BPH).

Action
Dilates both arteries and veins by blocking postsynaptic alpha$_1$-adrenergic receptors. **Therapeutic Effects:** Lowering of blood pressure. Increased urine flow and decreased symptoms of BPH.

Pharmacokinetics
Absorption: Well absorbed following oral administration.
Distribution: Probably enters breast milk; rest of distribution unknown.
Protein Binding: 98–99%.
Metabolism and Excretion: Extensively metabolized by the liver.
Half-life: 22 hr.

TIME/ACTION PROFILE

ROUTE	ONSET	PEAK	DURATION
PO†	1–2 hr	2–6 hr	24 hr
PO-XL‡	5 wk	unknown	unknown

† Antihypertensive effect
‡ Improved urinary flow and BPH symptoms

Contraindications/Precautions
Contraindicated in: Hypersensitivity.
Use Cautiously in: Hepatic dysfunction; Gastrointestinal narrowing (XL only); Geri: Appears on Beers list. Geriatric patients are at ↑ risk for hypotension; OB, Lactation, Pedi: Safety not established; Patients undergoing cataract surgery (↑ risk of intraoperative floppy iris syndrome).

Adverse Reactions/Side Effects
CNS: <u>dizziness</u>, <u>headache</u>, depression, drowsiness, fatigue, nervousness, weakness. **EENT:** abnormal vision, blurred vision, conjunctivitis, epistaxis, intraoperative floppy iris syndrome. **Resp:** dyspnea. **CV:** <u>first-dose orthostatic hypotension</u>, arrhythmias, chest pain, edema, palpitations. **GI:** abdominal discomfort, constipation, diarrhea, dry mouth, flatulence, nausea, vomiting. **GU:** ↓ libido, sexual dysfunction. **Derm:** flushing, rash, urticaria. **MS:** arthralgia, arthritis, gout, myalgia.

Interactions
Drug-Drug: ↑ risk of hypotension with **sildenafil**, **tadalafil**, **vardenafil**, other **antihypertensives**, **nitrates**, or acute ingestion of **alcohol**. **NSAIDs**, **sympathomimetics**, or **estrogens** may ↓ effects of antihypertensive therapy.

Route/Dosage
Hypertension
PO (Adults): —1 mg once daily, may be gradually ↑ at 2-wk intervals to 2–16 mg/day; incidence of postural hypotension greatly ↑ at doses >4 mg/day. *BPH*— 1 mg once daily, may be gradually increased to 8 mg/day.

Benign Prostatic Hyperplasia
PO (Adults): *Immediate release*— 1 mg once daily, may be ↑ every 1–2 wk up to 8 mg/day; *Extended release*— 4 mg once daily (with breakfast), may be ↑ in 3–4 wk to 8 mg/day.

Availability (generic available)
Tablets: 1 mg, 2 mg, 4 mg, 8 mg. **Cost:** *Generic*— 1 mg $49.97/90, 2 mg $43.97/90, 4 mg $59.97/90, 8 mg $62.99/90. **Extended-release tablets:** 4 mg, 8 mg.

NURSING IMPLICATIONS
Assessment
- Monitor blood pressure and pulse 2–6 hr after first dose, with each increase in dose, and periodically during therapy. Report significant changes.
- Assess for first-dose orthostatic hypotension and syncope. Incidence may be dose related. Observe patient closely during this period and take precautions to prevent injury.
- Monitor intake and output ratios and daily weight, and assess for edema daily, especially at beginning of therapy. Report weight gain or edema.
- **BPH:** Assess patient for symptoms of prostatic hyperplasia (urinary hesitancy, feeling of incomplete bladder emptying, interruption of urinary stream, impairment of size and force of urinary stream, terminal urinary dribbling, straining to start flow, dysuria, urgency) prior to and periodically during therapy.

Potential Nursing Diagnoses
Impaired urinary elimination (Indications)
Risk for injury (Side Effects)

Implementation
- Do not confuse Cardura (doxazosin) with Cardene (nicardipine) or Ridaura (auranofin).
- **PO:** Administer daily dose at bedtime.
- XL tablets should be swallowed whole; do not break, crush, or chew.
- **Hypertension:** May be administered concurrently with a diuretic or other antihypertensive.

Patient/Family Teaching
- Emphasize the importance of continuing to take this medication, even if feeling well. Instruct patient to take medication at the same time each day. Take missed doses as soon as remembered unless almost time for next dose. Do not double doses.
- May cause drowsiness or dizziness. Advise patient to avoid driving or other activities requiring alertness until response to medication is known.
- Caution patient to change positions slowly to decrease orthostatic hypotension.
- Advise patient to consult health care professional before taking any cough, cold, or allergy remedies or herbal products.
- Emphasize the importance of follow-up visits to determine effectiveness of therapy.
- **Hypertension:** Instruct patient and family on proper technique for blood pressure monitoring. Advise them to check blood pressure at least weekly and report significant changes.
- Encourage patient to comply with additional interventions for hypertension (weight reduction, low-sodium diet, smoking cessation, moderation of alcohol consumption, regular exercise, and stress management).

Evaluation/Desired Outcomes
- Decrease in blood pressure without appearance of side effects.
- Decrease in urinary symptoms of BPH.

---

doxepin (dox-e-pin)
Sinequan, ✣Triadapin, Zonalon

Classification
Therapeutic: antianxiety agents, antidepressants, antihistamines (topical)
Pharmacologic: tricyclic antidepressants

Pregnancy Category C

Indications
PO: Depression. **Topical:** Short-term control of pruritus associated with: Eczematous dermatitis, Lichen simplex chronicus. **Unlabeled Use: PO:** Chronic pain syndromes: Pruritus, Dermatitis, Anxiety, Insomnia.

Action
PO: Prevents the reuptake of norepinephrine and serotonin by presynaptic neurons; resultant accumulation of neurotransmitters potentiates their activity. Also possesses significant anticholinergic properties. **Topical:** Antipruritic action due to antihistaminic properties. **Therapeutic Effects: PO:** Relief of depression. Decreased anxiety.
Topical: Decreased pruritus.

Pharmacokinetics

Absorption: Well absorbed from the GI tract, although much is metabolized on first pass through the liver. Some systemic absorption follows topical application.

Distribution: Widely distributed. Enters breast milk; probably crosses the placenta.

Metabolism and Excretion: Metabolized by the liver. Some conversion to active antidepressant compound. May re-enter gastric juice via secretion from enterohepatic circulation, where more absorption may occur.

Half-life: 8–25 hr.

TIME/ACTION PROFILE (antidepressant activity)

ROUTE	ONSET	PEAK	DURATION
PO	2–3 wk	up to 6 wk	days–weeks

Contraindications/Precautions

Contraindicated in: Hypersensitivity; Some products contain bisulfites and should be avoided in patients with known intolerance; Untreated angle-closure glaucoma; Period immediately after myocardial infarction; history of QTc prolongation, heart failure, cardiac arrhythmia.

Use Cautiously in: Geri: Pre-existing cardiovascular disease (increased risk of adverse reactions); Prostatic enlargement (more susceptible to urinary retention); Seizures; OB: Use during pregnancy only if potential maternal benefit outweighs risks to fetus; use during lactation may result in neonatal sedation. Recommend discontinue drug or bottle-feed; Pedi: May ↑ risk of suicide attempt/ideation especially during dose early treatment or dose adjustment; risk may be greater in children or adolescents; Pedi: Safety not established in children <12 yr); Geri: Appears on *Beers list* and is associated with increased falls risk secondary to anticholinergic and sedative effects. Geriatric patients should have initial dosage reduction.

Adverse Reactions/Side Effects

CNS: fatigue, sedation, agitation, confusion, hallucinations. **EENT:** blurred vision, increased intraocular pressure. **CV:** hypotension, arrhythmias, ECG abnormalities. **GI:** constipation, dry mouth, hepatitis, increased appetite, weight gain, nausea, paralytic ileus. **GU:** urinary retention, decreased libido. **Derm:** photosensitivity, rashes. **Hemat:** blood dyscrasias. **Misc:** hypersensitivity reactions.

Interactions

Apply to both topical and oral use.

Drug-Drug: Doxepin is metabolized in the liver by the cytochrome P450 2D6 enzyme and its action may be affected by drugs that compete for metabolism by this enzyme including other **antidepressants**, **phenothiazines**, **carbamazepine**, **class 1C antiarrhythmics** (**propafenone**, **flecainide**); when used concurrently, dosage ↓ of one or the other or both may be necessary. Concurrent use of other drugs that inhibit the activity of the enzyme, including **cimetidine**, **quinidine**, **amiodarone**, and **ritonavir**, may result in ↑ effects of doxepin. May cause hypotension, tachycardia, and potentially fatal reactions when used with **MAO inhibitors** (avoid concurrent use—discontinue 2 wk prior to doxepin). Concurrent use with **SSRI antidepressants** may result in ↑ toxicity and should be avoided (fluoxetine should be stopped 5 wk before). Concurrent use with **clonidine** may result in hypertensive crisis and should be avoided. Concurrent use with **levodopa** may result in delayed/ ↓ absorption of levodopa or hypertension. Blood levels and effects may be ↓ by **rifamycins**. ↑ CNS depression with other **CNS depressants** including **alcohol**, **antihistamines**, **clonidine**, **opioid analgesics**, and **sedative/hypnotics**. **Barbiturates** may alter blood levels and effects. **Adrenergic** and **anticholinergic** side effects may be ↑ with other **agents having these properties**. **Phenothiazines** or **hormonal contraceptives** ↑ levels and may cause toxicity. **Smoking** may increase metabolism and alter effects.

Drug-Natural Products: Concomitant use of **kava-kava**, **valerian**, or **chamomile** can increase CNS depression. Increased anticholinergic effects with **jimson weed** and **scopolia**.

Route/Dosage

PO (Adults): *Antidepressant/antianxiety*—25 mg 3 times daily, may be increased as needed (up to 150 mg/day in outpatients or 300 mg/day in inpatients; some patients may require only 25–50 mg/day). Once stabilized, entire daily dose may be given at bedtime. *Antipruritic*—10 mg at bedtime initially, may be increased up to 25 mg.

PO (Geriatric Patients): *Antidepressant*— 25–50 mg/day initially, may be increased as needed.

Topical (Adults): Apply 4 times daily (wait 3–4 hr between applications) for up to 8 days.

Availability (generic available)
Capsules: 10 mg, 25 mg, 50 mg, 75 mg, 100 mg, 150 mg. **Oral concentrate:** 10 mg/mL. **Topical cream:** 5%.

NURSING IMPLICATIONS
Assessment
- Monitor blood pressure and pulse rate prior to and during initial therapy. Patients taking high doses or with a history of cardiovascular disease should have ECG monitored prior to and periodically during therapy.
- Assess for sexual dysfunction (decreased libido; erectile dysfunction).
- Assess weight and BMI initially and throughout treatment. Obtain FBS and cholesterol levels in overweight/obese individuals.
- Geri: Assess falls risk and institute fall prevention strategies. Assess for anticholinergic effects.
- **Depression:** Assess mental status (orientation, mood, behavior) frequently. Confusion, agitation, and hallucinations may occur during initiation of therapy and may require dosage reduction. Assess for suicidal tendencies, especially during early therapy. Restrict amount of drug available to patient.
- **Anxiety:** Assess degree and manifestations of anxiety prior to and during therapy.
- **Pain:** Assess the type, location, and severity of pain prior to and periodically during therapy. Use pain scale to assess effectiveness of therapy.
- **Topical:** Assess pruritic area prior to and periodically during therapy.
- *Lab Test Considerations:* Monitor WBC and differential blood counts, hepatic function, and serum glucose periodically. May cause ↑ serum bilirubin and alkaline phosphatase levels. May cause bone marrow depression. Serum glucose may be ↑ or ↓.

Potential Nursing Diagnoses
Ineffective coping (Indications)
Risk for injury (Side Effects)
Sexual dysfunction (Side Effects)

Implementation
- Do not confuse doxepin with doxycycline.
- May be given as a single dose at bedtime to minimize sedation during the day. Dose increases should be made at bedtime because of sedation. Dose titration is a slow process; may take weeks to months.
- To avoid withdrawal, taper by 50% for 3 days, then 50% again for 3 days, then discontinue.
- **PO:** Administer medication with or immediately following a meal to minimize gastric irritation. Capsules may be opened and mixed with foods or fluids if patient has difficulty swallowing.
- Oral concentrate must be diluted in at least 120 mL of water, milk, or fruit juice. Do not mix with carbonated beverages or grape juice. Use calibrated measuring device to ensure accurate amount.
- **Topical:** Apply thin film of doxepin cream only to affected areas, and rub in gently. Apply only to affected skin; not for ophthalmic, oral, or intravaginal use.

Patient/Family Teaching
- Inform patient that systemic side effects may occur with oral or topical use.
- May cause drowsiness and blurred vision. Caution patient to avoid driving and other activities requiring alertness until response to the medication is known.
- Orthostatic hypotension, sedation, and confusion are common during early therapy, especially in geriatric patients. Protect patient from falls. Institute fall precautions. Advise patient to change positions slowly.
- Advise patient to avoid alcohol or other CNS depressant drugs during and for at least 3–7 days after therapy has been discontinued.
- Instruct patient to notify health care professional if urinary retention occurs or if dry mouth or constipation persists. Sugarless candy or gum may diminish dry mouth, and an increase in fluid intake or bulk may prevent constipation. If symptoms persist, dose reduction or discontinuation may be necessary. Consult health care professional if dry mouth persists for more than 2 wk.
- Advise patient to notify health care professional of medication regimen prior to treatment or surgery.
- **PO:** Instruct patient to take medication as directed. Take missed doses as soon as possible unless almost time for next dose; if regimen is a single dose at bedtime, do not take in the morning because of side effects. Advise patient that drug effects may not be noticed for at least 2 wk. Abrupt discontinuation may cause nausea, vomiting, diarrhea, headache, trouble sleeping with vivid dreams, and irritability.
- Refer appropriate individuals for weight management.
- Caution patient to use sunscreen and protective clothing to prevent photosensitivity reactions.

- Inform patient that urine may turn blue-green in color.
- Inform patient of need to monitor dietary intake. Increase in appetite is possible and may lead to undesired weight gain.
- Therapy for depression is usually prolonged. Emphasize the importance of follow-up exams to monitor effectiveness and side effects.
- Refer patient to psychotherapy to improve coping skills and to local support group.
- **Topical:** Instruct patient to apply a thin film of medication exactly as directed; do not use more medication than directed, apply to a larger area than directed, use more often than directed, or use longer than 8 days.
- Inform patient that topical preparation may cause burning, stinging, swelling, increased itching, or worsening of eczema. Notify health care professional if these symptoms become bothersome.
- Caution patient not to use occlusive dressings; may increase systemic absorption.
- Advise patient to notify health care professional if excessive drowsiness occurs with topical application. Number of applications per day, amount of cream applied, or area of application may be reduced. May require discontinuation of therapy.

Evaluation/Desired Outcomes
- Increased sense of well-being.
- Renewed interest in surroundings.
- Increased appetite.
- Improved energy level.
- Improved sleep.
- Decrease in anxiety.
- Decrease in chronic pain. Patients may require 2–6 wk of oral therapy before full therapeutic effects of medication are evident.
- Decrease in pruritus associated with eczema.

doxercalciferol, See VITAMIN D COMPOUNDS.

HIGH ALERT

DOXOrubicin
(dox-oh-**roo**-bi-sin)
Adriamycin PFS, Adriamycin RDF, Rubex

Classification
Therapeutic: antineoplastics
Pharmacologic: anthracyclines

Pregnancy Category D

Indications
Alone or with other modalities in the treatment of various solid tumors including: Breast, Ovarian, Bladder, Bronchogenic carcinoma, Malignant lymphomas and leukemias.

Action
Inhibits DNA and RNA synthesis by forming a complex with DNA; action is cell-cycle S-phase–specific. Also has immunosuppressive properties.
Therapeutic Effects: Death of rapidly replicating cells, particularly malignant ones.

Pharmacokinetics
Absorption: Administered IV only, resulting in complete bioavailability.
Distribution: Widely distributed; does not cross the blood-brain barrier; extensively bound to tissues.
Metabolism and Excretion: Mostly metabolized by the liver. Converted by liver to an active compound. Excreted predominantly in the bile, 50% as unchanged drug. Less than 5% eliminated unchanged in the urine.
Half-life: 16.7 hr.

TIME/ACTION PROFILE (effect on blood counts)

ROUTE	ONSET	PEAK	DURATION
IV	10 days	14 days	21–24 days

Contraindications/Precautions
Contraindicated in: Hypersensitivity; OB, Lactation: Pregnancy or lactation.
Use Cautiously in: History of cardiac disease or high cumulative doses of anthracyclines; Depressed bone marrow reserve; Liver impairment (reduce dose if serum bilirubin >1.2 mg/dL); Children, geriatric patients, mediastinal radiation, concurrent cyclophosphamide (risk of cardiotoxicity); OB: Patients with childbearing potential.

Adverse Reactions/Side Effects
Resp: recall pneumonitis. **CV:** CARDIOMYOPATHY, ECG changes. **GI:** diarrhea, esophagitis, nausea, stomatitis, vomiting. **GU:** red urine. **Derm:** alopecia, photosensitivity. **Endo:** sterility, prepubertal growth failure with temporary gonadal impairment (children only). **Hemat:** anemia, leuko-

penia, thrombocytopenia. **Local:** phlebitis at IV site, tissue necrosis. **Metab:** hyperuricemia. **Misc:** hypersensitivity reactions.

Interactions
Drug-Drug: ↑ bone marrow depression with other **antineoplastics** or **radiation therapy**. Pediatric patients who have received concurrent doxorubicin and **dactinomycin** have an ↑ risk of recall pneumonitis at variable times following local radiation therapy. May ↑ skin reactions at previous **radiation therapy** sites. If **paclitaxel** is administered first, clearance of doxorubicin is ↓ and the incidence and severity of neutropenia and stomatitis are ↑ (problem is diminished if doxorubicin is administered first). Hematologic toxicity is ↑ and prolonged by concurrent use of **cyclosporine**; risk of coma and seizures is also ↑. Incidence and severity of neutropenia and thrombocytopenia are ↑ by concurrent **progesterone**. **Phenobarbital** may ↑ clearance and decrease effects of doxorubicin. Doxorubicin may ↓ metabolism and ↑ effects of **phenytoin**. **Streptozocin** may ↑ the half-life of doxorubicin (dosage ↓ of doxorubicin recommended). May ↑ risk of hemorrhagic cystitis from **cyclophosphamide** or hepatitis from **mercaptopurine**. Cardiac toxicity may be ↑ by **radiation therapy** or **cyclophosphamide**. May ↓ antibody response to **live-virus vaccines** and ↑ risk of adverse reactions.

Route/Dosage
Other regimens are used.
IV (Adults): 60–75 mg/m² daily, repeat q 21 days; or 25–30 mg/m² daily for 2–3 days, repeat q 3–4 wk or 20 mg/m²/wk. Total cumulative dose should not exceed 550 mg/m² without monitoring of cardiac function or 400 mg/m² in patients with previous chest radiation or other cardiotoxic chemotherapy.
IV (Children): 30 mg/m²/day for 3 days every 4 wk.

Hepatic Impairment
IV (Adults): Serum bilirubin 1.2–3mg/dL—50% of usual dose; serum bilirubin 3.1–5 mg/dL—25% of usual dose.

Availability (generic available)
Powder for injection: 10-mg, 20-mg, 50-mg, 100-mg, 150-mg vials. **Injection:** 2 mg/mL.

NURSING IMPLICATIONS
Assessment
- Monitor blood pressure, pulse, respiratory rate, and temperature frequently during administration. Report significant changes.
- Monitor for bone marrow depression. Assess for bleeding (bleeding gums, bruising, petechiae, guaiac stools, urine, and emesis) and avoid IM injections and taking rectal temperatures if platelet count is low. Apply pressure to venipuncture sites for 10 min. Assess for signs of infection during neutropenia. Anemia may occur. Monitor for increased fatigue, dyspnea, and orthostatic hypotension.
- Monitor intake and output ratios, and report occurrence of significant discrepancies. Encourage fluid intake of 2000–3000 mL/day. Allopurinol and alkalinization of the urine may be used to decrease serum uric acid levels and to help prevent urate stone formation.
- Severe and protracted nausea and vomiting may occur as early as 1 hr after therapy and may last 24 hr. Administer parenteral antiemetics 30–45 min prior to therapy and routinely around the clock for the next 24 hr as indicated. Monitor amount of emesis and notify physician or other health care professional if emesis exceeds guidelines to prevent dehydration.
- Monitor for development of signs of cardiac toxicity, which may be either acute and transient (ST segment depression, flattened T wave, sinus tachycardia, and extrasystoles) or late onset (usually occurs 1–6 mo after initiation of therapy) and characterized by intractable CHF (peripheral edema, dyspnea, rales/crackles, weight gain). Chest x-ray, echocardiography, ECGs, and radionuclide angiography may be ordered prior to and periodically during therapy. Cardiotoxicity is more prevalent in children younger than 2 yr and geriatric patients. Dexrazoxane may be used to prevent cardiotoxicity in patients receiving cumulative doses of >300 mg/m².
- Assess injection site frequently for redness, irritation, or inflammation. Doxorubicin is a vesicant but may infiltrate painlessly even if blood returns on aspiration of infusion needle. Severe tissue damage may occur if doxorubicin extravasates. If extravasation occurs, stop infusion immediately, restart, and complete dose in another vein. Local infiltration of antidote is not recommended. Apply ice packs and elevate and rest extremity for 24–48 hr to reduce swelling, then resume normal activity as tolerated. If swelling, redness, and/or pain persists beyond 48 hr, immediate consultation for possible debridement is indicated.
- Assess oral mucosa frequently for development of stomatitis. Increased dosing interval and/or

decreased dosing is recommended if lesions are painful or interfere with nutrition.
- **Lab Test Considerations:** Monitor CBC and differential prior to and periodically during therapy. The WBC nadir occurs 10–14 days after administration, and recovery usually occurs by the 21st day. Thrombocytopenia and anemia may also occur. Increased dosing interval and/or decreased dose is recommended if ANC is <1000 cells/mm³ and/or platelet count is <50,000 cells/mm³.
- Monitor renal (BUN and creatinine) and hepatic (AST, ALT, LDH, and serum bilirubin) function prior to and periodically during therapy. Dose reduction is required for bilirubin >1.2 mg/dL or serum creatinine >3 mg/dL.
- May cause ↑ serum and urine uric acid concentrations.

Potential Nursing Diagnoses
Risk for infection (Adverse Reactions)
Decreased cardiac output (Adverse Reactions)

Implementation
- ***High Alert:*** Fatalities have occurred with incorrect administration of chemotherapeutic agents. Before administering, clarify all ambiguous orders; double check single, daily, and course-of-therapy dose limits; have second practitioner independently double check original order, calculations and infusion pump settings. Do not confuse doxorubicin hydrochloride (Adriamycin, Rubex) with doxorubicin hydrochloride liposome (Doxil) or with daunorubicin hydrochloride (Cerubidine) or daunorubicin citrate liposome (DaunoXome) or with idarubicin.. Do not confuse adriamycin with idamycin. Clarify orders that do not include generic and brand names.
- Solution should be prepared in a biologic cabinet. Wear gloves, gown, and mask while handling medication. Discard IV equipment in specially designated containers (see Appendix L).
- Aluminum needles may be used to administer doxorubicin but should not be used during storage, because prolonged contact results in discoloration of solution and formation of a dark precipitate. Solution is red.

IV Administration
- **Direct IV:** ***Diluent:*** Dilute each 10 mg with 5 mL of 0.9% NaCl (nonbacteriostatic) for injection. Shake to dissolve completely. Do not add to IV solution. Reconstituted medication is stable for 24 hr at room temperature and 48 hr if refrigerated. Protect from sunlight. ***Concentration:*** 2 mg/mL. ***Rate:*** Administer each dose over 3–5 minutes through Y-site of a free-flowing infusion of 0.9% NaCl or D5W. Facial flushing and erythema along involved vein frequently occur when administration is too rapid.
- **Y-Site Compatibility:** alfentanil, amifostine, anidulafungin, aztreonam, bivalirudin, bleomycin, bumetanide, buprenorphine, butorphanol, calcium chloride, calcium gluconate, carboplatin, caspofungin, ceftizoxime, chlorpromazine, cimetidine, ciprofloxacin, cisplatin, cladribine, clindamycin, cyclophosphamide, cyclosporine, cytarabine, dactinomycin, daptomycin, dexamethasone, dexmedetomidine, dexrazoxane, diltiazem, diphenhydramine, dobutamine, docetaxel, dolasetron, dopamine, doripenem, doxycycline, droperidol, enalaprilat, ephedrine, epinephrine, erythromycin, esmolol, etoposide, etoposide phosphate, famotidine, fenoldopam, fentanyl, filgrastim, fluconazole, fludarabine, gemcitabine, gentamicin, granisetron, haloperidol, hydrocortisone, hydromorphone, ifosfamide, imipenem cilastatin, inamrinone, isoproterenol, ketorolac, labetalol, leucovorin calcium, levorphanol, lidocaine, linezolid, lorazepam, mannitol, mechlorethamine, melphalan, meperidine, mesna, methotrexate, metoclopramide, metoprolol, metronidazole, midazolam, milrinone, mitomycin, morphine, nalbuphine, naloxone, nesiritide, nicardipine, nitroglycerin, nitroprusside, octreotide, ofloxacin, ondansetron, oxaliplatin, paclitaxel, palonosetron, pancuronium, phenylephrine, potassium chloride, procainamide, prochlorperazine, promethazine, propranolol, quinupristin/dalfopristin, ranitidine, sargramostim, sodium acetate, tacrolimus, teniposide, theophylline, thiotepa, ticarcillin/clavulanate, tigecycline, tirofiban, tobramycin, topotecan, trastuzumab, trimethobenzamide, vancomycin, vasopression, vecuronium, verapamil, vinblastine, vincristine, vinorelbine, zidovudine.
- **Y-Site Incompatibility:** acyclovir, allopurinol, aminophylline, amiodarone, amphotericin B cholesteryl, amphotericin B colloidal, amphotericin B liposome, ampicillin, ampicillin/sulbactam, cefazolin, cefepime, cefoperazone, cefotaxime, cefotetan, cefoxitin, ceftazidime, ceftriaxone, cefuroxime, diazepam, digoxin, er-

tapenem, foscarnet, fosphenytoin, ganciclovir, magnesium sulfate, meropenem, methohexital, pantoprazole, pemetrexed, pentamidine, pentobarbital, phenobarbital, phenytoin, piperacillin/tazobactam, potassium phosphates, propofol, rituximab, sodium phosphates, thiopental, trimethoprim/sufamethoxazole, voriconazole.

Patient/Family Teaching
- Instruct patient to notify health care professional promptly if fever; sore throat; signs of infection; bleeding gums; bruising; petechiae; blood in stools, urine, or emesis; increased fatigue; dyspnea; or orthostatic hypotension occurs. Caution patient to avoid crowds and persons with known infections. Instruct patient to use soft toothbrush and electric razor and to avoid falls. Caution patient not to drink alcoholic beverages or take medication containing aspirin or NSAIDs, because these may precipitate gastric bleeding.
- Instruct patient to report pain at injection site immediately.
- Instruct patient to inspect oral mucosa for erythema and ulceration. If ulceration occurs, advise patient to use sponge brush, rinse mouth with water after eating and drinking, and confer with health care professional if mouth pain interferes with eating. Pain may require treatment with opioid analgesics. The risk of developing stomatitis is greatest 5–10 days after a dose; the usual duration is 3–7 days.
- Advise patient that this medication may have teratogenic effects. Contraception should be used during and for at least 4 mo after therapy is concluded. Inform patient before initiating therapy that this medication may cause irreversible gonadal suppression.
- Instruct patient to notify health care professional immediately if irregular heartbeat, shortness of breath, swelling of lower extremities, or skin irritation (swelling, pain, or redness of feet or hands) occurs.
- Discuss the possibility of hair loss with patient. Explore methods of coping. Regrowth usually occurs 2–3 mo after discontinuation of therapy.
- Instruct patient not to receive any vaccinations without advice of health care professional.
- Inform patient that medication may cause urine to appear red for 1–2 days.
- Instruct patient to notify health care professional if skin irritation occurs at site of previous radiation therapy.
- Advise family and/or caregivers to take precautions (i.e., latex gloves) in handling body fluids for at least 5 days posttreatment.
- Emphasize the need for periodic lab tests to monitor for side effects.

Evaluation/Desired Outcomes
- Decrease in size or spread of malignancies in solid tumors.
- Improvement of hematologic status in leukemias.

HIGH ALERT

DOXOrubicin, liposomal
(dox-oh-**roo**-bi-sin **lye**-poe-sohm-al)
Doxil

Classification
Therapeutic: antineoplastics
Pharmacologic: anthracyclines

Pregnancy Category D

Indications
AIDS-related Kaposi's sarcoma (KS) in patients who cannot tolerate or fail conventional therapy. Ovarian carcinoma. Multiple myeloma with bortezomib in patients who have not previously received bortezomib and have received at least one prior therapy.

Action
Inhibits DNA and RNA synthesis by forming a complex with DNA; action is cell-cycle S-phase–specific. Also has immunosuppressive properties. Encapsulation in a liposome increases uptake by tumors, prolongs action, and may decrease some toxicity. **Therapeutic Effects:** Death of rapidly replicating cells, particularly malignant ones.

Pharmacokinetics
Absorption: Administered IV only, resulting in complete bioavailability.
Distribution: Widely distributed; does not cross the blood-brain barrier; extensively bound to tissues (↑ concentrations delivered to KS lesions due to liposomal carrier).
Metabolism and Excretion: Mostly metabolized by the liver with conversion to an active compound. Excreted mostly in bile, 50% as unchanged drug. <5% eliminated unchanged in the urine.
Half-life: 55 hr.

DOXOrubicin, liposomal **483**

TIME/ACTION PROFILE (effect on blood counts)

ROUTE	ONSET	PEAK	DURATION
IV	10 days	14 days	21–24 days

Contraindications/Precautions
Contraindicated in: Hypersensitivity; OB: Pregnancy or lactation.
Use Cautiously in: Pre-existing cardiac disease or ↑ cumulative doses of anthracyclines; Depressed bone marrow reserve; Liver impairment (dose reduction required if serum bilirubin >1.2 mg/dL); Geri, Pedi: Children, geriatric patients, prior mediastinal radiation, concurrent cyclophosphamide (increased risk of cardiotoxicity); OB: Patients with childbearing potential.

Adverse Reactions/Side Effects
CNS: weakness. **CV:** CARDIOMYOPATHY. **GI:** nausea, diarrhea, increased alkaline phosphatase, moniliasis, stomatitis, vomiting. **Derm:** alopecia, palmar-plantar erythrodysesthesia. **Hemat:** anemia, leukopenia, thrombocytopenia. **Local:** injection site reactions. **Misc:** ANAPHYLACTOID ALLERGIC REACTIONS, acute infusion-related reactions, fever.

Interactions
Drug-Drug: ↑ bone marrow depression with other **antineoplastics** or **radiation therapy**. Pediatric patients who have received concurrent doxorubicin and **dactinomycin** have ↑ risk of recall pneumonitis following local radiation therapy. May ↑ skin reactions at previous **radiation therapy** sites. If **paclitaxel** is administered first, clearance of doxorubicin is ↓ and incidence and severity of neutropenia and stomatitis are ↑ (problem is less if doxorubicin is administered first). Hematologic toxicity is ↑ by concurrent use of **cyclosporine**; risk of coma and seizures is also ↑. Incidence and severity of neutropenia and thrombocytopenia are ↑ by concurrent **progesterone**. **Phenobarbital** may ↑ clearance and ↓ effects of doxorubicin. Doxorubicin may ↓ metabolism and ↑ effects of **phenytoin**. **Streptozocin** may ↑ the half-life of doxorubicin (dose reduction of doxorubicin recommended). May ↑ risk of hemorrhagic cystitis from **cyclophosphamide** or hepatitis from **mercaptopurine**. Cardiac toxicity may be ↑ by **radiation therapy** or **cyclophosphamide**. May ↓ antibody response to **live-virus vaccines** and ↑ risk of adverse reactions.

Route/Dosage
Other regimens are used.
IV (Adults): *AIDS-related KS*—20 mg/m² every 3 wk; *Metastatic ovarian cancer*—40–50 mg/m² every 4 wk; *Multiple myeloma*—30 mg/m² on day 4 after following borezomib for up to 8 cycles.

Availability
Liposomal dispersion for injection: 20 mg/10 mL in 10-mL and 25-mL vials.

NURSING IMPLICATIONS
Assessment
- Monitor blood pressure, pulse, respiratory rate, and temperature frequently during administration. Report significant changes.
- Monitor for acute infusion-related reactions consisting of flushing, shortness of breath, facial swelling, headache, chills, chest pain, back pain, chest or throat tightness, fever, tachycardia, pruritus, rash, cyanosis, syncope, bronchospasm, asthma, apnea, which may be accompanied by hypotension. Reactions usually resolve over 1 day and are usually limited to first dose. Slowing infusion rate may minimize this reaction. Reaction is thought to be due to liposome.
- Observe for signs and symptoms of anaphylaxis (rash, pruritus, laryngeal edema, wheezing). Discontinue doxorubicin and notify health care professional immediately if these problems occur. Keep epinephrine, an antihistamine, and resuscitation equipment close by in case of an anaphylactic reaction.
- Monitor for bone marrow depression. Assess for bleeding (bleeding gums, bruising, petechiae, guaiac stools, urine, and emesis) and avoid IM injections and taking rectal temperatures if platelet count is low. Apply pressure to venipuncture sites for 10 min. Assess for signs of infection during neutropenia. Anemia may occur. Monitor for increased fatigue, dyspnea, and orthostatic hypotension.
- Monitor intake and output ratios, and report occurrence of significant discrepancies. Encourage fluid intake of 2000–3000 mL/day. Allopurinol and alkalinization of the urine may be used to decrease serum uric acid levels and to help prevent urate stone formation.
- Severe and protracted nausea and vomiting may occur as early as 1 hr after therapy and may last 24 hr. Administer parenteral antiemetics 30–45 min prior to therapy and routinely

✶ = Canadian drug name. ✇ = Genetic implication.
*CAPITALS indicates life-threatening; underlines indicate most frequent.

around the clock for the next 24 hr as indicated. Monitor amount of emesis and notify health care professional if emesis exceeds guidelines to prevent dehydration.
- Monitor for development of signs of cardiac toxicity, which may be either acute and transient (ST segment depression, flattened T wave, sinus tachycardia, and extrasystoles) or late onset (usually occurs 1–6 mo after initiation of therapy) and characterized by intractable CHF (peripheral edema, dyspnea, rales/crackles, weight gain); occurs more frequently in patients receiving a cumulative dose of ≥550 mg/m^2. Chest x-ray, echocardiography, ECGs, and radionuclide angiography may be ordered prior to and periodically during therapy. Cardiotoxicity is more prevalent in children younger than 2 yr and geriatric patients. Dexrazoxane may be used to prevent cardiotoxicity in patients receiving cumulative doses of >300 mg/m^2.
- Assess injection site frequently for redness, irritation, or inflammation. Doxorubicin is a vesicant but may infiltrate painlessly even if blood returns on aspiration of infusion needle. Severe tissue damage may occur if doxorubicin extravasates. If extravasation occurs, stop infusion immediately, restart, and complete dose in another vein. Local infiltration of antidote is not recommended. Apply ice packs and elevate and rest extremity for 24–48 hr to reduce swelling, then resume normal activity as tolerated. If swelling, redness, and/or pain persists beyond 48 hr, immediate consultation for possible debridement is indicated.
- Assess oral mucosa frequently for development of stomatitis. Increased dosing interval and/or decreased dose is recommended if lesions are painful or interfere with nutrition.
- Monitor for skin toxicity with prolonged use; palmar-plantar erythrodysesthesia usually occurs after 6 wk of treatment and consists of swelling, pain, and erythema of the hands and feet. This may progress to desquamation but usually regresses after 2 wk. In severe cases, modification and delay of future doses of doxorubicin liposome may be necessary.
- **Lab Test Considerations:** Monitor CBC and differential prior to and periodically during therapy. The WBC nadir occurs 10–14 days after administration, and recovery usually occurs by the 21st day. Thrombocytopenia and anemia may also occur. ↑ dosing interval and/or ↓ dose is recommended if ANC is <1000 cells/mm^3 and/or platelet count is <50,000 cells/mm^3.
- Monitor renal (BUN and creatinine) and hepatic (AST, ALT, LDH, and serum bilirubin) function prior to and periodically during therapy. Dose reduction is required for bilirubin >1.2 mg/dL or serum creatinine >3 mg/dL.
- May cause ↑ serum and urine uric acid concentrations.

Potential Nursing Diagnoses
Risk for infection (Adverse Reactions)
Decreased cardiac output (Adverse Reactions)

Implementation
- ***High Alert:*** Fatalities have occurred with incorrect administration of chemotherapeutic agents. Before administering, clarify all ambiguous orders; double check single, daily, and course-of-therapy dose limits; have second practitioner independently double check original order, calculations, and infusion pump settings. Do not confuse doxorubicin hydrochloride liposome (Doxil) with doxorubicin hydrochloride (Adriamycin, Rubex) or with daunorubicin hydrochloride (Cerubidine) or daunorubicin citrate liposome (DaunoXome). Clarify orders that do not include generic and brand names.
- Prepare solution in a biologic cabinet. Wear gloves, gown, and mask while handling medication. Discard IV equipment in specially designated containers.
- Aluminum needles may be used to administer doxorubicin but should not be used during storage, because prolonged contact results in discoloration of solution and formation of a dark precipitate. Solution is red.

IV Administration
- **Intermittent Infusion:** ***Diluent:*** Dilute dose, up to 90 mg, in 250 mL of D5W. Do not dilute with other diluents or diluents containing a bacteriostatic agent. Solution is not clear, but a translucent red liposomal dispersion. Do not use in-line filters. Refrigerate diluted solutions and administer within 24 hr of dilution. ***Concentration:*** 0.36 mg/mL. ***Rate:*** Initial rate of infusion should be 1 mg/min to minimize risk of infusion reactions. If no reactions occur, increase rate to complete administration within 1 hr. Do not administer as a bolus or undiluted solution. Rapid infusion may increase infusion-related reactions.
- **Y-Site Compatibility:** acyclovir, allopurinol, aminophylline, ampicillin, aztreonam, bleomycin, butorphanol, calcium gluconate, carboplatin, cefazolin, cefepime, cefoxitin, ceftizoxime, ceftriaxone, chlorpromazine, cimetidine, cip-

rofloxacin, cisplatin, clindamycin, cyclophosphamide, cytarabine, dacarbazine, dexamethasone sodium phosphate, diphenhydramine, dobutamine, dopamine, droperidol, enalaprilat, etoposide, famotidine, fluconazole, fluorouracil, furosemide, ganciclovir, gentamicin, granisetron, haloperidol, heparin, hydrocortisone sodium succinate, hydromorphone, ifosfamide, leucovorin, lorazepam, magnesium sulfate, mesna, methotrexate, methylprednisolone sodium succinate, metronidazole, ondansetron, piperacillin, potassium chloride, prochlorperazine, ranitidine, ticarcillin/clavulanate, tobramycin, trimethoprim/sulfamethoxazole, vancomycin, vinblastine, vincristine, vinorelbine, zidovudine.

- **Y-Site Incompatibility:** amphotericin B, amphotericin B cholesteryl sulfate complex, buprenorphine, cefoperazone, ceftazidime, docetaxel, mannitol, meperidine, metoclopramide, mitoxantrone, morphine, ofloxacin, paclitaxel, piperacillin/tazobactam, promethazine, sodium bicarbonate.
- **Additive Incompatibility:** Do not admix with other solutions or medications.

Patient/Family Teaching

- Instruct patient to notify health care professional promptly if fever; sore throat; signs of infection; bleeding gums; bruising; petechiae; blood in stools, urine, or emesis; increased fatigue; dyspnea; or orthostatic hypotension occurs. Caution patient to avoid crowds and persons with known infections. Instruct patient to use soft toothbrush and electric razor and to avoid falls. Caution patient not to drink alcoholic beverages or take medication containing aspirin or NSAIDs; may precipitate gastric bleeding.
- Instruct patient to report pain at injection site immediately.
- Instruct patient to inspect oral mucosa for erythema and ulceration. If ulceration occurs, advise patient to use sponge brush, rinse mouth with water after eating and drinking, and confer with health care professional if mouth pain interferes with eating. Pain may require treatment with opioid analgesics. The risk of developing stomatitis is greatest 5–10 days after a dose; the usual duration is 3–7 days.
- Advise patient that this medication may have teratogenic effects. Contraception should be used during and for at least 4 mo after therapy is concluded. Inform patient before initiating therapy that this medication may cause irreversible gonadal suppression.
- Instruct patient to notify health care professional immediately if irregular heartbeat, shortness of breath, swelling of lower extremities, or skin irritation (swelling, pain, or redness of feet or hands) occurs.
- Discuss the possibility of hair loss with patient. Explore methods of coping. Regrowth usually occurs 2–3 mo after discontinuation of therapy.
- Instruct patient not to receive any vaccinations without advice of health care professional.
- Inform patient that medication may cause urine to appear red for 1–2 days.
- Instruct patient to notify health care professional if skin irritation occurs at site of previous radiation therapy.
- Advise family and/or caregivers to take precautions (i.e., latex gloves) in handling body fluids for at least 5 days posttreatment.
- Emphasize the need for periodic lab tests to monitor for side effects.

Evaluation/Desired Outcomes

- Decrease in size or spread of malignancies.
- Arrested progression of KS in patients with HIV infection.

---

doxycycline, See TETRACYCLINES.

---

dronedarone (dro-ned-a-rone)
Multaq

Classification
Therapeutic: antiarrhythmics
Pharmacologic: benzofurans

Pregnancy Category X

Indications
Reduces the risk of hospitalization in patients with paroxysmal or persistent atrial fibrillation (AF) or atrial flutter (AFL), who have had a recent episode of AF/AFL and have other cardiovascular risk factors and are currently in sinus rhythm or plan to be cardioverted.

Action
Has several antiarrhythmic properties; prolongs PR and QTc intervals. **Therapeutic Effects:** Suppression of AF/AFL.

dronedarone

Pharmacokinetics
Absorption: Poor bioavailability (4%) due to extensive first pass hepatic metabolism (4%) food increases bioavailability (15%).
Distribution: Unknown.
Protein Binding: >98%.
Metabolism and Excretion: Undergoes extensive first pass hepatic metabolism; mostly by the CYP3A enzyme system. 6% excreted in urine as metabolites, 84% was excreted in feces as metabolites. Minimal elimination as unchanged drug.
Half-life: 13–19 hr.

TIME/ACTION PROFILE (antiarrhythmic effect)

ROUTE	ONSET	PEAK	DURATION
PO	unknown†	3–6 hr‡	12 hr

† Steady state blood levels are attained at 4–8 days
‡ Peak levels after individual doses

Contraindications/Precautions
Contraindicated in: Class IV heart failure or Class II–III heart failure with recent decompensation; Second- or third-degree atrioventricular (AV) block or sick sinus syndrome (unless a pacemaker is present); Heart rate <50 bpm; Concurrent use of strong CYP3A inhibitors or drugs/herbal products that prolong the QT interval; QTc interval ≥500 ms; Concurrent use of Class I or III antiarrhythmics including amiodarone, flecainide, propafenone, quinidine, disopyramide, dofetilide and sotalol; must be discontinued prior to treatment; Severe hepatic impairment; OB: Pregnancy (may cause fetal harm); Lactation: Avoid use during lactation.
Use Cautiously in: New/worsening heart failure; Hypokalemia or hypomagnesemia (may ↑ risk of arrhythmias); Mild or moderate hepatic impairment; OB: Women with childbearing potential; contraception should be used; Pedi: Safey and effectiveness in patients <18 yr not established.

Adverse Reactions/Side Effects
CNS: weakness. **CV:** CHF, QTc prolongation. **GI:** abdominal pain, diarrhea, nausea, taste abnormality, vomiting. **Derm:** photosensitivity.

Interactions
Drug-Drug: Dronedarone is metabolized by CYP-3A and is a moderate inhibitor of CYP3A and CYP2D6 enzyme systems; interactions may occur with other drugs that are substrates for or are metabolized by theses systems. Dronedarone also inhibits P-gP, which can result in ↑ absorption of certain drugs. Concurrent use of **strong CYP3A inhibitors** including **ketoconazole, itraconazole, voriconazole, cyclosporine, telithromycin, clarithromycin, nefazodone,** and **ritonavir** or **drugs that prolong the QT interval** including **phenothiazine antipsychotics, tricyclic antidepressants,** some oral **macrolide antibiotics** and other **Class I and III antiarrhythmics** ↑ risk of serious adverse cardiovascular reactions and should be avoided. Concurrent use of CYP3A4 inducers including **rifampin, phenobarbital, carbamazepine,** or **phenytoin** ↓ blood levels and effectiveness and should be avoided. ↑ **digoxin** levels and the risk of toxicity (discontinue or ↓ dose by 50% before treatment and monitor carefully). Avoid concurrent use of other **antiarrhythmics,** including **amiodarone, flecainide, propafenone, quinidine, disopyramide, dofetilide,** and **sotalol** due to ↑ risk of adverse cardiovascular reactions; discontinue prior to dronedarone therapy (concurrent use is contraindicated). Concurrent use of **calcium channel blockers** ↑ risk of adverse cardiovascular reactions (initiate at lower dose and increase only after ECG evaluation). Concurrent use of **betablockers** ↑ risk of bradycardia (initiate at lower dose and increase only after ECG evaluation). May also ↑ levels and effects of **tricyclic antidepressants,** and **selective serotonin reuptake inhibitors (SSRIs).** May ↑ levels and risk of toxicity of some **HMG-CoA reductase inhibitors (statins),** see recommendations for specific agents. Concurrent use with **CYP 3A substrates** including **sirolimus** and **tacrolimus** may ↑ risk of serious adverse reactions; monitor and adjust dosage carefully.
Drug-Natural Products: St. John's wort ↓ blood levels and may ↓ effectiveness; avoid concurrent use.
Drug-Food: Grapefruit juice may ↑ levels and the risk of toxicity; avoid concurrent ingestion.

Route/Dosage
PO (Adults): 400 mg twice daily.

Availability
Tablets: 400 mg.

NURSING IMPLICATIONS

Assessment
- Assess for signs and symptoms of atrial fibrillation or atrial flutter (palpitations, abnormal ECG) periodically during therapy.
- Monitor ECG periodically during therapy. If QTc ≥500 ms discontinue therapy.
- *Lab Test Considerations:* Monitor serum potassium and magnesium levels during therapy and maintain within normal range. May cause hypokalemia and hypomagnesemia.

droperidol **487**

- Serum creatinine levels increase by about 0.1 mg/dL following initiation of therapy with a rapid onset and plateau after 7 days; reversible with discontinuation. If increase and plateau occurs, use increased value as new baseline.

Potential Nursing Diagnoses
Decreased cardiac output (Indications)

Implementation
- **PO:** Administer twice daily with morning and evening meals.

Patient/Family Teaching
- Instruct patient to take dronederone as directed. Do not stop taking dronederone, even if feeling better without consulting health care professional. If a dose is missed, omit and take next dose at regularly scheduled time; do not double dose. Advise patient to read *Medication Guide* before starting therapy and with each Rx refill; there may be new information.
- Advise patient to avoid grapefruit juice during therapy.
- Advise patient to notify health care professional if signs and symptoms of heart failure (weight gain, dependent edema, increasing shortness of breath) occur.
- Advise patient to consult health care professional before taking other Rx, OTC, or herbal products, especially St. John's wort.
- May be teratogenic. Caution female patients of childbearing yr to use effective contraception during therapy and to notify health care professional if pregnancy is planned or suspected or if breastfeeding.

Evaluation/Desired Outcomes
- Reduction in hospitalization of patients with paroxysmal or persistent atrial fibrillation or atrial flutter.

---

droperidol (droe-**per**-i-dole)
Inapsine

Classification
Therapeutic: sedative/hypnotics
Pharmacologic: butyrophenones

Pregnancy Category C

Indications
Used to produce tranquilization and as an adjunct to general and regional anesthesia. **Unlabeled Use:** Useful in decreasing postoperative or postprocedure nausea and vomiting.

Action
Similar to haloperidol—alters the action of dopamine in the CNS. **Therapeutic Effects:** Tranquilization. Suppression of nausea and vomiting in selected situations.

Pharmacokinetics
Absorption: Well absorbed following IM administration.
Distribution: Appears to cross the blood-brain barrier and placenta.
Metabolism and Excretion: Mainly metabolized by the liver. Only 10% excreted unchanged by the kidneys.
Half-life: 2.2 hr.

TIME/ACTION PROFILE (sedation)

ROUTE	ONSET	PEAK	DURATION*
IM, IV	3–10 min	30 min	2–4 hr

*Listed as duration of tranquilization; alterations in consciousness may last up to 12 hr

Contraindications/Precautions
Contraindicated in: Hypersensitivity; Known intolerance; Angle-closure glaucoma; Bone marrow depression; CNS depression; Severe liver or cardiac disease; Known or suspected QT prolongation.
Use Cautiously in: Geriatric, debilitated, or severely ill patients (smaller doses should be used); Diabetic patients; Respiratory insufficiency; Prostatic hyperplasia; CNS tumors; Intestinal obstruction; Seizures (may lower seizure threshold); Severe liver disease; Pregnancy, lactation, and children <2 yr (although safety not established, droperidol has been used during cesarean section without respiratory depression in the newborn); Age >65 yr, concurrent benzodiazepines, volatile anesthetics, IV opioids (may increase risk of serious arrhythmias); use lower initial doses.
Exercise Extreme Caution in: Patients with risk factors for prolonged QT syndrome (CHF, bradycardia, diuretic use, cardiac hypertrophy, hypokalemia, hypomagnesema) or other drugs known to prolong QT interval.

Adverse Reactions/Side Effects
CNS: SEIZURES, <u>extrapyramidal reactions</u>, abnormal EEG, anxiety, confusion, dizziness, excessive sedation, hallucinations, hyperactivity, mental depression, nightmares, restlessness, tardive dyskinesia. **CV:** ARRHYTHMIAS (including torsades de pointes), QT prolongation. **EENT:** blurred vision, dry eyes. **Resp:** bronchospasm, laryngospasm.

✶ = Canadian drug name. ▓ = Genetic implication.
*CAPITALS indicates life-threatening; <u>underlines</u> indicate most frequent.

CV: hypotension, tachycardia. **GI:** constipation, dry mouth. **Misc:** chills, facial sweating, shivering.

Interactions
Drug-Drug: Additive hypotension with **antihypertensives** or **nitrates**. Additive CNS depression with other **CNS depressants**, including **alcohol**, **antihistamines**, **antidepressants**, **opioid analgesics**, and other **sedatives**. Concurrent use of **drugs known to prolong QT interval** (↑ risk of potentially life-threatening arrhythmias).
Drug-Natural Products: Concomitant use of **kava-kava**, **valerian**, **chamomile**, or **hops** can ↑ CNS depression.

Route/Dosage

Premedication/Use Without Premedication in Diagnostic Procedures
IV, IM (Adults): 2.5 – initially, 30 – 60 min prior to induction of anesthesia; additional doses of 1.25 mg IV may be needed, but should be undertaken with caution.
IM, IV (Children 2 – 12 yr): 0.1 mg/kg maximum initial dose.

Adjunct to General Anesthesia
IV (Adults): 2.5 mg additional doses of 1.25 mg IV may be needed, but should be undertaken with caution.
IM, IV (Children 2 – 12 yr): 0.1 mg/kg maximum initial dose.

Adjunct in Regional Anesthesia
IM, IV (Adults): 2.5 mg.

Antiemetic
IV (Adults): 0.5 – 1.25 mg q 4 hr as needed (unlabeled).

Availability (generic available)
Injection: 2.5 mg/mL.

NURSING IMPLICATIONS

Assessment
- Monitor blood pressure and heart rate frequently during therapy. Report significant changes immediately. Hypotension may be treated with parenteral fluids if hypovolemia is a causal factor. Vasopressors (norepinephrine, phenylephrine) may be needed. Avoid use of epinephrine, because droperidol reverses its pressor effects and may cause paradoxical hypotension.
- Assess 12-lead ECG in all patients prior to administration to determine if prolonged QT interval is present. Do not administer to patients with a prolonged QT interval. Monitor ECG prior to, during, and for 2 – 3 hr after treatment to monitor for arrhythmias.
- Assess patient for level of sedation following administration.
- Observe patient for extrapyramidal symptoms (dystonia, oculogyric crisis, extended neck, flexed arms, tremor, restlessness, hyperactivity, anxiety) throughout therapy. Notify physician or other health care professional should these occur. An anticholinergic antiparkinsonian agent may be used to treat these symptoms.
- **Nausea and Vomiting:** Assess nausea, vomiting, hydration status, bowel sounds, and abdominal pain prior to and following administration.

Potential Nursing Diagnoses
Risk for injury (Side Effects)

Implementation

IV Administration
- **Direct IV:** *Diluent:* Administer undiluted. *Concentration:* 2.5 mg/mL. *Rate:* Administer each dose slowly over 30 – 60 sec.
- **Intermittent Infusion:** *Diluent:* May be added to D5W, 0.9% NaCl, or LR. *Rate:* Administer by slow IV infusion. Titrate according to patient response.
- **Syringe Compatibility:** atropine, bleomycin, butorphanol, chlorpromazine, cimetidine, cisplatin, cyclophosphamide, dimenhydrinate, diphenhydramine, doxorubicin, fentanyl, glycopyrrolate, hydroxyzine, meperidine, metoclopramide, midazolam, mitomycin, morphine, nalbuphine, pentazocine, perphenazine, prochlorperazine, promethazine, scopolamine, vinblastine, vincristine.
- **Syringe Incompatibility:** fluorouracil, furosemide, heparin, leucovorin calcium, methotrexate, ondansetron , pentobarbital.
- **Y-Site Compatibility:** amifostine, azithromycin, aztreonam, bivalirudin, bleomycin, buprenorphine, cisatracurium, cladribine, cisplatin, cyclophosphamide, cytarabine, dexmedetomidine, docetaxel, doxorubicin, doxorubicin liposome, etoposide, famotidine, fenoldopam, filgrastim, fluconazole, fludarabine, gemcitabine, granisetron, hydrocortisone sodium succinate, idarubicin, linezolid, melphalan, meperidine, metoclopramide, mitomycin, ondansetron, oxaliplatin, paclitaxel, potassium chloride, propofol, remifentanil, sargramostim, teniposide, thiotepa, vinblastine, vincristine, vinorelbine, vitamin B complex with C.

- **Y-Site Incompatibility:** allopurinol sodium, amphotericin B cholesteryl sulfate complex, cefepime, fluorouracil, foscarnet, furosemide, lansoprazole, leucovorin calcium, nafcillin, pemetrexed, piperacillin/tazobactam.
- **Additive Incompatibility:** barbiturates.

Patient/Family Teaching
- Caution patient to change positions slowly to minimize orthostatic hypotension.
- Medication causes drowsiness. Advise patient to call for assistance during ambulation and transfer.

Evaluation/Desired Outcomes
- General quiescence and reduced motor activity.
- Decreased nausea and vomiting.

drotrecogin (dro-tre-**coe**-gin)
Xigris

Classification
Therapeutic: anti-infectives
Pharmacologic: activated protein C, human

Pregnancy Category C

Indications
To reduce mortality in adult patients with sepsis.

Action
Probably acts by suppressing widespread inflammation associated with sepsis. **Therapeutic Effects:** Decrease mortality due to sepsis.

Pharmacokinetics
Absorption: IV administration results in complete bioavailability.
Distribution: Unknown.
Metabolism and Excretion: Unknown.
Half-life: Unknown.

TIME/ACTION PROFILE (activity)

ROUTE	ONSET	PEAK	DURATION
IV	unknown	end of infusion	unknown

Contraindications/Precautions
Contraindicated in: Hypersensitivity; Patients with a high risk of bleeding, including those with: active internal bleeding, recent (within 3 months) stroke, recent (within 2 months) intracranial or intraspinal injury or severe head trauma, any trauma associated with an increased risk of life-threatening bleeding, presence of an epidural catheter, intracranial neoplasm/mass lesion/cerebral herniation; Patients not expected to survive due to pre-existing medical condition(s); HIV-positive patients with CD-4 cell counts ≤50/mm^3; Chronic dialysis patients; Patients who have undergone bone marrow, lung, liver, pancreas or small bowel transplantation; OB: Lactation.
Use Cautiously in: Concurrent therapeutic heparin therapy (≥15 units/kg/hr), recent (within 3 days) thrombolytic therapy, recent (within 7 days) oral anticoagulants or glycoprotein IIb/IIIa inhibitors, recent (within 7 days) aspirin therapy > 650 mg/day or other platelet inhibitors; Platelet count <30,000 x 10^6/L; Prothrombin time—INR >3.0; Recent (within 6 wk) GI bleeding; Recent (within 3 mos) ischemic stroke; Intracranial arteriovenous malformation or aneurysm; Known bleeding diathesis; Chronic severe hepatic disease; Any other serious bleeding risk; Surgical procedures (discontinue 2 hr before; resume 12 hr after if hemostasis is achieved); OB: Pregnancy (use only if clearly needed); Pedi: Children (safety not established).

Adverse Reactions/Side Effects
Hemat: BLEEDING.

Interactions
Drug-Drug: Risk of serious bleeding may be ↑ by **antiplatelet agents**, **anticoagulants**, **thrombolytic agents**, or **other agents that may affect coagulation**.
Drug-Natural Products: Risk of bleeding may be ↑ by **arnica**, **chamomile**, **clove**, **dong quai**, **feverfew**, **garlic**, **ginger**, **gingko**, **Panax ginseng**, and others.

Route/Dosage
IV (Adults): 24 mcg/kg/hr for 96 hr.

Availability
Powder for intravenous infusion (requires reconstitution): 5-mg vial, 20-mg vial.

NURSING IMPLICATIONS

Assessment
- Assess for signs of bleeding and hemorrhage (bleeding gums; nosebleed; unusual bruising; tarry, black stools; hematuria; fall in hematocrit or blood pressure; guaiac-positive stools, urine, or nasogastric aspirate) throughout therapy. If clinically important bleeding occurs, stop drotrecogin infusion immediately. Assess other agents used that may affect coagulation.

Once hemostasis is achieved, reinstitution of drotrecogin may be reconsidered.
- Assess patient for infection (vital signs; appearance of wound, sputum, urine, and stool; WBC) at beginning of and during therapy.
- **Lab Test Considerations:** Most patients with severe sepsis have coagulopathy prolonging activated partial thromboplastin time (aPTT) and prothrombin time (PT). Drotrecogin may also affect aPTT, but has minimal effect on PT. Use PT to monitor coagulation status of patients receiving drotrecogin.

Potential Nursing Diagnoses
Ineffective tissue perfusion, impaired (Indications)

Implementation
- Drotrecogin should be discontinued 2 hr prior to invasive surgical procedures or procedures with a risk of bleeding. Once hemostasis is achieved, drotrecogin may be started 12 hr after the procedure.

IV Administration
- **Intermittent Infusion:** Calculate dose and number of 5-mg or 20-mg vials needed (vials contain excess to facilitate delivery). Reconstitute 5-mg vials with 2.5 mL and 20-mg vials with 10 mL sterile water for injection for a concentration of 2 mg/mL. Add sterile water slowly to vial; avoid inverting or shaking. Gently swirl until powder is completely dissolved. *Diluent:* Reconstituted solution must be diluted further with 0.9% NaCl. Withdraw amount of reconstituted solution needed from vial and add to infusion bag of 0.9% NaCl; direct stream to side of the bag to avoid agitating solution. Gently invert bag to mix. Reconstituted solution must be used within 3 hr and IV administration must be completed within 14 hr of preparation of IV solution. Do not administer if discolored or contains particulate matter. If infusion is interrupted, restart at initial infusion rate and continue to complete recommended infusion. *Concentration:* 100–1000 mcg/mL. When using low concentrations (<200 mcg/mL) at low flow rates (<5 mL/hr), prime infusion set for approximately 15 min at a flow rate of 5 mL/hr. *Rate:* Administer at a rate of 24 mcg/kg/hr for 96 hr. Do not use bolus dosing or dose escalation.
- **Y-Site Incompatibility:** Administer via a dedicated IV line or a dedicated lumen of a multilumen central venous catheter.
- **Solution Compatibility:** May be administered only with 0.9% NaCl, LR, dextrose or dextrose/saline combinations.

Patient/Family Teaching
- Explain purpose of medication to patient.

Evaluation/Desired Outcomes
- Reduction of mortality in adult patients with severe sepsis.

---

duloxetine (do-lox-e-teen)
Cymbalta

Classification
Therapeutic: antidepressants
Pharmacologic: selective serotonin/norepinephrine reuptake inhibitors

Pregnancy Category C

Indications
Major depressive disorder. Diabetic peripheral neuropathic pain. Generalized anxiety disorder. Fibromyalgia. **Unlabeled Use:** Stress urinary incontinence.

Action
Inhibits serotonin and norepinephrine reuptake in the CNS. Both antidepressant and pain inhibition are centrally mediated. **Therapeutic Effects:** Decreased depressive symptomatology. Decreased neuropathic pain. Decreased symptoms of anxiety. Decreased pain.

Pharmacokinetics
Absorption: Well absorbed following oral administration.
Distribution: Unknown.
Protein Binding: Highly (> 90%) protein-bound.
Metabolism and Excretion: Mostly metabolized, primarily by the CYP2D6 and CYP1A2 enzyme pathways.
Half-life: 12 hr.

TIME/ACTION PROFILE (blood levels)

ROUTE	ONSET	PEAK	DURATION
PO	unknown	6 hr	12 hr

Contraindications/Precautions
Contraindicated in: Hypersensitivity; Concurrent MAO inhibitor therapy; Uncontrolled angle-closure glaucoma; End-stage renal disease; Chronic hepatic impairment or substantial alcohol use (increased risk of hepatitis); Lactation: May enter breast milk; discontinue or bottle-feed.
Use Cautiously in: History of suicide attempt or ideation; History of mania (may activate mania/hypomania); Concurrent use of other centrally acting drugs (↑ risk of adverse reactions); History of seizure disorder; Controlled angle-closure

duloxetine

glaucoma; Diabetic patients and those with renal impairment (consider lower initial dose with gradual increase); OB: Use during 3rd trimester may result in neonatal serotonin syndrome requiring prolonged hospitalization, respiratory and nutritional support; Pedi: May ↑ risk of suicide attempt/ideation especially during dose early treatment or dose adjustment; risk may be greater in children or adolescents (safe use in children/adolescents not established).

Adverse Reactions/Side Effects
CNS: NEUROLEPTIC MALIGNANT SYNDROME, SEIZURES, SUICIDAL THOUGHTS, fatigue, drowsiness, insomnia, activation of mania, dizziness, nightmares. **EENT:** blurred vision, ↑ intraocular pressure. **CV:** ↑ blood pressure. **GI:** HEPATOTOXICITY, ↓ appetite, constipation, dry mouth, nausea, diarrhea, ↑ liver enzymes, gastritis, vomiting. **F and E:** hyponatremia. **GU:** dysuria, abnormal orgasm, erectile dysfunction, ↓ libido, urinary retention. **Derm:** ↑ sweating, pruritus, rash. **Neuro:** tremor. **Misc:** SEROTONIN SYNDROME.

Interactions
Drug-Drug: Concurrent use with **MAO inhibitors** may result in serious potentially fatal reactions (do not use within 14 days of discontinuing MAOI. Wait at least 5 days after stopping duloxetine to start MAOI). ↑ risk of hepatotoxicity with chronic **alcohol** abuse. Drugs that affect serotonergic neurotransmitter systems, including **linezolid**, **tramadol**, and **triptans** ↑ risk of serotonin syndrome. **Drugs that inhibit CYP1A2**, including **fluvoxamine** and some **fluoroquinolones** ↑ levels of duloxetine and should be avoided. **Drugs that inhibit CYP2D6**, including **paroxetine**, **fluoxetine** and **quinidine** ↑ levels of duloxetine and may increase the risk of adverse reactions. Duloxetine also inhibits CYP2D6 and may ↑ levels of drugs metabolized by CYP2D6, including **tricyclic antidepressants**, **phenothiazines** and **class 1C antiarrhythmics** (**propafenone** and **flecainide**); concurrent use should be undertaken with caution. ↑ risk of serious arrhythmias with **thioridazine**; avoid concurrent use. ↑ risk of bleeding with **aspirin**, **NSAIDs**, or **warfarin**.
Drug-Natural Products: Use with **St. John's wort** ↑ of serotonin syndrome.

Route/Dosage
PO (Adults): *Antidepressant* — 20–30 mg twice daily; *Neuropathic pain or generalized anxiety disorder* — 60 mg once daily; *Fibromyalgia* - 30 mg once daily for 1 wk, then ↑ to 60 mg once daily.

Renal Impairment
PO (Adults): start with lower dose and ↑ gradually.

Availability
Capsules: 20 mg, 30 mg, 60 mg. **Cost:** 20 mg $320.96/90, 30 mg $345.99/90, 60 mg $347.98/90.

NURSING IMPLICATIONS

Assessment
- Assess for sexual dysfunction (erectile dysfunction; decreased libido).
- Monitor blood pressure before and periodically during therapy. Sustained hypertension may be dose related; decrease dose or discontinue therapy if this occurs.
- Monitor appetite and nutritional intake. Weigh weekly. Report continued weight loss. Adjust diet as tolerated to support nutritional status.
- Monitor closely for notable changes in behavior that could indicate the emergence or worsening of suicidal thoughts or behavior or depression. Risk may be increased in children, adolescents, and adults ≤24 yr.
- **Depression:** Assess mental status (orientation, mood, and behavior). Inform health care professional if patient demonstrates significant increase in anxiety, nervousness, or insomnia.
- Assess suicidal tendencies in both adults and children, especially in early therapy or during dose changes. Restrict amount of drug available to patient.
- **Pain and Fibromyalgia:** Assess intensity, quality, and location of pain periodically during therapy. Use pain scale. May require several weeks for effects to be seen.
- *Lab Test Considerations:* May cause ↑ ALT, AST, bilirubin, CPK, and alkaline phosphatase.

Potential Nursing Diagnoses
Ineffective coping (Indications)
Risk for suicide (Adverse Reactions)
Chronic pain (Indications)

Implementation
- **PO:** May be administered without regard to meals. Capsules should be swallowed whole. Do not crush, chew, or open and sprinkle con-

tents on food or liquids; may affect enteric coating.

Patient/Family Teaching
- Instruct patient to take duloxetine as directed at the same time each day. Take missed doses as soon as possible unless time for next dose. Do not stop abruptly; must be decreased gradually.
- Encourage patient and family to be alert for emergence of anxiety, agitation, panic attacks, insomnia, irritability, hostility, impulsivity, akathisia, hypomania, mania, worsening of depression and suicidal ideation, especially during early antidepressant therapy. If these symptoms occur, notify health care professional.
- May cause drowsiness. Caution patient to avoid driving or other activities requiring alertness until response to medication is known.
- Advise patient to consult health care professional prior to taking any Rx, OTC, or herbal products.
- Instruct patient to notify health care professional if signs of serotonin syndrome (mental status changes: agitation, hallucinations, coma; autonomic instability: tachycardia, labile blood pressure, hyperthermia; neuromuscular aberrations: hyperreflexia, incoordination; and/or gastrointestinal symptoms: nausea, vomiting, diarrhea) or liver damage (pruritus, dark urine, jaundice, right upper quadrant tenderness, unexplained "flu-like" symptoms) occur.
- Advise patient to avoid taking alcohol during duloxetine therapy.
- Instruct patient to notify health care professional if pregnancy is planned or suspected or if breastfeeding.
- Refer patient/family to local support group.

Evaluation/Desired Outcomes
- Increased sense of well-being.
- Renewed interest in surroundings. Need for therapy should be periodically reassessed. Patients may notice improvement within 1–4 wk, but should be advised to continue therapy as directed. Therapy is usually continued for several months.
- Decrease in neuropathic pain associated with diabetic peripheral neuropathy.
- Decrease in pain and soreness associated with fibromyalgia.

dutasteride (doo-tas-te-ride)
Avodart

Classification
Therapeutic: benign prostatic hyperplasia (BPH) agents
Pharmacologic: androgen inhibitors

Pregnancy Category X

Indications
Management of the symptoms of benign prostatic hyperplasia (BPH) in men with an enlarged prostate gland (alone or with tamsulosin).

Action
Inhibits the enzyme 5-alpha-reductase, which is responsible for converting testosterone to its potent metabolite 5-alpha-dihydrotestosterone in the prostate gland and other tissues. 5-Alpha-dihydrotestosterone is partly responsible for prostatic hyperplasia. **Therapeutic Effects:** Reduced prostate size with associated decrease in urinary symptoms.

Pharmacokinetics
Absorption: Well absorbed (60%) following oral administration; also absorbed through skin.
Distribution: 11.5% of serum concentration partitions into semen.
Protein Binding: 99% bound to albumin; 96.6% bound to alpha-1 glycoprotein.
Metabolism and Excretion: Mostly metabolized by the liver via the CYP3A4 metabolic pathway; metabolites are excreted in feces.
Half-life: 5 wk.

TIME/ACTION PROFILE (reduction in dihydrotestosterone levels†)

ROUTE	ONSET	PEAK	DURATION
PO	unknown	1-2 wk	unknown

†Symptoms may only improve over 3–12 mo

Contraindications/Precautions
Contraindicated in: Hypersensitivity; Cross-sensitivity with other 5-alpha-reductase inhibitors may occur; Women; Pedi: Children.
Use Cautiously in: Hepatic impairment.

Adverse Reactions/Side Effects
GU: decreased libido, ejaculation disorders, erectile dysfunction. **Endo:** gynecomastia. **Derm:** rash, urticaria. **Misc:** ALLERGIC REACTIONS, ANGIOEDEMA.

Interactions
Drug-Drug: Blood levels and effects may be increased by **ritonavir**, **ketoconazole**, **verapamil**, **diltiazem**, **cimetidine**, **ciprofloxacin**, or other **CYP3A4 enzyme inhibitors**.

Route/Dosage
PO (Adults): 0.5 mg once daily (with or without tamsulosin).

Availability
Soft gelatin capsules: 0.5 mg. **Cost:** $269.97/90.

NURSING IMPLICATIONS

Assessment
- Assess patient for symptoms of prostatic hyperplasia (urinary hesitancy, feeling of incomplete bladder emptying, interruption of urinary stream, impairment of size and force of urinary stream, terminal urinary dribbling, straining to start flow, dysuria, urgency) before and periodically during therapy.
- Digital rectal examinations should be performed before and periodically during therapy for BPH.
- ***Lab Test Considerations:*** Serum prostate-specific antigen (PSA) concentrations, which are used to screen for prostate cancer, decrease by about 20% within the 1st mo of therapy and stabilize at about 50% of the pretreatment level within 6 mo. New baseline PSA concentrations should be established at 3 and 6 mo of therapy and evaluated periodically during therapy.

Potential Nursing Diagnoses
Impaired urinary elimination (Indications)

Implementation
- **PO:** Administer once daily with or without meals. Do not break, crush, or chew capsule.

Patient/Family Teaching
- Instruct patient to take dutasteride at the same time each day as directed, even if symptoms improve or are unchanged. Take missed doses as soon as remembered later in the day or omit dose. Do not make up by taking double doses the next day.
- Caution patient that sharing of dutasteride may be dangerous.
- Inform patient that the volume of ejaculate may be decreased during therapy but that this will not interfere with normal sexual function.
- Caution patient that dutasteride poses a potential risk to a male fetus. Women who are pregnant or may become pregnant should avoid exposure to semen of a partner taking dutasteride and should not handle dutasteride because of the potential for absorption.
- Advise patient to avoid donating blood for at least 6 mo after last dose of dutasteride to prevent a pregnant female from receiving dutasteride through a blood transfusion.
- Emphasize the importance of periodic follow-up exams to determine whether a clinical response has occurred.

Evaluation/Desired Outcomes
- Decrease in urinary symptoms of BPH.

econazole, See **ANTIFUNGALS (TOPICAL).**

---

efavirenz (e-fa-veer-enz)
Sustiva

Classification
Therapeutic: antiretrovirals
Pharmacologic: non-nucleoside reverse transcriptase inhibitors

Pregnancy Category D

Indications
HIV infection (in combination with one or more other antiretroviral agents).

Action
Inhibits HIV reverse transcriptase, which results in disruption of DNA synthesis. **Therapeutic Effects:** Slowed progression of HIV infection and decreased occurrence of sequelae. Increases CD4 cell counts and decreases viral load.

Pharmacokinetics
Absorption: 50% absorbed when ingested following a high-fat meal.
Distribution: 99.5–99.75% bound to plasma proteins; enters CSF.
Metabolism and Excretion: Mostly metabolized by the liver.
Half-life: *Following single dose*—52–76 hr. *Following multiple doses*—40–55 hr.

TIME/ACTION PROFILE (blood levels)

ROUTE	ONSET	PEAK	DURATION
PO	rapid	3–5 hr	24 hr

Contraindications/Precautions
Contraindicated in: Hypersensitivity; Concurrent pimozide, midazolam, triazolam, voriconazole (standard doses), St. John's wort, or ergot derivatives.
Use Cautiously in: History of mental illness or substance abuse (↑ risk of psychiatric symptomatology); History of hepatic impairment (including hepatitis B or C infection or concurrent therapy with hepatotoxic agents); History of seizure disorders (↑ risk of seizures); OB: Use in pregnancy only if other options have been exhausted; Lactation: Breastfeeding not recommended for HIV-infected mothers; Pedi: ↑ incidence of rash; Geri: Cautious initial dosing due to ↑ incidence of renal or cardiac dysfunction.

Adverse Reactions/Side Effects
CNS: abnormal dreams, depression, dizziness, drowsiness, fatigue, headache, impaired concentration, insomnia, nervousness, psychiatric symptomatology. **GI:** nausea, abdominal pain, anorexia, diarrhea, dyspepsia, flatulence. **GU:** hematuria, renal calculi. **Derm:** RASH, sweating, pruritus. **Endo:** hypercholesterolemia, hypertriglyceridemia. **Neuro:** hypoesthesia. **Misc:** fat redistribution.

Interactions
Drug-Drug: ↑ levels of **pimozide, midazolam, triazolam,** or **ergot alkaloids** when used concurrently; may result in potentially serious adverse reactions including arrhythmias, CNS, and respiratory depression (concurrent use contraindicated). Induces (stimulates) the hepatic cytochrome P450 3A4 enzyme system and would be expected to influence the effects of other drugs that are metabolized by this system; efavirenz itself is also metabolized by this system. ↑ risk of CNS depression with other **CNS depressants**, including **alcohol, antidepressants, antihistamines,** and **opioid analgesics**. Concurrent use with **ritonavir** ↑ levels of both agents and the likelihood of adverse reactions, especially hepatotoxicity. May alter the effectiveness of **hormonal contraceptives**. Use with **voriconazole** significantly ↓ voriconazole levels and ↑ efavirenz levels; concurrent use with standard doses of voriconazole is contraindicated; if used together, ↑ dose of voriconazole to 400 mg q 12 hr and ↓ dose of efavirenz to 300 mg daily. ↓ **indinavir** blood levels (indinavir dose ↑ recommended). ↓ **saquinavir** blood levels (avoid using saquinavir as the only protease inhibitor with efavirenz). May alter the effects of **warfarin**.
Drug-Natural Products: Use with **St. John's wort** may cause ↓ levels and effectiveness, including development of drug resistance (concurrent use contraindicated).
Drug-Food: Ingestion following a high-fat meal ↑ absorption by 50%.

Route/Dosage
PO (Adults and Children >40 kg): 600 mg once daily.
PO (Children 32.5–40 kg): 400 mg once daily.
PO (Children 25–32.5 kg): 350 mg once daily.
PO (Children 20–25 kg): 300 mg once daily.
PO (Children 15–20 kg): 250 mg once daily.

PO (Children 10–15 kg): 200 mg once daily.

Availability
Capsules: 50 mg, 200 mg. **Tablets:** 600 mg. *In combination with:* emtricitabine and tenofovir (Atripla) (See Appendix B).

NURSING IMPLICATIONS

Assessment
- Assess for change in severity of HIV symptoms and for symptoms of opportunistic infections during therapy.
- Assess for rash, especially during 1st mo of therapy. Onset is usually within 2 wk and resolves with continued therapy within 1 mo. May range from mild maculopapular with erythema and pruritus to exfoliative dermatitis and Stevens-Johnson syndrome. Occurs more often and may be more severe in children. If rash is severe or accompanied by blistering, desquamation, mucosal involvement, or fever, therapy must be discontinued immediately. Efavirenz may be reinstated concurrently with antihistamines or corticosteroids in patients discontinuing due to rash.
- Assess patient for CNS and psychiatric symptoms (dizziness, impaired concentration, somnolence, abnormal dreams, insomnia) during therapy. Symptoms usually begin during 1st or 2nd day of therapy and resolve after 2–4 wk. Administration at bedtime may minimize symptoms. Concurrent use with alcohol or psychoactive agents may cause additive CNS symptoms.
- *Lab Test Considerations:* Monitor viral load and CD4 cell count regularly during therapy.
- Monitor liver function tests in patients with a history of hepatitis B or C. May cause ↑ serum AST, ALT, and GGT concentrations. If moderate to severe liver function test abnormalities occur, efavirenz doses should be held until levels return to normal. Discontinue if liver function abnormalities recur when therapy is resumed.
- May cause ↑ in total cholesterol and serum triglyceride levels.
- May cause false-positive urine cannabinoid results.

Potential Nursing Diagnoses
Risk for infection (Indications)
Noncompliance (Patient/Family Teaching)

Implementation
- **PO:** Administer on an empty stomach, preferably at bedtime to minimize nervous system side effects Avoid taking with a high-fat meal. Do not break tablets.

Patient/Family Teaching
- Emphasize the importance of taking efavirenz as directed. It must always be used in combination with other antiretroviral drugs. Do not take more than prescribed amount, and do not stop taking without consulting health care professional. Take missed doses as soon as remembered; do not double doses.
- Instruct patient that efavirenz should not be shared with others.
- May cause dizziness, impaired concentration, or drowsiness. Caution patient to avoid driving or other activities requiring alertness until response to medication is known.
- Instruct patient to notify health care professional immediately if rash occurs.
- Inform patient that efavirenz does not cure AIDS or prevent associated or opportunistic infections. Efavirenz does not reduce the risk of transmission of HIV to others through sexual contact or blood contamination. Caution patient to use a condom and to avoid sharing needles or donating blood to prevent spreading the AIDS virus to others. Advise patient that the long-term effects of efavirenz are unknown at this time.
- Advise patient to avoid taking other Rx, OTC, or herbal products without consulting health care professional.
- Advise patients taking oral contraceptives to use a nonhormonal method of birth control during efavirenz therapy and for at least 12 wk following discontinuation and to notify health care professional if they become pregnant while taking efavirenz.
- Inform patient that redistribution and accumulation of body fat may occur, causing central obesity, dorsocervical fat enlargement (buffalo hump), peripheral wasting, breast enlargement, and cushingoid appearance. The cause and long-term effects are not known.
- Emphasize the importance of regular follow-up exams and blood counts to determine progress and monitor for side effects.

Evaluation/Desired Outcomes
- Delayed progression of AIDS and decreased opportunistic infections in patients with HIV.
- Decrease in viral load and increase in CD4 cell counts.

eletriptan (e-le-trip-tan)
Relpax

eletriptan

Classification
Therapeutic: vascular headache suppressants
Pharmacologic: 5-HT$_1$ agonists

Pregnancy Category C

Indications
Acute treatment of migraine headache.

Action
Acts as an agonist at specific 5-hydroxy-tryptamine receptor sites in intracranial blood vessels and sensory trigeminal nerves. **Therapeutic Effects:** Cranial vessel vasoconstriction with resultant decrease in migraine headache.

Pharmacokinetics
Absorption: 50% absorbed after oral administration.
Distribution: Enters breast milk.
Metabolism and Excretion: Mostly metabolized by the liver via the CYP3A4 enzyme system.
Half-life: 4 hr.

TIME/ACTION PROFILE (decreased migraine pain)

ROUTE	ONSET	PEAK	DURATION
PO	within 2 hr	2 hr	up to 24 hr

Contraindications/Precautions
Contraindicated in: Hypersensitivity; Hemiplegic or basilar migraine; Ischemic cardiovascular, cerebrovascular, or peripheral vascular syndromes (including ischemic bowel disease); History of significant cardiovascular disease; Uncontrolled hypertension; Severe hepatic impairment; Should not be used within 24 hr of other 5-HT$_1$ agonists or ergot-type compounds (dihydroergotamine); Should not be used within 72 hr of potent CYP3A4 inhibitors including ketoconazole, itraconazole, nefazodone, clarithromycin, ritonavir, and nelfinavir.
Use Cautiously in: OB: Use during pregnancy only if potential benefits justify potential risk to fetus; Lactation: Doses up to 80 mg daily not expected to cause adverse effects in breastfed infants >2 mo (NIH); Pedi: Children <18 yr (safety not established); Geri: ↑ risk of ↑ blood pressure.
Exercise Extreme Caution in: Cardiovascular risk factors (hypertension, hypercholesterolemia, cigarette smoking, obesity, diabetes, strong family history, menopausal women or men >40 yr); use only if cardiovascular status has been evaluated and determined to be safe and 1st dose is administered under supervision.

Adverse Reactions/Side Effects
CNS: dizziness, drowsiness, weakness. **CV:** chest tightness/pressure. **GI:** abdominal pain, dry mouth, dysphagia, nausea. **Neuro:** paresthesia.

Interactions
Drug-Drug: Blood levels and risk of adverse reactions are increased by potent **CYP3A4 inhibitors** (including **ketoconazole**, **itraconazole**, **nefazodone**, **clarithromycin**, **ritonavir**, and **nelfinavir**); use within 72 hr is contraindicated. Concurrent use (within 24 hr of each other) with ergot-containing drugs (**dihydroergotamine**) may result in prolonged vasospastic reactions and should be avoided.

Route/Dosage
PO (Adults): 20 or 40 mg; may be repeated in 2 hr if initial response is inadequate (not to exceed 80 mg/24 hr or treatment of 3 headaches/mo).

Availability
Tablets: 20 mg, 40 mg. **Cost:** 20 mg $113.61/6, 40 mg $113.99/6.

NURSING IMPLICATIONS

Assessment
- Assess pain location, intensity, character, duration and associated symptoms (photophonia, phonophobia, nausea, vomiting) during migraine attack.

Potential Nursing Diagnoses
Acute pain (Indications)

Implementation
- **PO:** Administer at the first sign of a headache. If after the initial dose, headache improves but then returns, dose may be repeated at least 2 hr after initial dose. If initial dose is ineffective, second dose is unlikely to be effective.

Patient/Family Teaching
- Instruct patient that eletriptan should only be used during a migraine attack. Eletriptan is used for treatment of a migraine attack, not for prevention.
- Instruct patient to take eletriptan at the first sign of a migraine, but may be administered at any time during attack. Allow at least 2 hr between doses and do not use more than 80 mg/day or 3 attacks/mo.
- Caution patient not to take eletriptan within 24 hr of other vascular headache suppressants.

✦ = Canadian drug name. ❚ = Genetic implication.
*CAPITALS indicates life-threatening; underlines indicate most frequent.

- Advise patient that lying down in a darkened room after eletriptan administration may further help relieve headache.
- Advise patient to notify health care professional if she plans or suspects pregnancy, or if breastfeeding.
- Advise patient to notify health care professional before next dose of eletriptan if pain or tightness in the chest occurs. If chest pain is severe or does not subside, notify health care professional immediately. If feelings of tingling, heat, flushing, heaviness, pressure, drowsiness, dizziness, tiredness, or sickness develop, discuss with health care provider at next visit.
- May cause drowsiness or dizziness. Caution patient to avoid driving or other activities requiring alertness until response to medication is known.
- Advise patient to avoid alcohol, which aggravates headaches, during therapy.

Evaluation/Desired Outcomes
- Relief of migraine attack.

---

emtricitabine
(em-tri-**si**-ti-been)
Emtriva

Classification
Therapeutic: antiretrovirals
Pharmacologic: nucleoside reverse transcriptase inhibitors

Pregnancy Category B

Indications
HIV infection (with other antiretrovirals).

Action
Phosphorylated intracellularly where it inhibits HIV reverse transcriptase, resulting in viral DNA chain termination. **Therapeutic Effects:** Slowed progression of HIV infection and decreased occurrence of sequelae. Increases CD4 cell counts and decreases viral load.

Pharmacokinetics
Absorption: Rapidly and extensively absorbed; 93% bioavailable.
Distribution: Unknown.
Metabolism and Excretion: Some metabolism, 86% renally excreted, 14% fecal excretion.
Half-life: 10 hr.

TIME/ACTION PROFILE (blood levels*)

ROUTE	ONSET	PEAK	DURATION
PO	rapid	1–2 hr	24 hr

*Normal renal function

Contraindications/Precautions
Contraindicated in: Hypersensitivity; Lactation: Breastfeeding not recommended in HIV-infected patients.
Use Cautiously in: Hepatitis B infection (may exacerbate following discontinuation); Renal impairment; OB: Use only if clearly needed; Geri: May be at ↑ risk for adverse effects.

Adverse Reactions/Side Effects
CNS: dizziness, headache, insomnia, weakness, depression, nightmares. **GI:** abdominal pain, diarrhea, nausea, SEVERE HEPATOMEGALY WITH STEATOSIS, dyspepsia,, vomiting. **Derm:** rash, skin discoloration. **F and E:** LACTIC ACIDOSIS. **MS:** arthralgia, myalgia. **Neuro:** neuropathy, paresthesia. **Resp:** cough, rhinitis. **Misc:** fat redistribution.

Interactions
Drug-Drug: None noted.

Route/Dosage
PO (Adults ≥18 yr): 200 mg once daily.

Renal Impairment
PO (Adults ≥18 yr): *CCr 30–49 mL/min*— 200 mg every 48 hr; *CCr 15–29 mL/min*—200 mg every 72 hr; *CCr <15 mL/min*—200 mg every 96 hr.

Availability
Capsules: 200 mg. **Oral solution (cotton candy flavor):** 10 mg/mL. *In combination with:* efavirenz and tenofovir (Atripla); tenofovir (Truvada). See Appendix B.

NURSING IMPLICATIONS

Assessment
- Assess patient for change in severity of HIV symptoms and for symptoms of opportunistic infections during therapy.
- May cause lactic acidosis and severe hepatomegaly with steatosis. These events are more likely to occur if patients are female, obese, or receiving nucleoside analogue medications for extended periods of time. Monitor patient for signs (increased serum lactate levels, elevated liver enzymes, liver enlargement on palpation). Therapy should be suspended if clinical or laboratory signs occur.
- Test patients for chronic hepatitis B virus (HBV) before initiating therapy. Emtricitabine is not indicated for treatment of HBV. Exacerbations of HBV have occurred upon discontinuation of emtricitabine.
- *Lab Test Considerations:* Monitor viral load and CD4 cell count regularly during therapy.

- May cause ↑ AST, ALT, bilirubin, creatine kinase, serum amylase, serum lipase, and triglycerides. May cause ↑ or ↓ serum glucose. May cause ↓ neutrophil count.

Potential Nursing Diagnoses
Risk for infection (Indications)
Noncompliance (Patient/Family Teaching)

Implementation
- **PO:** May be administered with or without food.

Patient/Family Teaching
- Emphasize the importance of taking emtricitabine as directed. It must always be used in combination with other antiretroviral drugs. Do not take more than prescribed amount and do not stop taking without consulting health care professional. Take missed doses as soon as remembered, but not if almost time for next dose; do not double doses.
- Instruct patient that emtricitabine should not be shared with others.
- Inform patient that emtricitabine does not cure AIDS or prevent associated or opportunistic infections. Emtricitabine does not reduce the risk of transmission of HIV to others through sexual contact or blood contamination. Caution patient to use a condom and to avoid sharing needles or donating blood to prevent spreading the AIDS virus to others. Advise patient that the long-term effects of emtricitabine are unknown at this time.
- Instruct patient to notify health care professional immediately if symptoms of lactic acidosis (tiredness or weakness, unusual muscle pain, trouble breathing, stomach pain with nausea and vomiting, cold especially in arms or legs, dizziness, fast or irregular heartbeat) or if signs of hepatotoxicity (yellow skin or whites of eyes, dark urine, light colored stools, lack of appetite for several days or longer, nausea, abdominal pain) occur. These symptoms may occur more frequently in patients that are female, obese, or have been taking medications like emtricitabine for a long time.
- Inform patient that redistribution of body fat (central obesity, dorsocervical fat enlargement or buffalo hump, peripheral and facial wasting, breast enlargement, cushingoid appearance) and skin discoloration (hyperpigmentation on palms and soles) may occur.
- Advise patient to notify health care professional if she plans or suspects pregnancy or is breastfeeding.
- Emphasize the importance of regular follow-up exams and blood counts to determine progress and monitor for side effects.

Evaluation/Desired Outcomes
- Delayed progression of AIDS and decreased opportunistic infections in patients with HIV.
- Decrease in viral load and increase in CD4 cell counts.

---

enalapril/enalaprilat, See **ANGIOTENSIN-CONVERTING ENZYME (ACE) INHIBITORS.**

---

enoxaparin, See **HEPARINS (LOW MOLECULAR WEIGHT).**

---

entacapone (en-tak-a-pone)
Comtan

Classification
Therapeutic: antiparkinson agents
Pharmacologic: catechol-*O*-methyltransferase inhibitors

Pregnancy Category C

Indications
With levodopa/carbidopa to treat idiopathic Parkinson's disease when signs and symptoms of end-of-dose "wearing-off" (so-called fluctuating patients) occur.

Action
Acts as a selective and reversible inhibitor of the enzyme catechol *O*-methyltransferase (COMT). Inhibition of this enzyme prevents the breakdown of levodopa, increasing availability to the CNS.
Therapeutic Effects: Prolongs duration of response to levodopa with end-of-dose motor fluctuations. Decreased signs and symptoms of Parkinson's disease.

Pharmacokinetics
Absorption: 35% absorbed following oral administration; absorption is rapid.
Distribution: Unknown.
Protein Binding: 98%.
Metabolism and Excretion: Minimal amounts excreted unchanged; highly metabolized followed by biliary excretion.
Half-life: *Initial phase*—0.4–0.7 hr; *second phase*—2.4 hr.

entecavir

TIME/ACTION PROFILE (inhibition of COMT)

ROUTE	ONSET	PEAK	DURATION
PO	unknown	unknown	up to 8 hr

Contraindications/Precautions
Contraindicated in: Hypersensitivity; Concurrent nonselective MAO inhibitor therapy.
Use Cautiously in: Hepatic impairment; Concurrent use of drugs that are metabolized by COMT; OB, Lactation: Safety not established; Pedi: No identified use in children.

Adverse Reactions/Side Effects
CNS: NEUROLEPTIC MALIGNANT SYNDROME, dizziness, hallucinations, syncope, urges (gambling, sexual). **Resp:** pulmonary infiltrates, pleural effusion, pleural thickening. **CV:** hypotension. **Derm:** melanoma. **GI:** abdominal pain, diarrhea, nausea (during initiation), retroperitoneal fibrosis. **GU:** brownish-orange discoloration of urine. **MS:** RHABDOMYOLYSIS. **Neuro:** dyskinesia.

Interactions
Drug-Drug: Concurrent use with selective **MAO inhibitors** is not recommended; both agents inhibit the metabolic pathways of catecholamines. Concurrent use of drugs that are metabolized by COMT such as **isoproterenol**, **epinephrine**, **norepinephrine**, **dopamine**, **dobutamine**, and **methyldopa** may ↑ risk of tachycardia, ↑ blood pressure, and arrhythmias. **Probenecid**, **cholestyramine**, **erythromycin**, **rifampin**, **ampicillin**, and **chloramphenicol** may interfere with biliary elimination of entacapone; use concurrently with caution.

Route/Dosage
PO (Adults): 200 mg with each dose of levodopa/carbidopa up to a maximum of 8 times daily.

Availability
Tablets: 200 mg. *In combination with:* levodopa/carbidopa (Stalevo), see Appendix B.

NURSING IMPLICATIONS

Assessment
- Assess parkinsonian and extrapyramidal symptoms (restlessness or desire to keep moving, rigidity, tremors, pill rolling, mask-like face, shuffling gait, muscle spasms, twisting motions, difficulty speaking or swallowing, loss of balance control) prior to and during therapy. Dyskinesia may increase with therapy.
- Monitor patient for development of diarrhea. Usually occurs within 4 to 12 wk of start of therapy, but may occur as early as the first week and as late as months after initiation of therapy.
- Monitor patient for signs similar to neuroleptic malignant syndrome (elevated temperature, muscular rigidity, altered consciousness, elevated CPK). Symptoms have been associated with rapid dose reduction or withdrawal of other dopaminergic drugs. Withdrawal should be gradual.

Potential Nursing Diagnoses
Impaired physical mobility (Indications)
Risk for injury (Indications)

Implementation
- **PO:** Always administer entacapone with levodopa/carbidopa. Entacapone has no antiparkinsonism effects of its own.

Patient/Family Teaching
- Encourage patient to take entacapone as directed. Take missed doses as soon as possible, up to 2 hr before the next dose. Taper gradually when discontinuing or a withdrawal reaction may occur.
- May cause dizziness or hallucinations. Advise patient to avoid driving or other activities that require alertness until response to the drug is known.
- Inform patient that nausea may occur, especially at initiation of therapy. Therapy may cause change in urine color to brownish orange.
- Caution patient to change positions slowly to minimize orthostatic hypotension.
- Advise patient to notify health care professional if suspicious or unusual skin changes, hallucinations, or new or increased gambling, sexual, or other intense urges occur.
- Instruct patient to notify health care professional if pregnancy is planned or suspected.
- Emphasize the importance of routine follow-up exams.

Evaluation/Desired Outcomes
- Decreased signs and symptoms of Parkinson's disease.

---

entecavir (en-tek-Aveer)
Baraclude

Classification
Therapeutic: antivirals
Pharmacologic: nucleoside analogues

Pregnancy Category C

Indications
Chronic hepatitis B infection with evidence of active disease.

Action
Phosphorylated intracellularly to active form which acts as an analogue of guanosine, interfering with viral DNA synthesis. **Therapeutic Effects:** Decreased hepatic damage due to chronic hepatitis B infection.

Pharmacokinetics
Absorption: Well absorbed following oral administration.
Distribution: Extensive tissue distribution.
Metabolism and Excretion: 62–73% excreted unchanged by kidneys.
Half-life: Plasma—128–149 hr; intracellular—15 hr.

TIME/ACTION PROFILE (blood levels)

ROUTE	ONSET	PEAK	DURATION
PO	rapid	0.5–1 hr	24 hr

Contraindications/Precautions
Contraindicated in: Hypersensitivity; Lactation: Potential for serious adverse effects in infant.
Use Cautiously in: Renal impairment (dose reduction recommended if CCr <50 mL/min; Liver transplant recipients (careful monitoring of renal function recommended); Patients co-infected with HIV (unless receiving highly active antiretroviral therapy; at ↑ risk for resistance); OB: Use only if clearly needed, considering benefits and risks; Pedi: Safety not established in children <16 yr; Geri: ↑ risk of toxicity due to age-related ↓ in renal function.

Adverse Reactions/Side Effects
CNS: dizziness, fatigue, headache. **GI:** HEPATOMEGALY (WITH STEATOSIS), dyspepsia, nausea. **F and E:** LACTIC ACIDOSIS. **Derm:** alopecia, rash.

Interactions
Drug-Drug: Concurrent use of drugs which may impair renal function may ↑ blood levels and risk of toxicity.

Route/Dosage
PO (Adults and Children >16 yr): 0.5 mg once daily; *history of lamivudine resistance*—1 mg once daily.

Renal Impairment
PO (Adults and Children >16 yr): *CCr 30–50 mL/min*—0.25 mg once daily, *history of lamivudine resistance*—0.5 mg once daily; *CCr 10–<30 mL/min*—0.15 mg once daily, *history of lamivudine resistance*—0.3 mg once daily; *CCr <10 mL/min*—0.05 mg once daily, *history of lamivudine resistance*—0.1 mg once daily.

Availability
Tablets: 0.5 mg, 1 mg. **Oral solution (orange):** 0.05 mg/mL.

NURSING IMPLICATIONS

Assessment
- Monitor signs of hepatitis (jaundice, fatigue, anorexia, pruritus) during and for several months following discontinuation of therapy. Exacerbations may occur when therapy is discontinued.
- May cause lactic acidosis and severe hepatomegaly with steatosis. Monitor patient for signs (increased serum lactate levels, elevated liver enzymes, liver enlargement on palpation). Therapy should be suspended if clinical or laboratory signs occur.
- *Lab Test Considerations:* Monitor liver function closely during and for several months following discontinuation of therapy. May cause ↑ AST, ALT, bilirubin, amylase, lipase, creatinine and serum glucose. May cause ↓ serum albumin.

Potential Nursing Diagnoses
Risk for infection (Indications)
Noncompliance (Patient/Family Teaching)

Implementation
- **PO:** Administer on an empty stomach at least 2 hr before or after a meal. Oral solution is ready to use and should not be diluted or mixed with water or any other liquid. Hold spoon in a vertical position and fill gradually to mark corresponding to the prescribed dose. Rinse dosing spoon with water after each daily dose. Store in outer carton at room temperature. After opening, solution can be used until expiration date on bottle.

Patient/Family Teaching
- Instruct patient to read the *Patient Information* with each refill and to take entecavir as directed. Take missed doses as soon as possible unless almost time for next dose. Do not run out of entecavir, get more when supply runs low. Do not double doses. Emphasize the importance of compliance with full course of therapy, not taking more than the prescribed

amount, and not discontinuing without consulting health care professional. Inform patient that hepatitis exacerbation may occur upon discontinuation of therapy. Caution patient not to share medication with others.
- Inform patient that entecavir does not cure HBV disease, but may lower the amount of HBV in the body, lower the ability of HBV to multiply and infect new liver cells, and may improve the condition of the liver. Entecavir does not reduce the risk of transmission of HBV to others through sexual contact or blood contamination. Caution patient to use a condom during sexual contact and avoid sharing needles or donating blood to prevent spreading HBV to others.
- Advise patient to notify health care professional promptly if signs of lactic acidosis (weakness or tiredness; unusual muscle pain; trouble breathing; stomach pain with nausea and vomiting; feeling cold, especially in arms or legs; dizziness, fast or irregular heartbeat) or hepatotoxicity (jaundice, dark urine, light-colored bowel movements, anorexia, nausea, lower stomach pain) occur.
- May cause dizziness. Caution patient to avoid driving or other activities requiring alertness until response to medication is known.
- Advise patient to consult health care professional before taking other Rx, OTC, or herbal products with entecavir.
- Discuss the possibility of hair loss with patient. Explore methods of coping.
- Advise patient to notify health care professional if pregnancy is planned or suspected or if breastfeeding.
- Emphasize the importance of regular follow-up exams and blood tests to determine progress and monitor for side effects.

Evaluation/Desired Outcomes
- Decreased hepatic damage due to chronic hepatitis B infection.

EPIDURAL LOCAL ANESTHETICS

bupivacaine (byoo-**pi**-vi-kane)
Marcaine, Sensorcaine

ropivacaine (**roe**-pi-vi-kane)
Naropin

Classification
Therapeutic: epidural local anesthetics, anesthetics (topical/local)

Pregnancy Category B (ropivacaine), C (bupivacaine)

Indications
Local or regional anesthesia or analgesia for surgical, obstetric, or diagnostic procedures.

Action
Local anesthetics inhibit initiation and conduction of sensory nerve impulses by altering the influx of sodium and efflux of potassium in neurons, slowing or stopping pain transmission. Epidural administration allows action to take place at the level of the spinal nerve roots immediately adjacent to the site of administration. The catheter is placed as close as possible to the dermatomes (skin surface areas innervated by a single spinal nerve or group of spinal nerves) that, when blocked, will produce the most effective spread of analgesia for the site of injury. **Therapeutic Effects:** Decreased pain or induction of anesthesia; low doses have minimal effect on sensory or motor function; higher doses may produce complete motor blockade.

Pharmacokinetics
Absorption: Systemic absorption follows epidural administration, but amount absorbed depends on dose.
Distribution: Agents are lipid soluble, which selectively keeps them in the epidural space and limits systemic absorption. If systemic absorption occurs, these agents are widely distributed and cross the placenta.
Metabolism and Excretion: Small amounts that may reach systemic circulation are mostly metabolized by the liver. Very little excreted unchanged in the urine.
Half-life: *Bupivacaine*—1.5–5 hr (after epidural use); *ropivacaine*—4.2 hr (after epidural use).

TIME/ACTION PROFILE (analgesia)

ROUTE	ONSET	PEAK	DURATION
Epidural	10–30 min	unknown	2-8 hr†

†Duration of anesthetic block

Contraindications/Precautions
Contraindicated in: Hypersensitivity; cross-sensitivity with other amide local anesthetics may occur (lidocaine, mepivacaine, prilocaine); Bupivacaine contains bisulfites and should be avoided in patients with known intolerance; OB: Bupivacaine

only—Do not use 0.75% concentration. Only 0.5% and 0.25% concentrations should be used for obstetrical anesthesia due to reports of cardiac arrest and difficult resuscitation with the 0.75% concentration ; Lactation: Discontinue nursing.
Use Cautiously in: Concurrent use of other local anesthetics; Liver disease; Concurrent use of anticoagulants (including low-dose heparin and low-molecular-weight heparins/heparinoids) ; ↑ the risk of spinal/epidural hematomas; OB: Bupivacaine and ropivacaine—both agents rapidly cross the placenta with obstetrical paracervical block anesthesia and can result in maternal, fetal, or neonatal toxicity with cardiac, central nervous system, or vascular tone abnormalities. May cause maternal hypotension. ; Pedi: Bupivacaine—safety not established in children <12 yr. Ropivacaine—safety not established in chlidren <18 yr; Geri: May require lower doses due to ↑ risk of hypotension and/or ↑ risk of toxicity due to age-related decline in renal function.

Adverse Reactions/Side Effects
CNS: SEIZURES, anxiety, dizziness, headache, irritability. **EENT:** blurred vision, tinnitus. **CV:** CARDIOVASCULAR COLLAPSE, arrhythmias, bradycardia, hypotension, tachycardia. **GI:** nausea, vomiting. **GU:** urinary retention. **Derm:** pruritus. **F and E:** metabolic acidosis. **Neuro:** circumoral tingling/numbness, tremor. **Misc:** allergic reactions, fever.

Interactions
Drug-Drug: Additive toxicity may occur with concurrent use of other **amide local anesthetics** (including **lidocaine**, **mepivacaine**, and **prilocaine**). Use of bupivacaine solution containing epinephrine with **MAO inhibitors** may cause hypertension. **Fluvoxamine**, **amiodarone**, **ciprofloxacin**, and **propofol** may ↑ effects of ropivacaine.

Route/Dosage
Solutions containing preservatives should not be used for caudal or epidural blocks.

Bupivacaine
Epidural (Adults and Children > 12 yr): 10–20 mL of 0.25% (partial to moderate block), 0.5% (moderate to complete block), or 0.75% (complete block) solution. Administer in increments of 3–5 mL allowing sufficient time to detect toxic signs/symptoms of inadvertent IV or IT administration. A test dose of 2–3 mL of 0.5% with epinephrine solution is recommended prior to epidural blocks.

Ropivacaine
Surgical Anesthesia
Epidural (Adults): *Lumbar epidural*-15–30 mL of 0.5% solution or 15–25 mL of 0.75% solution or 15–20 mL of 1% solution; *Lumbar epidural for cesarean section*-20–30 mL of 0.5% solution or 15–20 mL of 0.75% solution; *Thoracic epidural*-5–15 mL of 0.5–0.75% solution.

Labor Pain
Epidural (Adults): *Lumbar epidural*-10–20 mL of 0.2% solution initially, then continuous infusion of 6–14 mL/hr of 0.2% solution with incremental injection of 10–15 mL/hr of 0.2% solution.

Postoperative Pain
Epidural (Adults): *Lumbar or thoracic epidural*-Continuous infusion of 6–14 mL/hr of 0.2% solution.

Availability (generic available)
Bupivacaine
Solution for injection (preservative-free): 0.25%, 0.5%, 0.75%. *In combination with:* epinephrine 1:200,000.

Ropivacaine
Solution for injection (preservative-free): 0.2%, 0.5%, 0.75%, 1%.

NURSING IMPLICATIONS
Assessment
- Monitor for sensation during procedure and return of sensation after procedure.
- **Systemic Toxicity:** Assess for systemic toxicity (circumoral tingling and numbness, ringing in ears, metallic taste, dizziness, blurred vision, tremors, slow speech, irritability, twitching, seizures, cardiac dysrhythmias) each shift. Report to physician or other health care professional.
- **Orthostatic Hypotension:** Monitor blood pressure, heart rate, and respiratory rate continuously while patient is receiving this medication. Mild hypotension is common because of the effect of local anesthetic block of nerve fibers on the sympathetic nervous system, causing vasodilation. Significant hypotension and bradycardia may occur, especially when rising from a prone position or following large dose increases or boluses. Treatment of unresolved

hypotension may include hydration, decreasing the epidural infusion rate, and/or removal of local anesthetic from analgesic solution.
- **Unwanted Motor and Sensory Deficit:** The goal of adding low-dose local anesthetics to epidural opioids for pain management is to provide analgesia, not to produce anesthesia. Patients should be able to ambulate if their condition allows, and epidural analgesic should not hamper this important recovery activity. However, many factors, including location of the epidural catheter, local anesthetic dose, and variability in patient response, can result in patients experiencing unwanted motor and sensory deficits. Pain is the first sensation lost, followed by temperature, touch, proprioception, and skeletal muscle tone.
- Assess for sensory deficit every shift. Ask patient to point to numb and tingling skin areas (numbness and tingling at the incision site is common and usually normal). Notify physician or other health care professional of unwanted motor and sensory deficits.
- Unwanted motor and sensory deficits often can be corrected with simple treatment. For example, a change in position may relieve temporary sensory loss in an extremity. Minor extremity muscle weakness is often treated by decreasing the epidural infusion rate and keeping the patient in bed until the weakness resolves. Sometimes removing the local anesthetic from the analgesic solution is necessary, such as when signs of local anesthetic toxicity are detected or when simple treatment of motor and sensory deficits has been unsuccessful.

Potential Nursing Diagnoses
Acute pain, acute (Indications)
Impaired physical mobility (Side Effects)

Implementation
- See Route and Dosage section.

Patient/Family Teaching
- Instruct patient to notify nurse if signs or symptoms of systemic toxicity occur.
- Advise patient to request assistance during ambulation until orthostatic hypotension and motor deficits are ruled out.

Evaluation/Desired Outcomes
- Decrease in postoperative pain without unwanted sensory or motor deficits.

HIGH ALERT

epinephrine (e-pi-**nef**-rin)
Adrenalin, Ana-Guard, AsthmaHaler Mist, AsthmaNefrin (racepinephrine), EpiPen, microNefrin, Nephron, Primatene, Sus-Phrine, S-2

Classification
Therapeutic: antiasthmatics, bronchodilators, vasopressors
Pharmacologic: adrenergics

Pregnancy Category C
See Appendix C for ophthalmic use

Indications
Subcut, IV, Inhaln: Management of reversible airway disease due to asthma or COPD. **Subcut, IM, IV:** Management of severe allergic reactions. **IV, Intracardiac, Intratracheal, Intraosseous (part of advanced cardiac life support [ACLS] and pediatric advanced life support [PALS] guidelines):** Management of cardiac arrest (unlabeled). **Inhaln:** Management of upper airway obstruction and croup (racemic epinephrine). **Local/Spinal:** Adjunct in the localization/prolongation of anesthesia.

Action
Results in the accumulation of cyclic adenosine monophosphate (cAMP) at beta-adrenergic receptors. Affects both beta$_1$(cardiac)-adrenergic receptors and beta$_2$(pulmonary)-adrenergic receptor sites. Produces bronchodilation. Also has alpha-adrenergic agonist properties, which result in vasoconstriction. Inhibits the release of mediators of immediate hypersensitivity reactions from mast cells. **Therapeutic Effects:** Bronchodilation. Maintenance of heart rate and blood pressure. Localization/prolongation of local/spinal anesthetic.

Pharmacokinetics
Absorption: Well absorbed following subcut administration; some absorption may occur following repeated inhalation of large doses.
Distribution: Does not cross the blood-brain barrier; crosses the placenta and enters breast milk.
Metabolism and Excretion: Action is rapidly terminated by metabolism and uptake by nerve endings.
Half-life: Unknown.

TIME/ACTION PROFILE (bronchodilation)

ROUTE	ONSET	PEAK	DURATION
Inhaln	1 min	unknown	1–3 hr
Subcut	5–10 min	20 min	<1–4 hr
IM	6–12 min	unknown	<1–4 hr
IV	rapid	20 min	20–30 min

epinephrine

Contraindications/Precautions
Contraindicated in: Hypersensitivity to adrenergic amines; Cardiac arrhythmias; Some products may contain bisulfites or fluorocarbons (in some inhalers) and should be avoided in patients with known hypersensitivity or intolerance.
Use Cautiously in: Cardiac disease (angina, tachycardia, MI); Hypertension; Hyperthyroidism; Diabetes; Cerebral arteriosclerosis; Glaucoma (except for ophthalmic use); Excessive use may lead to tolerance and paradoxical bronchospasm (inhaler); OB: Use only if potential maternal benefit outweighs potential risks to fetus; Lactation: High intravenous doses of epinephrine might ↓ milk production or letdown. Low-dose epidural, topical, inhaled or ophthalmic epinephrine are unlikely to interfere with breastfeeding (NIH); Geri: More susceptible to adverse reactions; may require ↓ dose.

Adverse Reactions/Side Effects
CNS: nervousness, restlessness, tremor, headache, insomnia. **Resp:** paradoxical bronchospasm (excessive use of inhalers). **CV:** angina, arrhythmias, hypertension, tachycardia. **GI:** nausea, vomiting. **Endo:** hyperglycemia.

Interactions
Drug-Drug: Concurrent use with other **adrenergic agents** will have additive adrenergic side effects. Use with **MAO inhibitors** may lead to hypertensive crisis. **Beta blockers:** may negate therapeutic effect. **Tricyclic antidepressants** enhance pressor response to epinephrine.
Drug-Natural Products: Use with caffeine-containing herbs (**cola nut**, **guarana**, **mate**, **tea**, **coffee**) ↑ stimulant effect.

Route/Dosage
Subcut, IM (Adults): *Anaphylactic reactions/asthma*—0.1–0.5 mg (single dose not to exceed 1 mg); may repeat q 10–15 min for anaphylactic shock or q 20 min–4 hr for asthma.
Subcut (Children > 1 month): *Anaphylactic reactions/asthma*—0.01 mg/kg (not to exceed 0.5 mg/dose) q 15 min for 2 doses, then q 4 hr.
IV (Adults): *Severe anaphylaxis*—0.1–0.25 mg q 5–15 min; may be followed by 1–4 mcg/min continuous infusion; *cardiopulmonary resuscitation (ACLS guidelines)*—1 mg q 3–5 min; *bradycardia (ACLS guidelines)*—2–10 mcg/min).
IV (Children): *Severe anaphylaxis*—0.1 mg (less in younger children); may be followed by 0.1 mcg/kg/min continuous infusion (may be increased up to 1.5 mcg/kg/min); *symptomatic bradycardia/pulseless arrest (PALS guidelines)*—0.01 mg/kg, may be repeated q 3–5 min higher doses (up to 0.1–0.2 mg/kg) may be considered; may also be given by the intraosseous route. May also be given by the endotracheal route in doses of 0.1–0.2 mg/kg diluted to a volume of 3–5 mL with normal saline followed by several positive pressure ventilations.
Inhaln (Adults): *Metered-dose inhaler*—1 inhalation (160–250 mcg), may be repeated after 1–2 min; additional doses may be repeated q 3 hr; *inhalation solution*—1 inhalation of 1% solution; may be repeated after 1–2 min; additional doses may be given q 3 hr; *racepinephrine*—Via hand nebulizer, 2–3 inhalations of 2.25% solution; may repeat in 5 min with 2–3 more inhalations, up to 4–6 times daily.
Inhaln (Children > 1 month): 0.25–0.5 mL of 2.25% racemic epinephrine solution diluted in 3 mL normal saline.
IV, Intratracheal (Neonates): 0.01–0.03 mg/kg q 3–5 min as needed.
IM (Children > 1 month < 30 kg): 0.15 mg (EpiPen Jr); > 30 kg: 0.3 mg (EpiPen).
Intracardiac (Adults): 0.3–0.5 mg.
Endotracheal (Adults): *Cardiopulmonary resuscitation (ACLS guidelines)*—2–2.5 mg.
Topical (Adults and Children ≥6 yr): *Nasal decongestant*—Apply 1% solution as drops, spray, or with a swab.
Intraspinal (Adults and Children): 0.2–0.4 mL of 1:1000 solution.
With Local Anesthetics (Adults and Children): Use 1:200,000 solution with local anesthetic.

Availability (generic available)
Inhalation aerosol: 0.125% (≥300 inhalations/15 mL)^OTC, 0.5% (≥300 inhalations/15 mL)^OTC, 300 mcg/spray (≥300 inhalations/15 mL)^OTC. **Inhalation solution:** 1%^OTC. **Injection:** 0.1 mg/mL (1:10,000), 1 mg/mL (1:1000). **Autoinjector (EpiPen):** 0.15 mg/0.3 mL (1:2000), 0.3 mg/0.3 mL (1:1000). **Cost:** 0.15 mg $56.48/syringe, 0.3 mg $58.99/syringe. **Topical solution:** 0.1%.

NURSING IMPLICATIONS

Assessment
- **Bronchodilator:** Assess lung sounds, respiratory pattern, pulse, and blood pressure before administration and during peak of medication. Note amount, color, and character of sputum

produced, and notify health care professional of abnormal findings.
- Monitor pulmonary function tests before and periodically during therapy.
- Observe for paradoxical bronchospasm (wheezing). If condition occurs, withhold medication and notify health care professional immediately.
- Observe patient for drug tolerance and rebound bronchospasm. Patients requiring more than 3 inhalation treatments in 24 hr should be under close supervision. If minimal or no relief is seen after 3–5 inhalation treatments within 6–12 hr, further treatment with aerosol alone is not recommended.
- Assess for hypersensitivity reaction (rash; urticaria; swelling of the face, lips, or eyelids). If condition occurs, withhold medication and notify health care professional immediately.
- **Vasopressor:** Monitor blood pressure, pulse, ECG, and respiratory rate frequently during IV administration. Continuous ECG, hemodynamic parameters, and urine output should be monitored continuously during IV administration.
- Monitor for chest pain, arrhythmias, heart rate > 110 bpm, and hypertension. Consult physician for parameters of pulse, blood pressure, and ECG changes for adjusting dosage or discontinuing medication.
- **Shock:** Assess volume status. Hypovolemia should be corrected prior to administering epinephrine IV.
- **Nasal Decongestant:** Assess patient for nasal and sinus congestion prior to and periodically during therapy.
- *Lab Test Considerations:* May cause transient ↓ in serum potassium concentrations with nebulization or at higher than recommended doses.
- May cause an ↑ in blood glucose and serum lactic acid concentrations.
- *Toxicity and Overdose:* Symptoms of overdose include persistent agitation, chest pain or discomfort, decreased blood pressure, dizziness, hyperglycemia, hypokalemia, seizures, tachyarrhythmias, persistent trembling, and vomiting.
- Treatment includes discontinuing adrenergic bronchodilator and other beta-adrenergic agonists and symptomatic, supportive therapy. Cardioselective beta blockers are used cautiously-because they may induce bronchospasm.

Potential Nursing Diagnoses
Ineffective airway clearance (Indications)
Ineffective tissue perfusion (Indications)

Implementation
- *High Alert:* Patient harm or fatalities have occurred from medication errors with epinephrine. Epinephrine is available in various concentrations, strengths, and percentages and used for different purposes. Packaging labels may be easily confused or products incorrectly diluted. Dilutions should be prepared by a pharmacist. IV doses should be expressed in milligrams not ampules, concentration or volume. Prior to administration, have second practitioner independently check original order, dose calculations, concentration, route of administration, and infusion pump settings.
- Medication should be administered promptly at the onset of bronchospasm.
- Use a tuberculin syringe with a 26-gauge ½-in. needle for subcut injection to ensure that correct amount of medication is administered.
- Tolerance may develop with prolonged or excessive use. Effectiveness may be restored by discontinuing for a few days and then readministering.
- Do not use solutions that are pinkish or brownish or that contain a precipitate.
- For anaphylactic shock, volume replacement should be administered concurrently with epinephrine. Antihistamines and corticosteroids may be used in conjunction with epinephrine.
- **IM, Subcut:** Medication can cause irritation of tissue. Rotate injection sites to prevent tissue necrosis. Massage injection sites well after administration to enhance absorption and to decrease local vasoconstriction. Avoid IM administration in gluteal muscle.

IV Administration
- **Direct IV:** *Diluent:* The 1:10,000 solution can be administered undiluted. Dilute 1 mg (1 mL) of a 1:1000 solution in 9 mL of 0.9% NaCl to prepare a 1:10,000 solution. *Concentration:* 0.1 mg/mL (1:10,000). *Rate:* Administer each 1 mg (10 mL) of a 1:10,000 solution over at least 1 min; more rapid administration may be used during cardiac resuscitation. Follow each dose with 20 mL IV saline flush.
- **Continuous Infusion:** *Diluent:* Dilute 1 mg (1 mL) of a 1:1000 solution in 250 mL of D5W or 0.9% NaCl. Protect from light. Infusion stable for 24 hr. *Concentration:* 4 mcg/mL. *Rate:* See Route/Dosage section. Titrate to response (blood pressure, heart rate, respiratory rate).
- **Y-Site Compatibility:** alfentanil, amikacin, amiodarone, amphotericin B liposome, anidulafungin, ascorbic acid, atropine, aztreonam,

benztropine, bivalirudin, bumetanide, buprenorphine, butorphanol, calcium chloride, calcium gluconate, carboplatin, caspofungin, cefazolin, cefoperazone, cefotaxime, cefotetan, cefoxitin, ceftazidime, ceftizoxime, ceftriaxone, cefuroxime, chloramphenicol , chlorpromazine, cimetidine, cisatracurium, cisplatin, clindamycin, cyanocobalamin, cyclophosphamide, cyclosporine, cytarabine, dactinomycin, daptomycin, dexamethasone sodium phosphate, dexmedetomidine, digoxin, diltiazem, diphenhydramine, dobutamine, docetaxel, dopamine, doxorubicin, doxycycline, enalaprilat, epirubicin, epoetin alfa, ertapenem, erythromycin, esmolol, etoposide, etoposide phosphate, famotidine, fenoldopam, fentanyl, fluconazole, fludarabine, folic acid, furosemide, gemcitabine, gentamicin, glycopyrrolate, granisetron, heparin, hydrocortisone sodium succinate, hydromorphone, ifosfamide, imipenem/cilastatin, isoproterenol, ketorolac, labetalol, levofloxacin, lidocaine, linezolid, lorazepam, magnesium sulfate, mannitol, mechlorethamine, meperidine, metaraminol, methicillin, methotrexate, methoxamine, methyldopa, methylprednisolone sodium succinate, metoclopramide, metoprolol, metronidazole, midazolam, milrinone, minocycline, mitoxantrone, morphine, multiple vitamins, nafcillin, nalbuphine, naloxone, nicardipine, nitroglycerin, nitroprusside, norepinephrine, octreotide, ondansetron, oxacillin, oxaliplatin, oxytocin, paclitaxel, palonosetron, pancuronium, pantoprazole, pemetrexed, penicillin G potassium, pentamidine, pentazocine, phentolamine, phenylephrine, phytonadione, piperacillin/tazobactam, potassium chloride, procainamide, prochlorperazine, promethazine, propofol, propranolol, protamine, pyridoxime, quinupristin/dalfopristin, ranitidine, remifentanil, ritodrine, rocuronium, sodium acetate, streptokinase, streptomycin, succinylcholine, sufentanil, tacrolimus, teniposide, theophylline, thiamine, thiotepa, ticarcillin/clavulanate, tigecycline, tirofiban, tobramycin, tolazoline, trimethophan, urokinase, vancomycin, vasopressin, vecuronium, verapamil, vincristine, vinorelbine, vitamin B complex with C, voriconazole, warfarin.
- **Y-Site Incompatibility:** acyclovir, aminophylline, azathioprine, dantrolene, diazepam, diazoxide, fluorouracil, ganciclovir, indomethacin, micafungin, pentobarbital, phenobarbital, phenytoin, sodium bicarbonate, thiopental, trimethoprim/sulfamethoxazole.
- **Inhaln:** When using epinephrine inhalation solution, 10 drops of 1% base solution should be placed in the reservoir of the nebulizer.
- The 2.25% inhalation solution of racepinephrine must be diluted for use in the combination nebulizer/respirator.
- Allow 1–2 min to elapse between inhalations of epinephrine inhalation solution, epinephrine inhalation aerosol, or epinephrine bitartrate inhalation aerosol to make certain the second inhalation is necessary.
- When epinephrine is used concurrently with corticosteroid or ipratropium inhalations, administer bronchodilator first and other medications 5 min apart to prevent toxicity from inhaled fluorocarbon propellants.
- **Endotracheal:** Epinephrine can be injected directly into the bronchial tree via the endotracheal tube if the patient has been intubated. Perform 5 rapid insufflations; forcefully administer 10 mL containing 2–2.5 mg epinephrine (1 mg/mL) directly into tube; follow with 5 quick insufflations.

Patient/Family Teaching

- Instruct patient to take medication exactly as directed. If on a scheduled dosing regimen, take a missed dose as soon as possible; space remaining doses at regular intervals. Do not double doses. Caution patient not to exceed recommended dose; may cause adverse effects, paradoxical bronchospasm, or loss of effectiveness of medication.
- Instruct patient to contact health care professional immediately if shortness of breath is not relieved by medication or is accompanied by diaphoresis, dizziness, palpitations, or chest pain.
- Advise patient to consult health care professional before taking any OTC medications or alcoholic beverages concurrently with this therapy. Caution patient also to avoid smoking and other respiratory irritants.
- **Inhaln:** Review correct administration technique (aerosolization, IPPB, metered-dose inhaler) with patient. See Appendix D for administration with metered-dose inhaler. Wait 1–5 min before administering next dose. Mouthpiece should be washed after each use.
- Do not spray inhaler near eyes.
- Instruct patient to save inhaler; refill canisters may be available.

- Advise patients to use bronchodilator first if using other inhalation medications, and allow 5 min to elapse before administering other inhalant medications, unless otherwise directed.
- Advise patient to rinse mouth with water after each inhalation dose to minimize dry mouth.
- Advise patient to maintain adequate fluid intake (2000–3000 mL/day) to help liquefy tenacious secretions.
- Advise patient to consult health care professional if respiratory symptoms are not relieved or worsen after treatment or if chest pain, headache, severe dizziness, palpitations, nervousness, or weakness occurs.
- Instruct patient to notify health care professional if contents of one canister are used up in less than 2 wk.
- **Autoinjector:** Instruct patients using auto-injector for anaphylactic reactions to remove gray safety cap, placing black tip on thigh at right angle to leg. Press hard into thigh until auto-injector functions, hold in place for 10 seconds, remove, and discard properly. Massage injected area for 10 sec. Pedi: Teach parents or caregivers signs and symptoms of anaphlyaxis, how to use auto-injector safely, and to get the child to a hospital as soon as possible. Instruct parents or caregivers to teach child how to manage his or her allergy, how to self-inject, and what to do in an emergency. For children too young to self-inject and who will be separated from parent, tell parents to always discuss allergy and use of auto-injector with responsible adult.

Evaluation/Desired Outcomes
- Prevention or relief of bronchospasm.
- Increase in ease of breathing.
- Prevention of bronchospasm or reduction of frequency of acute asthma attacks in patients with chronic asthma.
- Prevention of exercise-induced asthma.
- Reversal of signs and symptoms of anaphylaxis.
- Increase in cardiac rate and output, when used in cardiac resuscitation.
- Increase in blood pressure, when used as a vasopressor.
- Localization of local anesthetic.
- Decrease in sinus and nasal congestion.

HIGH ALERT

epirubicin (ep-i-roo-bi-sin)
Ellence

Classification
Therapeutic: antineoplastics
Pharmacologic: anthracyclines

Pregnancy Category D

Indications
A component of adjuvant therapy for evidence of axillary tumor involvement following resection of primary breast cancer.

Action
Inhibits DNA and RNA synthesis by forming a complex with DNA. **Therapeutic Effects:** Death of rapidly replicating cells, particularly malignant ones.

Pharmacokinetics
Absorption: IV administration results in complete bioavailability.
Distribution: Rapidly and widely distributed; concentrates in RBCs.
Metabolism and Excretion: Extensively and rapidly metabolized by the liver and other tissues.
Half-life: 35 hr.

TIME/ACTION PROFILE (effect on WBCs)

ROUTE	ONSET	PEAK	DURATION
IV	unknown	10–14 days	21 days

Contraindications/Precautions
Contraindicated in: Hypersensitivity to epirubicin, other anthracyclines, or related compounds; Baseline neutrophil count <1500 cells/mm^3; Severe myocardial insufficiency or recent MI; Previous anthracyclines up to the maximum cumulative dose; Severe hepatic dysfunction; Concurrent cimetidine therapy; OB, Lactation: Significant risk for fetal or infant harm.
Use Cautiously in: Severe renal impairment (serum creatinine >5 mg/dL); consider ↓ dose; Hepatic impairment (dose ↓ recommended for bilirubin >1.2 mg/dL or AST >2–4 times upper limit of normal); Depressed bone marrow reserve; OB: Warn patients with childbearing potential to avoid pregnancy during treatment; Pedi: Safety not established; ↑ risk of acute cardiotoxicity and chronic CHF; Geri: ↑ risk of toxicity in female patients ≥70 yr.

Adverse Reactions/Side Effects
CNS: lethargy. **CV:** CARDIOTOXICITY (dose-related). **GI:** nausea, vomiting, anorexia, diarrhea, mucositis. **Derm:** alopecia, flushing, itching, photosensitivity, radiation-recall reaction, rash, skin/nail hyperpigmentation. **Endo:** gonadal suppression. **Hemat:** LEUKOPENIA, anemia, thrombocytopenia, treatment-related leukemia/myelodysplas-

tic syndromes. **Local:** injection site reactions, phlebitis at IV site, tissue necrosis. **Metab:** hot flashes, hyperuricemia. **Misc:** ANAPHYLAXIS, INFECTION.

Interactions
Drug-Drug: Cimetidine ↑ blood levels and risk of serious toxicity; avoid concurrent use. Additive hematologic and gastrointestinal toxicity with other **antineoplastics** or **radiation therapy**. May ↓ antibody response to **live-virus vaccines** and ↑ risk of adverse reactions.

Route/Dosage
IV (Adults): 100–120 mg/m² repeated in 3–4 wk cycles (total dose may be given on day 1 or split and given in equally divided doses on day 1 and day 8 of each cycle (combination regimens may employ concurrent 5-fluorouracil and cyclophosphamide).

Hepatic Impairment
IV (Adults): *Bilirubin 1.2–3 mg/dL or AST 2–4 times upper limit of normal*—use 50% of recommended starting dose; *bilirubin >3 mg/dL or AST >4 times upper limit of normal*—use 25% of recommended starting dose.

Availability (generic available)
Solution for injection (red): 50-mg/25-mL single-use vial, 200-mg/100-mL single-use vial.

NURSING IMPLICATIONS

Assessment
- Monitor for bone marrow depression. Assess for bleeding (bleeding gums, bruising, petechiae, guaiac stools, urine, and emesis) and avoid IM injections and taking rectal temperatures if platelet count is low. Apply pressure to venipuncture sites for 10 min. Assess for signs of infection during neutropenia. Anemia may occur. Monitor for increased fatigue, dyspnea, and orthostatic hypotension.
- Severe nausea and vomiting may occur. Administer parenteral antiemetic agents 30–45 min prior to therapy and routinely around the clock for the next 24 hr as indicated. Monitor amount of emesis and notify health care professional if emesis exceeds guidelines to prevent dehydration.
- Measure cardiac function, using ECG and a multigated radionuclide angiography (MUGA) scan or an ECHO, prior to therapy. Perform repeated evaluations of left ventricular ejection fraction during therapy. Monitor for development of signs of cardiac toxicity, which may occur early (ST-T wave changes, sinus tachycardia, and extrasystoles) or late (may occur months to yr after termination of therapy). Delayed cardiac toxicity is characterized by cardiomyopathy, tachycardia, peripheral edema, dyspnea, rales/crackles, weight gain, hepatomegaly, ascites, pleural effusion. Toxicity is usually dependent on cumulative dose.
- Assess injection site frequently for redness, irritation, or inflammation. Burning or stinging during infusion may indicate infiltration and infusion should be discontinued and restarted in another vein. Epirubicin is a vesicant but may infiltrate painlessly even if blood returns on aspiration of infusion needle. Severe tissue damage may occur if epirubicin extravasates. If extravasation occurs, stop infusion immediately, restart, and complete dose in another vein.
- Assess oral mucosa frequently for development of stomatitis (pain, burning, erythema, ulcerations, bleeding, infection). Increased dosing interval and/or decreased dosing is recommended if lesions are painful or interfere with nutrition.
- *Lab Test Considerations:* Monitor CBC and differential before and during each cycle of therapy. Epirubicin should not be administered to patients with a baseline neutrophil count <1500 cells/mm³. The WBC nadir occurs 10–14 days after administration, and recovery usually occurs by the 21st day. Severe thrombocytopenia and anemia may also occur.
- Monitor renal (BUN and creatinine) and hepatic (AST, ALT, LDH, and serum bilirubin) function prior to and periodically during therapy. Dose reduction is required for bilirubin >1.2 mg/dL, AST 2–4 times the upper limit of normal, or serum creatinine >5 mg/dL.

Potential Nursing Diagnoses
Risk for infection (Adverse Reactions)
Decreased cardiac output (Adverse Reactions)

Implementation
- *High Alert:* Fatalities have occurred with incorrect administration of chemotherapeutic agents. Before administering, clarify ambiguous orders; double check single, daily, and course-of-therapy dose limits; have second practitioner independently double check original order, calculations and infusion pump settings. Epirubicin should be administered only under the supervision of a physician experi-

enced in the use of cancer chemotherapeutic agents.
- Prepare solution in a biologic cabinet. Wear gloves, gown, and mask while handling medication. Discard IV equipment in specially designated containers.
- Administer prophylactic anti-infective therapy with trimethoprim/sulfamethoxazole or a fluoroquinolone and antiemetic therapy prior to administration of epirubicin.
- Do not administer subcut or IM.

IV Administration

- **Intermittent Infusion:** *Diluent:* Administer undiluted. Solution is clear red. Use epirubicin within 24 hr of penetration of rubber stopper. Discard unused solution. *Concentration:* 2 mg/mL. *Rate:* Administer initial dose of 100–120 mg/m^2 over 15–20 min through Y-site of a free-flowing infusion of 0.9% NaCl or D5W. Lower doses may be infused for shorter periods, but not less than over 3 min. Do not administer via direct IV push. Facial flushing and erythema along involved vein frequently occur when administration is too rapid. Venous sclerosis may result from injection into a small vein or repeated injections into the same vein. Avoid veins over joints or in extremities with compromised venous or lymphatic drainage.
- **Syringe Incompatibility:** Do not mix in syringe with other drugs or with alkaline solutions, fluorouracil, heparin, ifosfamide.
- **Y-Site Compatibility:** alfentanil, amifostine, amikacin, aminocaproic acid, atracurium, aztreonam, bivalirudin, bretylium, bumetanide, buprenorphine, butorphanol, calcium chloride, calcium gluconate, carboplatin, caspofungin, cefazolin, cefotaxime, ceftizoxime, chlorpromazine, cimetidine, ciprofloxacin, cisatracurium, cisplatin, clindamycin, cyclophosphamide, cyclosporine, daptomycin, dexrazoxane, digoxin, diltiazem, diphenhydramine, docetaxel, dolasetron, dopamine, doxacurium, doxacycline, droperidol, enalaprilat, ephedrine, epinephrine, erythromycin, etoposide, etoposide phosphate, famotidine, fenoldopam, fentanyl, fluconazole, gemcitabine, gentamicin, granisetron, haloperidol, hydrocortisone sodium succinate, hydromorphone, ifosfamide, imipenem cilastatin, inamrinone, insulin, isoproterenol, labetalol, levofloxacin, levorphanol, lidocaine, linezolid, lorazepam, mannitol, meperidine, mesna, methotrexate, metoclopramide, metoprolol, metronidazole, midazolam, milrinone, monocycline, mitomycin, mivacurium, morphine, nalbuphine, naloxone, nesiritide, nicardipine, nitroglycerin, nitroprusside, norepinephrine, octreotide, ondansetron, oxaliplatin, paclitaxel, palonosetron, pancuronium, pentamidine, pentazocine, phenylephrine, potassium chloride, procainamide, prochlorperazine, promethazine, propranolol, quinapristin/dalfopristin, ranitidine, remifentanil, rocuronium, sodium acetate, succinylcholine, sufentanil, tacrolimus, teniposide, theophylline, thiotepa, tirofiban, tobramycin, trimethobenzamide, vancomycin, vasopressin, vecuronium, verapamil, vinblastine, vincristine, vinorelbine, voriconazole, zidovudine.
- **Y-Site Incompatibility:** acyclovir, allopurinol, aminophylline, amphotericin B colloidal, amphotericin B liposome, ampicillin, ampicillin/sulbactam, azithromycin, cefepime, cefoperazone, cefotetan, cefoxitin, ceftazidime, ceftriaxone, cefuroxime, dexamethasone sodium phosphate, diazepam, ertapenem, fluorouracil, foscarnet, fosphenytoin, furosemide, ganciclovir, heparin, hydrocortisone sodium phosphate, ketorolac, leucovorin, magnesium sulfate, meropenem, methohexital, methylprednisolone, nafcillin, pantoprazole, pemetrexed, pentobarbital, phenobarbital, phenytoin, piperacillin/tazobactam, potassium phosphates, sodium bicarbonate, sodium phosphates, thiopental, ticarcillin/clavulanate, tigecycline, trimethoprim/sulfamethoxazole.

Patient/Family Teaching

- Instruct patient to notify health care professional promptly if fever; sore throat; signs of infection; bleeding gums; bruising; petechiae; blood in stools, urine, or emesis; increased fatigue; dyspnea; or orthostatic hypotension occurs. Caution patient to avoid crowds and persons with known infections. Instruct patient to use soft toothbrush and electric razor and to avoid falls. Patient should be cautioned not to drink alcoholic beverages or take medication containing aspirin or NSAIDs, because these may precipitate gastric bleeding.
- Instruct patient to report pain at injection site immediately.
- Instruct patient to inspect oral mucosa for erythema and ulceration. If ulceration occurs, advise patient to use sponge brush, rinse mouth with water after eating and drinking, and confer with health care professional if mouth pain interferes with eating. Pain may require treatment with opioid analgesics. Patients usually recover by the third week of therapy.

- Advise patient that this medication may have teratogenic effects. Contraception should be used during and for at least 4 mo after therapy is concluded. Inform patient before initiating therapy that this medication may cause irreversible gonadal suppression.
- Instruct patient to avoid taking cimetidine, OTC or Rx, during therapy, and to consult health care professional prior to taking other Rx, OTC, or herbal products.
- Instruct patient to notify health care professional immediately if vomiting, dehydration, fever, evidence of infection, symptoms of CHF, or pain at injection site occurs. Patients should be informed of the risk of irreversible cardiac damage and treatment-related leukemia.
- Discuss the possibility of hair loss with patient. Explore methods of coping. Regrowth usually occurs 2–3 mo after discontinuation of therapy.
- Instruct patient not to receive any vaccinations without advice of health care professional.
- Inform patient that medication may cause urine to appear red for 1–2 days.
- Instruct patient to notify health care professional if skin irritation occurs at site of previous radiation therapy. May cause hyperpigmentation of the skin and nails. Advise patient to use sunscreen and protective clothing to prevent photosensitivity reactions.
- Emphasize the need for periodic lab tests to monitor for side effects.

Evaluation/Desired Outcomes
- Decrease in size or spread of malignancies in patients with axillary node tumor involvement following resection of primary breast cancer.

---

eplerenone (e-ple-re-none)
Inspra

Classification
Therapeutic: antihypertensives
Pharmacologic: aldosterone antagonists

Pregnancy Category B

Indications
Hypertension (alone, or with other agents). LV systolic dysfunction and evidence of HF post-MI.

Action
Blocks the effects of aldosterone by attaching to mineralocorticoid receptors. **Therapeutic Effects:** Lowering of blood pressure. Improves survival in patients with evidence of HF post-MI.

Pharmacokinetics
Absorption: Well absorbed following oral administration.
Distribution: Unknown.
Metabolism and Excretion: Mostly metabolized by the liver (CYP3A4 enzyme system); <5% excreted unchanged by the kidneys.
Half-life: 4–6 hr.

TIME/ACTION PROFILE (antihypertensive effect)

ROUTE	ONSET	PEAK	DURATION
PO	Unknown	4 wk	Unknown

Contraindications/Precautions
Contraindicated in: Serum potassium >5.5 mEq/L; Type 2 diabetes with microalbuminuria (for patients with HTN; ↑ risk of hyperkalemia); Serum creatinine >2 mg/dL in males or >1.8 mg/dL in females (for patients with HTN); CCr ≤30 mL/min (for all patients); CCr <50 mL/min (for patients with HTN); Concurrent use of potassium supplements or potassium-sparing diuretics (for patients with HTN); Concurrent use of strong inhibitors of the CYP3A4 enzyme system (ketoconazole, itraconazole, nefazodone, clarithromycin, ritonavir, or nelfinavir); Lactation: Lactation.
Use Cautiously in: Severe hepatic impairment; OB: Use only if clearly needed; Pedi: Safety not established.

Adverse Reactions/Side Effects
CNS: dizziness, fatigue. **GI:** abnormal liver function tests, abdominal pain, diarrhea. **GU:** albuminuria. **Endo:** abnormal vaginal bleeding, gynecomastia. **F and E:** HYPERKALEMIA. **Metab:** hypercholesterolemia, hypertriglyceridemia. **Misc:** flu-like symptoms.

Interactions
Drug-Drug: Concurrent use of strong inhibitors of the CYP3A4 enzyme system (**ketoconazole**, **itraconazole**, **nefazodone**, **clarithromycin**, **ritonavir**, or **nelfinavir**) significantly ↑ effects of eplerenone; concurrent use contraindicated. Concurrent use of weak inhibitors of the CYP3A4 enzyme system (**erythromycin**, **saquinavir**, **fluconazole**, **verapamil**) may ↑ effects of eplerenone; initial dose of eplerenone should be ↓ by 50%. **NSAIDs** may ↓ antihypertensive effects. Concurrent use of **ACE inhibitors** or **Angioten-**

sin II receptor blockers may ↑ risk of hyperkalemia.

Route/Dosage
Hypertension
PO (Adults): 50 mg daily initially; may be increased to 50 mg twice daily; *Patients receiving concurrent moderate CYP3A4 inhibitors (erythromycin, saquinavir, verapamil, fluconazole)*—25 mg once daily initially.

HF Post-MI
PO (Adults): 25 mg daily initially; increase in 4 wk to 50 mg daily; subsequent dose adjustments may need to be made based on serum potassium concentrations.

Availability
Tablets: 25 mg, 50 mg.

NURSING IMPLICATIONS
Assessment
- Monitor blood pressure periodically during therapy.
- Monitor prescription refills to determine adherence.
- *Lab Test Considerations:* May cause hyperkalemia. Monitor serum potassium levels prior to starting therapy, within the first wk, at 1 month following start of therapy or dose adjustmentand periodically thereafter. Monitor serum potassium and serum creatinine in 3-7 days in patients who start taking a moderate CYP3A4 inhibitor.
- May cause ↓ serum sodium and ↑ serum triglyceride, cholesterol, ALT, GGT, creatinine, and uric acid levels.

Potential Nursing Diagnoses
Decreased cardiac output (Indications)
Noncompliance (Patient/Family Teaching)

Implementation
- **PO:** Administer once daily. May be increased to twice daily if response is inadequate.

Patient/Family Teaching
- Instruct patient to take medication as directed at the same time each day, even if feeling well.
- Encourage patient to comply with additional interventions for hypertension (weight reduction, discontinuation of smoking, moderation of alcohol consumption, regular exercise, stress management). Medication controls, but does not cure, hypertension.
- Instruct patient and family on correct technique for monitoring blood pressure. Advise them to monitor blood pressure at least weekly, and notify health care professional of significant changes.
- Inform patient not to use potassium supplements, salt substitutes containing potassium, or other Rx, OTC, or herbal products without consulting health care professional.
- May cause dizziness. Caution patient to avoid driving or other activities requiring alertness until response to medication is known.
- Advise patient to notify health care professional if dizziness, diarrhea, vomiting, rapid or irregular heartbeat, lower extremity edema, or difficulty breathing occur.
- Advise patient to inform health care professional of treatment regimen prior to treatment or surgery.
- Advise patient to notify health care professional if pregnancy is planned or suspected. Advise patient to avoid breastfeeding during therapy.
- Emphasize the importance of follow-up exams to check serum potassium.

Evaluation/Desired Outcomes
- Decrease in blood pressure without appearance of side effects.
- Improvement in survival in patients with evidence of HF post-MI.

---

epoetin (e-poe-e-tin)
Epogen, EPO, ✤Eprex, erythropoietin, Procrit

Classification
Therapeutic: antianemics
Pharmacologic: hormones

Pregnancy Category C

Indications
Anemia associated with chronic renal failure. Anemia secondary to zidovudine (AZT) therapy in HIV-infected patients. Anemia from chemotherapy in patients with nonmyeloid malignancies. Reduction of need for transfusions after surgery. **Unlabeled Use:** Anemia of prematurity.

Action
Stimulates erythropoiesis (production of red blood cells). **Therapeutic Effects:** Maintains and may elevate RBCs, decreasing the need for transfusions.

Pharmacokinetics
Absorption: Well absorbed after subcut administration.
Distribution: Unknown.
Metabolism and Excretion: Unknown.

epoetin

Half-life: *Children and Adults*—4–13 hr; *Neonates*—11–17 hr.

TIME/ACTION PROFILE (increase in RBCs)

ROUTE	ONSET†	PEAK	DURATION
IV, subcut	7–10 days	within 2 mos	2 wk‡

†Increase in reticulocytes
‡After discontinuation

Contraindications/Precautions
Contraindicated in: Hypersensitivity to albumin or mammalian cell-derived products; Uncontrolled hypertension; Patients with erythropoietin levels >200 mUnits/mL; Patients receiving chemotherapy when anticipated outcome is cure; Neutropenia in newborns.

Use Cautiously in: History of seizures; History of porphyria; OB: Evidence of fetal harm in animal studies—use only if potential benefit outweighs potential risk to fetus; OB, Lactation: Little published information, however, erythropoetin alfa is a normal constituent of breastmilk; Pedi: Multidose vials contain benzyl alcohol, which can cause potentially fatal gasping syndrome in neonates.

Adverse Reactions/Side Effects
CNS: SEIZURES, headache. **CV:** CHF, MI, STROKE, THROMBOTIC EVENTS (especially with hemoglobin >12 g/dL), hypertension. **Derm:** transient rashes. **Endo:** restored fertility, resumption of menses. **Misc:** ↑ mortality and ↑ tumor growth (with hemoglobin ≥12 g/dL).

Interactions
Drug-Drug: May ↑ requirement for **heparin** anticoagulation during hemodialysis.

Route/Dosage
(Use lowest dose that will gradually increase hemoglobin level and avoid RBC transfusion).

Anemia of Chronic Renal Failure
Subcut, IV (Adults): 50–100 units/kg 3 times weekly initially; adjust dose to attain target hemoglobin of 10–12 g/dL.
Subcut, IV (Children): 50 units/kg 3 times weekly initially; adjust dose to attain target hemoglobin of 10–12 g/dL.

Anemia Secondary to AZT Therapy
Subcut, IV (Adults): 100 units/kg 3 times weekly for 8 wk; if inadequate response, may increase by 50–100 units/kg every 4–8 wk (max: 300 units/kg 3 times weekly).
Subcut, IV (Children 8 mo-17 yr): 50–400 units/kg 2–3 times weekly.

Anemia from Chemotherapy
(Use only for chemotherapy-related anemia and discontinue when chemotherapy course is completed; do not initiate if hemoglobin ≥10 g/dL).
Subcut (Adults): 150 units/kg 3 times weekly or 40,000 units weekly; adjust dose to maintain lowest hemoglobin level sufficient to avoid blood transfusions (do not exceed hemoglobin of 12 g/dL).
IV (Children 6 mo—18 yr): 600 units/kg 3 times weekly; adjust dose to maintain lowest hemoglobin level sufficient to avoid blood transfusions (do not exceed hemoglobin of 12 g/dL).

Surgery
Subcut (Adults): 300 units/kg/day for 10 days before surgery, day of surgery, and 4 days after *or* 600 units/kg 21, 14, and 7 days before surgery and on day of surgery.

Anemia of Prematurity
IV, Subcut (Neonates): 25–100 units/kg/dose 3 times weekly or 100 units/kg/dose 5 times weekly or 200 units/kg/dose every other day for 10 doses.

Availability
Injection: 2000 units/mL, 3000 units/mL, 4000 units/mL, 10,000 units/mL, 20,000 units/mL, 40,000 units/mL.

NURSING IMPLICATIONS

Assessment
- Monitor blood pressure before and during therapy. Inform health care professional if severe hypertension is present or if blood pressure begins to increase. Additional antihypertensive therapy may be required during initiation of therapy.
- Monitor for symptoms of anemia (fatigue, dyspnea, pallor).
- Monitor dialysis shunts (thrill and bruit) and status of artificial kidney during hemodialysis. Heparin dose may need to be increased to prevent clotting. Patients with underlying vascular disease should be monitored for impaired circulation.
- **Lab Test Considerations:** May cause ↑ in WBCs and platelets. May ↓ bleeding times.
- Serum ferritin, transferrin, and iron levels should also be monitored to assess need for concurrent iron therapy. Transferrin saturation should be at least 20% and ferritin should be at least 100 ng/mL.

- **Anemia of Chronic Renal Failure:** Monitor hematocrit before and twice weekly during initial therapy, for 2–6 wk after a change in dose, and regularly after target range (30–36%) has been reached and maintenance dose is determined. Monitor other hematopoietic parameters (CBC with differential and platelet count) before and periodically during therapy. If hemoglobin ↑ and approached 12 g/dL or ↑ by more than 1 g/dL in a 2-wk period, ↓ dose by 25% and monitor hemoglobin twice weekly for 2–6 wk. If ↑ in hemoglobin continues and exceeds 12 g/dL, dose should be withheld until hemoglobin begins to ↓; epoetin is then reinitiated at a dose 25% lower than previous dose. If hemoglobin ↑ by <1 g/dL over 4 wk (and iron stores are adequate), ↑ dose by 25%; monitor hemoglobin twice weekly for 2–6 wk; further dose ↑ may be made at 4–wk intervals until desired response attained.
- Monitor renal function studies and electrolytes closely; resulting increased sense of well-being may lead to decreased compliance with other therapies for renal failure. Increases in BUN, creatinine, uric acid, phosphorus, and potassium may occur.
- **Anemia Secondary to Zidovudine Therapy:** Before initiating therapy, determine serum erythropoietin level before transfusion. Patients receiving zidovudine with endogenous serum erythropoietin levels >500 mUnits/mL may not respond to therapy. Monitor hemoglobin weekly during dosage adjustment. If response does not reduce transfusion requirements or increase hemoglobin effectively after 8 wk of therapy, dose may be ↑ by 50–100 units/kg 3 times weekly. Evaluate response and adjust dose by 50–100 units/kg every 4–8 wk thereafter. If a satisfactory response is not obtained with a dose of 300 units/kg 3 times weekly, it is unlikely that a higher dose will produce a response. Once the desired response is attained, maintenance dose is titrated based on variations of zidovudine dose and intercurrent infections. If hemoglobin exceeds 12 g/dL, discontinue dose until hemoglobin drops to <11 g/dL, then ↓ dose by 25%.
- **Anemia from Chemotherapy:** Monitor hemoglobin weekly until stable. Do not initiate if hemoglobin ≥10 g/dL. Patients with lower baseline serum erythropoietin levels may respond more rapidly; not recommended if levels >200 mUnits/mL. If hemoglobin exceeds 12 g/dL, withhold dose until hemoglobin approaches level where transfusions may be required and then reinitiate at a dose 25% lower than previous dose. If hemoglobin ↑ by >1 g/dL in any 2–wk period, ↓ dose by 25%. For 3 times weekly dosing regimens, if response is not adequate (no ↓ in transfusion requirements or no ↑ in hemoglobin) after 8 wk of therapy, dose may be ↑ up to 300 units/kg 3 times weekly. If no response is obtained to this dose, it is unlikely that higher doses will produce a response. For weekly dosing regimens, if response is not adequate (no ↑ in hemoglobin by ≥1 g/dL after 4 wk in absence of RBC transfusion), ↑ dose to 60,000 units weekly (adults) or 900 units/kg (max: 60,000 units) (children).
- **Surgery:** Determine that hemoglobin is >10 to ≤13 g/dL before therapy.

Potential Nursing Diagnoses
Activity intolerance (Indications)
Noncompliance (Patient/Family Teaching)

Implementation

<u>IV Administration</u>

- Transfusions are still required for severe symptomatic anemia. Supplemental iron should be initiated with epoetin and continued throughout therapy.
- Institute seizure precautions in patients who experience greater than a 4-point increase in hematocrit in a 2-wk period or exhibit any change in neurologic status. Risk of seizures is greatest during the first 90 days of therapy.
- Do not shake vial; inactivation of medication may occur. Discard vial immediately after withdrawing dose from single-use 1-mL vial. Refrigerate multidose 2-mL vial; stable for 21 days after initial entry.
- **Subcut:** This route is often used for patients not requiring dialysis.
- May be admixed in syringe immediately before administration with 0.9% NaCl with benzyl alcohol 0.9% in a 1:1 ratio to prevent injection site discomfort.
- **Direct IV: *Diluent:*** Administer undiluted or dilute with an equal amount of 0.9% NaCl. ***Concentration:*** 1000–40000 units/mL. ***Rate:*** May be administered as direct injection or bolus over 1–3 minutes into IV tubing or via venous line at end of dialysis session.

Patient/Family Teaching
- Advise patient to read the *Medication Guide* prior to initiating therapy and with each Rx refill.
- Explain rationale for concurrent iron therapy (increased red blood cell production requires iron).

- Discuss possible return of menses and fertility in women of childbearing age. Patient should discuss contraceptive options with health care professional.
- Discuss ways of preventing self-injury in patients at risk for seizures. Driving and activities requiring continuous alertness should be avoided.
- Inform patient that use of epoetin may result in shortened overall survival and/or ↓ time to tumor progression.
- Advise patient to notify health care professional immediately if signs of blood clots (chest pain, trouble breathing or shortness of breath, pain in the legs, with or without swelling; a cool or pale arm or leg, sudden confusion, trouble speaking or trouble understanding others' speech, sudden numbness or weakness in the face, arm, or leg, especially on one side of the body, sudden trouble seeing, sudden trouble walking, dizziness, loss of balance or coordination, loss of consciousness or fainting, hemodialysis vascular access stops working) occur.
- Advise patient to inform health care professional of medication prior to treatment or surgery.
- **Anemia of Chronic Renal Failure:** Stress importance of compliance with dietary restrictions, medications, and dialysis. Foods high in iron and low in potassium include liver, pork, veal, beef, mustard and turnip greens, peas, eggs, broccoli, kale, blackberries, strawberries, apple juice, watermelon, oatmeal, and enriched bread. Epoetin will result in increased sense of well-being, but it does not cure underlying disease.
- **Home Care Issues:** Home dialysis patients determined to be able to safely and effectively administer epoetin should be taught proper dosage, administration technique, and disposal of equipment. *Information for Home Dialysis Patients* should be provided to patient along with medication.

Evaluation/Desired Outcomes
- Increase in hematocrit to 30–36% with improvement in symptoms of anemia in patients with chronic renal failure.
- Increase in hematocrit in anemia secondary to zidovudine therapy.
- Increase in hematocrit in patients with anemia resulting from chemotherapy.
- Reduction of need for transfusions after surgery.

eprosartan, See ANGIOTENSIN II RECEPTOR ANTAGONISTS.

HIGH ALERT

eptifibatide (ep-ti-fib-a-tide)
Integrilin

Classification
Therapeutic: antiplatelet agents
Pharmacologic: glycoprotein IIb/IIIa inhibitors

Pregnancy Category B

Indications
Acute coronary syndrome (unstable angina/non–Q-wave MI), including patients who will be managed medically and those who will undergo percutaneous coronary intervention (PCI) that may consist of percutaneous transluminal angioplasty (PCTA) or atherectomy. Treatment of patients undergoing PCI. Usually used concurrently with aspirin and heparin.

Action
Decreases platelet aggregation by reversibly antagonizing the binding of fibrinogen to the glycoprotein IIb/IIIa binding site on platelet surfaces. **Therapeutic Effects:** Inhibition of platelet aggregation resulting in decreased incidence of new MI, death, or refractory ischemia, reducing the need for repeat urgent cardiac intervention.

Pharmacokinetics
Absorption: IV administration results in complete bioavailability.
Distribution: Unknown.
Metabolism and Excretion: 50% excreted by the kidneys.
Half-life: 2.5 hr.

TIME/ACTION PROFILE (effects on platelet function)

ROUTE	ONSET	PEAK	DURATION
IV	immediate	following bolus	brief†

†Inhibition is reversible following cessation of infusion

Contraindications/Precautions
Contraindicated in: Hypersensitivity; Active internal bleeding or history of bleeding within previous 30 days; Severe uncontrolled hypertension (systolic BP >200 mm Hg and/or diastolic BP

>110 mm Hg); Major surgical procedure within 6 wk; History of hemorrhagic stroke or other stroke within 30 days; Concurrent use of other glycoprotein IIb/IIIa receptor antagonists; Platelet count <100,000/mm^3; Severe renal insufficiency (serum creatinine ≥4 mg/dL) or dependency on renal dialysis.

Use Cautiously in: Geri: ↑ risk of bleeding; Renal insufficiency (↓ infusion rate if CCr < 50 mL/min); OB, Pedi: Pregnancy, lactation, or children (safety not established; use in pregnancy only if clearly needed).

Adverse Reactions/Side Effects
Noted for patients receiving heparin and aspirin in addition to eptifibatide.
CV: hypotension. **Hemat:** BLEEDING (including GI and intracranial bleeding, hematuria, and hematomas).

Interactions
Drug-Drug: ↑ risk of bleeding with other drugs that affect hemostasis (**heparins**, **warfarin**, **NSAIDs**, **thrombolytic agents**, **abciximab**, **dipyridamole**, **ticlopidine**, **clopidogrel**, some **cephalosporins**, **valproates**).
Drug-Natural Products: ↑ bleeding risk with **arnica**, **chamomile**, **clove**, **dong quai**, **feverfew**, **garlic**, **ginger**, **ginkgo**, and **Panax ginseng**.

Route/Dosage
Acute Coronary Syndrome
IV (Adults ≤121 kg): 180 mcg/kg as a bolus dose, followed by 2 mcg/kg/min until hospital discharge or surgical intervention (up to 72 hr).

Percutaneous Coronary Intervention
IV (Adults): 180 mcg/kg as a bolus dose, immediately before PCI, followed by 2 mcg/kg/min infusion; a second bolus of 180 mcg/kg is given 10 min after first bolus; infusion should continue for 18–24 or hospital discharge (minimum of 12 hr).

Renal Impairment
(Adults CCr <50 mL/min): 180 mcg/kg bolus followed by 1 mcg/kg/min infusion; second bolus of 180 mcg/kg is given 10 min after first bolus for patients undergoing PCI.

Availability
Solution for injection: 20 mg/10 mL, 75 mg/100 mL, 200 mg/100 mL.

NURSING IMPLICATIONS
Assessment
- Assess for bleeding. Most common sites are arterial access site for cardiac catheterization or GI or GU tract. Arterial and venous punctures, IM injections, and use of urinary catheters, nasotracheal intubation, and NG tubes should be minimized. Noncompressible sites for IV access should be avoided. If bleeding cannot be controlled with pressure, discontinue eptifibatide and heparin immediately.
- *Lab Test Considerations:* Prior to eptifibatide therapy, assess hemoglobin or hematocrit, platelet count, serum creatinine, and PT/aPTT. Activated clotting time (ACT) should also be measured in patients undergoing PCI.
- Maintain the aPTT between 50 and 70 sec unless PCI is to be performed. Maintain ACT between 300 and 350 sec during PCI.
- Arterial sheath should not be removed unless aPTT <45 sec.
- If platelet count decreases to <100,000 and is confirmed, eptifibatide and heparin should be discontinued and condition monitored and treated.

Potential Nursing Diagnoses
Ineffective tissue perfusion (Indications)

Implementation
- *High Alert:* Accidental overdose of antiplatelet medications has resulted in patient harm or death from internal hemorrhage or intracranial bleeding. Have second practitioner independently check original order, dose calculations, and infusion pump settings.
- Most patients receive heparin and aspirin concurrently with eptifibatide.
- After PCI, femoral artery sheath may be removed during eptifibatide treatment only after heparin has been discontinued and its effects mostly reversed.
- Do not administer solutions that are discolored or contain particulate matter. Discard unused portion.

IV Administration
- **Direct IV:** *High Alert: Diluent:* Withdraw appropriate loading dose from bolus vial (20 mg/10-mL vial) into a syringe. Administer undiluted. *Concentration:* 2 mg/mL. *Rate:* Administer over 1–2 min.
- **Continuous Infusion:** *Diluent:* Administer undiluted directly from the 100-mL vial via an infusion pump. *Concentration:* 0.75 mg/mL or 2 mg/mL (depends on vial used). *Rate:* Based on patient's weight (see Route/Dosage section).
- **Y-Site Compatibility:** alteplase, amiodarone, argatroban, atropine, bivalirudin, daptomycin, dobutamine, ertapenem, heparin, lidocaine,

meperidine, metoprolol, micafungin, midazolam, morphine, nitroglycerin, palonosetron, potassium chloride, verapamil.
- **Y-Site Incompatibility:** furosemide.
- **Solution Compatibility:** 0.9% NaCl, D5/0.9% NaCl.

Patient/Family Teaching
- Inform patient of the purpose of eptifibatide.
- Instruct patient to notify health care professional immediately if any bleeding is noted.

Evaluation/Desired Outcomes
- Inhibition of platelet aggregation, resulting in decreased incidence of new MI, death, or refractory ischemia with the need for repeat urgent cardiac intervention.

---

ergocalciferol, See VITAMIN D COMPOUNDS.

---

ergonovine (er-goe-noe-veen)
ergometrine, Ergotrate

Classification
Therapeutic: none assigned
Pharmacologic: oxytocics

Pregnancy Category UK

Indications
Prevention and treatment of postpartum or postabortion hemorrhage caused by uterine atony or involution. **Unlabeled Use:** As a diagnostic agent to provoke coronary artery spasm.

Action
Directly stimulates uterine and vascular smooth muscle. **Therapeutic Effects:** Uterine contraction.

Pharmacokinetics
Absorption: Well absorbed after oral or IM administration.
Distribution: Unknown.
Metabolism and Excretion: Unknown. Probably metabolized by the liver.
Half-life: Unknown.

TIME/ACTION PROFILE (uterine contractions)

ROUTE	ONSET	PEAK	DURATION
PO	5–15 min	unknown	≥3 hr
IM	2–5 min	unknown	≥3 hr
IV	immediate	unknown	45 min

Contraindications/Precautions
Contraindicated in: Hypersensitivity; Avoid chronic use; Should not be used to induce labor.
Use Cautiously in: Hypertensive or eclamptic patients (increased susceptibility to hypertensive and arrhythmogenic side effects); Severe hepatic or renal disease; Sepsis; Third stage of labor.

Adverse Reactions/Side Effects
CNS: dizziness, headache. **EENT:** tinnitus. **Resp:** dyspnea. **CV:** arrhythmias, chest pain, hypertension, palpitations. **GI:** nausea, vomiting. **Derm:** sweating. **Misc:** allergic reactions.

Interactions
Drug-Drug: Excessive vasoconstriction may result when used with other **vasopressors**, such as **dopamine** or **nicotine**. May ↑ the risk of adverse reactions with **bromocriptine**.

Route/Dosage
Oxytocic
PO, SL (Adults): 0.2–0.4 mg q 6–12 hr (usual course is 48 hr).
IM, IV (Adults): 200 mcg (0.2 mg) q 2–4 hr for up to 5 doses.

Provocative Agent for Coronary Artery Spasm
IV (Adults): 50 mcg (0.05 mg) q 5 min until chest pain occurs or a total dose of 400 mcg (0.4 mg) has been given (unlabeled).

Availability
Tablets: 0.2 mg. Injection: 0.2 mg/mL, ✤ 0.25 mg/mL.

NURSING IMPLICATIONS
Assessment
- Monitor blood pressure, pulse, and respirations every 15–30 min until transfer to the postpartum unit, then every 1–2 hr. Report hypertension, chest pain, arrhythmias, headache, or change in neurologic status.
- Monitor amount and type of vaginal discharge. Report symptoms of hemorrhage (increased bleeding, hypotension, pallor, tachycardia) immediately.

- Palpate uterine fundus; note position and consistency. Notify physician or other health care professional if fundus fails to contract in response to ergonovine. Assess patient for severe cramping; dose may be decreased.
- Assess for signs of ergotism (cold, numb fingers and toes; nausea; vomiting; diarrhea; headache; muscle pain; weakness).
- If patient fails to respond to ergonovine, check serum calcium level. Correction of hypocalcemia may restore responsiveness.
- *Lab Test Considerations:* May cause ↓ serum prolactin level, which inhibits synthesis of breast milk.
- *Toxicity and Overdose:* Toxicity, initially manifested as ergotism, may cause seizures and gangrene. Seizures are treated with anticonvulsants. Vasodilators and heparin may be ordered to improve circulation to extremities.

Potential Nursing Diagnoses
Ineffective tissue perfusion (Indications)
Risk for injury (Side Effects)

Implementation
- Do not administer solution that is discolored or contains a precipitate.
- **PO:** Administration is usually limited to 48 hr postpartum, by which time the danger of hemorrhage from uterine atony has passed.
- Tablets may be administered SL.
- **IM:** The preferred route is IM. Firm uterine contractions are produced within a few minutes. Dose may need to be repeated every 2–4 hr for full therapeutic effect.

IV Administration
- **Direct IV:** The IV route is reserved for severe uterine bleeding. **Diluent:** Dilute with 5 mL of 0.9% NaCl. **Rate:** Administer slow IV push over at least 1 min through Y-site injection of an IV of D5W or 0.9% NaCl.

Patient/Family Teaching
- Review symptoms of toxicity with patient. Instruct the patient to report occurrence of these immediately.
- Inform patient that uterine cramping demonstrates effectiveness of therapy.
- Explain need for pad count to determine degree of bleeding. Instruct patient to report immediately an increase in degree of bleeding or passage of clots.
- Instruct patient to report breastfeeding difficulties.
- Caution patient not to smoke while receiving ergonovine; nicotine is also a vasoconstrictor.

Evaluation/Desired Outcomes
- Uterine contraction and cramping in the prevention or cessation of uterine hemorrhage after delivery or abortion.
- Vasoconstriction of the coronary arteries when used as a diagnostic agent.

---

ergotamine (er-**got**-a-meen)
Ergomar

dihydroergotamine
(dye-hye-droe-er-**got**-a-meen)
D.H.E. 45, Migranal

Classification
Therapeutic: vascular headache suppressants
Pharmacologic: ergot alkaloids

Pregnancy Category X

Indications
Treatment of vascular headaches including: Migraine with or without aura, Cluster headaches.

Action
Vasoconstriction of dilated blood vessels by stimulating alpha-adrenergic and serotonergic (5-HT) receptors. Larger doses may produce alpha-adrenergic blockade and vasodilation. **Therapeutic Effects:** Constriction of dilated carotid artery bed with resolution of vascular headache.

Pharmacokinetics
Absorption: *Ergotamine*—Unpredictably absorbed (60%) from the GI tract (may be enhanced by caffeine). Sublingual absorption is very poor. *Dihydroergotamine*—rapidly absorbed after IM and subcut administration, 32% absorbed from nasal mucosa.
Distribution: Ergotamine crosses the blood-brain barrier and enters breast milk.
Protein Binding: *Dihydroergotamine*—90%; *ergotamine*—93–98%.
Metabolism and Excretion: Both ergotamine and dihydroergotamine are 90% metabolized by the liver (CYP3A4 enzyme system). Some metabolites are active.
Half-life: *Ergotamine*—1.5–2.5 hr. *Dihydroergotamine*—9–10 hr.

TIME/ACTION PROFILE (relief of headache)

ROUTE	ONSET	PEAK	DURATION
PO	1–2 hr (variable)	1–5 hr	unknown
Nasal	within 30 min	unknown	unknown
SL	unknown	unknown	unknown

ergotamine **519**

IM, subcut	15–30 min	15 min–2 hr	8 hr
IV	<5 min	15 min–2 hr	8 hr

Contraindications/Precautions
Contraindicated in: Peripheral vascular disease; Ischemic heart disease; Uncontrolled hypertension; Severe renal or liver disease; Malnutrition; Known alcohol intolerance (dihydroergotamine injection only); OB, Lactation: Pregnancy and lacation; Concurrent use of CYP3A4 inhibitors (protease inhibitors and macrolide anti-infectives).

Use Cautiously in: Illnesses associated with peripheral vascular pathology such as diabetes mellitus; Concurrent administration of other vasoconstrictor agents; Pedi: Children (safety not established).

Adverse Reactions/Side Effects
CNS: dizziness. **EENT:** rhinitis (nasal). **CV:** MI, hypertension, angina pectoris, arterial spasm, intermittent claudication. **GI:** abdominal pain, nausea, vomiting, altered taste (nasal), diarrhea, polydipsia. **MS:** extremity stiffness, muscle pain, stiff neck, stiff shoulders. **Neuro:** leg weakness, numbness or tingling in fingers or toes. **Misc:** fatigue.

Interactions
Drug-Drug: Concurrent use of potent inhibitors of the CYP3A4 enzyme system, including protease inhibitors (**ritonavir**, **nelfinavir**, and **indinavir**) some macrolide anti-infectives (**erythromycin**, **clarithromycin**, and **troleandomycin**) and some azole antifungals (**ketoconazole**, **itraconazole**) may produce serious life-threatening peripheral ischemia and is contraindicated. Concurrent use with **beta blockers**, **hormonal contraceptives**, or **nicotine** (heavy smoking) may ↑ risk of peripheral vasoconstriction. Dihydroergotamine antagonizes the antianginal effects of **nitrates**. Concurrent use with **vasoconstrictors** may have ↑ effects (avoid concurrent use). Concurrent use with **almotriptan**, **frovatriptan**, **naratriptan**, **rizatriptan**, **sumatriptan**, and **zolmitriptan** may result in prolonged vasoconstriction (allow 24 hr between use).

Route/Dosage
Ergotamine
PO, SL (Adults): 1–2 mg initially, then 1–2 mg q 30 min until attack subsides or a total of 6 mg has been given. Should not be used more than twice weekly, with at least 5 days between courses; 1–2 mg PO at bedtime daily for 10–14 days have been used to terminate series of cluster headaches.

Dihydroergotamine
IM, Subcut (Adults): 1 mg; may repeat in 1 hr to a total of 3 mg (not to exceed 3 mg/day or 6 mg/wk).
IV (Adults): 0.5 mg; may repeat in 1 hr (not to exceed 2 mg/day or 6 mg/wk). For chronic intractable headache, 0.5–1 mg q 8 hr may be given until relief is obtained (not to exceed 6 mg/wk).
Intranasal (Adults): 1 spray (0.5 mg) in each nostril, repeat after 15 min (2 mg total dose); not to exceed 3 mg/24 hr or 4 mg/wk.

Availability
Ergotamine
Sublingual tablets: 2 mg. *In combination with:* caffeine, barbiturates, and belladonna alkaloids in preparations for vascular headaches. See Appendix B.

Dihydroergotamine
Injection: 1 mg/mL (contains alcohol). **Nasal spray:** 4 mg/1 mL in 1-mL ampules with nasal spray applicator. *In combination with:* Ergotamine—caffeine, barbiturates, and belladonna alkaloids in preparations for vascular headaches. See Appendix B.

NURSING IMPLICATIONS
Assessment
- Assess frequency, location, duration, and characteristics (pain, nausea, vomiting, visual disturbances) of chronic headaches. During acute attack, assess type, location, and intensity of pain before and 60 min after administration.
- Monitor blood pressure and peripheral pulses periodically during therapy. Report any increases in blood pressure.
- Assess for signs of ergotism (cold, numb fingers and toes; nausea; vomiting; headache; muscle pain; weakness).
- Assess for nausea and vomiting. Ergotamine stimulates the chemoreceptor trigger zone. Metoclopramide or a phenothiazine antiemetic may be given orally as prophylaxis 1 hr before administration of dihydroergotamine IV. Oral administration may decrease risk of extrapyramidal reactions and other side effects encountered with IV administration.

- **Toxicity and Overdose:** Toxicity is manifested by severe ergotism (chest pain, abdominal pain, persistent paresthesia in the extremities) and gangrene. Vasodilators, dextran, or heparin may be ordered to improve circulation.

Potential Nursing Diagnoses
Acute pain (Indications)
Risk for injury (Side Effects)
Deficient knowledge, related to medication regimen (Patient/Family Teaching)

Implementation
- Do not confuse Cafergot (ergotamine/caffeine) with Carafate (sucralfate).
- Administer as soon as patient reports prodromal symptoms or headache.
- **SL:** Allow tablet to dissolve under tongue. Do not allow patient to eat, drink, or smoke while tablet is dissolving.

IV Administration
- **Direct IV:** *Diluent:* Dihydroergotamine may be administered undiluted. *Concentration:* 1 mg/mL. *Rate:* Administer over 1 min.

Patient/Family Teaching
- Instruct patient to take ergotamine at the first sign of an impending headache and not to exceed the maximum dose prescribed.
- Encourage patient to rest in a quiet, dark room after taking ergotamine.
- Review symptoms of toxicity. Instruct patient to report these promptly.
- Caution patient not to smoke and to avoid exposure to cold; these vasoconstrictors may further impair peripheral circulation.
- May cause dizziness. Caution patient to avoid driving and other activities requiring alertness until response to the drug is known.
- Advise patient to avoid alcohol, which may precipitate vascular headaches.
- Instruct female patients to inform health care professional if they plan or suspect pregnancy. Ergotamine should not be taken during pregnancy.
- **Subcut, IM:** Inject at the first sign of a headache and repeat at 1-hr intervals up to 3 doses. Once minimal effective dose is determined, adjust dose for subsequent attacks.
- **Intranasal:** Instruct patient in proper use of nasal spray. Prime nasal sprayer 4 times before dose. Administer 1 spray to each nostril followed in 15 min by an additional spray in each nostril for a total of 4 sprays. Do not tilt head or sniff after spray. Do not use more than amount instructed. Discard ampule within 8 hr of opening. Do not refrigerate. Assembly may be used for 4 treatments; then discard.
- Advise patient not to use *Migranal* to prevent a headache if there are no symptoms or if headache is different from typical migraine.
- Instruct patient to notify health care professional if numbness or tingling in fingers or toes; pain, tightness, or discomfort in chest; muscle pain or cramps in arms or legs; weakness in legs; temporary speeding or slowing of heart rate; or swelling or itching occurs.

Evaluation/Desired Outcomes
- Relief of pain from vascular headaches.

---

erlotinib (er-lo-ti-nib)
Tarceva

Classification
Therapeutic: antineoplastics
Pharmacologic: enzyme inhibitors

Pregnancy Category D

Indications
Locally advanced/metastatic non-small cell lung cancer, which has not responded to previous chemotherapy. First-line therapy for locally advanced, surgically unresectable, or metastatic pancreatic cancer (with gemcitabine).

Action
Inhibits the enzyme tyrosine kinase, which is associated with human epidermal growth factor receptor (EGFR); blocks growth stimulation signals in cancer cells. **Therapeutic Effects:** Decreased spread of lung or pancreatic cancer with increased survival.

Pharmacokinetics
Absorption: 60% absorbed; bioavailability ↑ to 100% with food.
Distribution: Unknown.
Protein Binding: 93% protein bound.
Metabolism and Excretion: Mostly metabolized by the liver (CYP3A4 enzyme system).
Half-life: 36 hr.

TIME/ACTION PROFILE (blood levels)

ROUTE	ONSET	PEAK	DURATION
Oral	unknown	4 hr	24 hr

Contraindications/Precautions
Contraindicated in: OB, Lactation: Pregnancy or lactation.
Use Cautiously in: Hepatic impairment; Previous chemotherapy/radiation, pre-existing lung disease, metastatic lung disease (may ↑ risk of

erlotinib **521**

interstitial lung disease); Patients with child-bearing potential; Pedi: Safety not established.

Adverse Reactions/Side Effects
CNS: CEREBROVASCULAR ACCIDENT (pancreatic cancer patients), fatigue. **CV:** MYOCARDIAL INFARCTION/ISCHEMIA (pancreatic cancer patients). **EENT:** conjunctivitis, corneal perforation, corneal ulceration. **Resp:** INTERSTITIAL LUNG DISEASE, dyspnea, cough. **GI:** HEPATOTOXICITY, GI PERFORATION, diarrhea, abdominal pain, anorexia, nausea, stomatitis, vomiting, ↑ liver enzymes. **Derm:** BULLOUS AND EXFOLIATIVE SKIN DISORDERS, rash, dry skin, pruritus. **GU:** RENAL FAILURE. **Hemat:** microangiopathic hemolytic anemia with thrombocytopenia (pancreatic cancer patients).

Interactions
Drug-Drug: Strong inhibitors of CYP3A4, including **atazanavir**, **clarithromycin**, **indinavir**, **itraconazole**, **ketoconazole**, **nefazodone**, **nelfinavir**, **ritonavir**, **saquinavir**, **telithromycin**, or **voriconazole** ↑ levels and the risk of toxicity; consider dose reduction. Strong inducers of CYP3A4, including **rifampin** ↓ levels and may ↓ response; alternative therapy or ↑ dose should be considered. **Ciprofloxacin** may ↑ levels and the risk of toxicity. **Smoking** may ↓ levels and may ↓ response; may consider ↑ dose if smoking continues. May ↑ risk of bleeding with **warfarin**. ↓ levels with **proton pump inhibitors** and **H₂ blockers**; avoid concurrent use.

Route/Dosage
PO (Adults): *Non-small cell lung cancer*—150 mg daily taken at least 1 hr before or 2 hr after food; *Pancreatic cancer*—100 mg daily taken at least 1 hr before or 2 hr after food.

Availability
Tablets: 25 mg, 100 mg, 150 mg.

NURSING IMPLICATIONS

Assessment
- Assess respiratory status prior to and periodically during therapy. If dyspnea, cough or fever occur, discontinue erlotinib, assess for interstitial lung disease, and institute treatment as needed.
- Assess for diarrhea. Usually responds to loperamide but may require dose reduction or discontinuation of therapy if patient becomes dehydrated.
- Assess skin throughout therapy. If bullous, blistering, and exfoliative skin conditions, including Stevens-Johnson syndrome/toxic epidermal necrolysis, occur, interrupt or discontinue treatment. Skin rash may require treatment with corticosteroids or anti-infectives with anti-inflammatory properties; acne treatments may aggravate dry skin and erythema.
- Assess eyes periodically during therapy. If acute or worsening eye disorders or pain occur, interrupt or discontinue therapy.
- Assess for GI pain. Patients receiving concomitant anti-angiogenic agents, corticosteroids, NSAIDs, and/or taxane-based chemotherapy, or who have prior history of peptic ulceration or diverticular disease, are at increased risk for GI perforation. Permanently discontinue erlotinib in patients who develop gastrointestinal perforation.
- *Lab Test Considerations:* Monitor liver function tests (AST, ALT, bilirubin, alkaline phosphatase) periodically during therapy. Dose reduction or discontinuation of therapy should be considered if severe changes in liver function (total bilirubin ≥3 times upper limit of normal and/or transaminases ≥ 5 times upper limit of normal) occur.
- Monitor renal function and electrolytes in patients at risk for dehydration. Withhold therapy if dehydration occurs.
- Monitor INR regularly in patients taking warfarin. May cause ↑ INR.

Potential Nursing Diagnoses
Ineffective breathing pattern (Side Effects)

Implementation
- **PO:** Administer at least 1 hr before or 2 hr after food.

Patient/Family Teaching
- Instruct patient to take erlotinib as directed.
- Caution patient to use contraceptive during and for at least 2 wk after completion of therapy. Advise female patients to notify health care professional if pregnancy is planned or suspected or if breastfeeding.
- Advise patient to notify health care professional if severe or persistent diarrhea, nausea, anorexia, vomiting, onset or worsening of skin rash, unexplained dyspnea or cough, or eye irritation occur.
- Advise patient to wear sunscreen and protective clothing to decrease skin reactions.

- Instruct patient to discontinue smoking during therapy; smoking decreases blood levels of erlotinib.

Evaluation/Desired Outcomes
- Decrease in spread of non–small cell lung or pancreatic cancer with increased survival.

---

ertapenem (er-ta-pen-em)
Invanz

Classification
Therapeutic: anti-infectives
Pharmacologic: carbapenems

Pregnancy Category B

Indications
Moderate to severe: complicated intra-abdominal infections, complicated skin and skin structure infections, community acquired pneumonia, complicated urinary tract infections (including pyelonephritis), acute pelvic infections including postpartum endomyometritis, septic abortion, and post surgical gynecologic infections. Prophylaxis of surgical site infection following elective colorectal surgery.

Action
Therapeutic Effects: Bactericidal action against susceptible bacteria. **Spectrum:** Active against the following aerobic gram-positive organisms *Staphylococcus aureus* (methicillin-susceptible strains only), *Staphylococcus epidermidis*, *Streptococcus agalactiae*, *S. pneumoniae* (penicillin-susceptible strains only), and *S. pyogenes*. Also active against the following gram-negative aerobic organisms *Escherichia coli*, *Haemophilus influenzae* (beta-lactamase negative strains), *Klebsiella pneumonia*, and *Moraxella catarrhalis*, *Providencia rettgeri*. Addition anaerobic spectrum includes *Bacteroides fragilis*, *B. distasonis*, *B. ovatus*, *B. thetaiotamicron*, *B. uniformis*, *B. vulgatis*, *Clostridium clostrioforme*, *Eubacterium lentum*, *Peptostreptococcus*, *Porphyromonas asaccharolytica*, and *Prevotella bivia*.

Pharmacokinetics
Absorption: 90% after IM administration; IV administration results in complete bioavailability.
Distribution: Enters breast milk.
Metabolism and Excretion: Mostly excreted by the kidneys.
Half-life: 1.8 hr (increased in renal impairment).

TIME/ACTION PROFILE (blood levels)

ROUTE	ONSET	PEAK	DURATION
IM	rapid	2 hr	24 hr
IV	rapid	end of infusion	24 hr

Contraindications/Precautions
Contraindicated in: Hypersensitivity; Cross-sensitivity may occur with penicillins, cephalosporins and other carbapenems; Hypersensitivity to lidocaine (may be used as a diluent for IM administration).
Use Cautiously in: History of multiple hypersensitivity reactions; Seizure disorders; Renal impairment; OB: Use in pregnancy only if clearly needed; Lactation: Not expected to cause adverse effects in breast-fed infants (NIH); Pedi: Safety not established in children <18 yr ; Geri: ↑ sensitivity due to age-related ↓ in renal function.

Adverse Reactions/Side Effects
CNS: SEIZURES, headache. **GI:** PSEUDOMEMBRANOUS COLITIS, diarrhea, nausea, vomiting. **GU:** vaginitis. **Local:** phlebitis at IV site, pain at IM site. **Misc:** hypersensitivity reaction including ANAPHYLAXIS.

Interactions
Drug-Drug: Probenecid ↓ excretion and ↑ blood levels. May ↓ serum **valproate** levels (↑ risk of seizures).

Route/Dosage
IV, IM (Adults and Children 13 yrs or older): 1 g once daily for up to 14 days (IV) or 7 days (IM).
IV, IM (Children 3 months–12 yrs): 15 mg/kg twice daily (not to exceed 1 g/day) for up to 14 days (IV) or 7 days (IM).

Renal Impairment
IM, IV (Adults): *CCr ≤30 mL/min/1.73m² — 500 mg once daily.*

Availability
Powder for injection: 1 g/vial.

NURSING IMPLICATIONS

Assessment
- Assess for infection (vital signs; appearance of wound, sputum, urine, and stool; WBC) at beginning of and during therapy.
- Obtain a history before initiating therapy to determine previous use of and reactions to penicillins, cephalosporins or carbapenems. Persons with a negative history of penicillin sensitivity may still have an allergic response.

ERYTHROMYCIN 523

- Obtain specimens for culture and sensitivity before initiating therapy. First dose may be given before receiving results.
- Observe patient for signs and symptoms of anaphylaxis (rash, pruritus, laryngeal edema, wheezing). Discontinue the drug and notify the physician immediately if these occur. Have epinephrine, an antihistamine, and resuscitative equipment close by in the event of an anaphylactic reaction.
- *Lab Test Considerations:* May cause ↑ AST, ALT, serum alkaline phosphatase levels.
- May cause ↑ platelet and eosinophil counts.

Potential Nursing Diagnoses
Risk for infection (Indications, Side Effects)

Implementation
- **IM:** Reconstitute 1-g vial with 3.2 mL of 1% lidocaine without epinephrine. Shake well to form solution. Immediately withdraw contents and inject deep into large muscle mass. Use reconstituted solution within 1 hr.

IV Administration
- **Intermittent Infusion:** *Diluent:* Reconstitute 1-g vial with 10 mL of sterile water for injection or 0.9% NaCl and shake well. Further dilute in 50 mL of 0.9% NaCl. Administer within 6 hr of reconstitution. *Rate:* Infuse over 30 min.
- **Y-Site Compatibility:** acyclovir, amikacin, aminophylline, amphotericin B liposome, argatroban, azithromycin, aztreonam, bumetanide, calcium chloride, calcium gluconate, chloramphenicol, cimetidine, ciprofloxacin, cisatracurium, cyclosporine, daptomycin, dexamethasone sodium phosphate, digoxin, diltiazem, diphenhydramine, dolasetron, dopamine, doxycycline, enalaprilat, epinephrine, eptifibatide, erythromycin, esmolol, famotidine, fenoldopam, fluconazole, furosemide, ganciclovir, gentamicin, granisetron, haloperidol, heparin, hydromorphone, insulin, isoproterenol, ketorolac, labetalol, levofloxacin, lidocaine, linezolid, lorazepam, magnesium sulfate, meperidine, methylprednisolone sodium succinate, metoclopramide, metronidazole, milrinone, morphine, nesiritide, nitroglycerin, nitroprusside, norepinephrine, pancuronium, pantoprazole, phenylephrine, potassium chloride, potassium phosphate, procainamide, propranolol, ranitidine, sodium bicarbonate, tacrolimus, tigecycline, tirofiban, tobramycin, trimethoprim/sulfamethoxazole, vancomycin, vasopressin, vecuronium, voriconazole, zoledronic acid.
- **Y-Site Incompatibility:** amiodarone, anidulafungin, caspofungin, diazepam, dobutamine, droperidol, hydralazine, hydroxyzine, midazolam, nicardipine, ondansetron, phenytoin, prochlorperazine, promethazine, quinupristin/dalfopristin, verapamil.

Patient/Family Teaching
- Advise patient to report the signs of superinfection (black, furry overgrowth on the tongue; vaginal itching or discharge; loose or foul-smelling stools) and allergy.
- Caution patient to notify health care professional if fever and diarrhea occur, especially if stool contains blood, pus, or mucus. Advise patient not to treat diarrhea without consulting health care professional. May occur up to several weeks after discontinuation of medication. Consult health care professional before treating with antidiarrheals.

Evaluation/Desired Outcomes
- Resolution of the signs and symptoms of infection. Length of time for complete resolution depends on the organism and site of infection.

ERYTHROMYCIN†
(eh-rith-roe-**mye**-sin)

erythromycin base
✤ Apo-Erythro-EC, E-Mycin, ✤ Erybid, Eryc, Ery-Tab, ✤ Erythromid, ✤ Novo-rythro, PCE

erythromycin ethylsuccinate
✤ Apo-Erythro-ES, E.E.S, EryPed

erythromycin lactobionate
Erythrocin

erythromycin stearate
Erythrocin, ✤ Novo-rythro

erythromycin (topical)
Akne-Mycin, Erygel, ✤ Sans-Acne

Classification
Therapeutic: anti-infectives
Pharmacologic: macrolides

Pregnancy Category B
†See Appendix C for ophthalmic use

✤ = Canadian drug name. 🧬 = Genetic implication.
*CAPITALS indicates life-threatening; <u>underlines</u> indicate most frequent.

ERYTHROMYCIN

Indications
IV, PO: Infections caused by susceptible organisms including: Upper and lower respiratory tract infections, Otitis media (with sulfonamides), Skin and skin structure infections, Pertussis, Diphtheria, Erythrasma, Intestinal amebiasis, Pelvic inflammatory disease, Nongonococcal urethritis, Syphilis, Legionnaires' disease, Rheumatic fever. Useful when penicillin is the most appropriate drug but cannot be used because of hypersensitivity, including: Streptococcal infections, Treatment of syphilis or gonorrhea. **Topical:** Treatment of acne.

Action
Suppresses protein synthesis at the level of the 50S bacterial ribosome. **Therapeutic Effects:** Bacteriostatic action against susceptible bacteria. **Spectrum:** Active against many gram-positive cocci, including: Streptococci, Staphylococci. Gram-positive bacilli, including: *Clostridium*, *Corynebacterium*. Several gram-negative pathogens, notably: *Neisseria*, *Legionella pneumophila*. *Mycoplasma* and *Chlamydia* are also usually susceptible.

Pharmacokinetics
Absorption: Variable absorption from the duodenum after oral administration (dependent on salt form). Absorption of enteric-coated products is delayed. Minimal absorption may follow topical or ophthalmic use.
Distribution: Widely distributed. Minimal CNS penetration. Crosses placenta; enters breast milk.
Protein Binding: 70–80%.
Metabolism and Excretion: Partially metabolized by the liver, excreted mainly unchanged in the bile; small amounts excreted unchanged in the urine.
Half-life: Neonates: 2.1 hr; Adults: 1.4–2 hr.

TIME/ACTION PROFILE (blood levels)

ROUTE	ONSET	PEAK	DURATION
PO	1 hr	1–4 hr	6–12 hr
IV	rapid	end of infusion	6–12 hr

Contraindications/Precautions
Contraindicated in: Hypersensitivity; Concurrent pimozide; Known alcohol intolerance (most topicals); Tartrazine sensitivity (some products contain tartrazine—FDC yellow dye #5); Products containing benzyl alcohol should be avoided in neonates.
Use Cautiously in: Liver/renal disease; **OB:** May be used in pregnancy to treat chlamydial infections or syphilis; Geri: ↑ risk of ototoxicity if parenteral dose >4 g/day, ↑ risk of QTc prolongation.

Adverse Reactions/Side Effects
CNS: seizures (rare). **EENT:** ototoxicity. **CV:** QTC PROLONGATION (may result in torsades de pointes), VENTRICULAR ARRHYTHMIAS. **GI:** nausea, vomiting, abdominal pain, cramping, diarrhea, drug-induced hepatitis, infantile hypertrophic pyloric stenosis, drug-induced pancreatitis (rare). **Derm:** rashes. **Local:** phlebitis at IV site. **Misc:** allergic reactions, superinfection.

Interactions
Drug-Drug: Concurrent use with **pimozide** ↑ risk of serious arrhythmias (concurrent use contraindicated); similar effects may occur with **diltiazem, verapamil, ketoconazole, itraconazole, nefazodone,** and **protease inhibitors**; avoid concurrent use. Concurrent use with **verapamil** ↑ risk of hypotension, bradycardia, and lactic acidosis. ↑ blood levels and effects of **sildenafil, tadalafil** and **vardenafil**; use lower doses. Concurrent **rifabutin** or **rifampin** may ↓ effect of erythromycin and ↑ risk of adverse GI reactions. ↑ levels and risk of toxicity from **alfentanil, alprazolam, buspirone, clozapine, bromocriptine, theophylline, carbamazepine, cyclosporine, cilostazol diazepam disopyramide, ergot alkaloids, felodipine, warfarin, methylprednisolone, midazolam, quinidine, rifabutin, tacrolimus, triazolam,** or **vinblastine**. Concurrent **HMG-CoA reductase inhibitors** ↑ risk of myopathy/rhabdomyolysis. May ↑ serum **digoxin** levels in a few patients. **Theophylline** may ↓ blood levels. Beneficial effects may be ↓ by **clindamycin** or **lincomycin**.

Route/Dosage
250 mg of erythromycin base or stearate = 400 mg of erythromycin ethylsuccinate.

Most Infections
PO (Adults): *Base, stearate*—250 mg q 6 hr, *or* 333 mg q 8 hr, *or* 500 mg q 12 hr. *Ethylsuccinate*—400 mg q 6 hr *or* 800 mg q 12 hr.
PO (Children >1 mo): *Base and ethylsuccinate*—30–50 mg/kg/day divided q 6–8 hr (maximum 2 g/day as base or 3.2 g/day as ethylsuccinate). *Stearate*—30–50 mg/kg/day divided q 6 hr (maximum 2 g/day).
PO (Neonates): *Ethylsuccinate*—20–50 mg/kg/day divided q 6–12 hr.
IV (Adults): 250–500 mg (up to 1 g) q 6 hr.
IV (Children > 1 mo): 15–50 mg/kg/day divided q 6 hr, maximum 4 g/day.

Acne
Topical (Adults and Children >12 yr): 2% ointment, gel, or solution bid.

Availability (generic available)
Erythromycin Base
Enteric-coated tablets: 250 mg, 333 mg. Tablets with polymer-coated particles: 333 mg, 500 mg. Film-coated tablets: 500 mg. Delayed-release capsules: 250 mg.

Erythromycin Ethylsuccinate
Chewable tablets (fruit flavor): 200 mg. Tablets: 400 mg. Oral suspension (fruit flavor, cherry): 200 mg/5 mL. Oral suspension (orange, banana flavors): 400 mg/5 mL. Drops (fruit flavor): 100 mg/2.5 mL.

Erythromycin Lactobionate
Powder for injection: 500 mg, 1 g.

Erythromycin Stearate
Film-coated tablets: 250 mg.

Topical Preparations
Ointment: 2%. Gel: 2%. Solution: 2%. *In combination with:* sulfisoxazole (generic only) and benzoyl peroxide (Benzamycin). See Appendix B.

NURSING IMPLICATIONS

Assessment
- Assess for infection (vital signs; appearance of wound, sputum, urine, and stool; WBC) at beginning of and during therapy.
- Obtain specimens for culture and sensitivity before initiating therapy. First dose may be given before receiving results.
- *Lab Test Considerations:* Monitor liver function tests periodically on patients receiving high-dose, long-term therapy.
- May cause ↑ serum bilirubin, AST, ALT, and alkaline phosphatase concentrations.
- May cause false ↑ of urinary catecholamines.

Potential Nursing Diagnoses
Risk for infection (Indications, Side Effects)
Noncompliance (Patient/Family Teaching)

Implementation
- Do not confuse erythromycin with azithromycin.
- **PO:** Administer around the clock. *Erythromycin film-coated tablets (base and stearate)* are absorbed better on an empty stomach, at least 1 hr before or 2 hr after meals; may be taken with food if GI irritation occurs. *Enteric-coated erythromycin (base)* may be taken without regard to meals. *Erythromycin ethylsuccinate* is best absorbed when taken with meals. Take each dose with a full glass of water.
- Use calibrated measuring device for liquid preparations. Shake well before using.
- Chewable tablets should be crushed or chewed and not swallowed whole.
- Do not crush or chew delayed-release capsules or tablets; swallow whole. *Erythromycin base delayed-release capsules* may be opened and sprinkled on applesauce, jelly, or ice cream immediately before ingestion. Entire contents of the capsule should be taken.

IV Administration

- **IV:** Add 10 mL of sterile water for injection without preservatives to 250- or 500-mg vials and 20 mL to 1-g vial. Solution is stable for 7 days after reconstitution if refrigerated.
- **Intermittent Infusion:** *Diluent:* Dilute in 0.9% NaCl or D5W. *Concentration:* 1–5 mg/mL. *Rate:* Administer slowly over 20–60 min to avoid phlebitis. Assess for pain along vein; slow rate if pain occurs; apply ice and notify health care professional if unable to relieve pain.
- **Continuous Infusion:** May also be administered as an infusion in a dilution of 1 g/L of 0.9% NaCl, D5W, or LR over 4 hr.

Erythromycin Lactobionate
- **Y-Site Compatibility:** acyclovir, alfentanil, amikacin, aminophylline, amiodarone, anidulafungin, atracurium, atropine, azathioprine, benztropine, bivalirudin, bumetanide, buprenorphine, butorphanol, calcium chloride, calcium gluconate, carboplatin, caspofungin, cefotaxime, ceftriaxone, cefuroxime, chlorpromazine, cimetidine, cisplatin, cyanocobalamin, cyclophosphamide, cyclosporine, cytarabine, dactinomycin, daptomycin, dexmedetomidine, digoxin, diltiazem, diphenhydramine, dobutamine, docetaxel, dopamine, doxacurium, doxapram, doxorubicin, enalaprilat, ephedrine, epinephrine, epirubicin, epoetin alfa, eftifibatide, ertapenem, esmolol, etoposide, etoposide phosphate, famotidine, fenoldopam, fentanyl, fluconazole, fludarabine, fluorouracil, folic acid, foscarnet, gemcitabine, gentamicin, glycopyrrolate, granisetron, hydrocortisone, hydromorphone, idarubicin, ifos-

famide, imipenem/cilastatin, insulin, isoproterenol, labetalol, levofloxacin, lidocaine, lorazepam, mannitol, mechlorethamine, meperidine, methotrexate, methoxamine, methyldopa, methylprednisolone, metoclopramide, metronidazole, miconazole, midazolam, milrinone, mitoxantrone, morphine, multivitamins, nafcillin, nalbuphine, naloxone, nesiritide, nicardipine, nitroglycerin, norepinephrine, octreotide, ondansetron, oxaliplatin, oxytocin, paclitaxel, palonosetron, papaverine, pentamidine, pentazocine, perphenazine, phentolamine, phenylephrine, phytonadione, piperacillin/tazobactam, procainamide, prochlorperazine, promethazine, propranolol, protamine, pyridoxine, ranitidine, sodium acetate, sodium bicarbonate, streptokinase, succinylcholine, sufentanil, tacrolimus, teniposide, theophylline, thiamine, thiotepa, tigecycline, tirofiban, tobramycin, tolazoline, trimethaphan, urokinase, vancomycin, vasopressin, vecuronium, verapamil, vincristine, vinorelbine, vitamin B complex with C, voriconazole, zidovudine.

- **Y-Site Incompatibility:** amphotericin B colloidal, amphotericin B liposome, ascorbic acid, aztreonam, cefazolin, cefepime, cefotetan, cefoxitin, ceftizoxime, chloramphenicol, dantrolene, dexamethasone, diazepam, diazoxide, doxycycline, furosemide, ganciclovir, indomethacin, ketorolac, metaraminol, nitroprusside, penicillin G, pentobarbital, phenobarbital, phenytoin, ticarcillin/clavulanate, trimethoprim/sulfamethoxazole.
- **Topical:** Cleanse area before application. Wear gloves during application.

Patient/Family Teaching

- Instruct patient to take medication around the clock and to finish the drug completely as directed, even if feeling better. Take missed doses as soon as remembered, with remaining doses evenly spaced throughout day. Advise patient that sharing of this medication may be dangerous.
- May cause nausea, vomiting, diarrhea, or stomach cramps; notify health care professional if these effects persist or if severe abdominal pain, yellow discoloration of the skin or eyes, darkened urine, pale stools, or unusual tiredness develops. May cause infantile hypertrophic pyloric stenosis in infants; notify health care professional if vomiting and irritability occur.
- Advise patient to report signs of superinfection (black, furry overgrowth on the tongue; vaginal itching or discharge; loose or foul-smelling stools).
- Instruct patient to notify health care professional if symptoms do not improve.

Evaluation/Desired Outcomes

- Resolution of the signs and symptoms of infection. Length of time for complete resolution depends on the organism and site of infection.
- Improvement of acne lesions.

---

escitalopram
(ess-sit-**al**-o-pram)
Lexapro

Classification
Therapeutic: antidepressants
Pharmacologic: selective serotonin reuptake inhibitors (SSRIs)

Pregnancy Category C

Indications
Major depressive disorder. Generalized anxiety disorder (GAD). **Unlabeled Use:** Panic disorder. Obsessive-compulsive disorder (OCD). Post-traumatic stress disorder (PTSD). Social anxiety disorder (social phobia). Premenstrual dysphoric disorder (PMDD).

Action
Selectively inhibits the reuptake of serotonin in the CNS. **Therapeutic Effects:** Antidepressant action.

Pharmacokinetics
Absorption: 80% absorbed following oral administration.
Distribution: Enters breast milk.
Metabolism and Excretion: Mostly metabolized by the liver (primarily CYP3A4 and CYP2C19 isoenzymes); 7% excreted unchanged by kidneys.
Half-life: ↑ in geriatric patients and patients with hepatic impairment.

TIME/ACTION PROFILE (antidepressant effect)

ROUTE	ONSET	PEAK	DURATION
PO	within 1–4 wk	Unknown	Unknown

Contraindications/Precautions
Contraindicated in: Hypersensitivity; Concurrent MAO inhibitor or pimozide therapy; Concurrent use of citalopram.
Use Cautiously in: History of mania (may activate mania/hypomania); History of seizures; Patients at risk for suicide; Hepatic impairment (dose ↓ recommended); Severe renal impairment; **OB:** Neonates exposed to SSRIs in the 3rd

escitalopram

trimester may develop drug discontinuation syndrome manifested by respiratory distress, feeding difficulty, and irritability; Lactation: May cause adverse effects in infant; consider risk/benefit; Pedi: May ↑ risk of suicide attempt/ideation especially during early treatment or dose adjustment; safety not established in children <12 yr; Geri: ↓ doses recommended due to ↓ drug clearance in older patients.

Adverse Reactions/Side Effects
CNS: NEUROLEPTIC MALIGNANT SYNDROME, SUICIDAL THOUGHTS, insomnia, dizziness, drowsiness, fatigue. **GI:** diarrhea, nausea, abdominal pain, constipation, dry mouth, indigestion. **GU:** anorgasmia, ↓ libido, ejaculatory delay, erectile dysfunction. **Derm:** sweating. **Endo:** syndrome on inappropriate secretion of antidiuretic hormone (SIADH). **F and E:** hyponatremia. **Metab:** SEROTONIN SYNDROME, ↑ appetite.

Interactions
Drug-Drug: May cause serious, potentially fatal reactions when used with **MAO inhibitors**; allow at least 14 days between escitalopram and **MAO inhibitors**. Concurrent use with **pimozide** may result in prolongation of the QTc interval and is contraindicated. Use cautiously with other **centrally acting drugs** (including **alcohol**, **antihistamines**, **opioid analgesics**, and **sedative/hypnotics**; concurrent use with **alcohol** is not recommended). Drugs that affect serotonergic neurotransmitter systems, including **linezolid**, **tramadol**, and **triptans** ↑ risk of serotonin syndrome. **Cimetidine** may ↑ levels. Serotonergic effects may be ↑ by **lithium** (concurrent use should be carefully monitored). **Carbamazepine** may ↓ levels. May ↑ levels of **metoprolol**. Use cautiously with **tricyclic antidepressants** due to unpredictable effects on serotonin and norepinephrine reuptake. ↑ risk of bleeding with **aspirin**, **NSAIDs**, **clopidogrel**, or **warfarin**.
Drug-Natural Products: ↑ risk of serotonin syndrome with **St. John's wort** and **SAMe**.

Route/Dosage
PO (Adults): *Depression and GAD* – 10 mg once daily, may be ↑ to 20 mg once daily after 1 wk.

Hepatic Impairment
PO (Adults): 10 mg once daily.
PO (Geriatric Patients): 10 mg once daily.
PO (Children ≥12 yr): *Depression* — 10 mg once daily, may be ↑ to 20 mg once daily after 3 wk.

Availability
Tablets: 5 mg, 10 mg, 20 mg. **Cost:** 5 mg $214.97/90, 10 mg $228.97/90, 20 mg $239.97/90. **Oral solution (peppermint):** 1 mg/mL. **Cost:** $131.64/240 mL.

NURSING IMPLICATIONS

Assessment
- Monitor mood changes and level of anxiety during therapy.
- Assess for suicidal tendencies, especially during early therapy. Restrict amount of drug available to patient. Risk may be increased in children, adolescents, and adults ≤24 yr. After starting therapy, children, adolescents, and young adults should be seen by health care professional at least weekly for 4 wk, every 3 wk for next 4 wk, and on advice of health care professional thereafter.
- Assess for sexual dysfunction (erectile dysfunction; decreased libido).
- Assess for serotonin syndrome (mental changes [agitation, hallucinations, coma], autonomic instability [tachycardia, labile blood pressure, hyperthermia], neuromuscular aberrations [hyperreflexia, incoordination], and/or GI symptoms [nausea, vomiting, diarrhea]), especially in patients taking other serotonergic drugs (SSRIs, SNRIs, triptans).

Potential Nursing Diagnoses
Ineffective coping (Indications)
Risk for injury (Side Effects)
Sexual dysfunction (Side Effects)

Implementation
- Do not administer escitalopram and citalopram concomitantly. Taper to avoid potential withdrawal reactions. Reduce dose by 50% for 3 days, then again by 50% for 3 days, then discontinue.
- **PO:** Administer as a single dose in the morning or evening without regard to meals.

Patient/Family Teaching
- Instruct patient to take escitalopram as directed. Take missed doses on the same day as soon as remembered and consult health care professional. Resume regular dosing schedule next day. Do not double doses. Do not stop abruptly, should be discontinued gradually.
- May cause dizziness. Caution patient to avoid driving or other activities requiring alertness until response to medication is known.

- Advise patient, family, and caregivers to look for suicidality, especially during early therapy or dose changes. Notify health care professional immediately if thoughts about suicide or dying, attempts to commit suicide, new or worse depression or anxiety, agitation or restlessness, panic attacks, insomnia, new or worse irritability, aggressiveness, acting on dangerous impulses, mania, or other changes in mood or behavior or if symptoms of serotonin syndrome occur.
- Advise patient to avoid alcohol and other CNS-depressant drugs during therapy and to consult health care professional before taking other Rx, OTC, or herbal products.
- Instruct female patients to notify health care professional if pregnancy is planned or suspected or if they plan to breastfeed. If used during pregnancy, should be tapered during 3rd trimester to avoid neonatal serotinin syndrome.
- Caution patients that escitalopram should not be used for at least 14 days after discontinuing MAO inhibitors, and at least 14 days should be allowed after stopping escitalopram before starting an MAO inhibitor.
- Emphasize importance of follow-up exams to monitor progress.

Evaluation/Desired Outcomes
- Increased sense of well-being.
- Renewed interest in surroundings. May require 1–4 wk of therapy to obtain antidepressant effects. Full antidepressant effects occur in 4–6 wk.
- Decrease in anxiety.

HIGH ALERT

esmolol (es-moe-lole)
Brevibloc

Classification
Therapeutic: antiarrhythmics (class II)
Pharmacologic: beta blockers

Pregnancy Category C

Indications
Management of sinus tachycardia and supraventricular arrhythmias.

Action
Blocks stimulation of beta$_1$(myocardial)-adrenergic receptors. Does not usually affect beta$_2$(pulmonary, vascular, or uterine)-receptor sites. **Therapeutic Effects:** Decreased heart rate. Decreased AV conduction.

Pharmacokinetics
Absorption: IV administration results in complete bioavailability.
Distribution: Rapidly and widely distributed.
Metabolism and Excretion: Metabolized by enzymes in RBCs and liver.
Half-life: 9 min.

TIME/ACTION PROFILE (antiarrhythmic effect)

ROUTE	ONSET	PEAK	DURATION
IV	within minutes	unknown	1–20 min

Contraindications/Precautions
Contraindicated in: Uncompensated CHF; Pulmonary edema; Cardiogenic shock; Bradycardia or heart block; Known alcohol intolerance.
Use Cautiously in: Geri: ↑ sensitivity to the effects of beta blockers; Thyrotoxicosis (may mask symptoms); Diabetes mellitus (may mask symptoms of hypoglycemia); Patients with a history of severe allergic reactions (intensity of reactions may be increased); OB, Lactation, Pedi: Safety not established; neonatal bradycardia, hypotension, hypoglycemia, and respiratory depression may occur rarely.

Adverse Reactions/Side Effects
CNS: fatigue, agitation, confusion, dizziness, drowsiness, weakness. **CV:** hypotension, peripheral ischemia. **GI:** nausea, vomiting. **Derm:** sweating. **Local:** injection site reactions.

Interactions
Drug-Drug: General anesthesia, IV **phenytoin**, and **verapamil** may cause additive myocardial depression. Additive bradycardia may occur with **digoxin**. Additive hypotension may occur with other **antihypertensives**, acute ingestion of **alcohol**, or **nitrates**. Concurrent use with **amphetamine**, **cocaine**, **ephedrine**, **epinephrine**, **norepinephrine**, **phenylephrine**, or **pseudoephedrine** may result in unopposed alpha-adrenergic stimulation (excessive hypertension, bradycardia). Concurrent **thyroid hormone** administration may ↓ effectiveness. May alter the effectiveness of **insulins** or **oral hypoglycemic agents** (dose adjustments may be necessary). May ↓ effectiveness of **theophylline**. May ↓ beneficial beta cardiovascular effects of **dopamine** or **dobutamine**. Use cautiously within 14 days of **MAO inhibitor** therapy (may result in hypertension).

Route/Dosage
IV (Adults): *Antiarrhythmic*—500-mcg/kg loading dose over 1 min initially, followed by 50-mcg/kg/min infusion for 4 min; if no response

within 5 min, give 2nd loading dose of 500 mcg/kg over 1 min, then ↑ infusion to 100 mcg/kg/min for 4 min. If no response, repeat loading dose of 500 mcg/kg over 1 min and ↑ infusion rate by 50-mcg/kg/min increments (not to exceed 200 mcg/kg/min for 48 hr). As therapeutic end point is achieved, eliminate loading doses and decrease dose increments to 25 mg/kg/min. *Intraoperative antihypertensive/antiarrhythmic*—250–500-mcg/kg loading dose over 1 min initially, followed by 50-mcg/kg/min infusion for 4 min; if no response within 5 min, give 2nd loading dose of 250–500 mcg/kg over 1 min, then ↑ infusion to 100 mcg/kg/min for 4 min. If no response, repeat loading dose of 250–500 mcg/kg over 1 min and ↑ infusion rate by 50-mcg/kg/min increments (not to exceed 200 mcg/kg/min for 48 hr).

IV (Children): *Antiarrhythmic*—50 mcg/kg/min, may be ↑ q 10 min up to 300 mcg/kg/min.

Availability
Solution for injection (prediluted for use as loading dose): 10 mg/mL, 20 mg/mL. **Premixed infusion:** 2000 mg/100 mL, 2500 mg/250 mL.

NURSING IMPLICATIONS

Assessment
- Monitor blood pressure, ECG, and pulse frequently during dose adjustment period and periodically during therapy. The risk of hypotension is greatest within the first 30 min of initiating esmolol infusion.
- Monitor intake and output ratios and daily weights. Assess routinely for signs and symptoms of CHF (dyspnea, rales/crackles, weight gain, peripheral edema, jugular venous distention).
- Assess infusion site frequently throughout therapy. Concentrations >10 mg/mL may cause redness, swelling, skin discoloration, and burning at the injection site. Do not use butterfly needles for administration. If venous irritation occurs, stop the infusion and resume at another site.
- *Toxicity and Overdose:* Monitor patients receiving esmolol for signs of overdose (bradycardia, severe dizziness or fainting, severe drowsiness, dyspnea, bluish fingernails or palms, seizures).
- IV glucagon and symptomatic care are used in the treatment of esmolol overdose. Because of the short action of esmolol, discontinuation of therapy may relieve acute toxicity.

Potential Nursing Diagnoses
Decreased cardiac output (Side Effects)

Implementation
- *High Alert:* IV vasoactive medications are inherently dangerous. Esmolol is available in different concentrations; fatalities have occurred when loading dose vial is confused with concentrated solution for injection, which contains 2500 mg in 10 mL (250 mg/mL) and must be diluted. Before administering, have second practitioner independently check original order, dose calculations, and infusion pump settings.
- *High Alert:* Do not confuse Brevibloc (esmolol) with Brevital (methohexital). If both are available as floor stock, store in separate areas.
- To convert to other antiarrhythmics following esmolol administration, administer the 1st dose of the antiarrhythmic agent and decrease the esmolol dose by 50% after 30 min. If an adequate response is maintained for 1 hr following the 2nd dose of the antiarrhythmic agent, discontinue esmolol.

IV Administration
- **Direct IV:** *Diluent:* The 10 mg/mL and 20 mg/mL vials should be used for the loading dose. These vials are already diluted. No further dilution is needed. *Concentration:* Avoid concentrations >10 mg/mL. *Rate:* Administer over 1 min.
- **Continuous Infusion:** *Diluent:* Premixed infusions are already diluted and ready to use. Solution is clear, colorless to light yellow. *Concentration:* 10 mg/mL. *Rate:* Based on patient's weight (see Route/Dosage section). Titration of dose is based on desired heart rate or undesired decrease in blood pressure. Esmolol infusions should not be abruptly discontinued; the infusion rate should be tapered.
- **Y-Site Compatibility:** alfentanil, amikacin, aminophylline, amiodarone, amphotericin B liposome, anidulafungin, ascorbic acid, atracurium, atropine, aztreonam, benztropine, bivalirudin, bleomycin, bumetanide, buprenorphine, butorphanol, calcium chloride, calcium gluconate, carboplatin, caspofungin, cefazolin, cefotaxime, cefoxitin, ceftazidime, ceftizoxime, ceftriaxone, cefuroxime, chlorpromazine, cimetidine, cisatracurium, cisplatin, clindamy-

cin, cyanocobalamin, cyclophosphamide, cyclosporine, cytarabine, dactinomycin, daptomycin, dexmedetomidine, digoxin, diltiazem, diphenhydramine, dobutamine, docetaxel, dopamine, doriopenem, doxorubicin, doxycycline, enalaprilat, ephedrine, epinephrine, epoetin alfa, eftifibatide, ertapenem, erythromycin, etoposide, etoposide phosphate, famotidine, fenoldopam, fentanyl, fluconazole, fludarabine, fluorouracil, folic acid, gemcitabine, gentamicin, glycopyrrolate, granisetron, hetastarch, hydromorphone, idarubicin, ifosfamide, imipenem/cilastatin, insulin, isoproterenol, labetalol, levofloxacin, lidocaine, linezolid, lorazepam, magnesium sulfate, mannitol, mechlorethamine, meperidine, metaraminol, methotrexate, methoxamine, methyldopate, metoclopramide, metoprolol, metronidazole, micafungin, midazolam, mitoxantrone, morphine, multivitamins, nalbuphine, naloxone, nesiritide, nicardipine, nitroglycerin, nitroprusside, norepinephrine, octreotide, ondansetron, oxaliplatin, oxytocin, paclitaxel, palonosetron, pancuronium, papaverine, pemetrexed, penicillin G, pentamidine, pentazocine, phentolamine, phenylephrine, phytonadione, piperacillin/tazobactam, potassium chloride, potassium phosphates, procainamide, prochlorperazine, promethazine, propofol, propranolol, protamine, pyridoxime, quinupristin/dalfopristin, ranitidine, remifentanil, rocuronium, sodium acetate, sodium bicarbonate, streptokinase, succinylcholine, sufentanil, tacrolimus, teniposide, theophylline, thiamine, thiotepa, ticarcillin/clavulanate, tigecycline, tirofiban, tobramycin, tolazoline, trimetaphan, urokinase, vancomycin, vasopressin, vecuronium, verapamil, vincristine, voriconazole.

- **Y-Site Incompatibility:** acyclovir, amphotericin B cholesteryl, amphotericin B colloidal, azathioprine, cefotetan, dantrolene, dexamethasone, diazepam, diazoxide, furosemide, ganciclovir, inamrinone, indomethacin, ketorolac, milrinone, oxacillin, pantoprazole, phenobarbital, phentolamine, warfarin.

Patient/Family Teaching
- May cause drowsiness. Caution patients receiving esmolol to call for assistance during ambulation or transfer.
- Advise patients to change positions slowly to minimize orthostatic hypotension.
- Patients with diabetes should closely monitor blood glucose, especially if weakness, malaise, irritability, or fatigue occurs. Medication does not block dizziness or sweating as signs of hypoglycemia.

Evaluation/Desired Outcomes
- Control of arrhythmias without appearance of detrimental side effects.

esomeprazole
(es-o-**mep**-ra-zole)
Nexium

Classification
Therapeutic: antiulcer agents
Pharmacologic: proton-pump inhibitors

Pregnancy Category B

Indications
GERD/erosive esophagitis. Hypersecretory conditions, including Zollinger-Ellison syndrome. With amoxicillin and clarithromycin to eradicate *Helicobacter pylori* in duodenal ulcer disease or history of duodenal ulcer disease. Decrease risk of gastric ulcer during continuous NSAID therapy.

Action
Binds to an enzyme on gastric parietal cells in the presence of acidic gastric pH, preventing the final transport of hydrogen ions into the gastric lumen. **Therapeutic Effects:** Diminished accumulation of acid in the gastric lumen with lessened gastroesophageal reflux. Healing of duodenal ulcers. Decreased incidence of gastric ulcer during continuous NSAID therapy.

Pharmacokinetics
Absorption: 90% absorbed following oral administration; food ↓ absorption.
Distribution: Unknown.
Protein Binding: 97%.
Metabolism and Excretion: Extensively metabolized by the liver (cytochrome P450 [CYP450] system, primarily CYP2C19 isoenzyme, but also the CYP3A4 isoenzyme) ▓ (the CYP2C19 enzyme system exhibits genetic polymorphism; 15–20% of Asian patients and 3–5% of Caucasian and Black patients may be poor metabolizers and may have significantly ↑ esomeprazole concentrations and an ↑ risk of adverse effects); <1% excreted unchanged in urine.
Half-life: 1.0–1.5 hr.

TIME/ACTION PROFILE (blood levels*)

ROUTE	ONSET	PEAK	DURATION
PO	rapid	1.6 hr	24 hr
IV	rapid	end of infusion	24 hr

*Resolution of symptoms takes 5–8 days

Contraindications/Precautions

Contraindicated in: Hypersensitivity; Lactation: Not recommended; Concurrent use of **atazanavir** or **nelfinavir**.

Use Cautiously in: Severe hepatic impairment; Geri: ↑ risk of hip fractures in patients using high-doses for >1 year; OB: Use only if clearly needed; Pedi: Children <1 yr (safety not established).

Adverse Reactions/Side Effects

CNS: headache. **GI:** abdominal pain, constipation, diarrhea, dry mouth, flatulence, nausea.

Interactions

Drug-Drug: May ↓ levels of **atazanavir** and **nelfinavir** (avoid concurrent use with either of these antiretrovirals). May ↑ levels and risk of toxicity of **saquinavir** (may need to ↓ dose of saquinavir). May ↓ absorption of drugs requiring acid pH, including **ketoconazole**, **itraconazole**, **atazanavir**, **ampicillin**, and **iron salts**. May ↑ risk of bleeding with **warfarin** (monitor INR and PT). **Voriconazole** may ↑ levels. May ↓ the antiplatelet effects of **clopidogrel**.

Route/Dosage

Gastroesophageal Reflux Disease

PO (Adults): *Healing of erosive esophagitis*—20 mg or 40 mg once daily for 4–8 wk; *maintenance of healing of erosive esophagitis*—20 mg once daily; *symptomatic GERD*—20 mg once daily for 4 wk (additional 4 wk may be considered for nonresponders).

PO (Children 12–17 yrs): *Short-term treatment of GERD*—20–40 mg once daily up to 8 wk.

PO (Children 1–11 yrs): *Short-term treatment of GERD*—10 mg once daily up to 8 wk; *Healing of erosive esophagitis*—<20 kg: 10 mg once daily for 8 wk; ≥20 kg: 10–20 mg daily for 8 wk.

IV (Adults): 20 or 40 mg once daily.

H. pylori Eradication to Reduce the Risk of Duodenal Ulcer Recurrence (Triple Therapy)

PO (Adults): 40 mg once daily for 10 days with amoxicillin 1000 mg twice daily for 10 days and clarithromycin 500 mg twice daily for 10 days.

Decrease Gastric Ulcer During Continuous NSAID Therapy

PO (Adults): 20 or 40 mg once daily for up to 6 mo.

Pathological Hypersecretory Conditions Including Zollinger-Ellison Syndrome

PO (Adults): 40 mg twice daily.

Hepatic Impairment

PO, IV (Adults): *Severe hepatic impairment*—Dose should not exceed 20 mg/day.

Availability

Delayed-release capsules: 20 mg, 40 mg. **Cost:** 20 mg $430.97/90, 40 mg $425.97/90. **Delayed-release oral suspension packets:** 10 mg, 20 mg, 40 mg. **Powder for injection (requires reconstitution):** 20 mg/vial, 40 mg/vial.

NURSING IMPLICATIONS

Assessment

- Assess patient routinely for epigastric or abdominal pain and frank or occult blood in the stool, emesis, or gastric aspirate.
- *Lab Test Considerations:* May cause ↑ serum creatinine, uric acid, total bilirubin, alkaline phosphatase, AST, and ALT.
- May alter hemoglobin, WBC, platelets, serum sodium, potassium, and thyroxine levels.

Potential Nursing Diagnoses

Acute pain (Indications)

Implementation

- Antacids may be used while taking esomeprazole.
- **PO:** Administer at least 1 hr before meals. Capsules should be swallowed whole.
- *Delayed-release capsules:* For patients with difficulty swallowing, place 1 tbsp of applesauce in an empty bowl. Open capsule and carefully empty the pellets inside onto applesauce. Mix pellets with applesauce and swallow immediately. Applesauce should not be hot and should be soft enough to swallow without chewing. Do not store applesauce mixture for future use. Tap water, orange juice, apple juice, and yogurt have also been used. Do not crush or chew pellets.
- *For patients with an NG tube,* delayed-release capsules can be opened and intact granules emptied into a 60-mL syringe and mixed with 50 mL of water. Replace plunger and shake syringe vigorously for 15 sec. Hold syringe with tip up and check for granules in tip. Attach syringe to NG tube and administer solution. After administering, flush syringe with additional water. Do not administer if granules have dis-

solved or disintegrated. Administer immediately after mixing.
- For *Delayed-release oral suspension:* Mix contents of packet with 1 tbsp (15 mL) of water, leave 2–3 min to thicken, stir and drink within 30 minutes.
- For *Delayed-Release Oral Suspension Nasogastric or Gastric Tube:* Add 15 mL of water to a syringe and then add contents of packet. Shake the syringe, leave 2–3 min to thicken. Shake the syringe and inject through the nasogastric or gastric tube within 30 min.

IV Administration
- **Direct IV:** Reconstitute each vial with 5 mL of 0.9% NaCl, LR, or D5W. Do not administer solutions that are discolored or contain a precipitate. Stable at room temperature for up to 12 hr. *Rate:* Administer over at least 3 min.
- **Intermittent Infusion:** *Diluent:* Dilute reconstituted solution to a volume of 50 mL. Solutions diluted with 0.9% NaCl or LR are stable for 12 hr and those diluted with D5W are stable for 6 hr at room temperature. *Rate:* Administer over 10–30 min.
- **Y-Site Incompatibility:** Do not administer with other medications or solutions. Flush line with 0.9% NaCl, LR, or D5W before and after administration.

Patient/Family Teaching
- Instruct patient to take medication as directed for the full course of therapy, even if feeling better. Take missed doses as soon as remembered but not if almost time for next dose. Do not double doses.
- Advise patient to avoid alcohol, products containing aspirin or NSAIDs, and foods that may cause an increase in GI irritation.
- Advise patient to report onset of black, tarry stools; diarrhea; abdominal pain; or persistent headache to health care professional promptly.

Evaluation/Desired Outcomes
- Decrease in abdominal pain or prevention of gastric irritation and bleeding. Healing of duodenal ulcers can be seen on x-ray examination or endoscopy.
- Decrease in symptoms of GERD and erosive esophagitis. Sustained resolution of symptoms usually occurs in 5–8 days. Therapy is continued for 4–8 wk after initial episode.
- Decreased incidence of gastric ulcer during continuous NSAID therapy.
- Eradication of H. Pylori in duodenal ulcer disease.
- Decrease in symptoms of hypersecretory conditions, including Zollinger-Ellison.

ESTRADIOL (es-tra-**dye**-ole)
Estrace

estradiol acetate
Femtrace

estradiol cypionate
Depo-Estradiol

estradiol valerate
Delestrogen, ✦Femogex

estradiol topical emulsion
Estrasorb

estradiol topical gel
Divigel, Elestrin, EstroGel

estradiol transdermal spray
EvaMist

estradiol transdermal system
Alora, Climara, Estraderm, Menostar, Vivelle-Dot

estradiol vaginal tablet
Vagifem

estradiol vaginal ring
Femring, Estring

Classification
Therapeutic: hormones
Pharmacologic: estrogens

Pregnancy Category X

Indications
PO, IM, Topical, Transdermal: Replacement of estrogen (HRT) to diminish moderate to severe vasomotor symptoms of menopause and of various estrogen deficiency states including: Female hypogonadism, Ovariectomy, Primary ovarian failure. Treatment and prevention of postmenopausal osteoporosis (not vaginal dose forms). **PO:** Inoperable metastatic postmenopausal breast or prostate carcinoma. **Vag:** Management of atrophic vaginitis that may occur with menopause (low dose), bothersome systemic symptoms of menopause (higher dose). Concurrent use of progestin is recommended during cyclical therapy to decrease the risk of endometrial carcinoma in patients with an intact uterus.

Action
Estrogens promote growth and development of female sex organs and the maintenance of secondary sex characteristics in women. Metabolic effects include reduced blood cholesterol, protein synthesis, and sodium and water retention.

ESTRADIOL

Therapeutic Effects: Restoration of hormonal balance in various deficiency states, including menopause. Treatment of hormone-sensitive tumors.

Pharmacokinetics

Absorption: Well absorbed after oral administration. Readily absorbed through skin and mucous membranes.
Distribution: Widely distributed. Crosses the placenta and enters breast milk.
Metabolism and Excretion: Mostly metabolized by the liver and other tissues. Enterohepatic recirculation occurs, and more absorption may occur from the GI tract.
Half-life: Gel: 36 hr.

TIME/ACTION PROFILE (estrogenic effects)

ROUTE	ONSET	PEAK	DURATION
PO	unknown	unknown	unknown
IM	unknown	unknown	unknown
TD	unknown	unknown	3–4 days (Estraderm), 7 days (Climara)
Topical	unknown	unknown	uknown
Vaginal ring	unknown	unknown	90 days
Vaginal tablet	unknown	unknown	3–4 days

Contraindications/Precautions

Contraindicated in: Thromboembolic disease; Undiagnosed vaginal bleeding; OB: Positive evidence of fetal risk.
Use Cautiously in: Underlying cardiovascular disease; Severe hepatic or renal disease; May ↑ the risk of endometrial carcinoma; History of porphyria; Lactation: Usually compatible with breast feeding (AAP).

Adverse Reactions/Side Effects

CNS: headache, dizziness, lethargy. **EENT:** intolerance to contact lenses, worsening of myopia or astigmatism. **CV:** MI, THROMBOEMBOLISM, edema, hypertension. **GI:** nausea, weight changes, anorexia, ↑ appetite, jaundice, vomiting. **GU:** women—amenorrhea, dysmenorrhea, breakthrough bleeding, cervical erosions, loss of libido, vaginal candidiasis;; men, erectile dysfunction, testicular atrophy. **Derm:** oily skin, acne, pigmentation, urticaria. **Endo:** gynecomastia (men), hyperglycemia. **F and E:** hypercalcemia, sodium and water retention. **MS:** leg cramps. **Misc:** breast tenderness.

Interactions

Drug-Drug: May alter requirement for **warfarin**, **oral hypoglycemic agents**, or **insulins**. **Barbiturates** or **rifampin** may ↓ effectiveness. **Smoking** ↑ risk of adverse CV reactions.

Route/Dosage

Estrogens should be used in the lowest doses for the shortest period of time consistent with desired therapeutic outcome.

Symptoms of Menopause, Atrophic Vaginitis, Female Hypogonadism, Ovarian Failure/Osteoporosis

PO (Adults): 0.45–2 mg daily or in a cycle.
IM (Adults): 1–5 mg monthly (estradiol cypionate) *or* 10–20 mg (estradiol valerate) monthly.
Topical Emulsion *(Estrasorb)* **(Adults):** Apply two 1.74 g pouches (4.35 mg estradiol) daily.
Gel (Adults): Apply contents of one packet *(Divigel)* or one actuation from pump *(EstroGel, Elestrin)* daily.
Spray *EvaMist* **(Adults):** 1 spray daily, may be increased to 2–3 sprays daily.
Transdermal (Adults): *Alora*—25–50mcg/24-hr transdermal patch applied twice weekly. *Estraderm*—50–mcg/24-hr transdermal patch applied twice weekly. *Climara*—25-mcg/24-hr patch applied weekly. *Vivelle-Dot*—25–50–mcg/24-hr transdermal patch applied twice weekly. *Menostar*—14-mcg/24-hr patch applied q 7 days. Progestin may be administered for 10–14 days of each month.
Vag (Adults): *Cream*—2–4 g (0.2–0.4 mg estradiol) daily for 1–2 wk, then decrease to 1–2 g/day for 1–2 wk; then maintenance dose of 1 g 1–3 times weekly for 3 wk, then off for 1 wk; then repeat cycle once vaginal mucosa has been restored; *Vaginal ring (Estring)*—2-mg (releases 7.5 mcg estradiol/24 hr) q 3 mo; *Vaginal ring (Femring)*—12.4 mg (releases 50 mcg estradiol/24 hr) q 3 mo or 24.8 mg (releases 100 mcg estradiol/24 hr) q 3 mo (*Femring* requires concurrent progesterone) *Vaginal tablet*—25-mcg once daily for 2 wk, then twice weekly.

Postmenopausal Breast Carcinoma

PO (Adults): 10 mg 3 times daily.

Prostate Carcinoma

PO (Adults): 1–2 mg 3 times daily.
IM (Adults): 30 mg q 1–2 wk (estradiol valerate).

Availability (generic available)

Tablets: 0.45 mg, 0.5 mg, 0.9 mg, 1 mg, 1.8 mg, 2 mg. **Cost:** *Generic*—0.5 mg $22.17/100, 1 mg $15.52/100, 2 mg $33.30/100. **Injection (val-**

erate in oil): 10 mg/mL, 20 mg/mL, 40 mg/mL. **Injection (cypionate in oil):** 5 mg/mL. **Topical emulsion:** 4.35 mg/1.74 g pouch in boxes of 14 pouches in a 1-month supply carton of 56 pouches. **Topical gel packet:** 0.25 mg/packet, 0.5 mg/packet, 1 mg/packet. **Topical gel pump (0.06%):** 0.52 mg/actuation, 0.75 mg/actuation. **Transdermal Spray:** 1.53 mg/spray. **Transdermal system:** 14 mcg/24-hr release rate, 25 mcg/24-hr release rate, 37.5 mcg/24-hr release rate, 50 mcg/24-hr release rate, 60 mcg/24-hr release rate, 75 mcg/24-hr release rate, 100 mcg/24-hr release rate. **Cost:** *Generic*—25 mcg/24-hr release rate $36.99/4 patches, 37.5 mcg/24-hr release rate $39.35/4 patches, 50 mcg/24-hr release rate $29.97/4 patches, 60 mcg/24-hr release rate $39.99/4 patches, 75 mcg/24-hr release rate $35.99/4 patches, 100 mcg/24-hr release rate $31.46/4 patches. **Vaginal cream:** 100 mcg/g. **Vaginal ring (Estring):** 2 mg (releases 7.5 mcg/day over 90 days). **Vaginal ring (Femring):** 12.4 mg (releases 50 mcg/day over 90 days), 24.8 mg (releases 100 mcg/day over 90 days). **Vaginal tablet:** 25 mcg. **Cost:** $75.81/18 tablets.

NURSING IMPLICATIONS

Assessment
- Assess blood pressure before and periodically during therapy.
- Monitor intake and output ratios and weekly weight. Report significant discrepancies or steady weight gain.
- **Menopause:** Assess frequency and severity of vasomotor symptoms.
- *Lab Test Considerations:* May cause ↑ HDL, phospholipids, and triglycerides and ↓ serum LDL and total cholesterol concentrations.
- May cause ↑ serum glucose, sodium, cortisol, prolactin, prothrombin, and factor VII, VIII, IX, and X levels. May ↓ serum folate, pyridoxine, antithrombin III, and urine pregnanediol concentrations.
- Monitor hepatic function before and periodically during therapy.
- May cause false interpretations of thyroid function tests, false ↑ in norepinephrine platelet-induced aggregability, and false ↓ in metyrapone tests.
- May cause hypercalcemia in patients with metastatic bone lesions.

Potential Nursing Diagnoses
Sexual dysfunction (Indications)

Implementation
- **PO:** Administer with or immediately after food to reduce nausea.
- **Vag:** Manufacturer provides applicator with cream. Dose is marked on the applicator. Wash applicator with mild soap and warm water after each use.
- **Transdermal:** When switching from PO form, begin transdermal therapy 1 wk after the last dose or when symptoms reappear.
- **Topical:** In a comfortable position, apply *Estrasorb* to clean, dry skin of thighs each morning. Open each foil pouch individually. Cut or tear the first pouch at the notches near the top of the pouch. Apply the contents of the pouch to the top of the left thigh; push entire contents from bottom through neck of pouch. Using one or both hands rub the emulsion into the thigh and calf for 3 min until completely absorbed. Rub any excess remaining on hands into buttocks. Repeat procedure with second pouch on right leg. Allow application sites to dry completely before covering with clothing to prevent transfer. Wash hands with soap and water to remove residual estradiol.
- Apply *Divigel* individual-use once-daily packets of quick drying gel to an area measuring 5 inches by 7 inches (size of 2 palm prints) on the thigh. Do not wash area for at least 1 hr after gel has dried.
- Spray *EvaMist* on inside of forearm at the same time each day. Do not massage or rub the spray into the skin. Allow to dry for 2 min before dressing and 30 min before washing. Never spray *EvaMist* around breast or vagina Do not use more than 56 doses, even if fluid remains in pump.
- **IM:** Injection has oil base. Roll syringe to ensure even dispersion. Administer deep IM. Avoid IV administration.

Patient/Family Teaching
- Instruct patient on correct method of administration. Instruct patient to take medication as directed. Take missed doses as soon as remembered as long as it is not just before next dose. If a dose of *EvaMist* is missed, apply if more than 12 hr before next dose; if less than 12 hr, omit dose and return to regular schedule. Do not double doses.
- Explain dose schedule and maintenance routine. Discontinuing medication suddenly may cause withdrawal bleeding.
- If nausea becomes a problem, advise patient that eating solid food often provides relief.

- Advise patient to report signs and symptoms of fluid retention (swelling of ankles and feet, weight gain), thromboembolic disorders (pain, swelling, tenderness in extremities, headache, chest pain, blurred vision), mental depression, or hepatic dysfunction (yellowed skin or eyes, pruritus, dark urine, light-colored stools) to health care professional.
- Instruct patient to stop taking medication and notify health care professional if pregnancy is planned or suspected.
- Advise patient to notify health care professional of medication regimen before treatment or surgery.
- Caution patient that cigarette smoking during estrogen therapy may cause increased risk of serious side effects, especially for women over age 35.
- Caution patient to use sunscreen and protective clothing to prevent increased pigmentation.
- Advise patient treated for osteoporosis that exercise has been found to arrest and reverse bone loss. The patient should discuss any exercise limitations with health care professional before beginning program.
- Inform patient that estrogens should not be used to decrease risk of cardiovascular disease. Estrogens may increase risk of cardiovascular disease and breast cancer.
- Emphasize the importance of routine follow-up physical exams, including blood pressure; breast, abdomen, and pelvic examinations; Papanicolaou smears every 6–12 mo; and mammogram every 12 mo or as directed. Health care professional will evaluate possibility of discontinuing medication every 3–6 mo. If on continuous (not cyclical) therapy or without concurrent progestins, endometrial biopsy may be recommended, if uterus is intact.
- **Vag:** Instruct patient in the correct use of applicator. Patient should remain recumbent for at least 30 min after administration. May use sanitary napkin to protect clothing, but do not use tampon. If a dose is missed, do not use the missed dose, but return to regular dosing schedule.
- Instruct patient to use applicator provided with vaginal tablet. Insert as high up in the vagina as comfortable, without using force.
- **Vaginal Ring:** Instruct patient to press ring into an oval and insert into the upper third of the vaginal vault. Exact position is not critical. Once ring is inserted, patient should not feel anything. If discomfort is felt, ring is probably not in far enough; gently push farther into vagina. Leave in place continuously for 90 days. Ring does not interfere with sexual intercourse. If straining at defecation makes ring move to lower vagina, push up with finger. If expelled totally, rinse ring with lukewarm water and reinsert. To remove, hook a finger through the ring and pull it out.
- **Transdermal:** Instruct patient to wash and dry hands first. Apply disc to intact skin on hairless portion of abdomen (do not apply to breasts or waistline). Press disc for 10 sec to ensure contact with skin (especially around edges). Avoid areas where clothing may rub disc loose. Change site with each administration to prevent skin irritation. Do not reuse site for 1 wk; disc may be reapplied if it falls off.
- Advise patient referred for MRI test to discuss patch with referring health care professional and MRI facility to determine if removal of patch is necessary prior to test and for directions for replacing patch.

Evaluation/Desired Outcomes

- Resolution of menopausal vasomotor symptoms.
- Decreased vaginal and vulvar itching, inflammation, or dryness associated with menopause.
- Normalization of estrogen levels in patients with ovariectomy or hypogonadism.
- Control of the spread of advanced metastatic breast or prostate cancer.
- Prevention of osteoporosis.

---

estrogens, conjugated (equine) (ess-troe-jenz)
✦ C.E.S, ✦ Congest, Premarin

estrogens, conjugated (synthetic, A)
Cenestin

estrogens, conjugated (synthetic, B)
Enjuvia

Classification
Therapeutic: hormones
Pharmacologic: estrogens

Pregnancy Category X

✦ = Canadian drug name. 🧬 = Genetic implication.
*CAPITALS indicates life-threatening; underlines indicate most frequent.

Indications
PO: Treatment of moderate to severe vasomotor symptoms of menopause. Estrogen deficiency states, including: Female hypogonadism, Ovariectomy, Primary ovarian failure. Prevention of postmenopausal osteoporosis. Advanced inoperable metastatic breast and prostatic carcinoma. **IM, IV:** Uterine bleeding resulting from hormonal imbalance. **Vag:** Atrophic vaginitis. Moderate to severe dyspareunia due to menopause. Concurrent use of progestin is recommended during cyclical therapy to decrease the risk of endometrial carcinoma in patients with an intact uterus.

Action
Estrogens promote the growth and development of female sex organs and the maintenance of secondary sex characteristics in women. **Therapeutic Effects:** Restoration of hormonal balance in various deficiency states and treatment of hormone-sensitive tumors.

Pharmacokinetics
Absorption: Well absorbed after oral administration. Readily absorbed through skin and mucous membranes.
Distribution: Widely distributed. Crosses placenta and enters breast milk.
Metabolism and Excretion: Mostly metabolized by liver and other tissues. Enterohepatic recirculation occurs, with more absorption from GI tract.
Half-life: Unknown.

TIME/ACTION PROFILE (estrogenic effects†)

ROUTE	ONSET	PEAK	DURATION
PO	rapid	unknown	24 hr
IM	delayed	unknown	6–12 hr
IV	rapid	unknown	6–12 hr

†Tumor response may take several weeks

Contraindications/Precautions
Contraindicated in: Thromboembolic disease (e.g., DVT, PE, MI, stroke); Undiagnosed vaginal bleeding; History of breast cancer; History of estrogen-dependent cancer; Liver dysfunction; OB: May result in harm to the fetus; Lactation: Negatively affects quantity and quality of breast milk.
Use Cautiously in: Long-term use (more than 4–5 yr); may ↑ risk of myocardial infarction, stroke, invasive breast cancer, pulmonary emboli, deep vein thrombosis and dementia in postmenopausal women; Underlying cardiovascular disease; Hypertriglyceridemia; May ↑ risk of endometrial carcinoma.

Adverse Reactions/Side Effects
(Systemic use) **CNS:** headache, dizziness, insomnia, lethargy, mental depression. **CV:** MI, THROMBOEMBOLISM, edema, hypertension. **GI:** nausea, weight changes, anorexia, increased appetite, jaundice, vomiting. **GU:** *women*—amenorrhea, breakthrough bleeding, dysmenorrhea, cervical erosion, loss of libido, vaginal candidiasis; *men*, erectile dysfunction, testicular atrophy. **Derm:** acne, oily skin, pigmentation, urticaria. **Endo:** gynecomastia (men), hyperglycemia. **F and E:** hypercalcemia, sodium and water retention. **MS:** leg cramps. **Misc:** breast tenderness.

Interactions
Drug-Drug: May alter requirement for **warfarin**, **oral hypoglycemic agents**, or **insulins**. **Barbiturates**, **carbamazepine**, or **rifampin** may ↓ effectiveness. **Smoking** ↑ risk of adverse CV reactions. **Erythromycin**, **clarithromycin**, **itraconazole**, **ketoconazole**, and **ritonavir** may ↑ risk of adverse effects.
Drug-Natural Products: Grapefruit juice may ↑ risk of adverse effects.

Route/Dosage
Estrogens should be used in the lowest doses for the shortest period of time consistent with desired therapeutic outcome.

Ovariectomy, Primary Ovarian Failure
PO (Adults): 1.25 mg daily administered cyclically (3 wk on, 1 wk off).

Osteoporosis/Menopausal Symptoms
PO (Adults): 0.3–1.25 mg daily or in a cycle.

Female Hypogonadism
PO (Adults): 0.3–0.625 mg daily administered cyclically (3 wk on, 1 wk off).

Inoperable Breast Carcinoma—Men and Postmenopausal Women
PO (Adults): 10 mg 3 times daily.

Inoperable Prostate Carcinoma
PO (Adults): 1.25–2.5 mg 3 times daily.

Uterine Bleeding
IM, IV (Adults): 25 mg, may repeat in 6–12 hr if necessary.

Atrophic Vaginitis
PO (Adults): 0.3–1.25 mg daily.
Vag (Adults): *Conjugated estrogens (equine)*– 0.5–2 g cream (0.3125 mg–1.25 g conjugated estrogens) daily for 3 wk, off for 1 wk, then repeat; *Synthetic conjugated estrogens, A*-1 g cream (0.3125 mg synthetic conjugated estrogens, A) daily for 1 wk, then twice weekly.

estrogens, conjugated (equine) **537**

Moderate to Severe Dyspareunia
Vag (Adults): *Conjugated estrogens (equine)* – 0.5 g cream (0.3125 mg conjugated estrogens) twice weekly continuously or daily for 3 wk, off for 1 wk, then repeat; *Synthetic conjugated estrogens, A*-1 g cream (0.3125 mg synthetic conjugated estrogens, A) daily for 1 wk, then twice weekly.

Availability (generic available)
Tablets: 0.3 mg, 0.45 mg, 0.625 mg, 0.9 mg, 1.25 mg. **Cost:** *Premarin*—0.3 mg $166.63/100, 0.45 mg $139.97/100, 0.625 mg $136.95/100, 0.9 mg $139.97/100, 1.25 mg $126.46/100. **Powder for injection:** 25 mg/vial. **Vaginal cream:** 0.625 mg/g. **Cost:** $85.99/42.5-g tube. *In combination with:* medroxyprogesterone (Prempro and Premphase [compliance package]). See Appendix B.

NURSING IMPLICATIONS

Assessment
- Assess blood pressure before and periodically during therapy.
- Monitor intake and output ratios and weekly weight. Report significant discrepancies or steady weight gain.
- **Menopause:** Assess frequency and severity of vasomotor symptoms.
- *Lab Test Considerations:* May cause ↑ HDL and triglycerides, and ↓ serum LDL and total cholesterol concentrations.
- May cause ↑ serum glucose, sodium, cortisol, prolactin, prothrombin, and factor VII, VIII, IX, and X levels. May ↓ serum folate, pyridoxine, antithrombin III, and urine pregnanediol concentrations.
- Monitor hepatic function before and periodically during therapy.
- May cause false interpretations of thyroid function tests.
- May cause hypercalcemia in patients with metastatic bone lesions.

Potential Nursing Diagnoses
Sexual dysfunction (Indications)

Implementation
- Estrogens should be used in the lowest doses for the shortest period of time consistent with desired therapeutic outcome.
- **PO:** Administer with or immediately after food to reduce nausea.
- **Vag:** Manufacturer provides applicator with cream. Dose is marked on the applicator. Wash applicator with mild soap and warm water after each use.
- **IM:** To reconstitute, withdraw at least 5 mL of air from dry container and then slowly introduce the sterile diluent (bacteriostatic water for injection) against the container side. Gently agitate container to dissolve; do not shake vigorously. Solution is stable for 60 days if refrigerated. Do not use if precipitate is present or if solution is darkened.
- IV is preferred parenteral route because of rapid response.

IV Administration
- **Direct IV:** *Diluent:* Reconstitute as for IM. Inject into distal port tubing of free-flowing IV of 0.9% NaCl, D5W, or lactated Ringer's solution. *Concentration:* 5 mg/mL. *Rate:* Administer slowly (no faster than 5 mg/min) to prevent flushing.
- **Y-Site Compatibility:** heparin, hydrocortisone sodium succinate, potassium chloride, vitamin B complex with C.

Patient/Family Teaching
- Instruct patient to take oral medication as directed. Take missed doses as soon as remembered, but not just before next dose. Do not double doses.
- Explain dose schedule and maintenance routine. Discontinuing medication suddenly may cause withdrawal bleeding. Bleeding is anticipated during the week when conjugated estrogens are withheld.
- If nausea becomes a problem, advise patient that eating solid food often provides relief.
- Advise patient to report signs and symptoms of fluid retention (swelling of ankles and feet, weight gain), thromboembolic disorders (pain, swelling, tenderness in extremities; headache; chest pain; blurred vision), depression, hepatic dysfunction (yellowed skin or eyes, pruritus, dark urine, light-colored stools), or abnormal vaginal bleeding to health care professional.
- Instruct patient to stop taking medication and notify health care professional if pregnancy is suspected.
- Caution patient that cigarette smoking during estrogen therapy may increase risk of serious side effects, especially for women over age 35.
- Caution patient to use sunscreen and protective clothing to prevent increased pigmentation.

- Advise patient to notify health care professional of medication regimen before treatment or surgery.
- Advise patient treated for osteoporosis that exercise has been found to arrest and reverse bone loss. The patient should discuss any exercise limitations with health care professional before beginning program.
- Emphasize the importance of routine follow-up physical exams, including blood pressure; breast, abdomen, and pelvic examinations; Papanicolaou smears every 6–12 mo; and mammogram every 12 mo or as directed. Health care professional will evaluate possibility of discontinuing medication every 3–6 mo. If on continuous (not cyclical) therapy or without concurrent progestins, endometrial biopsy may be recommended if uterus is intact.
- Inform patient that estrogens should not be used to decrease risk of cardiovascular disease. Estrogens may increase risk of cardiovascular disease and breast cancer.
- **Vag:** Instruct patient in the correct use of applicator. Patient should remain recumbent for at least 30 min after administration. May use sanitary napkin to protect clothing, but do not use tampon. If a dose is missed, do not use the missed dose, but return to regular dosing schedule.

Evaluation/Desired Outcomes
- Resolution of menopausal vasomotor symptoms.
- Decreased vaginal and vulvar itching, inflammation, or dryness associated with menopause.
- Normalization of estrogen levels in patients with ovariectomy or hypogonadism.
- Control of the spread of advanced metastatic breast or prostate cancer.
- Prevention of osteoporosis.
- Relief of moderate to severe dyspareunia due to menopause.

---

eszopiclone (es-zop-i-klone)
Lunesta

Classification
Therapeutic: sedative/hypnotics
Pharmacologic: cyclopyrrolones

Schedule IV

Pregnancy Category C

Indications
Insomnia.

Action
Interacts with GABA-receptor complexes; not a benzodiazepine. **Therapeutic Effects:** Improved sleep with decreased latency and increased maintenance of sleep.

Pharmacokinetics
Absorption: Rapidly absorbed after oral administration.
Distribution: Unknown.
Metabolism and Excretion: Extensively metabolized by the liver (CYP3A4 and CYP2E1 enzyme systems); metabolites are renally excreted, <10% excreted unchanged in urine.
Half-life: 6 hr.

TIME/ACTION PROFILE (blood levels)

ROUTE	ONSET	PEAK	DURATION
PO	rapid	1 hr	6 hr

Contraindications/Precautions
Contraindicated in: Hypersensitivity.
Use Cautiously in: Debilitated patients may have ↓ metabolism or increased sensitivity; use lower initial dose; Conditions that may alter metabolic or hemodynamic function; Severe hepatic impairment (use lower initial dose); OB, Pedi:Safety not established in pregnancy or in children < 18 yr ; Lactation:Occasional use while breastfeeding an older infant should pose little risk (NIH); Geri: May impair motor and/or cognitive performance; see dosing guidelines.

Adverse Reactions/Side Effects
CNS: abnormal thinking, behavior changes, depression, hallucinations, headache, sleep-driving. **CV:** chest pain, peripheral edema. **GI:** dry mouth, unpleasant taste. **Derm:** rash.

Interactions
Drug-Drug: ↑ risk of CNS depression with other **CNS depressants** including **antihistamines**, **antidepressants**, **opioids**, **sedative/hypnotics** and **antipsychotics**. ↑ levels and risk of CNS depression with **drugs that inhibit the CYP3A4 enzyme system**, including **ketoconazole**, **itraconazole**, **clarithromycin**, **nefazodone**, **ritonavir** and **nelfinavir**. Levels and effectiveness may be ↓ by **drugs that induce the CYP3A4 enzyme system**, including **rifampicin**.

Route/Dosage
PO (Adults): 2 mg immediately before bedtime, may be raised to 3 mg if needed (3 mg dose is more effective for sleep maintenance); *geriatric patients*—1 mg immediately before bedtime for

patients with difficulty falling asleep, 2 mg for patients who difficulty staying asleep.

Hepatic Impairment
PO (Adults): *Severe hepatic impairment*—1 mg immediately before bedtime.
PO (Adults receiving concurrent CYP3A4 inhibitors): 1 mg immediately before bedtime, may be raised to 2 mg if needed.

Availability
Tablets: 1 mg, 2 mg, 3 mg. **Cost:** 1 mg $136.69/30, 2 mg $139.97/30, 3 mg $139.98/30.

NURSING IMPLICATIONS

Assessment
- Assess sleep patterns prior to and during administration. Continued insomnia after 7–10 days of therapy may indicate primary psychiatric or mental illness.
- Assess mental status and potential for abuse prior to administration. Prolonged use of >7–10 days may lead to physical and psychological dependence. Limit amount of drug available to the patient.

Potential Nursing Diagnoses
Insomnia (Indications)

Implementation
- **PO:** Onset is rapid. Administer immediately before going to bed or after patient has gone to bed and has experienced difficulty falling asleep, only on nights when patient is able to get 8 or more hours of sleep before being active again.
- Swallow tablet whole; do not break, crush, or chew.
- Eszopiclone is more effective if not taken with or before a high-fat, heavy meal.

Patient/Family Teaching
- Instruct patient to take eszopiclone immediately before going to bed, as directed. Taking prior to going to bed may result in short-term memory impairment, hallucinations, impaired coordination, and dizziness. Do not increase dose or discontinue without notifying health care professional. Dose may need to be decreased gradually to minimize withdrawal symptoms. Rebound insomnia may occur upon discontinuation and usually resolves within 1–2 nights.
- May cause daytime drowsiness. Caution patient to avoid driving or other activities requiring alertness until response to medication is known.
- Advise patient to notify health care professional before taking any Rx, OTC, or herbal products with eszopiclone.
- Caution patient to avoid concurrent use of alcohol or other CNS depressants.
- Advise patient to notify health care professional if pregnancy is planned or suspected.

Evaluation/Desired Outcomes
- Decreased sleep latency and improved sleep maintenance.

---

etanercept (e-tan-er-sept)
Enbrel

Classification
Therapeutic: antirheumatics (DMARDs)
Pharmacologic: anti-TNF agents

Pregnancy Category B

Indications
To decrease progression, signs and symptoms of rheumatoid arthritis, juvenile arthritis, ankylosing spondylitis, psoriatic arthritis or plaque psoriasis when response has been inadequate to other disease-modifying agents. May be used with other agents.

Action
Binds to tumor necrosis factor (TNF), making it inactive. TNF is a mediator of inflammatory response. **Therapeutic Effects:** Decreased inflammation and slowed progression of arthritis, spondylitis or psoriasis.

Pharmacokinetics
Absorption: 60% absorbed after subcut administration.
Distribution: Unknown.
Metabolism and Excretion: Unknown.
Half-life: 115 hr (range 98–300 hr).

TIME/ACTION PROFILE (symptom reduction)

ROUTE	ONSET	PEAK	DURATION
Subcut	2–4 wk	unknown	unknown

Contraindications/Precautions
Contraindicated in: Hypersensitivity; Sepsis; Lactation: Lactation; Untreated infections; Wegener's granulomatosis (receiving immunosuppressive agents); Concurrent cyclophosphamide or anakinra.
Use Cautiously in: Pre-existing or recent demyelinating disorders (multiple sclerosis, myelitis,

540   etanercept

optic neuritis); History of tuberculosis (increased risk of reactivation); Underlying chronic diseases which may predispose to infections (advanced or poorly-controlled diabetes mellitus); Latex allergy (needle cover of diluent syringe contains latex); Geri: May have ↑ risk of infection; Pedi: Children with significant exposure to varicella virus (temporarily discontinue etanercept; consider varicella zoster immune globulin); ↑ risk of lymphoma, leukemia, and other malignancies; OB: Use only if needed.

Adverse Reactions/Side Effects
CNS: headache, dizziness, weakness. **EENT:** rhinitis, pharyngitis. **Resp:** upper respiratory tract infection, cough, respiratory disorder. **GI:** abdominal pain, dyspepsia. **Derm:** psoriasis, rash. **Hemat:** LEUKEMIA, pancytopenia. **Local:** injection site reactions. **Misc:** INFECTIONS (including reactivation tuberculosis and invasive fungal infections), MALIGNANCY.

Interactions
Drug-Drug: Concurrent use with **anakinra** ↑ risk of serious infections (not recommended). Concurrent use of **cyclophosphamide** may ↑ risk of malignancies. May ↓ antibody response to **live-virus vaccine** and ↑ risk of adverse reactions (do not administer concurrently).

Route/Dosage
Subcut (Adults): *Adult rheumatoid arthritis, ankylosing spondylitis, psoriatic arthritis*—50 mg once weekly; *adult plaque psoriasis*—50 mg twice weekly for 3 mos, then 50 mg once weekly, may also be given as 25–50 mg once weekly as an initial dose.
Subcut (Children 4–17 yr): *>63 kg*—0.8 mg/kg/wk (up to 50 mg) as a single injection; *31–62 kg*—0.8 mg/kg/wk either as two injections on the same day or divided and given on two separate days 3–4 days apart; *<31 kg*—0.8 mg/kg/wk as a single injection.

Availability
Pre-filled syringes: 50 mg/mL. **Powder for injection:** 25 mg/vial.

NURSING IMPLICATIONS

Assessment
- Assess range of motion, degree of swelling, and pain in affected joints before and periodically during therapy.
- Assess patient for injection site reaction (erythema, pain, itching, swelling). Reactions are usually mild to moderate and last 3–5 days after injection.
- Monitor patients who develop a new infection while taking etanercept closely. Discontinue therapy in patients who develop a serious infection or sepsis. Do not initiate therapy in patients with active infections.
- Assess for signs and symptoms of systemic fungal infections (fever, malaise, weight loss, sweats, cough, dypsnea, pulmonary infiltrates, serious systemic illness with or without concomitant shock). Ascertain if patient lives in or has traveled to areas of endemic mycoses. Consider empiric antifungal treatment for patients at risk of histoplasmosis and other invasive fungal infections until the pathogens are identified. Consult with an infectious diseases specialist. Consider stopping etanercept until the infection has been diagnosed and adequately treated.
- ***Lab Test Considerations:*** Monitor CBC with differential periodically during therapy. May cause leukopenia, neutropenia, thrombocytopenia, and pancytopenia. Discontinue etanerceptif symptoms of blood dyscrasias (persistent fever) occur.

Potential Nursing Diagnoses
Impaired physical mobility (Indications)
Acute pain (Indications)

Implementation
- Administer a tuberculin skin test prior to administration of etanercept. Patients with active latent TB should be treated for TB prior to therapy.
- Needle cover of the pre-filled syringe contains latex and should not be handled by people with latex allergies.
- **Subcut:** Prepare injection with single dose pre-filled syringe or multi-dose vial for reconstitution.
- Solution in pre-filled syringe may be allowed to reach room temperature (15–30 min); do not remove needle cap during this time.
- For multi-dose vial, reconstitute with 1 mL of the bacteriostatic sterile water supplied by manufacturer for a concentration of 25 mg/mL. If the vial is used for multiple doses, use a 25–gauge needle for reconstituting and withdrawing solution and apply "Mixing Date" sticker with date of reconstitution entered. Inject diluent slowly into vial to avoid foaming. Some foaming will occur. Swirl gently for dissolution; do not shake or vigorously agitate to prevent excess foaming. Solution should be clear and colorless; do not administer solution that is discolored or contains particulate matter. Dissolution usually takes <10 min. Withdraw solution into syringe. Some foam may remain in

vial. Amount in syringe should approximate 1 mL. Do not filter reconstituted solution during preparation or administration. Attach a 27 gauge needle to inject. Administer as soon as possible after reconstitution; stable up to 6 hr if refrigerated. Solution and pre-filled syringes are stable if refrigerated and used within 14 days.
- May be injected into abdomen, thigh, or upper arm. Rotate sites. Do not administer within 1 inch of an old site or into area that is tender, red, hard, or bruised.
- **Syringe Incompatibility:** Do not mix with other solutions or dilute with other diluents.

Patient/Family Teaching
- Instruct patient on self-administration technique, storage, and disposal of equipment. First injection should be administered under the supervision of health care professional. Provide patient with a puncture-proof container for used equipment.
- Advise patient not to receive live vaccines during therapy. Parents should be advised that children should complete immunizations to date before initiation of etanercept. Patients with significant exposure to varicella virus (chickenpox) should temporarily discontinue therapy and varicella immune globulin should be considered.
- Advise patient that methotrexate, analgesics, NSAIDs, corticosteroids, and salicylates may be continued during therapy.
- Instruct patient to notify health care professional if upper respiratory or other infections occur. Therapy may need to be discontinued if serious infection occurs.

Evaluation/Desired Outcomes
- Reduction in symptoms of rheumatoid arthritis. Symptoms may return within 1 mo of discontinuation of therapy.

---

ethambutol (e-tham-byoo-tole)
✦ Etibi, Myambutol

Classification
Therapeutic: antituberculars

Pregnancy Category C

Indications
Active tuberculosis or other mycobacterial diseases (with at least one other drug).

Action
Inhibits the growth of mycobacteria. **Therapeutic Effects:** Tuberculostatic effect against susceptible organisms.

Pharmacokinetics
Absorption: Rapidly and well absorbed (80%) from the GI tract.
Distribution: Widely distributed; crosses blood-brain barrier in small amounts; crosses placenta and enters breast milk.
Metabolism and Excretion: 50% metabolized by the liver, 50% eliminated unchanged by the kidneys.
Half-life: 3.3 hr (increased in renal or hepatic impairment).

TIME/ACTION PROFILE (blood levels)

ROUTE	ONSET	PEAK	DURATION
PO	rapid	2–4 hr	24 hr

Contraindications/Precautions
Contraindicated in: Hypersensitivity; Optic neuritis.
Use Cautiously in: Renal and severe hepatic impairment (dosage reduction required); OB: Although safety not established, ethambutol has been used with isoniazid in pregnant women without fetal adverse effects; Lactation: Usually compatible with breastfeeding (AAP); Pedi: Safety not established in children <13 yr.

Adverse Reactions/Side Effects
CNS: confusion, dizziness, hallucinations, headache, malaise. **EENT:** optic neuritis. **GI:** HEPATITIS, abdominal pain, anorexia, nausea, vomiting. **Metab:** hyperuricemia. **MS:** joint pain. **Neuro:** peripheral neuritis. **Misc:** anaphylactoid reactions, fever.

Interactions
Drug-Drug: Neurotoxicity may be ↑ with other **neurotoxic agents**.

Route/Dosage
PO (Adults and Children >13 yr): 15–25 mg/kg/day (maximum 2.5 g/day) *or* 50 mg/kg (up to 2.5 g) twice weekly *or* 25–30 mg/kg (up to 2.5 g) 3 times weekly.

Availability (generic available)
Tablets: 100 mg, 400 mg.

NURSING IMPLICATIONS
Assessment
- Mycobacterial studies and susceptibility tests should be performed before and periodically during therapy to detect possible resistance.
- Assess lung sounds and character and amount of sputum periodically during therapy.
- Assessments of visual function should be made frequently during therapy. Advise patient to report blurring of vision, constriction of visual fields, or changes in color perception immediately. Visual impairment, if not identified early, may lead to permanent sight impairment.
- **Lab Test Considerations:** Monitor renal and hepatic functions, CBC, and uric acid levels routinely therapy. Frequently causes elevated uric acid concentrations, which may precipitate an attack of gout.

Potential Nursing Diagnoses
Risk for infection (Indications)
Disturbed sensory perception (Side Effects)

Implementation
- Ethambutol is given as a single daily dose and should be taken at the same time each day. Some regimens require dosing 2–3 times/week. Usually administered concurrently with other antitubercular medications to prevent development of bacterial resistance.
- **PO:** Administer with food or milk to minimize GI irritation.

Patient/Family Teaching
- Instruct patient to take medication as directed. Take missed doses as soon as possible unless almost time for next dose; do not double up on missed doses. A full course of therapy may take months to yr. Do not discontinue without consulting health care professional, even though symptoms may disappear.
- Advise patient to notify health care professional if pregnancy is suspected.
- Instruct patient to notify health care professional if no improvement is seen in 2–3 wk. Health care professional should also be notified if unexpected weight gain or decreased urine output occurs.
- Emphasize the importance of routine exams to evaluate progress and ophthalmic examinations if signs of optic neuritis occur.

Evaluation/Desired Outcomes
- Resolution of clinical symptoms of tuberculosis.
- Decrease in acid-fast bacteria in sputum samples.
- Improvement seen in chest x-rays. Therapy for tuberculosis is usually continued for at least 1–2 yr.

---

ethinyl estradiol/desogestrel, See CONTRACEPTIVES, HORMONAL.

---

ethinyl estradiol/drospirenone, See CONTRACEPTIVES, HORMONAL.

---

ethinyl estradiol/ethynodiol, See CONTRACEPTIVES, HORMONAL.

---

ethinyl estradiol/etonogestrel, See CONTRACEPTIVES, HORMONAL.

---

ethinyl estradiol/levonorgestrel, See CONTRACEPTIVES, HORMONAL.

---

ethinyl estradiol/norelgestromin, See CONTRACEPTIVES, HORMONAL.

---

ethinyl estradiol/norethindrone, See CONTRACEPTIVES, HORMONAL.

---

ethinyl estradiol/norgestimate, See CONTRACEPTIVES, HORMONAL.

---

ethinyl estradiol/norgestrel, See CONTRACEPTIVES, HORMONAL.

---

etidronate (eh-tih-**droe**-nate)
✦Didrocal, Didronel

Classification
Therapeutic: bone resorption inhibitors, hypocalcemics
Pharmacologic: biphosphonates

Pregnancy Category B (oral)

Indications
Treatment of Paget's disease of bone. Treatment and prophylaxis of heterotopic calcification associated with total hip replacement or spinal cord injury.

Action
Blocks the growth of calcium hydroxyapatite crystals by binding to calcium phosphate. **Therapeutic Effects:** Decreased bone resorption and turnover.

Pharmacokinetics
Absorption: Absorption is generally poor (1–6%) after oral administration.
Distribution: Half of the absorbed dose is bound to hydroxyapatite crystals in areas of increased osteogenesis.
Metabolism and Excretion: Unabsorbed drug is eliminated in the feces; 50% of the absorbed dose is excreted unchanged by the kidneys.
Half-life: 5–7 hr.

TIME/ACTION PROFILE

ROUTE	ONSET	PEAK	DURATION
PO (Paget's disease)	1 mo†	unknown	1 yr
PO (heterotopic calcification)	unknown	unknown	several months

†As measured by decreased urinary hydroxyproline

Contraindications/Precautions
Contraindicated in: Hypersensitivity; Overt osteomalacia.
Use Cautiously in: Hypocalcemia; Hypovitaminosis D; Renal impairment (dosage reduction may be needed); Dental surgery (may ↑ risk of jaw osteonecrosis); OB, Lactation, Pedi: Safety not established.

Adverse Reactions/Side Effects
GI: <u>diarrhea</u>, <u>nausea</u>, esophagitis, esophageal cancer, esophageal ulcer. **MS:** <u>musculoskeletal pain</u>, microfractures, osteonecrosis (primarily of jaw).

Interactions
Drug-Drug: Antacids, **mineral supplements**, or **buffers** (as in **didanosine**) containing **calcium**, **aluminum**, **iron**, or **magnesium** may ↓ absorption of etidronate. Hypocalcemic effect may be additive with **calcitonin**.
Drug-Food: Foods containing large amounts of **calcium**, **aluminum**, **iron**, or **magnesium** may ↓ absorption of etidronate.

Route/Dosage
Paget's Disease
PO (Adults): 5–10 mg/kg/day single dose for up to 6 mo *or* 11–20 mg/kg/day for not more than 3 mo.

Heterotopic Ossification (Hip Replacement)
PO (Adults): 20 mg/kg/day for 1 mo before and 3 mo after surgery.

Heterotopic Ossification (Spinal Cord Injury)
PO (Adults): 20 mg/kg/day for 2 wk, then decreased to 10 mg/kg/day for 10 wk.

Availability (generic available)
Tablets: 200 mg, 400 mg.

NURSING IMPLICATIONS
Assessment
- Assess patient for bone pain, weakness, or loss of function before and throughout therapy. Bone pain may persist or increase in patients with Paget's disease; usually subsides days to months after therapy is discontinued. Confer with health care professional regarding analgesic to control pain.
- **Heterotopic Ossification:** Monitor for inflammation and pain at the site and loss of function if ossification occurs near a joint.
- *Lab Test Considerations:* Etidronate interferes with bone uptake of technetium 99 in diagnostic scans.
- *Paget's disease:* ↓ urinary excretions of hydroxyproline and serum alkaline phosphatase are often the first clinical signs of effectiveness; monitor every 3 mo. Treatment is restarted when levels return to 75% of pretreatment values. Monitor serum phosphate levels before and 4 wk after beginning therapy. Dose may be reduced if serum phosphate is elevated without corresponding decrease in urinary excretion of hydroxyproline or serum alkaline phosphatase.

Potential Nursing Diagnoses
Acute pain (Indications, Side Effects)
Risk for injury (Indications)

Implementation
- Do not confuse etidronate with etomidate.
- **PO:** Administer on empty stomach, because food decreases absorption. Tablet should be swallowed whole; do not break, crush, or chew.

Patient/Family Teaching
- Advise patient to take as directed. Take missed doses as soon as remembered unless almost time for next dose. Do not double up on doses. Dose should not be taken within 2 hr of eating

(especially products high in calcium) or taking vitamins or antacids, because absorption will be impaired.
- Instruct patient to notify health care professional if diarrhea occurs. Health care professional may divide the dose throughout the day to control diarrhea.
- Encourage patients to comply with diet recommendations. Diet should contain adequate amounts of calcium and vitamin D (see Appendix M).
- Inform patient that severe musculoskeletal pain may occur within days, months, or yr after starting etidronate. Symptoms my resolve completely after discontinuation or slow or incomplete resolution may occur. Notify health care professional if severe pain occurs.
- Emphasize need for keeping follow-up appointments to monitor progress, even after medication is discontinued, to detect relapse.
- Advise patient to inform health care professional of etidronate therapy prior to dental surgery.

Evaluation/Desired Outcomes
- Decreased bone pain and fractures in Paget's disease.
- Prevention or treatment of heterotopic ossification. Normal serum calcium levels are usually attained in 2–8 days in hypercalcemia associated with bony metastasis. Therapy may be repeated once after 1 wk.

---

etodolac (ee-toe-doe-lak)
Lodine, Lodine XL

Classification
Therapeutic: antirheumatics, nonopioid analgesics
Pharmacologic: pyranocarboxylic acid

Pregnancy Category C

Indications
Osteoarthritis. Rheumatoid arthritis. Mild to moderate pain (not XL tablets).

Action
Inhibits prostaglandin synthesis. Also has uricosuric action. **Therapeutic Effects:** Suppression of inflammation. Decreased severity of pain.

Pharmacokinetics
Absorption: Well absorbed after oral administration.
Distribution: Widely distributed.
Protein Binding: >99%.

Metabolism and Excretion: Mostly metabolized by the liver; <1% excreted unchanged in urine.
Half-life: 6–7 hr (single dose); 7.3 hr (chronic dosing).

TIME/ACTION PROFILE (analgesic effect)

ROUTE	ONSET	PEAK	DURATION
PO (analgesic)	0.5 hr	1–2 hr	4–12 hr
PO (anti-inflammatory)	days–wk	unknown	6–12 hr†

†Up to 24 hr as XL (extended-release) tablet

Contraindications/Precautions
Contraindicated in: Hypersensitivity; Active GI bleeding or ulcer disease; Cross-sensitivity may exist with other NSAIDs, including aspirin; OB: Use during second half of pregnancy can result in premature closure of ductus arteriosis.
Use Cautiously in: Cardiovascular disease or risk factors for cardiovascular disease (may ↑ risk of serious cardiovascular thrombotic events, myocardial infarction, and stroke, especially with prolonged use) Renal or hepatic disease; History of ulcer disease; Lactation: Limited information available; use other safer NSAID; Pedi: Safety not established; Geri: Increased risk of GI bleeding.

Adverse Reactions/Side Effects
CNS: depression, dizziness, drowsiness, insomnia, malaise, nervousness, syncope, weakness. **EENT:** blurred vision, photophobia, tinnitus. **Resp:** asthma. **CV:** CHF, edema, hypertension, palpitations. **GI:** GI BLEEDING, dyspepsia, abdominal pain, constipation, diarrhea, drug-induced hepatitis, dry mouth, flatulence, gastritis, nausea, stomatitis, thirst, vomiting. **GU:** dysuria, renal failure, urinary frequency. **Derm:** EXFOLIATIVE DERMATITIS, STEVENS-JOHNSON SYNDROME, TOXIC EPIDERMAL NECROLYSIS, ecchymoses, flushing, hyperpigmentation, pruritus, rashes, sweating. **Hemat:** anemia, prolonged bleeding time, thrombocytopenia. **Misc:** allergic reactions including ANAPHYLAXIS, ANGIOEDEMA, chills, fever.

Interactions
Drug-Drug: Concurrent use with **aspirin** may ↓ effectiveness. ↑ adverse GI effects with **aspirin**, other **NSAIDs**, **potassium supplements**, **corticosteroids**, **antiplatelet agents**, or **alcohol**. Chronic use with **acetaminophen** may ↑ risk of adverse renal reactions. May ↓ effectiveness of **diuretic** or **antihypertensive** therapy. May ↑ serum **lithium** levels and ↑ risk of toxicity. ↑ risk of toxicity from **methotrexate**. ↑

risk of bleeding with **cefotetan**, **cefoperazone**, **valproic acid**, **thrombolytics**, **antiplatelet agents**, or **anticoagulants**. Increased risk of adverse hematologic reactions with **antineoplastics** or **radiation therapy**. May increase the risk of nephrotoxicity from **cyclosporine**.
Drug-Natural Products: ↑ risk of bleeding with **arnica**, **chamomile**, **clove**, **dong quai**, **fever few**, **garlic**, **ginko**, and **Panax ginseng**.

Route/Dosage
PO (Adults): *Analgesia*—200–400 mg q 6–8 hr (not to exceed 1200 mg/day). *Osteoarthritis/rheumatoid arthritis*—300 mg 2–3 times daily, 400 mg twice daily, or 500 mg twice daily; may also be given as 400–1200 mg once daily as XL tablets.

Availability (generic available)
Capsules: 200 mg, 300 mg. **Tablets:** 400 mg, 500 mg. **Extended-release tablets (XL):** 400 mg, 600 mg.

NURSING IMPLICATIONS
Assessment
- Patients who have asthma, aspirin-induced allergy, and nasal polyps are at increased risk for developing hypersensitivity reactions. Monitor for rhinitis, asthma, and urticaria.
- **Osteoarthritis/Rheumatoid Arthritis:** Assess pain and range of movement before and 1–2 hr after administration.
- **Pain:** Assess location, duration, and intensity of the pain before and 60 min after administration.
- *Lab Test Considerations:* May cause ↓ hemoglobin, hematocrit, leukocyte, and platelet counts.
- Monitor liver function tests within 8 wk of initiating etodolac therapy and periodically during therapy. May cause ↑ serum alkaline phosphatase, LDH, AST, and ALT concentrations.
- Monitor BUN, serum creatinine, and electrolytes periodically during therapy. May cause ↑ BUN, serum creatinine, and electrolyte concentrations and ↓ urine electrolyte concentrations.
- May cause ↓ serum and ↑ urine uric acid concentrations.

Potential Nursing Diagnoses
Acute pain (Indications)
Impaired physical mobility (Indications)

Implementation
- Do not confuse Lodine (etodolac) with codeine or iodine.
- Administration in higher-than-recommended doses does not provide increased effectiveness but may cause increased side effects.
- Use lowest effective dose for shortest period of time.
- **PO:** For rapid initial effect, administer 30 min before or 2 hr after meals. May be administered with food, milk, or antacids containing aluminum or magnesium to decrease GI irritation.
- Do not break, crush, or chew extended-release tablets.

Patient/Family Teaching
- Advise patients to take etodolac with a full glass of water and to remain in an upright position for 15–30 min after administration.
- Instruct patient to take medication as directed. Take missed doses as soon as possible within 1–2 hr if taking twice/day, or unless almost time for next dose if taking more than twice/day. Do not double doses.
- Etodolac may occasionally cause drowsiness or dizziness. Advise patient to avoid driving or other activities requiring alertness until response to the medication is known.
- Caution patient to avoid the concurrent use of alcohol, aspirin, acetaminophen, NSAIDs, or other OTC medications without consultation with health care professional.
- Advise patient to inform health care professional of medication regimen before treatment or surgery.
- Advise patient to consult health care professional if rash, itching, visual disturbances, tinnitus, weight gain, edema, black stools, persistent headache, or influenza-like syndrome (chills, fever, muscle aches, pain) occurs.

Evaluation/Desired Outcomes
- Decreased severity of pain.
- Improved joint mobility. Patients who do not respond to one NSAID may respond to another. May require 2 wk or more for maximum anti-inflammatory effects.

---

etonorgestrel, See **CONTRACEPTIVES, HORMONAL.**

ETOPOSIDES (e-toe-poe-sides)

HIGH ALERT

etoposide
VePesid, VP-16

etoposide phosphate
Etopophos

Classification
Therapeutic: antineoplastics
Pharmacologic: podophyllotoxin derivatives

Pregnancy Category D

Indications
Refractory testicular neoplasms (used in combination with other chemotherapeutic agents in patients who have already received chemotherapy, surgery, or radiation) (IV only). Small cell lung carcinoma (first-line therapy, used in combination with other chemotherapeutic agents) (oral and IV). **Unlabeled Use:** Lymphomas and some leukemias. Uterine cancer. Brain tumors.

Action
Damages DNA before mitosis (cycle-dependent and phase-specific). **Therapeutic Effects:** Death of rapidly replicating cells, particularly malignant ones.

Pharmacokinetics
Absorption: Variably absorbed after oral administration. After IV administration, etoposide phosphate is rapidly converted to etoposide.
Distribution: Rapidly distributed, poorly enters the CSF; probably crosses placenta; enters breast milk.
Protein Binding: 97%.
Metabolism and Excretion: Some metabolism by the liver with biliary excretion, 44% excreted in feces; 45% excreted unchanged by the kidneys.
Half-life: 4–11 hr.

TIME/ACTION PROFILE (noted as effects on blood counts)

ROUTE	ONSET	PEAK	DURATION
Etoposide PO	unknown	7–14 days (granulocytes); 9–16 days (platelets)	20 days
Etoposide IV	7–14 days	7–14 days granulocytes; 9–16 days (platelets)	20 days
Etoposide phosphate IV	Unknown	12–19 days (granulocytes); 10–15 days (platelets)	21 days

Contraindications/Precautions
Contraindicated in: Hypersensitivity; Known intolerance to benzyl alcohol, polysorbate 80, polyethylene glycol (IV etoposide only), or dextran (IV etoposide phosphate only); OB: Teratogenic in animal studies; Lactation: Antineoplastic therapy can cause adverse effects in the breastfed infant.
Use Cautiously in: Patients with childbearing potential; Active infections; Decreased bone marrow reserve; Hypoalbuminemia; Renal/hepatic impairment (dosage modification may be necessary); Other chronic debilitating illnesses; OB: Women of childbearing age should use two forms of contraception; Pedi: Safety and effectiveness not established; Geri: ↑ risk for adverse effects.

Adverse Reactions/Side Effects
CNS: dizziness, drowsiness, fatigue. **CV:** hypotension (IV). **GI:** anorexia, diarrhea, nausea, vomiting, abdominal pain, stomatitis, taste alteration. **Derm:** alopecia, pruritus, rashes, urticaria. **Endo:** sterility. **Hemat:** anemia, leukopenia, thrombocytopenia. **Local:** phlebitis at IV site. **Neuro:** peripheral neuropathy. **Misc:** allergic reactions including ANAPHYLAXIS, fever.

Interactions
Drug-Drug: ↑ bone marrow depression with other **antineoplastics** or **radiation therapy**. May alter immune response to **live-virus vaccines** and ↑ risk of adverse reactions.

Route/Dosage
Other regimens are used. Dosages below are expressed as the desired etoposide dosage.

Testicular Neoplasms
IV (Adults): Dosage ranges from 50–100 mg/m² daily for 5 days to 100 mg/m² on days 1, 3, and 5; repeat at 3–4 wk intervals.

Small-Cell Carcinoma of the Lung
PO (Adults): Dosage ranges from 70 mg/m² (rounded to the nearest 50 mg) daily for 4 days to 100 mg/m² (rounded to the nearest 50 mg) daily for 5 days; repeat at 3–4 wk intervals.
IV (Adults): Dosages range from 35 mg/m² daily for 4 days to 50 mg/m² daily for 5 days; repeat at 3–4 wk intervals.

Availability

Etoposide (generic available)
Capsules: 50 mg. **Injection:** 20 mg/mL.

Etoposide Phosphate
Powder for injection: 100 mg/vial (with dextran).

NURSING IMPLICATIONS
Assessment
- Monitor blood pressure before and every 15 min during infusion. If hypotension occurs, stop infusion and notify physician or other health care professional. After stabilizing blood pressure with IV fluids and supportive measures, infusion may be resumed at slower rate.
- Monitor for hypersensitivity reaction (fever, chills, dyspnea, pruritus, urticaria, bronchospasm, tachycardia, hypotension). If these occur, stop infusion and notify physician. Keep epinephrine, an antihistamine, corticosteroids, volume expanders, and resuscitative equipment close by in the event of an anaphylactic reaction.
- Assess for signs of infection (fever, chills, cough, hoarseness, lower back or side pain, sore throat, difficult or painful urination). Notify physician if these symptoms occur.
- Assess for bleeding (bleeding gums, bruising, petechiae, guaiac test stools, urine, and emesis). Avoid IM injections and taking rectal temperatures. Apply pressure to venipuncture sites for 10 min.
- Monitor intake and output, appetite, and nutritional intake. Etoposide causes mild-to-moderate nausea and vomiting. Prophylactic antiemetics may ↓ frequency and duration of nausea and vomiting.
- Adjust diet as tolerated to help maintain fluid and electrolyte balance and nutritional status.
- **Lab Test Considerations:** Monitor CBC and differential before and periodically during therapy. The nadir of leukopenia occurs in 7–14 days (etoposide) or 12–19 days (etoposide phosphate). Notify physician if leukocyte count is <1000/mm³. The nadir of thrombocytopenia occurs in 9–16 days. Notify physician if the platelet count is <75,000/mm³. Recovery of leukopenia and thrombocytopenia occurs in 20 days.
- Monitor liver function studies (AST, ALT, LDH, bilirubin) and renal function studies (BUN, creatinine) before and periodically during therapy to detect hepatotoxicity and nephrotoxicity.

Potential Nursing Diagnoses
Risk for injury (Side Effects)
Risk for infection (Side Effects)

Implementation
- **High Alert:** Fatalities have occurred with incorrect administration of chemotherapeutic agents. Before administering, clarify all ambiguous orders; double check single, daily, and course-of-therapy dose limits; have second practitioner independently double check original order, calculations, and infusion pump settings. Do not confuse VePesid (etoposide) with Versed (midazolam). Do not confuse etoposide (VePesid) with etoposide phosphate (Etopophos).
- Solution should be prepared in a biologic cabinet. Wear gloves, gown, and mask while handling medication. Discard equipment in designated containers.
- Avoid contact with skin. Use Luer-Lok tubing to prevent accidental leakage. If contact with skin occurs, immediately wash skin with soap and water.
- **PO:** Capsules should be refrigerated. Capsules are stable for 24 mo when refrigerated.

Etoposide (VePesid)
IV Administration
- **Intermittent Infusion: *Diluent:*** Dilute 5-mL vial with D5W or 0.9% NaCl. ***Concentration:*** 200–400 mcg/mL. The 200-mcg/mL solution is stable for 96 hr. The 400-mcg/mL solution is stable for 48 hr. Concentrations >400 mcg/mL are not recommended, because crystallization is likely. Discard solution if crystals are present. ***Rate:*** Infuse slowly over 30–60 min. Temporary hypotension may occur with infusion rates shorter than 30 min.
- **Y-Site Compatibility:** allopurinol, amifostine, aztreonam, cladribine, doxorubicin liposome, fludarabine, gemcitabine, granisetron, melphalan, methotrexate, mitoxandrone, ondansetron, paclitaxel, piperacillin/tazobactam, sargramostim, sodium bicarbonate, teniposide, thiotepa, topotecan, vinorelbine.
- **Y-Site Incompatibility:** cefepime, filgrastim, idarubicin.
- **Additive Compatibility:** carboplatin, cisplatin, cytarabine, floxuridine, fluorouracil, ifosfamide, mitoxantrone, ondansetron.

✤ = Canadian drug name.   ♊ = Genetic implication.
*CAPITALS indicates life-threatening; underlines indicate most frequent.

Etoposide phosphate (Etopophos)

IV Administration

- **Intermittent Infusion:** Reconstitute each vial with 5 or 10 mL of sterile water, D5W, or 0.9% NaCl for a concentration of 20 or 10 mg/mL, respectively.
- **Diluent:** May be administered undiluted or diluted with D5W or 0.9% NaCl. **Concentration:** Undiluted: 10–20 mg/mL; Diluted: as low as 0.1 mg/mL, Reconstituted solutions are stable for 24 hr at room temperature or if refrigerated. **Rate:** Administer over 5–210 min.
- **Y-Site Compatibility:** acyclovir, amikacin, aminophylline, ampcillin, ampicillin/sulbactam, aztreonam, bleomycin, bumetanide, buprenorphine, butorphanol, calcium gluconate, carboplatin, carmustine, cefazolin, cefotaxime, cefotetan, cefoxitin, ceftazidime, ceftizoxime, ceftriaxone, cefuroxime, cimetidine, ciprofloxacin, cisplatin, clindamycin, cyclophosphamide, cytarabine, dacarbazine, dactinomycin, daunorubicin, dexamethasone sodium phosphate, diphenhydramine, dobutamine, dopamine, doxorubicin, doxycycline, droperidol, enalaprilat, famotidine, floxuridine, fluconazole, fludarabine, fluorouracil, furosemide, ganciclovir, gemcitabine, gentamicin, granisetron, haloperidol, heparin, hydrocortisone, hydromorphone, idarubicin, ifosfamide, leucovorin calcium, linezolid, lorazepam, magnesium sulfate, mannitol, meperidine, mesna, methotrexate, metoclopramide, metronidazole, mitoxantrone, morphine, nalbuphine, ofloxacin, ondansetron, oxaliplatin, paclitaxel, piperacillin, piperacillin/tazobactam, potassium chloride, promethazine, ranitidine, sodium bicarbonate, streptozocin, teniposide, thiotepa, ticarcillin/clavulanate, tobramycin, trimethoprim/sulfamethoxazole, vancomycin, vinblastine, vincristine, zidovudine.
- **Y-Site Incompatibility:** amphotericin B, cefepime, chlorpromazine, imipenem/cilastatin, lansoprazole, methylprednisolone, mitomycin, prochlorperazine.

Patient/Family Teaching

- Instruct patient to take etoposide exactly as directed, even if nausea or vomiting occurs. If vomiting occurs shortly after dose is taken, consult physician. If a dose is missed, do not take at all.
- Advise patient to notify health care professional if fever; chills; sore throat or other signs of infection; bleeding gums; bruising; petechiae; or blood in urine, stool, or emesis occurs. Caution patient to avoid crowds and persons with known infections. Instruct patient to use soft toothbrush and electric razor. Caution patient not to drink alcoholic beverages or take products containing aspirin or NSAIDs.
- Instruct patient to notify health care professional if rapid heartbeat, difficulty breathing, abdominal pain, yellow skin, weakness, paresthesia, or gait disturbances occur.
- Instruct patient to inspect oral mucosa for redness and ulceration. If mouth sores occur, advise patient to use sponge brush and rinse mouth with water after eating and drinking. Viscous lidocaine swishes may be used if pain interferes with eating. Stomatitis pain may require treatment with opioid analgesics.
- Discuss with patient the possibility of hair loss. Explore coping strategies.
- Advise patient to use contraception.
- Instruct patient not to receive any vaccinations without advice of physician.
- Emphasize the need for periodic lab tests to monitor for side effects.

Evaluation/Desired Outcomes

- Decrease in size or spread of testicular or small cell lung cancer.

---

etravirine (e-tra-veer-een)
Intelence

Classification
Therapeutic: antiretrovirals
Pharmacologic: non-nucleoside reverse transcriptase inhibitors

Pregnancy Category B

Indications
HIV infection (with other antiretrovirals).

Action
Binds to the enzyme reverse transcriptase, which results in disrupted viral DNA synthesis. **Therapeutic Effects:** Evidence of decreased viral replication and reduced viral load with slowed progression of HIV and its sequelae.

Pharmacokinetics
Absorption: Well absorbed following oral administration. Food enhances absorption.
Distribution: Unknown.
Protein Binding: 99.9%.
Metabolism and Excretion: Mostly metabolized by the liver (CYP3A4, CYP2C9, and CYP2C19 enzyme systems); minimal renal excretion; mostly eliminated in feces as unchanged drug and metabolites.

etravirine

Half-life: 41 hr.

TIME/ACTION PROFILE (blood levels)

ROUTE	ONSET	PEAK	DURATION
PO	unknown	2.5–4 hr	12 hr

Contraindications/Precautions
Contraindicated in: Concurrent use with other non-nucleoside reverse transcriptase inhibitors (NNRTIs), rifampin, rifapentine, St. John's wort.
Use Cautiously in: Concurrent use of antiarrhythmics, anticonvulsants, antifungals, clarithromycin, rifabutin, diazepam, dexamethasone, HMG CoA reductase inhibitors (statins), immunosuppressants; **Geri:** Consider age-related ↓ in organ function and body mass, concurrent disease states and medications; **Pedi, OB, Lactation:** Safety not established, breast-feeding not recommended in HIV-infected women.

Adverse Reactions/Side Effects
CNS: SEIZURES, anxiety, confusion, fatigue, headache, insomnia, sleep disorders. **EENT:** blurred vision, vertigo. **CV:** MYOCARDIAL INFARCTION, angina pectoris, atrial fibrillation, hypertension. **GI:** HEPATIC FAILURE, nausea, abdominal pain, anorexia, dry mouth, hepatitis, stomatitis, vomiting. **GU:** renal failure. **Endo:** gynecomastia, hyperglycemia, hyperlipidemia. **Hemat:** anemia, hemolytic anemia. **Derm:** ERYTHEMA MULTIFORME, STEVENS JOHNSON SYNDROME, TOXIC EPIDERMAL NECROLYSIS, rash. **Metab:** fat redistribution. **Neuro:** peripheral neuropathy. **MS:** hemarthrosis. **Misc:** allergic reactions including, IMMUNE RECONSTITUTION SYNDROME.

Interactions
Drug-Drug: Etravirine is a substrate of the **CYP3A4**, **CYP2C9**, and **CYP2C19** enzyme systems; other medications that induce or inhibit these systems may be expected to alter the response to etravirine. Etravirine is an inducer of **CYP3A4** and an inhibitor of **CYP2C9** and **CYP2C19**. The effects of medications that are substrates of these enzyme systems may be altered by concurrent use. Concurrent use with other **NNRTIs** including **efavirenz**, **nevirapine**, and **delavirdine** may lead to ↓ effectiveness and should be avoided. Concurrent use with **protease inhibitors (PIs)** including **atazanavir, fosamprenavir, nelfinavir,** and **indinavir** may lead to altered plasma levels and should be undertaken with concurrent low dose **ritonavir**. Concurrent use with higher dose **ritonavir**, combination **tipranavir/ritonavir, fosamprenavir/ritonavir, atazanavir/ritonavir** alter levels and effectiveness of etravirine and should be avoided. Concurrent use of the combination **saquinavir/ritonavir** should be undertake cautiously. ↓ blood levels and effectiveness of **antiarrhythmics** including **amiodarone, bepridil, disopyramide, flecainide, lidocaine, mexiletine, quinidine, propafenone,** and **quinidine**; blood level monitoring recommended. Blood levels and effects may be ↓ by anticonvulsants including **carbamazepine, phenobarbital,** and **phenytoin**. Concurrent use with **voriconazole** may ↑ levels of both drugs; ↓ levels of **itraconazole** and **ketoconazole** (dose adjustments may be necessary). May alter levels and response to **clarithromycin**; other agents should be considered. **Rifampin** and **rifapentine** ↓ blood levels and effectiveness and should be avoided; **rifabutin** should only be used without a protease inhibitor/ritonavir combination. May ↑ blood levels and sedation from **diazepam**, monitor for effects. Levels and effectiveness may be ↓ by **dexamethasone** use cautiously and consider alternatives. May alter blood levels and effects of **fluvastatin, lovastatin,** and **simvastatin** (dose adjustments may be necessary. May alter blood levels and effects of **cyclosporine, sirolimus,** and **tacrolimus**; careful monitoring required.
Drug-Natural Products: St. John's wort may ↓ blood levels and effectiveness; avoid concurrent use.

Route/Dosage
PO (Adults): 200 mg twice daily.

Availability
Tablets: 100 mg.

NURSING IMPLICATIONS

Assessment
- Assess for change in severity of HIV symptoms and for symptoms of opportunistic infections during therapy.
- Assess patient for rash (mild to moderate rash usually occurs in the 2nd wk of therapy and resolves within 1–2 wk of continued therapy). If rash is severe (extensive erythematous or maculopapular rash with moist desquamation or angioedema) or accompanied by systemic symptoms (serum sickness-like reaction, Stevens-Johnson syndrome, toxic epidermal necrolysis), therapy must be discontinued immediately.

550   exenatide

- ***Lab Test Considerations:*** Monitor viral load and CD4 cell count regularly during therapy.
- Monitor liver function tests periodically during therapy. May cause ↑ serum AST, ALT concentrations.
- May cause ↑ pancreatic amylase and lipase.
- May cause ↑ in total cholesterol, low density lipoprotein, serum triglyceride, and glucose levels.
- May cause ↑ serum creatinine.
- May cause ↓ neutrophils, ↓ platelet count, anemia and hemolytic anemia.

Potential Nursing Diagnoses
Risk for infection (Indications)
Noncompliance (Patient/Family Teaching)

Implementation
- **PO:** Administer 2 tablets twice daily following a meal; type of food does not matter. Swallow tablet whole, do not break, crush, or chew. If patient has difficulty swallowing, may disperse tablet in a glass of water. Once dispersed, patient should stir well and drink immediately; rinse glass with water and drink several times to ensure entire dose is consumed.

Patient/Family Teaching
- Emphasize the importance of taking etravirine as directed, at the same time each day. It must always be used in combination with other antiretroviral drugs. Do not take more than prescribed amount and do not stop taking without consulting health care professional. Take missed doses following a meal if remembered within 6 hr of the time its usually taken, then return to regular schedule. If more than 6 hr from time dose is usually taken, omit dose and resume dosing schedule; do not double doses.
- Instruct patient that etravirine should not be shared with others.
- Inform patient that etravirine does not cure AIDS or prevent associated or opportunistic infections. Etravirine does not reduce the risk of transmission of HIV to others through sexual contact or blood contamination. Caution patient to use a condom and to avoid sharing needles or donating blood to prevent spreading the AIDS virus to others. Advise patient that the long-term effects of etravirine are unknown at this time.
- May cause dizziness, impaired concentration, or drowsiness. Caution patient to avoid driving or other activities requiring alertness until response to medication is known.
- Instruct patient to notify health care professional immediately if rash, signs of hypersensitivity (fever, generally ill feeling, extreme tiredness, muscle or joint aches, blisters, oral lesions, eye inflammation, facial swelling), signs and symptoms of liver problems (yellowing of skin or whites of eyes, dark or tea colored urine, pale colored stools/bowel movements, nausea, vomiting, loss of appetite, or pain, aching or sensitivity on right side below ribs), or signs of Immune Reconstitution Syndrome (signs and symptoms of an infection) occur.
- Advise patient to avoid taking other Rx, OTC, vitamins, or herbal products, especially St. John's wort, without consulting health care professional.
- Inform patient that changes in body fat (increased fat in upper back and neck, breast, and around back, chest, and stomach area, loss of fat from legs, arms, and face) may occur.
- Advise patients taking oral contraceptives to use a nonhormonal method of birth control during etravirine therapy and to notify health care professional if they become pregnant or plan to breastfeed while taking etravirine.
- Emphasize the importance of regular follow-up exams and blood counts to determine progress and monitor for side effects.

Evaluation/Desired Outcomes
- Delayed progression of AIDS and decreased opportunistic infections in patients with HIV.
- Decrease in viral load and increase in CD4 cell counts.

---

exenatide (ex-en-a-tide)
Byetta

Classification
Therapeutic: antidiabetics
Pharmacologic: incretin mimetic agents

Pregnancy Category C

Indications
Type 2 diabetes uncontrolled by metformin, a sulfonylurea, or a thiazolidinedione (or a combination of these agents).

Action
Mimics the action of incretin which promotes endogenous insulin secretion and promotes other mechanisms of glucose-lowering. **Therapeutic Effects:** Improved control of blood glucose.

Pharmacokinetics
Absorption: Well absorbed following subcutaneous administration.

Distribution: Unknown.
Metabolism and Excretion: Excreted mostly by glomerular filtration followed by degradation.
Half-life: 2.4 hr.

TIME/ACTION PROFILE (effects on postprandial blood glucose)

ROUTE	ONSET	PEAK	DURATION
subcut	within 30 min	2.1 hr	8 hr

Contraindications/Precautions
Contraindicated in: Hypersensitivity; Type 1 diabetes or diabetic ketoacidosis; End-stage renal disease (CCr <30 mL/min); Severe gastrointestinal disease; OB: Has caused fetal physical defects and neonatal death in animal studies; Lactation: Excretion into breast milk unknown.
Use Cautiously in: Pedi: Safety not established.

Adverse Reactions/Side Effects
CV: dizziness, headache, jitteriness, weakness. **GI:** PANCREATITIS, diarrhea, nausea, vomiting, dyspepsia, gastrointestinal reflux. **Derm:** hyperhydrosis. **Metab:** ↓ appetite, weight loss.

Interactions
Drug-Drug: Concurrent use with **sulfonlyureas** may ↑ risk of hypoglycemia (↓ dose of **sulfonylurea** if hypoglycemia occurs). Due to slowed gastric emptying, may decrease absorption of **orally administered medications**, especially those requiring rapid GI absorption or require a specific level for efficacy (**anti-infectives**, **oral contraceptives**).

Route/Dosage
Subcut (Adults): 5 mcg within 60 min before morning and evening meal; after 1 month, dose may be increased to 10 mcg depending on response.

Availability
Solution for subcutaneous injection: 250 mcg/mL in prefilled pen-injector that delivers either 5 mcg/dose (1.2-mL pen) or 10 mcg/dose (2.4-mL pen) for 60 doses (30 days of twice daily dosing). **Cost:** $200.98/1.2-mL pen, $225.99/2.4-mL pen.

NURSING IMPLICATIONS

Assessment
- Observe for signs and symptoms of hypoglycemic reactions (abdominal pain, sweating, hunger, weakness, dizziness, headache, drowsiness, tremor, tachycardia, anxiety, confusion, irritability, jitteriness), especially when combined with oral sulfonylureas.
- *Lab Test Considerations:* Monitor serum glucose and glycosylated hemoglobin periodically during therapy to evaluate effectiveness of therapy.

Potential Nursing Diagnoses
Imbalanced nutrition: more than body requirements (Indications)
Noncompliance (Patient/Family Teaching)

Implementation
- Some medications may need to be taken 1 hr before exenatide.
- Patients stabilized on a diabetic regimen who are exposed to stress, fever, trauma, infection, or surgery may require administration of insulin.
- **Subcut:** Follow directions for *New Pen Setup* in *Information for Patient* prior to use of each new pen. Administer exenatide in thigh, abdomen, or upper arm at any time within the 60–min period **before** the morning and evening meals. Do not administer after a meal. Solution should be clear and colorless; do not administer solutions that are discolored or contain particulate matter. Refrigerate; discard pen 30 days after 1st use, even if some drug remains in pen. Do not freeze. Do not store pen with needle attached; medication may leak from pen or air bubbles may form in the cartridge.

Patient/Family Teaching
- Instruct patient to take exenatide as directed within 60 min before a meal. Do not take after a meal. If a dose is missed, skip the dose and take the next dose at the prescribed time. Do not take an extra dose or increase the amount of the next dose to make up for missed dose.
- Instruct patient in proper technique for administration, timing of dose and concurrent oral medications, storage of medication and disposal of used needles. Patients should read the *Information for Patient* insert prior to initiation of therapy and with each Rx refill. Advise patient that *New Pen Setup* should be done only with each new pen, not with each dose.
- Inform patient that pen needles are not included with pen and must be purchased separately. Advise patient which needle length and gauge should be used. Caution patient not to share pen and needles.

- Explain to patient that exenatide helps control hyperglycemia but does not cure diabetes. Therapy is usually long term.
- Encourage patient to follow prescribed diet, medication, and exercise regimen to prevent hyperglycemic or hypoglycemic episodes.
- Review signs of hypoglycemia and hyperglycemia with patient. If hypoglycemia occurs, advise patient to take a glass of orange juice or 2–3 tsp of sugar, honey, or corn syrup dissolved in water, and notify health care professional. Risk of hypoglycemia is increased if sulfonureas are taken concurrently with exenatide.
- Advise patient to notify health care professional immediately if symptoms of pancreatitis (unexplained, persistent, severe abdominal pain which may or may not be accompanied by vomiting) occur.
- Inform patient that therapy may result in reduction of appetite, food intake, and/or body weight. Dose modification is not necessary. Nausea is more common at initiation of therapy and usually decreases over time.
- Advise patient to notify health care professional before taking any Rx, OTC, and herbal products. Exenatide delays stomach emptying. Some medications (such as anti-infectives and oral contraceptives) may need to be taken 1 hr before exenatide injection.
- Instruct patient in proper testing of blood glucose and urine ketones. These tests should be monitored closely during periods of stress or illness and health care professional notified if significant changes occur.
- Advise patient to notify health care professional if pregnancy is suspected or planned.
- Advise patient to inform health care professional of medication regimen before treatment or surgery.
- Advise patient to carry a form of sugar (sugar packets, candy) and identification describing disease process and medication regimen at all times.
- Emphasize the importance of routine follow-up exams and regular testing of blood glucose and glycosylated hemoglobin.

Evaluation/Desired Outcomes
- Control of blood glucose levels without the appearance of hypoglycemic or hyperglycemic episodes.

---

ezetimibe (e-zet-i-mibe)
★ Ezetrol, Zetia

Classification
Therapeutic: lipid-lowering agents
Pharmacologic: cholesterol absorption inhibitors

Pregnancy Category C

Indications
Alone or with other agents (HMG-CoA reductase inhibitors) in the management of dyslipidemias including primary hypercholesterolemia, homozygous familial hypercholesterolemia and homozygous sitosterolemia.

Action
Inhibits absorption of cholesterol in the small intestine. **Therapeutic Effects:** Lowering of cholesterol, a known risk factor for atherosclerosis.

Pharmacokinetics
Absorption: Following absorption, rapidly converted to ezetimibe-glucaronide, which is active. Bioavailability is variable.
Distribution: Unknown.
Metabolism and Excretion: Undergoes enterohepatic recycling, mostly eliminated in feces, minimal renal excretion.
Half-life: 22 hr.

TIME/ACTION PROFILE

ROUTE	ONSET	PEAK	DURATION
PO	unknown	unknown	unknown

Contraindications/Precautions
Contraindicated in: Hypersensitivity; Acute liver disease or unexplained laboratory evidence of liver disease (when used with HMG-CoA reductase inhibitor); Moderate or severe hepatic insufficiency; Concurrent use of fibrates; OB: May cause fetal harm by interfering with cholesterol synthesis and, possibly, biologically active substances derived from cholesterol; Potential for adverse effects in nursing infant.
Use Cautiously in: Pedi: Safety not established in children <10 yr.

Adverse Reactions/Side Effects
GI: cholecystitis, cholelithiasis, ↑ hepatic transaminases (with HMG-CoA reductase inhibitors), nausea, pancreatitis. **Derm:** rash. **Misc:** ANGIOEDEMA.

Interactions
Drug-Drug: Effects may be ↓ by **cholestyramine** or other **bile acid sequestrants**. Concurrent use of **fibrates** may ↑ blood levels of ezetimibe and also ↑ the risk of cholelithiasis. **Cyclosporine** may ↑ ezetimibe levels. May ↑

risk of rhabdomyolysis when used with **HMG CoA-reductase inhibitors**.

Route/Dosage
PO (Adults): 10 mg once daily.

Availability
Tablets: 10 mg. **Cost:** $265.98/90. *In combination with:* simvastatin (Vytorin); see Appendix B.

NURSING IMPLICATIONS

Assessment
- Obtain a diet history, especially with regard to fat consumption.
- *Lab Test Considerations:* Evaluate serum cholesterol and triglyceride levels before initiating, after 2–4 wk of therapy, and periodically thereafter.
- May cause ↑ liver transaminases when administered with HMG-CoA reductase inhibitors. Monitor liver enzymes prior to initiation and during therapy according to recommendations of HMG-CoA reductase inhibitor. Elevations are usually asymptomatic and return to baseline with continued therapy.

Potential Nursing Diagnoses
Noncompliance, related to diet and medication regimen (Patient/Family Teaching)

Implementation
- **PO:** Administer without regard to meals. May be taken at the same time as HMG-CoA reductase inhibitors.

Patient/Family Teaching
- Instruct patient to take medication as directed, at the same time each day, even if feeling well. Take missed doses as soon as remembered, but do not take more than 1 dose/day. Medication helps control but does not cure elevated serum cholesterol levels.
- Advise patient that this medication should be used in conjunction with diet restrictions (fat, cholesterol, carbohydrates, alcohol), exercise, and cessation of smoking. Ezetimibe does not assist with weight loss.
- Instruct female patients to notify health care professional promptly if pregnancy is planned or suspected or if breast feeding. If regimen includes HMG-CoA reductase inhibitors, they are contraindicated in pregnancy.
- Instruct patient to notify health care professional if unexplained muscle pain, tenderness, or weakness occur. Risk may increase when used with HMG CoA reductase inhibitors.
- Advise patient to avoid taking OTC medications or natural/herbal products without consulting health care professional.
- Advise patient to notify health care professional of medication regimen prior to treatment or surgery.
- Emphasize the importance of follow-up exams to determine effectiveness and to monitor for side effects.

Evaluation/Desired Outcomes
- Decrease in serum LDL and total cholesterol levels.
- Increase in HDL cholesterol levels.

famciclovir (fam-**sye**-kloe-veer)
Famvir

Classification
Therapeutic: antivirals

Pregnancy Category B

Indications
Acute herpes zoster infections (shingles). Treatment/suppression of recurrent herpes genitalis in immunocompetent patients. Treatment of recurrent herpes labialis (cold sores) in immunocompetent patients. Treatment of recurrent mucocutaneous herpes simplex virus (HSV) infection in HIV-infected patients.

Action
Inhibits viral DNA synthesis in herpes-infected cells only. **Therapeutic Effects:** Decreased duration of herpes zoster infection with decreased duration of viral shedding. Decreased time to healing for cold sores. Decreased lesion formation and improved healing in recurrent HSV infection.

Pharmacokinetics
Absorption: Following absorption, famciclovir is rapidly converted in the intestinal wall to penciclovir, the active compound.
Distribution: Unknown.
Metabolism and Excretion: Penciclovir is mostly excreted by the kidneys.
Half-life: *Penciclovir*—2.1–3 hr (↑ in renal impairment).

TIME/ACTION PROFILE (penciclovir blood levels)

ROUTE	ONSET	PEAK	DURATION
PO	rapid	0.9 hr	8–12 hr

Contraindications/Precautions
Contraindicated in: Hypersensitivity.
Use Cautiously in: Patients with impaired renal function (↑ dose interval/↓ dose recommended if CCr <40–60 mL/min); OB, Lactation: Limited information; use only if maternal benefit clearly outweighs potential risks to fetus or infant; Pedi: Safety not established in children <18 yr; Geri: Consider age-related ↓ in renal function when prescribing.

Adverse Reactions/Side Effects
CNS: headache, dizziness, fatigue. **GI:** diarrhea, nausea, vomiting.

Interactions
Drug-Drug: Probenecid ↑ plasma concentrations of penciclovir.

Route/Dosage

Herpes Zoster
PO (Adults): 500 mg q 8 hr for 7 days.

Renal Impairment
PO (Adults): *CCr 40–59 mL/min*—500 mg q 12 hr; *CCr 20–39mL/min*—500 mg q 24 hr; *CCr <20 mL/min*—250 mg q 24 hr; *Hemodialysis*—250 mg after each dialysis.

Recurrent Genital Herpes Simplex Infections
PO (Adults): 1000 mg twice daily for one day.

Renal Impairment
PO (Adults): *CCr 40–59 mL/min*—500 mg twice daily for 1 day; *CCr 20–39 mL/min*—500 mg as a single dose; *CCr <20 mL/min*—250 mg as a single dose; *Hemodialysis*—250 mg as a single dose after dialysis.

Suppression of Recurrent Herpes Simplex Infections
PO (Adults): 250 mg q 12 hr for up to 1 yr.

Renal Impairment
PO (Adults): *CCr 20–39 mL/min*—125 mg q 12 hr for 5 days; *CCr <20 mL/min*—125 mg q 24 hr for 5 days; *Hemodialysis*—125 mg after each dialysis.

Recurrent Herpes Labialis Infections (cold sores)
PO (Adults): 1500 mg as a single dose.

Renal Impairment
PO (Adults): *CCr 40–59 mL/min*—750 mg as a single dose; *CCr 20–39 mL/min*—500 mg as a single dose; *CCr <20 mL/min*—250 mg as a single dose; *Hemodialysis*—250 mg as a single dose after dialysis.

Herpes Simplex in HIV-Infected Patients
PO (Adults): 500 mg q 12 hr for 7 days.

Renal Impairment
PO (Adults): *CCr 20–39 mL/min*—500 mg q 24 hr for 7 days; *CCr <20 mL/min*—250 mg q 24 hr for 7 days; *Hemodialysis*—250 mg after each dialysis.

Availability (generic available)
Tablets: 125 mg, 250 mg, 500 mg.

NURSING IMPLICATIONS
Assessment
- Assess lesions prior to and daily during therapy.
- Assess patient for postherpetic neuralgia periodically during and following therapy.

Potential Nursing Diagnoses
Risk for impaired skin integrity (Indications)
Risk for infection (Indications, Patient/Family Teaching)

Implementation
- Famciclovir therapy should be started as soon as herpes zoster is diagnosed, at least within 72 hr, preferably within 48 hr.
- **PO:** Famciclovir may be administered without regard to meals.

Patient/Family Teaching
- Instruct patient to take famciclovir as directed for the full course of therapy. Take missed doses as soon as remembered, if not just before next dose.
- Inform patient that famciclovir does not prevent the spread of infection to others. Until all lesions have crusted, precautions should be taken around others who have not had chickenpox or varicella vaccine or people who are immunosuppressed.
- Advise patient that condoms should be used during sexual contact and that no sexual contact should be made while lesions are present.
- May cause dizziness. Caution patient to avoid driving and other activities requiring alertness until response to medication is known.
- Instruct women with genital herpes to have yearly Papanicolaou smears because these women may be more likely to develop cervical cancer.

Evaluation/Desired Outcomes
- Decrease in time to full crusting, loss of vesicles, loss of ulcers, and loss of crusts in patients with acute herpes zoster (shingles).
- Crusting over and healing of lesions in herpes labialis, genital herpes and in recurrent mucocutaneous HSV infection in HIV-infected patients.
- Prevention of recurrence of herpes genitalis.
- Decreased time to healing for cold sores.

---

famotidine, See HISTAMINE H₂ ANTAGONISTS.

---

febuxostat (fe-bux-o-stat)
Uloric

Classification
Therapeutic: antigout agents
Pharmacologic: xanthine oxidase inhibitors

Pregnancy Category C

Indications
Chronic management of hyperuricemia in patients with a history of gout.

Action
Decreases production of uric acid by inhibiting xanthine oxidase. **Therapeutic Effects:** Lowering of serum uric acid levels with resultant decrease in gouty attacks.

Pharmacokinetics
Absorption: Well absorbed (49%) following oral administration.
Distribution: Unknown.
Protein Binding: 99.2%.
Metabolism and Excretion: Extensively metabolized by the liver; minimal renal excretion of unchanged drug, 45% eliminated in feces as unchanged drug, remainder is eliminated in urine and feces as inactive metabolites.
Half-life: 5–8 hr.

TIME/ACTION PROFILE (blood levels)

ROUTE	ONSET	PEAK	DURATION
PO	rapid	1–1.5 hr*	24 hr

*Maximum lowering of uric acid may take 2 wk

Contraindications/Precautions
Contraindicated in: Concurrent azathioprine, mercaptopurine, or theophylline.
Use Cautiously in: Severe renal impairment (CCr <30 mL/min); Severe hepatic impairment; OB: Use in pregnancy only when potential maternal benefit outweighs potential fetal risk; Pedi: Safety in children <18 yr not established.

Adverse Reactions/Side Effects
GI: liver function abnormalities, nausea. **Derm:** rash. **MS:** gout flare, arthralgia.

Interactions
Drug-Drug: Significantly ↑ blood levels of, and risk of serious toxicity from, **azathioprine**, **mercaptopurine**, and **theophylline**; concurrent use is contraindicated.

Route/Dosage
PO (Adults): 40 mg once daily initially; if serum uric acid does not drop to <6 mg/dL dose should be increased to 80 mg daily.

Availability
Tablets: 40 mg, 80 mg.

NURSING IMPLICATIONS
Assessment
- Assess for joint pain and swelling, especially during early therapy. Changing serum uric acid levels from mobilization of urate from tissue deposits may cause gout flares. Use prophylactic NSAID or colchicine therapy for up to 6 months. If a gout flare occurs, continue febuxostat therapy and treat flare concurrently.
- Monitor for signs and symptoms of MI and stroke.
- **Lab Test Considerations:** Monitor serum uric acid levels prior to, 2 wk after intitiating, and periodically thereafter. If serum uric acid levels are ≥6 mg/dL after 2 wk of daily 40 mg therapy, increase dose to 80 mg daily.
- Monitor liver function at 2 and 4 months of therapy and periodically thereafter. May cause ↑ AST, ALT, CPK, LDH, alkaline phosphatase and creatine.
- May cause prolonged aPTT and PT, and ↓ hematocrit, hemoglobin, RBC, platelet count, and lymphocyte, neutrophil counts. May cause ↑ or ↓ WBC.
- May cause ↓ serum bicarbonate and ↑ serum sodium, glucose, potassium, and TSH levels.
- May cause ↑ serum cholesterol, triglycerides, amylase, and LDL levels.
- May cause ↑ BUN and serum creatinine and proteinuria.

Potential Nursing Diagnoses
Chronic pain (Indications)

Implementation
- **PO:** May be taken with or without food and with antacids.

Patient/Family Teaching
- Instruct patient to take febuxostat as directed. If a gout flare occurs, continue febuxostat and consult health care professional; medications to manage gout flare may be added.
- Advise patient to notify health care professional if rash, chest pain, shortness of breath, or stroke symptoms (weakness, headache, confusion, slurred speech) occur or if side effects are persistent or bothersome.
- Instruct patient to consult health care professional prior to taking any other Rx, OTC, or herbal products.
- Advise female patient to notify health care professional if pregnancy is planned or suspected or if breastfeeding.
- Emphasize the importance of follow-up lab tests to monitor therapy.

Evaluation/Desired Outcomes
- Reduction in serum uric acid levels and resultant gout attacks.

---

felodipine (fe-loe-di-peen)
✤Renedil

Classification
Therapeutic: antianginals, antihypertensives
Pharmacologic: calcium channel blockers

Pregnancy Category C

Indications
Management of hypertension, angina pectoris, and vasospastic (Prinzmetal's) angina.

Action
Inhibits the transport of calcium into myocardial and vascular smooth muscle cells, resulting in inhibition of excitation-contraction coupling and subsequent contraction. **Therapeutic Effects:** Systemic vasodilation resulting in decreased blood pressure. Coronary vasodilation resulting in decreased frequency and severity of attacks of angina.

Pharmacokinetics
Absorption: Well absorbed after oral administration, but extensively metabolized, resulting in ↓ bioavailability.
Distribution: Unknown.
Protein Binding: >99%.
Metabolism and Excretion: Mostly metabolized; minimal amounts excreted unchanged by kidneys.
Half-life: 11–16 hr.

TIME/ACTION PROFILE (antihypertensive effect)

ROUTE	ONSET	PEAK	DURATION
PO	1 hr	2–4 hr	up to 24 hr

Contraindications/Precautions
Contraindicated in: Hypersensitivity (cross-sensitivity may occur); Sick sinus syndrome; 2nd- or 3rd-degree AV block (unless an artificial pacemaker is in place); Systolic blood pressure <90 mm Hg.

✤ = Canadian drug name.   ⊞ = Genetic implication.
*CAPITALS indicates life-threatening; underlines indicate most frequent.

Use Cautiously in: Severe hepatic impairment (dose ↓ recommended); Geri: Dose ↓ recommended; ↑ risk of hypotension; Severe renal impairment; History of serious ventricular arrhythmias or CHF; OB, Lactation, Pedi: Safety not established.

Adverse Reactions/Side Effects
CNS: headache, abnormal dreams, anxiety, confusion, dizziness, drowsiness, nervousness, psychiatric disturbances, weakness. **EENT:** blurred vision, disturbed equilibrium, epistaxis, tinnitus. **Resp:** cough, dyspnea. **CV:** ARRHYTHMIAS, CHF, peripheral edema, chest pain, hypotension, palpitations, syncope, tachycardia. **GI:** anorexia, constipation, diarrhea, dry mouth, dysgeusia, dyspepsia, ↑ liver function tests, nausea, vomiting. **GU:** dysuria, nocturia, polyuria, sexual dysfunction, urinary frequency. **Derm:** dermatitis, erythema multiforme, flushing, ↑ sweating, photosensitivity, pruritus/urticaria, rash. **Endo:** gynecomastia, hyperglycemia. **Hemat:** anemia, leukopenia, thrombocytopenia. **Metab:** weight gain. **MS:** joint stiffness, muscle cramps. **Neuro:** paresthesia, tremor. **Misc:** STEVENS-JOHNSON SYNDROME, gingival hyperplasia.

Interactions
Drug-Drug: Additive hypotension may occur when used concurrently with **fentanyl**, other **antihypertensives**, **nitrates**, acute ingestion of **alcohol**, or **quinidine**. Antihypertensive effects may be ↓ by concurrent use of **NSAIDs**. **Ketoconazole**, **itraconazole**, **propranolol** and **erythromycin** ↓ metabolism, ↑ blood levels and the risk of toxicity (dose ↓ may be necessary).
Drug-Food: Grapefruit juice ↑ serum levels and effect.

Route/Dosage
PO (Adults): 5 mg/day (2.5 mg/day in geriatric patients); may ↑ q 2 wk (range 5–10 mg/day; not to exceed 10 mg/day).

Availability (generic available)
Extended-release tablets: 2.5 mg, 5 mg, 10 mg. **Cost:** *Generic*—2.5 mg $89.96/90, 5 mg $85.97/90, 10 mg $139.97/90.

NURSING IMPLICATIONS

Assessment
- Monitor blood pressure and pulse before therapy, during dosage titration, and periodically during therapy. Monitor ECG periodically during prolonged therapy.
- Monitor intake and output ratios and daily weight. Assess for signs of CHF (peripheral edema, rales/crackles, dyspnea, weight gain, jugular venous distention).
- **Angina:** Assess location, duration, intensity, and precipitating factors of patient's anginal pain.
- **Hypertension:** Check frequency of refills to monitor adherence.
- *Lab Test Considerations:* Total serum calcium concentrations are not affected by calcium channel blockers.
- Monitor serum potassium periodically. Hypokalemia ↑ risk of arrhythmias and should be corrected.
- Monitor renal and hepatic functions periodically during long-term therapy. May cause ↑ in hepatic enzymes after several days of therapy, which return to normal upon discontinuation of therapy.

Potential Nursing Diagnoses
Ineffective tissue perfusion (Indications)
Acute pain (Indications)

Implementation
- **PO:** May be administered without regard to meals. May be administered with meals if GI irritation becomes a problem.
- Swallow tablets whole; do not break, crush, or chew. Empty tablets that appear in stool are not significant.

Patient/Family Teaching
- Advise patient to take medication as directed, even if feeling well. If a dose is missed, take as soon as possible unless almost time for next dose; do not double doses. May need to be discontinued gradually.
- Instruct patient on correct technique for monitoring pulse. Instruct patient to contact health care professional if heart rate is <50 bpm.
- Advise patient to avoid grapefruit or grapefruit juice during therapy.
- Caution patient to change positions slowly to minimize orthostatic hypotension.
- May cause drowsiness or dizziness. Advise patient to avoid driving or other activities requiring alertness until response to the medication is known.
- Instruct patient on importance of maintaining good dental hygiene and seeing dentist frequently for teeth cleaning to prevent tenderness, bleeding, and gingival hyperplasia (gum enlargement).
- Instruct patient to avoid concurrent use of alcohol or other Rx, OTC, or herbal products, especially cold preparations, without consulting health care professional.

- Advise patient to notify health care professional if irregular heartbeat, dyspnea, swelling of hands and feet, pronounced dizziness, nausea, constipation, rash, or hypotension occurs or if headache is severe or persistent.
- Caution patient to wear protective clothing and to use sunscreen to prevent photosensitivity reactions.
- Advise patient to inform health care professional of medication regimen before treatment or surgery.
- **Angina:** Instruct patient on concurrent nitrate or beta-blocker therapy to continue taking both medications as directed and to use SL nitroglycerin as needed for anginal attacks.
- Advise patient to contact health care professional if chest pain does not improve or worsens after therapy, occurs with diaphoresis or shortness of breath, or if severe, persistent headache occurs.
- Caution patient to discuss exercise restrictions with health care professional before exertion.
- **Hypertension:** Encourage patient to comply with other interventions for hypertension (weight reduction, low-sodium diet, smoking cessation, moderation of alcohol consumption, regular exercise, and stress management). Medication controls but does not cure hypertension.
- Instruct patient and family in proper technique for monitoring blood pressure. Advise patient to take blood pressure weekly and to report significant changes.

Evaluation/Desired Outcomes
- Decrease in blood pressure.
- Decrease in frequency and severity of anginal attacks.
- Decrease in need for nitrate therapy.
- Increase in activity tolerance and sense of well-being.

---

fenofibrate (fen-o-fi-brate)
Antara, Fenoglide, Lipofen, ✤Lipidil Micro, ✤Lipidil Supra, Lofibra, Tricor, Triglide

Classification
Therapeutic: lipid-lowering agents
Pharmacologic: fibric acid derivatives

Pregnancy Category C

Indications
With dietary therapy to decrease LDL cholesterol, total cholesterol, triglycerides, and apolipoprotein B in adult patients with hypercholesterolemia or mixed dyslipidemia. With dietary management in the treatment of hypertriglyceridemia (types IV and V hyperlipidemia) in patients who are at risk for pancreatitis and do not respond to nondrug therapy.

Action
Fenofibric acid primarily inhibits triglyceride synthesis. **Therapeutic Effects:** Lowering of cholesterol and triglycerides with subsequent decreased risk of pancreatitis.

Pharmacokinetics
Absorption: Well absorbed (60%) after oral administration; absorption ↑ by food.
Distribution: Unknown.
Protein Binding: 99%.
Metabolism and Excretion: Rapidly converted to fenofibric acid, which is the active metabolite; fenofibric acid is metabolized by the liver. Fenofibric acid and its metabolites are primarily excreted in urine (60%).
Half-life: 20 hr.

TIME/ACTION PROFILE (lowering of triglycerides)

ROUTE	ONSET	PEAK	DURATION
PO	unknown	2 wk	unknown

Contraindications/Precautions
Contraindicated in: Hypersensitivity; Hepatic impairment (including primary biliary cirrhosis); Pre-existing gallbladder disease; Severe renal impairment; Concurrent use of HMG-CoA reductase inhibitors; Lactation: Potential for tumorigenicity noted in animal studies; discontinue breastfeeding.
Use Cautiously in: Concurrent warfarin therapy; OB: Embryocidal and teratogenic in animal studies; use only if potential benefits outweigh risks to the fetus; Pedi: Safety not established in children <18 yr; Geri: Age-related decline in renal function may make older patients more susceptible to adverse reactions.

Adverse Reactions/Side Effects
CNS: fatigue/weakness, headache. **CV:** PULMONARY EMBOLISM, arrhythmias, deep vein thrombosis. **GI:** cholelithiasis, pancreatitis. **Derm:** rash, urticaria. **MS:** rhabdomyolysis. **Misc:** hypersensitivity reactions.

fenofibrate

Interactions
Drug-Drug: ↑ anticoagulant effects of **warfarin**. Concurrent use with **HMG-CoA reductase inhibitors** ↑ risk of rhabdomyolysis (combined use should be avoided). Absorption is ↓ by **bile acid sequestrants** (fenofibrate should be given 1 hr before or 4–6 hr after). ↑ risk of nephrotoxicity with **cyclosporine**.

Route/Dosage

Primary hypercholesterolemia/mixed dyslipidemia
PO (Adults): *Antara*—130 mg/day initially; *Fenoglide*—120 mg/day; *Lofibra*—200 mg/day initially; *Tricor*—145 mg/day initially; *Triglide*—160 mg/day initially; *Lipofen*—50 mg daily; *Lipidil Supra*—160 mg daily.

Hypertriglyceridemia
PO (Adults): *Antara*—43–130 mg/day ; *Fenoglide*—40–120 mg/day; *Lofibra*—67–200 mg/day initially; *Tricor*—48–145 mg/day initially; *Triglide*—50–160 mg/day initially; *Lipofen*—50 mg daily; *Lipidil Supra*—160 mg daily.

Renal impairment/Geriatric patients
PO (Adults): *Antara*—43 mg/day; *Fenoglide*—start at 40 mg/day; *Lofibra*—67 mg/day; *Tricor*—48mg/day.

Availability
Tablets (Tricor): 48 mg, 145 mg. **Cost:** 48 mg $109.97/90, 145 mg $299.96/90. **Tablets (Fenoglide):** 40 mg, 120 mg. **Tablets (Triglide):** 50 mg, 160 mg. **Micronized tablets (Lofibra):** 54 mg, 160 mg. **Cost:** 160 mg $189.97/90. **Micro-coated tablets (Lipidil Supra):** 100 mg, 160 mg. **Micronized capsules (Antara):** 43 mg, 130 mg. **Cost:** 43 mg $116.96/90, 130 mg $318.93/90. **Capsules (Lipofen):** 50 mg, 100 mg, 150 mg. **Micronized capsules (Lofibra):** 67 mg, 134 mg, 200 mg. **Cost:** *Generic*—67 mg $76.39/90, 134 mg $147.00/90, 200 mg $226.87/90. **Micronized capsules (Lipidil Micro):** 67 mg, 200 mg.

NURSING IMPLICATIONS

Assessment
- Obtain a diet history, especially with regard to fat consumption. Every attempt should be made to obtain normal serum triglyceride levels with diet, exercise, and weight loss in obese patients before fenofibrate therapy is instituted.
- Assess patient for cholelithiasis. If symptoms occur, gallbladder studies are indicated. Therapy should be discontinued if gallstones are found.
- ***Lab Test Considerations:*** Monitor serum lipids before therapy to determine consistent elevations, then monitor periodically during therapy.
- Monitor serum AST and ALT periodically during therapy. May cause ↑ levels. Therapy should be discontinued if levels rise >3 times the normal limit.
- If patient develops muscle tenderness during therapy, CPK levels should be monitored. If CPK levels are markedly ↑ or myopathy occurs, therapy should be discontinued.
- May cause mild to moderate ↓ in hemoglobin, hematocrit, and WBCs. Monitor periodically during first 12 mo of therapy. Levels usually stabilize during long-term therapy.
- Patients taking anticoagulants concurrently should have prothrombin levels monitored frequently until levels stabilize.

Potential Nursing Diagnoses
Noncompliance (Patient/Family Teaching)

Implementation
- Patients should be placed on a triglyceride-lowering diet before therapy and remain on this diet throughout therapy.
- Dose may be increased after repeated serum triglyceride levels every 4–8 wk.
- Brands are not interchangeable.
- **PO:** Administer *Antara, Fenoglide, Lipofen, Lipidil Micro, Lipidil Supra, Lofibra,* and *Tricor* products with meals. *Triglide* formulation may be taken without regard to meals.

Patient/Family Teaching
- Instruct patient to take medication as directed, not to skip doses or double up on missed doses. Medication helps control but does not cure elevated serum triglyceride levels.
- Advise patient that this medication should be used in conjunction with diet restrictions (fat, cholesterol, carbohydrates, alcohol), exercise, and cessation of smoking.
- Instruct patient to notify health care professional if unexplained muscle pain, tenderness, or weakness occurs, especially if accompanied by fever or malaise.
- Instruct female patients to notify health care professional promptly if pregnancy is planned or suspected.
- Advise patient to notify health care professional of medication regimen before treatment or surgery.
- Emphasize the importance of follow-up exams to determine effectiveness and to monitor for side effects.

Evaluation/Desired Outcomes
- Decrease in serum triglycerides and cholesterol to normal levels. Therapy should be discontinued in patients who do not have an adequate response in 2 months of therapy.

fenofibric acid
(feen-oh**fye**-brik **as**-id)
Tri-Lipix

Classification
Therapeutic: lipid-lowering agents
Pharmacologic: fibric acid derivatives

Indications
With a statin to reduce triglycerides (TG) and increase high density lipoprotein-C (HDL-C) in patients with mixed dyslipidemias and CHD or a CHD risk equivalent who are on statin therapy to achieve their low-density lipoprotein-C (LDL-C) goal. As monotherapy to reduce TG in patients with severe hypertriglyceridemia. As monotherapy to reduce elevated LDL-C, total cholesterol (Total-C), TG and apolipoprotein B (Apo B), and increase HDL-C in patients with primary hyperlipidemia or mixed dyslipidemia. Part of a comprehensive program to decrease cardiovascular risk factors.

Action
Activates the peroxisome proliferator activated receptor α (PPARα), resulting in increased lipolysis and elimination of triglycerides from plasma. Activation of PPARα also increases production of HDL. **Therapeutic Effects:** Improvement in lipid profile with lowered triglycerides and LDL cholesterol, and increased HDL cholesterol.

Pharmacokinetics
Absorption: Well absorbed following oral administration.
Distribution: Unknown.
Protein Binding: 99%.
Metabolism and Excretion: Fenofibric acid is the active metabolite of fenofibrate. Fenofibric acid is mostly metabolized by glucuronidation and the metabolites are mostly excreted by the kidneys.
Half-life: 20 hr.

TIME/ACTION PROFILE (effects on blood lipids)

ROUTE	ONSET	PEAK	DURATION
PO	unknown	4–5 hr†	unknown

†Blood levels

Contraindications/Precautions
Contraindicated in: Hypersensitivity to fenofibric acid, choline fenofibrate or fenofibrate; Severe renal impairment (CCr <30 mL/min); Active liver or gallbladder disease; Lactation: Avoid use during breastfeeding.

Use Cautiously in: Mild/moderate renal impairment (dose reduction required for CCr 30–80 mL/min); Concurrent use with statins in elderly patients, patients with diabetes, renal failure, or hypothyroidism (↑ risk of myopathy/rhabdomyolysis); Geri: Consider age-related decrease in renal function, concurrent illnesses and drug therapy; OB: Use during pregnancy only if the potential benefit justifies the potential risk to the fetus.; Pedi: Safe and effective use in children has not been established.

Adverse Reactions/Side Effects
CNS: headache. **GI:** diarrhea, nausea, cholelithiasis, ↑ liver enzymes, pancreatitis. **GU:** ↑ creatinine. **MS:** MYOPATHY/RHABDOMYOLYSIS, myalgia, back pain.

Interactions
Drug-Drug: ↑ effects and risk of bleeding with **coumadin**; monitor prothrombin time/INR. **Bile acid sequestrants** may ↓ absorption and effectiveness; administer at least 1 hr before or 4–6 hr after a bile acid sequestrant. Concurrent use with **nephrotoxic drugs** including **cyclosporine** may impair renal function and excretion, ↑ risk of adverse reactions.

Route/Dosage
PO (Adults): *Mixed dyslipidemia*—135 mg once daily; *Hypertriglyceridemia*—45–135 mg once daily.

Renal Impairment
PO (Adults): *CCr 30–80 mL/min*—45 mg once daily.

Availability
Delayed-release capsules (choline fenofibrate): 45 mg, 135 mg.

NURSING IMPLICATIONS

Assessment
- Obtain a diet history, especially with regard to fat consumption. Every attempt should be made to obtain normal serum triglyceride levels with diet, exercise, and weight loss in obese patients before fenofibric acid therapy is instituted.
- Assess patient for cholelithiasis. If symptoms occur, gallbladder studies are indicated. Ther-

apy should be discontinued if gallstones are found.
- **Lab Test Considerations:** Monitor serum lipids before therapy to determine consistent elevations, then monitor periodically during therapy.
- Monitor serum AST and ALT periodically during therapy. May cause ↑ levels. Therapy should be discontinued if levels rise >3 times the normal limit.
- If patient develops muscle tenderness during therapy, CPK levels should be monitored. If CPK levels are markedly ↑ or myopathy occurs, therapy should be discontinued.
- May cause reversible ↑ in serum creatinine. Monitor renal function in patients at risk for renal insufficiency (elderly, diabetics).
- May cause mild to moderate ↓ in hemoglobin, hematocrit, and WBCs. Monitor periodically during first 12 mo of therapy. Levels usually stabilize during long-term therapy.
- Patients taking anticoagulants concurrently should have prothrombin time and INR monitored frequently until levels stabilize.

Potential Nursing Diagnoses
Noncompliance (Patient/Family Teaching)

Implementation
- Patients should be placed on a triglyceride-lowering diet before therapy and remain on this diet throughout therapy.
- **PO:** Administer without regard to meals. Swallow capsules whole; do not open, crush, or chew. May be administered at same time as statin dose.

Patient/Family Teaching
- Instruct patient to take medication as directed. Take missed doses as soon as remembered; if time for next dose, skip dose and take next dose at regular time. Do not double doses. Medication helps control but does not cure elevated serum triglyceride levels. Advise patient to read *Medication Guide* before starting and with each Rx refill, new information may be available.
- Advise patient that this medication should be used in conjunction with diet restrictions (fat, cholesterol, carbohydrates, alcohol), exercise, and cessation of smoking.
- Instruct patient to notify health care professional if unexplained muscle pain, tenderness, weakness, tiredness, fever, nausea, vomiting, or abdominal pain occurs, especially if accompanied by fever or malaise.
- Instruct female patients to notify health care professional promptly if pregnancy is planned or suspected.
- Advise patient to consult health care professional before taking any other Rx, OTC, or herbal products.
- Advise patient to notify health care professional of medication regimen before treatment or surgery.
- Emphasize the importance of follow-up exams to determine effectiveness and to monitor for side effects.

Evaluation/Desired Outcomes
- Decrease in serum triglycerides and LDL cholesterol to normal levels with an increase in HDL levels.

---

fenoldopam (fen-**ole**-doe-pam)
Corlopam

Classification
Therapeutic: antihypertensives
Pharmacologic: vasodilators

Pregnancy Category B

Indications
Short-term (<48 hr), in-hospital management of hypertensive emergencies, including malignant hypertension with end-organ deterioration.

Action
Acts as an agonist at dopamine d_1-like receptors. Also binds to alpha-adrenergic receptors. Acts as a vasodilator. **Therapeutic Effects:** Rapid lowering of blood pressure.

Pharmacokinetics
Absorption: IV administration results in complete bioavailability.
Distribution: Unknown.
Metabolism and Excretion: Mostly metabolized by the liver; 90% of metabolites are excreted in urine, 10% in feces.
Half-life: 5–10 min.

TIME/ACTION PROFILE (effect on blood pressure)

ROUTE	ONSET	PEAK	DURATION
IV	rapid	15 min	1–4 hr

Contraindications/Precautions
Contraindicated in: Hypersensitivity to fenoldopam or sulfites; Concurrent beta blocker therapy (will prevent reflex tachycardia).

Use Cautiously in: Glaucoma or intraocular hypertension; OB, Lactation, Pedi: Safety not established.

Adverse Reactions/Side Effects
CNS: headache, nervousness/anxiety, dizziness. **CV:** hypotension, tachycardia, ECG changes, peripheral edema. **GI:** nausea, abdominal pain, constipation, diarrhea, vomiting. **Derm:** flushing, sweating. **F and E:** hypokalemia. **Local:** injection site reactions. **MS:** back pain.

Interactions
Drug-Drug: Concurrent use with **beta blockers** may result in excessive hypotension (concurrent use should be avoided).

Route/Dosage
IV (Adults): 0.01–1.6 mcg/kg/min.

Availability
Concentrate for injection: 10 mg/mL in 1- and 2-mL single-use ampules (with sodium metabisulfite).

NURSING IMPLICATIONS

Assessment
- Monitor blood pressure, heart rate, and ECG frequently throughout therapy; continuous monitoring is preferred. Consult physician for parameters.
- *Lab Test Considerations:* Monitor serum potassium concentrations every 6 hr during therapy. May cause hypokalemia. Treat with oral or IV potassium supplementation.

Potential Nursing Diagnoses
Ineffective tissue perfusion (Indications)

Implementation

IV Administration

- Administer via continuous infusion; do not use bolus doses. Avoid hypotension and rapid decreases in blood pressure. Initial dose titration should occur no more frequently than every 15 min and less frequently as desired blood pressure is reached. Increments of 0.05 to 0.1 mcg/kg/min are recommended for titration. Lower initial doses (0.03 to 0.1 mcg/kg/min) titrated slowly have been associated with less reflex tachycardia than higher initial doses.
- Infusion can be abruptly discontinued or gradually tapered before discontinuation. Oral therapy with other antihypertensives can begin anytime after the blood pressure is stable. Do not administer beta blockers concurrently with fenoldopam.
- **Continuous Infusion:** *Diluent:* Dilute 4 mL (40 mg of drug) with 1000 mL, 2 mL (20 mg of drug) with 500 mL, or 1 mL (10 mg of drug) with 250 mL of 0.9% NaCl or D5W. Infusion is stable for 24 hr at room temperature. *Concentration:* 40 mcg/mL. *Rate:* Based on patient's weight (see Route/Dosage section). Titrate to desired effect. Administer via infusion pump to ensure accurate dosage rate.
- **Y-Site Compatibility:** alfentanil, amikacin, aminocaproic acid, amiodarone, ampicillin/sulbactam, argatroban, atracurium, atropine, azithromycin, aztreonam, butorphanol, calcium chloride, calcium gluconate, caspofungin, cefazolin, cefepime, cefotaxime, ceftazidime, ceftizoxime, ceftriaxone, cefuroxime, chloramphenicol, cimetidine, ciprofloxacin, cisatracurium, clindamycin, cyclosporine, daptomycin, dexmedetomidine, digoxin, diltiazem, diphenhydramine, dobutamine, dolasetron, dopamine, doxycycline, droperidol, enalaprilat, epinephrine, ertapenem, erythromycin, esmolol, famotidine, fentanyl, fluconazole, gentamicin, granisetron, haloperidol, heparin, hydralazine, hydrocortisone sodium succinate, hydromorphone, imipenem/cilastatin, inamrinone, insulin, isoproterenol, labetalol, levofloxacin, lidocaine, linezolid, lorazepam, magnesium sulfate, mannitol, meperidine, metoclopramide, metoprolol, metronidazole, micafungin, midazolam, milrinone, morphine, nafcillin, nalbuphine, naloxone, nicardipine, nitroglycerin, nitroprusside, norepinephrine, ondansetron, palonosetron, pancuronium, phenylephrine, piperacillin/tazobactam, potassium chloride, potassium phosphate, procainamide, promethazine, propofol, propranolol, quinupristin/dalfopristin, ranitidine, remifentanil, rocuronium, sufentanil, tacrolimus, theophylline, ticarcillin/clavulanate, tirofiban, tobramycin, trimethoprim/sulfamethoxazole, vancomycin, vasopressin, vecuronium, verapamil, voriconazole.
- **Y-Site Incompatibility:** acyclovir, aminophylline, amphotericin B, ampicillin, bumetanide, cefoxitin, dexamethasone sodium phosphate, diazepam, fosphenytoin, furosemide, ganciclovir, ketorolac, meropenem, methohexital, methylprednisolone sodium succinate, pantoprazole, pentobarbital, phenytoin, prochlorperazine, sodium bicarbonate, thiopental.

Patient/Family Teaching
- Explain purpose of medication to patient.
- Advise patient to report headache or pain at the injection site.

Evaluation/Desired Outcomes
- Decrease in blood pressure without the appearance of side effects.

---

fentanyl buccal/transmucosal (fen-ta-nil)
Actiq, Fentora, Onsolis

Classification
Therapeutic: opioid analgesics
Pharmacologic: opioid agonists

Schedule II

Pregnancy Category C

Indications
Management of breakthrough pain in cancer patients already receiving and tolerant to around-the-clock opioid therapy for persistent cancer pain (60 mg/day of oral morphine or equivalent).

Action
Binds to opiate receptors in the CNS, altering the response to and perception of pain. **Therapeutic Effects:** Decrease in severity of breakthrough pain.

Pharmacokinetics
Absorption: *Buccal tablets*–65% absorbed from buccal mucosa; 50% is absorbed transmucosally, remainder is swallowed and is absorbed slowly from the GI tract. Buccal absorption is enhanced by an effervescent reaction in the dose form. Bioavailability is greater than transmucosal fentanyl; *Buccal soluble film*—51% absorbed from buccal mucosa and remaining 49% is swallowed (20% of which becomes systemically available); bioavailability is greater than transmucosal fentanyl; *Transmucosal*—Initial rapid absorption (25%) from buccal mucosa is followed by more prolonged absorption (25%) from GI tract (combined bioavailability 50%).
Distribution: Readily crosses the placenta and enters breast milk.
Protein Binding: 80–85%.
Metabolism and Excretion: >90% metabolized by the liver and intestinal mucosa (CYP3A4 enzyme system); <7% excreted unchanged in urine.
Half-life: *100 mcg tablet*—2.6 hr; *200 mcg tablet*—4.4 hr; *100 mcg tablet*—2.6 hr; *400 mcg tablet*—11.0 hr; *800 mcg tablet*—11.7 hr; *Buccal soluble film*—14 hr; *Transmucosal*—7 hr.

TIME/ACTION PROFILE (decreased pain)

ROUTE	ONSET	PEAK	DURATION
Buccal tablet	15 min	40–60 min	60 min
Buccal soluble film	15–30 min	1 hr	2–6 hr
Transmucosal	rapid	15–30 min	several hr

Contraindications/Precautions
Contraindicated in: Known intolerance or hypersensitivity; Acute/postoperative pain; Opioid-naive (non-tolerant) patients; OB: Labor and delivery; Lactation: Lactation.
Use Cautiously in: Chronic obstructive pulmonary disease; Concurrent use of CNS active drugs; History of substance abuse; Severe renal/hepatic impairment (use lowest effective starting dose); Concurrent use of CYP3A4 inhibitors (use lowest effective dose); Bradyarrhythmias; OB, Lactation: Short-term use at lower doses may be acceptable (AAP); Geri: May be more sensitive to effects and may have an ↑ risk of adverse reactions; titrate dosage carefully; Pedi: Safety not established.
Exercise Extreme Caution in: Head injuries/ ↑ intracranial pressure.

Adverse Reactions/Side Effects
Opioid side effects ↑ with increased dosage.
CNS: dizziness, drowsiness, headache, confusion, depression, fatigue, hallucinations, headache, insomnia, weakness. **Resp:** RESPIRATORY DEPRESSION, dyspnea. **CV:** hypotension. **GI:** constipation, nausea, vomiting, abdominal pain, anorexia, dry mouth. **Misc:** physical dependence, psychological dependence.

Interactions
Drug-Drug: Should not be used within 14 days of **MAO inhibitors** because of possible severe and unpredictable reactions. **CNS depressants**, including other **opioids**, **sedative/hypnotics**, **general anesthetics**, **phenothiazines**, **skeletal muscle relaxants**, **sedating antihistamines**, and **alcohol** may ↑ CNS depression, hypoventilation and hypotension. Concurrent use with **CYP3A4 inhibitors** including **ritonavir**, **ketoconazole**, **itraconazole**, **clarithromycin**, **nelfinavir**, **nefazodone**, **diltiazem**, **erythromycin**, **aprepitant**, **fluconazole**, **fosamprenavir**, and **verapamil** may significantly ↑ blood levels and ↑ risk of respiratory and CNS depression; careful monitoring and dose adjustment is recommended. Concurrent use of **agents that induce CYP3A4 enzyme activity** may ↓ analgesia. Administration of **partial-antagonist**

opioid analgesics or **opioid antagonists** will precipitate withdrawal in physically dependent patients.

Drug-Food: Grapefruit juice is a moderate inhibitor of the CYP3A4 enzyme system; concurrent use may ↑ blood levels and the risk of respiratory and CNS depression. Careful monitoring and dose adjustment is recommended.

Route/Dosage
Buccal (Adults): *Tablets*–100 mcg, then titrated to dose that provides adequate analgesia with tolerable side effects; *Soluble film*—200 mcg, then titrated to dose that provides adequate analgesia with tolerable side effects; doses >1200 mcg should not be used.

Transmucosal (Adults): *Dose titration*—One 200 mcg unit dissolved in mouth (see Implementation section) over 15 min; additional unit may be used 15 min after first unit is completed. If more than one unit is required per episode (as evaluated over several episodes), dose may be increased as required to control pain. Optimal usage/titration should result in using no more than 4 units/day.

Availability
Buccal tablets (Fentora): 100 mcg, 200 mcg, 300 mcg, 400 mcg, 600 mcg, 800 mcg. **Buccal soluble film (Onsolis):** 200 mcg, 400 mcg, 600 mcg, 800 mcg, 1200 mcg. **Transmucosal lozenge on a stick (Actiq) (berry flavor-sugar free):** 200 mcg, 400 mcg, 600 mcg, 800 mcg, 1200 mcg, 1600 mcg.

NURSING IMPLICATIONS

Assessment
- Monitor type, location, and intensity of pain before and 15–30 min after administration of buccal fentanyl.
- Assess blood pressure, pulse, and respirations before and periodically during administration. If respiratory rate is <10 min, assess level of sedation. Physical stimulation may be sufficient to prevent hypoventilation. Subsequent doses may need to be decreased. Patients tolerant to opioid analgesics are usually tolerant to the respiratory depressant effects also.
- Monitor for application site reactions (paresthesia, ulceration, bleeding, pain, ulcer, irritation). Reactions are usually self-limited and rarely require discontinuation.
- *Toxicity and Overdose:* If an opioid antagonist is required to reverse respiratory depression or coma, naloxone (Narcan) is the antidote. Dilute the 0.4-mg ampule of naloxone in 10 mL of 0.9% NaCl and administer 0.5 mL (0.02 mg) by direct IV push every 2 min. For patients weighing <40 kg, dilute 0.1 mg of naloxone in 10 mL of 0.9% NaCl for a concentration of 10 mcg/mL and administer 0.5 mcg every 2 min. Use extreme caution when titrating dose in patients physically dependent on opioid analgesics to avoid withdrawal, seizures, and severe pain. Duration of respiratory depression may be longer than duration of opioid antagonist, requiring repeated doses.

Potential Nursing Diagnoses
Acute pain (Indications)
Risk for injury (Adverse Reactions)

Implementation
- *High Alert:* Accidental overdosage of opioid analgesics has resulted in fatalities. Before administering, clarify all ambiguous orders; have second practitioner independently check original order and dose calculations.
- Patients considered opioid-tolerant are those who are taking ≥60 mg of oral morphine/day, at least 25 mcg transdermal fentanyl/hr, 30 mg of oxycodone/day, 8 mg of hydromorphone/day or an equianalgesic dose of another opioid for ≥1 wk.
- *High Alert:* Dose may be lethal to a child; keep out of reach of children.
- Do not substitute fentanyl buccal products *(Actiq, Fentora, or Onsolis)*; doses are not equivalent.
- **Actiq (Transmucosal):** Open the foil package immediately before use. Instruct patient to place unit in the mouth between the cheek and lower gum, moving it from one side to the other using the handle. Patient should suck, not chew, the lozenge. If it is chewed and swallowed, lower peak concentrations and lower bioavailability may occur. Instruct patient to consume lozenge over 15-min period; longer or shorter periods may be less efficacious. If signs of excessive opioid effects occur, remove from patient's mouth immediately and decrease future doses.
- Initial dose for breakthrough pain should be 200 mcg. Six 200-mcg units should be prescribed and should be used before increasing to a higher dose. If one unit is ineffective, a second unit may be started 15 min after the completion of the first unit. Do not use more than 2

units during a single episode of breakthrough pain during titration phase. With each new dose during titration, 6 units should be prescribed, allowing treatment of several episodes of breakthrough pain. Adequate dose is determined based on effective analgesia with acceptable side effects. Side effects during titration period are usually greater than after effective dose is determined.
- Once an effective dose is determined, instruct patient to limit dose to 4 units/day. If >4 units/day are required, consider increasing the dose of the long-acting opioid.
- Discontinue with a gradual decrease in dose to prevent signs and symptoms of abrupt withdrawal.
- To dispose of remaining unit, using wire-cutting pliers cut off the drug matrix end so that it falls into the toilet. Flush remaining drug matrix down toilet. Drug remaining on handle may be removed by placing under running warm water until dissolved. Dispose of drug-free handle according to institutional protocol. ***High Alert:*** *Partially consumed units are no longer protected by child-resistant pouch; dose may still be fatal. A temporary child-resistant storage bottle is provided for partially consumed units that cannot be disposed of properly.*
- **Buccal: Fentora**: Do not attempt to push tablet through blister, may cause damage to tablet. Open by tearing along perforations to separate from blister card. Then bend blister unit on line where indicated. Blister backing should then be peeled to expose tablets. Use immediately; do not store, may damage integrity of tablet. Tablets are not to be sucked, chewed or swallowed whole; this will reduce medication effectiveness. Place between cheek and gum above a molar and allow medication to dissolve, usually 14–25 min. May cause bubbling sensation between teeth and gum while tablet dissolves. Do not attempt to split tablet. After 30 min, if remnants of tablet remain, swallow with glass of water.
- For patients not previously using transmucosal fentanyl, initial dose should be 100 mcg. Titrate to provide adequate relief while minimizing side effects. For patients switching from oral transmucosal fentanyl to fentanyl buccal, if transmucosal dose is 200–400 mcg, switch to 100 mcg buccal; if transmucosal dose is 600–800 mcg, switch to 200 mcg buccal; if transmucosal dose is 1200–1600 mcg, switch to 400 mcg buccal fentanyl.
- Dose may be repeated once during a single episode of breakthrough pain if not adequately relieved. Re-dose may occur 30 min after start of administration of fentanyl buccal and the same dose should be used.
- If more than one dose is required per breakthrough pain episode for several consecutive episodes, dose of maintenance opioid and fentanyl buccal should be adjusted. To increase dose, use multiples of 100 mcg tablet, use two 100 mcg tablets (one on each side of mouth in buccal cavity). If unsuccessful in controlling breakthrough pain episode, two 100 mcg tablets may be placed on each side of mouth in buccal cavity (four 100 mcg tablets). Titrate above 400 mcg by 200 mcg increments. To reduce risk of overdose, patients should have only one strength available at any one time.
- Once a successful dose has been established, if more than 4 breakthrough pain episodes/day occur, re-evaluate opioid dose for persistent pain.
- Inform patient if medication is no longer needed they should contact Cephalon at 1-800-896-5855 or remove from blister pack and flush any remaining product down toilet.
- **Buccal: Onsolis**: Available only through FOCUS, a restricted distribution program. Only prescribers and pharmacies registered in the program and patients enrolled in the program have access. Program provides education, counseling, and facilitated distribution of the medication. To enroll in the FOCUS Program call 1–877–4ONSOLIS or visit www.OnsolisFocus.com.
- Use tongue to wet inside of cheek or rinse mouth with water to wet area for placement of film. Open package immediately prior to use. Place entire film near tip of dry finger with pink side facing up and hold in place. Place pink side of film against inside of cheek. Press and hold film in place for 5 seconds. Film should stay in place on its own after this period. May consume liquids after 5 min. Do not cut or tear film prior to use. Film should dissolve within 15–30 min after application. Do not manipulate with tongue or fingers; avoid eating food until film has dissolved.
- If film is chewed or swallowed, lower peak concentration and lower bioavailability may result.
- Dose must be started with one 200 mcg film; do not convert patients on a mcg/mcg basis. If adequate relief is not achieved with one 200 mcg film, titrate using multiples of the 200 mcg film to provide adequate relief while minimizing side effects. Do not use more than 4 of the 200 mcg films simultaneously. Do not place on

top of each other; use both sides of the mouth. If adequate pain relief is not achieved after 800 mcg (four 200 mcg films) and patient tolerated 800 mcg dose, treat next episode with one 1200 mcg film. Do not use doses above 1200 mcg.
- Single doses should be separated by at least 2 hr. Use fentanyl buccal film only once per breakthrough pain episode; do not redose. Other rescue medications may be used as directed.
- Once a successful dose has been established, if more than 4 breakthrough pain episodes/day occur, re-evaluate opioid dose for persistent pain.
- To dispose of unneeded films, open foil packets, drop films into toilet and flush.

Patient/Family Teaching
- Instruct patient to take fentanyl buccal exactly as directed. Do not take more often than prescribed, keep out of reach of children, protect it from being stolen, and do not share with others, even if they have the same symptoms. Open only when ready to administer. Advise patient to review *Medication Guide* each time fentanyl buccal is dispensed; new information may be available. Advise patient to notify health care professional if breakthrough pain is not alleviated, worsens, if >4 units/day are required to control pain, or if excessive opioid effects occur.
- Advise patient to avoid grapefruit juice during therapy.
- Caution patient to make position changes slowly to minimize orthostatic hypotension.
- Medication causes dizziness and drowsiness. Advise patient to call for assistance during ambulation and transfer, and to avoid driving or other activities requiring alertness until response to medication is known.
- Instruct patient to avoid concurrent use of alcohol or other CNS depressants, such as sleep aids.
- Advise patient to notify health care professional if sores on gums or inside cheek become a problem.
- Instruct patient to notify health care professional before taking Rx, OTC, or herbal products.
- Advise patient to notify health care professional if pregnancy is planned or suspected or if breastfeeding.

- **Actiq:** Inform patient that this drug may contain sugar and may cause dry mouth. Advise patient to maintain good oral hygiene regular dental exams.
- **Onsolis:** Explain FOCUS Program to patient and caregiver, including receipt of medication via a traceable courier and need of adult signature upon delivery.

Evaluation/Desired Outcomes
- Decrease in severity of pain during episodes of breakthrough pain in patients receiving long-acting opioids.

HIGH ALERT

fentanyl (parenteral)
(**fen**-ta-nil)
Sublimaze

Classification
Therapeutic: opioid analgesics
Pharmacologic: opioid agonists

Schedule II

Pregnancy Category C

Indications
Analgesic supplement to general anesthesia; usually with other agents (ultra–short-acting barbiturates, neuromuscular blocking agents, and inhalation anesthetics) to produce balanced anesthesia. Induction/maintenance of anesthesia (with oxygen or oxygen/nitrous oxide and a neuromuscular blocking agents). Neuroleptanalgesia/neuroleptanesthesia (with or without nitrous oxide). Supplement to regional/local anesthesia. Preoperative and postoperative analgesia. **Unlabeled Use:** Continuous IV infusion as part of PCA.

Action
Binds to opiate receptors in the CNS, altering the response to and perception of pain. Produces CNS depression. **Therapeutic Effects:** Supplement in anesthesia. Decreased pain.

Pharmacokinetics
Absorption: Well absorbed after IM administration.
Distribution: Unknown.
Metabolism and Excretion: Mostly metabolized by the liver, 10–25% excreted unchanged by the kidneys.
Half-life: Children: Bolus dose—2.4 hr, long-term continuous infusion—11–36 hr; Adults:

fentanyl (parenteral)

2–4 hr (increased after cardiopulmonary bypass and in geriatric patients).

TIME/ACTION PROFILE (analgesia*)

ROUTE	ONSET	PEAK	DURATION
IM	7–15 min	20–30 min	1–2 hr
IV	1–2 min	3–5 min	0.5–1 hr

*Respiratory depression may last longer than analgesia

Contraindications/Precautions
Contraindicated in: Hypersensitivity; cross-sensitivity among agents may occur; Known intolerance.
Use Cautiously in: Geri: Geriatric, debilitated, or critically ill patients; Diabetes; Severe renal, pulmonary or hepatic disease; CNS tumors; ↑ intracranial pressure; Head trauma; Adrenal insufficiency; Undiagnosed abdominal pain; Hypothyroidism; Alcoholism; Cardiac disease (arrhythmias); OB, Lactation: Pregnancy and lactation.

Adverse Reactions/Side Effects
CNS: confusion, paradoxical excitation/delirium, postoperative depression, postoperative drowsiness. **EENT:** blurred/double vision. **Resp:** APNEA, LARYNGOSPASM, allergic bronchospasm, respiratory depression. **CV:** arrhythmias, bradycardia, circulatory depression, hypotension. **GI:** biliary spasm, nausea/vomiting. **Derm:** facial itching. **MS:** skeletal and thoracic muscle rigidity (with rapid IV infusion).

Interactions
Drug-Drug: Avoid use in patients who have received **MAO inhibitors** within the previous 14 days (may produce unpredictable, potentially fatal reactions). Concomitant use of **CYP3A4 inhibitors** including **ritonavir**, **ketoconazole**, **itraconazole**, **clarithromycin**, **nelfinavir**, **nefazodone**, **diltiazem**, **aprepitant**, **fluconazole**, **fosamprenavir**, **verapamil**, and **erythromycin** may result in ↑ plasma levels and ↑ risk of CNS and respiratory depression. Additive CNS and respiratory depression with other **CNS depressants**, including **alcohol**, **antihistamines**, **antidepressants**, other **sedative/hypnotics**, and other **opioid analgesics**. ↑ risk of hypotension with **benzodiazepines**. **Nalbuphine**, **buprenorphine**, or **pentazocine** may ↓ analgesia.
Drug-Food: **Grapefruit juice** is a moderate inhibitor of the CYP3A4 enzyme system; concurrent use may ↑ blood levels and the risk of respiratory and CNS depression. Careful monitoring and dose adjustment is recommended.

Route/Dosage
Preoperative Use
IM, IV (Adults and Children > 12 yr): 50–100 mcg 30–60 min before surgery.

Adjunct to General Anesthesia
IM, IV (Adults and Children > 12 yr): *Low dose–minor surgery*—2 mcg/kg. *Moderate dose–major surgery*—2–20 mcg/kg. *High dose–major surgery*—20–50 mcg/kg.

Adjunct to Regional Anesthesia
IM, IV (Adults and Children > 12 yr): 50–100 mcg.

Postoperative Use (Recovery Room)
IM, IV (Adults and Children > 12 yr): 50–100 mcg; may repeat in 1–2 hr.

General Anesthesia
IV (Adults and Children > 12 yr): 50–100 mcg/kg (up to 150 mcg/kg).
IV (Children 1–12 yr): 2–3 mcg/kg.

Sedation/Analgesia
IV (Adults and Children > 12 yr): 0.5–1 mcg/kg/dose, may repeat after 30–60 min.
IV (Children 1–12 yr): *Bolus*—1–2 mcg/kg/dose, may repeat at 30–60 min intervals. *Continuous infusion*—1–5 mcg/kg/hr following bolus dose.
IV (Neonates): *Bolus*—0.5–3 mcg/kg/dose. *Continuous infusion*—0.5–2 mcg/kg/hr following bolus dose. *Continuous infusion during ECMO*—5–10 mcg/kg bolus followed by 1–5 mcg/kg/hr, may require up to 20 mcg/kg/hr after 5 days of therapy.

Availability (generic available)
Injection: 0.05 mg/mL.

NURSING IMPLICATIONS
Assessment
- Monitor respiratory rate and blood pressure frequently throughout therapy. Report significant changes immediately. The respiratory depressant effects of fentanyl may last longer than the analgesic effects. Initial doses of other opioids should be reduced by 25–33% of the usually recommended dose. Monitor closely.
- Geri: Opioids have been associated with increased risk of falls in geriatric patients. Assess risk and implement fall prevention strategies.
- **IV, IM:** Assess type, location, and intensity of pain before and 30 min after IM administration or 3–5 min after IV administration when fentanyl is used to treat pain.

fentanyl (parenteral)

- **Lab Test Considerations:** May cause ↑ serum amylase and lipase concentrations.
- **Toxicity and Overdose:** Symptoms of toxicity include respiratory depression, hypotension, arrhythmias, bradycardia, and asystole. Atropine may be used to treat bradycardia. If respiratory depression persists after surgery, prolonged mechanical ventilation may be required. If an opioid antagonist is required to reverse respiratory depression or coma, naloxone (Narcan) is the antidote. Dilute the 0.4-mg ampule of naloxone in 10 mL of 0.9% NaCl and administer 0.5 mL (0.02 mg) by direct IV push every 2 min. Pedi: For children and patients weighing <40 kg, dilute 0.1 mg of naloxone in 10 mL of 0.9% NaCl for a concentration of 10 mcg/mL and administer 0.5 mcg/kg every 2 min. Titrate dose to avoid withdrawal, seizures, and severe pain. Administration of naloxone in these circumstances, especially in cardiac patients, has resulted in hypertension and tachycardia, occasionally causing left ventricular failure and pulmonary edema.

Potential Nursing Diagnoses
Acute pain (Indications)
Ineffective breathing pattern (Adverse Reactions)
Risk for injury (Side Effects)

Implementation
- **High Alert:** Accidental overdosage of opioid analgesics has resulted in fatalities. Before administering, clarify all ambiguous orders; have second practitioner independently check original order, dose calculations, route of administration, and infusion pump programming. Do not confuse fentanyl with alfentanil or sufentanil.
- Benzodiazepines may be administered before or after administration of fentanyl to reduce the induction dose requirements, decrease the time to loss of consciousness, and produce amnesia. This combination may also increase the risk of hypotension.
- **High Alert:** Opioid antagonists, oxygen, and resuscitative equipment should be readily available during the administration of fentanyl. Fentanyl derivatives should be administered IV only in monitored anesthesia care settings (operating room, emergency department, ICU) with immediate access to life-support equipment and should be administered only by personnel trained in resuscitation and emergency airway management.

IV Administration
- **Direct IV:** *Diluent:* Administer undiluted. *Concentration:* 50 mcg/mL. *Rate:* Injections should be administered slowly over 1–3 min. Administer doses > 5 mcg/kg over 5–10 min. Slow IV administration may reduce the incidence and severity of muscle rigidity, bradycardia, or hypotension. Neuromuscular blocking agents may be administered concurrently to decrease chest wall muscle rigidity.
- **Intermittent Infusion:** *Diluent:* May be diluted in D5W or 0.9% NaCl. *Concentration:* Up to 50 mcg/mL. *Rate:* see Direct IV.
- **Y-Site Compatibility:** acyclovir, alfentanil, alprostadil, amikacin, aminophylline, amiodarone, amphotericin cholesteryl, amphotericin B liposome, anidulafungin, argatroban, ascorbic acid, atracurium, atropine, azathioprine, aztreonam, benztropine, bivalirudin, bumetanide, calcium chloride, calcium gluconate, carboplatin, caspofungin, cefazolin, cefonocid, cefoperazone, cefotaxime, cefotetan, cefoxitin, ceftazidime, ceftozoxime, ceftriaxone, cefuroxime, chloramphenicol, chlorpromazine, cimetidine, cisatracurium, cisplatin, clindamycin, cyanocobalamin, cyclophosphamide, cyclosporine, cytarabine, dactinomycin, daptomycin, dexamethasone, dexmedetomidine, digoxin, diltiazem, diphenhydramine, dobutamine, docetaxel, dopamine, doripenem, doxacurium, doxapram, doxorubicin, doxycycline, enalaprilat, ephedrine, epinephrine, epirubicin, epoetin alfa, eptifibatide, erythromycin, esmolol, etomidate, etoposide, etoposide phosphate, famotidine, fenoldopam, fluconazole, fludarabine, fluorouracil, folic acid, furosemide, ganciclovir, gemcitabine, gentamicin, glycopyrrolate, granisetron, heparin, hetastarch, hydrocortisone, hydromorphone, idarubicin, ifosfamide, imipenem/cilastatin, inamrinone, insulin, isoproterenol, ketorolac, labetalol, levofloxacin, lidocaine, linezolid, lorazepam, magnesium sulfate, mannitol, mechlorethamine, meperidine, metaraminol, methotrexate, methotrimeprazine, methoxamine, methyldopate, methylpresnisolone, metoclopramide, metoprolol, metronidazole, midazolam, milrinone, mitoxantrone, morphine, multivitamins, nafcillin, naloxone, nesiritide, nicardipine, nitroglycerin, nitroprusside, norepinephrine, octreotide, ondansetron, oxacillin, oxaliplatin, oxytocin, paclitaxel, palonosetron, pancuronium, papaverine, pemetrexed,

✱ = Canadian drug name. ▤ = Genetic implication.
*CAPITALS indicates life-threatening; underlines indicate most frequent.

fentanyl (transdermal)

penicillin G, pentamidine, pentobarbital, phenobarbital, phentolamine, phenylephrine, phytonadione, pipercaillin/tazobactam, potassium chloride, procainamide, prochlorperazine, promethazine, propofol, propranolol, protamine, quinupristin/dalfopristin, ranitidine, remifentanil, rituximab, rocuronium, sargramostim, scopolamine, sodium acetate, sodium bicarbonate, streptokinase, succinylcholine, sufentanil, tacrolimus, teniposide, theophylline, thiamine, thiopental, thiotepa, ticarcillin/clavulanate, tigecycline, tirofiban, tobramycin, tolazoline, trastuzumab, trimetaphan, urokinase, vancomycin, vasopressin., vecuronium, verapamil, vincristine, vinorelbine, vitamin B complex with C, voriconazole.

- **Y-Site Incompatibility:** azithromycin, dantrolene, diazoxide, pantoprazole, phenytoin, trimethoprim/sulfamethoxazole.
- **Additive Compatibility:** bupivacaine, caffeine citrate, ropivacaine.

Patient/Family Teaching
- Discuss the use of anesthetic agents and the sensations to expect with the patient before surgery.
- Explain pain assessment scale to patient.
- Caution patient to change positions slowly to minimize orthostatic hypotension. Geri: Geriatric patients may be a greater risk for orthostatic hypotension and, consequently, falls. Teach patient to take precautions until drug effects have completely resolved.
- Medication causes dizziness and drowsiness. Advise patient to call for assistance during ambulation and transfer and to avoid driving or other activities requiring alertness for 24 hr after administration during outpatient surgery.
- Instruct patient to avoid alcohol or other CNS depressants for 24 hr after administration for outpatient surgery.

Evaluation/Desired Outcomes
- General quiescence.
- Reduced motor activity.
- Pronounced analgesia.

HIGH ALERT

fentanyl (transdermal)
(fen-ta-nil)
Duragesic

Classification
Therapeutic: opioid analgesics, anesthetic adjuncts
Pharmacologic: opioid agonists

Schedule II

Pregnancy Category C

Indications
Moderate to severe chronic pain requiring continuous opioid analgesic therapy for an extended time at a dose of 25 mcg/hr or more of the transdermal system. Transdermal fentanyl is not recommended for the control of postoperative, mild, or intermittent pain, nor should it be used for short-term pain relief.

Action
Binds to opiate receptors in the CNS, altering the response to and perception of pain. **Therapeutic Effects:** Decrease in severity of chronic pain.

Pharmacokinetics
Absorption: Well absorbed (92% of dose) through skin surface under transdermal patch, creating a depot in the upper skin layers. Release from transdermal system into systemic circulation ↑ gradually to a constant rate, providing continuous delivery for 72 hr.
Distribution: Crosses the placenta; enters breast milk.
Metabolism and Excretion: Mostly metabolized by the liver (CYP3A4 enzyme system); 10–25% excreted unchanged by the kidneys.
Half-life: 17 hr after removal of a single application patch, ↑ to 21 hr after removal of multiple patches (because of continued release from deposition of drug in skin layers).

TIME/ACTION PROFILE (decreased pain)

ROUTE	ONSET	PEAK	DURATION
Transdermal	6 hr†	12–24 hr	72 hr‡

†Achievement of blood levels associated with analgesia. Maximal response and dose titration may take up to 6 days
‡While patch is worn

Contraindications/Precautions
Contraindicated in: Hypersensitivity to fentanyl or adhesives; Known intolerance; Acute pain (onset not rapid enough); Postoperative pain; Mild or intermittent pain; Alcohol intolerance (small amounts of alcohol released into skin); OB: Not recommended during labor and delivery; Lactation: May cause adverse affects in infant.
Use Cautiously in: Diabetes; Patients with severe pulmonary or hepatic disease; CNS tumors; ↑ intracranial pressure; Head trauma; Adrenal

fentanyl (transdermal)

insufficiency; Undiagnosed abdominal pain; Hypothyroidism; Alcoholism; Cardiac disease (particularly bradyarrhythmias); Fever or situations that increase body temperature (↑ release of fentanyl from delivery system); Titration period (additional analgesics may be required); Cachectic or debilitated patients (dose reduction suggested because of altered drug disposition); Pedi: Safety not established for children <2 yr; pediatric patients initiating therapy at 25 mcg/hr should be opioid tolerant and receiving at least 60 mg oral morphine equivalents per day; Geri: Dose reduction suggested due to altered drug disposition.

Adverse Reactions/Side Effects
CNS: confusion, sedation, weakness, dizziness, restlessness. **Resp:** APNEA, bronchoconstriction, laryngospasm, respiratory depression. **CV:** bradycardia. **GI:** anorexia, constipation, dry mouth, nausea, vomiting. **Derm:** sweating, erythema. **Local:** application site reactions. **MS:** skeletal and thoracic muscle rigidity. **Misc:** physical dependence, psychological dependence.

Interactions
Drug-Drug: Avoid use in patients who have received **MAO inhibitors** within the previous 14 days (may produce unpredictable, potentially fatal reactions). Concomitant use of **CYP3A4 inhibitors** including **ritonavir, ketoconazole, itraconazole, clarithromycin, nelfinavir, nefazodone, diltiazem, aprepitant, fluconazole, fosamprenavir, verapamil,** and **erythromycin** may result in ↑ plasma levels and ↑ risk of CNS and respiratory depression. Levels and effectiveness may be ↓ by **drugs that induce the CYP3A4 enzyme.** ↑ CNS and respiratory depression with other **CNS depressants**, including **alcohol, antihistamines, antidepressants, sedative/hypnotics,** and other **opioids.**
Drug-Natural Products: Concomitant use of **kava-kava, valerian,** or **chamomile** can ↑ CNS depression.
Drug-Food: Grapefruit juice is a moderate inhibitor of the CYP3A4 enzyme system; concurrent use may ↑ blood levels and the risk of respiratory and CNS depression. Careful monitoring and dose adjustment is recommended.

Route/Dosage
Transdermal (Adults): 25 mcg/hr is the initial dose; patients who have not been receiving opioids should receive not more that 25 mcg/hr. To calculate the dose of transdermal fentanyl required in patients who are already receiving opioid analgesics, assess the 24-hr requirement of currently used opioid. Using the equianalgesic table in Appendix K, convert this to an equivalent amount of morphine/24 hr. Conversion to fentanyl transdermal may be accomplished by using the fentanyl conversion table (Appendix K). During dose titration, additional short-acting opioids should be available for any breakthrough pain that may occur. Morphine 10 mg IM or 60 mg PO q 4 hr (60 mg/24 hr IM or 360 mg/24 hr PO) is considered to be approximately equivalent to transdermal fentanyl 100 mcg/hr. Transdermal patch lasts 72 hr in most patients. Some patients require a new patch every 48 hr.

Transdermal (Adults >60 yr, Debilitated, or Cachectic Patients): Initial dose should be 25 mcg/hr unless previous opioid use was >135 mg morphine PO/day (or other opioid equivalent).

Availability (generic available)
Transdermal systems: 12 mcg/hr, 25 mcg/hr, 50 mcg/hr, 75 mcg/hr, 100 mcg/hr.

NURSING IMPLICATIONS

Assessment
- Assess type, location, and intensity of pain before and 24 hr after application and periodically during therapy. Monitor pain frequently during initiation of therapy and dose changes to assess need for supplementary analgesics for breakthrough pain.
- Assess blood pressure, pulse, and respirations before and periodically during administration. If respiratory rate is <10/min, assess level of sedation. Physical stimulation may be sufficient to prevent significant hypoventilation. Dose may need to be decreased by 25–50%. Initial drowsiness will diminish with continued use.
- Prolonged use may lead to physical and psychological dependence and tolerance. This should not prevent patient from receiving adequate analgesia. Most patients who receive opioid analgesics for pain do not develop psychological dependence.
- Progressively higher doses may be required to relieve pain with long-term therapy. It may take up to 6 days after increasing doses to reach equilibrium, so patients should wear higher dose through 2 applications before increasing dose again.
- Assess bowel function routinely. Prevent constipation with increased intake of fluids and bulk, and laxatives to minimize constipating effects.

Administer stimulant laxatives routinely if opioid use exceeds 2–3 days, unless contraindicated.
- **Lab Test Considerations:** May ↑ plasma amylase and lipase levels.
- **Toxicity and Overdose:** If an opioid antagonist is required to reverse respiratory depression or coma, naloxone (Narcan) is the antidote. Dilute the 0.4-mg ampule of naloxone in 10 mL of 0.9% NaCl and administer 0.5 mL (0.02 mg) by direct IV push every 2 min. For patients weighing <40 kg, dilute 0.1 mg of naloxone in 10 mL of 0.9% NaCl for a concentration of 10 mcg/mL and administer 0.5 mcg/kg every 2 min. Titrate dose to avoid withdrawal, seizures, and severe pain. Monitor patient closely; dose may need to be repeated or may need to be administered as an infusion because of long duration of action despite removal of patch.

Potential Nursing Diagnoses
Chronic pain (Indications)
Risk for injury (Side Effects)

Implementation
- **High Alert:** Accidental overdose of opioid analgesics has resulted in fatalities. Before administering, confirm patient is opioid tolerant and clarify ambiguous orders; have second practitioner independently check original order and dose calculations.
- Duragesic-12 delivers 12.5 mcg/hr of fentanyl. Use supplemental doses of short-acting opioid analgesics to manage pain until relief is obtained with the transdermal system. Patients may continue to require supplemental opioids for breakthrough pain. If >100 mcg/hr is required, use multiple transdermal systems.
- Titrate dose based on patient's report of pain until adequate analgesia (50% reduction in patient's pain rating on numerical or visual analogue scale or patient reports satisfactory relief) is attained. Determine dose by calculating the previous 24-hr analgesic requirement and converting to the equianalgesic morphine dose using Appendix K. The conversion ratio from morphine to transdermal fentanyl is conservative; 50% of patients may require a dose increase after initial application. Increase after 3 days based on required daily doses of supplemental analgesics. Increases should be based on ratio of 45 mg/24 hr of oral morphine to 12.5 mcg/hr increase in transdermal fentanyl dose.
- Coadministration with nonopioid analgesics may have additive analgesic effects and permit lower opioid doses.
- To convert to another opioid analgesic, remove transdermal fentanyl system and begin treatment with half the equianalgesic dose of the new analgesic in 12–18 hr.
- Medication should be discontinued gradually after long-term use to prevent withdrawal symptoms.
- **Transdermal:** Apply system to flat, nonirritated, and nonirradiated site such as chest, back, flank, or upper arm. If skin preparation is necessary, use clear water and clip, do not shave, hair. Allow skin to dry completely before application. Apply immediately after removing from package. Do not alter the system (i.e., cut) in any way before application. Remove liner from adhesive layer and press firmly in place with palm of hand for 30 sec, especially around the edges, to make sure contact is complete. Remove used system and fold so that adhesive edges are together. Flush system down toilet immediately on removal. Apply new system to a different site.

Patient/Family Teaching
- Instruct patient in how and when to ask for and take pain medication.
- Instruct patient in correct method for application and disposal of transdermal system. Fatalities have occurred from children having access to improperly discarded patches. May be worn while bathing, showering, or swimming.
- May cause drowsiness or dizziness. Caution patient to call for assistance when ambulating or smoking and to avoid driving or other activities requiring alertness until response to medication is known.
- Advise patient to change positions slowly to minimize dizziness.
- Caution patient to avoid concurrent use of alcohol or other CNS depressants with this medication.
- Advise patient that fever, electric blankets, heating pads, saunas, hot tubs, and heated water beds increase the release of fentanyl from the patch.
- Advise patient that good oral hygiene, frequent mouth rinses, and sugarless gum or candy may decrease dry mouth.
- Advise patient referred for MRI test to discuss patch with referring health care professional and MRI facility to determine if removal of patch is necessary prior to test and for directions for replacing patch.

Evaluation/Desired Outcomes
- Decrease in severity of pain without a significant alteration in level of consciousness, respiratory status, or blood pressure.

---

ferrous fumarate, See IRON SUPPLEMENTS.

---

ferrous gluconate, See IRON SUPPLEMENTS.

---

ferrous sulfate, See IRON SUPPLEMENTS.

---

ferumoxytol (fer-u-mox-y-tole)
Feraheme

Classification
Therapeutic: antianemics
Pharmacologic: iron supplements

Pregnancy Category C

Indications
Treatment of iron deficiency anemia in adult patients with chronic kidney disease (CKD).

Action
Consists of a superparamagnetic iron oxide coated with a carbohydrate shell; when the iron-carbohydrate complex enters the reticuloendothelial system (RES), iron is released from the iron-carbohydrate complex within macrophages. This iron can either enter the intracellular storage iron pool or be transferred to erythroid precursor cells for incorporation into hemoglobin. **Therapeutic Effects:** Improvement in anemia in patients with chronic kidney disease.

Pharmacokinetics
Absorption: IV administration results in complete bioavailability of iron-carboydrate complex, however iron is not liberated until incorporation into RES.
Distribution: Taken up by RES.
Metabolism and Excretion: Iron can either become part of intracellular ferritin or be transferred to erythroid precursor cells.
Half-life: 15 hr.

TIME/ACTION PROFILE (effect on anemia)

ROUTE	ONSET	PEAK	DURATION
IV	unknown	unknown	up to 1 mo

Contraindications/Precautions
Contraindicated in: Hypersensitivity; Evidence of iron overload; Anemia not due to iron deficiency; Lactation: Avoid use during breastfeeding.
Use Cautiously in: MRI; Geri: Consider age-related decrease in hepatic, renal, or cardiac function, and concurrent diseases or other drug therapy; dose cautiously; OB: Use during pregnancy only if potential benefit justifies potential risk to the fetus.; Pedi: Safe and effective use in patients <18 yr not established.

Adverse Reactions/Side Effects
CNS: dizziness. **CV:** hypertension, hypotension, peripheral edema. **GI:** constipation, diarrhea, nausea. **Hemat:** iron overload. **Misc:** hypersensitivity reactions including ANAPHYLAXIS AND ANAPHYLACTOID REACTIONS.

Interactions
Drug-Drug: May ↓ absorption of concurrently administered **oral iron preparations**.

Route/Dosage
IV (Adults ≥ 18yr): 510 mg initially, followed by a second 510-mg IV injection 3 to 8 days later. Course may be repeated after 1 mo.

Availability
Aqueous colloid for intravenous injection: 510-mg elemental iron/17 mL (30 mg/mL) vials.

NURSING IMPLICATIONS
Assessment
- Assess nutritional status and dietary history to determine need for patient teaching.
- Assess bowel function for constipation or diarrhea. Notify health care professional and use appropriate measures should these occur.
- Monitor blood pressure frequently following administration until stable. May cause hypotension. For patients receiving hemodialysis, administer ferumoxytol once the blood pressure is stable and at least 1 hr of hemodialysis has been completed.
- Observe patient for signs and symptoms of anaphylaxis (rash, pruritus, urticaria, laryngeal edema, wheezing) for at least 30 min following injection. Notify health care professional immediately if these occur. Keep epinephrine and re-

suscitation equipment close by in the event of an anaphylactic reaction.
- Conduct MRI studies prior to administration. Alteration of MRI studies may persist for up to 3 mo following a dose; if imaging is required within 3 mo after administration, use T1- or proton density-weighted MR pulse sequences to decrease effects; MRI using T2-weighted pulse sequences should not be performed earlier than 4 weeks after administration; maximum alteration of vascular MRI is evident for 1–2 days after dose. Ferumoxytol does not interfere with x-ray, computed tomography (CT), or positron emission tomography (PET), single photon emission computed tomography (SPECT), ultrasound, or nuclear imaging.
- *Lab Test Considerations:* Monitor hemoglobin, ferritin, iron and transferrin saturation prior to and at least 1 mo following second dose and regularly thereafter. Iron and transferrin bound iron may be overestimated within first 24 hr by measuring iron in the *Fereheme* complex.

Potential Nursing Diagnoses
Activity intolerance

Implementation
- **Intermittent Infusion:** Administer undiluted. Do not administer solutions that are discolored or contain particulate matter. Solution may be stored at room temperature. *Rate:* Administer at a rate of 1 mL/sec (30 mg/sec).

Patient/Family Teaching
- Explain purpose of iron therapy to patient.
- Advise patients to avoid MRI studies during and for 3 mo following ferumoxytol therapy.
- May cause dizziness. Caution patient to avoid driving or other activities requiring alertness until response to medication is known.
- Advise patient to report signs and symptoms of hypersensitivity reactions (rash, itching, dizziness, swelling, and breathing problems) to health care professional immediately.

Evaluation/Desired Outcomes
- Improvement in iron deficiency anemia.

---

fesoterodine
(fee-soe-**ter**-o-deen)
Toviaz

Classification
Therapeutic: urinary tract antispasmodics
Pharmacologic: anticholinergics

Pregnancy Category C

Indications
Treatment of overactive bladder function that results in urinary frequency, urgency, or urge incontinence.

Action
Acts as a competitive muscarinic receptor antagonist resulting in inhibition of cholinergically mediated bladder contraction. **Therapeutic Effects:** Decreased urinary frequency, urgency, and urge incontinence.

Pharmacokinetics
Absorption: Rapidly absorbed following oral administration, but is rapidly converted to its active metabolite (bioavailability of metabolite 52%; further metabolism occurs in the liver via CYP2D6 and CYP3A4 enzyme systems. 16% of active metabolite is excreted in urine, most of the remainder of inactive metabolites are renally excreted. 7% excreted in feces.
Distribution: Unknown.
Metabolism and Excretion: Rapidly converted by esterases to active metabolite.
Half-life: 7 hr (following oral administration).

TIME/ACTION PROFILE (active metabolite)

ROUTE	ONSET	PEAK	DURATION
PO	rapid	5 hr	24 hr

Contraindications/Precautions
Contraindicated in: Hypersensitivity; Urinary retention; Gastric retention; Severe hepatic impairment; Uncontrolled narrow-angle glaucoma.
Use Cautiously in: Significant bladder outlet obstruction (↑ risk of retention); Severe renal insufficiency (dose adjustment required); Decreased GI motility including severe constipation; Treated narrow-angle glaucoma (use only if benefits outweigh risks); Myasthenia gravis; Severe renal impairment (dose should not exceed 4 mg/day); Geri: ↑ risk of anticholinergic side effects in patients >75 yr; OB, Lactation: Avoid using unless potential benefits outweighs potential risk to fetus/neonate; Pedi: Safety in children not established.

Adverse Reactions/Side Effects
CV: tachycardia (dose related). **GI:** dry mouth, constipation, nausea, upper abdominal pain. **GU:** dysuria, urinary retention. **MS:** back pain.

Interactions
Drug-Drug: Concurrent use of **potent CYP3A4 enzyme inhibitors** including **ketoconazole**, **itraconazole**, and **clarithromycin** ↑ blood levels and risk of toxicity; daily dose should not exceed 4 mg. Use **less potent inhibitors of**

CYP3A4 (such as **erythromycin**) with caution; escalate dose carefully. Anticholinergic effects may alter the GI absorption of other drugs.

Route/Dosage
PO (Adults): 4 mg once daily initially may be increased to 8 mg/daily; *concurrent potent CYP3A4 inhibitors or CCr <30 mL/min*—dose should not exceed 4 mg/day.

Availability
Extended-release tablets: 4 mg, 8 mg.

NURSING IMPLICATIONS

Assessment
- Assess patient for urinary urgency, frequency, and urge incontinence periodically throughout therapy.
- *Lab Test Considerations:* May cause ↑ ALT and GGT.

Potential Nursing Diagnoses
Impaired urinary elimination (Indications)
Urinary retention (Indications)

Implementation
- **PO:** Administer without regard to food.
- Extended-release tablets should be swallowed whole; do not break, crush, or chew.

Patient/Family Teaching
- Instruct patient to take fesoterodine as directed. If a dose is missed, omit and begin taking again the next day; do not take 2 doses the same day. Advise patient to read the *Patient Information* sheet prior to initiation of therapy and with each Rx refill.
- May cause drowsiness and blurred vision. Caution patient to avoid driving or other activities requiring alertness until response to medication is known.
- Advise patient to avoid alcohol; may increase drowsiness.
- Advise patient to use caution in hot environments; may cause decreased sweating and severe heat illness.
- Instruct patient to consult health care professional before taking other Rx, OTC, or herbal products.
- Advise patient to notify health care professional if pregnancy is planned or suspected or if breastfeeding.

Evaluation/Desired Outcomes
- Decreased urinary frequency, urgency, and urge incontinence.

fexofenadine 575

fexofenadine
(fex-oh-**fen**-a-deen)
Allegra

Classification
Therapeutic: allergy, cold, and cough remedies, antihistamines

Pregnancy Category C

Indications
Relief of symptoms of seasonal allergic rhinitis. Management of chronic idiopathic urticaria.

Action
Antagonizes the effects of histamine at peripheral histamine–1 (H_1) receptors, including pruritus and urticaria. Also has a drying effect on the nasal mucosa. **Therapeutic Effects:** Decreased sneezing, rhinorrhea, itchy eyes, nose, and throat associated with seasonal allergies. Decreased urticaria.

Pharmacokinetics
Absorption: Rapidly absorbed after oral administration.
Distribution: Unknown.
Metabolism and Excretion: 80% excreted in urine, 11% excreted in feces.
Half-life: 14.4 hr (increased in renal impairment).

TIME/ACTION PROFILE (antihistaminic effect)

ROUTE	ONSET	PEAK	DURATION
PO	within 1 hr	2–3 hr	12–24 hr

Contraindications/Precautions
Contraindicated in: Hypersensitivity.
Use Cautiously in: Impaired renal function (increased dosing interval recommended); OB: use only if maternal benefit outweighs potential risk to fetus; Lactation: Usually compatible with breastfeeding (AAP).

Adverse Reactions/Side Effects
CNS: drowsiness, fatigue. **GI:** dyspepsia. **Endo:** dysmenorrhea.

Interactions
Drug-Drug: Magnesium and aluminum-containing **antacids** ↓ absorption and may decrease effectiveness.
Drug-Food: Apple, **orange**, and **grapefruit juice** ↓ absorption and may decrease effectiveness.

✦ = Canadian drug name. ▒ = Genetic implication.
*CAPITALS indicates life-threatening; underlines indicate most frequent.

576   filgrastim

Route/Dosage
PO (Adults and Children ≥12 yr): 60 mg twice daily, or 180 mg once daily.
PO (Children 2–11 yr): 30 mg twice daily.
PO (Children 6 mo–2 yr): 15 mg twice daily.

Renal Impairment
PO (Adults): 60 mg once daily as a starting dose.
PO (Children 6–11 yr): 30 mg once daily as a starting dose.

Availability (generic available)
Tablets: 30 mg, 60 mg, 180 mg. **Cost:** *Generic*—30 mg $49.97/90, 60 mg $99.97/90, 180 mg $161.97/90. **Suspension (raspberry–cream):** 30 mg/5 mL in 30-mL and 300-mL bottles. **Cost:** $59.07/300 mL. *In combination with:* pseudoephedrine (Allegra-D). See Appendix B.

NURSING IMPLICATIONS

Assessment
- Assess allergy symptoms (rhinitis, conjunctivitis, hives) before and periodically during therapy.
- Assess lung sounds and character of bronchial secretions. Maintain fluid intake of 1500–2000 mL/day to decrease viscosity of secretions.
- *Lab Test Considerations:* Will cause false-negative reactions on allergy skin tests; discontinue 3 days before testing.

Potential Nursing Diagnoses
Ineffective airway clearance (Indications)
Risk for injury (Adverse Reactions)

Implementation
- **PO:** Administer with food or milk to decrease GI irritation. Capsules and tablets should be taken with water or milk, not juice.

Patient/Family Teaching
- Instruct patient to take medication as directed. Take missed doses as soon as remembered unless almost time for next dose.
- Inform patient that drug may cause drowsiness, although it is less likely to occur than with other antihistamines. Avoid driving or other activities requiring alertness until response to drug is known.
- Instruct patient to contact health care professional if symptoms persist.

Evaluation/Desired Outcomes
- Decrease in allergic symptoms.
- Decrease in urticaria.

filgrastim (fil-gra-stim)
Neupogen, G-CSF, granulocyte colony stimulating factor

Classification
Therapeutic: colony-stimulating factors

Pregnancy Category C

Indications
Prevention of febrile neutropenia and associated infection in patients who have received bone marrow–depressing antineoplastics for the treatment of nonmyeloid malignancies. Reduction of time for neutrophil recovery and duration of fever in patients undergoing induction and consolidation chemotherapy for acute myelogenous leukemia. Reduction of time to neutrophil recovery and sequelae of neutropenia in patients with nonmyeloid malignancies undergoing myeloablative chemotherapy followed by bone marrow transplantation. Mobilization of hematopoietic progenitor cells into peripheral blood for collection by leukapheresis. Management of severe chronic neutropenia. **Unlabeled Use:** Neutropenia associated with HIV infection. Neonatal neutropenia.

Action
A glycoprotein, filgrastim binds to and stimulates immature neutrophils to divide and differentiate. Also activates mature neutrophils. **Therapeutic Effects:** Decreased incidence of infection in patients who are neutropenic from chemotherapy or other causes. Improved harvest of progenitor cells for bone marrow transplantation.

Pharmacokinetics
Absorption: Well absorbed after subcut administration.
Distribution: Unknown.
Metabolism and Excretion: Unknown.
Half-life: *Adults*–3.5 hr; *Neonates*-4.4 hr.

TIME/ACTION PROFILE

ROUTE	ONSET	PEAK	DURATION
IV, subcut	unknown	unknown	4 days†

†Return of neutrophil count to baseline

Contraindications/Precautions
Contraindicated in: Hypersensitivity to filgrastim or *Escherichia coli*–derived proteins.
Use Cautiously in: Malignancy with myeloid characteristics; Pre-existing cardiac disease; OB: Use only potential benefit justifies potential risk to fetus; Lactation: Unlikely to adversely affect breastfed infant (NIH).

Adverse Reactions/Side Effects
Hemat: excessive leukocytosis. **Local:** pain, redness at subcut site. **MS:** <u>medullary bone pain</u>.

Interactions
Drug-Drug: Simultaneous use with **antineoplastics** may have adverse effects on rapidly proliferating neutrophils—avoid use for 24 hr before and 24 hr after chemotherapy. **Lithium** may potentiate the release of neutrophils; concurrent use should be undertaken cautiously.

Route/Dosage
After Myelosuppressive Chemotherapy
IV, Subcut (Adults and Children): 5 mcg/kg/day as a single injection daily for up to 2 wk. Dosage may be increased by 5 mcg/kg during each cycle of chemotherapy, depending on blood counts.

After Bone Marrow Transplantation
IV, Subcut (Adults): 10 mcg/kg/day as a 4- or 24-hr IV infusion or as a continuous subcut infusion; initiate at least 24 hr after chemotherapy and at least 24 hr after bone marrow transplantation. Subsequent dosage is adjusted according to blood counts.

Peripheral Blood Progenitor Cell Collection and Therapy
Subcut (Adults): 10 mcg/kg/day as a bolus or continuous infusion for at least 4 days before first leukapheresis and continued until last leukapheresis; dosage modification suggested if WBC >100,000 cells/mm^3.

Severe Chronic Neutropenia
Subcut (Adults): *Congenital neutropenia*—6 mcg/kg twice daily. *Idiopathic/cyclical neutropenia*—5 mcg/kg daily (decrease if ANC remains >10,000/mm^3).

Neonatal neutropenia
IV, Subcut (Neonates): 5–10 mcg/kg/day once daily for 3–5 days.

Availability
Injection: 300 mcg/mL in 1- and 1.6-mL vials.

NURSING IMPLICATIONS

Assessment
- Monitor heart rate, blood pressure, and respiratory status before and periodically during therapy.
- Assess bone pain throughout therapy. Pain is usually mild to moderate and controllable with nonopioid analgesics, but may require treatment with opioid analgesics, especially in patients receiving high-dose IV therapy.
- ***Lab Test Considerations:*** *After chemotherapy,* obtain a CBC with differential, including examination for the presence of blast cells, and platelet count before chemotherapy and twice weekly during therapy to avoid leukocytosis. Monitor ANC. A transient rise is seen 1–2 days after initiation of therapy, but therapy should not be discontinued until ANC >10,000/mm^3.
- *After bone marrow transplant,* the daily dose is titrated by the neutrophil response. When the ANC is >1000/mm^3 for 3 consecutive days, the dose should be reduced by 5 mcg/kg/day. If the ANC remains >1000/mm^3 for 3 or more consecutive days, filgrastim is discontinued. If the ANC decreases to <1000/mm^3, filgrastim should be resumed at 5 mcg/kg/day.
- *For chronic severe neutropenia,* monitor CBC with differential and platelet count twice weekly during initial 4 wk of therapy and during 2 wk after any dose adjustment.
- May cause ↓ platelet count and transient increases in uric acid, LDH, and alkaline phosphatase concentrations.

Potential Nursing Diagnoses
Risk for infection (Indications)
Acute pain (Side Effects)

Implementation
- Administer no earlier than 24 hr after cytotoxic chemotherapy, at least 24 hr after bone marrow infusion, and not during the 24 hr before administration of chemotherapy.
- Refrigerate; do not freeze. Do not shake. May warm to room temperature for up to 6 hr before injection. Discard if left at room temperature for >6 hr. Vial is for 1-time use only.
- **Subcut:** If dose requires >1 mL of solution, may be divided into 2 injection sites.
- May also be administered as a continuous subcut infusion over 24 hr after bone marrow transplantation.

IV Administration
- **Continuous Infusion:** ***Diluent:*** Dilute in D5W. Refrigerate; do not freeze. Do not shake. May warm to room temperature for up to 6 hr before injection. Vial is for 1-time use only.
Concentration: Dilute to a final concentration of at least 15 mcg/mL. If the final concen-

tration is <15 mcg/mL, human albumin in a concentration of 2 mg/mL must be added to D5W before filgrastim to prevent adsorption of the components of the drug delivery system.
Rate: *After chemotherapy* dose is administered via infusion over 15–60 min.
- *After chemotherapy* dose may also be administered as a continuous infusion.
- *After bone marrow transplant,* dose should be administered as an infusion over 4 or 24 hr.
- **Y-Site Compatibility:** acyclovir, allopurinol, amikacin, aminophylline, ampicillin, ampicillin/sulbactam, aztreonam, bleomycin, bumetanide, buprenorphine, butorphanol, calcium gluconate, carboplatin, carmustine, cefazolin, cefotetan, ceftazidime, chlorpromazine, cimetidine, cisplatin, cyclophosphamide, cytarabine, dacarbazine, daunorubicin, dexamethasone, diphenhydramine, doxorubicin, doxycycline, droperidol, enalaprilat, famotidine, floxuridine, fluconazole, fludarabine, ganciclovir, granisetron, haloperidol, hydrocortisone, hydromorphone, idarubicin, ifosfamide, leucovorin calcium, lorazepam, mechlorethamine, melphalan, meperidine, mesna, methotrexate, metoclopramide, mitoxantrone, morphine, nalbuphine, ondansetron, potassium chloride, promethazine, ranitidine, sodium bicarbonate, streptozocin, ticarcillin/clavulanate, tobramycin, trimethoprim/sulfamethoxazole, vancomycin, vinblastine, vincristine, vinorelbine, zidovudine.
- **Y-Site Incompatibility:** amphotericin B, cefepime., cefotaxime, cefoxitin, ceftizoxime, ceftriaxone, cefuroxime, clindamycin, dactinomycin, etoposide, fluorouracil, furosemide, heparin, mannitol, methylprednisolone sodium succinate, metronidazole, mitomycin, piperacillin, prochlorperazine, thiotepa.

Patient/Family Teaching
- **Home Care Issues:** Instruct patient on correct technique and proper disposal for home administration. Caution patient not to reuse needle, vial, or syringe. Provide patient with a puncture-proof container for needle and syringe disposal.

Evaluation/Desired Outcomes
- Decreased incidence of infection in patients who receive bone marrow–depressing antineoplastics.
- Reduction of duration and sequelae of neutropenia after bone marrow transplantation.
- Reduction of the incidence and duration of sequelae of neutropenia in patients with severe chronic neutropenia.

- Improved harvest of progenitor cells for bone marrow transplantation.

finasteride (fi-**nas**-teer-ide)
Propecia, Proscar

Classification
Therapeutic: hair regrowth stimulants
Pharmacologic: androgen inhibitors

Pregnancy Category X

Indications
Benign prostatic hyperplasia (BPH); can be used with doxazosin. Androgenetic alopecia (male pattern baldness) in men only.

Action
Inhibits the enzyme 5-alpha-reductase, which is responsible for converting testosterone to its potent metabolite 5-alpha-dihydrotestosterone in prostate, liver, and skin; 5-alpha-dihydrotestosterone is partially responsible for prostatic hyperplasia and hair loss. **Therapeutic Effects:** Reduced prostate size with associated decrease in urinary symptoms. Decreases hair loss; promotes hair regrowth.

Pharmacokinetics
Absorption: Well absorbed after oral administration (63%).
Distribution: Enters prostatic tissue and crosses the blood-brain barrier. Remainder of distribution not known.
Protein Binding: 90%.
Metabolism and Excretion: Mostly metabolized; 39% excreted in urine as metabolites; 57% excreted in feces.
Half-life: 6 hr (range 6–15 hr; slightly increased in patients >70 yr).

TIME/ACTION PROFILE (reduction in dihydrotestosterone levels†)

ROUTE	ONSET	PEAK	DURATION
PO	rapid	8 hr	2 wk

†Clinical effects as noted by urinary tract symptoms and hair regrowth may not be evident for several months and remain for 4 mo after discontinuation

Contraindications/Precautions
Contraindicated in: Hypersensitivity; Women.
Use Cautiously in: Patients with hepatic impairment or obstructive uropathy.

Adverse Reactions/Side Effects
GU: decreased libido, decreased volume of ejaculate, erectile dysfunction.

Interactions
Drug-Drug: None noted.

Route/Dosage
PO (Adults): *BPH*—5 mg once daily (Proscar); *androgenetic alopecia*—1 mg/day (Propecia).

Availability (generic available)
Tablets: 1 mg (Propecia), 5 mg (Proscar). **Cost:** *Propecia*—1 mg $177.97/90; *Generic*—5 mg $199.98/90.

NURSING IMPLICATIONS
Assessment
- Assess for symptoms of prostatic hyperplasia (urinary hesitancy, feeling of incomplete bladder emptying, interruption of urinary stream, impairment of size and force of urinary stream, terminal urinary dribbling, straining to start flow, dysuria, urgency) before and periodically during therapy.
- Digital rectal examinations should be performed before and periodically during therapy for BPH.
- **Lab Test Considerations:** Serum prostate-specific antigen (PSA) concentrations, which are used to screen for prostate cancer, may be evaluated before and periodically during therapy. Finasteride may cause a ↓ in serum PSA levels.

Potential Nursing Diagnoses
Impaired urinary elimination (Indications)

Implementation
- **PO:** Administer once daily with or without meals.

Patient/Family Teaching
- Instruct patient to take finasteride as directed, even if symptoms improve or are unchanged. At least 6–12 mo of therapy may be necessary to determine whether or not an individual will respond to finasteride.
- Inform patient that the volume of ejaculate may be decreased during therapy but that this will not interfere with normal sexual function. Sexual dysfunction side effects will diminish over time.
- Caution patient that finasteride poses a potential risk to a male fetus. Women who are pregnant or may become pregnant should avoid exposure to semen of a partner taking finasteride and should not handle crushed finasteride because of the potential for absorption.
- Emphasize the importance of periodic follow-up exams to determine whether a clinical response has occurred.

Evaluation/Desired Outcomes
- Decrease in urinary symptoms of benign prostatic hyperplasia.
- Hair regrowth in androgenetic alopecia. Evidence of hair growth usually requires 3 mo or longer. Continued use is recommended to sustain benefit. Withdrawal leads to reversal of effect within 12 mo.

---

flecainide (flek-a-nide)
Tambocor

Classification
Therapeutic: antiarrhythmics (class IC)

Pregnancy Category C

Indications
Life-threatening ventricular arrhythmias, including ventricular tachycardia. Supraventricular tachyarrhythmias including: Paroxysmal supraventricular tachycardia (PSVT), Paroxysmal atrial fibrillation/flutter (PAF). **Unlabeled Use:** Single dose treatment of atrial fibrillation.

Action
Slows conduction in cardiac tissue by altering transport of ions across cell membranes. **Therapeutic Effects:** Suppression of arrhythmias.

Pharmacokinetics
Absorption: Well absorbed from the GI tract following oral administration.
Distribution: Widely distributed.
Metabolism and Excretion: Mostly metabolized by liver; 30% excreted unchanged by kidneys.
Half-life: 11–14 hr.

TIME/ACTION PROFILE (antiarrhythmic effects)

ROUTE	ONSET	PEAK	DURATION
PO	days	days–weeks	12 hr

Contraindications/Precautions
Contraindicated in: Hypersensitivity; Cardiogenic shock.
Use Cautiously in: CHF (dosage reduction may be required); Pre-existing sinus node dysfunction or 2nd- or 3rd-degree heart block (without a pacemaker); Renal impairment (dosage reduc-

flecainide

tion required if CCr <35 mL/min); OB: Teratogenic in animal studies; use only if potential benefit justifies potential risk to fetus; Lactation: Usually compatible with breast feeding (AAP).

Adverse Reactions/Side Effects
CNS: dizziness, anxiety, fatigue, headache, mental depression. **EENT:** blurred vision, visual disturbances. **CV:** ARRHYTHMIAS, CHEST PAIN, CHF. **GI:** anorexia, constipation, drug-induced hepatitis, nausea, stomach pain, vomiting. **Derm:** rashes. **Neuro:** tremor.

Interactions
Drug-Drug: ↑ risk of arrhythmias with other **antiarrhythmics**, including **calcium channel blockers**. **Disopyramide**, **beta blockers**, or **verapamil** may have ↑ myocardial depressant effects; combination use should be undertaken cautiously. **Amiodarone** doubles serum flecainide levels (↓ flecainide dose by 50%). Increases serum **digoxin** levels by a small amount (15–25%). Concurrent **beta blocker** therapy may cause ↑ levels of beta blocker and flecainide. **Alkalinizing agents** promote reabsorption, ↑ blood levels, and may cause toxicity. **Acidifying agents** ↑ renal elimination and may ↓ effectiveness of flecainide (if urine pH <5).
Drug-Food: Foods that ↑ urine pH to >7 result in ↑ levels (strict **vegetarian diet**). Foods or beverages that ↓ urine pH to <5 ↑ renal elimination and may ↓ effectiveness of flecainide (**acidic juices**).

Route/Dosage
Ventricular Tachycardia
PO (Adults): 100 mg q 12 hr initially, increased by 50 mg bid until response is obtained or maximum total daily dose of 400 mg is reached. Some patients may require q 8 hr dosing.

Renal Impairment
PO (Adults): *CCr <35 mL/min*—100 mg once a day or 50 mg q 12 hr initially; further dosing on the basis of frequent blood level monitoring.

PSVT/PAF
PO (Adults): 50 mg q 12 hr initially, increased by 50 mg bid until response is obtained or maximum total daily dose of 300 mg is reached. Some patients may require q 8 hr dosing.

Atrial Fibrillation (unlabeled)
PO (Adults): 200 mg or 300 mg single dose.

Availability (generic available)
Tablets: 50 mg, 100 mg, 150 mg.

NURSING IMPLICATIONS
Assessment
- Monitor ECG or Holter monitor prior to and periodically during therapy. May cause QRS widening, PR prolongation, and QT prolongation.
- Monitor blood pressure and pulse periodically during therapy.
- Monitor intake and output ratios and daily weight. Assess patient for signs of CHF (peripheral edema, rales/crackles, dyspnea, weight gain, jugular venous distention).
- *Lab Test Considerations:* Evaluate renal, pulmonary, and hepatic functions and CBC periodically on patients receiving long-term therapy. Flecainide should be discontinued if bone marrow depression occurs.
- May cause ↑ in serum alkaline phosphatase during prolonged therapy.
- *Toxicity and Overdose:* Therapeutic blood levels range from 0.2 to 1.0 mcg/mL. Monitor plasma trough levels frequently during dose adjustment in patients with severe renal or hepatic disease or in patients with CHF and moderate renal impairment.

Potential Nursing Diagnoses
Decreased cardiac output (Adverse Reactions)

Implementation
- Previous antiarrhythmic therapy (except lidocaine) should be withdrawn 2–4 half-lives before starting flecainide.
- Therapy should be initiated in a hospital setting to monitor for increase in arrhythmias.
- Dose adjustments should be at least 4 days apart because of the long half-life of flecainide.
- **PO:** May be administered with meals if GI irritation becomes a problem.

Patient/Family Teaching
- Instruct patient to take medication around the clock as directed at evenly spaced intervals, even if feeling better. Take missed doses as soon as remembered if within 6 hr; omit if remembered later. Gradual dosage reduction may be necessary.
- May cause dizziness or visual disturbances. Caution patient to avoid driving and other activities requiring alertness until response to medication is known.
- Advise patient to notify health care professional of medication regimen prior to treatment or surgery.
- Instruct patient to notify health care professional if chest pain, shortness of breath, or diaphoresis occurs.

fluconazole **581**

- Advise patient to carry identification describing disease process and medication regimen at all times.
- Emphasize the importance of follow-up exams to monitor progress.

TIME/ACTION PROFILE (blood levels)

ROUTE	ONSET	PEAK	DURATION
PO	unknown	2–4 hr	24 hr
IV	rapid	end of infusion	24 hr

Evaluation/Desired Outcomes

- Decrease in frequency of life-threatening ventricular arrhythmias.
- Decrease in supraventricular tachyarrhythmias.

Contraindications/Precautions

Contraindicated in: Hypersensitivity to fluconazole or other azole antifungals; Concurrent use with pimozide.
Use Cautiously in: Renal impairment (dose reduction required if CCr <50 mL/min); Underlying liver disease; OB: Safety not established; Lactation: Usually compatible with breastfeeding (AAP); Geri: Increased risk of adverse reactions (rash, vomiting, diarrhea, seizures); consider age-related decrease in renal function in determining dose.

fluconazole (floo-**kon**-a-zole)
Diflucan

Classification
Therapeutic: antifungals (systemic)

Pregnancy Category C

Indications
PO, IV: Fungal infections caused by susceptible organisms, including: Oropharyngeal or esophageal candidiasis, Serious systemic candidal infections, Urinary tract infections, Peritonitis, Cryptococcal meningitis. Prevention of candidiasis in patients who have undergone bone marrow transplantation. **PO:** Single-dose oral treatment of vaginal candidiasis. **Unlabeled Use:** Prevention of recurrent vaginal yeast infections.

Action
Inhibits synthesis of fungal sterols, a necessary component of the cell membrane. **Therapeutic Effects:** Fungistatic action against susceptible organisms. May be fungicidal in higher concentrations. **Spectrum:** *Cryptococcus neoformans. Candida* spp.

Pharmacokinetics
Absorption: Well absorbed after oral administration.
Distribution: Widely distributed, good penetration into CSF, saliva, sputum, vaginal fluid, skin, eye, and peritoneum. Excreted in breast milk.
Metabolism and Excretion: >80% excreted unchanged by the kidneys; <10% metabolized by the liver.
Half-life: Premature neonates: 46–74 hr; Children: 19–25 hr (PO) and 15–17 hr (IV); Adults: 30 hr (increased in renal impairment).

Adverse Reactions/Side Effects
Incidence of adverse reactions is increased in HIV patients.
CNS: headache, dizziness, seizures. **GI:** HEPATOTOXICITY, abdominal discomfort, diarrhea, nausea, vomiting. **Derm:** exfoliative skin disorders including STEVENS-JOHNSON SYNDROME. **Endo:** hypokalemia, hypertriglyceridemia. **Misc:** allergic reactions, including ANAPHYLAXIS.

Interactions
Drug-Drug: ↑ activity of **warfarin**. **Rifampin, rifabutin,** and **isoniazid** ↓ levels. Fluconazole at doses >200 mg/day may inhibit the CYP3A4 enzyme system and effect the activity of drugs metabolized by this system. ↑ hypoglycemic effects of **tolbutamide, glyburide,** or **glipizide.** ↑ levels and risk of toxicity from **cyclosporine, rifabutin, tacrolimus, theophylline, zidovudine, alfentanil,** and **phenytoin.** ↑ levels and effects of **benzodiazepines, zolpidem, bispirone, nisoldipine, tricyclic antidepressants,** and **losartan**. May ↑ risk of bleeding with **warfarin**. May antagonize effects of **amphotericin B**.

Route/Dosage
Oropharyngeal Candidiasis
PO, IV (Adults): 200 mg initially, then 100 mg daily for at least 2 wk.
PO, IV (Children >14 days): 6 mg/kg initially, then 3 mg/kg/day for at least 2 wk.
PO, IV (Neonates < 14 days, 30–36 weeks gestation): same dose as older children except frequency is q 48 hr; Premature neonates < 29 weeks gestation: 5–6 mg/kg/dose q 48–72 hr.

✦ = Canadian drug name. 🧬 = Genetic implication.
*CAPITALS indicates life-threatening; underlines indicate most frequent.

fluconazole

Esophageal Candidiasis
PO, IV (Adults): 200 mg initially, then 100 mg once daily for at least 3 wk (up to 400 mg/day).
PO, IV (Children >14 days): 6 mg/kg initially, then 3–12 mg/kg/day for at least 3 wk.
PO, IV (Neonates < 14 days, 30–36 weeks gestation): same dose as older children except frequency is q 48 hr; Premature neonates < 29 weeks gestation: 5–6 mg/kg/dose q 48–72 hr.

Vaginal Candidiasis
PO (Adults): 150-mg single dose; prevention of recurrence (unlabeled)—150 mg daily for 3 days then weekly for 6 mo.

Systemic Candidiasis
PO, IV (Adults): 400 mg/day initially, then 200–800 mg/day for 28 days.
PO, IV (Children > 14 days): 6–12 mg/kg/day for 28 days.
PO, IV (Neonates < 14 days, 30–36 weeks gestation): same dose as older children except frequency is q 48 hr; Premature neonates <29 weeks gestation: 5–6 mg/kg/dose q 48–72 hr.

Cryptococcal Meningitis
PO, IV (Adults): *Treatment*—400 mg once daily until favorable clinical response, then 200–800 mg once daily for at least 10–12 wk after clearing of CSF; change to oral therapy as soon as possible. *Suppressive therapy*—200 mg once daily.
PO, IV (Children >14 days): 12 mg/kg/day initially, then 6–12 mg/kg/day for at least 10–12 wk after clearing of CSF; change to oral therapy as soon as possible. *Suppressive therapy*—6 mg/kg/day.
PO, IV (Neonates < 14 days, 30–36 weeks gestation): same dose as older children except frequency is q 48 hr; Premature neonates <29 weeks gestation: 5–6 mg/kg/dose q 48–72 hr.

Prevention of Candidiasis after Bone Marrow Transplant
PO, IV (Adults): 400 mg once daily; begin several days before procedure if severe neutropenia is expected, and continue for 7 days after ANC >1000 /mm³.
PO, IV (Children >14 days): 10–12 mg/kg/day, not to exceed 600 mg/day.

Renal Impairment
PO, IV (Adults): *CCr 11–50 mL/min*—50% of the usual dose.

Availability (generic available)
Tablets: 50 mg, 100 mg, 150 mg, 200 mg. **Cost:** *Generic*—100 mg $109.99/30, 150 mg $167.19/12, 200 mg $247.57/30. **Oral suspension (orange flavor):** 10 mg/mL in 35-mL bottle, 40 mg/mL in 35-mL bottle. **Cost:** $25.99/35 mL. **Premixed infusion:** 2 mg/mL in 100- or 200-mL bottles/containers.

NURSING IMPLICATIONS

Assessment
- Assess infected area and monitor CSF cultures before and periodically during therapy.
- Specimens for culture should be taken before instituting therapy. Therapy may be started before results are obtained.
- *Lab Test Considerations:* Monitor BUN and serum creatinine before and periodically during therapy; patients with renal dysfunction will require dose adjustment.
- Monitor liver function tests before and periodically during therapy. May cause ↑ AST, ALT, serum alkaline phosphate, and bilirubin concentrations.

Potential Nursing Diagnoses
Risk for infection (Indications)

Implementation
- Do not confuse Diflucan (fluconazole) with Diprivan (propofol).
- **PO:** Shake oral suspension well before administration.

IV Administration
- **Intermittent Infusion:** *Diluent:* Premixed infusions are pre-diluted and ready to use. Do not unwrap until ready to use. Do not administer solution that is cloudy or has a precipitate. Check for leaks by squeezing inner bag. If leaks are found, discard container as unsterile. *Concentration:* 2 mg/mL. *Rate:* Infuse over 1–2 hr. Do not exceed a rate of 200 mg/hr. Pedi: For children receiving doses > 6 mg/kg/day, give over 2 hr.
- **Y-Site Compatibility:** acyclovir, aldesleukin, amifostine, amikacin, aminophylline, amiodarone, anidulafungin, ampicillin/sulbactam, atropine, aztreonam, benztropine, bivalirudin, bumetanide, calcium chloride, caspofungin, cefazolin, cefepime, cefoxitin, ceftizoxime, cimetidine, cisatracurium, cyclosporine, daptomycin, dexamethasone sodium phosphate, dexmedetomidine, diltiazem, diphenhydramine, dobutamine, docetaxel, dopamine, doxorubicin liposome, doxycycline, droperidol, drotrecogin, enalaprilat, epinephrine, ertapenem, esmolol, etoposide phosphate, famotidine, fenoldopam, fentanyl, filgrastim, fludarabine, foscarnet, ganciclovir, gemcitabine,

gentamicin, granisetron, heparin, hydrocortisone, hydromorphone, insulin, isoproterenol, immune glogulin, ketorolac, labetalol, lansoprazole, leucovorin, levofloxacin, lidocaine, linezolid, lorazepam, melphanan, magnesium sulfate, meperidine, meropenem, methylprednisolone sodium succinate, metoclopramide, metoprolol, metronidazole, midazolam, morphine, nafcillin, nitroglycerin, nitroprusside, norepinephrine, ondansetron, paclitaxel, palonosetron, pancuronium, pemetrexed, penicillin G potassium, phenytoin, phytonadione, piperacillin/tazobactam, potassium chloride, procainamide, prochlorperazine, promethazine, propofol, propranolol, quinapristin-dalfopristin, ranitidine, remifentanil, sargramostim, sodium bicarbonate, tacrolimus, teniposide, theophylline, thiotepa, ticarcillin/clavulanate, tigecycline, tirofiban, tobramycin, vancomycin, vasopressin, vecuronium, verapamil, vinorelbine, voriconazole, zidovudine.

- **Y-Site Incompatibility:** amphotericin B, amphotericin B cholesteryl sulfate, ampicillin, calcium gluconate, cefotaxime, ceftriaxone, cefuroxime, chloramphenicol, clindamycin, diazepam, digoxin, furosemide, haloperidol, hydroxyzine, imipenem/cilastatin, pantoprazole, pentamidine, trimethoprim/sulfamethoxazole.

Patient/Family Teaching
- Instruct patient to take medication as directed, even if feeling better. Doses should be taken at the same time each day. Take missed doses as soon as remembered, but not if almost time for next dose. Do not double doses.
- Instruct patient to notify health care professional if skin rash, abdominal pain, fever, or diarrhea becomes pronounced, if signs and symptoms of liver dysfunction (unusual fatigue, anorexia, nausea, vomiting, jaundice, dark urine, or pale stools) occur, if unusual bruising or bleeding occur, or if no improvement is seen within a few days of therapy.

Evaluation/Desired Outcomes
- Resolution of clinical and laboratory indications of fungal infections. Full course of therapy may require weeks or months of treatment after resolution of symptoms.
- Prevention of candidiasis in patients who have undergone bone marrow transplantation.
- Decrease in skin irritation and vaginal discomfort in patients with vaginal candidiasis. Diagnosis should be reconfirmed with smears or cultures before a second course of therapy to rule out other pathogens associated with vulvovaginitis. Recurrent vaginal infections may be a sign of systemic illness.

HIGH ALERT

fludarabine (floo-**dar**-a-been)
Fludara, Oforta

Classification
Therapeutic: antineoplastics
Pharmacologic: antimetabolites

Pregnancy Category D

Indications
B-cell chronic lymphocytic leukemia unresponsive to standard therapy. **Unlabeled Use:** Non-Hodgkin's lymphoma.

Action
Converted intracellularly to an active phosphorylated metabolite that inhibits DNA synthesis. **Therapeutic Effects:** Death of rapidly replicating cells, particularly malignant ones.

Pharmacokinetics
Absorption: Bioavailability of active metabolite, 2–fluoro-ara-A, is 50–65%.
Distribution: Extensively distributed.
Metabolism and Excretion: Following administration, rapidly converted to an active metabolite (2–fluoro-ara-A), which, when phosphorylated intracellularly, exerts antineoplastic activity; 40% of initial active metabolite excreted unchanged by the kidneys.
Half-life: 20 hr (for initial active metabolite).

TIME/ACTION PROFILE (effects on blood counts)

ROUTE	ONSET	PEAK	DURATION
PO	unknown	13–16 days	unknown
IV	7 wk†	13–16 days	unknown

†Median time to response

Contraindications/Precautions
Contraindicated in: Hypersensitivity to fludarabine, mannitol, or sodium hydroxide; Patients taking pentostatin; OB, Lactation: Pregnancy or lactation; Severe renal impairment (CCr <30 mL/min) (for intravenous).
Use Cautiously in: Moderate renal impairment (↓ dose if CCr <70 mL/min); OB: Patients with childbearing potential; Bone marrow depression; Pedi: Safety not established.

✦ = Canadian drug name. **𝐆** = Genetic implication.
*CAPITALS indicates life-threatening; underlines indicate most frequent.

fludarabine

Adverse Reactions/Side Effects
CNS: NEUROTOXICITY, fatigue, agitation, coma, confusion, headache, malaise, weakness. **EENT:** hearing loss, visual disturbances. **Resp:** PULMONARY HYPERSENSITIVITY, cough, pneumonia, dyspnea, sinusitis. **CV:** edema. **GI:** GI BLEEDING, diarrhea, nausea, anorexia, esophagitis, mucositis, stomatitis, vomiting. **GU:** dysuria, hematuria, urinary tract infection. **Derm:** rashes. **Endo:** gonadal suppression. **Hemat:** PANCYTOPENIA, anemia, leukopenia, thrombocytopenia, hemolytic anemia. **MS:** myalgia. **Neuro:** peripheral neuropathy. **Misc:** fever, tumor lysis syndrome.

Interactions
Drug-Drug: ↑ bone marrow suppression with other **antineoplastics** or **radiation therapy**. Concomitant use with **pentostatin** ↑ risk of potentially fatal pulmonary toxicity (concurrent use not recommended).

Route/Dosage
PO (Adults): 40 mg/m^2 daily for 5 days; repeat course every 28 days.
IV (Adults): 25 mg/m^2 daily for 5 days; repeat course every 28 days.

Renal Impairment
PO, IV (Adults): *CCr 30–70 mL/min*— ↓ dose by 20%.

Renal Impairment
PO (Adults): *CCr <30 mL/min*— ↓ dose by 50%.

Availability
Tablets: 10 mg. **Powder for injection:** 50 mg/vial. **Solution for injection:** 25 mg/mL.

NURSING IMPLICATIONS

Assessment
- Assess patient for visual changes, weakness, confusion, and changes in level of consciousness during and for 60 days following therapy, as neurologic effects resulting in blindness, coma, and death have been reported. Therapy may be delayed or discontinued if neurotoxicity occurs.
- Monitor for bone marrow depression. Assess for bleeding (bleeding gums, bruising, petechiae, guaiac stools, urine, and emesis) and avoid IM injections and rectal temperatures if platelet count is low. Apply pressure to venipuncture sites for 10 min. Assess for signs of infection during neutropenia. Anemia may occur. Monitor for increased fatigue, dyspnea, and orthostatic hypotension.
- Monitor respiratory status, intake and output ratios, and daily weights. Report significant changes or symptoms of pulmonary hypersensitivity (cough, fever, shortness of breath).
- Assess nutritional status. Administering an antiemetic prior to and periodically during therapy and adjusting diet as tolerated may help maintain fluid and electrolyte balance and nutritional status.
- May cause tumor lysis syndrome, resulting in hyperuricemia, hyperphosphatemia, hypocalcemia, metabolic acidosis, hyperkalemia, hematuria, urate crystalluria, and renal failure. Monitor for flank pain and hematuria. Uric acid nephropathy may be prevented by adequate oral hydration. Allopurinol and alkalization of the urine may also be used to treat elevated uric acid concentrations.
- ***Lab Test Considerations:*** Monitor CBC with differential prior to and frequently during therapy. The nadir for leukopenia occurs in 13 days (range 3–25 days) and for thrombocytopenia in 16 days (range 2–32 days) after administration.
- Monitor serum uric acid concentrations periodically during therapy; may be ↑ as part of tumor lysis in patients with large tumor burdens.
- May cause ↑ AST and serum alkaline phosphatase concentrations.

Potential Nursing Diagnoses
Risk for infection (Adverse Reactions)
Risk for injury (Side Effects)

Implementation
- ***High Alert:*** Fatalities have occurred with incorrect administration of chemotherapeutic agents. Before administering, clarify all ambiguous orders; double check single, daily, and course-of-therapy dose limits; have second practitioner independently double check original order, calculations, and infusion pump settings.
- PO and IV doses are different.
- **PO:** Administer daily without regard to food for 5 days every 28 days. Swallow tablets whole; do not break, crush, or chew. Avoid handling tablets directly.

IV Administration
- Prepare solution in a biologic cabinet. Wear gloves, gown, and mask while handling IV medication. Discard IV equipment in specially designated containers (see Appendix L). Unopened vials should be refrigerated. The 5-day course of therapy is continued every 28 days

until patient is in complete remission or until neurotoxicity develops.
- **IV:** Reconstitute with 2 mL of sterile water for injection; solid cake should dissolve in <15 sec. *Concentration:* 25 mg/mL. Reconstituted solution is stable for 8 hr.
- **Intermittent Infusion:** *Diluent:* Dilute further in 100–125 mL of 0.9% NaCl or D5W. *Rate:* Infuse over 15–30 min.
- **Y-Site Compatibility:** alfentanil, allopurinol, amifostine, amikacin, aminocaproic acid, aminophylline, amphotericin B liposome, ampicillin, ampicillin/sulbactam, amsacrine, atracurium, aztreonam, bivalirudin, bleomycin, bumetanide, buprenorphine, butorphanol, calcium acetate, calcium chloride, calcium gluconate, carboplatin, carmustine, caspofungin, cefazolin, cefepime, cefoperazone, cefotaxime, cefotetan, cefoxitin, ceftazidime, ceftizoxime, ceftriaxone, cefuroxime, chloramphenicol, cimetidine, ciprofloxacin, cisatracurium, cisplatin, clindamycin, cyclophosphamide, cyclosporine, cytarabine, dacarbazine, dactinomycin, daptomycin, dexamethasone, dexmedetomidine, dexrazoxane, digoxin, diltiazem, diphenhydramine, dobutamine, docetaxel, dopamine, doxacurium, doxorubicin hydrochloride, doxycycline, droperidol, enalaprilat, ephedrine, epinephrine, ertapenem, erythromycin, esmolol, etoposide, etoposide phosphate, famotidine, fenoldopam, fentanyl, filgrastim, floxuridine, fluconazole, fluorouracil, foscarnet, fosphenytoin, furosemide, gemcitabine, gentamicin, glycopyrrolate, granisetron, haloperidol, heparin, hetastarch, hydrocortisone, hydromorphone, ifosfamide, imipenem/cilastatin, inamrinone, insulin, isoproterenol, ketorolac, labetalol, leucovorin, levofloxacin, lidocaine, linezolid, lorazepam, magnesium sulfate, mannitol, mechlorethamine, melphalan, meperidine, meropenem, mesna, metaraminol, methohexital, methotrexate, methyldopa, methylprednisolone sodium succinate, metoclopramide, metoprolol, metronidazole, midazolam, milrinone, minocycline, mitoxantrone, mivacurium, morphine, multivitamins, nafcillin, nalbuphine, naloxone, nesiritide, nitroglycerin, nitroprusside, norepinephrine, octreotide, ondansetron, oxaliplatin, paclitaxel, palonosetron, pancuronium, pemetrexed, pentamidine, pentazocine, pentobarbital, pentostatin, phenobarbital, phentolamine, phenylephrine, piperacillin/tazobactam, potassium chloride, potassium phosphate, procainamide, promethazine, propranolol, ranitidine, remifentanil, rituximab, rocuronium, sodium acetate, sodium bicarbonate, sodium phosphate, succinylcholine, sufentanil, tacrolimus, teniposide, theophylline, thiopental, thiotepa, ticarcillin/clavulanate, tigecycline, tirofiban, tobramycin, tolazoline, trimethoprim/sulfamethoxazole, vancomycin, vasopressin, vecuronium, verapamil, vinblastine, vincristine, vinorelbine, voriconazole, zidovudine.
- **Y-Site Incompatibility:** acyclovir, amiodarone, amphotericin B colloidal, chlorpromazine, dantrolene, daunorubicin hydrochloride, diazepam, ganciclovir, hydroxyzine, pantoprazole, phenytoin, prochlorperazine, quinapristin/dalfopristin, trastuzumab.

Patient/Family Teaching
- Instruct patient to take fludarabine as directed. Avoid handling tablets; wash hands with soap and water if touching tablet or powder from tablets. Notify health care professional if a dose is missed.
- Caution patient to avoid crowds and persons with known infections. Health care professional should be informed immediately if symptoms of infection (chills, cough, or burning pain on urination) occur.
- Instruct patient to report unusual bleeding. Advise patient of thrombocytopenia precautions (use soft toothbrush and electric razor; avoid contact sports and other situations in which injury might occur). Do not drink alcoholic beverages or take medication containing aspirin or NSAIDs; may precipitate gastric bleeding.
- Instruct patient to inspect oral mucosa for redness and ulceration. If mouth sores occur, advise patient to use sponge brush and rinse mouth with water after eating and drinking. Consult health care professional if pain interferes with eating. Stomatitis pain treatment may require opioid analgesics.
- Advise patient that this medication may have teratogenic effects. Contraception should be used during therapy and for at least 6 mo after therapy is concluded.
- Emphasize the need for periodic lab tests to monitor for side effects.

Evaluation/Desired Outcomes
- Improvement of hematopoietic values in leukemias.

fludrocortisone
(floo-droe-**kor**-ti-sone)

Classification
Therapeutic: hormones
Pharmacologic: corticosteroids (mineralocorticoid)

Pregnancy Category C

Indications
Sodium loss and hypotension associated with adrenocortical insufficiency (given with hydrocortisone or cortisone). Management of sodium loss due to congenital adrenogenital syndrome (congenital adrenal hyperplasia). **Unlabeled Use:** Idiopathic orthostatic hypotension (with increased sodium intake). Type IV renal tubular acidosis.

Action
Causes sodium reabsorption, hydrogen and potassium excretion, and water retention by its effects on the distal renal tubule. **Therapeutic Effects:** Maintenance of sodium balance and blood pressure in patients with adrenocortical insufficiency.

Pharmacokinetics
Absorption: Well absorbed following oral administration.
Distribution: Widely distributed; probably enters breast milk.
Protein Binding: High.
Metabolism and Excretion: Mostly metabolized by the liver.
Half-life: 3.5 hr.

TIME/ACTION PROFILE (mineralocorticoid activity)

ROUTE	ONSET	PEAK	DURATION
PO	unknown	unknown	1–2 days

Contraindications/Precautions
Contraindicated in: Hypersensitivity.
Use Cautiously in: CHF; Addison's disease (patients may have exaggerated response); OB, Lactation, Pedi: Safety not established.

Adverse Reactions/Side Effects
CNS: dizziness, headache. **CV:** CHF, arrhythmias, edema, hypertension. **GI:** anorexia, nausea. **Endo:** adrenal suppression, weight gain. **F and E:** hypokalemia, hypokalemic alkalosis. **MS:** arthralgia, muscular weakness, tendon contractures. **Neuro:** ascending paralysis. **Misc:** hypersensitivity reactions.

Interactions
Drug-Drug: Use with **thiazide or loop diuretics, piperacillin**, or **amphotericin B** may ↑ risk of hypokalemia. Hypokalemia may ↑ risk of **digoxin** toxicity. May produce prolonged neuromuscular blockade following the use of **nondepolarizing neuromuscular blocking agents**. **Phenobarbital** or **rifampin** may ↑ metabolism and ↓ effectiveness of fludrocortisone.
Drug-Food: Large amounts of **salt** or **sodium-containing foods** may cause excessive sodium retention and potassium loss.

Route/Dosage
PO (Adults): *Adrenocortical insufficiency*—100 mcg/day (range 100 mcg 3 times weekly—200 mcg daily). Doses as small as 50 mcg daily may be required by some patients. Use with 10–37.5 mg cortisone daily or 10–30 mg hydrocortisone daily. *Adrenogenital syndrome*—100–200 mcg/day. *Idiopathic hypotension*—50–200 mcg/day (unlabeled).
PO (Children): 50–100 mcg/day.

Availability (generic available)
Tablets: 100 mcg (0.1 mg).

NURSING IMPLICATIONS

Assessment
- Monitor blood pressure periodically during therapy. Report significant changes. Hypotension may indicate insufficient dose.
- Monitor for fluid retention (weigh daily, assess for edema, and auscultate lungs for rales/crackles).
- Monitor patients with Addison's disease closely and stop treatment if a significant increase in weight or blood pressure, edema, or cardiac enlargement occurs. Patients with Addison's disease are more sensitive to the action of fludrocortisone and may have an exaggerated response.
- *Lab Test Considerations:* Monitor serum electrolytes periodically during therapy. Fludrocortisone causes ↓ serum potassium levels.

Potential Nursing Diagnoses
Deficient fluid volume (Indications)
Excess fluid volume (Side Effects)

Implementation
- **PO:** Tablets are scored and may be broken if dose adjustment is necessary.

Patient/Family Teaching
- Instruct patient to take medication as directed. Take missed doses as soon as remembered but

not just before next dose is due. Explain that lifelong therapy may be necessary and that abrupt discontinuation may lead to addisonian crisis. Patient should keep an adequate supply available at all times.
- Advise patient to follow dietary modification prescribed by health care professional. Instruct patient to follow a diet high in potassium (see Appendix M). Amount of sodium allowed in diet varies with pathophysiology.
- Instruct patient to inform health care professional if weight gain or edema, muscle weakness, cramps, nausea, anorexia, or dizziness occurs.
- Advise patient to carry identification at all times describing disease process and medication regimen.

Evaluation/Desired Outcomes
- Normalization of fluid and electrolyte balance without the development of hypokalemia or hypertension.

---

flumazenil (flu-maz-e-nil)
※ Anexate, Romazicon

Classification
Therapeutic: antidotes
Pharmacologic: benzodiazepines

Pregnancy Category C

Indications
Complete/partial reversal of effects of benzodiazepines used as general anesthetics, or during diagnostic or therapeutic procedures. Management of intentional or accidental overdose of benzodiazepines.

Action
Flumazenil is a benzodiazepine derivative that antagonizes the CNS depressant effects of benzodiazepine compounds. It has no effect on CNS depression from other causes, including opioids, alcohol, barbiturates, or general anesthetics.
Therapeutic Effects: Reversal of benzodiazepine effects.

Pharmacokinetics
Absorption: IV administration results in complete bioavailability.
Distribution: Unknown.
Protein Binding: 50% primarily to albumin.
Metabolism and Excretion: Metabolism of flumazenil occurs primarily in the liver.

Half-life: Children: 20–75 min; Adults: 41–79 min.

TIME/ACTION PROFILE (reversal of benzodiazepine effects)

ROUTE	ONSET	PEAK	DURATION
IV	1–2 min	6–10 min	1–2 hr†

†Depends on dose/concentration of benzodiazepine and dose of flumazenil

Contraindications/Precautions
Contraindicated in: Hypersensitivity to flumazenil or benzodiazepines; Patients receiving benzodiazepines for life-threatening medical problems, including status epilepticus or increased intracranial pressure, should not be given flumazenil; Serious cyclic antidepressant overdosage.
Use Cautiously in: Mixed CNS depressant overdose (effects of other agents may emerge when benzodiazepine effect is removed); History of seizures (seizures are more likely to occur in patients who are experiencing sedative/hypnotic withdrawal, who have recently received repeated doses of benzodiazepines, or who have a previous history of seizure activity); Head injury (may increase intracranial pressure and risk of seizures); Severe hepatic impairment; OB, Lactation: Safety not established; Pedi: Safety not established in children <1 yr.

Adverse Reactions/Side Effects
CNS: SEIZURES, dizziness, agitation, confusion, drowsiness, emotional lability, fatigue, headache, sleep disorders. **EENT:** abnormal hearing, abnormal vision, blurred vision. **CV:** arrhythmias, chest pain, hypertension. **GI:** nausea, vomiting, hiccups. **Derm:** flushing, sweating. **Local:** pain/injection-site reactions, phlebitis. **Neuro:** paresthesia. **Misc:** rigors, shivering.

Interactions
Drug-Drug: None significant.

Route/Dosage

Reversal of Conscious Sedation or General Anesthesia
IV (Adults): 0.2 mg. Additional doses may be given at 1-min intervals until desired results are obtained, up to a total dose of 1 mg. If resedation occurs, regimen may be repeated at 20-min intervals, not to exceed 3 mg/hr.
IV (Children): 0.01 mg/kg (up to 0.2 mg); if the desired level of consciousness is not obtained after waiting an additional 45 sec, further injections

of 0.01 mg/kg (up to 0.2 mg) can be administered and repeated at 60-sec intervals when necessary (up to a maximum of 4 additional times) to a maximum total dose of 0.05 mg/kg or 1 mg, whichever is lower. The dose should be individualized based on the patient's response.

Suspected Benzodiazepine Overdose
IV (Adults): 0.2 mg. Additional 0.3 mg may be given 30 sec later. Further doses of 0.5 mg may be given at 1-min intervals, if necessary, to a total dose of 3 mg. Usual dose required is 1–3 mg. If resedation occurs, additional doses of 0.5 mg/min for 2 min may be given at 20-min intervals (given no more than 1 mg at a time, not to exceed 3 mg per hr).
IV (Children): *Unlabeled*—0.01 mg/kg (maximum dose 0.2 mg) with repeat doses every minute up to a cumulative dose of 1 mg. As an alternative to repeat doses, continuous infusions of 0.005–0.01 mg/kg/hr have been used.

Availability (generic available)
Injection: 0.1 mg/mL in 5- and 10-mL vials.

NURSING IMPLICATIONS

Assessment
- Assess level of consciousness and respiratory status before and during therapy. Observe patient for at least 2 hr after administration for the appearance of resedation. Hypoventilation may occur.
- **Overdose:** Attempt to determine time of ingestion and amount and type of benzodiazepine taken. Knowledge of agent ingested allows an estimate of duration of CNS depression.

Potential Nursing Diagnoses
Risk for injury (Indications)
Risk for poisoning (Indications)

Implementation
- Ensure that patient has a patent airway before administration of flumazenil.
- Observe IV site frequently for redness or irritation. Administer through a free-flowing IV infusion into a large vein to minimize pain at the injection site.
- Optimal emergence should be undertaken slowly to decrease undesirable effects including confusion, agitation, emotional lability, and perceptual distortion.
- Institute seizure precautions. Seizures are more likely to occur in patients who are experiencing sedative/hypnotic withdrawal, patients who have recently received repeated doses of benzodiazepines, or those who have a previous history of seizure activity. Seizures may be treated with benzodiazepines, barbiturates, or phenytoin. Larger than normal doses of benzodiazepines may be required.
- **Suspected Benzodiazepine Overdose:** If no effects are seen after administration of flumazenil, consider other causes of decreased level of consciousness (alcohol, barbiturates, opioid analgesics).

IV Administration
- **Direct IV:** ***Diluent:*** May be administered undiluted or diluted in syringe with D5W, 0.9% NaCl, or LR. Diluted solution should be discarded after 24 hr. ***Concentration:*** Up to 0.1 mg/mL. ***Rate:*** Administer each dose over 15–30 sec into free-flowing IV in a large vein. Do not exceed 0.2 mg/min in children or 0.5 mg/min in adults.

Patient/Family Teaching
- Flumazenil does not consistently reverse the amnestic effects of benzodiazepines. Provide patient and family with written instructions for postprocedure care. Inform family that patient may appear alert at the time of discharge but the sedative effects of the benzodiazepine may recur. Instruct patient to avoid driving or other activities requiring alertness for at least 24 hr after discharge.
- Instruct patient not to take any alcohol or nonprescription drugs for at least 18–24 hr after discharge.
- Resumption of usual activities should occur only when no residual effects of the benzodiazepine remain.

Evaluation/Desired Outcomes
- Improved level of consciousness.
- Decrease in respiratory depression caused by benzodiazepines.

flunisolide, See CORTICOSTEROIDS (INHALATION).

flunisolide, See CORTICOSTEROIDS (NASAL).

fluocinolone, See CORTICOSTEROIDS (TOPICAL/LOCAL).

fluocinonide, See CORTICOSTEROIDS (TOPICAL/LOCAL).

FLUOROQUINOLONES
(floor-oh-**kwin**-oh-lones)

ciprofloxacin†
(sip-roe-**flox**-a-sin)
✤ Apo-Ciprofox, Cipro, Cipro XR, Proquin XR

gemifloxacin (gem-i-**flox**-a-sin)
Factive

levofloxacin (le-voe-**flox**-a-sin)
Levaquin, ✤ Novo-Levofloxacin

moxifloxacin† (mox-i-**flox**-a-sin)
Avelox

norfloxacin† (nor-**flox**-a-sin)
✤ Apo-Norfloxacin, ✤ Co-Norfloxacin, Noroxin, ✤ Novo-Norfloxacin, ✤ PMS-Norfloxacin, ✤ Riva-Norfloxacin

ofloxacin† (oh-**flox**-a-sin)
✤ Apo-Ofloxacin, Floxin

Classification
Therapeutic: anti-infectives
Pharmacologic: fluoroquinolones

Pregnancy Category C
†See Appendix C for ophthalmic use

Indications
PO, IV: Treatment of the following bacterial infections: Urinary tract infections including cystitis and prostatitis (ciprofloxacin, levofloxacin, norfloxacin, ofloxacin), Gonorrhea (may not be considered first-line agents due to increasing resistance), Gynecologic infections (ciprofloxacin, norfloxacin, ofloxacin), Respiratory tract infections including acute sinusitis, acute exacerbations of chronic bronchitis, and pneumonia (not norfloxacin), Skin and skin structure infections (levofloxacin, moxifloxacin, ciprofloxacin, ofloxacin), Bone and joint infections (ciprofloxacin), Infectious diarrhea (ciprofloxacin), Intra-abdominal infections (ciprofloxacin, moxifloxacin). Febrile neutropenia (ciprofloxacin). Post-exposure treatment of inhalational anthrax (ciprofloxacin, levofloxacin).

Action
Inhibit bacterial DNA synthesis by inhibiting DNA gyrase. **Therapeutic Effects:** Death of susceptible bacteria. **Spectrum:** Broad activity includes many gram-positive pathogens: Staphylococci including methicillin-resistant *Staphylococcus aureus*, *Staphylococcus epidermidis*, *Staphylococcus saprophyticus*, *Streptococcus pneumoniae*, *Streptococcus pyogenes*, and *Bacillus anthracis*. Gram-negative spectrum notable for activity against: *Escherichia coli*, *Klebsiella*, *Enterobacter*, *Salmonella*, *Shigella*, *Proteus*, *Providencia*, *Morganella morganii*, *Pseudomonas aeruginosa*, *Serratia*, *Haemophilus*, *Acinetobacter*, *Neisseria gonorrhoeae*, *Moraxella catarrhalis*, *Campylobacter*. Additional spectrum includes: *Chlamydia pneumoniae*, *Legionella pneumoniae*, and *Mycoplasma pneumoniae*.

Pharmacokinetics
Absorption: Well absorbed after oral administration (*ciprofloxacin*—70%; *moxifloxacin*—90%; *gemifloxacin*—71%; *levofloxacin*—99%; *norfloxacin*—30–40%; *ofloxacin*—98%.
Distribution: Widely distributed. High tissue and urinary levels are achieved. All agents appear to cross the placenta. *Ciprofloxacin* and *ofloxacin* enter breast milk.
Metabolism and Excretion: *Ciprofloxacin*—15% metabolized by the liver, 40–50% excreted unchanged by the kidneys; *gemifloxacin*—Minimal metabolism, 61% excreted unchanged in feces, 36% excreted unchanged in urine; *levofloxacin*—87% excreted unchanged in urine, small amounts metabolized; *moxifloxacin*—mostly metabolized by the liver, 20% excreted unchanged in urine, 25% excreted unchanged in feces; *norfloxacin*—10% metabolized by the liver, 30% excreted unchanged by the kidneys, 30% excreted unchanged in feces; *ofloxacin*—70–80% excreted unchanged by the kidneys.
Half-life: *Ciprofloxacin*—4 hr; *gemifloxacin*—7 hr; *levofloxacin*—8 hr; *moxifloxacin*—12 hr; *norfloxacin*—6.5 hr; *ofloxacin*—5–7 hr (all are ↑ in renal impairment).

TIME/ACTION PROFILE (blood levels)

ROUTE	ONSET	PEAK	DURATION
Ciprofloxacin—PO	rapid	1–2 hr	12 hr
Ciprofloxacin—PO-ER	rapid	1–4 hr	24 hr
Ciprofloxacin—IV	rapid	end of infusion	12 hr
Gemifloxacin—PO	rapid	0.5—2 hr	24 hr
Levofloxacin—PO	rapid	1–2 hr	24 hr
Levofloxacin—IV	rapid	end of infusion	24 hr

✤ = Canadian drug name. 🧬 = Genetic implication.
*CAPITALS indicates life-threatening; underlines indicate most frequent.

590　FLUOROQUINOLONES

Moxifloxacin—PO	within 1 hr	1–3 hr	24 hr
Moxifloxacin—IV	rapid	end of infusion	24 hr
Norfloxacin—PO	rapid	2–3 hr	12 hr
Ofloxacin—PO	rapid	1–2 hr	12 hr
Ofloxacin—IV	rapid	end of infusion	12 hr

Contraindications/Precautions

Contraindicated in: Hypersensitivity. Cross-sensitivity among agents within class may occur; **Gemifloxacin and moxifloxacin:** Concurrent use of Class IA antiarrhythmics (disopyramide, quinidine, procainamide) or Class III antiarrhythmics (amiodarone, sotalol) (↑ risk of QTc prolongation and torsades de pointes); Known QT prolongation or concurrent use of agents causing prolongation; OB: Do not use unless potential benefit outweighs potential fetal risk; Pedi: Use only for treatment of anthrax and complicated UTIs in children 1–17 yrs due to possible arthropathy.

Use Cautiously in: Known or suspected CNS disorder; Renal impairment (dosage reduction if CCr ≤50 mL/min for ciprofloxacin, levofloxacin, ofloxacin; ≤30 mL/min for norfloxacin; <40 mL/min for gemifloxacin); Cirrhosis (levofloxacin, moxifloxacin, or norfloxacin); **Gemifloxacin and moxifloxacin:** Concurrent use of erythromycin, antipsychotics, and tricyclic antidepressants (↑ risk of QTc prolongation and torsades de pointes); **Gemifloxacin and moxifloxacin:** Bradycardia; **Gemifloxacin and moxifloxacin:** Acute myocardial ischemia; Concurrent use of corticosteroids (↑ risk of tendinitis/tendon rupture); Kidney, heart, or lung transplant patients (↑ risk of tendinitis/tendon rupture); Lactation: Safety not established except for treatment of anthrax; Geri: ↑ risk of adverse reactions.

Adverse Reactions/Side Effects

CNS: SEIZURES, dizziness, headache, insomnia, acute psychoses, agitation, confusion, drowsiness. **CV:** *gemifloxacin, levofloxacin, moxifloxacin, norfloxacin*—ARRHYTHMIAS, QT prolongation, vasodilation. **GI:** HEPATOTOXICITY (NORFLOXACIN), PSEUDOMEMBRANOUS COLITIS, diarrhea, nausea, abdominal pain, increased liver function tests (ciprofloxacin, moxifloxacin), vomiting. **GU:** vaginitis. **Derm:** photosensitivity, rash. **Endo:** hyperglycemia, hypoglycemia. **Local:** phlebitis at IV site. **MS:** tendinitis, tendon rupture. **Misc:** hypersensitivity reactions including ANAPHYLAXIS, STEVENS-JOHNSON SYNDROME.

Interactions

Drug-Drug: ↑ risk of QTc prolongation and life-threatening arrhythmias with concurrent use of gemifloxacin, moxifloxacin, and norfloxacin and **amiodarone**, **disopyramide**, **erythromycin**, **pentamidine**, **phenothiazines**, **procainamide**, **quinidine**, **sotalol**, and **tricyclic antidepressants** (concurrent use should be avoided). ↑ serum **theophylline** levels and may lead to toxicity. Administration with **magnesium and aluminum-containing antacids**, **iron salts**, **bismuth subsalicylate**, **sucralfate**, **didanosine**, and **zinc salts** ↓ absorption of fluoroquinolones. May ↑ the effects of **warfarin**. Ciprofloxacin may ↓ blood levels and effectiveness of **phenytoin**. Serum levels of fluoroquinolones may be ↓ by **antineoplastics**. **Cimetidine** may interfere with elimination of fluoroquinolones. Beneficial effects of ciprofloxacin may be antagonized by **nitrofurantoin**. **Probenecid** ↓ renal elimination of fluoroquinolones. May ↑ risk of nephrotoxicity from **cyclosporine**. Concurrent use of ciprofloxacin with **foscarnet** may ↑ risk of seizures. Concurrent therapy with **corticosteroids** may ↑ the risk of tendon rupture. May ↑ risk of hypoglycemia when used with **antidiabetic agents**.
Drug-Natural Products: Fennel ↓ the absorption of ciprofloxacin.
Drug-Food: Absorption is impaired by **concurrent tube feeding** (because of metal cations). Absorption is ↓ if taken with **dairy products** or calcium-fortified juices.

Route/Dosage

Ciprofloxacin

PO (Adults): *Most infections*—500–750 mg q 12 hr. *Complicated urinary tract infections*—500 mg q 12 hr for 7–14 days (immediate-release); *or* 1000 mg q 24 hr for 7–14 days (extended-release). *Uncomplicated urinary tract infections*—250 mg every 12 hr for 3 days (immediate-release) *or* 500 mg every 24 hr for 3 days (extended-release). *Gonorrhea*—250-mg single dose. *Inhalational anthrax (post exposure) or cutaneous anthrax*—500 mg every 12 hr for 60 days.

PO (Children 1–17 yr): *Complicated urinary tract infections*—10–15 mg/kg q 12 hr (not to exceed 750 mg/dose) for 10–21 days. *Inhalational anthrax (post-exposure) or cutaneous anthrax*—10–15 mg/kg q 12 hr (not to exceed 500 mg/dose) for 60 days.

FLUOROQUINOLONES

IV (Adults): *Most infections*—400 mg q 12 hr. *Complicated urinary tract infections*—400 mg q 12 hr for 7–14 days. *Uncomplicated urinary tract infections*—200 mg q 12 hr for 7–14 days. *Inhalational anthrax (post exposure)*—400 mg q 12 hr for 60 days.
IV (Children 1–17 yr): *Inhalational anthrax (post exposure)*—10 mg/kg q 12 hr (not to exceed 400 mg/dose) for 60 days; *Complicated urinary tract infections*—6–10 mg/kg q 8 hr (not to exceed 400 mg/dose) for 10–21 days.

Renal Impairment
PO (Adults): *CCr 30–50 mL/min*—250–500 mg q 12 hr; *CCr 5–29 mL/min*—250–500 mg q 18 hr (immediate-release) *or* 500 mg q 24 hr (extended-release).
IV (Adults): *CCr 5–29 mL/min*—200–400 mg q 18–24 hr.

Gemifloxacin
PO (Adults): *Acute bacterial exacerbation of chronic bronchitis*—320 mg once daily for 5 days; *Community-acquired pneumonia (CAP) caused by Klebsiella pneumoniae, Moraxella catarrhalis, and multidrug resistant strains of S. pneumonia*—320 mg once daily for 7 days. *Community-acquired-pneumonia (CAP) caused by S. pneumonia, Haemophilus influenzae, Mycoplasma pneumoniae, or Chlamydia pneumonia, and multidrug resistant strains of S. pneumonia*—320 mg once daily for 5 days.

Renal Impairment
PO (Adults): *CCr ≤40 mL/min*—160 mg once daily for 5 days.

Levofloxacin
PO, IV (Adults): *Most infections*—250–750 mg q 24 hr; *inhalational anthrax (post-exposure)*—500 mg once daily for 60 days.

Renal Impairment
PO, IV (Adults): *Normal renal function dosing of 750 mg/day: CCr 20–49 mL/min*—750 mg q 48 hr; *CCr 10–19 mL/min*—750 mg initially, then 500 mg q 48 hr; *Normal renal function dosing of 500 mg/day: CCr 20–49 mL/min*—500 mg initially then 250 mg q 24 hr; *CCr 10–19 mL/min*—500 mg initially then 250 mg q 48 hr. *Normal renal function dosing of 250 mg/day: CCr 10–19 mL/min*—250 mg q 48 hr.

Moxifloxacin
PO, IV (Adults): *Bacterial sinusitis*—400 mg once daily for 10 days; *Community-acquired pneumonia*—400 mg once daily for 7–14 days. *Acute bacterial exacerbation of chronic bronchitis*—400 mg once daily for 5 days. *Complicated intra-abdominal infection*—400 mg once daily for 5–14 days. *Urethritis/cervicitis*—300 mg q 12 hr for 7 days. *Skin/skin structure infections*—400 mg/day for 7–21 days.

Norfloxacin
PO (Adults): *Uncomplicated urinary tract infections*—400 mg q 12 hr for 3–14 days. *Complicated urinary tract infections*—400 mg q 12 hr for 10–21 days. *Gonorrhea*—800-mg single dose. *Prostatitis*—400 mg q 12 hr for 4–6 wk.

Renal Impairment
PO (Adults): *CCr ≤30 mL/min*—400 mg once daily.

Ofloxacin
PO (Adults): *Most infections*—400 mg q 12 hr. *Prostatitis*—300 mg q 12 hr for 6 wk. *Uncomplicated urinary tract infections*—200 mg q 12 hr for 3–7 days. *Complicated urinary tract infections*—200 mg q 12 hr for 10 days. *Gonorrhea*—400-mg single dose.
Otic (Adults and Children ≥6 mo): *Otitis Externa 6 months to 13 yr*—5 drops instilled into affected ear once daily for 7 days; *Otitis Externa ≥13 yr*—10 drops instilled into affected ear once daily for 7 days. *Acute Otitis Media in pediatric patients 1–12 yr old with tympanostomy tubes*—5 drops instilled into the affected ear twice daily for 10 days. *Chronic Suppurative Otitis Media with perforated tympanic membranes in patients ≥12 yr*—10 drops instilled into the affected ear twice daily for 14 days.

Renal Impairment
PO, IV (Adults): *CCr 20–50 mL/min*—100% of the usual dose q 24 hr; *CCr <20 mL/min*—50% of the usual dose q 24 hr.

Availability

Ciprofloxacin (generic available)
Tablets: 100 mg, 250 mg, 500 mg, 750 mg. **Extended-release tablets:** 500 mg, 1000 mg. **Oral suspension (strawberry flavor):** 250 mg/5 mL, 500 mg/5 mL. **Solution for injection:** 10 mg/mL. **Premixed infusion:** 200 mg/100 mL D5W, 400 mg/200 mL D5W. ***In combination with:*** hydrocortisone (Cipro HC) (see Appendix B).

Gemifloxacin
Tablets: 320 mg.

Levofloxacin (generic available)
Tablets: 250 mg, 500 mg, 750 mg. **Cost:** 250 mg $199.98/20, 500 mg $231.98/20, 750 mg $429.99/20. **Oral solution:** 25 mg/mL. **Solution for injection:** 25 mg/mL. **Premixed infusion:** 250 mg/50 mL D5W, 500 mg/100 mL D5W, 750 mg/150 mL D5W.

Moxifloxacin
Tablets: 400 mg. **Cost:** $160.21/14. **Premixed infusion:** 400 mg/250 mL 0.8% NaCl.

Norfloxacin
Tablets: 400 mg.

Ofloxacin (generic available)
Tablets: 200 mg, 300 mg, 400 mg. **Cost:** Generic—200 mg $77.13/20, 300 mg $91.42/20, 400 mg $83.33/20. **Otic solution:** 0.3% in 5- and 10-mL dropper bottles and 0.25 mL single-dispensing containers. **Cost:** Generic—$55.99/5 mL, $92.99/10 mL.

NURSING IMPLICATIONS
Assessment
- Assess for infection (vital signs; appearance of wound, sputum, urine, and stool; WBC; urinalysis; frequency and urgency of urination; cloudy or foul-smelling urine) prior to and during therapy.
- Obtain specimens for culture and sensitivity before initiating therapy. First dose may be given before receiving results.
- Observe for signs and symptoms of anaphylaxis (rash, pruritus, laryngeal edema, wheezing). Discontinue drug and notify physician or other health care professional immediately if these problems occur. Keep epinephrine, an antihistamine, and resuscitation equipment close by in case of an anaphylactic reaction. Patients taking gemifloxacin who are at greater risk for rash are those receiving gemifloxacin for >7 days, <40 yr of age, females, and postmenopausal females receiving hormone replacement therapy.
- Monitor bowel function. Diarrhea, abdominal cramping, fever, and bloody stools should be reported to health care professional promptly as a sign of pseudomembranous colitis. May begin up to several weeks following cessation of therapy.
- *Lab Test Considerations:* May cause ↑ serum AST, ALT, LDH, bilirubin, and alkaline phosphatase.
- May also cause ↑ or ↓ serum glucose.
- Moxifloxacin may cause hyperglycemia, hyperlipidemia, and altered prothrombin time. It may also cause ↑ WBC; ↑ serum calcium, chloride, albumin, and globulin; and ↓ glucose, hemoglobin, RBCs, neutrophils, eosinophils, and basophils.
- Monitor prothrombin time closely in patients receiving fluoroquinolones and warfarin; may enhance the anticoagulant effects of warfarin.

Potential Nursing Diagnoses
Risk for infection (Patient/Family Teaching)

Implementation
- Do not confuse norfloxacin with Norflex (orphenadrine).
- **PO:** Administer *norfloxacin and ofloxacin* on an empty stomach 1 hr before or 2 hr after meals, with a full glass of water. *Moxifloxacin, levofloxacin,* and *gemifloxacin* may be administered without regard to meals. Should be taken at least 2 hr (3 hr for gemifloxacin, 4 hr for moxifloxacin) before or 2 hr (8 hr for moxifloxacin) after antacids or other products containing calcium, iron, zinc, magnesium, or aluminum.
- If gastric irritation occurs, ciprofloxacin may be administered with meals.
- Ciprofloxacin 5% and 10% oral suspension should not be administered through a feeding tube (may ↓ absorption). Shake solution for 15 seconds prior to administration.
- *Gemifloxacin* and *ciprofloxacin extended-release tablets* should be swallowed whole; do not break, crush, or chew.

Ciprofloxacin
IV Administration
- **Intermittent Infusion:** *Diluent:* Dilute with 0.9% NaCl or D5W. Stable for 14 days at refrigerated or room temperature. *Concentration:* 1–2 mg/mL. *Rate:* Administer over 60 min into a large vein to minimize venous irritation.
- **Y-Site Compatibility:** amifostine, amiodarone, anakinra, anidulafungin, aztreonam, bivalirudin, calcium gluconate, carboplatin, caspofungin, ceftazidime, cisatracurium, cisplatin, cyclophosphamide, cytarabine, dactinomycin, daptomycin, dexmedetomidine, digoxin, diltiazem, diphenhydramine, dobutamine, docetaxel, dopamine, doxacurium, doxarubicin, doxorubicin liposome, epirubicin, ertapenem, etoposide, etoposide phosphate, fenoldopam, fludarabine, gemcitabine, gentamicin, granisetron, hydromorphone, ifosfamide, lidocaine, linezolid, lorazepam, LR, mechlorethamine, meperidine, methotrexate, metoclopramide, metronidazole, midazolam, midodrine, milri-

none, mitoxantrone, nesiritide, octreotide, ondansetron, oxaliplatin, oxytocin, paclitaxel, palonosetron, potassium acetate, potassium chloride, promethazine, quinupristin-dalfopristin, ranitidine, remifentanil, rocuronium, sodium acetate, 0.9% NaCL, tacrolimus, teniposide, thiotepa, tigecycline, tirofiban, tobramycin, trastuzumab, vasopressin, vecuronium, verapamil, vincristine, vinorelbine, voriconazole.

- **Y-Site Incompatibility:** Manufacturer recommends temporarily discontinuing other solutions when administering ciprofloxacin, acyclovir, aminophylline, amphotericin B liposome, ampicillin/sulbactam, azithromycin, cefepime, dexamethasone, drotrecogin, fluorouracil, furosemide, heparin, hydrocortisone, magnesium sulfate, methylprednisolone, pantoprazole, pemetrexed, phenytoin, piperacillin/tazobactam, potassium phosphates, propofol, rituxumab, sodium phosphates, warfarin.

Levofloxacin

IV Administration

- **Intermittent Infusion:** *Diluent:* Dilute with 0.9% NaCl, D5W, dextrose/saline combinations, 5% sodium bicarbonate, Plasmalyte 56, or sodium lactate. Also available in premixed bottles and flexible containers with D5W, which need no further dilution. *Concentration:* 5 mg/mL Discard unused solution. Diluted solution is stable for 72 hr at room temperature and 14 days if refrigerated. *Rate:* Administer by infusion over at least 60 min for 250 mg or 500 mg doses and over 90 min for 750 mg dose. Avoid rapid bolus injection to prevent hypotension.
- **Y-Site Compatibility:** alfentanil, amifostine, amikacin, aminophylline, ampicillin, ampicillin/sulbactam, anidulafungin, atracurium, aztreonam, bivalirudin, bleomycin, bumetanide, buprenorphine, busulfan, butorphanol, caffeine citrate, calcium gluconate, carboplatin, carmustine, caspofungin, cefepime, cefotetan, ceftazidime, ceftizoxime, ceftriaxone, cefuroxime, chlorpromazine, cimetidine, cisatracurium, cisplatin, clindamycin, cyclophosphamide, cyclosporine, cytarabine, dactomycin, daptomycin, dexamethasone, dexmedetomidine, dexrazoxane, digoxin, diltiazem, diphenhydramine, dobutamine, docetaxel, dolasetron, dopamine, doripenem, doxacurium, doxycycline, droperidol, enalaprilat, ephedrine, epinephrine, epirubicin, ertapenem, erythromycin, esmolol, etoposide, etoposide phosphate, famotidine, fenoldopam, fentanyl, filgrastim, floxuridine, fluconazole, fludarabine, fosphenytoin, gemcitabine, gentamicin, granisetron, haloperidol, hydrocortisone, hydromorphone, idarubicin, ifosfamide, imipenem/cilastatin, isoproterenol, labetalol, leucovorin, levorphanol, lidocaine, linezolid, magnesium sulfate, mannitol, mechlorethamine, meperidine, mesna, methylprednisolone, metoclopramide, metronidazole, midazolam, milrinone, mitomycin, mitoxantrone, morphine, nalbuphine, naloxone, nesiritide, octreotide, ondansetron, oxacillin, oxaliplatin, oxytocin, paclitaxel, palonosetron, pancuronium, pemetrexed, penicillin G sodium, pentamidine, phenylephrine, plicamycin, potassium chloride, promethazine, propranolol, quinupristin/dalfopristin, ranitidine, remifentanil, rocuronium, sargramostim, sodium acetate, sodium bicarbonate, succinylcholine, sufentanil, tacrolimus, teniposide, theophylline, thiotepa, ticarcillin/clavulanate, tigecycline, tirofiban, tobramycin, trimethoprim/sulfamethoxazole, vancomycin, vasopressin, vecuronium, verapamil, vinblastine, vincristine, vinorelbine, voriconazole, zidovudine.
- **Y-Site Incompatibility:** acyclovir, alprostadil, amiodarone, amphotericin B colloidal, amphotericin B liposome, cefazolin, cefoperazone, cefoxitin, daunorubicin hydrochloride, diazepam, drotrecogin, fluorouracil, furosemide, ganciclovir, heparin, inamrinone, indomethacin, ketorolac, labetalol, methotrexate, nitroglycerin, nitroprusside, pentobarbital, phenytoin, piperacillin/tazobactam, prochlorperazine, propofol, rituximab, streptozocin, thiopental, trastuzumab.

Moxifloxacin

IV Administration

- **Intermittent Infusion:** *Diluent:* Premixed bags are diluted in sodium chloride 0.8% and should not be further diluted. Use transfer set whose piercing pin does not require excessive force; insert with a gentle twisting motion until pin is firmly seated. *Concentration:* 1.6 mg/mL. *Rate:* Administer over 60 min. Avoid rapid or bolus infusion.
- **Y-Site Compatibility:** bivalirudin, caspofungin, daptomycin, doripenem, ertapenem, nesiritide, octreotide, oxytocin, palonosetron, pemetrexed, tigecycline, tirofiban, vasopressin.

- **Y-Site Incompatibility:** furosemide, voriconazole.
- **Solution Compatibility:** 0.9% NaCl, D5W, D10W, LR.

Patient/Family Teaching
- Instruct patient to take medication as directed at evenly spaced times and to finish drug completely, even if feeling better. Take missed doses as soon as possible, unless almost time for next dose. Do not double doses. Advise patient that sharing of this medication may be dangerous.
- Advise patients to notify health care professional immediately if they are taking theophylline.
- Encourage patient to maintain a fluid intake of at least 1500–2000 mL/day to prevent crystalluria.
- Advise patient that antacids or medications containing iron or zinc will decrease absorption. *Ciprofloxacin, levofloxacin, norfloxacin,* and *ofloxacin* should be taken at least 2 hr before (3 hr for *gemifloxacin,* 4 hr for *moxifloxacin*) or 2 hr after (8 hr for *moxifloxacin*) these products.
- May cause dizziness and drowsiness. Caution patient to avoid driving or other activities requiring alertness until response to medication is known.
- Caution patient to use sunscreen and protective clothing to prevent phototoxicity reactions during and for 5 days after therapy. Notify health care professional if a sunburn-like reaction or skin eruption occurs.
- Instruct patients being treated for gonorrhea that partners also must be treated.
- Instruct patient to consult health care professional before taking any other Rx, OTC, or herbal products.
- Advise patient to report signs of superinfection (furry overgrowth on the tongue, vaginal itching or discharge, loose or foul-smelling stools).
- Instruct patient to notify health care professional if fever and diarrhea develop, especially if stool contains blood, pus, or mucus. Advise patient not to treat diarrhea without consulting health care professional.
- Instruct patient to notify health care professional immediately if rash, jaundice, signs of hypersensitivity, or tendon (shoulder, hand, Achilles, and other) pain, swelling, or inflammation occur. If tendon symptoms occur, avoid exercise and use of the affected area. Increased risk in >65 yrs old, kidney, heart and lung transplant recipients, and patients taking corticosteroids concurrently. Therapy should be discontinued.

Evaluation/Desired Outcomes
- Resolution of the signs and symptoms of infection. Time for complete resolution depends on organism and site of infection.
- Post exposure treatment of inhalational anthrax or cutaneous anthrax (ciprofloxacin and levofloxacin).

HIGH ALERT

fluorouracil
(flure-oh-**yoor**-a-sill)
Carac, Efudex, Fluoroplex, 5-FU

Classification
Therapeutic: antineoplastics
Pharmacologic: antimetabolites

Pregnancy Category D

Indications
IV: Used alone and in combination with other modalities (surgery, radiation therapy, other antineoplastics) in the treatment of: Colon cancer, Breast cancer, Rectal cancer, Gastric cancer, Pancreatic carcinoma. **Topical:** Management of multiple actinic (solar) keratoses and superficial basal cell carcinomas.

Action
Inhibits DNA and RNA synthesis by preventing thymidine production (cell-cycle S-phase–specific). **Therapeutic Effects:** Death of rapidly replicating cells, particularly malignant ones.

Pharmacokinetics
Absorption: Minimal absorption (5–10%) after topical application.
Distribution: Widely distributed; concentrates and persists in tumors.
Metabolism and Excretion: Metabolized by dihydropyrimidine dehydrogenase to a less toxic compound; inactive metabolites are excreted primarily in urine.
Half-life: 20 hr.

fluorouracil

TIME/ACTION PROFILE (IV = effects on blood counts, Top = dermatologic effects)

ROUTE	ONSET	PEAK	DURATION
IV	1–9 days	9–21 days (nadir)	30 days
Top	2–3 days	2–6 wk	1–2 mo

Contraindications/Precautions
Contraindicated in: Hypersensitivity; ▓ Dihydropyrimidine dehydrogenase deficiency (patients at ↑ risk of 5–FU toxicity); OB, Lactation: Pregnancy or lactation.
Use Cautiously in: Infections; Depressed bone marrow reserve; Other chronic debilitating illnesses; Obese patients, patients with edema or ascites (dose should be based on ideal body weight).

Adverse Reactions/Side Effects
More likely to occur with systemic use than with topical use.
CNS: acute cerebellar dysfunction. **GI:** diarrhea, nausea, stomatitis, vomiting. **Derm:** alopecia, maculopapular rash, local inflammatory reactions (topical only), melanosis of nails, nail loss, palmar-plantar erythrodysesthesia, phototoxicity. **Endo:** sterility. **Hemat:** anemia, leukopenia, thrombocytopenia. **Local:** thrombophlebitis. **Misc:** fever.

Interactions
Drug-Drug: Combination chemotherapy with **irinotecan** may produce unacceptable toxicity (dehydration, neutropenia, sepsis). Additive bone marrow depression with other **bone marrow depressants**, including other **antineoplastics** and **radiation therapy**. May ↓ antibody response to **live-virus vaccines** and ↑ risk of adverse reactions.

Route/Dosage
Doses may vary greatly, depending on tumor, patient condition, and protocol used.

Advanced Colorectal Cancer
IV (Adults): 370 mg/m^2 preceded by leucovorin *or* 425 mg/m^2 preceded by leucovorin daily for 5 days. May be repeated q 4–5 wk.

Other Tumors
IV (Adults): *Initial dose*—12 mg/kg/day for 4 days, then 1 day of rest, then 6 mg/kg every other day for 4–5 doses *or* 7–12 mg/kg/day for 4 days followed by 3-day rest, then 7–10 mg/kg q 3–4 days for 3 doses. *Maintenance*—7–12 mg/kg q 7–10 days *or* 300–500 mg/m^2/day for 4–5 days, repeated monthly (no single daily dose should exceed 800 mg). **Poor-Risk Patients:** 3–6 mg/kg/day on days 1–3, 3 mg/kg/day on days 5, 7, 9 (not to exceed 400 mg/dose). Doses of 370–425 mg/m^2/day for 5 days have been used in combination with leucovorin.

Actinic (Solar) Keratoses
Topical (Adults): *Carac*—Apply 0.5% cream to lesions once daily for up to 4 wk; *Efudex*—Apply 2% or 5% solution or cream to lesions twice daily for 2–4 wk; *Fluoroplex*—Apply 1% cream to lesions twice daily for 2–6 wk.

Superficial Basal Cell Carcinomas
Topical (Adults): *Efudex*—Apply 5% solution or cream to lesions twice daily for 3–6 wk (up to 12 wk).

Availability (generic available)
Injection: 50 mg/mL. **Cream:** 0.5%, 1%, 5%. **Solution:** 2%, 5%.

NURSING IMPLICATIONS

Assessment
- Monitor vital signs before and frequently during therapy.
- Assess mucous membranes, number and consistency of stools, and frequency of vomiting. Assess for signs of infection (fever, chills, sore throat, cough, hoarseness, pain in lower back or side, difficult or painful urination). Assess for bleeding (bleeding gums; bruising; petechiae; and guaiac test stools, urine, and emesis). Avoid IM injections and taking rectal temperatures. Apply pressure to venipuncture sites for 10 min. Notify health care professional if symptoms of toxicity (stomatitis or esophagopharyngitis, uncontrollable vomiting, diarrhea, GI bleeding, myocardial ischemia, leukocyte count <3500/mm^3, platelet count <100,000/mm^3, or hemorrhage from any site) occur; drug will need to be discontinued. May be reinitiated at a lower dose when side effects have subsided.
- Assess IV site frequently for inflammation or infiltration. Patient should notify nurse if pain or irritation at injection site occurs. May cause thrombophlebitis. If extravasation occurs, infusion must be stopped and restarted in another vein to avoid damage to subcut tissue. Report immediately. Standard treatment includes application of ice compresses.
- Assess skin for palmar-plantar erythrodysesthesia (tingling of hands and feet followed by

pain, erythema, and swelling) throughout therapy.
- Monitor intake and output, appetite, and nutritional intake. GI effects usually occur on 4th day of therapy. Adjusting diet as tolerated may help maintain fluid and electrolyte balance and nutritional status.
- Monitor patient for cerebellar dysfunction (weakness, ataxia, dizziness). This may persist after discontinuation of therapy.
- **Topical:** Inspect involved skin before and throughout therapy.
- *Lab Test Considerations:* May cause ↓ in plasma albumin.
- Monitor hepatic (AST, ALT, LDH, and serum bilirubin), renal, and hematologic (hematocrit, hemoglobin, leukocyte, platelet count) functions before and periodically during therapy. Monitor CBC daily during IV therapy. Report WBC of <3500/mm³ or platelets <100,000/mm³ immediately; they are criteria for discontinuation. Nadir of leukopenia usually occurs in 9–14 days, with recovery by day 30. May also cause thrombocytopenia.
- May cause ↑ in urine excretion of 5-hydroxyindoleacetic acid (5-HIAA).

Potential Nursing Diagnoses
Risk for infection (Side Effects)
Imbalanced nutrition: less than body requirements (Side Effects)

Implementation
- *High Alert:* Fatalities have occurred with incorrect administration of chemotherapeutic agents. Before administering, clarify all ambiguous orders; double check single, daily, and course-of-therapy dose limits; have second practitioner independently double check original order, calculations and infusion pump settings. The number 5 in 5-fluorouracil is part of the drug name and does not refer to the dose.
- Do not confuse Carac with Kuric (ketoconazole).
- Prepare solution in a biologic cabinet. Wear gloves, gown, and mask while handling IV medication. Discard IV equipment in specially designated containers.

IV Administration
- **Direct IV:** *Diluent:* May be administered undiluted. *Concentration:* 50 mg/mL. *Rate:* Rapid IV push administration (over 1–2 min) is most effective, but there is a more rapid onset of toxicity.
- **Intermittent Infusion:** *Diluent:* May be diluted with D5W or 0.9% NaCl.
- Use plastic IV tubing and IV bags to maintain greater stability of medication. Solution is stable for 24 hr at room temperature; do not refrigerate. Solution is colorless to faint yellow. Discard highly discolored or cloudy solution. If crystals form, dissolve by warming solution to 140°F, shaking vigorously, and cooling to body temperature. *Concentration:* Up to 50 mg/mL. *Rate:* Onset of toxicity is greatly delayed by administering an infusion over 2–8 hr.
- **Y-Site Compatibility:** acyclovir, alfentanil, allopurinol, amifostine, amikacin, aminophylline, amphotericin B liposome, ampicillin, ampicillin/sulbactam, anidulafungin, azithromycin, aztreonam, bivalirudin, bleomycin, bumetanide, butorphanol, calcium gluconate, carboplatin, cefazolin, cefepime, cefoperazone, cefotaxime, cefotetan, cefoxitin, ceftazidime, ceftriaxone, cefuroxime, cimetidine, cisatracurium, cisplatin, clindamycin, codeine, cyclophosphamide, cyclosporine, daptomycin, dexamethasone, dexmedetomidine, dexrazoxane, digoxin, docetaxel, dopamine, doripenem, doxorubicin liposome, enalaprilat, ephedrine, ertapenem, erythromycin, esmolol, etoposide phosphate, famotidine, fenoldopam, fentanyl, fluconazole, fludarabine, foscarnet, fosphenytoin, furosemide, ganciclovir, gemcitabine, gentamicin, granisetron, heparin, hetastarch, hydrocortisone, hydromorphone, ifosfamide, imipenem/cilastatin, inamrinone, isoproterenol, ketorolac, labetalol, leucovorin, levorphanol, lidocaine, linezolid, magnesium sulfate, mannitol, melphalan, meperidine, meropenem, mesna, methohexital, methotrexate, methylprednisolone, metoprolol, metronidazole, milrinone, mitomycin, mitoxantrone, morphine, nalbuphine, naloxone, nesiritide, nitroglycerin, nitroprusside, octreotide, paclitaxel, palonosetron, pancuronium, pantoprazole, pemetrexed, pentobarbital, phenobarbital, phenylephrine, piperacillin/tazobactam, potassium chloride, potassium phosphate, procainamide, propofol, propranolol, ranitidine, remifentanil, rituximab, sargramostim, sodium acetate, sodium bicarbonate, sodium phosphates, succinylcholine, sufentanil, teniposide, theophylline, thiopental, thiotepa, ticarcillin/clavulanate, tigecycline, tirofiban, tobramycin, trastuzumab, vasopressin, vecuronium, vinblastine, vincristine, vitamin B complex with C, voriconazole, zidovudine.
- **Y-Site Incompatibility:** aldesleukin, amiodarone, amphotericin B cholesteryl, amphotericin B colloidal, buprenorphine, calcium chloride, caspofungin, chlorpromazine,

ciprofloxacin, diazepam, diltiazem, diphenhydramine, dobutamine, doxycycline, droperidol, epinephrine, epirubicin, filgrastim, haloperidol, hydroxyzine, idarubicin, levofloxacin, lorazepam, midazolam, nicardipine, ondansetron, pentamidine, phenytoin, prochlorperazine, promethazine, quinapristin/dalfopristin, topotecan, trimethobenzamide, vancomycin, verapamil, vinorelbine.

- **Topical:** Consult health care professional before administering topical preparations to determine which skin preparation regimen should be followed. Tight occlusive dressings are not advised because of irritation to surrounding healthy tissue. A loose gauze dressing for cosmetic purposes is usually preferred. Wear gloves when applying medication. Do not use metallic applicator.

Patient/Family Teaching

- Instruct patient to notify health care professional if fever; chills; sore throat; signs of infection; yellowing of skin or eyes; abdominal pain; joint or flank pain; swelling of feet or legs; bleeding gums; bruising; petechiae; or blood in urine, stool, or emesis occurs. Caution patient to avoid crowds and persons with known infections. Instruct patient to use soft toothbrush and electric razor. Patients should be cautioned not to drink alcoholic beverages or take products containing aspirin or NSAIDs.
- Advise patient to rinse mouth with clear water after eating and drinking and to avoid flossing to minimize stomatitis. Viscous lidocaine may be used if mouth pain interferes with eating. Stomatitis pain may require treatment with opioid analgesics.
- Discuss with patient the possibility of hair loss. Explore methods of coping.
- Review with patient the need for contraception during therapy.
- Caution patient to use sunscreen and protective clothing to prevent phototoxicity reactions.
- Instruct patient not to receive any vaccinations without advice of health care professional.
- Emphasize the importance of routine follow-up lab tests to monitor progress and to check for side effects.
- **Topical:** Instruct patient in correct application of solution or cream. Emphasize importance of avoiding the eyes; caution should also be used when applying medication near mouth and nose. If patient uses clean finger to self-administer, emphasize importance of washing hands thoroughly after application. Explain that erythema, scaling, and blistering with pruritus and burning sensation are expected. Advise patient to avoid sunlight or ultraviolet light (tanning booths) as much as possible; may increase side effects. Therapy is discontinued when erosion, ulceration, and necrosis occur in 2–6 wk (10–12 wk for basal cell carcinomas). Skin heals 4–8 wk later.

Evaluation/Desired Outcomes

- Tumor regression.
- Removal of solar keratoses or superficial basal cell skin cancers.

fluoxetine (floo-ox-uh-teen)
Prozac, Prozac Weekly, Sarafem

Classification
Therapeutic: antidepressants
Pharmacologic: selective serotonin reuptake inhibitors (SSRIs)

Pregnancy Category B

Indications
Major depressive disorder. Obsessive compulsive disorder (OCD). Bulimia nervosa. Panic disorder. Depressive episodes associated with bipolar I disorder (when used with olanzapine). Treatment-resistant depression (when used with olanzapine). **Sarafem:** Premenstrual dysphoric disorder (PMDD). **Unlabeled Use:** Anorexia nervosa: ADHD, Diabetic neuropathy, Fibromyalgia, Obesity, Raynaud's phenomenon, Social anxiety disorder (social phobia), Post-traumatic stress disorder (PTSD).

Action
Selectively inhibits the reuptake of serotonin in the CNS. **Therapeutic Effects:** Antidepressant action. Decreased behaviors associated with: panic disorder, bulimia. Decreased mood alterations associated with PMDD.

Pharmacokinetics
Absorption: Well absorbed after oral administration.
Distribution: Crosses the blood-brain barrier.
Protein Binding: 94.5%.
Metabolism and Excretion: Converted by the liver to norfluoxetine (primarily by CYP2D6 isoenzyme), another antidepressant compound; the CYP2D6 enzyme system exhibits genetic polymorphism (~7% of population may be poor

metabolizers and may have significantly ↑ fluoxetine concentrations and an ↑ risk of adverse effects). Fluoxetine and norfluoxetine are mostly metabolized by the liver; 12% excreted by kidneys as unchanged fluoxetine, 7% as unchanged norfluoxetine.

Half-life: 1–3 days (norfluoxetine 5–7 days).

TIME/ACTION PROFILE (antidepressant effect)

ROUTE	ONSET	PEAK	DURATION
PO	1–4 wk	unknown	2 wk

Contraindications/Precautions
Contraindicated in: Hypersensitivity; Concurrent use or use within 14 days of discontinuing MAO inhibitors (fluoxetine should be discontinued at least 5 wk before MAO therapy is initiated); Concurrent use of pimozide; Concurrent use of thioridazine (fluoxetine should be discontinued at least 5 wk before thioridazine therapy is initiated).
Use Cautiously in: Severe hepatic or renal impairment (lower/less frequent dose may be necessary); History of seizures; Debilitated patients (↑ risk of seizures); Diabetes mellitus; Patients with concurrent chronic illness or multiple drug therapy (dose adjustments may be necessary); Patients with impaired hepatic function (↓ doses/ ↑ dosing interval may be necessary); May ↑ risk of suicide attempt/ideation especially during early treatment or dose adjustment; OB: Use during third trimester may result in neonatal serotonin syndrome requiring prolonged hospitalization, respiratory and nutritional support. May cause sedation in infant; Lactation: May cause sedation in infant; discontinue drug or bottle-feed; Pedi: Risk of suicide ideation or attempt may be greater in children or adolescents (safe use in children <8 yr not established); Geri: Appears on Beers list. Geriatric patients are at ↑ risk for excessive CNS stimulation, sleep disturbances, and agitation.

Adverse Reactions/Side Effects
CNS: NEUROLEPTIC MALIGNANT SYNDROME, SEIZURES, SUICIDAL THOUGHTS, anxiety, drowsiness, headache, insomnia, nervousness, abnormal dreams, dizziness, fatigue, hypomania, mania, weakness. **EENT:** stuffy nose, visual disturbances. **Resp:** cough. **CV:** chest pain, palpitations. **GI:** diarrhea, abdominal pain, abnormal taste, anorexia, constipation, dry mouth, dyspepsia, nausea, vomiting, weight loss. **GU:** sexual dysfunction, urinary frequency. **Derm:** ↑ sweating, pruritus, erythema nodusum, flushing, rashes. **Endo:** dysmenorrhea. **F and E:** hyponatremia. **MS:** arthralgia, back pain, myalgia. **Neuro:** tremor. **Misc:** SEROTONIN SYNDROME, allergic reactions, fever, flu-like syndrome, hot flashes, sensitivity reaction.

Interactions
Drug-Drug: Discontinue use of **MAO inhibitors** for 14 days before fluoxetine therapy; combined therapy may result in confusion, agitation, seizures, hypertension, and hyperpyrexia (serotonin syndrome). Fluoxetine should be discontinued for at least 5 wk before MAO inhibitor therapy is initiated. Concurrent use with **pimozide** may ↑ risk of QT interval prolongation. ↑ levels of **thioridazine** may ↑ risk of QT interval prolongation (concurrent use contraindicated; fluoxetine should be discontinued for at least 5 wk before thioridazine is initiated). Inhibits the activity of cytochrome P450 2D6 enzyme in the liver and ↑ effects of drugs metabolized by this enzyme system. **Medications that inhibit the P450 enzyme system** (including **ritonavir**, **saquinavir**, and **efavirenz**) may ↑ risk of developing the serotonin syndrome). For concurrent use with **ritonavir** ↓ fluoxetine dose by 70%; if initiating fluoxetine, start with 10 mg/day dose. ↓ metabolism and ↑ effects of **alprazolam** (decrease alprazolam dose by 50%). Drugs that affect serotonergic neurotransmitter systems, including **linezolid**, **tramadol**, and **triptans**, ↑ risk of serotonin syndrome. ↑ CNS depression with **alcohol**, **antihistamines**, other **antidepressants**, **opioid analgesics**, or **sedative/hypnotics**. ↑ risk of side effects and adverse reactions with other **antidepressants**, **risperidone**, or **phenothiazines**. May ↑ effectiveness/risk of toxicity from **carbamazepine**, **clozapine**, **digoxin**, **haloperidol**, **phenytoin**, **lithium**, or **warfarin**. May ↓ the effects of **buspirone**. **Cyproheptadine** may ↓ or reverse effects of fluoxetine. May ↑ sensitivity to **adrenergics** and increase the risk of serotonin syndrome. May alter the activity of other **drugs that are highly bound to plasma proteins**. ↑ risk of serotonin syndrome with **5HT$_1$ agonists**. ↑ risk of bleeding with **NSAIDS**, **aspirin**, **clopidogrel**, or **warfarin**.
Drug-Natural Products: ↑ risk of serotonin syndrome with **St. John's wort** and **SAMe**.

Route/Dosage
PO (Adults): *Depression, OCD*— 20 mg/day in the morning. After several weeks, may ↑ by 20 mg/day at weekly intervals. Doses greater than 20 mg/day should be given in 2 divided doses, in the morning and at noon (not to exceed 80 mg/day). Patients who have been stabilized on the 20 mg/

fluoxetine

day dose may be switched over to delayed-release capsules (Prozac Weekly) at dose of 90 mg weekly, initiated 7 days after the last 20–mg dose. *Panic disorder*— 10 mg/day initially, may ↑ after 1 week to 20 mg/day (usual dose is 20 mg, but may be ↑ as needed/tolerated up to 60 mg/day). *Bulimia nervosa*— 60 mg/day (may need to titrate up to dosage over several days). *PMDD*— 20 mg/day (not to exceed 80 mg/day) *or* 20 mg/day starting 14 days prior to expected onset on menses, continued through first full day of menstruation, repeated with each cycle. *Depressive episodes associated with bipolar I disorder*-20 mg/day with olanzapine 5 mg/day (both given in evening); may ↑ fluoxetine dose up to 50 mg/day and olanzapine dose up to 12.5 mg/day; *Treatment-resistant depression*-20 mg/day with olanzapine 5 mg/day (both given in evening); may ↑ fluoxetine dose up to 50 mg/day and olanzapine dose up to 20 mg/day.

PO (Geriatric Patients): *Depression*— 10 mg/day in the morning initially, may be ↑ (not to exceed 60 mg/day).

PO (Children 7–17 yr): *Adolescents and higher weight children*— 10 mg/day may be ↑ after 2 wk to 20 mg/day; additional increases may be made after several more weeks (range 20–60 mg/day); *Lower-weight children*— 10 mg/day initially, may be ↑ after several more weeks (range 20–30 mg/day).

Availability (generic available)
Tablets: 10 mg, 20 mg. **Cost:** *Generic*— 10 mg $47.98/90, 20 mg $62.97/90. **Capsules:** 10 mg, 20 mg, 40 mg. **Cost:** *Generic*— 10 mg $48.97/90, 20 mg $26.99/90, 40 mg $119.97/90. **Delayed-release capsules (Prozac Weekly):** 90 mg. **Cost:** $110.99/4. **Oral solution (mint flavor):** 20 mg/5 mL. **Cost:** *Generic*—$72.98/120 mL. *In combination with:* olanzapine (Symbyax; see Appendix B).

NURSING IMPLICATIONS

Assessment
- Monitor mood changes. Inform health care professional if patient demonstrates significant increase in anxiety, nervousness, or insomnia.
- Assess for suicidal tendencies, especially during early therapy. Restrict amount of drug available to patient. Risk may be increased in children, adolescents, and adults ≤24 yr. After starting therapy, children, adolescents, and young adults should be seen by health care professional at least weekly for 4 wk, every 3 wk for next 4 wk, and on advice of health care professional thereafter.
- Monitor appetite and nutritional intake. Weigh weekly. Notify health care professional of continued weight loss. Adjust diet as tolerated to support nutritional status.
- Assess patient for sensitivity reaction (urticaria, fever, arthralgia, edema, carpal tunnel syndrome, rash, hives, lymphadenopathy, respiratory distress) and notify health care professional if present; symptoms usually resolve by stopping fluoxetine but may require administration of antihistamines or corticosteroids.
- Assess for sexual side effects (erectile dysfunction; decreased libido).
- Assess for serotonin syndrome (mental changes [agitation, hallucinations, coma], autonomic instability [tachycardia, labile blood pressure, hyperthermia], neuromuscular aberrations [hyperreflexia, incoordination], and/or GI symptoms [nausea, vomiting, diarrhea]), especially in patients taking other serotonergic drugs (SSRIs, SNRIs, triptans).
- **OCD:** Assess patient for frequency of obsessive-compulsive behaviors. Note degree to which these thoughts and behaviors interfere with daily functioning.
- **Bulimia Nervosa:** Assess frequency of binge eating and vomiting during therapy.
- **PMDD:** Monitor patient's mood prior to and periodically during therapy.
- *Lab Test Considerations:* Monitor CBC and differential periodically during therapy. Notify health care professional if leukopenia, anemia, thrombocytopenia, or increased bleeding time occurs.
- Proteinuria and mild ↑ in AST may occur during sensitivity reactions.
- May cause ↑ in serum alkaline phosphatase, ALT, BUN, creatine phosphokinase; hypouricemia, hypocalcemia, hypoglycemia or hyperglycemia, and hyponatremia.

Potential Nursing Diagnoses
Ineffective coping (Indications)
Risk for injury (Side Effects)
Sexual dysfunction (Side Effects)

Implementation
- Do not confuse Sarafem (fluoxetine) with Serophene (clomiphene).
- **PO:** Administer as a single dose in the morning. Some patients may require increased

amounts, in divided doses, with a 2nd dose at noon.
- May be administered with food to minimize GI irritation. Do not open or crush ER preparations.

Patient/Family Teaching
- Instruct patient to take fluoxetine as directed. If a dose is missed, omit and return to regular schedule. Do not double doses or discontinue without consulting health care professional; discontinuation may cause anxiety, insomnia, nervousness.
- May cause drowsiness, dizziness, impaired judgment, and blurred vision. Caution patient to avoid driving and other activities requiring alertness until response to the drug is known.
- Advise patient, family and caregivers to look for suicidality, especially during early therapy or dose changes. Notify health care professional immediately if thoughts about suicide or dying, attempts to commit suicide, new or worse depression or anxiety, agitation or restlessness, panic attacks, insomnia, new or worse irritability, aggressiveness, acting on dangerous impulses, mania, or other changes in mood or behavior or if symptoms of serotonin syndrome occur.
- Advise patient to avoid alcohol or other CNS depressant drugs during therapy and to consult health care professional before taking other medications or natural/herbal products with fluoxetine.
- Caution patient to change positions slowly to minimize dizziness.
- Inform patient that frequent mouth rinses, good oral hygiene, and sugarless gum or candy may minimize dry mouth. If dry mouth persists for more than 2 wk, consult health care professional regarding use of saliva substitute.
- Instruct female patients to inform health care professional if pregnancy is planned or suspected.
- Caution patient to wear protective clothing and use sunscreen to prevent photosensitivity reactions.
- Inform patient that medication may cause decreased libido.
- Advise patient to notify health care professional if symptoms of sensitivity reaction occur or if headache, nausea, anorexia, anxiety, or insomnia persists.
- Emphasize the importance of follow-up exams to monitor progress. Encourage patient participation in psychotherapy to improve coping skills.

Evaluation/Desired Outcomes
- Increased sense of well-being.
- Renewed interest in surroundings. May require 1–4 wk of therapy to obtain antidepressant effects.
- Decrease in obsessive-compulsive behaviors.
- Decrease in binge eating and vomiting in patients with bulimia nervosa.
- Decreased incidence frequency of panic attacks.
- Decreased mood alterations associated with PMDD.

---

fluphenazine (floo-fen-a-zeen)
✦ Apo-Fluphenazine,
✦ Modecate Concentrate,
✦ PMS-Fluphenazine, Prolixin, Prolixin Decanoate

Classification
Therapeutic: antipsychotics
Pharmacologic: phenothiazines

Pregnancy Category C

Indications
Acute and chronic psychoses.

Action
Alters the effects of dopamine in the CNS. Has anticholinergic and alpha-adrenergic blocking activity. **Therapeutic Effects:** Diminished signs and symptoms of psychoses.

Pharmacokinetics
Absorption: Well absorbed after PO/IM administration. Decanoate salt in sesame oil has delayed onset and prolonged action because of delayed release from oil vehicle and subsequent delayed release from fatty tissues.
Distribution: Widely distributed. Crosses the blood-brain barrier. Crosses the placenta; enters breast milk.
Protein Binding: ≥90%.
Metabolism and Excretion: Highly metabolized by the liver; undergo enterohepatic recirculation.
Half-life: *Fluphenazine hydrochloride*—33 hr; *fluphenazine decanoate*—6.8–9.6 days.

TIME/ACTION PROFILE (antipsychotic activity)

ROUTE	ONSET	PEAK	DURATION
PO hydrochloride	1 hr	unknown	6–8 hr
IM decanoate	24–72 hr	48–96 hr	≥4 wk

Contraindications/Precautions

Contraindicated in: Hypersensitivity; Cross-sensitivity with other phenothiazines may exist; Subcortical brain damage; Severe CNS depression; Coma; Bone marrow depression; Liver disease; Hypersensitivity to sesame oil (decanoate salt); Some products contain alcohol or tartrazine and should be avoided in patients with known intolerance; Concurrent use of drugs that prolong the QT interval; Pedi: Safety not established in children <6 mo.

Use Cautiously in: Cardiovascular disease; Parkinson's disease; Angle-closure glaucoma; Myasthenia gravis; Prostatic hypertrophy; Seizure disorders; OB: Use only if potential benefit justifies potential risk to fetus; Lactation: Enters breast milk, not recommended; Geri: Initial dose reduction may be necessary in geriatric or debilitated patients; ↑ risk of mortality in elderly patients treated for dementia-related psychosis.

Adverse Reactions/Side Effects

CNS: NEUROLEPTIC MALIGNANT SYNDROME, extrapyramidal reactions, sedation, tardive dyskinesia. **EENT:** blurred vision, dry eyes. **CV:** hypertension, hypotension, tachycardia. **GI:** anorexia, constipation, drug-induced hepatitis, dry mouth, ileus, nausea, weight gain. **GU:** urinary retention. **Derm:** photosensitivity, pigment changes, rashes. **Endo:** galactorrhea. **Hemat:** AGRANULOCYTOSIS, leukopenia, thrombocytopenia. **Misc:** allergic reactions.

Interactions

Drug-Drug: Concurrent use with drugs that prolong the QT interval, including **antiarrhythmics**, **pimozide**, **erythromycin**, **clarithromycin**, **fluoroquinolones**, **methadone**, and **tricyclic antidepressants** may ↑ the risk for arrhythmias; concurrent use should be avoided. Additive hypotension with **antihypertensives**. Additive CNS depression with other **CNS depressants**, including **alcohol**, **antidepressants**, **antihistamines**, **opioids**, **sedative/hypnotics**, or **general anesthetics**. **Phenobarbital** may increase metabolism and decrease effectiveness of fluphenazine. May ↑ the risk of **lithium** toxicity. **Aluminum-containing antacids** may decrease oral absorption of fluphenazine. May decrease anti-Parkinson activity of **levodopa** and **bromocriptine**. May decrease the vasopressor response to **epinephrine** and **norepinephrine**. **Beta blockers**, **chlorpromazine**, **chloroquine**, **delavirdine**, **fluoxetine**, **paroxetine**, **quinidine**, **quinine**, **ritonavir**, and **ropinirole** may ↑ the effects of fluphenazine. Increased risk of anticholinergic effects with other **agents having anticholinergic properties**, including **antihistamines**, **tricyclic antidepressants**, **disopyramide**, or **quinidine**. **Metoclopramide** may ↑ the risk of extrapyramidal reactions.

Route/Dosage

Fluphenazine Decanoate

IM (Adults): 12.5–25 mg initially; may be repeated q 3 wk. Dose may be slowly increased as needed (not to exceed 100 mg/dose).

Fluphenazine Hydrochloride

PO (Adults): 0.5–10 mg/day in divided doses q 6–8 hr (maximum dose = 40 mg/day).
PO (Geriatric Patients or Debilitated Patients): 1–2.5 mg/day initially; increase dose every 4–7 days by 1–2.5 mg/day as needed (max dose = 20 mg/day).
IM (Adults): 1.25–2.5 mg q 6–8 hr.

Availability (generic available)

Fluphenazine decanoate injection: 25 mg/mL, ✦ 100 mg/mL. **Fluphenazine hydrochloride tablets:** 1 mg, 2.5 mg, 5 mg, 10 mg. **Fluphenazine hydrochloride elixir (orange flavor):** 2.5 mg/5 mL. **Fluphenazine hydrochloride concentrate:** 5 mg/mL. **Fluphenazine hydrochloride injection:** 2.5 mg/mL.

NURSING IMPLICATIONS

Assessment

- Assess patient's mental status (orientation, mood, behavior) before and periodically during therapy.
- Monitor blood pressure (sitting, standing, lying), ECG, pulse, and respiratory rate before and frequently during the period of dose adjustment. May cause Q-wave and T-wave changes in ECG.
- Observe patient carefully when administering oral medication to ensure that medication is actually taken and not hoarded.
- Assess fluid intake and bowel function. Increased bulk and fluids in the diet help minimize constipation.
- Monitor patient for onset of akathisia (restlessness or desire to keep moving) and extrapyramidal side effects (*parkinsonian*—diffi-

culty speaking or swallowing, loss of balance control, pill rolling, mask-like face, shuffling gait, rigidity, tremors; *dystonic*—muscle spasms, twisting motions, twitching, inability to move eyes, weakness of arms or legs) every 2 mo during therapy and 8–12 wk after therapy has been discontinued. Reduction in dose or discontinuation of medication may be necessary. Benztropine or diphenhydramine may be used to control these symptoms.
- Monitor for tardive dyskinesia (uncontrolled rhythmic movement of mouth, face, and extremities; lip smacking or puckering; puffing of cheeks; uncontrolled chewing; rapid or worm-like movements of tongue). Report immediately; may be irreversible.
- Monitor for development of neuroleptic malignant syndrome (fever, respiratory distress, tachycardia, seizures, diaphoresis, arrhythmias, hypertension or hypotension, pallor, tiredness, severe muscle stiffness, loss of bladder control). Report immediately.
- **Lab Test Considerations:** Evaluate CBC, liver function tests, and ocular examinations periodically during therapy. May cause ↓ hematocrit, hemoglobin, leukocytes, granulocytes, and platelets. May cause ↑ bilirubin, AST, ALT, and alkaline phosphatase. Agranulocytosis may occur after 4–10 wk of therapy with recovery 1–2 wk after discontinuation. May recur if medication is restarted. Liver function abnormalities may require discontinuation of therapy.

Potential Nursing Diagnoses
Disturbed thought process (Indications)
Noncompliance (Patient/Family Teaching)

Implementation
- Slight yellow to amber color does not alter potency.
- To prevent contact dermatitis, avoid getting liquid preparations on hands and wash hands thoroughly if spillage occurs.
- Injectable forms must be drawn up with a dry syringe and dry 21-gauge needle to prevent clouding of the solution.
- **PO:** Dilute concentrate just before administration in 120–240 mL of water, milk, carbonated beverage, soup, or tomato or fruit juice. Do not mix with beverages containing caffeine (cola, coffee), tannics (tea), or pectinates (apple juice).
- **Subcut:** Fluphenazine decanoate is dissolved in sesame oil for long duration of action. It may be administered subcut or IM. 12.5 mg of fluphenazine decanoate given every 3 wk is approximately equivalent to 10 mg/day orally of fluphenazine hydrochloride.
- **IM:** IM dose of fluphenazine hydrochloride is usually 30–50% of oral dose. Because fluphenazine hydrochloride has a shorter duration of action, it is used initially to determine the patient's response to the drug and to treat the acutely agitated patient.
- Administer deep IM, using a dry syringe and 21-gauge needle, into dorsal gluteal site. Instruct patient to remain recumbent for 30 min to prevent hypotension.
- **Syringe Compatibility:** Fluphenazine hydrocholride is compatible in syringe with, benztropine, diphenhydramine, hydroxyzine.

Patient/Family Teaching
- Advise patient to take medication as directed and not to skip doses or double up on missed doses. If a dose is missed, take within 1 hr or skip dose and return to regular schedule if taking more than 1 dose/day; take as soon as possible unless almost time for next dose if taking 1 dose/day. Abrupt withdrawal may lead to gastritis, nausea, vomiting, dizziness, headache, tachycardia, and insomnia.
- Inform patient of possibility of extrapyramidal symptoms and tardive dyskinesia. Caution patient to report these symptoms immediately to health care professional.
- Advise patient to change positions slowly to minimize orthostatic hypotension.
- Medication may cause drowsiness. Caution patient to avoid driving or other activities requiring alertness until response to medication is known.
- Caution patient to avoid taking alcohol or other CNS depressants concurrently with this medication.
- Advise patient to use sunscreen and protective clothing when exposed to the sun. Exposed surfaces may develop a blue-gray pigmentation, which may fade after discontinuation of the medication. Extremes of temperature should also be avoided because this drug impairs body temperature regulation.
- Advise patient that good oral hygiene, frequent rinsing of mouth with water, and sugarless gum or candy may help relieve dry mouth. Health care professional should be notified if dry mouth persists beyond 2 wk.
- Instruct patient to notify health care professional promptly if sore throat, fever, unusual bleeding or bruising, rash, weakness, tremors, visual disturbances, dark-colored urine, or clay-colored stools occur.

- Advise patient to notify health care professional of medication regimen before treatment or surgery.
- Emphasize the importance of routine follow-up exams, including ocular exams, with long-term therapy and continued participation in psychotherapy.

Evaluation/Desired Outcomes
- Decrease in excitable, paranoic, or withdrawn behavior.

flurandrenolide, See CORTICOSTEROIDS (TOPICAL/LOCAL).

flurazepam (flur-az-e-pam)
✤Apo-Flurazepam, Dalmane, ✤Novoflupam, ✤Somnol

Classification
Therapeutic: sedative/hypnotics
Pharmacologic: benzodiazepines

Schedule IV

Pregnancy Category UK

Indications
Short-term management of insomnia (<4 wk).

Action
Depresses the CNS, probably by potentiating GABA, an inhibitory neurotransmitter. **Therapeutic Effects:** Relief of insomnia.

Pharmacokinetics
Absorption: Well absorbed after oral administration.
Distribution: Widely distributed; crosses blood-brain barrier. Probably crosses the placenta and enters breast milk. Accumulation of drug occurs with chronic dosing.
Protein Binding: 97% (one of the active metabolites).
Metabolism and Excretion: Metabolized by the liver; some metabolites have hypnotic activity.
Half-life: 2.3 hr (half-life of active metabolite may be 30–200 hr).

TIME/ACTION PROFILE (hypnotic activity)

ROUTE	ONSET	PEAK	DURATION
PO	15–45 min	0.5–1 hr	7–8 hr

Contraindications/Precautions
Contraindicated in: Impaired respiratory function; Impaired respiratory function; Sleep apnea; Hypersensitivity; Cross-sensitivity with other benzodiazepines may exist; Pre-existing CNS depression; Severe uncontrolled pain; Angle-closure glaucoma; OB: Chronic use during pregnancy may cause withdrawal effects in neonates; Lactation: Enters breast milk; discontinue or bottle-feed.
Use Cautiously in: Hepatic dysfunction (dosage reduction may be necessary); History of suicide attempt or drug dependence; Debilitated patients (initial dose reduction may be necessary); Pedi: Safety not established in children <15 yr; Geri: Appears on Beer's list and is associated with increased falls risk in geriatric patients.

Adverse Reactions/Side Effects
CNS: abnormal thinking, behavior changes, confusion, daytime drowsiness, decreased concentration, dizziness, hallucinations, headache, lethargy, mental depression, paradoxical excitation, sleep—driving. **EENT:** blurred vision. **GI:** constipation, diarrhea, nausea, vomiting. **Derm:** rashes. **Neuro:** ataxia. **Misc:** physical dependence, psychological dependence, tolerance.

Interactions
Drug-Drug: Concurrent use with **alcohol**, **antidepressants**, **antihistamines**, and **opioids** may result in additive CNS depression. **Cimetidine**, **hormonal contraceptives**, **disulfiram**, **fluoxetine**, **isoniazid**, **ketoconazole**, **metoprolol**, **propoxyphene**, **propranolol**, or **valproic acid** may ↓ metabolism of flurazepam, enhancing its actions. May ↓ efficacy of **levodopa**. **Rifampin** or **barbiturates** may ↑ metabolism and decrease ↓ effectiveness of flurazepam. Sedative effects may be ↓ by **theophylline**.
Drug-Natural Products: Concomitant use of **kava-kava**, **valerian**, **chamomile**, or **hops** can ↑ CNS depression.

Route/Dosage
PO (Adults): 15–30 mg at bedtime.
PO (Geriatric Patients or Debilitated Patients): 15 mg initially, may be increased.

Availability (generic available)
Capsules: 15 mg, 30 mg. **Tablets:** 15 mg, 30 mg.

NURSING IMPLICATIONS
Assessment
- Assess sleep patterns before and periodically throughout therapy.
- Assess mental status (orientation, mood, behavior) and potential for abuse prior to administering medication.
- Prolonged use may lead to psychological or physical dependence. Restrict amount of drug available to patient, especially if patient is depressed, suicidal, or has a history of addiction.
- Geri: Assess fall risk and institute prevention strategies.

Potential Nursing Diagnoses
Insomnia (Indications)
Ineffective coping (Indications)
Sleep deprivation (Indications)
Risk for falls (Side Effects)
Acute confusion (Side Effects)
Risk for injury (Side Effects)

Implementation
- Do not confuse flurazepam with temazepam.
- Supervise ambulation and transfer of patients after administration. Remove cigarettes. Two side rails should be raised and call bell within reach at all times.
- When discontinuing, taper to decrease chance of withdrawal effects (may take months in some patients).
- **PO:** Capsules may be opened and mixed with food or fluids for patients having difficulty swallowing.

Patient/Family Teaching
- Advise patient to take medication exactly as directed.
- Teach sleep hygiene techniques (dark room, quiet, bedtime ritual, limit daytime napping, avoidance of nictotine and caffeine).
- Maximum hypnotic properties are apparent 2–3 nights after initiating therapy and may last 1–2 nights after therapy is discontinued.
- Medication may cause daytime drowsiness. Caution patient to avoid driving and other activities requiring alertness until response to medication is known.
- Caution patient to avoid taking alcohol or other CNS depressants concurrently with this medication.
- Refer for psychotherapy if ineffective coping is basis for sleep pattern disturbance.
- OB: Instruct patient to contact health care professional immediately if pregnancy is planned or suspected.
- Geri: Caution patient or family to institute fall prevention strategies at home.
- Instruct patient to contact health care professional immediately if pregnancy is planned or suspected.

Evaluation/Desired Outcomes
- Improvement in sleep patterns (decreased number of night time awakenings, improved sleep onset, and increased total sleep time).

---

fluticasone, See CORTICOSTEROIDS (INHALATION).

---

fluticasone, See CORTICOSTEROIDS (NASAL).

---

fluticasone, See CORTICOSTEROIDS (TOPICAL/LOCAL).

---

fluvastatin, See HMG-CoA REDUCTASE INHIBITORS (statins).

---

fluvoxamine
(floo-**voks**-a-meen)
Luvox, Luvox CR

Classification
Therapeutic: antidepressants, antiobsessive agents
Pharmacologic: selective serotonin reuptake inhibitors (SSRIs)

Pregnancy Category C

Indications
Obsessive-compulsive disorder (OCD) (immediate and controlled-release). Social anxiety disorder (SAD) (controlled-release only). **Unlabeled Use:** Depression. Generalized anxiety disorder (GAD). Post-traumatic stress disorder (PSTD).

Action
Inhibits the reuptake of serotonin in the CNS. **Therapeutic Effects:** Decrease in obsessive-compulsive behaviors. Decrease in symptoms of social anxiety disorder.

Pharmacokinetics
Absorption: 53% absorbed after oral administration.
Distribution: Excreted in breast milk; enters the CNS. Remainder of distribution not known.
Metabolism and Excretion: Eliminated mostly by the kidneys.

fluvoxamine

Half-life: 13.6–15.6 hr.

TIME/ACTION PROFILE (improvement on obsessive-compulsive behaviors)

ROUTE	ONSET	PEAK	DURATION
PO	within 2–3 wk	several mo	unknown

Contraindications/Precautions

Contraindicated in: Hypersensitivity to fluvoxamine or other SSRIs; Concurrent use or use within 14 days of discontinuing MAOIs, alosetron, pimozide, thioridazine, or tizanidine.
Use Cautiously in: Impaired hepatic function; May ↑ risk of suicide attempt/ideation especially during early treatment or dose adjustment; risk may be greater in children or adolescents; OB: Neonates exposed to SSRI in third trimester may develop drug discontinuation syndrome including respiratory distress, feeding difficulty, and irritability; Lactation: Discontinue drug or bottle-feed; Pedi: Safety not established in children <8 yr (for immediate-release); Geri: May have ↑ sensitivity; recommend lower initial dose and slower dosage titration.

Adverse Reactions/Side Effects

CNS: NEUROLEPTIC MALIGNANT SYNDROME, SUICIDAL THOUGHTS, sedation, dizziness, drowsiness, headache, insomnia, nervousness, weakness, agitation, anxiety, apathy, emotional lability, manic reactions, mental depression, psychotic reactions, syncope. **EENT:** sinusitis. **Resp:** cough, dyspnea. **CV:** edema, hypertension, palpitations, postural hypotension, tachycardia, vasodilation. **GI:** constipation, diarrhea, dry mouth, dyspepsia, nausea, anorexia, dysphagia, ↑ liver enzymes, flatulence, weight gain (unusual), vomiting. **GU:** ↓ libido/sexual dysfunction. **Derm:** ↑ sweating. **Metab:** weight gain, weight loss. **MS:** hypertonia, myoclonus/twitching. **Neuro:** hypokinesia/hyperkinesia, tremor. **Misc:** SEROTONIN SYNDROME, allergic reactions, chills, flu-like symptoms, tooth disorder/caries, yawning.

Interactions

Drug-Drug: Serious, potentially fatal reactions (serotonin syndrome) may occur with **MAO inhibitors**. **Smoking** may ↓ effectiveness of fluvoxamine. Concurrent use with **tricyclic antidepressants** may ↑ plasma levels of fluvoxamine. Drugs that affect serotonergic neurotransmitter systems, including **linezolid**, **tramadol**, and **triptans**, ↑ risk of serotonin syndrome. ↓ metabolism and may ↑ effects of some **beta blockers** (**propranolol**), **alosetron** (avoid concurrent use), some **benzodiazepines** (avoid concurrent **diazepam**), **carbamazepine**, **methadone**, **lithium**, **theophylline** (↓ dose to 33% of usual dose), **ramelteon** (avoid concurrent use), **warfarin**, and **L-tryptophan**. ↑ risk of bleeding with **NSAIDS**, **aspirin**, **clopidogrel**, or **warfarin**. ↑ blood levels and risk of toxicity from **clozapine** (dosage adjustments may be necessary).

Route/Dosage

PO (Adults): *Immediate release (OCD only)*— 50 mg daily at bedtime; ↑ by 50 mg q 4–7 days until desired effect is achieved. If daily dose >100 mg, give in two equally divided doses or give a larger dose at bedtime (not to exceed 300 mg/day); *Controlled release (OCD and SAD)*—100 mg at bedtime; ↑ by 50 mg q 7 days until desired effect is achieved, not to exceed 300 mg/day.
PO (Children 8–17 yr): *Immediate release (OCD only)*—25 mg at bedtime, may ↑ by 25 mg/day q 4–7 days (not to exceed 200 mg/day; daily doses >50 mg should be given in divided doses with a larger dose at bedtime).

Hepatic Impairment

PO (Adults): 25 mg daily at bedtime initially, slower titration and longer dosing intervals should be used.

Availability

Tablets: 25 mg, 50 mg, 100 mg. **Controlled-release capsules:** 100 mg, 150 mg.

NURSING IMPLICATIONS

Assessment

- Monitor mood changes. Assess patient for frequency of obsessive-compulsive behaviors. Note degree to which these thoughts and behaviors interfere with daily functioning. Inform health care professional if patient demonstrates significant increase in anxiety, nervousness, or insomnia.
- Assess for suicidal tendencies, especially during early therapy. Restrict amount of drug available to patient. Risk may be increased in children, adolescents, and adults ≤24 yrs. After starting therapy, children, adolescents, and young adults should be seen by health care professional at least weekly for 4 wk, every 3 wk for next 4 wk, and on advice of health care professional thereafter.
- Monitor appetite and nutritional intake. Weigh weekly. Report significant changes in weight.

606 folic acid

Adjust diet as tolerated to support nutritional status.
- Assess for serotonin syndrome (mental changes [agitation, hallucinations, coma], autonomic instability [tachycardia, labile blood pressure, hyperthermia], neuromuscular aberations [hyperreflexia, incoordination], and/or GI symptoms [nausea, vomiting, diarrhea]), especially in patients taking other serotonergic drugs (SSRIs, SNRIs, triptans).
- *Toxicity and Overdose:* Common symptoms of toxicity include drowsiness, vomiting, diarrhea, and dizziness. Coma, tachycardia, bradycardia, hypotension, ECG abnormalities, liver function abnormalities, and convulsions may also occur. Treatment is symptomatic and supportive.

Potential Nursing Diagnoses
Ineffective coping (Indications)
Risk for injury (Side Effects)

Implementation
- Taper to avoid withdrawal effects. Reduce dose by 50% for 3 days, then reduce by 50% for 3 days, then discontinue.
- **PO:** Initial therapy is administered as a single bedtime dose. May be increased every 4–7 days as tolerated.
- Fluvoxamine may be given without regard to meals. Do not open, break, crush, or chew controlled-release capsules.

Patient/Family Teaching
- Instruct patient to take fluvoxamine as directed. Do not skip or double up on missed doses. Improvement in symptoms may be noticed in 2–3 wk, but medication should be continued as directed.
- May cause drowsiness and dizziness. Caution patient to avoid driving and other activities requiring alertness until response to medication is known.
- Advise patient, family, and caregivers to look for suicidality, especially during early therapy or dose changes. Notify health care professional immediately if thoughts about suicide or dying, attempts to commit suicide, new or worse depression or anxiety, agitation or restlessness, panic attacks, insomnia, new or worse irritability, aggressiveness, acting on dangerous impulses, mania, or other changes in mood or behavior or if symptoms of serotonin syndrome occur.
- Advise patient to avoid alcohol or other CNS depressants during therapy and to consult health care professional before taking other medications with fluvoxamine.
- Instruct female patients to notify health care professional if breastfeeding or if pregnancy is planned or suspected.
- Advise patient to notify health care professional if rash or hives occur or if headache, nausea, anorexia, anxiety, or insomnia persists.
- Advise patient to avoid use of caffeine (chocolate, tea, cola).
- Emphasize the importance of follow-up exams to monitor progress.

Evaluation/Desired Outcomes
- Decrease in symptoms of obsessive-compulsive disorder.
- Decrease in symptoms of social anxiety disorder.

---

folic acid (foe-lika-sid)
✹ Apo-Folic, folate, Folvite,
✹ Novofolacid, vitamin B

Classification
Therapeutic: antianemics, vitamins
Pharmacologic: water soluble vitamins

Pregnancy Category A

Indications
Prevention and treatment of megaloblastic and macrocytic anemias. Given during pregnancy to promote normal fetal development.

Action
Required for protein synthesis and red blood cell function. Stimulates the production of red blood cells, white blood cells, and platelets. Necessary for normal fetal development. **Therapeutic Effects:** Restoration and maintenance of normal hematopoiesis.

Pharmacokinetics
Absorption: Well absorbed from the GI tract and IM and subcut sites.
Distribution: Half of all stores are in the liver. Enters breast milk. Crosses the placenta.
Protein Binding: Extensive.
Metabolism and Excretion: Converted by the liver to its active metabolite, dihydrofolate reductase. Excess amounts are excreted unchanged by the kidneys.
Half-life: Unknown.

TIME/ACTION PROFILE (↑ in reticulocyte count)

ROUTE	ONSET	PEAK	DURATION
PO, IM, subcut, IV	30–60 min	1 hr	unknown

Contraindications/Precautions
Contraindicated in: Uncorrected pernicious, aplastic, or normocytic anemias (neurologic damage will progress despite correction of hematologic abnormalities); Pedi: Preparations containing benzyl alcohol should not be used in newborns.
Use Cautiously in: Undiagnosed anemias.

Adverse Reactions/Side Effects
Derm: rash. **CNS:** irritability, difficulty sleeping, malaise, confusion. **Misc:** fever.

Interactions
Drug-Drug: Pyrimethamine, methotrexate, trimethoprim, and triamterene prevent the activation of folic acid (leucovorin should be used instead to treat overdoses of these drugs). Absorption of folic acid is ↓ by sulfonamides (including sulfasalazine), antacids, and cholestyramine. Folic acid requirements are ↑ by estrogens, phenytoin, phenobarbital, primidone, carbamazepine, or corticosteroids. May ↓ phenytoin levels.

Route/Dosage
Therapeutic Dose (Folic acid deficiency)
PO, IM, IV, Subcut (Adults and Children >11 yr): 1 mg/day initial dose then 0.5 mg/day maintenance dose.
PO, IM, IV, Subcut (Children >1 yr): 1 mg/day initial dose then 0.1–0.4 mg/day maintenance dose.
PO, IM, IV, Subcut (Infants): 15 mcg/kg/dose daily or 50 mcg/day.

Recommended Daily Allowance
PO (Adults and Children >15 yr): 0.2 mg/day.
PO (Adults): *Females of childbearing potential*—0.4–0.8 mg/day.
PO (Children 11–14 yr): 0.15 mg/day.
PO (Children 7–10 yr): 0.1 mg/day.
PO (Children 4–6 yr): 0.075 mg/day.
PO (Infants 6 mo–3 yr): 0.05 mg/day.

Availability (generic available)
Tablets: 0.4 mg, 0.8 mg, 1 mg, ✱ 5 mg. **Injection:** 5 mg/mL. *In combination with:* other vitamins and minerals as multiple vitamins[Rx, OTC].

NURSING IMPLICATIONS

Assessment
- Assess patient for signs of megaloblastic anemia (fatigue, weakness, dyspnea) before and periodically throughout therapy.
- **Lab Test Considerations:** Monitor plasma folic acid levels, hemoglobin, hematocrit, and reticulocyte count before and periodically during therapy.
- May cause ↓ serum concentrations of other B complex vitamins when given in high continuous doses.

Potential Nursing Diagnoses
Imbalanced nutrition: less than body requirements (Indications)
Activity intolerance (Indications)

Implementation
- Do not confuse folic acid with folinic acid (leucovorin calcium).
- Because of infrequency of solitary vitamin deficiencies, combinations are commonly administered (see Appendix B).
- May be given subcut, deep IM, or IV when PO route is not feasible.
- **PO:** Antacids should be given at least 2 hr after folic acid; folic acid should be given 2 hr before or 4–6 hr after cholestyramine. A 50-mcg/mL oral solution may be extemporaneously prepared by pharmacy for use in neonates and infants.
- **IV:** Solution ranges from yellow to orange-yellow in color.

IV Administration
- **Direct IV:** *Diluent:* Dilute with dextrose or 0.9%NaCl. *Concentration:* 0.1 mg/mL. *Rate:* 5 mg/min.
- **Continuous Infusion:** May be added to hyperalimentation solution.
- **Y-Site Compatibility:** alfentanil, aminophylline, ascorbic acid, atracurium, atropine, azathioprine, aztreonam, benztropine, bumetanide, calcium gluconate, cefazolin, cefonocid, cefoperazone, cefotexime, cefotetan, cefoxitin, ceftazidime, ceftizoxime, ceftriaxone, cefuroxime, chloramphenicol, cimetidine, clindamycin, cyanocobalamin, cyclosporine, dexamethasone, digoxin, diphenhydramine, dopamine, enelaprilat, ephedrine, epinephrine, epoetin alfa, erythromycin, esmolol, famotidine, fentanyl, fluconazole, furosemide, ganciclovir, glycopyrrolate, heparin, hydrocortisone, imipenem/cilastatin, indomethacin, insulin, ketorolac, labetalol, lidocaine, magnesium sulfate, mannitol, meperidine, methylprednisolone, metoclopramide, metoprolol, midazolam, multivitamins, naloxone, nitroglycerin,

nitroprusside, ondansetron, oxacillin, penicillin G, pentobarbital, phenobarbital, phentolamine, phenylephrine, phytonadione, potassium chloride, procainamide, propranolol, ranitidine, sodium bicarbonate, streptokinase, succinylcholine, sufentanil, theophylline, ticarcillin/clavulanate, trimetaphan, urokinase, vancomycin, vasopressin.
- **Y-Site Incompatibility:** amikacin, calcium chloride, chlorpromazine, dantrolene, diazepam, diazoxide, dobutamine, doxycycline, gentamicin, haloperidol, hydralazine, inamrinone, metaraminol, methoxamine, methyldopate, morphine, nafcillin, nalbuphine, norepinephrine, pentamidine, pentazocine, phenytoin, prochlorperazine, promethazine, protamine, pyridoxime, tacrolimus, thiamine, tobramycin, tolazoline, trimethoprim/sulfamethoxazole, verapamil.

Patient/Family Teaching
- Encourage patient to comply with diet recommendations of health care professional. Explain that the best source of vitamins is a well-balanced diet with foods from the four basic food groups. A diet low in vitamin B and folate will be used to diagnose folic acid deficiency without concealing pernicious anemia.
- Folic acid in early pregnancy is necessary to prevent neural tube defects.
- Foods high in folic acid include vegetables, fruits, and organ meats; heat destroys folic acid in foods.
- Patients self-medicating with vitamin supplements should be cautioned not to exceed RDA. The effectiveness of megadoses for treatment of various medical conditions is unproven and may cause side effects.
- Explain that folic acid may make urine more intensely yellow.
- Instruct patient to notify health care professional if rash occurs, which may indicate hypersensitivity.
- Emphasize the importance of follow-up exams to evaluate progress.

Evaluation/Desired Outcomes
- Reticulocytosis 2–5 days after beginning therapy.
- Resolution of symptoms of megaloblastic anemia.
- Prevention of neural tube defects.

HIGH ALERT

fondaparinux
(fon-da-**par**-i-nux)
Arixtra

Classification
Therapeutic: anticoagulants
Pharmacologic: active factor X inhibitors

Pregnancy Category B

Indications
Prevention and treatment of deep vein thrombosis and pulmonary embolism. **Unlabeled Use:** Systemic anticoagulation for other diagnoses.

Action
Binds selectively to antithrombin III (AT III). This binding potentiates the neutralization (inactivation) of active factor X (Xa). **Therapeutic Effects:** Interruption of the coagulation cascade resulting in inhibition of thrombus formation. Prevention of thrombus formation decreases the risk of pulmonary emboli.

Pharmacokinetics
Absorption: 100% absorbed following subcutaneous administration.
Distribution: Distributes mainly throughout the intravascular space.
Metabolism and Excretion: Eliminated mainly unchanged in urine.
Half-life: 17–21 hr.

TIME/ACTION PROFILE (anticoagulant effect)

ROUTE	ONSET	PEAK	DURATION
Subcut	rapid	3 hr	24 hr

Contraindications/Precautions
Contraindicated in: Hypersensitivity; Severe renal impairment (CCr <30 mL/min; ↑ risk of bleeding); Body weight <50 kg in patients undergoing hip replacement (markedly ↑ risk of bleeding); Active major bleeding; Bacterial endocarditis; Thrombocytopenia due to fonaparinux antibodies.
Use Cautiously in: Mild-to-moderate renal impairment; Retinopathy (hypertensive or diabetic); Untreated hypertension; Recent history of ulcer disease; History of congenital or acquired bleeding disorder; Geri: Patients >65 yr (↑ risk of bleeding); Malignancy; History of heparin-induced thrombocytopenia; OB, Lactation, Pedi: Safety not established; use during pregnancy only if clearly needed.
Exercise Extreme Caution in: Severe uncontrolled hypertension; Bleeding disorders; GI bleeding/ulceration/pathology; Hemorrhagic stroke; Recent CNS or ophthalmologic surgery; Active GI bleeding/ulceration; Spinal/epidural anesthesia or spinal puncture (↑ risk of spinal/epidural hematoma that may lead to long-term or permanent paralysis).

fondaparinux

Adverse Reactions/Side Effects
CNS: confusion, dizziness, headache, insomnia. **CV:** edema, hypotension. **GI:** constipation, diarrhea, dyspepsia, ↑ serum aminotransferases, nausea, vomiting. **GU:** urinary retention. **Derm:** bullous eruption, hematoma, purpura, rash. **Hemat:** <u>bleeding</u>, thrombocytopenia. **F and E:** hypokalemia. **Misc:** fever, ↑ wound drainage.

Interactions
Drug-Drug: Risk of bleeding may be ↑ by concurrent use of **warfarin** or **drugs that affect platelet function**, including **aspirin**, **NSAIDs**, **dipyridamole**, some **cephalosporins**, **valproates**, **clopidogrel**, **ticlopidine**, **abciximab**, **eptifibatide**, **tirofiban**, and **dextran**. **Drug-Natural Products:** ↑ risk of bleeding with **arnica**, **chamomile**, **clove**, **dong quai**, **feverfew**, **garlic**, **ginger**, **gingko**, **Panax ginseng**, and others.

Route/Dosage

Treatment of DVT/PE
Subcut (Adults): <*50 kg*—5 mg once daily for at least 5 days until therapeutic anticoagulation with warfarin is achieved (INR >2 for 2 consecutive days); warfarin may be started withing 72 hr of fondaparinux (has been used for up to 26 days); *50–100 kg*—7.5 mg once daily for at least 5 days until therapeutic anticoagulation with warfarin is achieved (INR >2 for 2 consecutive days); *>100 kg*—10 mg once daily for at least 5 days until therapeutic anticoagulation with warfarin is achieved (INR >2 for 2 consecutive days); warfarin may be started within 72 hr of fondaparinux.

Prevention of DVT/PE
Subcut (Adults): 2.5 mg once daily, starting 6–8 hr after surgery, continuing for 5–9 days (up to 11 days) following abdominal surgery or knee/hip replacement or continuing for 24 days following hip fracture surgery (up to 32 days).

Availability
Solution for subcut injection: 2.5 mg/0.5 mL in prefilled syringes, 5 mg/0.4 mL in prefilled syringes, 7.5 mg/0.6 mL in prefilled syringes, 10 mg/0.8 mL in prefilled syringes.

NURSING IMPLICATIONS

Assessment
- Assess for signs of bleeding and hemorrhage (bleeding gums; nosebleed; unusual bruising; black, tarry stools; hematuria; fall in hematocrit; sudden drop in blood pressure; guaiac positive stools); bleeding from surgical site. Notify health care professional if these occur.
- Assess for evidence of additional or increased thrombosis. Symptoms will depend on area of involvement. Monitor neurological status frequently for signs of impairment, especially in patients with indwelling epidural catheters for administration of analgesia or with concomitant use of drugs affecting hemostasis (NSAIDs, platelet inhibitors, other anticoagulants). Risk is increased by traumatic or repeated epidural or spinal puncture. May require urgent treatment.
- *Lab Test Considerations:* Monitor platelet count closely; may cause thrombocytopenia. If platelet count is <100,000/mm³, discontinue fondaparinux.
- Fondaparinux is not accurately measured by prothrombin time (PT), activated thromboplastin time (aPTT), or international standards of heparin or low molecular weight heparins. If unexpected changes in coagulation parameters or major bleeding occurs, discontinue fondaparinux.
- Monitor CBC, serum creatinine levels, and stool occult blood tests routinely during therapy.
- May cause asymptomatic ↑ in AST and ALT. Elevations are fully reversible and not associated with ↑ in bilirubin.
- May cause ↑ aPTT temporally associated with bleeding with or without concomitant administration of other anticoagulants and thrombocytopenia with thrombosis similar to heparin-induced thrombocytopenia, with or without exposure to heparin or low-molecular-weight heparin.

Potential Nursing Diagnoses
Ineffective tissue perfusion (Indications)
Risk for injury (Side Effects)

Implementation
- Fondaparinux cannot be used interchangeably with heparin, low-molecular-weight heparins, or heparinoids as they differ in manufacturing process, anti-Xa and anti-IIa activity, units, and dosage. Each of these medications has its own instructions for use.
- Initial dose should be administered 6-8 hr after surgery. Administration before 6 hr after surgery has been associated with risk of major bleeding.

✱ = Canadian drug name.　 = Genetic implication.
*CAPITALS indicates life-threatening; <u>underlines</u> indicate most frequent.

610 formoterol

- **Subcut:** Administer subcut only into fatty tissue, alternating sites between right and left anterolateral or posterolateral abdominal wall. Inject entire length of needle at a 45° or 90° angle into a skin fold held between thumb and forefinger; hold skin fold throughout injection. Do not aspirate or massage. Rotate sites frequently. Do not administer IM because of danger of hematoma formation. Solution should be clear; do not inject solution containing particulate matter. Do not mix with other injections.
- Fondaparinux is provided in a single-dose prefilled syringe with an automatic needle protection system. Do not expel air bubble from prefilled syringe before injection to prevent loss of drug.

Patient/Family Teaching
- Advise patient to report any symptoms of unusual bleeding or bruising, dizziness, itching, rash, fever, swelling, or difficulty breathing to health care professional immediately.
- Instruct patient not to take aspirin or NSAIDs without consulting health care professional during therapy.

Evaluation/Desired Outcomes
- Prevention and treatment of deep vein thrombosis and pulmonary embolism.

---

formoterol (for-**mo**-te-role)
Foradil, Perforomist

Classification
Therapeutic: bronchodilators
Pharmacologic: adrenergics

Pregnancy Category C

Indications
Long-term maintenance treatment of asthma. Prevention of bronchospasm in reversible obstructive airways disease, including. Long-term management of bronchoconstriction associated with COPD including chronic bronchitis and emphysema. Acute prevention of exercise-induced bronchospasm, when used on an occasional, as needed, basis.

Action
Produces accumulation of cyclic adenosine monophosphate (cAMP) at beta-adrenergic receptors, resulting in relaxation of airway smooth muscle. Relatively specific for beta$_2$ (pulmonary) receptors. **Therapeutic Effects:** Bronchodilation.

Pharmacokinetics
Absorption: Following inhalation, majority of inhaled drug is swallowed and absorbed.
Distribution: Unknown.
Metabolism and Excretion: Mostly metabolized by the liver; 10–18% excreted unchanged in urine.
Half-life: 10 hr.

TIME/ACTION PROFILE (bronchodilation)

ROUTE	ONSET	PEAK	DURATION
inhalation	15 min	1–3 hr	12 hr

Contraindications/Precautions
Contraindicated in: Hypersensitivity; Acute attack of asthma (onset of action is delayed).
Use Cautiously in: Cardiovascular disease (including angina and hypertension); Diabetes; Glaucoma; Hyperthyroidism; Pheochromocytoma; Excessive use (may lead to tolerance and paradoxical bronchospasm); OB, Lactation, Pedi: Pregnancy, lactation, or children <5 yr (may inhibit contractions during labor; use only if potential benefits outweigh risks).

Adverse Reactions/Side Effects
CNS: dizziness, fatigue, headache, insomnia, malaise, nervousness. **Resp:** PARADOXICAL BRONCHOSPASM. **CV:** angina, arrhythmias, hypertension, hypotension, palpitations, tachycardia. **GI:** dry mouth, nausea. **F and E:** hypokalemia. **Metab:** hyperglycemia, metabolic acidosis. **MS:** muscle cramps. **Neuro:** tremor. **Misc:** allergic reactions including ANAPHYLAXIS.

Interactions
Drug-Drug: Concurrent use with **MAO inhibitors**, **tricyclic antidepressants**, or other **agents that may prolong the QTc interval** may result in serious arrhythmias and should be undertaken with extreme caution. ↑ risk of hypokalemia with **theophylline**, **corticosteroids**, **potassium-losing diuretics**. **Beta blockers** may ↓ therapeutic effects of formoterol. ↑ adrenergic effects may occur with concurrent use of **adrenergics**.

Route/Dosage

Maintenance Treatment of Asthma
Inhaln (Adults and Children ≥ 5 yr): 1 capsule (12 mcg) every 12 hr using the Aerolizer Inhaler.

Prevention of Exercise-Induced Bronchospasm
Inhaln (Adults and Children ≥12 yr): 1 capsule (12 mcg) at least 15 min before exercise on an occasional as-needed basis.

Maintenance Treatment of COPD (Emphysema and Chronic Bronchitis)
Inhaln (Adults): 20 mcg/2 mL-unit-dose vial twice daily via jet nebulizer.

Availability
Capsule for Aerolizer use: 12 mcg. **Vials for nebulization:** 20 mcg/2 mL. *In combination with:* budesonide (Symbicort; see Appendix B).

NURSING IMPLICATIONS
Assessment
- Assess lung sounds, pulse, and blood pressure before administration and during peak of medication. Note amount, color, and character of sputum produced. Closely monitor patients on higher dose for adverse effects.
- Monitor pulmonary function tests before initiating and periodically therapy to determine effectiveness.
- Observe for paradoxical bronchospasm (wheezing). If condition occurs, withhold medication and notify health care provider immediately.
- Monitor ECG periodically during therapy. May cause prolonged QTc interval.
- Monitor patient for signs of anaphylaxis (dyspnea, rash, laryngeal edema) throughout therapy.
- *Lab Test Considerations:* May cause ↑ serum glucose and decreased serum potassium.

Potential Nursing Diagnoses
Ineffective airway clearance (Indications)

Implementation
- **Inhaln:** *For use with inhaler:* Place capsule in the well of the *Aerolizer Inhaler* with dry hands; do not expose to moisture. The capsule is pierced by pressing and releasing the buttons on the side of the device. Medication is dispersed into the air stream when patient inhales rapidly and deeply through mouthpiece. Capsules are only to be used with *Aerolizer Inhaler* and should not be taken orally. Store capsules in the blister and only remove immediately before use. Store inhaler in a level, horizontal position. *Aerolizer Inhaler* should never be washed and should be kept dry.
- Do not use a spacer with formoterol.
- To use, pull off the *Aerolizer* cover. Hold the base of the inhaler firmly, and twist mouthpiece in the direction of the arrow to open. Push the buttons in to make sure four pins are visible in the capsule well on each side. Remove capsule from blister pack immediately before use. Separate one blistered capsule by tearing at perforations. With foil-side up, fold back along perforation and flatten. Starting at slit, tear off corner; separate and peel foil from paper backing and remove capsule. Place capsule in the capsule chamber in the base of the *Aerolizer Inhaler*. Never place a capsule directly into the mouthpiece. Twist the mouthpiece back to the closed position. With the mouthpiece upright, simultaneously press both buttons only once. A click should be heard as the capsule is being pierced. Release buttons; if buttons stick in depressed position grasp wings on buttons and retract before inhalation. With patient sitting or standing in a comfortable upright position, exhale fully. Do not exhale into the device. Tilt head back slightly and breathe in rapidly but steadily. A sweet taste will be experienced and a whirring noise heard. If no whirring is heard, the capsule may be stuck. Open inhaler and loosen capsule allowing it to spin freely. Do not repeatedly press buttons to loosen capsule. Hold breath for as long as comfortably possible after removing inhaler from mouth. Open inhaler to see if any powder is still in capsule. If powder is found, repeat inhalation steps. After use, open, remove and discard empty capsule.
- **Inhaln:** *For use with nebulizer:* Administer via standard jet nebulizer via mouthpiece or face mask. Remove vial from foil immediately prior to use and discard via after use. May be stored in refrigerator for up to 3 months.

Patient/Family Teaching
- Instruct patient to take fomoterol as directed. Do not discontinue therapy without discussing with health care professional, even if feeling better. If on a scheduled dosing regimen, take a missed dose as soon as remembered, spacing remaining doses at regular intervals. Do not double doses. Use a rapid-acting bronchodilator if symptoms occur before next dose is due. Caution patient not to use more than 2 times a day or less than 12 hr apart; may cause adverse effects, paradoxical bronchospasm, or loss of effectiveness of medication Instruct patient to review medication guide with each Rx refill.
- Advise patient to have a rapid-acting bronchodilator available for use at all times for symptomatic relief of acute asthma attacks.

- Instruct patient to contact health care professional immediately if shortness of breath is not relieved by medication or nausea, vomiting, shakiness, headache, fast or irregular heartbeat, or sleeplessness occur.
- Instruct patient to notify health care professional if there is no response to the usual dose of formoterol. Asthma and treatment regimen should be re-evaluated and corticosteroids should be considered. Need for increased use to treat symptoms indicates decrease in asthma control and need to reevaluate therapy.
- Advise patient to consult health care professional before taking any Rx, OTC, or herbal products or alcohol concurrently with this therapy. Caution patient also to avoid smoking and other respiratory irritants.
- Advise patient to notify health care professional if pregnancy is planned or suspected, or if nursing.
- **Inhaler:** Instruct patient on correct technique for use of *Aerolizer Inhaler*. Advise patient always to use new *Aerolizer Inhaler* that comes with each refill. Take sticker with "use by" date written by pharmacist from the outside of the box and place it on the *Aerolizer Inhaler* cover. If the date is blank, count 4 months from the date of purchase and write date on sticker. Use new inhaler and blister pack following the "use by" date.
- Inform patient that in rare cases capsule might break into small pieces. These pieces should be retained by the screen in the inhaler, however in rare instances tiny pieces may reach mouth or throat after inhalation. Shattering of capsule is less likely to happen if storage conditions are strictly followed, capsules removed from blister immediately before use, and capsules are only pierced once.

Evaluation/Desired Outcomes
- Prevention of bronchospasm.

---

fosamprenavir
(fos-am-**pren**-a-veer)
Lexiva, ✦Telzir

Classification
Therapeutic: antiretrovirals
Pharmacologic: protease inhibitors

Pregnancy Category C

Indications
With other antiretrovirals in the management of HIV infection.

Action
Inhibits the action of HIV protease and prevents the cleavage of viral polyproteins. **Therapeutic Effects:** Increased CD4 cell counts and decreased viral load with subsequent slowed progression of HIV and its sequelae.

Pharmacokinetics
Absorption: Fosamprenavir is a prodrug. Following oral administration, it is rapidly converted to amprenavir by the gut lining during absorption.
Distribution: Penetration into RBCs is concentration dependent.
Metabolism and Excretion: Mostly metabolized the liver (CYP3A4 enzyme system). Minimal renal excretion.
Half-life: 7.7 hr.

TIME/ACTION PROFILE (blood levels)

ROUTE	ONSET	PEAK	DURATION
PO	rapid	1.5–4 hr	12–24 hr

Contraindications/Precautions
Contraindicated in: Hypersensitivity, sulfonamide/sulfa hypersensitivity; Severe hepatic impairment; Concurrent use of flecainide, propafenone, rifampin, ergot derivatives, St. John's wort, lovastatin, simvastatin, pimozide, delavirdine, midazolam or triazolam.
Use Cautiously in: Geri: Consider age-related ↓ in body mass, cardiac/hepatic/renal impairment, concurrent illness and medications; Hepatic impairment; Concurrent use of medications handled by or affecting the CYP3A4 enzyme system (may require serum level monitoring, dose or dosing interval alterations); OB, Lactation, Pedi: Pregnancy, lactation, children <2 yr (safety not established; breast feeding not recommended in HIV-infected patients).

Adverse Reactions/Side Effects
Reflects use with other antiretrovirals.
CNS: headache, fatigue, mood disorders. **GI:** diarrhea, nausea, vomiting, abdominal pain, ↑ liver enzymes. **Derm:** rash. **Endo:** glucose intolerance. **GU:** nephrolithiasis. **Hemat:** neutropenia. **Metab:** ↑ cholesterol, fat redistribution, ↑ triglycerides. **Misc:** allergic reactions including STEVENS-JOHNSON SYNDROME, ANGIOEDEMA, inflammatory response to opportunistic infection.

Interactions
Drug-Drug: Amprenavir, the active moiety of fosamprenavir is metabolized by **CYP3A4**; it also inhibits and induces this enzyme system. The action of any other medication that is also handled by or affects this system may be altered by concurrent

fosamprenavir

use. Concurrent use of **flecainide**, **propafenone**, **rifampin**, **ergot derivatives** (**dihydroergotamine**, **ergotamine**, **ergonovine**, **methylergonovine**), **fluticasone**, **lovastatin**, **simvastatin**, **pimozide**, **delavirdine**, **midazolam**, or **triazolam** may result in serious, potentially life-threatening adverse reactions including arrhythmias, excessive sedation, myopathy or loss of virologic response and is contraindicated. Blood levels are ↓ by **efavirenz** (additional ritonavir may be required when used together), **nevirapine**, **lopinavir/ritonavir**, **saquinavir**, **carbamazepine**, **phenobarbital**, **phenytoin**, **dexamethasone**, **histamine H$_2$-receptor antagonists**, and **proton-pump inhibitors**; monitor for ↓ antiretroviral activity. Levels are ↑ by **indinavir** and **nelfinavir**. May ↓ **methadone** and **paroxetine** levels. ↑ levels and risk of toxicity from **amiodarone**, **lidocaine**, **quinidine** (monitor blood levels), **ketoconazole**, and **itraconazole** (dose of itraconazole or ketoconazole should not exceed 200 mg/day when fosamprenavir is used with ritonavir or 400 mg/day when used without), **rifabutin** (monitor for neutropenia, ↓ rifabutin dose by 50% when used with fosamprenavir or by 75% when used with fosamprenavir with ritonavir), **atorvastatin** and **rosuvastatin** (dose not to exceed 20 mg/day or consider other HMG-CoA reductase inhibitors), **cyclsosporine** or **tacrolimus** (monitor blood levels of immunosuppressants), **calcium channel blockers** (clinical monitoring recommended), some **benzodiazepines** (**alprazolam**, **clorazepate**, **diazepam**, **flurazepam**; dose reduction of benzodiazepine may be needed), **sildenafil**, **tadalafil**, and **vardenafil** (use cautiously; ↓ dose of sildenafil to 25 mg every 48 hr, for tadalafil single dose should not exceed 10 mg in any 72 hr period, dose of vardenafil should not exceed 2.5 mg every 24 hr if used without ritonavir or 2.5 mg every 72 hr with ritonavir with monitoring for toxicity) and **tricyclic antidepressants** (blood level monitoring recommended). May alter the effects of **warfarin** (monitor INR) or **hormonal contraceptives** (use alternative method of contraception).
Drug-Natural Products: Concurrent use of **St. John's wort** is contraindicated; ↓ blood levels and may lead to ↓ virologic response.

Route/Dosage
PO (Adults): *Treatment-naive patients without ritonavir*—1400 mg twice daily; *Treatment-naive patients with ritonavir*—1400 mg once daily with ritonavir 100 or 200 mg once daily, or 700 mg twice daily with ritonavir 100 mg twice daily. *Protease inhibitor–experienced patients*—700 mg twice daily with ritonavir 100 mg twice daily. If efavirenz is added to a once daily regimen using both fosamprenavir and ritonavir, an additional 100 mg of ritonavir (total of 300 mg) should be given.
PO (Children 2–5 yr): *Treatment-naive*—30 mg/kg twice daily, not to exceed 1400 mg twice daily.
PO (Children ≥6 yr): *Treatment-naive*—30 mg/kg twice daily, not to exceed 1400 mg twice daily, or 18 mg/kg twice daily (not to exceed 700 mg twice daily) with ritonavir 3 mg/kg twice daily (not to exceed 100 mg twice daily); *Protease inhibitor-experienced*— 18 mg/kg twice daily (not to exceed 700 mg twice daily) with ritonavir 3 mg/kg twice daily (not to exceed 100 mg twice daily). When used without ritonavir in children ≥47 kg, may use adult regimen of 1400 mg twice daily.

Hepatic Impairment
PO (Adults): *Mild hepatic impairment*–700 mg twice daily without ritonavir (therapy-naive) or 700 mg twice daily with ritonavir 100 mg once daily (therapy-naive or protease inhibitor experienced); *Moderate hepatic impairment*-700 mg twice daily without ritonavir (therapy-naive) or 450 mg twice daily with ritonavir 100 mg once daily (therapy-naive or protease inhibitor experienced); *Severe hepatic impairment*—350 mg twice daily without ritonavir (therapy-naive) or 300 mg twice daily with ritonavir 100 mg once daily (therapy-naive or protease inhibitor experienced).

Availability
Tablets: 700 mg. **Oral suspension:** 50 mg/mL.

NURSING IMPLICATIONS
Assessment
- Assess patient for change in severity of HIV symptoms and for symptoms of opportunistic infections throughout therapy.
- Assess patient for allergy to sulfonamides. May exhibit cross-sensitivity.
- Assess patient for skin reactions throughout therapy. Reactions may be severe and life threatening. Discontinue therapy if severe reactions or moderate rashes with systemic symptoms occur.

- **Lab Test Considerations:** Monitor viral load and CD4 cell count regularly during therapy.
- May cause ↑ serum glucose cholesterol, and triglyceride levels.
- May cause ↑ AST and ALT levels.
- May cause neutropenia.

Potential Nursing Diagnoses
Risk for infection (Indications)
Noncompliance (Patient/Family Teaching)

Implementation
- **PO:** Tablets may be administered with or without food. Oral suspension should be taken without food in adults and with food in children. If emesis occurs within 30 minutes after dosing, re-dose.

Patient/Family Teaching
- Emphasize the importance of taking fosamprenavir as directed. Advise patient to read the *Patient Information* that comes with the prescription prior to initiation of therapy and with each prescription refill. Fosamprenavir must always be used in combination with other antiretroviral drugs. Do not take more than prescribed amount and do not stop taking without consulting health care professional. Take missed doses as soon as remembered, then return to regular schedule. If a dose is skipped, do not double the next doses.
- Instruct patient that fosamprenavir should not be shared with others.
- Inform patient that fosamprenavir does not cure AIDS or prevent associated or opportunistic infections. Fosamprenavir does not reduce the risk of transmission of HIV to others through sexual contact or blood contamination. Caution patient to use a condom and to avoid sharing needles or donating blood to prevent spreading the AIDS virus to others. Advise patient that the long-term effects of fosamprenavir are unknown at this time.
- Emphasize the importance of providing health care professional with accurate current drug history and notifying health care professional before taking any Rx, OTC, or herbal products because of potentially serious drug interactions.
- May decrease effectiveness of hormonal contraceptives; advise patient to use a nonhormonal form of contraception during therapy.
- Instruct patient to notify health care professional if nausea, vomiting, diarrhea, or rash occurs.
- Inform patient that redistribution and accumulation of body fat may occur, causing central obesity, dorsocervical fat enlargement (buffalo hump), peripheral wasting, breast enlargement, and cushingoid appearance. The cause and long-term effects are not known.
- Emphasize the importance of regular follow-up exams and blood counts to determine progress and monitor for side effects.

Evaluation/Desired Outcomes
- Delayed progression of AIDS and decreased opportunistic infections in patients with HIV.
- Decrease in viral load and increase in CD4 cell counts.

---

foscarnet (foss-kar-net)

Classification
Therapeutic: antivirals

Pregnancy Category C

Indications
Treatment of cytomegalovirus (CMV) retinitis in HIV-infected patients (alone or with ganciclovir). Treatment of acyclovir-resistant mucocutaneous herpes simplex virus (HSV) infections in immunocompromised patients.

Action
Prevents viral replication by inhibiting viral DNA-polymerase and reverse transcriptase. **Therapeutic Effects:** Virustatic action against susceptible viruses including CMV.

Pharmacokinetics
Absorption: IV administration results in complete bioavailability.
Distribution: Variable penetration into CSF. May concentrate in and be slowly released from bone.
Metabolism and Excretion: 80–90% excreted unchanged in urine.
Half-life: 3 hr (in patients with normal renal function); longer half-life of 90 hr may reflect release of drug from bone.

TIME/ACTION PROFILE

ROUTE	ONSET	PEAK	DURATION
IV	rapid	end of infusion	8–24 hr

Contraindications/Precautions
Contraindicated in: Hypersensitivity.
Use Cautiously in: Renal impairment (dose reduction required if CCr ≤1.4–1.6 mL/min/kg; see product information); History of seizures; OB, Lactation, Pedi: Safety not established.

foscarnet 615

Adverse Reactions/Side Effects
CNS: SEIZURES, headache, anxiety, confusion, dizziness, fatigue, malaise, mental depression, weakness. **EENT:** conjunctivitis, eye pain, vision abnormalities. **Resp:** coughing, dyspnea. **CV:** chest pain, ECG abnormalities, edema, palpitations. **GI:** diarrhea, nausea, vomiting, abdominal pain, abnormal taste sensation, anorexia, constipation, dyspepsia. **GU:** renal failure, albuminuria, dysuria, nocturia, polyuria, urinary retention. **Derm:** increased sweating, pruritus, rash, skin ulceration. **F and E:** hypocalcemia, hypokalemia, hypomagnesemia, hyperphosphatemia, hypophosphatemia. **Hemat:** anemia, granulocytopenia, leukopenia. **Local:** pain/inflammation at injection site. **MS:** arthralgia, myalgia, back pain, involuntary muscle contraction. **Neuro:** ataxia, hypoesthesia, neuropathy, paresthesia, tremor. **Misc:** fever, chills, flu-like syndrome, lymphoma, sarcoma.

Interactions
Drug-Drug: Concurrent use with parenteral **pentamidine** may result in severe, life-threatening hypocalcemia. Risk of nephrotoxicity may be ↑ by concurrent use of other **nephrotoxic agents** (**amphotericin B**, **aminoglycosides**).

Route/Dosage
IV (Adults): *CMV retinitis*—60 mg/kg q 8 hr or 90 mg/kg q 12 hr for 2–3 wk, then 90–120 mg/kg/day as a single dose. Dosage reduction required for any degree of renal impairment; *HSV*—40 mg/kg q 8–12 hr for 2–3 wk or until healing occurs.

Availability (generic available)
Injection: 6000 mg/250 mL, 12,000 mg/500 mL.

NURSING IMPLICATIONS

Assessment
- **CMV Retinitis:** Diagnosis of CMV retinitis should be determined by ophthalmoscopy before treatment with foscarnet. Ophthalmologic examinations should also be performed at the conclusion of induction and every 4 wk during maintenance therapy.
- Culture for CMV (urine, blood, throat) may be taken before administration. However, a negative CMV culture does not rule out CMV retinitis.
- **HSV Infections:** Assess lesions before and daily during therapy.
- *Lab Test Considerations:* Monitor serum creatinine before and 2–3 times weekly during induction therapy and at least once every 1–2 wk during maintenance therapy. Monitor 24-hr CCr before and periodically throughout therapy. If CCr drops below 0.4 mL/min/kg, discontinue foscarnet.
- Monitor serum calcium, magnesium, potassium, and phosphorus before and 2–3 times weekly during induction therapy and at least weekly during maintenance therapy. May cause ↓ concentrations.
- May cause anemia, granulocytopenia, leukopenia, and thrombocytopenia. May cause ↑ AST and ALT levels and abnormal A-G ratios.

Potential Nursing Diagnoses
Risk for infection (Indications)

Implementation
- Adequately hydrate patient with 750–1000 mL of 0.9% NaCl or D5W before first infusion to establish diuresis, then administer 750–1000 mL with 120 mg/kg of foscarnet or 500 mL with 40–60 mg/kg of foscarnet with each dose to prevent renal toxicity.

IV Administration
- **Intermittent Infusion:** *Diluent:* May be administered via central line undiluted. If administered via peripheral line, *must* be diluted with D5W or 0.9% NaCl to prevent vein irritation. Do not administer solution that is discolored or contains particulate matter. Use diluted solution within 24 hr. *Concentration:* Undiluted: 24 mg/mL; Diluted: 12 mg/mL.
- Dose is based on patient weight; excess solution may be discarded from bottle before administration to prevent overdosage.
- Patients who experience progression of CMV retinitis during maintenance therapy may be retreated with induction therapy followed by maintenance therapy. *Rate:* Administer at a rate not to exceed 1 mg/kg/min.
- Infuse solution via infusion pump to ensure accurate infusion rate.
- **Y-Site Compatibility:** aldesleukin, amikacin, aminophylline, ampicillin, aztreonam, bivalirudin, carboplatin, cefazolin, cefoperazone, cefoxitin, ceftazidime, ceftizoxime, ceftriaxone, cefuroxime, chloramphenicol, cimetidine, cisplatin, clindamycin, cyclophosphamide, cytarabine, dactinomycin, daptomycin, dexamethasone sodium phosphate, dexmedetomidine, diltiazem, docetaxel, dopamine, doripenem, ertapenem, erythromycin lactobionate, etopo-

✸ = Canadian drug name. ⚜ = Genetic implication.
CAPITALS indicates life-threatening; underlines indicate most frequent.

side, etoposide phosphate, fenoldopam, fluconazole, flucytosine, fludarabine, fluorouracil, furosemide, gemcitabine, gentamicin, granisetron, heparin, hydrocortisone, hydromorphone, ifosfamide, imipenen-cilastatin, linezolid, mechlorethamine, methotrexate, metoclopramide, metronidazole, morphine, nafcillin, nesiritide, octreotide, oxacillin, oxaliplatin, oxytocin, paclitaxel, palonosetron, pantoprazole, pemetrexed, penicillin G potassium, phenytoin, piperacillin/tazobactam, ranitidine, tacrolimus, teniposide, thiotepa, ticarcillin/clavulanate, tigecycline, tirofiban, tobramycin, vincristine, voriconazole.

- **Y-Site Incompatibility:** Manufacturer recommends that foscarnet not be administered concurrently with other drugs or solutions in the same IV catheter except D5W or 0.9% NaCl, acyclovir, amphotericin B colloidal, caspofungin, diazepam, digoxin, diphenhydramine, dobutamine, doxorubicin, droperidol, epirubicin, ganciclovir, haloperidol, leucovorin, midazolam, mitoxantrone, pentamidine, prochlorperazine, promethazine, trimetrexate, vinorelbine.

Patient/Family Teaching
- Inform patient that foscarnet is not a cure for CMV retinitis. Progression of retinitis may continue in immunocompromised patients during and after therapy. Advise patients to have regular ophthalmologic exams.
- Advise patient to notify health care professional immediately if perioral tingling or numbness in the extremities or paresthesia occurs during or after infusion. If these signs of electrolyte imbalance occur during administration, infusion should be stopped and lab samples for serum electrolyte concentrations obtained immediately.
- Emphasize the importance of frequent follow-up exams to monitor renal function and electrolytes.

Evaluation/Desired Outcomes
- Management of the symptoms of CMV retinitis in patients with AIDS.
- Crusting over and healing of skin lesions in HSV infections.

---

fosinopril, See ANGIOTENSIN-CONVERTING ENZYME (ACE) INHIBITORS.

---

fosphenytoin
(foss-**fen**-i-toyn)
Cerebyx

Classification
Therapeutic: anticonvulsants

Pregnancy Category D

Indications
Short-term (<5 day) parenteral management of generalized, convulsive status epilepticus when use of phenytoin is not feasible. Treatment and prevention of seizures during neurosurgery when use of phenytoin is not feasible.

Action
Limits seizure propagation by altering ion transport. May also decrease synaptic transmission. Fosphenytoin is rapidly converted to phenytoin, which is responsible for its pharmacologic effects. **Therapeutic Effects:** Diminished seizure activity.

Pharmacokinetics
Absorption: Rapidly converted to phenytoin after IV administration and completely absorbed after IM administration.
Distribution: Distributes into CSF and other body tissues and fluids. Enters breast milk; crosses the placenta, achieving similar maternal/fetal levels. Preferentially distributes into fatty tissue.
Protein Binding: *Fosphenytoin*—95–99%; *phenytoin*—90–95%.
Metabolism and Excretion: Mostly metabolized by the liver; minimal amounts excreted in the urine.
Half-life: *Fosphenytoin*—15 min; *phenytoin*—22 hr (range 7–42 hr).

TIME/ACTION PROFILE (anticonvulsant effect)

ROUTE	ONSET	PEAK	DURATION
IM	unknown	30 min	up to 24 hr
IV	15–45 min	15–60 min	up to 24 hr

Contraindications/Precautions
Contraindicated in: Hypersensitivity; Sinus bradycardia, sinoatrial block, 2nd- or 3rd-degree AV heart block or Adams-Stokes syndrome.
Use Cautiously in: Hepatic or renal disease (↑ risk of adverse reactions; dose reduction recommended for hepatic impairment); OB: Safety not established; may result in fetal hydantoin syndrome if used chronically or hemorrhage in the newborn if used at term; Lactation: Safety not established.

fosphenytoin

Exercise Extreme Caution in: ▸ Patients positive for HLA-B*1502 allele (unless exceptional circumstances exist where benefits clearly outweigh the risks).

Adverse Reactions/Side Effects
CNS: dizziness, drowsiness, nystagmus, agitation, brain edema, headache, stupor, vertigo. **EENT:** amblyopia, deafness, diplopia, tinnitus. **CV:** hypotension (with rapid IV administration), tachycardia. **GI:** dry mouth, nausea, taste perversion, tongue disorder, vomiting. **Derm:** pruritus, rash, STEVENS-JOHNSON SYMDROME. **MS:** back pain. **Neuro:** ataxia, dysarthria, extrapyramidal syndrome, hypesthesia, incoordination, paresthesia, tremor. **Misc:** pelvic pain.

Interactions
Drug-Drug: **Disulfiram**, acute ingestion of **alcohol**, **amiodarone**, **ethosuximide**, **isoniazid**, **chloramphenicol**, **sulfonamides**, **fluoxetine**, **gabapentin**, **H2 antagonists**, **benzodiazepines**, **omeprazole**, **ketoconazole**, **fluconazole**, **estrogens**, **succinamides**, **halothane**, **methylphenidate**, **phenothiazines**, **salicylates**, **ticlopidine**, **tolbutamide**, **topiramate**, **trazodone**, **felbamate**, and **cimetidine** may ↑ phenytoin blood levels. **Barbiturates**, **carbamazepine**, **reserpine**, and chronic ingestion of **alcohol** may ↓ phenytoin blood levels. Phenytoin may ↓ the effects of **amiodarone**, **benzodiazepines**, **carbamazepine**, **chloramphenicol**, **corticosteroids**, **disopyramide**, **warfarin**, **felbamate**, **doxycycline**, **lamotrigine**, **oral contraceptives**, **paroxetine**, **propafenone**, **rifampin**, **ritonavir**, **quinidine**, **tacrolimus**, **theophylline**, **topiramate**, **tricyclic antidepressants**, **zonisamide**, **methadone**, **cyclosporine**, and **estrogens**. IV phenytoin and **dopamine** may cause additive hypotension. Additive CNS depression with other **CNS depressants**, including **alcohol**, **antihistamines**, **antidepressants**, **opioids**, and **sedative/hypnotics**. **Antacids** may ↓ absorption of orally administered phenytoin. ↑ systemic clearance of antileukemic drugs **teniposide** and **methotrexate** which has been associated with a worse event-free survival, phenytoin use is not recommended in children undergoing chemotherapy for acute lymphocytic leukemia. **Calcium** and **sucralfate** ↓ phenytoin absorption.

Route/Dosage
Note: Doses of fosphenytoin are expressed as phenytoin sodium equivalents [PE].

Status Epilepticus
IV (Adults): 15–20 mg PE/kg.

Nonemergent and Maintenance Dosing
IV, IM (Adults and Children > 16 yr): *Loading dose*—10–20 mg PE/kg. *Maintenance dose*—4–6 mg PE/kg/day.
IV, IM (Children 10–16 yr): 6–7 mg PE/kg/day.
IV, IM (Children 7–9 yr): 7–8 mg PE/kg/day.
IV, IM (Children 4–6 yr): 7.5–9 mg PE/kg/day.
IV, IM (Children 0.5–3 yr): 8–10 mg PE kg/day.
IV, IM (Infants): 5 mg PE kg/day.
IV, IM (Neonates): 5–8 mg PE/kg/day.

Availability (generic available)
Injection: 50 mgPE/mL.

NURSING IMPLICATIONS

Assessment
- **Seizures:** Assess location, duration, frequency, and characteristics of seizure activity. EEG may be monitored periodically during therapy.
- Monitor blood pressure, ECG, and respiratory function continuously during administration of fosphenytoin and during period when peak serum phenytoin levels occur (15–30 min after administration).
- Observe patient for development of rash. Discontinue fosphenytoin at the first sign of skin reactions. Serious adverse reactions such as exfoliative, purpuric, or bullous rashes or the development of lupus erythematosus, Stevens-Johnson syndrome, or toxic epidermal necrolysis preclude further use of phenytoin or fosphenytoin. ▸ Stevens-Johnson syndrome and toxic epidermal necrolysis are significantly more common in patients with a particular human leukocyte antigen (HLA) allele, HLA-B*1502 (occurs almost exclusively in patients with Asian ancestry, including including Han Chinese, Filipinos, Malaysians, South Asian Indians, and Thais). Avoid using phenytoin or fosphenytoin as alternatives to carbamazepine for patients who test positive. If less serious skin eruptions (measles-like or scarlatiniform) occur, fosphenytoin may be resumed after

---
✦ = Canadian drug name. ▸ = Genetic implication.
*CAPITALS indicates life-threatening; underlines indicate most frequent.

complete clearing of the rash. If rash reappears, further use of fosphenytoin or phenytoin should be avoided.
- **Lab Test Considerations:** Fosphenytoin contains 0.0037 mmol phosphate per mg PE. Monitor serum phosphate concentrations in patients with renal insufficiency; may cause ↑ phosphate concentrations.
- May cause ↑ serum alkaline phosphatase, GTT, and glucose levels.
- Fosphenytoin therapy may be monitored using phenytoin levels. Optimal total plasma phenytoin concentrations are typically 10–20 mcg/mL (unbound plasma phenytoin concentrations of 1–2 mcg/mL).
- *Toxicity and Overdose:* Serum phenytoin levels should not be monitored until complete conversion from fosphenytoin to phenytoin has occurred (2 hr after IV or 4 hr after IM administration).
- Initial signs and symptoms of phenytoin toxicity include nystagmus, ataxia, confusion, nausea, slurred speech, and dizziness.

Potential Nursing Diagnoses
Risk for injury (Indications)
Deficient knowledge, related to medication regimen (Patient/Family Teaching)

Implementation
- Do not confuse fosphenytoin (Cerebyx) with celocoxib (Celebrex) or citalopram (Celexa).
- Implement seizure precautions.
- When substituting *fosphenytoin* for oral *phenytoin* therapy, the same total daily dose may be given as a single dose. Unlike parenteral phenytoin, fosphenytoin may be given safely by the IM route.
- The anticonvulsant effect of fosphenytoin is not immediate. Additional measures (including parenteral benzodiazepines) are usually required in the immediate management of status epilepticus. Loading dosage of *fosphenytoin* should be followed with the institution of maintenance anticonvulsant therapy.

IV Administration
- **Direct IV:** *Diluent:* D5W or 0.9% NaCl. *Concentration:* 1.5–25 mg PE/mL May be refrigerated for up to 48 hr. *Rate:* Administer at a rate of <150 mg PE/min in adults and <3 mg/kg/min in children to minimize risk of hypotension.
- **Y-Site Compatibility:** amphotericin B liposome, bivalirudin, carboplatin, caspofungin, cisplatin, cyclophosphamide, cytarabine, dactinomycin, daptomycin, dexmedetomidine, diltiazem, docetaxel, doxacurium, ertapenem, etoposide, etoposide phosphate, fludarabine, fluorouracil, gemcitabine, granisetron, ifosfamide, levofloxacin, linezolid, lorazepam, mechlorethamine, meperidine, methotrexate, metronidazole, nesiritide, octreotide, oxaliplatin, oxytocin, paclitaxel, palonosetron, pantoprazole, pemetrexed, phenobarbital, piperacillin/tazobactam, rocuronium, sodium acetate, tacrolimus, teniposide, thiotepa, tigecycline, tirofiban, vincristine, vinorelbine, voriconazole.
- **Y-Site Incompatibility:** caspofungin, doxorubicin hydrochloride, epirubicin, fenoldopam, midazolam, mitoxantrone, quinapristin/dalfopristin.
- **Additive Incompatibility:** Information unavailable. Do not admix with other solutions or medications.

Patient/Family Teaching
- May cause drowsiness or dizziness. Caution patient to avoid driving or other activities requiring alertness until response to medication is known. Do not resume driving until physician gives clearance based on control of seizure disorder.
- Advise patient to carry identification describing disease process and medication regimen at all times.
- Advise patient to notify health care professional if skin rash, severe nausea or vomiting, drowsiness, slurred speech, unsteady gait, swollen glands, bleeding or tender gums, yellow skin or eyes, joint pain, fever, sore throat, unusual bleeding or bruising, or persistent headache occurs.
- Advise female patients to use an additional non-hormonal method of contraception during therapy and until next menstrual period. Instruct patient to notify health care professional if pregnancy is planned or suspected.
- Emphasize the importance of routine exams to monitor progress. Patient should have routine physical exams, especially monitoring skin and lymph nodes, and EEG testing.

Evaluation/Desired Outcomes
- Decrease or cessation of seizures without excessive sedation.

frovatriptan (froe-va-**trip**-tan)
Frova

frovatriptan 619

Classification
Therapeutic: vascular headache suppressants
Pharmacologic: 5-HT₁ agonists

Pregnancy Category C

Indications
Acute treatment of migraine headache.

Action
Acts as an agonist at specific 5-HT receptor sites in intracranial blood vessels and sensory trigeminal nerves. **Therapeutic Effects:** Cranial vessel vasoconstriction with associated decrease in release of neuropeptides and resultant decrease in migraine headache.

Pharmacokinetics
Absorption: 20–30% following oral administration.
Distribution: Unknown.
Metabolism and Excretion: Mostly metabolized by the liver (P450 1A2 enzyme system); some metabolites eliminated in urine, <10% excreted unchanged.
Half-life: 26 hr.

TIME/ACTION PROFILE (blood levels)

ROUTE	ONSET	PEAK	DURATION
PO	unknown	2–4 hr	unknown

Contraindications/Precautions
Contraindicated in: Hypersensitivity; History, symptoms or findings consistent with: ischemic heart disease, coronary artery vasospasm, other significant underlying cardiovascular disease; Cerebrovascular syndromes including: strokes of any type, transient ischemic attacks; Uncontrolled hypertension; Hemiplegic or basilar migraine; Peripheral vascular disease, including ischemic bowel disease; Should not be used within 24 hr of any other 5-HT agonist or ergot-type compounds (e.g. dihydroergotamine, ergotamine); Pedi: Children <18 yr.
Use Cautiously in: Concurrent use of SSRIs or SNRIs (↑ risk of serotonin syndrome); Geri: May be more susceptible to adverse cardiovascular effects; OB, Lactation: Safety not established.
Exercise Extreme Caution in: Cardiovascular risk factors (hypertension, hypercholesterolemia, cigarette smoking, obesity, diabetes, strong family history, menopausal women or men >40 yr); use only if cardiovascular status has been evaluated and determined to be safe and first dose is administered under supervision.

Adverse Reactions/Side Effects
CNS: dizziness, drowsiness, fatigue. **CV:** CORONARY ARTERY VASOSPASM, MI, VENTRICULAR FIBRILLATION, VENTRICULAR TACHYCARDIA, chest pain, myocardial ischemia. **GI:** dry mouth, dyspepsia, nausea. **Derm:** flushing. **MS:** skeletal pain. **Neuro:** paresthesia. **Misc:** pain.

Interactions
Drug-Drug: **Hormonal contraceptives** or **propranolol** may ↑ levels. ↑ risk of serious vasospastic reactions with **dihydroergotamine** or **ergotamine** (concurrent use contraindicated). ↑ risk of serotonin syndrome when used with **fluoxetine, paroxetine, sertraline, fluvoxamine, citalopram, escitalopram, venlafaxine,** or **duloxetine**.

Route/Dosage
PO (Adults): 2.5 mg; if there has been initial relief, a second tablet may be taken after at least 2 hr (daily dose should not exceed 3 tablets and should not be used to treat more than 4 attacks/30 day period).

Availability
Tablets: 2.5 mg.

NURSING IMPLICATIONS

Assessment
- Assess pain location, intensity, duration, and associated symptoms (photophobia, phonophobia, nausea, vomiting) during migraine attack.

Potential Nursing Diagnoses
Acute pain (Indications)

Implementation
- **PO:** Tablets may be administered at any time after the headache starts.

Patient/Family Teaching
- Inform patient that frovatriptan should be used only during a migraine attack. It is meant to be used to relieve migraine attack but not to prevent or reduce the number of attacks.
- Instruct patient to administer frovatriptan as soon as symptoms appear, but it may be administered any time during an attack. If migraine symptoms return, a second dose may be used. Allow at least 2 hr between doses, and do not use more than 3 tablets in any 24-hr period.

✦ = Canadian drug name.   = Genetic implication.
*CAPITALS indicates life-threatening; underlines indicate most frequent.

- If dose does not relieve headache, additional frovatriptan doses are not likely to be effective; notify health care professional.
- Advise patient that lying down in a darkened room following frovatriptan administration may further help relieve headache.
- Caution patient not to use frovatriptan if she is pregnant, suspects she is pregnant, plans to become pregnant, or is breastfeeding. Adequate contraception should be used during therapy.
- May cause dizziness or drowsiness. Caution patient to avoid driving or other activities requiring alertness until response to medication is known.
- Advise patient to notify health care professional prior to next dose of frovatriptan if pain or tightness in the chest occurs during use. If pain is severe or does not subside, notify health care professional immediately. If wheezing; heart throbbing; swelling of eyelids, face, or lips; skin rash; skin lumps; or hives occur, notify health care professional immediately and do not take more frovatriptan without approval of health care professional. If feelings of tingling, heat, flushing, heaviness, pressure, drowsiness, dizziness, tiredness, or sickness develop, discuss with health care professional at next visit.
- Advise patient to avoid alcohol, which aggravates headaches, during frovatriptan use.

Evaluation/Desired Outcomes
- Relief of migraine attack.

---

furosemide (fur-oh-se-mide)
✥ Apo-Furosemide, Lasix,
✥ Lasix Special, ✥ Novosemide,
✥ Nu-Furosemide, ✥ PMS-Furosemide

Classification
Therapeutic: diuretics
Pharmacologic: loop diuretics

Pregnancy Category C

Indications
Edema due to heart failure, hepatic impairment or renal disease. Hypertension.

Action
Inhibits the reabsorption of sodium and chloride from the loop of Henle and distal renal tubule. Increases renal excretion of water, sodium, chloride, magnesium, potassium, and calcium. Effectiveness persists in impaired renal function.
Therapeutic Effects: Diuresis and subsequent mobilization of excess fluid (edema, pleural effusions). Decreased blood pressure.

Pharmacokinetics
Absorption: 60–67% absorbed after oral administration (↓ in acute CHF and in renal failure); also absorbed from IM sites.
Distribution: Crosses placenta, enters breast milk.
Protein Binding: 91–99%.
Metabolism and Excretion: Minimally metabolized by liver, some nonhepatic metabolism, some renal excretion as unchanged drug.
Half-life: 30–60 min (↑ in renal impairment).

TIME/ACTION PROFILE (diuretic effect)

ROUTE	ONSET	PEAK	DURATION
PO	30–60 min	1–2 hr	6–8 hr
IM	10–30 min	unknown	4–8 hr
IV	5 min	30 min	2 hr

Contraindications/Precautions
Contraindicated in: Hypersensitivity; Cross-sensitivity with thiazides and sulfonamides may occur; Hepatic coma or anuria; Some liquid products may contain alcohol, avoid in patients with alcohol intolerance.
Use Cautiously in: Severe liver disease (may precipitate hepatic coma; concurrent use with potassium-sparing diuretics may be necessary); Electrolyte depletion; Diabetes mellitus; Increasing azotemia; OB, Lactation: Safety not established; Pedi: Increased risk for renal calculi and patent ductus arteriosis in premature neonates; Geri: Geriatric patients may have increased risk of side effects, especially hypotension and electrolyte imbalance, at usual doses.

Adverse Reactions/Side Effects
CNS: blurred vision, dizziness, headache, vertigo. **EENT:** hearing loss, tinnitus. **CV:** hypotension. **GI:** anorexia, constipation, diarrhea, dry mouth, dyspepsia, nausea, pancreatitis, vomiting. **GU:** excessive urination. **Derm:** photosensitivity, pruritis, rash. **Endo:** hyperglycemia, hyperuricemia. **F and E:** dehydration, hypocalcemia, hypochloremia, hypokalemia, hypomagnesemia, hyponatremia, hypovolemia, metabolic alkalosis. **Hemat:** APLASTIC ANEMIA, AGRANULOCYTOSIS, hemolytic anemia, leukopenia, thrombocytopenia. **MS:** muscle cramps. **Neuro:** paresthesia. **Misc:** fever, increased BUN, nephrocalcinosis.

Interactions
Drug-Drug: ↑ hypotension with **antihypertensives**, **nitrates**, or acute ingestion of **alcohol**. ↑ risk of hypokalemia with other **diuretics**, **amphotericin B**, **stimulant laxatives**, and **corticosteroids**. Hypokalemia may ↑ risk of **digoxin** toxicity and ↑ risk of arrhythmia in

furosemide 621

patients taking drugs that prolong the QT interval. ↓ **lithium** excretion, may cause **lithium** toxicity. ↑ risk of ototoxicity with **aminoglycosides**. **NSAIDS** ↓ effects of furosemide. ↓ effects of furosemide when given at same time as **sucralfate**, **cholestyramine**, or **colestipol**. ↑ risk of **salicylate** toxicity (with use of high-dose **salicylate** therapy).

Route/Dosage
Edema
PO (Adults): 20–80 mg/day as a single dose initially, may repeat in 6–8 hr; may increase dose by 20–40 mg q 6–8 hr until desired response. Maintenance doses may be given once or twice daily (doses up to 2.5 g/day have been used in patients with congestive heart failure or renal disease). *Hypertension*—40 twice daily initially (when added to regimen, decrease dose of other antihypertensives by 50%); adjust further dosing based on response; *Hypercalcemia*—120 mg/day in 1–3 doses.

PO (Children > 1 month): 2 mg/kg as a single dose; may be increased by 1–2 mg/kg q 6–8 hr (maximum dose = 6 mg/kg).

PO (Neonates): 1–4 mg/kg/dose 1–2 times/day.

IM, IV (Adults): 20–40 mg, may repeat in 1–2 hr and increase by 20 mg every 1–2 hr until response is obtained, maintenance dose may be given q 6–12 hr; *Continuous infusion*—Bolus 0.1 mg/kg followed by 0.1 mg/kg/hr, double q 2 hr to a maximum of 0.4 mg/kg/hr.

IM, IV (Children): 1–2 mg/kg/dose q 6–12 hr *Continuous infusion*—0.05 mg/kg/hr, titrate to clinical effect.

IM, IV (Neonates): 1–2 mg/kg/dose q 12–24 hr.

Hypertension
PO (Adults): 40 twice daily initially (when added to regimen, decrease dose of other antihypertensives by 50%); adjust further dosing based on response.

Availability (generic available)
Tablets: 20 mg, 40 mg, 80 mg, ✱500 mg. **Cost:** *Generic*—20 mg $10.99/100, 40 mg $8.99/100, 80 mg $16.99/100. **Oral solution (10 mg/mL—orange flavor, 8 mg/mL—pineapple—peach flavor):** 8 mg/mL, 10 mg/mL. **Cost:** *Generic*—10 mg/mL $13.99/60 mL. **Solution for injection:** 10 mg/mL.

NURSING IMPLICATIONS
Assessment
- Assess fluid status. Monitor daily weight, intake and output ratios, amount and location of edema, lung sounds, skin turgor, and mucous membranes. Notify physician or other health care professional if thirst, dry mouth, lethargy, weakness, hypotension, or oliguria occurs.
- Monitor blood pressure and pulse before and during administration. Monitor frequency of prescription refills to determine compliance in patients treated for hypertension.
- Geri: Diuretic use is associated with increased risk for falls in older adults. Assess falls risk and implement fall prevention strategies.
- Assess patients receiving digoxin for anorexia, nausea, vomiting, muscle cramps, paresthesia, and confusion. Patients taking digoxin are at increased risk of digoxin toxicity because of the potassium-depleting effect of the diuretic. Potassium supplements or potassium-sparing diuretics may be used concurrently to prevent hypokalemia.
- Assess patient for tinnitus and hearing loss. Audiometry is recommended for patients receiving prolonged high-dose IV therapy. Hearing loss is most common after rapid or high-dose IV administration in patients with decreased renal function or those taking other ototoxic drugs.
- Assess for allergy to sulfonamides.
- ***Lab Test Considerations:*** Monitor electrolytes, renal and hepatic function, serum glucose, and uric acid levels before and periodically throughout therapy. Commonly ↓ serum potassium. May cause ↓ serum sodium, calcium, and magnesium concentrations. May also cause ↑ BUN, serum glucose, creatinine, and uric acid levels.

Potential Nursing Diagnoses
Excess fluid volume (Indications)
Deficient fluid volume (Side Effects)

Implementation
- Do not confuse furosemide with torsemide.
- If administering twice daily, give last dose no later than 5 pm to minimize disruption of sleep cycle.
- IV route is preferred over IM route for parenteral administration.
- PO: May be taken with food or milk to minimize gastric irritation. Tablets may be crushed if patient has difficulty swallowing.

✱ = Canadian drug name. ▮ = Genetic implication.
*CAPITALS indicates life-threatening; underlines indicate most frequent.

furosemide

- Do not administer discolored solution or tablets.

IV Administration

- **Direct IV:** *Diluent:* Administer undiluted (larger doses may be diluted and administered as intermittent infusion [see below]). *Concentration:* 10 mg/mL. *Rate:* Administer at a rate of 20 mg/min. **Pedi:** Administer at a maximum rate of 0.5 mg/kg/min (for doses <120 mg) or 4 mg/min (for doses >120 mg).
- **Intermittent Infusion:** *Diluent:* Dilute larger doses in 50 mL of D5W or 0.9% NaCl. Infusion stable for 24 hr at room temperature. Do not refrigerate. Protect from light. *Concentration:* Final concentration should not exceed 10 mg/mL. *Rate:* Administer at a rate not to exceed 4 mg/min (for doses > 120 mg) in adults to prevent ototoxicity. Use an infusion pump to ensure accurate dosage.
- **Continuous Infusion:** *Diluent:* May dilute in D5W or 0.9% NaCl. May also administer as undiluted drug. Protect from light. *Concentration:* Final concentration should not exceed 10 mg/mL. *Rate:* See Route/Dosage section.
- **Y-Site Compatibility:** acyclovir, amikacin, aminophylline, amphotericin B cholesteryl sulfate, anidulafungin, argatroban, atropine, aztreonam, bivalirudin, calcium chloride, calcium gluconate, cefazolin, cefepime, cefotaxime, cefoxitin, ceftazidime, ceftizoxime, ceftriaxone, cefuroxime, chloramphenicol, clindamycin, cyclosporine, daptomycin, dexamethasone, digoxin, enalaprilat, epinephrine, ertapenem, fentanyl, ganciclovir, granisetron, heparin, hydrocortisone sodium succinate, hydromorphone, imipenem, insulin, ketorolac, lidocaine, linezolid, lorazepam, meropenem, methylprednisolone, metoprolol, metronidazole, micafungin, nafcillin, nitroglycerin, nitroprusside, palonosetron, pantoprazole, penicillin G potassium, phytonadione, piperacillin/tazobactam, potassium chloride, procainamide, propofol, propranolol, ranitidine, sodium bicarbonate, tacrolimus, thiopental, ticarcillin/clavulanate, tirofiban, tobramycin, vitamin B complex with C, voriconazole.
- **Y-Site Incompatibility:** azithromycin, caspofungin, cimetidine, ciprofloxacin, diazepam, diltiazem, diphenhydramine, doxycycline, droperidol, eptifibatide, erythromycin, esmolol, fenoldopam, filgrastim, hydroxyzine, labetalol, lansoprazole, levofloxacin, midazolam, milrinone, nesiritide, nicardipine, ondansetron, phenytoin, prochlorperazine, promethazine, protamine, quinupristin/dalfopristin, sulfamethoxazole/trimethoprim, vecuronium, vinblastine, vincristine, vinorelbine.

Patient/Family Teaching

- Instruct patient to take furosemide as directed. Take missed doses as soon as possible; do not double doses.
- Caution patient to change positions slowly to minimize orthostatic hypotension. Caution patient that the use of alcohol, exercise during hot weather, or standing for long periods during therapy may enhance orthostatic hypotension.
- Instruct patient to consult health care professional regarding a diet high in potassium (see Appendix M).
- Advise patient to contact health care professional of weight gain more than 3 lbs in 1 day.
- Advise patient to consult health care professional before taking OTC medication or herbal products concurrently with this therapy.
- Instruct patient to notify health care professional of medication regimen before treatment or surgery.
- Caution patient to use sunscreen and protective clothing to prevent photosensitivity reactions.
- Advise patient to contact health care professional immediately if muscle weakness, cramps, nausea, dizziness, numbness, or tingling of extremities occurs.
- Advise diabetic patients to monitor blood glucose closely; may cause increased blood glucose levels.
- Emphasize the importance of routine follow-up examinations.
- **Geri:** Caution older patients or their caregivers about increased risk for falls. Suggest strategies for fall prevention.
- **Hypertension:** Advise patients on antihypertensive regimen to continue taking medication even if feeling better. Furosemide controls but does not cure hypertension.
- Reinforce the need to continue additional therapies for hypertension (weight loss, exercise, restricted sodium intake, stress reduction, regular exercise, moderation of alcohol consumption, cessation of smoking).

Evaluation/Desired Outcomes

- Decrease in edema.
- Decrease in abdominal girth and weight.
- Increase in urinary output.
- Decrease in blood pressure.

gabapentin (ga-ba-**pen**-tin)
Neurontin

Classification
Therapeutic: analgesic adjuncts, therapeutic, anticonvulsants, mood stabilizers

Pregnancy Category C

Indications
Partial seizures (adjunct treatment). Post-herpetic neuralgia. **Unlabeled Use:** Neuropathic pain. Prevention of migraine headache. Bipolar disorder. Anxiety. Diabetic peripheral neuropathy.

Action
Mechanism of action is not known. May affect transport of amino acids across and stabilize neuronal membranes. **Therapeutic Effects:** Decreased incidence of seizures. Decreased post-herpetic pain.

Pharmacokinetics
Absorption: Well absorbed after oral administration by active transport. At larger doses, transport becomes saturated and absorption decreases (bioavailability ranges from 60% for a 300-mg dose to 35% for a 1600-mg dose).
Distribution: Crosses blood-brain barrier; enters breast milk.
Metabolism and Excretion: Eliminated mostly by renal excretion of unchanged drug.
Half-life: *Adults*—5–7 hr (normal renal function); up to 132 hr in anuria; *Children*—4.7 hr.

TIME/ACTION PROFILE (blood levels)

ROUTE	ONSET	PEAK	DURATION
PO	rapid	2–4 hr	8 hr

Contraindications/Precautions
Contraindicated in: Hypersensitivity.
Use Cautiously in: All patients (may ↑ risk of suicidal thoughts/behaviors); Renal insufficiency (↓ dose and/or ↑ dosing interval if CCr ≤60 mL/min); OB, Pedi: Safety not established for children <3 yr and pregnant women; Lactation: Discontinue drug or bottle-feed; Geri: May be more susceptible to toxicity due to age-related ↓ in renal function.

Adverse Reactions/Side Effects
CNS: SUICIDAL THOUGHTS, confusion, , depression, drowsiness, sedation, anxiety, concentration difficulties (children), dizziness, emotional lability (children), hostility, hyperkinesia (children), malaise, vertigo, weakness. **EENT:** abnormal vision, nystagmus. **CV:** hypertension. **GI:** weight gain, anorexia, flatulence, gingivitis. **MS:** arthralgia. **Neuro:** ataxia, altered reflexes, hyperkinesia, paresthesia. **Misc:** facial edema.

Interactions
Drug-Drug: **Antacids** may ↓ absorption of gabapentin. ↑ risk of CNS depression with other **CNS depressants**, including **alcohol**, **antihistamines**, **opioids**, and **sedative/hypnotics**. **Morphine** ↑ gabapentin levels and may ↑ risk of toxicity, dosage adjustments may be required.
Drug-Natural Products: **Kava-kava**, **valerian**, or **chamomile** can ↑ CNS depression.

Route/Dosage

Epilepsy
PO (Adults and Children >12 yr): 300 mg 3 times daily initially. Titration may be continued until desired (range is 900–1800 mg/day in 3 divided doses; doses should not be more than 12 hr apart). Doses up to 2400–3600 mg/day have been well tolerated.

PO (Children ≥5–12 yr): 10–15 mg/kg/day in 3 divided doses initially titrated upward over 3 days to 25–35 mg/kg/day in 3 divided doses; dosage interval should not exceed 12 hr (doses up to 50 mg/kg/day have been used).

PO (Children 3–4 yrs): 10–15 mg/kg/day in 3 divided doses initially titrated upward over 3 days to 40 mg/kg/day in 3 divided doses; dosage interval should not exceed 12 hr (doses up to 50 mg/kg/day have been used).

Neuropathic Pain
PO (Adults): 100 mg 3 times daily initially. Titrate weekly by 300 mg/day up to 900–2400 mg/day (maximum: 3600 mg/day).

PO (Children): 5 mg/kg/dose at bedtime initially then increase to 5 mg/kg BID on day 2 and 5 mg/kg TID on day 3. Titrate to effect up to 8–35 mg/kg/day in 3 divided doses.

Renal Impairment
PO (Adults and Children >12 yr): *CCr 30–60 mL/min*—300 mg 2 times daily; *CCr 15–30 mL/min*—300 mg once daily; *CCr <15 mL/min*—300 mg once every other day; further adjustments are based on clinical response.

Post-Herpetic Neuralgia
PO (Adults): 300 mg once daily on first day, 300 mg 2 times daily on second day, then 300 mg 3

times/day on day 3, may then be titrated upward as needed up to 600 mg 3 times/day.

Availability (generic available)
Capsules: 100 mg, 300 mg, 400 mg. **Cost:** *Generic*— 100 mg $64.96/270, 300 mg $169.97/270, 400 mg $209.98/270. **Tablets:** 100 mg, 300 mg, 400 mg, 600 mg, 800 mg. **Cost:** *Generic*— 600 mg $229.96/270, 800 mg $199.96/270. **Oral solution (cool strawberry anise flavor):** 250 mg/5 mL. **Cost:** $130.10/470 mL.

NURSING IMPLICATIONS
Assessment
- Monitor closely for notable changes in behavior that could indicate the emergence or worsening of suicidal thoughts or behavior or depression.
- **Seizures:** Assess location, duration, and characteristics of seizure activity.
- **Post-herpetic Neuralgia & Neuropathic Pain:** Assess location, characteristics, and intensity of pain periodically during therapy.
- **Migraine Prophylaxis:** Monitor frequecy and intensity of pain on pain scale.
- *Lab Test Considerations:* May cause false-positive readings when testing for urinary protein with *Ames N-Multistix SG* dipstick test; use sulfosalicylic acid precipitation procedure.
- May cause leukopenia.

Potential Nursing Diagnoses
Risk for injury (Side Effects)
Chronic pain (Indications)
Ineffective coping (Indications)

Implementation
- **PO:** May be administered without regard to meals.
- 600 mg and 800 mg tablets are scored and can be broken to administer a half-tablet. If half-tablet is used, administer other half at the next dose. Discard half-tablets not used within several days.
- Gabapentin should be discontinued gradually over at least 1 wk. Abrupt discontinuation may cause increase in seizure frequency.

Patient/Family Teaching
- Instruct patient to take medication exactly as directed. Patients on tid dosing should not exceed 12 hr between doses. Take missed doses as soon as possible; if less than 2 hr until next dose, take dose immediately and take next dose 1–2 hr later, then resume regular dosing schedule. Do not double dose. Do not discontinue abruptly; may cause increase in frequency of seizures. Instruct patient to read the *Medication Guide* before starting and with each Rx refill, changes may occur.
- Advise patient not to take gabapentin within 2 hr of an antacid.
- Gabapentin may cause dizziness and drowsiness. Caution patient to avoid driving or activities requiring alertness until response to medication is known. Seizure patients should not resume driving until physician gives clearance based on control of seizure disorder.
- Advise patient and family to notify health care professional if thoughts about suicide or dying, attempts to commit suicide; new or worse depression; new or worse anxiety; feeling very agitated or restless; panic attacks; trouble sleeping; new or worse irritability; acting aggressive; being angry or violent; acting on dangerous impulses; an extreme increase in activity and talking, other unusual changes in behavior or mood occur.
- Advise female patient to notify health care professional if pregnancy is planned or suspected or if breastfeeding.
- Instruct patient to notify health care professional of medication regimen before treatment or surgery.
- Advise patient to carry identification describing disease process and medication regimen at all times.

Evaluation/Desired Outcomes
- Decreased frequency of or cessation of seizures.
- Decreased post-herpetic neuralgia pain.
- Decreased intensity of neuropathic pain.
- Decreased frequency of migraine headaches.
- Increased mood stability.

---

galantamine (ga-lant-a-meen)
Razadyne, Razadyne ER

Classification
Therapeutic: anti-Alzheimer's agents
Pharmacologic: cholinergics (cholinesterase inhibitors)

Pregnancy Category B

Indications
Mild to moderate dementia of the Alzheimer's type.

Action
Enhances cholinergic function by reversible inhibition of cholinesterase. **Therapeutic Effects:** Decreased dementia (temporary) associated with Alzheimer's disease. Cognitive enhancer.

Pharmacokinetics
Absorption: Well absorbed (90%) following oral administration.
Distribution: Unknown.
Metabolism and Excretion: Mostly metabolized by the liver; 20% excreted unchanged in urine.
Half-life: 7 hr.

TIME/ACTION PROFILE (antihcholinesterase activity)

ROUTE	ONSET	PEAK	DURATION
PO	unknown	1 hr	12 hr
PO-ER	unknown	1 hr	24 hr

Contraindications/Precautions
Contraindicated in: Hypersensitivity; Severe hepatic or renal impairment; Pedi, Lactation: Children or lactation.
Use Cautiously in: Patients with supraventricular cardiac conduction defects or concurrent use of drugs that may slow heart rate (↑ risk of bradycardia); History of ulcer disease/GI bleeding/concurrent NSAID use; Severe asthma or obstructive pulmonary disease; Mild to moderate renal impairment (avoid use if CCr <9 mL/min); Mild to moderate hepatic impairment (cautious dose titration recommended); May ↑ risk of cardiovascular mortality; OB: Use only if potential benefit outweighs potential risk to fetus.

Adverse Reactions/Side Effects
CNS: fatigue, dizziness, headache, syncope. **CV:** bradycardia, chest pain. **GI:** anorexia, diarrhea, dyspepsia, flatulence, nausea, vomiting. **GU:** bladder outflow obstruction, incontinence. **Neuro:** tremor. **Misc:** weight loss.

Interactions
Drug-Drug: Will ↑ neuromuscular blockade from **succinylcholine-type neuromuscular blocking agents**. May ↑ effects of other **cholinesterase inhibitors** or other **cholinergic agonists**, including **bethanechol**. May ↓ effectiveness of **anticholinergic medications**. Blood levels and effects may be ↑ by **ketoconazole**, **paroxetine**, **amitriptyline**, **fluvoxamine**, or **quinidine**.

Route/Dosage
PO (Adults): *Immediate-release tablets* 4 mg twice daily initially, dose increments of 4 mg should be made at 4 wk intervals, up to 12 mg twice daily. Doses up to 16 mg twice daily have been used (range 16–32 mg/day; *Extended-release capsules*—8mg/day as a single dose in the morning, may be ↑ to 16 mg/day after 4 wk, then up to 24 mg/day after 4 wk, increments based on benefit/tolerability.

Renal Impairment
PO (Adults): *Moderate renal impairment*—Daily dose should not exceed 16 mg.

Hepatic Impairment
PO (Adults): *Moderate hepatic impairment*—Daily dose should not exceed 16 mg.

Availability (generic available)
Immediate-release tablets: 4 mg, 8 mg, 12 mg. **Extended-release capsules:** 8 mg, 16 mg, 24 mg. **Oral solution:** 4 mg/mL.

NURSING IMPLICATIONS

Assessment
- Assess cognitive function (memory, attention, reasoning, language, ability to perform simple tasks) periodically during therapy.
- Monitor heart rate periodically during therapy. May cause bradycardia.

Potential Nursing Diagnoses
Disturbed thought process (Indications)
Risk for injury (Indications)
Impaired environmental interpretation syndrome (Indications)

Implementation
- Patient should be maintained on a stable dose for a minimum of 4 weeks prior to increasing dose.
- If dose has been interrupted for several days or longer, restart at the lowest dose and escalate to the current dose.
- **PO:** Administer twice daily, preferably with morning and evening meal. Administration with food, the use of antiemetic medications, and ensuring adequate fluid intake may decrease nausea and vomiting.
- Administer extended-release capsules in the morning, preferably with food. Swallow whole; do not open, crush, or chew.
- Use pipette provided with oral solution to administer accurate amount.

Patient/Family Teaching
- Emphasize the importance of taking galantamine daily, as directed. Instruct patient and/or caregiver in correct use of pipette if using oral solution. Skip missed doses and return to regular schedule the following day; do not double

doses. Do not discontinue abruptly; although no increase in frequency of adverse events may occur, beneficial affects of galantamine are lost when the drug is discontinued.
- Caution patient and caregiver that galantamine may cause dizziness.
- Advise patient and caregiver to notify health care professional if nausea or vomiting persists beyond 7 days or if new symptoms occur or previously noted symptoms increase in severity.
- Advise patient and caregiver to notify health care professional of medication regimen prior to treatment or surgery.
- Emphasize the importance of follow-up exams to monitor progress.
- Teach patient and caregivers that improvements in cognitive functioning may take weeks to months to stabilize.
- Caution that disease is not cured and degenerative process is not reversed.

Evaluation/Desired Outcomes
- Improvement in cognitive function (memory, attention, reasoning, language, ability to perform simple tasks) in patients with Alzheimer's disease.

ganciclovir (gan-sye-kloe-vir)
Cytovene, Vitrasert

Classification
Therapeutic: antivirals

Pregnancy Category C

Indications
IV: Treatment of cytomegalovirus (CMV) retinitis in immunocompromised patients, including HIV-infected patients (may be used with foscarnet). Prevention of CMV infection in transplant patients at risk. **PO:** Maintenance treatment of stable CMV retinitis in immunocompromised patients after initial IV treatment and prevention of CMV retinitis in patients with advanced HIV infection.

Action
CMV converts ganciclovir to its active form (ganciclovir phosphate) inside the host cell, where it inhibits viral DNA polymerase. **Therapeutic Effects:** Antiviral effect directed preferentially against CMV-infected cells.

Pharmacokinetics
Absorption: 5–9% absorbed after oral administration. IV administration results in complete bioavailability. Action of intravitreal implant is local.
Distribution: Widely distributed; enters CSF.

Metabolism and Excretion: 90% excreted unchanged by the kidneys.
Half-life: 2.9 hr (↑ in renal impairment).

TIME/ACTION PROFILE (antiviral levels)

ROUTE	ONSET	PEAK	DURATION
PO	rapid	1.8–3 hr	3–8 hr
IV	rapid	end of infusion	12–24 hr
Intravitreal	rapid	unknown	5–8 mo

Contraindications/Precautions
Contraindicated in: Hypersensitivity to ganciclovir or acyclovir.
Use Cautiously in: Renal impairment (dose ↓ required if CCr <80 mL/min); Geri: Dose ↓ recommended; Bone marrow depression or immunosuppression; OB, Lactation, Pedi: Safety not established.

Adverse Reactions/Side Effects
CNS: SEIZURES, abnormal dreams, coma, confusion, dizziness, drowsiness, headache, malaise, nervousness. **EENT:** retinal detachment; *intravitreal only*, ↓ visual acuity, vitreous hemorrhage, hyphema, intraocular pressure spikes, lens opacities, macular abnormalities, optic nerve changes, uveitis. **Resp:** dyspnea. **CV:** arrhythmias, edema, hypertension, hypotension. **GI:** GI BLEEDING, abdominal pain, ↑ liver enzymes, nausea, vomiting. **GU:** gonadal suppression, hematuria, renal toxicity. **Derm:** alopecia, photosensitivity, pruritus, rash, urticaria. **Endo:** hypoglycemia. **Hemat:** neutropenia, thrombocytopenia, anemia, eosinophilia. **Local:** pain/phlebitis at IV site. **Neuro:** ataxia, tremor. **Misc:** fever.

Interactions
Drug-Drug: ↑ risk of bone marrow depression with **antineoplastics**, **radiation therapy**, or **zidovudine**. Toxicity may be ↑ by **probenecid**. ↑ risk of seizures with **imipenem/cilastatin**. Concurrent use of other **nephrotoxic drugs**, **cyclosporine**, or **amphotericin B** ↑ risk of nephrotoxicity.

Route/Dosage
IV (Adults): *Induction*—5 mg/kg q 12 hr for 14–21 days. *Maintenance regimen*—5 mg/kg/day or 6 mg/kg for 5 days of each week. If progression occurs, ↑ to q 12 hr regimen. *Prevention*—5 mg/kg q 12 hr for 7–14 days, then 5 mg/kg/day or 6 mg/kg for 5 days of each week.
PO (Adults): *Maintenance regimen*—1000 mg 3 times daily (with food) or 500 mg 6 times daily; *Prevention of CMV retinitis in advanced HIV infection*—1000 mg 3 times daily.
Intravitreal (Adults): 4.5 mg implant.

ganciclovir

Availability (generic available)
Capsules: 250 mg, 500 mg. **Powder for injection:** 500 mg/vial. **Intravitreal insert:** 4.5 mg.

NURSING IMPLICATIONS
Assessment
- Diagnosis of CMV retinitis should be determined by ophthalmoscopy before treatment with ganciclovir.
- Culture for CMV (urine, blood, throat) may be taken before administration. However, a negative CMV culture does not rule out CMV retinitis. If symptoms do not respond after several weeks, resistance to ganciclovir may have occurred. Ophthalmologic exams should be performed weekly during induction and every 2 wk during maintenance or more frequently if the macula or optic nerve is threatened. Progression of CMV retinitis may occur during or after ganciclovir treatment.
- Assess for signs of infection (fever, chills, cough, hoarseness, lower back or side pain, sore throat, difficult or painful urination). Notify health care professional if these symptoms occur.
- Assess for bleeding (bleeding gums, bruising, petechiae; guaiac stools, urine, and emesis). Avoid IM injections and taking rectal temperatures. Apply pressure to venipuncture sites for 10 min.
- **Lab Test Considerations:** Monitor neutrophil and platelet count at least every 2 days during bid therapy and weekly thereafter. Granulocytopenia usually occurs during the first 2 wk of treatment but may occur anytime during therapy. Do not administer if neutrophil count <500/mm³ or platelet count <25,000/mm³. Recovery begins within 3–7 days of discontinuation of therapy.
- Monitor BUN and serum creatinine at least once every 2 wk throughout therapy.
- Monitor liver function tests (AST, ALT, serum bilirubin, alkaline phosphatase) periodically during therapy. May cause ↑ levels.
- May cause ↓ blood glucose.

Potential Nursing Diagnoses
Risk for infection (Indications, Patient/Family Teaching)

Implementation
- Do not confuse Cytovene (ganciclovir) with Cytosar (cytarabine).
- Prepare solution in a biologic cabinet. Wear gloves, gown, and mask while handling medication. Discard IV equipment in specially designated containers.
- Do not administer subcut or IM; severe tissue irritation may result.
- **PO:** Administer capsules with food. Swallow capsules whole; do not open, crush, or chew.
- **IV:** Observe infusion site for phlebitis. Rotate infusion site to prevent phlebitis.
- Maintain adequate hydration throughout therapy.

IV Administration
- **Intermittent Infusion:** Reconstitute 500 mg with 10 mL of sterile water for injection for a concentration of 50 mg/mL. Do not reconstitute with bacteriostatic water with parabens; precipitation will occur. Shake well to dissolve completely. Discard vial if particulate matter or discoloration occurs. Reconstituted solution is stable for 12 hr at room temperature; do not refrigerate.
- ***Diluent:*** Dilute in 100 mL of D5W, 0.9% NaCl, Ringer's or LR. Once diluted for infusion, solution should be used within 24 hr. Refrigerate but do not freeze. ***Concentration:*** 10 mg/mL. ***Rate:*** Administer slowly, via infusion pump, over 1 hr using an in-line filter. Rapid administration may increase toxicity.
- **Y-Site Compatibility:** alfentanyl, allopurinol, amphotericin B cholesteryl, anidulafungin, atropine, bivalirudin, calcium gluconate, carboplatin, caspofungin, cisplatin, cyanocobalamin, cyclophosphamide, cyclosporine, dactinomycin, daptomycin, dexamethasone, dexmedetomidine, digoxin, docetaxel, doxacurium, doxorubicin liposome, enalaprilat, epoetin alfa, eptifibatide, ertapenem, etoposide, etoposide phosphate, fentanyl, filgrastim, fluconazole, fluorouracil, folic acid, furosemide, glycopyrrolate, granisetron, heparin, hetastarch, hydromorphone, ifosfamide, indomethacin, insulin, labetalol, linezolid, lorazepam, mannitol, mechlorethamine, melphalan, methotrexate, metoprolol, milrinone, mitoxantrone, nafcillin, naloxone, nesiritide, nitroglycerin, nitroprusside, octreotide, oxytocin, paclitaxel, pancuronium, pantoprazole, pemetrexed, pentobarbital, phenobarbital, phytonadione, potassium chloride, propofol, propranolol, protamine, ranitidine, remifentanil, rituximab, rocuronium, sodium acetate, sufentanil, teniposide, thi-

otepa, tigecycline, tirofiban, trastuzumab, trimetaphan, vasopressin, vincristine, voriconazole.
- **Y-Site Incompatibility:** aldesleukin, amifostine, amikacin, aminophylline, amphotericin B colloidal, ampicillin, ampicillin/sulbactam, amsacrine, ascorbic acid, atracurium, azathioprine, aztreonam, bumetanide, butorphanol, cefazolin, cefepime, cefonocid, cefoperazone, cefotaxime, cefotetan, cefoxitin, ceftazidime, ceftizoxime, ceftriaxone, cefuroxime, chloramphenicol, chlorpromazine, cimetidine, clindamycin, cytarabine, dantrolene, diazepam, diazoxide, diltiazem, diphenhydramine, dobutamine, dopamine, doxorubicin, doxycycline, ephedrine, epinephrine, epirubicin, erythromycin, esmolol, famotidine, fenoldopam, fludarabine, foscarnet, gemcitabine, gentamicin, haloperidol, hydralazine, hydrocortisone, hydroxyzine, idarubicin, imipenem/cilastatin, inamrinone, isorpoterenol, isoproterenol, ketorolac, levofloxacin, lidocaine, meperidine, metaraminol, methoxamine, methyldoapte, methylprednisolone, metoclopramide, metronidazole, midazolam, morphine, multivitamins, nalbuphine, norepinephrine, ondansetron, palonosetron, penicillin G, pentazocine, phentolamine, phenylephrine, phenytoin, piperacillin/tazobactam, procainamide, prochlorperazine, promethazine, pyridoxime, quinupristin/dalfopristin, sargramostim, sodium bicarbonate, streptokinase, succinylcholine, tacrolimus, theophylline, thiamine, ticarcillin/clavulanate, tobramycin, tolazoline, trimethoprim/sulfamethoxazone, vancomycin, verapamil, vinorelbine.

Patient/Family Teaching
- Instruct patient to take ganciclovir with food, as directed.
- Inform patient that ganciclovir is not a cure for CMV retinitis. Progression of retinitis may continue in immunocompromised patients during and after therapy. Advise patients to have regular ophthalmic exams at least every 6 wk. Duration of therapy for CMV prevention is based on the duration and degree of immunosuppression.
- Advise patient to notify health care professional if fever; chills; sore throat; other signs of infection; bleeding gums; bruising; petechiae; or blood in urine, stool, or emesis occurs. Caution patient to avoid crowds and persons with known infections. Instruct patient to use soft toothbrush and electric razor. Patient should be cautioned not to drink alcoholic beverages or take products containing aspirin or NSAIDs.
- Advise patient that ganciclovir may have teratogenic effects. A nonhormonal method of contraception should be used during and for at least 90 days after therapy.
- Caution patient to use sunscreen and protective clothing to prevent photosensitivity reactions.
- Emphasize the importance of frequent follow-up exams to monitor blood counts.

Evaluation/Desired Outcomes
- Management of the symptoms of CMV retinitis in immunocompromised patients.
- Prevention of CMV retinitis in transplant patients at risk.

gefitinib (je-fit-in-ib)
Iressa

Classification
Therapeutic: antineoplastics
Pharmacologic: enzyme inhibitors

Pregnancy Category D

Indications
Patients who are currently benefiting from or have benefited from gefitinib in the past for treatment of non-small cell lung cancer.

Action
Inhibits activation of kinases found in transmembrane cell surface receptors, including epidermal growth factor receptor (EGFR-TK). **Therapeutic Effects:** Death of rapidly replicating cells, particularly malignant ones.

Pharmacokinetics
Absorption: 60% absorbed following oral administration.
Distribution: Extensively distributed.
Metabolism and Excretion: Mostly metabolized by the liver (CYP3A4 enzyme system); excreted in feces, <4% excreted in urine.
Half-life: 48 hr.

TIME/ACTION PROFILE

ROUTE	ONSET	PEAK	DURATION
PO	unknown	unknown	unknown

Contraindications/Precautions
Contraindicated in: Hypersensitivity; OB, Lactation, Pedi: Pregnancy, lactation, children.
Use Cautiously in: Idiopathic pulmonary fibrosis (↑ risk of pulmonary toxicity); Concurrent use of strong inhibitors of the CYP3A4 enzyme system (may ↑ risk of toxicity).

Adverse Reactions/Side Effects
CNS: weakness. **EENT:** aberrant eyelash, conjunctivitis, corneal erosion/ulcer, eye pain, ↓ vision. **CV:** peripheral edema. **Resp:** PULMONARY TOXICITY, dyspnea. **GI:** diarrhea, nausea, vomiting, anorexia, hepatotoxicity, mouth ulceration. **Derm:** acne, dry skin, rash, pruritus. **Metab:** weight loss. **Misc:** allergic reactions including ANGIOEDEMA.

Interactions
Drug-Drug: Strong inducers of the CYP3A4 enzyme system, including **rifampin** and **phenytoin** ↓ blood levels and effects (consider ↑ dose of gefitinib to 500 mg/day). Strong inhibitors of the CYP3A4 enzyme system, including **ketoconazole** and **itraconazole** ↑ blood levels and effects (use with caution). Absorption and efficacy may be ↓ by **drugs that** ↑ **gastric pH** including **cimetidine** and **ranitidine**. May ↑ the risk of bleeding with **warfarin**. Concurrent use with **vinorelbine** may ↑ risk/severity of neutropenia.

Route/Dosage
PO (Adults): 250 mg once daily.

Availability
Tablets: 250 mg.

NURSING IMPLICATIONS

Assessment
- Assess for signs of pulmonary toxicity (dyspnea, cough, fever). If interstitial lung disease is confirmed, discontinue gefitinib and treat appropriately.
- Assess patient for eye symptoms such as pain during therapy. May require interruption of therapy and removal of aberrant eyelash. After symptoms and eye changes have resolved, may reinstate therapy.
- *Lab Test Considerations:* Monitor liver function tests periodically. May cause ↑ transaminases, bilirubin, and alkaline phosphatase. Discontinue gefitinib if elevations are severe.
- Monitor for changes in prothrombin time and INR in patients taking warfarin. May cause ↑ levels.

Potential Nursing Diagnoses
Diarrhea (Adverse Reactions)
Impaired skin integrity (Side Effects)
Ineffective breathing pattern (Adverse Reactions)

Implementation
- Available only through the *Iressa Access Program*. Patients must be currently on the medication or in an approved study and must sign the Patient Consent Form. Physicians and prescribers must enroll in program.
- **PO:** Administer one tablet daily without regard to food. Tablets can also be dispersed in half a glass of drinking water (non-carbonated). No other liquids should be used. Drop the tablet in the water, without crushing it, stir until the tablet is dispersed (approximately 10 minutes) and drink the liquid immediately. Rinse the glass with half a glass of water and drink. The liquid can also be administered through a nasogastric tube.
- May interrupt therapy briefly (14 days) for patients with poorly tolerated diarrhea with dehydration or skin adverse reactions. Follow by restarting 250 mg dose.

Patient/Family Teaching
- Instruct patient to take gefitinib as directed. Advise patient to read the *Instruction Sheet* with each Rx refill; new information may be available.
- Advise patient to notify health care professional promptly if severe persistent diarrhea, nausea, vomiting, or anorexia occur; if shortness of breath or cough occur or worsen; or if eye irritation or other new symptoms develop.
- Instruct patient to notify health care professional if pregnancy is planned or suspected or if breastfeeding.

Evaluation/Desired Outcomes
- Decrease in size and spread of tumors in non-small cell lung cancer.

HIGH ALERT

gemcitabine (jem-site-a-been)
Gemzar

Classification
Therapeutic: antineoplastics
Pharmacologic: antimetabolites, nucleoside analogues

Pregnancy Category D

Indications
Pancreatic cancer (locally advanced or metastatic). Inoperable locally advanced/metastatic non-small cell lung cancer (with cisplatin). Metastatic breast cancer (with paclitaxel). Advanced ovarian cancer that has relapsed 6 months after completion of platinum-based therapy (with carboplatin).

✦ = Canadian drug name. ✇ = Genetic implication.
*CAPITALS indicates life-threatening; underlines indicate most frequent.

630 gemcitabine

Action
Interferes with DNA synthesis (cell-cycle phase–specific). **Therapeutic Effects:** Death of rapidly replicating cells, particularly malignant ones.

Pharmacokinetics
Absorption: IV administration results in complete bioavailability.
Distribution: Unknown.
Metabolism and Excretion: Converted in cells to active diphosphate and triphosphate metabolites; these are excreted primarily by the kidneys.
Half-life: 32–94 min.

TIME/ACTION PROFILE (effect on blood counts)

ROUTE	ONSET	PEAK	DURATION
IV	unknown	unknown	unknown

Contraindications/Precautions
Contraindicated in: Hypersensitivity; OB: Can cause fetal malformation; Lactation: Can expose infant to serious adverse effects. Bottle feed if gemcitabine therapy is necessary.
Use Cautiously in: History of cardiovascular disease; Impaired hepatic or renal function (increased risk of toxicity); Other chronic debilitating illness; OB: Patients with childbearing potential.

Adverse Reactions/Side Effects
Resp: PULMONARY TOXICITY, dyspnea, bronchospasm. **CV:** ARRHYTHMIAS, CEREBROVASCULAR ACCIDENT, MI, edema, hypertension. **GI:** HEPATOTOXICITY, diarrhea, nausea, stomatitis, transient elevation of hepatic transaminases, vomiting. **GU:** HEMOLYTIC UREMIC SYNDROME, hematuria, proteinuria. **Derm:** alopecia, rash. **Hemat:** anemia, leukopenia, thrombocytopenia. **Local:** injection site reactions. **Neuro:** paresthesias. **Misc:** flu-like symptoms, fever, anaphylactoid reactions.

Interactions
Drug-Drug: ↑ bone marrow depression with other **antineoplastics** or **radiation therapy**. May ↓ antibody response to **live virus vaccines** and ↑ risk of adverse reactions.

Route/Dosage
Other regimens are used.

Pancreatic Cancer
IV (Adults): 1000 mg/m^2 once weekly for 7 wk, followed by a week of rest. May be followed by cycles of once-weekly administration for 3 wk followed by a week of rest.

Non-Small Cell Lung Cancer (with Cisplatin)
IV (Adults): 1000 mg/m^2 on days 1, 8, and 15 of each 28-day cycle (cisplatin is also given on day 1) *or* 1250 mg/m^2 on days 1 and 8 of each 21-day cycle (cisplatin is also given on day 1).

Breast Cancer
IV (Adults): 1250 mg/m^2 on days 1 and 8 of each 21-day cycle (paclitaxel is also given on day 1).

Ovarian Cancer
IV (Adults): 1000 mg/m^2 on days 1 and 8 of each 21-day cycle.

Availability
Powder for injection: 200 mg in 10-mL vial, 1 g in 50-mL vial. **Cost:** 200 mg $117.95/10-mL vial, 1 g $589.90/50-mL vial.

NURSING IMPLICATIONS

Assessment
- Monitor vital signs before and frequently during therapy.
- Assess injection site during administration. Although gemcitabine is not considered a vesicant, local reactions may occur.
- Monitor for bone marrow depression. Assess for bleeding (bleeding gums, bruising, petechiae; guaiac stools, urine, and emesis) and avoid IM injections and taking rectal temperatures if platelet count is low. Apply pressure to venipuncture sites for 10 min. Assess for signs of infection during neutropenia. Anemia may occur. Monitor for increased fatigue, dyspnea, and orthostatic hypotension.
- Monitor intake and output, appetite, and nutritional intake. Mild to moderate nausea and vomiting occur frequently. Antiemetics may be used prophylactically.
- *Lab Test Considerations:* Monitor CBC, including differential and platelet count, before each dose. Dose guidelines are based on the CBC. *For single-agent use:* If the absolute granulocyte count is >1000 and platelet count is >100,000, the full dose may be administered. If the absolute granulocyte count is 500–999 or platelet count is 50,000–99,000, 75% of the dose may be given. If the absolute granulocyte count is <500 or the platelet count is <50,000, withhold further doses. *For gemcitabine with paclitaxel (breast cancer):* If the absolute granulocyte count is >1200 and platelet count is >75,000, the full dose may be administered. If the absolute granulocyte count is

1000–1199 or platelet count is 50,000–75,000, 75% of the dose may be given. If the absolute granulocyte count is 700–999 or platelet count is ≥50,000, 50% of the dose may be given. If the absolute granulocyte count is <700 or the platelet count is <50,000, withhold further doses.
- Monitor serum creatinine, potassium, calcium, and magnesium in patients taking cisplatin with gemcitabine. *For gemcitabine with carboplatin (ovarian cancer):* If the absolute granulocyte count is >1500 and platelet count is >100,000, the full dose may be administered. If the absolute granulocyte count is 1000–1499 or platelet count is 75,000–99,000, 75% of the dose may be given. If the absolute granulocyte count is <1000 or the platelet count is <75,000, withhold further doses.
- Monitor hepatic and renal function before and periodically during therapy. May cause transient ↑ in serum AST, ALT, alkaline phosphatase, and bilirubin concentrations.
- May also cause ↑ BUN and serum creatinine concentrations, proteinuria, and hematuria.

Potential Nursing Diagnoses
Risk for infection (Adverse Reactions)

Implementation
- **High Alert:** Fatalities have occurred with incorrect administration of chemotherapeutic agents. Before administering, clarify all ambiguous orders; double-check single, daily, and course-of-therapy dose limits; have second practitioner independently double-check original order, calculations, and infusion pump settings.
- Solution should be prepared in a biologic cabinet. Wear gloves, gown, and mask while handling IV medication. Discard IV equipment in specially designated containers.

IV Administration
- **Intermittent Infusion:** To reconstitute, add 5 mL of 0.9% NaCl without preservatives to 200-mg vial or 25 mL of 0.9% NaCl to the 1-g vial of gemcitabine for a concentration of 40 mg/mL. Incomplete dissolution may result in concentrations greater than 40 mg/mL. *Diluent:* May be further diluted with 0.9% NaCl. Solution is colorless to light straw color. Do not administer solutions that are discolored or contain particulate matter. Solution is stable for 24 hr at room temperature. Discard unused portions. Do not refrigerate; crystallization may occur. *Concentration:* 0.1–38 mg/mL. *Rate:* Administer dose over 30 min. Infusions longer than 60 min have a greater incidence of toxicity.
- **Y-Site Compatibility:** amifostine, amikacin, aminophylline, ampicillin, ampicillin/sulbactam, aztreonam, bleomycin, bumetanide, buprenorphine, butorphanol, calcium gluconate, carboplatin, carmustine, cefazolin, cefotetan, cefoxitin, ceftazidime, ceftizoxime, ceftriaxone, cefuroxime, chlorpromizine, cimetidine, ciprofloxacin, cisplatin, clindamycin, cyclophosphamide, cytarabine, dactinomycin, daunorubicin, dexrazoxane, diphenhydramine, dobutamine, docetaxel, dopamine, doxorubicin, doxycycline, droperidol, enalaprilat, etoposide, etoposide phosphate, famotidine, floxuridine, fluconazole, fludarabine, fluorouracil, gentamicin, granisetron, haloperidol, heparin, hydrocortisone, hydromorphone, idarubicin, ifosfamide, leucovorin, linezolid, lorazepam, mannitol, meperidine, mesna, metoclopramide, metronidazole, mitoxantrone, morphine, nalbuphine, ofloxacin, ondansetron, oxaliplatin, paclitaxel, potassium chloride, promethazine, ranitidine, sodium bicarbonate, streptozocin, teniposide, thiotepa, ticarcillin/clavulanate, tobramycin, topotecan, trimethoprim/sulfamethoxazole, vancomycin, vinblastine, vincristine, vinorelbine, zidovudine.
- **Y-Site Incompatibility:** acyclovir, amphotericin B, cefotaxime, furosemide, ganciclovir, imipenem-cilastatin, irinotecan, lansoprazole, methotrexate, methoprednisolone, mitomycin, pemetrexed, piperacillin, piperacillin/tazobactam, prochlorperazine.

Patient/Family Teaching
- Instruct patient to notify health care professional if fever; chills; sore throat; signs of infection; bleeding gums; bruising; petechiae; or blood in urine, stool, or emesis occurs. Caution patient to avoid crowds and persons with known infections. Instruct patient to use soft toothbrush and electric razor. Patient should be cautioned not to drink alcoholic beverages or take products containing aspirin or NSAIDs.
- Instruct patient to inspect oral mucosa for erythema and ulceration. If ulceration occurs, advise patient to use sponge brush and rinse mouth with water after eating and drinking. Stomatitis pain may require management with opioid analgesics.

- Instruct patient to notify health care professional if flu-like symptoms (fever, anorexia, headache, cough, chills, myalgia), swelling of the feet or legs, or shortness of breath occurs.
- Discuss with patient the possibility of hair loss. Explore methods of coping.
- Advise patient that this medication may have teratogenic effects. Contraception should be used during therapy.
- Instruct patient not to receive any vaccinations without advice of health care professional.
- Emphasize the need for periodic lab tests to monitor for side effects.

Evaluation/Desired Outcomes
- Palliative, symptomatic improvement in patients with pancreatic cancer.
- Decrease in size and spread of malignancy in lung, ovarian, and breast cancer.

---

gemfibrozil (gem-**fye**-broe-zil)
Lopid

Classification
Therapeutic: lipid-lowering agents
Pharmacologic: fibric acid derivatives

Pregnancy Category C

Indications
Management of type II-b hyperlipidemia (decreased HDLs, increased LDLs, increased triglycerides) in patients who do not yet have clinical coronary artery disease and have failed therapy with diet, exercise, weight loss, or other agents (niacin, bile acid sequestrants).

Action
Inhibits peripheral lipolysis. Decreases triglyceride production by the liver. Decreases production of the triglyceride carrier protein. Increases HDL. **Therapeutic Effects:** Decreased plasma triglycerides and increased HDL.

Pharmacokinetics
Absorption: Well absorbed after oral administration.
Distribution: Unknown.
Metabolism and Excretion: Some metabolism by the liver, 70% excreted by the kidneys (mostly unchanged), 6% excreted in feces.
Half-life: 1.3–1.5 hr.

TIME/ACTION PROFILE (triglyceride-VLDL–lowering effect)

ROUTE	ONSET	PEAK	DURATION
PO	2–5 days	4 wk	several mo

Contraindications/Precautions
Contraindicated in: Hypersensitivity; Primary biliary cirrhosis; Concurrent use of HMG-CoA reductase inhibitors or repaglinide.
Use Cautiously in: Gallbladder disease; Liver disease; Severe renal impairment; OB, Lactation, Pedi: Safety not established.

Adverse Reactions/Side Effects
CNS: dizziness, headache. **EENT:** blurred vision. **GI:** <u>abdominal pain</u>, <u>diarrhea</u>, epigastric pain, flatulence, gallstones, heartburn, nausea, vomiting. **Derm:** alopecia, rashes, urticaria. **Hemat:** anemia, leukopenia. **MS:** myositis.

Interactions
Drug-Drug: May ↑ the effects of **warfarin** or **sulfonylurea oral hypoglycemic agents**. Concurrent use with **HMG-CoA reductase inhibitors** may ↑ the risk of rhabdomyolysis (avoid concurrent use). Concurrent use with **repaglinide** may ↑ the risk of severe hypoglycemia (avoid concurrent use). May ↓ the effect of **cyclosporine**.

Route/Dosage
PO (Adults): 600 mg twice daily 30 min before breakfast and dinner.

Availability (generic available)
Tablets: 600 mg. Cost: *Generic*—$45.97/180.
Capsules: 300 mg.

NURSING IMPLICATIONS

Assessment
- Obtain patient's diet history, especially regarding fat and alcohol consumption.
- ***Lab Test Considerations:*** Monitor serum triglyceride and cholesterol levels before and periodically during therapy. Assess LDL and VLDL levels before and periodically during therapy. Discontinue gemfibrozil if paradoxical ↑ in lipid levels occurs.
- Assess liver function tests before and periodically during therapy. May cause ↑ serum bilirubin, alkaline phosphatase, CK, LDH, AST, and ALT. If hepatic function tests rise significantly, therapy should be discontinued and not resumed.
- Evaluate CBC and electrolytes every 3–6 mo and then yearly during therapy. May cause mild ↓ in hemoglobin, hematocrit, and leukocyte counts. May cause ↓ serum potassium concentrations.
- May cause slight ↑ in serum glucose.

Potential Nursing Diagnoses
Noncompliance (Patient/Family Teaching)

Implementation
- Do not confuse Lopid (gemfibrozil) with Levbid (hyoscyamine).
- **PO:** Administer 30 min before breakfast or dinner.

Patient/Family Teaching
- Instruct patient to take medication as directed, not to skip doses or double up on missed doses. Take missed doses as soon as remembered unless almost time for next dose.
- Advise patient that this medication should be used in conjunction with dietary restrictions (fat, cholesterol, carbohydrates, alcohol), exercise, and cessation of smoking.
- Instruct patient to notify health care professional promptly if any of the following symptoms occur: severe stomach pains with nausea and vomiting, fever, chills, sore throat, rash, diarrhea, muscle cramping, general abdominal discomfort, or persistent flatulence.

Evaluation/Desired Outcomes
- Decrease in serum triglyceride and cholesterol levels and improved HDL to total cholesterol ratios. If response is not seen within 3 mo, medication is usually discontinued.

HIGH ALERT

gemtuzumab ozogamicin
(gem-**tu**-zoo-mab o-zo-ga-**my**-sin)
Mylotarg

Classification
Therapeutic: antineoplastics
Pharmacologic: monoclonal antibodies, antitumor antibiotics

Pregnancy Category D

Indications
Treatment of patients with patients with CD33 positive acute myeloid leukemia in first relapse who are ≥60 yr old and who are not considered to be candidates for cytotoxic chemotherapy.

Action
The antibody portion (gemtuzumab) attaches to the CD33 antigen on the surface of acute myeloid leukemic cells. Binding produces a complex that is internalized by the leukemic cells. Once internalized the antitumor antibiotic portion of the drug (ozogamicin, also know as calicheamicin) is released and binds to DNA resulting in breaks in double strand DNA and cell death. **Therapeutic Effects:** Death of acute myeloid leukemic cells.

Pharmacokinetics
Absorption: IV administration results in complete bioavailability.
Distribution: Binds to CD33 receptor sites, is then internalized by leukemic cells, releasing ozogamicin.
Metabolism and Excretion: Ozogamicin is probably metabolized by the liver.
Half-life: *Total ozogamicin*—45 hr (↑ with second dose); *unconjugated ozogamicin*—100 hr.

TIME/ACTION PROFILE

ROUTE	ONSET	PEAK	DURATION
IN	rapid	following infusion	2 wk

Contraindications/Precautions
Contraindicated in: Hypersensitivity; OB: Pregnancy; Lactation: Lactation.
Use Cautiously in: Patients with hepatic impairment; Pedi: Children (safety not established).

Adverse Reactions/Side Effects
CNS: headache. **Resp:** dyspnea, hypoxia. **CV:** hypotension, hypertension. **GI:** mucositis, nausea, vomiting, hepatotoxicity. **Derm:** rash. **Endo:** hyperglycemia. **F and E:** hypokalemia. **Hemat:** NEUTROPENIA, anemia, bleeding, thrombocytopenia. **Misc:** chills, fever, postinfusion reaction, allergic reactions, infection, tumor lysis syndrome.

Interactions
Drug-Drug: None reported to date.

Route/Dosage
IV (Adults ≥60 yr): 9 mg/m^2 as a 2-hr infusion followed by a second dose 14 days later.

Availability
Powder for injection (requires reconstitution): 5 mg/vial.

NURSING IMPLICATIONS

Assessment
- Prophylactically treat patient with diphenhydramine 50 mg PO, and acetaminophen 650–1000 mg PO 1 hr prior to administration, with 2 additional doses of acetaminophen 650–1000 mg PO every 4 hr as needed. Assess patient for postinfusion symptom complex (fever, chills, nausea, vomiting, headache, hypotension, hypertension, dyspnea, hyperglycemia), which may occur within the first 24 hr following administration and usually resolve after 2–

4 hr with supportive therapy. Fewer infusion-related events occur with second dose.
- Monitor vital signs during infusion and for 4 hr after infusion.
- Monitor for development of tumor lysis syndrome. May require hydration and allopurinol to prevent hyperuricemia.
- **Lab Test Considerations:** Monitor hematologic status (electrolytes, hepatic function, CBC, platelet counts) during therapy. Severe myelosuppression (anemia, thrombocytopenia) will occur in all patients given the recommended dose of gemtuzumab. Full recovery from hematologic toxicities is not required before second infusion.
- May cause ↑ AST and ALT levels which are transient and usually reversible.

Potential Nursing Diagnoses
Deficient knowledge, related to medication regimen (Patient/Family Teaching)

Implementation
- *High Alert:* Fatalities have occurred with incorrect administration of chemotherapeutic agents. Before administering, clarify all ambiguous orders; double check single, daily, and course-of-therapy dose limits; have second practitioner independently double check original order, calculations, and infusion pump settings. Gemtuzumab should be administered under the supervision of a physician experienced in the use of cancer chemotherapeutic agents. May be administered in a outpatient setting. Do not administer by intravenous push or bolus.
- Protect medication from direct and indirect light and unshielded fluorescent lights during preparation and administration. Must be prepared under a biologic safety hood with the fluorescent light off.

IV Administration
- **Intermittent Infusion:** Prior to reconstitution, allow drug to come to room temperature. Reconstitute each vial with 5 ml of sterile water for injection. Gently swirl each vial and inspect for particulate matter. Reconstituted drug may be stored refrigerated for up to 8 hr. *Diluent:* To dilute for administration, withdraw desired volume from each vial and inject into 100 mL IV bag of 0.9% NaCl and place into a UV protectant bag. Use diluted solution immediately. *Concentration:* Concentration in vial will be 1 mg/mL. *Rate:* Infuse over 2 hr via a separate IV line with a low protein-binding 1.2-micron terminal filter. May be administered through peripheral or central line.

Patient/Family Teaching
- Explain purpose of gemtuzumab to patient.

Evaluation/Desired Outcomes
- Remission in patients with leukemia.

---

gentamicin, See AMINOGLYCOSIDES.

---

glimepiride, See SULFONYLUREAS.

---

glipiZIDE, See SULFONYLUREAS.

---

glucagon (gloo-ka-gon)
GlucaGen

Classification
Therapeutic: hormones
Pharmacologic: pancreatics

Pregnancy Category B

Indications
Acute management of severe hypoglycemia when administration of glucose is not feasible. Facilitation of radiographic examination of the GI tract. **Unlabeled Use:** Antidote to: Beta blockers, Calcium channel blockers.

Action
Stimulates hepatic production of glucose from glycogen stores (glycogenolysis). Relaxes the musculature of the GI tract (stomach, duodenum, small bowel, and colon), temporarily inhibiting movement. Has positive inotropic and chronotropic effects. **Therapeutic Effects:** Increase in blood glucose. Relaxation of GI musculature, facilitating radiographic examination.

Pharmacokinetics
Absorption: Well absorbed following IM and subcut administration.
Distribution: Unknown.
Metabolism and Excretion: Extensively metabolized by the liver, plasma, and kidneys.
Half-life: 8–18 min.

glucagon

TIME/ACTION PROFILE

ROUTE	ONSET	PEAK	DURATION
IM (hyperglycemic action)	within 10 min	30 min	12–27 min
IV (hyperglycemic action)	1 min	5 min	9–17 min
Subcut (hyperglycemic action)	within 10 min	30–45 min	60–90 min
IV (effect on GI musculature)	45 sec (for 0.25–2-mg dose)	unknown	9–17 min (0.25–0.5-mg dose); 22–25 min (2-mg dose)
IM (effect on GI musculature)	8–10 min (1-mg dose); 4–7 min (2-mg dose)	unknown	9–27 min (1-mg dose); 21–32 min (2-mg dose)

Contraindications/Precautions
Contraindicated in: Hypersensitivity; Pheochromocytoma; Some products contain glycerin and phenol—avoid use in patients with hypersensitivities to these ingredients.
Use Cautiously in: History suggestive of insulinoma or pheochromocytoma; Prolonged fasting, starvation, adrenal insufficiency or chronic hypoglycemia (low levels of releasable glucose); When used to inhibit GI motility, use cautiously in geriatric patient with cardiac disease or diabetics; OB: Should be used during pregnancy only if clearly needed; Lactation: Safety not established.

Adverse Reactions/Side Effects
CV: hypotension. **GI:** nausea, vomiting. **Misc:** hypersensitivity reactions including ANAPHYLAXIS.

Interactions
Drug-Drug: Large doses may enhance the effect of **warfarin**. Negates the response to **insulin** or **oral hypoglycemic agents**. **Phenytoin** inhibits the stimulant effect of glucagon on insulin release. Hyperglycemic effect is intensified and prolonged by **epinephrine**. Patients on concurrent **beta blocker** therapy may have a greater increase in heart rate and blood pressure.

Route/Dosage

Hypoglycemia
IV, IM, Subcut (Adults and Children ≥20 kg): 1 mg; may be repeated in 15 min if necessary.

IV, IM, Subcut (Children <20 kg): 0.5 mg or 0.02–0.03 mg/kg; may be repeated in 15 min if necessary.

Radiographic Examination of the GI Tract
IM, IV (Adults): 0.25–2 mg; depending on location and duration of examination (0.5 mg IV or 2 mg IM for relaxation of stomach, for examination of the colon 2 mg IM 10 min before procedure).

Antidote (unlabeled)
IV (Adults): *To beta blockers*—50–150 mcg (0.05–0.15 mg)/kg, followed by 1–5 mg/hr infusion. *To calcium channel blockers*—2 mg; additional doses determined by response.

Availability
Powder for injection: 1-mg (equivalent to 1 unit) vials as an emergency kit for low blood glucose and a diagnostic kit.

NURSING IMPLICATIONS

Assessment
- Assess for signs of hypoglycemia (sweating, hunger, weakness, headache, dizziness, tremor, irritability, tachycardia, anxiety) prior to and periodically during therapy.
- Assess neurologic status throughout therapy. Institute safety precautions to protect patient from injury caused by seizures, falling, or aspiration. For insulin shock therapy, 0.5–1 mg is administered after 1 hr of coma; patient usually awakens in 10–25 min. If no response occurs, repeat the dose. Feed patient supplemental carbohydrates orally to replenish liver glycogen and prevent secondary hypoglycemia as soon as possible after awakening, especially pediatric patients.
- Assess nutritional status. Patients who lack liver glycogen stores (starvation, chronic hypoglycemia, adrenal insufficiency) will require glucose instead of glucagon.
- Assess for nausea and vomiting after administration of dose. Protect patients with depressed level of consciousness from aspiration by positioning on side; ensure that a suction unit is available. Notify health care professional if vomiting occurs; patient will require parenteral glucose to prevent recurrent hypoglycemia.
- *Lab Test Considerations:* Monitor serum glucose levels throughout episode, during treatment, and for 3–4 hr after patient regains consciousness. Use of bedside fingerstick

✱ = Canadian drug name. ▌ = Genetic implication.
*CAPITALS indicates life-threatening; underlines indicate most frequent.

blood glucose determination methods is recommended for rapid results. Follow-up lab results may be ordered to validate fingerstick values, but do not delay treatment while awaiting lab results, as this could result in neurologic injury or death.
- Large doses of glucagon may cause a ↓ in serum potassium concentrations.

Potential Nursing Diagnoses
Risk for injury (Indications)
Noncompliance (Patient/Family Teaching)

Implementation
- May be given subcut, IM, or IV. Reconstitute with diluent supplied in kit by manufacturer. Inspect solution prior to use; use only clear, water-like solution. Solution is stable for 48 hr if refrigerated, 24 hr at room temperature. Unmixed medication should be stored at room temperature.
- Administer supplemental carbohydrates IV or orally to facilitate increase of serum glucose levels.

IV Administration
- **Direct IV:** *Diluent:* Reconstitute each vial with 1 mL of an appropriate diluent. For doses ≤2 mg, use diluent provided by manufacturer. For doses >2 mg, use sterile water for injection instead of diluent supplied by manufacturer to minimize risk of thrombophlebitis, CNS toxicity, and myocardial depression from phenol preservative in diluent supplied by manufacturer. Reconstituted vials should be used immediately. *Concentration:* Not exceed 1 mg/mL. *Rate:* Administer at a rate not exceeding 1 mg/min. May be administered through IV line containing D5W.
- **Continuous Infusion:** *Diluent:* Reconstitute vials as per directions above (use sterile water for injection). Further dilute 10 mg of glucagon in 100 mL of D5W. *Concentration:* 0.1 mg/mL. *Rate:* See Route/Dosage section.
- **Y-Site Compatibility:** No information available.

Patient/Family Teaching
- Teach patient and family signs and symptoms of hypoglycemia. Instruct patient to take oral glucose as soon as symptoms of hypoglycemia occur—glucagon is reserved for episodes when patient is unable to swallow because of decreased level of consciousness.
- **Home Care Issues:** Instruct family on correct technique to prepare, draw up, and administer injection. Health care professional must be contacted immediately after each dose for orders regarding further therapy or adjustment of insulin dose or diet.
- Advise family that patient should receive oral glucose when alertness returns.
- Instruct family to position patient on side until fully alert. Explain that glucagon may cause nausea and vomiting. Aspiration may occur if patient vomits while lying on back.
- Instruct patient to check expiration date monthly and to replace outdated medication immediately.
- Review hypoglycemic medication regimen, diet, and exercise programs.
- Patients with diabetes mellitus should carry a source of sugar (such as a packet of sugar or candy) and identification describing disease process and treatment regimen at all times.

Evaluation/Desired Outcomes
- Increase of serum glucose to normal levels with improved level of consciousness.
- Smooth muscle relaxation of the stomach, duodenum, and small and large intestine in patients undergoing radiologic examination of the GI tract.

---

glyBURIDE, See SULFONYLUREAS.

---

glycopyrrolate
(glye-koe-**pye**-roe-late)
Robinul, Robinul-Forte

Classification
Therapeutic: antispasmodics
Pharmacologic: anticholinergics

Pregnancy Category B

Indications
Inhibits salivation and excessive respiratory secretions when given preoperatively. Reverses some of the secretory and vagal actions of cholinesterase inhibitors used to treat nondepolarizing neuromuscular blockade (cholinergic adjunct). Adjunctive management of peptic ulcer disease.

Action
Inhibits the action of acetylcholine at postganglionic sites located in smooth muscle, secretory glands, and the CNS (antimuscarinic activity). Low doses decrease sweating, salivation, and respiratory secretions. Intermediate doses result in increased heart rate. Larger doses decrease GI and GU tract motility. **Therapeutic Effects:** Decreased GI and respiratory secretions.

Pharmacokinetics
Absorption: Incompletely absorbed (10%) after oral administration. Well absorbed after IM administration.
Distribution: Distribution not fully known. Does not significantly cross the blood-brain barrier or eye. Crosses the placenta.
Metabolism and Excretion: Eliminated primarily unchanged in the feces, via biliary excretion.
Half-life: 1.7 hr (0.6–4.6 hr).

TIME/ACTION PROFILE (anticholinergic effects)

ROUTE	ONSET	PEAK	DURATION
PO	1 hr	unknown	8–12 hr
IM	15–30 min	30–45 min	2–7 hr*
IV	1–10 min	unknown	2–7 hr*

*Antisecretory effect lasts up to 7 hr; vagal blockade lasts 2–3 hr

Contraindications/Precautions
Contraindicated in: Hypersensitivity; Angle-closure glaucoma; Acute hemorrhage; Tachycardia secondary to cardiac insufficiency or thyrotoxicosis; Pedi: Injection contains benzyl alcohol and should not be given to neonates; Myasthenia gravis; Obstructive uropathy; Paralytic ileus.
Use Cautiously in: Patients who may have intra-abdominal infections; Prostatic hyperplasia; Chronic renal, hepatic, pulmonary, or cardiac disease; Down syndrome and children with spastic paralysis or brain damage (may be hypersensitive to antimuscarinic effects); OB, Lactation: Safety not established; Pedi: ↑ sensitivity to anticholinergic effects and adverse reactions; Geri: ↑ sensitivity to anticholinergic effects and adverse reactions.

Adverse Reactions/Side Effects
CNS: confusion, drowsiness. **EENT:** blurred vision, cycloplegia, dry eyes, mydriasis. **CV:** tachycardia, orthostatic hypotension, palpitations. **GI:** dry mouth, constipation. **GU:** urinary hesitancy, retention.

Interactions
Drug-Drug: Additive anticholinergic effects with other **anticholinergics**, including **antihistamines**, **phenothiazines**, **meperidine**, **amantadine**, **tricyclic antidepressants**, **quinidine**, and **disopyramide**. May alter the absorption of other **orally administered drugs** by slowing motility of the GI tract. **Antacids** or **adsorbent antidiarrheal agents** ↓ absorption of anticholinergics. May ↑ GI mucosal lesions in patients taking oral **potassium chloride** tablets. ↑ risk of adverse cardiovascular reactions with **cyclopropane** anesthesia. Concurrent use may ↓ absorption of **ketoconazole** (administer 2 hr after ketoconazole).

Route/Dosage
Control of Secretions during Surgery
IM (Adults): 4.4 mcg/kg 30–60 min preop (not to exceed 0.1 mg).
IM (Children > 2 yr): 4.4 mcg/kg 30–60 min preop.
IM (Children < 2 yr): 4.4–8.8 mcg/kg 30–60 min preop.

Control of Secretions (chronic)
IM, IV (Children): 4–10 mcg/kg/dose q 3–4 hr.
PO (Children): 40–100 mcg/kg/dose 3–4 times/day.

Cholinergic Adjunct
IV (Adults and Children): 200 mcg for each 1 mg of neostigmine or 5 mg of pyridostigmine given at the same time.

Antiarrhythmic
IV (Adults): 100 mcg, may be repeated q 2–3 min.
IV (Children): 4.4 mcg/kg (up to 100 mcg); may be repeated q 2–3 min.

Peptic Ulcer
PO (Adults): 1–2 mg 2–3 times daily. An additional 2 mg may be given at bedtime; may be decreased to 1 mg twice daily (not to exceed 8 mg/day).
IM, IV (Adults): 100–200 mcg q 4 hr up to 4 times daily.

Availability (generic available)
Tablets: 1 mg, 2 mg. **Injection:** 200 mcg (0.2 mg)/mL.

NURSING IMPLICATIONS
Assessment
- Assess heart rate, blood pressure, and respiratory rate before and periodically during parenteral therapy.
- Pedi: Assess for hyperexcitability, a paradoxical response that may occur in children.
- Monitor intake and output ratios in geriatric or surgical patients; glycopyrrolate may cause uri-

nary retention. Instruct patient to void before parenteral administration.
- Assess patient routinely for abdominal distention and auscultate for bowel sounds. If constipation becomes a problem, increasing fluids and adding bulk to the diet may help alleviate the constipating effects of the drug.
- Periodic intraocular pressure determinations should be made for patients receiving long-term therapy.
- **Lab Test Considerations:** Antagonizes effects of pentagastrin and histamine during the gastric acid secretion test. Avoid administration for 24 hr preceding the test.
- May cause ↓ uric acid levels in patients with gout or hyperuricemia.
- **Toxicity and Overdose:** If overdosage occurs, neostigmine is the antidote.

Potential Nursing Diagnoses
Impaired oral mucous membrane (Side Effects)
Constipation (Side Effects)

Implementation
- Do not administer cloudy or discolored solution.
- **PO:** Administer 30–60 min before meals to maximize absorption.
- Do not administer within 1 hr of antacids or antidiarrheal medications.
- Oral dose is 10 times the parenteral dose.
- **IM:** May be administered undiluted (200 mcg/mL).

IV Administration
- **Direct IV:** *Diluent:* May be given undiluted through Y-site. *Concentration:* 200 mcg/mL. *Rate:* Administer at a maximum rate of 20 mcg over 1 min.
- **Syringe Compatibility:** chlorpromazine, cimetidine, codeine, diphenhydramine, droperidol, hydromorphone, hydroxyzine, levorphanol, lidocaine, meperidine, midazolam, morphine, nalbuphine, neostigmine, ondansetron, oxymorphone, prochlorperazine, promethazine, pyridostigmine, ranitidine, triflupromazine.
- **Syringe Incompatibility:** chloramphenicol, dexamethasone, diazepam, dimenhydrinate, methohexital, pentazocine, pentobarbital, secobarbital, sodium bicarbonate, thiopental.
- **Y-Site Compatibility:** propofol.
- **Solution Compatibility:** D5/0.45% NaCl, D5W, 0.9% NaCl, Ringer's solution. Administer immediately after admixing.
- **Additive Incompatibility:** methylprednisolone sodium succinate.

Patient/Family Teaching
- Instruct patient to take glycopyrrolate exactly as directed and not to take more than the prescribed amount. Take missed doses as soon as remembered if not just before next dose.
- Medication may cause drowsiness and blurred vision. Caution patient to avoid driving or other activities requiring alertness until response to the medication is known.
- Inform patient that frequent oral rinses, sugarless gum or candy, and good oral hygiene may help relieve dry mouth. Consult health care professional regarding use of saliva substitute if dry mouth persists for more than 2 wk.
- Advise patient to change positions slowly to minimize the effects of drug-induced orthostatic hypotension.
- Caution patient to avoid extremes of temperature. This medication decreases the ability to sweat and may increase the risk of heat stroke.
- Advise patient to notify health care professional immediately if eye pain or increased sensitivity to light occurs. Emphasize the importance of routine eye exams throughout therapy.
- Advise patient to consult health care professional before taking any OTC medications concurrently with this therapy.
- Geri: Advise geriatric patients about increased susceptibility to side effects and to call health care professional immediately if they occur.

Evaluation/Desired Outcomes
- Mouth dryness preoperatively.
- Reversal of cholinergic medications.
- Decrease in GI motility and pain in patients with peptic ulcer disease.

---

golimumab (go-li-mu-mab)
Simponi

Classification
Therapeutic: antirheumatics
Pharmacologic: DMARDs, monoclonal antibodies, anti-TNF agents

Pregnancy Category B

Indications
Treatment of moderately to severely active rheumatoid arthritis (with methotrexate). Treatment of active psoriatic arthritis (alone or with methotrexate). Treatment of active ankylosing spondylitis.

Action
Inhibits binding of TNFα to receptors inhibiting activity and resulting in anti-iflammatory and anti-proliferative activity. **Therapeutic Effects:** De-

creased pain and swelling with decreased joint destruction in patients with rheumatoid arthritis, psoriatic arthritis and ankylosing spondylitis.

Pharmacokinetics
Absorption: Well absorbed following subcutaneous administration.
Distribution: Distributed primarily in the circulatory system with limited extravascular distribution.
Metabolism and Excretion: Unknown.
Half-life: 2 wk.

TIME/ACTION PROFILE (improvement)

ROUTE	ONSET	PEAK	DURATION
Subcut	within 3 mo	2–7 days†	unknown

† Blood levels

Contraindications/Precautions
Contraindicated in: Active infection; Concurrent use of abatacept or anakinra (↑ risk of infections); Lactation: Avoid during breastfeeding.
Use Cautiously in: Past history of latent or active tuberculosis when adequate treatment cannot be confirmed; antitubercular therapy should be considered; Negative test for latent tuberculosis with risk factors for tuberculosis infection; consider treatment with antituberculars; History of CHF (may worsen); History of central nervous system demyelinating disorders (may worsen); History of psoriasis (may exacerbate); Hepatitis B virus carriers (risk of reactivation); Geri: Use cautiously in elderly patients due to ↑ risk of infection; OB: Use during pregnancy only if clearly needed; Pedi: Safety not established; ↑ risk of lymphoma, leukemia, and other malignancies.

Adverse Reactions/Side Effects
CNS: CENTRAL NERVOUS SYSTEM DEMYELINATING DISORDERS. **EENT:** nasopharyngitis. **Resp:** upper respiratory tract infection. **CV:** CONGESTIVE HEART FAILURE, hypertension. **GI:** ↑ liver enzymes. **Derm:** psoriasis. **Hemat:** aplastic anemia, leukopenia, neutropenia, pancytopenia, thrombocytopenia. **Local:** injection site reactions. **Neuro:** paresthesia. **Misc:** INFECTIONS (including reactivation tuberculosis, invasive fungal infections, and hepatitis B virus), ↑ RISK OF LYMPHOMA/MALIGNANCIES, fever.

Interactions
Drug-Drug: Abatacept, **anakinra**, **corticosteroids** or **methotrexate** ↑ risk of serious infections; concurrent use with anakinra or abatacept is not recommended. ↓ antibody response and ↑ risk of adverse reactions with **live virus vaccines**. May normalize previously suppressed levels of CYP450 enzymes, following initiation or discontinuation of golimumab, effects of substrates of this system may be altered and should be monitored, including **warfarin**, **theophylline**, and **cyclosporine**.

Route/Dosage
Subcut (Adults): 50 mg once monthly.

Availability
Solution for subcutaneous injection: 50 mg/0.5 mL in single-dose prefilled syringes and Smartject autoinjectors.

NURSING IMPLICATIONS
Assessment
- Assess pain and range of motion before and periodically during therapy.
- Assess for signs and symptoms of infection (fever, dyspnea, flu-like symptoms, frequent or painful urination, redness or swelling at the site of a wound) prior to, during, and after therapy. Discontinue therapy if serious or opportunistic infection or sepsis occurs. If new infection develops during therapy, assess patient and institute antimicrobial therapy. Patients who tested negative for latent tuberculosis (TB) prior to therapy may develop TB during therapy. Initiate treatment for latent TB prior to initiating therapy.
- Monitor carriers of HBV for signs of reactivation during and for several months after therapy. If reactivation occurs, discontinue golimumab and institute antiviral therapy.
- Monitor patients with CHF for new or worsening symptoms. Discontinue therapy if symptoms occur.
- Assess for exacerbations and new onset psoriasis. Discontinue therapy of these occur.
- Assess patient for latex allergy. Needle cover of syringe contains latex and should not be handled by persons sensitive to latex.
- Assess for signs and symptoms of systemic fungal infections (fever, malaise, weight loss, sweats, cough, dypsnea, pulmonary infiltrates, serious systemic illness with or without concomitant shock). Ascertain if patient lives in or has traveled to areas of endemic mycoses. Consider empiric antifungal treatment for patients at risk of histoplasmosis and other invasive fungal infections until the pathogens are identified. Consult with an infectious diseases specialist.

Consider stopping golimumab until the infection has been diagnosed and adequately treated.
- **Lab Test Considerations:** Monitor liver function tests periodically during therapy. May cause ↑ serum AST and ALT.
- Monitor CBC with differential periodically during therapy. May cause leukopenia, neutropenia, thrombocytopenia, and pancytopenia. Discontinue golimumab if symptoms of blood dyscrasias (persistent fever) occur.

Potential Nursing Diagnoses
Chronic pain (Indications)
Risk for infection (Adverse Reactions)

Implementation
- Administer a tuberculin skin test prior to administration of golimumab.
- Initial injection should be supervised by health care professional.
- Refrigerate solution; do not freeze. Allow prefilled syringe or auto-injector to sit at room temperature for 30 min prior to injection; do not warm in any other way. Do not shake. Solution is clear to slightly opalescent and colorless to light yellow. Do not administer solutions that are discolored, cloudy, or contain particulate matter. Discard unused solution.
- **Subcut:** Remove the needle cover or autoinjector cap just prior to injection. Inject into front of middle thigh, lower part of abdomen 2 inches from navel, or caregiver may administer into outer area of upper arm. Do not inject in areas where skin is tender, bruised, red, scaly, or hard; avoid scars or stretch marks. Press a cotton ball or gauze over injection site for 10 seconds; do not rub.
- *Autoinjector:* Press open end of autoinjector against skin at 90° angle. Use free hand to pinch and hold skin at injection site. Press button with fingers or thumb; button will stay pressed and does not need to be held. Injection will begin following a loud click. Keep holding the auto injector against skin until a second loud click is heard (usually 3–6 seconds, but may take up to 15 seconds). Lift autoinjector from skin following second click. Yellow indicator in viewing window indicates autoinjector worked correctly. If yellow does not appear in viewing window call 1-800-457-6399 for help.
- *Prefilled syringe:* Hold body of syringe between thumb and index finger. Do not pull back on plunger at any time. Pinch skin. Using a dart-like motion, insert needle into pinched skin at 45° angle. Inject all medication by pushing plunger until plunger head is between needle guard wings. Take needle out of skin and let go of skin. Slowly take thumb off plunger to allow empty syringe to move up until entire needle is covered by needle guard.

Patient/Family Teaching
- Instruct patient on correct technique for administration. Review patient information sheet, preparation of dose, administration sites and technique, and disposal of equipment into a puncture-resistant container. Advise patient of risks and benefits of golimumab therapy. Inject missed doses as soon as remembered, then return to regular schedule. Instruct patient to read *Medication Guide* before starting therapy and with each Rx refill; new information may be available.
- Caution patient not to share this medication with others, even with the same symptoms; may be harmful.
- Caution patient to notify health care professional if any signs of infection, including TB, invasive fungal infections (fever, malaise, weight loss, sweats, cough, dypsnea, pulmonary infiltrates, serious systemic illness with or without concomitant shock), or reactivation of HBV, develop.
- Advise patient to notify health care professional before taking other Rx, OTC, or herbal products.
- Inform patient to avoid receiving live vaccinations; other vaccinations may be given.
- Advise patient to notify health care professional of pregnancy is planned or suspected or if breastfeeding.

Evaluation/Desired Outcomes
- Decreased pain and swelling with decreased rate of joint destruction in patients with rheumatoid arthritis.
- Decreased signs and symptoms, slowed progression of joint destruction, and improved physical function in patients with psoriatic arthritis.
- Reduced signs and symptoms of ankylosing spondylitis.

goserelin (goe-se-rel-lin)
Zoladex

goserelin 641

Classification
Therapeutic: antineoplastics, hormones
Pharmacologic: gonadotropin-releasing hormones

Pregnancy Category D (breast cancer), X (endometriosis)

Indications
Prostate cancer in patients who cannot tolerate orchiectomy or estrogen therapy (palliative). With flutamide and radiation therapy in the treatment of locally confined stage T2b–T4 (stage B2–C) prostate cancer. Advanced breast cancer in peri- and postmenopausal women (palliative). Endometriosis. Produces thinning of the endometrium before endometrial ablation for dysfunctional uterine bleeding.

Action
Acts as a synthetic form of luteinizing hormone–releasing hormone (LHRH, GnRH). Inhibits the production of gonadotropins by the pituitary gland. Initially, levels of luteinizing hormone (LH), follicle-stimulating hormone (FSH), and testosterone increase. Continued administration leads to decreased production of testosterone and estradiol. **Therapeutic Effects:** Decreased spread of cancer of the prostate or breast. Regression of endometriosis with decreased pain. Thinning of the endometrium.

Pharmacokinetics
Absorption: Well absorbed from subcut implant. Absorption is slower in first 8 days, then is faster and continuous for remainder of 28-day dosing cycle.
Distribution: Unknown.
Metabolism and Excretion: Some metabolism by the liver (<10%), some excretion by kidneys (>90%, only 20% as unchanged drug).
Half-life: 4.2 hr.

TIME/ACTION PROFILE (↓ in serum testosterone levels)

ROUTE	ONSET	PEAK	DURATION
Subcut	unknown	2–4 wk	length of therapy

Contraindications/Precautions
Contraindicated in: Hypersensitivity; Undiagnosed vaginal bleeding; OB, Lactation: Pregnancy or lactation.
Use Cautiously in: Pedi: Safety not established.

Adverse Reactions/Side Effects
CNS: headache, anxiety, depression, dizziness, fatigue, insomnia, weakness. **Resp:** dyspnea. **CV:** CEREBROVASCULAR ACCIDENT, MYOCARDIAL INFARCTION, vasodilation, chest pain, hypertension, palpitations. **GI:** anorexia, constipation, diarrhea, nausea, ulcer, vomiting. **GU:** renal insufficiency, urinary obstruction. **Derm:** sweating, rash. **Endo:** ↓ libido, erectile dysfunction, breast swelling, breast tenderness, infertility, ovarian cysts, ovarian hyperstimulation syndrome (with gonadotropins). **F and E:** peripheral edema. **Hemat:** anemia. **Metab:** gout, hyperglycemia, ↑ lipids. **MS:** ↑ bone pain, arthralgia, ↓ bone density. **Misc:** hot flashes, chills, fever, weight gain.

Interactions
Drug-Drug: None significant.

Route/Dosage
Subcut (Adults): 3.6 mg every 4 wk or 10.8 mg q 12 wk. *Endometrial thinning*—1 or 2 depots given 4 wk apart; if 1 depot used, surgery is performed at 4 wk; if 2 depots used, surgery is performed 2–4 wk after 2nd depot.

Availability
Implant: 3.6 mg, 10.8 mg.

NURSING IMPLICATIONS

Assessment
- **Cancer:** Monitor patients with vertebral metastases for increased back pain and decreased sensory/motor function.
- Monitor intake and output ratios and assess for bladder distention in patients with urinary tract obstruction during initiation of therapy.
- **Endometriosis:** Assess patient for signs and symptoms of endometriosis before and periodically during therapy. Amenorrhea usually occurs within 8 wk of initial administration and menses usually resume 8 wk after completion.
- *Lab Test Considerations:* Initially ↑, then ↓ LH and FSH. This leads to castration levels of testosterone in men 2–4 wk after initial increase in concentrations.
- Monitor serum acid phosphatase and prostate-specific antigen concentrations periodically during therapy. May cause transient ↑ in serum acid phosphatase concentrations, which usually return to baseline by the 4th wk of therapy and may ↓ to below baseline or return to baseline if elevated before therapy.

♦ = Canadian drug name. ❖ = Genetic implication.
*CAPITALS indicates life-threatening; underlines indicate most frequent.

- May cause hypercalcemia in patients with breast or prostate cancer with bony metastases.
- May cause an ↑ in serum HDL, LDL, and triglycerides.

Potential Nursing Diagnoses
Sexual dysfunction (Side Effects)

Implementation
- **Subcut:** Implant is inserted in upper subcut tissue of upper abdominal wall every 28 days. Local anesthesia may be used before injection.
- If the implant needs to be removed for any reason, it can be located by ultrasound.

Patient/Family Teaching
- Advise patient that bone pain may increase at initiation of therapy. This will resolve with time. Patient should discuss use of analgesics to control pain with health care professional.
- Advise female patients to notify health care professional if regular menstruation persists.
- Inform diabetic patients of potential for hyperglycemia. Encourage close monitoring of serum glucose.
- Advise patient that medication may cause hot flashes. Notify health care professional if these become bothersome. Hormone replacement therapy may be added to decrease vasomotor symptoms and vaginal dryness without compromising beneficial effect.
- Instruct patient to notify health care professional promptly if difficulty urinating occurs.
- Advise premenopausal women to notify health care professional if pregnancy is planned or suspected of if breastfeeding. Effective contraception should be used during and for 12 wk after treatment ends.
- Emphasize the importance of adhering to the schedule of monthly or every-3-month administration.

Evaluation/Desired Outcomes
- Decrease in the spread of prostate cancer.
- Reduction of symptoms of advanced breast cancer in peri- and postmenopausal women.
- Decrease in the signs and symptoms of endometriosis. Symptoms are usually reduced within 4 wk of implantation.
- Thinning of the endometrium before endometrial ablation for dysfunctional uterine bleeding.

---

granisetron (oral and IV)
(gra-**nees**-e-tron)
Kytril

granisetron (transdermal)

Sancuso

Classification
Therapeutic: antiemetics
Pharmacologic: 5-HT$_3$ antagonists

Pregnancy Category B

Indications
PO: Prevention of nausea and vomiting due to emetogenic chemotherapy or radiation therapy. Prevention and treatment of postoperative nausea and vomiting. **Transdermal:** Prevention of nausea and vomiting due to moderately/highly emetogenic chemotherapy.

Action
Blocks the effects of serotonin at receptor sites (selective antagonist) located in vagal nerve terminals and in the chemoreceptor trigger zone in the CNS. **Therapeutic Effects:** Decreased incidence and severity of nausea and vomiting following emetogenic chemotherapy, radiation therapy or surgery.

Pharmacokinetics
Absorption: 50% absorbed following oral administration; transdermal enters systemic circulation via passive diffusion through intact skin.
Distribution: Distributes into erythrocytes; remainder of distribution is unknown.
Metabolism and Excretion: Mostly metabolized by the liver; 12% excreted unchanged in urine.
Half-life: *Patients with cancer*—8–9 hr (range 0.9–31.1 hr); *healthy volunteers*—4.9 hr (range 0.9–15.2 hr); *geriatric patients*—7.7 hr (range 2.6–17.7 hr).

TIME/ACTION PROFILE

ROUTE	ONSET	PEAK	DURATION
PO	rapid	60 min	24 hr
IV	rapid	30 min	up to 24 hr
TD*	unknown	48 hr	unknown

* Blood levels

Contraindications/Precautions
Contraindicated in: Hypersensitivity; Some products contain benzyl alcohol; avoid use in neonates.
Use Cautiously in: OB, Lactation: Safety not established; Pedi: Safe use of IV route not established in children <2 yr ; safe use of PO or transdermal route not established in children <18 yr.

Adverse Reactions/Side Effects
CNS: headache, agitation, anxiety, CNS stimulation, drowsiness, weakness. **CV:** hypertension. **GI:** constipation, diarrhea, elevated liver enzymes,

taste disorder. **Derm:** *Topical*—application site reactions, photosensitivity. **Misc:** anaphylactoid reactions, fever.

Interactions
Drug-Drug: ↑ risk of extrapyramidal reactions with other **agents causing extrapyramidal reactions**.

Route/Dosage

Prevention of Nausea and Vomiting Due to Emetogenic Chemotherapy
PO (Adults): 1 mg twice daily; 1st dose given at least 60 min prior to chemotherapy and 2nd dose 12 hr later only on days when chemotherapy is administered; may also be given as 2 mg once daily at least 60 min prior to chemotherapy.
IV (Adults and Children 2–16 yr): 10 mcg/kg within 30 min prior to chemotherapy.
Transdermal (Adults): One 34.3 mg patch (delivers 3.1 mg/24 hr) applied up to 48 hr prior to chemotherapy, leave in place for at least 24 hr following chemotherapy, may be left in place for a total of 7 days.

Prevention of Nausea and Vomiting Associated with Radiation Therapy
PO (Adults): 2 mg taken once daily within 1 hr of radiation therapy.

Prevention and Treatment of Postoperative Nausea and Vomiting
IV (Adults): *Prevention*—1 mg prior to induction of anesthesia or just prior to reversal of anesthesia; *Treatment*—1 mg.

Availability (generic available)
Tablets: 1 mg. **Cost:** $131.99/2. **Oral solution (orange flavor):** 2 mg/10 mL in 30-mL bottles. **Solution for injection:** 1 mg/mL. **Transdermal patch:** Each patch contains 34.3 mg/52 cm^2 (delivers 3.1 mg/24 hr).

NURSING IMPLICATIONS

Assessment
- Assess patient for nausea, vomiting, abdominal distention, and bowel sounds prior to and following administration.
- Assess for extrapyramidal symptoms (involuntary movements, facial grimacing, rigidity, shuffling walk, trembling of hands) during therapy. This occurs rarely and is usually associated with concurrent use of other drugs known to cause this effect.
- **Transdermal:** Monitor application site. If allergic, erythematous, macular, or papular rash or pruritus occurs, remove patch.
- *Lab Test Considerations:* May cause ↑ AST and ALT levels.

Potential Nursing Diagnoses
Imbalanced nutrition: less than body requirements (Indications)

Implementation
- For chemotherapy or radiation, granisetron is administered only on the day(s) chemotherapy or radiation is given. Continued treatment when not on chemotherapy or radiation therapy has not been found to be useful.
- **PO:** Administer 1st dose up to 1 hr before chemotherapy or radiation therapy and 2nd dose 12 hr after the first.
- 2 tsp oral solution are equal to 2 mg granisetron.

IV Administration
- **Direct IV:** *Diluent:* May be administered undiluted or diluted in 20–50 mL of 0.9% NaCl or D5W. Solution should be prepared at time of administration but is stable for 24 hr at room temperature. *Concentration:* Up to 1 mg/mL. *Rate:* Administer undiluted granisetron over 30 sec or as a diluted solution over 5 min.
- **Syringe Compatibility:** dexamethasone, methylprednisolone.
- **Y-Site Compatibility:** acyclovir, alfentanil, allopurinol, amifostine, amikacin, aminophylline, amiodarone, amphotericin B cholesteryl, amphotericin B liposome, ampicillin, ampicillin-sulbactam, amsacrine, atracurium, aztreonam, bleomycin, bumetanide, buprenorphine, busulfan, butorphanol, calcium acetate, calcium chloride, calcium gluconate, carboplatin, carmustine, caspofungin, cefazolin, cefepime, cefoperazone, cefotaxime, cefotetan, cefoxitin, ceftazidime, ceftizoxime, ceftriaxone, cefuroxime, chloramphenicol, chlorpromazine, cimetidine, ciprofloxacin, cisatracurium, cisplatin, cladribine, clindamycin, cyclophosphamide, cyclosporine, cytarabine, dacarbazine, dactinomycin, daunorubicin, dexamethasone, dexmedetomidine, dexrazoxane, digoxin, diltiazem, diphenhydramine, dobutamine, docetaxel, dopamine, doripenem, doxacurium, doxorubicin hydrochloride, doxorubicin liposome, doxycycline, droperidol, enalaprilat, ephedrine, epinephrine, epirubicin, ertape-

nem, erythromycin, esmolol, etoposide, etoposide phosphate, famotidine, fenoldopam, fentanyl, filgrastim, floxuridine, fluconazole, fludarabine, fluorouracil, foscarnet, fosphenytoin, furosemide, ganciclovir, gemcitabine, gentamicin, glycopyrrolate, haloperidol, heparin, hetastarch, hydrocortisone, hydromorphone, idarubicin, ifosfamide, imipenem/cilastatin, inamrinone, insulin, isoproterenol, ketorolac, labetalol, leucovorin, levofloxacin, lidocaine, linezolid, lorazepam, magnesium sulfate, mannitol, mechlorethamine, melphalan, meperidine, meropenem, mesna, metaraminol, methotrexate, methyldopate, methylprednisolone, metoclopramide, metoprolol, metronidazole, midazolam, milrinone, mitomycin, mitoxantrone, morphine, nafcillin, nalbuphine, naloxone, nesiritide, nitroglycerin, nitroprusside, norepinephrine, octreotide, oxaliplatin, oxytocin, paclitaxel, pancuronium, pantoprazole, pemetrexed, pentamidine, pentazocine, pentobarbital, phenobarbital, phentolamine, phenylephrine, piperacillin-tazobactam, plicamycin, potassium chloride, potassium phosphates, procainamide, prochlorperazine, promethazine, propofol, propranolol, quinupristin/dalfopristin, ranitidine, remifentanil, rituximab, rocuronium, sargramostim, sodium acetate, sodium bicarbonate, sodium phosphates, streptozocin, succinylcholine, sufentanil, tacrolimus, teniposide, theophylline, thiopental, thiotepa, ticarcillin/clavulanate, tigecycline, tirofiban, tobramycin, topotecan, trastuzumab, trimethobenzamide, trimethoprim/sulfamethoxazole, vancomycin, vasopressin, vecuronium, verapamil, vinblastine, vincristine, vinorelbine, voriconazole, zidovudine.

- **Y-Site Incompatibility:** amphotericin B colloidal, dantrolene, diazepam, phenytoin.
- **Additive Incompatibility:** Granisetron should not be admixed with other medications.
- **Transdermal:** Apply system clear, dry, intact healthy skin on upper outer arm 24–48 hr before chemotherapy. Do not use creams, lotions, or oils that may keep patch from sticking. Do not apply to skin that is red, irritated, or damaged. Apply immediately after removing from package. Do not cut patch into pieces. Remove liner from adhesive layer and press firmly in place with palm of hand for 30 sec, especially around the edges, to make sure contact is complete. Patch should be worn throughout chemotherapy. If patch does not stick, bandages or medical adhesive tape may be applied on edges of patch; do not cover patch with tape or bandages or wrap completely around arm. Patient may shower and wash normally while wearing patch; avoid swimming, strenuous exercise, sauna, or whirlpool during patch use. Remove patch gently at least 24 hr after completion of chemotherapy; may be worn for up to 7 days. Fold so that adhesive edges are together. Throw away in garbage out of reach of children and pets on removal. Do not re-use patch. Use soap and water to remove remaining adhesive; do not use alcohol or acetone.

Patient/Family Teaching

- Instruct patient to take granisetron as directed.
- Advise patient to notify health care professional immediately if involuntary movement of eyes, face, or limbs occurs.
- May cause dizziness and drowsiness. Caution patient to avoid driving and other activities requiring alertness until response to medication is known.
- Advise patient to consult health care professional prior to taking any other Rx, OTC, or herbal products.
- Advise female patient to notify health care professional if pregnancy is planned or suspected or if breastfeeding.
- **Transdermal:** Instruct patient on correct application, removal, and disposal of patch. Advise patient to read *Patient Information* sheet prior to using and with each Rx refill in case of new information. Inform patient that additional granisetron should not be taken during patch application unless directed by health care professional.
- Advise patient referred for MRI test to discuss patch with referring health care professional and MRI facility to determine if removal of patch is necessary prior to test and for directions for replacing patch.
- Advise patient to cover patch application site with clothing to avoid exposure to sunlight, sunlamp, or tanning beds during and for 10 days following removal of patch.
- Instruct patient to notify health care professional if pain or swelling in the abdomen occurs or if redness at patch removal site remains for more than 3 days.

Evaluation/Desired Outcomes

- Prevention of nausea and vomiting associated with emetogenic cancer chemotherapy or radiation therapy.
- Prevention and treatment of postoperative nausea and vomiting.

GROWTH HORMONES

somatropin (recombinant)
(soe-ma-**troe**-pin)
Genotropin, Humatrope, Nordiflex, Norditropin, Nutropin, Nutropin AQ, Omnitrope, Saizen, Serostim, Serostim LQ, Tev-Tropin, Zorbtive

Classification
Therapeutic: hormones
Pharmacologic: growth hormones

Pregnancy Category B (Omnitrope, Serostim, and Zorbtive), C (all others)

Indications
Growth failure in children due to chronic renal insufficiency. Growth failure in children due to deficiency of growth hormone. Short stature associated with Turner's syndrome. Short stature associated with or Noonan's syndrome (Norditropin only). Children with short stature born small for gestational age with no catch-up growth by age 2–4 yr (Norditropin only). Growth hormone deficiency in adults (Humatrope, Nutropin, Norditropin, Omnitrope). Idiopathic short stature syndrome (Genotropin, Humatrope, Nutropin, Nutropin AQ). AIDS wasting or cachexia (Serostim only). Increases spinal bone density in childhood–onset growth hormone–deficient patients (somatropin). As part of a comprehensive treatment program for Short Bowel Syndrome (Zorbtive).

Action
Produce growth (skeletal and cellular). Metabolic actions include: Increased protein synthesis, Increased carbohydrate metabolism, Lipid mobilization, Retention of sodium, phosphorus, and potassium. Somatropin has the same amino acid sequence as naturally occurring growth hormone; somatrem has 1 additional amino acid. Both are produced by recombinant DNA techniques. Growth hormone enhances GI tract mucosal transport of water, electrolytes, and nutrients.
Therapeutic Effects: Increased skeletal growth in children with growth hormone deficiency. Replacement of somatropin in deficient adults. Decreased wasting in patients with AIDS. Increased bone density in adult growth hormone–deficient patients. Enhanced GI absorption of water, electrolytes and nutrients in short bowel syndrome.

Pharmacokinetics
Absorption: Well absorbed.
Distribution: Localize to highly perfused organs (liver, kidneys).
Metabolism and Excretion: Broken down in renal cells to amino acids that are recirculated; some liver metabolism.
Half-life: *Subcut*—3.8 hr; *IM*—4.9 hr.

TIME/ACTION PROFILE (growth)

ROUTE	ONSET	PEAK	DURATION
IM, subcut	within 3 mo	unknown	12–48 hr

Contraindications/Precautions
Contraindicated in: Closure of epiphyses; Active neoplasia; Hypersensitivity to growth hormone, *m*-cresol or glycerin (somatropin) or benzyl alcohol (Zorbtive); Acute critical illness (therapy should not be initiated) or respiratory failure; Diabetic retinopathy; Prader-Willi syndrome with obesity and respiratory impairment (risk of fatal complications; can be used only if growth hormone deficiency is documented); OB: Use only if clearly needed.
Use Cautiously in: Growth hormone deficiency due to intracranial lesion; Coexisting adrenocorticotropic hormone (ACTH) deficiency; Diabetes (may cause insulin resistance); Thyroid dysfunction; Lactation: Safety not established; Geri: ↑ sensitivity, ↑ risk of adverse reactions; use lower starting dose and smaller dose increments.

Adverse Reactions/Side Effects
CV: edema of the hands and feet. **Endo:** hyperglycemia, hypothyroidism, insulin resistance. **Local:** pain at injection site. **MS:** arthralgia; *Serostim only*, carpal tunnel syndrome, musculoskeletal pain.

Interactions
Drug-Drug: Excessive **corticosteroid** use (equivalent to 10–15 mg/m^2/day) may ↓ response to somatropin.

Route/Dosage

Somatrem (Protropin)
IM, Subcut (Children): Up to 0.3 mg (0.9 unit)/kg weekly; subcut route is preferred.

Somatropin (Genotropin)
Subcut (Children): 0.16–0.48 mg/kg/wk divided in 6–7 daily doses.
Subcut (Adults): 0.04–0.8 mg/kg/wk divided in 6–7 daily doses.

Somatropin (Humatrope)
Subcut (Adults): 0.018 unit/kg/day (up to 0.0375 unit/kg/day).
IM, Subcut (Children): 0.18 mg/kg (0.54 unit/kg)/wk given in divided doses on 3 alternating days or 6 times weekly (up to 0.3 mg/kg or 0.9 unit/kg/wk).

Somatropin (Nutropin/Nutropin AQ)
Subcut (Children): *Growth hormone inadequacy*—0.3 mg/kg. *Chronic renal insufficiency*—0.35 mg/kg (1.05 units/kg)/wk given as daily injections. *Turner's syndrome*—≤0.375 mg/kg (1.125 units/kg)/wk in 3–7 divided doses.
Subcut (Adults): <0.006 mg/kg daily; may be ↑ to 0.025 mg/kg/day in patients <35 yrs or 0.0125 mg/kg in patients >35 yrs.

Somatropin (Norditropin)
Subcut (Adults): 0.004 mg/kg/day, may be increased to 0.016 mg/kg/day after 6 wk or 0.2 mg/day starting dose (without consideration of body weight) then gradually increase by 0.1–0.2 mg/day q 1–2 months until clinical response achieved.
Subcut (Children): *Growth hormone inadequacy*—0.024–0.034 mg/kg 6–7 times weekly; *Short stature associated with Noonan's syndrome*—Up to 0.066 mg/kg/day; *Short stature associated with Turner's syndrome or short stature born small for gestational age*-Up to 0.067 mg/kg/day.

Somatropin (Omnitrope)
Subcut (Adults): 0.04 mg/kg/wk given in 7 divided doses; may be ↑ at 4–8 wk intervals (up to 0.08 mg/kg/wk).
Subcut (Children): 0.16–0.24 mg/kg/wk given in 6–7 divided doses.

Somatropin (Saizen)
Subcut, IM (Children): 0.06 mg (0.18 unit/kg) 3 times weekly.

Somatropin (Serostim)
Subcut (Adults): *>55 kg*—6 mg once daily; *45–55 kg*—5 mg once daily; *35–45 kg*—4 mg once daily; *<35 kg*—0.1 mg/kg once daily.

Somatropin (Tev-Tropin)
Subcut (Children): up to 0.1 mg/kg 3 times weekly.

Somatropin (Zorbtive)
Subcut (Adults): 0.1 mg/kg/day for 4 wk (not to exceed 8 mg/dose), dose may be stopped for 5 days and resumed at half dose for fluid retention or arthalgias.

Availability
Genotropin
Powder for injection: 1.5-mg intra-mix cartridge (delivers 1.3 mg), 5.8-mg intra-mix cartridge (delivers 5 mg), 5.8-mg intra-mix cartridge (delivers 5 mg) as Pen 5 system, 13.8-mg intra-mix cartridge (delivers 12 mg), 13.8-mg intra-mix cartridge (delivers 12 mg) as Pen 12 system, MiniQuick system 0.2 mg, MiniQuick system 0.4 mg, MiniQuick system 0.6 mg, MiniQuick system 0.8 mg, MiniQuick system 1 mg, MiniQuick system 1.4 mg, MiniQuick system 1.6 mg, MiniQuick system 1.8 mg, MiniQuick system 2 mg.

Humatrope
Powder for injection: 5-mg/vial.

Norditropin
Cartridges for injection (using Nordipen): 5 mg/1.5 mL (orange), 15 mg/1.5 mL (green).
Prefilled pens for injection (Nordiflex): 5 mg/1.5 mL (orange), 10 mg/1.5 mL (blue), 15 mg/1.5 mL (green).

Nutropin
Powder for injection: 5-mg (13 units)/vial, 10-mg (26 units)/vial.

Nutropin AQ
Solution for injection (AQ): 5 mg (15 units)/mL in 2-mL vial.

Omnitrope
Powder for injection: 1.5 mg/vial, 5.8 mg/vial.
Cartridges for injection (using Omnitrope Pen 5 or 10): 5 mg/1.5 mL, 10 mg/1.5 mL.

Saizen
Powder for injection: 5-mg (15 units)/vial, 8.8-mg (26.4 units)/vial.

Serostim
Powder for injection: 6-mg (15 units)/vial.
Liquid for injection: 6–mg/0.5 mL cartridge.

Tev-Tropin
Powder for injection: 5-mg (15 units)/vial.

Zorbtive
Powder for injection: 4-, 5- or 6-mg vials, 8.8-mg multidose vials.

NURSING IMPLICATIONS
Assessment
- Assess for fluid retention (edema, arthralgia, carpal tunnel syndrome) especially in adults. May occur frequently; reduce dose as necessary.

- **Growth Failure:** Monitor bone age annually and growth rate determinations, height, and weight every 3–6 mo during therapy.
- **AIDS Wasting/Cachexia:** Re-evaluate treatment in patients who continue to lose weight in first 2 wk of treatment.
- **Lab Test Considerations:** Monitoring serum insulin-like growth factor I (IGF-I) levels may be useful during dose titration.
- Monitor thyroid function prior to and during therapy. May ↓ T^4, radioactive iodine uptake, and thyroxine-binding capacity. Hypothyroidism necessitates concurrent thyroid replacement for growth hormone to be effective. Serum inorganic phosphorus, alkaline phosphatase, and parathyroid hormone may ↑ with somatropin therapy.
- Monitor blood glucose periodically during therapy. Diabetic patients may require ↑ insulin dose.
- Monitor for development of neutralizing antibodies if growth rate does not exceed 2.5 cm/6 mo.
- Monitor alkaline phosphatase closely in patients with adult growth hormone deficiency.

Potential Nursing Diagnoses
Disturbed body image (Indications)

Implementation
- Rotate injection sites with each injection.
- **Somatropin:** Reconstitute 5-mg vial with 1.5–5 mL of sterile water for injection provided by manufacturer (contains preservative *m*-cresol), aiming the liquid against glass vial wall. Do not shake; swirl gently to dissolve. Solution is clear; do not use solutions that are cloudy or contain a precipitate. Stable for 14 days when refrigerated; do not freeze.
- *Genotropin intra-mix:* Dissolve powder with solution provided with 2-chamber cartridge as directed. Gently tip cartridge upside down a few times until contents are completely dissolved. The 1.5-mg cartridge is stable following dilution for 24 hr if refrigerated. The 5.8-mg and 13.8-mg cartridges contain preservatives and are stable for 14 days if refrigerated.
- *Genotropin Pen:* Prepare and administer as directed in patient instruction insert. Store in the refrigerator.
- *Genotropin MiniQuick:* For single use only. Inject immediately after reconstitution; may be refrigerated for 24 hr after reconstitution. Follow directions on patient package insert for reconstitution and administration.
- *Humatrope:* Reconstitute each 5-mg vial with 1.5–5 mL of diluent provided. Stable for 14 days if refrigerated.
- *Norditropin:* Reconstitute each 4-mg or 8-mg vial with 2 mL of diluent. Use reconstituted vials within 14 days. If using cartridges for the *Nordipen*, each cartridge has a corresponding color-coded pen which is graduated to deliver the appropriate dose based on the concentration of norditropin in the cartridge. Color coding of cartridge and pen must match. *Nordiflex* prefilled pens contain multiple doses. After initial injection, use within 4 weeks if stored in refrigerator or within 3 weeks if stored at room temperature.
- *Nutropin/Nutropin AQ:* Reconstitute 5-mg vial with 1–5 mL and 10-mg vial with 1–10 mL of bacteriostatic water for injection. Reconstituted vials are stable for 14 days (Nutropin) or 28 days (Nutropin AQ) if refrigerated.
- *Omnitrope Pen:* Insert cartridge into corresponding *Omnitrope Pen 5 delivery system*. Follow instructions in booklet provided by manufacturer. Solution is light sensitive; store in carton in refrigerator for up to 21 days.
- *Omnitrope vials:* Reconstitute with provided Sterile Water for Injection diluent. Do not shake. Do not administer solutions that are cloudy or contain a precipitate. 1.5 mg vial may be stored in refrigerator for 24 hr after reconstitution. 5.8 mg vial may be stored in carton in refrigerator up to 3 wk.
- *Saizen:* Reconstitute each 5-mg vial with 1–3 mL of bacteriostatic water for injection. Reconstituted vials are stable for 14 days if refrigerated. To use cool.click needle-free injector, wind the device to energize the spring, and draw medication into the Crystal Check nozzle. Using firm pressure at the injection site, hold the injector at a 90° angle and press the blue actuator button.
- *Serostim:* Reconstitute each vial with 1 mL of sterile water for injection. Use within 24 hr of reconstitution.
- *Tev-tropin:* Reconstitute with 1–5 mL or 0.9% NaCl. May be cloudy if refrigerated. Allow to warm to room temperature. If remains solution cloudy or contains particulate matter, do not use.
- *Zorbtive:* Reconstitute each 4-, 5-, or 6-mg vial with 0.5–1 mL of sterile water for injection and

each 8.8-mg vial with 1 or 2 mL bacteriostatic water for injection. Solution should be clear upon reconstitution. Do not administer if cloudy upon reconstitution (4-, 5-, or 6-mg vials) or after refrigeration (8.8-mg vial). After refrigeration may contain small particles which should disappear when allowed to warm to room temperature. Solution reconstituted with bacteriostatic water is stable for 14 days if refrigerated.
- **Subcut:** Injection volume for *somatropin* should not exceed 1 mL.

Patient/Family Teaching
- Instruct patient and parents on correct procedure for reconstituting medication, site selection, technique for IM or subcut injection, and disposal of needles and syringes. Review dose schedule. Parents should report persistent pain or edema at injection site.
- Explain rationale for prohibition of use for increasing athletic performance. Administration to persons without growth hormone deficiency or after epiphyseal closure may result in acromegaly (coarsening of facial features; enlarged hands, feet, and internal organs; increased blood glucose; hypertension).
- Emphasize need for regular follow-up with endocrinologist to ensure appropriate growth rate, to evaluate lab work, and to determine bone age by x-ray exam.
- Assure parents and child that these dose forms are synthetic and therefore not capable of transmitting Creutzfeldt-Jakob disease, as was the original somatropin, which was extracted from human cadavers.

Evaluation/Desired Outcomes
- Child's attainment of adult height in growth failure secondary to pituitary growth hormone deficiency. Therapy is limited to period before closure of epiphyseal plates (approximately up to 14–15 yr in girls, 15–16 yr in boys). Failure to increase growth rate, particularly during the first year of therapy, indicates the need for close assessment of compliance and evaluation for other causes of growth failure (hypothyroidism, undernutrition, advanced bone age, antibodies to recombinant human GH).
- Replacement of somatropin in deficient adults.
- Decreased wasting in patients with AIDS.
- Enhanced GI absorption of water, electrolytes and nutrients in short bowel syndrome.

---

guaifenesin (gwye-fen-e-sin)
Alfen Jr, Altarussin, ✤Benylin-E, Breonesin, ✤Calmylin Expectorant, Diabetic Tussin, Ganidin NR, Guiatuss, Hytuss, Hytuss-2X, Mucinex, Naldecon Senior EX, Organidin NR, ✤Resyl, Robitussin, Scot-tussin Expectorant, Siltussin SA, Siltussin DAS

Classification
Therapeutic: allergy, cold, and cough remedies, expectorant

Pregnancy Category C

Indications
Coughs associated with viral upper respiratory tract infections.

Action
Reduces viscosity of tenacious secretions by increasing respiratory tract fluid. **Therapeutic Effects:** Mobilization and subsequent expectoration of mucus.

Pharmacokinetics
Absorption: Well absorbed after oral administration.
Distribution: Unknown.
Metabolism and Excretion: Renally excreted as metabolites.
Half-life: Unknown.

TIME/ACTION PROFILE (expectorant action)

ROUTE	ONSET	PEAK	DURATION
PO	30 min	unknown	4–6 hr
PO-ER	unknown	unknown	12 hr

Contraindications/Precautions
Contraindicated in: Hypersensitivity; Some products contain alcohol; avoid in patients with known intolerance; Some products contain aspartame and should be avoided in patients with phenylketonuria.
Use Cautiously in: Cough lasting >1 wk or accompanied by fever, rash, or headache; Patients receiving disulfiram (liquid products may contain alcohol); Diabetic patients (some products may contain sugar); OB: Although safety has not been established, guaifenesin has been used without adverse effects; Pedi: OTC cough and cold products containing this medication should be avoided in children <4 yr.

Adverse Reactions/Side Effects
CNS: dizziness, headache. **GI:** nausea, diarrhea, stomach pain, vomiting. **Derm:** rashes, urticaria.

Interactions
Drug-Drug: None significant.

guaifenesin

Route/Dosage
PO (Adults): 200–400 mg q 4 hr or 600–1200 mg q 12 hr as extended-release product (not to exceed 2400 mg/day).
PO (Children 6–12 yr): 100–200 mg q 4 hr or 600 mg q 12 hr as extended-release product (not to exceed 1200 mg/day).
PO (Children 4–6 yr): 50–100 mg q 4 hr (not to exceed 600 mg/day).

Availability (generic available)
Syrup: 100 mg/5 mL^OTC. **Oral solution:** 100 mg/5 mL^{Rx, OTC}, 200 mg/5 mL^OTC. **Capsules:** 200 mg^OTC. **Tablets:** 100 mg^OTC, 200 mg^{Rx, OTC}, 1200 mg. **Extended-release tablets (Mucinex):** 600 mg, 1200 mg. *In combination with:* analgesics/antipyretics, antihistamines, decongestants, and cough suppressants^{Rx, OTC}.

NURSING IMPLICATIONS

Assessment
- Assess lung sounds, frequency and type of cough, and character of bronchial secretions periodically during therapy. Maintain fluid intake of 1500–2000 mL/day to decrease viscosity of secretions.

Potential Nursing Diagnoses
Ineffective airway clearance (Indications)

Implementation
- **PO:** Administer each dose of guaifenesin followed by a full glass of water to decrease viscosity of secretions.
- Extended-release tablets should be swallowed whole; do not open, break, crush, or chew.

Patient/Family Teaching
- Instruct patient to cough effectively. Patient should sit upright and take several deep breaths before attempting to cough.
- Caution parents to avoid OTC cough and cold products while breastfeeding or to children <4 yrs.
- Inform patient that drug may occasionally cause dizziness. Avoid driving or other activities requiring alertness until response to drug is known.
- Advise patient to limit talking, stop smoking, maintain moisture in environmental air, and take some sugarless gum or hard candy to help alleviate the discomfort caused by a chronic nonproductive cough.
- Instruct patient to contact health care professional if cough persists longer than 1 wk or is accompanied by fever, rash, or persistent headache or sore throat.

Evaluation/Desired Outcomes
- Easier mobilization and expectoration of mucus from cough associated with upper respiratory infection.

halcinonide, See **CORTICOSTEROIDS (TOPICAL/LOCAL).**

halobetasol, See **CORTICOSTEROIDS (TOPICAL/LOCAL).**

haloperidol (ha-loe-per-i-dole)
✱ Apo-Haloperidol, Haldol, Haldol Decanoate, ✱ Haldol LA, ✱ Novo-Peridol, ✱ Peridol, ✱ PMS Haloperidol

Classification
Therapeutic: antipsychotics
Pharmacologic: butyrophenones

Pregnancy Category C

Indications
Acute and chronic psychotic disorders including: schizophrenia, manic states, drug-induced psychoses. Schizophrenic patients who require long-term parenteral (IM) antipsychotic therapy. Also useful in managing aggressive or agitated patients. Tourette's syndrome. Severe behavioral problems in children which may be accompanied by: unprovoked, combative, explosive hyperexcitability, hyperactivity accompanied by conduct disorders (short-term use when other modalities have failed). Considered second-line treatment after failure with atypical antipsychotic. **Unlabeled Use:** Nausea and vomiting from surgery or chemotherapy.

Action
Alters the effects of dopamine in the CNS. Also has anticholinergic and alpha-adrenergic blocking activity. **Therapeutic Effects:** Diminished signs and symptoms of psychoses. Improved behavior in children with Tourette's syndrome or other behavioral problems.

Pharmacokinetics
Absorption: Well absorbed following PO/IM administration. Decanoate salt is slowly absorbed and has a long duration of action.
Distribution: Concentrates in liver. Crosses placenta; enters breast milk.
Protein Binding: 90%.
Metabolism and Excretion: Mostly metabolized by the liver.
Half-life: 21–24 hr.

TIME/ACTION PROFILE (antipsychotic activity)

ROUTE	ONSET	PEAK	DURATION
PO	2 hr	2–6 hr	8–12 hr
IM	20–30 min	30–45 min	4–8 hr†
IM (decanoate)	3–9 days	unknown	1 mo

†Effect may persist for several days

Contraindications/Precautions
Contraindicated in: Hypersensitivity; Angle-closure glaucoma; Bone marrow depression; CNS depression; Severe liver or cardiovascular disease (QT interval prolonging conditions); Some products contain tartrazine, sesame oil, or benzyl alcohol and should be avoided in patients with known intolerance or hypersensitivity.
Use Cautiously in: Debilitated patients (dose ↓ required); Cardiac disease; Diabetes; Respiratory insufficiency; Prostatic hyperplasia; CNS tumors; Intestinal obstruction; Seizures; OB: Safety not established; Lactation: Discontinue drug or bottle-feed; Geri: Dose ↓ required due to ↑ sensitivity; ↑ risk of mortality in elderly patients treated for dementia-related psychosis.

Adverse Reactions/Side Effects
CNS: SEIZURES, extrapyramidal reactions, confusion, drowsiness, restlessness, tardive dyskinesia. **EENT:** blurred vision, dry eyes. **Resp:** respiratory depression. **CV:** hypotension, tachycardia. **GI:** constipation, dry mouth, anorexia, drug-induced hepatitis, ileus, weight gain. **GU:** impotence, urinary retention. **Derm:** diaphoresis, photosensitivity, rashes. **Endo:** amenorrhea, galactorrhea, gynecomastia. **Hemat:** AGRANULOCYTOSIS, anemia, leukopenia, neutropenia. **Metab:** hyperpyrexia. **Misc:** NEUROLEPTIC MALIGNANT SYNDROME, hypersensitivity reactions.

Interactions
Drug-Drug: ↑ hypotension with **antihypertensives**, **nitrates**, or acute ingestion of **alcohol**. ↑ anticholinergic effects with **drugs having anticholinergic properties**, including **antihistamines**, **antidepressants**, **atropine**, **phenothiazines**, **quinidine**, and **disopyramide**. ↑ CNS depression with other **CNS depressants**, including **alcohol**, **antihistamines**, **opioid analgesics**, and **sedative/hypnotics**. Concurrent use with **epinephrine** may result in severe hypotension and tachycardia. May ↓ therapeutic effects of **levodopa**. Acute encephalopathic syndrome may occur when used with **lithium**. Dementia may occur with **methyldopa**.

652 haloperidol

Drug-Natural Products: Kava-kava, **valerian**, or **chamomile** can ↑ CNS depression.

Route/Dosage
Haloperidol
PO (Adults): 0.5–5 mg 2–3 times daily. Patients with severe symptoms may require up to 100 mg/day.
PO (Geriatric Patients or Debilitated Patients): 0.5–2 mg twice daily initially; may be gradually ↑ as needed.
PO (Children 3–12 yr or 15–40 kg): 50 mcg/kg/day in 2–3 divided doses; may ↑ by 500 mcg (0.5 mg)/day q 5–7 days as needed (up to 75 mcg/kg/day for nonpsychotic disorders or Tourette's syndrome or 150 mcg/kg/day for psychoses).
IM (Adults): 2–5 mg q 1–8 hr (not to exceed 100 mg/day).
IV (Adults): 0.5–5 mg, may be repeated q 30 min (unlabeled).

Haloperidol Decanoate
IM (Adults): 10–15 times the previous daily PO dose but not to exceed 100 mg initially, given monthly (not to exceed 300 mg/mo).

Availability (generic available)
Tablets: 0.5 mg, 1 mg, 2 mg, 5 mg, 10 mg, 20 mg. **Oral concentrate:** 2 mg/mL. **Haloperidol injection:** 5 mg/mL. **Haloperidol decanoate injection:** 50 mg/mL, 100 mg/mL.

NURSING IMPLICATIONS
Assessment
- Assess mental status (orientation, mood, behavior) prior to and periodically during therapy.
- Assess positive (hallucination, delusions) and negative (social isolation) symptoms of schizophrenia.
- Monitor blood pressure (sitting, standing, lying) and pulse prior to and frequently during the period of dose adjustment. May cause QT interval changes on ECG.
- Observe patient carefully when administering medication, to ensure that medication is actually taken and not hoarded.
- Monitor intake and output ratios and daily weight. Assess patient for signs and symptoms of dehydration (decreased thirst, lethargy, hemoconcentration), especially in geriatric patients.
- Assess fluid intake and bowel function. Increased bulk and fluids in the diet help minimize constipating effects.
- Monitor patient for onset of akathisia (restlessness or desire to keep moving), which may appear within 6 hr of 1st dose and may be difficult to distinguish from psychotic agitation. Benztropine may be used to differentiate agitation from akathisia. Observe closely for extrapyramidal side effects (*parkinsonian*—difficulty speaking or swallowing, loss of balance control, pill rolling of hands, mask-like face, shuffling gait, rigidity, tremors; and *dystonic*—muscle spasms, twisting motions, twitching, inability to move eyes, weakness of arms or legs). Trihexyphenidyl or Benztropine may be used to control these symptoms. Benzodiazepines may alleviate akathisia.
- Monitor for tardive dyskinesia (uncontrolled rhythmic movement of mouth, face, and extremities; lip smacking or puckering; puffing of cheeks; uncontrolled chewing; rapid or worm-like movements of tongue, excessive eye blinking). Report immediately; may be irreversible.
- Monitor for symptoms related to hyperprolactinemia (menstrual abnormalities, galactorrhea, sexual dysfunction).
- Monitor for development of neuroleptic malignant syndrome (fever, respiratory distress, tachycardia, seizures, diaphoresis, hypertension or hypotension, pallor, tiredness, severe muscle stiffness, loss of bladder control). Report symptoms immediately. May also cause leukocytosis, elevated liver function tests, elevated CPK.
- **Lab Test Considerations:** Monitor CBC with differential and liver function tests periodically during therapy.
- Monitor serum prolactin prior to and periodically during therapy. May cause ↑ serum prolactin levels.

Potential Nursing Diagnoses
Disturbed thought process (Indications)
Disturbed sensory perception (specify: visual, auditory, kinesthetic, gustatory, tactile, olfactory) (Indications)

Implementation
- Avoid skin contact with oral solution; may cause contact dermatitis.
- **PO:** Administer with food or full glass of water or milk to minimize GI irritation.
- Use calibrated measuring device for accurate dosage. Do not dilute concentrate with coffee or tea; may cause precipitation. May be given undiluted or mixed with water or juice.
- **IM:** Inject slowly, using 2-in., 21-gauge needle into well-developed muscle via Z-track technique. Do not exceed 3 mL per injection site.

haloperidol 653

Slight yellow color does not indicate altered potency. Keep patient recumbent for at least 30 min following injection to minimize hypotensive effects.

IV Administration

- **IV:** Haloperidol decanoate should not be administered IV.
- **Direct IV:** *Diluent:* May be administered undiluted for rapid control of acute psychosis or delirium. *Concentration:* 5 mg/mL. *Rate:* Administer at a rate of 5 mg/min.
- **Intermittent Infusion:** *Diluent:* May be diluted in 30–50 mL of D5W. *Rate:* Infuse over 30 min.
- **Y-Site Compatibility:** amifostine, amphotericin B liposome, amsacrine, bivalirudin, carboplatin, caspofungin, cisatracurium, cisplatin, cladribine, cyclophosphamide, cytarabine, dactinomycin, daptomycin, dexmedetomidine, diltiazem, docetaxel, doxacurium, doxorubicin hydrochloride, doxorubicin liposome, epirubicin, ertapenem, etoposide, etoposide phosphate, fenoldopam, filgrastim, fludarabine, gemcitabine, granisetron, hetastarch, hydromorphone, ifosfamide, levofloxacin, linezolid, lorazepam, mechlorethamine, melphalan, methadone, metronidazole, milrinone, mitoxantrone, nesiritide, octreotided, oxaliplatin, paclitaxel, palonosetron, pemetrexed, propofol, quinupristin/dalfopristin, remifentanil, rituximab, rocuronium, sodium acetate, tacrolimus, teniposide, thiotepa, tigecycline, tirofiban, trastuzumab, vecuronium, vincristine, vinorelbine, voriconazole.
- **Y-Site Incompatibility:** acyclovir, allopurinol, aminophylline, amphotericin B cholesteryl, amphotericin B colloidal, ampicillin, ampicillin/sulbactam, azathioprine, bumetanide, calcium chloride, cefazolin, cefepime, cefonocid, cefoperazone, cefotaxime, cefotetan, cefoxitin, ceftazidime, ceftizoxime, ceftriaxone, cefuroxime, chloramphenicol, clindamycin, dantrolene, dexamethasone sodium phosphate, diazepam, diazoxide, epoetin alfa, fluorouracil, folic acid, foscarnet, furosemide, ganciclovir, heparin, hydralazine, hydrocortisone, imipenem/cilastatin, indomethacin, ketorolac, magnesium sulfate, methylprednisolone sodium succinate, nafcillin, oxacillin, pantoprazole, penicillin G potassium, pentobarbital, phenobarbital, phenytoin, piperacillin/tazobactam, potassium chloride, sargramostim, sodium bicarbonate, ticarcillin/clavulanate, trimethoprim/sulfamethoxazole.

Patient/Family Teaching

- Advise patient to take medication as directed. Take missed doses as soon as remembered, with remaining doses evenly spaced throughout the day. May require several weeks to obtain desired effects. Do not increase dose or discontinue medication without consulting health care professional. Abrupt withdrawal may cause dizziness; nausea; vomiting; GI upset; trembling; or uncontrolled movements of mouth, tongue, or jaw.
- Inform patient of possibility of extrapyramidal symptoms and tardive dyskinesia. Caution patient to report symptoms immediately.
- Advise patient to change positions slowly to minimize orthostatic hypotension.
- May cause drowsiness. Caution patient to avoid driving or other activities requiring alertness until response to medication is known.
- Caution patient to avoid taking alcohol or other CNS depressants concurrently with this medication.
- Advise patient to use sunscreen and protective clothing when exposed to the sun to prevent photosensitivity reactions. Extremes of temperature should also be avoided, because this drug impairs body temperature regulation.
- Instruct patient to use frequent mouth rinses, good oral hygiene, and sugarless gum or candy to minimize dry mouth.
- Advise patient to notify health care professional of medication regimen prior to treatment or surgery.
- Instruct patient to notify health care professional promptly if weakness, tremors, visual disturbances, dark-colored urine or clay-colored stools, sore throat, fever, menstrual abnormalities, galactorrhea or sexual dysfunction occur.
- Emphasize the importance of routine follow-up exams to monitor response to medication and detect side effects.

Evaluation/Desired Outcomes

- Decrease in hallucinations, insomnia, agitation, hostility, and delusions.
- Decreased tics and vocalization in Tourette's syndrome.
- Improved behavior in children with severe behavioral problems. If no therapeutic effects are seen in 2–4 wk, dosage may be increased.

heparin (hep-a-rin)

HIGH ALERT

♣Calcilean, ♣Calciparine, ♣Hepalean, ♣Heparin Leo, Hep-Lock, Hep-Lock U/P

Classification
Therapeutic: anticoagulants
Pharmacologic: antithrombotics

Pregnancy Category C

Indications
Prophylaxis and treatment of various thromboembolic disorders including: Venous thromboembolism, Pulmonary emboli, Atrial fibrillation with embolization, Acute and chronic consumptive coagulopathies, Peripheral arterial thromboembolism. Used in very low doses (10–100 units) to maintain patency of IV catheters (heparin flush).

Action
Potentiates the inhibitory effect of antithrombin on factor Xa and thrombin. In low doses, prevents the conversion of prothrombin to thrombin by its effects on factor Xa. Higher doses neutralize thrombin, preventing the conversion of fibrinogen to fibrin. **Therapeutic Effects:** Prevention of thrombus formation. Prevention of extension of existing thrombi (full dose).

Pharmacokinetics
Absorption: Erratically absorbed following subcut or IM administration.
Distribution: Does not cross the placenta or enter breast milk.
Protein Binding: Very high (to low-density lipoproteins, globulins, and fibrinogen).
Metabolism and Excretion: Probably removed by the reticuloendothelial system (lymph nodes, spleen).
Half-life: 1–2 hr (↑ with increasing dose); affected by obesity, renal and hepatic function, malignancy, presence of pulmonary embolism, and infections.

TIME/ACTION PROFILE (anticoagulant effect)

ROUTE	ONSET	PEAK	DURATION
Heparin subcut	20–60 min	2 hr	8–12 hr
Heparin IV	immediate	5–10 min	2–6 hr

Contraindications/Precautions
Contraindicated in: Hypersensitivity; Uncontrolled bleeding; Severe thrombocytopenia; Open wounds (full dose); Avoid use of products containing benzyl alcohol in premature infants.
Use Cautiously in: Severe liver or kidney disease; Retinopathy (hypertensive or diabetic); Untreated hypertension; Ulcer disease; Spinal cord or brain injury; History of congenital or acquired bleeding disorder; Malignancy; OB: May be used during pregnancy, but use with caution during the last trimester and in the immediate postpartum period; Geri: Women >60 yr have ↑ risk of bleeding.
Exercise Extreme Caution in: Severe uncontrolled hypertension; Bacterial endocarditis, bleeding disorders; GI bleeding/ulceration/pathology; Hemorrhagic stroke; Recent CNS or ophthalmologic surgery; Active GI bleeding/ulceration; History of thrombocytopenia related to heparin.

Adverse Reactions/Side Effects
GI: drug-induced hepatitis. **Derm:** alopecia (long-term use), rashes, urticaria. **Hemat:** BLEEDING, anemia, thrombocytopenia (can occur up to several weeks after discontinuation of therapy). **Local:** pain at injection site. **MS:** osteoporosis (long-term use). **Misc:** fever, hypersensitivity.

Interactions
Heparin is frequently used concurrently or sequentially with other agents affecting coagulation. The risk of potentially serious interactions is greatest with full anticoagulation.

Drug-Drug: Risk of bleeding may be ↑ by concurrent use of **drugs that affect platelet function**, including **aspirin**, **NSAIDs**, **clopidogrel**, **dipyridamole**, some **penicillins**, **ticlopidine**, **abciximab**, **eptifibitide**, **tirofiban**, and **dextran**. Risk of bleeding may be ↑ by concurrent use of **drugs that cause hypoprothrombinemia**, including **quinidine**, **cefoperazone**, **cefotetan**, and **valproic acid**. Concurrent use of **thrombolytics** ↑ risk of bleeding. Heparins affect the prothrombin time used in assessing the response to **warfarin**. **Digoxin**, **tetracyclines**, **nicotine**, and **antihistamines** may ↓ anticoagulant effect of heparin. **Streptokinase** may be followed by relative resistance to heparin.
Drug-Natural Products: ↑ risk of bleeding with **arnica, anise, chamomile, clove, dong quai, fever few, garlic, ginger,** and **Panax ginseng**.

Route/Dosage

Therapeutic Anticoagulation
IV (Adults): *Intermittent bolus*—10,000 units, followed by 5000–10,000 units q 4–6 hr. *Continuous infusion*—5000 units (35–70 units/

kg), followed by 20,000–40,000 units infused over 24 hr (approx. 1000 units/hr or 15–18 units/kg/hr).
IV (Children > 1 yr): *Intermittent bolus*—50–100 units/kg, followed by 50–100 units/kg q 4 hr. *Continuous infusion*—Loading dose 75 units/kg, followed by 20 units/kg/hr, adjust to maintain aPTT of 60–85 sec.
IV (Neonates and Infants < 1 yr): *Continuous infusion*—Loading dose 75 units/kg, followed by 28 units/kg/hr, adjust to maintain aPTT of 60–85 sec.
Subcut (Adults): 5000 units IV, followed by initial subcut dose of 10,000–20,000 units, then 8000–10,000 units q 8 hr or 15,000–20,000 units q 12 hr.

Prophylaxis of Thromboembolism
Subcut (Adults): 5000 units q 8–12 hr (may be started 2 hr prior to surgery).

Cardiovascular Surgery
IV (Adults): At least 150 units/kg (300 units/kg if procedure <60 min; 400 units/kg if >60 min).
Intraarterial (Neonates, Infants, and Children): 100–150 units/kg via an artery prior to cardiac catheterization.

Line Flushing
IV (Adults and Children): 10–100 units/mL (10 units/mL for infants <10 kg, 100 units/mL for all others) solution to fill heparin lock set to needle hub; replace after each use.

Total Parenteral Nutrition
IV (Adults and Children): 05–1 units/mL (final solution concentration) to maintain line patency.

Arterial Line Patency
Intraarterial (Neonates): 0.5–2 units/mL.

Availability (generic available)
Heparin Sodium
Solution for injection: 10 units/mL, 100 units/mL, 1000 units/mL, 5000 units/mL, 7500 units/mL, 10,000 units/mL, 20,000 units/mL, 40,000 units/mL. **Premixed solution:** 1000 units/500 mL, 2000 units/1000 mL, 12,500 units/250 mL, 25,000 units in 250 and 500 mL.

NURSING IMPLICATIONS
Assessment
- Assess for signs of bleeding and hemorrhage (bleeding gums; nosebleed; unusual bruising; black, tarry stools; hematuria; fall in hematocrit or blood pressure; guaiac-positive stools). Notify health care professional if these occur.
- Assess patient for evidence of additional or increased thrombosis. Symptoms will depend on area of involvement.
- Monitor patient for hypersensitivity reactions (chills, fever, urticaria).
- **Subcut:** Observe injection sites for hematomas, ecchymosis, or inflammation.
- *Lab Test Considerations:* Monitor activated partial thromboplastin time (aPTT) and hematocrit prior to and periodically during therapy. When *intermittent IV* therapy is used, draw aPTT levels 30 min before each dose during initial therapy and then periodically. During *continuous* administration, monitor aPTT levels every 4 hr during early therapy. For *Subcut* therapy, draw blood 4–6 hr after injection.
- Monitor platelet count every 2–3 days throughout therapy. May cause mild thrombocytopenia, which appears on 4th day and resolves despite continued heparin therapy. Heparin-induced thrombocytopenia (HIT), a more severe form which necessitates discontinuing medication, may develop on 8th day of therapy; may reduce platelet count to as low as 5000/mm^3 and lead to increased resistance to heparin therapy. HIT may progress to development of venous and arterial thrombosis (HITT) and may occur up to several wk after discontinuation. Patients who have received a previous course of heparin may be at higher risk for severe thrombocytopenia for several months after the initial course.
- May cause hyperkalemia and ↑ AST and ALT levels.
- *Toxicity and Overdose:* Protamine sulfate is the antidote. Due to short half-life, overdose can often be treated by withdrawing the drug.

Potential Nursing Diagnoses
Ineffective tissue perfusion (Indications)
Risk for injury (Side Effects)

Implementation
- *High Alert:* Fatal hemorrhages have occurred in pediatric patients due to errors in which heparin sodium injection vials were confused with heparin flush vials. Carefully examine all heparin sodium injection vials to confirm the correct vial choice prior to administration. Have second practitioner independently check original order, dose calculation, and infusion

pump settings. Unintended concomitant use of two heparin products (unfractionated heparin and LMW heparins) has resulted in serious harm or death. Review patients' recent (emergency department, operating room) and current medication administration records before administering any heparin or LMW heparin product. Do not confuse heparin with Hespan (hetastarch in sodium chloride). Do not confuse vials of heparin with vials of insulin.

- Inform all personnel caring for patient of anticoagulant therapy. Venipunctures and injection sites require application of pressure to prevent bleeding or hematoma formation. Avoid IM injections of other medications; hematomas may develop.
- In patients requiring long-term anticoagulation, oral anticoagulant therapy should be instituted 4–5 days prior to discontinuing heparin therapy.
- Solution is colorless to slightly yellow.

IV Administration

- **Subcut:** Administer deep into subcut tissue. Alternate injection sites between arm and the left and right abdominal wall above the iliac crest. Inject entire length of needle at a 45°- or 90°-angle into a skin fold held between thumb and forefinger; hold skin fold throughout injection. Do not aspirate or massage. Rotate sites frequently. Do not administer IM because of danger of hematoma formation. Solution should be clear; do not inject solution containing particulate matter.
- **Direct IV:** *Diluent:* Administer loading dose undiluted. *Concentration:* Varies depending upon vial used. *Rate:* Administer over at least 1 min. Loading dose given before continuous infusion.
- **Continuous Infusion:** *Diluent:* Dilute 25,000 units of heparin in 250–500 mL of 0.9% NaCl or D5W. Premixed infusions are already diluted and ready to use. Admixed solutions stable for 24 hr at room temperature or if refrigerated. Premixed infusion stable for 30 days once overwrap removed. *Concentration:* 50–100 units/mL. *Rate:* See Route/Dosage section. Adjust to maintain therapeutic aPTT. Use an infusion pump to ensure accuracy.
- **Flush:** To prevent clot formation in intermittent infusion (heparin lock) sets, inject dilute heparin solution of 10–100 units/0.5–1 mL after each medication injection or every 8–12 hr. To prevent incompatibility of heparin with medication, flush lock set with sterile water or 0.9% NaCl for injection before and after medication is administered.
- **Y-Site Compatibility:** acyclovir, alfentanil, allopurinol, amifostine, aminophylline, amphotericin B liposome, anidulafungin, ascorbin acid, atenolol, atropine, azathioprine, aztreonam, benztropine, betamethasone, bivalirudin, bleomycin, bretylium, bumetanide, buprenorphine, butorphanol, calcium chloride, calcium gluconate, carboplatin, cefazolin, cefonicid, cefoperazone, cefotaxime, cefotetan, cefoxitin, ceftazidime, ceftizoxime, ceftriaxone, cefuroxime, chloramphenicol, chlordiazepoxide, cimetidine, cisplatin, cladribine, clindamycin, cyanocobalamin, cyclosporine, cytarabine, daptomycin, dexamethasone, dexmedetomidine, digoxin, docetaxel, dopamine, doripenem, doxacurium, doxapram, doxorubicin liposome, edrophonium, enalaprilat, ephedrine, epinephrine, epoetin, eptifibatide, ertapenem, estrogens, conjugated, ethacrynate, etoposide, etoposide phosphate, famotidine, fenoldopam, fentanyl, fluconazole, fludarabine, flumazenil, fluorouracil, folic acid, foscarnet, furosemide, gallium nitrate, ganciclovir, gemcitabine, glycopyrrolate, granisetron, hydrocortisone, hydromorphone, ifosfamide, imipenem/cilastatin, indomethacin, insulin, isoproterenol, kanamycin, ketorolac, lansoprazole, leucovorin, lidocaine, linezolid, lorazepam, magnesium sulfate, mannitol, mechlorethamine, melphalan, meropenem, metaraminol, methicillin, methotrexate, methoxamine, methyldopate, methylergonovine, metoclopramide, metoprolol, metronidazole, mezlocillin, micafungin, miconazole, midazolam, milrinone, minocycline, mitomycin, morphine, multiple vitamins, nafcillin, nalbuphine, naloxone, neostigmine, nitroglycerin, nitroprusside, norepinephrine, octreotide, ondansetron, oxacillin, oxaliplatin, oxytocin, paclitaxel, palonosetron, pancuronium, pantoprazole, pemetrexed, penicillin G potassium, pentobarbital, phenobarbital, phentolamine, phenylephrine, phytonadione, piperacillin/tazobactam, potassium chloride, procainamide, propofol, propranolol, pyridostigmine, pyridoxine, ranitidine, remifentanil, ritodrine, rituximab, rocuronium, sargramostim, scopolamine, sodium acetate, sodium bicarbonate, streptokinase, succinylcholine, sufentanil, tacrolimus, teniposide, thiotepa, ticarcillin/clavulanate, tigecycline, tirofiban, tolazoline, trastuzumab, trimethoprim, trimethobenazamide, urokinse, vasopressin, vecuronium, verapamil, vinblas-

tine, vincristine, voriconazole, warfarin, zidovudine.
- **Y-Site Incompatibility:** alteplase, amikacin, amiodarone, amphotericin B cholesteryl sulfate, amsacrine, caspofungin, ciprofloxacin, dantrolene, diazepam, diazoxide, doxycycline, epirubicin, filgrastim, gentamicin, haloperidol, hydroxyzine, idarubicin, inamrinone, levofloxacin, methotrimeprazine, mitoxandrone, netilmicin, palifermin, papaverine, pentamidine, phenytoin, protamine, quinupristin/dalfopristin, reteplase, trimethoprim/sulfamethoxazole, tobramycin, vancomycin.
- **Additive Compatibility:** It is recommended that heparin not be mixed in solution with other medications when given for anticoagulation, even those that are compatible, because changes in rate of heparin infusion may be required that would also affect admixtures.

Patient/Family Teaching
- Advise patient to report any symptoms of unusual bleeding or bruising to health care professional immediately.
- Instruct patient not to take medications containing aspirin or NSAIDs while on heparin therapy.
- Caution patient to avoid IM injections and activities leading to injury and to use a soft toothbrush and electric razor during heparin therapy.
- Advise patient to inform health care professional of medication regimen prior to treatment or surgery.
- Patients on anticoagulant therapy should carry an identification card with this information at all times.

Evaluation/Desired Outcomes
- Prolonged partial thromboplastin time (PTT) of 1.5–2.5 times the control, without signs of hemorrhage.
- Prevention of deep vein thrombosis and pulmonary emboli.
- Patency of IV catheters.

HIGH ALERT

HEPARINS (LOW MOLECULAR WEIGHT)

dalteparin (dal-**te**-pa-rin)
Fragmin

enoxaparin (e-nox-a-**pa**-rin)
Lovenox

tinzaparin (tin-za-**pa**-rin)
Innohep

Classification
Therapeutic: anticoagulants
Pharmacologic: antithrombotics

Pregnancy Category B

Indications
Enoxaparin and dalteparin: Prevention of venous thromboembolism (VTE) (deep vein thrombosis (DVT) and/or pulmonary embolism (PE)) in surgical or medical patients. **Dalteparin only:** Extended treatment of symptomatic DVT and/or PE in patients with cancer. **Enoxaparin and tinzaparin:** Treatment of DVT with or without PE (with warfarin). **Enoxaparin and dalteparin only:** Prevention of ischemic complications (with aspirin) from unstable angina and non-ST-segment-elevation MI. **Enoxaparin only:** Treatment of acute ST-segment-elevation MI (with thrombolytics or percutaneous coronary intervention).

Action
Potentiate the inhibitory effect of antithrombin on factor Xa and thrombin. **Therapeutic Effects:** Prevention of thrombus formation.

Pharmacokinetics
Absorption: Well absorbed after subcut administration (87% for dalteparin and tinzaparin, 92% for enoxaparin).
Distribution: Unknown.
Metabolism and Excretion: *Dalteparin*—unknown; *enoxaparin*—primarily eliminated renally; *tinzaparin*—partially metabolized, elimination is primarily renal.
Half-life: *Dalteparin*—2.1–2.3 hr; *enoxaparin*—3–6 hr; *tinzaparin*—3.9 hr (all are ↑ in renal insufficiency).

TIME/ACTION PROFILE (anticoagulant effect)

ROUTE	ONSET	PEAK	DURATION
Dalteparin subcut	rapid	4 hr	up to 24 hr
Enoxaparin subcut	unknown	3–5 hr	12 hr
Tinzaparin subcut	rapid	4–6 hr	24 hr

Contraindications/Precautions
Contraindicated in: Hypersensitivity to specific agents or pork products; cross-sensitivity may occur; Some products contain sulfites or benzyl alcohol and should be avoided in patients with

known hypersensitivity or intolerance; Active major bleeding; History of heparin-induced thrombocytopenia; *Dalteparin*—regional anesthesia during treatment for unstable angina/non–Q-wave MI.

Use Cautiously in: Severe liver or kidney disease (adjust dose of enoxaparin if CCr <30 mL/min); Women <45 kg or men <57 kg; Retinopathy (hypertensive or diabetic); Untreated hypertension; Geri: May have ↑ risk of bleeding due to age-related decrease in renal function; *Dalteparin*-Geri: ↑ mortality in patients > 70 yrs with renal insufficiency; Recent history of ulcer disease; History of congenital or acquired bleeding disorder; OB, Lactation, Pedi: Safety not established; should not be used in pregnant patients with prosthetic heart valves without careful monitoring.

Exercise Extreme Caution in: Spinal/epidural anesthesia (increased risk of spinal/epidural hematomas, especially with concurrent NSAIDs, repeated or traumatic epidural puncture, or indwelling epidural catheter); Severe uncontrolled hypertension; Bacterial endocarditis, bleeding disorders.

Adverse Reactions/Side Effects

CNS: dizziness, headache, insomnia. **CV:** edema. **GI:** constipation, nausea, reversible ↑ in liver enzymes, vomiting. **GU:** urinary retention. **Derm:** ecchymoses, pruritus, rash, urticaria. **Hemat:** BLEEDING, anemia, thrombocytopenia. **Local:** erythema at injection site, hematoma, irritation, pain. **Misc:** fever.

Interactions

Drug-Drug: Risk of bleeding may be ↑ by concurrent use of **drugs that affect platelet function and coagulation**, including **warfarin, aspirin, NSAIDs, dipyridamole, clopidogrel, ticlopidine, abciximab, eptifibatide, tirofiban,** and **thrombolytics.**

Drug-Natural Products: ↑ bleeding risk with, **arnica, chamomile, clove, feverfew, garlic, ginger, ginkgo, Panax ginseng,** and others.

Route/Dosage

Dalteparin

Subcut (Adults): *Prophylaxis of DVT following abdominal surgery*—2500 IU 1–2 hr before surgery, then once daily for 5–10 days; *Prophylaxis of VTE in high-risk patients undergoing abdominal surgery*—5000 IU evening before surgery, then once daily for 5–10 days *or* in patients with malignancy, 2500 IU 1–2 hr before surgery, another 2500 IU 12 hr later, then 5000 IU once daily for 5–10 days; *Prophylaxis of VTE in patients undergoing hip replacement surgery*—2500 IU within 2 hr before surgery, then 2500 IU 4–8 hr after surgery, then 5000 IU once daily (start at least 6 hr after postsurgical dose) for 5–10 days *or* 5000 IU evening before surgery (10–14 hr before surgery), then 5000 IU 4–8 hr after surgery, then 5000 IU once daily for 5–10 days *or* 2500 IU 4–8 hr after surgery, then 5000 IU once daily (start at least 6 hr after postsurgical dose); *Prophylaxis of VTE in medical patients with severely restricted mobility during acute illness:* 5000 IU once daily for 12 to 14 days. *Unstable angina/non–ST-segment-elevation MI*—120 IU/kg (not to exceed 10,000 IU) q 12 hr for 5–8 days with concurrent aspirin; *Extended treatment of symptomatic VTE in cancer patients*—200 IU/kg (not to exceed 18,000 IU) once daily for first 30 days, followed by 150 IU/kg (not to exceed 18,000 IU) once daily for months 2–6.

Renal Impairment
Subcut (Adults): *Cancer patients receiving extended treatment of symptomatic VTE with CCr <30 mL/min*—Monitor anti-Xa levels (target 0.5–1.5 IU/mL).

Enoxaparin

Subcut (Adults): *VTE prophylaxis in patients undergoing knee replacement surgery*—30 mg q 12 hr starting 12–24 hr postop for 7–10 days; *VTE prophylaxis in patients undergoing hip replacement surgery*—30 mg q 12 hr starting 12–24 hr postop *or* 40 mg once daily starting 12 hr before surgery (either dose may be continued for 7–14 days; continued prophylaxis with 40 mg once daily may be continued for up to 3 wk); *VTE prophylaxis following abdominal surgery*—40 mg once daily starting 2 hr before surgery and then continued for 7–12 days or until ambulatory (up to 14 days); *VTE prophylaxis in medical patients with acute illness*—40 mg once daily for 6–14 days; *Treatment of DVT/PE (outpatient)*—1 mg/kg q 12 hr. Warfarin should be started within 72 hr; enoxaparin may be continued for a minimum of 5 days and until therapeutic anticoagulation with warfarin is achieved (INR >2 for 2 consecutive days); *Treatment of DVT/PE (inpatient)*—1 mg/kg q 12 hr *or* 1.5 mg/kg once daily. Warfarin should be started within 72 hr; enoxaparin may be continued for a minimum of 5 days and until therapeutic anticoagulation with warfarin is achieved (INR >2 for two consecutive days); *Unstable angina/non—ST-segment-elevation MI*—1 mg/kg q 12 hr for 2–8 days (with aspirin).

HEPARINS (LOW MOLECULAR WEIGHT)

IV, Subcut (Adults <75 yr): *Acute ST–segment-elevation MI*—Administer single IV bolus of 30 mg plus 1 mg/kg subcut dose (maximum of 100 mg for first 2 doses only), followed by 1 mg/kg subcut q 12 hr. The usual duration of treatment is 2–8 days. In patients undergoing percutaneous coronary intervention, if last subcut dose was <8 hr before balloon inflation, no additional dosing needed; if last subcut dose was ≥8 hr before balloon inflation, administer single IV bolus of 0.3 mg/kg.

Subcut (Adults ≥75 yr): *Acute ST-segment-elevation MI*—0.75 mg/kg every 12 hr (no IV bolus needed) (maximum of 75 mg for first 2 doses only; no initial bolus). The usual duration of treatment is 2–8 days.

Renal Impairment
Subcut (Adults CCr <30 mL/min): *VTE prophylaxis for abdominal or knee/hip replacement surgery*—30 mg once daily. *Treatment of DVT/PE*—1 mg/kg once daily. *Unstable angina/non-ST-segment-elevation MI*—1 mg/kg once daily. *Acute ST-segment-elevation MI (patients <75 yr)*—Single IV bolus of 30 mg plus 1 mg/kg subcut dose, followed by 1 mg/kg subcut once daily. *Acute ST-segment-elevation MI (patients ≥75 yr)*—1 mg/kg once daily (no initial bolus).

Tinzaparin
Subcut (Adults): *Treatment of deep vein thrombosis*—175 anti-Xa IU/kg once daily for at least 6 days and until adequate anticoagulation is achieved with warfarin (INR >2 for 2 consecutive days).

Availability
Dalteparin
Solution for injection (prefilled syringes): 2500 IU/0.2 mL, 5000 IU/0.2 mL, 7500 IU/0.3 mL, 10,000 IU/0.4 mL, 10,000 IU/1 mL, 12,500 IU/0.5 mL, 15,000 IU/0.6 mL, 18,000 IU/0.72 mL. **Solution for injection (multidose vials):** 10,000 IU/mL in 9.5-mL vials, 25,000 IU/mL in 3.8-mL vials.

Enoxaparin
Solution for injection (prefilled syringes): 30 mg/0.3 mL, 40 mg/0.4 mL, 60 mg/0.6 mL, 80 mg/0.8 mL, 100 mg/1 mL, 120 mg/0.8 mL, 150 mg/mL. **Solution for injection (multidose vials):** 300 mg/3 mL.

Tinzaparin
Solution for injection: 20,000 anti-Xa units/mL in 2-mL vials.

NURSING IMPLICATIONS
Assessment
- Assess for signs of bleeding and hemorrhage (bleeding gums; nosebleed; unusual bruising; black, tarry stools; hematuria; fall in hematocrit or blood pressure; guaiac-positive stools); bleeding from surgical site. Notify health care professional if these occur.
- Assess for evidence of additional or increased thrombosis. Symptoms depend on area of involvement. Monitor neurological status frequently for signs of neurological impairment. May require urgent treatment.
- Monitor for hypersensitivity reactions (chills, fever, urticaria). Report signs to health care professional.
- Monitor patients with epidural catheters frequently for signs and symptoms of neurologic impairment.
- **Subcut:** Observe injection sites for hematomas, ecchymosis, or inflammation.
- **Lab Test Considerations:** Monitor CBC, platelet count, and stools for occult blood periodically during therapy. If thrombocytopenia occurs (platelet count <100,000/mm³), discontinue therapy. If hematocrit ↓ unexpectedly, assess patient for potential bleeding sites. For *dalteparin* use for extended treatment of symptomatic VTE in cancer patients, if platelets ↓ to 50,000–100,000/mm³, reduce dose to 2500 IU once daily until recovery to ≥100,000/mm³; if platelets <50,000/mm³, discontinue until count returns to ≥50,000/mm³.
- Special monitoring of aPTT is not necessary. Monitoring of anti-Xa levels may be considered in patients who are obese or have renal dysfunction (for *enoxaparin*, obtain 4 hr after injection).
- May cause ↑ in AST and ALT levels.
- ***Toxicity and Overdose:*** For *enoxaparin* overdose, protamine sulfate 1 mg for each mg of *enoxaparin* should be administered by slow IV injection. For *dalteparin* overdose, protamine sulfate 1 mg for each 100 anti-factor Xa IU of *dalteparin* should be administered by slow IV injection. If the aPTT measured 2–4 hr after protamine administration remains prolonged, a 2nd infusion of protamine 0.5 mg/

= Canadian drug name. = Genetic implication.
*CAPITALS indicates life-threatening; underlines indicate most frequent.

100 anti-factor Xa IU of *dalteparin* may be administered.

Potential Nursing Diagnoses
Ineffective tissue perfusion (Indications)
Risk for injury (Side Effects)

Implementation
- **High Alert:** Unintended concomitant use of two heparin products (unfractionated heparin and LMW heparins) has resulted in serious harm and death. Review patients' recent and current medication administration records before administering any heparin or low-molecular-weight heparin product.
- Cannot be used interchangeably (unit for unit) with unfractionated heparin or other low-molecular-weight heparins.
- **Subcut:** Administer deep into subcut tissue. Alternate injection sites daily between the left and right anterolateral and left and right posterolateral abdominal wall, the upper thigh, or buttocks. Inject entire length of needle at a 45° or 90° angle into a skin fold held between thumb and forefinger; hold skin fold throughout injection. Do not aspirate or massage. Rotate sites frequently. Do not administer IM because of danger of hematoma formation. Solution should be clear; do not inject solution containing particulate matter.
- If excessive bruising occurs, ice cube massage of site before injection may lessen bruising.
- **Enoxaparin:** To avoid the loss of drug, do not expel the air bubble from the syringe before the injection.
- **Subcut:** Per manufacturer's recommendations, to enhance absorption, inject enoxaparin into left or right anterolateral or posterolateral abdominal wall only.
- To minimize risk of bleeding after vascular instrumentation for unstable angina, recommended intervals between doses should be followed closely. Leave vascular access sheath in place for 6–8 hr after enoxaparin dose. Give next enoxaparin dose ≥6–8 hr after sheath removal. Observe site for bleeding or hematoma formation.
- **Direct IV:** Use multidose vial for bolus injections. Administer through a pre-exsting IV line. Flush line with 0.9% NaCl or D5W before and after administration.
- **Tinzaparin:** Tinzaparin should be administered daily for at least 6 days and until patient is adequately anticoagulated with warfarin (INR at least 2.0 for 2 consecutive days). Warfarin therapy should be started within 1–3 days of tinzaparin initiation.

Patient/Family Teaching
- Advise patient to report any symptoms of unusual bleeding or bruising, dizziness, itching, rash, fever, swelling, or difficulty breathing to health care professional immediately.
- Instruct patient not to take aspirin or NSAIDs without consulting health care professional while on therapy.

Evaluation/Desired Outcomes
- Prevention of DVT and pulmonary emboli (enoxaparin and dalteparin only).
- Resolution of DVT and pulmonary embolism (enoxaparin and tinzaparin only).
- Prevention of ischemic complications (with aspirin) in patients with unstable angina or non–ST—segment—elevation MI (enoxaparin and dalteparin only).
- Prevention of recurrent MI or death in patients with acute ST-segment-elevation MI (enoxparin only).

HISTAMINE H₂ ANTAGONISTS

cimetidine (sye-**me**-ti-deen)
✤Apo-Cimetidine, ✤Dom-Cimetidine, ✤Gen-Cimetidine, ✤Novo-Cimetine, ✤Nu-Cimet, ✤PMS-Cimetidine, Tagamet, Tagamet HB

famotidine (fa-**moe**-ti-deen)
✤Acid Control, ✤Apo-Famotidine, ✤Gen-Famotidine, ✤Novo-Famotidine, ✤Nu-Famotidine, Pepcid, Pepcid AC, ✤Ulcidine

nizatidine (ni-**za**-ti-deen)
✤Apo-Nizatidine, Axid, Axid AR, ✤Dom-Nizatidine, ✤Gen-Nizatidine, ✤Novo-Nizatidine, ✤PHL-Nizatidine, ✤PMS-Nizatidine

ranitidine (ra-**ni**-ti-deen)
✤Apo-Ranitidine, ✤Dom-Ranitidine, ✤Gen-Ranitidine, ✤Novo-Ranitidine, ✤Nu-Ranitidine, ✤PHL-Ranitidine, ✤PMS-Ranitidine, ✤Ratio-Ranitidine, ✤Riva-Ranitidine, Zantac, Zantac EFFERdose, Zantac 75, Zantac 150

Classification
Therapeutic: antiulcer agents
Pharmacologic: histamine H₂ antagonists

Pregnancy Category B

HISTAMINE H₂ ANTAGONISTS 661

Indications
Short-term treatment of active duodenal ulcers and benign gastric ulcers. Maintenance therapy for duodenal and gastric ulcers after healing of active ulcers. Management of GERD. Treatment of heartburn, acid indigestion, and sour stomach (OTC use). **Cimetidine, famotidine, ranitidine:** Management of gastric hypersecretory states (Zollinger-Ellison syndrome). **Cimetidine, famotidine, ranitidine IV:** Prevention and treatment of stress-induced upper GI bleeding in critically ill patients. **Ranitidine:** Treatment of and maintenance therapy for erosive esophagitis.
Unlabeled Use: Management of GI symptoms associated with the use of NSAIDs. Prevention of acid inactivation of supplemental pancreatic enzymes in patients with pancreatic insufficiency. Management of urticaria.

Action
Inhibits the action of histamine at the H₂-receptor site located primarily in gastric parietal cells, resulting in inhibition of gastric acid secretion.
Therapeutic Effects: Healing and prevention of ulcers. Decreased symptoms of gastroesophageal reflux. Decreased secretion of gastric acid.

Pharmacokinetics
Absorption: *Cimetidine*—well absorbed after oral and IM administration. *Famotidine*—40-45% absorbed after oral administration. *Nizatidine*—70-95% absorbed after oral administration. *Ranitidine*—50% absorbed after PO and IM administration.
Distribution: All agents enter breast milk and cerebrospinal fluid.
Metabolism and Excretion: *Cimetidine*—30% metabolized by the liver; remainder is eliminated unchanged by the kidneys. *Famotidine*—up to 70% excreted unchanged by the kidneys, 30-35% metabolized by the liver. *Nizatidine*—60% excreted unchanged by the kidneys; some hepatic metabolism; at least 1 metabolite has histamine-blocking activity. *Ranitidine*—metabolized by the liver, mostly on first pass; 30% excreted unchanged by the kidneys after PO administration, 70% after parenteral administration.
Half-life: *Cimetidine*—2 hr; *famotidine*—2.5-3.5 hr; *nizatidine*—1.6 hr; *ranitidine*—2-2.5 hr (all are ↑ in renal impairment).

TIME/ACTION PROFILE

ROUTE	ONSET	PEAK	DURATION
Cimetidine PO	30 min	45-90 min	4-5 hr
Cimetidine IM, IV	10 min	30 min	4-5 hr
Famotidine PO	within 60 min	1-4 hr	6-12 hr
Famotidine IV	within 60 min	0.5-3 hr	8-15 hr
Nizatidine PO	unknown	unknown	8-12 hr
Ranitidine PO	unknown	1-3 hr	8-12 hr
Ranitidine IM	unknown	15 min	8-12 hr
Ranitidine IV	unknown	15 min	8-12 hr

Contraindications/Precautions
Contraindicated in: Hypersensitivity; Some products contain alcohol and should be avoided in patients with known intolerance; Some products contain aspartame and should be avoided in patients with phenylketonuria.
Use Cautiously in: Renal impairment (more susceptible to adverse CNS reactions; ↑ dose interval recommended for *cimetidine* and *nizatidine* if CCr ≤ 50 mL/min, and for *famotidine* and *ranitidine* if CCr <50 mL/min; Hepatic impairment (for *ranitidine*); Acute porphyria (for *ranitidine*); Geri: More susceptible to adverse CNS reactions; dose ↓ recommended; OB, Lactation: Pregnancy or lactation.

Adverse Reactions/Side Effects
CNS: <u>confusion</u>, dizziness, drowsiness, hallucinations, headache. **CV:** ARRHYTHMIAS. **GI:** constipation, diarrhea, drug-induced hepatitis (nizatidine, cimetidine), nausea. **GU:** ↓ sperm count, erectile dysfunction (cimetidine). **Endo:** gynecomastia. **Hemat:** AGRANULOCYTOSIS, APLASTIC ANEMIA, anemia, neutropenia, thrombocytopenia. **Local:** pain at IM site. **Misc:** hypersensitivity reactions, vasculitis.

Interactions
Drug-Drug: Cimetidine is a moderate inhibitor of the CYP1A2, CYP2C9, CYP2D6, and CYP3A4 isoenzymes in the liver; may lead to ↑ levels and toxicity with **benzodiazepines** (especially **chlordiazepoxide, diazepam,** and **midazolam**), some **beta blockers (labetalol, metoprolol, propranolol), caffeine, calcium channel blockers, carbamazepine, cyclosporine, dofetilide, lidocaine, metronidazole, mexiletine, nefazodone, pentoxifylline, phenytoin, procainamide, propafenone, quinidine, metformin, risperidone, ritonavir, ropinirole, selective serotonin reuptake inhibitors, sildenafil, sulfo-

nylureas, **tacrolimus**, **theophylline**, **tricyclic antidepressants**, **venlafaxine**, and **warfarin**. Famotidine, nizatidine, and ranitidine have a much smaller and less significant effect on the metabolism of other drugs. Cimetidine may ↑ myelosuppressive effects of **carmustine** (avoid concurrent use). All may ↓ absorption of **ketoconazole, itraconazole, atazanavir, delavirdine,** and **geftinib**. Ranitidine may ↑ absorption of **triazolam, midazolam,** and **glipizide**. Ranitidine may ↑ **procainamide** levels. Ranitidine may ↑ the effects of **warfarin**.

Route/Dosage

Cimetidine
PO (Adults): *Short-term treatment of active ulcers*—300 mg 4 times daily *or* 800 mg at bedtime *or* 400–600 mg twice daily (not to exceed 2.4 g/day) for up to 8 wk. *Duodenal ulcer prophylaxis*—300 mg twice daily *or* 400 mg at bedtime. *GERD*—400 mg q 6 hr *or* 800 mg twice daily for 12 wk. *Gastric hypersecretory conditions*—300–600 mg q 6 hr (up to 2400 mg/day). *OTC use*—up to 200 mg may be taken twice daily (for not more than 2 wk).
PO (Children): *Short-term treatment of active ulcers*—5–10 mg/kg q 6 hr.
IM, IV (Adults): *Short-term treatment of active ulcers*—300 mg q 6 hr (not to exceed 2.4 g/day). *Continuous IV infusion*—900 mg infused over 24 hr (37.5 mg/hr); may be preceded by a 150-mg bolus dose. *Gastric hypersecretory conditions*—300–600 mg q 6 hr (not to exceed 2.4 g/day). *Prevention of upper GI bleeding in critically ill patients*—50 mg/hr.
IM, IV (Children): *Short-term treatment of active ulcers*—5–10 mg/kg q 6 hr.

Renal Impairment
IV, PO (Adults): *CCr 10–50 mL/min*—Administer 50% of normal dose; *CCr <10 mL/min*—Administer 25% of normal dose; *prevention of upper GI bleeding in critically ill patients if CCr <30 mL/min*—25 mg/hr.

Renal Impairment
PO (Children): 10–15 mg/kg/day.

Famotidine
PO (Adults): *Short-term treatment of active duodenal ulcers*—40 mg/day at bedtime or 20 mg twice daily for up to 8 wk. *Treatment of benign gastric ulcers*—40 mg/day at bedtime. *Maintenance treatment of duodenal ulcers*—20 mg once daily at bedtime. *GERD*—20 mg twice daily for up to 6 wk; up to 40 mg twice daily for up to 12 wk for esophagitis with erosions, ulcerations, and continuing symptoms. *Gastric hypersecretory conditions*—20 mg q 6 hr initially, up to 160 mg q 6 hr. *OTC use*—10 mg for relief of symptoms; for prevention—10 mg 60 min before eating or take 10 mg as chewable tablet 15 minutes before heartburn-inducing foods or beverages (not to exceed 20 mg/24 hr for up to 2 wk).
PO, IV (Children 1–16 yr): *Peptic ulcer*—0.5 mg/kg/day as a single bedtime dose or in 2 divided doses (up to 40 mg daily); *GERD*—1 mg/kg/day in 2 divided doses (up to 80 mg twice daily).
PO (Infants >3 mo–1 yr): *GERD*—0.5 mg/kg/dose twice daily.
PO (Infants and neonates <3 mo): *GERD*—0.5 mg/kg/dose once daily.
IV (Adults): 20 mg q 12 hr.

Renal Impairment
PO (Adults): *CCr <50 mL/min*—administer normal dose q 36–48 hr *or* 50% of normal dose at normal dosing interval. *CCr <10 mL/min*—dosing interval may need to be ↑ to q 36–48 hr.

Nizatidine
PO (Adults): *Short-term treatment of active duodenal or benign gastric ulcers*—300 mg once daily at bedtime. *Maintenance treatment of duodenal ulcers*—150 mg once daily at bedtime. *GERD*—150 mg twice daily. *OTC use*—75 mg twice daily given 30–60 min before foods or beverages expected to cause symptoms.

Renal Impairment
PO (Adults): *Short-term treatment of active ulcers*—*CCr 20–50 mL/min*—150 mg once daily; *CCr <20 mL/min*—150 mg every other day. *Maintenance treatment of duodenal ulcers*—*CCr 20–50 mL/min*—150 mg every other day; *CCr <20 mL/min*—150 mg every 3 days.

Ranitidine
PO (Adults): *Short-term treatment of active duodenal of benign gastric ulcers*—150 mg twice daily *or* 300 mg once daily at bedtime. *Maintenance treatment of duodenal or gastric ulcers*—150 mg once daily at bedtime. *GERD*—150 mg twice daily. *Erosive esophagitis*—150 mg 4 times daily initially, then 150 mg twice daily as maintenance. *Gastric hypersecretory conditions*—150 mg twice daily initially; up to 6 g/day have been used. *OTC use*—75 mg 30–60 min before foods or beverages expected to cause symptoms (up to twice daily) (not to be used for more than 2 wk).

HISTAMINE H₂ ANTAGONISTS 663

PO (Children 1 mo-16 yr): *Treatment of gastric/duodenal ulcers*—2–4 mg/kg/day in 2 divided doses (up to 300 mg/day); *Maintenance treatment of ulcers*—2–4 mg/kg once daily (up to 150 mg/day); *GERD/erosive esophagitis*—5–10 mg/kg/day in 2 divided doses (up to 300 mg/day for GERD or 600 mg/day for erosive esophagitis).
PO (Neonates): 2 mg/kg/day in 2 divided doses.
IV, IM (Adults): 50 mg q 6–8 hr. *Continuous IV infusion*—6.25 mg/hr. *Gastric hypersecretory conditions*—1 mg/kg/hr; may be ↑ by 0.5 mg/kg/hr (not to exceed 2.5 mg/kg/hr).
IV, IM (Children 1 mo-16 yr): *Treatment of gastric/duodenal ulcers*—2–4 mg/kg/day divided q 6–8 hr (up to 200 mg/day). *Continuous infusion*—1 mg/kg/dose followed by 0.08–0.17 mg/kg/hr.
IV (Neonates): 1.5 mg/kg/dose load, then in 12 hr start maintenance of 1.5–2 mg/kg/day divided q 12 hr. *Continuous IV infusion*—1.5 mg/kg/dose load followed by 0.04–0.08 mg/kg/hr infusion.

Renal Impairment
PO (Adults): *CCr<50 mL/min*—150 mg q 24 hr.

Renal Impairment
IV (Adults): *CCr<50 mL/min*—50 mg q 24 hr.

Availability

Cimetidine (generic available)
Tablets: 200 mg^(Rx, OTC), 300 mg, 400 mg, ✦600 mg, 800 mg. **Oral liquid (mint-peach flavor):** 200 mg/5 mL^(OTC), 300 mg/5 mL. **Premixed infusion:** 300 mg/50 mL 0.9% NaCl. **Solution for injection:** 150 mg/mL.

Famotidine (generic available)
Tablets: 10 mg^(OTC), 20 mg^(Rx, OTC), 40 mg. **Gelcaps:** 10 mg^(OTC). **Oral suspension (cherry-banana-mint flavor):** 40 mg/5 mL. **Premixed infusion:** 20 mg/50 mL 0.9% NaCl. **Solution for injection:** 10 mg/mL. *In combination with:* calcium carbonate and magnesium hydroxide^(OTC) (Pepcid Complete, see Appendix B).

Nizatidine (generic available)
Tablets: 75 mg^(OTC). **Capsules:** 150 mg, 300 mg. **Oral solution (bubble gum flavor):** 15 mg/mL.

Ranitidine (generic available)
Tablets: 75 mg^(OTC), 150 mg, 300 mg. **Cost:** *Generic*—150 mg $23.99/180, 300 mg $24.84/90.

Capsules: 150 mg, 300 mg. **Cost:** *Generic*—150 mg $89.95/180, 300 mg $79.99/90. **Effervescent tablets (EFFERdose):** 25 mg. **Syrup (peppermint flavor):** 15 mg/mL. **Cost:** $330.01/473 mL. **Premixed infusion:** 50 mg/50 mL 0.45% NaCl. **Solution for injection:** 25 mg/mL.

NURSING IMPLICATIONS

Assessment
- Assess for epigastric or abdominal pain and frank or occult blood in the stool, emesis, or gastric aspirate.
- **Geri:** Assess geriatric and debilitated patients routinely for confusion. Report promptly.
- ***Lab Test Considerations:*** Monitor CBC with differential periodically during therapy.
- Antagonize effects of pentagastrin and histamine during gastric acid secretion testing. Avoid administration for 24 hr before the test.
- May cause false-negative results in skin tests using allergenic extracts. Histamine H₂ antagonists should be discontinued 24 hr before the test.
- May cause ↑ in serum transaminases and serum creatinine.
- Serum prolactin concentration may be ↑ after IV bolus of *cimetidine*. May also cause ↓ parathyroid concentrations.
- *Nizatidine* may cause ↑ alkaline phosphatase concentrations.
- *Ranitidine* and *famotidine* may cause false-positive results for urine protein; test with sulfosalicylic acid.

Potential Nursing Diagnoses
Acute pain (Indications)

Implementation
- **PO:** Administer with meals or immediately afterward and at bedtime to prolong effect.
- If antacids or sucralfate are used concurrently for relief of pain, avoid administration of antacids within 30 min-1 hr of the H₂ antagonist and take sucralfate 2 hr after H₂ antagonist; may ↓ absorption of H₂ antagonist.
- Doses administered once daily should be administered at bedtime to prolong effect.
- Shake oral suspension before administration. Discard unused suspension after 30 days.
- Remove foil from *ranitidine effervescent tablets* and dissolve in 6–8 oz water before drinking.

✦ = Canadian drug name. ❀ = Genetic implication.
*CAPITALS indicates life-threatening; underlines indicate most frequent.

Cimetidine

IV Administration

- **Direct IV:** *Diluent:* Dilute each 300 mg in 20 mL of 0.9% NaCl for injection. *Concentration:* Final concentration will be 13.7 mg/mL. *Rate:* Administer over at least 5 min. Rapid administration may cause hypotension and arrhythmias.
- **Intermittent Infusion:** *Diluent:* Dilute each 300 mg in 50 mL of 0.9% NaCl, D5W, D10W, D5/LR, D5/0.9% NaCl, D5/0.45% NaCl, D5/0.25% NaCl, Ringer's or lactated Ringer's solution, or sodium bicarbonate. *Concentration:* Final concentration will be 5.8 mg/mL. Diluted solution is stable for 48 hr at room temperature. Refrigeration may cause cloudiness but will not affect potency. Do not use solution that is discolored or contains precipitate. *Rate:* Administer over 15–20 min.
- **Continuous Infusion:** Dilute cimetidine 900 mg in 100–1000 mL of compatible solution (see Direct IV).
- **Rate:** Usually infused at a rate of 37.5 mg/hr or greater but should be individualized.
- **Y-Site Compatibility:** acyclovir, alfentanil, amifostine, amikacin, aminophylline, amphotericin B liposome, anikinra, anidulafungin, ascorbic acid, atracurium, atropine, aztreonam, bivalirudin, bumetanide, buprenorphine, butorphanol, calcium chloride, calcium gluconate, carboplatin, caspofungin, cefazolin, cefonocid, cefotaxime, cefotetan, cefoxitin, ceftazidime, ceftizoxime, ceftriaxone, cefuroxime, chlorpromazine, cisatracurium, cisplatin, cladribine, clindamycin, cyanocobalamin, cyclophosphamide, cyclosporine, cytarabine, dactinomycin, daptomycin, ddexamethasone, dexmedetomidine, digoxin, diltiazem, diphenhydramine, dobutamine, docetaxel, dopamine, doripenem, doxacurium, doxorubicin hydrochloride, doxorubicin liposome, doxycycline, enalaprilat, ephedrine, epinephrine, epirubicin, epoetin alfa, ertapenem, erythromycin, esmolol, etoposide, etoposide phosphate, famotidine, fenoldopam, fentanyl, filgrastim, fluconazole, fludarabine, fluorouracil, folic acid, foscarnet, gemcitabine, gentamicin, glycopyrrolate, granisetron, heparin, hetastarch, hydrocortisone, hydromorphone, idarubicin, ifosfamide, imipenem/cilastatin, isoproterenol, ketorolac, labetalol, levofloxacin, lidocaine, linezolid, lorazepam, magnesium sulfate, mannitol, mechlorethamine, melphalan, meperidine, meropenem, metaraminol, methotrexate, methoxamine, methyldopate, methylprednisolone, metoclopramide, metoprolol, metronidazole, midazolam, milrinone, mitoxantrone, morphine, multivitamins, nafcillin, nalbuphine, naloxone, nesiritide, nicardipine, nitroglycerin, nitroprusside, norepinephrine, octreotide, ondansetron, oxacillin, oxaliplatin, oxytocin, paclitaxel, palonosetron, pancuronium, papaverine, pemetrexed, penicillin G, pentamidine, pentazocine, phentolamine, phenylephrine, phytonadione, piperacillin/tazobactam, potassium chloride, procainamide, prochlorperazine, promethazine, propofol, propranolol, protamine, pyridoxime, quniupristin/dalfopristin, ranitidine, remifentanil, rituximab, rocuronium, sargramostim, sodium acetate, sodium bicarbonate, streptokinase, succinylcholine, sufentanil, tacrolimus, teniposide, theophylline, thiamine, thiotepa, ticarcillin/clavulanate, tigecycline, tirofiban, tobramycin, tolazoline, topotecan, trastuzumab, trimetaphan, urokinase, vancomycin, vecuronium, verapamil, vincristine, vinorelbine, voriconazole, zidovudine.
- **Y-Site Incompatibility:** allopurinol, amphotericin B cholesteryl, amphotericin B colloidal, amsacrine, azathioprine, cefepime, cefoperazone, chloramphenicol, dantrolene, diazepam, diazoxide, furosemide, ganciclovir, indomethacin, pantoprazole, pentobarbital, phenobarbital, phenytoin, trimethoprim/sulfamethoxazole, warfarin.

Famotidine

IV Administration

- **Direct IV:** *Diluent:* 0.9% NaCl, D5W, D10W, or LR. *Concentration:* 4 mg/mL. *Rate:* Administer at a rate of 10 mg/min. Rapid administration may cause hypotension.
- **Intermittent Infusion:** *Diluent:* Dilute each 20 mg in 100 mL of 0.9% NaCl, D5W, D10W, or LR. Diluted solution is stable for 48 hr at room temperature. Do not use solution that is discolored or contains a precipitate. *Concentration:* 0.2 mg/mL. *Rate:* Administer over 15–30 min.
- **Y-Site Compatibility:** acyclovir, alfentanil, allopurinol, amifostine, amikacin, aminophylline, amiodarone, amphotericin B liposome, amsacrine, anakinra, anidulafungin, ascorbic acid, atracurium, atropine, aztreonam, benztropine, bivalirudin, bleomycin, bumetanide, buprenorphine, butorphanol, calcium chloride, calcium gluconate, carboplatin, caspofungin, cefonocid, cefotaxime, cefotetan, cefoxitin, ceftazidime, cefuroxime, chlorpromazine, cimetidine, cisatracurium, cisplatin, cladribine,

HISTAMINE H₂ ANTAGONISTS

clindamycin, codeine, cyanocobalamin, cyclophosphamide, cyclosporine, cytarabine, dactinomycin, daptomycin, dexamethasone, dexmedetomidine, dextran 40, digoxin, diltiazem, diphenhydramine, dobutamine, docetaxel, dopamine, doripenem, doxacurium, doxorubicin, doxorubicin liposome, doxycycline, droperidol, enalaprilat, ephedrine, epinephrine, epirubicin, epoetin alfa, eftifibitide, ertapenem, erythromycin lactobionate, esmolol, etoposide, etoposide phosphate, fenoldopam, fentanyl, filgrastim, fluconazole, fludarabine, fluorouracil, folic acid, gemcitabine, gentamicin, glycopyrrolate, granisetron, heparin, hetastarch, hydrocortisone, hydromorphone, idarubicin, ifosfamide, imipenem/cilastatin, isoproterenol, ketorolac, labetalol, levofloxacin, lidocaine, linezolid, lorazepam, magnesium sulfate, mannitol, melphalan, meperidine, metaraminol, methotrexate, methoxamine, methyldopate, methylprednisolone, metoclopramide, metoprolol, metronidazole, midazolam, milrinone, mitoxantrone, morphine, multivitamins, nafcillin, nalbuphine, naloxone, nesiritide, nicardipine, nitroglycerin, nitroprusside, norepinephrine, octreotide, ondansetron, oxacillin, oxaliplatin, oxytocin, paclitaxel, palonosetron, pancuronium, papaverine, pemetrexed, penicillin G, pentamidine, pentazocine, pentobarbital, perphenazine, phenobarbital, phentolamine, phenylephrine, phenytoin, phytonadione, potassium chloride, potassium phosphates, procainamide, prochlorperazine, promethazine, propofol, propranolol, protamine, pyridoxime, ranitidine, remifentanil, rituximab, sargramostim, sodium acetate, sodium bicarbonate, streptokinase, succinylcholine, sufentanil, tacrolimus, teniposide, theophylline, thiamine, thiotepa, ticarcillin/clavulanate, tigecycline, tirofiban, tobramycin, tolazoline, trastuzumab, trimetaphan, urokinase, vancomycin, vasopressin, vecuronium, verapamil, vincristine, vinorelbine, voriconazole.

- **Y-Site Incompatibility:** amphotericin B cholesteryl, amphotericin B colloidal, azathioprine, azithromycin, cefepime, cefapirin, chloramphenicol, dantrolene, diazepam, diazoxide, ganciclovir, indomethacin, pantoprazole, piperacillin/tazobactam, trimethoprim/sulfamethoxazole.

Ranitidine

IV Administration

- **Direct IV:** *Diluent:* 0.9% NaCl or D5W for injection. *Concentration:* 2.5 mg/mL. *Rate:* Administer over at least 5 min not to exceed 10 mg/min. Rapid administration may cause hypotension and arrhythmias.
- **Intermittent Infusion:** *Diluent:* Dilute each 50 mg in 100 mL of 0.9% NaCl or D5W. Diluted solution is stable for 48 hr at room temperature. Do not use solution that is discolored or that contains precipitate. *Concentration:* 0.5 mg/mL. *Rate:* Administer over 15–30 min.
- **Continuous Infusion:** *Diluent:* D5W. *Concentration:* 150 mg/250 mL (no greater than 2.5 mg/mL for Zollinger-Ellison patients). *Rate:* Administer at a rate of 6.25 mg/hr. In patients with Zollinger-Ellison syndrome, start infusion at 1 mg/kg/hr. If gastric acid output is >10 mEq/hr or patient becomes symptomatic after 4 hr, adjust dose by 0.5 mg/kg/hr increments and remeasure gastric output.
- **Y-Site Compatibility:** acyclovir, aldesleukin, alfentanil, allopurinol, amifostine, amikacin, aminophylline, amphotericin B liposome, amsacrine, anikinra, anidulafungin, ascorbic acid, atracurium, atropine, aztreonam, bivalirudin, bumetanide, buprenorphine, butorphanol, calcium chloride, calcium gluconate, carboplatin, cefazolin, cefepime, cefonicid, cefoperazone, cefotaxime, cefotetan, cefoxitin, ceftazidime, ceftizoxime, ceftriaxone, cefuroxime, chloramphenicol, chlorpromazine, cimetidine, ciprofloxacin, cisatracurium, cisplatin, clindamycin, cyanocobalamin, cyclophosphamide, cyclosporine, cytarabine, dactinomycin, daptomycin, dexamethasone, dexmedetomidine, digoxin, diltiazem, dobutamine, docetaxel, dopamine, doripenem, doxacurium, doxapram, doxorubicin hydrochloride, doxorubicin liposome, doxycycline, enalaprilat, ephedrine, epinephrine, epirubicin, epoetin alfa, ertapenem, erythromycin, esmolol, etoposide, etoposide phosphate, famotidine, fenoldopam, fentanyl, filgrastim, fluconazole, fludarabine, fluorouracil, folic acid, foscarnet, furosemide, ganciclovir, gemcitabine, gentamicin, glycopyrrolate, granisetron, heparin, hydrocortisone, hydromorphone, idarubicin, ifosfamide, imipenem/cilastatin, inamrinone, indomethacin, isoproterenol, ketorolac, labetalol, levofloxacin, lidocaine, linezolid, lorazepam, magnesium

✱ = Canadian drug name.   H = Genetic implication.
*CAPITALS indicates life-threatening; underlines indicate most frequent.

sulfate, mannitol, mechlorethamine, melphalan, meperidine, metaraminol, methotrexate, methoxamine, methyldopa, methylprednisolone, metoclopramide, metoprolol, metronidazole, midazolam, milrinone, mitoxantrone, morphine, multivitamin, nalbuphine, naloxone, nesiritide, nicardipine, nitroglycerin, nitroprusside, norepinephrine, octreotide, ondansetron, oxacillin, oxaliplatin, oxytocin, paclitaxel, palonosetron, pancuronium, papaverine, pemetrexed, penicillin G, pentamidine, pentazocine, pentobarbital, phenobarbital, phentolamine, phenylephrine, phytonadione, piperacillin/tazobactam, potassium chloride, procainamide, prochlorperazine, promethazine, propofol, propranolol, protamine, pyridoxime, remifentanil, rituximab, rocuronium, sargramostim, sodium acetate, sodium bicarbonate, strepotkinase, succinylcholine, sufentanil, tacrolimus, teniposide, theophylline, thiamine, thiopental, thiotepa, ticarcillin/clavulanate, tigecycline, tirofiban, tobramycin, tolazoline, trastuzumab, trimethaphan, urokinase, vancomycin, vecuronium, vincristine, vinorelbine, warfarin, zidovudine.

- **Y-Site Incompatibility:** amphotericin B cholesteryl, caspofungin, diazepam, diazoxide, insulin, pantoprazole, phenytoin, quinupristin/dalfopristin, trimethoprim/sulfamethoxazole.

Patient/Family Teaching

- Instruct patient to take medication as directed for the full course of therapy, even if feeling better. Take missed doses as soon as remembered but not if almost time for next dose. Do not double doses.
- Advise patients taking OTC preparations not to take the maximum dose continuously for more than 2 wk without consulting health care professional. Notify health care professional if difficulty swallowing occurs or abdominal pain persists.
- Inform patient that smoking interferes with the action of histamine antagonists. Encourage patient to quit smoking or at least not to smoke after last dose of the day.
- May cause drowsiness or dizziness. Caution patient to avoid driving or other activities requiring alertness until response to the drug is known.
- Advise patient to avoid alcohol, products containing aspirin or NSAIDs, and foods that may cause an increase in GI irritation.
- Inform patient that increased fluid and fiber intake and exercise may minimize constipation.
- Advise patient to report onset of black, tarry stools; fever; sore throat; diarrhea; dizziness; rash; confusion; or hallucinations to health care professional promptly.

Evaluation/Desired Outcomes

- Decrease in abdominal pain.
- Treatment and prevention of gastric or duodenal irritation and bleeding. Healing of duodenal ulcers can be seen by x-rays or endoscopy. Therapy is continued for at least 6 wk in treatment of ulcers but not usually longer than 8 wk.
- Decreased symptoms of esophageal reflux.
- Treatment of heartburn, acid indigestion, and sour stomach (OTC use).

HMG-CoA REDUCTASE INHIBITORS (statins)

atorvastatin (a-**tore**-va-stat-in)
Lipitor

fluvastatin (**floo**-va-sta-tin)
Lescol, Lescol XL

lovastatin (**loe**-va-sta-tin)
Altoprev, Mevacor

pitavastatin (pi-**tav**a-sta-tin)
Livalo

pravastatin (**pra**-va-sta-tin)
Pravachol

rosuvastatin (roe-**soo**-va-sta-tin)
Crestor

simvastatin (**sim**-va-sta-tin)
Zocor

Classification
Therapeutic: lipid-lowering agents
Pharmacologic: HMG-CoA reductase inhibitors

Pregnancy Category X

Indications

Adjunctive management of primary hypercholesterolemia and mixed dyslipidemias. **Atorvastatin:** Primary prevention of cardiovascular disease (↓ risk of MI or stroke) in patients with multiple risk factors for coronary heart disease CHD or type 2 diabetes mellitus (also ↓ risk of angina or revascsularization procedures in patients with multiple risk factors for CHD). **Atorvastatin and Pravastatin:** Secondary prevention of cardiovascular disease (↓ risk of MI, stroke, revascularization procedures, angina, and hospitalizations

HMG-CoA REDUCTASE INHIBITORS (statins)

for CHF) in patients with clinically evident CHD. **Fluvastatin:** Secondary prevention of coronary revascularizations procedures in patients with clinically evident CHD. **Fluvastatin, lovastatin, and rosuvastatin:** Slow progression of coronary atherosclerosis in patients with CHD. **Lovastatin:** Primary prevention of CHD (↓ risk of MI, unstable angina, and coronary revascularization) in patients without symptomatic cardiovascular disease with ↑ total and low-density lipoprotein (LDL) cholesterol and ↓ high-density lipoprotein (HDL) cholesterol. **Pravastatin:** Primary prevention of CHD (↓ risk of MI, coronary revascularization, and cardiovascular mortality) in patients without clinically evident CHD. **Simvastatin:** Secondary prevention of cardiovascular events (↓ risk of MI, coronary revascularization, stroke, and cardiovascular mortality) in patients with clinically evident CHD or those at high-risk for CHD (history of diabetes, peripheral arterial disease, or stroke).

Action
Inhibit an enzyme, 3-hydroxy-3-methylglutaryl-coenzyme A (HMG-CoA) reductase, which is responsible for catalyzing an early step in the synthesis of cholesterol. **Therapeutic Effects:** Lowers total and LDL cholesterol and triglycerides. Slightly increase HDL. Slows of the progression of coronary atherosclerosis with resultant decrease in CHD-related events (all agents except rosuvastatin have indication for ↓ events).

Pharmacokinetics
Absorption: *Atorvastatin*—rapidly absorbed but undergoes extensive GI and hepatic metabolism, resulting in 14% bioavailability; *fluvastatin*—98% absorbed after oral administration, but undergoes extensive first-pass metabolism resulting in 24% bioavailability; *lovastatin, pravastatin*—poorly and variably absorbed after oral administration; *pitavastatin*-well absorbed (51%) after oral administration; *rosuvastatin*—20% absorbed following oral administration; *simvastatin*—85% absorbed but rapidly metabolized.

Distribution: *Atorvastatin*—probably enters breast milk. *Fluvastatin*—enters breast milk. *Lovastatin*—crosses the blood-brain barrier and placenta. *Pravastatin*—small amounts enter breast milk. *Pitavastatin, rosuvastatin, and simvastatin*—unknown.

Protein Binding: *Atorvastatin, fluvastatin, pitavastatin, and simvastatin*->98%.

Metabolism and Excretion: All agents are extensively metabolized by the liver; amount excreted unchanged in urine: *atorvastatin*—<2%, *lovastatin*—10%, *fluvastatin*—5%, *pitavastatin*-15%, *pravastatin*—20%, and *simvastatin*—13%.

Half-life: *Atorvastatin*—14 hr; *fluvastatin*—1.2 hr; *lovastatin*—3 hr; *pitavastatin*—12 hr; *pravastatin*—1.3–2.7 hr; *rosuvastatin*—19 hr; *simvastatin*—unknown.

TIME/ACTION PROFILE (cholesterol-lowering effect)

ROUTE	ONSET	PEAK	DURATION*
Atorvastatin	unknown	unknown	20–30 hr
Fluvastatin	1–2 wk	4–6 wk	unknown
Lovastatin	2 wk	4–6 wk	6 wk
Pitavastatin	within 4 wk	4 wk	unknown
Pravastatin	several days	2–4 wk	unknown
Rosuvastatin	unknown	2–4 wk	unknown
Simvastatin	several days	2–4 wk	unknown

*After discontinuation

Contraindications/Precautions
Contraindicated in: Hypersensitivity; Active liver disease or unexplained persistent ↑ in AST or ALT; Concurrent use of gemfibrozil or azole antifungals; Concurrent use of nelfinavir or ritonavir (with lovastatin or simvastatin); *Pitavastatin*—concurrent use of cyclosporine or lopinavir/ritonavir (with pitavastatin); *Pitavastatin*—severe renal impairment (CCr <30 mL/min); OB: Potential for fetal anomalies; Lactation: May disrupt infant lipid metabolism.

Use Cautiously in: History of liver disease; Alcoholism; ▨ *Rosuvastatin*—patients with Asian ancestry (may have ↑ blood levels and ↑ risk of rhabdomyolysis); *Atorvastatin, lovastatin, rosuvastatin, and simvastatin*—concurrent use of gemfibrozil, azole antifungals, macrolides, protease inhibitors, niacin, cyclosporine, amiodarone or verapamil (↑ risk of myopathy/rhabdomyolysis); *Pitavastatin*—Hypothyroidism, concurrent use of fibrates or lipid-lowering doses of niacin (↑ risk of myopathy); Renal impairment; Geri: *Pitavastatin*— ↑ risk of myopathy (age >65 yr); OB: Women of childbearing age; Pedi: Safety not established in children <8 yr (; some products approved for use in older children only.

Adverse Reactions/Side Effects
CNS: dizziness, headache, insomnia, weakness. **CV:** chest pain, peripheral edema. **EENT:** rhinitis; *lovastatin*, blurred vision. **Resp:** bronchitis. **GI:**

✦ = Canadian drug name. ▨ = Genetic implication.
*CAPITALS indicates life-threatening; underlines indicate most frequent.

abdominal cramps, constipation, diarrhea, flatus, heartburn, altered taste, drug-induced hepatitis, dyspepsia, elevated liver enzymes, nausea, pancreatitis. **GU:** erectile dysfunction. **Derm:** rashes, pruritus. **MS:** RHABDOMYOLYSIS, arthralgia, arthritis, myalgia, myositis. **Misc:** hypersensitivity reactions.

Interactions
Atorvastatin, lovastatin, simvastatin, and rosuvastatin are metabolized by the CYP3A4 metabolic pathway. Fluvastatin is metabolized by CYP 2C9. Pravastatin is not metabolized by the CYP P450 system.

Drug-Drug: Atorvastatin, lovastatin, and simvastatin may interact with **CYP3A4 inhibitors**. Bioavailability and effectiveness may be ↓ by **cholestyramine** and **colestipol**. Risk of myopathy with atorvastatin, lovastatin, and simvastatin is ↑ with **amiodarone, cyclosporine, gemfibrozil, clofibrate, diltiazem, verapamil, erythromycin, clarithromycin, telithromycin, nefazodone**, large doses of **niacin, azole antifungals, nelfinavir, saquinavir**, and **ritonavir**. Atorvastatin, fluvastatin, and simvastatin may slightly ↑ serum **digoxin** levels. Atorvastatin and rosuvastatin may ↑ levels of **hormonal contraceptives**. Atorvastatin, fluvastatin, lovastatin, rosuvastatin, and simvastatin may ↑ risk of bleeding with **warfarin**. **Isradipine** may ↓ the effectiveness of lovastatin. **Alcohol, cimetidine, ranitidine**, and **omeprazole** may ↑ fluvastatin levels. **Rifampin** may ↓ fluvastatin levels. **Antacids** ↓ absorption of rosuvastatin (administer 2 hr after rosuvastatin. **Lopinavir/ritonavir** may ↑ pitavastatin and rosuvastatin levels. **Cyclosporine** ↑ levels and risk of toxicity of pitavastatin and rosuvastatin (dosage adjustment of rosuvastatin required; avoid use with pitavastatin). Fluvastatin ↑ levels of **glyburide**; **glyburide** ↑ fluvastatin levels (monitoring of both agents recommended). Fluvastatin ↑ levels of **phenytoin**; **phenytoin** ↑ fluvastatin levels (monitoring of both agents recommended). **Erythromycin** and **rifampin** may ↑ blood levels of pitavastatin.
Drug-Natural Products: St. John's wort may ↓ levels and effectiveness (lovastatin and simvastatin).
Drug-Food: Large quantities of **grapefruit juice** ↑ blood levels and ↑ risk of rhabdomyolysis. **Food** enhances blood levels of lovastatin.

Route/Dosage

Atorvastatin
PO (Adults): 10–20 mg once daily initially (may start with 40 mg/day if LDL should be lowered by >45%); may be increased q 2–4 wk up to 80 mg/day.
PO (Children 10–17 yr): 10 mg/day initially, may be ↑ q 4 wk up to 20 mg/day.

Fluvastatin
PO (Adults): 20 mg (capsule) once daily at bedtime (may start with 40 mg once daily at bedtime if LDL needs to be lowered by ≥25%). May be ↑ to 80 mg once daily (as extended-release tablet) or 40 mg twice daily (capsule).

Lovastatin
PO (Adults): 20 mg once daily with evening meal. May be ↑ at 4-wk intervals to a maximum of 80 mg/day (immediate-release) or 60 mg/day (extended-release); initiate at 10 mg/day in patients receiving cyclosporine or other immunosuppressants and do not exceed 20 mg/day; should not exceed 40 mg/day (immediate-release) or 20 mg/day (extended-release) if receiving verapamil or amiodarone; should not exceed 20 mg/day if receiving danazol or niacin (>1 g/day).

Renal Impairment
PO (Adults): *CCr < 30 mL/min*—dosage should not exceed 20 mg/day unless carefully titrated.
PO (Children/Adolescents 10-17 yr): *Familial heterozygous hypercholesterolemia*—10-40 mg/day adjusted at 4-wk intervals.

Pitavastatin
PO (Adults): 2 mg once daily initially, may be increased up to 4 mg depending on response; *Concurrent erythromycin therapy*—daily dose should not exceed 1 mg; *Concurrent rifampin therapy*—daily dose should not exceed 2 mg.

Renal Impairment
PO (Adults): *CCr 30– <60 mL/min*—1 mg once daily initially, may be ↑ up to 2 mg daily.

Pravastatin
PO (Adults): 40 mg once daily at bedtime; may be ↑ at 4-wk intervals up to maximum of 80 mg/day. *Concurrent cyclosporine therapy*—initial dose is 10 mg/day and should not exceed 20 mg/day.
PO (Children 14-18 yrs): 40 mg once daily.
PO (Children 8-13 yrs): 20 mg once daily.

Hepatic/Renal Impairment
PO (Adults): 10–20 mg once daily at bedtime; ↑ at 4-wk intervals as needed (usual range = 10–20 mg/day).

Rosuvastatin

PO (Adults): 10 mg once daily initially (range 5–20 mg initially); dose may be adjusted at 2–4 wk intervals, some patients may require up to 40 mg/day (associated with ↑ risk of rhabdomyolysis); *Patients with Asian ancestry*—initial dose should not exceed 5 mg/day; *Concurrent cyclosporine therapy*—dose should not exceed 5 mg/day; *Concurrent gemfibrozil or lopinavir/ritonavir therapy*—dose should not exceed 10 mg/day (avoid if possible).

Renal Impairment
PO (Adults): *CCr <30 mL/min*—5 mg once daily intially; dose may be ↑ but should not exceed 10 mg/day.

Simvastatin

PO (Adults): 5–80 mg once daily in the evening. *Concurrent cyclosporine or danazol therapy*—Initiate at 5 mg once daily; dose should not exceed 10 mg/day. *Concurrent fibrate or niacin therapy*—Dose should not exceed 10 mg/day. *Concurrent amiodarone or verapamil therapy*—Dose should not exceed 20 mg/day.
PO (Children and Adolescents 10–17 yr): 10 mg once daily initially, may be ↑ at 4-wk intervals up to 40 mg/day (not to exceed 10 mg/day in patients receiving cyclosporine, danazol, fibrates, or niacin or 20 mg/day in patients receiving amiodarone or verapamil).

Renal Impairment
PO (Adults): *CCr <10 mL/min*—5 mg/day initially, titrate carefully.

Availability

Atorvastatin
Tablets: 10 mg, 20 mg, 40 mg, 80 mg. **Cost:** 10 mg $237.99/90, 20 mg $321.97/90, 40 mg $325.97/90, 80 mg $329.97/90. *In combination with:* amlodipine (Caduet); see Appendix B.

Fluvastatin
Capsules: 20 mg, 40 mg. **Cost:** 20 mg $205.97/90, 40 mg $205.97/90. **Extended-release tablets:** 80 mg. **Cost:** 80 mg $265.99/90.

Lovastatin (generic available)
Immediate-release tablets : 10 mg, 20 mg, 40 mg. **Cost:** 10 mg $89.70/60, 20 mg $158.19/60, 40 mg $284.76/60. **Extended-release tablets:** 10 mg, 20 mg, 40 mg, 60 mg. *In combination with:* Niacin (Advicor). See Appendix B.

Pitavastatin
Tablets: 1 mg, 2 mg, 4 mg.

Pravastatin (generic available)
Tablets: 10 mg, 20 mg, 40 mg, 80 mg. **Cost:** 10 mg $169.97/90, 20 mg $44.67/90, 40 mg $49.97/90, 80 mg $379.72/90.

Rosuvastatin
Tablets: 5 mg, 10 mg, 20 mg, 40 mg. **Cost:** 5 mg $275.96/90, 10 mg $275.96/90, 20 mg $275.96/90, 40 mg $278.96/90.

Simvastatin (generic available)
Tablets: 5 mg, 10 mg, 20 mg, 40 mg, 80 mg. **Cost:** *Generic*—5 mg $45.97/90, 10 mg $49.97/90, 20 mg $73.97/90, 40 mg $75.97/90, 80 mg $89.97/90. *In combination with:* Ezetimibe (Vytorin). See Appendix B.

NURSING IMPLICATIONS

Assessment
- Obtain a dietary history, especially with regard to fat consumption.
- *Lab Test Considerations:* Evaluate serum cholesterol and triglyceride levels before initiating, after 4–6 wk of therapy, and periodically thereafter.
- Monitor liver function tests, including AST, before, at 12 wk after initiation of therapy or after dose elevation, and then q 6 mo. If AST levels ↑ to 3 times normal, HMG-CoA reductase inhibitor therapy should be reduced or discontinued. May also cause ↑ alkaline phosphatase and bilirubin levels.
- If patient develops muscle tenderness during therapy, monitor CK levels. If CK levels are >10 times the upper limit of normal or myopathy occurs, therapy should be discontinued.

Potential Nursing Diagnoses
Noncompliance (Patient/Family Teaching)

Implementation
- Do not confuse Pravachol (pravastatin) with Prevacid (lansoprazole).
- **PO:** Administer *lovastatin* with food. Administration on an empty stomach decreases absorption by approximately 30%. Initial once-daily dose is administered with the evening meal.
- Administer extended-release tablets at bedtime. Extended-release tablets should be swallowed whole, do not break, crush, or chew.
- Administer *fluvastatin, pravastatin,* and *simvastatin* once daily in the evening. *Atorvasta-*

tin, *pitavastatin*, and *rosuvastatin* can be taken any time of day. May be administered without regard to food.
- Avoid large amounts of grapefruit juice during therapy; may ↑ risk of toxicity.
- If *fluvastatin* or *pravastatin* is administered in conjunction with bile acid sequestrants (cholestyramine, colestipol), administer at least 4 hr after bile acid sequestrant.
- If *rosuvastatin* is administered in conjunction with magnesium or aluminum-containing antacids, administer antacid at least 2 hr after *rosuvastatin*.

Patient/Family Teaching
- Instruct patient to take medication as directed and not to skip doses or double up on missed doses. Advise patient to avoid drinking more that 200 mL/day of grapefruit juice during therapy. Medication helps control but does not cure elevated serum cholesterol levels.
- Advise patient that this medication should be used in conjunction with diet restrictions (fat, cholesterol, carbohydrates, alcohol), exercise, and cessation of smoking.
- Instruct patient to notify health care professional if unexplained muscle pain, tenderness, or weakness occurs, especially if accompanied by fever or malaise.
- Advise patient to avoid taking Rx, OTC, or herbal products without consulting with a health care professional.
- Instruct female patients to notify health care professional promptly if pregnancy is planned or suspected. Advise women of childbearing age to use effective contraception during therapy and discuss plans to discontinue pitavastatin if trying to conceive. Advise patients to avoid breastfeeding during therapy.
- Advise patient to notify health care professional of medication regimen before treatment or surgery.
- Emphasize the importance of follow-up exams to determine effectiveness and to monitor for side effects.

Evaluation/Desired Outcomes
- Decrease in LDL and total cholesterol levels.
- Increase in HDL cholesterol levels.
- Decrease in triglyceride levels.
- Slowing of the progression of coronary artery disease.

human papillomavirus quadrivalent (types 6, 11, 16, and 18) vaccine, recombinant
(hyoo-man pa-pil-lo-ma)
Gardasil

Classification
Therapeutic: vaccines/immunizing agents

Indications
Prevention of cervical, vulvar, and vaginal cancers and genital warts (in females) and genital warts (in males).

Action
Vaccination results in antibodies to HPV viruses that are causative agents for cervical, vulvar, and vaginal cancers and genital warts. **Therapeutic Effects:** Prevention of cervical, vulvar, and vaginal cancers and genital warts.

Pharmacokinetics
Absorption: Well absorbed following IM administration.
Distribution: Unknown.
Metabolism and Excretion: Unknown.
Half-life: Unknown.

TIME/ACTION PROFILE (antibody response)

ROUTE	ONSET	PEAK	DURATION
IM	unknown	1 mo*	unknown

*After third vaccination

Contraindications/Precautions
Contraindicated in: Hypersensitivity; Thrombocytopenia/bleeding disorder; OB: Limited data available; use only if potential benefit justifies potential risk to fetus.
Use Cautiously in: Current/recent febrile illness; Immunosuppression may ↓ antibody response; Lactation: Excretion into breast milk unknown; Pedi: Safety not established in children <9 yr.

Adverse Reactions/Side Effects
Neuro: fainting. **Local:** injection site reactions. **Misc:** ANAPHYLAXIS (RARE).

Interactions
Drug-Drug: **Immunosuppressants** or **antineoplastics** may ↓ antibody response.

Route/Dosage
IM (Adults and Children — males and females 9–26 yr): Three 0.5 mL doses at 0, 2, and 6 mo.

Availability
Sterile preparation for intramuscular administration: 20 mcg of HPV 6 L1 protein, 40 mcg of HPV 11 L1 protein, 40 mcg of HPV 16 L1 protein, and 20 mcg of HPV 18 L1 protein/0.5-mL dose.

NURSING IMPLICATIONS
Assessment
- Assess vital signs prior to administration. Do not administer to patient with a current or recent febrile illness; low grade fever (<100°F) and mild upper respiratory infection are usually not contraindicated.
- Monitor patient for 15 min following injection for fainting. Patient should remain lying down or seated to prevent falls or injury.

Potential Nursing Diagnoses
Risk for infection (Indications)

Implementation
- Vaccine is not intended for treatment of active genital warts or cervical cancer and will not protect from diseases not caused by HPV.
- **IM:** Prefilled syringe is for single use; do not use for more than one person. Administer as supplied; do not dilute; administer full dose. Shake well prior to administration to maintain suspension of vaccine. Solution is cloudy and white; do not administer solution that is discolored or contains particulate matter. If using single-dose vial, withdraw 0.5 mL dose and administer entire contents of syringe. Administer intramuscularly in the deltoid or in the high anterolateral area of the thigh.

Patient/Family Teaching
- Provide information about vaccine and the importance of completing immunization series unless contraindicated to patient and guardian.
- Inform patient that vaccine does not replace routine cervical cancer screening or prevent other sexually transmitted diseases; such screening should be continued as usual.
- Advise patient to consult health care professional prior to taking Rx, OTC, or herbal products.
- Advise patient to notify health care professional if pregnancy is planned or suspected. Women exposed to vaccine during pregnancy are encouraged to call manufacturer pregnancy registry at 800-986-8999.
- Instruct patient to report any adverse reactions to health care professional.

Evaluation/Desired Outcomes
- Prevention of cervical cancer, genital warts, cervical adenocarcinoma in situ, cervical, vulvar, and vaginal intraepithelial neoplasia caused by HPV.

hydrALAZINE
(hye-**dral**-a-zeen)
Apresoline, ✦ Novo-Hylazin

Classification
Therapeutic: antihypertensives
Pharmacologic: vasodilators

Pregnancy Category C

Indications
Moderate to severe hypertension (with a diuretic). **Unlabeled Use:** CHF unresponsive to conventional therapy with digoxin and diuretics.

Action
Direct-acting peripheral arteriolar vasodilator.
Therapeutic Effects: Lowering of blood pressure in hypertensive patients and decreased afterload in patients with CHF.

Pharmacokinetics
Absorption: Rapidly absorbed following oral administration; well absorbed from IM sites.
Distribution: Widely distributed. Crosses the placenta; enters breast milk in minimal concentrations.
Metabolism and Excretion: Mostly metabolized by the GI mucosa and liver by N-acetyltransferase (rate of acetylation is genetically determined [slow acetylators have ↑ hydralazine levels and ↑ risk of toxicity; fast acetylators have ↓ hydralazine levels and ↓ response]).
Half-life: 2–8 hr.

TIME/ACTION PROFILE (antihypertensive effect)

ROUTE	ONSET	PEAK	DURATION
PO	45 min	2 hr	2–4 hr
IM	10–30 min	1 hr	3–8 hr
IV	5–20 min	15–30 min	2–6 hr

Contraindications/Precautions
Contraindicated in: Hypersensitivity; Some products contain tartrazine and should be avoided in patients with known intolerance.
Use Cautiously in: Cardiovascular or cerebrovascular disease; Severe renal and hepatic disease

✦ = Canadian drug name. = Genetic implication.
*CAPITALS indicates life-threatening; underlines indicate most frequent.

(dose modification may be necessary); OB, Lactation: Has been used safely during pregnancy.

Adverse Reactions/Side Effects
CNS: dizziness, drowsiness, headache. **CV:** <u>tachycardia</u>, angina, arrhythmias, edema, orthostatic hypotension. **GI:** diarrhea, nausea, vomiting. **Derm:** rashes. **F and E:** <u>sodium retention</u>. **MS:** arthralgias, arthritis. **Neuro:** peripheral neuropathy. **Misc:** <u>drug-induced lupus syndrome</u>.

Interactions
Drug-Drug: ↑ hypotension with acute ingestion of **alcohol**, other **antihypertensives**, or **nitrates**. **MAO inhibitors** may exaggerate hypotension. May ↓ pressor response to **epinephrine**. **NSAIDs** may ↓ antihypertensive response. **Beta blockers** ↓ tachycardia from hydralazine (therapy may be combined for this reason). **Metoprolol** and **propranolol** ↑ hydralazine levels. ↑ blood levels of **metoprolol** and **propranolol**.

Route/Dosage
PO (Adults): *Hypertension*—10 mg 4 times daily initially. After 2–4 days may ↑ to 25 mg 4 times daily for the rest of the 1st week; may then ↑ to 50 mg 4 times daily (up to 300 mg/day). Once maintenance dose is established, twice-daily dosing may be used. *CHF*—25–37.5 mg 4 times daily; may be ↑ up to 300 mg/day in 3–4 divided doses.

PO (Children > 1 mo): Initial—0.75–1 mg/kg/day in 2–4 divided doses, not to exceed 25 mg/dose; may ↑ gradually to 5 mg/kg/day in infants and 7.5 mg/kg/day in children (not to exceed 200 mg/day) in 2–4 divided doses.

IM, IV (Adults): *Hypertension*—5–40 mg repeated as needed. *Eclampsia*—5 mg q 15–20 min; if no response after a total of 20 mg, consider an alternative agent.

IM, IV (Children > 1 mo): Initial—0.1–0.2 mg/kg/dose (not to exceed 20 mg) q 4–6 hr as needed, up 1.7–3.5 mg/kg/day in 4–6 divided doses.

Availability (generic available)
Tablets: 10 mg, 25 mg, 50 mg, 100 mg. **Cost:** *Generic*—10 mg $23.30/100, 25 mg $22.90/100, 50 mg $23.30/100, 100 mg $66.65/100. **Injection:** 20 mg/mL. *In combination with:* isosorbide dinitrate (BiDil). See Appendix B.

NURSING IMPLICATIONS

Assessment
- Monitor blood pressure and pulse frequently during initial dose adjustment and periodically during therapy. About 50–65% of Caucasians, Black, South Indians, and Mexicans are slow acetylators at risk for toxicity, while 80–90% of Eskimos, Japanese, and Chinese are rapid acetylators at risk for decreased levels and treatment failure.
- Monitor frequency of prescription refills to determine adherence.
- *Lab Test Considerations:* Monitor CBC, electrolytes, LE cell prep, and ANA titer prior to and periodically during prolonged therapy.
- May cause a positive direct Coombs' test result.

Potential Nursing Diagnoses
Ineffective tissue perfusion (Indications)
Noncompliance (Patient/Family Teaching)

Implementation
- Do not confuse hydralazine with hydroxyzine.
- IM or IV route should be used only when drug cannot be given orally.
- May be administered concurrently with diuretics or beta blockers to permit lower doses and minimize side effects.
- **PO:** Administer with meals consistently to enhance absorption.
- Pharmacist may prepare oral solution from hydralazine injection for patients with difficulty swallowing.

IV Administration
- **Direct IV:** *Diluent:* Administer undiluted. Use solution as quickly as possible after drawing through needle into syringe. *Concentration:* 20 mg/mL. *Rate:* Administer over at least 1 min. Pedi: Administer at a rate of 0.2 mg/kg/min in children. Monitor blood pressure and pulse in all patients frequently after injection.
- **Y-Site Compatibility:** anidulafungin, bivalirudin, bleomycin, dactinomycin, daptomycin, diltiazem, docetaxel, etoposide, etoposide phosphate, fenoldopam, fludarabine, gemcitabine, granisetron, hetastarch, hydromorphone, idarubicin, linezolid, mechlorethamine, metronidazole, milrinone, mitoxantrone, octreotide, oxaliplatin, paclitaxel, palonosetron, pancuronium, potassium chloride, tacrolimus, teniposide, thiotepa, tirofiban, vecuronium, vinorelbine, vitamin B complex with C, voriconazole.
- **Y-Site Incompatibility:** acyclovir, aminophylline, amphotericin B colloidal, ampicillin/sulbactam, ascorbic acid, azathioprine, cefazolin, cefonocid, cefoperazone, cefotaxime, cefoxitin, ceftazidime, ceftizoxime, ceftriaxone, cefuroxime, chloramphenicol, chlorpromazine, dantrolene, diazepam, diazoxide, ertapenem, folic acid, ganciclovir, haloperidol, inamrinone, in-

hydralazine/isosorbide dinitrate 673

domethacin, lorazepam, methylprednisolone, multivitamins, nafcillin, nitroprusside, oxacillin, pantoprazole, pemetrexed, pentobarbital, phenytoin, piperacillin/tazobactam, procainamide, sodium acetate, tigecycline, trimethoprim/sulfamethoxazole, urokinase.

- **Solution Compatibility:** 0.45% NaCl, 0.9% NaCl, LR.
- **Solution Incompatibility:** D5W.

Patient/Family Teaching

- Emphasize the importance of continuing to take this medication, even if feeling well. Instruct patient to take medication at the same time each day; last dose of the day should be taken at bedtime. Take missed doses as soon as remembered; do not double doses. If more than 2 doses in a row are missed, consult health care professional. Must be discontinued gradually to avoid sudden increase in blood pressure. Hydralazine controls but does not cure hypertension.
- Encourage patient to comply with additional interventions for hypertension (weight reduction, low-sodium diet, smoking cessation, moderation of alcohol intake, regular exercise, and stress management). Instruct patient and family on proper technique for blood pressure monitoring. Advise them to check blood pressure at least weekly and report significant changes.
- Patients should weigh themselves twice weekly and assess feet and ankles for fluid retention.
- May occasionally cause drowsiness. Advise patient to avoid driving or other activities requiring alertness until response to medication is known.
- Caution patient to avoid sudden changes in position to minimize orthostatic hypotension.
- Advise patient to consult health care professional before taking any Rx, OTC, or herbal products, especially cough, cold, or allergy remedies.
- Instruct patient to notify health care professional of medication prior to treatment or surgery.
- Advise patient to notify health care professional immediately if general tiredness; fever; muscle or joint aching; chest pain; skin rash; sore throat; or numbness, tingling, pain, or weakness of hands and feet occurs. Vitamin B_6 (pyridoxine) may be used to treat peripheral neuritis.

- Emphasize the importance of follow-up exams to evaluate effectiveness of medication.

Evaluation/Desired Outcomes

- Decrease in blood pressure without appearance of side effects.
- Decreased afterload in patients with CHF.

---

hydralazine/isosorbide dinitrate
(hye-**dral**-a-zeen eye-so-**sor**-bide di-**ni**-trate)
BiDil

Classification
Therapeutic: vasodilators
Pharmacologic: vasodilators, nitrates

Pregnancy Category C

Indications
Management of heart failure in black patients.

Action
BiDil is a fixed-dose combination of **isosorbide dinitrate**, a vasodilator with effects on both arteries and veins, and **hydralazine**, a predominantly arterial vasodilator. **Therapeutic Effects:** Improved survival, increased time to hospitalization and decreased symptoms of heart failure in black patients.

Pharmacokinetics
See pharmacokinetic sections in hydralazine and isosorbide dinitrate monographs of Davis's Drug Guide for Nurses for more information.

Absorption: *Hydralazine*—10–26% absorbed in CHF patients, absorption can be saturated leading to large increases in absorption with higher doses; *isosorbide dinitrate*—variable absorbed (10–90%) reflecting first-pass hepatic metabolism.

Distribution: *Hydralazine*—widely distributed, crosses the placenta, minimal amounts in breast milk; *isosorbide dinitrate*—accumulates in muscle and venous wall.

Metabolism and Excretion: *Hydralazine*—mostly metabolized by GI mucosa and liver; *isosorbide dinitrate*—undergoes extensive first-pass metabolism in the liver mostly metabolized by the liver, some metabolites are vasodilators.

Half-life: *Hydralazine*—4 hr; *isosorbide dinitrate*—2 hr.

✱ = Canadian drug name. ≡ = Genetic implication.
*CAPITALS indicates life-threatening; underlines indicate most frequent.

hydralazine/isosorbide dinitrate

TIME/ACTION PROFILE (effect on blood pressure)

ROUTE	ONSET	PEAK	DURATION
hydralazine	45 min	2 hr	2–4 hr
isosorbide	15–40 min	unknown	4 hr

Contraindications/Precautions
Contraindicated in: Hypersensitivity to either component.
Use Cautiously in: Lactation, Pedi: Safety not established in children <18 yr or breastfed infants; **Hydralazine:** Cardiovascular or cerebrovascular disease; Severe renal/hepatic disease (dose modification may be necessary); OB: Has been used safely during pregnancy; Lactation: Usually compatible with breastfeeding (AAP); **isosorbide dinitrate:** Head trauma or cerebral hemorrhage; Geriatric patients (start with lower doses); OB: May compromise maternal/fetal circulation; Lactation: Safety not established.

Adverse Reactions/Side Effects
Hydralazine
CNS: dizziness, drowsiness, headache. **CV:** tachycardia, angina, arrhythmias, edema, orthostatic hypotension. **GI:** diarrhea, nausea, vomiting. **Derm:** rashes. **F and E:** sodium retention. **MS:** arthralgias, arthritis. **Neuro:** peripheral neuropathy. **Misc:** drug-induced lupus syndrome.

Isosorbide Dinitrate
CNS: dizziness, headache, apprehension, weakness. **CV:** hypotension, tachycardia, paradoxic bradycardia, syncope. **GI:** abdominal pain, nausea, vomiting. **Misc:** cross-tolerance, flushing, tolerance.

Interactions
Drug-Drug: ↑ risk of hypotension with **phosphodiesterase inhibitors** (**sildenafil**, **vardenafil**, or **tadalafil**) other **antihypertensives**, acute ingestion of **alcohol**, **beta blockers**, **calcium channel blockers**, and **phenothiazines**. **MAO inhibitors** may exaggerate hypotension. May reduce the pressor response to **epinephrine**. **Beta blockers** ↓ tachycardia from hydralazine (therapy may be combined for this reason). **Metoprolol** and **propranolol** increase hydralazine levels. Hydralazine ↑ blood levels of **metoprolol** and **propranolol**.

Route/Dosage
PO (Adults): 1 tablet 3 times daily, may be increased to 2 tablets 3 times daily.

Availability
Tablets: hydralazine 37.5 mg/isosorbide dinitrate 20 mg.

NURSING IMPLICATIONS
Assessment
- Monitor blood pressure and pulse routinely during period of dosage adjustment. Symptomatic hypotension may occur even with small doses. Use caution with patients who are volume depleted or hypotensive.
- *Lab Test Considerations:* If symptoms of systemic lupus erythematosus (SLE) occur obtain a CBC and ANA titer. If positive for SLE, carefully weigh risks/benefits of continued therapy.

Potential Nursing Diagnoses
Ineffective tissue perfusion (Indications)
Activity intolerance (Indications)

Implementation
- Dose may be titrated rapidly over 3–5 days, but may need to decrease if side effects occur. May decrease to one-half tablet 3 times daily if intolerable side effects occur. Titrate up as soon as side effects subside.

Patient/Family Teaching
- Instruct patient to take medication as directed on a regular schedule.
- Caution patient to make position changes slowly to minimize orthostatic hypotension.
- May cause dizziness. Caution patient to avoid driving or other activities requiring alertness until response to medication is known.
- Advise patient to avoid concurrent use of alcohol or medications for erectile dysfunction with this medication. Patient should also consult health care professional before taking Rx, OTC, or herbal products while taking this medication.
- Caution patient that inadequate fluid intake or excessive fluid loss from perspiration, diarrhea or vomiting may lead to a fall in blood pressure, dizziness or syncope. If syncope occurs, discontinue medication and notify health care professional promptly.
- Inform patient that headache is a common side effect that should decrease with continuing therapy. Aspirin or acetaminophen may be ordered to treat headache. Notify health care professional if headache is persistent or severe. Do not alter dose to avoid headache.
- Advise patient to notify health care professional if symptoms of systemic lupus erythematosus occur (arthralgia, fever, chest pain, prolonged malaise or other unexplained symptoms).

Evaluation/Desired Outcomes
- Improved survival, increased time to hospitalization and decreased symptoms of heart failure in black patients.

---

hydrochlorothiazide, See DIURETICS (THIAZIDE).

HIGH ALERT

hydrocodone
(hye-droe-**koe**-done)
Hycodan, Tussigon (U.S. antitussive formulations contain homatropine)

hydrocodone/acetaminophen
Anexsia, Co-Gesic, Lorcet-HD, Lortab, Norco, Vicodin, Zydone

hydrocodone/ibuprofen
Ibudone, Reprexain, Vicoprofen

Classification
Therapeutic: allergy, cold, and cough remedies (antitussive), opioid analgesics
Pharmacologic: opioid agonists/nonopioid analgesic combinations

Schedule III (in combination)

Pregnancy Category C

For information on the acetaminophen and ibuprofen components of these formulations, see the acetaminophen and ibuprofen monographs

Indications
Used mainly in combination with nonopioid analgesics (acetaminophen/ibuprofen) in the management of moderate to severe pain. Antitussive (usually in combination products with decongestants).

Action
Bind to opiate receptors in the CNS. Alter the perception of and response to painful stimuli while producing generalized CNS depression: Suppress the cough reflex via a direct central action. **Therapeutic Effects:** Decrease in severity of moderate pain. Suppression of the cough reflex.

Pharmacokinetics
Absorption: Well absorbed following oral administration.
Distribution: Unknown.

Metabolism and Excretion: Mostly metabolized by the liver; eliminated in the urine (50–60% as metabolites, 15% as unchanged drug).
Half-life: 2.2 hr.

TIME/ACTION PROFILE (analgesic effect)

ROUTE	ONSET	PEAK	DURATION
PO	10–30 min	30–60 min	4–6 hr

Contraindications/Precautions
Contraindicated in: Hypersensitivity to hydrocodone (cross-sensitivity may exist to other opioids); Hypersensitivity to acetaminophen/ibuprofen (for combination products); Ibuprofen-containing products should be avoided in patients with bleeding disorders or thrombocytopenia; Acetaminophen-containing products should be avoided in patients with severe hepatic or renal disease; Ibuprofen-containing products should be avoided in patients undergoing coronary artery bypass graft surgery; OB, Lactation: Avoid chronic use; Products containing alcohol, aspartame, saccharin, sugar, or tartrazine (FDC yellow dye #5) should be avoided in patients who have hypersensitivity or intolerance to these compounds.
Use Cautiously in: Head trauma; ↑ intracranial pressure; Severe renal, hepatic, or pulmonary disease; Cardiovascular disease (ibuprofen-containing products only); History of peptic ulcer disease (ibuprofen-containing products only); Alcoholism; Geri: Geriatric or debilitated patients (initial dosage ↓ required; more prone to CNS depression, constipation); Patients with undiagnosed abdominal pain; Prostatic hyperplasia; Pedi: Children (safety not established).

Adverse Reactions/Side Effects
Noted for hydrocodone only; see acetaminophen/ibuprofen monographs for specific information on individual components.
CNS: confusion, dizziness, sedation, euphoria, hallucinations, headache, unusual dreams.
EENT: blurred vision, diplopia, miosis. **Resp:** respiratory depression. **CV:** hypotension, bradycardia. **GI:** constipation, dyspepsia, nausea, vomiting. **GU:** urinary retention. **Derm:** sweating.
Misc: physical dependence, psychological dependence, tolerance.

Interactions
Drug-Drug: Use with extreme caution in patients receiving **MAO inhibitors** (may produce severe, unpredictable reactions—do not use within 14 days of each other). Additive CNS depression with

676 hydrocodone

alcohol, antihistamines, and sedative/hypnotics. Administration of partial antagonist opioids (buprenorphine, butorphanol, nalbuphine, or pentazocine) may ↓ analgesia or precipitate opioid withdrawal in physically dependent patients.

Drug-Natural Products: Concomitant use of **kava-kava**, **valerian**, **skullcap**, **chamomile**, or **hops** can ↑ CNS depression.

Route/Dosage
PO (Adults): *Analgesic*—2.5–10 mg q 3–6 hr as needed; if using combination products, acetaminophen dosage should not exceed 4 g/day and should not exceed 5 tablets/day of ibuprofen-containing products; *Antitussive*—5 mg q 4–6 hr as needed.

PO (Children): *Analgesic (2–13 yr)*—0.14 mg/kg q 4–6 hr. *Antitussive (6–12 yr)*—2.5 mg q 4–6 hr.

Availability
Hydrocodone
Hydrocodone tablets: ✱ 5 mg (Hycodan). Hydrocodone syrup: ✱ 5 mg/mL (Hycodan, Robidone).

Hydrocodone/Acetaminophen (generic available)
Tablets: 2.5 mg hydrocodone/500 mg acetaminophen, 5 mg hydrocodone/400 mg acetaminophen (Zydone), 5 mg hydrocodone/325 mg acetaminophen (Anexsia 5/325, Norco), 5 mg hydrocodone/500 mg acetaminophen (Anexsia 5/500, Co-Gesic, Lorcet, Lortab 5/500, Vicodin), 7.5 mg hydrocodone/325 mg acetaminophen (Anexsia 7.5/325, Norco), 7.5 mg hydrocodone/400 mg acetaminophen (Zydone), 7.5 mg hydrocodone/500 mg acetaminophen, 7.5 mg hydrocodone/650 mg acetaminophen (Anexsia 7.5/650), 7.5 mg hydrocodone/750 mg acetaminophen (Vicodin ES), 10 mg hydrocodone/325 mg acetaminophen (Norco), 10 mg hydrocodone/400 mg acetaminophen (Zydone), 10 mg hydrocodone/500 mg acetaminophen (Lortab 10/500), 10 mg hydrocodone/650 mg acetaminophen, 10 mg hydrocodone/660 mg acetaminophen (Vicodin HP), 10 mg hydrocodone/750 mg acetaminophen (Anexsia 10/750). **Capsules:** 5 mg hydrocodone/500 mg acetaminophen (Lorcet-HD). **Elixir/oral solution:** 2.5 mg hydrocodone plus 167 mg acetaminophen/5 mL.

Hydrocodone/Ibuprofen (generic available)
Tablets: 2.5 mg hydrocodone/200 mg ibuprofen (Reprexain), 5 mg hydrocodone/200 mg ibuprofen (Ibudone, Reprexain), 7.5 mg hydrocodone/200 mg ibuprofen (Reprexain, Vicoprofen), 10 mg hydrocodone/200 mg ibuprofen (Ibudone, Reprexain).

NURSING IMPLICATIONS
Assessment
- Assess blood pressure, pulse, and respirations before and periodically during administration. If respiratory rate is <10/min, assess level of sedation. Physical stimulation may be sufficient to prevent significant hypoventilation. Dose may need to be decreased by 25–50%. Initial drowsiness will diminish with continued use.
- Assess bowel function routinely. Prevention of constipation should be instituted with increased intake of fluids and bulk, and laxatives to minimize constipating effects. Stimulant laxatives should be administered routinely if opioid use exceeds 2–3 days, unless contraindicated.
- **Pain:** Assess type, location, and intensity of pain prior to and 1 hr (peak) following administration. When titrating opioid doses, increases of 25–50% should be administered until there is either a 50% reduction in the patient's pain rating on a numerical or visual analogue scale or the patient reports satisfactory pain relief. A repeat dose can be safely administered at the time of the peak if previous dose is ineffective and side effects are minimal.
- An equianalgesic chart (see Appendix K) should be used when changing routes or when changing from one opioid to another.
- Prolonged use may lead to physical and psychological dependence and tolerance. This should not prevent patient from receiving adequate analgesia. Most patients who receive opioids for pain do not develop psychological dependence. If progressively higher doses are required, consider conversion to a stronger opioid.
- **Cough:** Assess cough and lung sounds during antitussive use.
- *Lab Test Considerations:* May cause ↑ plasma amylase and lipase concentrations.
- *Toxicity and Overdose:* If an opioid antagonist is required to reverse respiratory depression or coma, naloxone (Narcan) is the antidote. Dilute the 0.4-mg ampule of naloxone in 10 mL of 0.9% NaCl and administer 0.5 mL (0.02 mg) by direct IV push every 2 min. For children and patients weighing <40 kg, dilute 0.1 mg of naloxone in 10 mL of 0.9% NaCl for a concentration of 10 mcg/mL and administer 0.5 mcg/kg every 2 min. Titrate dose to avoid withdrawal, seizures, and severe pain.

Potential Nursing Diagnoses
Acute pain (Indications)
Disturbed sensory perception (visual, auditory) (Side Effects)
Risk for injury (Side Effects)

Implementation
- *High Alert:* Accidental overdose of opioid analgesics has resulted in fatalities. Before administering, clarify all ambiguous orders; have second practitioner independently check original order and dose calculations. Do not confuse hydrocodone with hydrocortisone.
- Explain therapeutic value of medication prior to administration to enhance the analgesic effect.
- Regularly administered doses may be more effective than prn administration. Analgesic is more effective if given before pain becomes severe.
- Combination with nonopioid analgesics may have additive analgesic effects and permit lower doses. Maximum doses of nonopioid agents limit the titration of hydrocodone doses.
- Medication should be discontinued gradually after long-term use to prevent withdrawal symptoms.
- **PO:** May be administered with food or milk to minimize GI irritation.

Patient/Family Teaching
- Advise patient to take medication as directed and not to take more than the recommended amount. Severe and permanent liver damage may result from prolonged use or high doses of acetaminophen. Renal damage may occur with prolonged use of acetaminophen or ibuprofen. Doses of nonopioid agents should not exceed the maximum recommended daily dose.
- Instruct patient on how and when to ask for and take pain medication.
- May cause drowsiness or dizziness. Advise patient to call for assistance when ambulating or smoking. Caution patient to avoid driving or other activities requiring alertness until response to the medication is known.
- Advise patient to change positions slowly to minimize orthostatic hypotension.
- Caution patient to avoid concurrent use of alcohol or other CNS depressants with this medication.
- Encourage patient to turn, cough, and breathe deeply every 2 hr to prevent atelectasis.
- Advise patient that good oral hygiene, frequent mouth rinses, and sugarless gum or candy may decrease dry mouth.

Evaluation/Desired Outcomes
- Decrease in severity of pain without a significant alteration in level of consciousness or respiratory status.
- Suppression of nonproductive cough.

---

hydrocortisone, See CORTICOSTEROIDS (SYSTEMIC).

---

hydrocortisone, See CORTICOSTEROIDS (TOPICAL/LOCAL).

HIGH ALERT

hydromorphone
(hye-droe-**mor**-fone)
Dilaudid, Dilaudid-HP, Hydrostat IR, PMS Hydromorphone

Classification
Therapeutic: allergy, cold, and cough remedies (antitussives), opioid analgesics
Pharmacologic: opioid agonists

Schedule II

Pregnancy Category C

Indications
Moderate to severe pain (alone and in combination with nonopioid analgesics); extended release product for opioid-tolerant patients requiring around-the-clock management of persistent pain. Antitussive (lower doses).

Action
Binds to opiate receptors in the CNS. Alters the perception of and response to painful stimuli while producing generalized CNS depression. Suppresses the cough reflex via a direct central action. **Therapeutic Effects:** Decrease in moderate to severe pain. Suppression of cough.

Pharmacokinetics
Absorption: Well absorbed following oral, rectal, subcut, and IM administration. Extended-release product results in an initial release of drug, followed by a second sustained phase of absorption.
Distribution: Widely distributed. Crosses the placenta; enters breast milk.

✤ = Canadian drug name.   ✂ = Genetic implication.
*CAPITALS indicates life-threatening; underlines indicate most frequent.

hydromorphone

Metabolism and Excretion: Mostly metabolized by the liver.
Half-life: *Oral, immediate release, or injection*—2–4 hr.

TIME/ACTION PROFILE (analgesic effect)

ROUTE	ONSET	PEAK	DURATION
PO	30 min	30–90 min	4–5 hr
Subcut	15 min	30–90 min	4–5 hr
IM	15 min	30–60 min	4–5 hr
IV	10–15 min	15–30 min	2–3 hr
Rect	15–30 min	30–90 min	4–5 hr

Contraindications/Precautions
Contraindicated in: Hypersensitivity; Some products contain bisulfites and should be avoided in patients with known hypersensitivity; OB, Lactation: Avoid chronic use during pregnancy or lactation.
Use Cautiously in: Head trauma; Increased intracranial pressure; Severe renal, hepatic, or pulmonary disease; Hypothyroidism; Adrenal insufficiency; Alcoholism; Undiagnosed abdominal pain; Prostatic hypertrophy; Geri: Geriatric and debilitated patients may be more susceptible side effects; dose reduction recommended.

Adverse Reactions/Side Effects
CNS: confusion, sedation, dizziness, dysphoria, euphoria, floating feeling, hallucinations, headache, unusual dreams. **EENT:** blurred vision, diplopia, miosis. **Resp:** respiratory depression. **CV:** hypotension, bradycardia. **GI:** constipation, dry mouth, nausea, vomiting. **GU:** urinary retention. **Derm:** flushing, sweating. **Misc:** physical dependence, psychological dependence, tolerance.

Interactions
Drug-Drug: Exercise extreme caution with **MAO inhibitors** (may produce severe, unpredictable reactions—reduce initial dose of hydromorphone to 25% of usual dose, discontinue MAO inhibitors 2 wk prior to hydromorphone). ↑ risk of CNS depression with **alcohol**, **antidepressants**, **antihistamines**, and **sedative/hypnotics** including **benzodazepines** and **phenothiazines**. Administration of partial antagonists (**buprenorphine**, **butorphanol**, **nalbuphine**, or **pentazocine**) may precipitate opioid withdrawal in physically dependent patients. **Nalbuphine** or **pentazocine** may ↓ analgesia.
Drug-Natural Products: Concomitant use of **kava-kava**, **valerian**, **chamomile**, or **hops** can ↑ CNS depression.

Route/Dosage
Doses depend on level of pain and tolerance.

Analgesic
PO (Adults ≥50 kg): 4–8 mg q 3–4 hr initially (some patients may respond to doses as small as 2 mg initially).
PO (Adults and Children <50 kg): 0.06 mg/kg q 3–4 hr initially, younger children may require smaller initial doses of 0.03 mg/kg. Maximum dose 5 mg.
IV, IM, Subcut (Adults ≥50 kg): 1.5 mg q 3–4 hr as needed initially; may be increased.
IV, IM, Subcut (Adults and Children <50 kg): 0.015 mg/kg mg q 3–4 hr as needed initially; may be increased.
IV (Adults): *Continuous infusion (unlabeled)*—0.2–30 mg/hr depending on previous opioid use. An initial bolus of twice the hourly rate in mg may be given with subsequent breakthrough boluses of 50–100% of the hourly rate in mg.
Rect (Adults): 3 mg q 6–8 hr initially as needed.

Antitussive
PO (Adults and Children > 12 yr): 1 mg q 3–4 hr.
PO (Children 6–12 yr): 0.5 mg q 3–4 hr.

Availability (generic available)
Tablets: 2 mg, 3 mg, 4 mg, 8 mg. **Oral solution:** 5 mg/5 mL. **Injection:** 1 mg/mL, 2 mg/mL, 4 mg/mL, 10 mg/mL. **Suppositories:** 3 mg. *In combination with:* guaifenesin and alcohol (Dilaudid Cough Syrup). See Appendix B.

NURSING IMPLICATIONS
Assessment
- Assess blood pressure, pulse, and respirations before and periodically during administration. If respiratory rate is <10/min, assess level of sedation. Dose may need to be decreased by 25–50%. Initial drowsiness will diminish with continued use. Geri: Pedi: Assess geriatric and pediatric patients frequently; more sensitive to the effects of opioid analgesics and may experience side effects and respiratory complications more frequently.
- Assess bowel function routinely. Institute prevention of constipation with increased intake of fluids and bulk, and laxatives to minimize constipating effects. Administer stimulant laxatives routinely if opioid use exceeds 2–3 days, unless contraindicated.
- **Pain:** Assess type, location, and intensity of pain prior to and 1 hr following IM and 5 min (peak) following IV administration. When titrating opioid doses, increases of 25–50% should be administered until there is either a

hydromorphone

50% reduction in the patient's pain rating on a numerical or visual analogue scale or the patient reports satisfactory pain relief. When titrating doses of short-acting hydromorphone, a repeat dose can be safely administered at the time of the peak if previous dose is ineffective and side effects are minimal.
- Patients on a continuous infusion should have additional bolus doses provided every 15–30 min, as needed, for breakthrough pain. The bolus dose is usually set to the amount of drug infused each hour by continuous infusion.
- An equianalgesic chart (see Appendix K) should be used when changing routes or when changing from one opioid to another.
- Prolonged use may lead to physical and psychological dependence and tolerance. This should not prevent patient from receiving adequate analgesia. Most patients who receive hydromorphone for pain do not develop psychological dependence. Progressively higher doses may be required to relieve pain with long-term therapy.
- **Cough:** Assess cough and lung sounds during antitussive use.
- *Lab Test Considerations:* May ↑ plasma amylase and lipase concentrations.
- *Toxicity and Overdose:* If an opioid antagonist is required to reverse respiratory depression or coma, naloxone (Narcan) is the antidote. Dilute the 0.4-mg ampule of naloxone in 10 mL of 0.9% NaCl and administer 0.5 mL (0.02 mg) by direct IV push every 2 min. For children and patients weighing <40 kg, dilute 0.1 mg of naloxone in 10 mL of 0.9% NaCl for a concentration of 10 mcg/mL and administer 0.5 mcg every 2 min. Titrate dose to avoid withdrawal, seizures, and severe pain.

Potential Nursing Diagnoses
Acute pain (Indications)
Disturbed sensory perception (visual, auditory) (Side Effects)
Risk for injury (Side Effects)

Implementation
- *High Alert:* Accidental overdosage of opioid analgesics has resulted in fatalities. Before administering, clarify all ambiguous orders; have second practitioner independently check original order, dose calculations, and infusion pump settings. Do not confuse with meperidine or morphine; fatalities have occurred. Do not confuse high-potency (HP) dose forms with regular dose forms. Pedi: Medication errors with opioid analgesics are common in pediatric patients; do not misinterpret or miscalculate doses. Use appropriate measuring devices.
- Explain therapeutic value of medication prior to administration to enhance the analgesic effect.
- Regularly administered doses may be more effective than prn administration. Analgesic is more effective if given before pain becomes severe.
- Coadministration with nonopioid analgesics may have additive analgesic effects and permit lower opioid doses.
- Medication should be discontinued gradually after long-term use to prevent withdrawal symptoms.
- **PO:** May be administered with food or milk to minimize GI irritation.

IV Administration
- **Direct IV:** *Diluent:* Dilute with at least 5 mL of sterile water or 0.9% NaCl for injection. Inspect solution for particulate matter. Slight yellow color does not alter potency. Store at room temperature. *Rate:* Administer slowly, at a rate not to exceed 2 mg over 3–5 min. *High Alert:* Rapid administration may lead to increased respiratory depression, hypotension, and circulatory collapse.
- **Syringe Compatibility:** atropine, bupivacaine, ceftazidime, chlorpromazine, cimetidine, diphenhydramine, fentanyl, glycopyrrolate, hydroxyzine, lorazepam, metoclopramide, midazolam, pentobarbital, potassium chloride, prochlorperazine, promethazine, ranitidine, scopolamine, thiethylperazine.
- **Syringe Incompatibility:** ampicillin, diazepam, heparin, hyaluronidase, pantoprazole, phenobarbital, phenytoin.
- **Y-Site Compatibility:** acyclovir, allopurinol, amifostine, amikacin, amsacrine, atropine, aztreonam, bivalirudin, cefepime, cefoperazone, cefotaxime, cefoxitin, ceftazidime, ceftizoxime, cefuroxime, chloramphenicol, cisatracurium, cisplatin, cladribine, clindamycin, cyclophosphamide, cytarabine, dexamethasone, dexmedetomidine, diltiazem, diphenhydramine, dobutamine, docetaxel, dopamine, doxorubicin, doxorubicin liposome, doxycycline, epinephrine, erythromycin lactobionate, etoposide, famotidine, fenoldopam, fentanyl, filgrastim, fludarabine, foscarnet, furosemide, gemcita-

bine, gentamicin, granisetron, haloperidol, heparin, kanamycin, ketorolac, labetalol, linezolid, lorazepam, magnesium sulfate, melphalan, methotrexate, methotrimeprizine, metoclopramide, metronidazole, midazolam, milrinone, morphine, nafcillin, nitroglycerin, norepinephrine, ondansetron, oxaliplatin, paclitaxel, pemetrexed, penicillin G potassium, piperacillin/tazobactam, propofol, ranitidine, remifentanil, scopolamine, tacrolimus, teniposide, thiotepa, tobramycin, trimethoprim/sulfamethoxazole, vancomycin, vecuronium, vinorelbine.

- **Y-Site Incompatibility:** amphotericin B cholesteryl sulfate complex, lansoprazole, phenytoin, sargramostim, thiopental.
- **Additive Compatibility:** bupivicaine, clonidine, heparin, midazolam, ondansetron, potassium chloride.
- **Additive Incompatibility:** sodium bicarbonate, thiopental.
- **Solution Compatibility:** D5W, D5/0.45% NaCl, D5/0.9% NaCl, D5/LR, D5/Ringer's solution, 0.45% NaCl, 0.9% NaCl, Ringer's and LR.

Patient/Family Teaching
- Instruct patient on how and when to ask for pain medication.
- May cause drowsiness or dizziness. Advise patient to call for assistance when ambulating or smoking. Caution patient to avoid driving or other activities requiring alertness until response to medication is known.
- Advise patient to change positions slowly to minimize orthostatic hypotension.
- Instruct patient to avoid concurrent use of alcohol or other CNS depressants.
- Encourage patient to turn, cough, and breathe deeply every 2 hr to prevent atelectasis.
- **Home Care Issues:** Explain to patient and family how and when to administer hydromorphone and how to care for infusion equipment properly. Pedi: Teach parents or caregivers how to accurately measure liquid medication and to use only the measuring device dispensed with the medication.
- Emphasize the importance of aggressive prevention of constipation with the use of hydromorphone.

Evaluation/Desired Outcomes
- Decrease in severity of pain without a significant alteration in level of consciousness or respiratory status.
- Suppression of cough.

hydroxocobalamin, See VITAMIN B_{12} PREPARATIONS.

hydroxychloroquine
(hye-drox-ee-**klor**-oh-kwin)
Plaquenil

Classification
Therapeutic: antimalarials, antirheumatics (DMARDs)

Pregnancy Category C

Indications
Suppression/chemoprophylaxis of malaria. Treatment of severe rheumatoid arthritis/systemic lupus erythematosus.

Action
Inhibits protein synthesis in susceptible organisms by inhibiting DNA and RNA polymerase. **Therapeutic Effects:** Death of plasmodia responsible for causing malaria. Also has anti-inflammatory properties.

Pharmacokinetics
Absorption: Highly variable (31–100%) following oral administration.
Distribution: Widely distributed; high concentrations in RBCs; crosses the placenta; excreted into breast milk.
Metabolism and Excretion: Partially metabolized by the liver to active metabolites; partially excreted unchanged by the kidneys.
Half-life: 72–120 hr.

TIME/ACTION PROFILE (blood levels)

ROUTE	ONSET	PEAK	DURATION
PO	rapid†	1–2 hr	days–weeks

†Onset of antirheumatic action may take 6 wk

Contraindications/Precautions
Contraindicated in: Hypersensitivity to hydroxychloroquine or chloroquine; Previous visual damage from hydroxychloroquine or chloroquine.
Use Cautiously in: Concurrent use of hepatotoxic drugs; History of liver disease or alcoholism or renal impairment; Severe neurological disorders; Severe blood disorders; Retinal or visual field changes; G6PD deficiency; Psoriasis; Bone marrow depression; Obesity (determine dose by ideal body weight); OB, Lactation: Avoid use unless treating/preventing malaria or treating amebic abscess; Pedi: Long-term use may increase sensitivity to effects.

Adverse Reactions/Side Effects
CNS: SEIZURES, aggressiveness, anxiety, apathy, confusion, fatigue, headache, irritability, personality changes, psychoses. **EENT:** keratopathy, ototoxicity, retinopathy, tinnitus, visual disturbances. **CV:** ECG changes, hypotension. **GI:** abdominal cramps, anorexia, diarrhea, epigastric discomfort, nausea, vomiting, hepatic failure. **Derm:** bleaching of hair, alopecia, hyperpigmentation, photosensitivity, Stevens-Johnson syndrome. **Hemat:** AGRANULOCYTOSIS, APLASTIC ANEMIA, leukopenia, thrombocytopenia. **Neuro:** neuromyopathy, peripheral neuritis.

Interactions
Drug-Drug: May ↑ the risk of hepatotoxicity when administered with **hepatotoxic drugs**. May ↑ the risk of hematologic toxicity when administered with **penicillamine**. May ↑ risk of dermatitis when administered with other **agents having dermatologic toxicity**. May decrease serum titers of rabies antibody when given concurrently with **human diploid cell rabies vaccine**. **Urinary acidifiers** may ↑ renal excretion. May ↑ serum levels of **digoxin**.

Route/Dosage
Antimalarial doses expressed as mg of base; antirheumatic and lupus doses expressed as mg of hydroxychloroquine sulfate (200 mg hydroxychloroquine sulfate = 155 mg of hydroxychloroquine base).

Malaria
PO (Adults): *Suppression or chemoprophylaxis*—310 mg once weekly; start 1–2 wk prior to entering malarious area; continue for 4 wk after leaving area. *Treatment*—620 mg, then 310 mg at 6 hr, 24 hr, and 48 hr after initial dose.
PO (Children): *Suppression or chemoprophylaxis*—5 mg/kg once weekly; start 1–2 wk prior to entering malarious area; continue for 4 wk after leaving area. *Treatment*—10 mg/kg initially, then 5 mg/kg at 6–8 hr, 24 hr, and 48 hr after initial dose.

Rheumatoid Arthritis
PO (Adults): 400–600 mg once daily initially, maintenance 200–400 mg/day divided 1–2 times/day.
PO (Children): 3–5 mg/kg/day divided 1–2 times/day to a maximum of 400 mg/day; not to exceed 7 mg/kg/day.

Systemic Lupus Erythematosus
PO (Adults): 400 mg once or twice daily, maintenance 200–400 mg/day.
PO (Children): 3–5 mg/kg/day divided 1–2 times/day to a maximum of 400 mg/day; not to exceed 7 mg/kg/day.

Availability
Tablets: 200 mg (155-mg base).

NURSING IMPLICATIONS
Assessment
- Assess deep tendon reflexes periodically to determine muscle weakness. Therapy may be discontinued should this occur.
- Patients on prolonged high-dose therapy should have eye exams prior to and every 3–6 mo during therapy to detect retinal damage.
- **Malaria or Lupus Erythematosus:** Assess patient for improvement in signs and symptoms of condition daily throughout course of therapy.
- **Rheumatoid Arthritis:** Assess patient monthly for pain, swelling, and range of motion.
- *Lab Test Considerations:* Monitor CBC and platelet count periodically throughout therapy. May cause decreased RBC, WBC, and platelet counts. If severe decreases occur that are not related to the disease process, hydroxychloroquine should be discontinued.

Potential Nursing Diagnoses
Risk for infection (Indications)
Chronic pain (Indications)

Implementation
- **PO:** Administer with milk or meals to minimize GI distress.
- Tablets may be crushed and placed inside empty capsules for patients with difficulty swallowing. Contents of capsules may also be mixed with a teaspoonful of jam, jelly, or Jell-O prior to administration.
- **Malaria Prophylaxis:** Hydroxychloroquine therapy should be started 2 wk prior to potential exposure and continued for 4–6 wk after leaving the malarious area.

Patient/Family Teaching
- Instruct patient to take medication exactly as directed and continue full course of therapy even if feeling better. Missed doses should be taken as soon as remembered unless it is almost time for next dose. Do not double doses.

- Advise patients to avoid use of alcohol while taking hydroxychloroquine.
- Caution patient to keep hydroxychloroquine out of reach of children; fatalities have occurred with ingestion of 3 or 4 tablets.
- Explain need for periodic ophthalmic exams for patients on prolonged high-dose therapy. Advise patient that the risk of ocular damage may be decreased by the use of dark glasses in bright light. Protective clothing and sunscreen should also be used to reduce risk of dermatoses.
- Advise patient to notify health care professional promptly if sore throat, fever, unusual bleeding or bruising, blurred vision, visual changes, ringing in the ears, difficulty hearing, or muscle weakness occurs.
- **Malaria Prophylaxis:** Review methods of minimizing exposure to mosquitoes with patients receiving hydroxychloroquine prophylactically (use repellent, wear long-sleeved shirt and long trousers, use screen or netting).
- Advise patient to notify health care professional if fever develops while traveling or within 2 mo of leaving an endemic area.
- **Rheumatoid Arthritis:** Instruct patient to contact health care professional if no improvement is noticed within a few days. Treatment for rheumatoid arthritis may require up to 6 mo for full benefit.

Evaluation/Desired Outcomes
- Prevention or resolution of malaria.
- Improvement in signs and symptoms of rheumatoid arthritis.
- Improvement in symptoms of lupus erythematosus.

hydrOXYzine (hye-**drox**-i-zeen)
✜ Apo-Hydroxyzine, Atarax, Hyzine-50, ✜ Multipax, ✜ Novohydroxyzin, Vistaril

Classification
Therapeutic: antianxiety agents, antihistamines, sedative/hypnotics

Pregnancy Category C

Indications
Treatment of anxiety. Preoperative sedation. Antiemetic. Antipruritic. May be combined with opioid analgesics.

Action
Acts as a CNS depressant at the subcortical level of the CNS. Has anticholinergic, antihistaminic, and antiemetic properties. Blocks histamine 1 receptors. **Therapeutic Effects:** Sedation. Relief of anxiety. Decreased nausea and vomiting. Decreased allergic symptoms associated with release of histamine, including pruritus.

Pharmacokinetics
Absorption: Well absorbed following PO/IM administration.
Distribution: Unknown.
Metabolism and Excretion: Completely metabolized by the liver; eliminated in the feces via biliary excretion.
Half-life: 3 hr.

TIME/ACTION PROFILE (sedative, antiemetic, antipruritic effects)

ROUTE	ONSET	PEAK	DURATION
PO	15–30 min	2–4 hr	4–6 hr
IM	15–30 min	2–4 hr	4–6 hr

Contraindications/Precautions
Contraindicated in: Hypersensitivity; OB: Potential for congenital defects (oral clefts and hypoplasia of cerebral hemisphere; Lactation: Safety not established.
Use Cautiously in: Severe hepatic dysfunction; OB: Has been used safely during labor; Pedi: Injection contains benzyl alcohol, which can cause potentially fatal gasping syndrome in neonates; Geri: Appears on *Beers list*. Geriatric patients are more susceptible to adverse reactions due to anticholinergic effects; dosage reduction recommended.

Adverse Reactions/Side Effects
CNS: drowsiness, agitation, ataxia, dizziness, headache, weakness. **Resp:** wheezing. **GI:** dry mouth, bitter taste, constipation, nausea. **GU:** urinary retention. **Derm:** flushing. **Local:** pain at IM site, abscesses at IM sites. **Misc:** chest tightness.

Interactions
Drug-Drug: Additive CNS depression with other **CNS depressants**, including **alcohol**, **antidepressants**, **antihistamines**, **opioid analgesics**, and **sedative/hypnotics**. Additive anticholinergic effects with other **drugs possessing anticholinergic properties**, including **antihistamines, antidepressants, atropine, haloperidol, phenothiazines, quinidine**, and **disopyramide**. Can antagonize the vasopressor effects of **epinephrine**.
Drug-Natural Products: Concomitant use of **kava-kava**, **valerian**, or **chamomile** can increase CNS depression. Increased anticholinergic effects with **angel's trumpet**, **jimson weed**, and **scopolia**.

hydrOXYzine **683**

Route/Dosage
PO (Adults): *Antianxiety*—25–100 mg 4 times/day, not to exceed 600 mg/day. *Preoperative sedation*—50–100 mg single dose. *Antipruritic*—25 mg 3–4 times daily.
PO (Children): —2 mg/kg/day divided q 6–8 hr.
IM (Adults): *Preoperative sedation*—25–100 mg single dose. *Antiemetic, adjunct to opioid analgesics*—25–100 mg q 4–6 hr as needed.
IM (Children): —0.5–1 mg/kg/dose q 4–6 hr as needed.

Availability (generic available)
Tablets: 10 mg, 25 mg, 50 mg, 100 mg. **Capsules:** ✦ 10 mg, 25 mg, 50 mg, 100 mg. **Syrup:** 10 mg/5 mL. **Oral suspension:** 25 mg/5 mL. **Injection:** 25 mg/mL, 50 mg/mL.

NURSING IMPLICATIONS
Assessment
- Assess patient for profound sedation and provide safety precautions as indicated (side rails up, bed in low position, call bell within reach, supervision of ambulation and transfer). Geri: Older adults are more sensitive to CNS and anticholinergic effects (delirium, acute confusion, dizziness, dry mouth, blurred vision, urinary retention, constipation, tachycardia). Monitor for drowsiness, agitation, over sedation, and other systemic side effects. Assess falls risk and implement prevention strategies.
- **Anxiety:** Assess mental status (orientation, mood, and behavior).
- **Nausea and Vomiting:** Assess degree of nausea and frequency and amount of emesis.
- **Pruritus:** Assess degree of itching and character of involved skin.
- **Lab Test Considerations:** May cause false-negative skin test results using allergen extracts. Discontinue hydroxyzine at least 72 hr before test.

Potential Nursing Diagnoses
Anxiety (Indications)
Impaired skin integrity (Indications)
Risk for injury (Side Effects)
Ineffective coping (Side Effects)

Implementation
- Do not confuse hydroxyzine with hydralazine or Atarax (hydroxyzine) with Ativan (lorazepam).
- **PO:** Tablets may be crushed and capsules opened and administered with food or fluids for patients having difficulty swallowing.
- Shake suspension well before administration.
- **IM:** Administer *only* IM deep into well-developed muscle, preferably with Z-track technique. Injection is extremely painful. Do not use deltoid site. If must be administered to children, midlateral muscles of the thigh are preferred. Significant tissue damage, necrosis, and sloughing may result from subcut or intra-arterial injections. Hemolysis may result from IV injections. Rotate injection sites frequently.
- **Syringe Compatibility:** atropine, butorphanol, chlorpromazine, cimetidine, codeine, diphenhydramine, doxapram, droperidol, fentanyl, fluphenazine, glycopyrrolate, hydromorphone, lidocaine, meperidine, metoclopramide, midazolam, morphine, nalbuphine, oxymorphone, pentazocine, perphenazine, procaine, prochlorperazine, promethazine, scopolamine, sufentanil.
- **Syringe Incompatibility:** dimenhydrinate, haloperidol, heparin, ketorolac, pentobarbital, ranitidine.

Patient/Family Teaching
- Instruct patient to take medication exactly as directed. Missed doses should be taken as soon as remembered unless it is almost time for next dose; do not double doses.
- May cause drowsiness or dizziness. Caution patient to avoid driving and other activities requiring alertness until response to medication is known. Geri: Warn patients or caregivers that older adults are at increased risk for CNS effects and falls.
- Advise patient to avoid concurrent use of alcohol or other CNS depressants with this medication.
- Inform patient that frequent mouth rinses, good oral hygiene, and sugarless gum or candy may help decrease dry mouth. If dry mouth persists for more than 2 wk, consult dentist about saliva substitute.
- If used for anxiety, advise patient that psychotherapy is beneficial in addressing sources of anxiety and improving coping skills.
- Teach other methods to decrease anxiety, such as increased exercise, support groups, and relaxation techniques.

✦ = Canadian drug name. ᴴ = Genetic implication.
*CAPITALS indicates life-threatening; underlines indicate most frequent.

Evaluation/Desired Outcomes
- Decrease in anxiety.
- Relief of nausea and vomiting.
- Relief of pruritus.
- Sedation when used as a sedative/hypnotic.

---

hyoscyamine (hi-oh-si-a-meen)
Anaspaz, A-Spas S/L, Cystospaz, Cystospaz-M, Donnamar, ED-SPAZ, Gastrosed, Levsinex, Levsin, Levbid, L-hyoscyamine, NuLev

Classification
Therapeutic: antispasmodics
Pharmacologic: anticholinergics

Pregnancy Category C

Indications
Control of gastric secretion, visceral spasm, hypermotility in spastic colitis, spastic bladder, pylorospasm, and related abdominal cramps. Decreases symptoms of various functional intestinal disorders including mild dysenteries, diverticulitis, infant colic, biliary and renal colic. Adjunctive therapy in peptic ulcer disease, irritable bowel syndrome, neurogenic bowel disturbances. Decreases pain and hypersecretion associated with pancreatitis. Relief of symptoms of acute rhinitis. Decreases rigidity and tremors associated with parkinsonism and controls related sialorrhea and hyperhidrosis. May also be used to manage anticholinesterase poisoning. Management of cystitis or renal colic. Management of some forms of heart block due to vagal activity. **IM, IV, Subcut:** Facilitation of diagnostic hypotonic duodenography; may also increase radiologic visibility of the kidneys. Preoperative administration decreases secretions and blocks bradycardia associated with some forms of anesthesia and related surgical agents.

Action
Inhibits the muscarinic effect of acetylcholine in smooth muscle, secretory glands and the CNS. Small doses decrease salivary and bronchial secretions and decrease sweating; intermediate doses dilate the pupil, inhibit accommodation, increase heart rate (vagolytic action); large doses decrease GI and GU motility, further increase in dose decreases gastric acid secretion. **Therapeutic Effects:** Decreased secretions with decreased GI and GU symptomatology. Increased heart rate.

Pharmacokinetics
Absorption: Well absorbed; food does not affect absorption.
Distribution: Crosses the placenta and blood-brain barrier; enters breast milk.
Metabolism and Excretion: Excreted mostly unchanged by the kidneys.
Half-life: 3.5 hr.

TIME/ACTION PROFILE (GI effects)

ROUTE	ONSET	PEAK	DURATION
PO	20–30 min	unknown	4–6 hr
IM, IV, subcut	2–3 min	unknown	4–6 hr

Contraindications/Precautions
Contraindicated in: Hypersensitivity; Angle-closure glaucoma; Tachycardia or unstable cardiovascular status; GI obstructive disease, paralytic ileus, intestinal atony, severe ulcerative colitis; Obstructive uropathy; Myasthenia gravis; Lactation: Lactation; Pedi: Products containing benzyl alcohol should not be used in newborn or immature infants; Some products contain alcohol, sulfites, or tartrazine and should be avoided in patients with known intolerance/hypersensitivity; Phenylketonuria (NuLev contains aspartame).
Use Cautiously in: History of cardiovascular disease including CHF, arrhythmias, hypertension, tachycardia, or coronary artery disease; Renal or hepatic impairment; Prostatic hyperplasia; Early ileus or reflux esophagitis; Autonomic neuropathy; Hyperthyroidism; Geri: Appears on Beers list; ↑ sensitivity to anticholinergics; Pedi: Infants, small children, Down's syndrome, brain damage, or spastic paralysis (↑ sensitivity); OB: May cause fetal tachycardia; safety not established.

Adverse Reactions/Side Effects
CNS: confusion/excitement (especially in geriatric patients), dizziness, flushing, headache, insomnia, lightheadedness (IM, IV, subcut), nervousness. **EENT:** blurred vision, cycloplegia, ↑ intraocular pressure, mydriasis, photophobia. **CV:** palpitations, tachycardia. **GI:** dry mouth, altered taste perception, bloated feeling, constipation, nausea, paralytic ileus, vomiting. **GU:** erectile dysfunction, urinary hesitancy/retention. **Derm:** ↓ sweating, urticaria. **Local:** local irritation (IM, IV, subcut). **Misc:** allergic reactions including ANAPHYLAXIS, fever (especially in children), suppression of lactation.

Interactions
Drug-Drug: Concurrent administration with **amantadine** ↑ anticholinergic side effects (may require dose ↓). ↑ effects of **atenolol**. Concurrent use with **phenothiazines** may result in ↓ effect of phenothiazine and ↑ anticholinergic side effects (dose reduction may be necessary).

↑ anticholinergic side effects with **tricyclic antidepressants**.

Route/Dosage
PO, SL (Adults): 0.125–0.25 mg 3–4 times daily or 0.375–0.75 mg as sustained release form every 12 hr.

PO (Children 2–<12 yr): *orally disintegrating tablets (NuLev)*—0.0625–0.125 mg (1/2–1 tablet) every 4 hr, up to 6 times/day.

PO (Children 34–36 kg): 125–187 mcg every 4 hr as needed.

PO (Children 22.7–33 kg): 94–125 mcg every 4 hr as needed.

PO (Children 13.6–22.6 kg): 63 mcg every 4 hr as needed.

PO (Children 9.1–13.5 kg): 31.3 mcg every 4 hr as needed.

PO (Children 6.8–9 kg): 25 mcg every 4 hr as needed.

PO (Children 4.5–6.7 kg): 18.8 mcg every 4 hr as needed.

PO (Children 3.4–4.4 kg): 15.6 mcg every 4 hr as needed.

PO (Children 2.3–3.3 kg): 12.5 mcg every 4 hr as needed.

IM, IV, Subcut (Adults): *Gastrointestinal anticholinergic*—0.25–0.5 mg 3–4 times daily as needed; *preoperative prophylaxis of secretions*—0.5 mg or 0.005 mg/kg 30–60 min before anesthesia; *antiarrhythmic*—0.125 mg IV repeated as needed; *cholinergic adjunct (curariform block)*—0.2 mg for each 1 mg of neostigmine.

IM, IV, Subcut (Children ≥2 yr): *preoperative prophylaxis of secretions*—0.005 mg/kg 30–60 min before anesthesia.

Availability (generic available)
Tablets: 0.125 mg. **Sublingual tablets:** 0.125 mg. **Orally-disintegrating tablets (contains aspartame) (mint):** 0.125 mg. **Extended-release tablets:** 0.375 mg. **Timed-release capsules:** 0.375 mg. **Solution (drops) (orange):** 0.125 mg/mL. **Elixir (orange):** 0.125 mg/5 mL. **Injection:** 0.5 mg/mL.

NURSING IMPLICATIONS

Assessment
- Assess vital signs and ECG tracings frequently during IV drug therapy. Report any significant changes in heart rate or blood pressure, or increased ventricular ectopy or angina promptly.
- Monitor intake and output ratios in elderly or surgical patients because hyoscyamine may cause urinary retention.
- Assess patients routinely for abdominal distention and auscultate for bowel sounds. If constipation becomes a problem, increasing fluids and adding bulk to the diet may help alleviate constipation.
- ***Toxicity and Overdose:*** If overdose occurs, physostigmine is the antidote.

Potential Nursing Diagnoses
Decreased cardiac output (Indications)
Impaired oral mucous membrane (Side Effects)
Constipation (Side Effects)

Implementation
- Do not confuse Levbid (hyoscyamine) with Lithobid (lithium) or Lopid (gemfibrozil).
- **PO:** Oral doses are usually given 30 min before meals. Swallow extended-release and time-release products whole; do not open, break, crush, or chew.

IV Administration

- **Direct IV:** ***Diluent:*** May give IV undiluted or dilute in 10 mL of sterile water. ***Rate:*** No rate information available, administer slowly.

Patient/Family Teaching
- Instruct patient to take exactly as directed. Take missed doses as soon as remembered unless almost time for next dose. Do not double doses.
- May cause drowsiness. Caution patients to avoid driving or other activities requiring alertness until response to medication is known.
- Instruct patient that oral rinses, sugarless gum or candy, and frequent oral hygiene may help relieve dry mouth.
- Caution patients that hyoscyamine impairs heat regulation. Strenuous activity in a hot environment may cause heat stroke.
- Instruct patient to consult health care professional before taking any Rx, OTC, or herbal products concurrently with hyoscyamine.
- Inform male patients with benign prostatic hyperplasia that hyoscyamine may cause urinary hesitancy and retention. Changes in urinary stream should be reported to health care professional.

Evaluation/Desired Outcomes
- Increase in heart rate.
- Dryness of mouth.
- Reversal of muscarinic effects.

ibandronate (i-ban-dro-nate)
Boniva

Classification
Therapeutic: bone resorption inhibitors
Pharmacologic: biphosphonates

Pregnancy Category C

Indications
Treatment/prevention of postmenopausal osteoporosis.

Action
Inhibits resorption of bone by inhibiting ostoclast activity. **Therapeutic Effects:** Reversal/prevention of progression of osteoporosis with decreased fractures.

Pharmacokinetics
Absorption: 0.6% absorbed following oral administration (significantly decreased by food).
Distribution: Rapidly binds to bone.
Protein Binding: 90.9–99.5%.
Metabolism and Excretion: 50–60% excreted in urine; unabsorbed drug is eliminated in feces.
Half-life: *PO*—10–60 hr; *IV*—4.6–25.5 hr.

TIME/ACTION PROFILE

ROUTE	ONSET	PEAK	DURATION
PO	unknown	0.5–2 hr	up to 1 mo
IV	unknown	3 hr	up to 3 mo

Contraindications/Precautions
Contraindicated in: Hypersensitivity; Uncorrected hypocalcemia; Inability to stand/sit upright for at least 60 min; CCr <30 mL/min.
Use Cautiously in: Concurrent use of NSAIDs or aspirin; Concurrent dental surgery (may ↑ risk of jaw osteonecrosis); OB: Use only if potential benefit outweighs risks to mother and fetus; Lactation: Lactation; Pedi: Children <18 yr (safety not established); Geri: Consider age related ↓ in body mass, renal and hepatic function, concurrent disease states and drug therapy.

Adverse Reactions/Side Effects
GI: <u>diarrhea</u>, <u>dyspepsia</u>, dysphagia, esophageal cancer, esophagitis, esophageal/gastric ulcer. **MS:** <u>musculoskeletal pain</u>, <u>pain in arms/legs</u>, osteonecrosis (primarily of jaw). **Misc:** injection site reactions.

Interactions
Drug-Drug: **Calcium**-, **aluminum**-, **magnesium**-, and **iron**-containing products, including antacids ↓ absorption (ibandronate should be taken 60 min before). Concurrent use of **NSAIDs** including **aspirin**, may ↑ risk of gastric irritation.
Drug-Food: Milk and other foods ↓ absorption.

Route/Dosage
PO (Adults): 2.5 mg once daily or 150 mg once monthly.
IV (Adults): 3 mg every 3 months.

Availability
Tablets: 2.5 mg, 150 mg. **Cost:** 150 mg $254.00/3. **Injection:** 3 mg/3 mL in prefilled single-use syringe.

NURSING IMPLICATIONS

Assessment
- **Osteoporosis:** Assess patients for low bone mass before and periodically during therapy.
- *Lab Test Considerations:* Assess serum calcium before and periodically during therapy. Hypocalcemia and vitamin D deficiency should be treated before initiating ibandronate therapy.
- May cause ↓ total alkaline phosphatase levels.
- May cause hypercholesterolemia.

Potential Nursing Diagnoses
Risk for injury (Indications)

Implementation
- **PO:** Administer first thing in the morning with 6–8 oz plain water 30 min before other medications, beverages, or food. Tablet should be swallowed whole; do not break, crush, or chew.
- *Once-monthly tablet* should be administered on the same date each month.

IV Administration
- **IV:** Administer using prefilled syringe. Do not administer solution that is discolored or contain particulate matter. Administer IV only; other routes may cause tissue damage.
- *Rate:* Administer as a 15–30 second bolus.
- **Y-Site Incompatibility:** Do not administer with calcium-containing solutions or other IV drugs.

Patient/Family Teaching
- Advise patient to eat a balanced diet and consult health care professional about the need for supplemental calcium and vitamin D. Wait at

ibuprofen

least 60 min after administration before taking supplemental calcium and vitamin D.
- Encourage patient to participate in regular exercise and to modify behaviors that increase the risk of osteoporosis (stop smoking, reduce alcohol consumption).
- Inform patient that severe musculoskeletal pain may occur within days, months, or yr after starting ibandronate. Symptoms my resolve completely after discontinuation or slow or incomplete resolution may occur. Notify health care professional if sever pain occurs.
- Advise patient to inform health care professional of ibandronate therapy prior to dental surgery.
- Advise female patient to notify health care professional if pregnancy is planned or suspected or if she is breastfeeding.
- **PO:** Instruct patient on the importance of taking as directed, first thing in the morning, 60 min before other medications, beverages, or food. Ibandronate should be taken with 6–8 oz plain water (mineral water, orange juice, coffee, and other beverages decrease absorption). Do not chew or suck on tablet. If a dose is missed, skip dose and resume the next morning; do not double doses or take later in the day. If a once-monthly dose is missed and the next scheduled dose is >7 days away, take in the morning following the date it is remembered. Resume original schedule the following month. If the next dose is <7 days away, omit dose and take next scheduled dose. Do not discontinue without consulting health care professional.
- Caution patient to remain upright for 60 min following dose to facilitate passage to stomach and minimize risk of esophageal irritation.
- **IV:** Advice patient that IV doses should not be administered sooner that every 3 months. If a dose is missed, have health care professional administer as soon as possible; next injection should be scheduled 3 months from last injection.

Evaluation/Desired Outcomes
- Prevention of or decrease in the progression of osteoporosis in postmenopausal women.

ibuprofen (oral)
(eye-byoo-**proe**-fen)
✦ Actiprofen, Advil, Advil Migraine Liqui-Gels, ✦ Apo-Ibuprofen, Children's Advil, Children's Motrin, Excedrin IB, Genpril, Haltran, Junior Strength Advil, Menadol, Medipren, Midol Maximum Strength Cramp Formula, Motrin, Motrin Drops, Motrin IB, Motrin Junior Strength, Motrin Migraine Pain, ✦ Novo-Profen, Nu-Ibuprofen, Nuprin, PediaCare Children's Fever

ibuprofen (injection)
Caldolor

Classification
Therapeutic: antipyretics, antirheumatics, nonopioid analgesics, nonsteroidal anti-inflammatory agents
Pharmacologic: nonopioid analgesics

Pregnancy Category C (up to 30 wk gestation), D (starting at 30 wk gestation)

Indications
PO, IV: Treatment of: Mild to moderate pain, Fever. **PO:** Treatment of: Inflammatory disorders including rheumatoid arthritis (including juvenile) and osteoarthritis, Dysmenorrhea. **IV:** Moderate to severe pain with opioid analgesics.

Action
Inhibits prostaglandin synthesis. **Therapeutic Effects:** Decreased pain and inflammation. Reduction of fever.

Pharmacokinetics
Absorption: Oral formulation is well absorbed (80%) from the GI tract; IV administration results in complete bioavailability.
Distribution: Does not enter breast milk in significant amounts.
Protein Binding: 99%.
Metabolism and Excretion: Mostly metabolized by the liver; small amounts (1%) excreted unchanged by the kidneys.
Half-life: Children: 1–2 hr; Adults: 2–4 hr.

TIME/ACTION PROFILE

ROUTE	ONSET	PEAK	DURATION
PO (antipyretic)	0.5–2.5 hr	2–4 hr	6–8 hr
PO (analgesic)	30 min	1–2 hr	4–6 hr
PO (anti-inflammatory)	7 days	1–2 wk	unknown
IV (analgesic)	unknown	unknown	6 hr
IV (antipyretic)	within 2 hr	10–12 hr†	4–6 hr

† With repeated dosing

Contraindications/Precautions
Contraindicated in: Hypersensitivity (cross-sensitivity may exist with other NSAIDs, including

aspirin); Active GI bleeding or ulcer disease; Chewable tablets contain aspartame and should not be used in patients with phenylketonuria; Peri-operative pain from coronary artery bypass graft (CABG) surgery; OB: Avoid after 30 wk gestation (may cause premature closure of fetal ductus arteriosus).

Use Cautiously in: Cardiovascular disease (may ↑ risk of cardiovascular events); Renal or hepatic disease, dehydration, or patients on nephrotoxic drugs (may ↑ risk of renal toxicity); Aspirin triad patients (asthma, nasal polyps, and aspirin intolerance); can cause fatal anaphylactoid reactions; Geri: ↑ risk of adverse reactions secondary to age-related ↓ in renal and hepatic function, concurrent illnesses, and medications; Chronic alcohol use/abuse; Coagulation disorders; OB: Use cautiously up to 30 wk gestation; avoid after that; Lactation: Use cautiously; Pedi: Safety not established for infants <6 mo (oral) and children <17 yr (IV).

Exercise Extreme Caution in: History of GI bleeding or GI ulcer disease.

Adverse Reactions/Side Effects
CNS: headache, dizziness, drowsiness, psychic disturbances. **EENT:** amblyopia, blurred vision, tinnitus. **CV:** arrhythmias, edema, hypertension. **GI:** GI BLEEDING, HEPATITIS, constipation, dyspepsia, nausea, vomiting, abdominal discomfort. **GU:** cystitis, hematuria, renal failure. **Derm:** EXFOLIATIVE DERMATITIS, STEVENS-JOHNSON SYNDROME, TOXIC EPIDERMAL NECROLYSIS, rashes. **Hemat:** anemia, blood dyscrasias, prolonged bleeding time. **Misc:** allergic reactions including ANAPHYLAXIS.

Interactions
Drug-Drug: May limit the cardioprotective effects of low-dose **aspirin**. Concurrent use with **aspirin** may ↓ effectiveness of ibuprofen. Additive adverse GI side effects with **aspirin**, **oral potassium**, other **NSAIDs**, **corticosteroids**, or **alcohol**. Chronic use with **acetaminophen** may ↑ risk of adverse renal reactions. May ↓ effectiveness of **diuretics**, **ACE inhibitors**, or other **antihypertensives**. May ↑ hypoglycemic effects of **insulin** or **oral hypoglycemic agents**. May ↑ serum **lithium** levels and risk of toxicity. ↑ risk of toxicity from **methotrexate**. **Probenecid** ↑ risk of toxicity from ibuprofen. ↑ risk of bleeding with **cefotetan**, **cefoperazone**, **corticosteroids**, **valproic acid**, **thrombolytics**, **warfarin**, and **drugs affecting platelet func**tion including **clopidogrel**, **ticlopidine**, **abciximab**, **eptifibatide**, or **tirofiban**. ↑ risk of adverse hematologic reactions with **antineoplastics** or **radiation therapy**. ↑ risk of nephrotoxicity with **cyclosporine**.

Drug-Natural Products: ↑ bleeding risk with, **arnica**, **chamomile**, **feverfew**, **garlic**, **ginger**, **ginkgo**, **Panax ginseng**, and others.

Route/Dosage
Analgesia
PO (Adults): *Anti-inflammatory*—400–800 mg 3–4 times daily (not to exceed 3200 mg/day). *Analgesic/antidysmenorrheal/antipyretic*—200–400 mg q 4–6 hr (not to exceed 1200 mg/day).

PO (Children 6 mo–12 yr): *Anti-inflammatory*—30–50 mg/kg/day in 3–4 divided doses (maximum dose: 2.4 g/day). *Antipyretic*—5 mg/kg for temperature <102.5°F (39.17°C) or 10 mg/kg for higher temperatures (not to exceed 40 mg/kg/day); may be repeated q 4–6 hr. *Cystic fibrosis (unlabeled)*—20–30 mg/kg/day divided twice daily.

PO (Infants and Children): *Analgesic*—4–10 mg/kg/dose q 6–8 hr.

IV (Adults): *Analgesic*—400–800 mg q 6 hr as needed (not to exceed 3200 mg/day); *Antipyretic*—400 mg initially, then 400 mg q 4–6 hr or 100–200 mg q 4 hr as needed (not to exceed 3200 mg/day).

Pediatric OTC Dosing
PO (Children 11 yr/72–95 lb): 300 mg q 6–8 hr.

PO (Children 9–10 yr/60–71 lb): 250 mg q 6–8 hr.

PO (Children 6–8 yr/48–59 lb): 200 mg q 6–8 hr.

PO (Children 4–5 yr/36–47 lb): 150 mg q 6–8 hr.

PO (Children 2–3 yr/24–35 lb): 100 mg q 6–8 hr.

PO (Children 12–23 mo/18–23 lb): 75 mg q 6–8 hr.

PO (Infants 6–11 mo/12–17 lb): 50 mg q 6–8 hr.

Availability (generic available)
Tablets: 100 mg^OTC, 200 mg^OTC, 300 mg, 400 mg, 600 mg, 800 mg. **Capsules (liqui-gels):** 200 mg^OTC. **Chewable tablets (fruit, grape, orange, and citrus flavor):** 50 mg^OTC, 100 mg^OTC. **Liquid (berry flavor):** 100 mg/5 mL^OTC. **Oral**

690 ibuprofen

suspension (fruit, berry, grape flavor): 100 mg/5 mL^{OTC}, 100 mg/2.5 mL^{OTC}. **Pediatric drops (berry flavor):** 50 mg/1.25 mL^{OTC}. **Solution for injection:** 100 mg/mL. *In combination with:* decongestants, ^{OTC}, hydrocodone (Vicoprofen), oxycodone (Combunox). See Appendix B.

NURSING IMPLICATIONS

Assessment

- Patients who have asthma, aspirin-induced allergy, and nasal polyps are at increased risk for developing hypersensitivity reactions. Assess for rhinitis, asthma, and urticaria.
- Assess for signs and symptoms of GI bleeding (tarry stools, lightheadedness, hypotension), renal dysfunction (elevated BUN and creatinine levels, decreased urine output), and hepatic impairment (elevated liver enzymes, jaundice). Geri: Higher risk for poor outcomes or death from GI bleeding. Age-related renal impairment increases risk of hepatic and renal toxicity.
- Assess patient for skin rash frequently during therapy. Discontinue ibuprofen at first sign of rash; may be life-threatening. Stevens-Johnson syndrome or toxic epidermal necrolysis may develop. Treat symptomatically; may recur once treatment is stopped.
- **Pain:** Assess pain (note type, location, and intensity) prior to and 1–2 hr following administration.
- **Arthritis:** Assess pain and range of motion prior to and 1–2 hr following administration.
- **Fever:** Monitor temperature; note signs associated with fever (diaphoresis, tachycardia, malaise).
- *Lab Test Considerations:* BUN, serum creatinine, CBC, and liver function tests should be evaluated periodically in patients receiving prolonged therapy.
- Serum potassium, BUN, serum creatinine, alkaline phosphatase, LDH, AST, and ALT may show ↑ levels. Blood glucose, hemoglobin, and hematocrit concentrations, leukocyte and platelet counts, and CCr may be ↓.
- May cause prolonged bleeding time; may persist for <1 day following discontinuation.

Potential Nursing Diagnoses

Acute pain (Indications)
Impaired physical mobility (Indications)
Ineffective thermoregulation (Indications)

Implementation

- Administration of higher than recommended doses does not provide increased pain relief but may increase incidence of side effects.
- Patient should be well hydrated before administration to prevent renal adverse reactions.
- Use lowest effective dose for shortest period of time, especially in the elderly.
- Coadministration with opioid analgesics may have additive analgesic effects and may permit lower opioid doses.
- **PO:** For rapid initial effect, administer 30 min before or 2 hr after meals. May be administered with food, milk, or antacids to decrease GI irritation. Tablets may be crushed and mixed with fluids or food; 800-mg tablet can be dissolved in water.
- **Dysmenorrhea:** Administer as soon as possible after the onset of menses. Prophylactic treatment has not been shown to be effective.

IV Administration

- **Intermittent Infusion:** *Diluent:* 0.9% NaCl, D5W, or LR. *Concentration:* Dilute the 800 mg dose in at least 200 mL and the 400 mg dose in at least 100 mL for a concentration of 4 mg/mL. Do not administer solutions that are discolored or contain particulate matter. Stable for up to 24 hr at room temperature. *Rate:* Infuse over at least 30 min.

Patient/Family Teaching

- Advise patients to take ibuprofen with a full glass of water and to remain in an upright position for 15–30 min after administration.
- Instruct patient to take medication as directed. Take missed doses as soon as remembered but not if almost time for next dose. Do not double doses. Pedi: Teach parents and caregivers to calculate and measure doses accurately and to use measuring device supplied with product.
- May cause drowsiness or dizziness. Advise patient to avoid driving or other activities requiring alertness until response to medication is known.
- Caution patient to avoid the concurrent use of alcohol, aspirin, acetaminophen, and other OTC or herbal products without consulting health care professional.
- Advise patient to inform health care professional of medication regimen prior to treatment or surgery.
- Instruct patients not to take OTC ibuprofen preparations for more than 10 days for pain or more than 3 days for fever, and to consult health care professional if symptoms persist or worsen. Many OTC products contain ibuprofen; avoid duplication.
- Caution patient that use of ibuprofen with 3 or more glasses of alcohol per day may increase the risk of GI bleeding.

- Advise patient to consult health care professional if rash, itching, visual disturbances, tinnitus, weight gain, edema, epigastric pain, dyspepsia, black stools, hematemasis, persistent headache, or influenza-like syndrome (chills, fever, muscle aches, pain) occurs.
- Pedi: Advise parents or caregivers not to administer ibuprofen to children who may be dehydrated (can occur with vomiting, diarrhea, or poor fluid intake); dehydration increases risk of renal dysfuntion.
- Advise female patients to notify health care professional if pregnancy is planned or suspected.

Evaluation/Desired Outcomes
- Decrease in severity of pain.
- Improved joint mobility. Partial arthritic relief is usually seen within 7 days, but maximum effectiveness may require 1–2 wk of continuous therapy. Patients who do not respond to one NSAID may respond to another.
- Reduction in fever.

---

ibutilide (eye-**byoo**-ti-lide)
Corvert

Classification
Therapeutic: antiarrhythmics (class III)

Pregnancy Category C

Indications
Rapid conversion of recent-onset atrial flutter or fibrillation to normal sinus rhythm, including management of atrial flutter or fibrillation occurring within 1 wk of coronary artery bypass or cardiac valve surgery.

Action
Activates slow inward current of sodium in cardiac tissue, resulting in delayed repolarization, prolonged action potential duration, and increased refractoriness. Mildly slows sinus rate and AV conduction. **Therapeutic Effects:** Conversion to normal sinus rhythm.

Pharmacokinetics
Absorption: IV administration results in complete bioavailability.
Distribution: Unknown.
Metabolism and Excretion: Highly metabolized by the liver, 1 metabolite is active; metabolites excreted by kidneys.
Half-life: 6 hr (2–12 hr).

TIME/ACTION PROFILE (antiarrhythmic effect)

ROUTE	ONSET	PEAK	DURATION
IV	within 30–90 min	unknown	up to 24 hr

Contraindications/Precautions
Contraindicated in: Hypersensitivity.
Use Cautiously in: CHF or left ventricular dysfunction (↑ risk of more serious arrhythmias during infusion); OB, Lactation, Pedi: Pregnancy, lactation, or children <18 yr (safety not established).

Adverse Reactions/Side Effects
CNS: headache. **CV:** <u>arrhythmias</u>. **GI:** nausea.

Interactions
Drug-Drug: **Amiodarone**, **disopyramide**, **procainamide**, **quinidine**, and **sotalol** should not be given concurrently or within 4 hr because of additive effects on refractoriness. Proarrhythmic effects may be ↑ by **phenothiazines**, **tricyclic** and **tetracyclic antidepressants**, some **antihistamines**, and **histamine H$_2$-receptor blocking agents**; concurrent use should be avoided.

Route/Dosage
Atrial Fibrillation/Flutter
IV (Adults ≥60 kg): 1 mg infusion; may be repeated 10 min after end of first infusion.
IV (Adults <60 kg): 0.01 mg/kg infusion; may be repeated 10 min after end of first infusion.

Atrial Fibrillation/Flutter After Cardiac Surgery
IV (Adults ≥60 kg): 0.5 mg infusion, may be repeated once.
IV (Adults <60 kg): 0.005 mg/kg infusion, may be repeated once.

Availability
Solution for injection: 0.1 mg/mL.

NURSING IMPLICATIONS

Assessment
- Monitor ECG continuously throughout and for 4 hr after infusion or until QT interval normalizes. Discontinue if arrhythmia terminates or if sustained ventricular tachycardia, prolonged QT, or QT develops. Ibutilide may have proarrhythmic effects. These arrhythmias may be serious and potentially life threatening. Clinicians trained to treat ventricular arrhythmias, medications, and equipment (defibrillator/cardio-

verter) should be available during therapy and monitoring of patient.

Potential Nursing Diagnoses
Decreased cardiac output (Indications)

Implementation
- Oral antiarrhythmic therapy may be instituted 4 hr after ibutilide infusion.

IV Administration
- **Intermittent Infusion:** *Diluent:* May be administered undiluted or diluted in 50 mL of 0.9% NaCl or D5W. Diluted solution is stable for 24 hr at room temperature or 48 hr if refrigerated. *Concentration:* Undiluted: 0.1 mg/mL; Diluted: 0.017 mg/mL. *Rate:* Administer over 10 min.
- **Additive Incompatibility:** Information unavailable; do not admix with other solutions or medications.

Patient/Family Teaching
- Inform patient of the purpose of ibutilide.

Evaluation/Desired Outcomes
- Conversion of recent-onset atrial flutter or fibrillation to normal sinus rhythm.

---

idarubicin (eye-da-**roo**-bi-sin)
Idamycin

Classification
Therapeutic: antineoplastics
Pharmacologic: anthracyclines

Pregnancy Category D

Indications
Acute myelogenous leukemia in adults (with other agents).

Action
Inhibits nucleic acid synthesis. **Therapeutic Effects:** Death of rapidly replicating cells, particularly malignant ones.

Pharmacokinetics
Absorption: IV administration results in complete bioavailability.
Distribution: Rapidly distributed with extensive tissue binding. High degree of cellular uptake.
Metabolism and Excretion: Extensive hepatic and extrahepatic metabolism. One metabolite is active (idarubicinol). Primarily eliminated via biliary excretion.
Half-life: 22 hr (range 4–46 hr).

TIME/ACTION PROFILE (effects on blood counts)

ROUTE	ONSET	PEAK	DURATION
IV	Unknown	10–14 days	21 days

Contraindications/Precautions
Contraindicated in: OB, Lactation: Pregnancy or lactation.
Use Cautiously in: Patients with childbearing potential; Active infection; ↓ bone marrow reserve; Other chronic debilitating illnesses; Hepatic impairment (dose ↓ may be required; avoid if bilirubin ≥5 mg/dL); Renal impairment; Pre-existing cardiac disease; Previous daunorubicin or doxorubicin therapy; Pedi: Safety not established; Geri: ↑ incidence of side effects and adverse reactions.

Adverse Reactions/Side Effects
CNS: headache, mental status changes. **Resp:** pulmonary toxicity, pulmonary allergic reactions. **CV:** ARRHYTHMIAS, CARDIOTOXICITY, CHF. **GI:** abdominal cramps, diarrhea, mucositis, nausea, vomiting. **Derm:** alopecia, photosensitivity, rashes. **Endo:** gonadal suppression. **Hemat:** BLEEDING, anemia, leukopenia, thrombocytopenia. **Local:** phlebitis at IV site. **Metab:** hyperuricemia. **Neuro:** peripheral neuropathy. **Misc:** fever.

Interactions
Drug-Drug: ↑ myelosuppression with other **antineoplastics** or **radiation therapy**. May ↓ antibody response to and increase risk of adverse reactions from **live-virus vaccines**.

Route/Dosage
IV (Adults): 12 mg/m^2 daily for 3 days in combination with cytarabine.

Availability (generic available)
Powder for injection: 5 mg/vial, 10 mg/vial.

NURSING IMPLICATIONS

Assessment
- Monitor blood pressure, pulse, respiratory rate, and temperature frequently during administration. Report significant changes.
- Monitor for bone marrow depression. Assess for bleeding (bleeding gums, bruising, petechiae, guaiac stools, urine, and emesis) and avoid IM injections and taking rectal temperatures if platelet count is low. Apply pressure to venipuncture sites for 10 min. Assess for signs of infection during neutropenia. Anemia may occur. Monitor for increased fatigue, dyspnea, and orthostatic hypotension.

- Monitor intake and output ratios. Report significant discrepancies. Encourage fluid intake of 2000–3000 mL/day. Allopurinol and alkalinization of the urine may be used to decrease serum uric acid levels and to help prevent urate stone formation.
- Severe and protracted nausea and vomiting may occur as early as 1 hr after therapy and may last 24 hr. Parenteral antiemetics should be administered 30–45 min prior to therapy and routinely around the clock for the next 24 hr as indicated. Monitor amount of emesis; report emesis exceeding guidelines to prevent dehydration.
- Monitor for development of signs of myocardial toxicity manifested by life-threatening arrhythmias, cardiomyopathy, and CHF (peripheral edema, dyspnea, rales/crackles, weight gain). Chest x-ray, ECG, echocardiography, and radionuclide angiography determinations of ejection fraction should be monitored prior to and periodically during therapy.
- Assess injection site frequently for redness, irritation, or inflammation. May infiltrate painlessly. If extravasation occurs, infusion must be stopped and restarted elsewhere to avoid damage to subcut tissue. Treatment of extravasation includes rest and elevation of the extremity and application of intermittent ice packs (apply for 30 min immediately and 30 min qid for 3 days). If pain, erythema, or vesication persists longer than 48 hr, immediate plastic surgery may be warranted.
- **Lab Test Considerations:** Monitor CBC, differential, and platelet count prior to and frequently during therapy. Nadirs of leukopenia and thrombocytopenia are 10–14 days, with recovery occurring 21 days after a dose.
- Monitor renal and hepatic function prior to and periodically during therapy. Idarubicin may cause hyperuricemia. May also cause transient ↑ in AST, ALT, LDH, serum alkaline phosphatase, and bilirubin.

Potential Nursing Diagnoses
Risk for infection (Adverse Reactions)
Imbalanced nutrition: less than body requirements (Adverse Reactions)

Implementation
- Do not confuse Adriamycin (doxorubicin hydrochloride) with Idamycin (idarubicin).
- Solution should be prepared in a biologic cabinet. Wear gloves, gown, and mask while handling medication. Discard IV equipment in specially designated containers.
- See cytarabine monograph for specific information on administration of cytarabine with idarubicin.
- Do not administer subcut or IM and avoid extravasation; may cause severe tissue necrosis.

IV Administration
- **Direct IV:** *Diluent:* 0.9% NaCl (nonbacteriostatic) for injection. Reconstitute 5-mg and 10-mg vials with 5 mL and 10 mL, respectively. *Concentration:* 1 mg/mL. Vial contents are under pressure; use care when inserting needle.
- Reconstituted medication is stable for 72 hr at room temperature and 7 days if refrigerated. *Rate:* Administer each dose slowly over 10–30 min through Y-site of a free-flowing infusion of 0.9% NaCl or D5W. Tubing may be attached to a butterfly needle and injected into a large vein.
- **Y-Site Compatibility:** amifostine, amikacin, aztreonam, cimetidine, cladribine, cyclophosphamide, cytarabine, diphenhydramine, droperidol, erythromycin lactobionate, etoposide phosphate, filgrastim, gemcitabine, granisetron, imipenem/cilastatin, magnesium sulfate, mannitol, melphalan, metoclopramide, potassium chloride, ranitidine, sargramostim, thiotepa, vinorelbine.
- **Y-Site Incompatibility:** acyclovir, allopurinol, ampicillin/sulbactam, cefazolin, cefepime, ceftazidime, clindamycin, dexamethasone, etoposide, furosemide, gentamicin, heparin, hydrocortisone sodium succinate, lorazepam, meperidine, methotrexate, piperacillin/tazobactam, sodium bicarbonate, teniposide, vancomycin, vincristine.

Patient/Family Teaching
- Instruct patient to notify health care professional promptly if fever; sore throat; signs of infection; bleeding gums; bruising; petechiae; blood in stools, urine, or emesis; increased fatigue; dyspnea; or orthostatic hypotension occurs. Caution patient to avoid crowds and persons with known infections. Instruct patient to use soft toothbrush and electric razor and to avoid falls. Caution patient not to drink alcoholic beverages or take medication containing aspirin or NSAIDs, as these may precipitate gastric bleeding.

694 ifosfamide

- Instruct patient to report pain at injection site immediately.
- Instruct patient to inspect oral mucosa for erythema and ulceration. If ulceration occurs, advise patient to use sponge brush, rinse mouth with water after eating and drinking, and confer with health care professional if mouth pain interferes with eating. Further courses of idarubicin should be withheld until recovery from mucositis, and subsequent doses should be decreased by 25%. Stomatitis pain may require treatment with opioid analgesics.
- Advise patient that this medication may have teratogenic effects. Contraception should be practiced during and for at least 4 mo after therapy is concluded.
- Instruct patient to notify health care professional immediately if irregular heartbeat, shortness of breath, or swelling of lower extremities occurs.
- Advise patient to wear sunscreen and protective clothing to prevent photosensitivity reactions.
- Discuss with patient the possibility of hair loss. Explore methods of coping.
- Instruct patient not to receive any vaccinations without advice of health care professional.
- Inform patient that urine may turn a reddish color.
- Emphasize the need for periodic lab tests to monitor for side effects.

Evaluation/Desired Outcomes
- Improvement of hematologic status in leukemias.

---

ifosfamide (eye-foss-fam-ide)
Ifex

Classification
Therapeutic: antineoplastics
Pharmacologic: alkylating agents

Pregnancy Category D

Indications
Germ cell testicular carcinoma (with other agents). Used with mesna, which prevents ifosfamide-induced hemorrhagic cystitis.

Action
Following conversion to active compounds, interferes with DNA replication and RNA transcription, ultimately disrupting protein synthesis (cell-cycle phase–nonspecific). **Therapeutic Effects:** Death of rapidly replicating cells, particularly malignant ones.

Pharmacokinetics
Absorption: Administered IV only; inactive prior to conversion to metabolites.
Distribution: Excreted in breast milk.
Metabolism and Excretion: Metabolized by the liver to active antineoplastic compounds.
Half-life: 15 hr.

TIME/ACTION PROFILE (effects on blood counts)

ROUTE	ONSET	PEAK	DURATION
IV	unknown	7–14 days	21 days

Contraindications/Precautions
Contraindicated in: Hypersensitivity; OB, Lactation: Pregnancy or lactation.
Use Cautiously in: Patients with childbearing potential; Active infections; Decreased bone marrow reserve; Geri: Geriatric patients; Other chronic debilitating illness; Impaired renal function; Pedi: Children.

Adverse Reactions/Side Effects
CNS: <u>CNS toxicity</u> (somnolence, confusion, hallucinations, coma), cranial nerve dysfunction, disorientation, dizziness. **CV:** cardiotoxicity. **GI:** nausea, vomiting, anorexia, constipation, diarrhea, hepatotoxicity. **GU:** <u>hemorrhagic cystitis</u>, dysuria, sterility, renal toxicity. **Derm:** <u>alopecia</u>. **Hemat:** anemia, leukopenia, thrombocytopenia. **Local:** phlebitis. **Misc:** allergic reactions.

Interactions
Drug-Drug: ↑ myelosuppression with other **antineoplastics** or **radiation therapy**. Toxicity may be ↑ by **allopurinol** or **phenobarbital**. May ↓ antibody response to and ↑ risk of adverse reactions from **live-virus vaccines**.

Route/Dosage
Other Regimens are Used
IV (Adults): 1.2 g/m^2/day for 5 days; coadminister with mesna. May repeat cycle q 3 wk.

Availability (generic available)
Injection: 1 g/vial, 3 g/vial. *In combination with:* In a kit with mesna.

NURSING IMPLICATIONS

Assessment
- Monitor blood pressure, pulse, respiratory rate, and temperature frequently during administration. Report significant changes.
- Monitor urinary output frequently during therapy. Notify health care professional if hematuria occurs. To reduce the risk of hemorrhagic cystitis, fluid intake should be at least 3000 mL/

ifosfamide **695**

day for adults and 1000–2000 mL/day for children. Mesna is given concurrently to prevent hemorrhagic cystitis.
- Monitor neurologic status. Ifosfamide should be discontinued if severe CNS symptoms (agitation, confusion, hallucinations, unusual tiredness) occur. Symptoms usually abate within 3 days of discontinuation of ifosfamide but may persist for longer; fatalities have been reported.
- Assess nausea, vomiting, and appetite. Weigh weekly. Premedication with an antiemetic may be used to minimize GI effects. Adjust diet as tolerated.
- Monitor for bone marrow depression. Assess for bleeding (bleeding gums, bruising, petechiae, guaiac stools, urine, and emesis) and avoid IM injections and taking rectal temperatures if platelet count is low. Apply pressure to venipuncture sites for 10 min. Assess for signs of infection during neutropenia. Anemia may occur. Monitor for increased fatigue, dyspnea, and orthostatic hypotension.
- **Lab Test Considerations:** Monitor CBC, differential, and platelet count prior to and periodically during therapy. Withhold dose if WBC <2000/mm^3 or platelet count is <50,000/mm^3. Nadir of leukopenia and thrombocytopenia occurs within 7–14 days and usually recovers within 21 days of therapy.
- Urinalysis should be evaluated before each dose. Withhold dose until recovery if urinalysis shows >10 RBCs per high-power field.
- May cause ↑ in liver enzymes and serum bilirubin.
- Monitor AST, ALT, serum alkaline phosphatase, bilirubin, and LDH prior to and periodically during therapy. Ifosfamide may cause ↑ in liver enzymes and serum bilirubin.
- Monitor BUN, serum creatinine, phosphate, and potassium periodically during therapy. May cause hypokalemia.

Potential Nursing Diagnoses
Risk for infection (Side Effects)
Disturbed body image (Side Effects)

Implementation
- Prepare solution in a biologic cabinet. Wear gloves, gown, and mask while handling IV medication. Discard IV equipment in specially designated containers.

IV Administration
- **IV:** Prepare solution by diluting each 1-g vial with 20 mL of sterile water or bacteriostatic water for injection containing parabens. Use solution prepared without bacteriostatic water within 6 hr. Solution prepared with bacteriostatic water is stable for 1 wk at 30°C or 6 wk at 5°C.
- **Intermittent Infusion:** *Diluent:* May be further diluted in D5W, 0.9% NaCl, LR, or sterile water for injection. *Concentration:* 0.6 to 20 mg/mL (maximum 40 mg/mL). Dilute solution is stable for 7 days at room temperature or 6 wk if refrigerated. *Rate:* Administer over at least 30 min.
- **Continuous Infusion:** Has also been administered as a continuous infusion over 72 hr.
- **Y-Site Compatibility:** acyclovir, alfentanil, allopurinol, amifostine, amikacin, aminocaproic acid, aminophylline, amiodarone, amphotericin B cholesteryl, amphotericin B colloidal, amphotericin B liposome, ampicillin, ampicillin/sulbactam, anidulafungin, atracurium, aztreonam, bivalirudin, bleomycin, bumetanide, buprenorphine, butorphanol, calcium chloride, calcium gluconate, carboplatin, caspofungin, cafazolin, cefoperazone, cefotaxime, cefotetan, cefoxitin, ceftazidime, ceftizoxime, ceftriaxone, cefuroxime, chlorpromazine, cimetidine, ciprofloxacin, cisatracurium, cisplatin, clindamycin, codeine, cyclosporine, cytarabine, dactinomycin, daptomycin, dexamethasone, dexmedetomidine, dexrazoxane, digoxin, diltiazem, dipehnhydramine, dobutamine, docetaxel, dolasetron, dopamine, doripenem, doxacurium, doxorubicin, doxorubicin liposome, doxycycline, droperidol, enalaprilat, ephedrine, epinephrine, epirubicin, ertapenem, erythroycin, esmolol, etoposide, etoposide phosphate, famotidine, fenoldopam, fentanyl, filgrastim, fluconazole, fludarabine, fluorouracil, foscarnet, fosphenytoin, furosemide, ganciclovir, gemcitabine, gentamicin, granisetron, haloperidol, heparin, hetastarch, hydrocortisone, hydromorphone, idarubicin, imipenem/cilastatin, inamrinone, insulin, isoproterenol, ketorolac, labetalol, leucovorin, levofloxacin, levorphanol, lidocaine, linezolid, lorazepam, magnesium sulfate, mannitol, melphalan, meperidine, meropenem, mesna, methohexital, methylprednisolone, metoclopramide, metoprolol, metronidazole, midazolam, milrinone, mitoxantrone, morphine, nalbuphine, naloxone, nesiritide, nitroglycerin, nitroprusside, norepinephrine, octreotide, ondansetron, oxaliplatin, paclitaxel, palonose-

tron, pancuronium, pemetrexed, pentamidine, pentobarbital, phenobarbital, phenylephrine, piperacillin/tazobactam, potassium chloride, procainamide, prochlorperazine, promethazine, propofol, propranolol, quinupristin/dalfopristin, ranitidine, remifentanil, rocuronium, sargramostim, sodium acetate, sodium bicarbonate, sodium phosphates, succinylcholine, sufentanil, tacrolimus, teniposide, theophylline, thiopental, thiotepa, ticarcillin/clavulanate, tigecycline, tirofiban, tobramycin, topotecan, trastuzumab, trimethoprim/sulfamethoxazole, vancomycin, vecuronium, verapamil, vinblastine, vincristine, vinorelbine, voriconazole, zidovudine.

- **Y-Site Incompatibility:** cefepime, diazepam, methotrexate, pantoprazole, phenytoin, potassium phosphates.
- **Additive Compatibility:** carboplatin, cisplatin, epirubicin, etoposide, fluorouracil, mesna.

Patient/Family Teaching

- Emphasize need for adequate fluid intake throughout therapy. Patient should void frequently to decrease bladder irritation from metabolites excreted by the kidneys. Notify health care professional immediately if hematuria is noted.
- Instruct patient to drink at least 8 glasses of water/day during and for 3 days after completion of therapy.
- Instruct patient to notify health care professional promptly if fever; chills; cough; hoarseness; sore throat; signs of infection; lower back or side pain; painful or difficult urination; bleeding gums; bruising; petechiae; blood in urine, stool, or emesis; or confusion occurs.
- Caution patient to avoid crowds and persons with known infections. Instruct patient to use soft toothbrush and electric razor and to avoid falls. Patients should also be cautioned not to drink alcoholic beverages or to take products containing aspirin or NSAIDs, as these may precipitate GI hemorrhage.
- Review with patient the need for contraception during therapy.
- Discuss with patient the possibility of hair loss. Explore methods of coping.
- Advise patient to consult health care professional before taking any Rx, OTC, or herbal products.
- Instruct patient not to receive any vaccinations without advice of health care professional; ifosfamide may decrease antibody response to and increase risk of adverse reactions from live-virus vaccines.

Evaluation/Desired Outcomes

- Decrease in size or spread of malignant germ cell testicular carcinoma.

iloperidone (eye-loe-**per**-i-done)
Fanapt

Classification
Therapeutic: antipsychotics
Pharmacologic: benzisoxazoles

Pregnancy Category C

Indications
Acute management of schizophrenia.

Action
May act by antagonizing dopamine and serotonin in the CNS. **Therapeutic Effects:** Decreased symptoms of schizophrenia.

Pharmacokinetics
Absorption: Well absorbed (96%) following oral administration.
Distribution: Unknown.
Metabolism and Excretion: Extensively metabolized, primarily by CYP3A4 and CYP2D6 enzyme systems, with individual variability in metabolism (extensive metabolizers [EM] and poor metabolizers [PM] and some in-between; poor metabolizers account for less than 10% of the population). Two major metabolites (P88 and P95) may be partially responsible for pharmacologic activity. 58% excreted in urine as metabolites in EM and 45% in PM; respectively, with feces accounting 20% elimination for EM and 22.1% for PM.
Half-life: *Extensive metabolizers*—iloperidone–18 hr, P88–26 hr, P95–23 hr; *poor metabolizers*—iloperidone–33 hr, P88–37 hr, P95–31 hr.

TIME/ACTION PROFILE (antipsychotic effect)

ROUTE	ONSET	PEAK	DURATION
PO	2–4 wk	2–4 hr†	unknown

† Blood level

Contraindications/Precautions
Contraindicated in: Hypersensitivity; Concurrent use of drugs known to prolong QTc interval; Bradycardia, recent MI or uncompensated heart failure (↑ risk of serious arrhythmias); Congenital long QT syndrome, QTc >500 ms or history of cardiac arrhythmias; Hepatic impairment; Geri: Elderly patients with dementia-related psychoses (↑ risk of death, CVA or TIA); Lactation: Breastfeeding should be avoided.
Use Cautiously in: Known cardiovascular disease including heart failure, history of MI/ische-

mia, conduction abnormalities, cerebrovascular disease, or other conditions known to predispose to hypotension including dehydration, hypovolemia, concurrent antihypertensive therapy (↑ risk of orthostatic hypotension); Electrolyte abnormalities, especially hypomagnesemia or hypokalemia (correct prior to therapy); Concurrent use of inhibitors of the CYP3A4 or CYP2D6 enzyme systems; Known ↓ WBC or history of drug-induced leukopenia/neutropenia; Circumstances that may result in ↑ body temperature, including strenuous exercise, exposure to extreme heat, concurrent anticholinergic activity, or dehydration (may impair thermoregulation); Patients at risk for aspiration; Geri: May have ↑ sensitivity and risk of adverse reactions; OB: Use during pregnancy only if potential maternal benefit justifies potential fetal risk; Pedi: Safe and effective use in children/adolescents has not been established.

Adverse Reactions/Side Effects

CNS: NEUROLEPTIC MALIGNANT SYNDROME, dizziness, drowsiness, fatigue, agitation, delusion, restlessness, extrapyramidal disorders. **EENT:** nasal congestion. **CV:** orthostatic hypotension, tachycardia, palpitations, QTc prolongation. **GI:** dry mouth, nausea, abdominal discomfort, diarrhea. **GU:** priapism, urinary incontinence. **Endo:** hyperglycemia, hyperprolactinemia. **Neuro:** tardive dyskinesia. **Metab:** weight gain, weight loss. **MS:** ↓ bone density, musculoskeletal stiffness.

Interactions

Drug-Drug: Avoid use of drugs known to prolong QTc including the **antiarrhythmics quinidine**, **procainamide**, **amiodarone**, and **sotalol**; **antipsychotics** including **chlorpromazine** and **thioridazine**, the **antibiotics gatifloxacin**, **moxifloxacin**, or any other **medications known to prolong the QTc interval** including **pentamidine**, **levomethadyl**, and **methadone**; concurrent use may result in serious, life-threatening arrhythmias. Concurrent use of **CYP2D6 inhibitors** including **fluoxetine** and **paroxetine** ↑ levels and the risk of toxicity; dose reduction is required. A similar effect occurs with **CYP3A4 inhibitors** including **ketoconazole** and **clarithromycin**; dosage reduction is required. Concurrent use of **antihypertensives** including **diuretics** may ↑ risk of orthostatic hypotension. Concurrent **anticholinergics** may ↑ risk of impaired thermoregulation.

Route/Dosage

PO (Adults): Initiate treatment with 1 mg twice daily on the first day, then 2 mg twice daily the second day, then increase by 2 mg/day every day until a target dose of 12–24 mg/day given in two divided doses is reached; *Concurrent CYP2D6 or CYP3A4 inhibitors*—decrease dose by one-half, if inhibitor is withdrawn increase dose to previous amount. Re-titration is required if iloperidone is discontinued >3 days.

Availability

Tablets: 1 mg, 2 mg, 4 mg, 6 mg, 8 mg, 10 mg, 12 mg.

NURSING IMPLICATIONS

Assessment

- Monitor patient's mental status (delusions, hallucinations, and behavior) before and periodically during therapy.
- Monitor mood changes. Assess for suicidal tendencies, especially during early therapy. Restrict amount of drug available to patient.
- Monitor blood pressure (sitting, standing, lying down) and pulse before and periodically during therapy. May cause prolonged QT interval, tachycardia, and orthostatic hypotension.
- Observe patient when administering medication to ensure that medication is actually swallowed and not hoarded.
- Monitor patient for onset of extrapyramidal side effects (*akathisia*—restlessness; *dystonia*—muscle spasms and twisting motions; or *pseudoparkinsonism*—mask-like face, rigidity, tremors, drooling, shuffling gait, dysphagia). Report these symptoms; reduction of dose or discontinuation of medication may be necessary.
- Monitor for tardive dyskinesia (involuntary rhythmic movement of mouth, face, and extremities). Report immediately and discontinue therapy; may be irreversible.
- Monitor for development of neuroleptic malignant syndrome (fever, respiratory distress, tachycardia, seizures, diaphoresis, hypertension or hypotension, pallor, tiredness). Discontinue iloperidone and notify health care professional immediately if these symptoms occur.
- Monitor for symptoms related to hyperprolactinemia (menstrual abnormalities, galactorrhea, sexual dysfunction).

- **Lab Test Considerations:** Monitor fasting blood glucose before and periodically during therapy in diabetic patients.
- Monitor CBC frequently during initial months of therapy in patients with pre-existing or history of low WBC. May cause leukopenia, neutropenia, or agranulocytosis. Discontinue therapy if this occurs.
- Monitor serum potassium and magnesium levels in patients at risk for electrolyte disturbances.
- Monitor serum prolactin prior to and periodically during therapy. May cause ↑ serum prolactin levels.

Potential Nursing Diagnoses
Risk for self-directed violence (Indications)
Disturbed thought process (Indications)
Risk for injury (Side Effects)

Implementation
- **PO:** Administer twice daily without regard to food.

Patient/Family Teaching
- Instruct patient to take medication exactly as directed. Advise patient that appearance of tablets in stool is normal and not of concern.
- Inform patient of the possibility of extrapyramidal symptoms. Instruct patient to report these symptoms immediately to health care professional.
- Advise patient to change positions slowly to minimize orthostatic hypotension.
- May cause drowsiness. Caution patient to avoid driving or other activities requiring alertness until response to medication is known.
- Extremes in temperature should also be avoided; this drug impairs body temperature regulation.
- Caution patient to avoid concurrent use of alcohol, other CNS depressants, and Rx, OTC, or herbal products without consulting health care professional.
- Advise female patients to notify health care professional if pregnancy is planned or suspected or if they are breastfeeding or planning to breastfeed.
- Advise patient to notify health care professional of medication regimen before treatment or surgery.
- Instruct patient to notify health care professional promptly if sore throat, fever, unusual bleeding or bruising, rash, tremors, palpitations, fainting, menstrual abnormalities, galactorrhea or sexual dysfunction occur.
- Emphasize the need for continued follow-up for psychotherapy and monitoring for side effects.

Evaluation/Desired Outcomes
- Decrease in excited, paranoid, or withdrawn behavior.

HIGH ALERT

imatinib (i-mat-i-nib)
Gleevec

Classification
Therapeutic: antineoplastics
Pharmacologic: enzyme inhibitors

Pregnancy Category D

Indications
Newly diagnosed Philadelphia positive (Ph+) chronic myeloid leukemia (CML). CML in blast crisis, accelerated phase, or in chronic phase after failure of interferon-alpha treatment. Kit (CD117) positive metastatic/unresectable malignant gastrointestinal stomal tumors (GIST). Adjuvant treatment following resection of Kit (CD117) positive GIST. Pediatric patients with Ph+ CML after failure of bone marrow transplant or resistance to interferon-alpha. Adult patients with relapsed or refractory Ph+ acute lymphoblastic leukemia (ALL). Myelodysplastic/myelyproliferative disease (MDS/MPD). Aggressive systemic mastocytosis (ASM). Hypereosinophilic syndrome and/or chronic eosinophilic leukemia (HES/CEL). Unresectable, recurrent, or metastatic dermatofibrosarcoma protuberans (DFSP).

Action
Inhibits kinases which may be produced by malignant cell lines. **Therapeutic Effects:** Inhibits production of malignant cell lines with decreased proliferation of leukemic cells in CML, HES/CEL, and ALL and malignant cells in GIST, MDS/MPD, ASM, and DFSP.

Pharmacokinetics
Absorption: Well absorbed (98%) following oral administration.
Distribution: Unknown.
Protein Binding: 95%.
Metabolism and Excretion: Mostly metabolized by the CYP3A4 enzyme system to N-demethyl imatinib, which is as active as imatinib. Excreted mostly in feces as metabolites. 5% excreted unchanged in urine.
Half-life: *Imatinib*— 18 hr; *N-desmethyl imatinib*— 40 hr.

imatinib

TIME/ACTION PROFILE (blood levels of imatinib)

ROUTE	ONSET	PEAK	DURATION
PO	unknown	2–4 hr	24 hr

Contraindications/Precautions
Contraindicated in: Hypersensitivity; OB: Potential for fetal harm; Lactation: Potential for serious adverse reactions in nursing infants; breastfeeding should be avoided.
Use Cautiously in: Hepatic impairment (dose ↓ recommended if bilirubin >3 times normal or liver transaminases >5 times normal); Cardiac disease (severe congestive heart failure and left ventricular dysfunction may occur); Pedi: Children <3 yr (safety not established); Geri: ↑ risk of edema.

Adverse Reactions/Side Effects
CNS: fatigue, headache, weakness. **Resp:** cough, dyspnea, epistaxis, nasopharyngitis, pneumonia. **GI:** HEPATOTOXICITY, abdominal pain, anorexia, constipation, diarrhea, dyspepsia, nausea, vomiting. **Derm:** petechiae, pruritus, skin rash. **F and E:** edema (including pleural effusion, pericardial infusion, anasarca, superficial edema and fluid retention), hypokalemia. **Endo:** hypothyroidism. **Hemat:** BLEEDING, NEUTROPENIA, THROMBOCYTOPENIA. **Metab:** weight gain. **MS:** arthralgia, muscle cramps, musculoskeletal pain, myalgia. **Misc:** fever, night sweats.

Interactions
Drug-Drug: Blood levels and effects are ↑ by concurrent use of potent CYP3A4 inhibitors (e.g. **ketoconazole**, **itraconazole**, **clarithromycin**, **atazanavir**, **indinavir**, **nefazodone**, **nelfinavir**, **ritonavir**, **saquinavor**, **telithromycin**, or **voriconazole**). Blood levels and effects may be ↓ by potent CYP3A4 inducers (e.g., **dexamethasone**, **phenytoin**, **carbamazepine**, **rifampin**, **rifabutin**, and **phenobarbital**; if used concurrently, ↑ dose of imatinib by 50%. ↑ blood levels of **simvastatin**. Imatinib inhibits the following enzyme systems: CYP2C9, CYP2D6, CYP3A4/5 and may be expected to alter the effects of other drugs metabolized by these systems.
Drug-Food: Blood levels and effects are ↑ by **grapefruit juice**; concurrent use should be avoided.

Route/Dosage
Chronic Myeloid Leukemia
PO (Adults): *Chronic phase*—400 mg once daily, may be ↑ to 600 mg once daily; *accelerated phase or blast crisis*—600 mg once daily; may be ↑ to 800 mg/day given as 400 mg twice daily based on response and circumstances.
PO (Children): *Newly diagnosed Ph+ CML*-340 mg/m^2/day (not to exceed 600 mg); *CML recurrent after failure of bone marrow transplant or resistance to interferon-alpha*—260 mg/m^2/day.

Gastrointestinal Stromal Tumors
PO (Adults): *Metastatic or unresectable*—400 mg/day; may be ↑ to 400 mg twice daily if well tolerated and response insufficient; *Adjuvant treatment after resection*—400 mg/day.

Ph+ Acute Lymphoblastic Leukemia
PO (Adults): 600 mg/day.

Myelodysplastic/Myeloproliferative Diseases
PO (Adults): 400 mg/day.

Aggressive Systemic Mastocytosis
PO (Adults): 400 mg/day. *For patients with eosinophilia*—100 mg/day; ↑ to 400 mg/day if well tolerated and response insufficient.

Hypereosinophilic Syndrome and/or Chronic Eosinophilic Leukemia
PO (Adults): 400 mg/day. *For patients with FIP1L1-PDGFRa fusion kinase* 100 mg/day; increase to 400 mg/day if well tolerated and response insufficient.

Dermatofibrosarcoma Protuberans
PO (Adults): 800 mg/day.

Hepatic Impairment
PO (Adults): ↓ dose by 25% in severe hepatic impairment.

Renal Impairment
PO (Adults): *CCr 40–59 mL/min*—Do not exceed dose of 600 mg/day; *CCr 20–39 mL/min*—↓ initial dose by 50%; ↑ as tolerated.

Availability
Tablets: 100 mg, 400 mg.

imipenem/cilastatin

NURSING IMPLICATIONS
Assessment
* Monitor for fluid retention. Weigh regularly, and assess for signs of pleural effusion, pericardial effusion, pulmonary edema, ascites (dyspnea, periorbital edema, swelling in feet and ankles, weight gain). Evaluate unexpected weight gain. Edema is usually managed with diuretics. General fluid retention is usually dose related, more common in accelerated phase or blast crisis, and is more common in the elderly. Treatment usually involves diuretics, supportive therapy, and interruption of imatinib.
* Monitor vital signs; may cause fever.
* **Lab Test Considerations:** Monitor liver function before and monthly during treatment or when clinically indicated. May cause ↑ transamininases and bilirubin which usually lasts 1 wk and may require dose reduction or interruption. If bilirubin is >3 times the upper limit of normal or transaminases are >5 times the upper limit of normal withhold dose until bilirubin levels return to <1.5 times the upper limit of normal and transaminase levels to < 2.5 times the upper limit of normal. Treatment may then be continued at reduced levels (patients on 400 mg/day should receive 300 mg/day and patients receiving 600 mg/day should receive 400 mg/day).
* Monitor CBC weekly for the first month, biweekly for the second month, and periodically during therapy. May cause neutropenia and thrombocytopenia, usually lasting 2–3 wk or 3–4 wk, respectively, and anemia. Usually requires dose reduction, but may require discontinuation (see Implementation).
* May cause hypokalemia.

Potential Nursing Diagnoses
Risk for injury (Adverse Reactions)

Implementation
* **High Alert:** Fatalities have occurred with incorrect administration of chemotherapeutic agents. Before administering, clarify all ambiguous orders; double check single, daily, and course-of-therapy dose limits; have second practitioner independently double check original order and dose calculations. Therapy should be initiated by physician experienced in the treatment of patients with chronic myeloid leukemia.
* Patients requiring anticoagulation should receive low-molecular-weight or standard heparin, not warfarin.
* Treatment should be continued as long as patient continues to benefit.
* **PO:** Administer with food and a full glass of water to minimize GI irritation.
* Tablets may be dispersed in water or apple juice (50 mL for the 100 mg and 100 mL for the 400 mg tablet) and stirred with a spoon for patients unable to swallow pills. Administer immediately after suspension.
* Patients receiving *chronic phase, myelodysplastic/myeloproliferative disease, aggressive systemic mastocytosis, and hypereosinophilic syndrome and/or chronic eosinophilic leukemia* treatment who develop an ANC <1.0 × 10^9/L and/or platelets <50 × 10^9/L should stop imatinib until ANC ≥1.5 × 10^9/L and platelets are ≥75 × 10^9/L. Then resume imatinib treatment at 400 mg or 600 mg/day.
* *Patients receiving accelerated phase and blast crisis treatment or Ph+ acute lymphoblastic leukemia* who develop an ANC <0.5 × 10^9/L and/or platelets <10 × 10^9/L should determine if cytopenia is related to leukemia via marrow aspirate or biopsy. If cytopenia is unrelated to leukemia, reduce dose to 400 mg/day. If cytopenia persists for 2 wk, reduce dose to 300 mg/day. If cytopenia persists for 4 wk and is still unrelated to leukemia, stop imatinib until ANC ≥ 1 × 10^9/L and platelets are ≥ 20 × 10^9/L. Then resume imatinib treatment at 300 mg/day.
* *Patients receiving aggressive systemic mastocytosis with eosinophilia or hypereosinophilic syndrome and/or chronic eosinophilic leukemia with FIP1L1–PDGFRa fusion kinase*—who develop ANC <1.0 × 10^9/L and platelets <50 × 10^9/L should stop imatinib until ANC ≥1.5 × 10^9/L and platelets ≥75 × 10^9/L. Resume treatment at previous dose.

Patient/Family Teaching
* Explain purpose of imatinib to patient.
* Advise patient to avoid grapefruit and grapefruit juice during therapy.

Evaluation/Desired Outcomes
* Decrease in production of leukemic cells in patients with CML, HES/CEL, and ALL and malignant cells in GIST, MDS/MPD, ASM, and DFSP.

imipenem/cilastatin
(i-me-**pen**-em/sye-la-**stat**-in)
Primaxin

imipenem/cilastatin

Classification
Therapeutic: anti-infectives
Pharmacologic: carbapenems

Pregnancy Category C

Indications
Treatment of: Lower respiratory tract infections, Urinary tract infections, Abdominal infections, Gynecologic infections, Skin and skin structure infections, Bone and joint infections, Bacteremia, Endocarditis, Polymicrobic infections.

Action
Imipenem binds to the bacterial cell wall, resulting in cell death. Combination with cilastatin prevents renal inactivation of imipenem, resulting in high urinary concentrations. Imipenem resists the actions of many enzymes that degrade most other penicillins and penicillin-like anti-infectives.
Therapeutic Effects: Bactericidal action against susceptible bacteria. **Spectrum:** Spectrum is broad. Active against most gram-positive aerobic cocci: *Streptococcus pneumoniae*, Group A beta-hemolytic streptococci, *Enterococcus*, *Staphylococcus aureus*. Active against many gram-negative bacillary organisms: *Escherichia coli*, *Klebsiella*, *Acinetobacter*, *Proteus*, *Serratia*, *Pseudomonas aeruginosa*. Also displays activity against: *Salmonella*, *Shigella*, *Neisseria gonorrhoeae*, Numerous anaerobes.

Pharmacokinetics
Absorption: Well absorbed after IM administration (imipenem 95%, cilastatin 75%). IV administration results in complete bioavailability.
Distribution: Widely distributed. Crosses the placenta; enters breast milk.
Metabolism and Excretion: *Imipenem and cilastatin* —70% excreted unchanged by the kidneys.
Half-life: *Imipenem and cilastatin*—1 hr (↑ in renal impairment).

TIME/ACTION PROFILE (blood levels)

ROUTE	ONSET	PEAK	DURATION
IM	rapid	1–2 hr	12 hr
IV	rapid	end of infusion	6–8 hr

Contraindications/Precautions
Contraindicated in: Hypersensitivity; Cross-sensitivity may occur with penicillins and cephalosporins.
Use Cautiously in: Previous history of multiple hypersensitivity reactions; Seizure disorders; Renal impairment (dose ↓ required if CCr ≤70 mL/min/1.73 m²); OB, Lactation, Pedi: Safety not established; Geri: May be at ↑ risk for toxic reactions due to age-related ↑ in renal function.

Adverse Reactions/Side Effects
CNS: SEIZURES, dizziness, somnolence. **CV:** hypotension. **GI:** PSEUDOMEMBRANOUS COLITIS, diarrhea, nausea, vomiting. **Derm:** rash, pruritus, sweating, urticaria. **Hemat:** eosinophilia. **Local:** phlebitis at IV site. **Misc:** allergic reaction including ANAPHYLAXIS, fever, superinfection.

Interactions
Drug-Drug: Do not admix with **aminoglycosides** (inactivation may occur). **Probenecid** ↓ renal excretion and ↑ blood levels. ↑ risk of seizures with **ganciclovir** or **cyclosporine** (avoid concurrent use of ganciclovir). May ↓ serum **valproate** levels (↑ risk of seizures).

Route/Dosage
IV (Adults): *Mild infections*—250–500 mg q 6 hr. *Moderate infections*—500 mg q 6–8 hr or 1 g q 8 hr. *Serious infections*—500 mg q 6 hr to 1 g q 6–8 hr.
IV (Children ≥3 mo [non-CNS infections]): 15–25 mg/kg q 6 hr; higher doses have been used in older children with cystic fibrosis.
IV (Children 4 wk–3 mo): 25 mg/kg q 6 hr.
IV (Children 1–4 wk): 25 mg/kg q 8 hr.
IV (Children <1 wk): 25 mg/kg q 12 hr.
IM (Adults): 500–750 mg q 12 hr.
IM (Children): 10–15 mg/kg q 6 hr.

Renal Impairment
IV (Adults): If dose for normal renal function is 1 g/day *CCr 41–70 mL/min*—125–250 mg q 6–8 hr, *CCr 21–40 mL/min*—125–250 mg q 8–12 hr, *CCr 6–20 mL/min*—125–250 mg q 12 hr; **if dose for normal renal function is 1.5 g/day** *CCr 41–70 mL/min*—125–250 mg q 6–8 hr, *CCr 21–40 mL/min*—125–250 mg q 8–12 hr, *CCr 6–20 mL/min*—125–250 mg q 12 hr; **if dose for normal renal function is 2 g/day** *CCr 41–70 mL/min*—125–500 mg q 6–8 hr, *CCr 21–40 mL/min*—125–250 mg q 8–12 hr, *CCr 6–20 mL/min*—125–250 mg q 12 hr; **if dose for normal renal function is 3 g/day** *CCr 41–70 mL/min*—250–500 mg q 6–8 hr, *CCr 21–40 mL/min*—250–500 mg q 6–8 hr, *CCr 6–20 mL/min*—250–500 mg q 12 hr; **if dose for normal renal function is 4 g/day** *CCr 41–70 mL/min*—250–750 mg q 6–8 hr, *CCr 21–40 mL/min*—

imipenem/cilastatin

250–500 mg q 6–8 hr, *CCr 6–20 mL/min*—250–250 mg q 12 hr.

Availability
Powder for IV injection: 250 mg imipenem/250 mg cilastatin, 500 mg imipenem/500 mg cilastatin. **Powder for IM injection:** 500 mg imipenem/500 mg cilastatin, 750 mg imipenem/750 mg cilastatin.

NURSING IMPLICATIONS

Assessment
- Assess patient for infection (vital signs; appearance of wound, sputum, urine, and stool; WBC) at beginning of and throughout therapy.
- Obtain a history before initiating therapy to determine previous use of and reactions to penicillins. Persons with a negative history of penicillin sensitivity may still have an allergic response.
- Obtain specimens for culture and sensitivity before initiating therapy. First dose may be given before receiving results.
- Observe patient for signs and symptoms of anaphylaxis (rash, pruritus, laryngeal edema, wheezing). Discontinue the drug and notify the physician immediately if these occur. Have epinephrine, an antihistamine, and resuscitative equipment close by in the event of an anaphylactic reaction.
- **Lab Test Considerations:** BUN, AST, ALT, LDH, serum alkaline phosphatase, bilirubin, and creatinine may be transiently ↑.
- Hemoglobin and hematocrit concentrations may be ↓.
- May cause positive direct Coombs' test.

Potential Nursing Diagnoses
Risk for infection (Indications, Side Effects)

Implementation
- **IM: Only the IM formulation can be used for IM administration.** Reconstitute 500-mg vial with 2 mL and 750-mg vial with 3 mL of lidocaine without epinephrine. Shake well to form a suspension. Withdraw and inject entire contents of vial IM.

IV Administration
- **Intermittent Infusion: Only the IV formulation can be used for IV administration.** *Diluent:* Reconstitute each 250- or 500-mg vial with 10 mL of D5W or 0.9% NaCl and shake well. Further dilute in 100 mL of D5W or 0.9% NaCl. Solution may range from clear to yellow in color. Infusion is stable for 4 hr at room temperature and 24 hr if refrigerated. *Concentration:* 2.5 mg/mL (with 250–mg vial); 5 mg/mL (with 500-mg vial). *Rate:* Infuse doses ≤ 500 mg over 20–30 min. Infuse doses ≥ 750 mg over 40–60 min. Pedi: Infuse doses ≤ 500 mg over 15–30 min. Infuse doses > 500 mg over 40–60 min.
- Rapid infusion may cause nausea and vomiting. If these symptoms develop, slow infusion.
- **Y-Site Compatibility:** acyclovir, amifostine, amikacin, anidulafungin, atropine, aztreonam, bumetanide, caspofungin, cefazolin, cefepime, cefotaxime, cefoxitin, ceftazidime, ceftizoxime, cefuroxime, chloramphenicol, cimetidine, cisatracurium, clindamycin, cyclosporine, dexamethasone sodium phosphate, digoxin, diltiazem, diphenhydramine, docetaxel, dopamine, doxycycline, enalaprilat, epinephrine, erythromycin, esmolol, famotidine, fenoldopam, fentanyl, fludarabine, foscarnet, furosemide, gentamicin, granisetron, heparin, hydrocortisone sodium succinate, hydromorphone, idarubicin, insulin, isoproterenol, ketorolac, labetalol, levofloxacin, lidocaine, linezolid, magnesium sulfate, melphalan, methotrexate, methylprednisolone sodium succinate, metoclopramide, metoprolol, metronidazole, morphine, nafcillin, nitroglycerin, norepinephrine, ondansetron, pantoprazole, penicillin G potassium, phenylephrine, phytonadione, potassium chloride, propranolol, propofol, protamine, ranitidine, remifentanil, tacrolimus, teniposide, thiotepa, ticarcillin/clavulanate, tigecycline, tirofiban, tobramycin, vancomycin, vasopressin, verapamil, vinorelbine, voriconazole, zidovudine.
- **Y-Site Incompatibility:** allopurinol, amiodarone, amphotericin B cholesteryl sulfate, azithromycin, ceftriaxone, daptomycin, diazepam, drotrecogin, etoposide phosphate, fluconazole, gallium nitrate, ganciclovir, gemcitabine, haloperidol, lorazepam, meperidine, midazolam, milrinone, phenytoin, prochlorperazine, quinupristin/dalfopristin, sargramostim, sodium bicarbonate, trimethoprim/sulfamethoxazole.
- **Additive Incompatibility:** May be inactivated if administered concurrently with aminoglycosides. If administered concurrently, administer in separate sites, if possible, at least 1 hr apart. If second site is unavailable, flush lines between medications.

Patient/Family Teaching
- Advise patient to report the signs of superinfection (black, furry overgrowth on the tongue; vaginal itching or discharge; loose or foul-smelling stools) and allergy. Consult health

care professional before treating with antidiarrheals.
- Caution patient to notify health care professional if fever and diarrhea occur, especially if stool contains blood, pus, or mucus. Advise patient not to treat diarrhea without consulting health care professional. May occur up to several weeks after discontinuation of medication.

Evaluation/Desired Outcomes
- Resolution of the signs and symptoms of infection. Length of time for complete resolution depends on the organism and site of infection.

imipramine (im-ip-ra-meen)
✤ Apo-Imipramine, ✤ Impril, Norfranil, ✤ Novopramine, Tipramine, Tofranil, Tofranil PM

Classification
Therapeutic: antidepressants
Pharmacologic: tricyclic antidepressants

Pregnancy Category C

Indications
Various forms of depression. Enuresis in children. **Unlabeled Use:** Adjunct in the management of chronic pain, incontinence (in adults), vascular headache prophylaxis, cluster headache, insomnia.

Action
Potentiates the effect of serotonin and norepinephrine. Has significant anticholinergic properties. **Therapeutic Effects:** Antidepressant action that develops slowly over several weeks.

Pharmacokinetics
Absorption: Well absorbed from the GI tract.
Distribution: Widely distributed. Probably crosses the placenta and enters breast milk.
Protein Binding: 89–95%.
Metabolism and Excretion: Extensively metabolized by the liver, mostly on first pass; some conversion to active compounds. Undergoes enterohepatic recirculation and secretion into gastric juices.
Half-life: 8–16 hr.

TIME/ACTION PROFILE (antidepressant effect)

ROUTE	ONSET	PEAK	DURATION
PO, IM	hours	2–6 wk	weeks

Contraindications/Precautions
Contraindicated in: Hypersensitivity; Cross-sensitivity with other antidepressants may occur; Angle-closure glaucoma; Hypersensitivity to tartrazine or sulfites (in some preparations); Recent MI, known history of QTc prolongation, heart failure.
Use Cautiously in: Pre-existing cardiovascular disease; Seizures or history of seizure disorder; May ↑ risk of suicide attempt/ideation especially during early treatment or dose adjustment; OB: Drug is present in breast milk; discontinue imipramine or bottle feed; Pedi: Suicide risk may be greater in children or adolescents. Safety not established in children <6 yr; Geri: Geriatric patients (more susceptible to adverse reactions). Geriatric males with prostatic hyperplasia are more susceptible to urinary retention.

Adverse Reactions/Side Effects
CNS: drowsiness, fatigue, agitation, confusion, hallucinations, insomnia. **EENT:** blurred vision, dry eyes. **CV:** ARRHYTHMIAS, hypotension, ECG changes. **GI:** constipation, dry mouth, nausea, paralytic ileus, weight gain. **GU:** urinary retention, decreased libido. **Derm:** photosensitivity. **Endo:** gynecomastia. **Hemat:** blood dyscrasias.

Interactions
Drug-Drug: May cause hypotension, tachycardia, and potentially fatal reactions when used with **MAO inhibitors** (avoid concurrent use—discontinue 2 wk prior to imipramine). Concurrent use with **SSRI antidepressants** may result in increased toxicity and should be avoided (**fluoxetine** should be stopped 5 wk before). Concurrent use with **clonidine** may result in hypertensive crisis and should be avoided. Imipramine is metabolized in the liver by the **cytochrome P450 2D6 enzyme** and its action may be affected by drugs that compete for metabolism by this enzyme including **other antidepressants**, **phenothiazines**, **carbamazepine**, **class 1C antiarrhythmics** (**propafenone, flecainide**); when used concurrently, dose reduction of one or the other or both may be necessary. Concurrent use of other drugs that inhibit the activity of the enzyme, including **cimetidine, quinidine, amiodarone**, and **ritonavir**, may result in ↑ effects of imipramine. Concurrent use with **levodopa** may result in delayed/↓ absorption of levodopa or hypertension. Blood levels and effects may be ↓ by **rifamycins**. ↑ CNS depression with other CNS **depressants** including **alcohol, antihistamines,**

✤ = Canadian drug name. ᛜ = Genetic implication.
*CAPITALS indicates life-threatening; underlines indicate most frequent.

clonidine, opioids, and sedative/hypnotics. Barbiturates may alter blood levels and effects. Adrenergic and anticholinergic side effects may be ↑ with other agents having these properties. Phenothiazines or hormonal contraceptives ↑ levels and may cause toxicity. Cigarette smoking (nicotine) may increase metabolism and alter effects.
Drug-Natural Products: Concomitant use of kava-kava, valerian, or chamomile can increase CNS depression. ↑ anticholinergic effects with jimson weed and scopolia.

Route/Dosage
PO (Adults): 25–50 mg 3–4 times daily (not to exceed 300 mg/day); total daily dose may be given at bedtime.
PO (Geriatric Patients): 25 mg at bedtime initially, up to 100 mg/day in divided doses.
PO (Children >12 yr): *Antidepressant*—25–50 mg/day in divided doses (not to exceed 100 mg/day).
PO (Children 6–12 yr): *Antidepressant*—10–30 mg/day in 2 divided doses.
PO (Children ≥6 yr): *Enuresis*—25 mg once daily 1 hr before bedtime; increase if necessary by 25 mg at weekly intervals to 50 mg in children <12 yr, up to 75 mg in children >12 yr.
IM (Adults): Up to 100 mg/day in divided doses (not to exceed 300 mg/day).

Availability (generic available)
Tablets: 10 mg, 25 mg, 50 mg, ♣75 mg. **Capsules:** 75 mg, 100 mg, 125 mg, 150 mg. **Injection:** 12.5 mg/mL.

NURSING IMPLICATIONS

Assessment
- Monitor blood pressure and pulse rate prior to and during initial therapy.
- Monitor plasma levels in treatment-resisant patients.
- Monitor weight and BMI initially and periodically throughout therapy.
- For overweight/obese individuals, obtain FBS and cholesterol levels. Refer as appropriate for nutrition/weight management and medical management.
- Obtain weight and BMI initially and regularly throughout therapy.
- Assess for sexual dysfunction (decreased libido; erectile dysfunction).
- Pedi, Geri: Monitor baseline and periodic ECGs in elderly patients or patients with heart disease and before increasing dose with children treated for enuresis. May cause prolonged PR and QT intervals and may flatten T waves.
- **Depression:** Assess mental status (orientation, mood, behavior) frequently. Confusion, agitation, and hallucinations may occur during initiation of therapy and may require dosage reduction. Assess for suicidal tendencies, especially during early therapy. Restrict amount of drug available to patient.
- **Enuresis:** Assess frequency of bedwetting during therapy. Ask patient or caretaker to maintain diary.
- **Pain:** Assess location, duration, and severity of pain periodically during therapy. Use pain scale to monitor effectiveness of therapy.
- ***Lab Test Considerations:*** Assess leukocyte and differential blood counts and renal and hepatic functions prior to and periodically during prolonged or high-dose therapy.
- Serum levels may be monitored in patients who fail to respond to usual therapeutic dose. Therapeutic plasma concentration range for depression is 150–300 ng/mL.
- May cause alterations in blood glucose levels.
- ***Toxicity and Overdose:*** Symptoms of acute overdose include disturbed concentration, confusion, restlessness, agitation, seizures, drowsiness, mydriasis, arrhythmias, fever, hallucinations, vomiting, and dyspnea.
- Treatment of overdose includes gastric lavage, activated charcoal, and a stimulant cathartic. Maintain respiratory and cardiac function (monitor ECG for at least 5 days) and temperature. Medications may include digoxin for CHF, antiarrhythmics, and anticonvulsants.

Potential Nursing Diagnoses
Ineffective coping (Indications)
Chronic pain (Indications)
Impaired urinary elimination (Indications, Side Effects)
Sexual dysfunction (Side Effects)

Implementation
- Do not confuse imipramine with desipramine.
- Dose increases should be made at bedtime because of sedation. Dose titration is a slow process; may take weeks to months. May be given as a single dose at bedtime to minimize sedation during the day.
- Taper to avoid withdrawal effects. Reduce by 50% for 3 days, then reduce by 50% for 3 days, then discontinue.
- **PO:** Administer medication with or immediately following a meal to minimize gastric irritation.
- **IM:** May be slightly yellow or red in color. Crystals may develop if solution is cool; place

ampule under warm running water for 1 min to dissolve.

Patient/Family Teaching
- Instruct patient to take medication as directed. Take missed doses as soon as possible unless almost time for next dose; if regimen is a single dose at bedtime, do not take in the morning because of side effects. Advise patient that drug effects may not be noticed for at least 2 wk. Abrupt discontinuation may cause nausea, vomiting, diarrhea, headache, trouble sleeping with vivid dreams, and irritability.
- May cause drowsiness and blurred vision. Caution patient to avoid driving and other activities requiring alertness until response to drug is known.
- Instruct patient to notify health care professional if visual changes occur. Inform patient that periodic glaucoma testing may be needed during long-term therapy.
- Caution patient to change positions slowly to minimize orthostatic hypotension.
- Advise patient to avoid alcohol or other CNS depressant drugs during therapy and for at least 3–7 days after therapy has been discontinued.
- Instruct patient to notify health care professional if urinary retention, dry mouth, or constipation persists. Sugarless candy or gum may diminish dry mouth and an increase in fluid intake or bulk may prevent constipation. If symptoms persist, dose reduction or discontinuation may be necessary. Consult health care professional if dry mouth persists for more than 2 wk.
- Caution patient to use sunscreen and protective clothing to prevent photosensitivity reactions.
- Alert patient that urine may turn blue-green in color.
- Inform patient of need to monitor dietary intake, as possible increase in appetite may lead to undesired weight gain. Inform patient that increased amounts of riboflavin in the diet may be required; consult health care professional.
- Advise patient to notify health care professional of medication regimen prior to treatment or surgery.
- Therapy for depression is usually prolonged. Emphasize the importance of follow-up exams to evaluate progress and improve coping skills.
- Pedi: Inform parents that the side effects most likely to occur include nervousness, insomnia, unusual tiredness, and mild nausea and vomiting. Notify health care professional if these symptoms become pronounced.
- Advise parents to keep medication out of reach of children to prevent inadvertent overdose.
- Refer to local support group.

Evaluation/Desired Outcomes
- Increased sense of well-being.
- Renewed interest in surroundings.
- Increased appetite.
- Improved energy level.
- Pain relief.
- Diminished incidence of enuresis.
- Improved sleep in patients treated for depression. Patient may require 2–6 wk of therapy before full therapeutic effects of medication are noticeable.
- Control of bedwetting in children >6 yr.
- Decrease in chronic neurogenic pain.

imiquimod (i-mi-kwi-mod)
Aldara

Classification
Therapeutic: antivirals, immune modifiers
Pharmacologic: immune response modifiers

Pregnancy Category B

Indications
External genital or perianal warts/condylomata (condyloma acuminatum). Typical, nonhyperkeratotic, nonhypertrophic actinic keratoses on the face or scalp. Biopsy-confirmed, primary superficial basal cell carcinoma.

Action
May induce the formation of interferons that have antiproliferative and antiviral properties. **Therapeutic Effects:** Regression of external genital or perianal warts/condylomata, actinic keratoses, or basal cell carcinoma lesions.

Pharmacokinetics
Absorption: Minimal absorption.
Distribution: Action is primarily local.
Metabolism and Excretion: <0.9% excreted in urine and feces.
Half-life: Unknown.

TIME/ACTION PROFILE (regression of lesions)

ROUTE	ONSET	PEAK	DURATION
Topical	days–wk	10–16 wk	unknown

✦ = Canadian drug name.   ✦ = Genetic implication.
*CAPITALS indicates life-threatening; underlines indicate most frequent.

Contraindications/Precautions
Contraindicated in: None known.
Use Cautiously in: Previous treatment/surgery in affected area (area should be healed prior to use); Pre-existing inflammatory skin lesions (may be exacerbated); Immunocompromised patients (safety not established); OB, Lactation, Pedi: Pregnancy, lactation, or children <12 yr (safety not established).

Adverse Reactions/Side Effects
Local: irritation, pain, pruritus, burning, swelling, fungal infections (women).

Interactions
Drug-Drug: None known.

Route/Dosage
External Genital Warts
Topical (Adults and children > 12 yr): Apply thin layer to warts at bedtime every other day (3 times weekly); leave on for 6–10 hr, then rinse off with mild soap and water. Repeat until lesions are completely cleared or up to 16 wk.

Actinic Keratoses
Topical (Adults): Apply thin layer to clean, dry affected area twice weekly; leave on for 8 hr, then rinse off with mild soap and water. Continue for 16 wk.

Superficial Basal Cell Carcinoma
Topical (Adults): Apply thin layer to clean, dry affected area 5 times per week; leave on for 8 hr, then rinse off with mild soap and water. Continue for 6 wk.

Availability
Cream: 5% in single-use packets in boxes of 12. **Cost:** $185.59/box.

NURSING IMPLICATIONS

Assessment
- Assess affected area(s) prior to and periodically during therapy.

Potential Nursing Diagnoses
Risk for infection (Indications)
Risk for infection (Patient/Family Teaching)

Implementation
- **Topical:** Apply a thin film to clean and dry skin as directed prior to bedtime. Rub in well and leave on skin for time period specified. Remove by washing with mild soap and water. Discard unused cream from single-dose packet. A rest period of several days may be taken if required for patient comfort or severity of skin reaction. Resume therapy when reaction subsides.
- Do not use occlusive dressings. If covering is needed, use cotton gauze or cotton underclothes.

Patient/Family Teaching
- Instruct patient on proper application technique. Emphasize the importance of washing hands before and after application and avoiding contact with eyes. Advise patient not to use more cream than was prescribed. Missed doses should be applied as soon as possible; then return to regular schedule.
- Advise patient to delay next dose for several days when experiencing discomfort or severe reactions. Notify health care professional if severe reactions occur.
- Advise patient to avoid sharing this medication with others.
- Instruct patient to avoid contact with affected areas while the cream is on the skin. Wash cream off of genital areas before engaging in sexual activities. Inform patient that oils in the cream weaken latex contraceptive devices, such as cervical caps, condoms, and diaphragms.
- Advise patient to avoid use of other topical medications on same treatment area unless recommended by health care professional.

Evaluation/Desired Outcomes
- Healing of genital or perianal warts. Treatment is continued until wart is healed or up to 16 wk.
- Healing of actinic keratosis. Treatment is continued for 16 wk.
- Resolution of superficial basal cell carcinoma lesions. Treatment is continued for 6 wk.

---

indapamide (in-dap-a-mide)
♦ Lozide

Classification
Therapeutic: antihypertensives, diuretics
Pharmacologic: thiazide-like diuretics

Pregnancy Category B

Indications
Mild to moderate hypertension. Edema associated with CHF and other causes.

Action
Increases excretion of sodium and water by inhibiting sodium reabsorption in the distal tubule. Promotes excretion of chloride, potassium, magnesium, and bicarbonate. May produce arteriolar dilation. **Therapeutic Effects:** Lowering of

blood pressure in hypertensive patients and diuresis with subsequent mobilization of edema.

Pharmacokinetics
Absorption: Well absorbed from the GI tract after oral administration.
Distribution: Widely distributed.
Metabolism and Excretion: Mostly metabolized by the liver. Small amounts (7%) excreted unchanged by the kidneys.
Half-life: 14–18 hr.

TIME/ACTION PROFILE (antihypertensive effect)

ROUTE	ONSET	PEAK	DURATION
PO (single dose)	unknown	24 hr	unknown
PO (multiple dose)	1–2 wk	8–12 wk	up to 8 wk

Contraindications/Precautions
Contraindicated in: Hypersensitivity; Cross-sensitivity with sulfonamides may occur; Anuria.
Use Cautiously in: Renal or severe hepatic impairment; Lactation: May be taken while breastfeeding although higher doses followed by significant diuresis may ↓ milk production; Pedi: Safety not established; Geri: ↑ sensitivity to drug effects.

Adverse Reactions/Side Effects
CNS: dizziness, drowsiness, lethargy. **CV:** arrhythmias, hypotension. **GI:** anorexia, cramping, nausea, vomiting. **Derm:** photosensitivity, rashes. **Endo:** hyperglycemia. **F and E:** hypokalemia, dehydration, hypochloremic alkalosis, hyponatremia, hypovolemia. **Metab:** hyperuricemia. **MS:** muscle cramps.

Interactions
Drug-Drug: Additive hypotension with other **antihypertensives**, **nitrates**, or acute ingestion of **alcohol**. Additive hypokalemia with **corticosteroids**, **amphotericin B**, **piperacillin**, or **ticarcillin**. ↓ excretion of **lithium**; may cause toxicity. Hypokalemia may ↑ risk of **digoxin** toxicity.
Drug-Natural Products: **Licorice** and **stimulant laxative herbs** (**aloe**, **senna**) may ↑ risk of potassium depletion.

Route/Dosage
PO (Adults): *Hypertension*—1.25–5 mg once daily in the morning; may be ↑ at 4-wk intervals up to 5 mg/day. *Edema secondary to CHF*—2.5 mg once daily in the morning; may be ↑ after 1 wk to 5 mg/day.

Availability (generic available)
Tablets: 1.25 mg, 2.5 mg. **Cost:** *Generic*—1.25 mg $12.60/90, 2.5 mg $12.60/90.

NURSING IMPLICATIONS
Assessment
- Monitor blood pressure, intake and output, and daily weight and assess feet, legs, and sacral area for edema daily.
- Assess patient, especially if taking digoxin, for anorexia, nausea, vomiting, muscle cramps, paresthesia, and confusion; report signs of electrolyte imbalance. Patients taking digoxin have an increased risk of digitalis toxicity due to the potassium-depleting effect of the diuretic.
- Assess patient for allergy to sulfonamides.
- **Lab Test Considerations:** Monitor electrolytes (especially potassium), blood glucose, BUN, serum creatinine, and uric acid levels periodically during therapy. May cause ↓ potassium, sodium, and chloride concentrations. May ↑ serum glucose; diabetic patients may require ↑ oral hypoglycemic or insulin dose.
  ↑ uric acid level an average of 1.0 mg/100 mL; may precipitate an episode of gout.

Potential Nursing Diagnoses
Excess fluid volume (Indications)
Risk for deficient fluid volume (Side Effects)

Implementation
- Administer in the morning to prevent disruption of sleep cycle.
- PO: May be given with food or milk to minimize GI irritation.

Patient/Family Teaching
- Instruct patient to take this medication at the same time each day. Take missed doses as soon as remembered but not just before next dose is due. Do not double doses. Advise patients using indapamide for hypertension to continue taking the medication even if feeling well. Indapamide controls but does not cure hypertension.
- Caution patient to change positions slowly to minimize orthostatic hypotension. This may be potentiated by alcohol.
- Advise patient to use sunscreen (avoid those containing PABA) and protective clothing when in the sun to prevent photosensitivity reactions.

- Instruct patient to follow a diet high in potassium (see Appendix M).
- Advise patient to report muscle weakness, cramps, nausea, or dizziness to health care professional.
- Advise patient to consult health care professional before taking OTC medication concurrently with this therapy.
- Emphasize the importance of routine follow-up exams.
- **Hypertension:** Instruct patient and family on proper technique of blood pressure monitoring. Advise them to check blood pressure at least weekly and to report significant changes.
- Encourage patient to comply with additional interventions for hypertension (weight reduction, low-sodium diet, regular exercise, smoking cessation, moderation of alcohol consumption, and stress management).

Evaluation/Desired Outcomes
- Control of hypertension.
- Decrease in edema secondary to CHF.

---

indometacin
(in-doe-**meth**-a-sin)
✤Apo-Indomethacin, ✤Indameth, ✤Indocid, Indocin, Indocin I.V., ✤Indocin PDA, Indocin SR, ✤Novo-Methacin, ✤Nu-Indo

Classification
Therapeutic: antirheumatics, ductus arteriosus patency adjuncts (IV only), nonsteroidal anti-inflammatory agents

Pregnancy Category B (first trimester)

Indications
PO: Inflammatory disorders including: Rheumatoid arthritis, Gouty arthritis, Osteoarthritis, Ankylosing spondylitis. Generally reserved for patients who do not respond to less toxic agents. **IV:** Alternative to surgery in the management of patent ductus arteriosus (PDA) in premature neonates.

Action
Inhibits prostaglandin synthesis. **Therapeutic Effects: PO:** Suppression of pain and inflammation. **IV:** Closure of PDA.

Pharmacokinetics
Absorption: Well absorbed after oral administration in adults, incomplete oral absorption in neonates.
Distribution: Crosses the blood-brain barrier and the placenta. Enters breast milk.
Protein Binding: 99%.
Metabolism and Excretion: Mostly metabolized by the liver.
Half-life: Neonates <2 weeks: 20 hr; >2 weeks: 11 hr; Adults: 2.6–11 hr.

TIME/ACTION PROFILE

ROUTE	ONSET	PEAK	DURATION
PO (analgesic)	30 min	0.5–2 hr	4–6 hr
PO-ER (analgesic)	30 min	unknown	4–6 hr
PO (anti-inflammatory)	up to 7 days	1–2 wk	4–6 hr
PO-ER (anti-inflammatory)	up to 7 days	1–2 wk	4–6 hr
IV (closure of PDA)	up to 48 hr	unknown	unknown

Contraindications/Precautions
Contraindicated in: Hypersensitivity; Known alcohol intolerance (suspension); Cross-sensitivity may exist with other NSAIDs, including aspirin; Active GI bleeding; Ulcer disease; Proctitis or recent history of rectal bleeding; Intraventricular hemorrhage; Thrombocytopenia; Pedi: ↑ risk of necrotizing enterocolitis and bowel perforation in premature infants with PDA.
Use Cautiously in: Severe cardiovascular, renal, or hepatic disease; History of ulcer disease; Epilepsy; Hypertension; OB: Not recommended during 2nd half of pregnancy (potential for causing premature closure of ductus arteriosus); Lactation: Usually compatible with breastfeeding (AAP); Geri: ↑ risk of adverse reactions.

Adverse Reactions/Side Effects
CNS: dizziness, drowsiness, headache, psychic disturbances. **EENT:** blurred vision, tinnitus. **CV:** hypertension, edema. **GI:** *PO*— DRUG-INDUCED HEPATITIS, GI BLEEDING, constipation, dyspepsia, nausea, vomiting, discomfort, necrotizing enterocolitis. **GU:** cystitis, hematuria, renal failure. **Derm:** rashes. **F and E:** hyperkalemia; *IV*, dilutional hyponatremia; *IV*, hypoglycemia. **Hemat:** thrombocytopenia, blood dyscrasias, prolonged bleeding time. **Local:** phlebitis at IV site. **Misc:** allergic reactions including ANAPHYLAXIS.

Interactions
Drug-Drug: Concurrent use with **aspirin** may ↓ effectiveness. Additive adverse GI effects with **aspirin**, other **NSAIDs**, **corticosteroids**, or **alcohol**. Chronic use of **acetaminophen** ↑ risk of adverse renal reactions. May ↓ effectiveness of **diuretics** or **antihypertensives**. May ↑ hypo-

indomethacin

glycemia from **insulins** or **oral hypoglycemic agents**. May ↑ risk of toxicity from **lithium** or **zidovudine** (avoid concurrent use with zidovudine). ↑ risk of toxicity from **methotrexate**. **Probenecid** ↑ risk of toxicity from indomethacin. ↑ risk of bleeding with **cefotetan, cefoperazone, valproic acid, thrombolytics, warfarin,** and **drugs affecting platelet function** including **clopidogrel, ticlopidine, abciximab, eptifibatide,** or **tirofiban**. ↑ risk of adverse hematologic reactions with **antineoplastics** or **radiation therapy**. ↑ risk of nephrotoxicity with **cyclosporine**. Concurrent use with **potassium-sparing diuretics** may result in hyperkalemia. May ↑ levels of **digitalis glycosides, methotrexate, lithium,** and **aminoglycosides** when used IV in neonates.
Drug-Natural Products: ↑ bleeding risk with **anise, arnica, chamomile, clove, dong quai, feverfew, garlic, ginger, ginkgo, Panax ginseng**.

Route/Dosage
Anti-inflammatory

PO (Adults): *Antiarthritic*—25–50 mg 2–4 times daily *or* 75-mg extended-release capsule once or twice daily (not to exceed 200 mg or 150 mg of SR/day). A single bedtime dose of 100 mg may be used. *Antigout*—100 mg initially, followed by 50 mg 3 times daily for relief of pain, then ↓ further.

PO (Children >2 yr): 1–2 mg/kg/day in 2–4 divided doses (not to exceed 4 mg/kg/day or 150–200 mg/day).

PDA Closure

IV (Neonates): 0.2 mg/kg initially, then 2 subsequent doses at 12–24 hr intervals of 0.1 mg/kg if age <48 hr at time of initial dose; 0.2 mg/kg if 2–7 days at initial dose; 0.25 mg/kg if age >7 days at initial dose.

Availability (generic available)
Capsules: 25 mg, 50 mg. **Sustained-release capsules:** 75 mg. **Oral suspension (fruit mint, pineapple coconut mint flavors):** 25 mg/5 mL. **Powder for injection:** 1 mg/vial.

NURSING IMPLICATIONS
Assessment
- Patients who have asthma, aspirin-induced allergy, and nasal polyps are at increased risk for developing hypersensitivity reactions. Monitor for rhinitis, asthma, and urticaria.

- **Arthritis:** Assess limitation of movement and pain—note type, location, and intensity before and 1–2 hr after administration.
- **PDA:** Monitor respiratory status, heart rate, blood pressure, echocardiogram, and heart sounds routinely throughout therapy.
- Monitor intake and output. Fluid restriction is usually instituted throughout therapy.
- *Lab Test Considerations:* Evaluate BUN, serum creatinine, CBC, serum potassium levels, and liver function tests periodically in patients receiving prolonged therapy.
- Serum potassium, BUN, serum creatinine, AST, and ALT tests may show ↑ levels. Blood glucose concentrations may be altered. Hemoglobin and hematocrit concentrations, leukocyte and platelet counts, and CCr may be ↓.
- Urine glucose and urine protein concentrations may be ↑.
- Leukocyte and platelet count may be ↓. Bleeding time may be prolonged for several days after discontinuation.

Potential Nursing Diagnoses
Acute pain (Indications)
Impaired physical mobility (Indications)

Implementation
- If prolonged therapy is used, dose should be reduced to the lowest level that controls symptoms.
- **PO:** Administer after meals, with food, or with antacids to decrease GI irritation. Do not break, crush, or chew sustained-release capsules.
- Shake suspension before administration. Do not mix with antacid or any other liquid.

IV Administration
- **Direct IV:** *Diluent:* Preservative-free 0.9% NaCl or preservative-free sterile water. Reconstitute with 1 or 2 mL of diluent. *Concentration:* 0.5–1 mg/mL. Reconstitute immediately before use and discard any unused solution. Do not dilute further or admix. Do not administer via umbilical catheter into vessels near the superior mesenteric artery, as these can cause vasoconstriction and compromise blood flow to the intestines. Do not administer intra-arterially. *Rate:* Administer over 20–30 min. Avoid extravasation, as solution is irritating to tissues.
- **Y-Site Compatibility:** furosemide, insulin, nitroprusside, potassium chloride, sodium bicarbonate.

710 infliximab

- **Y-Site Incompatibility:** calcium gluconate, cimetidine, dobutamine, dopamine, gentamicin, levofloxacin, tobramycin, tolazoline.

Patient/Family Teaching
- Advise patient to take this medication with a full glass of water and to remain in an upright position for 15–30 min after administration.
- Instruct patient to take medication exactly as directed. Take missed doses as soon as remembered if not almost time for next dose. Do not double doses.
- May cause drowsiness or dizziness. Advise patient to avoid driving or other activities requiring alertness until response to medication is known.
- Caution patient to avoid the concurrent use of alcohol, aspirin, other NSAIDs, acetaminophen, or other OTC medications without consulting health care professional.
- Caution patient to wear sunscreen and protective clothing to prevent photosensitivity reactions.
- Advise patient to inform health care professional of medication regimen before treatment or surgery.
- Instruct patient to notify health care professional if rash, itching, chills, fever, muscle aches, visual disturbances, weight gain, edema, abdominal pain, black stools, or persistent headache occurs.
- **PDA:** Explain to parents the purpose of medication and the need for frequent monitoring.

Evaluation/Desired Outcomes
- Decrease in severity of moderate pain.
- Improved joint mobility. Partial arthritic relief is usually seen within 2 wk, but maximum effectiveness may require up to 1 mo of continuous therapy. Patients who do not respond to one NSAID may respond to another.
- Successful PDA closure.

---

infliximab (in-flix-i-mab)
Remicade

Classification
Therapeutic: antirheumatics (DMARDs), gastrointestinal anti-inflammatories
Pharmacologic: monoclonal antibodies

Pregnancy Category C

Indications
Active rheumatoid arthritis (moderate to severe, with methotrexate). Active Crohn's disease (moderate to severe). Active psoriatic arthritis. Active ankylosing spondylitis. Active ulcerative colitis (moderate to severe) with inadequate response to conventional therapy: reducing signs and symptoms, and inducing and maintaining clinical remission and mucosal healing, and eliminating corticosteroid use. Plaque psoriasis (chronic severe).

Action
Neutralizes and prevents the activity of tumor necrosis factor-alpha (TNF-alpha), resulting in anti-inflammatory and antiproliferative activity. **Therapeutic Effects:** Decreased pain and swelling, decreased rate of joint destruction and improved physical function in ankylosing spondylitis, rheumatoid or psoriatic arthritis. Reduction and maintenance of closure of fistulae in Crohn's disease. Decreased symptoms, maintaining remission and mucosal healing with decreased corticosteroid use in ulcerative Colitis. Decrease in induration, scaling and erythema of psoriatic lesions.

Pharmacokinetics
Absorption: IV administration results in complete bioavailability.
Distribution: Predominantly distributed within the vascular compartment.
Metabolism and Excretion: Unknown.
Half-life: 9.5 days.

TIME/ACTION PROFILE (symptoms of Crohn's disease)

ROUTE	ONSET	PEAK	DURATION
IV	1–2 wk	unknown	12–48 wk†

†After infusion

Contraindications/Precautions
Contraindicated in: Hypersensitivity to infliximab, murine (mouse) proteins, or other components in the formulation; Lactation: Lactation; CHF.
Use Cautiously in: Patients being retreated after 2 yr without treatment (↑ risk of adverse reactions); History of tuberculosis or exposure (latent tuberculosis should be treated prior to infliximab therapy); Chronic obstructive pulmonary disease (↑ risk of malignancy); Geri: Geriatric patients; OB: Use only if clearly needed; Pedi: Safety not established; ↑ risk of lymphoma, leukemia, and other malignancies.

Adverse Reactions/Side Effects
CNS: fatigue, headache, anxiety, depression, dizziness, insomnia. **EENT:** conjunctivitis. **Resp:** upper respiratory tract infection, bronchitis, cough, dyspnea, laryngitis, pharyngitis, respiratory tract allergic reaction, rhinitis, sinusitis. **CV:**

infliximab

chest pain, hypertension, hypotension, pericardial effusion, tachycardia, CHF. **GI:** HEPATOSPLENIC T-CELL LYMPHOMA, abdominal pain, nausea, vomiting, constipation, diarrhea, dyspepsia, flatulence, hepatotoxicity, intestinal obstruction, oral pain, tooth pain, ulcerative stomatitis. **GU:** dysuria, urinary frequency, urinary tract infection. **Derm:** acne, alopecia, dry skin, ecchymosis, eczema, erythema, flushing, hematoma, hot flushes, pruritus, psoriasis, rash, sweating, urticaria. **Hemat:** LEUKEMIA, neutropenia. **MS:** arthralgia, arthritis, back pain, involuntary muscle contractions, myalgia. **Neuro:** paresthesia. **Misc:** INFECTIONS (including reactivation tuberculosis, pneumonia, and invasive fungal infections), MALIGNANCY, fever, infusion reactions, chills, flu-like syndrome, herpes simplex, herpes zoster, hypersensitivity reactions, lupus-like syndrome, moniliasis, pain, peripheral edema, vasculitis.

Interactions
Drug-Drug: None significant.

Route/Dosage

Rheumatoid Arthritis
IV (Adults): 3 mg/kg followed by 3 mg/kg 2 and 6 wk after initial dose and then every 8 wk; dose may be adjusted in partial responders up to 10 mg/kg or treatment as often as every 4 wk (used with methotrexate).

Crohn's Disease
IV (Adults): *Moderate-to-severe Crohn's disease*—5 mg/kg as a single infusion. *Fistulizing Crohn's disease*—5 mg/kg repeated 2 and 6 wk after initial infusion; maintenance dose of 5 mg/kg may be given q 8 wk.

Ankylosing Spondylitis
IV (Adults): 5 mg/kg given as an infusion repeated 2 and 6 wk later, then every 6 wk.

Psoriatic Arthritis
IV (Adults): 5 mg/kg given as an infusion repeated 2 and 6 wk later, then every 8 wk thereafter (with or without methotrexate).

Ulcerative Colitis
IV (Adults): 5 mg/kg given as an infusion regimen at 0, 2, and 6 wk followed by a maintenance regimen of 5 mg/kg every 8 wk thereafter.

Psoriasis
IV (Adults): 5 mg/kg given as an infusion regimen at 0, 2, and 6 wk followed by a maintenance regimen of 5 mg/kg every 8 wk thereafter.

Availability
Powder for injection: 100 mg/vial.

NURSING IMPLICATIONS

Assessment
- Assess for infusion-related reactions (fever, chills, urticaria, pruritus) during and for 2 hr after infusion. Symptoms usually resolve when infusion is discontinued. Reactions are more common after 1st or 2nd infusion. Frequency of reactions may be reduced with immunosuppressant agents.
- Assess for signs and symptoms of systemic infections (fever, malaise, weight loss, sweats, cough, dyspnea, pulmonary infiltrates, serious systemic illness with or without concomitant shock). Ascertain if patient lives in or has traveled to areas of endemic mycoses. Consider empiric antifungal treatment for patients at risk of histoplasmosis and other invasive fungal infections until the pathogens are identified. Consult with an infectious diseases specialist. Consider stopping infliximab until the infection has been diagnosed and adequately treated.
- Assess for latent tuberculosis with a tuberculin skin test prior to initiation of therapy. Treatment of latent tuberculosis should be initiated prior to therapy with infliximab.
- Observe patient for hypersensitivity reactions (urticaria, dyspnea, hypotension) during infusion. Discontinue infliximab if severe reaction occurs. Have medications (antihistamines, acetaminophen, corticosteroids, epinephrine) and equipment readily available in the event of a severe reaction.
- **Rheumatoid Arthritis:** Assess pain and range of motion prior to and periodically during therapy.
- **Crohn's Disease and Ulcerative Colitis:** Assess for signs and symptoms before, during, and after therapy.
- **Psoriasis:** Assess lesions periodically during therapy.
- *Lab Test Considerations:* May cause ↑ in positive ANA. Frequency may be decreased with baseline immunosuppressant therapy.
- Monitor liver function tests periodically during therapy. May cause mild to moderate AST and

ALT ↑ without progressing to liver dysfunction. If patient develops jaundice or liver enzyme elevations ≥5 times the upper limits of normal, discontinue infliximab.
- Monitor CBC with differential periodically during therapy. May cause leukopenia, neutropenia, thrombocytopenia, and pancytopenia. Discontinue infliximab if symptoms of blood dyscrasias (persistent fever) occur.

Potential Nursing Diagnoses
Chronic pain (Indications)
Diarrhea (Indications)

Implementation

IV Administration

- **Intermittent Infusion:** Calculate the total number of vials needed. Reconstitute each vial with 10 mL of sterile water for injection using a syringe with a 21-gauge needle or smaller. Direct stream to sides of vial. Do not use if vacuum is not present in vial. Gently swirl solution by rotating vial to dilute; do not shake. May foam on reconstitution; allow to stand for 5 min. Solution is colorless to light yellow and opalescent; a few translucent particles may develop because infliximab is a protein. Do not use if opaque particles, discoloration, or other particles occur. **Diluent:** Withdraw volume of total infliximab dose from infusion container containing 250 mL with 0.9% NaCl. Slowly add total dose of infliximab. **Concentration:** 0.4 to 4 mg/mL. Mix gently. Infusion should begin within 3 hr of preparation. Solution is incompatible with polyvinyl chloride equipment. Prepare in glass infusion bottle or polypropylene or polyolefin bags. Do not reuse or store any portion of infusion solution. **Rate:** Administer over at least 2 hr through polyethylene-lined administration set with an in-line, sterile, non-pyrogenic, low protein-building filter with ≤1.2-micron pore size.
- **Y-Site Incompatibility:** Do not administer concurrently in the same line with any other agents.

Patient/Family Teaching
- Advise patient that adverse reactions (myalgia, rash, fever, polyarthralgia, pruritus) may occur 3–12 days after delayed (>2 yr) retreatment with infliximab. Symptoms usually decrease or resolve within 1–3 days. Instruct patient to notify health care professional if symptoms occur.
- May cause dizziness. Caution patient to avoid driving or other activities requiring alertness until response to medication is known.
- Advise patient to notify health care professional promptly if symptoms of fungal infection occur.

Evaluation/Desired Outcomes
- Decreased pain and swelling with decreased rate of joint destruction and improved physical function in patients with ankylosing spondylitis, psoriatic, or rheumatoid arthritis.
- Decrease in the signs and symptoms of Crohn's disease and a decrease in the number of draining enterocutaneous fistulas. Decreased symptoms, maintaining remission and mucosal healing with decreased corticosteroid use in ulcerative colitis.
- Decrease in induration, scaling and erythema of psoriatic lesions.

HIGH ALERT

INSULIN (mixtures) (in-su-lin)

insulin lispro protamine suspension/insulin lispro injection mixtures, rDNA origin
Humalog Mix 75/25, Humalog Mix 50/50

insulin aspart protamine suspension/insulin aspart injection mixtures, rDNA origin
NovoLog Mix 70/30, NovoLog Mix 50/50

NPH/regular insulin mixtures
Humulin 70/30, Novolin 70/30

Classification
Therapeutic: antidiabetics, hormones
Pharmacologic: pancreatics

Pregnancy Category B (insulin lispro protamine suspension/insulin lispro injection mixtures), C (insulin aspart protamine suspension/insulin aspart injection mixtures, NPH/regular insulin mixtures)

See Appendix N for more information concerning insulins

Indications
Control of hyperglycemia in patients with type 1 or type 2 diabetes mellitus.

Action
Lower blood glucose by: stimulating glucose uptake in skeletal muscle and fat, inhibiting hepatic glucose production. Other actions: inhibition of lipolysis and proteolysis, enhanced protein synthesis. **Therapeutic Effects:** Control of hyperglycemia in diabetic patients.

Pharmacokinetics
Absorption: Well absorbed from subcutaneous administration sites. Absorption rate is determined by type of insulin, injection site, volume of injectate, and other factors.
Distribution: Widely distributed.
Metabolism and Excretion: Metabolized by liver, spleen, kidney, and muscle.
Half-life: 5–6 min (prolonged in patients with diabetes; biologic half-life is 1–1.5 hr).

TIME/ACTION PROFILE (hypoglycemic effect)

ROUTE	ONSET	PEAK	DURATION
insulin lispro protamine suspension/insulin lispro injection mixture subcut	15–30 min	2.8 hr	24 hr
insulin aspart protamine suspension/insulin aspart injection mixture subcut	15 min	1–4 hr	18–24 hr
NPH/Regular Insulin mixture subcutaneous	30 min	4–8 hr	24 hr

Contraindications/Precautions
Contraindicated in: Hypoglycemia; Allergy or hypersensitivity to a particular type of insulin, preservatives, or other additives.
Use Cautiously in: Stress and infection (may temporarily ↑ insulin requirements); Renal/hepatic impairment (may ↓ insulin requirements); OB: Pregnancy may temporarily ↑ insulin requirements; Pedi: Safety of Humalog not established.

Adverse Reactions/Side Effects
Endo: HYPOGLYCEMIA. **Local:** erythema, lipodystrophy, pruritis, swelling. **Misc:** allergic reactions including ANAPHYLAXIS.

Interactions
Drug-Drug: Beta blockers, clonidine, and reserpine may mask some of the signs and symptoms of hypoglycemia. Corticosteroids, thyroid supplements, estrogens, isoniazid, niacin, phenothiazines, and rifampin may ↑ insulin requirements. Alcohol, ACE inhibitors, MAO inhibitors, octreotide, oral hypoglycemic agents, and salicylates, may ↓ insulin requirements.
Drug-Natural Products: Glucosamine may worsen blood glucose control. Fenugreek, chromium, and coenzyme Q-10 may produce additive hypoglycemic effects.

Route/Dosage
Dose depends on blood glucose, response, and many other factors.
Subcut (Adults and Children): 0.5–1 unit/kg/day. *Adolescents during rapid growth*—0.8–1.2 units/kg/day.

Availability
NPH insulin/regular insulin suspension mixture: 70 units NPH/30 units regular insulin/mL—Novolin 70/30, Humulin 70/30 (100 units/mL total) in 10-mL vials and 3 mL prefilled pens[OTC]. **Cost:** *Humulin 70/30 or Novolin 70/30*—$42.99/10-mL vial; *Humulin 70/30 pen (3 mL)*—$117.03/5 pens. **Insulin lispro protamine suspension/insulin lispro injection mixture:** 75% insulin lispro protamine suspension and 25% insulin lispro injection—Humalog Mix 75/25 100 units/mL in 10-mL vials and 3-mL disposable delivery devices, 50% insulin lispro protamine suspension and 50% insulin lispro injection—Humalog Mix 50/50 100 units/mL in 10-mL vials and 3-mL disposable delivery devices. **Cost:** $91.25/10-mL vial *Humalog Mix 75/25 Pens (3 mL)*—$147.50/5 pens. **Insulin aspart protamine suspension/insulin aspart injection mixture:** 70% insulin aspart protamine suspension and 30% insulin aspart inection—NovoLog Mix 70/30 100 units/mL in 10-mL vials and 3-mL disposable delivery devices, 50% insulin aspart protamine suspension and 50% insulin aspart injection—NovoLog Mix 50/50 100 units/mL in 3-mL disposable delivery devices. **Cost:** *Novolog Mix 70/30 Pens (3 mL)*—$166.38/5 pens.

NURSING IMPLICATIONS
Assessment
- Assess for symptoms of hypoglycemia (anxiety; restlessness; tingling in hands, feet, lips, or tongue; chills; cold sweats; confusion; cool, pale skin; difficulty in concentration; drowsiness; excessive hunger; headache; irritability; nightmares or trouble sleeping; nausea; nervousness; tachycardia; tremor; weakness; unsteady gait) and hyperglycemia (confusion,

drowsiness; flushed, dry skin; fruit-like breath odor; rapid, deep breathing, polyuria; loss of appetite; nausea; vomiting; unusual thirst) periodically during therapy.
- Monitor body weight periodically. Changes in weight may necessitate changes in insulin dose.
- **Lab Test Considerations:** May cause ↓ serum inorganic phosphate, magnesium, and potassium levels.
- Monitor blood glucose every 6 hr during therapy, more frequently in ketoacidosis and times of stress. A1C may also be monitored every 3–6 mo to determine effectiveness.
- **Toxicity and Overdose:** Overdose is manifested by symptoms of hypoglycemia. Mild hypoglycemia may be treated by ingestion of oral glucose. Severe hypoglycemia is a life-threatening emergency; treatment consists of IV glucose, glucagon, or epinephrine.

Potential Nursing Diagnoses
Noncompliance (Patient/Family Teaching)

Implementation
- **High Alert:** Insulin-related medication errors have resulted in patient harm and death. Clarify ambiguous orders; do not accept orders using the abbreviation "u" for units, (can be misread as a zero or the numeral 4; has resulted in tenfold overdoses).
- Insulins are available in different types and strengths. Check type, dose, and expiration date with another licensed nurse. Do not interchange insulins without consulting physician or other health care professional.
- Use *only* insulin syringes to draw up dose. The unit markings on the insulin syringe must match the insulin's units/mL.
- Store insulin in refrigerator. May also be kept at room temperature for up to 28 days. Do not use if cloudy, discolored, or unusually viscous. Humalog pens must be discarded after 2 wk.
- NPH insulins should not be used in the management of ketoacidosis.
- **Subcut:** Rotate injection sites.
- Administer into abdominal wall, thigh, or upper arm subcutaneously.

Patient/Family Teaching
- Instruct patient on proper technique for administration. Include type of insulin, equipment (syringe, cartridge pens, alcohol swabs), storage, and place to discard syringes. Discuss the importance of not changing brands of insulin or syringes, selection and rotation of injection sites, and compliance with therapeutic regimen. Caution patient that insulin pens should not be shared with others, even if clean needles are used.
- Explain to patient that this medication controls hyperglycemia but does not cure diabetes. Therapy is long term.
- Instruct patient in proper testing of serum glucose and ketones. These tests should be closely monitored during periods of stress or illness and health care professional notified of significant changes.
- Emphasize the importance of compliance with nutritional guidelines and regular exercise as directed by health care professional.
- Advise patient to consult health care professional prior to using alcohol or other Rx, OTC, or herbal products concurrently with insulin.
- Advise patient to notify health care professional of medication regimen prior to treatment or surgery.
- Advise patient to notify health care professional if nausea, vomiting, or fever develops, if unable to eat regular diet, or if blood glucose levels are not controlled.
- Instruct patient on signs and symptoms of hypoglycemia and hyperglycemia and what to do if they occur.
- Advise patient to notify health care professional if pregnancy is planned or suspected or if breastfeeding or planning to breastfeed.
- Patients with diabetes mellitus should carry a source of sugar (candy, glucose gel) and identification describing their disease and treatment regimen at all times.
- Emphasize the importance of regular follow-up, especially during first few weeks of therapy.

Evaluation/Desired Outcomes
- Control of blood glucose levels in diabetic patients without the appearance of hypoglycemic or hyperglycemic episodes.

HIGH ALERT

INSULINS (short acting)
(in-su-lin)

insulin, regular (injection, concentrated)
Humulin R, Humulin R U-500 (concentrated), ✤ Insulin-Toronto, Novolin R

Classification
Therapeutic: antidiabetics, hormones
Pharmacologic: pancreatics

Pregnancy Category B

See Appendix N for more information concerning insulins

INSULINS (short acting)

Indications
Control of hyperglycemia in patients with type 1 or type 2 diabetes; can be used to treat diabetic ketoacidosis. *Concentrated insulin U-500*: Only for use in patients with insulin requirements >200 units/day. **Unlabeled Use:** Treatment of hyperkalemia.

Action
Lower blood glucose by: stimulating glucose uptake in skeletal muscle and fat, inhibiting hepatic glucose production. Other actions: inhibition of lipolysis and proteolysis, enhanced protein synthesis. **Therapeutic Effects:** Control of hyperglycemia in diabetic patients.

Pharmacokinetics
Absorption: Rapidly absorbed from subcutaneous administration sites.
Distribution: Widely distributed.
Metabolism and Excretion: Metabolized by liver, spleen, kidney, and muscle.
Half-life: 30–60 min.

TIME/ACTION PROFILE (hypoglycemic effect)

ROUTE	ONSET	PEAK	DURATION
Regular insulin IV	10–30 min	15–30 min	30–60 min
Regular insulin subcut	30–60 min	2–4 hr	5–7 hr

Contraindications/Precautions
Contraindicated in: Hypoglycemia; Allergy or hypersensitivity to a particular type of insulin, preservatives, or other additives.
Use Cautiously in: Stress and infection (may temporarily ↑ insulin requirements); Renal/hepatic impairment (may ↓ insulin requirements); OB: Pregnancy may temporarily ↑ insulin requirements.

Adverse Reactions/Side Effects
Endo: HYPOGLYCEMIA. **Local:** erythema, lipodystrophy, pruritus, swelling. **Misc:** allergic reactions including ANAPHYLAXIS.

Interactions
Drug-Drug: Beta blockers, clonidine, and reserpine may mask some of the signs and symptoms of hypoglycemia. Corticosteroids, thyroid supplements, estrogens, isoniazid, niacin, phenothiazines, and rifampin may ↑ insulin requirements. Alcohol, ACE inhibitors, MAO inhibitors, octreotide, oral hypoglycemic agents, and salicylates, may ↓ insulin requirements.

Drug-Natural Products: Glucosamine may worsen blood glucose control. **Fenugreek, chromium,** and **coenzyme Q-10** may produce additive hypoglycemic effects.

Route/Dosage
Dose depends on blood glucose, response, and many other factors.

Ketoacidosis—Regular Insulin Only (100 units/mL)
IV (Adults): 0.1 unit/kg/hr as a continuous infusion.
IV (Children): Loading dose-0.1 unit/kg, then maintenance continuous infusion 0.05–0.2 unit/kg/hr, titrate to optimal rate of ↓ of serum glucose of 80–100 mg/dL/hr.

Maintenance Therapy
Subcut (Adults and Children): 0.5–1 unit/kg/day. *Adolescents during rapid growth*—0.8–1.2 units/kg/day.

Treatment of Hyperkalemia
Subcut, IV (Adults and Children): Dextrose 0.5–1 g/kg combined with insulin 1 unit for every 4–5 g dextrose given.

Availability
Insulin injection (regular insulin): 100 units/mL in 10-mL vials and 3-mL disposable delivery devices ᴼᵀᶜ. **Regular (concentrated) insulin injection:** 500 units/mL in 20 mL vials.

NURSING IMPLICATIONS

Assessment
- Assess for symptoms of hypoglycemia (anxiety; restlessness; tingling in hands, feet, lips, or tongue; chills; cold sweats; confusion; cool, pale skin; difficulty in concentration; drowsiness; nightmares or trouble sleeping; excessive hunger; headache; irritability; nausea; nervousness; tachycardia; tremor; weakness; unsteady gait) and hyperglycemia (confusion, drowsiness; flushed, dry skin; fruit-like breath odor; rapid, deep breathing, polyuria; loss of appetite; nausea; vomiting; unusual thirst) periodically during therapy.
- Monitor body weight periodically. Changes in weight may necessitate changes in insulin dose.
- *Lab Test Considerations:* May cause ↓ serum inorganic phosphate, magnesium, and potassium levels.

✦ = Canadian drug name. ⚠ = Genetic implication.
*CAPITALS indicates life-threatening; underlines indicate most frequent.

INSULINS (short acting)

- Monitor blood glucose every 6 hr during therapy, more frequently in ketoacidosis and times of stress. A1C may also be monitored every 3–6 mo to determine effectiveness.
- *Toxicity and Overdose:* Overdose is manifested by symptoms of hypoglycemia. Mild hypoglycemia may be treated by ingestion of oral glucose. Severe hypoglycemia is a life-threatening emergency; treatment consists of IV glucose, glucagon, or epinephrine.

Potential Nursing Diagnoses
Noncompliance (Patient/Family Teaching)

Implementation
- *High Alert:* Insulin-related medication errors have resulted in patient harm and death. Clarify ambiguous orders; do not accept orders using the abbreviation "u" for units, (can be misread as a zero or the numeral 4; has resulted in tenfold overdoses). Insulins are available in different types and strengths. Check type, dose, and expiration date with another licensed nurse. Do not interchange insulins without consulting physician or other health care professional. Do not confuse regular **concentrated (U-500)** insulin with regular insulin.
- Use *only* insulin syringes to draw up dose. The unit markings on the insulin syringe must match the insulin's units/mL. Special syringes for doses <50 units are available. Prior to withdrawing dose, rotate vial between palms to ensure uniform solution; do not shake.
- When mixing insulins, draw regular insulin into syringe first to avoid contamination of regular insulin vial. Mixed insulins should never be used in a pump or for IV infusion.
- Store insulin in refrigerator. May also be kept at room temperature for up to 28 days. Do not use if cloudy, discolored, or unusually viscous.
- **Subcut:** Rotate injection sites.
- Administer into abdominal wall, thigh, or upper arm subcutaneously.
- Administer *regular insulin* within 15–30 min before a meal.

IV Administration

- **IV:** Regular insulin is the *only* insulin that can be administered IV. *High Alert:* Regular (concentrated) insulin U-500 should not be given IV.
- **Direct IV:** May be administered IV undiluted directly into vein or through Y-site. *Rate:* Administer up to 50 units over 1 min.
- **Continuous Infusion:** *Diluent:* May be diluted in commonly used IV solutions as an infusion; however, insulin potency may be reduced by at least 20–80% by the plastic or glass container or tubing before reaching the venous system. *Concentration:* 0.2–1 unit/mL. *Rate:* Rate should be ordered by physician (usually 0.05–0.2 units/kg/hr), and infusion should be placed on an IV pump for accurate administration.
- Rate of administration should be decreased when serum glucose level reaches 250 mg/100 mL.
- **Y-Site Compatibility:** amiodarone, ampicillin, ampicillin-sulbactam, aztreonam, cefazolin, cefepime, ceftazidime, dobutamine, doxapram, esmolol, famotadine, gentamicin, heparin, imipenem/cilastatin, indomethacin, magnesium sulfate, meperidine, meropenem, midazolam, milrinone, morphine, nitroglycerin, nitroprusside, oxytocin, pantoprazole, pentobarbital, potassium chloride, propofol, ritodrine, sodium bicarbonate, tacrolimus, terbutaline, ticarcillin, ticarcillin/clavulanate, tobramycin, vancomycin, vitamin B complex with C.
- **Y-Site Incompatibility:** dopamine, drotrecogin, nafcillin, norepinephrine, ranitidine.
- **Additive Compatibility:** May be added to total parenteral nutrition (TPN) solutions.

Patient/Family Teaching
- Instruct patient on proper technique for administration. Include type of insulin, equipment (syringe, cartridge pens, alcohol swabs), storage, and place to discard syringes. Discuss the importance of not changing brands of insulin or syringes, selection and rotation of injection sites, and compliance with therapeutic regimen.
- Demonstrate technique for mixing insulins by drawing up regular insulin and rolling intermediate-acting insulin vial between palms to mix, rather than shaking (may cause inaccurate dose).
- Explain to patient that this medication controls hyperglycemia but does not cure diabetes. Therapy is long term.
- Instruct patient in proper testing of serum glucose and ketones. These tests should be closely monitored during periods of stress or illness and health care professional notified of significant changes.
- Emphasize the importance of compliance with nutritional guidelines and regular exercise as directed by health care professional.
- Advise patient to consult health care professional prior to using alcohol or other Rx, OTC, or herbal products concurrently with insulin.

- Advise patient to notify health care professional of medication regimen prior to treatment or surgery.
- Advise patient to notify health care professional if nausea, vomiting, or fever develops, if unable to eat regular diet, or if blood glucose levels are not controlled.
- Instruct patient on signs and symptoms of hypoglycemia and hyperglycemia and what to do if they occur.
- Advise patient to notify health care professional if pregnancy is planned or suspected or if breastfeeding or planning to breastfeed.
- Patients with diabetes mellitus should carry a source of sugar (candy, glucose gel) and identification describing their disease and treatment regimen at all times.
- Emphasize the importance of regular follow-up, especially during first few weeks of therapy.

Evaluation/Desired Outcomes
- Control of blood glucose levels in diabetic patients without the appearance of hypoglycemic or hyperglycemic episodes.

HIGH ALERT

INSULINS (intermediate-acting) (in-su-lin)

NPH insulin (isophane insulin suspension)
Humulin N, ✹Novolin ge NPH, Novolin N

Classification
Therapeutic: antidiabetics, hormones
Pharmacologic: pancreatics

Pregnancy Category B

See Appendix N for more information concerning insulins

Indications
Control of hyperglycemia in patients with type 1 or type 2 diabetes mellitus.

Action
Lower blood glucose by: stimulating glucose uptake in skeletal muscle and fat, inhibiting hepatic glucose production. Other actions: inhibition of lipolysis and proteolysis, enhanced protein synthesis. **Therapeutic Effects:** Control of hyperglycemia in diabetic patients.

Pharmacokinetics
Absorption: Well absorbed from subcutaneous administration sites; rate of absorption may vary by site or volume of injection and other factors.
Distribution: Widely distributed.
Metabolism and Excretion: Metabolized by liver, spleen, kidney, and muscle.
Half-life: 5–6 min (prolonged in patients with diabetes; biologic half-life is 1–1.5 hr).

TIME/ACTION PROFILE (hypoglycemic effect)

ROUTE	ONSET	PEAK	DURATION
NPH	1–2 hr	4–12 hr	18–24 hr

Contraindications/Precautions
Contraindicated in: Hypoglycemia; Allergy or hypersensitivity to a particular type of insulin, preservatives, or other additives.
Use Cautiously in: Stress and infection (may temporarily ↑ insulin requirements); Renal/hepatic impairment (may ↓ insulin requirements; OB: Pregnancy may temporarily ↑ insulin requirements.

Adverse Reactions/Side Effects
Endo: HYPOGLYCEMIA. **Local:** lipodystrophy, pruritus, erythema, swelling. **Misc:** allergic reactions including ANAPHYLAXIS.

Interactions
Drug-Drug: Beta blockers, clonidine, and reserpine may mask some of the signs and symptoms of hypoglycemia. Corticosteroids, thyroid supplements, estrogens, isoniazid, niacin, phenothiazines, and rifampin may ↑ insulin requirements. Alcohol, ACE inhibitors, MAO inhibitors, octreotide, oral hypoglycemic agents, and salicylates, may ↓ insulin requirements.
Drug-Natural Products: Glucosamine may worsen blood glucose control. Fenugreek, chromium, and coenzyme Q-10 may produce additive hypoglycemic effects.

Route/Dosage
Dose depends on blood glucose, response, and many other factors.

Subcut (Adults and Children): 0.5–1 unit/kg/day. *Adolescents during rapid growth*—0.8–1.2 units/kg/day.

Availability
Isophane insulin suspension (NPH insulin): 100 units/mL in 10-mL vials, 3 mL prefilled pens. **Cost:** $42.99/10-mL vial *Humulin N pen (3*

mL) —$124.90/5 pens. *In combination with:* regular insulin as 70/30 (NPH/Regular) mixture (Humulin 70/30, Novolin 70/30).

NURSING IMPLICATIONS
Assessment
- Assess for symptoms of hypoglycemia (anxiety; restlessness; mood changes; tingling in hands, feet, lips, or tongue; chills; cold sweats; confusion; cool, pale skin; difficulty in concentration; drowsiness; excessive hunger; headache; irritability; nightmares or trouble sleeping; nausea; nervousness; tachycardia; tremor; weakness; unsteady gait) and hyperglycemia (confusion, drowsiness; flushed, dry skin; fruit-like breath odor; rapid, deep breathing, polyuria; loss of appetite; nausea; vomiting; unusual thirst) periodically during therapy.
- Monitor body weight periodically. Changes in weight may necessitate changes in insulin dose.
- *Lab Test Considerations:* May cause ↓ serum inorganic phosphate, magnesium, and potassium levels.
- Monitor blood glucose every 6 hr during therapy, more frequently in ketoacidosis and times of stress. A1C may also be monitored every 3–6 mo to determine effectiveness.
- *Toxicity and Overdose:* Overdose is manifested by symptoms of hypoglycemia. Mild hypoglycemia may be treated by ingestion of oral glucose. Severe hypoglycemia is a life-threatening emergency; treatment consists of IV glucose, glucagon, or epinephrine.

Potential Nursing Diagnoses
Noncompliance (Patient/Family Teaching)

Implementation
- *High Alert:* Insulin-related medication errors have resulted in patient harm and death. Clarify ambiguous orders; do not accept orders using the abbreviation "u" for units, (can be misread as a zero or the numeral 4; has resulted in tenfold overdoses).
- Insulins are available in different types and strengths. Check type, dose, and expiration date with another licensed nurse. Do not interchange insulins without consulting health care professional.
- Use *only* insulin syringes to draw up dose. The unit markings on the insulin syringe must match the insulin's units/mL.
- When mixing insulins, draw regular insulin, insulin aspart, insulin glulisine, or insulin lispro into syringe first to avoid contamination of regular insulin vial. Mix insulin glulisine *only* with NPH insulin. Mixed insulins should never be used in a pump or for IV infusion.
- Store insulin vials in refrigerator. May also be kept at room temperature for up to 28 days. Humulin N pens should be kept at room temperature and should be discarded after 14 days. Do not use if cloudy, discolored, or unusually viscous.
- Because of short duration of *insulin lispro insulin glulisine* and *insulin aspart*, supplementation with longer-acting insulin may be necessary to control blood glucose levels.
- When transferring from once-daily NPH human insulin to *insulin glargine*, the dose usually remains unchanged. When transferring from twice-daily NPH human insulin to insulin glargine, the initial dose of insulin glargine is usually reduced by 20%.
- NPH insulin should not be used in the management of ketoacidosis.
- **Subcut:** Rotate injection sites.
- Administer into abdominal wall, thigh, or upper arm subcutaneously.
- Administer *NPH insulin* within 30–60 min before a meal.

Patient/Family Teaching
- Instruct patient on proper technique for administration. Include type of insulin, equipment (syringe, cartridge pens, alcohol swabs), storage, and place to discard syringes. Discuss the importance of not changing brands of insulin or syringes, selection and rotation of injection sites, and compliance with therapeutic regimen. Caution patient that insulin pens should not be shared with others, even if clean needles are used.
- Demonstrate technique for mixing insulins by drawing up regular insulin, insulin aspart, or insulin lispro first and rolling intermediate-acting insulin vial between palms to mix, rather than shaking (may cause inaccurate dose).
- Explain to patient that this medication controls hyperglycemia but does not cure diabetes. Therapy is long term.
- Instruct patient in proper testing of serum glucose and ketones. These tests should be closely monitored during periods of stress or illness and health care professional notified of significant changes.
- Emphasize the importance of compliance with nutritional guidelines and regular exercise as directed by health care professional.
- Advise patient to consult health care professional prior to using alcohol or other Rx, OTC, or herbal products concurrently with insulin.

- Advise patient to notify health care professional of medication regimen prior to treatment or surgery.
- Advise patient to notify health care professional if nausea, vomiting, or fever develops, if unable to eat regular diet, or if blood glucose levels are not controlled.
- Instruct patient on signs and symptoms of hypoglycemia and hyperglycemia and what to do if they occur.
- Advise patient to notify health care professional if pregnancy is planned or suspected or if breastfeeding or planning to breastfeed.
- Patients with diabetes mellitus should carry a source of sugar (candy, glucose gel) and identification describing their disease and treatment regimen at all times.
- Emphasize the importance of regular follow-up, especially during first few weeks of therapy.

Evaluation/Desired Outcomes
- Control of blood glucose levels in diabetic patients without the appearance of hypoglycemic or hyperglycemic episodes.

HIGH ALERT

INSULINS (long-acting)
(in-su-lin)

insulin detemir
Levemir

insulin glargine
Lantus

Classification
Therapeutic: antidiabetics, hormones
Pharmacologic: pancreatics

Pregnancy Category C

See Appendix N for more information concerning insulins

Indications
Control of hyperglycemia in patients with type 1 or type 2 diabetes mellitus.

Action
Lower blood glucose by: stimulating glucose uptake in skeletal muscle and fat, inhibiting hepatic glucose production. Other actions: inhibition of lipolysis and proteolysis, enhanced protein synthesis. **Therapeutic Effects:** Control of hyperglycemia in diabetic patients.

Pharmacokinetics
Absorption: Physiochemical characteristics of long-acting insulins result in delayed and prolonged absorption.
Distribution: Widely distributed.
Metabolism and Excretion: Metabolized by liver, spleen, kidney, and muscle.
Half-life: 5–6 min (prolonged in patients with diabetes); biologic half-life is 1–1.5 hr; *insulin detemir* 5–7 hr (dose-dependent).

TIME/ACTION PROFILE (hypoglycemic effect)

ROUTE	ONSET	PEAK	DURATION
Insulin detemir	3–4 hr	3–14 hr†	24 hr
Insulin glargine	3–4 hr	none†	24 hr

†Small amounts of insulin glargine and insulin detemir are slowly released resulting in a relatively constant effect over time

Contraindications/Precautions
Contraindicated in: Hypoglycemia; Allergy or hypersensitivity to a particular type of insulin, preservatives, or other additives.
Use Cautiously in: Stress and infection (may temporarily ↑ insulin requirements); Renal/hepatic impairment (may ↓ insulin requirements); OB: Pregnancy may temporarily ↑ insulin requirements; Pedi: Children <6 yr (safety not established).

Adverse Reactions/Side Effects
Endo: HYPOGLYCEMIA. **Local:** lipodystrophy, pruritis, erythema, swelling. **Misc:** allergic reactions including ANAPHYLAXIS.

Interactions
Drug-Drug: Beta blockers, **clonidine**, and **reserpine** may mask some of the signs and symptoms of hypoglycemia. **Corticosteroids, thyroid supplements, estrogens, isoniazid, niacin, phenothiazines**, and **rifampin** may ↑ insulin requirements. **Alcohol, ACE inhibitors, MAO inhibitors, octreotide, oral hypoglycemic agents**, and **salicylates**, may ↓ insulin requirements.
Drug-Natural Products: **Glucosamine** may worsen blood glucose control. **Fenugreek, chromium**, and **coenzyme Q-10** may produce additive hypoglycemic effects.

Route/Dosage

Insulin Detemir
Subcut (Adults and Children ≥6 yr): *Type 2 diabetes patients who are insulin-naive—*

0.1–0.2 units/kg once daily in the morning *or* 10 units once or twice daily. *Patients with type 1 or 2 diabetes receiving basal insulin or basal bolus therapy*—May substitute on an equivalent unit-per-unit basis.

Insulin Glargine

Subcut (Adults and Children ≥6 yr): *Type 1 diabetes*—Administer 50–75% of daily insulin requirements once daily. *Initiation in patients with type 2 diabetes already being treated with oral antidiabetic agents*—10 units once daily; then adjust on the basis of the patient's needs (range 2–100 units/day). *Patients already receiving insulin*—When switching from once daily NPH, same dose of insulin glargine can be administered once daily. When switching from twice daily NPH, use 80% of the total daily NPH dose and administer once daily. Dose can then be adjusted on the basis of the patient's needs.

Availability

Insulin detemir: 100 units/mL in 10-mL vials and 3-mL cartridges or prefilled syringes. **Cost:** $84.15/10-ml vial. **Insulin glargine:** 100 units/mL in 10-mL vials and 3-mL cartridges or prefilled disposable pens. **Cost:** $84.99/10-mL vial.

NURSING IMPLICATIONS

Assessment

- Assess patient for signs and symptoms of hypoglycemia (anxiety; restlessness; mood changes; tingling in hands, feet, lips, or tongue; chills; cold sweats; confusion; cool, pale skin; difficulty in concentration; drowsiness; nightmares or trouble sleeping; excessive hunger; headache; irritability; nausea; nervousness; tachycardia; tremor; weakness; unsteady gait) and hyperglycemia (confusion, drowsiness; flushed, dry skin; fruit-like breath odor; rapid, deep breathing, polyuria; loss of appetite; nausea; vomiting; tiredness; unusual thirst) periodically during therapy.
- Monitor body weight periodically. Changes in weight may necessitate changes in insulin dose.
- *Lab Test Considerations:* Monitor blood glucose every 6 hr during therapy, more frequently in ketoacidosis and times of stress. A1C may also be monitored every 3–6 mo to determine effectiveness.
- *Toxicity and Overdose:* Overdose is manifested by symptoms of hypoglycemia. Mild hypoglycemia may be treated by ingestion of oral glucose. Severe hypoglycemia is a life-threatening emergency; treatment consists of IV glucose, glucagon, or epinephrine. Recovery from hypoglycemia may be delayed due to the prolonged effect of long-acting insulins.

Potential Nursing Diagnoses

Noncompliance (Patient/Family Teaching)

Implementation

- **High Alert:** Insulin-related medication errors have resulted in patient harm and death. Clarify ambiguous orders; do not accept orders using the abbreviation "u" for units, (can be misread as a zero or the numeral 4; has resulted in tenfold overdoses).
- Insulins are available in different types and strengths. Check type, dose, and expiration date with another licensed nurse. Do not interchange insulins without consulting health care professional.
- Use *only* insulin syringes to draw up dose. The unit markings on the insulin syringe must match the insulin's units/mL. Special syringes for doses <50 units are available. Prior to withdrawing dose, rotate vial between palms to ensure uniform solution; do not shake.
- *High Alert:* Do not mix *insulin glargine or insulin detemir* with any other insulin or solution, or use syringes containing any other medicinal product or residue. If giving with a short-acting insulin, use separate syringes and different injection sites. Solution should be clear and colorless with no particulate matter.
- Do not use if cloudy, discolored, or unusually viscous. Store unopened vials and cartridges of *insulin glargine and insulin detemir* in the refrigerator; do not freeze. If unable to refrigerate, the 10-mL vial of *insulin glargine* can be kept in a cool place unrefrigerated for up to 28 days. Once the cartridge is placed in an OptiPen One, do not refrigerate. After initial use, *insulin detemir* vials, cartridges, or a prefilled syringe may be stored in a cool place for 42 days. Do not store in-use cartridges and pre-filled syringes in refrigerator or with needle in place. Keep away from direct heat and sunlight.
- When transferring from once-daily NPH human insulin to *insulin glargine*, the dose usually remains unchanged. When transferring from twice-daily NPH human insulin to insulin glargine, the initial dose of insulin glargine is usually reduced by 20%.
- **Subcut:** Rotate injection sites.
- Administer *insulin glargine* once daily at the same time each day.
- Administer *daily insulin detemir* with evening meal or at bedtime. With *twice daily insulin*

detemir, administer evening dose with evening meal, at bedtime, or 12 hr after morning dose.
- Do not administer *insulin detemir* or *insulin glargine* IV or in insulin pumps.

Patient/Family Teaching
- Instruct patient on proper technique for administration. Include type of insulin, equipment (syringe, cartridge pens, alcohol swabs), storage, and place to discard syringes. Discuss the importance of not changing brands of insulin or syringes, selection and rotation of injection sites, and compliance with therapeutic regimen. Patients taking insulin detemir should be given the *Patient Information* circular for this product.
- Explain to patient that this medication controls hyperglycemia but does not cure diabetes. Therapy is long term.
- Instruct patient in proper testing of serum glucose and ketones. These tests should be closely monitored during periods of stress or illness and health care professional notified of significant changes.
- Emphasize the importance of compliance with nutritional guidelines and regular exercise as directed by health care professional.
- Advise patient to consult health care professional prior to using alcohol or other Rx, OTC, or herbal products concurrently with insulin.
- Advise patient to notify health care professional of medication regimen prior to treatment or surgery.
- Advise patient to notify health care professional if nausea, vomiting, or fever develops, if unable to eat regular diet, or if blood glucose levels are not controlled.
- Instruct patient on signs and symptoms of hypoglycemia and hyperglycemia and what to do if they occur.
- Advise patient to notify health care professional if pregnancy is planned or suspected or if breastfeeding or planning to breastfeed.
- Patients with diabetes mellitus should carry a source of sugar (candy, glucose gel) and identification describing their disease and treatment regimen at all times.
- Emphasize the importance of regular follow-up, especially during first few weeks of therapy.

Evaluation/Desired Outcomes
- Control of blood glucose levels in diabetic patients without the appearance of hypoglycemic or hyperglycemic episodes.

HIGH ALERT

INSULINS (rapid acting)
(in-su-lin)

insulin aspart, rDNA origin
Novolog

insulin lispro, rDNA origin
Humalog

insulin glulisine
Apidra

Classification
Therapeutic: antidiabetics, hormones
Pharmacologic: pancreatics

Pregnancy Category B (insulin aspart, insulin lispro), C (insulin glulisine)

See Appendix N for more information concerning insulins

Indications
Control of hyperglycemia in patients with type 1 or type 2 diabetes mellitus.

Action
Lower blood glucose by: stimulating glucose uptake in skeletal muscle and fat, inhibiting hepatic glucose production. Other actions: inhibition of lypolysis and proteolysis, enhanced protein synthesis. These are rapid-acting insulins with a more rapid onset and shorter duration than regular insulin; should be used with an intermediate- or long-acting insulin. **Therapeutic Effects:** Control of hyperglycemia in diabetic patients.

Pharmacokinetics
Absorption: Very rapidly absorbed from subcut administration sites.
Distribution: Widely distributed.
Metabolism and Excretion: Metabolized by liver, spleen, kidney, and muscle.
Half-life: *Insulin aspart*—1–1.5 hr; *Insulin lispro*—1 hr; *insulin glulisine*—42 min.

TIME/ACTION PROFILE (hypoglycemic effect)

ROUTE	ONSET	PEAK	DURATION
Insulin aspart	10–20 min	1–3 hr	3–5 hr
Insulin glulisine	within 15 min	1 hr	2–4 hr
Insulin lispro	within 15 min	1–1.5 hr	3–4 hr

Contraindications/Precautions
Contraindicated in: Hypoglycemia; Allergy or hypersensitivity to a particular type of insulin, preservatives, or other additives.

INSULINS (rapid acting)

Use Cautiously in: Stress and infection (may temporarily ↑ insulin requirements); Renal/hepatic dysfunction (may ↓ insulin requirements); OB: Pregnancy may temporarily ↑ insulin requirements; Pedi: Safety not established in children <3 yr (for insulin lispro), <4 yr (insulin glulisine), <6 yr (for insulin aspart).

Adverse Reactions/Side Effects
Endo: HYPOGLYCEMIA. **Local:** erythema, lipodystrophy, pruritus, swelling. **Misc:** allergic reactions including ANAPHYLAXIS.

Interactions
Drug-Drug: Beta blockers, clonidine, and reserpine may mask some of the signs and symptoms of hypoglycemia. Corticosteroids, thyroid supplements, estrogens, isoniazid, niacin, phenothiazines, and rifampin may ↑ insulin requirements. Alcohol, ACE inhibitors, MAO inhibitors, octreotide, oral hypoglycemic agents, and salicylates, may ↓ insulin requirements.
Drug-Natural Products: Glucosamine may worsen blood glucose control. Fenugreek, chromium, and coenzyme Q-10 may produce additive hypoglycemic effects.

Route/Dosage
Dose depends on blood glucose, response, and many other factors. Only insulin aspart and insulin glulisine can be administered IV.
Subcut (Adults and Children): Total insulin dose determined by needs of patient; generally 0.5–1 unit/kg/day; 50–70% of this dose may be given as meal-related boluses of rapid-acting insulin, and the remainder as an intermediate or long-acting insulin. *Subcutaneous infusion pump*—~50% of total dose can be given as meal-related boluses and ~50% of total dose can be given as basal infusion.

Availability
Insulin aspart: 100 units/mL in 10 mL vials and 3 mL disposable delivery devices. **Cost:** $88.99/10–mL vial *NovoLog Pens (3 mL)*—$166.39/5 pens. *In combination with:* Insulin aspart 70/30 mix (Novolog Mix 70/30): 70% insulin aspart protamine suspension and 30% insulin aspart solution mix 100 units/mL in 10-mL vials and 3-mL disposable delivery devices. **Insulin aspart 50/50 mix (Novolog Mix 50/50):** 50% insulin aspart protamine suspension and 50% insulin aspart solution mix 100 units/mL in 3-mL disposable delivery devices. **Insulin glulisine:** 100 units/mL in 10-mL vials or 3-mL cartridges (for use with OptiClick Insulin Delivery Device), or 3-mL SoloStar prefilled pen. **Cost:** $79.99/10-mL vial. **Insulin lispro:** 100 units/mL in 10-mL vials and 3-mL disposable delivery device. **Cost:** $85.99/10-mL vial. *Humalog Pens (3 mL)*—$172.05/5 pens. *In combination with:* **Insulin lispro 75/25 mix (Humalog Mix 75/25):** 75% lispro insulin protamine suspension and 25% insulin lispro mix 100 units/mL in 10-mL vials and 3-mL disposable delivery devices. **Cost:** $91.25/10-mL vial. *Humalog Mix 75/25 Pens (3 mL)*—$147.50/5 pens. **Insulin lispro 50/50 mix (Humalog Mix 50/50):** 50% lispro insulin protamine suspension and 50% insulin lispro mix 100 units/mL in 10-mL vials and 3-mL disposable delivery devices.

NURSING IMPLICATIONS
Assessment
- Assess for symptoms of hypoglycemia (anxiety; restlessness; tingling in hands, feet, lips, or tongue; chills; cold sweats; confusion; cool, pale skin; difficulty in concentration; drowsiness; nightmares or trouble sleeping; excessive hunger; headache; irritability; nausea; nervousness; tachycardia; tremor; weakness; unsteady gait) and hyperglycemia (confusion, drowsiness; flushed, dry skin; fruit-like breath odor; rapid, deep breathing, polyuria; loss of appetite; nausea; vomiting; unusual thirst) periodically during therapy.
- Monitor body weight periodically. Changes in weight may necessitate changes in insulin dose.
- Assess patient for signs of allergic reactions (rash, shortness of breath, wheezing, rapid pulse, sweating, low blood pressure) during therapy.
- *Lab Test Considerations:* May cause ↓ serum inorganic phosphate, magnesium, and potassium levels.
- Monitor blood glucose every 6 hr during therapy, more frequently in ketoacidosis and times of stress. A1C may also be monitored every 3–6 mo to determine effectiveness.
- *Toxicity and Overdose:* Overdose is manifested by symptoms of hypoglycemia. Mild hypoglycemia may be treated by ingestion of oral glucose. Severe hypoglycemia is a life-threatening emergency; treatment consists of IV glucose, glucagon, or epinephrine. Early signs of hypoglycemia may be less pronounced by long duration of diabetes, diabetic nerve disease, and use of beta blockers; may result in loss of

INSULINS (rapid acting)

consciousness prior to patient's awareness of hypoglycemia.

Potential Nursing Diagnoses
Noncompliance (Patient/Family Teaching)

Implementation
- **High Alert:** Insulin-related medication errors have resulted in patient harm and death. Clarify ambiguous orders; do not accept orders using the abbreviation "u" for units, (can be misread as a zero or the numeral 4; has resulted in tenfold overdoses).
- Insulins are available in different types and strengths. Check type, dose, and expiration date with another licensed nurse. Do not interchange insulins without consulting physician or other health care professional.
- Use *only* insulin syringes to draw up dose. The unit markings on the insulin syringe must match the insulin's units/mL.
- *Insulin aspart, insulin glulisine,* and *insulin lispro* may be mixed with NPH insulin. When mixing insulins, draw insulin aspart, insulin glulisine, or insulin lispro into syringe first to avoid contamination of rapid-acting insulin vial. Mixed insulins should never be used in a pump or for IV infusion.
- Store vials in refrigerator. Vials may also be kept at room temperature for up to 28 days. Do not use if cloudy, discolored, or unusually viscous. Cartridges and pens should be stored at room temperature and used within 28 days. Never use the PenFill cartridge after the expiration date on the PenFill cartridge or on the box.
- Because of their short duration, *insulin lispro, insulin glulisine,* and *insulin aspart,* must be used with a longer-acting insulin or insulin infusion pump. In patients with type 2 diabetes, *insulin lispro* may be used without a longer-acting insulin when used in combination with an oral sulfonylurea agent.
- **Subcut:** Administer into abdominal wall, thigh, or upper arm subcut. Rotate injection sites.
- Administer *insulin aspart* within 5–10 min before a meal.
- When used as meal time insulin, administer *insulin glulisine* 15 min before or within 20 min after starting a meal.
- Administer *insulin lispro* within 15 min before or immediately after a meal.
- May also be administered subcut via external insulin pump. Do not mix with other insulins or solution when used with a pump. Change the solution in the reservoir at least every 6 days, change the infusion set, and the infusion set insertion site at least every 3 days. Do not mix with other insulins or with a diluent when used in the pump.

IV Administration
- **IV:** *Insulin aspart* and *insulin glulisine* may be administered IV in selected situations under appropriate medical supervision. **Diluent:** Dilute *insulin aspart* with 0.9% NaCl or D5W in infusion systems using polypropylene infusion bags. Dilute *insulin glulisine* with 0.9% NaCl, using polyvinyl chloride (PVC) Viaflex infusion bags and Polyvinyl chloride (PVC) tubing (Clearlink System Continu-Flo solution set) with a dedicated infusion line. **Concentration:** 0.05–1 unit/mL. *Insulin lispro* should not be administered IV.

Patient/Family Teaching
- Instruct patient on proper technique for administration. Include type of insulin, equipment (syringe, cartridge pens, external pump, alcohol swabs), storage, and place to discard syringes. Discuss the importance of not changing brands of insulin or syringes, selection and rotation of injection sites, and compliance with therapeutic regimen. Caution patient that insulin pens should not be shared with others, even if clean needles are used.
- Demonstrate technique for mixing insulins by drawing up insulin aspart, insulin glulisine, or insulin lispro first. Roll intermediate-acting insulin vial between palms to mix, rather than shaking (may cause inaccurate dose).
- Explain to patient that this medication controls hyperglycemia but does not cure diabetes. Therapy is long term.
- Instruct patient in proper testing of serum glucose and ketones. These tests should be closely monitored during periods of stress or illness and health care professional notified of significant changes.
- Emphasize the importance of compliance with nutritional guidelines and regular exercise as directed by health care professional.
- Advise patient to consult health care professional prior to using alcohol or other Rx, OTC, or herbal products concurrently with insulin.

✽ = Canadian drug name.   ≋ = Genetic implication.
*CAPITALS indicates life-threatening; underlines indicate most frequent.

724 INTERFERONS, ALPHA

- Advise patient to notify health care professional of medication regimen prior to treatment or surgery.
- Advise patient to notify health care professional if nausea, vomiting, or fever develops, if unable to eat regular diet, or if blood glucose levels are not controlled.
- Instruct patient on signs and symptoms of hypoglycemia and hyperglycemia and what to do if they occur.
- Advise patient to notify health care professional if pregnancy is planned or suspected or if breastfeeding or planning to breastfeed.
- Patients with diabetes mellitus should carry a source of sugar (candy, glucose gel) and identification describing their disease and treatment regimen at all times.
- Emphasize the importance of regular follow-up, especially during first few weeks of therapy.

Evaluation/Desired Outcomes
- Control of blood glucose levels without the appearance of hypoglycemic or hyperglycemic episodes.

INTERFERONS, ALPHA
(in-ter-**feer**-onz)

peginterferon alpha-2a
Pegasys

interferon alpha-2b (recombinant)
Intron A

peginterferon alpha-2b (pegylated)
Pegintron

interferon alpha-n3 (human)
Alferon N

Classification
Therapeutic: immune modifiers
Pharmacologic: interferons

Pregnancy Category C

Indications
Peginterferon alpha-2a: Treatment of: Chronic hepatitis C (alone or with ribavirin), Chronic hepatitis B. **Interferon alpha-2b:** Treatment of: Hairy cell leukemia, Malignant melanoma, AIDS-related Kaposi's sarcoma, Condylomata acuminata (intralesional), Chronic hepatitis B, Chronic hepatitis C (with oral ribavirin) which has relapsed following previous treatment with interferon alone, Follicular non-Hodgkin's lymphoma.
Peginterferon alpha–2b: Chronic hepatitis C (alone or with ribavirin). **Interferon alpha-n3:** Treatment of condylomata acuminata (intralesional).

Action
Interferons are proteins capable of modifying the immune response and have antiproliferative action against tumor cells. Interferon alpha-2b is produced by recombinant DNA techniques, peginterferon is a "pegylated" formulation of interferon alpha-2b formulated to have a longer duration of action; interferon alpha-n3 is from pooled human leukocytes. Interferons also have antiviral activity.
Therapeutic Effects: Antineoplastic, antiviral, and antiproliferative activity. Decreased progression of hepatic damage (for patients with hepatitis).

Pharmacokinetics
Absorption: Not absorbed orally. Well absorbed (>80%) following IM and subcut administration. Minimal systemic absorption follows intralesional administration.
Distribution: Unknown.
Metabolism and Excretion: Filtered by the kidneys and subsequently degraded in the renal tubule; *peginterferon alpha-2b*—30% renally excreted.
Half-life: *Peginterferon alpha-2a*—50–160 hr; *interferon alpha-2b*—2–3 hr; *peginterferon alpha-2b*—40 hr.

TIME/ACTION PROFILE (clinical effects)

ROUTE	ONSET	PEAK	DURATION
Interferon alpha-2b IM, subcut	1–3 mo	unknown	unknown (CR)
Interferon alpha-2b IM, subcut	unknown	3–5 days	3–5 days (BC)
Interferon alpha-2b IM, subcut	2 wk	unknown	unknown (LFT)
Interferon alpha-2b and n3	unknown	4–8 wk	unknown (IL)
Peginterferon alpha-2b subcut	unknown	6 mos or more	unknown

BC = effects on platelet counts; CR = clinical response; IL = regression of lesions; LFT = effects on liver function in patients with hepatitis

Contraindications/Precautions
Contraindicated in: Hypersensitivity to alpha interferons or human serum albumin; Autoimmune hepatitis; Hepatic decompensation (Child-Pugh class B and C) before or during therapy;

INTERFERONS, ALPHA

Pedi: Products containing benzyl alcohol should not be used in neonates.

Use Cautiously in: Severe cardiovascular, pulmonary, renal, or hepatic disease; Active infections; Underlying CNS pathology or psychiatric history; Decreased bone marrow reserve or underlying immunosuppression; Current history of chickenpox, herpes zoster, or herpes labialis (may reactivate or disseminate disease); Previous or concurrent radiation therapy; Autoimmune disorders (may ↑ risk of exacerbation); OB: ↑ risk of spontaneous abortion in animal studies; use only if potential fetal risks are outweighed by potential maternal benefit; women with childbearing potential should be advised of potential risk to fetus; Lactation: Usually compatible with breastfeeding (AAP); Pedi: Children <3 yr (safety not established); Geri: ↑ risk of adverse reactions.
Exercise Extreme Caution in: History of depression/suicide attempt.

Adverse Reactions/Side Effects

All are more prominent with subcut, IV, or IM administration.
CNS: NEUROPSYCHIATRIC DISORDERS, confusion, depression, dizziness, fatigue, headache, insomnia, irritability, anxiety. **EENT:** blurred vision, nose bleeds, rhinitis. **CV:** ISCHEMIC DISORDERS, arrhythmias, chest pain, edema. **GI:** COLITIS, PANCREATITIS, anorexia, abdominal pain, diarrhea, dry mouth, nausea, taste disorder, vomiting, weight loss, drug-induced hepatitis, flatulence. **Derm:** alopecia, dry skin, pruritus, rash, sweating. **Endo:** thyroid disorders. **Hemat:** LEUKOPENIA, THROMBOCYTOPENIA, anemia, hemolytic anemia (with ribavirin). **MS:** arthralgia, myalgia, leg cramps. **Neuro:** paresthesia. **Resp:** cough, dyspnea. **Local:** injection site reactions. **Misc:** AUTOIMMUNE DISORDERS, INFECTIOUS DISORDERS, allergic reactions including ANAPHYLAXIS, chills, fever, flu-like syndrome.

Interactions

Drug-Drug: Additive myelosuppression with other **antineoplastic agents** or **radiation therapy**. ↑ CNS depression may occur with **CNS depressants**, including **alcohol**, **antihistamines**, **sedative/hypnotics**, and **opioids**. May ↓ metabolism and ↑ blood levels and toxicity of **theophylline** and **methadone**. ↑ risk of adverse reactions with **zidovudine**. **Ribavirin** ↑ risk of hemolytic anemia, especially if CCr <50 mL/min (avoid if possible). May ↓ effects of **immunosuppressant agents**.

Route/Dosage

Peginterferon Alpha-2a

Subcut (Adults): *Chronic hepatitis C*—180 mcg once weekly for 48 wk for Genotypes 1,4 (24 wk for Genotypes 2,3). *Patients with chronic hepatitis C co-infected with HIV*-180 mcg once weekly for 48 wk.

Interferon Alpha-2b

IV (Adults): *Malignant melanoma (induction)*—20 million units/m² for 5 days of each week for 4 wk initially, followed by subcut maintenance dosing.
IM, Subcut (Adults): *Hairy cell leukemia*—2 million units/m² IM or subcut 3 times weekly for up to 6 mo. *Malignant melanoma (maintenance)*—10 million units/m² subcut 3 times weekly for 48 wk, following initial IV dosing. *AIDS-related Kaposi's sarcoma*—30 million units/m² IM or subcut 3 times weekly until disease progression or maximum response has been achieved after 16 wk. *Chronic hepatitis C*—3 million units IM or subcut 3 times weekly. If normalization of ALT occurs after 16 wk of therapy, continue treatment for total of 18–24 mo. If normalization of ALT does not occur after 16 wk of therapy, may consider discontinuing treatment. *Chronic hepatitis B*—5 million units/day IM or subcut *or* 10 million units IM or subcut 3 times weekly for 16 wk. *Follicular non-Hodgkin's lymphoma*—5 million units subcut 3 times weekly for up to 18 mo (to be used following completion of anthracycline-containing chemotherapy).
Subcut (Children > 3 yr): *Chronic hepatitis B*—3 million units/m² 3 times weekly for the first week of therapy then increase to 6 million units/m² 3 times weekly (not to exceed 10 million units/dose) for 16 to 24 weeks.
IL (Adults): *Condylomata acuminata*—1 million units/lesion 3 times weekly for 3 wk; treat only 5 lesions per course. An additional course of treatment may be initiated at 12–16 wk.

Peginterferon Alpha-2b

Monotherapy

Subcut (Adults): *137–160 kg*—150 mcg once weekly for 1 yr. *107–136 kg*—120 mcg once weekly for 1 yr. *89–106 kg*—96 mcg once weekly for 1 yr. *73–88 kg*—80 mcg once weekly for 1 year. *57–72 kg*—64 mcg once weekly for 1 yr. *46–56 kg*—50 mcg once weekly for 1 yr. *37–45 kg*—40 mcg once weekly for 1 yr.

INTERFERONS, ALPHA

In Combination with Ribavirin (Rebetol)
Subcut (Adults): *>85 kg*— 150 mcg once weekly. *76–85 kg*— 120 mcg once weekly. *61–75 kg*— 96 mcg once weekly. *51–60 kg*— 80 mcg once weekly. *40–50 kg*— 64 mcg once weekly. *<40 kg*— 50 mcg once weekly.
Subcut (Children 3–17 yr): 60 mcg/m² once weekly.

Interferon Alpha-n3
IL (Adults): 250,000 units/lesion twice weekly for up to 8 wk; for large lesions, divide dose and inject at several sites.

Availability

Peginterferon Alpha-2a
Solution for injection: 180 mcg/mL in single use vials. **Prefilled syringes:** 180 mcg/0.5 mL.

Interferon Alpha-2b
Powder for injection: 10-million-unit single-use vial, 18-million-unit single-use vial, 50-million-unit single-use vial. **Solution for injection:** 10-million-unit single-use vial, 18-million-unit single-use vial, 18-million-unit multidose pen, 25-million-unit multidose vial, 30-million-unit multidose pen, 60-million-unit multidose pen. *In combination with:* oral ribavarin (Rebetrol) as a combination package (Rebetron). See Appendix B (in various dosage packages).

Peginterferon Alpha-2b
Powder for injection (Redipen system or vials): 50 mcg/0.5 mL, 80 mcg/0.5 mL, 120 mcg/0.5 mL, 150 mcg/0.5 mL.

Interferon Alpha-n3
Solution for injection: 5 million units/mL.

NURSING IMPLICATIONS

Assessment
- Assess for signs of neuropsychiatric disorders (irritability, anxiety, depression, suicidal ideation, aggressive behavior). May require discontinuation of therapy.
- Monitor for signs of infection (vital signs, WBC) during therapy. Discontinue drug therapy in cases of severe infection, and antibiotic therapy instituted.
- Assess for cardiovascular disorders (pulse, blood pressure, chest pain). An ECG should be performed before and periodically during the course of therapy in patients with a history of cardiovascular disease.
- Assess for signs of colitis (abdominal pain, bloody diarrhea, fever) and pancreatitis (nausea, vomiting, abdominal pain) during therapy. Discontinue therapy if these occur; may be fatal. Colitis usually resolves within 1–3 wk of discontinuation.
- Assess for development of flu-like syndrome (fever, chills, myalgia, headache). Symptoms often appear suddenly 3–6 hr after therapy. Symptoms tend to decrease, even with continued therapy. Acetaminophen may be used for control of these symptoms.
- Monitor for bone marrow depression. Assess for bleeding (bleeding gums; bruising; petechiae; guaiac stools, urine, and emesis) and avoid IM injections and rectal temperatures if platelet count is low. Apply pressure to venipuncture sites for 10 min. Assess for signs of infection during neutropenia. Anemia may occur. Monitor for increased fatigue, dyspnea, and orthostatic hypotension.
- May cause nausea and vomiting. Antiemetics may be used prophylactically. Monitor intake and output, daily weight, and appetite. Adjust diet as tolerated for anorexia. Encourage fluid intake of at least 2 liters/day.
- Assess pulmonary status (lung sounds, respirations) periodically during therapy.
- Perform a baseline eye exam in all patients prior to initiation of therapy. Eye exams should be performed periodically during therapy in patients with pre-existing diabetic or hypertensive retinopathy. Discontinue therapy if patients develop new or worsening eye disorders.
- Assess for signs of thyroid dysfunction, as hypothyroidism or hyperthyroidism may occur. Discontinue therapy if the patient's thyroid function cannot be controlled with medications (e.g., thyroid hormone supplementation, antithyroid medications).
- **Kaposi's Sarcoma:** Monitor number, size, and character of lesions prior to and throughout therapy.
- *Lab Test Considerations:* Systemic: Monitor for CBC and differential prior to and periodically during therapy. May cause leukopenia, neutropenia, thrombocytopenia, decreased hemoglobin and hematocrit, and hemolytic anemia. The nadirs of leukopenia and thrombocytopenia occur in 3–5 days, with recovery 3–5 days after withdrawal of *interferon alpha-2b* For malignant melanoma, if granulocyte count >250/mm³ but <500/mm³, discontinue *interferon alpha-2b* until platelet or granulocyte counts return to normal or baseline levels, then reinstitute at 50% of dose. If granulocyte count <250/mm³ with *interferon alpha-2b*, discontinue permanently. For follicular non-Hodgkin's lymphoma, if granulocyte count <1000/

mm³ or platelet count <50,000/mm³, discontinue *interferon alpha-2b*. *Peginterferon alpha-2b* should be discontinued if granulocyte count <1000/mm³ or platelet count <50,000/mm³. *Peginterferon alpha-2a* should be discontinued if ANC<500/mm³ or platelet count <25,000/mm³ and then may be restarted at a lower dose if the ANC>1000/mm³.
- Platelet count should be ≥90,000 cells/mm³ and ANC ≥1500 cells/mm³ prior to initiation of peginterferon therapy. Commonly causes ↓ hemoglobin, hematocrit, WBC, ANC, lymphocytes and platelet counts within first 2 wk of therapy.
- Monitor liver function tests (AST, ALT, LDH, bilirubin, alkaline phosphatase), triglycerides, and renal function tests (BUN, creatinine, uric acid, urinalysis) prior to and periodically during therapy. CCr should be >50 mL/min prior to initiation of peginterferon therapy.
- Monitor TSH at baseline and if patients develop symptoms consistent with hypothyroidism or hyperthyroidism.
- **Hairy Cell Leukemia:** Monitor number of peripheral blood hairy cells and bone marrow hairy cells prior to and during therapy.

Potential Nursing Diagnoses
Risk for injury (Side Effects)
Risk for infection (Side Effects)

Implementation
- Solution should be prepared in a biologic cabinet. Wear gloves, gown, and mask while handling medication. Discard equipment in specially designated containers (see Appendix L).

Interferon Alpha-2b
- **IM, Subcut:** Subcut route is preferred for patients with a platelet count <50,000/mm³.
- Reconstitute 10-, 18-, and 50-million-unit vials with 1 mL of diluent provided by manufacturer (sterile water for injection). Agitate gently. Solution may be colorless to light yellow. Solution should be used immediately; stable for up to 24 hr if refrigerated.
- The solution for injection vials do not require reconstitution prior to use and may be used for IM, subcut, or intralesional administration.
- The solution for injection in multidose pens are for subcut use only. Only the needles provided in the package should be used with the pen. A new needle should be used with each dose.

Follow instructions in *Medication Guide* for use of multidose pens.
- **IL:** Reconstitute 10-million-unit vial with 1 mL of diluent provided by manufacturer (sterile water for injection). Use a TB syringe with 25–30-gauge needle to administer. Each 0.1-mL dose is injected into the center of the base of the wart using the intradermal injection approach. As many as 5 lesions can be treated at one time.

IV Administration
- **Intermittent Infusion:** (For Malignant Melanoma). *Diluent:* Add 1 mL of diluent provided by manufacturer (sterile water for injection) to vial. Further dilute appropriate dose in 100 mL of 0.9% NaCl. Solution should be used immediately; stable for 24 hr if refrigerated. The solution for injection vials are not recommended for IV administration. *Concentration:* Final concentration of infusion should not be less than 10 million units/100 mL. *Rate:* Infuse over 20 min.

Peginterferon Alpha–2a
- Vials and pre-filled syringes should be stored in refrigerator. Do not administer solution that is cloudy or contains a precipitate.
- Follow instructions in *Medication Guide* for use of pre-filled syringes.

Peginterferon Alpha–2b
- Reconstitute vial with 0.7 mL of diluent provided by manufacturer (sterile water for injection). Administer immediately; stable for 24 hr if refrigerated. Solution should be clear and colorless. Discard unused solution.
- *For PEG Intron Redipen*—To reconstitute the drug, hold the Redipen upright (dose button down) and press 2 halves of pen together until a click is heard. Gently invert the pen to mix the solution (do not shake). Solution should be clear and colorless. Follow instructions in *Medication Guide* for *RediPen* use. Dispose of *RediPen* and other materials in puncture-resistant container.

Interferon Alpha-n3
- Vials should be refrigerated.

Patient/Family Teaching
- Advise patient to take medication as directed. If a dose is missed, omit dose and return to the regular schedule. Notify health care professional if more than 1 dose is missed.

- **Home Care Issues:** Instruct patient and family on preparation and correct technique for administration of injection and care and disposal of equipment. Advise patient to read *Medication Guide* prior to administration and with each prescription refill to check for changes. Explain to patient that brands should not be switched without consulting health care professional; may result in a change of dose.
- Discuss possibility of flu-like reaction 3–6 hr after dose. Acetaminophen may be taken prior to injection and every 3–4 hr afterward as needed to control symptoms.
- Review side effects with patient. Interferon may be temporarily discontinued or dose decreased by 50% if serious side effects occur.
- Instruct patient to notify health care professional promptly if fever; chills; cough; hoarseness; sore throat; signs of infection; lower back or side pain; painful or difficult urination; bleeding gums; bruising; petechiae; blood in stools, urine, or emesis; increased fatigue; dyspnea; or orthostatic hypotension occurs. Caution patient to avoid crowds and persons with known infections. Instruct patient to use soft toothbrush and electric razor and to avoid falls. Caution patient not to drink alcoholic beverages or take medication containing aspirin or NSAIDs; may precipitate gastric bleeding.
- Inform patient of the potential for depression and advise patient to notify health care professional if depression occurs.
- Discuss with patient the possibility of hair loss. Explore coping strategies.
- Explain to patient that fertility may be impaired and that contraception is needed during treatment to prevent potential harm to the fetus.
- Instruct patient not to receive any vaccinations without advice of health care professional.
- Emphasize need for periodic lab tests to monitor for side effects.
- Inform patient that peginterferon alpha-2a may not reduce the risk of transmission of HCV to others or prevent cirrhosis, liver failure, or liver cancer.

Evaluation/Desired Outcomes
- Normalized blood parameters (hemoglobin, neutrophils, platelets, monocytes, and bone marrow and peripheral hairy cells) in hairy cell leukemia. Response may not be seen for 6 mo with *interferon alpha-2b*.
- Decrease in the size and number of lesions in Kaposi's sarcoma. Therapy may be required for 6 mo before full response is seen. Therapy is continued until disease progresses or a maximum response has been achieved after 4 mo of therapy.
- Improved hematologic parameters in patients with chronic myelogenous leukemia.
- Increase in time to relapse and overall survival in patients with malignant melanoma.
- Disappearance of or decrease in size and number of genital warts. Condylomata acuminata usually respond in 4–8 wk. A second course of therapy may be required if genital warts persist and laboratory values remain in acceptable limits.
- Decrease in symptoms and improvement in liver function tests and ↓ progression of hepatic damage in patients with hepatitis B or hepatitis C infection.

INTERFERONS, BETA
(in-ter-**feer**-on)

inteferon beta-1a
Avonex, Rebif

interferon beta-1b
Betaseron

Classification
Therapeutic: anti-multiple sclerosis agents, immune modifiers
Pharmacologic: interferons

Pregnancy Category C

Indications
Relapsing forms of multiple sclerosis.

Action
Antiviral and immunoregulatory properties produced by interacting with specific receptor sites on cell surfaces may explain beneficial effects. Produced by recombinant DNA technology. **Therapeutic Effects:** Reduce incidence of relapse (neurologic dysfunction) and slow physical disability.

Pharmacokinetics
Absorption: *Interferon beta-1b*—50% absorbed following subcut administration.
Distribution: Unknown.
Metabolism and Excretion: Unknown.
Half-life: *Interferon beta-1a*—69 hr (subcut), 10 hr (IM); *interferon beta-1b*—8 min–4.3 hr.

INTERFERONS, BETA

TIME/ACTION PROFILE (serum concentrations)

ROUTE	ONSET	PEAK	DURATION
Interferon beta-1a IM, subcut	unknown	3–15 h	unknown
Interferon beta-1b subcut	rapid	16 h	unknown

Contraindications/Precautions

Contraindicated in: Hypersensitivity to natural or recombinant interferon beta or human albumin.

Use Cautiously in: History of suicide attempt or depression; History of seizures (interferon beta-1a); Cardiovascular disease; Liver disease (interferon beta-1a); History of alcohol abuse (interferon beta-1a); Patients with childbearing potential; OB: May ↑ risk of spontaneous abortion; use only if potential maternal benefit outweighs potential fetal risk; Lactation: Safety not established; Pedi: Safety not established.

Adverse Reactions/Side Effects

CNS: SEIZURES (↑ WITH INTERFERON BETA-1A), depression, dizziness, fatigue, headache, insomnia, drowsiness, incoordination, rigors, suicidal ideation. **EENT:** sinusitis, vision abnormalities. **Resp:** dyspnea, upper respiratory tract infection. **CV:** chest pain, edema, hypertension. **GI:** constipation, nausea, vomiting, abdominal pain, autoimmune hepatitis, dry mouth, elevated liver function tests. **GU:** cystitis, erectile dysfunction, polyuria, urinary incontinence. **Derm:** rashes, alopecia. **Endo:** menstrual disorders, hyperthyroidism, hypothyroidism, menorrhagia, spontaneous abortion. **Hemat:** neutropenia, anemia, eosinophilia, thrombocytopenia. **Local:** injection-site reactions, injection site necrosis. **MS:** myalgia, arthralgia, muscle spasm. **Misc:** allergic reactions including ANAPHYLAXIS, chills, fever, flu-like symptoms, pain.

Interactions

(All interactions below are for Interferon beta-1b).

Drug-Drug: ↑ myelosuppression may occur with other myelosuppressives including **antineoplastics**. Concurrent use of **hepatotoxic agents** may ↑ the risk of hepatotoxicity (↑ liver enzymes).

Drug-Natural Products: Avoid concommitant use with immmunomodulating natural products such as **astragalus**, **echinacea**, and **melatonin**.

Route/Dosage

Interferon Beta-1a

IM (Adults): *Avonex*—30 mcg once weekly.
Subcut (Adults): *Rebif (target dose of 22 mcg 3 times/wk)*—Start with 4.4 mcg 3 times/wk for 2 wk, then ↑ to 11 mcg 3 times/wk for 2 wk, then ↑ to maintenance dose of 22 mcg 3 times/wk. *Rebif (target dose of 44 mcg 3 times/wk)*—Start with 8.8 mcg 3 times/wk for 2 wk, then ↑ to 22 mcg 3 times/wk for 2 wk, then ↑ to maintenance dose of 44 mcg 3 times/wk.

Interferon Beta-1b

Subcut (Adults): *Betaseron*—Initiate with 0.0625 mg (2 million units) every other day and then ↑ dose by 0.0625 mg q 2 wk over a 6-wk period up to target dose of 0.25 mg (8 million units) every other day.

Availability

Interferon Beta-1a (Avonex)

Powder for injection: 30 mcg/vial. **Prefilled syringes (Avonex):** 30 mcg/0.5 mL. **Pre-filled syringes (Rebif):** 22 mcg/0.5 mL, 44 mcg/0.5 mL, titration pack of 6 syringes prefilled with 8.8 mcg/0.2 mL and 6 syringes prefilled with 22 mcg/0.5 mL.

Interferon Beta-1b

Powder for injection (Betaseron): 0.3 mg (9.6 million units)/vial.

NURSING IMPLICATIONS

Assessment

- Assess frequency of exacerbations of symptoms of multiple sclerosis periodically during therapy.
- Monitor patient for signs of depression during therapy. If depression occurs, notify physician or other health care professional immediately.
- *Lab Test Considerations:* Monitor hemoglobin, WBC, platelets, and blood chemistries including liver function tests prior to and 1, 3, and 6 mo after initiation of therapy and periodically thereafter. Therapy may be temporarily discontinued if the absolute neutrophil count is <750/mm^3, if AST or ALT exceeds 10 times the upper limit of normal, or if serum bilirubin exceeds 5 times the upper limit of normal. Once

the absolute neutrophil count is >750/mm³ or the hepatic enzymes have returned to normal, therapy can be restarted at 50% of the original dose.
- Thyroid function tests should be monitored every 6 mo, especially in patients with a history of thyroid abnormalities.

Potential Nursing Diagnoses
Deficient knowledge, related to medication regimen (Patient/Family Teaching)

Implementation
- Do not confuse products. Interferon beta-1a and interferon beta-1b are not interchangeable.
- **Interferon Beta-1a:** *Avonex:* Reconstitute with 1.1 mL of diluent and swirl gently to dissolve. Do not shake the vial. Inject into the thigh or upper arm. Keep reconstituted solution in refrigerator; inject within 6 hr of reconstitution.
- *Rebif:* Administer subcut via pre-filled, single-use syringe at the same time (afternoon or evening) on the same days (Monday, Wednesday, Friday) at least 48 hr apart each wk. Rotate sites with each injection to minimize risk of injection site reactions. Discard unused portions. Store in refrigerator.
- **Interferon Beta-1b:** To reconstitute, inject 1.2 mL of diluent supplied into interferon beta-1b vial for a concentration of 0.25 mg/mL. Swirl gently to dissolve completely; do not shake. Do not use solutions that are discolored or contain particulate matter. Keep reconstituted solution refrigerated; inject within 3 hr of reconstitution.
- Following reconstitution, withdraw 1 mL into a syringe with a 27-gauge needle and inject subcut into arm, abdomen, hip, or thigh. Rotate sites with each injection to minimize risk of injection site reactions. Discard unused portion; vials are for single dose only.

Patient/Family Teaching
- **Home Care Issues:** Instruct patient in correct technique for injection and care and disposal of equipment. Caution patient not to reuse needles or syringes and provide patient with a puncture-resistant container for disposal.
- Instruct patient to take medication as directed; do not change dose or schedule without consulting health care professional. Patients should receive a medication guide with each product.
- Inform patient that flu-like symptoms (fever, chills, myalgia, sweating, malaise) may occur during therapy. Acetaminophen may be used for relief of fever and myalgias.
- Advise patient to notify health care professional if pregnancy is planned or suspected. May cause spontaneous abortion.

Evaluation/Desired Outcomes
- Decrease in the frequency of relapse (neurologic dysfunction) in patients with relapsing-remitting multiple sclerosis.

IODINE, IODIDE

potassium iodide†
Pima, SSKI, ThyroSafe, ThyroShield

strong iodine solution
Lugol's solution

Classification
Therapeutic: antithyroid agents
Pharmacologic: iodine containing agents

Pregnancy Category D

†For more information on potassium iodide as a radiation protectant see *Potassium Iodide as a Thyroid Blocking Agent in Radiation Emergencies* at www.fda.gov

Indications
Adjunct with other antithyroid drugs in preparation for thyroidectomy. Treatment of thyrotoxic crisis. Radiation protectant following radiation emergencies or administration of radioactive iodine.

Action
Rapidly inhibits the release and synthesis of thyroid hormones. Decreases the vascularity of the thyroid gland. Decreases thyroidal uptake of radioactive iodine following radiation emergencies or administration of radioactive isotopes of iodine. Iodine is a necessary component of thyroid hormone. **Therapeutic Effects:** Control of hyperthyroidism. Decreased bleeding during thyroid surgery. Decreased incidence of thyroid cancer following radiation emergencies.

Pharmacokinetics
Absorption: Converted in the GI tract and enters the circulation as iodine; also absorbed through skin and lungs; may also be obtained via recycling of iodothyronines.

Distribution: Concentrates in the thyroid gland and muscle; also found in skin, skeleton, breasts, and hair. Readily crosses the placenta; enters breast milk.

IODINE, IODIDE

Metabolism and Excretion: Taken up by the thyroid gland, then eliminated via kidneys, liver, skin, lungs, and intestines.
Half-life: Unknown.

TIME/ACTION PROFILE (effects on thyroid)

ROUTE	ONSET	PEAK	DURATION
PO	24 hr	10–15 days	variable†

†Radiation protection lasts 24 hr

Contraindications/Precautions
Contraindicated in: Hypersensitivity; Hyperkalemia; Pulmonary edema; Impaired renal function.
Use Cautiously in: Tuberculosis; Bronchitis; Cardiovascular disease; OB, Pedi: Pregnancy or lactation (although iodine is required during pregnancy, excess amounts may cause thyroid abnormalities/goiter in the newborn; excess use during lactation may cause skin rash or thyroid suppression in the infant).

Adverse Reactions/Side Effects
CNS: confusion, weakness. **GI:** GI BLEEDING, diarrhea, nausea, vomiting. **Derm:** acneiform eruptions. **Endo:** hypothyroidism, goiter, hyperthyroidism. **F and E:** hyperkalemia. **Neuro:** tingling. **MS:** joint pain. **Misc:** hypersensitivity, iodism.

Interactions
Drug-Drug: Use with **lithium** may cause ↑ hypothyroidism. ↑ antithyroid effect of **methimazole** and **propylthiouracil**. ↑ hyperkalemia may result from combined use with **potassium-sparing diuretics**, **ACE inhibitors**, **angiotensin II receptor antagonists** or **potassium supplements**.

Route/Dosage
Preparation for Thyroidectomy
PO (Adults and Children): *Strong iodine solution*—3–5 drops (0.1–0.3 mL) 3 times daily for 10 days prior to surgery. *Potassium iodide saturated solution* (SSKI)—1–5 drops (50–250 mg) 3 times daily for 10 days prior to surgery.

Hyperthyroidism
PO (Adults and Children): *Strong iodine solution*—1 mL in water 3 times daily. *Potassium iodide saturated solution* (SSKI)—6–10 drops (300–500 mg) 3 times daily.
PO (Infants <1 yr): 3–5 drops (150–250 mg) 3 times daily.

Radiation Protectant to Radioactive Isotopes of Iodine
PO (Adults): *Pima*—195 mg once daily for 10 days (start 24 hr prior to exposure (continue until risk of exposure has passed or other measures have been implemented).
PO (Children >1 yr): 130 mg once daily for 10 days (start 24 hr prior to exposure).
PO (Infants <1 yr): 65 mg once daily for 10 days (start 24 hr prior to exposure).

Reduction of Thyroid Cancer after Nuclear Accident
PO (Adults and Children >68 kg, including pregnant/lactating women): *Iosat, ThyroSafe, ThyroShield*—130 mg once daily (continue until risk of exposure has passed or other measures have been implemented).
PO (Children 3–18 yr): 65 mg once daily.
PO (Children 1 mo-3 yr): 32.5 mg once daily.
PO (Infants <1 mo): 16.25 mg once daily.

Availability
Potassium Iodide (generic available)
Oral solution: 65 mg/mL (ThyroShield), 1 g potassium iodide/mL (SSKI). **Syrup (Pima) (black-raspberry flavor):** 325 mg potassium iodide/5 mL. **Tablets:** 65 mg^{OTC}, 130 mg^{OTC} (available only through state and federal agencies).

Strong Iodine Solution (generic available)
Oral solution: Iodine 50 mg/mL plus potassium iodide 100 mg/mL.

NURSING IMPLICATIONS
Assessment
- Assess for signs and symptoms of iodism (metallic taste, stomatitis, skin lesions, cold symptoms, severe GI upset). Report these symptoms promptly.
- Monitor response symptoms of hyperthyroidism (tachycardia, palpitations, nervousness, insomnia, diaphoresis, heat intolerance, tremors, weight loss).
- Monitor for hypersensitivity reaction (rash, pruritus, laryngeal edema, wheezing). Discontinue drug and notify physician immediately if these problems occur.
- *Lab Test Considerations:* Monitor thyroid function before and periodically during therapy. May alter results of radionuclide thyroid imaging and may ↓ thyroidal uptake of ^{131}I,

^{123}I, and sodium pertechnetate ^{99m}Tc in thyroid uptake tests.
* Monitor serum potassium levels periodically during therapy.
* **Lab Test Considerations:** Monitor thyroid stimulating hormone (TSH) and free T$_4$ in neonates (within the first month of life) treated with potassium iodide for development of hypothyroidism. Thyroid hormone therapy should be instituted if hypothyroidism develops.

Potential Nursing Diagnoses
Deficient knowledge, related to medication regimen (Patient/Family Teaching)

Implementation
* Do not confuse iodine with Lodine (etodolac).
* For protection against inhaled radioiodines, administer potassium iodide prior to or immediately coincident with passage of the radioactive cloud, though a substantial protective effect lasts 3–4 hr after exposure.
* **PO:** Mix solutions in a full glass of fruit juice, water, broth, formula, or milk. Administer after meals to minimize GI irritation.
* Solution is normally clear and colorless. Darkening upon standing does not affect potency of drug. Solutions that are brownish yellow should be discarded.
* Crystals may form, especially if refrigerated, but redissolve upon warming and shaking.

Patient/Family Teaching
* Instruct patient to take medication as directed. Take missed doses as soon as possible but not just before next dose; do not double doses.
* Instruct patient to report suspected pregnancy to health care professional before therapy is initiated.
* Advise patient to consult health care professional about avoiding foods high in iodine (seafood, iodized salt, cabbage, kale, turnips) or potassium (see Appendix M).
* Advise patient to consult health care professional before using OTC or herbal cold remedies. Some cold remedies use iodide as an expectorant.
* **Hyperthyroidism:** Instruct patient to take medication as ordered. Missing a dose may precipitate hyperthyroidism.

Evaluation/Desired Outcomes
* Resolution of the symptoms of thyroid crisis.
* Decrease in size and vascularity of the gland before thyroid surgery. Use of iodides in the treatment of hyperthyroidism is usually limited to 2 wk.
* Protection of the thyroid gland from the effects of radioactive iodine.

---

ipratropium (i-pra-troe-pee-um)
Atrovent, Atrovent HFA

Classification
Therapeutic: allergy, cold, and cough remedies, bronchodilators
Pharmacologic: anticholinergics

Pregnancy Category B

Indications
Inhaln: Maintenance therapy of reversible airway obstruction due to COPD, including chronic bronchitis and emphysema. **Intranasal:** Rhinorrhea associated with allergic and nonallergic perennial rhinitis (0.03% solution) or the common cold (0.06% solution). **Unlabeled Use: Inhaln:** Adjunctive management of bronchospasm caused by asthma.

Action
Inhaln: Inhibits cholinergic receptors in bronchial smooth muscle, resulting in decreased concentrations of cyclic guanosine monophosphate (cGMP). Decreased levels of cGMP produce local bronchodilation. **Intranasal:** Local application inhibits secretions from glands lining the nasal mucosa. **Therapeutic Effects: Inhaln:** Bronchodilation without systemic anticholinergic effects. **Intranasal:** Decreased rhinorrhea.

Pharmacokinetics
Absorption: Minimal systemic absorption (2% for inhalation solution; 20% for inhalation aerosol; <20% following nasal use).
Distribution: 15% of dose reaches lower airways after inhalation.
Metabolism and Excretion: Small amounts absorbed are metabolized by the liver.
Half-life: 2 hr.

TIME/ACTION PROFILE (bronchodilation)

ROUTE	ONSET	PEAK	DURATION
Inhalation	1–3 min	1–2 hr	4–6 hr
Intranasal	15 min	unknown	6–12 hr

Contraindications/Precautions
Contraindicated in: Hypersensitivity to ipratropium, atropine, belladonna alkaloids, or bromide; Avoid use during acute bronchospasm; **Note: Atrovent HFA has replaced the discontinued Atrovent CFC (chlorofluorocarbon). Soy and CFC-allergic patients can now safely use the Atrovent HFA formulation. However,**

ipratropium

Combivent (ipratropium/albuterol combination) MDI does contain soya lecithin and is contraindicated in patients with a history of hypersensitivity to soy and peanuts.
Use Cautiously in: Patients with bladder neck obstruction, prostatic hyperplasia, glaucoma, or urinary retention; Geri: May be more sensitive to effects.

Adverse Reactions/Side Effects
CNS: dizziness, headache, nervousness. **EENT:** blurred vision, sore throat; *nasal only*, epistaxis, nasal dryness/irritation. **Resp:** bronchospasm, cough. **CV:** hypotension, palpitations. **GI:** GI irritation, nausea. **Derm:** rash. **Misc:** allergic reactions.

Interactions
Drug-Drug: ↑ anticholinergic effects with other **drugs having anticholinergic properties (antihistamines, phenothiazines, disopyramide).**

Route/Dosage
Inhaln (Adults and Children > 12 yr): *Metered-dose inhaler (nonacute)* — 2 inhalations 4 times daily (not to exceed 12 inhalations/24 hr or more frequently than q 4 hr). *Acute exacerbations* — 4–8 puffs using a spacer device as needed. *Via nebulization (nonacute)* — 500 mcg 3–4 times daily. *Via nebulization (acute exacerbations)* — 500 mcg q 30 min for 3 doses then q 2–4 hr as needed.
Inhaln (Children 5–12 yr): *Metered-dose inhaler (nonacute)* — 1–2 inhalations q 6 hr as needed (not to exceed 12 inhalations/24 hr). *Acute exacerbations* — 4–8 puffs as needed *Via nebulization (nonacute)* — 250–500 mcg 4 times daily given q 6 hr. *Acute exacerbations* — 250 mcg q 20 min for 3 doses then q 2–4 hr as needed.
Inhaln (Infants): *Nebulization* — 125–250 mcg 3 times a day.
Inhaln (Neonates): *Nebulization* — 25 mcg/kg/dose 3 times a day.
Intranasal (Adults and Children > 6 yr): *0.03% solution* — 2 sprays in each nostril 2–3 times daily (21 mcg/spray).
Inhaln (Adults and Children > 5 yr): *0.06% solution* — 2 sprays in each nostril 3–4 times daily (42 mcg/spray).

Availability (generic available)
Aerosol inhaler (HFA) (chlorofluorocarbon-free): 17 mcg/spray in 12.9-g canister (200 inhalations). **Inhalation solution:** ✱ 0.0125%, 0.02% in single-dose vials containing 500 mcg, ✱ 0.025%. **Nasal spray:** 0.03% solution — 21 mcg/spray in 30-mL bottle (345 sprays/bottle), 0.06% solution — 42 mcg/spray in 15-mL bottle (165 sprays). *In combination with:* albuterol (Combivent, Duoneb). See Appendix B.

NURSING IMPLICATIONS

Assessment
- Assess for allergy to atropine and belladonna alkaloids; patients with these allergies may also be sensitive to ipratropium. Atrovent HFA MDI does not contain CFC or soy and may be used safely in soy or CFC-allergic patients. However, Combivent MDI should be avoided in soy or peanut-allergic patients.
- **Inhaln:** Assess respiratory status (rate, breath sounds, degree of dyspnea, pulse) before administration and at peak of medication. Consult health care professional about alternative medication if severe bronchospasm is present; onset of action is too slow for patients in acute distress. If paradoxical bronchospasm (wheezing) occurs, withhold medication and notify health care professional immediately.
- **Nasal Spray:** Assess patient for rhinorrhea.

Potential Nursing Diagnoses
Ineffective airway clearance (Indications)
Activity intolerance (Indications)

Implementation
- Do not confuse Atrovent with Alupent (metaproterenol).
- **Inhaln:** See Appendix D for administration of inhalation medications.
- When ipratropium is administered concurrently with other inhalation medications, administer adrenergic bronchodilators first, followed by ipratropium, then corticosteroids. Wait 5 min between medications.
- Solution for *nebulization* can be diluted with preservative-free 0.9% NaCl. Diluted solution should be used within 24 hr at room temperature or 48 hr if refrigerated. Solution can be mixed with preservative-free albuterol, cromolyn, or metaproterenol if used within 1 hr of mixing.

Patient/Family Teaching
- Instruct patient in proper use of inhaler, nebulizer, or nasal spray and to take medication as directed. Take missed doses as soon as re-

membered unless almost time for the next dose; space remaining doses evenly during day. Do not double doses.
- Advise patient that rinsing mouth after using inhaler, good oral hygiene, and sugarless gum or candy may minimize dry mouth. Health care professional should be notified if stomatitis occurs or if dry mouth persists for more than 2 wk.
- **Inhalation:** Caution patient not to exceed 12 doses within 24 hr. Patient should notify health care professional if symptoms do not improve within 30 min after administration of medication or if condition worsens.
- Explain need for pulmonary function tests prior to and periodically during therapy to determine effectiveness of medication.
- Caution patient to avoid spraying medication in eyes; may cause blurring of vision or irritation.
- Advise patient to inform health care professional if cough, nervousness, headache, dizziness, nausea, or GI distress occurs.
- **Nasal Spray:** Instruct patient in proper use of nasal spray. Clear nasal passages gently before administration. Do not inhale during administration, so medication remains in nasal passages. Prime pump initially with 7 actuations. If used regularly, no further priming is needed. If not used in 24 hr, prime with 2 actuations. If not used for >7 days, prime with 7 actuations.
- Advise patient to contact health care professional if symptoms do not improve within 1–2 wk or if condition worsens.

Evaluation/Desired Outcomes
- Decreased dyspnea.
- Improved breath sounds.
- Decrease in rhinorrhea from perennial rhinitis or the common cold.

---

irbesartan, See ANGIOTENSIN II RECEPTOR ANTAGONISTS.

---

irinotecan
(eye-ri-noe-**tee**-kan)
Camptosar

Classification
Therapeutic: antineoplastics
Pharmacologic: enzyme inhibitors

Pregnancy Category D

Indications
Metastatic colorectal cancer (with 5-fluorouracil and leucovorin).

Action
Interferes with DNA synthesis by inhibiting the enzyme topoisomerase. **Therapeutic Effects:** Death of rapidly replicating cells, particularly malignant ones.

Pharmacokinetics
Absorption: IV administration results in complete bioavailability.
Distribution: Unknown.
Protein Binding: *Irinotecan*—30–68%; *SN-38 (active metabolite)*—95%.
Metabolism and Excretion: Converted by the liver to SN-38, its active metabolite, which is metabolized by the liver by UDP-glucuronosyl 111 transferase 1A1 (UGT1A1). Small amounts excreted by kidneys.
Half-life: 6 hr.

TIME/ACTION PROFILE (hematologic effects)

ROUTE	ONSET	PEAK	DURATION
IV	unknown	21–29 days	27–34 days

Contraindications/Precautions
Contraindicated in: Hypersensitivity; OB, Lactation: Pregnancy or lactation.
Use Cautiously in: Previous pelvic or abdominal irradiation or age ≥65 yr (↑ risk of myelosuppression); Presence of infection, underlying bone marrow depression, or concurrent chronic illness; History of prior pelvic/abdominal irradiation and serum bilirubin >1–2 mg/dL (initial dose reduction recommended); Geri: ↑ sensitivity to adverse effects (myelosuppression); initiate at lower dose; Previous severe myelosuppression or diarrhea (reinstitute at lower dose following resolution); Patients with genetically reduced UGT1A1 activity (↑ risk of neutropenia); OB: Patients with childbearing potential; Pedi: Safety not established.

Adverse Reactions/Side Effects
CNS: dizziness, headache, insomnia, weakness. **EENT:** rhinitis. **Resp:** coughing, dyspnea. **CV:** edema, vasodilation. **GI:** DIARRHEA, ↑ LIVER ENZYMES, abdominal pain/cramping, anorexia, constipation, dyspepsia, flatulence, nausea, stomatitis, vomiting, abdominal enlargement, colonic ulceration. **Derm:** alopecia, rash, sweating. **F and E:** dehydration. **Hemat:** anemia, leukopenia, neutropenia, thrombocytopenia. **Local:** injection site reactions. **Metab:** weight loss. **MS:** back pain. **Misc:** chills, fever.

Interactions
Drug-Drug: Combination with **fluorouracil** may result in serious toxicity (dehydration, neu-

tropenia, sepsis). ↑ bone marrow depression may occur with other **antineoplastics** or **radiation therapy**. **Laxatives** should be avoided (diarrhea may be ↑). **Diuretics** ↑ risk of dehydration (may discontinue during therapy). **Dexamethasone** used as an antiemetic ↑ risk of hyperglycemia and lymphocytopenia. **Prochlorperazine** given on the same day as irinotecan ↑ risk of akathisia.
Drug-Natural Products: St. John's wort ↑ increases levels and risk of toxicity.

Route/Dosage
Other regimens are used; careful modification required for all levels of toxicity/tolerance.

Single Agent
IV (Adults): *Weekly dosage schedule*—125 mg/m² once weekly for 4 wk, followed by a 2-wk rest period. Cycle may be repeated using doses which depend on patient tolerance and degree of toxicity encountered. *Once-every-3-wk schedule*—350 mg/m² once every 3 wk.
IV (Geriatric Patients >70 yr): Initiate at 300 mg/m² every 3 wk.

Hepatic Impairment
IV (Adults): *Bilirubin 1–2 mg/dL and history of prior pelvic/abdominal irradiation*— *Weekly dosage schedule*—Initiate therapy at lower dose (100 mg/m²); once weekly for 4 wk, followed by a 2-wk rest period. Cycle may be repeated with dose adjusted as tolerated. *Once-every-3-wk schedule*—300 mg/m² once every 3 wk, dose adjusted as tolerated as low as 200 mg/m² and further adjusted in 50-mg increments.

As Part of Combination Therapy with Leucovorin and 5-Fluorouracil
IV (Adults): *Regimen 1 (Bolus regimen)*— 125 mg/m² once weekly for 4 wk, followed by a 2-wk rest period. Cycle may be repeated using doses that depend on patient tolerance and degree of toxicity encountered; *Regimen 2 (Infusional regimen)*—180 mg/m² every 2 wk for 3 doses, followed by a 3-wk rest period. Cycle may be repeated using doses that depend on patient tolerance and degree of toxicity encountered.

Availability (generic available)
Solution for injection: 20 mg/mL.

NURSING IMPLICATIONS
Assessment
- Monitor vital signs frequently during administration.
- Monitor for bone marrow depression. Assess for bleeding (bleeding gums, bruising, petechiae, guaiac stools, urine, and emesis) and avoid IM injections and taking rectal temperatures if platelet count is low. Apply pressure to venipuncture sites for 10 min. Assess for signs of infection during neutropenia. Anemia may occur. Monitor for increased fatigue, dyspnea, and orthostatic hypotension.
- Monitor closely for the development of diarrhea. Two types may occur. The early type occurs within 24 hr of administration and may be preceded by cramps and sweating. Atropine 0.25–1 mg IV may be given to decrease symptoms. Potentially life-threatening diarrhea may occur more than 24 hr after a dose and may be accompanied by severe dehydration and electrolyte imbalance. Loperamide 4 mg initially, followed by 2 mg every 2 hr until diarrhea ceases for at least 12 hr (or 4 mg every 4 hr if given during sleeping hours) should be administered promptly to treat late-occurring diarrhea. Do not administer loperamide at these doses for >48 hr. Careful fluid and electrolyte replacement should be instituted to prevent complications. Subsequent doses should be delayed in patients with active diarrhea until diarrhea is resolved for 24 hr. If diarrhea is grade 2, 3, or 4, decrease subsequent doses of irinotecan.
- Nausea and vomiting are common. Pretreatment with dexamethasone 10 mg along with agents such as ondansetron or granisetron should be started on the same day as irinotecan at least 30 min before administration. Prochlorperazine may be used on subsequent days but may increase risk of akathisia if given on the same day as irinotecan.
- Assess IV site frequently for inflammation. Avoid extravasation. If extravasation occurs, infusion must be stopped and restarted in another vein to avoid damage to subcut tissue. Flushing site with sterile water and application of ice over the extravasated site are recommended.
- ***Lab Test Considerations:*** Monitor CBC with differential and platelet count prior to each dose. Temporarily discontinue irinotecan if ab-

solute neutrophil count is <500 cells/mm³ or if neutropenic fever occurs. Administration of a colony-stimulating factor may be considered if clinically significant decreases in WBC (<2000/mm³), neutrophil count (<1000/mm³), hemoglobin (<9 g/dL), or platelet count (<100,000 cells/mm³) occur.
- May cause ↑ serum alkaline phosphatase and AST concentrations.

Potential Nursing Diagnoses
Risk for infection (Adverse Reactions)

Implementation
- Prepare solution in a biologic cabinet. Wear gloves, gown, and mask while handling IV medication. Discard IV equipment in specially designated containers.

IV Administration
- **Intermittent Infusion:** *Diluent:* Dilute before infusion with D5W or 0.9% NaCl. Usual diluent is 500 mL of D5W. *Concentration:* 0.12–2.8 mg/mL. Solution is pale yellow. Do not administer solutions that are cloudy or contain particulate matter. Solution is stable for 24 hr at room temperature or 48 hr if refrigerated. To prevent microbial contamination, solutions should be used within 24 hr of dilution if refrigerated or 6 hr at room temperature. Do not refrigerate solutions diluted with 0.9% NaCl. *Rate:* Administer dose over 90 min.
- **Y-Site Compatibility:** anidulafungin, bivalirudin, caspofungin, daptomycin, docetaxel, ertapenem, fenoldopam, hetastarch, idarubicin, meperidine, nesiritide, octreotide, oxaliplatin, paclitaxel, palonosetron, pantoprazole, rituximab, teniposide, thiotepa, tigecycline, tirofiban, vinorelbine, voriconazole.
- **Y-Site Incompatibility:** gemcitabine, pemetrexed, trastuzumab.
- **Additive Incompatibility:** Information unavailable. Do not admix with other solutions or medications.

Patient/Family Teaching
- Instruct patient to report occurrence of diarrhea to health care professional immediately, especially if it occurs more than 24 hr after dose. Diarrhea may be accompanied by severe dehydration and electrolyte imbalance. It may be life-threatening and should be treated promptly.
- Instruct patient to notify health care professional promptly if fever; chills; sore throat; signs of infection; bleeding gums; bruising; petechiae; blood in urine, stool, or emesis occurs. Caution patient to avoid crowds and persons with known infections. Instruct patient to use soft toothbrush and electric razor. Caution patient not to drink alcoholic beverages or take products containing aspirin or other NSAIDs.
- Instruct patient to notify nurse of pain at injection site immediately.
- Instruct patient to notify health care professional if vomiting, fainting, or dizziness occurs.
- Discuss with patient possibility of hair loss. Explore methods of coping.
- Advise patient that this medication may have teratogenic effects. Contraception should be used during therapy.
- Instruct patient not to receive any vaccinations without consulting health care professional.
- Emphasize the need for periodic lab tests to monitor for side effects.

Evaluation/Desired Outcomes
- Decrease in size and spread of malignancy.

IRON SUPPLEMENTS

carbonyl iron (100%) (**kar**-bo-nil **eye**-ern)
Feosol, Icar

ferrous fumarate (33% elemental iron) (**fer**-us **fyoo**-ma-rate)
Femiron, Feostat, Fumasorb, Fumerin, Hemocyte, Neo-Fer, ✤ Nephro-Fer, ✤ Novofumar, ✤ Palafer, Span-FF

ferrous gluconate (12% elemental iron) (**fer**-us **gloo**-koe-nate)
✤ Apo-Ferrous Gluconate, Fergon, Ferralet, ✤ Fertinic, ✤ Novoferrogluc, Simron

ferrous sulfate (30% elemental iron) (**fer**-us **sul**-fate)
✤ Apo-Ferrous Sulfate, ED-IN-SOL, Fe50, Feosol, Feratab, Fer-gen-sol, Fer-In-Sol, Fer-Iron, ✤ Fero-Grad, ✤ Novoferrosulfa, ✤ PMS Ferrous Sulfate, Slow FE

iron dextran (eye-ern **dex**-tran)
DexFerrum, InFeD

iron polysaccharide (**eye**-ern poll-ee-**sak**-a-ride)
Hytinic, Niferex, Nu-Iron

iron sucrose (eye-ern su-krose)
Venofer

sodium ferric gluconate complex
(**so**-dee-yum **ferr**-ic **gloo**-ko-nate)
Ferrlecit

Classification
Therapeutic: antianemics
Pharmacologic: iron supplements

Pregnancy Category A (ferrous gluconate, ferrous sulfate, iron polysaccharide), B (sodium ferric gluconate, iron sucrose), C (iron dextran)

Indications
PO: Prevention/treatment of iron-deficiency anemia. **IM, IV:** *Iron dextran*—Treatment of iron-deficiency anemia in patients who cannot tolerate or receive oral iron. *Sodium ferric gluconate complex*—Treatment of iron deficiency in patients undergoing chronic hemodialysis or peritoneal dialysis who are concurrently receiving erythropoietin. Treatment of iron-deficiency anemia in patients with chronic kidney disease including patients who are not on dialysis (with or without erythropoietin) and patients dependent on dialysis (with erythropoietin).

Action
An essential mineral found in hemoglobin, myoglobin, and many enzymes. Enters the bloodstream and is transported to the organs of the reticuloendothelial system (liver, spleen, bone marrow), where it is separated out and becomes part of iron stores. **Therapeutic Effects:** Prevention/treatment of iron deficiency.

Pharmacokinetics
Absorption: 5–10% of dietary iron is absorbed (up to 30% in deficiency states). Therapeutically administered PO iron may be 60% absorbed via an active and passive transport process. Well absorbed following IM administration.
Distribution: Remains in the body for many months. Crosses the placenta; enters breast milk.
Protein Binding: ≥90%.
Metabolism and Excretion: Mostly recycled; small daily losses occurring via desquamation, sweat, urine, and bile.
Half-life: *Iron dextran, iron sucrose*—6 hr.

TIME/ACTION PROFILE (effects on erythropoiesis)

ROUTE	ONSET	PEAK	DURATION
PO	4 days	7–10 days	2–4 mo
IM, IV	4 days	1–2 wk	wk–mos

Contraindications/Precautions
Contraindicated in: Hemochromatosis, hemosiderosis, or other evidence of iron overload; Anemias not due to iron deficiency; Some products contain alcohol, tartrazine, or sulfites and should be avoided in patients with known intolerance or hypersensitivity.
Use Cautiously in: PO: Peptic ulcer; Ulcerative colitis or regional enteritis (condition may be aggravated); Alcoholism; Severe hepatic impairment; Severe renal impairment (oral products); Pre-existing cardiovascular disease (iron dextran) (may be exacerbated by adverse reactions to this drug); Significant allergies or asthma (iron dextran); Rheumatoid arthritis (iron dextran) (may have exacerbation of joint swelling); OB, Lactation: Pregnancy or lactation (safety of some parenteral products not established); Pedi: Safety not established for infants <4 mo (iron dextran) or children <6 yr (sodium ferric gluconate complex); safety may not be established for other products in the pediatric population.

Adverse Reactions/Side Effects
CNS: *IM, IV*— SEIZURES, dizziness, headache, syncope. **CV:** *IM, IV*—hypotension, hypertension, tachycardia. **GI:** nausea; *PO*, constipation, dark stools, diarrhea, epigastric pain, GI bleeding; *IM, IV*, taste disorder, vomiting. **Derm:** *IM, IV*—flushing, urticaria. **Resp:** *IV*—cough, dyspnea. **Local:** pain at IM site (iron dextran), phlebitis at IV site, skin staining at IM site (iron dextran). **MS:** *IM, IV*—arthralgia, myalgia. **Misc:** *PO*—staining of teeth (liquid preparations); *IM, IV*, allergic reactions including ANAPHYLAXIS, fever, lymphadenopathy, sweating.

Interactions
Drug-Drug: Oral iron supplements ↓ absorption of **tetracyclines**, **bisphosphonates**, **fluoroquinolones**, **levothyroxine**, **mycophenolate mofetil**, and **penicillamine** (simultaneous administration should be avoided). ↓ absorption of and may ↓ effects of **levodopa** and **methyldopa**. Concurrent administration of **H₂ antagonists**, **proton pump inhibitors**, and **cholestyramine** may ↓ absorption of iron. Doses of **ascorbic acid** ≥200 mg may ↑ absorption of iron up to ≥30%. **Chloramphenicol** and **vitamin E** may ↓ hematologic response to iron therapy.
Drug-Food: Iron absorption is ↓ 33–50% by concurrent administration of food.

Route/Dosage
Oral Iron Dosage for Iron Deficiency (expressed as mg elemental iron, note individual salt forms, multiple ones exist—see approximate equivalent doses below for dose conversions).

Approximate Equivalent Doses (mg of iron salt): *Ferrous fumarate*—197; *Ferrous gluconate*—560; *Ferrous sulfate*—324; *Ferrous sulfate, exsiccated*—217.

PO (Adults): *Deficiency*—120—240 mg/day (2–3 mg/kg/day) in 2–4 divided doses. *Prophylaxis*—60–100 mg/day.
PO (Infants and Children): *Severe deficiency*—4–6 mg/kg/day in 3 divided doses. *Mild to moderate deficiency*—3 mg/kg/day in 1–2 divided doses. *Prophylaxis*—1–2 mg/kg/day in 1–2 divided dose (maximum: 15 mg/day).
PO (Neonates, premature): 2–4 mg/kg/day in 1–2 divided doses, maximum: 15 mg/day.

Iron Dextran
IM, IV (Adults and Children): Test dose of 0.5 mL (25 mg) is given 1 hr prior to therapy.
IM, IV (Infants): Test dose of 0.25 mL (12.5 mg) is given 1 hr prior to therapy.
IM, IV (Adults and Children >15 kg): *Iron deficiency*—Total dose (mL) = 0.0442 × (desired Hgb– actual Hgb) × lean body weight (kg) + [0.26 × lean body weight (kg)]. Divided up and given in small daily doses until total is reached; not to exceed 100 mg/day. *Total dose IV infusion*—Total dose may be diluted and infused over 4–5 hr following a test dose of 10 drops (unlabeled).
IM, IV (Adults): *Blood loss*—Dose (mL) = (Blood loss [mL] × hematocrit) × 0.02.
IM, IV (Children 5–15 kg): *Iron deficiency*—Total dose (mL) = 0.042 (desried Hgb– actual Hgb) × weight (kg) + [0.26 × weight (kg)]. Divided up and given in small daily doses until total is reached; not to exceed 25 mg/day in children <5 kg; 50 mg/day in children 5–10 kg; or 100 mg/day in children > 10 kg.

Iron Polysaccharide Complex
PO (Adults): 50-100 mg twice daily of tablets/elixir or 150–300 mg/day of the capsules.
PO (Children >6yr): 50–100 mg/day (may be given in divided doses).
PO (Infants): 1–2 mg/kg/day.
PO (Adults —Pregnant Women): 30–60 mg/day.

Iron Sucrose
IV (Adults): *Hemodialysis dependent patients*—100 mg (5 mL) during each dialysis session for 10 doses (total of 1000 mg) additional smaller doses may be necessary; *Peritoneal dialysis dependent patients*—300 mg (15 mL) infusion, followed by another 300 mg (15 mL) infusion 14 days later, followed by 400 mg (20 mL) infusion 14 days later; *Non-dialysis dependent patients*—200 mg (10 mL) on 5 different days within a 14 day period to a total of 1000 mg, may also be given as infusion of 500 mg on day 1 and day 14.

Sodium Ferric Gluconate Complex
IV (Adults): 10 mL (125 mg elemental iron) repeated during 8 sequential dialysis treatments to a total cumulative dose of 1 g.
IV (Children >6 yr): 0.12 mL/kg (not to exceed 125 mg/dose) repeated during 8 sequential dialysis treatments.

Availability

Carbonyl Iron (100% Iron)
Tablets: 50 mg[OTC]. **Oral suspension:** 15 mg/1.25 mL[OTC].

Ferrous Fumarate (33% Elemental Iron) (generic available)
Tablets: 63 mg[OTC], 195 mg[OTC], 200 mg[OTC], 324 mg[OTC], 325 mg[OTC]. **Chewable tablets:** 100 mg[OTC]. **Controlled-release capsules:** 325 mg[OTC]. **Suspension (butterscotch flavor):** 100 mg/5 mL[OTC], ✱ 300 mg/5 mL[OTC]. **Drops:** 45 mg/0.6 mL[OTC], ✱ 60 mg/1 mL[OTC].

Ferrous Gluconate (11.6% Elemental Iron) (generic available)
Tablets: 300 mg[OTC], 320 mg[OTC], 325 mg[OTC]. **Sustained-release tablets:** 320 mg[OTC]. **Soft gelatin capsules:** 86 mg[OTC]. **Elixir:** 300 mg/5 mL[OTC]. **Syrup:** ✱ 300 mg/5 mL[OTC].

Ferrous Sulfate (20–30% Elemental Iron)
Tablets: 195 mg[OTC], 300 mg[OTC], 325 mg[OTC]. **Capsules:** 150 mg[OTC], 250 mg[OTC]. **Timed-release tablets:** 525 mg[OTC]. **Syrup:** 90 mg/5 mL[OTC]. **Elixir:** 220 mg/5 mL[OTC]. **Drops:** 75 mg/0.6 mL[OTC], 125 mg/1 mL[OTC].

Iron Dextran
Injection: 50 mg/mL.

Iron Polysaccharide (mg Iron)
Capsules: 150 mg[OTC]. **Elixir:** 100 mg/5 mL[OTC]. **Tablets:** 50 mg[OTC].

Iron Sucrose
Aqueous complex for injection: 20 mg/mL in 5 mL single-use vial (100 mg).

Sodium Ferric Gluconate Complex
Injection: 62.5 mg/5 mL.

NURSING IMPLICATIONS
Assessment
- Assess nutritional status and dietary history to determine possible cause of anemia and need for patient teaching.
- Assess bowel function for constipation or diarrhea. Notify health care professional and use appropriate nursing measures should these occur.
- **Iron Dextran, Iron Sucrose, and Sodium Ferric Gluconate Complex:** Monitor blood pressure and heart rate frequently following IV administration until stable. Rapid infusion rate may cause hypotension and flushing.
- Assess patient for signs and symptoms of anaphylaxis (rash, pruritus, laryngeal edema, wheezing). Notify physician immediately if these occur. Keep epinephrine and resuscitation equipment close by in the event of an anaphylactic reaction.
- *Lab Test Considerations:* Monitor hemoglobin, hematocrit, and reticulocyte values prior to and every 3 wk during the first 2 mo of therapy and periodically thereafter. Serum ferritin and iron levels may also be monitored to assess effectiveness of therapy.
- Occult blood in stools may be obscured by black coloration of iron in stool. Guaiac test results may occasionally be false-positive.
- **Iron Dextran:** Monitor hemoglobin, hematocrit, reticulocyte values, transferrin, ferritin, total iron-binding capacity, and plasma iron concentrations periodically during therapy. Serum ferritin levels peak in 7–9 days and return to normal in 3 wk. Serum iron determinations may be inaccurate for 1–2 wk after therapy with large doses; therefore, hemoglobin and hematocrit are used to gauge initial response.
- May impart a brownish hue to blood drawn within 4 hr of administration. May cause false ↑ in serum bilirubin and false decrease in serum calcium values.
- Prolonged PTT may be calculated when blood sample is anticoagulated with citrate dextrose solution; use sodium citrate instead.
- **Iron Sucrose:** Monitor hemoglobin, hematocrit, serum ferritin, and transferritin saturation prior to and periodically during therapy. Transferrin saturation values increase rapidly after IV administration; therefore, serum iron values may be reliably obtained 48 hr after IV administration. Withhold iron therapy if evidence of iron overload occurs.
- May cause ↑ liver enzymes.
- *Toxicity and Overdose:* Early symptoms of overdose include stomach pain, fever, nausea, vomiting (may contain blood), and diarrhea. Late symptoms include bluish lips, fingernails, and palms; drowsiness; weakness; tachycardia; seizures; metabolic acidosis; hepatic injury; and cardiovascular collapse. Patient may appear to recover prior to the onset of late symptoms. Therefore, hospitalization continues for 24 hr after patient becomes asymptomatic to monitor for delayed onset of shock or GI bleeding. Late complications of overdose include intestinal obstruction, pyloric stenosis, and gastric scarring.
- If patient is comatose or seizing, gastric lavage with sodium bicarbonate is performed. Deferoxamine is the antidote. Additional supportive treatments to maintain fluid and electrolyte balance and correction of metabolic acidosis are also indicated.
- If signs of overdose occur during IV administration of iron sucrose, treatment includes IV fluids, corticosteroids, and/or antihistamines. Administering at a slower rate usually relieves symptoms.

Potential Nursing Diagnoses
Activity intolerance (Indications)

Implementation
- Discontinue oral iron preparations prior to parenteral administration.
- Sodium ferric gluconate and iron sucrose are for IV use only.
- **PO:** Oral preparations are most effectively absorbed if administered 1 hr before or 2 hr after meals. If gastric irritation occurs, administer with meals. Take tablets and capsules with a full glass of water or juice. Do not crush or chew enteric-coated tablets and do not open capsules.
- Liquid preparations may stain teeth. Dilute in water or fruit juice, full glass (240 mL) for adults and ½ glass (120 mL) for children, and administer with a straw or place drops at back of throat.
- Avoid using antacids, coffee, tea, dairy products, eggs, or whole-grain breads with or within 1 hr after administration of ferrous salts. Iron absorption is decreased by 33% if iron and calcium are given with meals. If calcium supplementation is needed, calcium carbonate

does not decrease absorption of iron salts if supplements are administered between meals.
- **Iron Dextran:** The 2-mL ampule may be used for IM or IV administration.
- Prior to initial IM or IV dose, a test dose of 25 mg should be given by the same route as the dose will be given, to determine reaction. The IV test dose should be administered over 5 min. The IM dose should be administered in the same injection site and by same technique as the therapeutic dose. The remaining portion may be administered after 1 hr, if no adverse symptoms have occurred.
- **IM:** Inject deeply via Z-track technique into upper outer quadrant of buttock, never into arm or other exposed areas. Use a 2–3 in., 19- or 20-gauge needle. Change needles between withdrawal from container and injection to minimize staining of subcut tissues. Stains are usually permanent.

IV Administration

- **IV: Iron Dextran:** Following IV administration, patient should remain recumbent for at least 30 min to prevent orthostatic hypotension.
- **Direct IV:** *Diluent:* May administer undiluted or dilute in 0.9% NaCl or D5W. *Concentration:* 50 mg/mL. *Rate:* Administer slowly at a rate of 50 mg (1 mL) over at least 1 min.
- **Intermittent Infusion:** May be diluted in 200–1000 mL of 0.9% NaCl or D5W; 0.9% NaCl is the preferred diluent; dilution in D5W increases incidence of pain and phlebitis. *Rate:* Administer over 1–6 hr following a test dose of 10 drops/min for 10 min. Flush line with 10 mL of 0.9% NaCl at completion of infusion.
- **Y-Site Incompatibility:** Discontinue other IV solutions during infusion.
- **Additive Incompatibility:** Manufacturers recommend that iron dextran not be mixed with other solutions; however, iron dextran has been added to total parenteral nutrition solutions.
- **Sodium Ferric Gluconate Complex:** *Diluent:* Dilute test dose in 50 mL of 0.9% NaCl and administer IV over 60 min.
- To administer therapeutic dose of 10 mL (125 mg of elemental iron) dilute in 100 mL of 0.9% NaCl. Dialysis patients frequently require a cumulative dose of 1 g of elemental iron, administered over 8 sessions of sequential dialysis. *Concentration:* 12.5 mg/mL. *Rate:* Administer at a maximum rate of 12.5 mg/min.
- **Iron Sucrose:** Each 5-mL vial contains 100 mg of elemental iron.
- *Hemodialysis*—Most patients require a minimum cumulative dose of 1000 mg of elemental iron, administered over 10 sequential dialysis sessions, to achieve a favorable hemoglobin or hematocrit response.
- Solution is brown. Inspect for particulate matter or discoloration. Do not administer solutions that contain particulate matter or are discolored.
- **Direct IV:** May be administered undiluted by slow injection into dialysis line. *Rate:* Administer at a rate of 1 mL undiluted solution per minute, not to exceed one vial per injection. Discard any unused portion.
- **Intermittent Infusion:** May also be administered via infusion, into dialysis line for hemodialysis patients. May reduce risk of hypotensive episodes. *Diluent:* Each vial must be diluted in a maximum of 100 mL of 0.9% NaCl immediately prior to infusion. Unused diluted solution should be discarded. *Concentration:* 1–2 mg/mL. *Rate:* Infuse at a rate of 100 mg of iron over at least 15 min, large doses (500 mg) should be given over 3.5–4 hr.
- **Intermittent Infusion:** *For Peritoneal Dialysis Patients*—*Diluent:* Dilute each dose in a maximum of 250 mL of 0.9% NaCl. *Rate:* Administer doses of 300 mg over 1.5 hr and doses of 400 mg over 2.5 hr.
- **Direct IV:** *For Non-dialysis dependent patients*—May be administered as a slow injection of 200 mg undiluted. *Rate:* Administer over 2–5 min.
- **Intermittent Infusion:** Dilute 500 mg in 250 mL 0.9% NaCl. *Rate:* Infuse over 3.5–4 hr on days 1 and 14. May cause hypotension; monitor closely.
- **Additive Incompatibility:** Do not mix iron sucrose with other medications or add to parenteral nutrition solutions for IV infusion.

Patient/Family Teaching

- Explain purpose of iron therapy to patient.
- Encourage patient to comply with medication regimen. Take missed doses as soon as remembered within 12 hr; otherwise, return to regular dosing schedule. Do not double doses.
- Advise patient that stools may become dark green or black and that this change is harmless.
- Instruct patient to follow a diet high in iron (see Appendix M).
- Discuss with parents the risk of children's overdosing on iron. Medication should be stored in the original childproof container and kept out of reach of children. Do not refer to

vitamins as candy. In the event of a suspected overdose, parents or guardians should contact the poison control center (1-800-222-1222) or emergency medical services (911) immediately.
- **Iron Dextran:** Delayed reaction may occur 1–2 days after administration and last 3–4 days if IV route used, 3–7 days with IM route. Instruct patient to contact physician if fever, chills, malaise, muscle and joint aches, nausea, vomiting, dizziness, and backache occur.
- **Iron sucrose and sodium ferric gluconate complex:** Instruct patient to immediately report symptoms of hypersensitivity reaction to health care professional.

Evaluation/Desired Outcomes
- Increase in hemoglobin, which may reach normal parameters after 1–2 mo of therapy. May require 3–6 mo for normalization of body iron stores.
- Improvement in iron deficiency anemia or anemia of chronic renal failure.

isocarboxazid, See MONOAMINE OXIDASE (MAO) INHIBITORS.

isoniazid (eye-soe-nye-a-zid)
INH, ✤ Isotamine, ✤ PMS Isoniazid

Classification
Therapeutic: antituberculars

Pregnancy Category C

Indications
First-line therapy of active tuberculosis, in combination with other agents. Prevention of tuberculosis in patients exposed to active disease (alone).

Action
Inhibits mycobacterial cell wall synthesis and interferes with metabolism. **Therapeutic Effects:** Bacteriostatic or bactericidal action against susceptible mycobacteria.

Pharmacokinetics
Absorption: Well absorbed following PO/IM administration.
Distribution: Widely distributed; readily crosses the blood-brain barrier. Crosses the placenta; enters breast milk in concentrations equal to plasma.
Metabolism and Excretion: 50% metabolized by the liver by N-acetyltransferase ⚡ (rate of acetylation is genetically determined [slow acetylators have ↑ isoniazid levels and ↑ risk of toxicity; fast acetylators have ↓ isoniazid levels and ↑ risk for treatment failure]); 50% excreted unchanged by the kidneys.
Half-life: 1–4 hr in patients with normal renal and hepatic function; ⚡ 0.5–1.6 hr in fast acetylators; 2–5 hr in slow acetylators.

TIME/ACTION PROFILE (blood levels)

ROUTE	ONSET	PEAK	DURATION
PO	rapid	1–2 hr	up to 24 hr
IM	rapid	1–2 hr	up to 24 hr

Contraindications/Precautions
Contraindicated in: Hypersensitivity; Acute liver disease; Previous hepatitis from isoniazid.
Use Cautiously in: History of liver damage or chronic alcohol ingestion; Black and Hispanic women, women in the postpartum period, or patients >50 yr (↑ risk of drug-induced hepatitis); Severe renal impairment (dosage reduction may be necessary); Malnourished patients, patients with diabetes, or chronic alcoholics (↑ risk of neuropathy); OB, Lactation: Although safety is not established, isoniazid has been used with ethambutol to treat tuberculosis in pregnant women without harm to the fetus.

Adverse Reactions/Side Effects
CNS: psychosis, seizures. **EENT:** visual disturbances. **GI:** DRUG-INDUCED HEPATITIS, nausea, vomiting. **Derm:** rashes. **Endo:** gynecomastia. **Hemat:** blood dyscrasias. **Neuro:** <u>peripheral neuropathy</u>. **Misc:** fever.

Interactions
Drug-Drug: Additive CNS toxicity with other **antituberculars**. **BCG vaccine** may not be effective during isoniazid therapy. Isoniazid inhibits the metabolism of **phenytoin**. **Aluminum-containing antacids** may decrease absorption. Psychotic reactions and coordination difficulties may result with **disulfiram**. Concurrent administration of **pyridoxine** may prevent neuropathy. ↑ risk of hepatotoxicity with other **hepatotoxic agents** including **alcohol** and **rifampin**. Isoniazid may ↓ blood levels and effectiveness of **ketoconazole**. Concurrent use with **carbamazepine** ↑ carbamazepine blood levels and risk of hepatotoxicity.
Drug-Food: Severe reactions may occur with ingestion of foods containing high concentrations of **tyramine** (see Appendix M).

ISOSORBIDE

Route/Dosage
PO, IM (Adults): 300 mg/day (5 mg/kg) *or* 15 mg/kg (up to 900 mg) 2–3 times weekly.
PO, IM (Children): 10–20 mg/kg/day (up to 300 mg/day) *or* 20–40 mg/kg (up to 900 mg) 2–3 times weekly.

Availability (generic available)
Tablets: 100 mg, 300 mg. **Oral solution (orange, raspberry flavor):** 50 mg/5 mL. **Injection:** 100 mg/mL. *In combination with:* rifampin (Rifamate) or with rifampin and pyrazinamide (Rifater). See Appendix B.

NURSING IMPLICATIONS

Assessment
- Mycobacterial studies and susceptibility tests should be performed prior to and periodically throughout therapy to detect possible resistance. About 50% to 65% of Caucasians, Black, South Indians and Mexicans are slow acetylators at risk for toxicity, while 80 to 90% of Eskimos, Japanese, and Chinese are rapid acetylators at risk for decreased levels and treatment failure.
- *Lab Test Considerations:* Hepatic function should be evaluated prior to and monthly throughout therapy. Increased AST, ALT, and serum bilirubin may indicate drug-induced hepatitis. Black and Hispanic women, postpartal women, and patients >50 yr are at highest risk. The risk is lower in children; therefore, liver function tests are usually ordered less frequently for children.
- *Toxicity and Overdose:* If isoniazid overdosage occurs, treatment with pyridoxine (vitamin B) is instituted.

Potential Nursing Diagnoses
Risk for infection (Indications)
Noncompliance (Patient/Family Teaching)

Implementation
- **PO:** May be administered with food or antacids if GI irritation occurs, although antacids containing aluminum should not be taken within 1 hr of administration.
- **IM:** Medication may cause discomfort at injection site. Massage site after administration and rotate injection sites.
- Solution may form crystals at low temperatures; crystals will redissolve upon warming to room temperature.

Patient/Family Teaching
- Advise patient to take medication as directed. Take missed doses as soon as possible unless almost time for next dose; do not double up on missed doses. Emphasize the importance of continuing therapy even after symptoms have subsided. Therapy may be continued for 6 mo–2 yr.
- Advise patient to notify health care professional promptly if signs and symptoms of hepatitis (yellow eyes and skin, nausea, vomiting, anorexia, dark urine, unusual tiredness, or weakness) or peripheral neuritis (numbness, tingling, paresthesia) occur. Pyridoxine may be used concurrently to prevent neuropathy. Any changes in visual acuity, eye pain, or blurred vision should also be reported immediately.
- Caution patient to avoid the use of alcohol during this therapy, as this may increase the risk of hepatotoxicity. Ingestion of Swiss or Cheshire cheeses, fish (tuna, skipjack, and sardinella), and possibly tyramine-containing foods (see Appendix M) should also be avoided, as they may result in redness or itching of the skin; hot feeling; rapid or pounding heartbeat; sweating; chills; cold, clammy feeling; headache; or lightheadedness.
- Emphasize the importance of regular follow-up physical and ophthalmologic exams to monitor progress and to check for side effects.

Evaluation/Desired Outcomes
- Resolution of signs and symptoms of tuberculosis.
- Negative sputum cultures.
- Prevention of activation of tuberculosis in persons known to have been exposed.

ISOSORBIDE

isosorbide dinitrate
(eye-soe-**sor**-bide dye-**nye**-trate)
✽ Apo-ISDN, ✽ Cedocard-SR, ✽ Coronex, Dilatrate-SR, Isordil, ✽ Novosorbide, ✽ PMS-Isosorbide

isosorbide mononitrate
(eye-soe-**sor**-bide mo-noe-**nye**-trate)
✽ Apo-ISMN, IMDUR, ISMO, Monoket

Classification
Therapeutic: antianginals
Pharmacologic: nitrates

Pregnancy Category C

Indications
Acute treatment of anginal attacks (SL only). Prophylactic management of angina pectoris. Treatment of chronic CHF (unlabeled).

ISOSORBIDE

Action
Produce vasodilation (venous greater than arterial). Decrease left ventricular end-diastolic pressure and left ventricular end-diastolic volume (preload). Net effect is reduced myocardial oxygen consumption. Increase coronary blood flow by dilating coronary arteries and improving collateral flow to ischemic regions. **Therapeutic Effects:** Relief and prevention of anginal attacks.

Pharmacokinetics
Absorption: Isosorbide dinitrate undergoes extensive first-pass metabolism by the liver, resulting in 25% bioavailability; isosorbide mononitrate has 100% bioavailability (does not undergo first-pass metabolism).
Distribution: Unknown.
Metabolism and Excretion: Isosorbide dinitrate is metabolized by the liver to 2 active metabolites (5–mononitrate and 2–mononitrate). Isosorbide mononitrate is primarily meteabolized by the liver to inactive metabolites; primarily excreted in urine as metabolites.
Half-life: *Isosorbide dinitrate*—1 hr; *isosorbide mononitrate*—5 hr.

TIME/ACTION PROFILE (cardiovascular effects)

ROUTE	ONSET	PEAK	DURATION
ISDN-SL	2–10 min	unknown	1–2 hr
ISDN-PO	45–60 min	unknown	4 hr
ISDN-PO-ER	30 min	unknown	up to 12 hr
ISMN-PO	30–60 min	unknown	7 hr
ISMN-ER	unknown	unknown	12 hr

Contraindications/Precautions
Contraindicated in: Hypersensitivity; Concurrent use of sildenafil, vardenafil, or tadalafil.
Use Cautiously in: Volume depleted patients; Right ventricular infarction; Hypertrophic cardiomyopathy; OB: May compromise maternal/fetal circulation; Lactation: No data available; Pedi: Safety not established; Geri: Initial dose ↓ required due to ↑ potential for hypotension.

Adverse Reactions/Side Effects
CNS: dizziness, headache. **CV:** hypotension, tachycardia, paradoxic bradycardia, syncope. **GI:** nausea, vomiting. **Misc:** flushing, tolerance.

Interactions
Drug-Drug: Concurrent use of **sildenafil**, **tadalafil**, or **vardenafil** may result in significant and potentially fatal hypotension (do not use within 24 hr of isosorbide dinitrate or mononitrate). Additive hypotension with **antihypertensives**, acute ingestion of **alcohol**, **beta blockers**, **calcium channel blockers**, and **phenothiazines**.

Route/Dosage
Isosorbide Dinitrate
SL (Adults): *Acute attack of angina pectoris*—2.5–5 mg may be repeated q 5–10 min for 3 doses in 15–30 min. *Prophylaxis of angina pectoris*—2.5–5 mg given 15 min prior to activities known to provoke angina.
PO (Adults): *Prophylaxis of angina pectoris*—5–20 mg 2–3 times daily; usual maintenance dose is 10–40 mg q 6 hr (immediate-release) or 40–80 mg q 8–12 hr (sustained-release).

Isosorbide Mononitrate
PO (Adults): *ISMO, Monoket*—5–20 mg twice daily with the 2 doses given 7 hr apart. *Imdur*—30–60 mg once daily; may increase to 120 mg once daily (maximum dose = 240 mg/day).

Availability (generic available)
Isosorbide Dinitrate
Sublingual tablets: 2.5 mg, 5 mg. Cost: *Generic*—2.5 mg $39.16/100, 5 mg $18.59/100. **Tablets:** 5 mg, 10 mg, 20 mg, 30 mg, 40 mg. Cost: *Isordil*—40 mg $91.49/100; *Generic*—5 mg $31.23/100, 10 mg $35.45/100, 20 mg $18.85/100, 30 mg $23.32/100. **Extended-release tablets:** ✱ 20 mg, 40 mg. Cost: *Generic*—40 mg $71.29/100. **Sustained-release capsules:** 40 mg. *In combination with:* hydralazine (BiDil). See Appendix B.

Isosorbide Mononitrate (generic available)
Tablets (ISMO, Monoket): 10 mg, 20 mg. Cost: *Generic*—10 mg $45.99/180, 20 mg $48.98/180. **Extended-release tablets (Imdur):** 30 mg, 60 mg, 120 mg. Cost: *Generic*—30 mg $35.99/90, 60 mg $34.97/90, 120 mg $46.97/90.

NURSING IMPLICATIONS

Assessment
- Assess location, duration, intensity, and precipitating factors of anginal pain.
- Monitor blood pressure and pulse routinely during period of dosage adjustment.
- *Lab Test Considerations:* Excessive doses may ↑ methemoglobin concentrations.

♣ = Canadian drug name. ░ = Genetic implication.
*CAPITALS indicates life-threatening; underlines indicate most frequent.

Potential Nursing Diagnoses
Ineffective tissue perfusion (Indications)
Activity intolerance (Indications)

Implementation
Isosorbide Dinitrate
- **PO:** Extended-release capsules should be swallowed whole. Do not break, crush, or chew.
- **SL:** tablets should be held under tongue until dissolved.
- Avoid eating, drinking, or smoking until tablet is dissolved. Replace tablet if inadvertently swallowed.

Isosorbide Mononitrate
- Do not confuse Imdur with Imuran, Inderal, or K-Dur. Do not confuse Monoket with Monopril (fosinopril).
- **PO:** Extended-release tablets should be swallowed whole. Do not break, crush, or chew.

Patient/Family Teaching
- Instruct patient to take medication as directed, even if feeling better. Take missed doses as soon as remembered; doses of isosorbide dinitrate should be taken at least 2 hr apart (6 hr with extended-release preparations); daily doses of isosorbide mononitrate should be taken 7 hr apart. Do not double doses. Do not discontinue abruptly.
- Caution patient to make position changes slowly to minimize orthostatic hypotension.
- May cause dizziness. Caution patient to avoid driving or other activities requiring alertness until response to medication is known.
- Instruct patient to take last dose of day (when taking 2–4 doses/day) no later than 7 pm to prevent the development of tolerance.
- Advise patient to avoid concurrent use of alcohol with this medication. Patient should also consult health care professional before taking Rx, OTC, or herbal products while taking isosorbide.
- Inform patient that headache is a common side effect that should decrease with continuing therapy. Aspirin or acetaminophen may be ordered to treat headache. Notify health care professional if headache is persistent or severe. Do not alter dose to avoid headache.
- Advise patient to notify health care professional if dry mouth or blurred vision occurs.

Evaluation/Desired Outcomes
- Decrease in frequency and severity of anginal attacks.
- Increase in activity tolerance.

isotretinoin
(eye-soe-**tret**-i-noyn)
Amnesteem, Claravis, Sotret

Classification
Therapeutic: antiacne agents
Pharmacologic: retinoids

Pregnancy Category X

Indications
Management of severe nodular acne resistant to more conventional therapy, including topical therapy and systemic antibiotics. Not to be used under any circumstances in pregnant patients.

Action
A metabolite of vitamin A (retinol); reduces sebaceous gland size and differentiation. **Therapeutic Effects:** Diminution and resolution of severe acne. May also prevent abnormal keratinization.

Pharmacokinetics
Absorption: Rapidly absorbed following (23–25%) oral administration; absorption ↑ when taken with a high-fat meal.
Distribution: Appears to be widely distributed; crosses the placenta.
Protein Binding: 99.9%.
Metabolism and Excretion: Metabolized by the liver and excreted in the urine and feces.
Half-life: 10–20 hr.

TIME/ACTION PROFILE (diminution of acne)

ROUTE	ONSET	PEAK	DURATION
PO	unknown	up to 8 wk	unknown

Contraindications/Precautions
Contraindicated in: Hypersensitivity to retinoids, glycerin, soybean oil, or parabens; OB, Lactation: Pregnancy and lactation; Women of childbearing age who may become or who intend to become pregnant; Patients planning to donate blood.
Use Cautiously in: Pre-existing hypertriglyceridemia; Diabetes mellitus; History of alcohol abuse, psychosis, depression, or suicide attempt; Obese patients; Inflammatory bowel disease.

Adverse Reactions/Side Effects
CNS: SUICIDE ATTEMPT, behavior changes, depression, PSEUDOTUMOR CEREBRI, psychosis, suicidal ideation. **EENT:** conjunctivitis, epistaxis, blurred vision, contact lens intolerance, corneal opacities, decreased night vision, dry eyes. **CV:** edema. **GI:** cheilitis, dry mouth, nausea, vomiting, abdominal pain, anorexia, hepatitis, pancreatitis, ↑ appetite. **Derm:** pruritus, palmar desquamation, pho-

isotretinoin **745**

tosensitivity, skin infections, thinning of hair. **Hemat:** anemia. **Metab:** ↓ high-density lipoprotein cholesterol, hypercholesterolemia, hypertriglyceridemia, hyperglycemia, hyperuricemia. **MS:** arthralgia, back pain, muscle/bone pain (↑ in adolescents), hyperostosis. **Misc:** SEVERE BIRTH DEFECTS, ↑ thirst.

Interactions
Drug-Drug: Additive toxicity with **vitamin A** and **drugs having anticholinergic properties**. ↑ risk of pseudotumor cerebri with **tetracycline** or **minocycline**. Concurrent use with **alcohol** ↑ risk of hypertriglyceridemia. Drying effects ↑ by concurrent use of **benzoyl peroxide**, **sulfur**, **tretinoin**, and **other topical agents**.
Drug-Food: Excessive ingestion of **foods high in vitamin A** may result in additive toxicity.

Route/Dosage
PO (Adults): 0.5–1 mg/kg/day (up to 2 mg/kg/day) in 2 divided doses for 15–20 wk. Once discontinued, if relapse occurs, therapy may be reinstituted after an 8-wk rest period.

Availability (generic available)
Capsules: 10 mg, 20 mg, 30 mg, 40 mg.

NURSING IMPLICATIONS
Assessment
- Verify that patient receiving isotretinoin is registered with the iPLEDGE program and is completing all required interactions with their health care provider.
- Assess skin prior to and periodically during therapy. Transient worsening of acne may occur at initiation of therapy. Note number and severity of cysts, degree of skin dryness, erythema, and itching.
- Assess for allergy to parabens; capsules contain parabens as a preservative.
- Monitor patient for behavioral changes throughout therapy. May cause depression, psychosis, and suicide ideation. If behavioral changes occur, they usually resolve with discontinuation of therapy.
- *Lab Test Considerations:* Monitor liver function (AST, ALT, and LDH) prior to therapy, after 1 mo of therapy, and periodically thereafter. Inform health care professional if these values become ↑; therapy may need to be discontinued.
- Monitor blood lipids (cholesterol, HDL, triglycerides) under fasting conditions prior to beginning therapy, at 1–2 wk intervals until lipid response to isotretinoin is established (usually within 1 mo), and periodically thereafter. Report ↑ cholesterol and triglyceride levels or ↓ HDL.
- Obtain baseline and periodic CBC, urinalysis, and SMA-12. May cause ↑ blood glucose, CPK, platelet counts, and sedimentation rate. May ↓ RBC and WBC parameters. May cause proteinuria, red and white blood cells in urine, and ↑ uric acid.

Potential Nursing Diagnoses
Risk for impaired skin integrity (Indications, Side Effects)
Disturbed body image (Indications)

Implementation
- Isotretinoin is approved for marketing only under the iPLEDGE program, a special restricted distribution program approved by the FDA.
- Only patients who meet all requirements of the iPLEDGE program may receive isotretinoin.
- Isotretinoin may only be prescribed by health care providers registered and activated with the iPLEDGE program.
- Isotretinoin may only be dispensed by pharmacies registered with the iPLEDGE program.
- **PO:** Administer with meals. Do not crush or open capsules.

Patient/Family Teaching
- Explain the iPLEDGE program and its requirements to patient and parent.
- Instruct patient to take isotretinoin as directed. Do not take more than the amount prescribed. Take missed doses as soon as remembered if not almost time for next dose. Do not double doses. Patients must read *Medication Guide* and sign consent form prior to initiation of therapy.
- Explain to patient that a temporary worsening of acne may occur at beginning of therapy.
- Instruct female patients to use 2 forms of contraception 1 mo before therapy, throughout therapy, and for at least 1 mo after discontinuation of drug. This drug is contraindicated during pregnancy and may cause birth defects. Patient must have 2 negative serum or urine pregnancy tests with a sensitivity ≥25 mIU/mL before receiving initial prescription. First test is obtained by prescriber when decision is made to prescribe isotretinoin. Second pregnancy test should be done during first 5 days of menstrual period immediately preceding beginning

✽ = Canadian drug name. ▮ = Genetic implication.
*CAPITALS indicates life-threatening; underlines indicate most frequent.

of therapy. For patients with amenorrhea, second test should be done 11 days after last act of unprotected sexual intercourse. Each month of therapy patient must have a negative result from a urine or serum pregnancy test. Pregnancy test must be repeated every month prior to female patient receiving prescription. Manufacturer will make available pregnancy test kits to female patients. Patient should discontinue medication and inform health care professional immediately if pregnancy is suspected. Recommended consent form prepared by manufacturer stresses fetal risk. Parents of minors should also read and sign form. Yellow self-adhesive qualification stickers completed by prescriber must accompany prescription.
- May cause sudden decrease in night vision. Caution patient to avoid driving at night until response to the medication is known.
- Advise patient to consult with health care professional before using other acne preparations while taking isotretinoin. Soaps, cosmetics, and shaving lotion may also worsen dry skin.
- Inform patient that dry skin and chapped lips will occur. Lubricant to lips may help cheilitis.
- Instruct patient that oral rinses, good oral hygiene, and sugarless gum or candy may help minimize dry mouth. Notify health care professional if dry mouth persists for more than 2 wk.
- Discuss possibility of excessively dry eyes with patients who wear contact lenses. Patient should contact health care professional about eye lubricant. Patient may need to switch to glasses during course of therapy and for up to 2 wk following discontinuation.
- Advise patient to avoid alcoholic beverages while taking isotretinoin, as this may further increase triglyceride levels.
- Caution patient to use sunscreen and protective clothing to prevent photosensitivity reactions. Health care professional should be consulted about sunscreen, as some sunscreens may worsen acne.
- Instruct patient not to take vitamin A supplements and to avoid excessive ingestion of foods high in vitamin A (liver; fish liver oils; egg yolks; yellow-orange fruits and vegetables; dark green, leafy vegetables; whole milk; vitamin A–fortified skim milk; butter; margarine) while taking isotretinoin; this may result in hypervitaminosis.
- Advise patient not to donate blood while receiving this medication. After discontinuing isotretinoin, wait at least 1 mo before donating blood to prevent the possibility of a pregnant patient receiving the blood.
- Inform diabetic patients that difficulty controlling blood glucose may occur.
- Instruct patient to report burning of eyes, visual changes, rash, abdominal pain, diarrhea, headache, nausea, and vomiting to health care professional.
- Inform patient of need for medical follow-up. Periodic lab tests may be required.

Evaluation/Desired Outcomes
- Decrease in the number and severity of cysts in severe acne. Therapy may take 4–5 mo before full effects are seen. Therapy is discontinued when the number of cysts is reduced by 70% or after 5 mo. Improvement may occur after discontinuation of therapy; therefore, a delay of at least 8 wk is recommended before a second course of therapy is considered.

---

isradipine (is-ra-di-peen)
DynaCirc, DynaCirc CR

Classification
Therapeutic: antianginals, antihypertensives
Pharmacologic: calcium channel blockers

Pregnancy Category C

Indications
Management of hypertension, angina pectoris, and vasospastic (Prinzmetal's) angina.

Action
Inhibits the transport of calcium into myocardial and vascular smooth muscle cells, resulting in inhibition of excitation-contraction coupling and subsequent contraction. **Therapeutic Effects:** Systemic vasodilation resulting in decreased blood pressure. Coronary vasodilation resulting in decreased frequency and severity of attacks of angina.

Pharmacokinetics
Absorption: Well absorbed following oral administration but extensively metabolized, resulting in ↓ bioavailability.
Distribution: Unknown.
Protein Binding: 95%.
Metabolism and Excretion: Completely metabolized by the liver.
Half-life: 8 hr.

TIME/ACTION PROFILE (antihypertensive effects†)

ROUTE	ONSET	PEAK	DURATION
PO	<2 hr	2–3 hr	12 hr
PO-CR	2 hr	8–10 hr	24 hr

†For single doses, maximal antihypertensive effect during chronic dosing may take 2–4 wk

Contraindications/Precautions
Contraindicated in: Hypersensitivity; Sick sinus syndrome; 2nd- or 3rd-degree AV block (unless an artificial pacemaker is in place); Systolic blood pressure <90 mm Hg.
Use Cautiously in: Severe hepatic impairment (dose ↓ recommended); Geri: Dose ↓ recommended for most agents; ↑ risk of hypotension; Severe renal impairment; History of serious ventricular arrhythmias or CHF; OB, Lactation, Pedi: Safety not established.

Adverse Reactions/Side Effects
CNS: abnormal dreams, anxiety, confusion, dizziness, drowsiness, headache, nervousness, psychiatric disturbances, weakness. **EENT:** blurred vision, disturbed equilibrium, epistaxis, tinnitus. **Resp:** cough, dyspnea. **CV:** ARRHYTHMIAS, CHF, peripheral edema, bradycardia, chest pain, hypotension, palpitations, syncope, tachycardia. **GI:** ↑ liver enzymes, anorexia, constipation, diarrhea, dry mouth, dysgeusia, dyspepsia, nausea, vomiting. **GU:** dysuria, nocturia, polyuria, sexual dysfunction, urinary frequency. **Derm:** dermatitis, erythema multiforme, flushing, sweating, photosensitivity, pruritus/urticaria, rash. **Endo:** gynecomastia, hyperglycemia. **Hemat:** anemia, leukopenia, thrombocytopenia. **Metab:** weight gain. **MS:** joint stiffness, muscle cramps. **Neuro:** paresthesia, tremor. **Misc:** STEVENS-JOHNSON SYNDROME, gingival hyperplasia.

Interactions
Drug-Drug: Additive hypotension may occur when used concurrently with **fentanyl**, other **antihypertensives**, **nitrates**, acute ingestion of **alcohol**, or **quinidine**. Antihypertensive effects may be ↓ by concurrent use of **NSAIDs**. Concurrent use with **beta blockers**, **digoxin**, **disopyramide**, or **phenytoin** may result in bradycardia, conduction defects, or CHF.
Drug-Food: **Grapefruit juice** ↑ serum levels and effect.

Route/Dosage
PO (Adults): 2.5 mg twice daily; may be ↑ q 2–4 wk by 5 mg/day (not to exceed 20 mg/day) *or* 5 mg once daily as CR tablets; may be ↑ q 2–4 wk by 5 mg/day (not to exceed 20 mg/day).

Availability (generic available)
Capsules: 2.5 mg, 5 mg. **Controlled-release tablets:** 5 mg, 10 mg.

NURSING IMPLICATIONS
Assessment
- Monitor blood pressure and pulse prior to and periodically throughout therapy. Monitor ECG periodically in patients receiving prolonged therapy.
- Monitor intake and output ratios and daily weight. Assess patient for signs of CHF (peripheral edema, rales/crackles, dyspnea, weight gain, jugular venous distention).
- **Angina:** Assess location, duration, intensity, and precipitating factors of patient's anginal pain.
- *Lab Test Considerations:* Total serum calcium concentrations are not affected by calcium channel blockers.
- Monitor serum potassium periodically. Hypokalemia increases risk of arrhythmias; should be corrected.
- Monitor renal and hepatic functions periodically during long-term therapy. Several days of therapy may cause increase in hepatic enzymes, which return to normal upon discontinuation of therapy.

Potential Nursing Diagnoses
Decreased cardiac output (Side Effects)

Implementation
- **PO:** May be administered without regard to meals. May be administered with meals if GI irritation becomes a problem.
- Swallow controlled-release tablets whole; do not break, crush, or chew.

Patient/Family Teaching
- Advise patient to take medication as directed, even if feeling well. Take missed doses as soon as possible unless almost time for next dose; do not double doses. May need to be discontinued gradually.
- Advise patient to avoid drinking grapefruit juice during therapy.
- Caution patient to change positions slowly to minimize orthostatic hypotension.
- May cause dizziness. Advise patient to avoid driving or other activities requiring alertness until response to the medication is known.
- Instruct patient to avoid concurrent use of alcohol or other Rx, OTC, or herbal products without consulting health care professional.
- Caution patient to wear protective clothing and use sunscreen to prevent photosensitivity reactions.

- Advise patient to notify health care professional if irregular heartbeats, dyspnea, swelling of hands and feet, rash, pronounced dizziness, nausea, constipation, or hypotension occurs.
- **Angina:** Instruct patient on concurrent nitrate or beta-blocker therapy to continue taking both medications as directed and to use SL nitroglycerin as needed for anginal attacks.
- Inform patient that anginal attacks may occur 30 min after administration because of reflex tachycardia. This is usually temporary and is not an indication for discontinuation.
- Advise patient to contact health care professional if chest pain does not improve, worsens after therapy, or occurs with diaphoresis or if shortness of breath or persistent headache occurs.
- Caution patient to discuss exercise restrictions with health care professional prior to exertion.
- **Hypertension:** Encourage patient to comply with other interventions for hypertension (weight reduction, low-sodium diet, smoking cessation, moderation of alcohol consumption, regular exercise, and stress management). Medication controls but does not cure hypertension.
- Instruct patient and family in proper technique for monitoring BP. Advise patient to take BP weekly and to report significant changes to health care professional.

Evaluation/Desired Outcomes
- Decrease in blood pressure.
- Decrease in frequency and severity of anginal attacks.
- Decrease in need for nitrate therapy.
- Increase in activity tolerance and sense of well-being.

itraconazole (it-tra-kon-a-zole)
Sporanox

Classification
Therapeutic: antifungals (systemic)

Pregnancy Category C

Indications
Histoplasmosis. Blastomycosis. Aspergillosis. Dermatophyte infection of fingernails or toenails in nonimmunocompromised patients (oral capsules only). Oropharyngeal esophageal candidiasis.

Action
Inhibits enzymes necessary for integrity of the fungal cell membrane. **Therapeutic Effects:** Fungistatic effects against susceptible organisms.
Spectrum: Active against *Histoplasma capsulatum*, *Blastomyces dermatitidis*, *Cryptococcus neoformans*, *Aspergillus fumigatus*, *Trichophyton* spp., *Candida*, and *Tinea unguium*.

Pharmacokinetics
Absorption: Absorption is enhanced by food.
Distribution: Tissue concentrations are higher than plasma concentrations. Does not enter CSF; enters breast milk.
Protein Binding: *Itraconazole*—99.8%; *hydroxyitraconazole*—99.5%.
Metabolism and Excretion: Mostly metabolized by the liver and excreted in feces. Hydroxyitraconazole, the major metabolite, has antifungal activity.
Half-life: 21 hr.

TIME/ACTION PROFILE (blood levels)

ROUTE	ONSET	PEAK	DURATION
PO	rapid	4 hr	12–24 hr

Contraindications/Precautions
Contraindicated in: Hypersensitivity. Cross-sensitivity with other azole antifungals (**miconazole**, **ketoconazole**) may occur; Concurrent **quinidine**, **dofetilide**, **pimozide**, oral **midazolam**, **triazolam**, **nisoldipine**, **ergot alkaloids** (**dihydroergotamine**, **ergonovine**, **ergotamine**, **methylergonovine**), **simvastatin**, or **lovastatin**; Severe renal impairment (CCr <30 mL/min); CHF or other evidence of left ventricular dysfunction; Lactation: Lactation.
Use Cautiously in: Hepatic impairment (dose reduction may be required); Renal impairment; Achlorhydria or hypochlorhydria (absorption will be ↓); OB, Pedi: Safety not established; Geri: ↑ risk of hearing loss.

Adverse Reactions/Side Effects
CNS: dizziness, drowsiness, fatigue, headache, malaise. **EENT:** hearing loss, tinnitus. **CV:** CHF, edema, hypertension. **GI:** HEPATOTOXICITY, nausea, abdominal pain, anorexia, diarrhea, flatulence, vomiting. **GU:** albuminuria, ↓ libido, erectile dysfunction. **Derm:** TOXIC EPIDERMAL NECROLYSIS, photosensitivity, pruritus, rash. **Endo:** adrenal insufficiency. **F and E:** hypokalemia. **MS:** rhabdomyolysis. **Neuro:** neuropathy. **Misc:** allergic reactions including ANAPHYLAXIS, fever.

Interactions
Drug-Drug: Itraconazole is a potent inhibitor of the P450 3A hepatic enzyme, which can ↑ blood levels and effects of other drugs which are metabolized by this system. ↑ risk of potentially fatal

arrhythmias with **quinidine**, **dofetilide**, or **pimozide** (concurrent use is contraindicated and may result in QTc prolongation, torsades de pointes, ventricular arrhythmias, and sudden death).
↑ risk of excessive sedation with **midazolam** or **triazolam**, ↑ risk of adverse CNS reactions with **pimozide**, and ↑ risk of myopathy with **simvastatin** or **lovastatin** (concurrent use contraindicated). Concurrent use with **ergot alkaloids**, **(dihydroergotamine, ergonovine, ergotamine, methylergonovine)** ↑ risk of vasoconstriction and is contraindicated. Significantly ↑ **nisoldipine** levels (concurrent use contraindicated). May also ↑ blood levels and the risk of toxicity from **alprazolam, diazepam, atorvastatin, warfarin, ritonavir, indinavir, saquinavir, vinca alkaloids, busulfan, carbamazepine, cilostazol, diazepam, docetaxel, eletriptan, fentanyl, buspirone, cyclosporine, rifabutin, tacrolimus, sirolimus, clarithromycin, erythromycin, oral hypoglycemic agents, methylprednisolone, budesonide, dexamethasone, fluticasone, trimetrexate**, and **digoxin**. May ↑ levels and the negative inotropic effects of **calcium channel blockers**. Absorption ↓ by **antacids, histamine H₂ blockers, sucralfate, proton pump inhibitors**, or other **agents that increase gastric pH**, including the buffer in **didanosine** (take 2 hr after itraconazole). **Phenytoin, phenobarbital, nevirapine, isoniazid, rifampin, rifabutin**, and **carbamazepine** ↑ metabolism and ↓ blood levels of itraconazole (↑ dosage may be necessary). If hypokalemia occurs, the risk of **digoxin** toxicity is ↑.
Drug-Food: Food ↑ absorption.

Route/Dosage

Aspergillosis
PO (Adults): 200 mg once or twice daily for ≥3 mo.

Blastomycosis, Histoplasmosis
PO (Adults): 200 mg once daily; may be ↑ by 100 mg/day up to 200 mg twice daily.

Onychomycosis
PO (Adults): *Toenail fungus with or without fingernail fungus*—200 mg/day for 12 consecutive wk. *Fingernail fungus*—200 mg twice daily for 1 wk, then 3 wk without therapy, then 200 mg twice daily an additional wk—6 mo.

Candidiasis
PO (Adults): *Oropharyngeal candidiasis*—200 mg (20 mL) daily for 1–2 wk. *Oropharyngeal candidiasis unresponsive to fluconazole*—100 mg (10 mL) twice daily for at least 2–4 wk. *Esophageal candidiasis*—100 mg (10 mL) once daily for at least 3 wk.

Availability (generic available)
Capsules: 100 mg. **Oral solution (cherry caramel):** 10 mg/mL.

NURSING IMPLICATIONS

Assessment
- Assess for signs and symptoms of infection (vital signs, lung sounds, sputum, WBC, oral and pharyngeal mucosa, nail beds) before and periodically during therapy.
- Obtain specimens for culture before instituting therapy. Therapy may be started before results are obtained.
- *Lab Test Considerations:* Monitor hepatic function tests before and periodically during therapy, especially in patients with pre-existing hepatic function abnormalities. Discontinue itraconazole if abnormal values persist or worsen.
- Monitor serum potassium. May cause hypokalemia.

Potential Nursing Diagnoses
Risk for infection (Indications)
Noncompliance (Patient/Family Teaching)

Implementation
- Do not interchange capsules and oral solution. Only oral solution is effective for oropharyngeal candidiasis. Oral solution is not recommended for initial treatment of patients at risk for systemic candidiasis.
- **Capsules:** Administer with a full meal to minimize nausea and vomiting and to increase absorption.
- Do not administer with antacids or other medications that may increase gastric pH; may decrease absorption of itraconazole.
- **Oral Solution:** Administer without food if possible. Swish solution in mouth vigorously, 10 mL at a time, for several seconds, then swallow.

Patient/Family Teaching
- Instruct patient to take medication as directed, even if feeling better. Doses should be taken at the same time each day.

- May occasionally cause drowsiness. Caution patient to avoid driving or other activities requiring alertness until response to medication is known.
- Instruct patient to notify health care professional if signs and symptoms of liver dysfunction (unusual fatigue, anorexia, nausea, vomiting, jaundice, dark urine, or pale stools) or CHF (dyspnea, peripheral edema, weight gain) occur. If rash or signs of CHF occur, discontinue itraconazole and notify health care professional immediately.
- Advise patient to consult health care professional before taking any Rx, OTC, or herbal medications concurrently with itraconazole.
- Advise patient to use sunscreen and wear protective clothing to prevent photosensitivity reactions.

Evaluation/Desired Outcomes
- Resolution of clinical and laboratory indications of fungal infections. Minimal treatment for systemic fungal infections is 3 mo. Inadequate period of treatment may lead to recurrence of active infection.

ixabepilone (icks-a-bep-i-lone)
Ixempra

Classification
Therapeutic: antineoplastics
Pharmacologic: epothilone B analog

Pregnancy Category D

Indications
Combination use with capecitabine for the treatment of metastatic or locally advanced breast cancer currently resistant to a taxane and anthracycline or resistant to a taxane and cannot tolerate further anthracycline. May also be used as monotherapy for breast cancers that are not responding to anthracyclines, taxane, or capecitabine.

Action
Binds to β-tubulin subunits on microtubules; this action blocks cells in mitosis, leading to cell death. Also has antiangiogenic activity. **Therapeutic Effects:** Decreased spread of breast cancer.

Pharmacokinetics
Absorption: IV administration results in complete bioavailablity.
Distribution: Unknown.
Metabolism and Excretion: Extensively metabolized by the liver, primarily by the CYP3A4 enzyme system. Metabolites are not active and are excreted mainly by the kidneys.
Half-life: 52 hr.

TIME/ACTION PROFILE (blood levels)

ROUTE	ONSET	PEAK	DURATION
IV	unknown	end of infusion	unknown

Contraindications/Precautions
Contraindicated in: Previous hypersensitivity to any medications containing Cremophor EL or similar derivatives (polyoxyethylated castor oil); Neutrophils <1500 cells/m³ or platelets <100,000 cells/m³; Severe hepatic impairment; Use with capecitabine is contraindicated for hepatic impairment (AST or ALT >2.5 × upper limits of normal or bilirubin >1 × upper limit of normal) due to ↑ risk of toxicity and death associated with neutropenia; OB, Lactation: Pregnancy or lactation.

Use Cautiously in: Toxicity; dose adjustments may be required for neuropathy/arthralgia/myalgia/fatigue, neutropenia, thrombocytopenia, moderate hepatic impairment or palmar-plantar erythrodysesthesia; Diluent contains dehydrated alcohol; consider possible CNS effects; Diabetes or history of neuropathy (↑ risk of severe neuropathy); History of cardiac disease (may ↑ risk of myocardial ischemia or ventricular dysfunction; OB: Patients with childbearing potential.

Adverse Reactions/Side Effects
CNS: fatigue, weakness, dizziness, headache, insomnia. **EENT:** ↑ lacrimation. **CV:** chest pain, edema, myocardial ischemia, ventricular dysfunction. **Resp:** dyspnea. **GI:** abdominal pain, anorexia*, constipation, diarrhea, mucositis, nausea, stomatitis, vomiting, altered taste. **Derm:** alopecia, hyperpigmentation, nail disorder, palmar-plantar erythrodysesthesia (combination therapy with capecitabine), exfoliation, pruritus, rash, hot flushes. **Hemat:** MYELOSUPPRESSION. **MS:** arthralgia, musculoskeletal pain, myalgia. **Neuro:** peripheral neuropathy. **Misc:** hypersensitivity reactions.

Interactions
Drug-Drug: Strong CYP3A4 inhibitors including **ketoconazole**, **itraconazole**, **voriconazole**, **clarithromycin**, **telithromycin**, **atazanavir**, **delavirdine**, **ritonavir**, **saquinavir**, **nefazodone** ↑ blood levels and the risk of serious toxicities, concurrent use should be avoided if possible. If concurrent use is required, dose reduction of ixabepilone is recommended. Inducers of the **CYP3A4 enzyme system** including **dexa-**

mathasone, phenytoin, carbamazepine, phenobarbital, **rifampin**, **rifampicin**, or **rifabutin** may ↓ levels and effectiveness, avoid if possible.

Drug-Natural Products: St. John's wort may ↓ blood levels and should be avoided.

Drug-Food: Grapefruit juice may ↑ blood levels and toxicity; avoid concurrent use.

Route/Dosage
IV (Adults): 40 mg/m² every 3 wk; not to exceed dose greater than that calculated for 2.2 m² (88 mg/dose).

Hepatic Impairment
IV (Adults): *Moderate Impairment* — 20 mg/m² every 3 wk; not to exceed 30 mg/m².

Availability
Powder for injection (requires specific diluent for initial reconstitution): 15-mg vial (contains 16 mg ixabepilone to allow for withdrawal losses) with 8 mL of diluent in a separate vial as a kit, 45-mg vial (contains 47 mg ixabepilone to allow for withdrawal losses) with 23.5 mL of diluent in a separate vial.

NURSING IMPLICATIONS

Assessment
- Monitor for hypersensitivity reaction (flushing, rash, dyspnea, bronchospasm). If severe reactions occur stop infusion and provide aggressive supportive treatment with epinephrine and corticosteroids. In subsequent cycles, add corticosteroids to the premedication regimen.
- Monitor for myelosuppression frequently during therapy. Assess for signs of infection during neutropenia. Assess for bleeding (bleeding gums, bruising, petechiae, blood in stools, urine, and emesis) and avoid IM injections and taking rectal temperatures if platelet count is low. Apply pressure to venipuncture sites for 10 min.
- Assess patient for signs of peripheral neuropathy (burning sensation, hyperesthesia, hypoesthesia, paresthesia, discomfort, neuropathic pain); may occur early during treatment within the first 3 cycles. Patients experiencing new or worsening symptoms may require a reduction or delay in dose of ixabepilone. If neuropathy is Grade 2 (moderate) lasting for ≥7 days or Grade 3 (severe) lasting for <7 days decrease dose by 20%. If neuropathy is Grade 3 lasting ≥7 days or is disabling discontinue treatment.
- ***Lab Test Considerations:*** Monitor CBC and platelets frequently during therapy. If neutrophil count is <500 cells/mm³ for ≥7 days or patient has febrile neutropenia or if platelet count is <25,000/mm³ or platelets are <50,000/mm³ with bleeding decrease the dose by 20%. Begin new treatment cycle only if neutrophil count is at least 1500 cells/mm³ and nonhematologic toxicities have improved to Grade 1 (mild) or resolved. May also cause leukopenia and anemia.
- Monitor hepatic function prior to therapy. Patients with decreased hepatic function require a decreased dose. If AST and ALT ≤2.5 × the upper limits of normal (ULN) and bilirubin ≤1 × ULN administer ixabepilone at 40 mg/m². If AST and ALT ≤10 × the upper limits of normal (ULN) and bilirubin ≤1 X ULN administer ixabepilone at 32mg/m². If AST and ALT ≤10 × the upper limits of normal (ULN) and bilirubin >1.5 × ULN — ≤3 × ULN administer ixabepilone at 20–30 mg/m².

Potential Nursing Diagnoses
Risk for injury (Adverse Reactions)

Implementation
- Premedicate patient with an H₁ and an H₂ antagonist approximately 1 hr before ixabepilone infusion. Patients who experienced a hypersensitivity reaction in a previous ixabepilone cycle should also be premedicated with corticosteroids and extension of the infusion time should be considered.
- To minimize risk of dermal exposure, wear impervious gloves when handling ixabepilone vials regardless of setting (unpacking and inspection, transport within a facility, dose preparation and administration).

IV Administration
- **Intermittent Infusion:** Remove *Ixempra kit* (containing ixabepilone vial and diluent vial) from refrigerator and allow to stand at room temperature for 30 min prior to diluting. *Ixempra kit* must be stored in refrigerator. When vials are first removed from refrigerator, a white precipitate may be observed in the diluent vial; precipitate will dissolve to form a clear solution once diluent warms to room temperature. ***Diluent:*** Use only diluent supplied in kit for reconstitution. Reconstitute 15-mg vial with 8 mL and 45-mg vial with 23.5 mL of diluent. Gently swirl and invert vial until powder is com-

pletely dissolved. Prior to administration, dilute constituted solution further with only LR supplied in DEHP-free bags. Dilute as soon as possible after constitution, but may be stored at room temperature and room light for up to 1 hr. For most doses use 250 mL bag of LR, 0.9% NaCl (pH adjusted 6.0–9.0 with sodium bicarbonate), or Plasma-lyte A injection (pH 7.4).
Concentration: If final concentration is not between 0.2 mg/mL and 0.6 mg/mL add to appropriate size bag of LR. Thoroughly mix infusion bag by manual rotation. Diluted solution is stable for up to 6 hr at room temperature and room light; must complete infusion during 6-hr period. Administer through an in-line filter with a microporous membrane of 0.2–1.2 microns. DEHP-free infusion containers and administration sets must be used. Discard remaining solution. *Rate:* Infuse over 3 hr.

Patient/Family Teaching
- Advise patient to avoid grapefruit juice during therapy; may lead to increased levels and side effects.
- Solution contains alcohol and may cause drowsiness or dizziness. Caution patient to avoid driving and other activities requiring alertness until response to medication is known.
- Instruct patient to notify health care professional promptly if fever >100.5°F; chills; cough; hoarseness; sore throat; signs of infection; lower back or side pain; burning, painful or difficulty urination; bleeding gums; bruising; petechiae; blood in stools, urine, or emesis; increased fatigue; dyspnea; or orthostatic hypotension occurs. Caution patient to avoid crowds and persons with known infections. Instruct patients to use a soft toothbrush and electric razor and to avoid falls. Caution patient not to drink alcoholic beverages or take medication containing aspirin or NSAIDs; may precipitate bleeding.
- Instruct patient to notify health care professional promptly if signs and symptoms of hypersensitivity (hives, urticaria, pruritus, rash, flushing, swelling, dyspnea, chest tightness), peripheral neuropathy (numbness and tingling in hands and feet), or cardiac adverse reactions (chest pain, difficulty breathing, palpitations, unusual weight gain) occur.
- Advise patient to consult health care professional before taking any Rx, OTC, herbal, or vitamin products, especially St. John's wort, during therapy.
- Instruct patient not to receive any vaccinations without advice of health care professional.
- Discuss the possibility of hair loss with patient. Explore methods of coping. Regrowth usually occurs 2–3 mo after discontinuation of therapy.
- Advise women of childbearing potential to use effective contraception during therapy and to avoid breastfeeding during therapy.

Evaluation/Desired Outcomes
- Decreased progression of breast cancer.

kanamycin, See AMINOGLYCOSIDES.

ketoconazole (systemic)†
(kee-toe-**koe**-na-zole)
Nizoral

Classification
Therapeutic: antifungals (systemic)

Pregnancy Category C

†For topical use, see Antifungals (topical)

Indications
Treatment of: Candidiasis (disseminated and mucocutaneous), Chromomycosis, Coccidioidomycosis, Histoplasmosis, Paracoccidioidomycosis. **Unlabeled Use:** Treatment of advanced prostate cancer. Treatment of Cushing's syndrome.

Action
Disrupts fungal cell membrane. Interferes with fungal metabolism. Also inhibits the production of adrenal steroids. **Therapeutic Effects:** Fungistatic or fungicidal action against susceptible organisms, depending on organism and site of infection. **Spectrum:** Active against many pathogenic fungi, including: *Blastomyces*, *Candida*, *Coccidioides*, *Cryptococcus*, *Histoplasma*, many dermatophytes.

Pharmacokinetics
Absorption: Absorption from the GI tract is pH dependent; increasing pH decreases absorption.
Distribution: Widely distributed. CNS penetration is unpredictable and minimal. Crosses the placenta; enters breast milk.
Protein Binding: 99%.
Metabolism and Excretion: Partially metabolized by the liver. Excreted in feces via biliary excretion.
Half-life: 8 hr.

TIME/ACTION PROFILE (blood levels)

ROUTE	ONSET	PEAK	DURATION
PO	rapid	1–4 hr	24 hr

Contraindications/Precautions
Contraindicated in: Hypersensitivity; Concurrent triazolam; OB: Reported association with limb defects (1st trimester) and growth retardation (3rd trimester).
Use Cautiously in: History of liver disease; Achlorhydria or hypochlorhydria; Alcoholism; Lactation: Usually compatible with breastfeeding (AAP). Careful timing of dosage may ↓ infant exposure.

Adverse Reactions/Side Effects
CNS: dizziness, drowsiness. **EENT:** photophobia. **GI:** DRUG-INDUCED HEPATITIS, nausea, vomiting, abdominal pain, constipation, diarrhea, flatulence. **GU:** azoospermia, ↓ male libido, menstrual irregularities, oligospermia. **Derm:** rashes. **Endo:** gynecomastia.

Interactions
Drug-Drug: Ketoconazole inhibits the hepatic P450 3A4 enzyme system, which results in ↓ metabolism and possibly ↑ effects and/or toxicity from **cyclosporine**, **tacrolimus**, **corticosteroids** (dosage reduction may be necessary), **calcium channel blockers**, **sulfonylurea**, **oral hypoglycemic agents**, **quinidine**, **buspirone**, **clarithromycin**, **troleandomycin**, **erythromycin**, **cyclophosphamide**, **phenytoin**, **warfarin** (↑ risk of bleeding), **tamoxifen**, **tricyclic antidepressants**, **carbamazepine**, **nisoldipine**, **zolpidem**, **vinca alkaloids**, **ifosfamide**, some **benzodiazepines** (effect may persist for several days; use of triazolam is contraindicated), **alfentanil**, **fentanyl**, **sufentanil**, **donepezil**, **atorvastatin**, **lovastatin**, **simvastatin**, **amprenavir**, **indinavir** (dosage ↓ of indinavir recommended), **nelfinavir**, **ritonavir**, **saquinavir**, **quinidine**, **sildenafil** and **vardenafil** (dosage adjustments may be necessary). May alter the effectiveness of **hormonal contraceptives** (alternative method of contraception recommended). Drugs that ↑ gastric pH, including **antacids**, **histamine H₂ antagonists**, **didanosine** (chewable tablets, because of buffer), and **gastric acid–pump inhibitors** ↓ absorption (wait 2 hr before administration of ketoconazole). **Sucralfate** and **isoniazid** also ↓ bioavailability. ↑ hepatotoxicity with other **hepatotoxic agents**, including **alcohol**. Disulfiram-like reaction may occur with **alcohol**. **Rifampin** or **isoniazid** may ↓ levels and effectiveness. May ↓ absorption and effectiveness of **theophylline**.

Route/Dosage
PO (Adults): *Antifungal*—200–400 mg/day, single dose. *Prostate cancer*—400 mg 3 times daily (unlabeled).
PO (Children >2 yr): 3.3–6.6 mg/kg/day, single dose.

Availability (generic available)
Tablets: 200 mg. **Oral suspension:** ✽ 100 mg/5 mL.

NURSING IMPLICATIONS
Assessment
- Assess patient for symptoms of infection prior to and periodically during therapy.
- Specimens for culture should be taken prior to instituting therapy. Therapy may be started before results are obtained.
- ***Lab Test Considerations:*** Monitor hepatic function tests prior to and monthly for 3–4 mo and then periodically during therapy. May cause ↑ AST, ALT, serum alkaline phosphatase, and bilirubin concentrations. Ketoconazole should be discontinued if even minor abnormalities occur.
- May cause ↓ serum testosterone concentrations.

Potential Nursing Diagnoses
Risk for infection (Indications)
Noncompliance (Patient/Family Teaching)

Implementation
- Do not confuse Nizoral (ketoconazole) with Neoral (cyclosporine).
- **PO:** Administer with meals or snacks to minimize nausea and vomiting.
- Shake suspension well prior to administration.
- Do not administer histamine H_2 antagonists or antacids within 2 hr of ketoconazole.
- For patients with achlorhydria, dissolve each tablet in 4 mL of aqueous solution of 0.2 N hydrochloric acid. Use a glass or plastic straw to avoid contact with teeth and follow with a glass of water, swished in mouth and swallowed.

Patient/Family Teaching
- Instruct patient to take medication as directed, at the same time each day, even if feeling better. Take missed doses as soon as remembered; if almost time for next dose, space missed dose and next dose 10–12 hr apart.
- May cause dizziness or drowsiness. Caution patient to avoid driving or other activities requiring alertness until response to medication is known.
- Advise patient to avoid taking OTC antacids within 2 hr of ketoconazole.
- Caution patient to wear sunglasses and to avoid prolonged exposure to bright light to prevent photophobic reactions.
- Advise patient to use a nonhormonal form of contraception during ketoconazole therapy.
- Advise patient to avoid concurrent use of alcohol while taking ketoconazole; may cause a disulfiram-like reaction (flushing, rash, peripheral edema, nausea, headache) and increase the risk of hepatotoxicity.
- Instruct patient to notify health care professional if abdominal pain, fever, or diarrhea becomes pronounced or if signs and symptoms of liver dysfunction (unusual fatigue, anorexia, nausea, vomiting, jaundice, dark urine, or pale stools) occur.

Evaluation/Desired Outcomes
- Resolution of clinical and laboratory indications of fungal infections.
- Minimal treatment for candidiasis is 1–2 wk and for other systemic mycoses is 6 mo.
- Chronic mucocutaneous candidiasis usually requires maintenance therapy.

---

ketoconazole, See ANTIFUNGALS (TOPICAL).

---

ketoprofen (kee-toe-**proe**-fen)
✽ Apo-Keto, ✽ Apo-Keto-E, ✽ Orudis-E, ✽ Orudis-SR, ✽ Rhodis

Classification
Therapeutic: antipyretics, antirheumatics, nonopioid analgesics, nonsteroidal anti-inflammatory agents
Pharmacologic: nonopioid analgesics

Pregnancy Category B (first trimester)

Indications
Inflammatory disorders, including: Rheumatoid arthritis, Osteoarthritis. Mild to moderate pain, including dysmenorrhea and fever.

Action
Inhibits prostaglandin synthesis. **Therapeutic Effects:** Suppression of pain and inflammation. Reduction of fever.

Pharmacokinetics
Absorption: Well absorbed from the GI tract.
Distribution: Unknown.
Protein Binding: 99%.
Metabolism and Excretion: Mostly (60%) metabolized by the liver; some renal excretion.
Half-life: 2–4 hr.

ketoprofen

TIME/ACTION PROFILE

ROUTE	ONSET	PEAK	DURATION
PO (analgesic)	within 60 min	1 hr	4–6 hr
PO (anti-inflammatory)	few days–1 wk	unknown	up to 24 hr (SR products)

Contraindications/Precautions
Contraindicated in: Hypersensitivity; Cross-sensitivity may exist with other NSAIDs, including aspirin; Active GI bleeding; Ulcer disease; Some products contain tartrazine and should be avoided in patients with known intolerance; Perioperative pain from coronary artery bypass graft (CABG) surgery.
Use Cautiously in: Cardiovascular disease or risk factors for cardiovascular disease (may ↑ risk of serious cardiovascular thrombotic events, myocardial infarction, and stroke, especially with prolonged use); Severe renal, or hepatic disease; History of ulcer disease; Renal impairment (dosage reduction suggested); Geri: Extended-release product should not be used in geriatric patients, patients of small stature, or patients with renal impairment; ↑ risk of bleeding; Chronic alcohol use/abuse; OB, Lactation, Pedi: Safety not established; avoid use during 2nd half of pregnancy.

Adverse Reactions/Side Effects
CNS: drowsiness, headache, dizziness. **EENT:** blurred vision, tinnitus. **CV:** edema. **GI:** DRUG-INDUCED HEPATITIS, GI BLEEDING, constipation, diarrhea, dyspepsia, nausea, vomiting, anorexia, discomfort, flatulence. **GU:** cystitis, hematuria, renal failure. **Derm:** EXFOLIATIVE DERMATITIS, STEVENS-JOHNSON SYNDROME, TOXIC EPIDERMAL NECROLYSIS, photosensitivity, rashes. **Endo:** gynecomastia. **Hemat:** blood dyscrasias, prolonged bleeding time. **MS:** myalgia. **Misc:** allergic reactions including ANAPHYLAXIS, fever.

Interactions
Drug-Drug: **Aspirin** alters distribution, metabolism, and excretion of ketoprofen (concurrent use not recommended). ↑ adverse GI effects with other **NSAIDs**, **corticosteroids**, or **alcohol**. Chronic use with **acetaminophen** may ↑ risk of adverse renal reactions. May ↓ effectiveness of **diuretics** or **antihypertensives**. May ↑ hypoglycemic effects of **insulin** or sulfonylurea **oral hypoglycemic agents**. May ↑ serum **lithium** levels and increase the risk of toxicity. ↑ risk of toxicity from **methotrexate**. **Probenecid** ↑ risk of toxicity from ketoprofen (concurrent use not recommended). ↑ risk of bleeding with **cefotetan, cefoperazone, valproic acid, thrombolytic agents, clopidogrel, ticlopidine, eptifibatide, tirofiban,** or **anticoagulants**. ↑ risk of adverse hematologic reactions with **antineoplastics** or **radiation therapy**. ↑ risk of nephrotoxicity with **cyclosporine**.
Drug-Natural Products: ↑ bleeding risk with **arnica, chamomile, clove, dong quai, feverfew, garlic, ginger, ginkgo,** and **Panax ginseng**.

Route/Dosage
PO (Adults): *Anti-inflammatory*—150–300 mg/day in 3–4 divided doses or 150–200 mg once daily as extended-release product. *Analgesic*—25–50 mg q 6–8 hr.

Availability (generic available)
Capsules: 25 mg, 50 mg, 75 mg. **Extended-release capsules:** 100 mg, 150 mg, 200 mg.

NURSING IMPLICATIONS
Assessment
- Patients who have asthma, aspirin-induced allergy, and nasal polyps are at increased risk for developing hypersensitivity reactions. Assess for rhinitis, wheezing, and urticaria.
- **Arthritis:** Assess pain and range of motion prior to and 1 hr following administration.
- **Pain:** Assess pain (note type, location, and intensity) prior to and 1 hr following administration.
- **Fever:** Monitor temperature; note signs associated with fever (diaphoresis, tachycardia, malaise).
- *Lab Test Considerations:* Evaluate BUN, serum creatinine, CBC, and liver function tests periodically in patients receiving prolonged therapy.
- Serum potassium, BUN, serum creatinine, alkaline phosphatase, LDH, AST, and ALT tests may show ↑ levels. Blood glucose, hemoglobin and hematocrit concentrations, leukocyte and platelet counts, and CCr may be ↓.
- May prolong bleeding time by 3–4 min.
- May alter results of urine albumin, bilirubin, 17-ketosteroid, and 17-hydroxycorticosteroid determinations.

Potential Nursing Diagnoses
Acute pain (Indications)
Impaired physical mobility (Indications)

Implementation

- Administration in higher-than-recommended doses does not provide increased effectiveness but may cause increased side effects. Use lowest effective dose for shortest period of time.
- Coadministration with opioid analgesics may have additive analgesic effects and may permit lower opioid doses.
- Analgesic is more effective if given before pain becomes severe.
- **PO:** For rapid initial effect, administer 30 min before or 2 hr after meals. Capsules may be administered with food, milk, or antacids containing aluminum hydroxide and magnesium hydroxide to decrease GI irritation.
- Extended-release capsules should be swallowed whole; do not open or chew.
- **Dysmenorrhea:** Administer as soon as possible after the onset of menses. Prophylactic treatment has not been proved effective.

Patient/Family Teaching

- Advise patient to take this medication with a full glass of water and to remain in an upright position for 15–30 min after administration.
- Instruct patient to take medication exactly as directed. Take missed doses as soon as remembered but not if almost time for the next dose. Do not double doses.
- May cause drowsiness or dizziness. Advise patient to avoid driving or other activities requiring alertness until response to medication is known.
- Caution patient to avoid the concurrent use of alcohol, aspirin, acetaminophen, or other OTC medications without consulting health care professional.
- Advise patient to inform health care professional of medication regimen prior to treatment or surgery.
- Caution patient to wear sunscreen and protective clothing to prevent photosensitivity reactions.
- Instruct patients not to take OTC ketoprofen preparations for more than 10 days for pain or more than 3 days for fever and to consult health care professional if symptoms persist or worsen.
- Caution patient that use of ketoprofen with 3 or more glasses of alcohol may increase risk of GI bleeding.
- Advise patient to consult health care professional if rash, itching, visual disturbances, tinnitus, weight gain, edema, black stools, persistent headache, or influenza-like syndrome (chills, fever, muscle aches, pain) occurs.

Evaluation/Desired Outcomes

- Improved joint mobility.
- Decrease in severity of pain. Improvement in arthritis may be seen in a few days to 1 wk; 1–2 wk may be required for maximum effectiveness. Patients who do not respond to one NSAID may respond to another.
- Reduction of fever.

---

ketorolac† (kee-toe-role-ak)
◆ Toradol

Classification
Therapeutic: nonsteroidal anti-inflammatory agents, nonopioid analgesics
Pharmacologic: pyrroziline carboxylic acid

Pregnancy Category C

†See Appendix C for ophthalmic use

Indications
Short-term management of pain (not to exceed 5 days total for all routes combined).

Action
Inhibits prostaglandin synthesis, producing peripherally mediated analgesia. Also has antipyretic and anti-inflammatory properties. **Therapeutic Effects:** Decreased pain.

Pharmacokinetics
Absorption: Rapidly and completely absorbed following all routes of administration.
Distribution: Enters breast milk in low concentrations.
Metabolism and Excretion: <50% metabolized by the liver. Ketorolac and its metabolites are excreted primarily by the kidneys (92%); 6% excreted in feces.
Half-life: 4.5 hr (range 3.8–6.3 hr; ↑ in geriatric patients and patients with impaired renal function).

TIME/ACTION PROFILE (analgesic effects)

ROUTE	ONSET	PEAK	DURATION
PO	unknown	2–3 hr	4–6 hr or longer
IM, IV	10 min	1–2 hr	6 hr or longer

Contraindications/Precautions
Contraindicated in: Hypersensitivity; Cross-sensitivity with other NSAIDs may exist; Pre- or perioperative use; Known alcohol intolerance (injection only); Perioperative pain from coronary artery bypass graft (CABG) surgery; OB: Chronic use in 3rd trimester may cause constriction of ductus arteriosus. May inhibit labor and ↑ maternal bleeding at delivery; Lactation: Lactation.

Use Cautiously in: Cardiovascular disease or risk factors for cardiovascular disease (may ↑ risk of serious cardiovascular thrombotic events, myocardial infarction, and stroke, especially with prolonged use); History of GI bleeding; Renal impairment (dosage reduction may be required); Pedi: Safety not established; Geri: Appears on Beers list; ↑ risk of GI bleeding.

Adverse Reactions/Side Effects
CNS: drowsiness, abnormal thinking, dizziness, euphoria, headache. **Resp:** asthma, dyspnea. **CV:** edema, pallor, vasodilation. **GI:** GI BLEEDING, abnormal taste, diarrhea, dry mouth, dyspepsia, GI pain, nausea. **GU:** oliguria, renal toxicity, urinary frequency. **Derm:** EXFOLIATIVE DERMATITIS, STEVENS-JOHNSON SYNDROME, TOXIC EPIDERMAL NECROLYSIS, pruritus, purpura, sweating, urticaria. **Hemat:** prolonged bleeding time. **Local:** injection site pain. **Neuro:** paresthesia. **Misc:** allergic reactions including, anaphylaxis.

Interactions
Drug-Drug: Concurrent use with **aspirin** may ↓ effectiveness. ↑ adverse GI effects with **aspirin**, other **NSAIDs**, **potassium supplements**, **corticosteroids**, or **alcohol**. May ↓ effectiveness of **diuretics** or **antihypertensives**. May ↑ serum **lithium** levels and ↑ risk of toxicity. ↑ risk of toxicity from **methotrexate**. ↑ risk of bleeding with **cefotetan**, **cefoperazone**, **valproic acid**, **clopidogrel**, **ticlopidine**, **tirofiban**, **eptifibatide**, **thrombolytic agents**, or **anticoagulants**. ↑ risk of adverse hematologic reactions with **antineoplastics** or **radiation therapy**. May ↑ risk of nephrotoxicity from **cyclosporine**. **Probenecid** ↑ ketorolac blood levels and the risk of adverse reactions (concurrent use should be avoided).
Drug-Natural Products: ↑ bleeding risk with **arnica**, **chamomile**, **clove**, **dong quai**, **feverfew**, **garlic**, **ginger**, **ginkgo**, **Panax ginseng**.

Route/Dosage
Oral therapy is indicated only as a continuation of parenteral therapy; parenteral therapy should not exceed 20 doses/5 days. Total duration of therapy by all routes should not exceed 5 days.
PO (Adults <65 yr): 20 mg initially, followed by 10 mg q 4–6 hr as needed (not to exceed 40 mg/day).
PO (Adults ≥65 yr, <50 kg, or with renal impairment): 10 mg q 4–6 hr as needed (not to exceed 40 mg/day).
IM (Adults <65 yr): *Single dose*—60 mg. *Multiple dosing*—30 mg q 6 hr (not to exceed 120 mg/day).
IM (Adults ≥65 yr, <50 kg, or with renal impairment): *Single dose*—30 mg. *Multiple dosing*—15 mg q 6 hr (not to exceed 60 mg/day).
IV (Adults <65 yr): *Single dose*—30 mg. *Multiple dosing*—30 mg q 6 hr (not to exceed 120 mg/day).
IV (Adults ≥65 yr, <50 kg, or with renal impairment): *Single dose*—15 mg. *Multiple dosing*—15 mg q 6 hr (not to exceed 60 mg/day).

Availability (generic available)
Tablets: 10 mg. **Cost:** *Generic*—$16.66/20. **Injection:** 15 mg/mL, 30 mg/mL.

NURSING IMPLICATIONS
Assessment
- Patients who have asthma, aspirin-induced allergy, and nasal polyps are at increased risk for developing hypersensitivity reactions. Assess for rhinitis, asthma, and urticaria.
- **Pain:** Assess pain (note type, location, and intensity) prior to and 1–2 hr following administration.
- *Lab Test Considerations:* Evaluate liver function tests, especially AST and ALT, periodically in patients receiving prolonged therapy. May cause ↑ levels.
- May cause prolonged bleeding time that may persist for 24–48 hr following discontinuation of therapy.
- May cause ↑ BUN, serum creatinine, or potassium concentrations.

Potential Nursing Diagnoses
Acute pain (Indications)

Implementation
- Do not confuse Toradol (ketorolac) with tramadol (Ultram).
- Administration in higher-than-recommended doses does not provide increased effectiveness but may cause increased side effects. Duration of ketorolac therapy, by all routes combined, should not exceed 5 days Use lowest effective dose for shortest period of time.
- Coadministration with opioid analgesics may have additive analgesic effects and may permit lower opioid doses.
- **PO:** Ketorolac therapy should always be given initially by the IM or IV route. Use oral therapy *only* as a continuation of parenteral therapy.

ketorolac

IV Administration
- **Direct IV:** Administer undiluted. *Concentration:* 15–30 mg/mL. *Rate:* Administer over at least 15 sec.
- **Syringe Compatibility:** famotidine, metoclopramide, sufentanil.
- **Syringe Incompatibility:** haloperidol, hydroxyzine, nalbuphine, prochlorperazine, promethazine, thiethylperazine.
- **Y-Site Compatibility:** alfentanil, amikacin, aminophyllins, amphotericin B liposome, ascorbic acid, atracurium, atropine, aztreonam, bivalirudin, bumetanide, buprenorphine, butorphanol, carboplatin, cefazolin, cefonocid, cefoperazone, cefotaxime, cefotetan, cefoxitin, ceftazidime, ceftriaxone, cefuroxime, chloramphenicol, cimetidine, cisatracurium, cisplatin, clindamycin, cyanocobalamin, cyclophosphamide, cyclosporine, cytarabine, dactinomycin, daptomycin, dexamethasone, dexmedetomidine, digoxin, docetaxel, dopamine, doxacurium, doxorubicin hydrochloride, enalaprilat, ephedrine, epinephrine, epoetin alfa, ertapenem, etoposide, etoposide phosphate, famotidine, fentanyl, fluconazole, fludarabine, fluorouracil, folic acid, furosemide, gentamicin, glycopyrrolate, granisetron, heparin, hetastarch, hydrocortisone, hydromorphone, ifosfamide, imipenem/cilastatin, indomethacin, insulin, isoproterenol, lidocaine, linezolid, lorazepam, magnesium sulfate, mannitol, mechlorethamine, meperidine, methadone, methotrexate, metoprolol, metronidazole, milrinone, mitoxantrone, morphine, multivitamins, nafcillin, naloxone, nesiritide, nitroglycerin, nitroprusside, norepinephrine, octreotide, ondansetron, oxacillin, oxaliplatin, oxytocin, paclitaxel, palonosetron, pemetrexed, penicillin G, phenobarbital, phenylephrine, phytonadione, piperacillin/tazobactam, potassium chloride, procainamide, propranolol, ranitidine, remifentanil, sodium acetate, sodium bicarbonate, streptokinase, succinylcholine, sufentanil, sufentanil, tacrolimus, teniposide, theophylline, thiotepa, ticarcillin/clavulanate, tigecycline, tirofiban, tobramycin, trimethaphan, urokinase, vasopressin, verapamil, vincristine, voriconazole.
- **Y-Site Incompatibility:** acyclovir, amphotericin B colloidal, azathioprine, azithromycin, calcium chloride, caspofungin, chlorpromazine, dantrolene, diazepam, diazoxide, diltiazem, diphenhydramine, dobutamine, doxycycline, epirubicin, erythromycin, esmolol, fenoldopam, ganciclovir, gemcitabine, haloperidol, hydroxyzine, inamrinone, labetalol, metaraminol, methoxamine, midazolam, nalbuphine, pantoprazole, papaverine, pentamidine, pentazocine, phentolamine, phenytoin, prochlorperazine, promethazine, protamine, pyridoxime, quinupristin/dalfopristin, rocuronium, tolazoline, trimethoprim/sulfamethoxazole, vancomycin, vecuronium, vinorelbine.
- **Solution Compatibility:** D5/0.9% NaCl, D5W, Ringer's injection, lactated Ringer's injection, 0.9% NaCl.

Patient/Family Teaching
- Instruct patient on how and when to ask for and take pain medication.
- Instruct patient to take medication exactly as directed. Take missed doses as soon as remembered if not almost time for next dose. Do not double doses. Do not take more than prescribed or for longer than 5 days.
- May cause drowsiness or dizziness. Advise patient to avoid driving or other activities requiring alertness until response to the medication is known.
- Caution patient to avoid the concurrent use of alcohol, aspirin, NSAIDs, acetaminophen, or other OTC medications without consulting health care professional.
- Advise patient to inform health care professional of medication regimen prior to treatment or surgery.
- Advise patient to consult health care professional if rash, itching, visual disturbances, tinnitus, weight gain, edema, black stools, persistent headache, or influenza-like syndrome (chills, fever, muscle aches, pain) occurs.

Evaluation/Desired Outcomes
- Decrease in severity of pain. Patients who do not respond to one NSAID may respond to another.

labetalol (la-bet-a-lole)
Trandate

HIGH ALERT

Classification
Therapeutic: antianginals, antihypertensives
Pharmacologic: beta blockers

Pregnancy Category C

Indications
Management of hypertension.

Action
Blocks stimulation of beta$_1$ (myocardial)- and beta$_2$ (pulmonary, vascular, and uterine)-adrenergic receptor sites. Also has alpha$_1$-adrenergic blocking activity, which may result in more orthostatic hypotension. **Therapeutic Effects:** Decreased blood pressure.

Pharmacokinetics
Absorption: Well absorbed but rapidly undergoes extensive first-pass hepatic metabolism, resulting in 25% bioavailability.
Distribution: Some CNS penetration; crosses the placenta.
Metabolism and Excretion: Undergoes extensive hepatic metabolism.
Half-life: 3–8 hr.

TIME/ACTION PROFILE (cardiovascular effects)

ROUTE	ONSET	PEAK	DURATION
PO	20 min–2 hr	1–4 hr	8–12 hr
IV	2–5 min	5 min	16–18 hr

Contraindications/Precautions
Contraindicated in: Uncompensated CHF; Pulmonary edema; Cardiogenic shock; Bradycardia or heart block.
Use Cautiously in: Renal impairment; Hepatic impairment; Geriatric patients (increased sensitivity to beta blockers; initial dosage reduction recommended); Pulmonary disease (including asthma); Diabetes mellitus (may mask signs of hypoglycemia); Thyrotoxicosis (may mask symptoms); Patients with a history of severe allergic reactions (intensity of reactions may be increased); OB: May cause fetal/neonatal bradycardia, hypotension, hypoglycemia, or respiratory depression; Lactation: Usually compatible with breastfeeding (AAP); Pedi: Safety not established; Geri: ↑ risk of orthostatic hypotension.

Adverse Reactions/Side Effects
CNS: fatigue, weakness, anxiety, depression, dizziness, drowsiness, insomnia, memory loss, mental status changes, nightmares. **EENT:** blurred vision, dry eyes, nasal stuffiness. **Resp:** bronchospasm, wheezing. **CV:** ARRHYTHMIAS, BRADYCARDIA, CHF, PULMONARY EDEMA, orthostatic hypotension. **GI:** constipation, diarrhea, nausea. **GU:** erectile dysfunction, ↓ libido. **Derm:** itching, rashes. **Endo:** hyperglycemia, hypoglycemia. **MS:** arthralgia, back pain, muscle cramps. **Neuro:** paresthesia. **Misc:** drug-induced lupus syndrome.

Interactions
Drug-Drug: **General anesthesia** and **verapamil** may cause additive myocardial depression. Additive bradycardia may occur with **digoxin**, **verapamil**, or **diltiazem**. Additive hypotension may occur with other **antihypertensives**, acute ingestion of **alcohol**, or **nitrates**. Concurrent **thyroid** administration may ↓ effectiveness. May alter the effectiveness of **insulin** or **oral hypoglycemic agents** (dose adjustments may be necessary). May ↓ the effectiveness of **adrenergic bronchodilators** and **theophylline**. May ↓ beneficial beta cardiovascular effects of **dopamine** or **dobutamine**. Use cautiously within 14 days of **MAO inhibitor** therapy (may result in hypertension). Effects may be ↑ by **propranolol** or **cimetidine**. Concurrent **NSAIDs** may ↓ antihypertensive action.

Route/Dosage
PO (Adults): 100 mg twice daily initially, may be ↑ by 100 mg twice daily q 2–3 days as needed (usual range 400–800 mg/day in 2–3 divided doses; doses up to 1.2–2.4 g/day have been used).

IV (Adults): 20 mg (0.25 mg/kg) initially, additional doses of 40–80 mg may be given q 10 min as needed (not to exceed 300 mg total dose) *or* 2 mg/min infusion (range 50–300 mg total dose required).

Availability (generic available)
Tablets: 100 mg, 200 mg, 300 mg. **Cost:** *Generic*—100 mg $54.00/180, 200 mg $76.99/180, 300 mg $101.99/180. **Injection:** 5 mg/mL.

NURSING IMPLICATIONS

Assessment
- Monitor blood pressure and pulse frequently during dose adjustment and periodically dur-

760 labetalol

ing therapy. Assess for orthostatic hypotension when assisting patient up from supine position.
- Check frequency of refills to determine compliance.
- Patients receiving *labetalol IV* must be supine during and for 3 hr after administration. Vital signs should be monitored every 5–15 min during and for several hours after administration.
- Monitor intake and output ratios and daily weight. Assess patient routinely for evidence of fluid overload (peripheral edema, dyspnea, rales/crackles, fatigue, weight gain, jugular venous distention).
- *Lab Test Considerations:* May cause ↑ BUN, serum lipoprotein, potassium, triglyceride, and uric acid levels.
- May cause ↑ ANA titers.
- May cause ↑ in blood glucose levels.
- May cause ↑ serum alkaline phosphatase, LDH, AST, and ALT levels. Discontinue if jaundice or laboratory signs of hepatic function impairment occur.
- *Toxicity and Overdose:* Monitor patients receiving beta blockers for signs of overdose (bradycardia, severe dizziness or fainting, severe drowsiness, dyspnea, bluish fingernails or palms, seizures). Notify physician or other health care professional immediately if these signs occur.
- Glucagon has been used to treat bradycardia and hypotension.

Potential Nursing Diagnoses
Decreased cardiac output (Side Effects)
Noncompliance (Patient/Family Teaching)

Implementation
- *High Alert:* IV vasoactive medications are inherently dangerous. Before administering intravenously, have second practitioner independently check original order, dosage calculations, and infusion pump settings. Do not confuse labetalol with Lamictal.
- Discontinuation of concurrent clonidine should take place gradually, with beta blocker discontinued first. Then, after several days, discontinue clonidine.
- **PO:** Take apical pulse prior to administering. If <50 bpm or if arrhythmia occurs, withhold medication and notify physician or other health care professional.
- Administer with meals or directly after eating to enhance absorption.

IV Administration
- **Direct IV:** *Diluent:* Administer undiluted. *Concentration:* 5 mg/mL. *Rate:* Administer slowly over 2 min.
- **Continuous Infusion:** *Diluent:* Add 200 mg of labetalol to 160 mL of diluent. May also be administered as undiluted drug. Compatible diluents include D5W, 0.9% NaCl, D5/0.9% NaCl, and LR. *Concentration:* Diluted: 1 mg/mL; Undiluted: 5 mg/mL. *Rate:* Administer at a rate of 2 mg/min. Titrate for desired response. Infuse via infusion pump to ensure accurate dosage.
- **Y-Site Compatibility:** amikacin, aminophylline, amiodarone, atropine, aztreonam, ampicillin, bivalirudin, bumetanide, butorphanol, calcium chloride, calcium gluconate, caspofungin, cefazolin, ceftazidime, ceftizoxime, cimetidine, cyclosporine, daptomycin, digoxin, diltiazem, diphenhydramine, dobutamine, dopamine, doxycycline, enalaprilat, epinephrine, ertapenem, erythromycin lactobionate, esmolol, famotidine, fenoldopam, fentanyl, fluconazole, ganciclovir, gentamicin, granisetron, hydromorphone, imipenem/cilastatin, isoproterenol, levofloxacin, lidocaine, linezolid, lorazepam, magnesium sulfate, meperidine, methylprednisolone sodium succinate, metoclopramide, metronidazole, midazolam, milrinone, morphine, nicardipine, nitroglycerin, nitroprusside, norepinephrine, penicillin G, palonosetron, phenylephrine, phytonadione, potassium chloride, potassium phosphate, procainamide, prochlorperazine, promethazine, propofol, protamine, quinupristin/dalfopristin, ranitidine, sodium bicarbonate, tacrolimus, ticarcillin/clavulanate, tirofiban, tobramycin, trimethoprim/sulfamethoxazole, vancomycin, vasopressin, vecuronium, verapamil, voriconazole.
- **Y-Site Incompatibility:** acyclovir, amphotericin B cholesteryl sulfate complex, cefotaxime, cefoxitin, ceftriaxone, cefuroxime, dexamethasone sodium phosphate, diazepam, furosemide, hydrocortisone sodium succinate, insulin, ketorolac, lansoprazole, micafungin, nafcillin, pantoprazole, phenytoin, piperacillin/tazobactam, warfarin.

Patient/Family Teaching
- Instruct patient to take medication as directed, at the same time each day, even if feeling well; do not skip or double up on missed doses. Take missed doses as soon as possible up to 8 hr before next dose. Abrupt withdrawal may

precipitate life-threatening arrhythmias, hypertension, or myocardial ischemia.
- Advise patient to make sure enough medication is available for weekends, holidays, and vacations. A written prescription may be kept in wallet in case of emergency.
- Teach patient and family how to check pulse and blood pressure. Instruct them to check pulse daily and blood pressure biweekly. Advise patient to hold dose and contact health care professional if pulse is <50 bpm or blood pressure changes significantly.
- May cause drowsiness or dizziness. Caution patients to avoid driving or other activities that require alertness until response to the drug is known. Caution patients receiving labetalol IV to call for assistance during ambulation or transfer.
- Advise patients to make position changes slowly to minimize orthostatic hypotension, especially during initiation of therapy or when dose is increased. Patients taking oral labetalol should be especially cautious when drinking alcohol, standing for long periods, or exercising, and during hot weather, because orthostatic hypotension is enhanced.
- Caution patient that this medication may increase sensitivity to cold.
- Instruct patient to consult health care professional before taking any Rx, OTC, or herbal products, especially cold preparations, concurrently with this medication.
- Patients with diabetes should closely monitor blood glucose, especially if weakness, malaise, irritability, or fatigue occurs. Medication may mask tachycardia and increased blood pressure as signs of hypoglycemia, but dizziness and sweating may still occur.
- Advise patient to notify health care professional if slow pulse, difficulty breathing, wheezing, cold hands and feet, dizziness, light-headedness, confusion, depression, rash, fever, sore throat, unusual bleeding, or bruising occurs.
- Instruct patient to inform health care professional of medication regimen prior to treatment or surgery.
- Advise patient to carry identification describing disease process and medication regimen at all times.
- **Hypertension:** Reinforce the need to continue additional therapies for hypertension (weight loss, sodium restriction, stress reduction, regular exercise, moderation of alcohol consumption, and smoking cessation). Medication controls but does not cure hypertension.

Evaluation/Desired Outcomes
- Decrease in blood pressure.

---

lactulose (lak-tyoo-lose)
Cholac, Constilac, Constulose, Enulose, Generlac, Kristalose

Classification
Therapeutic: laxatives
Pharmacologic: osmotics

Pregnancy Category B

Indications
Treatment of chronic constipation. Adjunct in the management of portal-systemic (hepatic) encephalopathy (PSE).

Action
Increases water content and softens the stool. Lowers the pH of the colon, which inhibits the diffusion of ammonia from the colon into the blood, thereby reducing blood ammonia levels. **Therapeutic Effects:** Relief of constipation. Decreased blood ammonia levels with improved mental status in PSE.

Pharmacokinetics
Absorption: Less than 3% absorbed after oral administration.
Distribution: Unknown.
Metabolism and Excretion: Absorbed lactulose is excreted unchanged in the urine. Unabsorbed lactulose is metabolized by colonic bacteria to lactic, acetic, and formic acids.
Half-life: Unknown.

TIME/ACTION PROFILE (relief of constipation)

ROUTE	ONSET	PEAK	DURATION
PO	24–48 hr	unknown	unknown

Contraindications/Precautions
Contraindicated in: Patients on low-galactose diets.
Use Cautiously in: Diabetes mellitus; Excessive or prolonged use (may lead to dependence); OB, Lactation: Safety not established.

Adverse Reactions/Side Effects
GI: <u>belching</u>, <u>cramps</u>, distention, <u>flatulence</u>, diarrhea. **Endo:** hyperglycemia (diabetic patients).

Interactions
Drug-Drug: Should not be used with other **laxatives** in the treatment of hepatic encephalopathy (leads to inability to determine optimal dose of lactulose). **Anti-infectives** may ↓ effectiveness in treatment of hepatic encephalopathy.

Route/Dosage
Constipation
PO (Adults): 15–30 mL/day up to 60 mL/day as liquid or 10–20 g as powder for oral solution (up to 40 g /day has been used).
PO (Children): 7.5 mL daily after breakfast (unlabeled).

PSE
PO (Adults): 30–45 mL 3–4 times/day; may be given q 1–2 hr initially to induce laxation.
PO (Infants): 2.5–10 mL daily in 3–4 divided doses (unlabeled).
PO (Children and Adolescents): 40–90 mL daily in 3–4 divided doses (unlabeled).
Rect (Adults): 300 mL diluted and administered as a retention enema q 4–6 hr.

Availability (generic available)
Oral solution: 10 g lactulose/15 mL. **Rectal solution:** 10 g lactulose/15 mL. **Single-use packets (Kristalose):** 10 g (equal to 15 mL liquid lactulose), 20 g (equal to 30 mL liquid lactulose).

NURSING IMPLICATIONS
Assessment
- Assess patient for abdominal distention, presence of bowel sounds, and normal pattern of bowel function.
- Assess color, consistency, and amount of stool produced.
- **PSE:** Assess mental status (orientation, level of consciousness) before and periodically throughout course of therapy.
- *Lab Test Considerations:* ↓ blood ammonia concentrations by 25–50%.
- May cause ↑ blood glucose levels in diabetic patients.
- Monitor serum electrolytes periodically when used chronically. May cause diarrhea with resulting hypokalemia and hypernatremia.

Potential Nursing Diagnoses
Constipation (Indications)

Implementation
- When used in hepatic encephalopathy, adjust dose until patient averages 2–3 soft bowel movements per day. During initial therapy, 30–45 mL may be given hourly to induce rapid laxation.
- Darkening of solution does not alter potency.
- **PO:** Mix with fruit juice, water, milk, or carbonated citrus beverage to improve flavor. Administer with a full glass (240 mL) of water or juice. May be administered on an empty stomach for more rapid results.
- Dissolve single dose packets (Kristalose) in 4 oz of water. Solution should be colorless to slightly pale yellow.
- **Rect:** To administer enema, use rectal balloon catheter. Mix 300 mL of lactulose with 700 mL of water or 0.9% NaCl. Enema should be retained for 30–60 min. If inadvertently evacuated, may repeat administration.

Patient/Family Teaching
- Encourage patients to use other forms of bowel regulation, such as increasing bulk in the diet, increasing fluid intake, and increasing mobility. Normal bowel habits are individualized and may vary from 3 times/day to 3 times/wk.
- Caution patients that this medication may cause belching, flatulence, or abdominal cramping. Health care professional should be notified if this becomes bothersome or if diarrhea occurs.

Evaluation/Desired Outcomes
- Passage of a soft, formed bowel movement, usually within 24–48 hr.
- Clearing of confusion, apathy, and irritation and improved mental status in PSE. Improvement may occur within 2 hr after enema and 24–48 hr after oral administration.

---

lamivudine (la-mi-vyoo-deen)
Epivir, Epivir-HBV , 3TC

Classification
Therapeutic: antiretrovirals, antivirals
Pharmacologic: nucleoside reverse transcriptase inhibitors

Pregnancy Category C

Indications
HIV infection (with other antiretrovirals). Chronic hepatitis B infection. **Unlabeled Use:** Part of HIV-postexposure prophylaxis with zidovudine and indinavir.

Action
After intracellular conversion to its active form (lamivudine-5-triphosphate), inhibits viral DNA synthesis by inhibiting the enzyme reverse transcriptase. **Therapeutic Effects:** Slows the progression of HIV infection and decreases the occurrence of its sequelae. Increases CD4 cell

counts and decreases viral load. Protection from liver damage caused by chronic hepatitis B infection; decreases viral load.

Pharmacokinetics
Absorption: Well absorbed after oral administration (86% in adults, 66% in infants and children).
Distribution: Distributes into the extravascular space. Some penetration into CSF; remainder of distribution unknown.
Metabolism and Excretion: Mostly excreted unchanged in urine; <5% metabolized by the liver.
Half-life: *Adults*—3.7 hr; *children*—2 hr.

TIME/ACTION PROFILE (blood levels)

ROUTE	ONSET	PEAK	DURATION
PO	unknown	0.9 hr†	12 hr

†On an empty stomach; peak levels occur at 3.2 hr if lamivudine is taken with food. Food does not affect total amount of drug absorbed.

Contraindications/Precautions
Contraindicated in: Hypersensitivity; Lactation: Breastfeeding not recommended for HIV positive mothers.
Use Cautiously in: Impaired renal function (↑ dosing interval/ ↓ dose if CCr <50 mL/min); Women, prolonged exposure, obesity, history of liver disease (↑ risk of lactic acidosis and severe hepatomegaly with steatosis); Coinfection with hepatitis B (hepatitis may recur after discontinuation of lamivudine); OB, Pedi: Pregnancy or children <3 mo (safety not established); Geri: ↓ dosage may be necessary due to age-related ↓ in renal function.
Exercise Extreme Caution in: Pedi: Pediatric patients with a history of or significant risk factors for pancreatitis (use only if no alternative).

Adverse Reactions/Side Effects
Noted for combination of lamivudine plus zidovudine.
CNS: SEIZURES, fatigue, headache, insomnia, malaise, depression, dizziness. **Resp:** cough. **GI:** HEPATOMEGALY WITH STEATOSIS, PANCREATITIS (↑ in pediatric patients), anorexia, diarrhea, nausea, vomiting, abdominal discomfort, abnormal liver function studies, dyspepsia. **Derm:** alopecia, erythema multiforme, rashes, urticaria. **Endo:** hyperglycemia. **F and E:** lactic acidosis. **Hemat:** anemia, neutropenia, pure red cell aplasia. **MS:** musculoskeletal pain, arthralgia, muscle weakness, myalgia, rhabdomyolysis. **Neuro:** neuropathy. **Misc:** hypersensitivity reactions including ANAPHYLAXIS and STEVENS-JOHNSON SYNDROME.

Interactions
Drug-Drug: **Trimethoprim/sulfamethoxazole** ↑ lamivudine blood levels (dose alteration may be necessary in renal impairment). ↑ risk of pancreatitis with concurrent use of other **drugs causing pancreatitis**. ↑ risk of neuropathy with concurrent use of other **drugs causing neuropathy**. Combination therapy with **tenofovir** and **abacavir** may lead to virologic nonresponse and should not be used.

Route/Dosage
HIV infection
PO (Adults and Children >16 yr and ≥50 kg): 150 mg twice daily or 300 mg once daily.
PO (Adults <50 kg): 2 mg/kg twice daily.
PO (Children 3 mo–16 yr): *Oral solution*–4 mg/kg twice daily (up to 150 mg twice daily); *Tablets*—14–21 kg: 75 mg twice daily; 22–29 kg: 75 mg in AM, 150 mg in PM; ≥30 kg: 150 mg twice daily.

Renal Impairment
PO (Adults): *CCr 30–49 mL/min*—150 mg once daily; *CCr 15–29 mL/min*—150 mg first dose, then 100 mg once daily; *CCr 5–14 mL/min*—150 mg first dose, then 50 mg once daily; *CCr <5 mL/min*—50 mg first dose, then 25 mg once daily.

Chronic Hepatitis B
PO (Adults): 100 mg once daily.

Renal Impairment
PO (Adults): *CCr 30–49 mL/min*—100 mg first dose, then 50 mg once daily; *CCr 15–29 mL/min*—100 mg first dose, then 25 mg once daily; *CCr 5–14 mL/min*—35 mg first dose, then 15 mg once daily; *CCr <5 mL/min*—35 mg first dose, then 10 mg once daily.
PO (Children 2–17 yr): 3 mg/kg once daily (up to 100 mg/day).

Availability
Epivir
Tablets: 150 mg, 300 mg. **Oral solution (strawberry-banana flavor):** 10 mg/mL. *In combination with:* abacavir (Epzicom); zidovudine (Combivir); zidovudine and abacavir (Trizivir). See Appendix B.

Epivir-HBV
Tablets: 100 mg. **Oral solution (strawberry-banana flavor):** 5 mg/mL.

NURSING IMPLICATIONS
Assessment
- **HIV:** Assess patient for change in severity of symptoms of HIV infection and for symptoms of opportunistic infection during therapy.
- Monitor patient for signs and symptoms of peripheral neuropathy (tingling, burning, numbness, or pain in hands or feet); may be difficult to differentiate from peripheral neuropathy of severe HIV disease. May require discontinuation of therapy.
- **Assess patient, especially pediatric patients, for signs of pancreatitis (nausea, vomiting, abdominal pain) periodically during therapy. May require discontinuation of therapy.**
- **Chronic Hepatitis B Infection:** Monitor signs of hepatitis (jaundice, fatigue, anorexia, pruritus) during therapy.
- *Lab Test Considerations:* .
- Monitor viral load and CD4 levels before and periodically during therapy.
- Monitor serum amylase, lipase, and triglycerides periodically during therapy. Elevated serum levels may indicate pancreatitis and require discontinuation.
- Monitor liver function. May cause ↑ levels of AST, ALT, CPK, bilirubin, and alkaline phosphatase, which usually resolve after interruption of therapy. Lactic acidosis may occur with hepatic toxicity causing hepatic steatosis; may be fatal, especially in women.
- May rarely cause neutropenia and anemia.

Potential Nursing Diagnoses
Risk for infection (Indications)

Implementation
- Do not confuse lamivudine with lamotrigine. Do not confuse Epivir tablets and oral solution with Epivir-HBV tablets and oral solutions. Epivir Tablets and Oral Solution contain a higher dose of the same active ingredient (lamivudine) than in Epivir-HBV Tablets and Oral Solution. Epivir-HBV was developed for patients with hepatitis B and should not be used for patients dually infected with HIV and hepatitis B; use may lead to lamivudine-resistant HIV due to subtherapeutic dose.
- **PO:** May be administered without regard to food.

Patient/Family Teaching
- Instruct patient to take lamivudine as directed, every 12 hr. Explain the difference between Epivir and Epivir-HBV to patients. Emphasize the importance of compliance with full course of therapy, not taking more than the prescribed amount, and not discontinuing without consulting health care professional. Take missed doses as soon as possible unless almost time for next dose. Do not double doses. Caution patient not to share medication with others.
- Inform patient that lamivudine does not cure HIV disease or prevent associated or opportunistic infections. Lamivudine does not reduce the risk of transmission of HIV to others through sexual contact or blood contamination. Caution patient to use a condom during sexual contact and avoid sharing needles or donating blood to prevent spreading HIV to others. Advise patient that the long-term effects of lamivudine are unknown at this time.
- Instruct patient to notify health care professional promptly if signs of peripheral neuropathy or pancreatitis occur.
- Advise patient not to take other Rx, OTC, or herbal products without consulting health care professional.
- Emphasize the importance of regular follow-up exams and blood tests to determine progress and monitor for side effects.

Evaluation/Desired Outcomes
- Slowing of the progression of HIV infection and its sequelae.
- Decrease in viral load and improvement in CD4 levels in patients with advanced HIV infection.
- Protection from liver damage caused by chronic hepatitis B infection; decreases viral load.

---

lamotrigine (la-moe-tri-jeen)
Lamictal

Classification
Therapeutic: anticonvulsants

Pregnancy Category C

Indications
Adjunct treatment of partial seizures in adults with epilepsy (immediate-release, extended-release, chewable, and orally disintegrating tablets). Lennox-Gastaut syndrome (immediate-release, chewable, and orally disintegrating tablets only). Primary generalized tonic-clonic seizures in adults and children ≥2 yr (immediate-release, chewable, and orally disintegrating tablets only). Conversion to monotherapy in adults with partial seizures receiving a single enzyme-inducing

lamotrigine

antiepileptic drug (immediate-release, chewable, and orally disintegrating tablets only). Maintenance treatment of bipolar disorder (immediate-release, chewable, and orally disintegrating tablets only).

Action
Stabilizes neuronal membranes by inhibiting sodium transport. **Therapeutic Effects:** Decreased incidence of seizures. Delayed time to recurrence of mood episodes.

Pharmacokinetics
Absorption: 98% absorbed following oral administration.
Distribution: Enters breast milk. Highly bound to melanin-containing tissues (eyes, pigmented skin).
Metabolism and Excretion: Mostly metabolized by the liver to inactive metabolites; 10% excreted unchanged by the kidneys.
Half-life: Children taking enzyme–inducing antiepileptic drugs (AEDs): 7–10 hr; Children taking enzyme inducers and valproic acid: 15–27 hr; Children taking valproic acid: 44–94 hr; Adults: 25.4 hr (during chronic therapy of lamotrigine alone).

TIME/ACTION PROFILE (blood levels)

ROUTE	ONSET	PEAK	DURATION
PO	unknown	1.4–4.8 hr; 4–10 hr (XR)	unknown

Contraindications/Precautions
Contraindicated in: Hypersensitivity; Lactation: Lactation.
Use Cautiously in: All patients (may ↑ risk of suicidal thoughts/behaviors); Patients with renal dysfunction, impaired cardiac function, and hepatic dysfunction (lower maintenance doses may be required); Prior history of rash to lamotrigine; OB: Exposure during first trimester may ↑ risk of cleft lip/palate; Pedi: Immediate-release, chewable, and orally disintegrating tablets not safe for children <2 yr; extended-release tablets not approved for use in children <13 yr.

Adverse Reactions/Side Effects
CNS: SUICIDAL THOUGHTS, ataxia, dizziness, headache, behavior changes, depression, drowsiness, insomnia, tremor. **EENT:** blurred vision, double vision, rhinitis. **GI:** nausea, vomiting. **GU:** vaginitis. **Derm:** photosensitivity, rash (higher incidence in children, patients taking valproic acid, high initial doses, or rapid dose increases). **MS:** arthralgia. **Misc:** STEVENS-JOHNSON SYNDROME.

Interactions
Drug-Drug: Concurrent use with **carbamazepine** may result in ↓ levels of lamotrigine and ↑ levels of an active metabolite of carbamazepine. Lamotrigine levels are ↓ by concurrent use of **phenobarbital, phenytoin,** or **primidone**. Concurrent use with **valproic acid** results in a twofold ↑ in lamotrigine levels, ↑ incidence of rash, and a ↓ in valproic acid level (lamotrigine dose should be ↓ by at least 50%). **Oral contraceptives** may ↓ serum levels of lamotrigine (dose adjustments may be necessary when starting and stopping oral contraceptives).

Route/Dosage
Epilepsy
In Combination with Other Antiepileptic Agents
PO (Adults and Children > 12 yr; Immediate-release, chewable, or orally disintegrating tablets): *Patients taking anti-epileptic drugs other than carbamazepine, phenobarbital, phenytoin, primidone, or valproate*—25 mg daily for first 2 wk, then 50 mg daily for next 2 wk; then ↑ by 50 mg/day every 1–2 wk to maintenance dose of 225–375 mg/day (in 2 divided doses); *Patients taking carbamazepine, phenobarbital, phenytoin, or primidone (and not valproate)*—50 mg daily for first 2 wk, then 50 mg twice daily for next 2 wk; then ↑ by 100 mg/day every 1–2 wk to maintenance dose of 300–500 mg/day (in 2 divided doses); *Patients taking regimen containing valproate*—25 mg every other day for first 2 wk, then 25 mg daily for next 2 wk; then ↑ by 25–50 mg/day every 1–2 wk to maintenance dose of 100–400 mg/day (in 1–2 divided doses) (maintenance dose of 100–200 mg/day if receiving valproate alone).
PO (Adults and Children > 12 yr; Extended-release tablets): *Patients taking anti-epileptic drugs other than carbamazepine, phenobarbital, phenytoin, primidone, or valproate* -25 mg daily for first 2 wk, then 50 mg daily for next 2 wk; then 100 mg daily for 1 wk, then 150 mg daily for 1 wk, then 200 mg/day for 1 wk, then ↑ by 100 mg/day every week to maintenance dose of 300–400 mg daily; *Patients taking carbamazepine, phenobarbital, phenytoin, or primidone (and not valproate)*—50 mg daily for first 2 wk, then 100 mg daily for next 2 wk, then 200 mg daily for

1 wk, then 300 mg daily for 1 wk, then 400 mg daily for 1 wk, then ↑ by 100 mg/day every week to maintenance dose of 400–600 mg daily; *Patients taking regimen containing valproate*— 25 mg every other day for first 2 wk, then 25 mg daily for next 2 wk, then 50 mg daily for 1e wk, then 100 mg daily for 1 wk, then 150 mg daily for 1 wk, then maintenance dose of 200–250 mg daily.

PO (Children 2–12 yr; Immediate-release, chewable, or orally disintegrating tablets): *Patients taking anti-epileptic drugs other than carbamazepine, phenobarbital, phenytoin, primidone, or valproate* —0.3 mg/kg/day in 1–2 divided doses (rounded down to nearest whole tablet) for first 2 wk, then 0.6 mg/kg/day in 2 divided doses (rounded down to nearest whole tablet) for next 2 wk; then ↑ by 0.6 mg/kg/day (rounded down to nearest whole tablet) every 1–2 wk to maintenance dose of 4.5-7.5 mg/kg/day (not to exceed 300 mg/day in 2 divided doses); *Patients taking carbamazepine, phenobarbital, phenytoin, or primidone (and not valproate)*—0.6 mg/kg/day in 2 divided doses (rounded down to nearest whole tablet) for first 2 wk, then 1.2 mg/kg/day in 2 divided doses (rounded down to nearest whole tablet) for next 2 wk; then ↑ by 1.2 mg/kg/day (rounded down to nearest whole tablet) every 1–2 wk to maintenance dose of 5–15 mg/kg/day (not to exceed 400 mg/day in 2 divided doses). *Patients taking regimen containing valproate*—0.15 mg/kg/day in 1–2 divided doses (rounded down to nearest whole tablet) for first 2 wk, then 0.3 mg/kg in 1–2 divided doses (rounded down to nearest whole tablet) for next 2 wk; then ↑ by 0.3 mg/kg/day (rounded down to nearest whole tablet) every 1–2 wk to maintenance dose of 1–5 mg/kg/day (not to exceed 200 mg/day in 1–2 divided doses) (maintenance dose of 1–3 mg/kg/day if receiving valproate alone).

Conversion to Monotherapy
PO (Adults ≥ 16 yr): 50 mg/day for 2 wk, then 50 mg twice daily for 2 wk, then ↑ by 100 mg/day q 1–2 wk to maintenance dose of 300–500 mg/day in 2 divided doses; when target level is reached, ↓ other antiepileptics by 20% weekly over 4 wk.

Bipolar Disorder
Escalation Regimen
PO (Adults): *Patients not taking cabamazepine, phenobarbital, phenytoin, primidone, rifampin, or valproate*—25 mg daily for first 2 wk, then 50 mg daily for next 2 wk, then 100 mg daily for 1 wk, then 200 mg daily; *Patients taking valproate*—25 mg every other day for first 2 wk, then 25 mg daily for next 2 wk, then 50 mg daily for 1 wk, then 100 mg daily; *Patients taking carbamazepine, phenobarbital, phenytoin, primidone, or rifampin (and not valproate)* 50 mg daily for first 2 wk, then 100 mg/day (in divided doses) for next 2 wk, then 200 mg/day (in divided doses) for one wk, then 300 mg/day (in divided doses) for 1 wk, then up to 400 mg/day (in divided doses).

Dosage Adjustment Following Discontinuation of Other Psychotropics
PO (Adults): *Following discontinuation of valproate (if current dose 100 mg/day)*— ↑ to 150 mg/day for 1 wk, then 200 mg/day; *Following discontinuation of carbamazepine, phenobarbital, phenytoin, primidone, or rifampin (if current dose 400 mg/day)*—400 mg/day for 1 wk, then 300 mg/day for 1 wk, then 200 mg/day; *Following discontinuation of other psychotropics*—maintain previous dose.

Availability (generic available)
Immediate-release tablets: 25 mg, 100 mg, 150 mg, 200 mg. **Cost:** 25 mg $668.97/180, 100 mg $708.97/180, 150 mg $819.90/180, 200 mg $905.89/180. **Chewable dispersible tablets:** 2 mg, 5 mg, 25 mg. **Cost:** *Generic*—5 mg $453.96/180, 25 mg $489.92/180. **Orally disintegrating tablets:** 25 mg, 50 mg, 100 mg, 200 mg. **Extended-release tablets:** 25 mg, 50 mg, 100 mg, 200 mg.

NURSING IMPLICATIONS
Assessment
- Monitor closely for notable changes in behavior that could indicate the emergence or worsening of suicidal thoughts or behavior or depression.
- Assess patient for skin rash frequently during therapy. Discontinue lamotrigine at first sign of rash; may be life-threatening. Stevens-Johnson syndrome or toxic epidermal necrolysis may develop. Rash usually occurs during the initial 2–8 wk of therapy and is more frequent in patients taking multiple antiepileptic agents, especially valproic acid, and much more frequent in patients <16 yr.
- Monitor for hypersensitivity reactions (fever, lymphadenopathy with or without rash) If cause cannot be determined, discontinue lamotrigine immediately.
- **Seizures:** Assess location, duration, and characteristics of seizure activity.

- **Bipolar disorders:** Assess mood, ideation, and behaviors frequently. Initiate suicide precautions if indicated.
- ***Lab Test Considerations:*** Lamotrigine plasma concentrations may be monitored periodically during therapy, especially in patients concurrently taking other anticonvulsants. Therapeutic plasma concentration range has not been established, proposed therapeutic range: 1–5 mcg/mL.

Potential Nursing Diagnoses
Risk for impaired skin integrity (Adverse Reactions)
Risk for injury (Side Effects)

Implementation
- Do not confuse lamotrigine (Lamictal) with terbinafine (Lamisil), diphenoxylate/atropine (Lomotil), or lamivudine (Epivir).
- When converting from immediate-release to XR form, initial dose of XR should match the total daily dose of immediate-release lamotrigine; monitor closely and adjust and needed.
- **PO:** May be administered without regard to meals. Swallow XR tablets whole; do not break, crush, or chew.
- Lamotrigine should be discontinued gradually over at least 2 wk, unless safety concerns require a more rapid withdrawal. Abrupt discontinuation may cause increase in seizure frequency.
- **Orally Disintegrating Tablets:** Place on the tongue and move around the mouth. Tablet will rapidly disintegrate, can be swallowed with or without water, and can be taken with or without food.
- **Chewable/Dispersible Tablets:** May be swallowed whole, chewed, or dispersed in water or dispersed in fruit juice. If chewed, follow with water or fruit juice to aid in swallowing. Only use whole tablets, do not attempt to administer partial quantities of dispersible tablets.

Patient/Family Teaching
- Instruct patient to take medication exactly as directed. Take missed doses as soon as possible unless almost time for next dose. Do not double doses. Do not discontinue abruptly; may cause increase in frequency of seizures. Instruct patient to read the *Medication Guide* before starting and with each Rx refill, changes may occur.
- Advise patient to notify health care professional immediately if skin rash, fever, or swollen lymph glands occur or if frequency of seizures increases.
- May cause dizziness, drowsiness, and blurred vision. Caution patient to avoid driving or activities requiring alertness until response to medication is known. Do not resume driving until physician gives clearance based on control of seizure disorder.
- Caution patient to wear sunscreen and protective clothing to prevent photosensitivity reactions.
- Advise patient and family to notify health care professional if thoughts about suicide or dying, attempts to commit suicide; new or worse depression; new or worse anxiety; feeling very agitated or restless; panic attacks; trouble sleeping; new or worse irritability; acting aggressive; being angry or violent; acting on dangerous impulses; an extreme increase in activity and talking; other unusual changes in behavior or mood occur.
- Advise patient to notify health care professional if pregnancy is planned or suspected or if breastfeeding.
- Instruct patient to notify health care professional of medication regimen prior to treatment or surgery.
- Advise patient to carry identification at all times describing disease process and medication regimen.

Evaluation/Desired Outcomes
- Decrease in the frequency of or cessation of seizures.
- Decreased incidence of mood swings in bipolar disorders.

---

lansoprazole (lan-**soe**-pra-zole)
Prevacid, Prevacid 24 Hr

Classification
Therapeutic: antiulcer agents
Pharmacologic: proton-pump inhibitors

Pregnancy Category B

Indications
Erosive esophagitis. Duodenal ulcers (with or without anti-infectives for *Helicobacter pylori*). Active benign gastric ulcer. Short-term treatment of symptomatic GERD. Healing and risk reduction of NSAID-associated gastric ulcer. Pathologic hy-

persecretory conditions, including Zollinger-Ellison syndrome. **OTC:** Heartburn occurring ≥twice/wk.

Action
Binds to an enzyme in the presence of acidic gastric pH, preventing the final transport of hydrogen ions into the gastric lumen. **Therapeutic Effects:** Diminished accumulation of acid in the gastric lumen, with lessened acid reflux. Healing of duodenal ulcers and esophagitis.

Pharmacokinetics
Absorption: 80% absorbed after oral administration.
Distribution: Unknown.
Protein Binding: 97%.
Metabolism and Excretion: Extensively metabolized by the liver to inactive compounds. Converted intracellularly to at least two other antisecretory compounds.
Half-life: Children: 1.2–1.5 hr; Adults: 1.3–1.7 hr (↑ in geriatric patients and patients with impaired hepatic function).

TIME/ACTION PROFILE (acid suppression)

ROUTE	ONSET	PEAK	DURATION
PO	rapid	1.7 hr	more than 24 hr

Contraindications/Precautions
Contraindicated in: Hypersensitivity.
Use Cautiously in: Solutabs contain aspartame; use caution when used in phenylketonurics; Severe hepatic impairment (not to exceed 30 mg/day in these patients); OB, Lactation: Safety not established; Pedi: Safety not established in children <1 yr; Geri: Maintenance dose not to exceed 30 mg/day unless additional acid suppression is required.

Adverse Reactions/Side Effects
CNS: dizziness, headache. **GI:** diarrhea, abdominal pain, nausea. **Derm:** rash.

Interactions
Drug-Drug: Sucralfate ↓ absorption of lansoprazole (take 30 min before sucralfate). May ↓ absorption of drugs requiring acid pH, including **ketoconazole**, **itraconazole**, **atazanavir** **ampicillin**, **iron salts**, and **digoxin**. May ↑ risk of bleeding with **warfarin** (monitor INR/PT). May ↓ the anti-platelet effects of **clopidogrel**.

Route/Dosage
PO (Adults and children ≥12 yr): *Short-term treatment of duodenal ulcer*— 15 mg once daily for 4 wk; *H. pylori eradication to reduce the risk of duodenal ulcer recurrence*— 30 mg twice daily with clarithromycin 500 mg twice daily and amoxicillin 1000 mg twice daily for 10–14 days (triple therapy) or 30 mg 3 times daily with 1000 mg amoxicillin 3 times daily for 14 days (dual therapy); *maintenance of healed duodenal ulcers*—15 mg once daily; *short-term treatment of gastric ulcers/healing of NSAID-associated gastric ulcer*—30 mg once daily for up to 8 wk; *risk reduction of NSAID-associated gastric ulcer*—15 mg once daily for up to 12 wk; *short-term treatment of symptomatic GERD*—15 mg once daily for up to 8 wk; *short-term treatment of erosive esophagitis*—30 mg once daily for up to 8 wk (8 additional weeks may be necessary); *maintenance of healing of erosive esophagitis*—15 mg once daily; *pathologic hypersecretory conditions*—60 mg once daily intially, up to 90 mg twice daily (daily dose >120 mg should be given in divided doses).

PO (Adults): *OTC*—15 mg once daily for up to 14 days (14 day course may be repeated every 4 mo).

PO (Children 1–11 yr and >30 kg): *GERD*— 30 mg once to twice daily.

PO (Children 1–11 yr and 10–30 kg): *GERD*—15 mg once or twice daily.

PO (Children 1–11 yr and <10 kg): *GERD*— 7.5 mg once daily.

Availability (generic available)
Delayed-release capsules: 15 mg[Rx, OTC], 30 mg. **Cost:** 15 mg $136.28/30, 30 mg $444.38/100.
Delayed-release orally disintegrated tablets (SoluTabs): 15 mg, 30 mg. *In combination with:* amoxicillin and clarithromycin as part of a compliance package (Prevpac). See Appendix B.

NURSING IMPLICATIONS

Assessment
- Assess patient routinely for epigastric or abdominal pain and for frank or occult blood in stool, emesis, or gastric aspirate.
- *Lab Test Considerations:* May cause abnormal liver function tests, including ↑ AST, ALT, alkaline phosphatase, LDH, and bilirubin.
- May cause ↑ serum creatinine and ↑ or ↓ electrolyte levels.
- May alter RBC, WBC, and platelet levels.
- May also cause ↑ gastrin levels, abnormal A/G ratio, hyperlipidemia, and ↑ or ↓ cholesterol.
- Monitor INR and prothrombin time in patients taking warfarin.

Potential Nursing Diagnoses
Acute pain (Indications)

Implementation

- Do not confuse Prevacid (lansoprazole) with Pravachol (pravastatin).
- **PO:** Administer before meals. Capsules may be opened and sprinkled on 1 tbsp of applesauce, pudding, cottage cheese, or yogurt and swallowed immediately for patients with difficulty swallowing. Do not crush or chew capsule contents.
- For patients with an NG tube, capsules may be opened and intact granules may be mixed in 40 mL of apple, cranberry, grape, orange, pineapple, prune, or V8 vegetable juice and injected through the NG tube into stomach. Flush NG tube with additional apple juice to clear tube. If administered via jejunostomy tube, lansoprazole should be prepared as a suspension with 2.5 mL of 4.2% sodium bicarbonate and 2.5 mL water.
- *Orally disintegrating tablets* may be placed on tongue, allowed to disintegrate and swallowed with or without water. For administration via oral syringe or nasogastric tube, *Prevacid SoluTab* can be administered by placing a 15-mg tablet in oral syringe and drawing up 4 mL of water, or a 30-mg tablet in oral syringe and drawing up 10 mL of water. Shake gently to allow for a quick dispersal. After tablet has dispersed, administer the contents within 15 minutes. Refill syringe with 2 mL (5 mL for the 30-mg tablet) of water, shake gently, and administer any remaining contents and flush nasogastric tube.
- Antacids may be used concurrently.

Patient/Family Teaching

- Instruct patient to take medication as directed for the full course of therapy, even if feeling better.
- Advise patient to avoid alcohol, products containing aspirin or NSAIDs, and foods that may cause an increase in GI irritation.
- May occasionally cause dizziness. Caution patient to avoid driving and other activities that require alertness until response to medication is known.
- Advise patient to report onset of black, tarry stools; diarrhea; or abdominal pain to health care professional promptly.

Evaluation/Desired Outcomes

- Decrease in abdominal pain or prevention of gastric irritation and bleeding. Healing of duodenal ulcers can be seen on x-ray examination or endoscopy. Therapy is continued for at least 2–4 wk. Therapy for pathologic hypersecretory conditions may be long term.
- Healing in patients with erosive esophagitis. Therapy is continued for up to 8 wk, and an additional 8-wk course may be used for patients who do not heal in 8 wk or whose ulcer recurs.

lanthanum carbonate
(lan-than-um)
Fosrenol

Classification
Therapeutic: hypophosphatemics
Pharmacologic: phosphate binders

Pregnancy Category C

Indications
Reduction of serum phosphate levels associated with end-stage renal disease.

Action
Dissociates in the upper GI tract forming lanthanate ions, which form an insoluble complex with phosphate. **Therapeutic Effects:** Decreased serum phosphate levels.

Pharmacokinetics
Absorption: Negligible absorption.
Distribution: Stays within the GI tract.
Metabolism and Excretion: Eliminated almost entirely in feces.
Half-life: 53 hr (in plasma).

TIME/ACTION PROFILE (effect on phosphate levels)

ROUTE	ONSET	PEAK	DURATION
PO	unknown	2–3 wk	unknown

Contraindications/Precautions
Contraindicated in: OB: Congenital abnormalities noted in animal studies; Pedi: Potential negative effect on developing bone.
Use Cautiously in: Peptic ulcer disease, ulcerative colitis, Crohn's disease, any predisposition to bowel obstruction; Lactation: Safety not established.

Adverse Reactions/Side Effects
GI: nausea, vomiting, diarrhea.

Interactions
Drug-Drug: Drugs known to interact with **antacids** may interact with lanthanum carbonate; separate dosing by 2 hr.

Route/Dosage
PO (Adults): 750–1500 mg/day in divided doses; may be titrated upward every 2–3 wk in increments of 750 mg/day up to 3750 mg/day (usual range 1500–3000 mg/day).

Availability
Chewable tablets: 250 mg, 500 mg.

NURSING IMPLICATIONS

Assessment
- Assess patient for nausea and vomiting during therapy.
- **Lab Test Considerations:** Monitor serum phosphate levels prior to and periodically during therapy.

Potential Nursing Diagnoses
Nausea (Side Effects)

Implementation
- Divide total daily dose and administer with meals.
- **PO:** Administer with or immediately after meals. Tablets should be chewed completely before swallowing; intact tablets should not be swallowed.

Patient/Family Teaching
- Instruct patient to take lanthanum as directed.

Evaluation/Desired Outcomes
- Decrease in serum phosphate to below than 6.0 mg/dL in patients with end stage renal disease.

✠ lapatinib (la-pat-i-nib)
Tykerb

Classification
Therapeutic: antineoplastics
Pharmacologic: enzyme inhibitors, kinase inhibitors

Pregnancy Category D

Indications
✠ Advanced metastatic breast cancer with tumor overexpression of the Human Epidermal Receptor Type 2 (HER2) and past therapy with an anthracycline, a taxane and trastuzumab; used in combination with capecitabine (Xeloda).

Action
✠ Acts as an inhibitor of intracellular tyrosine kinase affecting Epidermal Growth Factor (EGFR, ErbB1) and HER2 (ErbB2). Inhibits the growth of ErbB-driven tumors. Effect is additive with capecitabine. **Therapeutic Effects:** Decreased/slowed spread of metastatic breast cancer.

Pharmacokinetics
Absorption: Incompletely and variably absorbed following oral administration blood levels are increased by food.
Distribution: Unknown.
Protein Binding: >99%.
Metabolism and Excretion: Extensively metabolized by, mostly by CYP3A4 and CYP3A5 enzyme systems; <2% excreted by kidneys.
Half-life: 24 hr.

TIME/ACTION PROFILE (blood levels)

ROUTE	ONSET	PEAK	DURATION
PO	unknown	4 hr	24 hr

Contraindications/Precautions
Contraindicated in: ↓ left ventricular ejection fraction (Grade 2 or greater); OB, Lactation: Pregnancy or lactation.
Use Cautiously in: Concurrent use of CYP3A4 inhibitors including ketoconazole, itraconazole, clarithromycin, atazanavir, indinavir, nefazodone, nelfinavir, ritoanvir, saquinavir, telithromycin, and voriconazole should be avoided (if necessary, dose reduction of lapatinib is required); Concurrent use of CYP3A4 inducers including dexamathasone, phenytoin, carbamazepine, rifampin, rifabutin, rifapentin and phenobarbital may decrease levels and effectiveness and should be avoided (if necassary, dose of lapatinib may be titrated upward to 4500 mg/day as tolerated); Severe hepatic impairment (dose reduction recommended for Child-Pugh Class C); Known QTc prolongation or co-existing risk factors of QTc prolongation including hypokalemia, hypomagnesemia, concurrent anti-arrhythmics or medications that are known to prolong QTc; Geri: May be more sensitive to effects; Pedi: Safety not established.

Adverse Reactions/Side Effects
CNS: fatigue, insomnia. **Resp:** dyspnea, interstitial lung disease, pneumonitis. **CV:** ↓ left ventricular ejection fraction. **GI:** HEPATOTOXICITY, diarrhea, nausea, vomiting, dyspepsia, ↑ liver enzymes, stomatitis. **Derm:** palmar-plantar erythrodysesthesia, rash, dry skin. **Hemat:** neutropenia. **MS:** back pain, extremity pain.

Interactions
Drug-Drug: Lapatinib inhibits CYP3A4, CYP28 and P-glycoprotein; concurrent use of drugs,

which are substrates for these enzyme should be undertaken with caution. Concurrent use of **CYP3A4 inhibitors** including **ketoconazole, itraconazole, clarithromycin, atazanavir, indinavir, nefazodone, nelfinavir, ritonavir, saquinavir, telithromycin,** and **voriconazole** may ↑ blood levels and the risk of toxicity. Concurrent use should be avoided, but if necessary dosage of lapatinib should be decreased. Concurrent use of **CYP3A4 inducers** including **dexamathasone, phenytoin, carbamazepine, rifampin, rifabutin, rifapentin,** and **phenobarbital** may ↓ blood levels and effectiveness and should be avoided. If necassary, dose of lapatinib may be titrated upward to 4500 mg/day as tolerated.

Drug-Food: Concurrent **grapefruit** may ↑ blood levels and the risk of toxicity and should be avoided.

Route/Dosage
PO (Adults): 1250 mg (5 tablets) once daily for 21 days.

Hepatic Impairment
PO (Adults): *Severe hepatic impairment—* 750 mg/day.

Availability
Tablets: 250 mg.

NURSING IMPLICATIONS

Assessment
- Evaluate left ventricular ejection fraction (LVEF) prior to therapy to determine if within institution's normal limits. Continue to monitor periodically during therapy to ensure it does not fall below limits. If LVEF decreases Grade 2 or greater discontinue therapy. If returns to normal and patient is asymptomatic after 2 wk, may restart therapy at a reduced dose of 1000 mg/day.
- Monitor ECG prior to and periodically during therapy to monitor QT.
- Monitor for respiratory status for symptoms of interstitial lung disease and pneumonitis (dyspnea, cough); may require discontinuation of therapy.
- *Lab Test Considerations:* Monitor liver function tests prior to initiation and every 4–6 wk during therapy and as clinically indicated. Discontinue and do not restart lapatinib if patients experience severe changes in liver function tests.
- Monitor serum potassium and magnesium prior to and periodically during therapy.

Potential Nursing Diagnoses
Diarrhea (Adverse Reactions)

Implementation
- Administer antidiarrheals prior to therapy to prevent severe diarrhea.
- Correct hypokalemia and hypomagnesemia prior to therapy.
- **PO:** Administer 5 tablets once daily at least 1 hr before or 1 hr after a meal for 21 days. Capecitabine is taken with food or 30 min after meals twice daily.

Patient/Family Teaching
- Instruct patient to take lapatinib as directed and to review the *Patient Information Sheet* prior to therapy and with each refill for new information If a dose is missed take as soon remembered that day. If a day is missed, skip the dose; do not double doses. Caution patient not to share this medication with others, even with same condition; may be harmful.
- Advise patient to avoid drinking grapefruit juice or eating grapefruit during therapy.
- Advise patient to report signs or decreased LVEF (shortness of breath, palpitations, fatigue) to health care professional promptly.
- Instruct patient to notify health care professional before taking any Rx, OTC, or herbal products during therapy.
- Advise patient that lapatinib may cause diarrhea, which may become severe. Instruct patient in how to prevent and manage diarrhea.
- Advise female patients to notify health care professional if pregnancy is planned or suspected; therapy may be teratogenic.

Evaluation/Desired Outcomes
- Decreased/slowed spread of metastatic breast cancer.

---

leflunomide (le-flu-noe-mide)
Arava

Classification
Therapeutic: antirheumatics (DMARDs)
Pharmacologic: immune response modifiers

Pregnancy Category X

Indications
Rheumatoid arthritis (disease-modifying agent).

leflunomide

Action
Inhibits an enzyme required for pyrimidine synthesis; has antiproliferative and anti-inflammatory effects. **Therapeutic Effects:** Decreased pain and inflammation, slowed structural progression and improved physical function.

Pharmacokinetics
Absorption: Tablets are 80% absorbed following oral administration; rapidly converted to the M1 metabolite, which is responsible for pharmacologic activity.
Distribution: Crosses the placenta.
Protein Binding: 99%.
Metabolism and Excretion: Extensively metabolized with metabolites excreted in urine (43%) and feces (48%). Also undergoes biliary recycling.
Half-life: 14–18 days.

TIME/ACTION PROFILE (antirheumatic effect)

ROUTE	ONSET	PEAK	DURATION
PO	1 mo	3–6 mo	wk–mos†

†Due to persistence of active metabolite

Contraindications/Precautions
Contraindicated in: Hypersensitivity; Compromised immune function, including bone marrow dysplasia or severe uncontrolled infection; Concurrent vaccination with live vaccines; OB: May cause fetal abnormalities or death. Contact Pregnancy Registry if accidental exposure occurs; Lactation: Lactation.
Use Cautiously in: Renal insufficiency; Pedi: Safety and effectiveness not established; OB: Women with childbearing potential must use two forms of birth control. Should not be used in men attempting to father a child.
Exercise Extreme Caution in: Significant hepatic impairment, including positive serology for hepatitis B or C; or concurrent use of other hepatotoxic agents (↑ risk of hepatotoxicity).

Adverse Reactions/Side Effects
CNS: headache, dizziness, weakness. **Resp:** INTERSTITIAL LUNG DISEASE, bronchitis, cough, pharyngitis, pneumonia, respiratory infection, rhinitis, sinusitis. **CV:** chest pain, hypertension. **GI:** diarrhea, nausea, abdominal pain, ↑ liver enzymes, hepatotoxicity (rare), anorexia, dyspepsia, gastroenteritis, mouth ulcers, vomiting. **GU:** urinary tract infection. **Derm:** alopecia, rash, dry skin, eczema, pruritus. **F and E:** hypokalemia. **Metab:** weight loss. **MS:** arthralgia, back pain, joint disorder, leg cramps, synovitis, tenosynovitis. **Neuro:** paresthesia. **Misc:** allergic reactions, flu syndrome, infections including sepsis and tuberculosis reactivation, pain.

Interactions
Drug-Drug: **Cholestyramine** and **activated charcoal** cause a rapid and significant ↓ in blood levels of active metabolite. Concurrent use of **methotrexate** and other **hepatotoxic drugs** ↑ risk of hepatotoxicity. Concurrent administration of **rifampin** ↑ blood levels of the active metabolite. May ↑ risk of bleeding with **warfarin**.

Route/Dosage
PO (Adults): *Loading dose*—100 mg daily for 3 days; *maintenance dosing*—20 mg/day (if intolerance occurs, dose may be ↓ to 10 mg/day).

Availability (generic available)
Tablets: 10 mg, 20 mg, 100 mg.

NURSING IMPLICATIONS

Assessment
- Assess range of motion and degree of swelling and pain in affected joints before and periodically during therapy.
- Monitor for signs and symptoms of interstitial lung disease (new onset or worsening cough or dyspnea, associated with fever). May require discontinuation of therapy; consider drug elimination procedure if needed.
- *Lab Test Considerations:* Monitor liver function throughout therapy. Assess ALT at baseline, then monthly during initial 6 mo of therapy, then every 6–8 wk. If given concurrently with methotrexate, monitor ALT, AST, and serum albumin monthly. May cause ↑ ALT and AST, which are usually reversible with reduction in dose or discontinuation, but may be fatal. If ALT is 2–3 times the upper limit of normal, reduce dose to 10 mg/day and continue therapy. Monitor closely after dose reduction; plasma levels may not ↓ for several weeks due to long half-life. If ALT ↑ of 2–3 times the upper limit of normal persists despite dose reduction or if ALT >3 times the upper limit of normal occurs, discontinue leflunomide and administer cholestyramine (see Toxicity and Overdose). Monitor closely and readminister cholestyramine as indicated.
- Monitor CBC with platelets monthly for 6 mo following initiation of therapy and every 6–8 wk thereafter. If used with methotrexate or other immunosuppressive therapy continue monitoring monthly. If bone marrow depression occurs, discontinue leflunomide and begin decreasing levels with cholestyramine (see Implementation).

- May rarely cause ↑ of alkaline phosphatase and bilirubin.
- ***Toxicity and Overdose:*** If overdose or significant toxicity occurs, cholestyramine 8 g 3 times a day for 24 hr, or activated charcoal orally or via nasogastric tube, 50 g every 6 hr for 24 hr, is recommended to accelerate elimination.

Potential Nursing Diagnoses
Impaired physical mobility (Indications)
Acute pain (Indications)

Implementation
- Administer a tuberculin skin test prior to administration of leflunomide. Patients with active latent TB should be treated for TB prior to therapy.
- **PO:** Initiate therapy with loading dose of 100 mg/day for 3 days, followed by 20 mg/day dose. May decrease to 10 mg/day if not well tolerated.
- **Drug Elimination Procedure:** Recommended to achieve nondectable plasma levels <0.02 mg/L after stopping treatment with leflunomide. Administer cholestyramine 8 g 3 times daily for 11 days. (Days do not need to be consecutive unless rapid lowering of levels is desired.) Verify plasma levels <0.02 mg/L by 2 separate tests at least 14 days apart. If plasma levels >0.02 mg/L, consider additional cholestyramine treatment. Plasma levels may take up to 2 yr to reach nondetectable levels without drug elimination procedure.

Patient/Family Teaching
- Instruct patient to take leflunomide as directed.
- May cause dizziness. Caution patient to avoid driving or other activities requiring alertness until response to medication is known.
- Caution patients of childbearing age that leflunomide has teratogenic effects. Women wishing to become pregnant must undergo the drug elimination procedure (see Implementation) and verify that the M1 metabolite plasma levels are <0.02 mg/L. Men wishing to father a child should also take cholestyramine 8 g 3 times daily for 11 days to minimize any possible risk.
- Advise patient to consult health care professional prior to taking other Rx, OTC, or herbal products concurrently with leflunomide. Aspirin, NSAIDs, or low-dose corticosteroids may be continued during therapy, but other agents for treatment of rheumatoid arthritis may require discontinuation.
- Discuss the possibility of hair loss with patient. Explore methods of coping.
- Advise patient to notify health care professional if rash, mucous membrane lesions, unusual tiredness, abdominal pain, jaundice, or symptoms of interstitial lung disease occur.
- Instruct patient to avoid vaccinations with live vaccines during and following therapy without consulting health care professional.

Evaluation/Desired Outcomes
- Decrease in signs and symptoms of rheumatoid arthritis and slowing of structural damage as evidenced by x-ray erosions and joint narrowings.
- Improved physical function.

HIGH ALERT

lepirudin (rDNA)
(le-**peer**-yoo-din)
Refludan

Classification
Therapeutic: anticoagulants
Pharmacologic: thrombin inhibitors

Pregnancy Category B

Indications
Management of thromboembolic disease and prevention of its complications in patients who have experienced heparin-induced thrombocytopenia.

Action
Acts as an anticoagulant by inhibiting the action of thrombin. Produced by recombinant DNA technology. **Therapeutic Effects:** Anticoagulation with prevention of thromboembolic complications.

Pharmacokinetics
Absorption: IV administration results in complete bioavailability.
Distribution: Distributes mainly to extracellular fluids.
Metabolism and Excretion: Metabolized by release of amino acids caused by breakdown of drug; 48% excreted unchanged in urine.
Half-life: 1.3 hr.

TIME/ACTION PROFILE (anticoagulant effect)

ROUTE	ONSET	PEAK	DURATION
IV	within 30–90 min	unknown	up to 24 hr

lepirudin (rDNA)

Contraindications/Precautions
Contraindicated in: Hypersensitivity; Severe renal impairment (CCr <15 mL/min or SCr >6 mg/dL).
Use Cautiously in: Recent puncture of large vessels/organ biopsy; Vessel/organ anomaly; Recent CVA, stroke, intracerebral surgery or other neuroaxial procedure; Severe uncontrolled hypertension; Bacterial endocarditis; Hemorrhagic diatheses; Recent major surgery; Recent major bleeding; Severe liver impairment; Moderate renal impairment (↓ bolus and maintenance infusion rate recommended if CCr ≤60 mL/min or SCr >1.5 mg/dL); OB: Lactation, Pedi: Safety not established.

Adverse Reactions/Side Effects
Hemat: BLEEDING. **Misc:** allergic reactions including ANAPHYLAXIS.

Interactions
Drug-Drug: ↑ risk of bleeding with **thrombolytic agents**, **NSAIDs**, **valproic acid**, **cefotetan**, **cefoperazone**, platelet aggregation inhibitors including **aspirin**, **dipyridamole**, **clopidogrel**, **ticlopidine**, **tirofiban**, and **eptifibatide**.

Route/Dosage
IV (Adults): 0.4 mg/kg (not to exceed 44 mg) as a bolus over 15–20 sec, followed by 0.15 mg/kg/hr (not to exceed 16.5 mg/hr) initially, further adjustments made on the basis of laboratory assessment (aPTT) but should not exceed infusion rate of 0.21 mg/kg/hr without checking for coagulation abnormalities.

Renal Impairment
IV (Adults): 0.2 mg/kg as a bolus over 15–20 sec, then if *CCr 45–60 mL/min (or SCr 1.6–2 mg/dL)*—0.075 mg/kg/hr; if *CCr 30–44 mL/min (or SCr 2.1–3 mg/dL)*—0.045 mg/kg/hr; if *CCr 15–29 mL/min (or SCr 3.1–6 mg/dL)*—0.0225 mg/kg/hr.

Availability
Powder for injection: 50 mg/vial.

NURSING IMPLICATIONS

Assessment
- Assess patient for signs of bleeding and hemorrhage (bleeding gums, nosebleed, unusual bruising, black tarry stools, hematuria, fall in hematocrit or blood pressure, guaiac-positive stools). Notify physician if these occur.
- Monitor patient for hypersensitivity reactions (chills, fever, urticaria). Report signs to physician.
- *Lab Test Considerations:* Dose is adjusted according to aPTT ratio (patient aPTT at a given time over aPTT reference value, usually median of laboratory normal range for aPTT). Target range for aPTT ratio during treatment should be 1.5–2.5.
- Determine baseline aPTT prior to therapy; therapy should not be started in patients with an aPTT ratio of >2.5.
- First aPTT should be drawn 4 hr after initiation of therapy, then at least daily during therapy. More frequent monitoring is required in patients with serious liver injury or renal impairment.
- If aPTT ratio is out of target range, confirm ratio before modifying dose, unless clinically necessitated. If the confirmed ratio is above the target range, stop infusion for 2 hr. Restart infusion at 50% of previous dose without bolus and determine aPTT ratio in 4 hr.
- If confirmed ratio is below target range, increase infusion in steps of 20% and determine ratio in 4 hr.
- *Toxicity and Overdose:* If life-threatening bleeding occurs and excessive plasma levels of lepirudin are suspected, immediately stop infusion, determine aPTT and other coagulation levels, determine hemoglobin and prepare for blood transfusion. No specific antidote for lepirudin is available.

Potential Nursing Diagnoses
Ineffective tissue perfusion (Indications)
Risk for injury (Side Effects)

Implementation
- Inform all personnel caring for patient of anticoagulant therapy. Venipunctures and injection sites require application of pressure to prevent bleeding or hematoma formation. IM injections of other medications should be avoided, as hematomas may develop.
- In patients scheduled to receive coumadin derivatives for oral anticoagulation, lepirudin dose should be gradually decreased to reach an aPTT ratio just above 1.5 before initiating oral anticoagulant therapy.

IV Administration
- **Direct IV:** *Diluent:* Reconstitute each vial with 1 mL of sterile water for injection or 0.9% NaCl. Shake gently. Transfer contents of vial into a 10-mL syringe and dilute to a total volume of 10 mL with sterile water for injection, 0.9% NaCl, or D5W. Clear, colorless solution should be obtained within a few seconds to 3 min. Do not use solutions that are cloudy or

contain particulate matter. Solution is stable for 24 hr at room temperature. *Concentration:* 5 mg/mL. *Rate:* Administer slowly over 15–20 sec.
- **Continuous Infusion:** *Diluent:* Reconstitute 2 vials (50 mg each) with 1 mL each of sterile water for injection or 0.9% NaCl. Transfer the contents into an infusion bag containing 500 mL or 250 mL of 0.9% NaCl or D5W. Solution is stable for 24 hr at room temperature. *Concentration:* 0.2–0.4 mg/mL. *Rate:* Based on patient's weight (see Route/Dosage section). Use an infusion pump to ensure accuracy.
- **Y-Site Compatibility:** amiodarone.

Patient/Family Teaching
- Advise patient to report any symptoms of unusual bleeding or bruising to health care professional immediately.
- Caution patient to avoid IM injections and activities leading to injury and to use a soft toothbrush and electric razor during therapy.

Evaluation/Desired Outcomes
- Range of aPTT ratio from 1.5–2.5, without signs of hemorrhage.
- Treatment and prevention of thromboembolic disease and its sequelae.

---

letrozole (let-roe-zole)
Femara

Classification
Therapeutic: antineoplastics
Pharmacologic: aromatase inhibitors

Pregnancy Category D

Indications
First-line treatment of postmenopausal women with hormone receptor positive or hormone receptor unknown metastatic or advanced breast cancer. Advanced breast cancer in postmenopausal patients with disease progression despite antiestrogen therapy. Extended adjuvant treatment of post-menopausal early breast cancer already treated with 5 yr of tamoxifen.

Action
Inhibits the enzyme aromatase, which is partially responsible for conversion of precursors to estrogen. **Therapeutic Effects:** Lowers levels of circulating estrogen, which may halt progression of estrogen-sensitive breast cancer. Decreased risk of recurrence/metastatic disease.

Pharmacokinetics
Absorption: Rapidly and completely absorbed.
Distribution: Unknown.
Metabolism and Excretion: Mostly metabolized by the liver.
Half-life: 2 days.

TIME/ACTION PROFILE (effect on lowering of serum estradiol levels)

ROUTE	ONSET	PEAK	DURATION
PO	unknown	2–3 days	unknown

Contraindications/Precautions
Contraindicated in: Hypersensitivity; Premenopausal women; OB: Potential for fetal harm.
Use Cautiously in: Severe hepatic impairment; Lactation, Pedi: Safety not established.

Adverse Reactions/Side Effects
CNS: anxiety, depression, dizziness, drowsiness, fatigue, headache, vertigo, weakness. **Resp:** coughing, dyspnea, pleural effusion. **CV:** chest pain, edema, hypertension, cerebrovascular events, thromboembolic events. **GI:** nausea, abdominal pain, anorexia, constipation, diarrhea, dyspepsia, vomiting. **Derm:** alopecia, hot flashes, increased sweating, pruritus, rash. **F and E:** hypercalcemia. **Metab:** hypercholesterolemia, weight gain. **MS:** musculoskeletal pain, arthralgia, fractures.

Interactions
Drug-Drug: None significant.

Route/Dosage
PO (Adults): 2.5 mg daily.

Availability
Tablets: 2.5 mg.

NURSING IMPLICATIONS

Assessment
- Assess patient for pain and other side effects periodically throughout therapy.
- *Lab Test Considerations:* May cause elevated GTT cholesterol levels.

Potential Nursing Diagnoses
Acute pain (Side Effects)

Implementation
- **PO:** May be taken without regard to food.

Patient/Family Teaching
- Instruct patient to take medication as directed.
- Inform patient of potential for adverse reactions and advise her to notify health care professional if side effects are problematic.

✦ = Canadian drug name. ≋ = Genetic implication.
*CAPITALS indicates life-threatening; underlines indicate most frequent.

- Caution women who are perimenopausal or who recently became menopausal to use adequate contraception during therapy; letrozole may cause fetal harm.

Evaluation/Desired Outcomes
- Slowing of disease progression in women with advanced breast cancer.
- Decreased risk of recurrence/metastatic disease.

---

leucovorin calcium
(loo-koe-**vor**-in)
folinic acid

Classification
Therapeutic: antidotes (for methotrexate), vitamins
Pharmacologic: folic acid analogues

Pregnancy Category C

Indications
Minimizes hematologic effects of high-dose methotrexate therapy (leucovorin rescue). Advanced colorectal carcinoma (with 5-fluorouracil). Management of overdoses/prevention of toxicity from folic acid antagonists (pyrimethamine, trimethoprim, trimetrexate). Folic acid deficiency (megaloblastic anemia) unresponsive to oral replacement.

Action
The reduced form of folic acid that serves as a cofactor in the synthesis of DNA and RNA. **Therapeutic Effects:** Reversal of toxic effects of folic acid antagonists. Reversal of folic acid deficiency.

Pharmacokinetics
Absorption: Well absorbed (38%) following PO administration. Bioavailability decreases with larger doses. Oral absorption is saturated at doses >25 mg.
Distribution: Widely distributed. Concentrates in the CNS and liver.
Metabolism and Excretion: Extensively converted to tetrahydrofolic derivatives, including 5-methyltetrahydrofolate, a major storage form.
Half-life: 3.5 hr.

TIME/ACTION PROFILE (serum folate levels)

ROUTE	ONSET	PEAK	DURATION
PO	20–30 min	unknown	3–6 hr
IM	10–20 min	unknown	3–6 hr
IV	<5 min	unknown	3–6 hr

Contraindications/Precautions
Contraindicated in: Hypersensitivity; Preparations containing benzyl alcohol should not be used in neonates.
Use Cautiously in: Undiagnosed anemia (may mask the progression of pernicious anemia); OB, Lactation: Safety not established but has been used safely to treat megaloblastic anemia in pregnancy; Coadministration with high-dose methotrexate requires crucial timing of dosing and knowledge of methotrexate levels; Ascites; Renal failure; Dehydration; Pleural effusions; Urine pH <7.

Adverse Reactions/Side Effects
Hemat: thrombocytosis (intra-arterial methotrexate only). **Misc:** allergic reactions (rash, urticaria, wheezing).

Interactions
Drug-Drug: May ↓ anticonvulsant effect of **barbiturates**, **phenytoin**, or **primidone**. High doses of the liquid contain significant **alcohol** and may cause ↑ CNS depression when used with **CNS depressants**. Concurrent use with **trimethoprim/sulfamethoxazole** may result in ↓ anti-infective efficacy and poor therapeutic outcome when used to treat *Pneumocystis jirovecii* pneumonia in HIV patients. May ↑ therapeutic effects and toxicity of **fluorouracil**; therapy may be combined for this purpose.

Route/Dosage

High-Dose Methotrexate—Leucovorin Rescue. Must start within 24 hr of methotrexate.
PO, IM, IV (Adults and Children): *Normal methotrexate elimination*—10 mg/m^2 q 6 hr (1st dose IV/IM, then change to PO) until methotrexate level is $<5 \times 10^{-8}$ M (0.05 micromolar). Larger doses/longer duration may be required in patients with aciduria, ascites, dehydration, renal impairment, GI obstruction, pleural/peritoneal effusions. Dose of leucovorin should be determined on the basis of plasma methotrexate levels.

Advanced Colorectal Cancer
IV (Adults): 200 mg/m^2 followed by 5-fluorouracil 370 mg/m^2 or leucovorin 20 mg/m^2 is followed by 5-fluorouracil 425 mg/m^2. Regimen is given daily for 5 days q 4–5 wk.

Prevention of Hematologic Toxicity from Trimetrexate
PO, IV (Adults and Children): 20 mg/m^2 q 6 hr continued for 72 hr after last trimetrexate dose (oral doses should be rounded up to the next 25

mg); both trimetrexate and leucovorin doses require adjustment for hematologic toxicity.

Prevention of Hematologic Toxicity from Pyrimethamine
PO, IV (Adults and Children): 5–15 mg/day.

Inadvertent Overdose of Folic Acid Antagonists
IM, IV (Adults and Children): *Methotrexate–large doses*—75 mg IV followed by 12 mg IM q 6 hr for 4 doses; *methotrexate–average doses*—6–12 mg IM q 6 hr for 4 doses; *other folic acid antagonists*—amount equal in mg to folic acid antagonist.

Megaloblastic Anemia
PO, IM, IV (Adults and Children): Up to 1 mg/day (up to 6 mg/day for dihydrofolate reductase deficiency).

Availability (generic available)
Tablets: 5 mg, 10 mg, 15 mg, 25 mg. **Solution for injection (preservative-free):** 10 mg/mL. **Powder for injection:** 50 mg, 100 mg, 200 mg, 350 mg.

NURSING IMPLICATIONS

Assessment
- Assess patient for nausea and vomiting secondary to methotrexate therapy or folic acid antagonists (pyrimethamine and trimethoprim) overdose. Parenteral route may be necessary to ensure that patient receives dose.
- Monitor for development of allergic reactions (rash, urticaria, wheezing). Notify health care professional if these occur.
- **Megaloblastic Anemia:** Assess degree of weakness and fatigue.
- **Lab Test Considerations:** Leucovorin rescue: Monitor serum methotrexate levels to determine dose and effectiveness of therapy. Leucovorin calcium levels should be equal to or greater than methotrexate level. Rescue continues until serum methotrexate level is <5 × 10M.
- Monitor CCr and serum creatinine prior to and every 24 hr during therapy to detect methotrexate toxicity. An increase >50% over the pretreatment concentration at 24 hr is associated with severe renal toxicity.
- Monitor urine pH every 6 hr during therapy; pH should be maintained >7 to decrease nephrotoxic effects of high-dose methotrexate. Sodium bicarbonate or acetazolamide may be ordered to alkalinize urine.
- *Megaloblastic anemia*—Monitor plasma folic acid levels, hemoglobin, hematocrit, and reticulocyte count prior to and periodically during therapy.

Potential Nursing Diagnoses
Risk for injury (Indications)
Imbalanced nutrition: less than body requirements (Indications)

Implementation
- Do not confuse folinic acid (leucovorin calcium) with folic acid. Do not confuse leucovorin with leukeran (chlorambucil) or leukine (sargramostim).
- Make sure leucovorin calcium is available before administering high-dose methotrexate. <u>Administration must be initiated within 24 hr of methotrexate therapy.</u>
- Administer as soon as possible after toxic dose of folic acid antagonists (pyrimethamine and trimethoprim). Effectiveness of therapy begins to decrease 1 hr after overdose.
- **PO:** Parenteral therapy should be used in patients with GI toxicity, with nausea and vomiting, or with doses >25 mg.
- **IM:** IM route is preferred for treatment of megaloblastic anemia. Ampules of leucovorin calcium injection for IM use do not require reconstitution.

IV Administration
- **Direct IV:** *Diluent:* Bacteriostatic water or sterile water. Do not use product containing benzyl alcohol. Use immediately if reconstituted with sterile water for injection. Stable for 7 days when reconstituted with bacteriostatic water. *Concentration:* reconstitute 50-mg, 100-mg, and 200-mg vials to a concentration of 10 mg/mL; reconstitute 350-mg vial to a concentration of 20 mg/mL. *Rate:* Administer by slow injection over a minimum of 3 min; not to exceed 160 mg/min.
- **Intermittent Infusion:** *Diluent:* May be diluted in 100–500 mL of D5W, D10W, 0.9% NaCl, Ringer's, or LR. Stable for 24 hr.
- **Y-Site Compatibility:** amifostine, anidulafungin, aztreonam, bivalirudin, bleomycin, caspofungin, cefepime, cisplatin, cladribine, codeine, cyclophosphamide, cytarabine, dactinomycin, daptomycin, dexamedetomidine, docetaxel, doxacurium, doxorubicin, doxoru-

bicin liposome, eptifibatide, ertapenem, etoposide, etoposide phosphate, fenoldopam, filgrastim, fluconazole, fludarabine, fluorouracil, furosemide, gemcitabine, granisetron, heparin, hetastarch, idarubicin, ifosfamide, levofloxacin, linezolid, mechlorethamine, meperidine, methotrexate, metoclopramide, mitomycin, mitoxantrone, nesiritide, octreotide, oxaliplatin, oxytocin, paclitaxel, palonosetron, pemetrexed, piperacillin/tazobactam, rituximab, sodium acetate, tacrolimus, teniposide, thiotepa, tigecycline, tirofiban, trastuzumab, vinblastine, vincristine, vinorelbine, voriconazole.

- **Y-Site Incompatibility:** amphotericin B cholesteryl, amphotericin B liposome, carboplatin, droperidol, epirubicin, foscarnet, pantoprazole, quinupristin/dalfopristin, sodium bicarbonate.

Patient/Family Teaching
- Explain purpose of medication to patient. Emphasize need to take exactly as ordered. Advise patient to contact health care professional if a dose is missed.
- **Leucovorin Rescue:** Instruct patient to drink at least 3 liters of fluid each day during leucovorin rescue.
- **Folic Acid Deficiency:** Encourage patient to eat a diet high in folic acid (meat proteins; bran; dried beans; and green, leafy vegetables).

Evaluation/Desired Outcomes
- Reversal of bone marrow and GI toxicity in patients receiving methotrexate or in overdose of folic acid antagonists.
- Increased sense of well-being and increased production of normoblasts in patients with megaloblastic anemia.

---

leuprolide (loo-**proe**-lide)
Eligard, Lupron, Lupron Depot, Lupron Depot-Ped, Lupron Depot-3 Month, Lupron Depot-4 Month

Classification
Therapeutic: antineoplastics
Pharmacologic: hormones, gonadotropin-releasing hormones

Pregnancy Category X

Indications
Advanced prostate cancer in patients who are unable to tolerate orchiectomy or estrogen therapy (may be used in combination with flutamide or bicalutamide). Central precocious puberty (CPP).

Endometriosis. Uterine fibroids (with iron therapy).

Action
A synthetic analogue of luteinizing hormone–releasing hormone (LHRH). Initially causes a transient increase in testosterone; however, with continuous administration, testosterone levels are decreased. Reduces gonadotropins, testosterone, and estradiol. **Therapeutic Effects:** Decreased testosterone levels and resultant decrease in spread of prostate cancer. Reduction of pain/lesions in endometriosis. Decreased growth of fibroids. Delayed puberty.

Pharmacokinetics
Absorption: Rapidly and almost completely absorbed following subcut administration. More slowly absorbed following IM administration of depot form.
Distribution: Unknown.
Metabolism and Excretion: Unknown.
Half-life: 3 hr.

TIME/ACTION PROFILE (effect on hormone levels)

ROUTE	ONSET†	PEAK‡	DURATION§
Subcut	within 1st week	2–4 wk	4–12 wk
IM	within 1st week	2–4 wk	4–12 wk
IM-depot	within 1st week	2–4 wk	4–12 wk

†Initial transient increase in testosterone and estradiol levels
‡Maximum decline in testosterone and estradiol levels
§Restoration of normal pituitary–gonadal function; in amenorrheic patients, normal menses usually returns 60–90 days after treatment is discontinued

Contraindications/Precautions
Contraindicated in: Intolerance to synthetic analogues of LHRH (GnRH); OB: Potential for fetal harm or spontaneous abortion; Lactation: Potential serious adverse effects.
Use Cautiously in: Hypersensitivity to benzyl alcohol (results in induration and erythema at subcut site).

Adverse Reactions/Side Effects
CNS: dizziness, headache, syncope; *Depot*—drowsiness, personality disorder; *Subcut*—anxiety, blurred vision, lethargy, memory disorder, mood swings. **EENT:** blurred vision; *Subcut*—hearing disorder. **Resp:** hemoptysis; *Depot*—epistaxis, throat nodules; *Subcut*—cough, pleural rub, pulmonary fibrosis, pulmonary infiltrate. **CV:** MI, PULMONARY EMBOLI, angina, arrhythmias; *Depot*—vasodilation; *Subcut*—transient ischemic attack/stroke. **GI:** anorexia, diarrhea, dysphagia, nausea, vomiting; *Depot*—gingivitis; *Subcut*—GI BLEEDING, hepatic dysfunction, pep-

tic ulcer, rectal polyps, taste disorders. **GU:** ↓ testicular size, dysuria, incontinence, testicular pain; *Depot*—cervix disorder; *Subcut*—bladder spasm, penile swelling, prostate pain, urinary obstruction. **Derm:** *Depot*—hair growth, rash; *Subcut*, dry skin, hair loss, pigmentation, skin cancer, skin lesions. **Endo:** breast swelling, breast tenderness, hyperglycemia. **F and E:** hypercalcemia, lower extremity edema. **Local:** burning, itching, swelling at injection site. **Metab:** *Depot*—hyperuricemia, ↑ bone density. **MS:** fibromyalgia, transient ↑ in bone pain (prostate cancer only); *Subcut*—ankylosing spondylitis, joint pain, pelvic fibrosis, temporal bone pain. **Neuro:** *Subcut*—peripheral neuropathy. **Misc:** hot flashes, chills, ↓ libido, fever; *Depot*—body odor, epistaxis.

Interactions
Drug-Drug: ↑ antineoplastic effects with **antiandrogens**, (**megestrol, flutamide**).

Route/Dosage
Prostate Cancer
Subcut (Adults): *Lupron*—1 mg/day *or Eligard*—7.5 mg once monthly, 22.5 mg every 3 mo, 30 mg q 4 mo or 45 mg q 6 mo.
IM (Adults): *Lupron Depot*—7.5 mg once monthly *or Lupron Depot-3 Month*—22.5 mg q 3 mo *or Lupron Depot-4 Month*—30 mg q 4 mo.

Endometriosis
IM (Adults): *Lupron Depot*—3.75 mg once monthly for up to 6 months *or Lupron Depot-3 Month*—11.25 mg q 3 mo for up to 2 doses.

Uterine Fibroids (with iron therapy)
IM (Adults): *Lupron Depot*—3.75 mg once monthly for up to 3 months *or Lupron Depot-3 Month*—11.25 mg single injection.

Central Precocious Puberty (CPP)
Subcut (Children): *Lupron*—50 mcg/kg/day, may be ↑ by 10 mcg/kg/day as required.
IM (Children >37.5 kg): *Lupron Depot-Ped*—15 mg q 4 wk; may be ↑ by 3.75 mg q 4 wk as required.
IM (Children 25–37.5 kg): *Lupron Depot-Ped*—11.25 mg q 4 wk; may be ↑ by 3.75 mg q 4 wk as required.
IM (Children ≤25 kg): *Lupron Depot-Ped*—7.5 mg q 4 wk; may be ↑ by 3.75 mg q 4 wk as required.

Availability (generic available)
Solution for subcut injection (Lupron): 5 mg/mL. **Lyophilized microspheres for depot injection (Lupron Depot):** 3.75 mg, 7.5 mg. **Lyophilized microspheres for pediatric depot injection (Lupron Depot-Ped):** 7.5 mg, 11.25 mg, 15-mg. **Lyophilized microspheres for 3-mo depot injection (Lupron Depot- 3 Month):** 11.25 mg, 22.5 mg. **Lyophilized microspheres for 4-mo depot injection (Lupron Depot-4 Month):** 30 mg. **Polymeric matrix injectable formulation for subcut injection (Eligard):** 7.5 mg, 22.5 mg, 30 mg, 45 mg.

NURSING IMPLICATIONS
Assessment
- **Prostate Cancer:** Assess patient for an increase in bone pain, especially during the first few weeks of therapy. Monitor patients with vertebral metastases for increased back pain and decreased sensory/motor function.
- Monitor intake and output ratios; assess for bladder distention in patients with urinary tract obstruction during initiation of therapy.
- **Fibroids:** Assess patient for severity of symptoms (bloating, pelvic pain, pressure, excessive vaginal bleeding) periodically during therapy.
- **Endometriosis:** Assess patient for endometrial pain prior to and periodically during therapy.
- **CPP:** Prior to therapy, diagnosis of CPP should be confirmed by onset of secondary sex characteristics in girls <8 yr or boys <9 yr; a complete physical and endocrinologic examination, including height, weight, hand and wrist x-ray; total sex steroid level (estradiol or testosterone); adrenal steroid level; beta human chorionic gonadotropin level; GnRH stimulation test; and computerized tomography of the head must be performed. These parameters are monitored after 1–2 mo and every 6–12 mo during therapy.
- Assess patient for signs of precocious puberty (menses, breast development, testicular growth) periodically during therapy. Dose is increased until no progression of the disease is noted either clinically or by lab test parameters, then usually maintained throughout therapy. Discontinuation of therapy should be considered before age 11 in girls and age 12 in boys.

- **Lab Test Considerations:** Initially ↑, then ↓ luteinizing hormone (LH) and follicle-stimulating hormone (FSH). This leads to castration levels of testosterone in boys 2–4 wk after initial increase in concentrations.
- Monitor testosterone, prostatic acid phosphate, and prostate-specific antigen (PSA) levels to evaluate response to therapy. Transient ↑ in levels may occur during the 1st month of therapy for prostate cancer.
- May cause ↑ BUN, serum calcium, uric acid, hypoproteinemia, LDH, alkaline phosphatase, AST, hyperglycemia, hyperlipidemia, hyperphosphatemia, WBC, PT, or PTT. May also cause ↓ platelets and serum potassium.

Potential Nursing Diagnoses
Sexual dysfunction (Side Effects)

Implementation
- Subcut *Eligard subcut formulation:* Bring to room temperature before mixing. Assemble the Eligard kit and reconstitute solution using syringes provided, as directed by manufacturer. Mix in syringes as directed by manufacturer, do not shake. Solution must reach room temperature before administration and must be administered within 30 min of mixing, or be discarded. Solution is light tan to tan in color. Inject into abdomen, upper buttocks, or anywhere that has adequate amounts of subcut tissue without excessive pigment, nodules, lesions, or hair. **Vary site with each injection.**
- IM: Use syringe supplied by manufacturer. Rotate sites.
- Leuprolide depot is *only* for IM injection.
- *Lupron Depot formulation:* To reconstitute a single vial, use a 22-gauge needle; withdraw 1 mL of diluent and inject into vial to mix. To mix 2 or more vials, withdraw 0.5 mL and inject into each vial for a total volume of 1 mL. Do not use vial if clumping or caking of microspheres (powder) is evident. Shake each vial well; suspension will appear milky. Withdraw entire contents of all vials into syringe and inject immediately. Patients may store medication at room temperature.
- Store at room temperature; stable for 24 hr following reconstitution.

Patient/Family Teaching
- Advise patient that medication may cause hot flashes. Notify health care professional if these become bothersome.
- Inform patient of the possibility of the development or worsening of depression and occurrence of memory disorders.
- **Prostate Cancer:** Instruct patient and family on subcut injection technique. Review patient insert provided with leuprolide patient-administration kit.
- Instruct patient to take medication exactly as directed. Take missed doses as soon as remembered unless not remembered until next day.
- Advise patient that bone pain may increase at initiation of therapy, but will resolve with time. Patient should discuss with health care professional use of analgesics to control pain.
- Instruct patient to notify health care professional promptly if difficulty urinating, weakness, or numbness occurs.
- **Endometriosis:** Advise patient to use a form of contraception other than oral contraceptives during therapy. Inform patient that amenorrhea is expected but does not guarantee contraception.
- **Central Precocious Puberty:** Instruct patient and family on the proper technique for subcut injection. Emphasize the importance of administering the medication at the same time each day. Rotate injection sites periodically.
- Inform patient and parents that if injections are not given daily, pubertal process may be reactivated.
- Advise patient and parents that during the first 2 mo of therapy patient may experience a light menstrual flow or spotting. Health care professional should be notified if this continues beyond 2nd mo.
- Instruct patient and parents to notify health care professional immediately if irritation at the injection site or unusual signs or symptoms occur.

Evaluation/Desired Outcomes
- Decrease in the spread of prostate cancer.
- Decrease in lesions and pain in endometriosis.
- Resolution of the signs of CPP.
- Improvement in preoperative hematologic parameters in patients with anemia from uterine fibroids.

---

levalbuterol
(leev-al-**byoo**-ter-ole)
Xopenex, Xopenex HFA

levalbuterol

Classification
Therapeutic: bronchodilators
Pharmacologic: adrenergics

Pregnancy Category C

Indications
Bronchospasm due to reversible airway disease (short-term control agent).

Action
R-enantiomer of racemic albuterol. Binds to beta-2 adrenergic receptors in airway smooth muscle leading to activation of adenylcyclase and increased levels of cyclic-3', 5'-adenosine monophosphate (cAMP). Increases in cAMP activate kinases, which inhibit the phosphorylation of myosin and decrease intracellular calcium. Decreased intracellular calcium relaxes bronchial smooth muscle. **Therapeutic Effects:** Relaxation of airway smooth muscle with subsequent bronchodilation. Relatively selective for beta-2 (pulmonary) receptors.

Pharmacokinetics
Absorption: Some absorption occurs following inhalation.
Distribution: Unknown.
Metabolism and Excretion: Metabolized in the liver to an inactive sulfate and 3–6% excreted unchanged in the urine.
Half-life: 3.3–4 hr.

TIME/ACTION PROFILE (bronchodilation)

ROUTE	ONSET	PEAK	DURATION
Inhaln	10–17 min	90 min	5–6 hr

Contraindications/Precautions
Contraindicated in: Hypersensitivity to levalbuterol or albuterol.
Use Cautiously in: Cardiovascular disorders (including coronary insufficiency, hypertension, and arrhythmias); History of seizures; Hypokalemia; Hyperthyroidism; Diabetes mellitus; Unusual sensitivity to adrenergic amines; OB, Lactation, Pedi: Pregnancy, lactation, or children <6 yr (for nebulized solution) or <4 yr (for metered-dose inhaler) (safety not established).
Exercise Extreme Caution in: Concurrent use or use within 2 weeks of **tricyclic antidepressants** or **MAO inhibitors** (may ↑ risk of adverse cardiovascular reactions).

Adverse Reactions/Side Effects
CNS: anxiety, dizziness, headache, nervousness. **Resp:** PARADOXICAL BRONCHOSPASM (excessive use of inhalers), increased cough, turbinate edema. **CV:** tachycardia. **GI:** dyspepsia, vomiting. **Endo:** hyperglycemia. **F and E:** hypokalemia. **Neuro:** tremor.

Interactions
Drug-Drug: Concurrent use or use within 2 weeks of **tricyclic antidepressants** or **MAO inhibitors** may ↑ risk of adverse cardiovascular reactions (use with extreme caution). **Beta blockers** block the beneficial pulmonary effects of adrenergic bronchodilators (choose cardioselective beta blockers if necessary and with caution). May ↑ risk of hypokalemia from **potassium-losing diuretics**. May ↓ serum **digoxin** levels. May ↑ risk of arrhythmias with **hydrocarbon inhalation anesthetics** or **cocaine**.
Drug-Natural Products: Use with caffeine-containing herbs (**guarana**, **tea**, **coffee**) ↑ stimulant effect.

Route/Dosage
Inhaln (Adults and Children ≥4 yr): 2 inhalations q 4–6 hr; some patients may respond to 1 inhalation q 4 hr.
Inhaln (Adults and Children > 12 yr): 0.63 mg via nebulization 3 times daily (every 6–8 hr); may be increased to 1.25 mg 3 times daily (every 6–8 hr).
Inhaln (Children 6–11 yr): 0.31 mg via nebulization 3 times daily (not to exceed 0.63 mg 3 times daily).

Availability (generic available)
Metered-dose inhaler: 45 mcg/actuation in 15-g (200 metered actuations) canisters. **Inhalation solution:** 0.31 mg/3 mL in green foil pouch containing 12 vials, 0.63 mg/3 mL in yellow foil pouch containing 12 vials, 1.25 mg/3 mL in red foil pouch containing 12 vials, 1.25 mg/0.5 mL in unit-dose vials. **Cost:** 0.31 mg/3 mL $83.76/24 vials, 0.63 mg/3 mL $84.15/24 vials, 1.25 mg/3 mL $85.00/24 vials.

NURSING IMPLICATIONS

Assessment
- Assess lung sounds, pulse, and blood pressure before administration and during peak of medication. Note amount, color, and character of sputum produced. Closely monitor patients on higher dose for adverse effects.
- Monitor pulmonary function tests before initiating therapy and periodically during course to determine effectiveness of medication.

✦ = Canadian drug name. ᴳ = Genetic implication.
*CAPITALS indicates life-threatening; underlines indicate most frequent.

- Observe for paradoxical bronchospasm (wheezing). If condition occurs, withhold medication and notify physician or other health care provider immediately.
- **Lab Test Considerations:** May cause ↑ serum glucose and ↓ serum potassium.

Potential Nursing Diagnoses
Ineffective airway clearance (Indications)

Implementation
- **Inhaln:** Allow at least 1 min between inhalations of aerosol medication.
- For nebulization, levalbuterol solution does not require dilution prior to administration. Once the foil pouch is opened, vials must be used within 2 weeks; open vials may be stored for 1 week. Discard vial if solution is not clear or colorless.

Patient/Family Teaching
- Instruct patient in the proper use of metered-dose inhaler and nebulizer (see Appendix D) and to take levalbuterol as directed. Caution patient not to exceed recommended dose; may cause adverse effects, paradoxical bronchospasm, or loss of effectiveness of medication.
- Advise patient to consult health care professional before taking any OTC medications or alcohol concurrently with this therapy. Caution patient to also avoid smoking and other respiratory irritants.
- Instruct patient to contact health care professional immediately if shortness of breath is not relieved by medication or is accompanied by diaphoresis, dizziness, palpitations, or chest pain.
- Advise patients to use levalbuterol first if using other inhalation medications, and allow 5 min to elapse before administering other inhalant medications unless otherwise directed.
- Advise patient to rinse mouth with water after each inhalation dose to minimize dry mouth.
- Instruct patient to notify health care professional if no response to the usual dose of levalbuterol.

Evaluation/Desired Outcomes
- Prevention or relief of bronchospasm.

---

levetiracetam
(le-ve-teer-**a**-se-tam)
Keppra, Keppra XR

Classification
Therapeutic: anticonvulsants
Pharmacologic: pyrrolidines

Pregnancy Category C

Indications
Partial onset seizures (adjunct). Primary generalized tonic-clonic seizures (adjunct) (immediate-release and injection only). Myoclonic seizures in patients with juvenile myoclonic epilepsy (adjunct) (immediate-release and injection only).

Action
Appears to inhibit burst firing without affecting normal neuronal excitability and may selectively prevent hypersynchronization of epileptiform burst firing and propagation of seizure activity. **Therapeutic Effects:** Decreased incidence and severity of seizures.

Pharmacokinetics
Absorption: Rapidly and completely absorbed following oral administration.
Distribution: Unknown.
Metabolism and Excretion: 66% excreted unchanged by the kidneys; some metabolism by the liver (metabolites inactive).
Half-life: 7.1 hr (↑ in renal impairment).

TIME/ACTION PROFILE (blood levels)

ROUTE	ONSET	PEAK	DURATION
PO	rapid	1–1.5 hr†‡	12 hr

† 1 hr in the fasting state, 1.5 hr when taken with food
‡ 4 hr with extended-release

Contraindications/Precautions
Contraindicated in: Hypersensitivity; Lactation: Lactation.
Use Cautiously in: All patients (may ↑ risk of suicidal thoughts/behaviors); Renal impairment (dose reduction recommended if CCr ≤80 mL/min); Pedi: Children <4 yr (safety not established); <16 yr (for extended-release and injection); OB: Use only during pregnancy if potential benefit justifies potential risk to fetus; Geri: ↓ renal elimination (dose ↓ may be necessary).

Adverse Reactions/Side Effects
CNS: SUICIDAL THOUGHTS, dizziness, fatigue/somnolence, weakness, behavioral abnormalities.
Neuro: coordination difficulties (adults only).

Interactions
Drug-Drug: None noted.

Route/Dosage

Partial Onset Seizures

PO, IV (Adults and Children ≥16 yr): 500 mg 2 times daily initially; may be ↑ by 1000 mg/day at 2-wk intervals up to 3000 mg/day; *Extended-release*—1000 mg daily; may ↑ by 1000 mg/day at 2-wk intervals up to 3000 mg/day.
PO (Children 4–15 yrs): 10 mg/kg twice daily; ↑ by 20 mg/kg/day at 2-wk intervals to recommended dose of 30 mg/kg twice daily.

Primary Generalized Tonic-Clonic Seizures

PO, IV (Adults and Children ≥16 yr): 500 mg 2 times daily initially; ↑ by 1000 mg/day at 2-wk intervals to recommended dose of 3000 mg/day.
PO (Children 6–15 yrs): 10 mg/kg twice daily; ↑ by 20 mg/kg/day at 2-wk intervals to recommended dose of 30 mg/kg 2 times daily.

Myoclonic Seizures

IV (Adults and Children ≥16 yr): 500 mg 2 times daily initially; ↑ by 1000 mg/day at 2-wk intervals to recommended dose of 3000 mg/day.
PO (Children ≥12 yrs): 500 mg twice daily initially; ↑ by 1000 mg/day at 2-wk intervals to recommended dose of 3000 mg/day.

Renal Impairment

PO, IV (Adults): *CCr 50–80 mL/min*—500–1000 mg q 12 hr (1000–2000 mg q 24 hr for extended-release); *CCr 30–50 mL/min*—250–750 mg q 12 hr (500–1500 mg q 24 hr for extended-release); *CCr <30 mL/min*—250–500 mg q 12 hr (500–1000 mg q 24 hr for extended-release); *Dialysis (immediate-release and injection)* 500–1000 mg q 24 hr with a 250–500-mg supplemental dose after dialysis.

Availability (generic available)

Tablets: 250 mg, 500 mg, 750 mg, 100 mg. **Cost:** 250 mg $385.94/180, 500 mg $519.93/180, 750 mg $699.95/180, 1000 mg $1,021.30/180. **Extended-release tablets:** 500 mg, 750 mg. **Oral solution (grape-flavored):** 100 mg/mL. **Cost:** $282.43/480 mL. **Injection:** 100 mg/mL.

NURSING IMPLICATIONS

Assessment

- Assess location, duration, and characteristics of seizure activity.
- Assess patient for CNS adverse effects throughout therapy. These adverse effects are categorized as somnolence and fatigue (asthenia), coordination difficulties (ataxia, abnormal gait, or incoordination), and behavioral abnormalities (agitation, hostility, anxiety, apathy, emotional lability, depersonalization, depression) and usually occur during the first 4 wk of therapy.
- ***Lab Test Considerations:*** May cause ↓ RBC and WBC and abnormal liver function tests.

Potential Nursing Diagnoses

Risk for injury (Side Effects)

Implementation

- Do not confuse Keppra with Kaletra (lopinavir/ritonavir).
- IV doses should be used temporarily when oral route is not feasible. To convert IV to PO, equivalent dose and frequency may be used.
- **PO:** May be administered without regard to meals.
- Administer tablets whole; do not administer partial tablets. Do not break, crush, or chew XR tablets.
- Pedi: Patients <20 kg should receive oral solution. Administer with calibrated measuring device for accurate dose.
- Discontinue gradually to minimize the risk of increase in seizure frequency.

IV Administration

- **Intermittent Infusion: *Diluent:*** Dilute dose in 100 mL of 0.9% NaCl, D5W, or LR. Do not administer solutions that are cloudy or contain particulate matter. ***Rate:*** Infuse over 15 min.
- **Y-Site Compatibility:** diazepam, lorazepam, valproate.

Patient/Family Teaching

- Instruct patient to take medication as directed. Pedi: Explain to parents the importance of using calibrated measuring device for accurate dosing. Take missed doses as soon as possible unless almost time for next dose. Do not double doses. Do not discontinue abruptly; may cause increase in frequency of seizures.
- May cause dizziness and somnolence. Caution patient to avoid driving or activities requiring alertness until response to medication is known. Do not resume driving until physician gives clearance based on control of seizure disorder.

- Advise female patients to notify health care professional if pregnancy is planned or suspected or if breast feeding. Encourage pregnant patients to enroll in the North American Antiepileptic Drug (NAAED) Pregnancy Registry by calling 1-888-233-2334; information is available at www.aedpregnancyregistry.org.
- Instruct patient to notify health care professional of medication regimen prior to treatment or surgery.
- Advise patient to carry identification describing disease process and medication regimen at all times.

Evaluation/Desired Outcomes
- Decrease in the frequency of or cessation of seizures.

---

levonorgestrel, See CONTRACEPTIVES, HORMONAL.

---

levothyroxine, See THYROID PREPARATIONS.

HIGH ALERT

LIDOCAINE

lidocaine (parenteral)
(**lye**-doe-kane)
LidoPen, Xylocaine, ✦ Xylocard

lidocaine (local anesthetic)
Xylocaine

lidocaine (mucosal)
Anestacon, Xylocaine Viscous

lidocaine patch
Lidoderm

lidocaine (topical)
L-M-X 4, L-M-X 5, Solarcaine Aloe Extra Burn Relief, Xylocaine, Zilactin-L

Classification
Therapeutic: anesthetics (topical/local), antiarrhythmics (class IB)

Pregnancy Category B

Indications
IV: Ventricular arrhythmias. **IM:** Self-injected or when IV unavailable (during transport to hospital facilities). **Local:** Infiltration/mucosal/topical anesthetic. **Patch:** Pain due to post-herpetic neuralgia.

Action
IV, IM: Suppresses automaticity and spontaneous depolarization of the ventricles during diastole by altering the flux of sodium ions across cell membranes with little or no effect on heart rate. **Local:** Produces local anesthesia by inhibiting transport of ions across neuronal membranes, thereby preventing initiation and conduction of normal nerve impulses. **Therapeutic Effects:** Control of ventricular arrhythmias. Local anesthesia.

Pharmacokinetics
Absorption: Well absorbed after administration into the deltoid muscle; some absorption follows local use.
Distribution: Widely distributed. Concentrates in adipose tissue. Crosses the blood-brain barrier and placenta; enters breast milk.
Metabolism and Excretion: Mostly metabolized by the liver; <10% excreted in urine as unchanged drug.
Half-life: Biphasic—initial phase, 7–30 min; terminal phase, 90–120 min; increased in CHF and liver impairment.

TIME/ACTION PROFILE (IV, IM = antiarrhythmic effects; local = anesthetic effects)

ROUTE	ONSET	PEAK	DURATION
IV	immediate	immediate	10–20 min (up to several hours after continuous infusion)
IM	5–15 min	20–30 min	60–90 min
Local	rapid	unknown	1–3 hr

Contraindications/Precautions
Applies mainly to systemic use
Contraindicated in: Hypersensitivity; cross-sensitivity may occur; Third-degree heart block.
Use Cautiously in: Liver disease, CHF, patients weighing <50 kg, and geriatric patients (reduce bolus and/or maintenance dose); Respiratory depression; Shock; Heart block; OB, Lactation: Safety not established; Pedi: Safety not established for transdermal patch.

Adverse Reactions/Side Effects
Applies mainly to systemic use.
CNS: SEIZURES, confusion, drowsiness, blurred vision, dizziness, nervousness, slurred speech, tremor. **EENT:** *mucosal use*— ↓ or absent gag reflex. **CV:** CARDIAC ARREST, arrhythmias, bradycardia, heart block, hypotension. **GI:** nausea, vomiting. **Resp:** bronchospasm. **Local:** stinging,

LIDOCAINE

burning, contact dermatitis, erythema. **Misc:** allergic reactions, including ANAPHYLAXIS.

Interactions

Applies mainly to systemic use.
Drug-Drug: ↑ cardiac depression and toxicity with **phenytoin, amiodarone, quinidine, procainamide,** or **propranolol**. **Cimetidine, azole antifungals, clarithromycin, erythromycin, fluoxetine, nefazodone, paroxetine, protease inhibitors, ritonavir, verapamil,** and **beta blockers** may ↓ metabolism and ↑ risk of toxicity. Lidocaine may ↑ levels of **calcium channel blockers**, certain **benzodiazepines, cyclosporine, fluoxetine, lovastatin, simvastatin, mirtazapine, paroxetine, ritonavir, tacrolimus, theophylline, tricyclic antidepressnts,** and **venlafaxine**. Effects of lidocaine may be ↓ by **carbamazepine, phenobarbital, phenytoin,** and **rifampin**.

Route/Dosage

Ventricular Tachycardia (with a Pulse) or Pulseless Ventricular Tachycardia/Ventricular Fibrillation

IV (Adults): 1–1.5 mg/kg bolus; may repeat doses of 0.5–0.75 mg/kg q 5–10 min up to a total dose of 3 mg/kg; may then start continuous infusion of 1–4 mg/min.

Endotracheal (Adults): Give 2–2.5 times the IV loading dose down the endotracheal tube, followed by a 10 mL saline flush.

IV (Children): 1 mg/kg bolus (not to exceed 100 mg), followed by 20–50 mcg/kg/min continuous infusion (range 20–50 mcg/kg/min); may administer second bolus of 0.5–1 mg/kg if delay between bolus and continuous infusion.

Endotracheal (Children): Give 2–3 mg/kg down the endotracheal tube followed by a 5 mL saline flush.

IM (Adults and Children ≥50 kg): 300 mg (4.5 mg/kg); may be repeated in 60–90 min.

Local

Infiltration (Adults and Children): Infiltrate affected area as needed (increased amount and frequency of use increases likelihood of systemic absorption and adverse reactions).

Topical (Adults): Apply to affected area 2–3 times daily.

Mucosal (Adults): *For anesthetizing oral surfaces*—20 mg as 2 sprays/quadrant (not to exceed 30 mg/quadrant) may be used. 15 mL of the viscous solution may be used q 3 hr for oral or pharyngeal pain. *For anesthetizing the female urethra*—3–5 mL of the jelly or 20 mg as 2% solution may be used. *For anesthetizing the male urethra*—5–10 mL of the jelly or 5–15 mL of 2% solution may be used before catheterization or 30 mL of jelly before cystoscopy or similar procedures. Topical solutions may be used to anesthetize mucous membranes of the larynx, trachea, or esophagus.

Patch (Adults): Up to 3 patches may be applied once for up to 12 hr in any 24-hr period; consider smaller areas of application in geriatric or debilitated patients.

Availability (generic available)

Autoinjector for IM injection: 300 mg/3 mL. **Direct IV injection:** 10 mg/mL (1%), 20 mg/mL (2%). **For IV admixture:** 100 mg/mL (10%). **Premixed solution for IV infusion:** 4 mg/mL (0.4%), 8 mg/mL (0.8%). **Injection for local infiltration/nerve block:** 0.5%, 1%, 2%, 4%. *In combination with:* epinephrine for local infiltration. **Cream:** 4% OTC. **Gel:** 0.5% OTC, 2.5% OTC. **Jelly:** 2%. **Liquid:** 5%. **Ointment:** 5%. **Transdermal system:** 5% patch. **Cost:** $189.98/box of 30 patches. **Solution:** 4%. **Spray:** 10%. **Viscous solution:** 2%. *In combination with:* prilocaine (as EMLA cream, Oraquix); with tetracaine (Synera); with bupivacaine (Duocaine); with epinephrine (LidoSite).

NURSING IMPLICATIONS

Assessment

- **Antiarrhythmic:** Monitor ECG continuously and blood pressure and respiratory status frequently during administration.
- **Anesthetic:** Assess degree of numbness of affected part.
- **Transdermal:** Monitor for pain intensity in affected area periodically during therapy.
- *Lab Test Considerations:* Serum electrolyte levels should be monitored periodically during prolonged therapy.
- IM administration may cause ↑ CPK levels.
- *Toxicity and Overdose:* Serum lidocaine levels should be monitored periodically during prolonged or high-dose IV therapy. Therapeutic serum lidocaine levels range from 1.5 to 5 mcg/mL.
- Signs and symptoms of toxicity include confusion, excitation, blurred or double vision, nausea, vomiting, ringing in ears, tremors, twitch-

LIDOCAINE

ing, seizures, difficulty breathing, severe dizziness or fainting, and unusually slow heart rate.
- If symptoms of overdose occur, stop infusion and monitor patient closely.

Potential Nursing Diagnoses
Decreased cardiac output (Indications)
Acute pain (Indications)

Implementation
- **High Alert:** Lidocaine is readily absorbed through mucous membranes. Inadvertent overdosage of lidocaine jelly and spray has resulted in patient harm or death from neurologic and/or cardiac toxicity. Do not exceed recommended doses.
- **Throat Spray:** Ensure that gag reflex is intact before allowing patient to drink or eat.
- **IM:** IM injections are recommended only when ECG monitoring is not available and benefits outweigh risks. Administer IM injections only into deltoid muscle while frequently aspirating to prevent IV injection.

IV Administration
- **Direct IV:** Only 1% and 2% solutions are used for direct IV injection. *Diluent:* Administer undiluted. *Rate:* Administer loading dose over 2–3 min. Follow by IV continuous infusion.
- **Continuous Infusion:** *Diluent:* Lidocaine vials need to be further diluted. Dilute 2 g of lidocaine in 250 mL or 500 mL of D5W or 0.9% NaCl. Admixed infusion stable for 24 hr at room temperature. Premixed infusions are already diluted and ready to use. *Concentration:* 4–8 mg/mL. *Rate:* See Route/Dosage section. Administer via infusion pump for accurate dose.
- **Y-Site Compatibility:** alteplase, amikacin, aminophylline, amiodarone, argatroban, atropine, aztreonam, bivalirudin, bumetanide, calcium chloride, calcium gluconate, cefazolin, cefotaxime, cefoxitin, ceftazidime, ceftizoxime, ceftriaxone, cefuroxime, chloramphenicol, cimetidine, ciprofloxacin, cisatracurium, clindamycin, cyclosporine, daptomycin, dexamethasone sodium phosphate, dexmedetomidine, digoxin, diltiazem, diphenhydramine, dobutamine, dopamine, doxycycline, enalaprilat, epinephrine, eptifibatide, ertapenem, erythromycin, esmolol, etomidate, famotidine, fenoldopam, fentanyl, fluconazole, furosemide, gentamicin, granisetron, haloperidol, heparin, hydrocortisone sodium succinate, imipenem/cilastatin, inamrinone, insulin, isoproterenol, ketorolac, labetalol, levofloxacin, linezolid, lorazepam, magnesium sulfate, meperidine, methylprednisolone sodium succinate, metoclopramide, metoprolol, metronidazole, micafungin, midazolam, morphine, nafcillin, nicardipine, nitroglycerin, nitroprusside, norepinephrine, ondansetron, palonosetron, penicillin G potassium, phenylephrine, phytonadione, piperacillin/tazobactam, potassium chloride, procainamide, prochlorperazine, promethazine, propofol, propranolol, protamine, quinupristin/dalfopristin, ranitidine, remifentanil, sodium bicarbonate, streptokinase, tacrolimus, theophylline, ticarcillin/clavulanate, tigecycline, tirofiban, tobramycin, vancomycin, vasopressin, verapamil, vitamin B complex with C, voriconazole, warfarin.
- **Y-Site Incompatibility:** acyclovir, amphotericin B cholesteryl sulfate complex, caspofungin, diazepam, ganciclovir, lansoprazole, pantoprazole, phenytoin, thiopental, trimethoprim/sulfamethoxazole.
- **Infiltration:** Lidocaine with epinephrine may be used to minimize systemic absorption and prolong local anesthesia.
- **Transdermal:** When used concomitantly with other products containing local anesthetic agents, consider amount absorbed from all formulations.

Patient/Family Teaching
- May cause drowsiness and dizziness. Advise patient to call for assistance during ambulation and transfer.
- **IM:** Available in LidoPen Auto-Injector for use outside the hospital setting. Advise patient to telephone health care professional immediately if symptoms of a heart attack occur. Do not administer unless instructed by health care professional. To administer, remove safety cap and place back end on thickest part of thigh or deltoid muscle. Press hard until needle prick is felt. Hold in place for 10 sec, then massage area for 10 sec. Do not drive after administration unless absolutely necessary.
- **Topical:** Apply *Lidoderm Patch* to intact skin to cover the most painful area. Patch may be cut to smaller sizes with scissors before removing release liner. Clothing may be worn over patch. If irritation or burning sensation occurs during application, remove patch until irritation subsides. Wash hands after application; avoid contact with eyes. Dispose of used patch to avoid access by children or pets.
- Caution women to consult health care professional before using a topical anesthetic for a mammogram or other procedures. If recom-

lidocaine/prilocaine 787

mended, use lowest drug concentration, and apply it sparingly. Do not apply to broken or irritated skin, do not wrap skin, and do not apply heat to area, to decrease chance that drug may be absorbed into the body. May result in seizures, cardiac arrhythmias, respiratory failure, coma, and death.
- Advise patient referred for MRI test to discuss patch with referring health care professional and MRI facility to determine if removal of patch is necessary prior to test and for directions for replacing patch.

Evaluation/Desired Outcomes
- Decrease in ventricular arrhythmias.
- Local anesthesia.

lidocaine/prilocaine
(lye-doe-kane/pri-loe-kane)
EMLA

Classification
Therapeutic: anesthetics (topical/local)

Pregnancy Category B

Indications
Produces local anesthesia prior to minor painful procedures including: Insertion of cannulae or needles, Arterial/venous/lumbar puncture, Intramuscular injections, Subcutaneous injections, Dermal procedures, Laser treatments, Circumcision. When applied to genital mucous membranes in preparation for superficial minor surgery or as preparation for infiltration anesthesia.

Action
Produces local anesthesia by inhibiting transport of ions across neuronal membranes, thereby preventing initiation and conduction of normal nerve impulses. Combination of two anesthetics is applied as a system consisting of a cream under an occlusive dressing. Active drug is released into the dermal and epidermal skin layers, resulting in accumulation of local anesthetic in the regions of dermal pain receptors and nerve endings. **Therapeutic Effects:** Anesthetic action localized to the area of the application.

Pharmacokinetics
Absorption: Small amounts are systemically absorbed during 4-hr placement of EMLA system.
Distribution: Small amounts absorbed are widely distributed and cross the placenta and blood-brain barrier.

Metabolism and Excretion: *Lidocaine*—mostly metabolized by the liver. *Prilocaine*—metabolized by the liver and kidneys.
Half-life: *Lidocaine*—7–30 min first phase, 90–120 min terminal phase: *Prilocaine*—10–50 min.

TIME/ACTION PROFILE (local anesthesia)

ROUTE	ONSET	PEAK	DURATION†
Top	15 min	3 hr	1–2 hr

†Following removal of occlusive dressing

Contraindications/Precautions
Contraindicated in: Hypersensitivity to lidocaine, prilocaine, or any other amide-type local anesthetic; Hypersensitivity to any other product in the formulation; Should not be applied to middle ear; Pedi: Congenital or idiopathic methemoglobinemia; Infants <6 mo receiving methemoglobin-inducing agents.
Use Cautiously in: Repeated use or use on large areas of skin (more likely to result in systemic absorption); Acutely ill, or debilitated patients (↑ risk of absorption and systemic effects); Severe liver disease; Any conditions associated with methemoglobinemia (including glucose-6-phosphate dehydrogenase deficiency); OB: Use only if clearly needed; Lactation: Usually compatible with breastfeeding (AAP); Pedi: Area/duration of treatment should be limited in neonates and children <20 kg or 37 weeks gestation (↑ susceptibility to methemoglobinemia); Geri: May have ↑ absorption and risk of systemic effects.

Adverse Reactions/Side Effects
Local: blanching, redness, alteration in temperature sensation, edema, itching, rash. **Misc:** allergic reactions including ANAPHYLAXIS.

Interactions
Drug-Drug: Concurrent use with class I antiarrhythmics including **mexiletine** may result in adverse cardiovascular effects. Concurrent use with other **local anesthetics** may result in ↑ toxicity. Concurrent use with **sulfonamides** in children ↑ the risk of methemoglobinemia (avoid concurrent use in children <12 mo).

Route/Dosage
Topical (Adults and Children): *Minor dermal procedures including venipuncture and IV cannulation*—2.5 g (½ of the 5-g tube) applied to 20–25 cm² (2 in. by 2 in.) area of skin, covered with an occlusive dressing applied for at least 1 hr. *Major dermal procedures including*

split-thickness skin graft harvesting—2 g/10 cm^2 area of skin, covered with an occlusive dressing for at least 2 hr. *Adult male genital skin*— as an adjunct prior to local anesthetic infiltration, apply a thick layer (1 g/10 cm^2) to skin surface for 15 min; local infiltration anesthesia should be performed immediately after removal of cream. *Adult female genital mucous membranes*—apply a thick layer (5–log) for 5–10 min.
Topical (Children 7–12 yr and >20 kg): Dose should not exceed 20 g over more than 200 cm^2 for more than 4 hr.
Topical (Children 1–6 yr and >10 kg): Dose should not exceed 10 g over more than 100 cm^2 for more than 4 hr.
Topical (Children 3 mo–12 mo and >5 kg): Dose should not exceed 2 g over more than 20 cm^2 for more than 4 hr.
Topical (Children 0–3 mo or <5 kg): Dose should not exceed 1 g over more than 10 cm^2 for more than 1 hr.

Availability (generic available)
Cream: 2.5% lidocaine with 2.5% prilocaine.

NURSING IMPLICATIONS
Assessment
- Assess application site for open wounds. Apply only to intact skin.
- Assess application site for anesthesia following removal of system and prior to procedure.

Potential Nursing Diagnoses
Acute pain (Indications)

Implementation
- **Topical:** When used for minor dermal procedures (venipuncture, IV cannulation, arterial puncture, lumbar puncture), apply the 2.5-g tube of cream (½ of the 5-g tube) to each 2 in. by 2 in. area of skin in a *thick* layer at the site of the impending procedure. Remove the center cutout piece from an occlusive dressing (supplied with the 5-g tube) and peel the paper liner from the paper-framed dressing. Cover the lidocaine/prilocaine cream so that there is a *thick* layer of cream underneath the occlusive dressing. Do not spread out or rub in the cream. Smooth the dressing edges carefully and ensure it is secure to avoid leakage. Remove the paper frame and mark the time of application on the occlusive dressing. Lidocaine/prilocaine cream must be applied *at least 1 hr* before the start of a minor dermal procedure (venipuncture, IV cannulation). Anesthesia may be more profound with 90 min–2 hr application. Remove the occlusive dressing and wipe off the lidocaine/prilocaine cream. Clean the entire area with antiseptic solution and prepare the patient for the procedure.
- For major dermal procedures (skin graft harvesting), follow the same procedure using larger amounts of lidocaine/prilocaine cream and the appropriate-size occlusive dressing. Lidocaine/prilocaine cream must be applied *at least 2 hr* before major dermal procedures.

Patient/Family Teaching
- Explain the purpose of cream and occlusive dressing to patient and parents. Inform the patient that lidocaine/prilocaine cream may block all sensations in the treated skin. Caution patient to avoid trauma to the area from scratching, rubbing, or exposure to extreme heat or cold temperatures until all sensation has returned.
- **Home Care Issues:** Instruct patient or parent in proper application. Provide a diagram of location for application.

Evaluation/Desired Outcomes
- Anesthesia in the area of application.

lindane (lin-dane)
gamma benzene hexachloride, ✦ GBH, ✦ Hexit, ✦ PMS Lindane

Classification
Therapeutic: pediculocides, scabicides

Pregnancy Category B

Indications
Second-line treatment of parasitic arthropod infestation (scabies and head, body, and crab lice) for use only in patients who are intolerant to or do not respond to less toxic agents.

Action
Causes seizures and death in parasitic arthropods.
Therapeutic Effects: Cure of infestation by parasitic arthropods.

Pharmacokinetics
Absorption: Significant systemic absorption (9–13%) greater with topical application to damaged skin.
Distribution: Stored in fat.
Metabolism and Excretion: Metabolized by the liver.
Half-life: 17–22 hr (infants and children).

TIME/ACTION PROFILE (antiparasitic action)

ROUTE	ONSET	PEAK	DURATION
Top	rapid	6 hr	190 min

Contraindications/Precautions

Contraindicated in: Hypersensitivity; Areas of skin rash, abrasion, or inflammation (absorption is increased); History of seizures; Lactation: Potentially toxic to infants; may ↓ milk supply; Pedi: Premature neonates (↑ risk of CNS toxicity).

Use Cautiously in: Patients with skin conditions (↑ risk of systemic absorption); OB: Do not exceed recommended dose; do not use >2 courses of therapy; Pedi, Geri: Children ≤2 yr and geriatric patients (↑ risk of systemic absorption and CNS side effects).

Adverse Reactions/Side Effects

All adverse reactions except dermatologic are signs of systemic absorption and toxicity. **CNS:** SEIZURES, headache. **CV:** tachycardia. **GI:** nausea, vomiting. **Derm:** contact dermatitis (repeated application), local irritation.

Interactions

Drug-Drug: Concurrent use of **medications that lower seizure threshold** (may ↑ risk of seizures). Simultaneous topical use of **skin, scalp,** or **hair** products may ↑ systemic absorption.

Route/Dosage

Scabies

Topical (Adults and Children > 1 month): 1% lotion applied to all skin surfaces from neck to toes; wash off 6 hr after application in infants, after 6–8 hr in children or after 8–12 hr in adults; may require a 2nd treatment 1 wk later.

Head Lice or Crab Lice

Topical (Adults and Children): 15–30 mL of shampoo applied and lathered for 4 min; may require a 2nd treatment 1 wk later.

Availability (generic available)

Lotion: 1%. **Shampoo:** 1%.

NURSING IMPLICATIONS

Assessment

- Assess skin and hair for signs of infestation before and after treatment.
- Examine family members and close contacts for infestation. When used in treatment of pediculosis pubis or scabies, sexual partners should receive concurrent prophylactic therapy.

Potential Nursing Diagnoses

Risk for impaired skin integrity (Indications)

Implementation

- Due to serious side effects, no more than 2 oz may be dispensed at a time and no refills are allowed.
- **Topical:** When applying medication to another person, wear gloves to prevent systemic absorption.
- Do not apply to open wounds (scratches, cuts, sores on skin or scalp) to minimize systemic absorption. Avoid contact with the eyes. If eye contact occurs, flush thoroughly with water and notify physician or other health care professional.
- Institute appropriate isolation techniques.
- **Lotion:** Instruct patient to bathe with soap and water. Dry skin well and allow to cool before application. Apply lotion in amount sufficient to cover entire body surface with a thin film from neck down (60 mL for an adult). Leave medication on for an age appropriate time frame (see dosing), then remove by washing. If rash, burning, or itching develops, wash off medication and notify physician or other health care professional.
- **Shampoo:** Use a sufficient amount of shampoo to wet hair and scalp (30 mL for short hair, 45 mL for medium hair, 60 mL for long hair). Rub thoroughly into hair and scalp and leave in place for 4 min. Then use enough water to work up a good lather; follow with thorough rinsing and drying. If applied in shower or bath, do not let shampoo run down on other parts of body or into water in which patient is sitting. When hair is dry, use fine-toothed comb to remove remaining nits or nit shells. Shampoo may also be used on combs and brushes to prevent spread of infestation.

Patient/Family Teaching

- Instruct patient on application technique and provide with a medication guide. Patient should repeat therapy only at the recommendation of health care professional. Discuss hygienic measures to prevent and to control infestation. Discuss potential for infectious contacts with patient. Explain why household members should be examined and sexual partners treated simultaneously.
- Instruct patient to wash all recently worn clothing and used bed linens and towels in very hot water or to dry clean to prevent reinfestation or spreading.

- Instruct patient not to apply other oils or creams during therapy; these increase the absorption of lindane and may lead to toxicity.
- Explain to patient that itching may persist after treatment; consult health care professional about use of topical hydrocortisone or systemic antihistamines.
- Advise patient that eyelashes can be treated by applying petroleum jelly 3 times/day for 1 wk.
- **Instruct patient not to reapply sooner than 1 week if live mites appear**.
- **Shampoo:** Advise patient that shampoo should not be used as a regular shampoo in the absence of infestation. Emphasize need to avoid contact with eyes.
- Pedi: Advise parents to monitor young children closely for evidence of CNS toxicity (seizures, dizziness, clumsiness, fast heartbeat, muscle cramps, nervousness, restlessness, irritability, nausea, vomiting) during and immediately after treatment.
- Pedi: Cover hands of young children to prevent accidental ingestion from thumbsucking.

Evaluation/Desired Outcomes
- Resolution of signs of infestation with scabies or lice.

---

linezolid (li-nez-o-lid)
Zyvox

Classification
Therapeutic: anti-infectives
Pharmacologic: oxazolidinones

Pregnancy Category C

Indications
Treatment of: Infections caused by vancomycin-resistant *Enterococcus faecium*, Nosocomial pneumonia caused by *Staphylococcus aureus* (methicillin-susceptible and -resistant strains), Complicated skin/skin structure infections caused by *Staphylococcus aureus* (methicillin-susceptible and -resistant strains), *Streptococcus pyogenes* or *Streptococcus agalactiae* (including diabetic foot infections), Uncomplicated skin/skin structure infections caused by *Staphylococcus aureus* (methicillin-susceptible and -resistant strains), *Streptococcus pyogenes*, Community-acquired pneumonia caused by *Streptococcus pneumoniae* (including multi-drug resistant strains) or *Staphylococcus aureus* (methicillin-susceptible strains only).

Action
Inhibits bacterial protein synthesis at the level of the 23S ribosome of the 50S subunit. **Therapeutic Effects:** Bactericidal action against streptococci; bacteriostatic action against enterococci and staphylococci.

Pharmacokinetics
Absorption: Rapidly and extensively (100%) absorbed following oral administration.
Distribution: Readily distributes to well-perfused tissues.
Metabolism and Excretion: 65% metabolized, mostly by the liver; 30% excreted unchanged by the kidneys.
Half-life: 6.4 hr.

TIME/ACTION PROFILE

ROUTE	ONSET	PEAK	DURATION
PO	rapid	1–2 hr	12 hr
IV	rapid	end of infusion	12 hr

Contraindications/Precautions
Contraindicated in: Hypersensitivity; Phenylketonuria (suspension contains aspartame); Uncontrolled HTN, pheochromocytoma, thyrotoxicosis, or concurrent use of sympathomimetic agents, vasopressors, or dopaminergic agents (↑ risk of hypertensive response); Concurrent or recent (< 2 wk) use of monoamine oxidase (MAO) inhibitors (↑ risk of hypertensive response); Carcinoid syndrome or concurrent use of SSRIs, TCAs, triptans, meperidine, or buspirone (↑ risk of serotonin syndrome).
Use Cautiously in: Thrombocytopenia, concurrent use of antiplatelet agents or bleeding diathesis (platelet counts should be monitored more frequently); OB: Safety not established; use only if maternal benefit outweighs potential risk to fetus; Lactation: Lactation.

Adverse Reactions/Side Effects
CV: headache, insomnia. **GI:** PSEUDOMEMBRANOUS COLITIS, diarrhea, ↑ liver function tests, nausea, taste alteration, vomiting. **F and E:** lactic acidosis. **Hemat:** thrombocytopenia. **Neuro:** optic neuropathy, peripheral neuropathy.

Interactions
Drug-Drug: ↑ risk of hypertensive response with **MAO inhibitors**, **sympathomimetics** (e.g., **pseudoephedrine**), **vasopressors** (e.g., **epinephrine**, **norepinephrine**), and **dopaminergic agents** (e.g., **dopamine**, **dobutamine**); concurrent or recent use should be avoided. ↑ risk of serotonin syndrome with **SSRIs**, **TCAs**, **5–HT₁ agonists**, **meperidine**, or **buspirone**; concurrent use should be avoided.
Drug-Food: Because of monoamine oxidase inhibitory properties, consumption of large

amounts of foods or beverages containing tyramine should be avoided (↑ risk of pressor response. See Appendix M).

Route/Dosage

Vancomycin-Resistant *Enterococcus faecium* Infections
PO, IV (Adults): 600 mg every 12 hr for 14–28 days.
PO, IV (Children birth-11 yr): (in the first week of life, pre-term neonates may initially receive 10 mg/kg every 12 hr).

Pneumonia, Complicated Skin/Skin Structure Infections
PO, IV (Adults): 600 mg every 12 hr for 10–14 days.
PO, IV (Children birth-11 yr): 10 mg/kg every 8 hr for 10–14 days (in the first week of life, pre-term neonates may initially receive 10 mg/kg every 12 hr).

Uncomplicated Skin/Skin Structure Infections
PO (Adults): 400 mg q 12 hr for 10–14 days.
PO, IV (Children 5-11 yr): 10 mg/kg every 12 hr for 10–14 days.
PO, IV (Children < 5 yr): 10 mg/kg every 8 hr for 10–14 days (in the first week of life, pre-term neonates may initially receive 10 mg/kg every 12 hr).

Availability (generic available)
Oral suspension: (orange): 20 mg/mL. **Tablets:** 400 mg, 600 mg. **Cost:** 600 mg $2,213.46/30. **Premixed infusion:** 200 mg/100 mL, 400 mg/200 mL, 600 mg/300 mL.

NURSING IMPLICATIONS

Assessment
- Assess for infection (vital signs; appearance of wound, sputum, urine, and stool; WBC) at beginning of and during therapy.
- Obtain specimens for culture and sensitivity prior to initiating therapy. First dose may be given before receiving.
- May cause lactic acidosis. Notify health care professional if recurrent nausea and vomiting, unexplained acidosis or low bicarbonate levels occur.
- Monitor visual function in patients receiving linezolid for ≥3 months or who report visual symptoms (changes in acuity or color vision, blurred vision, visual field defect) regardless of length of therapy. If optic neuropathy occurs therapy should be reconsidered.
- Monitor bowel function. Diarrhea, abdominal cramping, fever, and bloody stools should be reported to health care professional promptly as a sign of pseudomembranous colitis. May begin up to several weeks following cessation of therapy.
- *Lab Test Considerations:* May cause bone marrow suppression, anemia, leukopenia, pancytopenia. Monitor CBC and platelet count weekly, especially in patients at risk for increased bleeding, having pre-existing bone marrow suppression, receiving concurrent medications that may cause myelosuppression, or requiring >2 weeks of therapy. Discontinue therapy if bone marrow suppression occurs or worsens.
- May cause ↑ AST, ALT, LDH, alkaline phosphatase and BUN.

Potential Nursing Diagnoses
Risk for infection (Indications)

Implementation
- Dose adjustment is not necessary when switching from IV to oral dose.
- **PO:** May be administered with or without food.
- Before using oral solution gently invert 3–5 times to mix; do not shake. Store at room temperature.

IV Administration
- **Intermittent Infusion:** *Diluent:* Premixed infusions are already diluted and ready to use. Solution is yellowish in color which may intensify over time without affecting its potency. *Concentration:* 2 mg/mL. *Rate:* Infuse over 30–120 minutes. Flush line before and after infusion.
- **Y-Site Compatibility:** acyclovir, alfentanil, amikacin, aminophylline, amiodarone, ampicillin, ampicillin/sulbactam, anidulafungin, aztreonam, buprenorphine, butorphanol, bumetanide, calcium chloride, calcium gluconate, carboplatin, caspofungin, cefazolin, cefepime, cefotaxime, cefoxitin, ceftazidime, ceftizoxime, ceftriaxone, cefuroxime, chloramphenicol, cimetidine, ciprofloxacin, cisatracurium, cisplatin, clindamycin, cyclophosphamide, cyclosporine, cytarabine, daptomycin, dexamethasone sodium phosphate, dexmede-

tomidine, digoxin, diltiazem, diphenhydramine, dobutamine, dolasetron, dopamine, doxorubicin, doxycycline, droperidol, enalaprilat, epinephrine, ertapenem, esmolol, dexmedetomidine, etoposide phosphate, famotidine, fenoldopam, fentanyl, fluconazole, fluorouracil, furosemide, ganciclovir, gemcitabine, gentamicin, granisetron, haloperidol, heparin, hydralazine, hydrocortisone, hydromorphone, imipenem/cilastatin, insulin, isoproterenol, ketorolac, labetalol, leucovorin, levofloxacin, lidocaine, lorazepam, magnesium sulfate, mannitol, meperidine, meropenem, methotrexate, methylprednisolone, metoclopramide, metoprolol, metronidazole, midazolam, milrinone, morphine, nafcillin, nalbuphine, naloxone, nicardipine, nitroglycerin, nitroprusside, norepinephrine, ondansetron, paclitaxel, pentobarbital, phenobarbital, palonosetron, pancuronium, phenylephrine, piperacillin/tazobactam, potassium chloride, potassium phosphate, procainamide, prochlorperazine, promethazine, propranolol, quinupristin/dalfopristin, ranitidine, remifentanil, sodium bicarbonate, sufentanil, tacrolimus, theophylline, ticarcillin/clavulanate, tigecycline, tirofiban, tobramycin, trimethoprim/sulfamethoxazole, vancomycin, vasopressin, vecuronium, verapamil, vincristine, voriconazole, zidovudine.

- **Y-Site Incompatibility:** amphotericin B, chlorpromazine, diazepam, pantoprazole, pentamidine, phenytoin.

Patient/Family Teaching
- Advise patients taking oral linezolid to take as directed, for full course of therapy, even if feeling better. Take missed doses as soon as remembered unless almost time for next dose; do not double dose.
- Instruct patient to avoid large quantities of foods or beverages containing tyramine (See Appendix M). May cause hypertensive response.
- Instruct patient to notify health care professional if patient has a history of hypertension and before patient takes other Rx, OTC, or herbal products, especially cold remedies, decongestants, or antidepressants.
- Instruct patient to notify health care professional immediately if diarrhea, abdominal cramping, fever, or bloody stools occur and not to treat with antidiarrheals without consulting health care professionals.
- Advise patient to notify health care professional if no improvement is seen in a few days.

Evaluation/Desired Outcomes
- Resolution of signs and symptoms of infection. Length of time for complete resolution depends on organism and site of infection.

liothyronine, See THYROID PREPARATIONS.

liotrix, See THYROID PREPARATIONS.

lisinopril, See ANGIOTENSIN-CONVERTING ENZYME (ACE) INHIBITORS.

lithium (lith-ee-um)
♣ Carbolith, ♣ Duralith, Eskalith, ♣ Lithizine, Lithobid

Classification
Therapeutic: mood stabilizers

Pregnancy Category D

Indications
Manic episodes of manic depressive illness (treatment, maintenance, prophylaxis).

Action
Alters cation transport in nerve and muscle. May also influence reuptake of neurotransmitters.
Therapeutic Effects: Prevents/decreases incidence of acute manic episodes.

Pharmacokinetics
Absorption: Completely absorbed after oral administration.
Distribution: Widely distributed into many tissues and fluids; CSF levels are 50% of plasma levels. Crosses the placenta; enters breast milk.
Metabolism and Excretion: Excreted almost entirely unchanged by the kidneys.
Half-life: 20–27 hr.

TIME/ACTION PROFILE (antimanic effects)

ROUTE	ONSET	PEAK	DURATION
PO, PO–ER	5–7 days	10–21 days	days

Contraindications/Precautions
Contraindicated in: Hypersensitivity; Severe cardiovascular or renal disease; Dehydrated or debilitated patients; Should be used only where therapy, including blood levels, may be closely monitored; Some products contain alcohol or tartrazine and should be avoided in patients with

known hypersensitivity or intolerance; Lactation: Lactation.
Use Cautiously in: Any degree of cardiac, renal, or thyroid disease; Diabetes mellitus; OB: Fetal cardiac anomalies are associated with lithium use; however, potential maternal benefit may warrant use in some pregnant women; Geri: Initial dosage ↓ recommended.

Adverse Reactions/Side Effects
CNS: SEIZURES, fatigue, headache, impaired memory, ataxia, sedation, confusion, dizziness, drowsiness, psychomotor retardation, restlessness, stupor. **EENT:** aphasia, blurred vision, dysarthria, tinnitus. **CV:** ARRHYTHMIAS, ECG changes, edema, hypotension. **GI:** abdominal pain, anorexia, bloating, diarrhea, nausea, dry mouth, metallic taste. **GU:** polyuria, glycosuria, nephrogenic diabetes insipidus, renal toxicity. **Derm:** acneiform eruption, folliculitis, alopecia, diminished sensation, pruritus. **Endo:** hypothyroidism, goiter, hyperglycemia, hyperthyroidism. **F and E:** hyponatremia. **Hemat:** leukocytosis. **Metab:** weight gain. **MS:** muscle weakness, hyperirritability, rigidity. **Neuro:** tremors.

Interactions
Drug-Drug: May prolong the action of **neuromuscular blocking agents**. ↑ risk of neurologic toxicity with **haloperidol** or **molindone**. **Diuretics, methyldopa, probenecid, fluoxetine,** and **NSAIDs** may ↑ risk of toxicity. Blood levels may be ↑ by **ACE inhibitors**. Lithium may ↓ effects of **chlorpromazine**. **Chlorpromazine** may mask early signs of lithium toxicity. Hypothyroid effects may be additive with **potassium iodide** or **antithyroid agents**. **Aminophylline, phenothiazines,** and **drugs containing large amounts of sodium** ↑ renal elimination and ↓ effectiveness. **Psyllium** can ↓ **lithium** levels.
Drug-Natural Products: Caffeine-containing herbs (**cola nut, guarana, mate, tea, coffee**) may ↓ **lithium** serum levels and efficacy.
Drug-Food: Large changes in **sodium** intake may alter the renal elimination of lithium. ↑ sodium intake will ↑ renal excretion.

Route/Dosage
Precise dosing is based on serum lithium levels. 300 mg lithium carbonate contains 8–12 mEq lithium.
PO (Adults and children ≥12 yr): *Tablets/capsules*— 300–600 mg 3 times daily initially; usual maintenance dose is 300 mg 3–4 times daily. *Slow-release capsules*— 200–300 mg 3 times daily initially; increased up to 1800 mg/day in divided doses. Usual maintenance dose is 300–400 mg 3 times daily. *Extended-release tablets*— 450–900 mg twice daily *or* 300–600 mg 3 times daily initially; usual maintenance dose is 450 mg twice daily *or* 300 mg 3 times daily.
PO (Children <12 yr): 15–20 mg (0.4–0.5 mEq)/kg/day in 2–3 divided doses; dosage may be adjusted weekly.

Availability (generic available)
Capsules: 150 mg, 300 mg, 600 mg. **Cost:** *Generic*— 150 mg $18.88/100, 300 mg $17.77/100, 600 mg $42.30/100—$0. **Tablets:** 300 mg. **Controlled-release tablets:** 300 mg, 450 mg. **Cost:** *Generic*— 300 mg $39.97/100, 450 mg $48.32/100. **Slow-release tablets:** 300 mg. **Syrup:** 300 mg (8 mEq lithium)/5 mL. **Cost:** $60.00/500 mL.

NURSING IMPLICATIONS
Assessment
- Assess mental status (orientation, mood, behavior) initially and periodically. Assess manic symptoms with Young Mania Rating Scale (YMRS) at baseline and periodically through treatment in patients with mania. Initiate suicide precautions if indicated.
- Monitor intake and output ratios. Report significant changes in totals. Unless contraindicated, fluid intake of at least 2000–3000 mL/day should be maintained. Weight should also be monitored at least every 3 mo.
- *Lab Test Considerations:* Evaluate renal and thyroid function, WBC with differential, serum electrolytes, and glucose periodically during therapy.
- *Lab Test Considerations:* EKG for patients >50 yr old.
- *Toxicity and Overdose:* Monitor serum lithium levels twice weekly during initiation of therapy and every 2–3 mo during chronic therapy. Draw blood samples in the morning immediately before next dose. Therapeutic levels range from 0.5 to 1.5 mEq/L.
- Assess patient for signs and symptoms of lithium toxicity (vomiting, diarrhea, slurred speech, decreased coordination, drowsiness, muscle weakness, or twitching). If these occur, report before administering next dose.

Potential Nursing Diagnoses
Disturbed thought process (Indications)
Ineffective coping (Indications)
Imbalanced nutrition: risk for more than body requirements (Side Effects)

Implementation
- Do not confuse Lithobid (lithium) with Levbid (hyoscyamine).
- **PO:** Administer with food or milk to minimize GI irritation. Extended-release preparations should be swallowed whole; do not break, crush, or chew.

Patient/Family Teaching
- Instruct patient to take medication as directed, even if feeling well. Take missed doses as soon as remembered unless within 2 hr of next dose (6 hr if extended release).
- Lithium may cause dizziness or drowsiness. Caution patient to avoid driving or other activities requiring alertness until response to medication is known.
- Advise patient that psychotherapy is beneficial in improving coping skills.
- Low sodium levels may predispose patient to toxicity. Advise patient to drink 2000–3000 mL fluid each day and eat a diet with consistent and moderate sodium intake. Excessive amounts of coffee, tea, and cola should be avoided because of diuretic effect. Avoid activities that cause excess sodium loss (heavy exertion, exercise in hot weather, saunas). Notify health care professional of fever, vomiting, and diarrhea, which also cause sodium loss.
- Advise patient that weight gain may occur. Review principles of a low-calorie diet.
- Instruct patient to consult health care professional before taking OTC medications or herbal products concurrently with this therapy.
- Advise patient to use contraception and to consult health care professional if pregnancy is suspected.
- Review side effects and symptoms of toxicity with patient. Instruct patient to stop medication and report signs of toxicity to health care professional promptly.
- Explain to patients with cardiovascular disease or over 40 yr of age the need for ECG evaluation before and periodically during therapy. Patient should inform health care professional if fainting, irregular pulse, or difficulty breathing occurs.
- Emphasize the importance of periodic lab tests to monitor for lithium toxicity.

Evaluation/Desired Outcomes
- Resolution of the symptoms of mania (hyperactivity, pressured speech, poor judgment, need for little sleep).
- Decreased incidence of mood swings in bipolar disorders.
- Improved affect in unipolar disorders. Improvement in condition may require 1–3 wk.
- Remission of depressive symptoms.

---

loperamide (loe-**per**-a-mide)
Diar-aid Caplets, Imodium, Imodium A-D, Kaopectate II Caplets, Maalox Antidiarrheal Caplets, Neo-Diaral, Pepto Diarrhea Control

Classification
Therapeutic: antidiarrheals

Pregnancy Category B

Indications
Adjunctive therapy of acute diarrhea. Chronic diarrhea associated with inflammatory bowel disease. Decreases the volume of ileostomy drainage.

Action
Inhibits peristalsis and prolongs transit time by a direct effect on nerves in the intestinal muscle wall. Reduces fecal volume, increases fecal viscosity and bulk while diminishing loss of fluid and electrolytes. **Therapeutic Effects:** Relief of diarrhea.

Pharmacokinetics
Absorption: Not well absorbed following oral administration.
Distribution: Unknown. Does not cross the blood-brain barrier.
Protein Binding: 97%.
Metabolism and Excretion: Metabolized partially by the liver, undergoes enterohepatic recirculation; 30% eliminated in the feces. Minimal excretion in the urine.
Half-life: 10.8 hr.

TIME/ACTION PROFILE (relief of diarrhea)

ROUTE	ONSET	PEAK	DURATION
PO	1 hr	2.5–5 hr	10 hr

Contraindications/Precautions
Contraindicated in: Hypersensitivity; Patients in whom constipation must be avoided; Abdominal pain of unknown cause, especially if associated with fever; Alcohol intolerance (liquid only).
Use Cautiously in: Hepatic dysfunction; Lactation: Usually compatible with breastfeeding

(AAP); OB: Safety not established; Pedi: Children <2 yr (safety not established); Geri: ↑ sensitivity to effects.

Adverse Reactions/Side Effects
CNS: <u>drowsiness</u>, dizziness. **GI:** <u>constipation</u>, abdominal pain/distention/discomfort, dry mouth, nausea, vomiting. **Misc:** allergic reactions.

Interactions
Drug-Drug: ↑ CNS depression with other **CNS depressants**, including **alcohol**, **antihistamines**, **opioid analgesics**, and **sedative/hypnotics**. ↑ anticholinergic properties with other **drugs having anticholinergic properties**, including **antidepressants** and **antihistamines**.
Drug-Natural Products: Kava-kava, valerian, skullcap, chamomile, or hops can ↑ CNS depression.

Route/Dosage
PO (Adults): 4 mg initially, then 2 mg after each loose stool. Maintenance dose usually 4–8 mg/day in divided doses (not to exceed 8 mg/day for OTC use or 16 mg/day for Rx use).

PO (Children 9–11 yr or 30–47 kg): 2 mg initially; then 1 mg after each loose stool (not to exceed 6 mg/24 hr; OTC use should not exceed 2 days).

PO (Children 6–8 yr or 24–30 kg): 1 mg initially, then 1 mg after each loose stool (not to exceed 4 mg/24 hr; OTC use should not exceed 2 days).

Availability (generic available)
Tablets: 2 mg^{OTC}. **Capsules:** 2 mg. **Liquid (mint):** 1 mg/5 mL^{OTC}, 1 mg/7.5 mL^{OTC}. *In combination with:* simethicone (Immodium Advanced^{OTC}, see Appendix B).

NURSING IMPLICATIONS

Assessment
- Assess frequency and consistency of stools and bowel sounds prior to and during therapy.
- Assess fluid and electrolyte balance and skin turgor for dehydration.

Potential Nursing Diagnoses
Diarrhea (Indications)
Risk for injury (Side Effects)

Implementation
- **PO:** Administer with clear fluids to help prevent dehydration, which may accompany diarrhea.

Patient/Family Teaching
- Instruct patient to take medication as directed. Do not take missed doses, and do not double doses. In acute diarrhea, medication may be ordered after each unformed stool. Advise patient not to exceed the maximum number of doses.
- May cause drowsiness. Advise patient to avoid driving or other activities requiring alertness until response to drug is known.
- Advise patient that frequent mouth rinses, good oral hygiene, and sugarless gum or candy may relieve dry mouth.
- Caution patient to avoid using alcohol and other CNS depressants concurrently with this medication.
- Instruct patient to notify health care professional if diarrhea persists or if fever, abdominal pain, or distention occurs.

Evaluation/Desired Outcomes
- Decrease in diarrhea.
- In acute diarrhea, treatment should be discontinued if no improvement is seen in 48 hr.
- In chronic diarrhea, if no improvement has occurred after at least 10 days of treatment with maximum dose, loperamide is unlikely to be effective.

---

lopinavir/ritonavir
(loe-**pin**-a-veer/ri-**toe**-na-veer)
Kaletra

Classification
Therapeutic: antiretrovirals
Pharmacologic: protease inhibitors, metabolic inhibitors

Pregnancy Category C

Indications
HIV infection (with other antiretrovirals).

Action
Lopinavir: Inhibits HIV viral protease. **Ritonavir:** Although ritonavir has antiretroviral activity of its own (inhibits the action of HIV protease and prevents the cleavage of viral polyproteins), it is combined with lopinavir to inhibit the metabolism of lopinavir thus increasing its plasma levels.
Therapeutic Effects: Increased CD4 cell counts and decreased viral load with subsequent slowed progression of HIV infection and its sequelae.

796 lopinavir/ritonavir

Pharmacokinetics
Absorption: Well absorbed following oral administration; food enhances absorption.
Distribution: *Ritonavir*—poor CNS penetration.
Protein Binding: *Lopinavir*—98–99% bound to plasma proteins.
Metabolism and Excretion: *Lopinavir*—completely metabolized in the liver by cytochrome P450 P3A (CYP450 P3A); ritonavir is a potent inhibitor of this enzyme. *Ritonavir*—highly metabolized by the liver (by CYP450 P3A and CYP2D6 enzymes); one metabolite has antiretroviral activity; 3.5% excreted unchanged in urine.
Half-life: *Lopinavir*—5–6 hr *Ritonavir*—3–5 hr.

TIME/ACTION PROFILE (blood levels)

ROUTE	ONSET	PEAK	DURATION
Lopinavir PO	rapid	4 hr	12 hr
Ritonavir PO	rapid	4 hr*	12 hr

*Non-fasting

Contraindications/Precautions
Contraindicated in: Hypersensitivity; Concurrent use of dihydroergotamine, ergotamine, ergonovine, lovastatin, methylergonovine, midazolam (PO), pimozide, simvastatin, and triazolam (may result in serious and/or life-threatening events); Concurrent use with St. John's wort or rifampin (may lead to ↓ virologic response and possible resistance); Hypersensitivity or intolerance to alcohol or castor oil (present in liquid); Congenital long QT syndrome, concurrent use of QT-interval prolonging drugs, or hypokalemia (↑ risk of QT interval prolongation).
Use Cautiously in: Known alcohol intolerance (oral solution contains alcohol); Impaired hepatic function, history of hepatitis (for ritonavir content); Pre-existing conduction system disease (marked first-degree AV block or second- or third-degree AV block), ischemic heart disease, or concurrent use of other drugs that increase the PR interval (especially those metabolized by CYP3A4 including verapamil or diltiazem); OB, Lactation: Safety not established; breastfeeding not recommended in HIV-infected patients.

Adverse Reactions/Side Effects
CNS: headache, insomnia, weakness. **CV:** TORSADES DE POINTES, ↑ PR interval, heart block, QT interval prolongation. **GI:** HEPATOTOXICITY, PANCREATITIS, diarrhea (↑ in children), abdominal pain, nausea, taste aversion (in children), vomiting (↑ in children). **Derm:** rash.

Interactions
Drug-Drug: Concurrent use of **amiodarone**, **dihydroergotamine**, **ergonovine**, **ergotamine**, **methylergonovine**, **pimozide**, **simvastatin**, **lovastatin**, **midazolam** (oral), and **triazolam**, is contraindicated because of the risk of potentially serious, life-threatening drug interactions. Concurrent use of **rifampin** ↓ effectiveness of lopinavir/ritonavir (contraindicated). May ↑ levels of **sildenafil**, **vardenafil**, or **tadalafil**; may result in hypotension, syncope, visual changes, and prolonged erection (dose ↓ of sildenafil to 25 mg q 48 hr, vardenafil to 2.5 mg q 72 hr, and tadalafil to 10 mg q 72 hr recommended). ↑ risk of rhabdomyolysis with **atorvastatin** or **rosuvastatin** (alternatively consider using **pravastatin** or **fluvastatin**). Concurrent use with **efavirenz** or **nevirapine** ↓ lopinavir/ritonavir levels and effectiveness; dose ↑ recommended. **Delavirdine** ↑ lopinavir levels. ↑ **tenofovir** levels. ↓ **abacavir** and **zidovudine** levels. Concurrent use with **fosamprenavir** ↓ lopinavir and **fosamprenavir** levels. Concurrent use with **nelfinavir** ↓ lopinavir levels and ↑ **nelfinavir** levels. ↑ **indinavir** levels; indinavir dose should be ↓. ↑ **saquinavir** levels. **Tipranavir** ↓ lopinavir levels. ↑ **maraviroc** levels; maraviroc dose should be ↓ to 150 mg twice daily. ↑ levels of **amiodarone**, **lidocaine**, and **quinidine** (blood level monitoring recommended, if possible). Concurrent use of **carbamazepine**, **phenobarbital**, or **phenytoin** may ↓ effectiveness of lopinavir (blood level monitoring recommended); lopinavir may also ↓ **phenytoin** levels. May ↓ **bupropion** levels/effects. ↑ levels/effects of **trazodone**. ↑ levels of dihydropyridine calcium channel blockers including **felodipine**, **nifedipine**, **amlodipine**, and **nicardipine**. May alter levels and effectiveness of **warfarin**. ↑ levels of **clarithromycin** (dose ↓ recommended for patients with CCr ≤60 mL/min. ↑ blood levels of **itraconazole** and **ketoconazole** (high antifungal doses not recommended). ↓ levels of **voriconazole**; concurrent use not recommended. ↑ levels of **rifabutin** (dose ↓ recommended). ↓ levels of **atovaquone** (may require dosage ↑).
Dexamethasone ↓ levels/effectiveness of lopinavir. Oral solution contains alcohol may produce intolerance when administered with **disulfiram** or **metronidazole**. May ↑ levels and risk of toxicity with immunosuppressants including **cyclosporine**, **tacrolimus**, or **sirolimus** (blood level monitoring recommended). May ↓ levels and effects of **methadone** (dose of methadone may need to be ↑). May ↓ levels and contra-

ceptive efficacy of some estrogen-based **hormonal contraceptives** including **ethinyl estradiol** (alternative or additional methods of contraception recommended). ↑ levels of **fluticasone**; avoid concurrent use. ↑ **vincristine** and **vinblastine** levels. Concurrent use of other **drugs known to** ↑ **PR interval** may ↑ risk of heart block. Concurrent use of other **drugs known to** ↑ **QT interval** should be avoided. **Drug-Natural Products:** Concurrent use with **St. John's wort** may ↓ levels and beneficial effect of lopinavir/ritonavir (contraindicated).

Route/Dosage
PO (Adults and Children >40 kg): *Therapy-naive*—400/100 mg (two 200/50-mg tablets or 5 mL oral solution) twice daily *or* 800/200 mg (four 200/50–mg tablets or 10 mL oral solution) once daily; single dose approved for adults only; *Therapy-experienced*—400/100 mg (two 200/50-mg tablets or 5 mL oral solution) twice daily.
PO (Children 14 days–6 mo): *Oral solution*—16/4 mg/kg lopinavir/ritonavir content twice daily.
PO (Children ≥6 mo and 15–40 kg): *Oral solution*—10/2.5 mg/kg lopinavir/ritonavir content twice daily.
PO (Children ≥6 mo and <15 kg): *Oral solution*—12/3 mg/kg lopinavir/ritonavir content twice daily.
PO (Children ≥6 mo): *Tablets*—15–25 kg: Two 100/25-mg tablets twice daily; 26–35 kg: Three 100/25-mg tablets twice daily; >35 kg: Four 100/25-mg tablets or two 200/50-mg tablets twice daily.

With Concurrent Efavirenz, Nevirapine, Fosamprenavir, or Nelfinavir
PO (Adults and Children >40 kg): *Therapy-naive or therapy-experienced*—500/125 mg (two 200/50-mg tablets and one 100/25-mg tablet) twice daily *or* 533/133 mg (6.5 mL oral solution) twice daily.
PO (Children 14 days–6 mo): Not recommended for concomitant administration with these drugs.
PO (Children ≥6 mo and 15–45 kg): 11/2.75 mg/kg lopinavir/ritonavir content twice daily.
PO (Children ≥6 mo and <15 kg): 13/3.25 mg/kg lopinavir/ritonavir content twice daily.

Availability
Tablets: 100 mg lopinavir/25 mg ritonavir, 200 mg lopinavir/50 mg ritonavir. **Oral solution:** 80 mg lopinavir/20 mg ritonavir per mL (contains 42.4% alcohol).

NURSING IMPLICATIONS

Assessment
- Assess for change in severity of HIV symptoms and for symptoms of opportunistic infections during therapy.
- Assess patient for signs of pancreatitis (nausea, vomiting, abdominal pain, increased serum lipase or amylase) periodically during therapy. May require discontinuation of therapy.
- *Lab Test Considerations:* Monitor viral load and CD4 counts regularly during therapy.
- Monitor triglyceride and cholesterol levels prior to initiating therapy and periodically during therapy.
- May cause hyperglycemia.
- Monitor liver function before and during therapy, especially in patients with underlying hepatic disease, including hepatitis B and hepatitis C, or marked transaminase elevations. May cause ↑ serum AST, ALT, GGT, and total bilirubin concentrations.
- Monitor serum lipase and amylase levels during therapy.

Potential Nursing Diagnoses
Risk for infection (Indications)
Noncompliance (Patient/Family Teaching)

Implementation
- Do not confuse Kaletra (lopinavir/ritonavir) with Keppra (levetiracetam).
- Patients taking didanosine with Kaletra solution should take didanosine 1 hr before or 2 hr after taking lopinavir/ritonavir.
- **PO:** Tablets may be administered with or without food. Swallow whole, do not break, crush, or chew. Oral solution must be taken with food.
- Oral solution is light yellow to orange.
- Oral solution are stable if refrigerated until expiration date on label or 2 months at room temperature.

Patient/Family Teaching
- Emphasize the importance of taking lopinavir/ritonavir as directed, at evenly spaced times throughout day. Do not take more than prescribed amount, and do not stop taking this or other antiretrovirals without consulting health care professional. Take missed doses as soon as remembered; do not double doses. Advise patient to read the *Patient Information* prior

- to taking this medication and with each Rx refill in case of changes.
- Instruct parent/patient to measure oral solution carefully.
- Instruct patient that lopinavir/ritonavir should not be shared with others.
- Advise patient to avoid taking other medications, RX, OTC, or herbal products, especially St. John's wort, without consulting health care professional.
- Inform patient that lopinavir/ritonavir does not cure AIDS or prevent associated or opportunistic infections. Lopinavir/ritonavir does not reduce the risk of transmission of HIV to others through sexual contact or blood contamination. Caution patient to use a condom during sexual contact and to avoid sharing needles or donating blood to prevent spreading the AIDS virus to others. Advise patient that the long-term effects of lopinavir/ritonavir are unknown at this time.
- Instruct patient to notify health care professional immediately if symptoms of lactic acidosis (tiredness or weakness, unusual muscle pain, trouble breathing, stomach pain with nausea and vomiting, cold especially in arms or legs, dizziness, fast or irregular heartbeat) or if signs of hepatotoxicity (yellow skin or whites of eyes, dark urine, light-colored stools, lack of appetite for several days or longer, nausea, abdominal pain) occur.
- Inform patient that lopinavir/ritonavir may cause hyperglycemia. Advise patient to notify health care professional if increased thirst or hunger; unexplained weight loss; or increased urination occurs.
- Advise patients taking oral contraceptives to use a nonhormonal method of birth control during lopinavir/ritonavir therapy.
- Caution patients taking sildenafil, vardenafil, or tadalafil of increased risk of associated side effects (hypotension, visual changes, sustained erection). Notify health care professional promptly if these occur.
- Inform patient that redistribution and accumulation of body fat may occur causing central obesity, dorsocervical fat enlargement (buffalo hump), peripheral wasting, breast enlargement, and cushingoid appearance. The cause and long-term effects are not known.
- Instruct patient to notify health care professional if pregnancy is planned or suspected of if breastfeeding an infant.
- Emphasize the importance of regular follow-up exams and blood counts to determine progress and monitor for side effects.

Evaluation/Desired Outcomes
- Delayed progression of AIDS and decreased opportunistic infections in patients with HIV.
- Decrease in viral load and improvement in CD4 cell counts.

loratadine (lor-a-ta-deen)
Alavert, Claritin, Claritin 24-Hour Allergy, Claritin Hives Relief, Children's Loratidine, Claritin Reditabs, Clear-Atadine, Dimetapp Children's ND Non-Drowsy Allergy, Non-Drowsy Allergy Relief for Kids, Tavist ND

Classification
Therapeutic: antihistamines

Pregnancy Category B

Indications
Relief of symptoms of seasonal allergies. Management of chronic idiopathic urticaria. Management of hives.

Action
Blocks peripheral effects of histamine released during allergic reactions. **Therapeutic Effects:** Decreased symptoms of allergic reactions (nasal stuffiness; red, swollen eyes, itching).

Pharmacokinetics
Absorption: Rapidly absorbed after oral administration (80%).
Distribution: Unknown.
Protein Binding: *Loratadine*—97%; *descarboethoxyloratadine*—73–77%.
Metabolism and Excretion: Rapidly and extensively metabolized during first pass through the liver. Much is converted to descarboethoxyloratadine, an active metabolite.
Half-life: *Loratadine*—7.8–11 hr; *descarboethoxyloratadine*—20 hr.

TIME/ACTION PROFILE (antihistaminic effects)

ROUTE	ONSET	PEAK	DURATION
PO	1–3 hr	8–12 hr	>24 hr

Contraindications/Precautions
Contraindicated in: Hypersensitivity.
Use Cautiously in: Patients with hepatic impairment or CCr <30 mL/min (↓ dose to 10 mg every other day); Patients receiving drugs known to affect hepatic metabolism of drugs; Lactation: Usually compatible with breastfeeding (AAP); OB, Pedi: Pregnancy or children <2 yr (safety not established); Geri: ↑ risk of adverse reactions.

Adverse Reactions/Side Effects
CNS: confusion, drowsiness (rare), paradoxical excitation. **EENT:** blurred vision. **GI:** dry mouth, GI upset. **Derm:** photosensitivity, rash. **Metab:** weight gain.

Interactions
Drug-Drug: The following interactions may occur, but are less likely to occur with loratidine than with more sedating antihistamines. **MAO inhibitors** may intensify and prolong effects of antihistamines. ↑ CNS depression may occur with other **CNS depressants**, including **alcohol**, **antidepressants**, **opioid analgesics**, and **sedative/hypnotics**.
Drug-Natural Products: Kava-kava, valerian, or chamomile can ↑ CNS depression.

Route/Dosage
PO (Adults and Children ≥6 yr): 10 mg once daily.
PO (Children ≥2–5 yr): 5 mg once daily.

Renal Impairment
PO (Adults): *CCr <30 mL/min*— 10 mg every other day.

Hepatic Impairment
PO (Adults): 10 mg every other day.

Availability (generic available)
Rapidly disintegrating tablets (mint): 5 mg, 10 mg^{OTC}. **Tablets:** 10 mg^{OTC}, ✹10 mg. **Capsules:** 10 mg^{OTC}. **Chewable tablets:** 5 mg^{OTC} (grape flavored). **Syrup (grape, fruit):** 5 mg/5 mL^{OTC}. *In combination with:* pseudoephedrine (Claritin-D)^{OTC}. See Appendix B.

NURSING IMPLICATIONS
Assessment
- Assess allergy symptoms (rhinitis, conjunctivitis, hives) before and periodically during therapy.
- Assess lung sounds and character of bronchial secretions. Maintain fluid intake of 1500–2000 mL/day to decrease viscosity of secretions.
- *Lab Test Considerations:* May cause false-negative result on allergy skin testing.

Potential Nursing Diagnoses
Ineffective airway clearance (Indications)
Risk for injury (Adverse Reactions)

Implementation
- **PO:** Administer once daily.
- *For rapidly disintegrating tablets (Alavert, Claritin Reditabs)*—place on tongue. Tablet disintegrates rapidly. May be taken with or without water.

Patient/Family Teaching
- Instruct patient to take medication as directed.
- May cause dizziness or drowsiness. Caution patient to avoid driving or other activities requiring alertness until response to medication is known.
- Caution patient to use sunscreen and protective clothing to prevent photosensitivity reactions.
- Advise patient to avoid taking alcohol or other CNS depressants concurrently with this drug.
- Advise patient that good oral hygiene, frequent rinsing of mouth with water, and sugarless gum or candy may minimize dry mouth. Patient should notify dentist if dry mouth persists >2 wk.
- Instruct patient to contact health care professional immediately if dizziness, fainting, or fast or irregular heartbeat occurs or if symptoms persist.

Evaluation/Desired Outcomes
- Decrease in allergic symptoms.
- Management of chronic idiopathic urticaria.
- Management of hives.

---

lorazepam (lor-az-e-pam)
✹Apo-Lorazepam, Ativan, ✹Novo-Lorazem, ✹Nu-Loraz

Classification
Therapeutic: anesthetic adjuncts, antianxiety agents, sedative/hypnotics
Pharmacologic: benzodiazepines

Schedule IV

Pregnancy Category D

Indications
Anxiety disorder (oral). Preoperative sedation (injection). Decreases preoperative anxiety and provides amnesia. **Unlabeled Use: IV:** Antiemetic prior to chemotherapy. Insomnia, panic disorder, as an adjunct with acute mania or acute psychosis.

✹ = Canadian drug name. ❖ = Genetic implication.
*CAPITALS indicates life-threatening; underlines indicate most frequent.

lorazepam

Action
Depresses the CNS, probably by potentiating GABA, an inhibitory neurotransmitter. **Therapeutic Effects:** Sedation. Decreased anxiety. Decreased seizures.

Pharmacokinetics
Absorption: Well absorbed following oral administration. Rapidly and completely absorbed following IM administration. Sublingual absorption is more rapid than oral and is similar to IM.
Distribution: Widely distributed. Crosses the blood-brain barrier. Crosses the placenta; enters breast milk.
Metabolism and Excretion: Highly metabolized by the liver.
Half-life: Full-term neonates: 18–73 hr; Older children: 6–17 hr; Adults: 10–16 hr.

TIME/ACTION PROFILE (sedation)

ROUTE	ONSET	PEAK	DURATION
PO	15–60 min	1–6 hr	8–12 hr
IM	30–60 min	1–2 hr†	8–12 hr
IV	15–30 min	15–20 min	8–12 hr

†Amnestic response

Contraindications/Precautions
Contraindicated in: Hypersensitivity; Cross-sensitivity with other benzodiazepines may exist; Comatose patients or those with pre-existing CNS depression; Uncontrolled severe pain; Angle-closure glaucoma; Severe hypotension; Sleep apnea; OB: Use in pregnancy and lactation may cause CNS depression, flaccidity, feeding difficulties, hypothermia, seizures, and respiratory problems in the neonate; Lactation: Recommend to discontinue drug or bottle-feed.
Use Cautiously in: Severe hepatic/renal/pulmonary impairment; Myasthenia gravis; Depression; Psychosis; History of suicide attempt or drug abuse; COPD; Sleep apnea; Pedi: Use cautiously in children under 12 yr. In ↑ doses, benzyl alcohol in injection may cause potentially fatal "gasping syndrome" in neonates; Geri: Lower doses recommended for geriatric or debilitated patients; Hypnotic use should be short-term; **OVERDOSE:** Administer Flumazenil (do not use with patients with seizure disorder. May induce seizures).

Adverse Reactions/Side Effects
CNS: dizziness, drowsiness, lethargy, hangover, headache, ataxia, slurred speech, forgetfulness, confusion, mental depression, rhythmic myoclonic jerking in pre-term infants, paradoxical excitation. **EENT:** blurred vision. **Resp:** respiratory depression. **CV:** *rapid IV use only*—APNEA, CARDIAC ARREST, bradycardia, hypotension. **GI:** constipation, diarrhea, nausea, vomiting, weight gain (unusual). **Derm:** rashes. **Misc:** physical dependence, psychological dependence, tolerance.

Interactions
Drug-Drug: Additive CNS depression with other **CNS depressants** including **alcohol**, **antihistamines**, **antidepressants**, **opioid analgesics**, **clozapine**, and other **sedative/hypnotics** including other benzodiazepines. May ↓ the efficacy of **levodopa**. **Smoking** may ↑ metabolism and ↓ effectiveness. **Valproate** can ↑ serum concentrations and ↓ clearance (↓ dose by 50%). **Probenecid** may ↓ metabolism of lorazepam, enhancing its actions (↓ dose by 50%). **Oral contraceptives** may increase clearance and decrease concentration of lorazepam.
Drug-Natural Products: Concomitant use of **kava-kava**, **valerian**, or **chamomile** can ↑ CNS depression.

Route/Dosage
PO (Adults): *Anxiety*—1–3 mg 2–3 times daily (up to 10 mg/day). *Insomnia*—2–4 mg at bedtime.
PO (Geriatric Patients or Debilitated Patients): *Anxiety*—0.5–2 mg/day in divided doses initially. *Insomnia*—0.25–1 mg initially, increased as needed.
PO (Children): *Anxiety/sedation*—0.02–0.1 mg/kg/dose (not to exceed 2 mg) q 4–8 hr. *Preoperative sedation*—0.02–0.09 mg/kg/dose.
PO (Infants): *Anxiety/sedation*—0.02–0.1 mg/kg/dose (not to exceed 2 mg) q 4–8 hr. *Preoperative sedation*—0.02–0.09 mg/kg/dose.
SL (Adults and adolescents > 18 yr): *Anxiety*—2–3 mg/day in divided doses, not to exceed 6 mg/day; *preoperative sedation*—0.05 mg/kg, up to 4 mg total given 1–2 hr before surgery.
SL (Geriatric Patients and debilitated patients): 0.5 mg/day, dose may be adjusted as necessary.
IM (Adults): *Preoperative sedation*—50 mcg (0.05 mg)/kg 2 hr before surgery (not to exceed 4 mg).
IM (Children): *Preoperative sedation*—0.02–0.09 mg/kg/dose.
IM (Infants): *Preoperative sedation*—0.02–0.09 mg/kg/dose.
IV (Adults): *Preoperative sedation*—44 mcg (0.044 mg)/kg (not to exceed 2 mg) 15–20 min before surgery. *Operative amnestic effect*—up to 50 mcg/kg (not to exceed 4 mg). *Antiemetic*—2 mg 30 min prior to chemotherapy; may be repeated q 4 hr as needed (unlabeled).

Anticonvulsant—50 mcg (0.05 mg)/kg, up to 4 mg; may be repeated after 10–15 min (not to exceed 8 mg/12 hr; unlabeled).

IV (Children): *Preoperative sedation*—0.02–0.09 mg/kg/dose; may use smaller doses (0.01–0.03 mg/kg) and repeat q 20 min. *Antiemetic*—Single dose: 0.04–0.08 mg/kg/dose prior to chemotherapy (not to exceed 4 mg). Multiple doses: 0.02–0.05 mg/kg/dose q 6 hr prn (not to exceed 2 mg). *Anxiety/sedation*—0.02–0.1 mg/kg (not to exceed 2 mg) q 4–8 hr. *Status epilepticus*-0.1 mg/kg over 2–5 min (not to exceed 4 mg); may repeat with 0.05 mg/kg if needed.

IV (Infants): *Preoperative sedation:*—0.02–0.09 mg/kg/dose; may use smaller doses (0.01–0.03 mg/kg) and repeat q 20 min. *Anxiety/sedation*—0.02–0.1 mg/kg/dose (not to exceed 2 mg) q 4–8 hr. *Status epilepticus*—0.1 mg/kg over 2–5 min (not to exceed 4 mg); may repeat with 0.05 mg/kg if needed.

IV (Neonates): *Status epilepticus*—0.05 mg/kg over 2–5 min; may repeat in 10–15 min.

Availability (generic available)
Tablets: 0.5 mg, 1 mg, 2 mg. **Concentrated oral solution:** 0.5 mg/5 mL, 2 mg/mL. **Sublingual tablets :** ✽0.5 mg, ✽1 mg, ✽2 mg. **Injection:** 2 mg/mL, 4 mg/mL.

NURSING IMPLICATIONS
Assessment
- Conduct regular assessment of continued need for treatment.
- Pedi: Assess neonates for prolonged CNS depression related to inability to metabolize lorazepam.
- Geri: Assess geriatric patients carefully for CNS reactions as they are more sensitive to these effects. Assess falls risk.
- **Anxiety:** Assess degree and manifestations of anxiety and mental status (orientation, mood, behavior) prior to and periodically throughout therapy.
- Prolonged high-dose therapy may lead to psychological or physical dependence. Restrict amount of drug available to patient.
- **Status Epilepticus:** Assess location, duration, characteristics, and frequency of seizures. Institute seizure precautions.
- *Lab Test Considerations:* Patients on high-dose therapy should receive routine evaluation of renal, hepatic, and hematologic function.

Potential Nursing Diagnoses
Anxiety (Indications)
Risk for injury (Indications, Side Effects)

Implementation
- Do not confuse Ativan (lorazepam) with Atarax (hydroxyzine).
- Following parenteral administration, keep patient supine for at least 8 hr and observe closely.
- **PO:** Tablet may also be given sublingually (unlabeled) for more rapid onset.
- Take concentrated liquid solution with water, soda, pudding, or applesauce.
- **IM:** Administer IM doses deep into muscle mass at least 2 hr before surgery for optimum effect.

IV Administration
- **Direct IV:** *Diluent:* Dilute immediately before use with an equal amount of sterile water for injection, D5W, or 0.9% NaCl for injection. Pedi: To decrease the amount of benzyl alcohol delivered to neonates, dilute the 4 mg/mL injection with preservative-free sterile water for injection to make a 0.4 mg/mL dilution for IV use. Do not use if solution is colored or contains a precipitate. *Rate:* Administer at a rate not to exceed 2 mg/min or 0.05 mg/kg over 2–5 min. Rapid IV administration may result in apnea, hypotension, bradycardia, or cardiac arrest.
- **Y-Site Compatibility:** acyclovir, albumin, allopurinol, amifostine, amikacin, amiodarone, amphotericin B cholesteryl sulfate complex, amsacrine, anakinra, argatroban, atracurium, bivalirudin, bumetanide, calcium chloride, calcium gluconate, cefazolin, cefepime, cefotaxime, cefoxitin, ceftazidime, ceftizoxime, ceftriaxone, cefuroxime, chloramphenicol, cimetidine, ciprofloxacin, cisatracurium, clindamycin, cyclosporine, clindamycin, cladribine, clonidine, cyclophosphamide, cytarabine, daptomycin, dexamethasone sodium phosphate, dexmedetomidine, diltiazem, diphenhydramine, dobutamine, docetaxel, dopamine, doxorubicin, doxorubicin liposome, doxycycline, droperidol, enalaprilat, epinephrine, ertapenem, erythromycin lactobionate, esmolol, etomidate, etoposide phosphate, famotidine, fenoldopam, fentanyl, filgrastim, fluconazole, fludarabine, fosphenytoin, furosemide, gemcitabine, gentamicin, granisetron, haloperidol, heparin, hydrocortisone sodium succinate, hy-

dromorphone, hydroxyzine, insulin, isoproterenol, ketorolac, labetalol, levofloxacin, linezolid, magnesium sulfate, melphalan, meropenem, methadone, methotrexate, methylprednisolone sodium succinate, metoclopramide, metoprolol, metronidazole, micafungin, midazolam, milrinone, morphine, nafcillin, nicardipine, nitroglycerin, nitroprusside, norepinephrine, oxaliplatin, paclitaxel, palonosetron, pancuronium, pemetrexed, phenylephrine, piperacillin/tazobactam, potassium chloride, procainamide, prochlorperazine, promethazine, propofol, propranolol, quinupristin/dalfopristin, ranitidine, remifentanil, sodium bicarbonate, tacrolimus, teniposide, thiotepa, ticarcillin/clavulanate, tirofiban, tobramycin, trimethoprim/sulfamethoxazole, vancomycin, vasopressin, vecuronium, verapamil, vinorelbine, voriconazole, zidovudine.

- **Y-Site Incompatibility:** aldesleukin, ampicillin, ampicillin/sulbactam, aztreonam, caspofungin, hydralazine, idarubicin, imipenem/cilastatin, lansoprazole, omeprazole, ondansetron, pantoprazole, phenytoin, potassium phosphate, sargramostim, sufentanil.

Patient/Family Teaching
- Instruct patient to take medication exactly as directed and not to skip or double up on missed doses. If medication is less effective after a few weeks, check with health care professional; do not increase dose.
- Advise patient that lorazepam is usually prescribed for short-term use and does not cure underlying problem.
- Advise patient to taper lorazepam by 0.05 mg q 3 days to decrease withdrawal symptoms; abrupt withdrawal may cause tremors, nausea, vomiting, and abdominal and muscle cramps.
- Teach other methods to decrease anxiety, such as increased exercise, support groups, relaxation techniques. Emphasize that psychotherapy is beneficial in addressing source of anxiety and improving coping skills.
- May cause drowsiness or dizziness. Advise patient to avoid driving or other activities requiring alertness until response to medication is known.
- Caution patient to avoid taking alcohol or other CNS depressants concurrently with this medication.
- Instruct patient to contact health care professional immediately if pregnancy is planned or suspected.
- Emphasize the importance of follow-up exams to determine effectiveness of the medication.

Evaluation/Desired Outcomes
- Increase in sense of well-being.
- Decrease in subjective feelings of anxiety without excessive sedation.
- Reduction of preoperative anxiety.
- Postoperative amnesia.
- Improvement in sleep patterns.

---

losartan, See ANGIOTENSIN II RECEPTOR ANTAGONISTS.

---

lovastatin, See HMG-CoA REDUCTASE INHIBITORS (statins).

magaldrate, See **MAGNESIUM AND ALUMINUM SALTS.**

MAGNESIUM AND ALUMINUM SALTS

magaldrate (with simethicone) (**mag**-al-drate)
Riopan Plus,
❋Riopan Plus Double Strength

magnesium hydroxide/aluminum hydroxide
(mag-**nee**-zhum hye-**drox**-ide/ a-**loo**-mi-num hye-**drox**-ide)
Alamag, ❋Diovol Ex,
❋Gelusil Extra Strength, Maalox,
❋Mylanta, Rulox

Classification
Therapeutic: antiulcer agents
Pharmacologic: antacids

Pregnancy Category C

Indications
Useful in a variety of GI complaints, including: Hyperacidity, Indigestion, GERD, Heartburn.

Action
Neutralize gastric acid following dissolution in gastric contents. Inactivate pepsin if pH is raised to ≥4. **Therapeutic Effects:** Neutralization of gastric acid with healing of ulcers and decrease in associated pain.

Pharmacokinetics
Absorption: During routine use, antacids are nonabsorbable. With chronic use, 15–30% of magnesium and smaller amounts of aluminum may be absorbed.
Distribution: Small amounts absorbed are widely distributed, cross the placenta, and appear in breast milk. Aluminum concentrates in the CNS.
Metabolism and Excretion: Excreted by the kidneys.
Half-life: Unknown.

TIME/ACTION PROFILE (effect on gastric pH)

ROUTE	ONSET	PEAK	DURATION
Aluminum PO	slightly delayed	30 min	30 min–1 hr (empty stomach); 3 hr (after meals)
Magnesium PO	slightly delayed	30 min	30 min–1 hr (empty stomach); 3 hr (after meals)

Contraindications/Precautions
Contraindicated in: Severe abdominal pain of unknown cause, especially if accompanied by fever; Renal failure (CrCl <30 mL/min); Products containing tartrazine or sugar in patients with known intolerance.
Use Cautiously in: Antacids containing magnesium in patients with any degree of renal insufficiency; Decreased bowel motility; Dehydration; Upper GI hemorrhage; Pedi: Children <12 yr (safety not established).

Adverse Reactions/Side Effects
GI: *aluminum salts*—constipation; *magnesium salts*, diarrhea. **F and E:** *magnesium salts*—hypermagnesemia; *aluminum salts*, hypophosphatemia.

Interactions
Drug-Drug: Absorption of **tetracyclines**, **phenothiazines**, **ketoconazole**, **itraconazole**, **iron salts**, **fluoroquinolones**, and **isoniazid** may be decreased (separate by at least 2 hr).

Route/Dosage
Magaldrate/Simethicone
PO (Adults): 5–10 mL (540–1080 mg) between meals and at bedtime.

Magnesium Hydroxide/Aluminum Hydroxide
PO (Adults and Children ≥12 yr): 5–30 mL or 1–2 tablets 1–3 hr after meals and at bedtime.

Availability
Magaldrate/Simethicone (generic available)
Suspension: 540 mg magaldrate/20 mg simethicone/5 mL[OTC], 1080 mg magaldrate/40 mg simethicone/5 mL[OTC].

❋ = Canadian drug name. ▤ = Genetic implication.
*CAPITALS indicates life-threatening; underlines indicate most frequent.

Magnesium Hydroxide/Aluminum Hydroxide (generic available)

Chewable Tablets: 300 mg aluminum hydroxide/150 mg magnesium hydroxide[OTC]. **Suspension:** 225 mg aluminum hydroxide/200 mg magnesium hydroxide/5 mL[OTC], 500 mg aluminum hydroxide/500 mg magnesium hydroxide/5 mL[OTC]. *In combination with:* simethicone[OTC]. See Appendix B.

NURSING IMPLICATIONS

Assessment
- **Antacid:** Assess for heartburn and indigestion as well as location, duration, character, and precipitating factors of gastric pain.
- *Lab Test Considerations:* Monitor serum phosphate, potassium, and calcium levels periodically during chronic use. May cause increased serum calcium and decreased serum phosphate concentrations.

Potential Nursing Diagnoses
Acute pain (Indications)

Implementation
- Magnesium and aluminum are combined as antacids to balance the constipating effects of aluminum with the laxative effects of magnesium.
- **PO:** To prevent tablets from entering small intestine in undissolved form, they must be chewed thoroughly before swallowing. Follow with ½ glass of water.
- Shake suspensions well before administration.
- For an antacid effect, administer 1–3 hr after meals and at bedtime.

Patient/Family Teaching
- Caution patient to consult health care professional before taking antacids for more than 2 wk if problem is recurring, if relief is not obtained, or if symptoms of gastric bleeding (black, tarry stools; coffee-ground emesis) occur.
- Advise patient not to take this medication within 2 hr of taking other medications.
- Pedi: Aluminum- or magnesium-containing medicines can cause serious side effects in children, especially when given to children with renal disease or dehydration. Advise parents or caregivers not to administer OTC antacids to children without a doctor's order.

Evaluation/Desired Outcomes
- Relief of gastric pain and irritation.

---

magnesium salicylate, See **SALICYLATES.**

MAGNESIUM SALTS (ORAL)

magnesium chloride (12% Mg; 9.8 mEq Mg/g)
(mag-**nee**-zhum **klor**-ide)
Chloromag, Slo-Mag

magnesium citrate (16.2% Mg; 4.4 mEq Mg/g)
(mag-**nee**-zhum **si**-trate)
Citrate of Magnesia, Citroma, ✦ Citromag

magnesium gluconate (5.4 % Mg; 4.4 mEq/g)
Magtrate, Magonate

magnesium hydroxide (41.7% Mg; 34.3 mEq Mg/g)
(mag-**nee**-zhum hye-**drox**-ide)
Dulcolax Magnesia Tablets, Phillips Magnesia Tablets, Phillips Milk of Magnesia, MOM

magnesium oxide (60.3% Mg; 49.6 mEq Mg/g)
(mag-**nee**-zhum **ox**-ide)
Mag-Ox 400, Uro-Mag

Classification
Therapeutic: mineral and electrolyte replacements/supplements, laxatives
Pharmacologic: salines

Pregnancy Category UK

Indications
Treatment/prevention of hypomagnesemia. As a: Laxative, Bowel evacuant in preparation for surgical/radiographic procedures. Milk of Magnesia has also been used as an antacid.

Action
Essential for the activity of many enzymes. Play an important role in neurotransmission and muscular excitability. Are osmotically active in GI tract, drawing water into the lumen and causing peristalsis. **Therapeutic Effects:** Replacement in deficiency states. Evacuation of the colon.

MAGNESIUM SALTS (ORAL) 805

Pharmacokinetics
Absorption: Up to 30% may be absorbed orally.
Distribution: Widely distributed. Cross the placenta and are present in breast milk.
Metabolism and Excretion: Excreted primarily by the kidneys.
Half-life: Unknown.

TIME/ACTION PROFILE (laxative effect)

ROUTE	ONSET	PEAK	DURATION
PO	3–6 hr	unknown	unknown

Contraindications/Precautions
Contraindicated in: Hypermagnesemia; Hypocalcemia; Anuria; Heart block; OB: Unless used for preterm labor, use during active labor or within 2 hr of delivery may ↑ potential for magnesium toxicity in newborn.
Use Cautiously in: Any degree of renal insufficiency.

Adverse Reactions/Side Effects
GI: diarrhea. **Derm:** flushing, sweating.

Interactions
Drug-Drug: Potentiates **neuromuscular blocking agents**. May ↓ absorption of **fluoroquinolones**, **nitrofurantoin**, and **tetracyclines** and **penicillamine**.

Route/Dosage
Prevention of Deficiency (in mg of Magnesium)
PO (Adults and Children >10 yr): *Adolescent and adult men*—270–400 mg/day; *adolescent and adult women*—280–300 mg/day; *pregnant women*—320 mg/day; *breastfeeding women*—340–355 mg/day.
PO (Children 7–10 yr): 170 mg/day.
PO (Children 4–6 yr): 120 mg/day.
PO (Children birth–3 yr): 40–80 mg/day.

Treatment of Deficiency (Expressed as mg of Magnesium)
PO (Adults): 200–400 mg/day in 3–4 divided doses.
PO (Children 6–11 yr): 3–6 mg/kg/day in 3–4 divided doses.

Laxative
PO (Adults): *Magnesium citrate*—240 mL; *magnesium hydroxide (Milk of Magnesia)*—30–60 mL single or divided dose or 10–20 mL as concentrate.

PO (Children 6–12 yr): *Magnesium citrate*—100 mL; *magnesium hydroxide (Milk of Magnesia)*—15–30 mL single or divided dose.
PO (Children 2–5 yr): *magnesium hydroxide (Milk of Magnesia)*—5–15 mL single or divided dose.

Availability
Magnesium Chloride (generic available)
Sustained-release tablets: 535 mg (64 mg magnesium)[OTC]. **Enteric-coated tablets:** 833 mg (100 mg magnesium)[OTC].

Magnesium Citrate (generic available)
Oral solution: 240-, 296-, and 300-mL bottles (77 mEq magnesium/100 mL)[OTC].

Magnesium Gluconate (generic available)
Tablets: 500 mg[OTC]. **Liquid:** 54 mg/5 mL[OTC].

Magnesium Hydroxide (generic available)
Liquid: 400 mg/5 mL (164 mg magnesium/5 mL)[OTC]. **Concentrated liquid:** 800 mg/5 mL (328 mg magnesium/5 mL)[OTC]. **Chewable tablets:** 300 mg (130 mg magnesium)[OTC], 600 mg (260 mg magnesium)[OTC].

Magnesium Oxide (generic available)
Tablets: 400 mg (241.3 mg magnesium)[OTC].
Capsules: 140 mg (84.5 mg magnesium)[OTC].

NURSING IMPLICATIONS

Assessment
- **Laxative:** Assess patient for abdominal distention, presence of bowel sounds, and usual pattern of bowel function.
- Assess color, consistency, and amount of stool produced.
- **Antacid:** Assess for heartburn and indigestion as well as location, duration, character, and precipitating factors of gastric pain.

Potential Nursing Diagnoses
Constipation (Indications)

Implementation
- **PO:** To prevent tablets entering small intestine in undissolved form, they must be chewed thoroughly before swallowing. Follow with ½ glass of water.
- *Magnesium citrate:* Refrigerate solutions to ensure they retain potency and palatability. May be served over ice. Magnesium citrate in an open container will lose carbonation upon

standing; this will not affect potency but may reduce palatability.
- *Magnesium hydroxide:* Shake solution well before administration.
- **Antacid:** Administer 1–3 hr after meals and at bedtime.
- Powder and liquid forms are considered more effective than tablets.
- **Laxative:** Administer on empty stomach for more rapid results. Follow all oral laxative doses with a full glass of liquid to prevent dehydration and for faster effect. Do not administer at bedtime or late in the day.

Patient/Family Teaching
- Advise patient not to take this medication within 2 hr of taking other medications, especially fluoroquinolones, nitrofurantoin, and tetracyclines.
- **Antacids:** Caution patient to consult health care professional before taking antacids for more than 2 wk if problem is recurring, if relief is not obtained, or if symptoms of gastric bleeding (black, tarry stools; coffee-ground emesis) occur.
- **Laxatives:** Advise patient that laxatives should be used only for short-term therapy. Long-term therapy may cause electrolyte imbalance and dependence.
- Encourage patient to use other forms of bowel regulation, such as increasing bulk in the diet, fluid intake, and mobility. Normal bowel habits are individualized; frequency of bowel movement may vary from 3 times/day to 3 times/wk.
- Advise patient to notify health care professional if unrelieved constipation, rectal bleeding, or symptoms of electrolyte imbalance (muscle cramps or pain, weakness, dizziness) occur.

Evaluation/Desired Outcomes
- Relief of gastric pain and irritation.
- Passage of a soft, formed bowel movement, usually within 3–6 hr.
- Prevention and treatment of magnesium deficiency.

HIGH ALERT

magnesium sulfate (IV, parenteral) (9.9% Mg; 8.1 mEq Mg/g)
(mag-**nee**-zhum **sul**-fate)

Classification
Therapeutic: mineral and electrolyte replacements/supplements
Pharmacologic: minerals/electrolytes

Pregnancy Category D

Indications
Treatment/prevention of hypomagnesemia. Treatment of hypertension. Anticonvulsant associated with severe eclampsia, pre-eclampsia, or acute nephritis. **Unlabeled Use:** Preterm labor. Treatment of torsade de pointes. Adjunctive treatment for bronchodilation in moderate to severe acute asthma.

Action
Essential for the activity of many enzymes. Plays an important role in neurotransmission and muscular excitability. **Therapeutic Effects:** Replacement in deficiency states. Resolution of eclampsia.

Pharmacokinetics
Absorption: IV administration results in complete bioavailability; well absorbed from IM sites.
Distribution: Widely distributed. Crosses the placenta and is present in breast milk.
Metabolism and Excretion: Excreted primarily by the kidneys.
Half-life: Unknown.

TIME/ACTION PROFILE (anticonvulsant effect)

ROUTE	ONSET	PEAK	DURATION
IM	60 min	unknown	3–4 hr
IV	immediate	unknown	30 min

Contraindications/Precautions
Contraindicated in: Hypermagnesemia; Hypocalcemia; Anuria; Heart block; OB: Unless used for preterm labor, avoid continuous use during active labor or within 2 hr of delivery due to potential for magnesium toxicity in newborn.
Use Cautiously in: Any degree of renal insufficiency; Geri: May require ↓ dosage due to age-related ↓ in renal function.

Adverse Reactions/Side Effects
CNS: drowsiness. **Resp:** ↓ respiratory rate. **CV:** arrhythmias, bradycardia, hypotension. **GI:** diarrhea. **MS:** muscle weakness. **Derm:** flushing, sweating. **Metab:** hypothermia.

Interactions
Drug-Drug: May potentiate **calcium channel blockers** and **neuromuscular blocking agents.**

magnesium sulfate (IV, parenteral) 807

Route/Dosage

Treatment of Deficiency (Expressed as mg of Magnesium)
IM, IV (Adults): *Severe deficiency*—8–12 g/day in divided doses; *mild deficiency*—1 g q 6 hr for 4 doses or 250 mg/kg over 4 hr.
IM, IV (Children > 1 month): 25–50 mg/kg/dose q 4–6 hr for 3–4 doses, maximum single dose: 2 g.
IV (Neonates): 25–50 mg/kg/dose q 8–12 hr for 2–3 doses.

Seizures/Hypertension
IM, IV (Adults): 1 g q 6 hr for 4 doses as needed.
IM, IV (Children): 20–100 mg/kg/dose q 4–6 hr as needed, may use up to 200 mg/kg/dose in severe cases.

Torsade de Pointes
IV (Infants and Children): 25–50 mg/kg/dose, maximum dose: 2 g.

Bronchodilation
IV (Adults): 2 g single dose.
IV (Children): 25 mg/kg/dose, maximum dose: 2 g.

Eclampsia/Pre-Eclampsia
IV, IM (Adults): 4–5 g by IV infusion, concurrently with up to 5 g IM in each buttock; then 4–5 g IM q 4 hr *or* 4 g by IV infusion followed by 1–2 g/hr continuous infusion (not to exceed 40 g/day or 20 g/48 hr in the presence of severe renal insufficiency).

Part of Parenteral Nutrition
IV (Adults): 4–24 mEq/day.
IV (Children): 0.25–0.5 mEq/kg/day.

Availability (generic available)
Injection: 500 mg/mL (50%). **Premixed infusion:** 1 g/100 mL, 2 g/100 mL, 4 g/50 mL, 4 g/100 mL, 20 g/500 mL, 40 g/1000 mL.

NURSING IMPLICATIONS

Assessment
- **Hypomagnesemia/Anticonvulsant:** Monitor pulse, blood pressure, respirations, and ECG frequently throughout administration of parenteral magnesium sulfate. Respirations should be at least 16/min before each dose.
- Monitor neurologic status before and throughout therapy. Institute seizure precautions. Patellar reflex (knee jerk) should be tested before each parenteral dose of magnesium sulfate. If response is absent, no additional doses should be administered until positive response is obtained.
- Monitor newborn for hypotension, hyporeflexia, and respiratory depression if mother has received magnesium sulfate.
- Monitor intake and output ratios. Urine output should be maintained at a level of at least 100 mL/4 hr.
- **Lab Test Considerations:** Monitor serum magnesium levels and renal function periodically throughout administration of parenteral magnesium sulfate.

Potential Nursing Diagnoses
Risk for injury (Indications, Side Effects)

Implementation
- **High Alert:** Accidental overdosage of IV magnesium has resulted in serious patient harm and death. Have second practitioner independently double check original order, dose calculations, and infusion pump settings. Do not confuse milligram (mg), gram (g), or milliequivalent (mEq) dosages.
- **IM:** Administer deep IM into gluteal sites. Administer subsequent injections in alternate sides. Dilute to a concentration of 200 mg/mL prior to injection.

IV Administration
- **Direct IV:** *Diluent:* 50% solution must be diluted in 0.9% NaCl or D5W to a concentration of ≤20% prior to administration. *Concentration:* ≤20%. *Rate:* Administer at a rate not to exceed 150 mg/min.
- **Continuous Infusion:** *Diluent:* Dilute in D5W, 0.9% NaCl, or LR. *Concentration:* 0.5 mEq/mL (60 mg/mL) (may use maximum concentration of 1.6 mEq/mL (200 mg/mL) in fluid-restricted patients). *Rate:* Infuse over 2-4 hr. Do not exceed a rate of 1 mEq/kg/hr (125 mg/kg/hr). When rapid infusions are needed (severe asthma or torsade de pointes) may infuse over 10–20 min.
- **Y-Site Compatibility:** acyclovir, aldesleukin, amifostine, amikacin, ampicillin, atropine, aztreonam, bivalirudin, bumetanide, calcium gluconate, caspofungin, cefazolin, cefotaxime, cefoxitin, ceftazidime, ceftizoxime, chloramphenicol, cimetidine, cisatracurium, clindamycin, daptomycin, cefazolin, cefo-

---

✦ = Canadian drug name. ✚ = Genetic implication.
*CAPITALS indicates life-threatening; underlines indicate most frequent.

taxime, dexmedetomidine, digoxin, diltiazem, diphenhydramine, dobutamine, cefazolin, cefotaximedocetaxel, dopamine, cefazolin, cefotaxime, doxorubicin liposome, doxycycline, enalaprilat, epinephrine, cefazolin, cefotaximeerythromycin, ertapenem, esmolol, cefazolin, cefotaximeetoposide phosphate, famotidine, fenoldopam, fentanyl, fluconazole, fludarabine, gentamicin, granisetron, heparin, hydromorphone, hydroxyzine, idarubicin, imipenem/cilastatin, insulin, isoproterenol, ketorolac, labetalol, levofloxacin, lidocaine, linezolid, lorazepam, meperidine, metoclopramide, metoprolol, metronidazole, micafungin, midazolam, milrinone, morphine, nafcillin, nicardipine, nitroglycerin, nitroprusside, norepinephrine, ondansetron, oxaliplatin, paclitaxel, palonosetron, pantoprazole, penicillin G potassium, phenylephrine, piperacillin/tazobactam, potassium chloride, procainamide, prochlorperazine, promethazine, propofol, propranolol, protamine, quinupristin/dalfopristin, ranitidine, remifentanil, sargramostim, sodium bicarbonate, tacrolimus, thiotepa, ticarcillin/clavulanate, tirofiban, tobramycin, trimethoprim/sulfamethoxazole, vancomycin, vasopressin, verapamil, vitamin B complex with C, voriconazole.
- **Y-Site Incompatibility:** aminophylline, amphotericin B cholesteryl sulfate complex, calcium chloride, cefepime, ceftriaxone, cefuroxime, ciprofloxacin, dexamethasone sodium phosphate, diazepam, drotrecogin, haloperidol, lansoprazole, methylprednisolone sodium succinate, phenytoin, phytonadione.

Patient/Family Teaching
- Explain purpose of medication to patient and family.

Evaluation/Desired Outcomes
- Normal serum magnesium concentrations.
- Control of seizures associated with toxemias of pregnancy.

---

mannitol (man-i-tol)
Osmitrol, Resectisol

Classification
Therapeutic: diuretics
Pharmacologic: osmotic diuretics

Pregnancy Category C

Indications
IV: Adjunct in the treatment of: Acute oliguric renal failure, Edema, Increased intracranial or intraocular pressure, Toxic overdose. **GU irrigant:** During transurethral procedures (2.5–5% solution only).

Action
Increases the osmotic pressure of the glomerular filtrate, thereby inhibiting reabsorption of water and electrolytes. Causes excretion of: Water, Sodium, Potassium, Chloride, Calcium, Phosphorus, Magnesium, Urea, Uric acid. **Therapeutic Effects:** Mobilization of excess fluid in oliguric renal failure or edema. Reduction of intraocular or intracranial pressure. Increased urinary excretion of toxic materials. Decreased hemolysis when used as an irrigant after transurethral prostatic resection.

Pharmacokinetics
Absorption: IV administration produces complete bioavailability. Some absorption may follow use as a GU irrigant.
Distribution: Confined to the extracellular space; does not usually cross the blood-brain barrier or eye.
Metabolism and Excretion: Excreted by the kidneys; minimal liver metabolism.
Half-life: 100 min.

TIME/ACTION PROFILE (diuretic effect)

ROUTE	ONSET	PEAK	DURATION
IV	30–60 min	1 hr	6–8 hr

Contraindications/Precautions
Contraindicated in: Hypersensitivity; Anuria; Dehydration; Active intracranial bleeding.
Use Cautiously in: OB, Lactation: Safety not established).

Adverse Reactions/Side Effects
CNS: confusion, headache. **EENT:** blurred vision, rhinitis. **CV:** transient volume expansion, chest pain, CHF, pulmonary edema, tachycardia. **GI:** nausea, thirst, vomiting. **GU:** renal failure, urinary retention. **F and E:** dehydration, hyperkalemia, hypernatremia, hypokalemia, hyponatremia. **Local:** phlebitis at IV site.

Interactions
Drug-Drug: Hypokalemia ↑ the risk of **digoxin** toxicity.

Route/Dosage
IV (Adults): *Edema, oliguric renal failure—* 50–100 g as a 5–25% solution; may precede with a test dose of 0.2 g/kg over 3–5 min. *Reduc-*

tion of intracranial/intraocular pressure—0.25–2 g/kg as 15–25% solution over 30–60 min (500 mg/kg may be sufficient in small or debilitated patients). *Diuresis in drug intoxications*—50–200 g as a 5–25% solution titrated to maintain urine flow of 100–500 mL/hr.
IV (Children): *Edema, oliguric renal failure*—0.25–2 g/kg (60 g/m^2) as a 15–20% solution over 2–6 hr; may precede with a test dose of 0.2 g/kg over 3–5 min. *Reduction of intracranial/intraocular pressure*—1–2 g/kg (30–60 g/m^2) as a 15–20% solution over 30–60 min (500 mg/kg may be sufficient in small or debilitated patients). *Diuresis in drug intoxications*—up to 2 g/kg (60 g/m^2) as a 5–10% solution.

Availability (generic available)
IV injection: 5%, 10%, 15%, 20%. **GU irrigant:** 5%. *In combination with:* sorbitol for GU irrigation.

NURSING IMPLICATIONS
Assessment
- Monitor vital signs, urine output, CVP, and pulmonary artery pressures (PAP) before and hourly throughout administration. Assess patient for signs and symptoms of dehydration (decreased skin turgor, fever, dry skin and mucous membranes, thirst) or signs of fluid overload (increased CVP, dyspnea, rales/crackles, edema).
- Assess patient for anorexia, muscle weakness, numbness, tingling, paresthesia, confusion, and excessive thirst. Report signs of electrolyte imbalance.
- **Increased Intracranial Pressure:** Monitor neurologic status and intracranial pressure readings in patients receiving this medication to decrease cerebral edema.
- **Increased Intraocular Pressure:** Monitor for persistent or increased eye pain or decreased visual acuity.
- *Lab Test Considerations:* Renal function and serum electrolytes should be monitored routinely throughout course of therapy.

Potential Nursing Diagnoses
Excess fluid volume (Indications)
Risk for deficient fluid volume (Side Effects)

Implementation
- Observe infusion site frequently for infiltration. Extravasation may cause tissue irritation and necrosis.
- Do not administer electrolyte-free mannitol solution with blood. If blood must be administered simultaneously with mannitol, add at least 20 mEq NaCl to each liter of mannitol.
- Confer with physician regarding placement of an indwelling Foley catheter (except when used to decrease intraocular pressure).
- **IV:** Administer by IV infusion undiluted. If solution contains crystals, warm bottle in hot water and shake vigorously. Do not administer solution in which crystals remain undissolved. Cool to body temperature. Use an in-line filter for 15%, 20%, and 25% infusions.
- **Test Dose:** Administer over 3–5 min to produce a urine output of 30–50 mL/hr. If urine flow does not increase, administer 2nd test dose. If urine output is not at least 30–50 mL/hr for 2–3 hr after 2nd test dose, patient should be re-evaluated.
- **Oliguria:** Administration rate should be titrated to produce a urine output of 30–50 mL/hr. Administer child's dose over 2–6 hr.
- **Increased Intracranial Pressure:** Infuse dose over 30–60 min in adults and children.
- **Intraocular Pressure:** Administer dose over 30 min. When used preoperatively, administer 60–90 min before surgery.
- **Y-Site Compatibility:** amifostine, aztreonam, fludarabine, fluorouracil, idarubicin, linezolid, melphalan, ondansetron, paclitaxel, piperacillin/tazobactam, sargramostim, teniposide, thiotepa, vinorelbine.
- **Y-Site Incompatibility:** cefepime, filgrastim.
- **Irrigation:** Add contents of two 50-mL vials of 25% mannitol to 900 mL of sterile water for injection for a 2.5% solution for irrigation. Use only clear solutions.

Patient/Family Teaching
- Explain purpose of therapy to patient.

Evaluation/Desired Outcomes
- Urine output of at least 30–50 mL/hr or an increase in urine output in accordance with parameters set by physician.
- Reduction in intracranial pressure.
- Reduction of intraocular pressure.
- Excretion of certain toxic substances.
- Irrigation during transurethral prostate resection.

maraviroc (ma-ra-vi-rok)
Selzentry

Classification
Therapeutic: antiretrovirals
Pharmacologic: CCR5 co-receptor antagonists

Pregnancy Category B

Indications
HIV infection (with other antiretrovirals), specifically in patients with only CCR5–tropic HIV-1 detectable, with evidence of viral replication and HIV-1 strains displaying multiple resistance to other antiretrovirals. Use should be determined by treatment history and tropism testing.

Action
Blocks a specific receptor on CD-4 and T-cell surfaces which prevents CCR5–tropic HIV-1 from entering. **Therapeutic Effects:** Decreased invasion of CD-4 and T-cells by CCR5–tropic HIV-1 virus resulting in viral replication.

Pharmacokinetics
Absorption: 2–33% absorbed following oral administration.
Distribution: Unknown.
Metabolism and Excretion: Mostly metabolized by the liver (CYP3A enzyme system); 8% renal excretion as unchanged drug.
Half-life: 14–18 hr.

TIME/ACTION PROFILE (blood levels)

ROUTE	ONSET	PEAK	DURATION
PO	unknown	0.5–4 hr	1–2 hr

Contraindications/Precautions
Contraindicated in: Dual/mixed or CXCR4–tropic HIV-1; OB: Lactation (breastfeeding not recommended for HIV-infected patients).
Use Cautiously in: Pre-existing liver disease including hepatitis B or C (may ↑ risk of hepatotoxicity); Cardiovascular disease or risk factors (↑ risk of cardiovascular events); Hepatic impairment; Renal impairment (if CCr <50 mL/min and using a CYP3A inhibitor, use only if necessary); Treatment-naive adults (safety/efficacy not established); Geri: Consider age-related decrease in renal/hepatic function, concurrent drug therapy and concomittant disease; OB: Use only if clearly needed; Pedi: Safety not established in children <16 yr.

Adverse Reactions/Side Effects
CNS: dizziness. **CV:** myocardial ischemia/infarction. **Resp:** cough, upper respiratory tract infection. **GI:** abdominal pain, appetite disorder, HEPATOTOXICITY. **Derm:** RASH. **MS:** musculoskeletal pain. **Misc:** ALLERGIC REACTIONS, fever, immune reconstitution syndrome, ↑ risk of infection.

Interactions
Drug-Drug: Levels are ↑ by **CYP3A inhibitors** including **protease inhibitors** (excluding tipranavir/ritonavir), **delavirdine**, **ketoconazole**, **lopinavir/ritonavir**, **saquinavir**, and **atazanavir**. Levels are ↓ by **CYP3A inducers** including **efavirenz** and **rifampin**.

Route/Dosage
PO (Adults): *Concurrent CYP3A inhibitors (except tipranavir/ritonavir) or delavirdine*—150 mg twice daily; *Concurrent NRTIs, tipranavir/ritonavir, nevirapine and other drugs that are not strong inhibitors/inducers of CYP3A*—300 mg twice daily; *Concurrent CYP3A inducers, including efavirenz*—600 mg twice daily.

Availability
Tablets: 150 mg, 300 mg.

NURSING IMPLICATIONS

Assessment
- Assess patient for change in severity of HIV symptoms and for symptoms of opportunistic infections throughout therapy.
- Assess for signs of hepatitis or allergic reaction (pruritic rash, jaundice, dark urine, vomiting, abdominal pain). If symptoms occur, discontinue maraviroc immediately.
- *Lab Test Considerations:* Testing for CCR5–tropic HIV-1 should be obtained prior to initiating therapy.
- Monitor viral load and CD4 cell count regularly during therapy.
- May cause ↑ AST, ALT, total bilirubin, amylase, and lipase.
- May cause ↓ absolute neutrophil count.

Potential Nursing Diagnoses
Risk for infection (Indications)
Deficient knowledge, related to medication regimen (Patient/Family Teaching)

Implementation
- **PO:** May be administered without regard to food. Tablets should be swallowed whole; do not break, crush, or chew.

Patient/Family Teaching
- Emphasize the importance of taking maraviroc as directed, at the same time each day. Advise patient to read the *Patient Information* that comes with the medication with each Rx is refill. Maraviroc must always be used in combi-

nation with other antiretroviral drugs. Do not take more than prescribed amount and do not stop taking without consulting health care professional. Take missed doses as soon as remembered, then return to regular dose schedule. If it is within 6 hr of next dose, omit dose and take next dose at regular time. Do not double doses.

- Instruct patient that maraviroc should not be shared with others.
- Inform patient that maraviroc does not cure AIDS or prevent associated or opportunistic infections. Maraviroc does not reduce the risk of transmission of HIV to others through sexual contact or blood contamination. Caution patient to use a condom and to avoid sharing needles or donating blood to prevent spreading the AIDS virus to others. The long-term effects of maraviroc are unknown at this time. If new symptoms of infection develop after starting maraviroc, notify health care professional.
- Advise patient to discontinue maraviroc and notify health care professional if chest pain, itchy rash, yellow colored skin or eyes, dark urine, vomiting, or abdominal pain occur.
- May cause dizziness. Caution patient to avoid driving and other activities requiring alertness until response to medication is known.
- Advise patient to make position changes slowly to minimize postural hypotension.
- Instruct patient to consult health care professional before taking any Rx, OTC, or herbal products, especially St. John's Wort; may decrease effectiveness of maraviroc.
- Advise patient to notify health care professional if pregnancy is planned or suspected or if breastfeeding.
- Emphasize the importance of regular follow-up exams and blood counts to determine progress and monitor for side effects.

Evaluation/Desired Outcomes
- Delayed progression of AIDS and decreased opportunistic infections in patients with HIV.
- Decrease in viral load and increase in CD4 cell counts.

meclizine (mek-li-zeen)
Antivert, ✽Bonamine, Bonine, Dramamine Less Drowsy Formula

Classification
Therapeutic: antiemetics, antihistamines

Pregnancy Category B

Indications
Management/prevention of: Motion sickness, Vertigo.

Action
Has central anticholinergic, CNS depressant, and antihistaminic properties. Decreases excitability of the middle ear labyrinth and depresses conduction in middle ear vestibular-cerebellar pathways. **Therapeutic Effects:** Decreased motion sickness. Decreased vertigo from vestibular pathology.

Pharmacokinetics
Absorption: Absorbed after oral administration.
Distribution: Unknown.
Metabolism and Excretion: Unknown.
Half-life: 6 hr.

TIME/ACTION PROFILE (antihistaminic effects)

ROUTE	ONSET	PEAK	DURATION
PO	1 hr	unknown	8–24 hr

Contraindications/Precautions
Contraindicated in: Hypersensitivity; OB: Has caused congenital malformations (cleft palate) in animal studies.
Use Cautiously in: Prostatic hyperplasia; Angle-closure glaucoma; Lactation: Occasional use may be acceptable; prolonged use may expose infant to drug effects or may interfere with milk supply; Pedi: Children <12 yr (safety not established); Geri: ↑ sensitivity and risk of adverse reactions.

Adverse Reactions/Side Effects
CNS: drowsiness, fatigue. **EENT:** blurred vision. **GI:** dry mouth.

Interactions
Drug-Drug: Additive CNS depression with other **CNS depressants**, including **alcohol**, other **antihistamines**, **opioid analgesics**, and **sedative/hypnotics**. Additive anticholinergic effects with other **drugs possessing anticholinergic properties**, including some **antihistamines**, **antidepressants**, **atropine**, **haloperidol**, **phenothiazines**, **quinidine**, and **disopyramide**.

Route/Dosage
PO (Adults and Children ≥12 yr): *Motion sickness*—25–50 mg 1 hr before exposure; may repeat in 24 hr; *vertigo*—25–100 mg/day in divided doses.

Availability (generic available)
Tablets: 12.5 mg, 25 mg[Rx, OTC], 50 mg. **Cost:** 12.5 mg $4.09/100, 25 mg $5.40/100, 50 mg $6.99/100. **Chewable tablets:** 25 mg[Rx, OTC].

NURSING IMPLICATIONS
Assessment
- Assess patient for level of sedation after administration.
- **Motion Sickness:** Assess patient for nausea and vomiting before and 60 min after administration.
- **Vertigo:** Assess degree of vertigo periodically in patients receiving meclizine for labyrinthitis.
- *Lab Test Considerations:* May cause false-negative results in skin tests using allergen extracts. Discontinue meclizine 72 hr before testing.

Potential Nursing Diagnoses
Risk for injury (Side Effects)

Implementation
- **PO:** Administer oral doses with food, water, or milk to minimize GI irritation. Chewable tablet may be chewed or swallowed whole.

Patient/Family Teaching
- Instruct patient to take meclizine exactly as directed. If a dose is missed, take as soon as possible unless almost time for next dose. Do not double doses.
- May cause drowsiness. Caution patient to avoid driving or other activities requiring alertness until response to the medication is known.
- Advise patient that frequent mouth rinses, good oral hygiene, and sugarless gum or candy may decrease dryness of mouth.
- Caution patient to avoid concurrent use of alcohol and other CNS depressants with this medication.
- **Motion Sickness:** When used as prophylaxis for motion sickness, advise patient to take medication at least 1 hr before exposure to conditions that may cause motion sickness.

Evaluation/Desired Outcomes
- Prevention and relief of symptoms in motion sickness.
- Prevention and treatment of vertigo due to vestibular pathology.

---

medroxyPROGESTERone†
(me-**drox**-ee-proe-jess-te-rone)
✱ Alti-MPA, Depo-Provera, Depo-Sub Q Provera 104, ✱ Gen-Medroxy, ✱ Novo-Medrone, Provera, ✱ Provera Pak, ✱ Ratio-MPA

Classification
Therapeutic: antineoplastics, contraceptive hormones
Pharmacologic: hormones, progestins

Pregnancy Category X

†For contraceptive use see Contraceptives, Hormonal monograph

Indications
To decrease endometrial hyperplasia in postmenopausal women receiving concurrent estrogen (0.625 mg/day conjugated estrogens). Treatment of secondary amenorrhea and abnormal uterine bleeding caused by hormonal imbalance. **IM:** Treatment of advanced unresponsive endometrial or renal carcinoma. Management of endometriosis-associated pain (Depo-Sub Q Provera 104 only). **Unlabeled Use:** Obesity-hypoventilation (pickwickian) syndrome, sleep apnea, hypersomnolence.

Action
A synthetic form of progesterone—actions include secretory changes in the endometrium, increases in basal body temperature, histologic changes in vaginal epithelium, relaxation of uterine smooth muscle, mammary alveolar tissue growth, pituitary inhibition, and withdrawal bleeding in the presence of estrogen. **Therapeutic Effects:** Decreased endometrial hyperplasia in postmenopausal women receiving concurrent estrogen (combination with estrogen decreases vasomotor symptoms and prevents osteoporosis). Restoration of hormonal balance with control of uterine bleeding. Management of endometrial or renal cancer. Prevention of pregnancy.

Pharmacokinetics
Absorption: 0.6–10% absorbed after oral administration.
Distribution: Enters breast milk.
Metabolism and Excretion: Metabolized by the liver.
Half-life: *1st phase*—52 min; *2nd phase*—230 min; *biological*—14.5 hr.

TIME/ACTION PROFILE (IM = antineoplastic effects)

ROUTE	ONSET	PEAK	DURATION
PO	unknown	unknown	unknown
IM	wk–mos	mo	unknown†
SC	unknown	1 wk	3 mo

†Contraceptive effect lasts 3 mo

Contraindications/Precautions
Contraindicated in: Hypersensitivity; Hypersensitivity to parabens (IM suspension only); Missed abortion; Thromboembolic disease; Cerebrovascular disease; Severe liver disease; Breast or genital cancer; Porphyria; OB: May ↑ risk of fetal genitourinary malformation.
Use Cautiously in: History of liver disease; Renal disease; Cardiovascular disease; Seizure disorders; Mental depression; Lactation: If used as a contraceptive, wait 6 wk after delivery if breastfeeding.

Adverse Reactions/Side Effects
CNS: depression. **EENT:** retinal thrombosis. **CV:** PULMONARY EMBOLISM, thromboembolism, thrombophlebitis. **GI:** drug-induced hepatitis, gingival bleeding. **GU:** cervical erosions. **Derm:** chloasma, melasma, rashes. **Endo:** amenorrhea, breakthrough bleeding, breast tenderness, changes in menstrual flow, galactorrhea, hyperglycemia, spotting. **F and E:** edema. **Metab:** bone loss. **Misc:** allergic reactions including ANAPHYLAXIS and ANGIOEDEMA, weight gain, weight loss.

Interactions
Drug-Drug: May ↓ effectiveness of **bromocriptine** when used concurrently for galactorrhea/amenorrhea. Contraceptive effectiveness may be ↓ by **carbamazepine**, **phenobarbital**, **phenytoin**, **rifampin**, or **rifabutin**. **Aminoglutethimide** may ↓ oral absorption.

Route/Dosage

Postmenopausal Women Receiving Concurrent Estrogen
PO (Adults): 2.5–5 mg daily concurrently with 0.625 mg conjugated estrogens (monophasic regimen) *or* 5 mg daily on days 15–28 of the cycle with 0.625 mg conjugated estrogens taken daily throughout cycle (biphasic regimen).

Secondary Amenorrhea
PO (Adults): 5–10 mg/day for 5–10 days; start at any time in cycle.

Dysfunctional Uterine Bleeding/Induction of Menses
PO (Adults): 5–10 mg/day for 5–10 days, starting on day 16 or day 21 of menstrual cycle.

Renal or Endometrial Carcinoma
IM (Adults): 400–1000 mg, may be repeated weekly; if improvement occurs, attempt to decrease dosage to 400 mg monthly.

Endometriosis-Associated Pain
Subcut (Adults): 104 mg every 12–14 wk (3 mo), beginning on day 5 of normal menses (not recommended for more than 2 yr).

Availability (generic available)
Tablets: 2.5 mg, 5 mg, 10 mg, ✺ 100 mg. **Suspension for depot injection:** ✺ 50 mg/mL, ✺ 100 mg/mL, 150 mg/mL, 400 mg/mL. **Suspension for subcutaneous injection (Depo-Sub Q Provera 104):** 104 mg/0.65 mL in single-use syringes. *In combination with:* conjugated estrogens as Prempro (single combination tablet of 0.626 mg conjugated estrogens plus 2.5 or 5 mg medroxyprogesterone) or Premphase (0.625 mg conjugated estrogens tablet for 14 days followed by combination tablet of 0.625 mg conjugated estrogens plus 5 mg medroxyprogesterone for days 15–28) in convenience packages. See Appendix B.

NURSING IMPLICATIONS

Assessment
- Monitor blood pressure periodically during therapy.
- Assess patient's usual menstrual history. Administration of drug may begin on any day of cycle in patients with amenorrhea and on day 16 or 21 of cycle in patients with dysfunctional bleeding.
- Monitor intake and output ratios and weekly weight. Report significant discrepancies or steady weight gain.
- *Lab Test Considerations:* Monitor hepatic function before and periodically during therapy.
- May cause ↑ alkaline phosphatase levels. May ↓ pregnanediol excretion concentrations.
- May cause ↑ serum LDL concentrations or ↓ HDL concentrations.
- May alter thyroid hormone assays.

Potential Nursing Diagnoses
Sexual dysfunction (Indications)
Ineffective tissue perfusion (Side Effects)

Implementation
- Do not confuse Provera (medroxyprogesterone) with Covera (verapamil).
- Only the 150 mg/mL vial should be used for contraception.
- Injectable medroxyprogesterone may lead to bone loss, especially in women younger than 21 yr. Injectable medroxyprogesterone should be used for >2 yr only if other methods of contraception are inadequate. If used long term, women should use supplemental calcium and vitamin D, and monitor bone mineral density.
- **Subcut:** Shake vigorously before use to form a uniform suspension. Inject slowly (over 5–7 seconds) at a 45° angle into fatty area of anterior thigh or abdomen every 12 to 14 wk. If more than 14 wk elapse between injections, rule out pregnancy prior to administration. **Do not rub area after injection.**
- When switching from other hormonal contraceptives, administer within dosing period (7 days after taking last active pill, removing patch or ring, or within the dosing period for IM injection).
- **IM:** Shake vial vigorously before preparing IM dose. Administer deep IM into gluteal or deltoid muscle. If period between injections is >14 wk, determine that patient is not pregnant before administering the drug.
- In patients with cancer, IM dose may initially be required weekly. Once stabilized, IM dose may be required only monthly.

Patient/Family Teaching
- Explain the dose schedule. Instruct patient to take medication at the same time each day. Take missed doses as soon as remembered, but do not double doses.
- Advise patients receiving medroxyprogesterone for menstrual dysfunction to anticipate withdrawal bleeding 3–7 days after discontinuing medication.
- Review patient package insert (PPI) with patient. Emphasize the importance of notifying health care professional if the following side effects occur: visual changes, sudden weakness, incoordination, difficulty with speech, headache, leg or calf pain, shortness of breath, chest pain, changes in vaginal bleeding pattern, yellow skin, swelling of extremities, depression, or rash. Patients receiving medroxyprogesterone for cancer may not receive PPI.
- Advise patient to keep a 1-mo supply of medroxyprogesterone available at all times.
- Instruct patient in correct method of monthly breast self-examination. Increased breast tenderness may occur.
- Advise patient that gingival bleeding may occur. Instruct patient to use good oral hygiene and to receive regular dental care and examinations.
- Instruct patient to notify health care professional if menstrual period is missed or if pregnancy is suspected. Patient should not attempt conception for 3 mo after discontinuing medication in order to decrease risk to fetus.
- Medroxyprogesterone may cause melasma (brown patches of discoloration) on face when patient is exposed to sunlight. Advise patient to avoid sun exposure and to wear sunscreen or protective clothing when outdoors.
- Emphasize the importance of routine follow-up physical exams, including blood pressure; breast, abdomen, and pelvic exams; and Papanicolaou smears every 6–12 mo.
- **IM, Subcut:** Advise patient to maintain adequate amounts of dietary calcium and vitamin D to help prevent bone loss.

Evaluation/Desired Outcomes
- Regular menstrual periods.
- Decrease in endometrial hyperplasia in postmenopausal women receiving concurrent estrogen.
- Control of the spread of endometrial or renal cancer.

medroxyprogesterone, See also **CONTRACEPTIVES, HORMONAL.**

---

megestrol (me-**jess**-trole)
Megace

Classification
Therapeutic: antineoplastics, hormones
Pharmacologic: progestins

Pregnancy Category D (tablets), X (suspension)

Indications
Palliative treatment of endometrial and breast carcinoma, either alone or with surgery or radiation (tablets only). Treatment of anorexia, weight loss, and cachexia associated with AIDS (oral suspension only).

Action
Antineoplastic effect may result from inhibition of pituitary function. **Therapeutic Effects:** Regres-

sion of tumor. Increased appetite and weight gain in patients with AIDS.

Pharmacokinetics
Absorption: Well absorbed from the GI tract.
Distribution: Unknown.
Protein Binding: ≥90%.
Metabolism and Excretion: Completely metabolized by the liver.
Half-life: 38 hr (range 13–104 hr).

TIME/ACTION PROFILE (antineoplastic activity)

ROUTE	ONSET	PEAK	DURATION
PO	wk–mos	2 mo	unknown

Contraindications/Precautions
Contraindicated in: Hypersensitivity; Undiagnosed vaginal bleeding; Severe liver disease; Suspension contains alcohol and should be avoided in patients with known intolerance; OB, Lactation: Pregnancy or lactation.
Use Cautiously in: Diabetes; Mental depression; Renal disease; History of thrombophlebitis; Cardiovascular disease; Seizure disorders.

Adverse Reactions/Side Effects
CV: THROMBOEMBOLISM, edema. **GI:** GI irritation. **Derm:** alopecia. **Endo:** asymptomatic adrenal suppression (chronic therapy). **Hemat:** thrombophlebitis. **MS:** carpal tunnel syndrome.

Interactions
Drug-Drug: None significant.

Route/Dosage
PO (Adults): *Breast carcinoma*— 160 mg/day single dose or divided doses; *endometrial/ovarian carcinoma*— 40–320 mg/day in divided doses; *anorexia associated with AIDS*— 800 mg day; may decrease to 400 mg/day after 1 mo (range 400–800 mg/day).

Availability (generic available)
Tablets: 20 mg, 40 mg. **Cost:** *Generic*— 20 mg $37.99/100, 40 mg $52.99/100. **Oral suspension (lemon-lime flavor):** 40 mg/mL, 125 mg/mL(Megace ES). **Cost:** *Generic*— 40 mg/mL $131.33/240 mL; *Megace ES*— 125 mg/mL $526.89/150 mL.

NURSING IMPLICATIONS

Assessment
- Assess patient for swelling, pain, or tenderness in legs. Report these signs of deep vein thrombophlebitis.
- **Anorexia:** Monitor weight, appetite, and nutritional intake in patients with AIDS.

Potential Nursing Diagnoses
Imbalanced nutrition: less than body requirements (Indications)

Implementation
- Because of high dose, suspension is most convenient form for patients with AIDS.
- Do not confuse Megace 800 mg/20 mL with Megace ES 625 mg/5 mL.
- **PO:** May be administered with meals if GI irritation becomes a problem.

Patient/Family Teaching
- Instruct patient to take medication exactly as directed; do not skip or double up on missed doses. Missed doses may be taken as long as it is not right before next dose. Gradually decrease dose prior to discontinuation.
- Advise patient to report to health care professional any unusual vaginal bleeding or signs of deep vein thrombophlebitis.
- Advise patient that this medication may have teratogenic effects. Contraception should be used during therapy and for at least 4 months after therapy is completed.
- Discuss with patient the possibility of hair loss. Explore methods of coping.

Evaluation/Desired Outcomes
- Slowing or arresting the spread of endometrial or breast malignancy. Therapeutic effects usually occur within 2 months of initiating therapy.
- Increased appetite and weight gain in patients with AIDS.

---

meloxicam (me-**lox**-i-kam)
Mobic

Classification
Therapeutic: nonsteroidal anti-inflammatory agents
Pharmacologic: nonopioid analgesics

Pregnancy Category C

Indications
Relief of signs and symptoms of osteoarthritis and rheumatoid arthritis (including juvenile rheumatoid arthritis).

meloxicam

Action
Inhibits prostaglandin synthesis, probably by inhibiting the enzyme cyclooxygenase. **Therapeutic Effects:** Decreased pain and inflammation associated with osteoarthritis. Also decreases fever.

Pharmacokinetics
Absorption: Well absorbed following oral administration.
Distribution: Unknown.
Protein Binding: 99.4%.
Metabolism and Excretion: Mostly metabolized to inactive metabolites by the liver via the P450 enzyme system; metabolites are excreted in urine and feces.
Half-life: 20.1 hr.

TIME/ACTION PROFILE

ROUTE	ONSET	PEAK†	DURATION
PO	unknown	5–6 hr	24 hr

†Blood levels

Contraindications/Precautions
Contraindicated in: Hypersensitivity; Cross-sensitivity may occur with other NSAIDs, including aspirin; Severe renal impairment (CCr ≤15 mL/min); Concurrent use of aspirin (increased risk of adverse reactions); Perioperative pain from coronary artery bypass graft (CABG) surgery; OB: Can cause premature closure of ductus arteriosus if used during third trimester.
Use Cautiously in: Cardiovascular disease or risk factors for cardiovascular disease (may ↑ risk of serious cardiovascular thrombotic events, myocardial infarction, and stroke, especially with prolonged use) Dehydration (correct deficits before initiating therapy); Impaired renal function, heart failure, liver dysfunction, concurrent ACE inhibitor or diuretic therapy (↑ risk of renal dysfunction); Coagulation disorders or concurrent anticoagulant therapy (may ↑ risk of bleeding); Lactation: Safety not established; Pedi: Children <2 yr (safety not established); Geri: ↑ risk of GI bleeding and renal dysfunction.

Adverse Reactions/Side Effects
CV: edema. **GI:** GI BLEEDING, ↑ liver function tests, diarrhea, dyspepsia, nausea. **Derm:** EXFOLIATIVE DERMATITIS, STEVENS-JOHNSON SYNDROME, TOXIC EPIDERMAL NECROLYSIS, pruritus. **Hemat:** anemia, leukopenia, thrombocytopenia.

Interactions
Drug-Drug: May ↓ antihypertensive effects of **ACE inhibitors**. May ↓ diuretic effects of **furosemide** or **thiazide diuretics**. Concurrent use with **aspirin** ↑ meloxicam blood levels and may ↑ risk of adverse reactions. Concurrent use with **cholestyramine** ↓ blood levels. ↑ plasma **lithium** levels (close monitoring recommended when meloxicam is introduced or withdrawn). May ↑ risk of bleeding with **anticoagulants**, including **warfarin**.

Route/Dosage
PO (Adults): 7.5 mg once daily; some patients may require 15 mg/day.
PO (Children 2–17 yr and > 12 kg): 0.125 mg/kg once daily up to 7.5mg/day.

Availability (generic available)
Tablets: 7.5 mg, 15 mg. **Cost:** *Generic*—7.5 mg $43.83/90, 15 mg $18.90/90. **Oral suspension (raspberry flavor):** 7.5 mg/5 mL.

NURSING IMPLICATIONS

Assessment
- Patients who have asthma, aspirin-induced allergy, and nasal polyps are at increased risk for developing hypersensitivity reactions. Assess for rhinitis, asthma, and urticaria.
- Assess pain and range of motion prior to and 1–2 hr following administration.
- *Lab Test Considerations:* Evaluate BUN, serum creatinine, CBC, and liver function periodically in patients receiving prolonged therapy. May cause anemia, thrombocytopenia, leukopenia, and abnormal liver or renal function tests.
- Bleeding time may be prolonged.

Potential Nursing Diagnoses
Acute pain (Indications)
Impaired physical mobility (Indications)

Implementation
- Administration in higher than recommended doses does not provide increased effectiveness but may cause increased side effects. Use lowest effective dose for shortest period of time.
- PO: May be administered without regard to food.
- Pedi: Use oral suspension to ensure accuracy of dosing in children.

Patient/Family Teaching
- Advise patient to take this medication with a full glass of water and to remain in an upright position for 15–30 min after administration.
- Instruct patient to take medication as directed. Take missed doses as soon as remembered but not if almost time for the next dose. Do not double doses.
- Caution patient to avoid the concurrent use of alcohol, aspirin, acetaminophen, or other OTC

medications without consulting health care professional.
- Advise patient to inform health care professional of medication regimen prior to treatment or surgery.
- Advise patient to consult health care professional if rash, itching, visual disturbances, weight gain, edema, black stools, or signs of hepatotoxicity (nausea, fatigue, lethargy, jaundice, upper right quadrant tenderness, flu-like symptoms) occur.

Evaluation/Desired Outcomes
- Relief of pain.
- Improved joint mobility. Patients who do not respond to one NSAID may respond to another.

---

melphalan (mel-fa-lan)
Alkeran, L-PAM, phenylalanine mustard

Classification
Therapeutic: antineoplastics
Pharmacologic: alkylating agents

Pregnancy Category D

Indications
Alone or with other therapies for: Multiple myeloma, Ovarian cancer. **Unlabeled Use:** Breast cancer. Prostate cancer. Testicular carcinoma. Chronic myelogenous leukemia. Osteogenic sarcoma.

Action
Inhibits DNA and RNA synthesis by alkylation (cell-cycle phase–nonspecific). **Therapeutic Effects:** Death of rapidly replicating cells, particularly malignant ones. Also has immunosuppressive properties.

Pharmacokinetics
Absorption: Incompletely and variably absorbed following oral administration.
Distribution: Rapidly distributed throughout total body water.
Protein Binding: ≤30%.
Metabolism and Excretion: Rapidly metabolized in the bloodstream. Small amounts (10%) excreted unchanged by the kidneys.
Half-life: 1.5 hr.

TIME/ACTION PROFILE (effects on blood counts)

ROUTE	ONSET	PEAK	DURATION
PO	5 days	2–3 wk	5–6 wk

Contraindications/Precautions
Contraindicated in: Hypersensitivity to melphalan or chlorambucil; OB, Lactation: Pregnancy or lactation.
Use Cautiously in: Active infections; ↓ bone marrow reserve; Impaired renal function (dose ↓ recommended if BUN ≥30 mg/dL); OB: Women with childbearing potential (should be counseled to avoid pregnancy during treatment); Pedi: Safety not established; Geri: Begin at lower end of dosing range due to potential for age-related ↓ in renal, hepatic, or cardiac function.

Adverse Reactions/Side Effects
Resp: bronchopulmonary dysplasia, pulmonary fibrosis. **GI:** diarrhea, hepatitis, nausea, stomatitis, vomiting. **GU:** infertility. **Derm:** alopecia, pruritus, rashes. **Endo:** menstrual irregularities. **Hemat:** leukopenia, thrombocytopenia, anemia. **Metab:** hyperuricemia. **Misc:** allergic reactions, including ANAPHYLAXIS (more common after IV use).

Interactions
Drug-Drug: ↑ bone marrow depression with other **antineoplastics** or **radiation therapy**. May ↓ antibody response to **live-virus vaccines** and ↑ risk of adverse reactions. May ↑ the risk of pulmonary toxicity with **carmustine**. Concurrent IV use with **cyclosporine** may ↑ risk of renal failure. Risk of enterocolitis may be ↑ with concurrent **nalidixic acid**.

Route/Dosage
Multiple Myeloma
PO (Adults): 150 mcg (0.15 mg)/kg/day for 7 days, followed by 3-wk rest, then 50 mcg (0.05 mg)/kg/day maintenance dose *or* 100–150 mcg/kg/day or 250 mcg (0.25 mg)/kg/day for 4 days followed by 2–4-wk rest, then 2–4 mg/day maintenance dose *or* 7 mg/m^2 *or* 250 mcg (0.25 mg)/kg daily for 5 days q 5–6 wk.
IV (Adults): 16 mg/m^2 q 2 wk for 4 doses, then q 4 wk.

Ovarian Carcinoma
PO (Adults): 200 mcg (0.2 mg)/kg/day for 5 days q 4–5 wk.

✶ = Canadian drug name.   ✇ = Genetic implication.
*CAPITALS indicates life-threatening; underlines indicate most frequent.

Availability
Tablets: 2 mg. **Powder for injection:** 50 mg.

NURSING IMPLICATIONS
Assessment
- Assess for signs of infection (fever, chills, sore throat, cough, hoarseness, lower back or side pain, difficult or painful urination). Notify health care professional if these symptoms occur.
- Assess for bleeding (bleeding gums, bruising, petechiae, guaiac stools, urine, and emesis). Avoid IM injections and taking rectal temperatures. Apply pressure to venipuncture sites for 10 min.
- May cause nausea and vomiting. Monitor intake and output, appetite, and nutritional intake. Prophylactic antiemetics may be used. Adjust diet as tolerated.
- Monitor for symptoms of gout (increased uric acid, joint pain, edema). Encourage patient to drink at least 2 L of fluid per day. Allopurinol may be given to decrease uric acid levels.
- Anemia may occur. Monitor for increased fatigue and dyspnea.
- Assess patient for allergy to chlorambucil. Patients may have cross-sensitivity.
- **Lab Test Considerations:** Monitor CBC and differential weekly during therapy. The nadir of leukopenia occurs in 2–3 wk. Notify physician if leukocyte count is <3000/mm³. The nadir of thrombocytopenia occurs in 2–3 wk. Notify physician if platelet count is <100,000/mm³. Recovery of leukopenia and thrombocytopenia occurs in 5–6 wk.
- Monitor liver function studies (AST, ALT, LDH, bilirubin) and renal function studies (BUN, creatinine) prior to and periodically during therapy to detect hepatotoxicity and nephrotoxicity.
- May cause ↑ uric acid. Monitor periodically during therapy.
- May cause ↑ 5-hydroxyindoleacetic acid (5-HIAA) concentrations as a result of tumor breakdown.

Potential Nursing Diagnoses
Risk for injury (Side Effects)
Risk for infection (Side Effects)

Implementation
- Solution should be prepared in a biologic cabinet. Wear gloves, gown, and mask while handling medication. Discard IV equipment in specially designated container.
- If solution contacts skin or mucosa, immediately wash skin or mucosa with soap and water.
- **PO:** May be ordered in divided doses or as a single daily dose.

IV Administration
- **Intermittent Infusion:** *Diluent:* Reconstitute with 10 mL of diluent supplied for a concentration of 5 mg/mL and shake vigorously until solution is clear. *Concentration:* Dilute dose immediately with 0.9% NaCl for a concentration not to exceed 2 mg/mL for central line or 0.45 mg/mL for a peripheral line. Administer within 60 min of reconstitution. *Rate:* Administer over at least 15 min (not to exceed 10 mg/min).
- **Y-Site Compatibility:** acyclovir, amikacin, aminophylline, ampicillin, aztreonam, bleomycin, bumetanide, buprenorphine, butorphanol, calcium gluconate, carboplatin, carmustine, cefazolin, cefepime, cefotaxime, ceftazidime, ceftizoxime, ceftriaxone, cefuroxime, cimetidine, cisplatin, clindamycin, cyclophosphamide, cytarabine, dacarbazine, dactinomycin, daunorubicin, dexamethasone, diphenhydramine, doxorubicin, doxycycline, droperidol, enalaprilat, etoposide, famotidine, filgrastim, floxuridine, fluconazole, fludarabine, fluorouracil, furosemide, ganciclovir, gentamicin, haloperidol, heparin, hydrocortisone, hydromorphone, idarubicin, ifosfamide, imipenem/cilastatin, lorazepam, mannitol, mechlorethamine, meperidine, mesna, methotrexate, methylprednisolone, metoclopramide, metronidazole, minocycline, mitomycin, mitoxantrone, morphine, nalbuphine, ondansetron, pentostatin, potassium chloride, prochlorperazine edisylate, promethazine, ranitidine, sodium bicarbonate, streptozocin, teniposide, thiotepa, ticarcillin/clavulanate, tobramycin, trimethoprim/sulfamethoxazole, vancomycin, vinblastine, vincristine, vinorelbine, zidovudine.
- **Y-Site Incompatibility:** amphotericin B, chlorpromazine.

Patient/Family Teaching
- Instruct patient to take melphalan as directed, even if nausea and vomiting occur. If vomiting occurs shortly after dose is taken, consult health care professional. If a dose is missed, do not take at all.
- Advise patient to notify health care professional if fever; chills; dyspnea; persistent cough; sore throat; signs of infection; bleeding gums; bruising; petechiae; or blood in urine, stool, or emesis occurs. Caution patient to avoid crowds and persons with known infections. Instruct patient to use soft toothbrush and electric ra-

zor. Caution patient not to drink alcoholic beverages or take products containing aspirin or other NSAIDs.
- Instruct patient to notify health care professional if rash, itching, joint pain, or swelling occurs.
- Instruct patient to inspect oral mucosa for redness and ulceration. If ulceration occurs, advise patient to use sponge brush and to rinse mouth with water after eating and drinking. Consult health care professional if pain interferes with eating. Stomatitis pain may require treatment with opioid analgesics.
- Advise patient that although fertility may be decreased, contraception should be used during melphalan therapy because of potential teratogenic effects on the fetus.
- Instruct patient not to receive any vaccinations without advice of health care professional.
- Emphasize need for periodic lab tests to monitor for side effects.

Evaluation/Desired Outcomes
- Decrease in size and spread of malignant tissue.

---

memantine (me-**man**-teen)
Namenda

Classification
Therapeutic: anti-Alzheimer's agents
Pharmacologic: N-methyl-D-aspartate antagonist

Pregnancy Category B

Indications
Moderate to severe Alzheimer's dementia.

Action
Binds to CNS N-methyl-D-aspartate (NMDA) receptor sites, preventing binding of glutamate, an excitatory neurotransmitter. **Therapeutic Effects:** Decreased symptoms of dementia. Does not slow progression. Cognitive enhancement. Does not cure disease.

Pharmacokinetics
Absorption: Well absorbed after oral administration.
Distribution: Unknown.
Metabolism and Excretion: 57–82% excreted unchanged in urine by active tubular secretion moderated by pH dependent tubular reabsorption. Remainder metabolized; metabolites are not pharmacologically active.

Half-life: 60–80 hr.

TIME/ACTION PROFILE (blood levels)

ROUTE	ONSET	PEAK	DURATION
PO	unknown	3–7 hr	12 hr

Contraindications/Precautions
Contraindicated in: Severe renal impairment.
Use Cautiously in: Moderate renal impairment (consider ↓ dose); Concurrent use of other NMDA antagonists (amantadine, rimantadine, ketamine, dextromethorphan); Concurrent use of drugs or diets that cause alkaline urine; Conditions that ↑ urine pH including severe urinary tract infections or renal tubular acidosis (lead to ↓ excretion and ↑ levels); OB, Lactation, Pedi: Safety not established.

Adverse Reactions/Side Effects
CNS: dizziness, fatigue, headache, sedation. **CV:** hypertension. **Derm:** rash. **GI:** weight gain. **GU:** urinary frequency. **Hemat:** anemia.

Interactions
Drug-Drug: Medications that ↑ urine pH lead to ↓ excretion and ↑ blood levels (**carbonic anhydrase inhibitors, sodium bicarbonate**).

Route/Dosage
PO (Adults): 5 mg once daily initially, increased at weekly intervals to 10 mg/day (5 mg twice daily), then 15 mg/day (5 mg once daily, 10 mg once daily as separate doses, then to target dose of 20 mg/day (as 10 mg twice daily).

Availability
Tablets: 5 mg, 10 mg, titration package containing twenty eight 5 mg tablets and twenty one 10 mg tablets. **Cost:** 5 mg $458.95/180, 10 mg $435.98/180. **Oral solution, sugar-free, alcohol-free (peppermint):** 2 mg/mL.

NURSING IMPLICATIONS

Assessment
- Assess cognitive function (memory, attention, reasoning, language, ability to perform simple tasks) periodically during therapy.
- **Lab Test Considerations:** May cause anemia.

Potential Nursing Diagnoses
Disturbed thought process (Indications)
Risk for injury (Side Effects)
Impaired environmental interpretation syndrome

Implementation
- Dose increases should occur no more frequently than weekly.
- **PO:** May be administered without regard to food.
- Administer oral solution using syringe provided. Do not dilute or mix with other fluids.

Patient/Family Teaching
- Instruct caregivers on how and when to administer memantine and how to titrate dose. Provide caregiver with *Patient Instructions* sheet.
- Caution patient and caregiver that memantine may cause dizziness.
- Teach patient and caregivers that improvement in cognitive functioning may take months; degenerative process is not reversed.

Evaluation/Desired Outcomes
- Improvement in cognitive function (memory, attention, reasoning, language, ability to perform simple tasks) in patients with Alzheimer's disease.

HIGH ALERT

meperidine (me-per-i-deen)
Demerol

Classification
Therapeutic: opioid analgesics
Pharmacologic: opioid agonists

Schedule II

Pregnancy Category C

Indications
Moderate or severe pain (alone or with nonopioid agents). Anesthesia adjunct. Analgesic during labor. Preoperative sedation. **Unlabeled Use:** Rigors.

Action
Binds to opiate receptors in the CNS. Alters the perception of and response to painful stimuli, while producing generalized CNS depression. **Therapeutic Effects:** Decrease in severity of pain.

Pharmacokinetics
Absorption: 50% from the GI tract; well absorbed from IM sites. Oral doses are about half as effective as parenteral doses.
Distribution: Widely distributed. Crosses the placenta; enters breast milk.
Protein Binding: Neonates: 52%; Infants 3–18 months: 85%; Adults: 60–80%.
Metabolism and Excretion: Mostly metabolized by the liver; some converted to normeperidine, which may accumulate and cause seizures. 5% excreted unchanged by the kidneys.
Half-life: Neonates: 12–39 hr; Infants 3–18 months: 2.3 hr; Children 5–8 yr: 3 hr; Adults: 2.5–4 hr (↑ in impaired renal or hepatic function [7–11 hr]).

TIME/ACTION PROFILE (analgesia)

ROUTE	ONSET	PEAK	DURATION
PO	15 min	60 min	2–4 hr
IM	10–15 min	30–50 min	2–4 hr
Subcut	10–15 min	40–60 min	2–4 hr
IV	immediate	5–7 min	2–3 hr

Contraindications/Precautions
Contraindicated in: Hypersensitivity; Hypersensitivity to bisulfites (some injectable products); Recent (14–21 days) MAO inhibitor therapy; OB: Chronic use may pose risk to the fetus including possible addiction; Lactation: Excreted in breast milk and can cause respiratory depression in the infant.
Use Cautiously in: Head trauma; ↑ intracranial pressure; Severe renal, hepatic, or pulmonary disease; Hypothyroidism; Adrenal insufficiency; Alcoholism; Debilitated patients (dose reduction suggested); Undiagnosed abdominal pain or prostatic hyperplasia; Patients with renal impairment, or extensive burns; High-dose or prolonged therapy (>600 mg/day or >2 days; increased risk of CNS stimulation and seizures due to accumulation of normeperidine); Sickle cell anemia (may require reduced initial doses); OB: Use during labor and delivery can cause respiratory depression in the newborn; Pedi: Syrup contains benzyl alcohol, which can cause "gasping syndrome" in neonates. Children have ↑ risk of seizures due to accumulation of normeperidine; Geri: Appears on Beers list; morphine recommended.

Adverse Reactions/Side Effects
CNS: SEIZURES, confusion, sedation, dysphoria, euphoria, floating feeling, hallucinations, headache, unusual dreams. **EENT:** blurred vision, diplopia, miosis. **Resp:** respiratory depression. **CV:** hypotension, bradycardia. **GI:** constipation, nausea, vomiting. **GU:** urinary retention. **Derm:** flushing, sweating. **Misc:** allergic reactions including ANAPHYLAXIS, physical dependence, psychological dependence, tolerance.

Interactions
Drug-Drug: Do not use in patients receiving **MAO inhibitors** or **procarbazine** (may cause fatal reaction—contraindicated within 14–21 days of MAO inhibitor therapy). ↑ CNS depression with **alcohol**, **antihistamines**, and **seda-**

meperidine **821**

tive/hypnotics. Administration of **agonist/antagonist opioid analgesics** may precipitate opioid withdrawal in physically dependent patients. **Nalbuphine** or **pentazocine** may ↓ analgesia. **Protease inhibitors** may ↑ effects and adverse reactions (concurrent use should be avoided). **Phenytoin** ↑ metabolism and may ↓ effects. **Chlorpromazine** and **thioridazine** may ↑ the risk of adverse reactions (concurrent use should be avoided). May aggravate side effects of **isoniazid**. **Acyclovir** may ↑ plasma concentrations of meperidine and normeperidine.
Drug-Natural Products: Concomitant use of **kava-kava**, **valerian**, or **chamomile** can ↓ CNS depression. **St. John's wort** may ↑ serious side effects, concurrent use is not recommended.

Route/Dosage
PO, IM, Subcut (Adults): *Analgesia*— 50 mg q 3-4 hr; may be ↑ as needed (not to exceed 600 mg/24 hr). *Analgesia during labor*— 50–100 mg IM or subcut when contractions become regular; may repeat q 1–3 hr. *Preoperative sedation*—50–100 mg IM or subcut 30–90 min before anesthesia.

PO, IM, Subcut (Children): *Analgesia*—1–1.5 mg/kg q 3–4 hr (should not exceed 100 mg/dose). *Preoperative sedation*—1–2 mg/kg 30–90 min before anesthesia (not to exceed adult dose).

IV (Adults): 15–35 mg/hr as a continuous infusion; *PCA*—10 mg initially; with a range of 1–5 mg/incremental dose, recommended lockout interval is 6–10 min (minimum 5 min).

IV (Children): *Continuous infusion*—0.5–1 mg/kg loading dose followed by 0.3 mg/kg/hr, titrate to effect up to 0.5–0.7 mg/kg/hr.

Availability (generic available)
Tablets: 50 mg, 100 mg. **Cost:** 50 mg $99.04/100, 100 mg $188.37/100. **Syrup (banana flavor):** 50 mg/5 mL. **Injection:** ✱ 10 mg/mL, 25 mg/0.5 mL, 25 mg/mL, 50 mg/mL, 75 mg/mL, 100 mg/mL.

NURSING IMPLICATIONS
Assessment
- Assess type, location, and intensity of pain prior to and 1 hr following PO, subcut, and IM doses and 5 min (peak) following IV administration. When titrating opioid doses, increases of 25–50% should be administered until there is either a 50% reduction in the patient's pain rating on a numerical or visual analogue scale or the patient reports satisfactory pain relief. A repeat dose can be safely administered at the time of the peak if previous dose is ineffective and side effects are minimal.
- An equianalgesic chart (see Appendix K) should be used when changing routes or when changing from one opioid to another.
- Assess blood pressure, pulse, and respirations before and periodically during administration. If respiratory rate is <10/min, assess level of sedation. Dose may need to be decreased by 25–50%. Initial drowsiness will diminish with continued use.
- Assess bowel function routinely. Prevention of constipation should be instituted with increased intake of fluids and bulk and with laxatives to minimize constipating effects. Stimulant laxatives should be administered routinely if opioid use exceeds 2–3 days, unless contraindicated.
- Prolonged use may lead to physical and psychological dependence and tolerance. This should not prevent patient from receiving adequate analgesia. Most patients who receive meperidine for pain do not develop psychological dependence. Progressively higher doses may be required to relieve pain with long-term therapy.
- Monitor patients on chronic or high-dose therapy for CNS stimulation (restlessness, irritability, seizures) due to accumulation of normeperidine metabolite. Risk of toxicity increases with doses >600 mg/24 hr, chronic administration (>2 days), and renal impairment.
- Geri: Meperidine has been reported to cause delirium in the elderly; older adults are at increased risk for normeperidine toxicity. Monitor frequently.
- Pedi: Assess pediatric patient frequently; neonates, infants, and children are more sensitive to the effects of opioid analgesics and may experience respiratory complications, excitability and restlessness more frequently.
- *Lab Test Considerations:* May ↑ plasma amylase and lipase concentrations.
- *Toxicity and Overdose:* If an opioid antagonist is required to reverse respiratory depression or coma, naloxone (Narcan) is the antidote. Dilute the 0.4-mg ampule of naloxone in 10 mL of 0.9% NaCl and administer 0.5 mL (0.02 mg) by direct IV push every 2 min. For children and patients weighing <40 kg, dilute 0.1 mg of naloxone in 10 mL of 0.9% NaCl for a

✱ = Canadian drug name.   = Genetic implication.
*CAPITALS indicates life-threatening; underlines indicate most frequent.

concentration of 10 mcg/mL and administer 0.5 mcg/kg every 2 min. Titrate dose to avoid withdrawal, seizures, and severe pain. In patients receiving meperidine chronically, naloxone may precipitate seizures by eliminating the CNS depressant effects of meperidine, allowing the convulsant activity of normeperidine to predominate. Monitor patient closely.

Potential Nursing Diagnoses
Acute pain (Indications)
Disturbed sensory perception (visual, auditory) (Side Effects)
Risk for injury (Side Effects)

Implementation
- **High Alert:** Accidental overdose of opioid analgesics has resulted in fatalities. Before administering, clarify all ambiguous orders; have second practitioner independently check original order, dose calculations, and infusion pump settings. Do not confuse with morphine or hydromorphone; fatalities have occurred. Pedi: Medication errors with opioid analgesics are common in the pediatric population and include misinterpretation or miscalculation of doses and use of inappropriate measuring devices.
- Explain therapeutic value of medication prior to administration to enhance the analgesic effect.
- Regularly administered doses may be more effective than prn administration. Analgesic is more effective if given before pain becomes severe.
- Coadministration with nonopioid analgesics may have additive analgesic effects and permit lower doses.
- Oral dose is <50% as effective as parenteral. When changing to oral administration, dose may need to be increased (see Appendix K).
- Medication should be discontinued gradually after long-term use to prevent withdrawal symptoms.
- May be administered via PCA pump.
- **PO:** Doses may be administered with food or milk to minimize GI irritation. Syrup should be diluted in half-full glass of water.
- **IM:** Administration of repeated subcut doses may cause local irritation.

IV Administration
- **Direct IV:** *Diluent:* Dilute with sterile water or 0.9% NaCl for injection. *Concentration:* ≤10 mg/mL. *Rate: High Alert:* Administer slowly over at least 5 min. Rapid administration may lead to increased respiratory depression, hypotension, and circulatory collapse.
- **Intermittent Infusion:** *Diluent:* Dilute with D5W, D10W, dextrose/saline combinations, dextrose/Ringer's or lactated Ringer's injection combinations, 0.45% NaCl, 0.9% NaCl, or Ringer's or LR. Administer via infusion pump. *Concentration:* 1 mg/mL. *Rate:* Administer over 15–30 min.
- **Syringe Compatibility:** atropine, chlorpromazine, cimetidine, dimenhydrinate, diphenhydramine, droperidol, glycopyrrolate, hydroxyzine, ketamine, metoclopramide, midazolam, ondansetron, perphenazine, prochlorperazine, promazine, promethazine, ranitidine, scopolamine.
- **Syringe Incompatibility:** heparin, morphine, pantoprazole, pentobarbital.
- **Y-Site Compatibility:** alfentanil, amifostine, amikacin, aminophylline, amiodarone, anidulafungin, ascorbic acid, atracurium, atropine, azithromycin, aztreonam, bivalirudin, bleomycin, bumetanide, busulfan, calcium chloride, calcium gluconate, carboplatin, carmustine, caspofungin, cefazolin, cefotaxime, cefoxitin, ceftazidime, ceftizoxime, ceftriaxone, cefuroxime, chlorpromazine, cimetidine, cisatracurium, cladribine, clindamycin, cyanocobalamin, cyclophosphamide, cyclosporine, cytarabine, dactinomycin, daptomycin, daunorubicin, daunorubicin liposome, dexmedetomidine, dexrazoxane, digoxin, diltiazem, diphenhydramine, dobutamine, docetaxel, dolasetron, dopamine, doripenem, doxacurium, doxorubicin hydrochloride, doxycycline, droperidol, enalaprilat, ephedrine, epinephrine, epirubicin, epoetin alfa, eftifibatide, ertapenem, erythromycin, esmolol, etoposide, etoposide phosphate, famotidine, fenoldopam, fentanyl, filgrastim, floxuridine, fluconazole, fludarabine, folic acid, fosphenytoin, gemcitabine, gentamicin, glycopyrrolate, granisetron, hetastarch, hydrocortisone sodium phosphate, ifosfamide, insulin, irinotecan, isoproterenol, kanamycin, ketorolac, labetalol, leucovorin, levofloxacin, lidocaine, linezolid, mannitol, melphalan, mesna, mataraminol, methotrexate, methyldopate, metoclopramide, metoprolol, metronidazole, midazolam, milrinone, mitomycin, mitoxantrone, mivacurium, morphine, multivitamins, naloxone, nitroglycerin, nitroprusside, norepinephrine, octreotide, ondansetron, oxacillin, oxaliplatin, oxytocin, paclitaxel, palonosetron, papaverine, pemetrexed, penicillin G, pentamidine, phentolamine, phenylephrine, phytonadione, piperacillin/tazobactam, plicamycin, potassium chloride, procainamide, prochlorperazine, prometha-

zine, propofol, propranolol, protamine, pyridoxime, quinupristin/dalfopristin, ranitidine, remifentanil, rituximab, rocuronium, sargramostim, sodium acetate, streptokinase, streoptzocin, succinylcholine, sufentanil, tacrolimus, teniposide, theophylline, thiamine, thiotepa, ticarcillin/clavulanate, tigecycline, tirofiban, tobramycin, tolazoline, topotecan, trastuzumab, trimethaphan, trimethobenzamide, urokinase, vancomycin, vasopressin, vecuronium, verapamil, vinblastine, vinorelbine, voriconazole, zidovudine.

- **Y-Site Incompatibility:** allopurinol, amphotericin B cholesteryl, amphotericin B colloidal, amphotericin B liposome, azathioprine, cefepime, cefonocid, cefoperazone, dantrolene, diazepam, diazoxide, ganciclovir, idarubicin, indomethacin, lorazepam, micafungin, nafcillin, pantoprazole, pentobarbital, phenobarbital, phenytoin, sodium bicarbonate, thiopental.

Patient/Family Teaching

- Instruct patient on how and when to ask for and take pain medication.
- Instruct patient to take meperidine as directed. If dose is less effective after a few weeks, do not increase dose without consulting health care professional. Pedi: Teach parents or caregivers how to accurately measure liquid medication and to use only the measuring device dispensed with the medication.
- May cause drowsiness or dizziness. Advise patient to call for assistance when ambulating or smoking. Caution patient to avoid driving or other activities requiring alertness until response to medication is known.
- Advise patient to change positions slowly to minimize orthostatic hypotension.
- Instruct patient to avoid concurrent use of alcohol or other CNS depressants.
- Advise ambulatory patients that nausea and vomiting may be decreased by lying down.
- Encourage patient to turn, cough, and breathe deeply every 2 hr to prevent atelectasis.

Evaluation/Desired Outcomes

- Decrease in severity of pain without a significant alteration in level of consciousness or respiratory status.

---

meropenem (mer-oh-**pen**-nem)
Merrem

meropenem 823

Classification
Therapeutic: anti-infectives
Pharmacologic: carbapenems

Pregnancy Category B

Indications
Treatment of: Intra-abdominal infections, Bacterial meningitis, Skin and skin structure infections. **Unlabeled Use:** Febrile neutropenia, Hospital-acquired pneumonia and sepsis.

Action
Binds to bacterial cell wall, resulting in cell death. Meropenem resists the actions of many enzymes that degrade most other penicillins and penicillin-like anti-infectives. **Therapeutic Effects:** Bactericidal action against susceptible bacteria. **Spectrum:** Active against the following gram-positive organisms: *Staphylococcus aureus*, *Streptococcus pneumoniae*, Viridans group streptococci, *Enterococcus faecalis*. Also active against the following gram-negative pathogens: *Escherichia coli*, *Haemophilus influenzae*, *Klebsiella pneumoniae*, *Neisseria meningitidis*, *Pseudomonas aeruginosa*, *Proteus mirabilis*. Active against the following anaerobes: *Bacteroides fragilis*, *Bacteroides fragilis* group, *Peptostreptococcus* species.

Pharmacokinetics
Absorption: IV administration results in complete bioavailability.
Distribution: Widely distributed into body tissues and fluids; enters CSF when meninges are inflamed.
Metabolism and Excretion: 65–83% excreted unchanged by the kidneys.
Half-life: Premature neonates: 3 hr; Term neonates: 2 hr; Infants 3 mo–2 yr: 1.4 hr; Children >2 yr and Adults: 1 hr (↑ in renal impairment).

TIME/ACTION PROFILE (blood levels)

ROUTE	ONSET	PEAK	DURATION
IV	rapid	end of infusion	8 hr

Contraindications/Precautions
Contraindicated in: Hypersensitivity to meropenem or imipenem; Serious hypersensitivity to other beta-lactams (penicillins or cephalosporins; cross-sensitivity may occur).
Use Cautiously in: Renal impairment (↑ risk of thrombocytopenia and seizures; dose reduction recommended if CCr <50 mL/min); History

✽ = Canadian drug name. ⚡ = Genetic implication.
*CAPITALS indicates life-threatening; underlines indicate most frequent.

824 meropenem

of seizures, brain lesions, or meningitis; OB, Lactation, Pedi: Pregnancy, lactation, or children <3 mo (safety not established).

Adverse Reactions/Side Effects
CNS: SEIZURES, dizziness, headache. **Resp:** APNEA. **GI:** PSEUDOMEMBRANOUS COLITIS, constipation, diarrhea, glossitis (↑ in children), nausea, thrush (↑ in children), vomiting. **Derm:** moniliasis (children only), pruritus, rash. **Local:** inflammation at injection site, phlebitis. **Misc:** allergic reactions including ANAPHYLAXIS.

Interactions
Drug-Drug: Probenecid ↓ renal excretion and increases blood levels (coadministration not recommended). May ↓ serum **valproate** levels (↑ risk of seizures).

Route/Dosage
IV (Adults): 0.5–1 g q 8 hr. *Meningitis*—2 g q 8 hr.
IV (Children ≥3 mo–12 yr): *Intra-abdominal infections*—20 mg/kg q 8 hr; *meningitis*—40 mg/kg q 8 hr (maximum 2 g q 8 hr).
IV (Neonates <7 days): 20 mg/kg/dose q 12 hr. *Neonates >7 days, 1200–2000 g*—20 mg/kg/dose q 12 hr. *Neonates >7 days, >2000 g*—20 mg/kg/dose q 8 hr.

Renal Impairment
IV (Adults): *CCr 26–50 mL/min*—1 g q 12 hr; *CCr 10–25 mL/min*—500 mg q 12 hr; *CCr <10 mL/min*—500 mg q 24 hr.

Availability
Powder for injection: 500 mg, 1 g.

NURSING IMPLICATIONS

Assessment
- Assess patient for infection (vital signs; appearance of wound, sputum, urine, and stool; WBC) at beginning of and throughout therapy.
- Obtain a history before initiating therapy to determine previous use of and reactions to penicillins. Persons with a negative history of penicillin sensitivity may still have an allergic response.
- Obtain specimens for culture and sensitivity prior to initiating therapy. First dose may be given before receiving results.
- Observe patient for signs and symptoms of anaphylaxis (rash, pruritus, laryngeal edema, wheezing). Discontinue the drug and notify physician immediately if these symptoms occur. Have epinephrine, an antihistamine, and resuscitative equipment close by in the event of an anaphylactic reaction.
- Assess injection site for phlebitis, pain, and swelling periodically during administration.
- **Lab Test Considerations:** Monitor hematologic, hepatic, and renal functions periodically during therapy.
- BUN, AST, ALT, LDH, serum alkaline phosphatase, bilirubin, and creatinine may be transiently ↑.
- Hemoglobin and hematocrit concentrations may be ↓.
- May cause positive direct or indirect Coombs' test.

Potential Nursing Diagnoses
Risk for infection (Indications, Side Effects)
Deficient knowledge, related to medication regimen (Patient/Family Teaching)

Implementation
IV Administration
- **Direct IV:** *Diluent:* Reconstitute 500-mg and 1-g vials with 10 mL and 20 mL, respectively, of sterile water for injection, 0.9% NaCl, or D5W. Vials reconstituted with sterile water for injection are stable for 2 hr at room temperature and 12 hr if refrigerated; if reconstituted with 0.9% NaCl, stable for 2 hr at room temperature and 18 hr if refrigerated; if reconstituted with D5W, stable for 1 hr at room temperature and 8 hr if refrigerated. *Concentration:* 50 mg/mL. *Rate:* Administer over 3–5 min.
- **Intermittent Infusion:** *Diluent:* Reconstitute 500-mg and 1-g vials with 10 mL and 20 mL, respectively, of sterile water for injection, 0.9% NaCl, or D5W. Further dilute in 0.9% NaCl or D5W to achieve concentration below. Infusions further diluted in 0.9% NaCl are stable for 4 hr at room temperature and 24 hr if refrigerated. Infusions further diluted in D5W are stable for 1 hr at room temperature and 4 hr if refrigerated. *Concentration:* Final concentration of infusion should be 1–20 mg/mL. *Rate:* Infuse over 15–30 min.
- **Y-Site Compatibility:** aminophylline, anidulafungin, atenolol, atropine, caspofungin, cimetidine, daptomycin, dexamethasone, digoxin, diltiazem, diphenhydramine, docetaxel, enalaprilat, fluconazole, furosemide, gentamicin, granisetron, heparin, hydromorphone, insulin, linezolid, lorazepam, metoclopramide, milrinone, morphine, norepinephrine, palonosetron, phenobarbital, potassium chloride, tacrolimus, tirofiban, vancomycin, vasopressin, voriconazole.
- **Y-Site Incompatibility:** amphotericin B, diazepam, fenoldopam, metronidazole, quinupristin/dalfopristin.

Patient/Family Teaching
- Advise patient to report the signs of superinfection (black, furry overgrowth on the tongue; vaginal itching or discharge; loose or foul-smelling stools) and allergy.
- May cause dizziness. Caution patient to avoid driving or other activities requiring alertness until response to drug is known.
- Caution patient to notify health care professional if fever and diarrhea occur, especially if stool contains blood, pus, or mucus. Advise patient not to treat diarrhea without consulting health care professional. May occur up to several weeks after discontinuation of medication.

Evaluation/Desired Outcomes
- Resolution of the signs and symptoms of infection. Length of time for complete resolution depends on the organism and site of infection.

---

mesalamine (me-sal-a-meen)
Apriso, Asacol, Asacol HD, Canasa, Lialda, Pentasa, Rowasa, ♣ Salofalk

Classification
Therapeutic: gastrointestinal anti-inflammatories

Pregnancy Category B

Indications
Inflammatory bowel diseases including: Ulcerative colitis, Proctitis, Proctosigmoiditis.

Action
Locally acting anti-inflammatory action in the colon, where activity is probably due to inhibition of prostaglandin synthesis. **Therapeutic Effects:** Reduction in the symptoms of inflammatory bowel disease.

Pharmacokinetics
Absorption: 28% absorbed following oral administration; 10–30% absorbed from the colon, depending on retention time, following rectal administration.
Distribution: Unknown.
Metabolism and Excretion: Some metabolism occurs, site unknown; mostly eliminated unchanged in the feces.
Half-life: 12 hr PO (range 2–15 hr); 0.5–1.5 hr rectal.

TIME/ACTION PROFILE (clinical improvement)

ROUTE	ONSET	PEAK	DURATION
PO	unknown	unknown	6–8 hr
Extended release	2 hr	9–12 hr	24 hr
Rectal	3–21 days	unknown	24 hr

Contraindications/Precautions
Contraindicated in: Hypersensitivity reactions to sulfonamides, salicylates, mesalamine, or sulfasalazine; Cross-sensitivity with furosemide, sulfonylurea hypoglycemic agents, or carbonic anhydrase inhibitors may exist; G6PD deficiency; Hypersensitivity to bisulfites (mesalamine enema only); Urinary tract or intestinal obstruction; Porphyria.
Use Cautiously in: Severe hepatic or renal impairment; OB: Safety not established; Lactation: Has caused side effects in some infants; careful observation required.

Adverse Reactions/Side Effects
CNS: headache, dizziness, malaise, weakness. **EENT:** pharyngitis, rhinitis. **CV:** pericarditis. **GI:** diarrhea, eructation (PO), flatulence, nausea, vomiting. **GU:** interstitial nephritis, pancreatitis, renal failure. **Derm:** hair loss, rash. **Local:** anal irritation (enema, suppository). **MS:** back pain. **Misc:** ANAPHYLAXIS, acute intolerance syndrome, fever.

Interactions
Drug-Drug: May ↓ metabolism and ↑ effects/toxicity of **mercaptopurine** or **thioguanine**.

Route/Dosage

One Asacol HD 800-mg tablet is NOT bioequivalent to two Asacol 400-mg tablets
PO (Adults): 800 mg (two 400-mg delayed–release tablets) 3 times daily for 6 wk *or* 1.6 g (two 800-mg delayed–release tablets) 3 times daily for 6 wk *or* 1 g 4 times daily as controlled-release capsules *or* two–four 1.2-g tablets once daily with a meal for a total daily dose of 2.4 or 4.8 g of *Lialda* or 1500 mg daily in morning of *Apriso*.
Rect (Adults): 4-g enema (60 mL) at bedtime, retained for 8 hr for 3–6 wk *or* 1 g at bedtime.

Availability (generic available)
Delayed-release tablets: ♣ 250 mg, 400 mg, ♣ 500 mg, 800 mg (Asacol HD), 1.2 g (Lialda).
Cost: 400 mg $132.01/180, 1.2 g $515.96/120.

Controlled-release capsules: 250 mg, 500 mg. **Cost:** 250 mg $387.98/480, 500 mg $351.32/240. **Extended-release capsules (Apriso):** 375 mg. **Suppositories:** 1 g. **Cost:** $326.96/30. **Rectal suspension:** 4 g/60 mL. **Cost:** *Generic*—$317.69/28 bottles.

NURSING IMPLICATIONS
Assessment
- Assess patient for allergy to sulfonamides and salicylates. Patients allergic to sulfasalazine may take mesalamine or olsalazine without difficulty, but therapy should be discontinued if rash or fever occurs.
- Monitor intake and output ratios. Fluid intake should be sufficient to maintain a urine output of at least 1200–1500 mL daily to prevent crystalluria and stone formation.
- **Inflammatory Bowel Disease:** Assess abdominal pain and frequency, quantity, and consistency of stools at the beginning of and during therapy.
- *Lab Test Considerations:* Monitor urinalysis, BUN, and serum creatinine prior to and periodically during therapy. Mesalamine may cause renal toxicity.
- Mesalamine may cause ↑ AST and ALT levels, serum alkaline phosphatase, GGTP, LDH, amylase, and lipase.

Potential Nursing Diagnoses
Acute pain (Indications)
Diarrhea (Indications)

Implementation
- Do not confuse Asacol (mesalamine) with Os-Cal (calcium carbonate).
- **PO:** Administer with a full glass of water. Tablets should be swallowed whole; do not break the outer coating, which is designed to remain intact. Take *Lialda* tablets with a meal. Take *Apriso* capsules in the morning without regard to meals. Do not co-administer with antacids; may effect dissolution of the coating of the granules in *Apriso* capsules. Intact or partially intact tablets may occasionally be found in the stool. If this occurs repeatedly, advise patient to notify health care professional.
- **Rect:** Patient should empty bowel prior to administration of rectal dose forms.
- Avoid excessive handling of *suppository*. Remove foil wrapper and insert pointed end first into rectum with gentle pressure. Suppository should be retained for 1–3 hr or more for maximum benefit.
- Administer 60-mL retention enema once daily at bedtime. Solution should be retained for approximately 8 hr. Prior to administration of *rectal suspension*, shake bottle well and remove the protective cap. Have patient lie on left side with the lower leg extended and the upper leg flexed for support or place the patient in knee-chest position. Gently insert the applicator tip into the rectum, pointing toward the umbilicus. Squeeze the bottle steadily to discharge most of the preparation.

Patient/Family Teaching
- Instruct patient on the correct method of administration. Advise patient to take medication as directed, even if feeling better. Take missed doses as soon as remembered unless almost time for next dose.
- May cause dizziness. Caution patient to avoid driving or other activities that require alertness until response to medication is known.
- Advise patient to notify health care professional if skin rash, sore throat, fever, mouth sores, unusual bleeding or bruising, wheezing, fever, or hives occur.
- Instruct patient to notify health care professional if symptoms do not improve after 1–2 months of therapy.
- Instruct patient to notify health care professional if symptoms worsen or do not improve. If symptoms of acute intolerance (cramping, acute abdominal pain, bloody diarrhea, fever, headache, rash) occur, discontinue therapy and notify health care professional immediately.
- Inform patient that proctoscopy and sigmoidoscopy may be required periodically during treatment to determine response.
- **Rect:** Instruct patient to use *rectal suspension* at bedtime and retain suspension all night for best results.
- Advise patient not to change brands of mesalamine without consulting health care professional.

Evaluation/Desired Outcomes
- Decrease in diarrhea and abdominal pain.
- Return to normal bowel pattern in patients with inflammatory bowel disease. Effects may be seen within 3–21 days. The usual course of therapy is 3–6 wk.
- Maintenance of remission in patients with inflammatory bowel disease.

mesna (mes-na)
Mesnex, ✦Uromitexan

Classification
Therapeutic: antidotes
Pharmacologic: ifosfamide detoxifying agents

Pregnancy Category B

Indications
Prevention of ifosfamide-induced hemorrhagic cystitis (see Ifosfamide monograph). **Unlabeled Use:** May also prevent hemorrhagic cystitis from cyclophosphamide.

Action
Binds to the toxic metabolites of ifosfamide in the kidneys. **Therapeutic Effects:** Prevents hemorrhagic cystitis from ifosfamide.

Pharmacokinetics
Absorption: IV administration results in complete bioavailability; 45–79% absorbed after oral administration. Following IV with PO dosing ↑ systemic exposure.
Distribution: Unknown.
Metabolism and Excretion: Rapidly converted to mesna disulfide, then back to mesna in the kidneys, where it binds to toxic metabolites of ifosfamide (18–26% excreted as free mesna in urine after IV and PO dosing).
Half-life: *Mesna*—0.36 hr (IV); 1.2—8.3 hr (IV followed by PO); *mesna disulfide*—1.17 hr.

TIME/ACTION PROFILE (detoxifying action)

ROUTE	ONSET	PEAK	DURATION
PO, IV	rapid	unknown	4 hr

Contraindications/Precautions
Contraindicated in: Hypersensitivity to mesna or other thiol (rubber) compounds.
Use Cautiously in: OB, Lactation: Safety not established.

Adverse Reactions/Side Effects
CNS: dizziness, drowsiness, headache. **GI:** anorexia, diarrhea, nausea, unpleasant taste, vomiting. **Derm:** flushing. **Local:** injection site reactions. **Misc:** flu-like symptoms.

Interactions
Drug-Drug: None significant.

Route/Dosage
IV (Adults): Give a dose of mesna equal to 20% of the ifosfamide dose at the same time as ifosfamide and 4 and 8 hr after.

PO, IV (Adults): Give a dose of IV mesna equal to 20% of the ifosfamide dose at the same time as ifosfamide; then give PO mesna equal to 40% of the ifosfamide dose 2 and 6 hours after ifosfamide (total mesna dose is 100% of ifosfamide dose).

Availability (generic available)
Tablets: 400 mg. **Injection:** 100 mg/mL. *In combination with:* In a kit with ifosfamide.

NURSING IMPLICATIONS

Assessment
- Monitor for development of hemorrhagic cystitis in patients receiving ifosfamide.
- *Lab Test Considerations:* Causes a false-positive result when testing urinary ketones.

Potential Nursing Diagnoses
Deficient knowledge, related to medication regimen (Patient/Family Teaching)

Implementation
- Initial IV bolus is to be given at time of ifosfamide administration.
- **PO:** If second and third doses are given orally, administer 2 and 6 hours after IV dose.
- If PO mesna is vomited within 2 hr of administration, repeat dose or use IV mesna.

IV Administration

- **Intermittent Infusion:** 2nd IV dose is given 4 hr later, 3rd dose is given 8 hr after initial dose. This schedule must be repeated with each subsequent dose of ifosfamide. *Diluent:* Dilute 2-, 4-, and 10-mL ampules, containing a concentration of 100 mg/mL in 8 mL, 16 mL, or 50 mL, respectively, of D5W, 0.9% NaCl, D5/0.9% NaCl, D5/0.2% NaCl, D5/0.33% NaCl, or LR. *Concentration:* 20 mg/mL. Refrigerate to store. Use within 6 hr. Discard unused solution. *Rate:* Administer over 15–30 min or as a continuous infusion.
- **Syringe Compatibility:** ifosfamide.
- **Y-Site Compatibility:** allopurinol, amifostine, aztreonam, cefepime, docetaxel, doxorubicin liposome, etoposide phosphate, filgrastim, fludarabine, gemcitabine, granisetron, linezolid, melphalan, methotrexate, ondansetron, oxaliplatin, paclitaxel, pemetrexed, piperacillin/tazobactam, sargramostim, sodium bicarbonate, teniposide, thiotepa, vinorelbine.
- **Y-Site Incompatibility:** amphotericin B cholesteryl complex, lansoprazole.
- **Additive Compatibility:** ifosfamide.
- **Additive Incompatibility:** carboplatin, cisplatin.

Patient/Family Teaching
- Inform patient that unpleasant taste may occur during administration.
- Advise patient to notify health care professional if nausea, vomiting, or diarrhea persists or is severe.

Evaluation/Desired Outcomes
- Prevention of hemorrhagic cystitis associated with ifosfamide therapy.

---

mestranol/norethindrone, See CONTRACEPTIVES, HORMONAL.

---

metaxalone (me-tax-a-lone)
Skelaxin

Classification
Therapeutic: skeletal muscle relaxants (centrally acting)

Pregnancy Category UK

Indications
Muscle spasm associated with acute painful musculoskeletal conditions (with rest and physical therapy).

Action
Skeletal muscle relaxation, probably as a result of CNS depression. **Therapeutic Effects:** Skeletal muscle relaxation.

Pharmacokinetics
Absorption: Well absorbed following oral administration.
Distribution: Unknown.
Metabolism and Excretion: Mostly metabolized by the liver; metabolites excreted in urine.
Half-life: 2–3 hr.

TIME/ACTION PROFILE

ROUTE	ONSET	PEAK	DURATION
PO	1 hr	2 hr	4–6 hr

Contraindications/Precautions
Contraindicated in: Hypersensitivity; Significant hepatic/renal impairment; History of drug-induced hemolytic anemia or other anemia.
Use Cautiously in: Hepatic impairment; History of seizures; OB, Lactation, Pedi: Pregnancy, lactation or children ≤12 yr (safety not established); Geri: Appears on Beers list. Poorly tolerated due to anticholinergic effects.

Adverse Reactions/Side Effects
CNS: <u>drowsiness</u>, <u>dizziness</u>, confusion, headache, irritability, nervousness. **GI:** <u>nausea</u>, anorexia, dry mouth, GI upset, vomiting. **GU:** urinary retention.

Interactions
Drug-Drug: ↑ CNS depression with other **CNS depressants** including **alcohol**, **antihistamines**, **opioid analgesics**, and **sedative/hypnotics**.
Drug-Natural Products: Concomitant use of **kava-kava**, **valerian**, or **chamomile** can ↑ CNS depression.

Route/Dosage
PO (Adults): 800 mg 3–4 times daily.

Availability
Tablets: 800 mg. **Cost:** $299.97/100.

NURSING IMPLICATIONS

Assessment
- Assess patient for pain, muscle stiffness, and range of motion before and periodically during therapy.
- Geri: Assess geriatric patients for anticholinergic effects (sedation and weakness).
- **Lab Test Considerations:** Monitor hepatic function tests closely in patients with pre-existing liver damage.
- May cause false-positive Benedict's tests.

Potential Nursing Diagnoses
Acute pain (Indications)
Impaired bed mobility (Indications)
Risk for injury (Side Effects)

Implementation
- Provide safety measures as indicated. Supervise ambulation and transfer of patients.
- PO: Administer 3–4 times daily.

Patient/Family Teaching
- Instruct patient to take medication as directed. Take missed doses within 1 hr; if not, return to regular dosing schedule. Do not double doses.
- Encourage patient to comply with additional therapies prescribed for muscle spasm (rest, physical therapy, heat).
- Medication may cause dizziness, drowsiness, and blurred vision. Advise patient to avoid driving and other activities requiring alertness until response to drug is known.
- Instruct patient to make position changes slowly to minimize orthostatic hypotension.
- Advise patient to avoid concurrent use of alcohol and other CNS depressants while taking this medication.

- Instruct patient to notify health care professional if skin rash or yellowish discoloration of the skin or eyes occurs.
- Emphasize the importance of routine follow-up exams to monitor progress.

Evaluation/Desired Outcomes
- Decreased musculoskeletal pain and muscle spasticity.
- Increased range of motion.

---

metformin (met-for-min)
Fortamet, Glumetza, Glucophage, Glucophage XR, ✸Novo-Metformin, Riomet

Classification
Therapeutic: antidiabetics
Pharmacologic: biguanides

Pregnancy Category B

Indications
Management of type 2 diabetes mellitus; may be used with diet, insulin, or sulfonylurea oral hypoglycemics.

Action
Decreases hepatic glucose production. Decreases intestinal glucose absorption. Increases sensitivity to insulin. **Therapeutic Effects:** Maintenance of blood glucose.

Pharmacokinetics
Absorption: 50–60% absorbed after oral administration.
Distribution: Enters breast milk in concentrations similar to plasma.
Metabolism and Excretion: Eliminated almost entirely unchanged by the kidneys.
Half-life: 17.6 hr.

TIME/ACTION PROFILE (blood levels)

ROUTE	ONSET	PEAK	DURATION
PO	unknown	unknown	12 hr
XR	unknown	4–8 hr	24 hr

Contraindications/Precautions
Contraindicated in: Hypersensitivity; Metabolic acidosis; Dehydration, sepsis, hypoxemia, hepatic impairment, excessive alcohol use (acute or chronic); Renal dysfunction (serum creatinine >1.5 mg/dL in men or >1.4 mg/dL in women); Radiographic studies requiring IV iodinated contrast media (withhold metformin); CHF.

Use Cautiously in: Concurrent renal disease; Geri: Geriatric/debilitated patients (↓ doses may be required; avoid in patients >80 yr unless renal function is normal); Chronic alcohol use/abuse; Serious medical conditions (MI, stroke); Patients undergoing stress (infection, surgical procedures); Hypoxia; Pituitary deficiency or hyperthyroidism; OB, Lactation, Pedi: Pregnancy, lactation, or children <10 yr (safety not established; extended release for use in patients >17 yr only).

Adverse Reactions/Side Effects
GI: abdominal bloating, diarrhea, nausea, vomiting, unpleasant metallic taste. **Endo:** hypoglycemia. **F and E:** LACTIC ACIDOSIS. **Misc:** decreased vitamin B_{12} levels.

Interactions
Drug-Drug: Acute or chronic **alcohol** ingestion or **iodinated contrast media** ↑ risk of lactic acidosis. **Amiloride, digoxin, morphine, procainamide, quinidine, ranitidine, triamterene, trimethoprim, calcium channel blockers,** and **vancomycin** may compete for elimination pathways with metformin. Altered responses may occur. **Cimetidine** and **furosemide** may ↑ effects of metformin. **Nifedipine** ↑ absorption and effects.
Drug-Natural Products: Glucosamine may worsen blood glucose control. **Chromium,** and **coenzyme Q-10** may produce ↑ hypoglycemic effects.

Route/Dosage
PO (Adults and children >17 yr): 500 mg twice daily; may ↑ by 500 mg at weekly intervals up to 2000 mg/day. If doses >2000 mg/day are required, give in 3 divided doses (not to exceed 2500 mg/day) or 850 mg once daily; may ↑ by 850 mg at 2-wk intervals (in divided doses) up to 2550 mg/day in divided doses (up to 850 mg 3 times daily); *Extended-release tablets*— 500–1000 mg once daily with evening meal, may ↑ by 500 mg at weekly intervals up to 2500 mg once daily. If 2000 mg once daily is inadequate, 1000 mg twice daily may be used.

PO (Children >10 yr): 500 mg twice daily, may be ↑ by 500 mg/day at 1-wk intervals, up to 2000 mg/day in 2 divided doses.

Availability (generic available)
Tablets: 500 mg, 850 mg, 1000 mg. **Cost:** 500 mg $86.72/100, 850 mg $149.95/100, 1000 mg $149.95/100. **Extended-release tablets (Fortamet, Glucophage XR, Glumetza):** 500 mg,

750 mg, 1000 mg. **Oral solution (cherry flavor):** 100 mg/mL. *In combination with:* glyburide (Glucovance) glipizide (Metaglip), pioglitazone (Actoplus Met, Actoplus Met XR), repaglinide (PrandiMet), rosiglitazone (Avandamet) and sitagliptin (Janumet). See Appendix B.

NURSING IMPLICATIONS

Assessment
- When combined with oral sulfonylureas, observe for signs and symptoms of hypoglycemic reactions (abdominal pain, sweating, hunger, weakness, dizziness, headache, tremor, tachycardia, anxiety).
- Patients who have been well controlled on metformin who develop illness or laboratory abnormalities should be assessed for ketoacidosis or lactic acidosis. Assess serum electrolytes, ketones, glucose, and, if indicated, blood pH, lactate, pyruvate, and metformin levels. If either form of acidosis is present, discontinue metformin immediately and treat acidosis.
- *Lab Test Considerations:* Monitor serum glucose and glycosylated hemoglobin periodically during therapy to evaluate effectiveness of therapy. May cause false-positive results for urine ketones.
- Monitor blood glucose concentrations routinely by patient and every 3 mo by health care professional to determine effectiveness of therapy.
- Assess renal function before initiating and at least annually during therapy. Discontinue metformin if renal impairment occurs.
- Monitor serum folic acid and vitamin B_{12} every 1–2 yr in long-term therapy. Metformin may interfere with absorption.

Potential Nursing Diagnoses
Imbalanced nutrition: more than body requirements (Indications)
Noncompliance (Patient/Family Teaching)

Implementation
- Patients stabilized on a diabetic regimen who are exposed to stress, fever, trauma, infection, or surgery may require administration of insulin. Withhold metformin and reinstitute after resolution of acute episode.
- Metformin therapy should be temporarily discontinued in patients requiring surgery involving restricted intake of food and fluids. Resume metformin when oral intake has resumed and renal function is normal.
- Withhold metformin before or at the time of studies requiring IV administration of iodinated contrast media and for 48 hr after study.
- **PO:** Administer metformin with meals to minimize GI effects.
- XR tablets must be swallowed whole; do not crush or chew.

Patient/Family Teaching
- Instruct patient to take metformin at the same time each day, as directed. Take missed doses as soon as possible unless almost time for next dose. Do not double doses.
- Explain to patient that metformin helps control hyperglycemia but does not cure diabetes. Therapy is usually long term.
- Encourage patient to follow prescribed diet, medication, and exercise regimen to prevent hyperglycemic or hypoglycemic episodes.
- Review signs of hypoglycemia and hyperglycemia with patient. If hypoglycemia occurs, advise patient to take a glass of orange juice or 2–3 tsp of sugar, honey, or corn syrup dissolved in water, and notify health care professional.
- Instruct patient in proper testing of blood glucose and urine ketones. These tests should be monitored closely during periods of stress or illness and health care professional notified if significant changes occur.
- Explain to patient the risk of lactic acidosis and the potential need for discontinuation of metformin therapy if a severe infection, dehydration, or severe or continuing diarrhea occurs or if medical tests or surgery is required. Symptoms of lactic acidosis (chills, diarrhea, dizziness, low blood pressure, muscle pain, sleepiness, slow heartbeat or pulse, dyspnea, or weakness) should be reported to health care professional immediately.
- Caution patient to avoid taking other Rx, OTC, herbal products, or alcohol during metformin therapy without consulting health care professional.
- Insulin is the recommended method of controlling blood glucose during pregnancy. Counsel female patients to use a form of contraception other than oral contraceptives and to notify health care professional promptly if pregnancy is planned or suspected.
- Inform patient that metformin may cause an unpleasant or metallic taste that usually resolves spontaneously.
- Inform patients taking XR tablets that inactive ingredients resembling XR tablet may appear in stools.
- Advise patient to inform health care professional of medication regimen before treatment or surgery.

- Advise patient to carry a form of sugar (sugar packets, candy) and identification describing disease process and medication regimen at all times.
- Advise patient to report the occurrence of diarrhea, nausea, vomiting, and stomach pain or fullness to health care professional.
- Emphasize the importance of routine follow-up exams and regular testing of blood glucose, glycosylated hemoglobin, renal function, and hematologic parameters.

Evaluation/Desired Outcomes
- Control of blood glucose levels without the appearance of hypoglycemic or hyperglycemic episodes. Control may be achieved within a few days, but full effect of therapy may be delayed for up to 2 wk. If patient has not responded to metformin after 4 wk of maximum dose therapy, an oral sulfonylurea may be added. If satisfactory results are not obtained with 1–3 months of concurrent therapy, oral agents may be discontinued and insulin therapy instituted.

HIGH ALERT

methadone (meth-a-done)
Methadose

Classification
Therapeutic: opioid analgesics
Pharmacologic: opioid agonists

Schedule II

Pregnancy Category C

Indications
Severe pain. Suppresses withdrawal symptoms in opioid detoxification. **Unlabeled Use:** Neonatal abstinence syndrome.

Action
Binds to opiate receptors in the CNS. Alters the perception of and response to painful stimuli, while producing generalized CNS depression. **Therapeutic Effects:** Decrease in severity of pain. Suppression of withdrawal symptoms during detoxification and maintenance from heroin and other opioids.

Pharmacokinetics
Absorption: Well absorbed from all sites (50% absorbed following oral administration).
Distribution: Widely distributed. Crosses the placenta; enters breast milk.
Protein Binding: High.
Metabolism and Excretion: Mostly metabolized by the liver; some metabolites are active and may accumulate with chronic administration.
Half-life: 15–25 hr; ↑ with chronic use.

TIME/ACTION PROFILE (analgesic effect)

ROUTE	ONSET	PEAK	DURATION
PO	30–60 min	90–120 min	4–12 hr
IM, subcut	10–20 min	60–120 min	4–6 hr

Contraindications/Precautions
Contraindicated in: Hypersensitivity; Known alcohol intolerance (some oral solutions); Concurrent MAO inhibitor therapy.
Use Cautiously in: Structural heart disease, concomitant diuretic use, hypokalemia, hypomagnesemia, history of arrhythmia/syncope, or other risk factors for arrhythmias; Concurrent use of drugs that prolong the QTc interval or are CYP3A4 inhibitors; Head trauma; Increased intracranial pressure; Severe renal, hepatic, or pulmonary disease; Hypothyroidism; Adrenal insufficiency; Alcoholism; Undiagnosed abdominal pain; Prostatic hyperplasia or ureteral stricture; OB: Use with addiction control: weigh risk against potential for illicit drug use. Counsel mother about potential harm to fetus; Lactation: Appears in breast milk. Weigh risks against potential for illicit drug use. Counsel mother about potential harm to infant and to wean breastfeeding slowly to prevent abstinence syndrome; Geri: Dose reduction suggested.

Adverse Reactions/Side Effects
CNS: confusion, sedation, dizziness, dysphoria, euphoria, floating feeling, hallucinations, headache, unusual dreams. **EENT:** blurred vision, diplopia, miosis. **Resp:** respiratory depression. **CV:** hypotension, bradycardia, QT prolongation, torsades de pointes. **GI:** constipation, nausea, vomiting. **GU:** urinary retention. **Derm:** flushing, sweating. **Misc:** physical dependence, psychological dependence, tolerance.

Interactions
Drug-Drug: Use with extreme caution in patients receiving **MAO inhibitors** (may result in severe, unpredictable reactions—reduce initial dose of methadone to 25% of usual dose). Use with extreme caution with any drug known to potentially prolong QT interval, including **class I and III antiarrhythmics**, some **neuroleptics** and **tricyclic antidepressants**, and **calcium channel blockers**. Use with extreme caution with CYP3A4

inhibitors, including **ketoconazole**, **itraconazole**, **erythromycin**, **clarithromycin**, **calcium channel blockers**, or **voriconazole**. Concurrent use with **laxatives**, **diuretics**, or **mineralocorticoids** may ↑ risk of hypomagnesemia or hypokalemia and ↑ risk of arrhythmias. ↑ CNS depression with **alcohol**, **antihistamines**, and **sedative/hypnotics**. Administration of **agonist/antagonist opioids** may precipitate opioid withdrawal in physically dependent patients. **Nalbuphine** or **pentazocine** may ↓ analgesia. **Interferons (alpha)** may ↓ metabolism and ↑ effects. **Nevirapine**, **efavirenz**, **ritonavir**, **ritonavir/lopinavir**, **phenobarbital**, **carbamazepine** **phenytoin**, and **rifampin** may ↑ metabolism and ↓ analgesia; withdrawal may occur. **Fluvoxamine** may ↑ CNS depression; with **fluvoxamine**, opioid withdrawal may occur. May ↑ blood levels and effects of **zidovudine** and **desipramine**. May ↓ level and effects of **didanosine** and **stavudine**.

Drug-Natural Products: St. John's wort ↑ metabolism and ↓ blood levels, concurrent use may result in withdrawal. **Kava-kava**, **valerian**, or **chamomile**, can ↑ CNS depression.

Route/Dosage
Larger doses may be required for analgesia during chronic therapy; interval may be ↓/dose ↑ if pain recurs.

PO (Adults and Children ≥ 50 kg): *Analgesic*— 20 mg q 6–8 hr. *Opioid detoxification*— 15–40 mg once daily or amount needed to prevent withdrawal. Dose may be decreased q 1–2 days; maintenance dose is determined on an individual basis.

PO (Adults and Children < 50 kg): *Analgesic*— 0.1 mg/kg/dose q 4 hr for 2–3 doses then q 6–8 hr prn; maximum: 10 mg/dose. *Iatrogenic narcotic dependency*— 0.05–0.1 mg/kg/dose q 6 hr; increase by 0.05 mg/kg/dose until withdrawal symptoms controlled; after 1–2 days lengthen dosing interval to q 12–24 hr; taper by decreasing dose by 0.05 mg/kg/day.

PO, IV (Neonates): Initial 0.05–0.2 mg/kg/dose q 12–24 hr or 0.5 mg/kg/day divided q 8 hr; taper dose by 10–20% per week over 1–1½ months.

IV, IM, Subcut (Adults and Children ≥50 kg): *Analgesic*— 10 mg q 6–8 hr. *Opioid detoxification*— 15–40 mg once daily or amount needed to prevent withdrawal. Dose may be ↓ q 1–2 days; maintenance dose is determined on an individual basis.

IV, IM, Subcut (Adults and Children <50 kg): *Analgesic*– 0.1 mg/kg q 6–8 hr; maximum: 10 mg/dose.

Availability (generic available)
Tablets: 5 mg, 10 mg. **Dispersible tablets (diskettes):** 40 mg (available only to licensed detoxification/maintenance programs). **Injection:** 10 mg/mL. **Oral solution (contains alcohol) (citrus):** 5 mg/5 mL, 10 mg/5 mL. **Oral concentrate (cherry and unflavored):** 10 mg/mL.

NURSING IMPLICATIONS
Assessment
- **Pain:** Assess type, location, and intensity of pain prior to and 1–2 hr (peak) following administration. When titrating opioid doses, increases of 25–50% should be administered until there is either a 50% reduction in the patient's pain rating on a numeric or visual analogue scale or the patient reports satisfactory pain relief. A repeat dose can be safely administered at the time of the peak if previous dose is ineffective and side effects are minimal. Cumulative effects of this medication may require periodic dose adjustments.
- Doses of methadone for patients on methadone maintenance only prevent withdrawal symptoms; *no analgesia is provided*. Additional opioid doses are required for treatment of pain.
- An equianalgesic chart (see Appendix K) should be used when changing routes or when changing from one opioid to another.
- Assess blood pressure, pulse, and respirations before and periodically during administration. If respiratory rate is < 10/min, assess level of sedation. Dose may need to be decreased by 25–50%. Initial drowsiness will diminish with continued use.
- Assess bowel function routinely. Prevention of constipation should be instituted with increased intake of fluids and bulk and with laxatives to minimize constipating effects. Stimulant laxatives should be administered routinely if opioid use exceeds 2–3 days, unless contraindicated.
- Prolonged use may lead to physical and psychological dependence and tolerance. This should not prevent patient from receiving adequate analgesia. Most patients who receive methadone for pain do not develop psychological dependence. Progressively higher doses may be required to relieve pain with long-term therapy.

methadone

- Assess for history of structural heart disease, arrhythmia, and syncope. Obtain a pretreatment ECG to measure QTc interval and follow-up ECG within 30 days and annually. Additional ECGs recommended if dose >100 mg/day or if patients have unexplained syncope or seizures. If QTc interval is >450 ms but <500 ms, discuss potential risks and benefits with patients and monitor more frequently. If the QTc interval >500 ms, consider discontinuing or reducing dose; eliminating contributing factors (drugs that promote hypokalemia) or using an alternative therapy.
- **Opioid Detoxification:** Assess patient for signs of opioid withdrawal (irritability, runny nose and eyes, abdominal cramps, body aches, sweating, loss of appetite, shivering, unusually large pupils, trouble sleeping, weakness, yawning). Methadone maintenance is undertaken only by federally approved treatment centers. This does not preclude maintenance for addicts hospitalized for other conditions and who require temporary maintenance during their care.
- *Lab Test Considerations:* May ↑ plasma amylase and lipase levels.
- *Toxicity and Overdose:* If an opioid antagonist is required to reverse respiratory depression or coma, naloxone (Narcan) is the antidote. Dilute the 0.4-mg ampule of naloxone in 10 mL of 0.9% NaCl and administer 0.5 mL (0.02 mg) by direct IV push every 2 min. For children and patients weighing < 40 kg, dilute 0.1 mg of naloxone in 10 mL of 0.9% NaCl for a concentration of 10 mcg/mL and administer 0.5 mcg/kg every 2 min. Titrate dose to avoid withdrawal, seizures, and severe pain.

Potential Nursing Diagnoses
Acute pain (Indications)
Disturbed sensory perception (visual, auditory) (Side Effects)
Risk for injury (Side Effects)

Implementation
- *High Alert:* Accidental overdosage of opioid analgesics has resulted in fatalities. Before administering, clarify all ambiguous orders; have second practitioner independently check original order and dose calculations.
- Explain therapeutic value of medication prior to administration to enhance the analgesic effect.
- Regularly administered doses may be more effective than prn administration. Analgesic is more effective if administered before pain becomes severe. For patients in chronic severe pain, the oral solution containing 5 or 10 mg/5 mL is recommended on a fixed dose schedule.
- Coadministration with nonopioid analgesics may have additive analgesic effects and may permit lower doses.
- Medication should be discontinued gradually after long-term use to prevent withdrawal symptoms.
- Diskettes (dispersible tablets) are to be dissolved and used for detoxification and maintenance treatment only.
- **PO:** Doses may be administered with food or milk to minimize GI irritation.
- Dilute each dose of 10 mg/mL oral concentrate with at least 30 mL of water or other liquid prior to administration.
- **Subcut, IM:** IM is the preferred parenteral route for repeated doses. Subcut administration may cause tissue irritation.

Patient/Family Teaching
- Instruct patient on how and when to ask for and take pain medication.
- Instruct patient to take methadone exactly as directed. If dose is less effective after a few weeks, do not increase dose without consulting health care professional.
- May cause drowsiness or dizziness. Advise patient to call for assistance when ambulating or smoking and to avoid driving or other activities requiring alertness until response to medication is known.
- Inform patient of the potential for arrhythmias and emphasize the importance of regular ECGs.
- Caution patient notify health care professional if signs of overdose (difficult or shallow breathing, extreme tiredness or sleepiness, blurred vision, inability to think, talk, or walk normally, and feelings of faintness, dizziness, or confusion) occur. Methadone has a prolonged action causing increased risk of overdose.
- Advise patient to change positions slowly to minimize orthostatic hypotension.
- Caution patient to avoid concurrent use of alcohol or other CNS depressants with this medication.
- Encourage patient to turn, cough, and breathe deeply every 2 hr to prevent atelectasis.

Evaluation/Desired Outcomes
- Decrease in severity of pain without a significant alteration in level of consciousness or respiratory status.
- Prevention of withdrawal symptoms in detoxification from heroin and other opioid analgesics.

---

methimazole (meth-im-a-zole)
Tapazole

Classification
Therapeutic: antithyroid agents

Pregnancy Category D

Indications
Palliative treatment of hyperthyroidism. Used as an adjunct to control hyperthyroidism in preparation for thyroidectomy or radioactive iodine therapy.

Action
Inhibits the synthesis of thyroid hormones. **Therapeutic Effects:** Decreased signs and symptoms of hyperthyroidism.

Pharmacokinetics
Absorption: Rapidly absorbed following oral administration.
Distribution: Crosses the placenta and enters breast milk in high concentrations.
Metabolism and Excretion: Mostly metabolized by the liver; <10% eliminated unchanged by the kidneys.
Half-life: 3–5 hr.

TIME/ACTION PROFILE (effect on thyroid function)

ROUTE	ONSET	PEAK	DURATION
PO	1 wk	4–10 wk	wk

Contraindications/Precautions
Contraindicated in: Hypersensitivity; Lactation: Lactation.
Use Cautiously in: Patients with ↓ bone marrow reserve; Patients >40 yr (↑ risk of agranulocytosis); OB: May be used cautiously; however, thyroid problems may occur in the fetus.

Adverse Reactions/Side Effects
CNS: drowsiness, headache, vertigo. **GI:** diarrhea, hepatotoxicity, loss of taste, nausea, parotitis, vomiting. **Derm:** rash, skin discoloration, urticaria. **Hemat:** AGRANULOCYTOSIS, anemia, leukopenia, thrombocytopenia. **MS:** arthralgia. **Misc:** fever, lymphadenopathy.

Interactions
Drug-Drug: Additive bone marrow depression with **antineoplastics** or **radiation therapy**. Antithyroid effect may be ↓ by **potassium iodide** or **amiodarone**. ↑ risk of agranulocytosis with **phenothiazines**. May alter response to **warfarin** and **digoxin**.

Route/Dosage
PO (Adults): *Thyrotoxic crisis*—15–20 mg q 4 hr during the first 24 hr (with other interventions). *Hyperthyroidism*—15–60 mg/day as a single dose or divided doses for 6–8 wk. *Maintenance*—5–30 mg/kg as a single dose or 2 divided doses.

PO (Children): *Initial*—400 mcg (0.4 mg)/kg/day in single dose or 2 divided doses. *Maintenance*—200 mcg/kg/day in single dose or 2 divided doses.

Availability (generic available)
Tablets: 5 mg, 10 mg.

NURSING IMPLICATIONS
Assessment
- Monitor response for symptoms of hyperthyroidism or thyrotoxicosis (tachycardia, palpitations, nervousness, insomnia, fever, diaphoresis, heat intolerance, tremors, weight loss, diarrhea).
- Assess patient for development of hypothyroidism (intolerance to cold, constipation, dry skin, headache, listlessness, tiredness, or weakness). Dose adjustment may be required.
- Assess patient for skin rash or swelling of cervical lymph nodes. Treatment may be discontinued if this occurs.
- *Lab Test Considerations:* Monitor thyroid function studies prior to therapy, monthly during initial therapy, and every 2–3 mo during therapy.
- Monitor WBC and differential counts periodically during therapy. Agranulocytosis may develop rapidly; usually occurs during the first 2 mo and is more common in patients over 40 yr and those receiving >40 mg/day. This necessitates discontinuation of therapy.
- May cause ↑ AST, ALT, LDH, alkaline phosphatase, serum bilirubin, and prothrombin time.

Potential Nursing Diagnoses
Noncompliance (Patient/Family Teaching)

Implementation
- **PO:** Administer at same time in relation to meals every day. Food may either increase or decrease absorption.

Patient/Family Teaching
- Instruct patient to take medication as directed, around the clock. Take missed doses as soon as remembered; take both doses together if almost time for next dose; check with health care professional if more than 1 dose is missed. Consult health care professional prior to discontinuing medication.
- Instruct patient to monitor weight 2–3 times weekly. Notify health care professional of significant changes.
- May cause drowsiness. Caution patient to avoid driving or other activities requiring alertness until response to medication is known.
- Advise patient to consult health care professional regarding dietary sources of iodine (iodized salt, shellfish).
- Advise patient to report sore throat, fever, chills, headache, malaise, weakness, yellowing of eyes or skin, unusual bleeding or bruising, rash, or symptoms of hyperthyroidism or hypothyroidism promptly.
- Instruct patient to consult health care professional before taking any OTC medications.
- Advise patient to carry identification describing medication regimen at all times.
- Advise patient to notify health care professional of medication regimen prior to treatment or surgery.
- Emphasize the importance of routine exams to monitor progress and to check for side effects.

Evaluation/Desired Outcomes
- Decrease in severity of symptoms of hyperthyroidism (lowered pulse rate and weight gain).
- Return of thyroid function studies to normal.
- May be used as short-term adjunctive therapy to prepare patient for thyroidectomy or radiation therapy or may be used in treatment of hyperthyroidism. Treatment from 6 mo to several yr may be necessary, usually averaging 1 yr.

---

methocarbamol
(meth-oh-**kar**-ba-mole)
Robaxin

Classification
Therapeutic: skeletal muscle relaxants (centrally acting)

Pregnancy Category C

Indications
Adjunctive treatment of muscle spasm associated with acute painful musculoskeletal conditions (with rest and physical therapy).

Action
Skeletal muscle relaxation, probably as a result of CNS depression. **Therapeutic Effects:** Skeletal muscle relaxation.

Pharmacokinetics
Absorption: Rapidly absorbed from the GI tract.
Distribution: Widely distributed. Crosses the placenta; enters breast milk in small amounts.
Metabolism and Excretion: Metabolized by the liver.
Half-life: 1–2 hr.

TIME/ACTION PROFILE (skeletal muscle relaxation)

ROUTE	ONSET	PEAK	DURATION
PO	30 min	2 hr	unknown
IM	rapid	unknown	unknown
IV	immediate	end of infusion	unknown

Contraindications/Precautions
Contraindicated in: Hypersensitivity; Hypersensitivity to polyethylene glycol (parenteral form); Renal impairment (parenteral form).
Use Cautiously in: Seizure disorders (parenteral form); OB, Lactation, Pedi: Safety not established; Geri: Appears on Beers list. Poorly tolerated due to anticholinergic effects.

Adverse Reactions/Side Effects
CNS: SEIZURES (IV, IM only), dizziness, drowsiness, light-headedness. **EENT:** blurred vision, nasal congestion. **CV:** *IV*—bradycardia, hypotension. **GI:** anorexia, GI upset, nausea. **GU:** brown, black, or green urine. **Derm:** flushing (IV only), pruritus, rashes, urticaria. **Local:** pain at IM site, phlebitis at IV site. **Misc:** allergic reactions including ANAPHYLAXIS (IM, IV use only), fever.

Interactions
Drug-Drug: Additive CNS depression with other **CNS depressants**, including **alcohol**, **antihistamines**, **opioid analgesics**, and **sedative/hypnotics**.
Drug-Natural Products: Concomitant use of **kava-kava**, **valerian**, **chamomile**, or **hops** can ↑ CNS depression.

Route/Dosage
PO (Adults): 1.5 g 4 times daily initially (up to 8 g/day) for 2–3 days, then 4–4.5 g/day in 3–6 di-

vided doses; may be followed by maintenance dosing of 750 mg q 4 hr or 1 g 4 times daily or 1.5 g 3 times daily.
IM, IV (Adults): 1–3 g/day for not more than 3 days; course may be repeated after a 48-hr rest.

Availability (generic available)
Tablets: 500 mg, 750 mg. **Injection:** 100 mg/mL.

NURSING IMPLICATIONS
Assessment
- Assess patient for pain, muscle stiffness, and range of motion before and periodically throughout therapy.
- Monitor pulse and blood pressure every 15 min during parenteral administration.
- Geri: Assess geriatric patients for anticholinergic effects (sedation and weakness).
- Assess patient for allergic reactions (skin rash, asthma, hives, wheezing, hypotension) after parenteral administration. Keep epinephrine and oxygen on hand in the event of a reaction.
- Monitor IV site. Injection is hypertonic and may cause thrombophlebitis. Avoid extravasation.
- *Lab Test Considerations:* Monitor renal function periodically during prolonged parenteral therapy (>3 days), because polyethylene glycol 300 vehicle is nephrotoxic.
- May cause falsely increased urinary 5-hydroxyindoleacetic acid (5-HIAA) and vanillylmandelic acid (VMA) determinations.

Potential Nursing Diagnoses
Acute pain (Indications)
Impaired physical mobility (Indications)
Risk for injury (Side Effects)

Implementation
- Provide safety measures as indicated. Supervise ambulation and transfer of patients.
- **PO:** May be administered with food to minimize GI irritation. Tablets may be crushed and mixed with food or liquids to facilitate swallowing. For administration via NG tube, crush tablet and suspend in water or saline.
- **IM:** Do not administer subcut. IM injections should contain no more than 5 mL (500 mg) at a time in the gluteal region.

IV Administration
- **Direct IV:** *Diluent:* Administer undiluted. *Concentration:* 100 mg/mL. *Rate:* Administer at a maximum rate of 180 mg/m2/min but not > 3 mL (300 mg)/min.
- **Intermittent Infusion:** *Diluent:* Dilute each dose in no more than 250 mL of 0.9% NaCl or D5W for injection. *Concentration:* 4 mg/mL for slower infusions. Do not refrigerate after dilution.
- Have patient remain recumbent during and for at least 10–15 min after infusion to avoid orthostatic hypotension.

Patient/Family Teaching
- Advise patient to take medication as directed. Take missed doses within 1 hr; if not, return to regular dosing schedule. Do not double doses.
- Encourage patient to comply with additional therapies prescribed for muscle spasm (rest, physical therapy, heat).
- May cause dizziness, drowsiness, and blurred vision. Advise patient to avoid driving and other activities requiring alertness until response to drug is known.
- Instruct patient to change positions slowly to minimize orthostatic hypotension.
- Advise patient to avoid concurrent use of alcohol and other CNS depressants.
- Inform patient that urine may turn black, brown, or green, especially if left standing.
- Instruct patient to notify health care professional if skin rash, itching, fever, or nasal congestion occurs.
- Emphasize the importance of routine follow-up exams to monitor progress.

Evaluation/Desired Outcomes
- Decreased musculoskeletal pain and muscle spasticity.
- Increased range of motion.

HIGH ALERT

methotrexate (meth-o-**trex**-ate)
Rheumatrex, Trexall

Classification
Therapeutic: antineoplastics, antirheumatics (DMARDs), immunosuppressants
Pharmacologic: antimetabolites

Pregnancy Category X

Indications
Alone or with other treatment modalities in the treatment of: Trophoblastic neoplasms (choriocarcinoma, chorioadenoma destruens, hydatidiform mole), Leukemias, Breast carcinoma, Head carcinoma, Neck carcinoma, Lung carcinoma. Treatment of severe psoriasis and rheumatoid arthritis unresponsive to conventional therapy. Treatment of mycosis fungoides (cutaneous T-cell lymphoma).

Action
Interferes with folic acid metabolism. Result is inhibition of DNA synthesis and cell reproduction (cell-cycle S-phase–specific). Also has immunosuppressive activity. **Therapeutic Effects:** Death of rapidly replicating cells, particularly malignant ones, and immunosuppression.

Pharmacokinetics
Absorption: Small doses are well absorbed from the GI tract. Larger doses incompletely absorbed.
Distribution: Actively transported across cell membranes, widely distributed. Does not reach therapeutic concentrations in the CSF. Crosses placenta; enters breast milk in low concentrations. Absorption in children is variable (23–95%) and dose-dependent.
Metabolism and Excretion: Excreted mostly unchanged by the kidneys.
Half-life: *Low dose*—3–10 hr; *high dose*—8–15 hr (↑ in renal impairment).

TIME/ACTION PROFILE (effects on blood counts)

ROUTE	ONSET	PEAK	DURATION
PO, IM, IV	4–7 days	7–14 days	21 days

Contraindications/Precautions
Contraindicated in: Hypersensitivity; OB, Lactation: Pregnancy or lactation; Pedi: Products containing benzyl alcohol should not be used in neonates.
Use Cautiously in: Renal impairment (CCr must be ≥60 mL/min prior to therapy); Patients with childbearing potential; Active infections; ↓ bone marrow reserve; Geri: May be more sensitive to toxicity and adverse events.

Adverse Reactions/Side Effects
CNS: arachnoiditis (IT use only), dizziness, drowsiness, headache, malaise. **EENT:** blurred vision, dysarthria transient blindness. **Resp:** PULMONARY FIBROSIS, intestinal pneumonitis. **GI:** anorexia, hepatotoxicity, nausea, stomatitis, vomiting. **GU:** infertility. **Derm:** alopecia, painful plaque erosions (during psoriasis treatment), photosensitivity, pruritus, rashes, skin ulceration, urticaria. **Hemat:** APLASTIC ANEMIA, anemia, leukopenia, thrombocytopenia. **Metab:** hyperuricemia. **MS:** osteonecrosis, stress fracture. **Misc:** nephropathy, chills, fever, soft tissue necrosis.

Interactions
Drug-Drug: The following drugs may ↑ hematologic toxicity of methotrexate: high-dose **salicylates**, **NSAIDs**, **oral hypoglycemic agents (sulfonylureas)**, **phenytoin**, **tetracyclines**, **probenecid**, **trimethoprim/sulfamethoxazole**, **pyrimethamine**, and **chloramphenicol**. ↑ hepatotoxicity with other **hepatotoxic drugs** including **azathioprine**, **sulfasalazine**, and **retinoids**. ↑ nephrotoxicity with other **nephrotoxic drugs**. ↑ bone marrow depression with other **antineoplastics** or **radiation therapy**. **Radiation therapy** ↑ risk of soft tissue necrosis and osteonecrosis. May ↓ antibody response to **live-virus vaccines** and ↑ risk of adverse reactions. ↑ risk of neurologic reactions with **acyclovir** (IT methotrexate only). **Asparaginase** may ↓ effects of methotrexate.
Drug-Natural Products: Concomitant use with **echinacea** and **melatonin** may interfere with immunosuppression. **Caffeine** may ↓ efficacy of methotrexate, similar effect may occur with **guarana**.

Route/Dosage
Trophoblastic Neoplasms
PO, IM (Adults): 15–30 mg/day for 5 days; repeat after 1 or more weeks for 3–5 courses.

Breast Cancer
IV (Adults): 40 mg/m² on days 1 and 8 (with other agents; many regimens are used).

Leukemia
PO (Adults): *Induction*—3.3 mg/m²/day, usually with prednisone.
PO, IM (Adults): *Maintenance*—20–30 mg/m² twice weekly.
IV (Adults): 2.5 mg/kg q 2 wk.
IT (Adults): 12 mg/m² or 15 mg.
IT (Children ≥3 yr): 12 mg.
IT (Children 2 yr): 10 mg.
IT (Children 1 yr): 8 mg.
IT (Children <1 yr): 6 mg.

Osteosarcoma
IV (Adults): 12 g/m² as a 4-hr infusion followed by leucovorin rescue, usually as part of a combination chemotherapeutic regimen (or increase dose until peak serum methotrexate level is 1×10^{-3} M/L but not to exceed 15 g/m²; 12 courses are given starting 4 wk after surgery and repeated at scheduled intervals.

Psoriasis
Therapy may be preceded by a 5- –10-mg test dose.

PO (Adults): 2.5–5 mg q 12 hr for 3 doses *or* q 8 hr for 4 doses once weekly (not to exceed 30 mg/wk).
PO, IM, IV (Adults): 10–25 mg/weekly (not to exceed 30 mg/wk).

Arthritis
Therapy may be preceded by a 5–10-mg test dose in adults.
PO (Adults): 7.5 mg weekly (2.5 mg q 12 hr for 3 doses or single dose, not to exceed 20 mg/wk); when response is obtained, dose should be ↓.
PO (Children): 10 mg/m^2 once weekly initially, may be ↑ up to 20–30 mg/m^2, however response may be better if doses >20 mg/m^2 are given IM or subcut.

Mycosis Fungoides
PO, IM, Subcut (Adults): 5–50 mg once weekly, if response is poor, dose may be changed to 15–37.5 mg twice weekly.
IM (Adults): 50 mg once weekly or 25 mg twice weekly.

Availability (generic available)
Tablets: 2.5 mg, 5 mg, 7.5 mg, 10 mg, 15 mg.
Injection: 25 mg/mL. **Powder for injection:** 1 g/vial. **Preservative-free injection:** 25 mg/mL.

NURSING IMPLICATIONS

Assessment
- Monitor vital signs periodically during administration. Report significant changes.
- Monitor for abdominal pain, diarrhea, or stomatitis; therapy may need to be discontinued.
- Monitor for bone marrow depression. Assess for bleeding (bleeding gums, bruising, petechiae, guaiac stools, urine, and emesis) and avoid IM injections and taking rectal temperatures if platelet count is low. Apply pressure to venipuncture sites for 10 min. Assess for signs of infection during neutropenia. Anemia may occur. Monitor for increased fatigue, dyspnea, and orthostatic hypotension.
- Monitor intake and output ratios and daily weights. Report significant changes in totals.
- Monitor for symptoms of pulmonary toxicity, which may manifest early as a dry, nonproductive cough.
- Monitor for symptoms of gout (increased uric acid, joint pain, edema). Encourage patient to drink at least 2 L of fluid each day. Allopurinol and alkalinization of urine may be used to decrease uric acid levels.
- Assess nutritional status. Administering an antiemetic prior to and periodically during therapy and adjusting diet as tolerated may help maintain fluid and electrolyte balance and nutritional status.
- **IT:** Assess for development of nuchal rigidity, headache, fever, confusion, drowsiness, dizziness, weakness, or seizures.
- **Rheumatoid Arthritis:** Assess patient for pain and range of motion prior to and periodically during therapy.
- **Psoriasis:** Assess skin lesions prior to and periodically during therapy.
- *Lab Test Considerations:* Monitor CBC and differential prior to and frequently during therapy. The nadir of leukopenia and thrombocytopenia occurs in 7–14 days. Leukocyte and thrombocyte counts usually recover 7 days after the nadirs. Notify health care professional of any sudden drop in values.
- Monitor renal (BUN and creatinine) and hepatic function (AST, ALT, bilirubin, and LDH) prior to and routinely during therapy. Urine pH should be monitored prior to high-dose methotrexate therapy and every 6 hr during leucovorin rescue. Urine pH should be kept above 7.0 to prevent renal damage.
- May cause ↑ serum uric acid concentrations, especially during initial treatment of leukemia and lymphoma.
- *Toxicity and Overdose:* Monitor serum methotrexate levels every 12–24 hr during high-dose therapy until levels are <5 × 10 M. This monitoring is essential to plan correct leucovorin dose and determine duration of rescue therapy.
- With high-dose therapy, patient must receive leucovorin rescue within 24–48 hr to prevent fatal toxicity. In cases of massive overdose, hydration and urinary alkalization may be required to prevent renal tubule damage. Monitor fluid and electrolyte status. Intermittent hemodialysis using a high-flux dialyzer may be used for clearance until levels are <0.05 micromolar.

Potential Nursing Diagnoses
Risk for infection (Adverse Reactions)
Imbalanced nutrition: less than body requirements (Adverse Reactions)

Implementation
- *High Alert:* Fatalities have occurred with chemotherapeutic agents. Before administering, clarify all ambiguous orders; double check single, daily, and course-of-therapy dose limits; have second practitioner independently double check original order, calculations and infusion pump settings. Methotrexate for non-oncologic use is given at a much lower dose and fre-

quency—often just once a week. Do not confuse non-oncologic dosing regimens with dosing regimens for cancer patients.
- Solutions for injection should be prepared in a biologic cabinet. Wear gloves, gown, and mask while handling medication. Discard equipment in specially designated containers (see Appendix L).

IV Administration

- **Direct IV:** *Diluent:* Reconstitute each vial with 25 mL of 0.9% NaCl. Use sterile preservative-free diluents for high-dose regimens to prevent complications from large amounts of benzyl alcohol. Do not use preparations that are discolored or that contain a precipitate. Reconstitute immediately before use. Discard unused portion. *Concentration:* < 25 mg/mL for direct IV and intermittent/continuous infusions. *Rate:* Administer at a rate of 10 mg/min into Y-site of a free-flowing IV.
- **Intermittent/Continuous Infusion:** *Diluent:* Doses >100–300 mg/m2 may also be diluted in D5W, D5/0.9% NaCl, or 0.9% NaCl and infused as intermittent or continuous infusion. *Rate:* Administration rates of 4–20 mg/hr have been used.
- **Syringe Compatibility:** bleomycin, cisplatin, cyclophosphamide, doxapram, doxorubicin, fluorouracil, furosemide, heparin, leucovorin, mitomycin, vinblastine, vincristine.
- **Syringe Incompatibility:** droperidol.
- **Y-Site Compatibility:** allopurinol, amifostine, amphotericin B cholesteryl sulfate, asparaginase, aztreonam, bleomycin, cefepime, ceftriaxone, cimetidine, cisplatin, cyclophosphamide, cytarabine, daunorubicin, diphenhydramine, doxorubicin, doxorubicin liposome, etoposide, etoposide phosphate, famotidine, filgrastim, fludarabine, fluorouracil, furosemide, ganciclovir, granisetron, heparin, hydromorphone, imipenem/cilastatin, lansoprazole, leucovorin, linezolid, lorazepam, melphalan, mesna, methylprednisolone sodium succinate, metoclopramide, mitomycin, morphine, ondansetron, oxaliplatin, paclitaxel, piperacillin/tazobactam, prochlorperazine, ranitidine, sargramostim, teniposide, thiotepa, vinblastine, vincristine, vinorelbine.
- **Y-Site Incompatibility:** chlorpromazine, gemcitabine, idarubicin, ifosfamide, midazolam, nalbuphine, promethazine, propofol.
- **Additive Compatibility:** cyclophosphamide, cytarabine, fluorouracil, mercaptopurine, ondansetron, sodium bicarbonate, vincristine.
- **Additive Incompatibility:** bleomycin.
- **IT:** Reconstitute preservative-free methotrexate with preservative-free 0.9% NaCl, Elliot's B solution, or patient's CSF to a concentration not greater than 2 mg/mL. May be administered via lumbar puncture or Ommaya reservoir. To prevent bacterial contamination, use immediately.

Patient/Family Teaching

- Instruct patient to take medication as directed. If a dose is missed, it should be omitted. Consult health care professional if vomiting occurs shortly after a dose is taken.
- Instruct patient to notify health care professional promptly if fever; chills; cough; hoarseness; sore throat; signs of infection; lower back or side pain; painful or difficult urination; bleeding gums; bruising; petechiae; blood in stools, urine, or emesis; increased fatigue; dyspnea; or orthostatic hypotension occurs. Caution patient to avoid crowds and persons with known infections. Instruct patient to use soft toothbrush and electric razor and to avoid falls. Caution patient not to drink alcoholic beverages or take medication containing aspirin or other NSAIDs; may precipitate gastric bleeding.
- Instruct patient to inspect oral mucosa for erythema and ulceration. If ulceration occurs, advise patient to use sponge brush and to rinse mouth with water after eating and drinking. Topical therapy may be used if mouth pain interferes with eating. Stomatitis pain may require treatment with opioid analgesics.
- Instruct patient to avoid the use of Rx, OTC, or herbal products without first consulting health care professional.
- Advise patient that this medication may have teratogenic effects. Contraception should be used during therapy and for at least 3 mo for men and 1 ovulatory cycle for women after completion of therapy.
- Discuss the possibility of hair loss with patient. Explore methods of coping.
- Instruct patient not to receive any vaccinations without advice of health care professional.
- Caution patient to use sunscreen and protective clothing to prevent photosensitivity reactions.
- Emphasize the need for periodic lab tests to monitor for side effects.

Evaluation/Desired Outcomes
- Improvement of hematopoietic values in leukemia.
- Decrease in symptoms of meningeal involvement in leukemia.
- Decrease in size and spread of non-Hodgkin's lymphomas and other solid cancers.
- Resolution of skin lesions in severe psoriasis.
- Decreased joint pain and swelling.
- Improved mobility in patients with rheumatoid arthritis.
- Regression of lesions in mycosis fungoides.

---

methyldopa (meth-ill-doe-pa)
♣Apo-Methyldopa, ♣Dopamet, ♣Novamedopa, ♣Nu-Medopa

Classification
Therapeutic: antihypertensives
Pharmacologic: centrally acting antiadrenergics

Pregnancy Category B

Indications
Management of moderate to severe hypertension (with other agents).

Action
Stimulates CNS alpha-adrenergic receptors, producing a decrease in sympathetic outflow to heart, kidneys, and blood vessels. Result is decreased blood pressure and peripheral resistance, a slight decrease in heart rate, and no change in cardiac output. **Therapeutic Effects:** Lowering of blood pressure.

Pharmacokinetics
Absorption: 50% absorbed from the GI tract. Parenteral form, methyldopate hydrochloride, is slowly converted to methyldopa.
Distribution: Crosses the blood-brain barrier. Crosses the placenta; small amounts enter breast milk.
Metabolism and Excretion: Partially metabolized by the liver, partially excreted unchanged by the kidneys.
Half-life: 1.7 hr.

TIME/ACTION PROFILE (antihypertensive effect)

ROUTE	ONSET	PEAK	DURATION
PO	4–6 hr	12–24 hr	24–48 hr
IV	4–6 hr	unknown	10–16 hr

Contraindications/Precautions
Contraindicated in: Hypersensitivity; Active liver disease.
Use Cautiously in: Previous history of liver disease; OB: Has been used safely (may be used for treatment of hypertension in pregnancy); Lactation: Usually compatible with breastfeeding; Geri: ↑ risk of adverse reactions; consider age-related impairment of hepatic, renal and cardiovascular function as well as other chronic illnesses. Appears on Beers list. May cause bradycardia and exacerbate depression.

Adverse Reactions/Side Effects
CNS: sedation, ↓ mental acuity, depression. **EENT:** nasal stuffiness. **CV:** MYOCARDITIS, bradycardia, edema, orthostatic hypotension. **GI:** DRUG-INDUCED HEPATITIS, diarrhea, dry mouth. **GU:** erectile dysfunction. **Hemat:** eosinophilia, hemolytic anemia. **Misc:** fever.

Interactions
Drug-Drug: Additive hypotension with other **antihypertensives**, acute ingestion of **alcohol**, **anesthesia**, and **nitrates**. **Amphetamines**, **barbiturates**, **tricyclic antidepressants**, **NSAIDs**, and **phenothiazines** may ↓ antihypertensive effect of methyldopa. ↑ effects and risk of psychoses with **haloperidol**. Excess sympathetic stimulation may occur with concurrent use of **MAO inhibitors** or other **adrenergics**. May ↑ **lithium** toxicity. Additive hypotension and CNS toxicity with **levodopa**. Additive CNS depression may occur with **alcohol**, **antihistamines**, **sedative/hypnotics**, some **antidepressants**, and **opioid analgesics**. Concurrent use with **nonselective beta blockers** may rarely cause paradoxical hypertension.

Route/Dosage
PO (Adults): 250–500 mg 2–3 times daily (not to exceed 500 mg/day if used with other agents); may be ↑ every 2 days as needed; usual maintenance dose is 500 mg–2 g/day (not to exceed 3 g/day).
PO (Children): 10 mg/kg/day (300 mg/m^2/day); may be ↑ every 2 days up to 65 mg/kg/day in divided doses (not to exceed 3 g/day).
IV (Adults): 250–500 mg q 6 hr (up to 1 g q 6 hr).
IV (Children): 5–10 mg/kg q 6 hr; up to 65 mg/kg/day in divided doses (not to exceed 3 g/day).

Availability (generic available)
Tablets: 250 mg, 500 mg. **Injection:** 50 mg/mL. *In combination with:* hydrochlorothiazide. See Appendix B.

methyldopa **841**

NURSING IMPLICATIONS
Assessment
- Monitor blood pressure and pulse frequently during initial dose adjustment and periodically during therapy. Report significant changes.
- Monitor frequency of prescription refills to determine compliance.
- Monitor intake and output ratios and weight and assess for edema daily, especially at beginning of therapy. Report weight gain or edema; sodium and water retention may be treated with diuretics.
- Assess patient for depression or other alterations in mental status. Notify health care professional promptly if these symptoms develop.
- Monitor temperature during therapy. Drug fever may occur shortly after initiation of therapy and may be accompanied by eosinophilia and hepatic function changes. Monitor hepatic function test if unexplained fever occurs.
- **Lab Test Considerations:** Monitor renal and hepatic function and CBC before and periodically during therapy.
- Monitor direct Coombs' test before and after 6 and 12 mo of therapy. May cause a positive direct Coombs' test, rarely associated with hemolytic anemia.
- May cause ↑ BUN, serum creatinine, potassium, sodium, prolactin, uric acid, AST, ALT, alkaline phosphatase, and bilirubin concentrations.
- May cause prolonged prothrombin times.
- May interfere with serum creatinine and AST measurements.

Potential Nursing Diagnoses
Risk for injury (Side Effects)
Noncompliance (Patient/Family Teaching)

Implementation
- Do not confuse methyldopa with levodopa or L-dopa.
- Fluid retention and expanded volume may cause tolerance to develop within 2–3 mo after initiation of therapy. Diuretics may be added to regimen at this time to maintain control.
- Dose increases should be made with the evening dose to minimize drowsiness.
- When changing from IV to oral forms, dose should remain consistent.
- **PO:** Shake suspension before administration.

IV Administration
- **Intermittent Infusion:** *Diluent:* Dilute in 100 mL of D5W, 0.9% NaCl, D5/0.9% NaCl, 5% sodium bicarbonate, or Ringer's solution. *Concentration:* ≤10 mg/mL. *Rate:* Infuse slowly over 30–60 min.
- **Y-Site Compatibility:** alfentanil, amikacin, aminophylline, anidulafungin, ascorbic acid, atracurium, atropine, aztreonam, benztropine, bivalirudin, bleomycin, bumetanide, buprenorphine, butorphanol, calcium chloride, calcium gluconate, caspofungin, cefazolin, cefonocid, cefotaxime, cefotetan, cefoxitin, ceftazidime, ceftizoxime, ceftriaxone, cefuroxine, chlorpromazine, cimetidine, clindamycin, cyanocobalamin, cyclosporine, dactinomycin, daptomycin, dexamethasone, digoxin, diltiazem, diphenhydramine, dobutamine, docetaxel, dopamine, doxycycline, enalaprilat, ephedrine, epinephrine, epoetin alfa, ertapenem, erythromycin, esmolol, etoposide, etoposide phosphate, famotidine, fenoldopam, fentanyl, fluconazole, fludarabine, gemcitabine, gentamicin, glycopyrrolate, granisetron, heparin, hetastarch, hydrocortisone, hydromorphone, idarubicin, insulin, isoproterenol, labetalol, lidocaine, linezolid, lorazepam, magnesium sulfate, mannitol, mechlorethamine, meperidine, metaraminol, methoxamine, methylprednisolone, metoclopramide, metoprolol, metronidazole, midazolam, milrinone, mitoxantrone, morphine, multivitamins, nafcillin, nalbuphine, naloxone, nitroglycerin, nitroprusside, norepinephrine, octreotide, ondansetron, oxacillin, oxaliplatin, oxytocin, paclitaxel, palonosetron, pancruonium, pantoprazole, papaverine, pemetrexed, penicillin G, pentazocine, phentolamine, phenylephrine, phytonadione, potassium chloride, procainamide, prochlorperazine, promethazine, propranolol, protamine, pyridoxime, ranitidine, sodium bicarbonate, streptokinase, succinylcholine, sufentanil, tacrolimus, teniposide, theophylline, thiamine, thiotepa, ticarcillin/clavulanate, tigecycline, tirofiban, tobramycin, tolazoline, trimetaphan, urokinase, vancomycin, vasopressin, vecuronium, verapamil, vinorelbine, voriconazole.
- **Y-Site Incompatibility:** acyclovir, amphotericin B colloidal, azathioprine, cefoperazone, chloramphenicol, dantrolene, diazepam, diazoxide, folic acid, furosemide, ganciclovir, imipenem/cilastatin, inamrinone, indomethacin,

✹ = Canadian drug name.   = Genetic implication.
*CAPITALS indicates life-threatening; underlines indicate most frequent.

pentamidine, pentobarbital, phenobarbital, phenytoin, trimethoprim/sulfamethoxazole, piperacillin/tazobactam.

Patient/Family Teaching
- Emphasize the importance of continuing to take this medication, even if feeling well. Instruct patient to take medication at the same time each day; last dose of the day should be taken at bedtime. Take missed doses as soon as remembered but not if almost time for next dose. Do not double doses.
- Encourage patient to comply with additional interventions for hypertension (weight reduction, low-sodium diet, smoking cessation, moderation of alcohol consumption, regular exercise, and stress management). Methyldopa controls but does not cure hypertension.
- Instruct patient and family on proper technique for monitoring blood pressure. Advise them to check blood pressure at least weekly and to report significant changes.
- Inform patient that urine may darken or turn red-black when left standing.
- May cause drowsiness. Advise patient to avoid driving or other activities requiring alertness until response to medication is known. Drowsiness usually subsides after 7–10 days of continuous use.
- Caution patient to avoid sudden changes in position to decrease orthostatic hypotension.
- Advise patient that frequent mouth rinses, good oral hygiene, and sugarless gum or candy may minimize dry mouth. Notify health care professional if dry mouth continues for >2 wk.
- Caution patient to avoid concurrent use of alcohol or other CNS depressants.
- Advise patient to consult health care professional before taking any Rx, OTC, or Herbal products, especially cough, cold, or allergy remedies.
- Advise patient to notify health care professional of medication regimen before treatment or surgery.
- Instruct patient to notify health care professional if fever, muscle aches, or flu-like syndrome occurs.

Evaluation/Desired Outcomes
- Decrease in blood pressure without appearance of side effects.

---

methylergonovine
(meth-ill-er-goe-**noe**-veen)
Methergine

Classification
Therapeutic: oxytocic
Pharmacologic: ergot alkaloids

Pregnancy Category C

Indications
Prevention and treatment of postpartum or postabortion hemorrhage caused by uterine atony or subinvolution.

Action
Directly stimulates uterine and vascular smooth muscle. **Therapeutic Effects:** Uterine contraction.

Pharmacokinetics
Absorption: Well absorbed following oral or IM administration.
Distribution: Unknown. Enters breast milk in small quantities.
Metabolism and Excretion: Probably metabolized by the liver.
Half-life: 30–120 min.

TIME/ACTION PROFILE (effects on uterine contractions)

ROUTE	ONSET	PEAK	DURATION
PO	5–15 min	unknown	3 hr
IM	2–5 min	unknown	3 hr
IV	immediate	unknown	45 min–3 hr

Contraindications/Precautions
Contraindicated in: Hypersensitivity; OB: Should not be used to induce labor.
Use Cautiously in: Hypertensive or eclamptic patients (more susceptible to hypertensive and arrhythmogenic side effects); Severe hepatic or renal disease; Sepsis.
Exercise Extreme Caution in: OB: Third stage of labor.

Adverse Reactions/Side Effects
CNS: dizziness, headache. **EENT:** tinnitus. **Resp:** dyspnea. **CV:** HYPERTENSION, arrhythmias, chest pain, palpitations. **GI:** nausea, vomiting. **GU:** cramps. **Derm:** diaphoresis. **Misc:** allergic reactions.

Interactions
Drug-Drug: Excessive vasoconstriction may result when used with heavy cigarette smoking (**nicotine**) or other **vasopressors**, such as **dopamine**.

Route/Dosage
PO (Adults): 200–400 mcg (0.4–0.6 mg) q 6–12 hr for 2–7 days.
IM, IV (Adults): 200 mcg (0.2 mg) q 2–4 hr for up to 5 doses.

Availability (generic available)
Tablets: 200 mcg (0.2 mg). **Injection:** 200 mcg (0.2 mg)/mL.

NURSING IMPLICATIONS
Assessment
- Monitor blood pressure, heart rate, and uterine response frequently during medication administration. Notify health care professional promptly if uterine relaxation becomes prolonged or if character of vaginal bleeding changes.
- Assess for signs of ergotism (cold, numb fingers and toes, chest pain, nausea, vomiting, headache, muscle pain, weakness).
- *Lab Test Considerations:* If no response to methylergonovine, calcium levels may need to be assessed. Effectiveness of medication is ↓ with hypocalcemia.
- May cause ↓ serum prolactin levels.

Potential Nursing Diagnoses
Acute pain (Side Effects)

Implementation
IV Administration
- **IV:** IV administration is used for emergencies only. Oral and IM routes are preferred.
- **Direct IV:** *Diluent:* May be given undiluted or diluted in 5 mL of 0.9% NaCl and administered through Y site. Do not add to IV solutions. Do not mix in syringe with any other drug. Refrigerate; stable for storage at room temperature for 60 days; deteriorates with age. Use only solution that is clear and colorless and that contains no precipitate. *Concentration:* 0.2 mg/mL. *Rate:* Administer at a rate of 0.2 mg over at least 1 min.
- **Y-Site Compatibility:** heparin, hydrocortisone sodium succinate, potassium chloride, vitamin B complex with C.

Patient/Family Teaching
- Instruct patient to take medication as directed; do not skip or double up on missed doses. If a dose is missed, omit it and return to regular dose schedule.
- Advise patient that medication may cause menstrual-like cramps.
- Caution patient to avoid smoking, because nicotine constricts blood vessels.
- Instruct patient to notify health care professional if infection develops, as this may cause increased sensitivity to the medication.

Evaluation/Desired Outcomes
- Contractions that maintain uterine tone and prevent postpartum hemorrhage.

---

methylnaltrexone
(me-thil-nal-**trex**-one)
Relistor

Classification
Therapeutic: laxatives
Pharmacologic: opioid antagonists

Pregnancy Category B

Indications
Treatment of constipation caused by opioid use in patients being treated palliatively, when laxative therapy has failed.

Action
Acts peripherally as mu-opioid receptor antagonist, blocking opioid effects on the GI tract. **Therapeutic Effects:** Blocks constipating effects of opioids on the GI tract without loss of analgesia.

Pharmacokinetics
Absorption: Absorption follows subcutaneous administration.
Distribution: Moderate tissue distribution, does not cross the blood-brain barrier.
Metabolism and Excretion: Some metabolism, 85% excreted unchanged in urine.
Half-life: 8 hr.

TIME/ACTION PROFILE

ROUTE	ONSET	PEAK	DURATION
Subcut	rapid	0.5 hr	24–48 hr

Contraindications/Precautions
Contraindicated in: Known/suspected mechanical GI obstruction.
Use Cautiously in: OB, Lactation: Use in pregnancy only if clearly needed; use cautiously during lactation; Pedi: Safety and efficacy not established.

Adverse Reactions/Side Effects
CNS: dizziness. **GI:** <u>abdominal pain</u>, diarrhea, <u>flatulence</u>, <u>nausea</u>. **Derm:** hyperhidrosis.

Interactions
Drug-Drug: None noted.

Route/Dosage
Subcut (Adults): *38– <62 kg*—8 mg every other day, not to exceed every 24 hr; *62–114*

844 methylphenidate (oral)

kg—12 mg every other day, not to exceed every 24 hr; *other weights*—0.15 mg/kg every other day, not to exceed every 24 hr.

Renal Impairment
(Adults): *CCr <30 mL/min*—use 50% of recommended dose based on weight.

Availability
Solution for subcutaneous injection: 12mg/0.6 mL single use vial.

NURSING IMPLICATIONS
Assessment
- Assess bowel sounds and frequency, quantity, and consistency of stools periodically during therapy.
- Monitor pain intensity during therapy. Methylnaltrexone does not affect pain or effects of opioid analgesics on pain control.

Potential Nursing Diagnoses
Constipation (Indications)
Diarrhea (Adverse Reactions)

Implementation
- **Subcut:** Pinch skin and administer in upper arm, abdomen, or thigh at a 45° angle using a 1-mL syring with a 27-gauge needle inserted the full length of the needle. Do not rub the injection site. Solution is clear and colorless to pale yellow. Do not administer solutions that are discolored or contain a precipitate. Solution is stable for 24 hr at room temperature. Protect vials from light. Do not freeze. Do not use single-use vials for more than 1 dose.

Patient/Family Teaching
- Instruct patient on administration of methylnaltrexone and disposal of supplies. Usual schedule is one dose every other day, as needed, but no more than one dose in a 24-hr period. Advise patient to read the *Patient Information* prior to starting therapy and with each Rx refill.
- Advise patient that laxation may occur within 30 min, so toilet facilities should be available following administration.
- May cause dizziness. Caution patient to avoid driving and other activities requiring alertness until response to medication is known.
- Advise patient to notify health care professional and discontinue therapy if severe or persistent diarrhea occurs or if abdominal pain, nausea, or vomiting persists or worsens.
- Instruct patient to stop taking methylnaltrexone if they stop taking opioid medications.
- Advise patient to consult health care professional prior to taking other Rx, OTC, or herbal products.
- Advise female patients to notify health care professional if pregnancy is planned or suspected or if breastfeeding.

Evaluation/Desired Outcomes
- Laxation and relief of opioid-induced constipation.

---

methylphenidate (oral)
(meth-ill-**fen**-i-date)
Concerta, Metadate CD, Metadate ER, Methylin, Methylin ER,
✤PMS-Methylphenidate,
✤Riphenidate, Ritalin, Ritalin LA, Ritalin-SR

methylphenidate (transdermal)
Daytrana

Classification
Therapeutic: central nervous system stimulants

Schedule II

Pregnancy Category C

Indications
Treatment of ADHD (adjunct). **Oral:** Symptomatic treatment of narcolepsy. **Unlabeled Use:** Management of some forms of refractory depression.

Action
Produces CNS and respiratory stimulation with weak sympathomimetic activity. **Therapeutic Effects:** Increased attention span in ADHD. Increased motor activity, mental alertness, and diminished fatigue in narcoleptic patients.

Pharmacokinetics
Absorption: Slow and incomplete after oral administration; absorption of sustained or extended-release tablet (SR) is delayed and provides continuous release; well absorbed from skin.
Metadate CD, Concerta, Ritalin LA—provides initial rapid release followed by a second continuous release (biphasic release).
Distribution: Unknown.
Metabolism and Excretion: Mostly metabolized (80%) by the liver.
Half-life: 2–4 hr.

TIME/ACTION PROFILE (CNS stimulation)

ROUTE	ONSET	PEAK	DURATION
PO	unknown	1–3 hr	4–6 hr
PO-ER	unknown	4–7 hr	3–12 hr†
Transdermal	unknown	unknown	12 hr

†Depends on formulation

methylphenidate

Contraindications/Precautions
Contraindicated in: Hypersensitivity; Hyperexcitable states; Hyperthyroidism; Patients with psychotic personalities or suicidal or homicidal tendencies; Personal or family history of Tourette's syndrome; Glaucoma; Motor tics; Concurrent use or use within 14 days of MAO inhibitors; Fructose intolerance, glucose-galactose malabsorption, or sucrose-isomaltase insufficiency; Surgery.
Use Cautiously in: History of cardiovascular disease (sudden death has occurred in children with structural cardiac abnormalities or other serious heart problems); Hypertension; Diabetes mellitus; History of contact sensitization with transdermal product (may be at ↑ risk for systemic sensitization reactions with oral products); Geri: Geriatric or debilitated patients; Continual use (may result in psychological or physical dependence); Seizure disorders (may lower seizure threshold); Concerta product should be used cautiously in patients with esophageal motility disorders or severe GI narrowing (may ↑ the risk of obstruction); OB, Lactation: Safety not established; Pedi: Growth suppression may occur in children with long term use; children <6 yr (transdermal only).

Adverse Reactions/Side Effects
CNS: hyperactivity, insomnia, restlessness, tremor, behavioral disturbances, dizziness, hallucinations, headache, irritability, mania, thought disorder. **EENT:** blurred vision. **CV:** SUDDEN DEATH, hypertension, palpitations, tachycardia, hypotension. **GI:** anorexia, constipation, cramps, diarrhea, dry mouth, metallic taste, nausea, vomiting. **Derm:** erythema, rashes. **Metab:** growth suppression, weight loss (may occur with prolonged use). **Neuro:** akathisia, dyskinesia, tics. **Misc:** fever, hypersensitivity reactions, physical dependence, psychological dependence, tolerance.

Interactions
Drug-Drug: ↑ sympathomimetic effects with other **adrenergics**, including **vasoconstrictors**, **decongestants**, and **halogenated anesthetics**. Use with **MAO inhibitors** or **vasopressors** may result in hypertensive crisis (concurrent use or use within 14 days of MAO inhibitors is contraindicated). Metabolism of **warfarin**, **phenytoin**, **phenobarbital**, **primidone**, **phenylbutazone**, **selective serotonin reuptake inhibitors**, and **tricyclic antidepressants** may be ↓ and effects ↑. Avoid concurrent use with **pimozide** (may mask cause of tics). Concurrent use with **clonidine** may result in serious ECG abnormalities (a 40% dose ↓ of oral methylphenidate is necessary).
Drug-Natural Products: Use with caffeine-containing herbs (**guarana**, **tea**, **coffee**) ↑ stimulant effect. **St. John's wort** may ↑ serious side effects (concurrent use is NOT recommended).
Drug-Food: Excessive use of **caffeine**-containing foods or beverages (**coffee**, **cola**, **tea**) may cause ↑ CNS stimulation.

Route/Dosage
PO (Adults): *ADHD*— 5–20 mg 2–3 times daily as prompt-release tablets. When maintenance dose is determined, may change to extended-release formulation. *Narcolepsy*— 10 mg 2–3 times/day; maximum dose 60 mg/day.

PO (Children >6 yr): *Prompt release tablets*— 0.3 mg/kg/dose or 2.5–5 mg before breakfast and lunch; ↑ by 0.1 mg/kg/dose or by 5–10 mg/day at weekly intervals (not to exceed 60 mg/day or 2 mg/kg/day). When maintenance dose is determined, may change to extended-release formulation. *Ritalin SR, Metadate ER*—may be used in place of the prompt-release tablets when the 8-hour dosage corresponds to the titrated 8-hour dosage of the prompt-release tablets; *Ritalin LA*— can be used in place of twice daily regimen given once daily at same total dose, or in place of SR product at same dose; *Concerta (patients who have not taken methylphenidate previously)*— 18 mg once daily in the morning initially, may be titrated as needed up to 54 mg/day. *Concerta (patients are currently taking other forms of methylphenidate)*— 18 mg once daily in the morning if previous dose was 5 mg 2–3 times daily or 20 mg daily as SR product, 36 mg once daily in the morning if previous dose was 10 mg 2–3 times daily or 40 mg daily as SR product, 54 mg once daily in the morning if previous dose was 15 mg 2–3 times daily or 60 mg once daily as SR product. *Metadate CD*— 20 mg once daily. Dosage may be adjusted in weekly 20-mg increments to a maximum of 60 mg/day taken once daily in the morning.

Transdermal (Children >6 yr): Apply one 10-mg patch initially (should be applied 2 hr before desired effect and removed 9 hr after application); may be titrated based on response and tolerability; may ↑ to 15-mg patch after 1 week, and then to 20-mg patch after another week, and then to 30-mg patch after another week.

Availability (generic available)
Immediate-release tablets: 5 mg, 10 mg, 20 mg. **Cost:** *Generic*—5 mg $37.90/100, 10 mg $52.90/100, 20 mg $74.90/100. **Extended-release tablets (Metadate ER, Methylin ER):** 10 mg, 20 mg. **Extended-release tablets (Concerta):** 18 mg, 27 mg, 36 mg, 54 mg. **Cost:** 18 mg $359.96/90, 27 mg $359.98/90, 36 mg $374.96/90, 54 mg $404.96/90. **Sustained-release tablets (Ritalin SR):** 20 mg. **Cost:** $173.96/90. **Extended-release capsules (Metadate CD):** 10 mg, 20 mg, 30 mg. **Cost:** 10 mg $236.97/90, 20 mg $299.99/90, 30 mg $299.95/90 $34.68/30. **Extended-release capsules (Ritalin LA):** 10 mg, 20 mg, 30 mg, 40 mg. **Cost:** 10 mg $299.97/90, 20 mg $299.97/90, 30 mg $299.95/90, 40 mg $299.95/90. **Chewable tablets (Methylin) (grape flavor):** 2.5 mg, 5 mg, 10 mg. **Oral solution (Methylin) (grape flavor):** 5 mg/5 mL, 10 mg/5 mL. **Transdermal system:** releases 10 mg/9 hr, releases 15 mg/9 hr, releases 20 mg/9 hr, releases 30 mg/9 hr.

NURSING IMPLICATIONS
Assessment
- Monitor blood pressure, pulse, and respiration before administering and periodically during therapy. Obtain a history (including assessment of family history of sudden death or ventricular arrhythmia), physical exam to assess for cardiac disease, and further evaluation (ECG and echocardiogram), if indicated. If exertional chest pain, unexplained syncope, or other cardiac symptoms occur, evaluate promptly.
- Monitor closely for behavior change.
- Pedi: Monitor growth, both height and weight, in children on long-term therapy.
- May produce a false sense of euphoria and well-being. Provide frequent rest periods and observe patient for rebound depression after the effects of the medication have worn off.
- Methylphenidate has high dependence and abuse potential. Tolerance to abuse of medication occurs rapidly; do not increase dose.
- **ADHD:** Assess children for attention span, impulse control, and interactions with others. Therapy may be interrupted at intervals to determine whether symptoms are sufficient to continue therapy.
- **Narcolepsy:** Observe and document frequency of episodes.
- **Transdermal:** Assess skin for signs of contact sensitization (erythema with edema, papules, or vesicles that does not improve within 48 hr or spreads beyond patch site) during therapy. May lead to systemic sensitization to other forms of methylphenidate (flare-up of previous dermatitis or prior positive patch-test sites, generalized skin eruptions, headache, fever, malaise, arthralgia, diarrhea, vomiting). If contact sensitization develops and oral methylphenidate is instituted, monitor closely.
- *Lab Test Considerations:* Monitor CBC, differential, and platelet count periodically in patients receiving prolonged therapy.

Potential Nursing Diagnoses
Disturbed thought process (Side Effects)

Implementation
- **PO:** Immediate and sustained-release tablets should be administered on an empty stomach (30–45 min before a meal). Sustained-release tablets should be swallowed whole; do not break, crush, or chew. Medate CD and Ritalin LA capsules may be opened and sprinkled on cool applesauce; entire mixture should be ingested immediately and followed by a drink of water. Do not store for future use. Concerta may be administered without regard to food, but must be taken with water, milk, or juice.
- **Transdermal:** Apply patch to a clean, dry site on the hip which is not oily, damaged, or irritated; do not apply to waistline where tight clothing may rub it. Press firmly in place with palm of hand for 30 seconds to make sure of good contact with skin, especially around edges. Alternate site daily. Apply patch 2 hr before desired effect and remove 9 hr after applied; effects last several more hours. Do not apply or reapply with dressings, tape, or other adhesives. Do not cut patches.
- If difficulty in separating patch from release liner, tearing, or other damage occurs during removal from liner, discard patch and apply a new patch. Inspect release liner to ensure no adhesive containing medication has transferred to liner; if transfer has occurred, discard patch. Avoid touching adhesive during application; wash hands immediately after application.
- If patch does not fully adhere or partially detaches, remove and replace with another patch. Wear patched for a total of 9 hr, regardless of number used. Exposure to water during bathing, swimming, or showering may affect patch adherence.
- Patches may be removed earlier before decreasing dose if an unacceptable loss of appetite or insomnia occurs.
- Store patches at room temperature in a safe place to prevent abuse and misuse; do not refrigerate or freeze.

Patient/Family Teaching

- Instruct patient to take medication as directed. If an oral dose is missed, take the remaining doses for that day at regularly spaced intervals; do not double doses. Take the last dose before 6 PM to minimize the risk of insomnia. Instruct patient not to alter dose without consulting health care professional. Abrupt cessation of high doses may cause extreme fatigue and mental depression. Instruct parent/caregiver to read the Medication Guide prior to use and with each Rx refill; new information may be available.
- Advise patient to check weight 2–3 times weekly and report weight loss to health care professional.
- May cause dizziness or blurred vision. Caution patient to avoid driving or activities requiring alertness until response to medication is known.
- Inform patient and/or parents that shell of *Concerta* tablet may appear in the stool. This is no cause for concern.
- Advise patient to avoid using caffeine-containing beverages concurrently with this therapy.
- Advise patient to notify health care professional if nervousness, insomnia, palpitations, vomiting, skin rash, or fever occurs.
- Advise patient and/or parents to notify health care professional of behavioral changes.
- Inform patient that health care professional may order periodic holidays from the drug to assess progress and to decrease dependence.
- Emphasize the importance of routine follow-up exams to monitor progress.
- **Transdermal:** Encourage parent or caregiver to use the administration chart included in package to monitor application and removal time and disposal method.
- Caution patient to avoid exposing patch to direct external heat sources (hair dryers, heating pads, electric blankets, heated water beds, etc). May increase rate and extent of absorption.
- Inform parent/caregiver that skin redness, itching and small bumps on the skin are common. If swelling or blistering occurs, the patch should not be worn and health care professional notified. Caution parent/caregiver not to apply hydrocortisone or other solutions, creams, ointments, or emollients prior to application.
- **Home Care Issues:** Pedi: Advise parents to notify school nurse of medication regimen.

Evaluation/Desired Outcomes

- Improved attention span and social interactions in ADHD.
- Decreased frequency of narcoleptic symptoms.

---

methylPREDNISolone, See CORTICOSTEROIDS (SYSTEMIC).

---

metoclopramide
(met-oh-**kloe**-pra-mide)
✽ Apo-Metoclop, ✽ Emex, ✽ Maxeran, Metozolv ODT, Reglan

Classification
Therapeutic: antiemetics

Pregnancy Category B

Indications
Prevention of chemotherapy-induced emesis. Treatment of postsurgical and diabetic gastric stasis. Facilitation of small bowel intubation in radiographic procedures. Management of gastroesophageal reflux. Treatment and prevention of postoperative nausea and vomiting when nasogastric suctioning is undesirable. **Unlabeled Use:** Treatment of hiccups. Adjunct management of migraine headaches.

Action
Blocks dopamine receptors in chemoreceptor trigger zone of the CNS. Stimulates motility of the upper GI tract and accelerates gastric emptying. **Therapeutic Effects:** Decreased nausea and vomiting. Decreased symptoms of gastric stasis. Easier passage of nasogastric tube into small bowel.

Pharmacokinetics
Absorption: Well absorbed from the GI tract, from rectal mucosa, and from IM sites.
Distribution: Widely distributed into body tissues and fluids. Crosses blood-brain barrier and placenta. Enters breast milk in concentrations greater than plasma.

✽ = Canadian drug name. ⚙ = Genetic implication.
*CAPITALS indicates life-threatening; underlines indicate most frequent.

metoclopramide

Metabolism and Excretion: Partially metabolized by the liver; 25% eliminated unchanged in the urine.
Half-life: 2.5–6 hr.

TIME/ACTION PROFILE (effects on peristalsis)

ROUTE	ONSET	PEAK	DURATION
PO	30–60 min	unknown	1–2 hr
IM	10–15 min	unknown	1–2 hr
IV	1–3 min	immediate	1–2 hr

Contraindications/Precautions

Contraindicated in: Hypersensitivity; Possible GI obstruction or hemorrhage; History of seizure disorders; Pheochromocytoma; Parkinson's disease.
Use Cautiously in: History of depression; Diabetes (may alter response to insulin); Renal impairment (reduce dose in CCr <50 mL/min); Chronic use > 3 mo (↑ risk for tardive dyskinesia); OB, Lactation: Safety not established; Pedi: Prolonged clearance in neonates can result in high serum concentrations and increase the risk for methemoglobinemia. Side effects are more common in children, especially extrapyramidal reactions; Geri: More susceptible to oversedation, extrapyramidal reactions, and tardive dyskinesia.

Adverse Reactions/Side Effects

CNS: drowsiness, extrapyramidal reactions, restlessness, NEUROLEPTIC MALIGNANT SYNDROME, anxiety, depression, irritability, tardive dyskinesia. **CV:** arrhythmias (supraventricular tachycardia, bradycardia), hypertension, hypotension. **GI:** constipation, diarrhea, dry mouth, nausea. **Endo:** gynecomastia. **Hemat:** methemoglobinemia, neutropenia, leukopenia, agranulocytosis.

Interactions

Drug-Drug: Additive CNS depression with other **CNS depressants**, including **alcohol**, **antidepressants**, **antihistamines**, **opioid analgesics**, and **sedative/hypnotics**. May ↑ absorption and risk of toxicity from **cyclosporine**. May affect the GI absorption of other **orally administered drugs** as a result of effect on GI motility. May exaggerate hypotension during **general anesthesia**. ↑ risk of extrapyramidal reactions with agents such as **haloperidol** or **phenothiazines**. **Opioids** and **anticholinergics** may antagonize the GI effects of metoclopramide. Use cautiously with **MAO inhibitors** (causes release of catecholamines). May ↑ neuromuscular blockade from **succinylcholine**. May ↓ effectiveness of **levodopa**. May ↑ **tacrolimus** serum levels.

Route/Dosage

Prevention of Chemotherapy-Induced Vomiting

PO, IV (Adults and Children): 1–2 mg/kg 30 min before chemotherapy. Additional doses of 1–2 mg/kg may be given q 2–4 hr, pretreatment with diphenhydramine will ↓ the risk of extrapyramidal reactions to this dosage.

Facilitation of Small Bowel Intubation

IV (Adults and Children > 14 yr): 10 mg over 1–2 min.
IV (Children 6–14 yr): 2.5–5 mg (dose should not exceed 0.5 mg/kg) over 1–2 min.
IV (Children <6 yr): 0.1 mg/kg over 1–2 min.

Diabetic Gastroparesis

PO, IV (Adults): 10 mg 30 min before meals and at bedtime for 2–8 weeks.

Gastroesophageal Reflux

PO, IM, IV (Adults): 10–15 mg 30 min before meals and at bedtime (not to exceed 0.5 mg/kg/day). A single dose of 20 mg may be given preventively. Some patients may respond to doses as small as 5 mg.
PO, IM, IV (Neonates, Infants, and Children): 0.4–0.8 mg/kg/day in 4 divided doses.

Postoperative Nausea/Vomiting

IM, IV (Adults and Children > 14 yr): 10 mg at the end of surgical procedure, repeat in 6–8 hr if needed.
IM, IV (Children < 14 yr): 0.1–0.2 mg/kg/dose, repeat in 6–8 hr if needed.

Treatment of Hiccups

PO, IM (Adults): 10–20 mg 4 times daily PO; may be preceded by a single 10-mg dose IM (unlabeled).

Availability (generic available)

Tablets: 5 mg, 10 mg. Cost: *Reglan*—5 mg $50.91/100, 10 mg $80.26/100; *generic*—5 mg $29.77/100, 10 mg $21.12/100. **Orally disintegrating tablets:** 5 mg, 10 mg. **Oral solution (apricot-peach flavor):** 5 mg/5 mL. **Injection:** 5 mg/mL.

NURSING IMPLICATIONS

Assessment

- Assess patient for nausea, vomiting, abdominal distention, and bowel sounds before and after administration.
- Assess patient for extrapyramidal side effects (*parkinsonian*—difficulty speaking or swallowing, loss of balance control, pill rolling,

metoclopramide

mask-like face, shuffling gait, rigidity, tremors; and *dystonic*—muscle spasms, twisting motions, twitching, inability to move eyes, weakness of arms or legs) periodically throughout course of therapy. May occur weeks to months after initiation of therapy and are reversible on discontinuation. Dystonic reactions may occur within minutes of IV infusion and stop within 24 hr of discontinuation of metoclopramide. May be treated with 50 mg of IM diphenhydramine or diphenhydramine 1 mg/kg IV may be administered prophylactically 15 min before metoclopramide IV infusion.
- Monitor for tardive dyskinesia (uncontrolled rhythmic movement of mouth, face, and extremities; lip smacking or puckering; puffing of cheeks; uncontrolled chewing; rapid or worm-like movements of tongue). Usually occurs after a year or more of continued therapy. Report immediately; may be irreversible.
- Monitor for neuroleptic malignant syndrome (hyperthermia, muscle rigidity, altered consciousness, irregular pulse or blood pressure, tachycardia, and diaphoresis).
- Assess patient for signs of depression periodically throughout therapy.
- **Lab Test Considerations:** May alter hepatic function test results.
- May cause ↑ serum prolactin and aldosterone concentrations.

Potential Nursing Diagnoses
Imbalanced nutrition: less than body requirements (Indications)
Risk for injury (Side Effects)

Implementation
- **PO:** Administer doses 30 min before meals and at bedtime.
- Do not to remove *orally disintegrating tablets* from the bottle until just prior to dosing. Remove tablet from bottle with dry hands and immediately place on tongue to disintegrate and swallow with saliva. Tablet typically disintegrates in 1–1 ½ minutes. Administration with liquid is not necessary.
- **IM:** For prevention of postoperative nausea and vomiting, inject IM near the end of surgery.

IV Administration
- **Direct IV:** Administer IV dose 30 min before administration of chemotherapeutic agent. *Rate:* Doses may be given slowly over 1–2 min. Rapid administration causes a transient but intense feeling of anxiety and restlessness followed by drowsiness.
- **Intermittent Infusion:** *Diluent:* May be diluted for IV infusion in 50 mL of D5W, 0.9% NaCl, D5/0.45% NaCl, Ringer's solution, or LR. Diluted solution is stable for 48 hr if protected from light or 24 hr under normal light. *Concentration:* May dilute to 0.2 mg/mL or give undiluted at 5 mg/mL. *Rate:* Infuse slowly (maximum rate 5 mg/min) over at least 15–30 min.
- **Y-Site Compatibility:** acyclovir, aldesleukin, alfentanil, amifostine, amikacin, aminophylline, ascorbic acid, atracurium, atropine, azathioprine, aztreonam, bivalirudin, bleomycin, bumetanide, buprenorphine, butorphanol, calcium chloride, calcium gluconate, carboplatin, caspofungin, cefazolin, cefonicid, cefoperazone, cefotaxime, cefotetan, cefoxitin, ceftazidime, ceftizoxime, ceftriaxone, cefuroxime, chloramphenicol, chlorpromazine, cimetidine, ciprofloxacin, cisatracurium, cisplatin, cladribine, clindamycin, cyanocobalamin, cyclophosphamide, cyclosporine, cytarabine, dactinomycin, daptomycin, dexamethasone, dexmedetomidine, digoxin, diltiazem, diphenhydramine, dobutamine, docetaxel, dopamine, doripenem, doxapram, doxorubicin hydrochloride, doxycycline, droperidol, enalaprilat, ephedrine, epinephrine, epirubicin, epoetin alfa, ertapenem, erythromycin, esmolol, etoposide, etoposide phosphate, famotidine, fenoldopam, fentanyl, filgrastim, fluconazole, fludarabine, folic acid, foscarnet, gallium nitrate, gemcitabine, gentamicin, glycopyrrolate, granisetron, heparin, hetastarch, hydrocortisone sodium succinate, hydromorphone, idarubicin, ifosfamide, imipenem/cilastatin, indomethacin, insulin, isoproterenol, ketorolac, labetalol, leucovorin, levofloxacin, lidocaine, linezolid, lorazepam, magnesium sulfate, mannitol, mechlorethamine, melphalan, meperidine, meropenem, metaraminol, methadone, methotrexate, methoxamine, methyldopate, methylprednisolone, metoprolol, metronidazole, miconazole, midazolam, milrinone, minocycline, mitomycin, morphine, moxalactam, multiple vitamins, nafcillin, nalbuphine, naloxone, nesiritide, nitroglycerin, nitroprusside, norepinephrine, octreotide, ondansetron, oxaliplatin, oxytocin, paclitaxel, palonosetron, pantoprazole, papaverine, pemetrexed, penicillin G, pentamidine, pentazocine, pentobarbital, phe-

---
♣ = Canadian drug name. ⚡ = Genetic implication.
*CAPITALS indicates life-threatening; underlines indicate most frequent.

nobarbital, phentolamine, phenylephrine, phytonadione, piperacillin/tazobactam, potassium chloride, procainamide, prochlorperazine, promethazine, propranolol, protamine, pyridoxine, quinupristin/dalfopristin, ranitidine, remifentanil, rituximab, rocuronium, sargramostim, sodium acetate, sodium bicarbonate, streptokinase, succinylcholine, sufentanil, tacrolimus, teniposide, theophylline, thiamine, thiotepa, ticarcillin/clavulanate, tigecycline, tirofiban, tobramycin, tolazoline, topotecan, trastuzumab, trimethaphan, urokinase, vancomycin, vasopressin, vecuronium, verapamil, vinblastine, vincristine, vinorelbine, voriconazole, zidovudine.

- **Y-Site Incompatibility:** amphotericin B cholesteryl, amphotericin B colloidal, amphotericin B liposome, amsacrine, cefepime, dantrolene, diazepam, diazoxide, doxorubicin liposome, ganciclovir, inamrinone, phenytoin, propofol, trimethoprim/sulfamethoxazole.

Patient/Family Teaching

- Instruct patient to take metoclopramide as directed. Take missed doses as soon as remembered if not almost time for next dose.
- Pedi: Unintentional overdose has been reported in infants and children with the use of metoclopramide oral solution. Teach parents how to accurately read labels and administer medication.
- May cause drowsiness. Caution patient to avoid driving or other activities requiring alertness until response to medication is known.
- Advise patient to avoid concurrent use of alcohol and other CNS depressants while taking this medication.
- Advise patient to notify health care professional immediately if involuntary or repetitive movements of eyes, face, or limbs occur.

Evaluation/Desired Outcomes

- Prevention or relief of nausea and vomiting.
- Decreased symptoms of gastric stasis.
- Facilitation of small bowel intubation.
- Decreased symptoms of esophageal reflux.

---

metolazone (me-tole-a-zone)
Zaroxolyn

Classification
Therapeutic: antihypertensives, diuretics
Pharmacologic: thiazide-like diuretics

Pregnancy Category B

Indications
Mild to moderate hypertension. Edema associated with CHF or the nephrotic syndrome.

Action
Increases excretion of sodium and water by inhibiting sodium reabsorption in the distal tubule. Promotes excretion of chloride, potassium, magnesium, and bicarbonate. May produce arteriolar dilation. **Therapeutic Effects:** Lowering of blood pressure in hypertensive patients. Diuresis with subsequent mobilization of edema. Effect may continue in renal impairment.

Pharmacokinetics
Absorption: Absorption is variable.
Distribution: Unknown.
Metabolism and Excretion: Excreted mainly unchanged by the kidneys.
Half-life: 8 hr.

TIME/ACTION PROFILE (diuretic effect†)

ROUTE	ONSET	PEAK	DURATION
PO	1 hr	2 hr	12–24 hr

†Full antihypertensive effect may take days–weeks

Contraindications/Precautions
Contraindicated in: Hypersensitivity; Cross-sensitivity with other sulfonamides may exist; Anuria; Lactation: Lactation .
Use Cautiously in: Severe hepatic impairment; OB: Safety not established; Pedi: Safety not established; may be more susceptible to diuretic and hypokalemic effects; Geri: ↑ sensitivity to drug effects.

Adverse Reactions/Side Effects
CNS: drowsiness, lethargy. **CV:** chest pain, hypotension, palpitations. **GI:** anorexia, bloating, cramping, drug-induced hepatitis, nausea, vomiting. **Derm:** photosensitivity, rashes. **Endo:** hyperglycemia. **F and E:** hypokalemia, dehydration, hypercalcemia, hypochloremic alkalosis, hypomagnesemia, hyponatremia, hypophosphatemia, hypovolemia. **Hemat:** blood dyscrasias. **Metab:** hyperuricemia. **MS:** muscle cramps. **Misc:** chills, pancreatitis.

Interactions
Drug-Drug: ↑ risk of hypotension with **nitrates**, acute ingestion of **alcohol**, or other **antihypertensives**. ↑ risk of hypokalemia with **corticosteroids**, **amphotericin B**, **piperacillin**, or **ticarcillin**. May ↑ the risk of **digoxin** toxicity. ↓ the excretion of **lithium**; may cause toxicity. May ↓ the effectiveness of **methenamine**. **Stimulant laxatives** (including **aloe**, **senna**) may ↑ risk of potassium depletion.

Drug-Food: Food may ↑ extent of absorption.

Route/Dosage
PO (Adults): *Hypertension*—2.5–5 mg/day; *edema*—5–20 mg/day.

Availability (generic available)
Tablets: 2.5 mg, 5 mg, 10 mg. **Cost:** *Generic*—2.5 mg $99.99/90, 5 mg $110.09/90, 10 mg $121.97/90.

NURSING IMPLICATIONS

Assessment
- Monitor blood pressure, intake and output, and daily weight, and assess feet, legs, and sacral area for edema daily.
- Assess patient, especially if taking digoxin, for anorexia, nausea, vomiting, muscle cramps, paresthesia, and confusion. Notify physician or other health care professional if these signs of electrolyte imbalance occur. Patients taking digoxin are at risk of digoxin toxicity because of the potassium-depleting effect of the diuretic.
- Assess patient for allergy to sulfonamides.
- **Hypertension:** Monitor blood pressure before and periodically during therapy.
- Monitor frequency of prescription refills to determine compliance.
- ***Lab Test Considerations:*** Monitor electrolytes (especially potassium), blood glucose, BUN, and serum creatinine and uric acid levels before and periodically during therapy.
- May cause ↑ in serum and urine glucose in diabetic patients.
- May cause an ↑ in serum bilirubin, calcium, creatinine, and uric acid, and a ↓ in serum magnesium, potassium, and sodium and urinary calcium concentrations.
- May cause ↓ serum protein-bound iodine (PBI) concentrations.
- May cause ↑ serum cholesterol, low-density lipoprotein, and triglyceride concentrations.

Potential Nursing Diagnoses
Excess fluid volume (Indications)
Risk for deficient fluid volume (Side Effects)

Implementation
- Administer in the morning to prevent disruption of sleep cycle.
- Intermittent dose schedule may be used for continued control of edema.
- **PO:** May give with food or milk to minimize GI irritation.

Patient/Family Teaching
- Instruct patient to take metolazone at the same time each day. Take missed doses as soon as remembered but not just before next dose is due. Do not double doses.
- Instruct patient to monitor weight biweekly and notify health care professional of significant changes.
- Caution patient to change positions slowly to minimize orthostatic hypotension; may be potentiated by alcohol.
- Advise patient to use sunscreen and protective clothing in the sun to prevent photosensitivity reactions.
- Instruct patient to discuss dietary potassium requirements with health care professional (see Appendix M).
- Instruct patient to notify health care professional of medication regimen before treatment or surgery.
- Advise patient to report muscle weakness, cramps, nausea, vomiting, diarrhea, or dizziness to health care professional.
- Emphasize the importance of routine follow-up exams.
- **Hypertension:** Advise patient to continue taking the medication even if feeling better. Medication controls but does not cure hypertension.
- Encourage patient to comply with additional interventions for hypertension (weight reduction, low-sodium diet, regular exercise, smoking cessation, moderation of alcohol consumption, and stress management).
- Instruct patient and family in correct technique for monitoring weekly blood pressure.
- Advise patient to consult health care professional before taking OTC medication, especially cough or cold preparations, concurrently with this therapy.

Evaluation/Desired Outcomes
- Decrease in blood pressure.
- Increase in urine output.
- Decrease in edema.

HIGH ALERT

metoprolol (me-**toe**-proe-lole)
✚ Beloc, ✚ Beloc-ZOK,
✚ Betaloc Durules, ✚ Betaloc-ZOK,
✚ Lopresor, ✚ Lopresor SR, Lopresor, ✚ Metoprol, ✚ Novo-metoprol,
✚ Seloken-ZOK, Toprol-XL

✚ = Canadian drug name. **H** = Genetic implication.
*CAPITALS indicates life-threatening; underlines indicate most frequent.

metoprolol

Classification
Therapeutic: antianginals, antihypertensives
Pharmacologic: beta blockers

Pregnancy Category C

Indications
Hypertension. Angina pectoris. Prevention of MI and decreased mortality in patients with recent MI. Management of stable, symptomatic (class II or III) heart failure due to ischemic, hypertensive or cardiomyopathc origin (may be used with ACE inhibitors, diuretics and/or digoxin; Toprol XL only). **Unlabeled Use:** Ventricular arrhythmias/tachycardia. Migraine prophylaxis. Tremors. Aggressive behavior. Drug-induced akathisia. Anxiety.

Action
Blocks stimulation of beta$_1$(myocardial)-adrenergic receptors. Does not usually affect beta$_2$(pulmonary, vascular, uterine)-adrenergic receptor sites. **Therapeutic Effects:** Decreased blood pressure and heart rate. Decreased frequency of attacks of angina pectoris. Decreased rate of cardiovascular mortality and hospitalization in patients with heart failure.

Pharmacokinetics
Absorption: Well absorbed after oral administration.
Distribution: Crosses the blood-brain barrier, crosses the placenta; small amounts enter breast milk.
Metabolism and Excretion: Mostly metabolized by the liver.
Half-life: 3–7 hr.

TIME/ACTION PROFILE (cardiovascular effects)

ROUTE	ONSET	PEAK	DURATION
PO†	15 min	unknown	6–12 hr
PO–ER	unknown	6–12 hr	24 hr
IV	immediate	20 min	5–8 hr

†Maximal effects on BP (chronic therapy) may not occur for 1 wk. Hypotensive effects may persist for up to 4 wk after discontinuation

Contraindications/Precautions
Contraindicated in: Uncompensated CHF; Pulmonary edema; Cardiogenic shock; Bradycardia or heart block.
Use Cautiously in: Renal impairment; Hepatic impairment; Geri: ↑ sensitivity to beta blockers; initial dose reduction recommended; Pulmonary disease (including asthma; beta$_1$ selectivity may be lost at higher doses); Diabetes mellitus (may mask signs of hypoglycemia); Thyrotoxicosis (may mask symptoms); Patients with a history of severe allergic reactions (intensity of reactions may be increased); Untreated pheochromocytoma (initiate only after alpha blocker therapy started); **OB, Lactation, Pedi:** Safety not established; all agents cross the placenta and may cause fetal/neonatal bradycardia, hypotension, hypoglycemia, or respiratory depression.

Adverse Reactions/Side Effects
CNS: fatigue, weakness, anxiety, depression, dizziness, drowsiness, insomnia, memory loss, mental status changes, nervousness, nightmares. **EENT:** blurred vision, stuffy nose. **Resp:** bronchospasm, wheezing. **CV:** BRADYCARDIA, CHF, PULMONARY EDEMA, hypotension, peripheral vasoconstriction. **GI:** constipation, diarrhea, drug-induced hepatitis, dry mouth, flatulence, gastric pain, heartburn, ↑ liver enzymes, nausea, vomiting. **GU:** erectile dysfunction, ↓ libido, urinary frequency. **Derm:** rashes. **Endo:** hyperglycemia, hypoglycemia. **MS:** arthralgia, back pain, joint pain. **Misc:** drug-induced lupus syndrome.

Interactions
Drug-Drug: General anesthesia, **IV phenytoin**, and **verapamil** may cause ↑ myocardial depression. ↑ bradycardia may occur with **digoxin**. ↑ hypotension may occur with other **antihypertensives**, acute ingestion of **alcohol**, or **nitrates**. Concurrent use with **amphetamines**, **cocaine**, **ephedrine**, **epinephrine**, **norepinephrine**, **phenylephrine**, or **pseudoephedrine** may result in unopposed alpha-adrenergic stimulation (excessive hypertension, bradycardia). Concurrent administration of **thyroid** administration may ↓ effectiveness. May alter the effectiveness of **insulins** or **oral hypoglycemic agents** (dosage adjustments may be necessary). May ↓ the effectiveness of **theophylline**. May ↓ the beneficial beta$_1$-cardiovascular effects of **dopamine** or **dobutamine**. Use cautiously within 14 days of **MAO inhibitor** therapy (may result in hypertension).

Route/Dosage
PO (Adults): *Antihypertensive/antianginal*—25–100 mg/day as a single dose initially or 2 divided doses; may be ↑ q 7 days as needed up to 450 mg/day (for angina, give in divided doses). Extended-release products are given once daily. *MI*—25–50 mg (starting 15 min after last IV dose) q 6 hr for 48 hr, then 100 mg twice daily for a minimum of 3 mo. *Heart failure*—12.5–25 mg once daily, can be doubled every 2 wk up to 200 mg/day. *Migraine prevention*—50–100 mg 2–4 times daily (unlabeled).

metoprolol

IV (Adults): *MI*—5 mg q 2 min for 3 doses, followed by oral dosing.

Availability (generic available)
Tablets (tartrate): 25 mg, 50 mg, 100 mg. **Cost:** *Generic*—25 mg $28.37/180, 50 mg $27.00/180, 100 mg $22.99/180. **Extended-release tablets (succinate; Toprol XL):** 25 mg, 50 mg, 100 mg, 200 mg. **Cost:** *Generic*—25 mg $66.97/90, 50 mg $73.97/90, 100 mg $99.92/90, 200 mg $176.98/90. **Injection:** 1 mg/mL. *In combination with:* hydrochlorothiazide (Lopressor HCT). See Appendix B.

NURSING IMPLICATIONS

Assessment
- Monitor blood pressure, ECG, and pulse frequently during dose adjustment and periodically during therapy.
- Monitor frequency of prescription refills to determine compliance.
- Monitor vital signs and ECG every 5–15 min during and for several hours after parenteral administration. If heart rate <40 bpm, especially if cardiac output is also decreased, administer atropine 0.25–0.5 mg IV.
- Monitor intake and output ratios and daily weights. Assess routinely for signs and symptoms of CHF (dyspnea, rales/crackles, weight gain, peripheral edema, jugular venous distention).
- **Angina:** Assess frequency and characteristics of anginal attacks periodically during therapy.
- *Lab Test Considerations:* May cause ↑ BUN, serum lipoprotein, potassium, triglyceride, and uric acid levels.
- May cause ↑ ANA titers.
- May cause ↑ in blood glucose levels.
- May cause ↑ serum alkaline phosphatase, LDH, AST, and ALT levels.

Potential Nursing Diagnoses
Decreased cardiac output (Side Effects)
Noncompliance (Patient/Family Teaching)

Implementation
- *High Alert:* IV vasoactive medications are inherently dangerous. Before administering intravenously, have second practitioner independently check original order and dose calculations.
- *High Alert:* Do not confuse metoprolol with misoprostol. Do not confuse Toprol-XL (metoprolol) with Topamax (topiramate) or Tegretol (carbamazepine).
- **PO:** Take apical pulse before administering. If <50 bpm or if arrhythmia occurs, withhold medication and notify health care professional.
- Administer metoprolol with meals or directly after eating.
- Extended-release tablets should be swallowed whole; do not break, crush, or chew.

IV Administration
- **Direct IV:** *Diluent:* Administer undiluted. *Concentration:* 1 mg/mL. *Rate:* Administer over 1 min.
- **Y-Site Compatibility:** acyclovir, alfentanil, alteplase, amikacin, aminophylline, amiodarone, amphotericin B liposome, anidulafungin, argatroban, ascorbic acid, atracurium, atropine, azathioprine, aztreonam, benztropine, bivalirudin, bleomycin, bumetanide, buprenorphine, butorphanol, calcium chloride, calcium gluconate, carboplatin, caspofungin, cefazolin, cefonocid, cefoperazone, cefotaxime, cefotetan, cefoxitin, ceftazidime, ceftizoxime, ceftriaxone, cefuroxime, chloramphenicol, chlorpromazine, cimetidine, cisplatin, clindamycin, cyanocobalamin, cyclophosphamide, cyclosporine, cytarabine, dactinomycin, daptomycin, dexamethasone, dexmedetomidine, digoxin, diltiazem, diphenhydramine, dobutamine, docetaxel, dopamine, doxacurium, doxorubicin, doxycycline, enalaprilat, ephedrine, epinephrine, epirubicin, epoetin alfa, eptifibatide, esmolol, etoposide, etoposide phosphate, famotidine, fenoldopam, fentanyl, fluconazole, fludarabine, fluorouracil, folic acid, furosemide, ganciclovir, gemcitabine, gentamicin, glycopyrrolate, granisetron, heparin, hetastarch, hydrocortisone, hydromorphone, idarubicin, ifosfamide, imipenem/cilastatin, indomethacin, insulin, isoproterenol, ketorolac, labetalol, linezolid, lorazepam, magnesium sulfate, mannitol, mechlorethamine, meperidine, metaraminol, methotrexate, methoxamine, methyldopate, methylprednisolone, metoclopramide, metronidazole, midazolam, milrinone, mitoxantrone, morphine, multivitamins, nafcillin, nalbuphine, naloxone, nitroprusside, norepinephrine, octreotide, ondansetron, oxacillin, oxaliplatin, oxytocin, paclitaxel, palonosetron, pancuronium, papaverine, pemetrexed, penicillin G, pentamidine, pentazocine, pentobarbital, phenobarbital, phentolamine, phenylephrine, phytonadione, piperacillin/tazobactam, potassium chloride, procainamide,

prochlorperazine, promethazine, propranolol, protamine, pyridoxime, quinupristin/dalfopristin, ranitidine, rocuronium, sodium bicarbonate, streptokinase, succinylcholine, sufentanil, tacrolimus, teniposide, theophylline, thiamine, thiotepa, ticarcillin/clavulanate, tigecycline, tirofiban, tobramycin, tolazoline, trimetaphan, urokinase, vancomycin, vasopressin, vecuronium, verapamil, vincristine, vinorelbine, voriconazole.

- **Y-Site Incompatibility:** allopruinol, amphotericin B cholesteryl, amphotericin B colloidal, dantrolene, diazepam, diazoxide, lepirudin, pantoprazole, phenytoin, trimethoprim/sulfamethoxazole.

Patient/Family Teaching

- Instruct patient to take medication as directed, at the same time each day, even if feeling well; do not skip or double up on missed doses. Take missed doses as soon as possible up to 8 hr before next dose. Abrupt withdrawal may precipitate life-threatening arrhythmias, hypertension, or myocardial ischemia.
- Teach patient and family how to check pulse daily and blood pressure biweekly and to report significant changes to health care professional.
- May cause drowsiness. Caution patient to avoid driving or other activities that require alertness until response to the drug is known.
- Advise patient to change positions slowly to minimize orthostatic hypotension.
- Caution patient that this medication may increase sensitivity to cold.
- Instruct patient to consult health care professional before taking other Rx, OTC, or herbal products, especially cold preparations, concurrently with this medication. Patients on antihypertensive therapy should also avoid excessive amounts of caffeinated coffee, tea, and cola.
- Diabetics should closely monitor blood glucose, especially if weakness, malaise, irritability, or fatigue occurs. Medication does not block sweating as a sign of hypoglycemia.
- Advise patient to notify health care professional if slow pulse, difficulty breathing, wheezing, cold hands and feet, dizziness, light-headedness, confusion, depression, rash, fever, sore throat, unusual bleeding, or bruising occurs.
- Instruct patient to inform health care professional of medication regimen before treatment or surgery.

- Advise patient to carry identification describing disease process and medication regimen at all times.
- **Hypertension:** Reinforce the need to continue additional therapies for hypertension (weight loss, sodium restriction, stress reduction, regular exercise, moderation of alcohol consumption, and smoking cessation). Medication controls but does not cure hypertension.

Evaluation/Desired Outcomes

- Decrease in blood pressure.
- Reduction in frequency of anginal attacks.
- Increase in activity tolerance.
- Prevention of MI.

---

metronidazole
(me-troe-**ni**-da-zole)

✦ Apo-Metronidazole, Flagyl, Flagyl ER, MetroCream, MetroGel, MetroGel-Vaginal, MetroLotion, Metro IV, ✦ Nidagel, Noritate, ✦ Novonidazol, ✦ Trikacide, Vandazole

Classification
Therapeutic: anti-infectives, antiprotozoals, antiulcer agents

Pregnancy Category B

Indications

PO, IV: Treatment of the following anaerobic infections: Intra-abdominal infections (may be used with a cephalosporin), Gynecologic infections, Skin and skin structure infections, Lower respiratory tract infections, Bone and joint infections, CNS infections, Septicemia, Endocarditis. **IV:** Perioperative prophylactic agent in colorectal surgery. **PO:** Amebicide in the management of amebic dysentery, amebic liver abscess, and trichomoniasis: Treatment of peptic ulcer disease caused by *Helicobacter pylori*. **Topical:** Treatment of acne rosacea. **Vag:** Management of bacterial vaginosis. **Unlabeled Use:** Treatment of giardiasis. Treatment of anti-infective associated pseudomembranous colitis.

Action

Disrupts DNA and protein synthesis in susceptible organisms. **Therapeutic Effects:** Bactericidal, trichomonacidal, or amebicidal action. **Spectrum:** Most notable for activity against anaerobic bacteria, including: *Bacteroides*, *Clostridium*. In addition, is active against: *Trichomonas vaginalis*, *Entamoeba histolytica*, *Giardia lamblia*, *H. pylori*, *Clostridium difficile*.

Pharmacokinetics

Absorption: 80% absorbed after oral administration. Minimal absorption after topical or vaginal application.
Distribution: Widely distributed into most tissues and fluids, including CSF. Crosses the placenta and enters fetal circulation rapidly; enters breast milk in concentrations equal to plasma levels.
Metabolism and Excretion: Partially metabolized by the liver (30–60%), partially excreted unchanged in the urine, 6–15% eliminated in the feces.
Half-life: Neonates: 25–75 hr; Children and adults: 6–12 hr.

TIME/ACTION PROFILE (PO, IV = blood levels; topical = improvement in rosacea)

ROUTE	ONSET	PEAK	DURATION
PO	rapid	1–3 hr	8 hr
PO-ER	rapid	unknown	up to 24 hr
IV	rapid	end of infusion	6–8 hr
Topical	3 wk	9 wk	12 hr
Vaginal	unknown	6–12 hr	12 hr

Contraindications/Precautions

Contraindicated in: Hypersensitivity; Hypersensitivity to parabens (topical only); OB: First trimester of pregnancy.
Use Cautiously in: History of blood dyscrasias; History of seizures or neurologic problems; Severe hepatic impairment (dose ↓ suggested); OB: Although safety not established, has been used to treat trichomoniasis in 2nd- and 3rd-trimester pregnancy—but not as single-dose regimen; Lactation: If needed, use single dose and interrupt nursing for 24 hr thereafter; Patients receiving corticosteroids or predisposed to edema (injection contains 28 mEq sodium/g metronidazole).

Adverse Reactions/Side Effects

CNS: SEIZURES, dizziness, headache, aseptic meningitis (IV), encephalopathy (IV). **EENT:** optical neuropathy, tearing (topical only). **GI:** abdominal pain, anorexia, nausea, diarrhea, dry mouth, furry tongue, glossitis, unpleasant taste, vomiting. **Derm:** STEVENS-JOHNSON SYNDROME, rash, urticaria; *topical only*, burning, mild dryness, skin irritation, transient redness. **Hemat:** leukopenia. **Local:** phlebitis at IV site. **Neuro:** peripheral neuropathy. **Misc:** superinfection.

Interactions

Drug-Drug: Cimetidine may ↓ metabolism. **Phenobarbital** and **rifampin** ↑ metabolism and may ↓ effectiveness. Metronidazole ↑ the effects of **phenytoin, lithium,** and **warfarin.** Disulfiram-like reaction may occur with **alcohol** ingestion. May cause acute psychosis and confusion with **disulfiram.** ↑ risk of leukopenia with **fluorouracil** or **azathioprine.**

Route/Dosage

PO (Adults): *Anaerobic infections*—7.5 mg/kg q 6 hr (not to exceed 4 g/day). *Trichomoniasis*—250 mg q 8 hr for 7 days *or* single 2-g dose *or* 1 g bid for 1 day. *Amebiasis*—500–750 mg q 8 hr for 5–10 days. *H. pylori*—250 mg 4 times daily *or* 500 mg twice daily for 1–2 wk (with other agents). *Bacterial vaginoses*—750 mg once daily as ER tablets for 7 days. *Antibiotic associated pseudomembranous colitis*—250–500 mg 3–4 times/day for 10–14 days.
PO (Infants and Children): *Anaerobic infections*-30 mg/kg/day divided q 6 hr, maximum dose: 4 g/day *Trichomoniasis*—15–30 mg/kg/day divided q 8 hr for 7–10 days. *Amebiasis*—35–50 mg/kg/day divided q 8 hr for 5–10 days (not to exceed 750 mg/dose). *Antibiotic associated pseudomembranous colitis*—30 mg/kg/day divided q 6 hr for 7–10 days. *H. pylori*—15–20 mg/kg/day divided twice daily for 4 weeks.
IV, PO (Neonates 0–4 weeks, <1200 g): 7.5 mg/kg q 48 hr. *Postnatal age <7 days, 1200–2000 g*—7.5 mg/kg/day q 24 hr. *Postnatal age <7 days, >2000 g*—15 mg/kg/day divided q 12 hr. *Postnatal age >7 days, 1200–2000 g*—15 mg/kg/day divided q 12 hr. *Postnatal age >7 days, >2000 g*—30 mg/kg/day divided q 12 hr.
IV (Adults): *Anaerobic infections*—Initial dose 15 mg/kg, then 7.5 mg/kg q 6–8 hr *or* 500 mg q 6–8 hr (not to exceed 4 g/day). *Perioperative prophylaxis*—Initial dose 15 mg/kg 1 hr before surgery, then 7.5 mg/kg 6 and 12 hr later. *Amebiasis*—500–750 mg q 8 hr for 5–10 days.
IV (Children): *Anaerobic infections*—30 mg/kg/day divided q 6 hr, maximum dose: 4 g/day.
Topical (Adults): *Acne rosacea*—Apply thin film to affected area bid.
Vag (Adults): *Bacterial vaginosis*—One applicatorful (5 g) 2 times daily for 5 days.

Availability (generic available)

Tablets: 250 mg, 500 mg. *Cost: Generic*—250 mg $16.99/30, 500 mg $9.99/30. **Extended-**

metronidazole

release (ER) tablets: 750 mg. Cost: $297.98/30. Capsules: 375 mg, ✤ 500 mg. Premixed injection: 500 mg/100 mL. Topical gel: 0.75%, 1%. Cost: $132.99/60 g. Topical cream: 0.75%, 1%. Cost: *Generic*—$59.99/45 g. Topical lotion: 0.75%. Cost: *Generic*—$79.99/59 mL. Vaginal gel: 0.75% (37.5 mg/5 g applicatorful). Cost: $32.22/70 g. *In combination with:* bismuth subsalicylate tablets and tetracycline capsules (Helidac) as part of a compliance package; bismuth subcitrate potassium and tetracycline (Pylera). See Appendix B.

NURSING IMPLICATIONS

Assessment
- Assess for infection (vital signs; appearance of wound, sputum, urine, and stool; WBC) at beginning of and throughout therapy.
- Obtain specimens for culture and sensitivity before initiating therapy. First dose may be given before receiving results.
- Monitor neurologic status during and after IV infusions. Inform physician if numbness, paresthesia, weakness, ataxia, or seizures occur.
- Monitor intake and output and daily weight, especially for patients on sodium restriction. Each 500 mg of Flagyl IV for dilution contains 5 mEq of sodium; each 500 mg of Flagyl RTU contains 14 mEq of sodium.
- **Giardiasis:** Monitor three stool samples taken several days apart, beginning 3–4 wk after treatment.
- *Lab Test Considerations:* May alter results of serum AST, ALT, and LDH tests.

Potential Nursing Diagnoses
Risk for infection (Indications)
Diarrhea (Indications)

Implementation
- **PO:** Administer on an empty stomach, or may administer with food or milk to minimize GI irritation. Tablets may be crushed for patients with difficulty swallowing. Swallow extended-release tablets whole; do not break, crush, or chew.

IV Administration
- **Intermittent Infusion:** *Diluent:* Administer premixed injection (500 mg/100 mL) undiluted. Do not refrigerate. Once taken out of overwrap, premixed infusion stable for 30 days at room temperature. *Concentration:* 5 mg/mL. *Rate:* Infuse over 30–60 min.
- **Y-Site Compatibility:** acyclovir, alfentanil, allopurinol, amifistine, amikacin, aminophylline, amiodarone, ampicillin, ampicillin/sulbactam, anidulafungin, atracurium, bivalirudin, bumetanide, buprenorphine, busulfan, butorphanol, calcium acetate, calcium chloride, calcium gluconate, carboplatin, cefazolin, cefepime, cefoperazone, cefotetan, cefotaxime, ceftriaxone, cefuroxime, chloramphenicol, chlorpromazine, cimetidine, ciprofloxacin, cisatracurium, cisplatin, clindamycin, codeine, cyclophosphamide, cyclosporine, cytarabine, dactinomycin, dexamethasone, dexmedetomidine, dexrazoxane, digoxin, diltiazem, dimenhydrinate, diphenhydramine, dobutamine, docetaxel, dopamine, doripenem, doxacurium, doxapram, doxorubicin, doxorubicin liposome, doxycycline, droperidol, enalaprilat, ephedrine, epinephrine, erirubicin, eptifibatide, ertapenem, erythromycin, esmolol, etoposide, etoposide phosphate, famotidine, fenoldopam, fentanyl, fluconazole, fludarabine, fluorouracil, foscarnet, fosphenytoin, furosemide, gemcitabine, gentamicin, glycopyrrolate, granisetron, haloperidol, heparin, hetastarch, hydralazine, hydrocortisone, hydromorphone, idarubicin, ifosfamide, imipenem/cilastatin, inamrinone, insulin, isoproterenol, ketorolac, labetalol, leucovorin, levofloxacin, lidocaine, linezolid, lorazepam, magnesium sulfate, mannitol, mechlorethamine, melphalan, meperidine, meropenem, mesna, metaraminol, methotrexate, methyldopate, methylprednisolone, metoclopramide, metoprolol, midazolam, milrinone, mitoxantrone, morphine, nafcillin, nalbuphine, naloxone, nesiritide, nicardipine, nitroglycerin, nitroprusside, norepinephrine, octreotide, ondansetron, oxaliplatin, oxytocin, paclitaxel, palonosetron, pancuronium, pentamidine, pentazocine, pentobarbital, perphenazine, phenobarbital, phentolamine, phenylephrine, piperacillin/tazobactam, potassium chloride, potassium phosphates, prochlorperazine, promethazine, propranolol, ranitidine, remifentanil, rituximab, rocuronium, sargramostim, sodium acetate, sodium bicarbonate, sodium phosphates, streptozocin, succinylcholine, sufentanil, tacrolimus, teniposide, theophylline, thiopental, thiotepa, ticarcillin/clavulanate, tigecycline, tirofiban, tobramycin, trastuzumab, trimethobenzamide, trimethoprim/sulfamethoxazole, vancomycin, vasopressin, vecuronium, verapamil, vincristine, vinorelbine, voriconazole, zidovudine.
- **Y-Site Incompatibility:** amphotericin B cholesteryl, amphotericin B colloidal, amphotericin B liposome, aztreonam, dantrolene, daptomycin, diazepam, drotrecogin, filgrastim,

ganciclovir, pantoprazole, pemetrexed, phenytoin, procainamide, quinupristin/dalfopristin.
• **Topical:** Cleanse affected area before application. Apply and rub in a thin film twice daily, morning and evening. Avoid contact with eyes.

Patient/Family Teaching
• Instruct patient to take medication as directed with evenly spaced times between doses, even if feeling better. Do not skip doses or double up on missed doses. Take missed doses as soon as remembered if not almost time for next dose.
• Advise patients treated for trichomoniasis that sexual partners may be asymptomatic sources of reinfection and should be treated concurrently. Patient should also refrain from intercourse or use a condom to prevent reinfection.
• Caution patient to avoid intake of alcoholic beverages or preparations containing alcohol during and for at least 3 days after treatment with metronidazole, including vaginal gel. May cause a disulfiram-like reaction (flushing, nausea, vomiting, headache, abdominal cramps).
• May cause dizziness or light-headedness. Caution patient to avoid driving or other activities requiring alertness until response to medication is known.
• Inform patient that medication may cause an unpleasant metallic taste.
• Advise patient not to take OTC medications concurrently without consulting health care professional.
• Advise patient that frequent mouth rinses, good oral hygiene, and sugarless gum or candy may minimize dry mouth. Notify health care professional if dry mouth persists for more than 2 wk.
• Advise patient to inform health care professional if pregnancy is suspected before taking this medication.
• Inform patient that medication may cause urine to turn dark.
• Advise patient to consult health care professional if no improvement in a few days or if signs and symptoms of superinfection (black, furry overgrowth on tongue; vaginal itching or discharge; loose or foul-smelling stools) develop.
• **Vag:** Instruct patient in correct technique for intravaginal instillation. Advise patient to avoid intercourse during treatment with vaginal gel.
• **Topical:** Instruct patient on correct technique for application of topical gel. Cosmetics may be used after application of gel.

Evaluation/Desired Outcomes
• Resolution of the signs and symptoms of infection. Length of time for complete resolution depends on organism and site of infection.
• Significant results should be seen within 3 wk of application of topical gel. Application may be continued for 9 wk.

---

micafungin (my-ka-fun-gin)
Mycamine

Classification
Therapeutic: antifungals
Pharmacologic: echinocandins

Pregnancy Category C

Indications
Esophageal candidiasis. Candidemia/acute disseminated candidiasis/Candidal peritonitis and abscesses. Prophylaxis of *Candida* infections during hematopoetic stem cell transplantation.

Action
Inhibits synthesis of glucan required for the formation of fungal cell wall. **Therapeutic Effects:** Death of susceptible fungi. **Spectrum:** Active against the following *Candida* spp.: *C. albicans*, *C. glabrata*, *C. krusei*, *C. parapsilosis*, *C. tropicalis*.

Pharmacokinetics
Absorption: IV administration results in complete bioavailability.
Distribution: Unknown.
Protein Binding: >99%.
Metabolism and Excretion: Mostly metabolized; 71% fecal elimination.
Half-life: 15 hr.

TIME/ACTION PROFILE

ROUTE	ONSET	PEAK	DURATION
IV	rapid	end of infusion	24 hr

Contraindications/Precautions
Contraindicated in: Hypersensitivity.
Use Cautiously in: Severe hepatic impairment; OB: Use only if clearly needed; Lactation, Pedi: Safety not established.

Adverse Reactions/Side Effects
GI: worsening hepatic function/hepatitis. **GU:** renal impairment. **Hemat:** hemolysis/hemolytic anemia. **Local:** injection site reactions. **Misc:** allergic reactions including ANAPHYLAXIS (rare).

Interactions
Drug-Drug: ↑ blood levels and risk of toxicity with **sirolimus** and **nifedipine** (dose adjustments may be necessary).

Route/Dosage
IV (Adults): *Esophageal candidiasis*—150 mg/day for 15 days (range 10–30 days); *Candidemia/acute disseminated candidiasis/Candida peritonitis and abscesses*—100 mg/day for 15 days (range 10–47 days) *Prevention of Candida infections in stem cell transplantation*—50 mg/day.

Availability
Lyophilized powder for injection: 50 mg/vial, 100 mg/vial.

NURSING IMPLICATIONS

Assessment
- Assess symptoms of esophageal candidiasis (dysphagia, odynophagia, retrosternal pain) prior to and during therapy.
- Monitor for signs of anaphylaxis (rash, pruritus, wheezing, laryngeal edema, abdominal pain). Discontinue micafungin and notify health care professional immediately if these occur.
- Assess for injection site reactions (phlebitis, thrombophlebitis) during therapy. These occur more frequently in patients receiving micafungin via peripheral IV infusion.
- *Lab Test Considerations:* May cause ↑ serum alkaline phosphatase, bilirubin, ALT, AST, and LDH levels. If elevations occur, monitor for worsening liver function; may require discontinuation of therapy.
- May cause ↑ BUN and serum creatinine.
- May cause leukopenia, neutropenia, thrombocytopenia, and anemia. Monitor for worsening levels; may require discontinuation of therapy.
- May cause hypokalemia, hypocalcemia, and hypomagnesemia.

Potential Nursing Diagnoses
Risk for infection (Indications)

Implementation
IV Administration

- **Intermittent Infusion:** *Diluent:* Reconstitute each 50-mg vial with 5 mL of 0.9% NaCl or D5W to achieve concentration of 10 mg/mL. Reconstitute each 100-mg vial with 5 mL of 0.9% NaCl or D5w to achieve concentration of 20 mg/mL. Dissolve by gently swirling vial; do not shake vigorously. Directions for further dilution based on indication for use. For prophylaxis of *Candida* infections, add 50 mg of micafungin to 100 mL of 0.9% NaCl or D5W. For treatment of esophageal candidiasis, add 150 mg of micafungin to 100 mL of 0.9% NaCl or D5W. Reconstituted vials and infusion are stable for 24 hr at room temperature. Protect diluted solution from light. *Concentration:* 0.5–1.5 mg/mL. *Rate:* Flush line with 0.9% NaCl prior to administration. Infuse over 1 hr. More rapid infusions may result in more frequent histamine mediated reactions.
- **Y-Site Compatibility:** aminophylline, bumetanide, calcium chloride, calcium gluconate, cyclosporine, dopamine, eptifibatide, esmolol, fenoldopam, furosemide, heparin, hydromorphone, lidocaine, lorazepam, magnesium sulfate, milrinone, nitroglycerin, nitroprusside, norepinephrine, phenylephrine, potassium chloride, potassium phosphate, tacrolimus, vasopressin.
- **Y-Site Incompatibility:** amiodarone, cisatracurium, diltiazem, dobutamine, epinephrine, insulin, labetalol, meperidine, midazolam, morphine, mycophenolate mofetil, nesiritide, nicardipine, octreotide, ondansetron, phenytoin, vecuronium.

Patient/Family Teaching
- Inform patient of the purpose of micafungin.
- Advise patient to notify health care professional immediately if signs of anaphylaxis occur.

Evaluation/Desired Outcomes
- Resolution of signs and symptoms of esophageal candidiasis, candidemia, acute disseminated candidiasis, candidal peritonitis and abscesses.
- Prevention of *Candida* infections during hematopoetic stem cell transplantation.

---

miconazole, See ANTIFUNGALS (TOPICAL).

---

miconazole, See ANTIFUNGALS (VAGINAL).

HIGH ALERT

midazolam (mid-ay-zoe-lam)
Versed

midazolam

Classification
Therapeutic: antianxiety agents, sedative/hypnotics
Pharmacologic: benzodiazepines

Schedule IV

Pregnancy Category D

Indications
PO: Preprocedural sedation and anxiolysis in pediatric patients. **IM, IV:** Preoperative sedation/anxiolysis/amnesia. **IV:** Provides sedation/anxiolysis/amnesia during therapeutic, diagnostic, or radiographic procedures (conscious sedation). Aids in the induction of anesthesia and as part of balanced anesthesia. As a continuous infusion, provides sedation of mechanically ventilated patients during anesthesia or in a critical care setting. Status epilepticus.

Action
Acts at many levels of the CNS to produce generalized CNS depression. Effects may be mediated by GABA, an inhibitory neurotransmitter. **Therapeutic Effects:** Short-term sedation. Postoperative amnesia.

Pharmacokinetics
Absorption: Rapidly absorbed following oral and nasal administration; undergoes substantial intestinal and first-pass hepatic metabolism. Well absorbed following IM administration; IV administration results in complete bioavailability.
Distribution: Crosses the blood-brain barrier and placenta; excreted in breast milk.
Protein Binding: 97%.
Metabolism and Excretion: Almost exclusively metabolized by the liver, resulting in conversion to hydroxymidazolam, an active metabolite, and 2 other inactive metabolites (metabolized by cytochrome P450 3A4 enzyme system); metabolites are excreted in urine.
Half-life: Preterm neonates: 2.6–17.7 hr; Neonates: 4–12 hr; Children: 3–7 hr; Adults: 2–6 hr (increased in renal impairment, CHF, or cirrhosis).

TIME/ACTION PROFILE (sedation)

ROUTE	ONSET	PEAK	DURATION
IN	5 min	10 min	30–60 min
IM	15 min	30–60 min	2–6 hr
IV	1.5–5 min	rapid	2–6 hr

Contraindications/Precautions
Contraindicated in: Hypersensitivity; Cross-sensitivity with other benzodiazepines may occur; Shock; Comatose patients or those with pre-existing CNS depression; Uncontrolled severe pain; Acute angle-closure glaucoma; OB: Benzodiazepine drugs may ↑ risk of congenital malformations; use in the last weeks of pregnancy has caused CNS depression in the neonate; Lactation: Lactation; Pedi: Products containing benzyl alcohol should not be used in neonates.
Use Cautiously in: Pulmonary disease; CHF; Renal impairment; Severe hepatic impairment; Obese pediatric patients (calculate dose on the basis of ideal body weight); Pedi: Rapid injection in neonates has caused severe hypotension and seizures, especially when used with fentanyl; Geri: Older patients (especially >70 yr) are more susceptible to cardiorespiratory depressant effects; dosage ↓ required.

Adverse Reactions/Side Effects
CNS: agitation, drowsiness, excess sedation, headache. **EENT:** blurred vision. **Resp:** APNEA, LARYNGOSPASM, RESPIRATORY DEPRESSION, bronchospasm, coughing. **CV:** CARDIAC ARREST, arrhythmias. **GI:** hiccups, nausea, vomiting. **Derm:** rashes. **Local:** phlebitis at IV site, pain at IM site.

Interactions
Drug-Drug: ↑ CNS depression with **alcohol**, **antihistamines**, **opioid analgesics**, and other **sedative/hypnotics** (↓ midazolam dose by 30–50% if used concurrently). ↑ risk of hypotension with **antihypertensives**, **opioid analgesics**, acute ingestion of **alcohol**, or **nitrates**. Midazolam is metabolized by the cytochrome P450 3A4 enzyme system; drugs that induce or inhibit this system may be expected to alter the effects of midazolam. **Carbamazepine**, **phenytoin**, **rifampin**, **rifabutin**, and **phenobarbital** ↓ levels. **Erythromycin**, **cimetidine**, **ranitidine**, **diltiazem**, **verapamil**, **fluconazole**, **itraconazole**, and **ketoconazole** ↓ metabolism and may ↑ risk of toxicity.
Drug-Natural Products: Concomitant use of **kava-kava**, **valerian**, or **chamomile** can ↑ CNS depression. Long term use of **St. John's wort** may significantly ↓ levels.
Drug-Food: Grapefruit juice ↓ metabolism and may ↑ risk of toxicity.

midazolam

Route/Dosage
Dose must be individualized, taking caution to reduce dose in geriatric patients and in those who are already sedated.

Preoperative Sedation/Anxiolysis/Amnesia
PO (Children 6 mo–16 yr): 0.25–0.5 mg/kg, may require up to 1 mg/kg (dose should not exceed 20 mg); *patients with cardiac/respiratory compromise or concurrent CNS depressants*— 0.25 mg/kg.
IM (Adults Otherwise Healthy and <60 yr): 0.07–0.08 mg/kg 1 hr before surgery (usual dose 5 mg).
IM (Adults ≥60 yr, Debilitated or Chronically Ill): 0.02–0.03 mg/kg 1 hr before surgery (usual dose 1–3 mg).
IM (Children): 0.1–0.15 mg/kg up to 0.5 mg/kg 30–60 min prior to procedure; not to exceed 10 mg/dose.

Conscious Sedation for Short Procedures
IV (Adults and Children Otherwise Healthy >12 yr and <60 yr): 1–2.5 mg initially; dosage may be ↑ further as needed. Total doses >5 mg are rarely needed (↓ dose by 50% if other CNS depressants are used). Maintenance doses of 25% of the dose required for initial sedation may be given as necessary.
IV (Children 6–12 yr): 0.025–0.05 mg/kg initially, then titrate dose carefully, may need up to 0.4 mg/kg total, maximum dose 10 mg.
IV (Children 6 months–5 yr): 0.05 mg/kg initially, then titrate dose carefully, may need up to 0.6 mg/kg total, maximum dose 6 mg.
IV (Geriatric Patients ≥60 yr, Debilitated or Chronically Ill): 1–1.5 mg initially; dose may be ↑ further as needed. Total doses >3.5 mg are rarely needed (↓ dose by 30% if other CNS depressants are used). Maintenance doses of 25% of the dose required for initial sedation may be given as necessary.
Intranasal (Children): 0.2–0.3 mg/kg, may repeat in 5–15 min.

Status Epilepticus
IV (Children >2 months): 0.15 mg/kg load followed by a continuous infusion of 1 mcg/kg/min. Titrate dose upward q 5 min until seizure controlled, range: 1–18 mcg/kg/min.

Induction of Anesthesia (Adjunct)
May give additional dose of 25% of initial dose if needed.
IV (Adults Otherwise Healthy and <55 yr): 300–350 mcg/kg initially (up to 600 mcg/kg total). If patient is premedicated, initial dose should be further ↓ .
IV (Geriatric Patients >55 yr): 150–300 mcg/kg as initial dose. If patient is premedicated, initial dose should be further ↓ .
IV (Adults —Debilitated): 150–250 mcg/kg initial dose. If patient is premedicated, initial dose should be further ↓ .

Sedation in Critical Care Settings
IV (Adults): 0.01–0.05 mg/kg (0.5–4 mg in most adults) initially if a loading dose is required; may repeat q 10–15 min until desired effect is obtained; may be followed by infusion at 0.02–0.1 mg/kg/hr (1–7 mg/hr in most adults).
IV (Children): *Intubated patients only*— 0.05–0.2 mg/kg initially as a loading dose; follow with infusion at 0.06–0.12 mg/kg/hr (1–2 mcg/kg/min), titrate to effect, range: 0.4–6 mcg/kg/min.
IV (Neonates >32 wk): *Intubated patients only*—0.06 mg/kg/hr (1 mcg/kg/min).
IV (Neonates <32 wk): *Intubated patients only*—0.03 mg/kg/hr (0.5 mcg/kg/min).

Availability (generic available)
Injection: 1 mg/mL, 5 mg/mL. **Syrup (cherry flavor):** 2 mg/mL.

NURSING IMPLICATIONS

Assessment
- Assess level of sedation and level of consciousness throughout and for 2–6 hr following administration.
- Monitor blood pressure, pulse, and respiration continuously during IV administration. Oxygen and resuscitative equipment should be immediately available.
- ***Toxicity and Overdose:*** If overdose occurs, monitor pulse, respiration, and blood pressure continuously. Maintain patent airway and assist ventilation as needed. If hypotension occurs, treatment includes IV fluids, repositioning, and vasopressors.
- The effects of midazolam can be reversed with flumazenil (Romazicon).

Potential Nursing Diagnoses
Ineffective breathing pattern (Adverse Reactions)
Risk for injury (Side Effects)

Implementation
- ***High Alert:*** Accidental overdose of oral midazolam syrup in children has resulted in serious harm or death. Do not accept orders prescribed by volume (5 mL, or 1 tsp); instead, request dose be expressed in milligrams. Have

second practitioner independently check original order and dose calculations. Midazolam syrup should only be administered by health care professionals authorized to administer conscious sedation. Do not confuse Versed (midazolam) with VePesid (etoposide).

- **PO:** To use the *Press-in Bottle Adaptor (PIBA)*, remove the cap and push bottle adaptor into neck of bottle. Close bottle tightly with cap. Solution is a clear red to purplish-red cherry-flavored syrup. Then remove cap and insert tip of oral dispenser in bottle adaptor. Push the plunger completely down toward tip of oral dispenser and insert firmly into bottle adaptor. Turn entire unit (bottle and oral dispenser) upside down. Pull plunger out slowly until desired amount of medication is withdrawn into oral dispenser. Turn entire unit right side up and slowly remove oral dispenser from the bottle. Tip of dispenser may be covered with tip of cap until time of use. Close bottle with cap after each use.
- Dispense directly into mouth. Do not mix with any liquid prior to dispensing.
- **Intranasal:** Administer using a 1 mL needleless syringe into the nares over 15 sec. Using the 5 mg/mL injection, administer half dose into each nare.
- **IM:** Administer IM doses deep into muscle mass, maximum concentration 1 mg/mL.

IV Administration

- **Direct IV:** *Diluent:* Administer undiluted or diluted with D5W or 0.9% NaCl. *Concentration:* Undiluted: 1 mg/mL or 5 mg/mL. Diluted: 0.03–3 mg/mL. *Rate:* Administer slowly over at least 2–5 min. Titrate dose to patient response. Rapid injection, especially in neonates, has caused severe hypotension.
- **Continuous Infusion:** *Diluent:* Dilute with 0.9% NaCl or D5W. *Concentration:* 0.5–1 mg/mL. *Rate:* Based on patient's weight (see Route/Dosage section). Titrate to desired level of sedation. Assess sedation at regular intervals and adjust rate up or down by 25–50% as needed. Dose should also be decreased by 10–25% every few hours to find minimum effective infusion rate, which prevents accumulation of midazolam and provides more rapid recovery upon termination.
- **Y-Site Compatibility:** abciximab, amikacin, amiodarone, anidulafungin, argatroban, atropine, aztreonam, bivalirudin, calcium gluconate, caspofungin, cefazolin, cefotaxime, cefoxitin, ceftizoxime, ceftriaxone, cimetidine, ciprofloxacin, cisatracurium, cyclosporine, daptomycin, digoxin, diltiazem, diphenhydramine, dopamine, doxycycline, enalaprilat, epinephrine, eptifibatide, erythromycin lactobionate, esmolol, etomidate, famotidine, fenoldopam, fentanyl, fluconazole, gentamicin, granisetron, heparin, hydromorphone, hydroxyzine, isoproterenol, labetalol, levofloxacin, lidocaine, linezolid, lorazepam, magnesium sulfate, meperidine, methylprednisolone, metoclopramide, metoprolol, metronidazole, milrinone, morphine, nicardipine, nitroglycerin, nitroprusside, norepinephrine, ondansetron, palonosetron, pancuronium, penicillin G potassium, phenylephrine, phytonadione, potassium chloride, procainamide, promethazine, propranolol, protamine, quinupristin/dalfopristin, ranitidine, rifampin, tobramycin, vancomycin, vecuronium.
- **Y-Site Incompatibility:** acyclovir, amphotericin B cholesteryl sulfate, aminophylline, ampicillin, ampicillin/sulbactam, bumetanide, cefepime, ceftazidime, cefuroxime, chloramphenicol, dexamethasone sodium phosphate, diazepam, ertapenem, furosemide, ganciclovir, ketorolac, lansoprazole, micafungin, pantoprazole, phenytoin, piperacillin/tazobactam, prochlorperazine, sodium bicarbonate, thiopental, trimethoprim/sulfamethoxazole.

Patient/Family Teaching

- Inform patient that this medication will decrease mental recall of the procedure.
- May cause drowsiness or dizziness. Advise patient to request assistance prior to ambulation and transfer and to avoid driving or other activities requiring alertness for 24 hr following administration.
- Instruct patient to inform health care professional prior to administration if pregnancy is suspected.
- Advise patient to avoid alcohol or other CNS depressants for 24 hr following administration of midazolam.

Evaluation/Desired Outcomes

- Sedation during and amnesia following surgical, diagnostic, and radiologic procedures.
- Sedation and amnesia for mechanically ventilated patients in a critical care setting.

mifepristone (mi-fe-**priss**-tone)
Mifeprex

Classification
Therapeutic: abortifacients
Pharmacologic: antiprogestational agents

Pregnancy Category UK

Indications
Medical termination of intrauterine pregnancy up to day 49 of pregnancy.

Action
Antagonizes endometrial and myometrial effects of progesterone. Sensitizes the myometrium to contraction-inducing activity of prostaglandins.
Therapeutic Effects: Termination of pregnancy.

Pharmacokinetics
Absorption: Rapidly absorbed following oral administration (69% bioavailability).
Distribution: Unknown.
Protein Binding: 98%.
Metabolism and Excretion: Mostly metabolized by the liver (cytochrome CYP450 3A4 [CYP450 3A4] enzyme system).
Half-life: 18 hr.

TIME/ACTION PROFILE (termination of pregnancy)

ROUTE	ONSET	PEAK	DURATION
PO	unknown	within 2 days	unknown

Contraindications/Precautions
Contraindicated in: Presence of an intrauterine device (IUD); Confirmed or suspected ectopic pregnancy; Undiagnosed adnexal mass; Chronic adrenal failure; Concurrent long-term corticosteroid therapy; Bleeding disorders or concurrent anticoagulant therapy; Inherited porphyrias.
Use Cautiously in: Chronic medical conditions such as cardiovascular, hypertensive, hepatic, renal, or respiratory disease (safety and efficacy not established); Women >35 yrs old or who smoke ≥10 cigarettes/day.

Adverse Reactions/Side Effects
CNS: dizziness, fainting, headache, weakness. **GI:** abdominal pain, diarrhea, nausea, vomiting. **GU:** uterine bleeding, uterine cramping, ruptured ectopic pregnancy, pelvic pain.

Interactions
Drug-Drug: Blood levels and therapeutic effectiveness may be ↑ by **ketoconazole**, **itraconazole**, and **erythromycin**. Blood levels and effects may be ↓ by **rifampin**, **dexamethasone**, **phenytoin**, **phenobarbital**, and **carbamazepine**. Mifepristone may ↓ metabolism and ↑ effects of other **drugs metabolized by the CYP 450 3A4 enzyme system**, including **some agents used during general anesthesia**.
Drug-Natural Products: Blood levels and effects may be ↓ by **St. John's wort**.
Drug-Food: Blood levels and effects may be ↑ by **grapefruit juice**.

Route/Dosage
PO (Adults): *Day 1*—600 mg (given as three 200 mg tablets) as a single dose, followed on *day 3* by 400 mcg misoprostol (Cytotec), unless abortion has occurred and has been confirmed by clinical or ultrasonographic examination (see misoprostol monograph).

Availability
Tablets: 200 mg.

NURSING IMPLICATIONS

Assessment
- Determine duration of pregnancy. Pregnancy is dated from the first day of the last menstrual period in a presumed 28-day cycle with ovulation occurring at mid-cycle and can be determined by menstrual history and clinical examination; use ultrasound if duration is uncertain or if ectopic pregnancy is suspected.
- Assess amount of bleeding and cramping during treatment. Determine if termination is complete on day 14.
- ***Lab Test Considerations:*** Decrease in hemoglobin, hematocrit, and RBCs may occur in women who bleed heavily.
- Changes in quantitative human chorionic gonadotropin (hCG) levels are not accurate until at least 10 days after mifepristone administration; complete termination of pregnancy must be confirmed by clinical examination.

Potential Nursing Diagnoses
Acute pain (Side Effects)

Implementation
- Mifepristone should be administered only by health care professionals who have read and understood the prescribing information, are able to assess gestational age of an embryo and diagnose ectopic pregnancies, and who are able to provide surgical intervention in cases of incomplete abortion or severe bleeding.
- Any IUD should be removed prior to mifepristone adminstration.
- Measures to prevent rhesus immunization, similar to those of surgical abortion, should be taken.

- **PO:** On *day 1*, after the patient has read the *Medication Guide* and signed the Patient Agreement, administer three 200 mg tablets of mifepristone as a single dose. On *day 3*, unless abortion has occurred and been confirmed by clinical examination or ultrasound, administer two 200-mcg tablets of misoprostol. On *day 14*, confirm that termination of pregnancy has occurred by clinical examination or ultrasound.

Patient/Family Teaching
- Advise patient of the treatment and its effects. Patients must be given a copy of the *Medication Guide and Patient Agreement.* Patient must understand the necessity of completing the treatment schedule of three office visits (day 1, day 3, and day 14).
- Inform patient that vaginal bleeding and uterine cramping will probably occur and that prolonged or heavy vaginal bleeding is not proof of complete expulsion. Bleeding or spotting occurs for an average of 9–16 days; but may continue for more than 30 days. Advise patient that if the treatment fails, there is a risk of fetal malformation; medical abortion failures are managed by surgical termination.
- Caution patient to notify health care professional immediately if she develops weakness, nausea, vomiting, diarrhea, with or without abdominal pain or fever more than 24 hr after taking mifepristone; may indicate life-threatening sepsis.
- Instruct patient in the steps to take in an emergency situation, including precise instructions and a telephone number to call if she has problems or concerns.
- May cause dizziness or fainting. Caution patient to avoid driving or other activities requiring alertness until response to medication is known.
- Caution patient that pregnancy can occur following termination of pregnancy and before resumption of normal menses. Contraception can be initiated as soon as pregnancy termination is confirmed, or before sexual intercourse is resumed.
- Advise patient to notify health care professional if she smokes at least 10 cigarettes a day.

Evaluation/Desired Outcomes
- Termination of an intrauterine pregnancy of less than 49 days' duration.

---

miglitol 863

miglitol (mi-gli-tole)
Glyset

Classification
Therapeutic: antidiabetics
Pharmacologic: alpha-glucosidase inhibitors

Pregnancy Category B

Indications
Management of non–insulin-dependent diabetes mellitus (type 2) in conjunction with dietary therapy; may be used concurrently with sulfonyl-urea oral hypoglycemic agents.

Action
Lowers blood glucose by inhibiting the enzyme alpha-glucosidase in the GI tract, resulting in delayed glucose absorption. **Therapeutic Effects:** Lowering of blood glucose in diabetic patients, especially postprandial hyperglycemia.

Pharmacokinetics
Absorption: Completely absorbed at lower doses (25 mg); 50–70% absorbed at higher doses (100 mg).
Distribution: Distributes primarily into extracellular fluid; small amounts enter breast milk.
Metabolism and Excretion: Not metabolized; action is primarily local in the GI tract; amounts that are absorbed are excreted mostly unchanged in urine.
Half-life: 2 hr.

TIME/ACTION PROFILE (effect on glucose absorption)

ROUTE	ONSET	PEAK	DURATION
PO	rapid	within 1 hr	unknown

Contraindications/Precautions
Contraindicated in: Hypersensitivity; Diabetic ketoacidosis; Inflammatory bowel disease or other chronic intestinal conditions resulting in impaired absorption or predisposition to obstruction; Lactation: Lactation.
Use Cautiously in: Patients with fever, infection, trauma, or stress (may cause hyperglycemia requiring alternate therapy); Renal impairment (use not recommended if creatinine >2 mg/dL); OB, Pedi: Safety not established.

Adverse Reactions/Side Effects
GI: <u>abdominal pain</u>, <u>diarrhea</u>, <u>flatulence</u>. **Hemat:** low serum iron.

Interactions
Drug-Drug: May ↓ absorption of **ranitidine** and **propranolol**. Effects may be ↓ by **intestinal adsorbents** (such as **charcoal**) and **digestive enzyme products**; concurrent use should be avoided.
Drug-Food: Concurrent **carbohydrates** may ↑ diarrhea.

Route/Dosage
PO (Adults): 25 mg 3 times daily; may begin with 25 mg once daily; may be ↑ up to 100 mg 3 times daily.

Availability
Tablets: 25 mg, 50 mg, 100 mg.

NURSING IMPLICATIONS

Assessment
- Observe patient for signs and symptoms of hypoglycemic reactions (sweating, hunger, weakness, dizziness, tremor, tachycardia, anxiety), especially when taking concurrently with other oral hypoglycemic agents.
- *Lab Test Considerations:* Serum glucose and glycosylated hemoglobin levels should be monitored periodically throughout therapy to evaluate effectiveness of therapy.
- ***Toxicity and Overdose:*** Symptoms of overdose are transient increase in flatulence, diarrhea, and abdominal discomfort. Miglitol alone does not cause hypoglycemia; however, other concurrently administered hypoglycemic agents may produce hypoglycemia requiring treatment. Mild hypoglycemia may be treated with administration of oral glucose.

Potential Nursing Diagnoses
Imbalanced nutrition: more than body requirements (Indications)
Noncompliance (Patient/Family Teaching)

Implementation
- Patients stabilized on a diabetic regimen who are exposed to stress, fever, trauma, infection, or surgery may require administration of insulin.
- Does not cause hypoglycemia when taken while fasting but may increase hypoglycemic effect of other hypoglycemic agents.
- **PO:** Administer miglitol 3 times daily with the first bite of each meal. Dose may be started lower and increased gradually to minimize GI effects.

Patient/Family Teaching
- Instruct patient to take miglitol at the same time each day, exactly as directed.
- Explain to patient that miglitol helps control hyperglycemia but does not cure diabetes. Therapy is usually long term.
- Encourage patient to follow prescribed diet, medication, and exercise regimen to prevent hyperglycemic or hypoglycemic episodes.
- Review signs of hypoglycemia and hyperglycemia with patient. If hypoglycemia occurs, advise patient to take a glass of orange juice, 2–3 tsp of sugar, honey, or corn syrup dissolved in water, and notify health care professional.
- Instruct patient in proper testing of blood glucose or urine ketones. These tests should be monitored closely during periods of stress or illness and health care professional notified of significant changes.
- Insulin is the recommended method of controlling blood glucose during pregnancy. Counsel female patients to use a form of contraception other than oral contraceptives and to notify health care professional promptly if pregnancy is planned or suspected.
- Advise patient to inform health care professional of medication regimen prior to treatment or surgery.
- Advise patient to carry a form of oral glucose (dextrose, D-glucose) and identification describing disease process and medication regimen at all times.
- Emphasize the importance of routine follow-up exams and regular testing of blood glucose and glycosylated hemoglobin.

Evaluation/Desired Outcomes
- Control of blood glucose levels without the appearance of hypoglycemic or hyperglycemic episodes.

---

milnacipran (mil-na-**sip**-ran)
Savella

Classification
Therapeutic: antifibromyalgia agents
Pharmacologic: selective norepinephrine reuptake inhibitors

Pregnancy Category C

Indications
Management of fibromyalgia.

Action
Inhibits neuronal reuptake of norepinephrine and serotonin. **Therapeutic Effects:** Decreased pain associated with fibromyalgia.

Pharmacokinetics

Absorption: 85–90% absorbed following oral administration.
Distribution: Unknown.
Metabolism and Excretion: Mostly excreted urine as unchanged drug (55%) and inactive metabolites.
Half-life: *D*-isomer 8–10 hr; *L*-isomer 4–6 hr.

TIME/ACTION PROFILE (decrease in pain)

ROUTE	ONSET	PEAK	DURATION
PO	1 wk	unknown	unknown

Contraindications/Precautions

Contraindicated in: Uncontrolled narrow-angle glaucoma; Concurrent use of or in close temporal proximity to MAO inhibitors; End-stage renal disease; Significant history of alcohol use/abuse; Chronic liver disease.

Use Cautiously in: History of suicide risk or attempt; History of seizures; Moderate-to-severe renal impairment; for CCr <30 mL/min reduced dose is required; Severe hepatic impairment; Obstructive uropathy (↑ risk of adverse genitourinary effects); Geri: Consider age-related decrease in renal function, chronic disease state and concurrent drug therapy; OB: Use only if clearly required during pregnancy weighing benefit to mother versus potential harm to fetus; Lactation: Potential for serious adverse reactions in infant; discontinue drug or discontinue breastfeeding; Pedi: Increased risk of suicidal thinking and behavior (suicidality) in adolescents and young adults up to 24 yrs with Major Depressive Disorder (MDD) and other psychiatric disorders.

Adverse Reactions/Side Effects

CNS: dizziness, headache, insomnia. **CV:** hypertension, tachycardia. **GI:** constipation, dry mouth, liver function abnormalities, nausea, vomiting. **Derm:** hot flushes, hyperhidrosis.

Interactions

Drug-Drug: Concurrent use with **MAO inhibitors** may result in serious, potentially fatal reactions; wait at least 14 days following discontinuation of MAO inhibitor before initiation of milnacipran. Wait at least 5 days after discontinuing milnacipran before initiation of MAO inhibitor. Concurrent use with **MAO inhibitors** may result in serious, potentially fatal reactions; wait at least 14 days following discontinuation of MAO inhibitor before initiation of milnacipran. Wait at least 5 days after discontinuing milnacipran before initiation of MAO inhibitor. Concurrent use of **serotonergic drugs** (including **triptans**, **lithium**, and **tramadol**) may ↑ the risk of serotinin syndrome; also ↑ risk of coronary vasoconstriction and hypertension. Concurrent use of **NSAIDs**, **aspirin**, or other **drugs that affect coagulation** may ↑ the risk of bleeding. May ↓ antihypertensive effectiveness of **clonidine**. ↑ risk of hypertension and arrhythmias with **epinephrine** or **norepinephrine**. ↑ risk of euphoria and hypotension when switching from **clomipramine**. Concurrent use with **digoxin** may result in adverse hemodynamics, including hypotension and tachycardia; avoid concurrent use with IV digoxin.

Route/Dosage

PO (Adults): *Day 1*—12.5 mg; *Day 2–3*—12.5 mg twice daily; *Day 4–7*—25 mg twice daily; *After Day 7*—50 mg twice daily. Some patients may be require up to 100 mg twice daily depending on response.

Renal Impairment

PO (Adults): *CCr 5–29 mL/min*—maintenance dose is 25 mg twice daily; some patients may be require up to 50 mg twice daily depending on response.

Availability

Tablets (contain tartrazine): 12.5 mg, 25 mg, 50 mg, 100 mg.

NURSING IMPLICATIONS

Assessment

- Assess intensity, quality, and location of pain periodically during therapy. May require several wk for effects to be seen.
- Monitor blood pressure and heart rate before and periodically during therapy. Treat pre-existing hypertension and cardiac disease prior to therapy. Sustained hypertension may be dose related; decrease dose or discontinue therapy if this occurs.
- Monitor closely for notable changes in behavior that could indicate the emergence or worsening of suicidal thoughts or behavior or depression.
- *Lab Test Considerations:* May cause ↑ ALT, AST, and bilirubin.

Potential Nursing Diagnoses

Chronic pain (Indications)
Risk for suicide (Adverse Reactions)

Implementation
- **PO:** May be administered without regard to meals; may be more tolerable if taken with food.

Patient/Family Teaching
- Instruct patient to take milnacipran as directed at the same time each day. Take missed doses as soon as possible unless time for next dose. Do not stop abruptly; must be decreased gradually. Advise patient to read the *Medication Guide* prior to therapy and with each Rx refill.
- Encourage patient and family to be alert for emergence of anxiety, agitation, panic attacks, insomnia, irritability, hostility, impulsivity, akathisia, hypomania, mania, worsening of depression and suicidal ideation, especially during early antidepressant therapy. Assess symptoms on a day-to-day basis as changes may be abrupt. If these symptoms occur, notify health care professional.
- May cause dizziness. Caution patient to avoid driving or other activities requiring alertness until response to medication is known.
- Advise patient to consult health care professional prior to taking any Rx, OTC, or herbal products. Avoid use of aspirin, NSAIDs, and warfarin due to increased risk for bleeding.
- Instruct patient to notify health care professional if signs of liver damage (pruritus, dark urine, jaundice, right upper quadrant tenderness, unexplained "flu-like" symptoms) or hyponatremia (headache, difficulty concentrating, memory impairment, confusion, weakness, unsteadiness) occur.
- Advise patient to avoid taking alcohol during milnacipran therapy.
- Instruct patient to notify health care professional if pregnancy is planned or suspected or if breastfeeding.
- Encourage patient to maintain routine follow-up visits with health care provider to determine effectiveness.

Evaluation/Desired Outcomes
- Reduction in pain and soreness associated with fibromyalgia.

HIGH ALERT

milnrinone (mill-ri-none)
Primacor

Classification
Therapeutic: inotropics

Pregnancy Category C

Indications
Short-term treatment of CHF unresponsive to conventional therapy with digoxin, diuretics, and vasodilators.

Action
Increases myocardial contractility. Decreases preload and afterload by a direct dilating effect on vascular smooth muscle. **Therapeutic Effects:** Increased cardiac output (inotropic effect).

Pharmacokinetics
Absorption: IV administration results in complete bioavailability.
Distribution: Unknown.
Metabolism and Excretion: 80–90% excreted unchanged by the kidneys.
Half-life: 2.3 hr (increased in renal impairment).

TIME/ACTION PROFILE (hemodynamic effects)

ROUTE	ONSET	PEAK	DURATION
IV	5–15 min	unknown	3–6 hr

Contraindications/Precautions
Contraindicated in: Hypersensitivity; Severe aortic or pulmonic valvular heart disease; Hypertrophic subaortic stenosis (may increase outflow tract obstruction).
Use Cautiously in: History of arrhythmias, electrolyte abnormalities, abnormal digoxin levels, or insertion of vascular catheters (↑ risk of ventricular arrhythmias); Renal impairment (↓ infusion rate if CCr is <50 mL/min); OB, Lactation: Pregnancy or lactation.

Adverse Reactions/Side Effects
CNS: headache, tremor. **CV:** VENTRICULAR ARRHYTHMIAS, angina pectoris, chest pain, hypotension, supraventricular arrhythmias. **CV:** skin rash. **GI:** ↑ liver function tests. **F and E:** hypokalemia. **Hemat:** thrombocytopenia.

Interactions
Drug-Drug: None significant.

Route/Dosage
IV (Adults): *Loading dose*—50 mcg/kg followed by *continuous infusion* at 0.5 mcg/kg/min (range 0.375–0.75 mcg/kg/min).
IV (Infants and Children): *Loading dose*—50 mcg/kg over 10 min followed by *continuous infusion* at 0.5 mcg/kg/min (range 0.25–0.75 mcg/kg/min).

Availability (generic available)
Injection: 1 mg/mL. **Premixed infusion:** 20 mg/100 mL, 40 mg/200 mL.

NURSING IMPLICATIONS
Assessment
- Monitor heart rate and blood pressure continuously during administration. Milrinone should be slowed or discontinued if blood pressure drops excessively.
- Monitor intake and output and daily weight. Assess patient for resolution of signs and symptoms of CHF (peripheral edema, dyspnea, rales/crackles, weight gain) and improvement in hemodynamic parameters (increase in cardiac output and cardiac index, decrease in pulmonary capillary wedge pressure). Correct effects of previous aggressive diuretic therapy to allow for optimal filling pressure.
- Monitor ECG continuously during infusion. Arrhythmias are common and may be life threatening. The risk of ventricular arrhythmias is increased in patients with a history of arrhythmias, electrolyte abnormalities, abnormal digoxin levels, or insertion of vascular catheters.
- **Lab Test Considerations:** Monitor electrolytes and renal function frequently during administration. Correct hypokalemia prior to administration to decrease the risk of arrhythmias.
- Monitor platelet count during therapy.
- ***Toxicity and Overdose: High Alert:*** Overdose manifests as hypotension. Dose should be decreased or discontinued. Supportive measures may be necessary.

Potential Nursing Diagnoses
Decreased cardiac output (Indications)

Implementation
- *High Alert:* Accidental overdose of milrinone can cause patient harm or death. Have second practitioner independently check original order, dose calculations, and infusion pump settings.

IV Administration
- **Direct IV:** *Diluent:* Loading dose may be administered undiluted. May also be diluted in 0.9% NaCl, 0.45% NaCl, or D5W for ease of administration. *Concentration:* 1 mg/mL. *Rate:* Administer the loading dose over 10 min.
- **Continuous Infusion:** *Diluent:* Milrinone drawn from vials must be diluted. Dilute 10 mg (10 mL) of milrinone in 40 mL of diluent or 20 mg (20 mL) of milrinone in 80 mL of diluent. Compatible diluents include 0.45% NaCl, 0.9% NaCl, and D5W. Premixed infusions are already diluted and ready to use. Admixed solutions are stable for 72 hr at room temperature. Stability of premixed infusions based on manufacturer's expiration date. Do not use solutions that are discolored or contain particulate matter. *Concentration:* 200 mcg/mL. *Rate:* Based on patient's weight (see Route/Dosage section). Titrate according to hemodynamic and clinical response.
- **Y-Site Compatibility:** acyclovir, amikacin, amiodarone, ampicillin, argatroban, bivalirudin, bumetanide, calcium chloride, calcium gluconate, caspofungin, cefazolin, cefepime, cefotaxime, ceftazidime, cefuroxime, cimetidine, ciprofloxacin, clindamycin, daptomycin, dexamethasone sodium phosphate, digoxin, diltiazem, dobutamine, dopamine, epinephrine, ertapenem, fenoldopam, fentanyl, gentamicin, granisetron, heparin, hydromorphone, insulin, isoproterenol, labetalol, levofloxacin, linezolid, lorazepam, magnesium sulfate, meropenem, methylprednisolone sodium succinate, metronidazole, micafungin, midazolam, morphine, nesiritide, nicardipine, nitroglycerin, nitroprusside, norepinephrine, palonosetron, pancuronium, piperacillin/tazobactam, potassium chloride, propofol, propranolol, quinupristin/dalfopristin, ranitidine, rocuronium, sodium bicarbonate, tacrolimus, theophylline, thiopental, tirofiban, tobramycin, torsemide, vancomycin, vasopressin, vecuronium, voriconazole.
- **Y-Site Incompatibility:** furosemide, imipenem/cilastatin, pantoprazole, procainamide.

Patient/Family Teaching
- Inform patient and family of reasons for administration. Milrinone is not a cure but is a temporary measure to control the symptoms of CHF.

Evaluation/Desired Outcomes
- Decrease in the signs and symptoms of CHF.
- Improvement in hemodynamic parameters.

---

minocycline, See **TETRACYCLINES.**

---

mirtazapine (meer-taz-a-peen)
Remeron, Remeron Soltabs

mirtazapine

Classification
Therapeutic: antidepressants
Pharmacologic: tetracyclic antidepressants

Pregnancy Category C

Indications
Major Depressive Disorder. **Unlabeled Use:** Panic Disorder. Generalized Anxiety Disorder (GAD). Post-traumatic Stress Disorder (PTSD).

Action
Potentiates the effects of norepinephrine and serotonin. **Therapeutic Effects:** Antidepressant action, which may develop only after several weeks.

Pharmacokinetics
Absorption: Well absorbed but rapidly metabolized, resulting in 50% bioavailability.
Distribution: Unknown.
Protein Binding: 85%.
Metabolism and Excretion: Extensively metabolized by the liver (P450 2D6, 1A2 and 3A enzymes involved); metabolites excreted in urine (75%) and feces (15%).
Half-life: 20–40 hr.

TIME/ACTION PROFILE (antidepressant effect)

ROUTE	ONSET	PEAK	DURATION
PO	1–2 wk	6 wk or more	unknown

Contraindications/Precautions
Contraindicated in: Hypersensitivity; Concurrent MAO inhibitor therapy.
Use Cautiously in: History of seizures; History of suicide attempt; May ↑ risk of suicide attempt/ideation especially during early treatment or dose adjustment; History of mania/hypomania; Patients with hepatic or renal impairment; OB: Safety not established; Lactation: Discontinue drug or bottle-feed; Pedi: Safety not established. Suicide risk may be greater in chilren or adolscents; Geri: ↑ sensitivity to CNS effects and oversedation. Begin at lower doses and titrate carefully.

Adverse Reactions/Side Effects
CNS: drowsiness, abnormal dreams, abnormal thinking, agitation, anxiety, apathy, confusion, dizziness, malaise, weakness. **EENT:** sinusitis. **Resp:** dyspnea, increased cough. **CV:** edema, hypotension, vasodilation. **GI:** constipation, dry mouth, increased appetite, abdominal pain, anorexia, elevated liver enzymes, nausea, vomiting. **GU:** urinary frequency. **Derm:** pruritus, rash. **F and E:** increased thirst. **Hemat:** AGRANULOCYTOSIS. **Metab:** weight gain, hypercholesterolemia, increased triglycerides. **MS:** arthralgia, back pain, myalgia. **Neuro:** hyperkinesia, hypesthesia, twitching. **Misc:** flu-like syndrome.

Interactions
Drug-Drug: May cause hypertension, seizures, and death when used with **MAO inhibitors**; do not use within 14 days of MAO inhibitor therapy. ↑ CNS depression with other **CNS depressants**, including **alcohol** and **benzodiazepines**. **Drugs affecting P450 enzymes, CYP2D6, CYP1A2,** and **CYP3A4** may alter the effects of mirtazapine.
Drug-Natural Products: Concomitant use of **kava-kava, valerian, skullcap, chamomile,** or **hops** can ↑ CNS depression. ↑ risk of serotinergic side effects including serotonin syndrome with **St. John's wort** and **SAMe**.

Route/Dosage
PO (Adults): 15 mg/day as a single bedtime dose initially; may be increased q 1–2 wk up to 45 mg/day.

Availability (generic available)
Tablets: 15 mg, 30 mg, 45 mg. **Cost:** *Generic*—15 mg $50.00/30, 30 mg $45.99/30, 45 mg $45.99/30. **Orally disintegrating tablets (orange flavor):** 15 mg, 30 mg, 45 mg. **Cost:** *Generic*—15 mg $70.38/30, 30 mg $65.99/30, 45 mg $71.49/30.

NURSING IMPLICATIONS

Assessment
- Assess mental status (orientation, mood, behavior) frequently. Assess for suicidal tendencies, especially during early therapy. Restrict amount of drug available to patient.
- Assess weight and BMI initially and throughout therapy.
- Monitor blood pressure and pulse rate periodically during initial therapy. Report significant changes.
- For overweight/obese individuals, obtain BFS and cholesterol levels. Refer as appropriate for nutritional/weight management and medical management.
- Monitor for seizure activity in patients with a history of seizures or alcohol abuse. Institute seizure precautions.
- *Lab Test Considerations:* Assess CBC and hepatic function before and periodically during therapy.

Potential Nursing Diagnoses
Ineffective coping (Indications)
Anxiety (Indications)
Imbalanced nutrition: risk for more than body requirements (Side Effects)

Implementation
- May be given as a single dose at bedtime to minimize excessive drowsiness or dizziness.
- May be taken without regard to food.
- For *orally disintegrating tablets*, do not attempt to push through foil backing; with dry hands, peal back backing and remove tablet. Immediately place tablet on tongue; tablet will dissolve in seconds, then swallow with saliva. Administration with liquid is not necessary.

Patient/Family Teaching
- Instruct patient to take mirtazapine as directed. Take missed doses as soon as remembered; if almost time for next dose, skip missed dose and return to regular schedule. If single bedtime dose regimen is used, do not take missed dose in morning, but consult health care professional. Do not discontinue abruptly; gradual dose reduction may be required.
- May cause drowsiness and dizziness. Caution patient to avoid driving and other activities requiring alertness until response to drug is known.
- Caution patient to change positions slowly to minimize orthostatic hypotension.
- Advise patient to avoid alcohol or other CNS depressant drugs during and for at least 3–7 days after therapy has been discontinued.
- Advise patient to notify health care professional if dry mouth, urinary retention, or constipation occurs. Frequent rinses, good oral hygiene, and sugarless candy or gum may diminish dry mouth. An increase in fluid intake, fiber, and exercise may prevent constipation.
- Inform patient of need to monitor dietary intake. Increase in appetite may lead to undesired weight gain.
- Advise patient to consult health care professional before taking any OTC cold remedies or herbal products with this medication.
- Advise patient to notify health care professional of medication regimen before treatment or surgery.
- Therapy for depression may be prolonged. Emphasize the importance of follow-up exam to monitor effectiveness and side effects.

Evaluation/Desired Outcomes
- Resolution of the symptoms of depression.
- Increased sense of well-being.
- Renewed interest in surroundings.
- Increased appetite.
- Improved energy level.
- Improved sleep.
- Therapeutic effects may be seen within 1 wk, although several wk are usually necessary before improvement is observed.

misoprostol
(mye-soe-**prost**-ole)
Cytotec

Classification
Therapeutic: antiulcer agents, cytoprotective agents
Pharmacologic: prostaglandins

Pregnancy Category X

Indications
Prevention of gastric mucosal injury from NSAIDs, including aspirin, in high-risk patients (geriatric patients, debilitated patients, or those with a history of ulcers). With mifepristone for termination of pregnancy. **Unlabeled Use:** Treatment of duodenal ulcers. Cervical ripening and labor induction.

Action
Acts as a prostaglandin analogue, decreasing gastric acid secretion (antisecretory effect) and increasing the production of protective mucus (cytoprotective effect). Causes uterine contractions. **Therapeutic Effects:** Prevention of gastric ulceration from NSAIDs. With mifepristone terminates pregnancy of less than 49 days.

Pharmacokinetics
Absorption: Well absorbed following oral administration and rapidly converted to its active form (misoprostol acid).
Distribution: Unknown.
Protein Binding: 85%.
Metabolism and Excretion: Undergoes some metabolism and is then excreted by the kidneys.
Half-life: 20–40 min.

TIME/ACTION PROFILE (effect on gastric acid secretion)

ROUTE	ONSET	PEAK	DURATION
PO	30 min	unknown	3–6 hr

Contraindications/Precautions
Contraindicated in: Hypersensitivity to prostaglandins; OB: Should not be used to prevent NSAID-induced gastric injury due to potential for fetal harm or death; Lactation: May cause severe diarrhea in the nursing infant.

Use Cautiously in: OB: Patients with childbearing potential should be counseled to avoid pregnancy during misoprostol therapy for prevention of NSAID-induced gastric injury. Pregnancy status should be determined before initiating therapy; Pedi: Safety not established in children <18 yr.
Exercise Extreme Caution in: When used for cervical ripening (unlabeled use) may cause uterine rupture (risk factors are late trimester pregnancy, previous caesarian section or uterine surgery or ≥ 5 previous pregnancies).

Adverse Reactions/Side Effects
CNS: headache. **GI:** abdominal pain, diarrhea, constipation, dyspepsia, flatulence, nausea, vomiting. **GU:** miscarriage, menstrual disorders.

Interactions
Drug-Drug: ↑ risk of diarrhea with **magnesium-containing antacids**.

Route/Dosage
PO (Adults): *Antiulcer*—200 mcg 4 times daily with or after meals and at bedtime, *or* 400 mcg twice daily, with the last dose at bedtime. If intolerance occurs, dose may be decreased to 100 mcg 4 times daily. *Termination of pregnancy*—400 mcg single dose 2 days after mifepristone if abortion has not occurred.
Intravaginally (Adults): 25 mcg (1/4 of 100-mcg tablet); may repeat q 3–6 hr, if needed.

Availability (generic available)
Tablets: 100 mcg (0.1 mg), 200 mcg (0.2 mg).
In combination with: 50 mg diclofenac/200 mcg misoprostol and 75 mg diclofenac/200 mcg misoprostol (Arthrotec). See Appendix B.

NURSING IMPLICATIONS

Assessment
- Assess patient routinely for epigastric or abdominal pain and for frank or occult blood in the stool, emesis, or gastric aspirate.
- Assess women of childbearing age for pregnancy. Misoprostol is usually begun on 2nd or 3rd day of menstrual period following a negative pregnancy test result.
- **Termination of pregnancy:** Monitor uterine cramping and bleeding during therapy.
- **Cervical Ripening:** Assess dilation of cervix periodically during therapy.

Potential Nursing Diagnoses
Acute pain (Indications)

Implementation
- Do not confuse Cytotec (misoprostol) with Cytoxan (cyclophosphamide).
- Misoprostol therapy should be started at the onset of treatment with NSAIDs.
- **PO:** Administer medication with meals and at bedtime to reduce severity of diarrhea.
- Antacids may be administered before or after misoprostol for relief of pain. Avoid those containing magnesium, because of increased diarrhea with misoprostol.

Patient/Family Teaching
- Instruct patient to take medication as directed for the full course of therapy, even if feeling better. Take missed doses as soon as possible unless next dose is due within 2 hr; do not double doses. Emphasize that sharing of this medication may be dangerous.
- Inform patient that misoprostol will cause spontaneous abortion. Women of childbearing age must be informed of this effect through verbal and written information and must use contraception throughout therapy. If pregnancy is suspected, the woman should stop taking misoprostol and immediately notify her health care professional.
- Inform patient that diarrhea may occur. Health care professional should be notified if diarrhea persists for more than 1 wk. Also advise patient to report onset of black, tarry stools or severe abdominal pain.
- Advise patient to avoid alcohol and foods that may cause an increase in GI irritation.

Evaluation/Desired Outcomes
- The prevention of gastric ulcers in patients receiving chronic NSAID therapy.
- Termination of pregnancy.
- Cervical ripening and induction of labor.

---

mitomycin (mye-toe-**mye**-sin)
Mutamycin

Classification
Therapeutic: antineoplastics
Pharmacologic: antitumor antibiotics

Pregnancy Category D

Indications
Used with other agents in the management of disseminated adenocarcinoma of the stomach or pancreas. **Unlabeled Use:** Palliative treatment of: Carcinoma of the colon or breast, Head and neck tumors, Advanced biliary, lung, and cervical squamous cell carcinomas.

Action
Primarily inhibits DNA synthesis by causing cross-linking; also inhibits RNA and protein synthesis

mitomycin

(cell-cycle phase–nonspecific but is most active in S and G phases). **Therapeutic Effects:** Death of rapidly replicating cells, particularly malignant ones.

Pharmacokinetics
Absorption: IV administration results in complete bioavailability.
Distribution: Widely distributed, concentrates in tumor tissue. Does not enter CSF.
Metabolism and Excretion: Mostly metabolized by the liver. Small amounts (<10%) excreted unchanged by the kidneys and in bile.
Half-life: 50 min.

TIME/ACTION PROFILE (effects on blood counts)

ROUTE	ONSET	PEAK	DURATION
IV	3–8 wk	4–8 wk	up to 3 mo

Contraindications/Precautions
Contraindicated in: Hypersensitivity; Pregnancy or lactation.
Use Cautiously in: Active infections; ↓ bone marrow reserve; Hepatic dysfunction; History of pulmonary problems; OB: Patients with childbearing potential should be counseled to avoid pregnancy during treatment; Geri: May have ↑ sensitivity to drug effects.

Adverse Reactions/Side Effects
Resp: PULMONARY TOXICITY. **CV:** edema. **GI:** nausea, vomiting, anorexia, stomatitis. **GU:** infertility, renal failure. **Derm:** alopecia, desquamation. **Hemat:** leukopenia, thrombocytopenia, anemia. **Local:** phlebitis at IV site. **Misc:** HEMOLYTIC UREMIC SYNDROME, fever, prolonged malaise.

Interactions
Drug-Drug: Additive bone marrow depression with other **antineoplastics** or **radiation therapy**. May ↓ antibody response to **live-virus vaccines** and ↑ risk of adverse reactions. Concurrent or sequential use with **vinca alkaloids** may result in respiratory toxicity.

Route/Dosage
IV (Adults): 20 mg/m^2 every 6–8 wk.

Availability (generic available)
Powder for injection: 5 mg/vial, 20 mg/vial, 40 mg/vial.

NURSING IMPLICATIONS
Assessment
- Monitor vital signs periodically during administration.
- Monitor for bone marrow depression. Assess for bleeding (bleeding gums, bruising, petechiae, guaiac stools, urine, and emesis) and avoid IM injections and taking rectal temperatures if platelet count is low. Apply pressure to venipuncture sites for 10 min. Assess for signs of infection during neutropenia. Anemia may occur. Monitor for increased fatigue, dyspnea, and orthostatic hypotension.
- Monitor intake and output, appetite, and nutritional intake. Nausea and vomiting usually occur within 1–2 hr. Vomiting may stop within 3–4 hr; nausea may persist for 2–3 days. Antiemetics may be administered prophylactically. Adjust diet as tolerated to help maintain fluid and electrolyte balance and nutritional status.
- Assess respiratory status and chest x-ray examination prior to and periodically throughout course of therapy. Cough, bronchospasm, hemoptysis, or dyspnea usually occurs after several doses and may be indicative of pulmonary toxicity, which may be life threatening.
- Monitor for potentially fatal hemolytic uremic syndrome in patients receiving long-term therapy. Symptoms include microangiopathic hemolytic anemia, thrombocytopenia, renal failure, and hypertension.
- **Lab Test Considerations:** Monitor CBC with differential, platelet count, and observation for fragmented RBCs on peripheral blood smears prior to and periodically throughout therapy and for several months following therapy.
- The nadirs of leukopenia and thrombocytopenia occur in 4–8 wk. Notify physician if leukocyte count is <4000/mm^3 or if platelet count is <150,000/mm^3 or is progressively declining. Recovery from leukopenia and thrombocytopenia occurs within 10 wk after cessation of therapy. Myelosuppression is cumulative and may be irreversible. Repeat courses of therapy are held until leukocyte count is >4000/mm^3 and platelet count is >100,000/mm^3.
- Monitor liver function studies (AST, ALT, LDH, bilirubin) and renal function studies (BUN, creatinine) prior to and periodically throughout therapy to detect hepatotoxicity and nephrotoxicity. Notify physician if creatinine is >1.7 mg/dL.

Potential Nursing Diagnoses
Risk for injury (Side Effects)
Risk for infection (Side Effects)
Disturbed body image (Side Effects)

Implementation
- Solution should be prepared in a biologic cabinet. Wear gloves, gown, and mask while handling medication. Discard equipment in designated containers.
- Ensure patency of IV. Extravasation may cause severe tissue necrosis. If patient complains of discomfort at IV site, discontinue immediately and restart infusion at another site. Promptly notify physician of extravasation.

IV Administration
- **Direct IV:** *Diluent:* Reconstitute 5-mg vial with 10 mL and 10-mg vial with 40 mL of sterile water for injection or 0.9% NaCl. Shake the vial; may need to stand at room temperature for additional time to dissolve. Final solution is blue-gray. Reconstituted solution is stable for 7 days at room temperature, 14 days if refrigerated. *Concentration:* Dilute drug in vial to a concentration of 0.5–1 mg/mL and then may further dilute to 20–40 mcg/mL for administration. *Rate:* May be administered IV push over 5–10 min through free-flowing IV of 0.9% NaCl or D5W.
- **Y-Site Compatibility:** amifostine, bleomycin, cisplatin, cyclophosphamide, doxorubicin, droperidol, fluorouracil, furosemide, granisetron, heparin, leucovorin, melphalan, methotrexate, metoclopramide, ondansetron, teniposide, thiotepa, vinblastine, vincristine.
- **Y-Site Incompatibility:** aztreonam, cefepime, etoposide phosphate, filgrastim, gemcitabine, piperacillin/tazobactam, sargramostim, topotecan, vinorelbine.

Patient/Family Teaching
- Instruct patient to notify health care professional promptly if fever; chills; cough; hoarseness; sore throat; signs of infection; lower back or side pain; painful or difficult urination; bleeding gums; bruising; petechiae; blood in stools, urine, or emesis; increased fatigue; dyspnea; or orthostatic hypotension occurs. Caution patient to avoid crowds and persons with known infections. Instruct patient to use soft toothbrush and electric razor and to avoid falls. Caution patient not to drink alcoholic beverages or take medication containing aspirin or NSAIDs; may precipitate gastric bleeding.
- Instruct patient to notify health care professional if decreased urine output, edema in lower extremities, shortness of breath, skin ulceration, or persistent nausea occurs.
- Instruct patient to inspect oral mucosa for redness and ulceration. If ulceration occurs, advise patient to use sponge brush and rinse mouth with water after eating and drinking. Topical agents may be used if pain interferes with eating. Stomatitis pain may require treatment with opioid analgesics.
- Discuss with patient the possibility of hair loss. Explore coping strategies.
- Advise patient that, although mitomycin may cause infertility, contraception during therapy is necessary because of teratogenic effects.
- Instruct patient not to receive any vaccinations without advice of health care professional.
- Emphasize need for periodic lab tests to monitor for side effects.

Evaluation/Desired Outcomes
- Decrease in size and spread of malignant tissue.

---

mitoxantrone
(mye-toe-**zan**-trone)
Novantrone

Classification
Therapeutic: antineoplastics, immune modifiers
Pharmacologic: antitumor antibiotics

Pregnancy Category D

Indications
Acute nonlymphocytic leukemia (ANLL) in adults (with other antineoplastics). Initial chemotherapy for patients with pain associated with advanced hormone-refractory prostate cancer. Secondary (chronic) progressive, progressive relapsing, or worsening relapsing-remitting multiple sclerosis (MS). **Unlabeled Use:** Breast cancer, liver cancer, and non-Hodgkin's lymphoma.

Action
Inhibits DNA synthesis (cell-cycle phase–nonspecific). **Therapeutic Effects:** Death of rapidly replicating cells, particularly malignant ones. Decreased pain in patients with advanced prostate cancer. Decreased disability and slowed progression of MS.

Pharmacokinetics
Absorption: IV administration results in complete bioavailability.
Distribution: Widely distributed; limited penetration of CSF.

mitoxantrone **873**

Metabolism and Excretion: Mostly eliminated by hepatobiliary clearance; <10% excreted unchanged by the kidneys.
Half-life: 5.8 days.

TIME/ACTION PROFILE (effects on blood counts)

ROUTE	ONSET	PEAK	DURATION
IV	unknown	10 days	21 days

Contraindications/Precautions
Contraindicated in: Hypersensitivity; Pregnancy or lactation.
Use Cautiously in: Previous cardiac disease; OB: Patients with childbearing potential; Active infection; ↓ bone marrow reserve; Previous mediastinal radiation; Impaired hepatobiliary function; Pedi: Safety not established; Geri: May have ↑ sensitivity to drug effects.

Adverse Reactions/Side Effects
CNS: SEIZURES, headache. **EENT:** blue-green sclera, conjunctivitis. **Resp:** cough, dyspnea. **CV:** CARDIOTOXICITY, arrhythmias, ECG changes. **GI:** abdominal pain, diarrhea, hepatic toxicity, nausea, stomatitis, vomiting. **GU:** blue-green urine, gonadal suppression, renal failure. **Derm:** alopecia, rashes. **Hemat:** anemia, leukopenia, secondary leukemia, thrombocytopenia. **Metab:** hyperuricemia. **Misc:** fever, hypersensitivity reactions.

Interactions
Drug-Drug: ↑ bone marrow depression with other **antineoplastics** or **radiation therapy**. Risk of cardiomyopathy ↑ by previous **anthracycline antineoplastics (daunorubicin, doxorubicin, idarubicin)** or **mediastinal radiation**. May ↓ antibody response to **live-virus vaccines** and ↑ risk of adverse reactions.

Route/Dosage
Acute Nonlymphatic Leukemia
IV (Adults): *Induction*— 12 mg/m² /day for 3 days (usually given with cytosine arabinoside 100 mg/m²/day for 7 days); if incomplete remission occurs, a 2nd induction may be given. *Consolidation*— 12 mg/m²/day for 2 days (usually given with cytosine arabinoside 100 mg/m²/day for 5 days), given 6 wk after induction with another course 4 wk later.

Advanced Prostate Cancer
IV (Adults): 12–14 mg/m² single dose as a short infusion (with corticosteroids).

Multiple Sclerosis
IV (Adults): 12 mg/m² q 3 mo.

Availability (generic available)
Solution for injection: 2 mg/mL.

NURSING IMPLICATIONS
Assessment
- Monitor for hypersensitivity reaction (rash, urticaria, bronchospasm, tachycardia, hypotension). If these occur, stop infusion and notify physician. Keep epinephrine, an antihistamine, and resuscitation equipment close by in the event of an anaphylactic reaction.
- Monitor for bone marrow depression. Assess for bleeding (bleeding gums, bruising, petechiae, guaiac stools, urine, and emesis) and avoid IM injections and taking rectal temperatures if platelet count is low. Apply pressure to venipuncture sites for 10 min. Assess for signs of infection during neutropenia. Anemia may occur. Monitor for increased fatigue, dyspnea, and orthostatic hypotension.
- Monitor intake and output, appetite, and nutritional intake. Assess patient for nausea and vomiting. Antiemetics may be administered prophylactically. Adjust diet as tolerated to help maintain fluid and electrolyte balance and nutritional status.
- Monitor chest x-ray, ECG, echocardiography or MUGA, and radionuclide angiography to determine ejection fraction prior to and periodically during therapy. Multiple sclerosis patients with baseline left ventricular ejection fraction (LVEF)<50% should not receive mitoxantrone. May cause cardiotoxicity, especially in patients who have received daunorubicin or doxorubicin. Assess for rales/crackles, dyspnea, edema, jugular vein distention, ECG changes, arrhythmias, and chest pain. Monitor LVEF with echocardiogram or MUGA if signs of CHF occur and prior to each dose in patients with multiple sclerosis. Potentially fatal CHF may occur during or for months or yr after therapy. Risk is greater in patients receiving a cumulative dose >140mg/m².
- Monitor for symptoms of gout (↑ uric acid levels and joint pain and swelling). Encourage patient to drink at least 2 L of fluid per day. Allopurinol may be given to decrease serum uric acid levels.

🍁 = Canadian drug name. 🧬 = Genetic implication.
*CAPITALS indicates life-threatening; underlines indicate most frequent.

- **Multiple sclerosis:** Asses frequency of exacerbations of symptoms of multiple sclerosis periodically during therapy.
- *Lab Test Considerations:* Monitor CBC with differential and platelet count prior to and periodically during therapy. The nadir of leukopenia usually occurs within 10 days, and recovery usually occurs within 21 days.
- Monitor liver function studies (AST, ALT, LDH, bilirubin) and renal function studies (BUN, creatinine) prior to and periodically during therapy to detect hepatotoxicity and nephrotoxicity.
- May cause ↑ uric acid concentrations. Monitor periodically during therapy.

Potential Nursing Diagnoses
Risk for injury (Side Effects)
Risk for infection (Side Effects)
Disturbed body image (Side Effects)

Implementation
- Solution should be prepared in a biologic cabinet. Wear gloves, gown, and mask while handling medication. Discard equipment in designated containers.
- Avoid contact with skin. Use Luer-Lok tubing to prevent accidental leakage. If contact with skin occurs, immediately wash skin with soap and water.
- Clean all spills with an aqueous solution of calcium hypochlorite. Mix solution by adding 5.5 parts (per weight) of calcium hypochlorite to 13 parts water.

IV Administration

- **IV:** Monitor IV site. If extravasation occurs, discontinue IV and restart at another site. Mitoxantrone is not a vesicant.
- **Direct IV:** *Diluent:* Dilute dark blue mitoxantrone solution in at least 50 mL of 0.9% NaCl or D5W. Discard unused solution appropriately. *Rate:* Administer slowly over at least 3 min into the tubing of a free-flowing IV of 0.9% NaCl or D5W.
- **Intermittent Infusion:** May be further diluted in D5W, 0.9% NaCl, or D5/0.9% NaCl and used immediately. *Concentration:* 0.02-0.5 mg/mL. *Rate:* Administer over 15–30 min.
- **Continuous Infusion:** May also be administered over 24 hr.
- **Y-Site Compatibility:** allopurinol, amifostine, cladribine, etoposide, etoposide phosphate, filgrastim, fludarabine, gemcitabine, granisetron, linezolid, melphalan, ondansetron, oxaliplatin, sargramostim, teniposide, thiotepa, vinorelbine.
- **Y-Site Incompatibility:** amphotericin B cholesteryl sulfate, aztreonam, cefepime, doxorubicin liposome, paclitaxel, pemetrexed, piperacillin/tazobactam, propofol.
- **Additive Compatibility:** cyclophosphamide, cytarabine, etoposide, fluorouracil, hydrocortisone sodium succinate, potassium chloride.
- **Additive Incompatibility:** heparin.

Patient/Family Teaching
- Instruct patient to notify health care professional promptly if fever; chills; cough; hoarseness; sore throat; signs of infection; lower back or side pain; painful or difficult urination; bleeding gums; bruising; petechiae; blood in stools, urine, or emesis; increased fatigue; dyspnea; or orthostatic hypotension occurs. Caution patient to avoid crowds and persons with known infections. Instruct patient to use soft toothbrush and electric razor and to avoid falls. Caution patient not to drink alcoholic beverages or take medication containing aspirin or NSAIDS; may precipitate gastric bleeding.
- Instruct patient to notify health care professional if abdominal pain, yellow skin, cough, diarrhea, or decreased urine output occurs.
- Inform patient that medication may cause the urine and sclera to turn blue-green.
- Instruct patient to inspect oral mucosa for redness and ulceration. If mouth sores occur, advise patient to use sponge brush and rinse mouth with water after eating and drinking. Topical agents may be used if pain interferes with eating. Stomatitis pain may require treatment with opioid analgesics.
- Discuss with patient the possibility of hair loss. Explore coping strategies.
- Advise patient that, although mitoxantrone may cause infertility, contraception during therapy is necessary because of possible teratogenic effects.
- Instruct patient not to receive any vaccinations without advice of health care professional.
- Emphasize need for periodic lab tests to monitor for side effects.

Evaluation/Desired Outcomes
- Decrease in the production and spread of leukemic cells.
- Decreased pain in patients with prostate cancer.
- Decrease in the frequency of relapse (neurologic dysfunction) in patients with relapsing-remitting multiple sclerosis.

modafinil (mo-daf-i-nil)
Provigil

modafinil

Classification
Therapeutic: central nervous system stimulants

Pregnancy Category C

Indications
To improve wakefulness in patients with excessive daytime drowsiness due to narcolepsy, obstructive sleep apnea, or shift work sleep disorder.

Action
Produces CNS stimulation. **Therapeutic Effects:** Decreased daytime drowsiness in patients with narcolepsy and obstructive sleep apnea. Decreased drowsiness during work in patients with shift work sleep disorder.

Pharmacokinetics
Absorption: Rapidly absorbed; bioavailability unknown.
Distribution: Well distributed; moderately (60%) bound to plasma proteins.
Metabolism and Excretion: Highly (90%) metabolized by the liver; <10% eliminated unchanged.
Half-life: 15 hr.

TIME/ACTION PROFILE (blood levels)

ROUTE	ONSET	PEAK	DURATION
PO	rapid	2–4 hr	24 hr

Contraindications/Precautions
Contraindicated in: Hypersensitivity; History of left ventricular hypertrophy or ischemic ECG changes, chest pain, arrhythmia, or other significant manifestations of mitral valve prolapse in association with CNS stimulant use.
Use Cautiously in: History of MI or unstable angina; Severe hepatic impairment with or without cirrhosis (dosage ↓ recommended); Concurrent use of MAO inhibitors; OB, Lactation, Pedi: Pregnancy, lactation, or children <16 yr (safety not established); Geri: Lower doses may be necessary due to ↑ sensitivity to drug effects.

Adverse Reactions/Side Effects
CNS: headache, amnesia, anxiety, cataplexy, confusion, depression, dizziness, insomnia, nervousness. **EENT:** rhinitis, abnormal vision, amblyopia, epistaxis, pharyngitis. **Resp:** dyspnea, lung disorder. **CV:** arrhythmias, chest pain, hypertension, hypotension, syncope, vasodilation. **GI:** nausea, ↑ liver function tests, anorexia, diarrhea, gingivitis, mouth ulcers, thirst, vomiting. **GU:** abnormal ejaculation, albuminuria, urinary retention. **Derm:** dry skin, herpes simplex. **Endo:** hyperglycemia. **Hemat:** eosinophilia. **MS:** joint disorder, neck pain. **Neuro:** ataxia, dyskinesia, hypertonia, paresthesia, tremor. **Misc:** infection.

Interactions
Drug-Drug: May ↓ the metabolism and ↑ the effects of **diazepam**, **phenytoin**, **propranolol**, or **tricyclic antidepressants** (dosage adjustments may be necessary). May ↑ the metabolism and ↓ the effects of **hormonal contraceptives**, **cyclosporine**, and **theophylline** (dosage adjustments or additional methods of contraception may be necessary).
Drug-Natural Products: Use with **caffeine-containing herbs** (**cola nut**, **guarana**, **mate**, **tea**, **coffee**) may ↑ stimulant effect.

Route/Dosage
PO (Adults): 200 mg/day as a single dose.

Hepatic Impairment
PO (Adults): *Severe hepatic impairment—100 mg/day as a single dose.*

Availability
Tablets: 100 mg, 200 mg. **Cost:** 100 mg $176.99/30, 200 mg $269.97/30.

NURSING IMPLICATIONS

Assessment
- Observe and document frequency of narcoleptic episodes.
- *Lab Test Considerations:* May cause elevated liver enzymes.

Potential Nursing Diagnoses
Disturbed thought process (Side Effects)
Deficient knowledge, related to medication regimen (Patient/Family Teaching)

Implementation
- **PO:** Administer as a single dose in the morning for patients with narcolepsy or obstructive sleep apnea. Administer 1 hour before the start of work shift for patients with shift work sleep disorder.

Patient/Family Teaching
- Instruct patient to take medication as directed.
- Medication may impair judgment. Advise patient to use caution when driving or during other activities requiring alertness.
- Nonhormonal methods of contraception should be used during and for 1 month following discontinuation of therapy. Instruct patient

= Canadian drug name. = Genetic implication.
*CAPITALS indicates life-threatening; underlines indicate most frequent.

to notify health care professional promptly if pregnancy is planned or suspected or if breastfeeding.
- Instruct patient to avoid taking other prescription or OTC medication without consulting health care professional. If alcohol is used during therapy, intake should be limited to moderate amounts.
- Instruct patient to notify physician if rash, hives, or other allergic reactions occur.

Evaluation/Desired Outcomes
- Decrease in narcoleptic symptoms and an enhanced ability to stay awake.

---

moexipril, See ANGIOTENSIN-CONVERTING ENZYME (ACE) INHIBITORS.

---

mometasone, See CORTICOSTEROIDS (INHALATION).

---

mometasone, See CORTICOSTEROIDS (NASAL).

---

mometasone, See CORTICOSTEROIDS (TOPICAL/LOCAL).

MONOAMINE OXIDASE (MAO) INHIBITORS

isocarboxazid
(eye-soe-kar-**boks**-a-zid)
Marplan

phenelzine (**fen**-el-zeen)
Nardil

tranylcypromine
(tran-ill-**sip**-roe-meen)
Parnate

Classification
Therapeutic: antidepressants
Pharmacologic: monamine oxidase (MAO) inhibitors

Pregnancy Category C

Indications
Depression in patients who have failed other modes of therapy (tricyclic antidepressants, SSRIs, SSNRIs or electroconvulsive therapy). **Unlabeled Use:** Treatment-resistant depression, panic disorder, social anxiety disorder (social phobia).

Action
Inhibit the enzyme monoamine oxidase, resulting in an accumulation of various neurotransmitters (dopamine, epinephrine, norepinephrine, and serotonin) in the body. **Therapeutic Effects:** Improved mood in depressed patients.

Pharmacokinetics
Absorption: *Phenelzine*—well absorbed from the GI tract; *isocarboxazid* and *tranylcypromine*—unknown.

Distribution: *Phenelzine* and *tranylcypromine*—cross the placenta and enter breast milk; *isocarboxazid*—unknown.

Metabolism and Excretion: *Phenelzine*—metabolized by the liver and excreted in urine as metabolites and unchanged drug; *isocarboxazid* and *tranylcypromine*-unknown.

Half-life: *Phenelzine*—12 hr; *tranylcypromine*—90–190 min; *isocarboxazid*—unknown.

TIME/ACTION PROFILE (antidepressant effect)

ROUTE	ONSET	PEAK	DURATION
Isocarboxazid	unknown	3–6 wk	unknown
Phenelzine	2–4 wk	3–6 wk	2 wk
Tranylcypromine	2 days–3 wk	2–3 wk	3–5 days

Contraindications/Precautions
Contraindicated in: Hypersensitivity; Liver disease; Severe renal disease; Cardiovascular disease; Uncontrolled hypertension; Cerebrovascular disease; Pheochromocytoma; CHF; History of severe or frequent headache; Patients undergoing elective surgery requiring anesthesia (should be discontinued at least days before surgery); Concurrent meperidine, SSRI antidepressants, SSNRI antidepressants, tricyclic antidepressants, tetracyclic antidepressants, nefazodone, trazodone, procarbazine, selegilene, linezolid, carbamazepine, cyclobenzaprine, bupropion, buspirone, sympathomimetics, dextromethorphan, narcotics, alcohol, anesthetics, diuretics, tryptophan, or antihistamines; Excessive consumption of caffeine; Concurrent use of food containing high concentrations of tyramine (see Appendix M); Lactation: Lactation.

Use Cautiously in: Patients who may be suicidal or have a history of drug dependency; Schizophrenia; Bipolar disorder; Diabetes mellitus (↑ risk of hypoglycemia); Hyperthyroidism; Seizure disorders; OB: Safety not established; Pedi: Safe use in children/adolescents not established. May ↑ risk of suicide attempt/ideation especially dur-

MONOAMINE OXIDASE (MAO) INHIBITORS

ing first early treatment or dose adjustments; risk may be greater in children or adolescents; Geri: ↑ risk of adverse reactions; begin therapy at lower end of dosage ranges.

Adverse Reactions/Side Effects
CNS: SEIZURES, dizziness, headache, anxiety, ataxia, confusion, drowsiness, euphoria, insomnia, restlessness, tremor, weakness. **EENT:** blurred vision, glaucoma, nystagmus. **CV:** HYPERTENSIVE CRISIS, arrhythmias, edema, orthostatic hypotension. **GI:** diarrhea, weight gain, abdominal pain, anorexia, constipation, dry mouth, ↑ liver function tests, nausea, vomiting. **GU:** dysuria, sexual dysfunction, urinary incontinence, urinary retention. **Derm:** pruritus, rashes. **Endo:** hypoglycemia. **MS:** arthralgia. **Neuro:** paresthesia.

Interactions
Drug-Drug: Serious, potentially fatal adverse reactions may occur with concurrent use of other **antidepressants (SSRIs, SSNRIs, buproprion, tricyclics, tetracyclics, nefazodone, trazodone), carbamazepine, cyclobenzaprine, sibutramine, linezolid, procarbazine,** or **selegiline**. Avoid using within 2 wk of each other (wait 5 wk from end of **fluoxetine** therapy). Hypertensive crisis may occur with **amphetamines, methyldopa, levodopa, dopamine, epinephrine, norepinephrine, methylphenidate, reserpine,** or **vasoconstrictors**. Hypertension or hypotension, coma, seizures, respiratory depression, and death may occur with **meperidine** (avoid using within 2–3 wk of MAO inhibitor therapy). Concurrent use with **dextromethorphan** may produce psychosis or bizarre behavior. Hypertension may occur with concurrent use of **buspirone**; avoid using within 10 days of each other. Additive hypotension may occur with **antihypertensives, spinal anesthesia, opioids,** or **barbiturates**. Additive hypoglycemia may occur with **insulins** or **oral hypoglycemic agents**. Risk of seizures may be ↑ with **tramadol**.
Drug-Natural Products: Serious, potentially fatal adverse effects (serotonin syndrome) may occur with concomitant use of **St. John's wort** and **SAMe**. Hypertensive crises may occur with large amounts of **caffeine**-containing herbs (**cola nut, guarana, malt, coffee, tea**). Insomnia, headache, tremor, hypomania may occur with **ginseng**. Hypertensive crises, disorientation, and memory impairment may occur with **tryptophan** or supplements containing **tyrosine** or **phenylalanine**.
Drug-Food: Hypertensive crisis may occur with ingestion of foods containing high concentrations of **tyramine** (see Appendix M). Consumption of foods or beverages with high **caffeine** content ↑ the risk of hypertension and arrhythmias.

Route/Dosage
Isocarboxazid
PO (Adults and Children ≥16 yr): 10 mg twice daily; may be ↑ every 2–4 days by 10 mg, up to 40 mg/day by the end of the first wk, then may ↑ by up to 20 mg every wk, up to 60 mg/day in 2–4 divided doses. After optimal response is obtained, dose should be slowly decreased to lowest effective amount (40 mg/day or less).

Phenelzine
PO (Adults): 15 mg 3 times daily; ↑ to 60–90 mg/day in divided doses; after maximal benefit achieved, gradually reduce to smallest effective dose (15 mg/day or every other day).

Tranylcypromine
PO (Adults): 30 mg/day in 2 divided doses (morning and afternoon); after 2 wk can ↑ by 10 mg/day, at 1–3 wk intervals, up to 60 mg/day.

Availability
Isocarboxazid
Tablets: 10 mg.
Phenelzine
Tablets: 15 mg.
Tranylcypromine
Tablets: 10 mg.

NURSING IMPLICATIONS
Assessment
- Assess mental status (orientation, mood, behavior) and anxiety level frequently. Assess for suicidal tendencies, especially during early therapy. Restrict amount of drug available to patient.
- Monitor blood pressure and pulse before and frequently during therapy. Report significant changes promptly. Headache is often first symptom of a hypertensive crisis.
- Monitor intake and output ratios and daily weight. Assess patient for urinary retention.
- Monitor weight and BMI initially and throughout treatment.

- For overweight/obese individuals, moitor fasting blood sugar and cholesterol levels.
- **Lab Test Considerations:** Assess hepatic function periodically during prolonged or high-dose therapy.
- Monitor serum glucose closely in diabetic patients; hypoglycemia may occur.
- ***Toxicity and Overdose:*** Concurrent ingestion of tyramine-rich foods and many medications may result in a life-threatening hypertensive crisis. Signs and symptoms of hypertensive crisis include chest pain, tachycardia, severe headache, nausea, vomiting, photosensitivity, neck stiffness, sweating, and enlarged pupils. Treatment includes IV phentolamine or a single dose of oral calcium channel blocker (nifedipine).
- Symptoms of overdose include anxiety, irritability, tachycardia, hypertension or hypotension, respiratory distress, dizziness, drowsiness, hallucinations, confusion, seizures, sluggish reflexes, fever, and diaphoresis. Treatment includes induction of vomiting or gastric lavage and supportive therapy as symptoms arise.

Potential Nursing Diagnoses
Ineffective coping (Indications)
Ineffective therapeutic regimen management (Patient/Family Teaching)
Risk for falls (Side Effects)
Imbalanced nutrition: more than body requirements (Side Effects)
Sexual dysfunction (Side Effects)
Impaired oral mucous membrane (Side Effects)

Implementation
- Do not administer these medications in the evening because the psychomotor stimulating effects may cause insomnia or other sleep disturbances.
- **PO:** Tablets may be crushed and mixed with food or fluids for patients with difficulty swallowing.

Patient/Family Teaching
- Instruct patient to take medication as directed. Take missed doses if remembered within 2 hr; otherwise, omit and return to regular dosage schedule. Do not discontinue abruptly as withdrawal symptoms (nausea, vomiting, malaise, nightmares, agitation, psychosis, seizures) may occur.
- Caution patient to avoid alcohol, CNS depressants, OTC drugs, and foods or beverages containing tyramine (see Appendix M) or excessive caffeine during and for at least 2 wk after therapy has been discontinued; they may precipitate a hypertensive crisis. Instruct patient to notify health care professional immediately if symptoms of hypertensive crisis (e.g., severe headache, palpitations, chest or throat tightness, sweating, dizziness, neck stiffness, nausea, or vomiting) develop.
- Instruct patient and caregivers to contact health care professional if child exhibits any suicidal thoughts or behaviors (e.g., worsening depression, new or worsening anxiety, agitation, panic attacks, insomnia, new or worsening irritability, violent behavior, impulsive actions, excessive talking, unusual changes in mood or behavior).
- May cause dizziness or drowsiness. Caution patient to avoid driving and other activities requiring alertness until response to medication is known.
- Caution patient to change positions slowly to minimize orthostatic hypotension. Geriatric patients are at increased risk for this side effect.
- Instruct patient to consult with health care professional before taking any new Rx, OTC, or herbal product.
- Advise patient to notify health care professional if dry mouth, urinary retention, or constipation occurs. Frequent rinses, good oral hygiene, and sugarless candy or gum may diminish dry mouth. An increase in fluid intake, fiber, and exercise may prevent constipation.
- Advise patient to notify health care professional of medication regimen before treatment or surgery. If possible, therapy should be discontinued at least 2 wk before surgery.
- Instruct patient to carry identification describing medication regimen at all times.
- Emphasize the importance of participation in psychotherapy to improve coping skills. Refer for ophthalmic testing periodically during long-term therapy.
- Advise patient of possibility of weight gain and cholesterol elevation and recommend appropriate nutritional, weight, or medical management.
- Refer patient/family to local support group.

Evaluation/Desired Outcomes
- Improved mood in depressed patients.
- Increased sense of well-being.
- Decreased anxiety.
- Increased appetite.
- Improved energy level.
- Improved sleep.
- Patients may require 3–6 wk of therapy before therapeutic effects of medication are seen.

montelukast (mon-te-loo-kast)
Singulair

Classification
Therapeutic: allergy, cold, and cough remedies, bronchodilators
Pharmacologic: leukotriene antagonists

Pregnancy Category B

Indications
Prevention and chronic treatment of asthma. Management of seasonal allergic rhinitis. Prevention of exercise-induced bronchoconstriction in patients 15 yr and older.

Action
Antagonizes the effects of leukotrienes, which mediate the following: Airway edema, Smooth muscle constriction, Altered cellular activity. Result is decreased inflammatory process, which is part of asthma and allergic rhinitis. **Therapeutic Effects:** Decreased frequency and severity of acute asthma attacks. Decreased severity of allergic rhinitis. Decreased attacks of exercise-induced bronchoconstriction.

Pharmacokinetics
Absorption: Rapidly absorbed (63–73%) following oral administration.
Distribution: Unknown.
Protein Binding: 99%.
Metabolism and Excretion: Mostly metabolized by the liver (by P450 3A4 and 2C9 enzyme systems); metabolites eliminated in feces via bile; negligible renal excretion.
Half-life: 2.7–5.5 hr.

TIME/ACTION PROFILE (improved symptoms of asthma)

ROUTE	ONSET	PEAK†	DURATION
PO (swallow)	within 24 hr	3–4 hr	24 hr
PO (chew)	within 24 hr	2–2.5 hr	24 hr

†Blood levels

Contraindications/Precautions
Contraindicated in: Hypersensitivity.
Use Cautiously in: Acute attacks of asthma; Phenylketonuria (chewable tablets contain aspartame); Hepatic impairment (may need lower doses); Reduction of corticosteroid therapy (may ↑ the risk of eosinophilic conditions); OB, Lactation, Pedi: Pregnancy, lactation, or children <1 yr (safety not established).

Adverse Reactions/Side Effects
CNS: SUICIDAL THOUGHTS, agitation, aggression, anxiety, depression, dream abnormalities, fatigue, hallucinations, headache, insomnia, irritability, restlessness, tremor, weakness. **EENT:** nosebleed, otitis (children), sinusitis (children). **Resp:** cough, rhinorrhea. **GI:** abdominal pain, diarrhea (children), dyspepsia, nausea (children), ↑ liver enzymes. **Neuro:** tremor. **Derm:** rash. **Misc:** eosinophilic conditions (including CHURG-STRAUSS SYNDROME), fever.

Interactions
Drug-Drug: Drugs which induce the CYP450 enzyme system (**phenobarbital** and **rifampin**) may ↓ the effects of montelukast.

Route/Dosage

Asthma and Allergic Rhinitis
PO (Adults and Children ≥14 yr): 10 mg once daily.
PO (Children 6–14 yr): 5 mg once daily (as chewable tablet).
PO (Children 2–5 yr): 4 mg once daily (as chewable tablet or granules).
PO (Children 6–23 months): 4 mg once daily (as oral granules).

Exercise-Induced Bronchoconstriction (EIB)
PO (Adults and Children ≥15 yrs): 10 mg at least 2 hr before exercise. Do not take within 24 hr of another dose; if taking daily doses, do not take dose for EIB.

Availability
Tablets: 10 mg. **Cost:** $302.99/90. **Chewable tablets (cherry flavor):** 4 mg, 5 mg. **Cost:** 4 mg $294.97/90, 5 mg $305.97/90. **Oral granules:** 4 mg/packet in 30-packet cartons. **Cost:** $110.00/carton.

NURSING IMPLICATIONS

Assessment
- Assess lung sounds and respiratory function prior to and periodically during therapy.
- Assess allergy symptoms (rhinitis, conjunctivitis, hives) before and periodically during therapy.
- Monitor closely for changes in behavior that could indicate the emergence or worsening of depression or suicidal thoughts.
- *Lab Test Considerations:* May cause ↑ AST and ALT concentrations.

Potential Nursing Diagnoses
Ineffective airway clearance (Indications)

Implementation
- Doses of inhaled corticosteroids may be gradually decreased with supervision of health care professional; do not discontinue abruptly.
- **PO:** For asthma, administer once daily in the evening. For allergic rhinitis, may be administered at any time of day.
- Administer granules directly into mouth or mixed in a spoonful of cold or room temperature foods (use only applesauce, mashed carrots, rice, or ice cream). Do not open packet until ready to use. After opening packet, administer full dose within 15 min. Do not store mixture. Discard unused portion. Do not dissolve granules in fluid, but fluid may be taken following administration. Granules may be administered without regard to meals.

Patient/Family Teaching
- Instruct patient to take medication daily in the evening, even if not experiencing symptoms of asthma. Do not double doses. Do not discontinue therapy without consulting health care professional.
- Instruct patient not to discontinue or reduce other asthma medications without consulting health care professional.
- Advise patient that montelukast is not used to treat acute asthma attacks, but may be continued during an acute exacerbation. Patient should carry rapid-acting therapy for bronchospasm at all times. Advise patient to notify health care professional if more than the maximum number of short-acting bronchodilator treatments prescribed for a 24-hr period are needed.
- Advise patient to notify health care professional of behavioral changes or thoughts of suicide.

Evaluation/Desired Outcomes
- Prevention of and reduction in symptoms of asthma.
- Decrease in severity of allergic rhinitis.
- Prevention of exercise-induced bronchoconstriction.

HIGH ALERT

morphine (mor-feen)
Astramorph, Astramorph PF, Avinza, DepoDur, Duramorph, Embeda, ✦ Epimorph, Infumorph, Kadian, ✦ M-Eslon, ✦ Morphine H.P, ✦ Morphitec, ✦ M.O.S, ✦ M.O.S.-S.R, MS Contin, ✦ MS • IR, MSIR, Oramorph SR, Roxanol, Roxanol Rescudose, Roxanol-T, ✦ Statex

Classification
Therapeutic: opioid analgesics
Pharmacologic: opioid agonists

Schedule II

Pregnancy Category C

Indications
Severe pain. Pulmonary edema. Pain associated with MI.

Action
Binds to opiate receptors in the CNS. Alters the perception of and response to painful stimuli while producing generalized CNS depression.
Therapeutic Effects: Decrease in severity of pain. Addition of naltrexone in *Embeda* product is designed to prevent abuse or misuse by altering the formulation. Naltrexone has no effect unless the capsule is crushed or chewed.

Pharmacokinetics
Absorption: Variably absorbed (about 30%) following oral administration. More reliably absorbed from rectal, subcut, and IM sites. Following epidural administration, systemic absorption and absorption into the intrathecal space via the meninges occurs.
Distribution: Widely distributed. Crosses the placenta; enters breast milk in small amounts.
Protein Binding: Premature infants: <20%; Adults: 35%.
Metabolism and Excretion: Mostly metabolized by the liver. Active metabolites excreted renally.
Half-life: Premature neonates: 10–20 hr; Neonates: 7.6 hr; Infants 1–3 mo: 6.2 hr; Children 6 mo–2.5 yr: 2.9 hr; Children 3–6 yr: 1–2 hr; Children 6–19 yr with sickle cell disease: 1.3 hr; Adults: 2–4 hr.

TIME/ACTION PROFILE (analgesia)

ROUTE	ONSET	PEAK	DURATION
PO	unknown	60 min	4–5 hr
PO-ER, SR	unknown	3–4 hr	8–24 hr
IM	10–30 min	30–60 min	4–5 hr
Subcut	20 min	50–90 min	4–5 hr
Rect	unknown	20–60 min	3–7 hr
IV	rapid	20 min	4–5 hr
Epidural	6–30 min	1 hr	up to 24 hr (48 hr for liposomal injection)
IT	rapid (min)	unknown	up to 24 hr

Contraindications/Precautions

Contraindicated in: Hypersensitivity; Some products contain tartrazine, bisulfites, or alcohol and should be avoided in patients with known hypersensitivity.

Use Cautiously in: Head trauma; ↑ intracranial pressure; Severe renal, hepatic, or pulmonary disease; Hypothyroidism; Adrenal insufficiency; History of substance abuse; Geri: Geriatric or debilitated patients (dose reduction suggested); Undiagnosed abdominal pain; Prostatic hyperplasia; Patients undergoing procedures that rapidly ↓ pain (cordotomy, radiation); long-acting agents should be discontinued 24 hr before and replaced with short-acting agents; OB, Lactation: Avoid chronic use; has been used during labor but may cause respiratory depression in the newborn; Pedi: Epidural liposomal injection only-not recommended; Pedi: Neonates and infants <3 mo (more susceptible to respiratory depression); Pedi: Neonates (oral solution contains sodium benzoate which can cause potentially fatal gasping syndrome).

Adverse Reactions/Side Effects

CNS: confusion, sedation, dizziness, dysphoria, euphoria, floating feeling, hallucinations, headache, unusual dreams. **EENT:** blurred vision, diplopia, miosis. **Resp:** RESPIRATORY DEPRESSION. **CV:** hypotension, bradycardia. **GI:** constipation, nausea, vomiting. **GU:** urinary retention. **Derm:** flushing, itching, sweating. **Misc:** physical dependence, psychological dependence, tolerance.

Interactions

Drug-Drug: Use with **extreme caution** in patients receiving **MAO inhibitors** within 14 days prior (may result in unpredictable, severe reactions— ↓ initial dose of morphine to 25% of usual dose). ↑ CNS depression with **alcohol, sedative/hypnotics, clomipramine, barbiturates, tricyclic antidepressants,** and **antihistamines**. Administration of **partial-antagonist opioid analgesics** may precipitate opioid withdrawal in physically dependent patients. **Buprenorphine, nalbuphine, butorphanol,** or **pentazocine** may ↓ analgesia. May ↑ the anticoagulant effect of **warfarin**. **Cimetidine** ↓ metabolism and may ↑ effects. Epidural test dose of lidocaine/epinephrine may alter release of liposomal injection.

Drug-Natural Products: Concomitant use of **kava-kava, valerian,** or **chamomile** can ↑ CNS depression.

Route/Dosage

Larger doses may be required during chronic therapy.

PO, Rect (Adults ≥50 kg): *Usual starting dose for moderate to severe pain in opioid-naive patients*—30 mg q 3–4 hr initially *or* once 24-hr opioid requirement is determined, convert to controlled-, extended-, *or* sustained-release morphine by administering total daily oral morphine dose every 24 hr (as *Kadian* or *Avinza*), 50% of the total daily oral morphine dose every 12 hr (as *Oramorph SR, Kadian, MS Contin*), or 33% of the total daily oral morphine dose every 8 hr (as *MS Contin*). See equianalgesic chart, Appendix K. *Avinza* dose should not exceed 1600 mg/day because of fumaric acid in formulation.

PO, Rect (Adults and Children <50 kg): *Usual starting dose for moderate to severe pain in opioid-naive patients*—0.3 mg/kg q 3–4 hr initially.

PO (Children >1 mo): *Prompt-release tablets and solution*—0.2–0.5 mg/kg/dose q 4–6 hr as needed. *Controlled-release tablet*—0.3–0.6 mg/kg/dose q 12 hr.

IM, IV, Subcut (Adults ≥50 kg): *Usual starting dose for moderate to severe pain in opioid-naive patients*—4–10 mg q 3–4 hr. *MI*—8–15 mg, for very severe pain additional smaller doses may be given every 3–4 hr.

IM, IV, Subcut (Adults and Children <50 kg): *Usual starting dose for moderate to severe pain in opioid-naive patients*—0.05–0.2 mg/kg q 3–4 hr, maximum: 15 mg/dose.

IM, IV, Subcut (Neonates): 0.05 mg/kg q 4–8 hr, maximum dose: 0.1 mg/kg. Use preservative-free formulation.

IV, Subcut (Adults): *Continuous infusion*—0.8–10 mg/hr; may be preceded by a bolus of 15 mg (infusion rates vary greatly; up to 400 mg/hr have been used).

IV, Subcut (Children >1 mo): *Continuous infusion, postoperative pain*—0.01–0.04 mg/kg/hr. *Continuous infusion, sickle cell or cancer pain*—0.02–2.6 mg/kg/hr.

IV (Neonates): *Continuous infusion*—0.01–0.03 mg/kg/hr.

Epidural (Adults): *Intermittent injection*—5 mg/day (initially); if relief is not obtained at 60 min, 1–2 mg increments may be made; (total dose not to exceed 10 mg/day). *Continuous infusion*—2–4 mg/24 hr; may increase by 1–2 mg/day (up to 30 mg/day); *single-dose extended-*

release liposomal injection—lower extremity orthopedic surgery: 15 mg, lower abdominal/pelvic surgery: 10–15 mg, cesarean section: 10 mg. Use preservative-free formulation.
Epidural (Children >1 mo): 0.03–0.05 mg/kg, maximum dose: 0.1 mg/kg or 5 mg/24 hr. Use preservative-free formulation.
IT (Adults): 0.2–1 mg. Use preservative-free formulation.

Availability (generic available)
Soluble tablets: 10 mg, 15 mg, 30 mg. **Tablets:** 15 mg, 30 mg. **Cost:** *MSIR*—15 mg $18.32/100, 30 mg $31.22/100. **Extended (controlled, sustained)-release tablets:** 15 mg, 30 mg, 60 mg, 100 mg, 200 mg. **Cost:** *MS Contin*—15 mg $99.63/100, 30 mg $189.34/100, 60 mg $369.44/100, 100 mg $546.99/100, 200 mg $1001.71/100; *Oramorph SR*—15 mg $90.03/100, 30 mg $171.09/100, 60 mg $333.83/100, 100 mg $511.24/100. **Sustained-release capsules (Kadian):** 10 mg, 20 mg, 30 mg, 50 mg, 60 mg, 80 mg, 200 mg. **Cost:** *Kadian*—20 mg $105.49/60, 30 mg $119.00/60, 50 mg $223.05/60, 60 mg $227.39/60, 100 mg $383.80/60. **Extended-release capsules (Avinza):** 30 mg, 60 mg, 90 mg, 120 mg. **Cost:** *Avinza*—30 mg $231.00/100, 60 mg $445.00/100, 90 mg $675.00/100, 120 mg $790.00/100. **Oral solution (Roxanol-T—20 mg/mL fruit and mint flavor; also unflavored):** 10 mg/5 mL, 20 mg/5 mL, 100 mg/5 mL, ✽ 2 mg/mL, ✽ 4 mg/mL, 20 mg/mL (concentrate). **Cost:** *Roxanol*—20 mg/mL $20.76/30 mL. **Rectal suppositories:** 5 mg, 10 mg, 20 mg, 30 mg. **Solution for IM, subcut, IV injection:** 1 mg/mL, 2 mg/mL, 4 mg/mL, 5 mg/mL, 8 mg/mL, 10 mg/mL, 15 mg/mL, 25 mg/mL, 50 mg/mL. **Solution for epidural, IV injection (preservative-free):** 0.5 mg/mL, 1 mg/mL. **Solution for epidural or IT use (continuous microinfusion device; preservative-free):** 10 mg/mL in 20-mL vial, 25 mg/mL in 20-mL vial. **Extended-release liposome injection for epidural use:** 10 mg/mL in 1–, 2.5– and 2-mL vials. **Solution for IV injection (PCA device):** 1 mg/mL, 2 mg/mL, 3 mg/mL, 5 mg/mL.

NURSING IMPLICATIONS
Assessment
- Assess type, location, and intensity of pain prior to and 1 hr following PO, subcut, IM, and 20 min (peak) following IV administration. When titrating opioid doses, increases of 25–50% should be administered until there is either a 50% reduction in the patient's pain rating on a numerical or visual analogue scale or the patient reports satisfactory pain relief. When titrating doses of short-acting morphine, a repeat dose can be safely administered at the time of the peak if previous dose is ineffective and side effects are minimal.
- Patients on a continuous infusion should have additional bolus doses provided every 15–30 min, as needed, for breakthrough pain. The bolus dose is usually set to the amount of drug infused each hour by continuous infusion.
- Patients taking sustained-release morphine may require additional short-acting opioid doses for breakthrough pain. Doses should be equivalent to 10–20% of 24 hr total and given every 2 hr as needed.
- An equianalgesic chart (see Appendix K) should be used when changing routes or when changing from one opioid to another.
- *High Alert:* Assess level of consciousness, blood pressure, pulse, and respirations before and periodically during administration. If respiratory rate is <10/min, assess level of sedation. Physical stimulation may be sufficient to prevent significant hypoventilation. Subsequent doses may need to be decreased by 25–50%. Initial drowsiness will diminish with continued use. Geri: Assess geriatric patients frequently; older adults are more sensitive to the effects of opioid analgesics and may experience side effects and respiratory complications more frequently. Pedi: Assess pediatric patient frequently; children are more sensitive to the effects of opioid analgesics and may experience respiratory complications, excitability and restlessness more frequently.
- Prolonged use may lead to physical and psychological dependence and tolerance. This should not prevent patient from receiving adequate analgesia. Most patients who receive morphine for pain do not develop psychological dependence. Progressively higher doses may be required to relieve pain with long-term therapy.
- Assess bowel function routinely. Institute prevention of constipation with increased intake of fluids and bulk and with laxatives to minimize constipating effects. Administer stimulant laxatives routinely if opioid use exceeds 2–3 days, unless contraindicated.
- *Lab Test Considerations:* May ↑ plasma amylase and lipase levels.
- *Toxicity and Overdose:* If an opioid antagonist is required to reverse respiratory depression or coma, naloxone (Narcan) is the anti-

dote. Dilute the 0.4-mg ampule of naloxone in 10 mL of 0.9% NaCl and administer 0.5 mL (0.02 mg) by direct IV push every 2 min. For children and adults weighing <40 kg, dilute 0.1 mg of naloxone in 10 mL of 0.9% NaCl for a concentration of 10 mcg/mL and administer 0.5 mcg/kg every 2 min. Titrate dose to avoid withdrawal, seizures, and severe pain.

Potential Nursing Diagnoses
Acute pain (Indications)
Disturbed sensory perception (visual, auditory) (Side Effects)
Risk for injury (Side Effects)

Implementation
- **High Alert:** Do not confuse morphine with hydromorphone or meperidine—errors have resulted in death. Other errors associated with morphine include overdose and infusion pump miscalculations, especially in children. Consider patients' previous analgesic use and current requirements, but clarify doses that greatly exceed normal range. Have second practitioner independently check original order, dose calculations, and infusion pump settings. Use only preservative-free formulations in neonates, and for epidural and intrathecal routes in all patients.
- Explain therapeutic value of medication prior to administration to enhance the analgesic effect.
- Regularly administered doses may be more effective than prn administration. Analgesic is more effective if given before pain becomes severe.
- Coadministration with nonopioid analgesics may have additive analgesic effects and may permit lower doses.
- When transferring from other opioids or other forms of morphine to extended-release tablets, administer a total daily dose of oral morphine equivalent to previous daily dose (see Appendix K) and divided every 8 hr (MS Contin), every 12 hr (Embeda, Kadian, MS Contin, Oramorph SR), every 24 hr (Kadian or Avinza).
- Morphine should be discontinued gradually to prevent withdrawal symptoms after long-term use.
- **PO:** Doses may be administered with food or milk to minimize GI irritation.
- Administer oral solution with properly calibrated measuring device; may be diluted in a glass of fruit juice just prior to administration to improve taste.
- Extended-release and controlled-release tablets should be swallowed whole; do not break, crush, dissolve, or chew (could result in rapid release and absorption of a potentially toxic dose).
- *Embeda, Kadian, and Avinza* capsules may be opened and the pellets sprinkled onto applesauce immediately prior to administration. Patients should rinse mouth and swallow to assure ingestion of entire dose. Pellets should not be chewed, crushed, or dissolved. *Kadian* capsules may also be opened and sprinkled on approximately 10 mL of water and flushed while swirling through a pre-wetted 16 French gastrostomy tube fitted with a funnel at the port end. Additional water should be used to transfer and flush any remaining pellets. *Kadian* should not be administered via a nasogastric tube.
- **Rect:** *MS Contin* and *Oramorph SR* have been administered rectally.
- **IM, Subcut:** Use IM route for repeated doses, because morphine is irritating to subcut tissues.

IV Administration
- **IV:** Solution is colorless; do not administer discolored solution.
- **Direct IV:** *Diluent:* Dilute with at least 5 mL of sterile water or 0.9% NaCl for injection. *Concentration:* 0.5–5 mg/mL. *Rate:* **High Alert:** Administer 2.5–15 mg over 5 min. Rapid administration may lead to increased respiratory depression, hypotension, and circulatory collapse.
- **Continuous Infusion:** *Diluent:* May be added to D5W, D10W, 0.9% NaCl, 0.45% NaCl, Ringer's or LR, dextrose/saline solution, or dextrose/Ringer's or LR. *Concentration:* 0.1–1 mg/mL or greater for continuous infusion. *Rate:* Administer via infusion pump to control the rate. Dose should be titrated to ensure adequate pain relief without excessive sedation, respiratory depression, or hypotension. May be administered via patient-controlled analgesia (PCA) pump.
- **Syringe Compatibility:** alfentanil, alprostadil, atropine, bupivacaine, caffeine citrate, chlorpromazine, cimetidine, clonidine, diphenhydramine, droperidol, fentanyl, glycopyrrolate, hydroxyzine, ketamine, lidocaine, metoclopra-

mide, milrinone, ondansetron, perphenazine, promazine, ranitidine, salbutamol, scopolamine, ziconatide.
- **Syringe Incompatibility:** meperidine, pantoprazole, thiopental.
- **Y-Site Compatibility:** aldesleukin, alfentanyl, allopurinol, amifostine, amikacin, aminophylline, amiodarone, amsacrine, anikinra, anidulafungin, argatroban, ascorbic acid, atracurium, atropine, aztreonam, bivalirudin, bumetanide, calcium chloride, calcium gluconate, carboplatin, caspofungin, cefazolin, cefonocid, cefotaxime, cefotetan, cefoxitin, ceftazidime, ceftizoxime, ceftriaxone, cefuroxime, chloramphenicol, chlorpromazine, cimetidine, cisatracurium, cladribine, clindamycin, cyanocobalamin, cyclophosphamide, cyclosporine, cytarabine, dactinomycin, daptomycin, dexamethasone, dexmedetomidine, digoxin, diltiazem, diphenhydramine, dobutamine, docetaxel, dopamine, doripemen, doxacurium, doxorubicin, doxycycline, enalaprilat, ephedrine, epinephrine, epirubicin, epoetin alfa, eftifibatide, ertapenem, erythromycin, esmolol, etomidate, etoposide, etoposide phosphate, famotidine, fenoldopam, fentanyl, filgrastim, fluconazole, fludarabine, fluorouracil, foscarnet, gemcitabine, gentamicin, glycopyrrolate, granisetron, heparin, hetastarch, hydrocortisone, hydromorphone, idarubicin, ifosfamide, imipenem/cilastatin, isoproterenol, kanamycin, ketorolac, labetalol, levofloxacin, lidocaine, linezolid, lorazepam, magnesium sulfate, mannitol, melphalan, meperidine, meropenem, metaraminol, methotrexate, methyldopate, methylprednisolone, metoclopramide, metoprolol, metronidazole, midazolam, milrinone, mitoxantrone, multivitamins, nafcillin, naloxone, nicardipine, nitroglycerin, nitroprusside, norepinephrine, octreotide, ondansetron, oxacillin, oxaliplatin, oxytocin, paclitaxel, palonosetron, pancuronium, pemetrexed, penicillin G, phenobarbital, phentolamine, phenylephrine, phytonadione, piperacillin/tazobactam, potassium chloride, procainamide, prochlorperazine, promethazine, propranolol, protamine, pyridoxine, quniupristin/dalfopristin, ranitidine, remifentanil, rituximab, rocuronium, scopolamine, sodium acetate, sodium bicarbonate, streptokinase, succinylcholine, sufentanil, tacrolimus, teniposide, theophylline, thiamine, thiotepa, ticarcillin/clavulanate, tigecycline, tirofiban, tobramycin, tolazoline, trtimetaphan, trimethoprim/sulfamethoxazole, vancomycin, vasopressin, vecuronium, verapamil, vincristine, vinorelbine, vitamin B complex with C, voriconazole, warfarin, zidovudine.
- **Y-Site Incompatibility:** amphotericin B cholesteryl, amphotericin B colloidal, amphotericin B liposome, azathioprine, azithromycin, dantrolene, diazoxide, doxorubicin liposome, folic acid, ganciclovir, inamrinone, indomethacin, micafungin, pentobarbital, phenytoin, sargramostim, trastuzumab.
- **Epidural:** Invert vial gently to re-suspend liposomal product immediately prior to administration; do not shake. Administer undiluted. If a lidocaine test dose is administered, flush catheter with 0.9% NaCl and wait 15 min before administration of *DepoDur*. Do not use an in-lint filter. Do not admix or administer other medications in epidural space for 48 hr after administration. Administer within 4 hr after removing from vial. Store in refrigerator; do not freeze.

Patient/Family Teaching
- Instruct patient how and when to ask for pain medication.
- **High Alert:** Instruct family not to administer PCA doses to the sleeping patient. Overmedication, sedation, and respiratory depression can result.
- May cause drowsiness or dizziness. Caution patient to call for assistance when ambulating or smoking and to avoid driving or other activities requiring alertness until response to medication is known.
- Advise patient to change positions slowly to minimize orthostatic hypotension.
- Caution patient to avoid concurrent use of alcohol or other CNS depressants with this medication.
- Encourage patients who are immobilized or on prolonged bedrest to turn, cough, and breathe deeply every 2 hr to prevent atelectasis.
- **Home Care Issues: High Alert:** Explain to patient and family how and when to administer morphine and how to care for infusion equipment properly. Pedi: Teach parents or caregivers how to accurately measure liquid medication and to use only the measuring device dispensed with the medication.
- Emphasize the importance of aggressive prevention of constipation with the use of morphine.

Evaluation/Desired Outcomes
- Decrease in severity of pain without a significant alteration in level of consciousness or respiratory status.
- Decrease in symptoms of pulmonary edema.

mupirocin (myoo-**peer**-oh-sin)
Bactroban, Bactroban Nasal

Classification
Therapeutic: anti-infectives

Pregnancy Category B

Indications
Topical: Treatment of: Impetigo, Secondarily infected traumatic skin lesions (up to 10 cm in length or 100 cm² area) caused by *Staphylococcus aureus* and *Streptococcus pyogenes*. **Intranasal:** Eradicates nasal colonization with methicillin-resistant *S. aureus*.

Action
Inhibits bacterial protein synthesis. **Therapeutic Effects:** Inhibition of bacterial growth and reproduction. **Spectrum:** Greatest activity against gram-positive organisms, including: *S. aureus*, Beta-hemolytic streptococci. Resolution of impetigo. Eradication of *S. aureus* carrier state.

Pharmacokinetics
Absorption: Minimal systemic absorption.
Distribution: Remains in the stratum corneum after topical use for prolonged periods of time (72 hr).
Metabolism and Excretion: Metabolized in the skin, removed by desquamation.
Half-life: 17–36 min.

TIME/ACTION PROFILE (anti-infective effect)

ROUTE	ONSET	PEAK	DURATION
Nasal	unknown	unknown	12 hr
Topical†	unknown	3–5 days	72 hr

†Resolution of lesions

Contraindications/Precautions
Contraindicated in: Hypersensitivity to mupirocin or polyethylene glycol.
Use Cautiously in: Impaired renal function; Burn patients; OB, Lactation: Safety not established.

Adverse Reactions/Side Effects
CNS: *nasal only*—headache. **EENT:** *nasal only*—cough, itching, pharyngitis, rhinitis, upper respiratory tract congestion. **GI:** nausea; *nasal only*, altered taste. **Derm:** *topical only*—burning, itching, pain, stinging.

Interactions
Drug-Drug: Nasal mupirocin should not be used concurrently with other **nasal products**.

Route/Dosage
Topical (Adults and Children ≥2 mo): Ointment: Apply 3–5 times daily for 5–14 days.
Topical (Adults and Children ≥3 mo): Cream: Apply small amount 3 times/day for 10 days.
Intranasal (Adults and Children ≥1 yr): Apply small amount nasal ointment to each nostril 2–4 times/day for 5–14 days.

Availability (generic available)
Ointment: 2%. Cost: *Generic*—$34.99/22 g.
Cream: 2%. Cost: $47.99/15 g, $77.13/30 g. **Nasal ointment:** 2% in 1-g single-use tubes.

NURSING IMPLICATIONS

Assessment
- Assess lesions before and daily during therapy.

Potential Nursing Diagnoses
Impaired skin integrity (Indications)
Risk for infection (Indications, Patient/Family Teaching)

Implementation
- **Topical:** Wash affected area with soap and water and dry thoroughly. Apply a small amount of mupirocin to the affected area 3 times daily and rub in gently. Treated area may be covered with gauze if desired.
- **Nasal:** Apply one half of the ointment from the single-use tube to each nostril twice daily (morning and evening) for 5 days. After application, close nostrils by pressing together and releasing sides of the nose repeatedly for 1 min.

Patient/Family Teaching
- Instruct patient on the correct application of mupirocin. Advise patient to apply medication exactly as directed for the full course of therapy. If a dose is missed, apply as soon as possible unless almost time for next dose. Avoid contact with eyes.
- **Topical:** Teach patient and family appropriate hygienic measures to prevent spread of impetigo.
- Instruct parents to notify school nurse for screening and prevention of transmission.
- Patient should consult health care professional if symptoms have not improved in 3–5 days.

Evaluation/Desired Outcomes
- Healing of skin lesions. If no clinical response is seen in 3–5 days, condition should be re-evaluated.
- Eradication of methicillin-resistant *S. aureus* carrier state in patients and health care workers during institutional outbreaks.

muromonab-CD3
(myoo-roe-**moe**-nab CD3)
Orthoclone OKT3

Classification
Therapeutic: immunosuppressants
Pharmacologic: monoclonal antibodies

Pregnancy Category C

Indications
Acute renal allograft rejection reactions in transplant patients that have occurred despite conventional antirejection therapy. Acute corticosteroid-resistant hepatic or cardiac allograft rejection reactions.

Action
A purified immunoglobulin antibody that acts as an immunosuppressant by interfering with normal T-cell function. **Therapeutic Effects:** Reversal of graft rejection in transplant patients.

Pharmacokinetics
Absorption: Administered IV only, resulting in complete bioavailability.
Distribution: Unknown.
Metabolism and Excretion: Eliminated by binding to T lymphocytes.
Half-life: 18 hr.

TIME/ACTION PROFILE (noted as levels of circulating CD3-positive T cells)

ROUTE	ONSET	PEAK	DURATION
IV	mins	2–7 days	1 wk

Contraindications/Precautions
Contraindicated in: Hypersensitivity to muromonab-CD3, murine (mouse) proteins, or polysorbate; Previous muromonab therapy; Fluid overload; Fever >37.8°C or 100°F; Chickenpox or recent exposure to chickenpox; Herpes zoster.
Use Cautiously in: Active infections; Depressed bone marrow reserve; Chronic debilitating illnesses; CHF; OB, Lactation, Pedi: Pregnancy, lactation, or children <2 yr (safety not established).

Adverse Reactions/Side Effects
CNS: tremor, aseptic meningitis, dizziness. **Resp:** PULMONARY EDEMA, dyspnea, shortness of breath, wheezing. **CV:** chest pain. **GI:** diarrhea, nausea, vomiting. **Misc:** CYTOKINE RELEASE SYNDROME, INFECTIONS, chills, fever, hypersensitivity reactions, ↑ risk of lymphoma.

Interactions
Drug-Drug: Additive immunosuppression with other **immunosuppressives**. Concurrent **prednisone** and **azathioprine** dosages should be ↓ during muromonab therapy (↑ risk of infection and lymphoproliferative disorders). **Cyclosporine** should be ↓ or discontinued during muromonab-CD3 therapy (↑ risk of infection and lymphoproliferative disorders). ↑ risk of adverse CNS reactions with **indomethacin**. May ↓ antibody response to and ↑ risk of adverse reactions from **live-virus vaccines**.
Drug-Natural Products: Concomitant use with **astragalus**, **echinacea**, and **melatonin** may interfere with immunosuppression.

Route/Dosage
IV (Adults): 5 mg/day for 10–14 days (pretreatment with corticosteroids, acetaminophen, and/or antihistamines recommended).
IV (Children): 0.1 mg (100 mcg)/kg/day for 10–14 days.

Availability
Solution for injection: 1 mg/mL.

NURSING IMPLICATIONS
Assessment
- Assess for fluid overload (monitor weight and intake and output, assess for edema and rales/crackles). Notify health care professional if patient has experienced 3% or more weight gain in the previous week. Chest x-ray examination should be obtained within 24 hr before beginning therapy. Fluid-overloaded patients are at high risk of developing pulmonary edema. Monitor vital signs and breath sounds closely.
- Assess for cytokine release syndrome (CRS), usually manifested by high fever and chills, headache, tremor, nausea and vomiting, chest pain, muscle and joint pain, generalized weakness, shortness of breath, dizziness, abdominal pain, malaise, diarrhea, and trembling of hands, but may occasionally cause a severe, life-threatening, shock-like reaction. The severity of this reaction is greatest with initial dose. Reaction occurs within 30–48 hr and may persist for up to 6 hr. Acetaminophen and antihistamines may be used to treat early reactions.

Patient temperature should be maintained below 37.8°C (100°F) at administration of each dose. Manifestations of CRS may be prevented or minimized by pretreatment with methylprednisolone sodium succinate 8 mg/kg IV given 1–4 hr before 1st dose of muromonab-CD3. Hydrocortisone 100 mg IV may also be given 30 min after the 1st and possibly 2nd dose to control respiratory side effects. Serious symptoms of CRS may require oxygen, IV fluids, corticosteroids, vasopressors, antihistamines, and intubation.
- Monitor for signs of anaphylactic or hypersensitivity reactions at each dose. Resuscitation equipment should be readily available.
- Monitor for infection (fever, chills, rash, sore throat, purulent discharge, dysuria). Notify physician immediately if these symptoms occur; may necessitate discontinuation of therapy.
- Monitor for development of aseptic meningitis. Onset is usually within 3 days of beginning therapy. Assess for fever, headache, nuchal rigidity, and photophobia.
- ***Lab Test Considerations:*** Monitor CBC with differential and platelet count before and periodically throughout therapy.
- Monitor assays of T cells (CD3, CD4, CD8); target CD3 is <25 cells/mm³ or plasma levels as determined by ELISA daily; target levels should be ≥800 ng/mL.
- Monitor BUN, serum creatinine, and hepatic enzymes (AST, ALT, alkaline phosphatase, bilirubin), especially during the first 1–3 days of therapy. May cause transient ↑.

Potential Nursing Diagnoses
Risk for infection (Side Effects)
Excess fluid volume (Side Effects)

Implementation
- Physician will reduce dose of corticosteroids and azathioprine and discontinue cyclosporine during 10–14-day course of muromonab-CD3. Cyclosporine may be resumed 3 days before end of therapy.
- Initial dose is administered during hospitalization; patient should be monitored closely for 48 hr. Subsequent doses may be administered on outpatient basis.
- Keep medication refrigerated at 2–8°C. Do not shake vial. Solution may contain a few fine translucent particles that do not affect potency. Discard unused portion.

IV Administration
- **Direct IV:** Draw solution into syringe via low-protein-binding 0.2- or 0.22-micrometer filter to ensure removal of translucent protein particles that may be present. Discard filter and attach 20-gauge needle for IV administration. ***Concentration:*** 1 mg/mL (undiluted). ***Rate:*** Administer IV push over <1 min. Do not administer as an infusion.
- **Y-Site Incompatibility:** Do not admix; do not administer in IV line containing other medications. If line must be used for other medications, flush with 0.9% NaCl before and after muromonab-CD3.

Patient/Family Teaching
- Explain purpose of medication to patient. Inform patient of possible initial-dose side effects, which are markedly reduced in subsequent doses. Explain that patient will need to resume lifelong therapy with other immunosuppressive drugs after completion of muromonab-CD3 course.
- Inform patient of potential for CRS. Describe reportable symptoms.
- Instruct patient to continue to avoid crowds and persons with known infections, as this drug also suppresses the immune system.
- Advise patient to notify health care professional at first sign of rash, urticaria, tachycardia, dyspnea, or difficulty swallowing.
- May cause dizziness. Caution patient to avoid driving or other activities requiring alertness until response is known.
- Instruct patient not to receive any vaccinations and to avoid contact with persons receiving oral polio vaccine without advice of health care professional.

Evaluation/Desired Outcomes
- Reversal of the symptoms of acute organ rejection.

---

mycophenolate mofetil
(mye-koe-**fee**-noe-late **moe**-fe-til)
CellCept

mycophenolic acid
(mye-koe-**fee**-noe-lik)
Myfortic

♦ = Canadian drug name. = Genetic implication.
*CAPITALS indicates life-threatening; underlines indicate most frequent.

mycophenolate mofetil

Classification
Therapeutic: immunosuppressants

Pregnancy Category D

Indications
Mycophenolate mofetil: Prevention of rejection in allogenic renal, hepatic, and cardiac transplantation (used concurrently with cyclosporine and corticosteroids). **Mycophenolic acid**: Prevention of rejection in allogenic renal transplantation (used concurrently with cyclosporine and corticosteroids).

Action
Inhibits the enzyme inosine monophosphate dehydrogenase, which is involved in purine synthesis. This inhibition results in suppression of T- and B-lymphocyte proliferation. **Therapeutic Effects:** Prevention of heart, kidney, or liver transplant rejection.

Pharmacokinetics
Absorption: Following oral and IV administration, mycophenolate mofetil is rapidly hydrolyzed to mycophenolic acid (MPA), the active metabolite. Absorption of enteric-coated mycophenolic acid (Myfortic) is delayed compared with mycophenolate mofetil (CellCept).
Distribution: Cross the placenta and enter breast milk.
Protein Binding: *MPA*—97%.
Metabolism and Excretion: MPA is extensively metabolized; <1% excreted unchanged in urine. Some enterohepatic recirculation of MPA occurs.
Half-life: *MPA*—8–18 hr.

TIME/ACTION PROFILE (blood levels of MPA)

ROUTE	ONSET	PEAK	DURATION
mycophenolate mofetil-PO	rapid	0.25–1.25 hr	N/A
mycophenolic acid	rapid	1.5–2.75 hr	N/A

Contraindications/Precautions
Contraindicated in: Hypersensitivity; Hypersensitivity to polysorbate 80 (for IV mycophenolate mofetil); OB, Lactation: ↑ risk of congenital anomalies or spontaneous abortion.
Use Cautiously in: Active serious pathology of the GI tract (including history of ulcer disease or GI bleeding); Phenylketonuria (oral suspension contains aspartame); Severe chronic renal impairment (dose not to exceed 1 g twice daily (CellCept) if CCr <25 mL/min/1.73 m^2); careful monitoring recommended; Delayed graft function following transplantation (observe for increased toxicity); Geri: ↑ risk of adverse reactions related to immunosuppression; OB: Patients with childbearing potential; Pedi: Mycophenolate mofetil approved in children ≥3 mo for renal transplant; mycophenolic acid approved in children ≥5 yr for renal transplant; safety not established for other age groups.

Adverse Reactions/Side Effects
CNS: PROGRESSIVE MULTIFOCAL LEUKOENCEPHALOPATHY, anxiety, dizziness, headache, insomnia, paresthesia, tremor. **CV:** edema, hypertension, hypotension, tachycardia. **Derm:** rashes. **Endo:** hypercholesterolemia, hyperglycemia, hyperkalemia, hypocalcemia, hypokalemia, hypomagnesemia. **GI:** GI BLEEDING, anorexia, constipation, diarrhea, nausea, vomiting, abdominal pain. **GU:** renal dysfunction. **Hemat:** leukocytosis, leukopenia, thrombocytopenia, anemia, pure red cell aplasia. **Resp:** cough, dyspnea. **Misc:** fever, infection (including activation of latent viral infections such as BK virus-associated nephropathy), ↑ risk of malignancy.

Interactions
Drug-Drug: Combined use with **azathioprine** is not recommended (effects unknown). **Acyclovir** and **ganciclovir** compete with MPA for renal excretion and, in patients with renal dysfunction, may ↑ each other's toxicity. **Magnesium and aluminum hydroxide** antacids ↓ the absorption of MPA (avoid simultaneous administration). **Cholestyramine** and **colestipol** ↓ the absorption of MPA (avoid concurrent use). May interfere with the action of **oral contraceptives** (additional contraceptive method should be used). May ↓ the antibody response to and ↑ risk of adverse reactions from **live-virus vaccines**, although influenza vaccine may be useful. **Amoxicillin/clavulanic acid** or **ciprofloxacin** may ↓ MPA trough levels.
Drug-Food: When administered with food, peak blood levels of MPA are significantly ↓ (should be administered on an empty stomach).

Route/Dosage

Mycophenolate Mofetil (CellCept)

Renal Transplantation
PO, IV (Adults): 1 g twice daily; IV should be started ≤24 hr after transplantation and switched to PO as soon as possible (IV not recommended for ≥14 days).

mycophenolate mofetil

PO (Children 3 mo–18 yr): 600 mg/m² twice daily (not to exceed 2 g/day).

Hepatic Transplantation
PO, IV (Adults): 1 g twice daily IV, or 1.5 g twice daily PO. IV should be started ≤24 hr after transplantation and switched to PO as soon as possible (IV not recommended for ≥14 days).

Cardiac Transplantation
PO, IV (Adults): 1.5 g twice daily; IV should be started ≤24 hr after transplantation and switched to PO as soon as possible (IV not recommended for ≥14 days).

Renal Impairment
PO, IV (Adults): *CCr <25 mL/min*—daily dose should not exceed 2 g.

Mycophenolic Acid (Myfortic)
Mycophenolate mofetil and mycophenolic acid should not be used interchangeably without the advice of a health care professional..

Renal Transplantation
PO (Adults): 720 mg twice daily.
PO (Children 5–16 yr and ≥1.19 m²): 400 mg/m² twice daily (not to exceed 720 mg twice daily).

Availability (generic available)
Mycophenolate Mofetil (CellCept)
Capsules: 250 mg. **Tablets:** 500 mg. **Oral suspension (fruit flavor):** 200 mg/mL in 225 mL bottles. **Powder for injection:** 500 mg vial.

Mycophenolic Acid (Myfortic)
Delayed-release tablets (Myfortic): 180 mg, 360 mg.

NURSING IMPLICATIONS

Assessment
- Assess for symptoms of organ rejection throughout therapy.
- Assess for signs of progressive multifocal leukoencephalopathy (hemiparesis, apathy, confusion, cognitive deficiencies, and ataxia) periodically during therapy.
- ***Lab Test Considerations:*** Monitor CBC with differential weekly during the 1st month, twice monthly for the 2nd and 3rd month of therapy, and then monthly during the 1st yr. Neutropenia occurs most frequently from 31–180 days post-transplant. If ANC is <1000/mm³, dose should be reduced or discontinued.
- Monitor hepatic and renal status and electrolytes periodically during therapy. May cause ↑ serum alkaline phosphatase, AST, ALT, LDH, BUN, and creatinine. May also cause hyperkalemia, hypokalemia, hypocalcemia, hypomagnesemia, hyperglycemia, and hyperlipidemia.

Potential Nursing Diagnoses
Risk for infection (Adverse Reactions)

Implementation
- The initial dose of mycophenolate (usually IV) should be given within 24 hr of transplant.
- Women of childbearing yr should have a negative serum or urine pregnancy test within 1 wk prior to initiation of therapy.
- **PO:** Administer on an empty stomach, 1 hr before or 2 hr after meals. Capsules and delayed-release tablets should be swallowed whole; do not open, crush, or chew. Mycophenolate may be teratogenic; contents of capsules should not be inhaled or come in contact with skin or mucous membranes.
- Do not administer mycophenolate concurrently with antacids containing magnesium or aluminum.

IV Administration

- **IV:** IV route should only be used for patients unable to take oral medication and should be switched to oral dose form as soon as patient can tolerate capsules or tablets.
- **Intermittent Infusion:** ***Diluent:*** Reconstitute each vial with 14 mL of D5W. Shake gently to dissolve. Solution is slightly yellow; discard if solution is discolored or contains particulate matter. Dilute contents of 2 vials (1-g dose) further with 140 mL of D5W or 3 vials (1.5-g dose) with 210 mL of D5W. ***Concentration:*** 6 mg/mL. Solution is stable for 4 hr. ***Rate:*** Administer via slow IV infusion over 2 hr. Do not administer as a bolus or via rapid infusion.
- **Y-Site Compatibility:** anidulafungin, bivalirudin, caspofungin, cefepime, daptomycin, dopamine, norepinephrine, octreotide, oxytocin, tacrolimus, tigecycline, tirofiban, vancomycin.
- **Y-Site Incompatibility:** mycafungin.

Patient/Family Teaching
- Instruct patient to take medication as directed, at the same time each day. Do not skip or double up on missed doses. Do not discontinue without consulting health care professional.

- Reinforce the need for lifelong therapy to prevent transplant rejection. Review symptoms of rejection for the transplanted organ, and stress need to notify health care professional immediately if signs of rejection or infection occur.
- Inform female patients of the importance of simultaneously using two reliable forms of contraception, unless abstinence is the chosen method, prior to beginning, during, and for 6 wk following discontinuation of therapy.
- Advise patient to avoid contact with persons with contagious diseases.
- Inform patient of the increased risk of lymphoma and other malignancies. Advise patient to use sunscreen and wear protective clothing to decrease risk of skin cancer.
- Advise patient to consult health care professional prior to taking other medications concurrently with mycophenolate.
- Emphasize the importance of routine follow-up laboratory tests.

Evaluation/Desired Outcomes
- Prevention of rejection of transplanted organs.

nabumetone (na-**byoo**-me-tone)
Relafen

Classification
Therapeutic: antirheumatics, nonsteroidal anti-inflammatory agents

Pregnancy Category C

Indications
Symptomatic management of rheumatoid arthritis and osteoarthritis.

Action
Inhibits prostaglandin synthesis. **Therapeutic Effects:** Suppression of pain and inflammation.

Pharmacokinetics
Absorption: Nabumetone (a prodrug) is 80% absorbed after oral administration; 35% is rapidly converted to 6-methoxy-2-naphthylacetic acid (6-MNA), which is the active drug.
Distribution: Unknown.
Protein Binding: >99%.
Metabolism and Excretion: 6-MNA is metabolized by the liver to inactive compounds.
Half-life: 24 hr (increased in severe renal impairment).

TIME/ACTION PROFILE (analgesia/anti-inflammatory effects)

ROUTE	ONSET	PEAK	DURATION
PO	1–2 days	few days–2 wk	12–24 hr

Contraindications/Precautions
Contraindicated in: Hypersensitivity; Use with other NSAIDs, including aspirin; cross-sensitivity may occur; Active GI bleeding or ulcer disease; Peri-operative pain from coronary artery bypass graft (CABG) surgery; Lactation: Lactation.
Use Cautiously in: Severe renal, or hepatic disease; History of ulcer disease; OB: Avoid using during 2nd half of pregnancy due to potential of NSAIDs to cause premature closure of ductus arteriosus; Pedi: Safety not established.

Adverse Reactions/Side Effects
CNS: agitation, anxiety, confusion, depression, dizziness, drowsiness, fatigue, headache, insomnia, malaise, weakness. **EENT:** abnormal vision, tinnitus. **Resp:** dyspnea, hypersensitivity pneumonitis. **CV:** edema, fluid retention, vasculitis. **GI:** GI BLEEDING, abdominal pain, diarrhea, ↑ liver function tests, anorexia, constipation, dry mouth, dyspepsia, flatulence, gastritis, gastroenteritis, ↑ appetite, nausea, stomatitis, vomiting. **GU:** albuminuria, azotemia, interstitial nephritis. **Derm:** EXFOLIATIVE DERMATITIS, STEVENS-JOHNSON SYNDROME, TOXIC EPIDERMAL NECROLYSIS, increased sweating, photosensitivity, pruritus, rash. **Hemat:** prolonged bleeding time. **Metab:** weight gain. **Neuro:** paresthesia, tremor. **Misc:** allergic reactions including ANAPHYLAXIS, ANGIONEUROTIC EDEMA.

Interactions
Drug-Drug: ↑ adverse GI effects with **aspirin**, other **NSAIDs**, **potassium supplements**, **corticosteroids**, or **alcohol**. Chronic use with **acetaminophen** may ↑ risk of adverse renal reactions. May ↓ effectiveness of **diuretics** or **antihypertensives**. May ↑ hypoglycemic effects of **insulins** or **oral hypoglycemic agents**. ↑ risk of toxicity from **methotrexate**. ↑ risk of bleeding with **cefotetan**, **cefoperazone**, **valproic acid**, **anticoagulants**, **ticlopidine**, **clopidogrel**, **eptifibatide**, **tirofiban**, or **thrombolytic agents**. ↑ risk of adverse hematologic reactions with **antineoplastics** or **radiation therapy**. Concurrent use with **cyclosporine** may ↑ risk of renal toxicity.

Route/Dosage
PO (Adults): 1000 mg/day as a single dose or divided dose twice daily; may be ↑ up to 2000 mg/day; use lowest effective dose during chronic therapy.

Availability (generic available)
Tablets: 500 mg, 750 mg.

NURSING IMPLICATIONS

Assessment
- Patients who have asthma, aspirin-induced allergy, and nasal polyps are at increased risk for developing hypersensitivity reactions. Monitor for rhinitis, asthma, and urticaria.
- Assess pain and range of motion before and periodically throughout therapy.
- ***Lab Test Considerations:*** Evaluate BUN, serum creatinine, CBC, and liver function periodically in patients receiving prolonged therapy.
- Serum potassium, BUN, serum creatinine, alkaline phosphatase, LDH, AST, and ALT tests may show ↑ levels. Blood glucose, hemoglobin, and hematocrit concentrations, leukocyte and platelet counts, and CCr may be ↓.
- May cause prolonged bleeding time.

Potential Nursing Diagnoses
Acute pain (Indications)
Impaired physical mobility (Indications)

Implementation
- Administration in higher than recommended doses does not provide increased effectiveness but may cause increased side effects. Use lowest effective dose for the shortest duration possible to minimize cardiac risks.
- **PO:** Administer with meals or antacids to decrease GI irritation and increase absorption.

Patient/Family Teaching
- Advise patient to take this medication with a full glass of water and to remain in an upright position for 15–30 min after administration.
- Instruct patient to take medication as directed. Take missed doses as soon as remembered but not if almost time for the next dose. Do not double doses.
- May cause drowsiness, dizziness, or visual disturbances. Advise patient to avoid driving or other activities requiring alertness until response to the medication is known.
- Advise patient to use sunscreen and protective clothing to prevent photosensitivity reactions.
- Caution patient to avoid the concurrent use of alcohol, aspirin, acetaminophen, or other OTC medications without consulting health care professional.
- Advise patient to inform health care professional of medication regimen before treatment or surgery.
- Advise patient to consult health care professional if rash, itching, visual disturbances, tinnitus, weight gain, edema, black stools, persistent headache, or influenza-like syndrome (chills, fever, muscle aches, pain) occurs.

Evaluation/Desired Outcomes
- Decreased pain and improved joint mobility. Partial arthritic relief is usually seen within 1 wk, but maximum effectiveness may require 2 wk or more of continuous therapy. Patients who do not respond to one NSAID may respond to another.

---

nadolol (nay-doe-lole)
Corgard, ✦ Syn-Nadolol

Classification
Therapeutic: antianginals, antihypertensives
Pharmacologic: beta blockers

Pregnancy Category C

Indications
Management of hypertension. Management of angina pectoris. **Unlabeled Use:** Arrhythmias. Migraine prophylaxis. Tremors (essential, lithium-induced, parkinsonian). Aggressive behavior. Antipsychotic-associated akathisia. Situational anxiety. Esophageal varices. Reduction of intraocular pressure.

Action
Blocks stimulation of $beta_1$ (myocardial) and $beta_2$ (pulmonary, vascular, and uterine) receptor sites. **Therapeutic Effects:** Decreased heart rate and blood pressure.

Pharmacokinetics
Absorption: 30% absorbed after oral administration.
Distribution: Minimal penetration of the CNS. Crosses the placenta and enters breast milk.
Metabolism and Excretion: 70% excreted unchanged by the kidneys.
Half-life: 10–24 hr (↑ in renal impairment).

TIME/ACTION PROFILE (antihypertensive effects)

ROUTE	ONSET	PEAK	DURATION
PO†	up to 5 days	6–9 days	24 hr

†With chronic dosing

Contraindications/Precautions
Contraindicated in: Uncompensated CHF; Pulmonary edema; Cardiogenic shock; Bradycardia or heart block.
Use Cautiously in: Renal impairment (CCr <50 mL/min); Hepatic impairment; Pulmonary disease (including asthma); Diabetes mellitus (may mask signs of hypoglycemia); Thyrotoxicosis (may mask symptoms); Patients with a history of severe allergic reactions (intensity of reactions may be ↑); OB: Crosses the placenta and may cause fetal/neonatal bradycardia, hypotension, hypoglycemia, or respiratory depression;); Lactation, Pedi: Safety not established; Geri: ↑ sensitivity to beta blockers; initial dose ↓ recommended.

Adverse Reactions/Side Effects
CNS: fatigue, weakness, anxiety, depression, dizziness, drowsiness, insomnia, memory loss, mental status changes, nightmares. **EENT:** blurred vision, dry eyes, nasal stuffiness. **Resp:** bronchospasm, wheezing. **CV:** ARRHYTHMIAS, BRADYCARDIA, CHF, PULMONARY EDEMA, orthostatic hypotension, peripheral vasoconstriction. **GI:** constipation, diarrhea, nausea. **GU:** erectile dysfunction, ↓ libido. **Derm:** itching, rashes. **Endo:** hyperglycemia, hypoglycemia. **MS:** ar-

thralgia, back pain, muscle cramps. **Neuro:** paresthesia. **Misc:** drug-induced lupus syndrome.

Interactions
Drug-Drug: General anesthesia, **IV phenytoin**, **diltiazem**, and **verapamil** may cause additive myocardial depression. Additive bradycardia may occur with **digoxin**. Additive hypotension may occur with other **antihypertensives**, acute ingestion of **alcohol**, or **nitrates**. Concurrent use with **amphetamines**, **cocaine**, **ephedrine**, **epinephrine**, **norepinephrine**, **phenylephrine**, or **pseudoephedrine** may result in unopposed alpha-adrenergic stimulation (excessive hypertension, bradycardia). Concurrent use with **clonidine** ↑ hypotension and bradycardia. Concurrent **thyroid** administration may ↓ effectiveness. May alter the effectiveness of **insulins** or **oral hypoglycemic agents** (dosage adjustments may be necessary). May ↓ the effectiveness of **theophylline**. May ↓ the effects of **dopamine** or **dobutamine**. Use cautiously within 14 days of **MAO inhibitor therapy** (may result in hypertension). Concurrent **NSAIDs** may ↓ antihypertensive action.

Route/Dosage
PO (Adults): *Antianginal*—40 mg once daily initially; may ↑ by 40–80 mg/day q 3–7 days as needed (up to 240 mg/day). *Antihypertensive*—40 mg once daily initially; may ↑ by 40–80 mg/day q 7 days as needed (up to 320 mg/day).

Renal Impairment
PO (Adults): *CCr 31–50 mL/min*— ↑ dosing interval to 24–36 hr; *CCr 10–30 mL/min*— ↑ dosing interval to 24–48 hr; *CCr <10 mL/min*— ↑ dosing interval to 40–60 hr.

Availability (generic available)
Tablets: 20 mg, 40 mg, 80 mg. *In combination with:* bendroflumethiazide (Corzide). See Appendix B.

NURSING IMPLICATIONS

Assessment
- Monitor blood pressure and pulse frequently during dose adjustment and periodically during therapy. Assess for orthostatic hypotension when assisting patient up from supine position.
- Monitor intake and output ratios and daily weight. Assess patient routinely for evidence of fluid overload (peripheral edema, dyspnea, rales/crackles, fatigue, weight gain, jugular venous distention).
- **Hypertension:** Check frequency of refills to determine compliance.
- **Angina:** Assess frequency and characteristics of angina periodically during therapy.
- *Lab Test Considerations:* May cause increased BUN, serum lipoprotein, potassium, triglyceride, and uric acid levels.
- May cause increased ANA titers.
- May cause increase in blood glucose levels.
- *Toxicity and Overdose:* Monitor patients receiving beta blockers for signs of overdose (bradycardia, severe dizziness or fainting, severe drowsiness, dyspnea, bluish fingernails or palms, seizures). Notify physician or other health care professional immediately if these signs occur.

Potential Nursing Diagnoses
Decreased cardiac output (Side Effects)
Noncompliance (Patient/Family Teaching)

Implementation
- Discontinuation of concurrent clonidine should be done gradually, with beta blocker discontinued first; then, after several days, discontinue clonidine.
- **PO:** Take apical pulse before administering. If <50 bpm or if arrhythmia occurs, withhold medication and notify physician or other health care professional.
- May be administered with food or on an empty stomach.
- Tablets may be crushed and mixed with food.

Patient/Family Teaching
- Instruct patient to take medication exactly as directed, at the same time each day, even if feeling well; do not skip or double up on missed doses. Take missed doses as soon as possible up to 8 hr before next dose. Abrupt withdrawal may precipitate life-threatening arrhythmias, hypertension, or myocardial ischemia.
- Advise patient to ensure that enough medication is available for weekends, holidays, and vacations. A written prescription may be kept in wallet for emergencies.
- Teach patient and family how to check pulse and blood pressure. Instruct them to check pulse daily and blood pressure biweekly. Advise patient to hold dose and contact health care professional if pulse is <50 bpm or if blood pressure changes significantly.
- May cause drowsiness or dizziness. Caution patients to avoid driving or other activities that re-

quire alertness until response to the drug is known.
- Advise patients to make position changes slowly to minimize orthostatic hypotension, especially during initiation of therapy or when dose is increased.
- Caution patient that this medication may increase sensitivity to cold.
- Instruct patient to consult health care professional before taking any OTC medications, especially cold preparations, concurrently with this medication.
- Patients with diabetes should closely monitor blood glucose, especially if weakness, malaise, irritability, or fatigue occurs. Medication may mask some signs of hypoglycemia, but dizziness and sweating may still occur.
- Advise patient to notify health care professional if slow pulse, difficulty breathing, wheezing, cold hands and feet, dizziness, confusion, depression, rash, fever, sore throat, unusual bleeding, or bruising occurs.
- Instruct patient to inform health care professional of medication regimen before treatment or surgery.
- Advise patient to carry identification describing disease process and medication regimen at all times.
- **Hypertension:** Reinforce the need to continue additional therapies for hypertension (weight loss, sodium restriction, stress reduction, regular exercise, moderation of alcohol consumption, and smoking cessation). Medication controls but does not cure hypertension.
- **Angina:** Caution patient to avoid overexertion with decrease in chest pain.

Evaluation/Desired Outcomes
- Decrease in blood pressure.
- Reduction in frequency of angina.
- Increase in activity tolerance. May require up to 5 days before therapeutic effects are seen.

---

nafarelin (na-fare-e-lin)
Synarel

Classification
Therapeutic: hormones
Pharmacologic: gonadotropin-releasing hormones

Pregnancy Category X

Indications
Management of endometriosis. Management of central precocious puberty (gonadotropin-dependent) in children.

Action
Acts as a synthetic analogue of gonadotropin-releasing hormone (GnRH). Initially increases pituitary production of luteinizing hormone (LH) and follicle-stimulating hormone (FSH), which cause ovarian steroid production. Chronic administration leads to decreased production of gonadotropins. Endometriotic lesions are sensitive to ovarian hormones. **Therapeutic Effects:** Reduction in lesions and associated pain in endometriosis. Arrest and regression of puberty in children with central precocious puberty.

Pharmacokinetics
Absorption: Well absorbed following intranasal administration.
Distribution: Unknown.
Metabolism and Excretion: 20–40% excreted in feces; 3% excreted unchanged by the kidneys.
Half-life: 3 hr.

TIME/ACTION PROFILE (decreased ovarian steroid production)

ROUTE	ONSET	PEAK	DURATION
Intranasal	within 4 wk	3–4 wk	3–6 mo†

†Relief of symptoms of endometriosis following discontinuation

Contraindications/Precautions
Contraindicated in: Hypersensitivity to GnRH, its analogues, or sorbitol; OB, Lactation: Pregnancy or lactation.
Use Cautiously in: Rhinitis.

Adverse Reactions/Side Effects
CNS: emotional instability, headaches, depression, insomnia. **EENT:** nasal irritation. **CV:** edema. **GU:** vaginal dryness. **Derm:** acne, hirsutism, seborrhea. **Endo:** cessation of menses, impaired fertility, ↓ breast size. **MS:** ↓ bone density, myalgia. **Misc:** ↓ libido, hot flashes, hypersensitivity reactions, weight gain.

Interactions
Drug-Drug: Concurrent **topical nasal decongestants** may ↓ absorption of nafarelin (administer decongestant at least 2 hr after nafarelin).

Route/Dosage
Intranasal (Adults): *Endometriosis*—1 spray (200 mcg) in 1 nostril in the morning and 1 spray in the other nostril in the evening (400 mcg/day). May be ↑ to 1 spray in each nostril in the morning and evening (800 mcg/day).

Intranasal (Children): *Central precocious puberty*—2 sprays in each nostril in the morning and in the evening (1600 mcg/day); may be ↑

up to 1800 mcg/day (3 sprays in alternating nostrils 3 times daily).

Availability
Nasal spray: 2 mg/mL (200 mcg/spray).

NURSING IMPLICATIONS
Assessment
- **Endometriosis:** Assess patient for endometriotic pain periodically throughout therapy.
- **Central Precocious Puberty:** Prior to therapy, a complete physical and endocrinologic examination including height, weight, hand and wrist x-ray, total sex steroid level (estradiol or testosterone), adrenal steroid level, beta human chorionic gonadotropin level, GnRH stimulation test, pelvic/adrenal/testicular ultrasound, and CT of the head must be performed. These parameters are monitored after 6–8 wk and every 3–6 mo during therapy.
- Assess patient for signs of precocious puberty (menses, breast development, testicular growth) periodically throughout therapy.
- Nafarelin is discontinued when the onset of normal puberty is desired. Monitor the onset of normal puberty and assess menstrual cycle, reproductive function, and final adult height.

Potential Nursing Diagnoses
Acute pain (Indications)
Sexual dysfunction (Indications, Side Effects)

Implementation
- **Endometriosis:** Treatment should be started between days 2 and 4 of the menstrual cycle and continued for up to 6 mo.

Patient/Family Teaching
- Instruct patient on the correct technique for nasal spray: The head should be tilted back slightly; wait 30 sec between sprays.
- Advise patient to consult health care professional if rhinitis occurs during therapy. If a topical decongestant is needed, do not use decongestant until 2 hr after nafarelin dosing. If possible, avoid sneezing during and immediately after nafarelin dose.
- **Endometriosis:** Inform patient that 1 spray should be administered into 1 nostril in the morning and 1 spray into the other nostril in the evening for the 400 mcg/day dose. If dose is increased to 800 mcg/day, administer 1 spray to each nostril (2 sprays) morning and evening; 1 bottle should provide a 30-day supply at the 400 mcg/day dose.
- Advise patient to use a form of contraception other than oral contraceptives during therapy. Inform patient that amenorrhea is expected. Instruct patient to notify health care professional if regular menstruation persists or if successive doses are missed.
- Advise patient that medication may cause hot flashes. Notify health care professional if these become bothersome.
- **Central Precocious Puberty:** Instruct patient on correct timing and number of sprays. The 1600 mcg/day dose is achieved by 2 sprays to each nostril in the morning (4 sprays) and 2 sprays to each nostril in the evening (4 sprays), for a total of 8 sprays. The 1800 mcg/day dose is achieved by 3 sprays into alternating nostrils 3 times per day, for a total of 9 sprays. Inform patient and parents that if doses are not taken as directed pubertal process may be reactivated. One bottle should provide a 7-day supply at the 1600 mcg/day dose.
- Advise patient and parents that during 1st mo of therapy some signs of puberty (vaginal bleeding, breast enlargement) may occur. These should resolve after the 1st mo of therapy. If these signs persist after the 2nd mo of therapy, notify health care professional.

Evaluation/Desired Outcomes
- Reduction in lesions and associated pain in endometriosis.
- Resolution of the signs of precocious puberty.

---

nafcillin, See PENICILLINS, PENICILLINASE RESISTANT.

---

naftifine, See ANTIFUNGALS (TOPICAL).

HIGH ALERT

nalbuphine (nal-byoo-feen)
Nubain

Classification
Therapeutic: opioid analgesics
Pharmacologic: opioid agonists/analgesics

Pregnancy Category C

✻ = Canadian drug name. ▓ = Genetic implication.
*CAPITALS indicates life-threatening; underlines indicate most frequent.

nalbuphine

Indications
Moderate to severe pain. Also provides: Analgesia during labor, Sedation before surgery, Supplement to balanced anesthesia.

Action
Binds to opiate receptors in the CNS. Alters the perception of and response to painful stimuli while producing generalized CNS depression. In addition, has partial antagonist properties, which may result in opioid withdrawal in physically dependent patients. **Therapeutic Effects:** Decreased pain.

Pharmacokinetics
Absorption: Well absorbed after IM and subcut administration.
Distribution: Probably crosses the placenta and enters breast milk.
Metabolism and Excretion: Mostly metabolized by the liver and eliminated in the feces via biliary excretion. Minimal amounts excreted unchanged by the kidneys.
Half-life: 5 hr.

TIME/ACTION PROFILE (analgesia)

ROUTE	ONSET	PEAK	DURATION
IM	<15 min	60 min	3–6 hr
Subcut	<15 min	unknown	3–6 hr
IV	2–3 min	30 min	3–6 hr

Contraindications/Precautions
Contraindicated in: Hypersensitivity to nalbuphine or bisulfites; Patients physically dependent on opioids and who have not been detoxified (may precipitate withdrawal).
Use Cautiously in: Head trauma; ↑ intracranial pressure; Severe renal, hepatic, or pulmonary disease; Hypothyroidism; Adrenal insufficiency; Alcoholism; Undiagnosed abdominal pain; Prostatic hyperplasia; Patients who have recently received opioid agonists; OB: Has been used during labor but may cause respiratory depression in the newborn; Lactation, Pedi: Safety not established; Geri: Dose ↓ suggested.

Adverse Reactions/Side Effects
CNS: dizziness, headache, sedation, confusion, dysphoria, euphoria, floating feeling, hallucinations, unusual dreams. **EENT:** blurred vision, diplopia, miosis (high doses). **Resp:** respiratory depression. **CV:** hypertension, orthostatic hypotension, palpitations. **GI:** dry mouth, nausea, vomiting, constipation, ileus. **GU:** urinary urgency. **Derm:** clammy feeling, sweating. **Misc:** physical dependence, psychological dependence, tolerance.

Interactions
Drug-Drug: Use with extreme caution in patients receiving **MAO inhibitors** (may result in unpredictable, severe reactions— ↓ initial dose of nalbuphine to 25% of usual dose). Additive CNS depression with **alcohol**, **antihistamines**, and **sedative/hypnotics**. May precipitate withdrawal in patients who are physically dependent on **opioid agonists**. Avoid concurrent use with other **opioid analgesic agonists** (may diminish analgesic effect).
Drug-Natural Products: Concomitant use of **kava-kava**, **valerian**, **skullcap**, **chamomile**, or **hops** can ↑ CNS depression.

Route/Dosage
Analgesia
IM, Subcut, IV (Adults): Usual dose is 10 mg q 3–6 hr (single dose not to exceed 20 mg; total daily dose not to exceed 160 mg).

Supplement to Balanced Anesthesia
IV (Adults): *Initial*—0.3–3 mg/kg over 10–15 min. *Maintenance*—0.25–0.5 mg/kg as needed.

Availability (generic available)
Injection: 10 mg/mL, 20 mg/mL.

NURSING IMPLICATIONS

Assessment
- Assess type, location, and intensity of pain before and 1 hr after IM or 30 min (peak) after IV administration. When titrating opioid doses, increases of 25–50% should be administered until there is either a 50% reduction in the patient's pain rating on a numeric or visual analogue scale or the patient reports satisfactory pain relief. A repeat dose can be safely administered at the time of the peak if previous dose is ineffective and side effects are minimal. Patients requiring doses higher than 20 mg should be converted to an opioid agonist. Nalbuphine is not recommended for prolonged use or as first-line therapy for acute or cancer pain.
- An equianalgesic chart (see Appendix K) should be used when changing routes or when changing from one opioid to another.
- Assess blood pressure, pulse, and respirations before and periodically during administration. If respiratory rate is <10/min, assess level of sedation. Physical stimulation may be sufficient to prevent significant hypoventilation. Dose may need to be decreased by 25–50%. Nalbuphine produces respiratory depression, but

this does not markedly increase with increased doses.
- Assess previous analgesic history. Antagonistic properties may induce withdrawal symptoms (vomiting, restlessness, abdominal cramps, and increased blood pressure and temperature) in patients physically dependent on opioids.
- Although this drug has a low potential for dependence, prolonged use may lead to physical and psychological dependence and tolerance. This should not prevent patient from receiving adequate analgesia. Most patients who receive nalbuphine for pain do not develop psychological dependence. If tolerance develops, changing to an opioid agonist may be required to relieve pain.
- *Lab Test Considerations:* May cause ↑ serum amylase and lipase concentrations.
- *Toxicity and Overdose:* If an opioid antagonist is required to reverse respiratory depression or coma, naloxone (Narcan) is the antidote. Dilute the 0.4-mg ampule of naloxone in 10 mL of 0.9% NaCl and administer 0.5 mL (0.02 mg) by direct IV push every 2 min. For children and patients weighing <40 kg, dilute 0.1 mg of naloxone in 10 mL of 0.9% NaCl for a concentration of 10 mcg/mL and administer 0.5 mcg/kg every 2 min. Titrate dose to avoid withdrawal, seizures, and severe pain.

Potential Nursing Diagnoses
Acute pain (Indications)
Risk for injury (Side Effects)
Disturbed sensory perception (visual, auditory) (Side Effects)

Implementation
- *High Alert:* Accidental overdose of opioid analgesics has resulted in fatalities. Before administering, clarify all ambiguous orders; have second practitioner independently check original order, dose calculations, and infusion pump settings.
- Explain therapeutic value of medication before administration to enhance the analgesic effect.
- Regularly administered doses may be more effective than prn administration. Analgesic is more effective if administered before pain becomes severe.
- Coadministration with nonopioid analgesics may have additive effects and permit lower opioid doses.
- **IM:** Administer deep into well-developed muscle. Rotate sites of injections.

IV Administration

- **Direct IV:** May give IV undiluted- *Concentration:* 10–20 mg/mL. *Rate:* Administer slowly, each 10 mg over 3–5 min.
- **Syringe Compatibility:** atropine, cimetidine, diphenhydramine, droperidol, glycopyrrolate, hydroxyzine, lidocaine, midazolam, prochlorperazine, ranitidine, scopolamine.
- **Syringe Incompatibility:** diazepam, ketorolac, pentobarbital.
- **Y-Site Compatibility:** amifostine, aztreonam, bivalirudin, cisatracurium, cladribine, dexmedetomidine, etoposide phosphate, fenoldopam, filgrastim, fludarabine, gemcitabine, granisetron, lansoprazole, linezolid, melphalan, oxaliplatin, paclitaxel, propofol, remifentanil, teniposide, thiotepa, vinorelbine.
- **Y-Site Incompatibility:** allopurinol, amphotericin B cholesteryl sulfate complex, cefepime, docetaxel, methotrexate, pemetrexed, piperacillin/tazobactam, sargramostim, sodium bicarbonate.

Patient/Family Teaching
- Instruct patient on how and when to ask for pain medication.
- May cause drowsiness or dizziness. Advise patient to call for assistance when ambulating and to avoid driving or other activities requiring alertness until response to the medication is known.
- Caution patient to change positions slowly to minimize orthostatic hypotension.
- Advise patient that frequent mouth rinses, good oral hygiene, and sugarless gum or candy may decrease dry mouth.
- Encourage patient to turn, cough, and breathe deeply every 2 hr to prevent atelectasis.
- Advise patient to avoid concurrent use of alcohol or other CNS depressants with this medication.

Evaluation/Desired Outcomes
- Decrease in severity of pain without significant alteration in level of consciousness or respiratory status.

naloxone (nal-ox-one)

Classification
Therapeutic: antidotes (for opioids)
Pharmacologic: opioid antagonists

Pregnancy Category B

Indications
Reversal of CNS depression and respiratory depression because of suspected opioid overdose. **Unlabeled Use:** Opioid-induced pruritus (low dose IV infusion). Management of refractory circulatory shock.

Action
Competitively blocks the effects of opioids, including CNS and respiratory depression, without producing any agonist (opioid-like) effects. **Therapeutic Effects:** Reversal of signs of opioid excess.

Pharmacokinetics
Absorption: Well absorbed after IM or subcut administration.
Distribution: Rapidly distributed to tissues. Crosses the placenta.
Metabolism and Excretion: Metabolized by the liver.
Half-life: 60–90 min (up to 3 hr in neonates).

TIME/ACTION PROFILE (reversal of opioid effects)

ROUTE	ONSET	PEAK	DURATION
IV	1–2 min	unknown	45 min
IM, Subcut	2–5 min	unknown	>45 min

Contraindications/Precautions
Contraindicated in: Hypersensitivity.
Use Cautiously in: Cardiovascular disease; Patients physically dependent on opioids (may precipitate severe withdrawal); OB: May cause acute withdrawal syndrome in mother and fetus if mother is opioid dependent; Lactation: Safety not established; Pedi: May cause acute withdrawal syndrome in neonates of opioid-dependent mothers.

Adverse Reactions/Side Effects
CV: VENTRICULAR ARRHYTHMIAS, hypertension, hypotension. **GI:** nausea, vomiting.

Interactions
Drug-Drug: Can precipitate withdrawal in patients physically dependent on **opioid analgesics**. Larger doses may be required to reverse the effects of **buprenorphine**, **butorphanol**, **nalbuphine**, **pentazocine**, or **propoxyphene**. Antagonizes postoperative **opioid analgesics**.

Route/Dosage
Postoperative Opioid-Induced Respiratory Depression
IV (Adults): 0.02–0.2 mg q 2–3 min until response obtained; repeat q 1–2 hr if needed.
IV (Children): 0.01 mg/kg; may repeat q 2–3 min until response obtained. Additional doses may be given q 1–2 hr if needed.
IM, IV, Subcut (Neonates): 0.01 mg/kg; may repeat q 2–3 min until response obtained. Additional doses may be given q 1–2 hr if needed.

Opioid-Induced Respiratory Depression During Chronic (>1 wk) Opioid Use
IV, IM, Subcut (Adults >40 kg): 20–40 mcg (0.02–0.04 mg) given as small, frequent (q min) boluses or as an infusion titrated to improve respiratory function without reversing analgesia.
IV, IM, Subcut (Adults and Children <40 kg): 0.005–0.02 mg/dose given as small, frequent (q min) boluses or as an infusion titrated to improve respiratory function without reversing analgesia.

Overdose of Opioids
IV, IM, Subcut (Adults): *Patients not suspected of being opioid dependent*—0.4 mg (10 mcg/kg); may repeat q 2–3 min (IV route is preferred). Some patients may require up to 2 mg. *Patients suspected to be opioid dependent*— Initial dose should be decreased to 0.1–0.2 mg q 2–3 min. May also be given by IV infusion at rate adjusted to patient's response.
IV, IM, Subcut (Children > 5 yr or > 20 kg): 2 mg/dose, may repeat q 2–3 min.
IV, IM, Subcut (Infants up to 5 yr or 20 kg): 0.1 mg/kg, may repeat q 2–3 min.

Opioid-Induced Pruritus
IV (Children): 2 mcg/kg/hr continuous infusion, may ↑ by 0.5 mcg/kg/hr every few hours if pruritus continues.

Availability (generic available)
Injection: 0.4 mg/mL, 1 mg/mL. *In combination with:* pentazocine (Talwin NX). See Appendix B.

NURSING IMPLICATIONS

Assessment
- Monitor respiratory rate, rhythm, and depth; pulse, ECG, blood pressure; and level of consciousness frequently for 3–4 hr after the expected peak of blood concentrations. After a moderate overdose of a short half-life opioid, physical stimulation may be enough to prevent

significant hypoventilation. The effects of some opioids may last longer than the effects of naloxone, and repeat doses may be necessary.
- Patients who have been receiving opioids for >1 wk are extremely sensitive to the effects of naloxone. Dilute and administer carefully.
- Assess patient for level of pain after administration when used to treat postoperative respiratory depression. Naloxone decreases respiratory depression but also reverses analgesia.
- Assess patient for signs and symptoms of opioid withdrawal (vomiting, restlessness, abdominal cramps, increased blood pressure, and temperature). Symptoms may occur within a few minutes to 2 hr. Severity depends on dose of naloxone, the opioid involved, and degree of physical dependence.
- Lack of significant improvement indicates that symptoms are caused by a disease process or other non-opioid CNS depressants not affected by naloxone.
- *Toxicity and Overdose:* Naloxone is a pure antagonist with no agonist properties and minimal toxicity.

Potential Nursing Diagnoses
Ineffective breathing pattern (Indications)
Ineffective coping (Indications)
Acute pain

Implementation
- Larger doses of naloxone may be necessary when used to antagonize the effects of buprenorphine, butorphanol, nalbuphine, pentazocine, and propoxyphene.
- Resuscitation equipment, oxygen, vasopressors, and mechanical ventilation should be available to supplement naloxone therapy as needed.
- Doses should be titrated carefully in postoperative patients to avoid interference with control of postoperative pain.

IV Administration
- **Direct IV:** *Diluent:* Administer undiluted for *suspected opioid overdose*. For *opioid-induced respiratory depression*, dilute with sterile water for injection. For children or adults weighing <40 kg, dilute 0.1 mg of naloxone in 10 mL of sterile water or 0.9% NaCl for injection. *Concentration:* 0.4 mg/mL, 1 mg/mL, or 10 mcg/mL (depending on preparation used). *Rate:* Administer over 30 seconds for patients with a *suspected opioid overdose*. For patients who develop *opioid-induced respiratory depression*, administer dilute solution of 0.4 mg/10 mL at a rate of 0.5 mL (0.02 mg) direct IV every 2 min. Titrate to avoid withdrawal and severe pain. Excessive dose in postoperative patients may cause excitement, pain, hypotension, hypertension, pulmonary edema, ventricular tachycardia and fibrillation, and seizures. For children and adults weighing <40 kg, administer 10 mcg/mL solution at a rate of 0.5 mcg/kg every 1–2 min.
- **Continuous Infusion:** *Diluent:* Dilute 2 mg of naloxone in 500 mL of 0.9% NaCl or D5W. Infusion is stable for 24 hr. *Concentration:* 4 mcg/mL. *Rate:* Titrate dose according to patient response.
- **Y-Site Compatibility:** acyclovir, amikacin, aminophylline, atropine, aztreonam, bumetanide, calcium chloride, calcium gluconate, caspofungin, cefazolin, cefotaxime, cefoxitin, ceftazidime, ceftizoxime, ceftriaxone, cefuroxime, chloramphenicol, cimetidine, clindamycin, cyclosporine, daptomycin, dexamethasone sodium phosphate, digoxin, diltiazem, diphenhydramine, dobutamine, dopamine, doxycycline, enalaprilat, epinephrine, ertapenem, erythromycin, esmolol, famotidine, fenoldopam, fentanyl, fluconazole, furosemide, ganciclovir, gentamicin, granisetron, heparin, hydrocortisone sodium succinate, hydroxyzine, imipenem/cilastatin, insulin, isoproterenol, ketorolac, labetalol, levofloxacin, lidocaine, linezolid, lorazepam, methylprednisolone sodium succinate, metoclopramide, metoprolol, metronidazole, midazolam, nafcillin, nitroglycerin, nitroprusside, norepinephrine, ondansetron, palonosetron, penicillin G potassium, phenylephrine, phytonadione, piperacillin/tazobactam, potassium chloride, procainamide, prochlorperazine, promethazine, propofol, propranolol, protamine, quinupristin/dalfopristin, ranitidine, sodium bicarbonate, tacrolimus, ticarcillin/clavulanate, tirofiban, tobramycin, vancomycin, vasopressin, verapamil, voriconazole.
- **Y-Site Incompatibility:** diazepam, lansoprazole, pantoprazole, phenytoin, trimethoprim/sulfamethoxazole.
- **Additive Incompatibility:** Incompatible with preparations containing bisulfite, sulfite, and solutions with an alkaline pH.

Patient/Family Teaching
- As medication becomes effective, explain purpose and effects of naloxone to patient.

Evaluation/Desired Outcomes
- Adequate ventilation.
- Alertness without significant pain or withdrawal symptoms.

---

naproxen (na-**prox**-en)
Aleve, Anaprox, Anaprox DS, ✤ Apo-Napro-Na, ✤ Apo-Naproxen, EC-Naprosyn, Naprelan, Naprosyn, ✤ Naprosyn-E, ✤ Naprosyn-SR, ✤ Naxen, ✤ Novo-Naprox, ✤ Novo-Naprox Sodium DS, ✤ Nu-Naprox, ✤ Synflex, ✤ Synflex DS

Classification
Therapeutic: nonopioid analgesics, nonsteroidal anti-inflammatory agents, antipyretics

Pregnancy Category B (first trimester)

Indications
Mild to moderate pain. Dysmenorrhea. Fever. Inflammatory disorders, including: Rheumatoid arthritis (adults and children), Osteoarthritis.

Action
Inhibits prostaglandin synthesis. **Therapeutic Effects:** Decreased pain. Reduction of fever. Suppression of inflammation.

Pharmacokinetics
Absorption: Completely absorbed from the GI tract. Sodium salt is more rapidly absorbed.
Distribution: Crosses the placenta; enters breast milk in low concentrations.
Protein Binding: >99%.
Metabolism and Excretion: Mostly metabolized by the liver.
Half-life: Children <8 yr: 8–17 hr; Children 8–14 yr: 8–10 hr; Adults: 10–20 hr.

TIME/ACTION PROFILE

ROUTE	ONSET	PEAK	DURATION
PO (analgesic)	1 hr	unknown	8–12 hr
PO (anti-inflammatory)	14 days	2–4 wk	unknown

Contraindications/Precautions
Contraindicated in: Hypersensitivity; Cross-sensitivity may occur with other NSAIDs, including aspirin; Active GI bleeding; Ulcer disease; Lactation: Passes into breast milk and should not be used by nursing mothers.

Use Cautiously in: Severe cardiovascular, renal, or hepatic disease; History of ulcer disease or any other history of gastrointestinal bleeding (may ↑ risk of GI bleeding); Underlying cardiovascular disease (may ↑ risk of MI or stroke); Chronic alcohol use/abuse; OB: Avoid using during third trimester; may cause premature closure of the ductus arteriosus; Pedi: Safety not established in children <2 yr; Geri: ↑ risk of adverse reactions.

Adverse Reactions/Side Effects
CNS: dizziness, drowsiness, headache. **EENT:** tinnitus, visual disturbances. **Resp:** dyspnea. **CV:** edema, palpitations, tachycardia. **GI:** DRUG-INDUCED HEPATITIS, GI BLEEDING, constipation, dyspepsia, nausea, anorexia, diarrhea, discomfort, flatulence, vomiting. **GU:** cystitis, hematuria, renal failure. **Derm:** photosensitivity, rashes, sweating, pseudoporphyria (12% incidence in children with juvenile rheumatoid arthritis—discontinue therapy if this occurs). **Hemat:** blood dyscrasias, prolonged bleeding time. **Misc:** allergic reactions including ANAPHYLAXIS and STEVENS-JOHNSON SYNDROME.

Interactions
Drug-Drug: Concurrent use with **aspirin** ↓ naproxen blood levels and may ↓ effectiveness. ↑ risk of bleeding with **anticoagulants**, **thrombolytic agents**, **eptifibatide**, **tirofiban**, **cefotetan**, **cefoperazone**, **valproic acid**, **corticosteroids**, **clopidogrel**, and **ticlopidine**. Additive adverse GI side effects with **aspirin**, **corticosteroids**, **alcohol**, and other **NSAIDs**. **Probenecid** ↑ blood levels and may ↑ toxicity. May ↑ risk of toxicity from **methotrexate**, **antineoplastics**, or **radiation therapy**. May ↑ serum levels and risk of toxicity from **lithium**. ↑ risk of adverse renal effects with **cyclosporine** or chronic use of **acetaminophen**. May ↓ response to **ACE Inhibitors**, **angiotensin II antagonists**, or **furosemide**. May ↑ risk of hypoglycemia with **insulin** or **oral hypoglycemic agents**. **Oral potassium supplements** may ↑ GI adverse effects.

Drug-Natural Products: ↑ anticoagulant effect and bleeding risk with **anise**, **arnica**, **chamomile**, **clove**, **dong quai**, **feverfew**, **garlic**, **ginger**, **ginkgo**, **Panax ginseng**, **licorice**, and others.

Route/Dosage
275 mg naproxen sodium is equivalent to 250 mg naproxen.

naproxen 901

Anti-Inflammatory/Analgesic/Antidysmenorrheal
PO (Adults): *Naproxen*—250–500 mg twice daily (up to 1.5 g/day). *Delayed-release naproxen*—375–500 mg twice daily. *Naproxen sodium*—275–550 mg twice daily (up to 1.65 g/day).

PO (Children >2 yr): *Analgesia:* 5–7 mg/kg/dose q 8–12 hr. *Inflammatory disease:* 10–15 mg/kg/day divided q 12 hr, maximum: 1000 mg/day.

Antigout
PO (Adults): *Naproxen*—750 mg naproxen initially, then 250 mg q 8 hr. *Naproxen sodium*—825 mg initially, then 275 mg q 8 hr.

OTC Use (naproxen sodium)
PO (Adults): 200 mg q 8–12 hr or 400 mg followed by 200 mg q 12 hr (not to exceed 600 mg/24 hr).

PO (Geriatric Patients >65 yr): Not to exceed 200 mg q 12 hr.

Availability
Naproxen (generic available)
Tablets (Naprosyn, Apo-Naproxen, Naxen, Novo-Naprox, Nu-Naprox): ✤ 125 mg, 250 mg, 375 mg, 500 mg. **Controlled-release tablets (Naprelan):** 375 mg, 500 mg. **Delayed-release tablets (EC-Naprosyn, Naprosyn-E):** ✤ 250 mg, 375 mg, 500 mg. **Extended-release tablets (Naprosyn-SR):** ✤ 750 mg. **Oral suspension (Naprosyn):** 125 mg/5 mL. **Suppositories (Naprosyn, Naxen):** ✤ 500 mg.

Naproxen Sodium (generic available)
Tablets (Aleve, Anaprox, Anaprox DS, Novo-Naprox Sodium, Novo-Naprox Sodium DS, Synaflex, Synaflex DS): 220 mg^OTC, 275 mg, 550 mg. *In combination with:* pseudoephedrine (Aleve Cold and Sinus Tablets, Aleve Sinus and Headache Tablets), sumatriptan (Treximet). See Appendix B.

NURSING IMPLICATIONS

Assessment
- Patients who have asthma, aspirin-induced allergy, and nasal polyps are at increased risk for developing hypersensitivity reactions. Assess for rhinitis, asthma, and urticaria.
- **Pain:** Assess pain (note type, location, and intensity) prior to and 1–2 hr following administration.
- **Arthritis:** Assess pain and range of motion prior to and 1–2 hr following administration.
- **Fever:** Monitor temperature; note signs associated with fever (diaphoresis, tachycardia, malaise).
- **Lab Test Considerations:** Evaluate BUN, serum creatinine, CBC, and liver function tests periodically in patients receiving prolonged therapy.
- May ↑ serum potassium, BUN, serum creatinine, alkaline phosphatase, LDH, AST, and ALT tests levels. May ↓ blood glucose, hemoglobin, and hematocrit concentrations, leukocyte and platelet counts, and CCr.
- Bleeding time may be prolonged up to 4 days following discontinuation of therapy.
- May alter test results for urine 5-HIAA and urine steroid determinations.

Potential Nursing Diagnoses
Acute pain (Indications)
Chronic pain (Indications)
Impaired physical mobility (Indications)

Implementation
- Administration in higher than recommended doses does not provide increased effectiveness but may cause increased side effects. Use lowest effective dose for the shortest duration possible to minimize cardiac risks.
- Coadministration with opioid analgesics may have additive analgesic effects and may permit lower opioid doses.
- Analgesic is more effective if given before pain becomes severe.
- **PO:** For rapid initial effect, administer 30 min before or 2 hr after meals. May be administered with food, milk, or antacids to decrease GI irritation. Food slows but does not reduce the extent of absorption. Do not mix suspension with antacid or other liquid prior to administration. Swallow extended-release, delayed-release, and controlled-release tablets whole; do not break, crush, or chew.
- **Dysmenorrhea:** Administer as soon as possible after the onset of menses. Prophylactic treatment has not been shown to be effective.

Patient/Family Teaching
- Advise patient to take this medication with a full glass of water and to remain in an upright position for 15–30 min after administration.
- Instruct patient to take medication as directed. Take missed doses as soon as remembered but

✤ = Canadian drug name.   ■ = Genetic implication.
*CAPITALS indicates life-threatening; underlines indicate most frequent.

- not if almost time for the next dose. Do not double doses.
- May cause drowsiness or dizziness. Advise patient to avoid driving or other activities requiring alertness until response to the medication is known.
- Caution patient to avoid the concurrent use of alcohol, aspirin, acetaminophen, or other OTC medications without consulting health care professional. Use of naproxen with 3 or more glasses of alcohol per day may increase risk of GI bleeding.
- Advise patient to inform health care professional of medication regimen prior to treatment or surgery.
- Caution patient to wear sunscreen and protective clothing to prevent photosensitivity reactions (especially in children with JRA).
- Instruct patients not to take OTC naproxen preparations for more than 3 days for fever and to consult health care professional if symptoms persist or worsen.
- Advise patient to consult health care professional if rash, itching, visual disturbances, tinnitus, weight gain, edema, black stools, persistent headache, or influenza-like syndrome (chills, fever, muscle aches, pain) occurs.

Evaluation/Desired Outcomes
- Relief of pain.
- Improved joint mobility. Partial arthritic relief is usually seen within 2 wk, but maximum effectiveness may require 2–4 wk of continuous therapy. Patients who do not respond to one NSAID may respond to another.
- Reduction of fever.

---

naratriptan (nar-a-trip-tan)
Amerge

Classification
Therapeutic: vascular headache suppressants
Pharmacologic: 5-HT$_1$ agonists

Pregnancy Category C

Indications
Acute treatment of migraine headache.

Action
Acts as an agonist at specific 5-HT$_1$ receptor sites in intracranial blood vessels and sensory trigeminal nerves. **Therapeutic Effects:** Cranial vessel vasoconstriction with resultant decrease in migraine headache.

Pharmacokinetics
Absorption: Well absorbed (70%) following oral administration.
Distribution: Unknown.
Metabolism and Excretion: 60% excreted unchanged in urine; 30% metabolized by the liver.
Half-life: 6 hr (↑ in renal impairment).

TIME/ACTION PROFILE (↓ migraine pain)

ROUTE	ONSET	PEAK	DURATION
PO	30–60 min	2–3 hr†	up to 24 hr

†3–4 hr during migraine attack

Contraindications/Precautions
Contraindicated in: Hypersensitivity; Ischemic cardiovascular, cerebrovascular, or peripheral vascular syndromes (including ischemic bowel disease); History of significant cardiovascular disease; Uncontrolled hypertension; Severe renal impairment (CCr <15 mL/min); Severe hepatic impairment; Should not be used within 24 hr of other 5-HT$_1$ agonists or ergot-type compounds (dihydroergotamine); Geri: Age-related ↓ in renal function and ↑ likelihood of CAD greatly ↑ risk of fatal adverse events.
Use Cautiously in: Mild to moderate renal or hepatic impairment (dose should not exceed 2.5 mg/24 hr; initial dose should be ↓); OB, Lactation, Pedi: Safety not established.
Exercise Extreme Caution in: Cardiovascular risk factors (hypertension, hypercholesterolemia, cigarette smoking, obesity, diabetes, strong family history, menopausal women or men >40 yr); use only if cardiovascular status has been evaluated and determined to be safe and 1st dose is administered under supervision.

Adverse Reactions/Side Effects
CNS: dizziness, drowsiness, malaise/fatigue. **CV:** CORONARY ARTERY VASOSPASM, MI, VENTRICULAR FIBRILLATION, VENTRICULAR TACHYCARDIA, myocardial ischemia. **GI:** nausea. **Neuro:** paresthesia. **Misc:** pain/pressure sensation in throat/neck.

Interactions
Drug-Drug: Concurrent use with **SSRI or SNRI antidepressants** may result in serotonin syndrome. **Cigarette smoking** ↑ the metabolism of naratriptan. Blood levels and effects are ↑ by **hormonal contraceptives**. Avoid concurrent use (within 24 hr of each other) with **ergot-containing drugs (dihydroergotamine)** may result in prolonged vasospastic reactions. Avoid concurrent (within 2 wk) use with **MAO inhibitors**; produces ↑ systemic exposure and risk of adverse reactions to naratriptan. Serotonin syndrome may occur with **sibutramine**.

Drug-Natural Products: ↑ risk of serotinergic side effects including serotonin syndrome with **St. John's wort** and **SAMe**.

Route/Dosage
PO (Adults): 1 or 2.5 mg; dose may be repeated in 4 hr if response is inadequate (not to exceed 5 mg/24 hr or treatment of more than 4 headaches/mo).

Availability
Tablets: 1 mg, 2.5 mg. **Cost:** 1 mg $210.69/9, 2.5 mg $210.97/9.

NURSING IMPLICATIONS

Assessment
- Assess pain location, character, intensity, and duration and associated symptoms (photophobia, phonophobia, nausea, vomiting) during migraine attack.
- Monitor for serotonin syndrome in patients taking SSRIs or SNRIs concurrently with naratriptan.

Potential Nursing Diagnoses
Acute pain (Indications)

Implementation
- **PO:** Tablets may be administered at any time after the headache starts.

Patient/Family Teaching
- Inform patient that naratriptan should be used only during a migraine attack. It is meant to be used for relief of migraine attacks but not to prevent or reduce the number of attacks.
- Instruct patient to administer naratriptan as soon as symptoms of a migraine attack appear, but it may be administered any time during an attack. If migraine symptoms return, a 2nd dose may be used. Allow at least 4 hr between doses, and do not use more than 2 tablets in any 24-hr period. Do not use to treat more than 4 headaches per month.
- Advise patient that lying down in a darkened room following naratriptan administration may further help relieve headache.
- Advise patient to notify health care professional prior to next dose of naratriptan if pain or tightness in the chest occurs during use. If pain is severe or does not subside, notify health care professional immediately. If wheezing; heart throbbing; swelling of eyelids, face, or lips; skin rash; skin lumps; or hives occur, notify health care professional immediately and do not take more naratriptan without approval of health care professional. If feelings of tingling, heat, flushing, heaviness, pressure, drowsiness, dizziness, tiredness, or sickness develop, discuss with health care professional at next visit.
- Instruct patient not to take additional naratriptan if no response is seen with initial dose without consulting health care professional. There is no evidence that 5 mg provides greater relief than 2.5-mg dose. Additional naratriptan doses are not likely to be effective and alternative medications, as previously discussed with health care professional, may be used.
- Naratriptan may cause dizziness or drowsiness. Caution patient to avoid driving or other activities requiring alertness until response to medication is known.
- Advise patient to avoid alcohol, which aggravates headaches, during naratriptan use.
- Advise patient to consult health care professional before taking other Rx, OTC, or herbal products concurrently with naratriptan. Patients concurrently taking SSRI or SNRI antidepressants should notify health care professional promptly if signs of serotonin syndrome (mental status changes: agitation, hallucinations, coma; autonomic instability: tachycardia, labile blood pressure, hyperthermia; neuromuscular aberrations: hyperreflexia, incoordination; and/or gastrointestinal symptoms: nausea, vomiting, diarrhea) occur.
- Caution patient not to use naratriptan if pregnancy is planned or suspected or if breastfeeding. Adequate contraception should be used during therapy.

Evaluation/Desired Outcomes
- Relief of migraine attack.

---

nateglinide (na-teg-li-nide)
Starlix

Classification
Therapeutic: antidiabetics
Pharmacologic: meglitinides

Pregnancy Category C

Indications
To improve glycemic control in patients with type 2 diabetes (with diet and exercise); may also be used with metformin or a thiazolidinedione (pioglitazone, rosiglitazone).

nateglinide

Action
Stimulates the release of insulin from pancreatic beta cells by closing potassium channels, which results in the opening of calcium channels in beta cells. This is followed by release of insulin. Requires functioning pancreatic beta cells. **Therapeutic Effects:** Lowering of blood glucose.

Pharmacokinetics
Absorption: Well absorbed (73%) following oral administration; absorption is rapid.
Distribution: Unknown.
Protein Binding: 98%.
Metabolism and Excretion: Mostly metabolized by the liver (cytochrome P2 C9 and P3 A4 [CYP2C9 and CYP3A4] enzyme systems); 16% excreted unchanged in urine.
Half-life: 1.5 hr.

TIME/ACTION PROFILE (effect on blood glucose)

ROUTE	ONSET	PEAK	DURATION
PO	within 20 min	1 hr	4 hr

Contraindications/Precautions
Contraindicated in: Hypersensitivity; Diabetic ketoacidosis; Type 1 diabetes; OB: Insulin recommended to control diabetes during pregnancy; Lactation: Effects on nursing infant unknown.
Use Cautiously in: Malnourished patients, patients with pituitary or adrenal insufficiency (↑ susceptibility to hypoglycemia); Strenuous physical exercise, insufficient caloric intake (increased risk of hypoglycemia); Autonomic neuropathy (hypoglycemia may be masked); Moderate to severe liver impairment; Fever, infection, trauma, or surgery (may lead to transient loss of glycemic control; insulin may be required); Pedi: Safety not established; Geri: May have ↑ sensitivity to drug effects (↑ risk of hypoglycemia).

Adverse Reactions/Side Effects
CNS: dizziness. **Resp:** bronchitis, coughing, upper respiratory infection. **GI:** diarrhea. **Endo:** HYPOGLYCEMIA. **MS:** arthropathy, back pain. **Misc:** flu symptoms.

Interactions
Drug-Drug: Concurrent use with **beta blockers** may mask hypoglycemia. **Alcohol**, combination with other **antidiabetics**, **NSAIDs**, **MAO inhibitors**, **nonselective beta blockers** may ↑ the risk of hypoglycemia. Hypoglycemic effects may be ↓ by **thiazide diuretics**, **corticosteroids**, **thyroid supplements**, or **sympathomimetic (adrenergic) agents**.

Drug-Food: Blood levels and effects are significantly ↓ when administered prior to a **liquid meal**.

Route/Dosage
PO (Adults): 120 mg 3 times daily before meals; patients who are approaching glycemic control may be started at 60 mg 3 times daily.

Availability (generic available)
Tablets: 60 mg, 120 mg.

NURSING IMPLICATIONS

Assessment
- Observe for signs and symptoms of hypoglycemic reactions (sweating, hunger, weakness, dizziness, tremor, tachycardia, anxiety).
- *Lab Test Considerations:* Monitor serum glucose and HbA$_{1c}$ periodically during therapy to evaluate effectiveness.
- May cause ↑ uric acid levels.
- *Toxicity and Overdose:* Overdose is manifested by symptoms of hypoglycemia. Mild hypoglycemia may be treated with administration of oral glucose. Severe hypoglycemia should be treated with IV D50W followed by continuous IV infusion of more dilute dextrose solution at a rate sufficient to keep serum glucose at approximately 100 mg/dL.

Potential Nursing Diagnoses
Imbalanced nutrition: more than body requirements (Indications)
Noncompliance (Patient/Family Teaching)

Implementation
- Patients stabilized on a diabetic regimen who are exposed to stress, fever, trauma, infection, or surgery may require administration of insulin.
- **PO:** Administer 1–30 min prior to meals.
- May be administered concurrently with metformin, pioglitazone, or rosiglitazole.

Patient/Family Teaching
- Instruct patient to take medication at same time each day. Take missed doses as soon as remembered unless almost time for next dose. Do not take if unable to eat.
- Explain to patient that this medication controls hyperglycemia but does not cure diabetes. Therapy is long term.
- Review signs of hypoglycemia and hyperglycemia with patient. If hypoglycemia occurs, advise patient to take a glass of orange juice or 2–3 tsp of sugar, honey, or corn syrup dissolved in water and notify health care professional.

- Encourage patient to follow prescribed diet, medication, and exercise regimen to prevent hypoglycemic or hyperglycemic episodes.
- Instruct patient in proper testing of serum glucose and ketones. These tests should be closely monitored during periods of stress or illness and health care professional notified if significant changes occur.
- May occasionally cause dizziness. Caution patient to avoid driving or other activities requiring alertness until response to medication is known.
- Caution patient to avoid other medications, especially aspirin and alcohol, while on this therapy without consulting health care professional.
- Insulin is the recommended method of controlling blood glucose during pregnancy. Counsel female patients to use a form of contraception other than oral contraceptives and to notify health care professional promptly if pregnancy is planned or suspected.
- Advise patient to inform health care professional of medication regimen prior to treatment or surgery.
- Advise patient to carry a form of sugar (sugar packets, candy) and identification describing disease process and medication regimen at all times.
- Emphasize the importance of routine follow-up exams.

Evaluation/Desired Outcomes
- Control of blood glucose levels without the appearance of hypoglycemic or hyperglycemic episodes.

---

nebivolol (ne-bi-vi-lole)
Bystolic

Classification
Therapeutic: antihypertensives
Pharmacologic: beta blockers (selective)

Pregnancy Category C

Indications
Hypertension (alone and with other antihypertensives).

Action
Blocks stimulation of beta adrenergic receptor sites; selective for beta$_1$ (myocardial) receptors in most patients. In some patients (poor metabolizers, higher blood levels may result in some beta$_2$ [pulmonary, vascular, uterine] adrenergic) blockade. **Therapeutic Effects:** Lowering of blood pressure.

Pharmacokinetics
Absorption: Well absorbed following oral administration.
Distribution: Unknown.
Protein Binding: 98%.
Metabolism and Excretion: Mostly metabolized by the liver, including the CYP2D6 enzyme system; some have antihypertensive action; minimal excretion of unchanged drug.
Half-life: *Extensive metabolizers*—12 hr; *poor metabolizers*—19 hr.

TIME/ACTION PROFILE (blood levels)

ROUTE	ONSET	PEAK	DURATION
PO	unknown	1.5–4 hr	24 hr

Contraindications/Precautions
Contraindicated in: Hypersensitivity; Severe bradycardia, heart block greater than first degree. cardiogenic shock, decompensated heart failure or sick sinus syndrome (without pacemaker); Severe hepatic impairment (Child-Pugh >B); Bronchospastic disease; OB: Lactation.
Use Cautiously in: Coronary artery disease (rapid cessation should be avoided); Compensated congestive heart failure; Major surgery (anesthesia may augment myocardial depression); Diabetes mellitus (may mask signs of hypoglycemia); Thyrotoxicosis (may mask symptoms); Moderate hepatic impairment (↓ metabolism); Severe renal impairment (↓ initial dose if CCr <30 mL/min); History of severe allergic reactions (↑ intensity of reactions); Pheochromocytoma (alpha blockers required prior to beta blockers); Geri: Consider increased sensitivity, concurrent chronic diseases, medications and presence of age-related decrease in clearance; OB: Use in pregnancy only if maternal benefit outweighs fetal risk; Pedi: Safe use in children <18 yr not established.

Adverse Reactions/Side Effects
CNS: dizziness, fatigue, headache.

Interactions
Drug-Drug: Drugs that affect the CYP2D6 enzyme system are expected to alter levels and possibly effects of nebivolol; dose alterations may be required. **Fluoxetine**, a known inhibitor of CYP2D6, ↑ levels and effects; similar effects may

be expected from **quinidine**, **propafenone**, and **paroxetine**. Blood levels are also ↑ by **cimetine**. **Anesthetic agents** including **ether**, **trichloroethylene**, and **cyclopropane** as well as **other myocardial depressants** or **inhibitors of AV conduction**, such as **diltiazem** and **verapamil** may ↑ risk of myocardial depression and bradycardia. Avoid concurrent use with **beta blockers**. Concurrent use with **reserpine** or **guanethidine** may excessively reduce sympathetic activity. If used concurrently with **clonidine**, nebivolol should be tapered and discontinued several days prior to gradual withdrawal of clonidine.

Route/Dosage
PO (Adults): 5 mg once daily initially, may increase at 2 wk intervals up to 40 mg/day.

Hepatic/Renal Impairment
PO (Adults): 2.5 mg once daily initially; titrate upward cautiously.

Availability
Tablets: 2.5, 5 mg, 10 mg.

NURSING IMPLICATIONS

Assessment
- Monitor blood pressure, ECG, and pulse prior to and periodically during therapy.
- Monitor intake and output ratios and daily weights. Assess routinely for signs and symptoms of CHF (dyspnea, rales/crackles, weight gain, peripheral edema, jugular venous distention).
- *Lab Test Considerations:* May cause ↑ BUN, uric acid, triglycerides and ↓ HDL cholesterol and platelet court.

Potential Nursing Diagnoses
Decreased cardiac output (Side Effects)

Implementation
- **PO:** May be administered without regard to food.
- When discontinuation is planned, observe patient carefully and advise to minimize physical activity. Taper over 1–2 wk when possible. If angina worsens or acute coronary insufficiency develops, reinstitute nebivolol promptly, at least temporarily.

Patient/Family Teaching
- Instruct patient to take nebivolol as directed, at the same time each day, even if feeling well. If a dose is missed, skip missed dose and take next scheduled dose; do not double doses. Do not discontinue without consulting health care professional. Abrupt withdrawal may precipitate life-threatening arrhythmias, hypertension, or myocardial ischemia.
- Advise patient to ensure that enough medication is available for weekends, holidays, and vacations. A written prescription may be kept in the wallet for emergencies.
- Reinforce the need to continue additional therapies for hypertension (weight loss, sodium restriction, stress reduction, regular exercise, moderation of alcohol consumption, and smoking cessation). Medication controls but does not cure hypertension.
- Teach patient and family how to check pulse and blood pressure. Instruct them to check pulse daily and blood pressure biweekly and to report significant changes to health care professional.
- Instruct patient to consult health care professional before taking any Rx, OTC, or herbal products, especially cold preparations, concurrently with this medication. Patients on antihypertensive therapy should also avoid excessive amounts of coffee, tea, and cola.
- May mask some signs of hypoglycemia, especially tachycardia. Diabetics should closely monitor blood sugar, especially if weakness, malaise, irritability, or fatigue occurs. Medication does not block dizziness or sweating as signs of hypoglycemia.
- May cause dizziness. Caution patients to avoid driving or other activities requiring alertness until response to medication is known.
- Advise patient to notify health care professional if difficulty breathing or signs and symptoms of worsening CHF (weight gain, increasing shortness or breath, excessive bradycardia) occur.
- Instruct patient to inform health care professional of medication regimen before treatment or surgery.
- Advise patient to carry identification describing disease process and medication regimen at all times.
- Advise female patients that breastfeeding should be avoided during nebivolol therapy.

Evaluation/Desired Outcomes
- Decrease in blood pressure.

---

nefazodone (neff-a-zoe-done)

Classification
Therapeutic: antidepressants

Pregnancy Category C

Indications
Major depression. **Unlabeled Use:** Panic disorder, post-traumatic stress disorder (PTSD).

Action
Inhibits the reuptake of serotonin and norepinephrine by neurons. Antagonizes alpha$_1$-adrenergic receptors. **Therapeutic Effects:** Antidepressant action, which may develop only after several weeks.

Pharmacokinetics
Absorption: Well absorbed but undergoes extensive and variable first-pass hepatic metabolism (bioavailability about 20%).
Distribution: Widely distributed; enters the CNS.
Protein Binding: ≥99%.
Metabolism and Excretion: Extensively metabolized. One metabolite (hydroxynefazodone) has antidepressant activity.
Half-life: *Nefazodone*—2–4 hr; *hydroxynefazodone*—1.5–4 hr.

TIME/ACTION PROFILE (antidepressant action)

ROUTE	ONSET	PEAK	DURATION
PO	days–wk	several wk	unknown

Contraindications/Precautions
Contraindicated in: Hypersensitivity; Concurrent MAO inhibitor therapy; Active liver disease or baseline elevated serum transaminases.
Use Cautiously in: May ↑ risk of suicide attempt/ideation especially during dose early treatment or dose adjustment; History of suicide attempt or drug abuse; Underlying cardiovascular or cerebrovascular disease; History of mania; OB: Safety no established; Lactation: Discontinue drug or bottle-feed; Pedi: Safety not established in children; suicide risk may be greater in children and adolescents ; Geri: Initiate therapy at lower doses.

Adverse Reactions/Side Effects
CNS: dizziness, insomnia, somnolence, agitation, confusion, weakness. **EENT:** abnormal vision, blurred vision, eye pain, tinnitus. **Resp:** dyspnea. **CV:** bradycardia, hypotension. **GI:** HEPATIC FAILURE, HEPATOTOXICITY, constipation, dry mouth, nausea, gastroenteritis. **GU:** erectile dysfunction. **Derm:** rashes. **Hemat:** decreased hematocrit.

Interactions
Drug-Drug: Serious, potentially fatal reactions may occur during concurrent use with **MAO inhibitors** (do not use concurrently or within 2 wk of MAO inhibitors; discontinue nefazodone at least 14 days before starting MAO inhibitor therapy). ↑ CNS depression with other CNS depressants including **alcohol**, **antihistamines**, **opioid analgesics**, and **sedative/hypnotics**. May ↑ blood levels and effects of **alprazolam** or **triazolam**. May increase serum **digoxin** levels. Additive hypotension may occur with **antihypertensives**, **nitrates**, or acute ingestion of **alcohol**. May ↑ risk of myopathy with **HMG-CoA reductase inhibitors**. Decreased antidepressant action with concomitant use of **carbamazepine**. May reduce clearance of **haloperidol**, so **haloperidol** dose may need to be decreased.
Drug-Natural Products: ↑ risk of seritonergic side effects including serotonin syndrome with **St. John's wort** and **SAMe**. **Kava-kava**, **valerian**, or **chamomile** can ↑ CNS depression.

Route/Dosage
PO (Adults): 100 mg twice daily initially; may be increased weekly up to 600 mg/day in 2 divided doses.
PO (Geriatric Patients): 50 mg twice daily initially; may be increased weekly as tolerated.

Availability (generic available)
Tablets: 50 mg, 100 mg, 150 mg, 200 mg, 250 mg.

NURSING IMPLICATIONS
Assessment
- Assess mental status (orientation, mood, behavior) frequently. Inform health care professional if patient demonstrates significant increase in anxiety, nervousness, or insomnia.
- Assess suicidal tendencies, especially in early therapy. Restrict amount of drug available to patient.
- Monitor blood pressure and pulse before and periodically during therapy.
- Monitor liver function tests prior to and routinely during therapy. Obtain LFTs at first sign of hepatic dysfunction (nausea, vomiting, abdominal pain, fatigue, anorexia, dark urine).
- Assess for sexual dysfunction throughout treatment.
- ***Lab Test Considerations:*** May cause decrease in hematocrit and leukopenia.
- Monitor liver function periodically. If serum AST or ALT levels are >3 times the upper limit of normal discontinue nefazodone.
- May also cause hypercholesterolemia and hypoglycemia.

Potential Nursing Diagnoses
Ineffective coping (Indications)
Risk for injury (Side Effects)

Implementation
- Discontinue nefazodone prior to elective surgery to prevent potential interactions with general anesthesia.
- **PO:** Administer doses twice daily.

Patient/Family Teaching
- Instruct patient to take medication as directed. Several weeks may be required to obtain a full antidepressant response. Once response is obtained, therapy should be continued for at least 6 mo. If a dose is missed, take as soon as possible unless almost time for next dose. Do not double doses.
- May cause drowsiness or dizziness. Caution patient to avoid driving or other activities requiring alertness until response to the drug is known.
- Advise patient to make position changes slowly to minimize orthostatic hypotension.
- Caution patient to avoid taking alcohol or other CNS depressant drugs during therapy and not to take other prescription, OTC medications, or herbal products without consulting health care professional.
- Advise patient to notify health care professional immediately if signs of liver dysfunction (jaundice, anorexia, GI complaints, malaise, dark urine) occur.
- Inform patient that frequent mouth rinses, good oral hygiene, and sugarless gum or candy may minimize dry mouth. If dry mouth persists for more than 2 wk, consult health care professional regarding use of saliva substitute.
- Instruct female patient to inform health care professional if pregnancy is planned or suspected or if breastfeeding.
- Instruct patient to notify health care professional of signs of allergy (rash, hives) or if agitation, blurred or other changes in vision, confusion, dizziness, unsteadiness, difficult or frequent urination, difficulty concentrating, or memory problems occur.
- Emphasize the importance of follow-up examinations to monitor progress. Encourage patient participation in psychotherapy.
- Refer to local support group.
- Inform patient that some side effects may go away with time.

Evaluation/Desired Outcomes
- Increased sense of well-being.
- Renewed interest in surroundings. May require several weeks of therapy to obtain full response. Need for therapy should be periodically reassessed. Therapy is usually continued for 6 months or more.

neomycin, See AMINOGLYCOSIDES.

neostigmine
(nee-oh-**stig**-meen)
Prostigmin

Classification
Therapeutic: antimyasthenics
Pharmacologic: cholinergics

Pregnancy Category C

Indications
Improvement in muscle strength in symptomatic treatment of myasthenia gravis. Prevention and treatment of postoperative bladder distention and urinary retention or ileus. Reversal of nondepolarizing neuromuscular blockers.

Action
Inhibits the breakdown of acetylcholine so that it accumulates and has a prolonged effect. Effects include miosis, increased intestinal and skeletal muscle tone, bronchial and ureteral constriction, bradycardia, increased salivation, lacrimation, and sweating. **Therapeutic Effects:** Improved muscular function in patients with myasthenia gravis, improved bladder-emptying in patients with urinary retention, or reversal of nondepolarizing neuromuscular blockers.

Pharmacokinetics
Absorption: Poorly absorbed following oral administration, necessitating large oral doses compared with parenteral doses.
Distribution: Probably does not cross the placenta or enter breast milk.
Metabolism and Excretion: Metabolized by plasma cholinesterases and the liver.
Half-life: *PO, IV*—40–60 min; *IM*—50–90 min.

TIME/ACTION PROFILE (cholinergic effects, increased muscle tone)

ROUTE	ONSET	PEAK	DURATION
PO	45–75 min	unknown	2–4 hr
IM	10–30 min	20–30 min	2–4 hr
IV	10–30 min	20–30 min	2–4 hr

Contraindications/Precautions
Contraindicated in: Hypersensitivity; Mechanical obstruction of the GI or GU tract; Lactation: Lactation.

neostigmine

Use Cautiously in: History of asthma; Ulcer disease; Cardiovascular disease; Epilepsy; Hyperthyroidism; OB: May cause uterine irritability after IV administration near term; newborns may display muscle weakness.

Adverse Reactions/Side Effects
CNS: SEIZURES, dizziness, weakness. **EENT:** lacrimation, miosis. **Resp:** bronchospasm, excess secretions. **CV:** bradycardia, hypotension. **GI:** abdominal cramps, diarrhea, excess salivation, nausea, vomiting. **Derm:** sweating, rash.

Interactions
Drug-Drug: Action may be antagonized by **drugs possessing anticholinergic properties**, including **antihistamines**, **antidepressants**, **atropine**, **haloperidol**, **phenothiazines**, **quinidine**, and **disopyramide**. Prolongs action of **depolarizing muscle-relaxing agents (succinylcholine, decamethonium)**.

Route/Dosage
Myasthenia Gravis
PO (Adults): 15 mg q 3–4 hr initially; ↑ at daily intervals until optimal response is achieved. Usual maintenance dose is 150 mg/day (up to 375 mg/day may be needed).
PO (Children): 2 mg/kg/day (60 mg/m^2) in 6–8 divided doses.
Subcut, IM (Adults): 0.5 mg.
Subcut, IM (Children): 10–40 mcg/kg q 2–3 hr; may give with 10 mcg/kg atropine.

Bladder Atony, Abdominal Distention: Prevention
IM, Subcut (Adults): 250 mcg q 4–6 hr for 2–3 days.

Bladder Atony, Abdominal Distention: Treatment
IM, Subcut (Adults): 500 mcg as needed; may repeat q 3 hr for 5 doses after bladder has been emptied for bladder atony.

Antidote for Nondepolarizing Neuromuscular Blockers
IV (Adults): 0.5–2 mg slowly; pretreat with 0.6–1.2 mg atropine IV (may be repeated to a total dose of 5 mg).
IV (Children): 40 mcg/kg with 20 mcg/kg atropine.

Availability (generic available)
Tablets: 15 mg. **Injection:** 0.5 mg/mL, 1 mg/mL.

NURSING IMPLICATIONS
Assessment
- Assess pulse, respiratory rate, and blood pressure prior to administration. Report significant changes in heart rate.
- **Myasthenia Gravis:** Assess neuromuscular status, including vital capacity, ptosis, diplopia, chewing, swallowing, hand grasp, and gait, prior to administering and at peak effect. Patients with myasthenia gravis may be advised to keep a daily record of their condition and the effects of this medication.
- Assess patient for overdose and underdose or resistance. Both have similar symptoms (muscle weakness, dyspnea, dysphagia), but symptoms of overdose usually occur within 1 hr of administration, whereas underdose symptoms occur 3 or more hr after administration. Overdose (cholinergic crisis) symptoms may also include increased respiratory secretions and saliva, bradycardia, nausea, vomiting, cramping, diarrhea, and diaphoresis. A Tensilon test (edrophonium chloride) may be used to distinguish between overdose and underdose.
- **Postoperative Ileus:** Monitor abdominal status (assess for distention, auscultate bowel sounds). A rectal tube may be inserted to facilitate expulsion of flatus.
- **Postoperative Urinary Retention:** Assess for bladder distention. Monitor intake and output. If patient is unable to void within 1 hr of neostigmine administration, consider catheterization.
- **Antidote to Nondepolarizing Neuromuscular Blocking Agents:** Monitor reversal of effects of neuromuscular blocking agents with a peripheral nerve stimulator. Recovery usually occurs consecutively in the following muscles: diaphragm, intercostal muscles, muscles of the glottis, abdominal muscles, limb muscles, muscles of mastication, and levator muscles of the eyelids. Closely observe the patient for residual muscle weakness and respiratory distress throughout the recovery period. Maintain airway patency and ventilation until recovery of normal respiration occurs.
- *Toxicity and Overdose:* If overdose occurs, atropine is the antidote.

Potential Nursing Diagnoses
Impaired physical mobility (Indications)
Ineffective breathing pattern (Indications)

✦ = Canadian drug name. = Genetic implication.
*CAPITALS indicates life-threatening; underlines indicate most frequent.

Implementation
- Oral and parenteral doses are not interchangeable.
- When used as an antidote to nondepolarizing neuromuscular blocking agents, atropine may be used prior to or concurrently with neostigmine to prevent or treat bradycardia.
- **PO:** Administer with food or milk to minimize side effects. For patients who have difficulty chewing, neostigmine may be taken 30 min before meals.

IV Administration
- **Direct IV:** Administer doses undiluted. May be given through Y-site of an IV of D5W, 0.9% NaCl, Ringer's solution, or LR. *Concentration:* 0.5–1 mg/mL. *Rate:* Administer each 0.5 mg over 1 min.
- **Syringe Compatibility:** glycopyrrolate, heparin, ondansetron, pentobarbital, thiopental.
- **Y-Site Compatibility:** heparin, hydrocortisone sodium succinate, potassium chloride, vitamin B complex with C.

Patient/Family Teaching
- Instruct patient to take medication exactly as directed. Do not skip or double up on missed doses. Patients with a history of dysphagia should have a nonelectric or battery-operated backup alarm clock to remind them of exact dosage time. Patients with dysphagia may not be able to swallow the medication if the dose is not taken exactly on time. Taking the dose late may result in myasthenic crisis. Taking the dose early may result in cholinergic crisis. Patients with myasthenia gravis must continue this regimen as lifelong therapy.
- Instruct patient with myasthenia gravis to space activities to avoid fatigue.
- Advise patient to carry identification describing disease and medication regimen at all times.

Evaluation/Desired Outcomes
- Relief of ptosis and diplopia.
- Improved chewing, swallowing, extremity strength, and breathing without the appearance of cholinergic symptoms in myasthenia gravis.
- Relief or prevention of postoperative gastrointestinal ileus.
- Relief of nonobstructive postoperative urinary retention.
- Reversal of nondepolarizing neuromuscular blocking agents in general anesthesia.

HIGH ALERT

nesiritide (ne-sir-i-tide)
Natrecor

Classification
Therapeutic: none assigned
Pharmacologic: vasodilators (human B-type natriuretic peptide)

Pregnancy Category C

Indications
Acutely decompensated CHF in hospitalized patients who have dyspnea at rest or with minimal activity; has been used with digoxin, diuretics, and ACE inhibitors. Should not be used for intermittent outpatient infusion, scheduled repetitive use, as a diuretic or to improve renal function.

Action
Binds to guanyl cyclase receptors in vascular smooth muscle and endothelial cells, producing increased intracellular guanosine 3'5'-cyclic monophosphate (cGMP) and smooth muscle cell relaxation. cGMP acts as a "second messenger" to dilate veins and arteries. **Therapeutic Effects:** Dose-dependent reduction in pulmonary capillary wedge pressure (PCWP) and systemic arterial pressure in patients with heart failure with resultant decrease in dyspnea.

Pharmacokinetics
Absorption: IV administration results in complete bioavailability.
Distribution: Unknown.
Metabolism and Excretion: Cleared from circulation by binding to cell surface clearance receptors resulting in cellular internalization and proteolysis, proteolytic breakdown by endopeptidases, and renal filtration.
Half-life: 18 min.

TIME/ACTION PROFILE (effects on cardiovascular parameters)

ROUTE	ONSET	PEAK	DURATION
IV	15 min	1 hr	60 min†

†Longer with higher than recommended doses

Contraindications/Precautions
Contraindicated in: Hypersensitivity; Cardiogenic shock; Systolic blood pressure <90 mm Hg; Low cardiac filling pressure, significant valvular stenosis, restrictive/subtractive cardiomyopathy, constrictive pericarditis/cardiac tamponade, or other conditions in which cardiac output is dependent on venous return.
Use Cautiously in: Heart failure where renal function is dependent on activity of the renin/an-

giotensin/aldosterone system (may cause azotemia); Cardiogenic shock (should not be used as primary therapy); OB, Lactation, Pedi: Pregnancy, lactation, or children (safety not established); Geri: May have ↑ sensitivity to effects.

Adverse Reactions/Side Effects
CNS: anxiety, confusion, dizziness, headache, hypotension (dose related), insomnia, drowsiness. **EENT:** amblyopia. **Resp:** APNEA, cough, hemoptysis. **CV:** hypotension, arrhythmias, bradycardia. **GI:** abdominal pain, nausea, vomiting. **GU:** ↑ creatinine, renal failure. **Derm:** itching, rash, sweating. **Hemat:** anemia. **Local:** injection site reactions. **MS:** back pain, leg cramps. **Neuro:** paresthesia, tremor. **Misc:** fever.

Interactions
Drug-Drug: None reported.

Route/Dosage
IV (Adults): 2 mcg/kg bolus followed by 0.01 mcg/kg/min as a continuous infusion. May ↑ by 0.005 mcg/kg/min every 3 hr up to a maximum infusion rate of 0.03 mcg/kg/min (based on response).

Availability
Powder for injection: 1.5 mg/vial.

NURSING IMPLICATIONS
Assessment
- Monitor blood pressure, pulse, ECG, respiratory rate, cardiac index, PCWP, and central venous pressure frequently during administration. May cause hypotension, especially in patients with a BP <100 mm Hg. Reduce dose or discontinue nesiritide if patient develops hypotension. Hypotension may cause renal compromise. Use IV fluids and changes in body position to support blood pressure if symptomatic hypotension occurs. Nesiritide may be restarted at a dose reduced by 30% with no bolus administration once patient is stabilized. Hypotension may be prolonged for hours, requiring a period of monitoring prior to restarting administration.
- Monitor intake and output and weigh daily. Assess for decrease in signs of CHF (dyspnea, rales/crackles, peripheral edema, weight gain).
- **Lab Test Considerations:** Monitor BUN and serum creatinine. May cause ↑ in serum creatinine; ↑ serum creatinine may be dose-related.

Potential Nursing Diagnoses
Decreased cardiac output (Indications)
Activity intolerance (Indications)
Excess fluid volume (Indications)

Implementation
- ***High Alert:*** Intravenous vasoactive medications have an increased potential for causing harm. Have second practitioner independently check original order, dose calculations, and infusion pump settings. Administer only in settings where blood pressure can be closely monitored.
- Prime the IV tubing with an infusion of 25 mL prior to connecting to the patient's vascular access port and prior to administering bolus or infusion. Flush catheter between administration of nesiritide and other medications. Do not administer through a central heparin-coated catheter as nesiritide binds to heparin. Concomitant administration of a heparin infusion through a separate catheter is acceptable.

IV Administration
- **Direct IV:** ***Diluent:*** Reconstitute 1.5-mg vial of nesiritide by adding 5 mL of diluent removed from a pre-filled 250-mL plastic IV bag containing D5W, 0.9% NaCl, D5/0.45% NaCl, or D5/0.2% NaCl. Do not shake vial; rock gently so all surfaces including stopper are in contact with diluent to ensure complete reconstitution. Withdraw entire content of reconstituted vial and add back to 250-mL plastic IV bag. Invert IV bag several times to ensure complete mixing of solution. Infusion stable for 24 hr. After preparation of infusion bag, withdraw bolus volume from infusion bag. To calculate amount: bolus volume (mL) = 0.33 × patient weight (kg). ***Concentration:*** 6 mcg/mL. *Rate:* Administer bolus over 60 seconds through a port in the IV tubing.
- **Intermittent Infusion:** ***Diluent:*** See Diluent section under Direct IV section above for preparation instructions for infusion bag. Immediately follow bolus with infusion. ***Concentration:*** 6 mcg/mL. *Rate:* Based on patient's weight (see Route/Dosage section).
- **Y-Site Compatibility:** amiodarone, argatroban, digoxin, diltiazem, metoprolol, milrinone, nicardipine, nitroglycerin, nitroprusside, palonosetron, propranolol, tirofiban, torsemide, verapamil.

- **Y-Site Incompatibility:** bumetanide, daptomycin, enalaprilat, ethacrynic acid, furosemide, heparin, hydralazine, insulin, micafungin.

Patient/Family Teaching
- Explain purpose of nesiritide to patient and family.

Evaluation/Desired Outcomes
- Improvement in dyspnea and reduction in mean PCWP in patients with decompensated CHF.

---

nevirapine (ne-**veer**-a-peen)
Viramune

Classification
Therapeutic: antiretrovirals
Pharmacologic: non-nucleoside reverse transcriptase inhibitors

Pregnancy Category C

Indications
Management of HIV infection in combination with a nucleoside analogue.

Action
Binds to the enzyme reverse transcriptase, which results in disruption of DNA synthesis. **Therapeutic Effects:** Slowed progression of HIV infection and decreased occurrence of sequelae.

Pharmacokinetics
Absorption: >90% absorbed after oral administration.
Distribution: Crosses placenta and enters breast milk; CSF levels are 45% of those in plasma.
Metabolism and Excretion: Mostly metabolized by the liver (CYP3A4 enzyme system); minor amounts excreted unchanged in urine.
Half-life: 25–30 hr (during multiple dosing).

TIME/ACTION PROFILE (blood levels)

ROUTE	ONSET	PEAK	DURATION
PO	rapid	4 hr	12 hr

Contraindications/Precautions
Contraindicated in: Hypersensitivity; Concurrent ketoconazole, rifampin, or St. John's wort; Moderate to severe hepatic impairment (Child-Pugh Class B or C); Women with CD4+ cell counts >250 cells/mm^3 (↑ risk of liver toxicity).
Use Cautiously in: Women (↑ risk of liver toxicity); Hepatic or renal impairment; Concurrent clarithromycin, fluconazole, methadone, or rifabutin (careful monitoring required; alternative therapy should be considered); OB, Lactation: Pedi: Safety not established; breastfeeding not recommended in HIV-infected patients.

Adverse Reactions/Side Effects
Reflects combination therapy.
CNS: headache. **GI:** HEPATOTOXICITY, elevated liver enzyme levels, nausea, abdominal pain, diarrhea, hepatitis, ulcerative stomatitis. **Derm:** RASH (MAY PROGRESS TO TOXIC EPIDERMAL NECROLYSIS). **Hemat:** granulocytopenia (increased in children). **MS:** myalgia. **Neuro:** paresthesia, peripheral neuropathy. **Misc:** STEVENS-JOHNSON SYNDROME, fever.

Interactions
Drug-Drug: Nevirapine induces the hepatic CYP3A4 enzyme system and can affect the behavior of drugs metabolized by this system. Significantly ↓ **ketoconazole** levels (concurrent use contraindicated). May induce **methadone** withdrawal within 2 weeks of starting therapy in patients physically dependent on methadone. May ↓ levels and effectiveness **hormonal contraceptives** (concurrent use of hormonal contraceptives should be avoided). **Rifampin** significantly ↓ levels and effectiveness of nevirapine (concurrent use contraindicated). ↓ Levels and effectiveness of **clarithromycin** (consider other agents). Also may ↓ levels and effectiveness of the following: **lopinavir, saquinavir, nelfnavir, indinavir, efavirenz, amiodarone, disopyramide, lidocaine, itraconazole, carbamazepine, clonazepam, ethosuximide, diltiazem, nifedipine, verapamil, cyclosporine, tacrolimus, sirolimus, cyclophosphamide, ergotamine fentanyl rifabutin** (use together only with careful monitoring). **Fluconazole** ↑ nevirapine levels and risk of toxcity. May ↑ risk of bleeding with **warfarin**. Use of **prednisone** during first 2 wk of therapy may ↑ risk of rash. Initiating other **drugs that often cause rash**, including **trimethoprim/sulfamethoxazole** and **abacavir** simultaneously with nevirapine may ↑ risk of rash.
Drug-Natural Products: St. John's wort may ↓ efficacy.

Route/Dosage
PO (Adults): 200 mg daily for the first 2 wk, then 200 mg twice daily (in combination with a nucleoside analogue antiretroviral).
PO (Children ≥15 days): 150 mg/m^2 once daily for first 2 wk, then 150 mg/m^2 twice daily.

Availability
Tablets: 200 mg. **Oral suspension:** 50 mg/5 mL.

NURSING IMPLICATIONS

Assessment
- Assess for change in severity of HIV symptoms and for symptoms of opportunistic infections throughout therapy.
- Assess for rash (mild to moderate rash = erythema or maculopapular rash; urticaria, pruritic raised rash with welts; constitutional symptoms—fever, blistering, oral erosive lesions, conjunctivitis, facial edema, myalgia, arthralgia), especially during 1st 6 wk of therapy. If rash is severe (extensive erythematous or maculopapular rash with moist desquamation or angioedema) or accompanied by systemic symptoms (serum sickness-like reaction, Stevens-Johnson syndrome, toxic epidermal necrolysis), therapy must be discontinued immediately. Prednisone and antihistamines are not effective in preventing or treating the rash. If mild to moderate rash occurs during 2 wk lead-in period, do not increase dose until rash resolves. If not resolved within 28 days, reconsider therapy.
- ***Lab Test Considerations:*** Monitor viral load and CD4 cell count regularly during therapy.
- Monitor for liver function at baseline and frequently during the first 18 wk for toxicity, especially during first 6 wk of therapy. May be asymptomatic with ↑ AST and ALT without clinical signs or symptoms, or symptomatic with ↑ liver enzymes and at least one symptom (rash, flu-like symptoms, fever). May progress to liver failure and dealth. If signs of liver toxicity occur, permanently discontinue nevirapine.
- Assess patient for hepatitis B and C. Patients with HBV and/or HCV are at risk for liver toxicity.

Potential Nursing Diagnoses
Risk for infection (Indications)
Noncompliance (Patient/Family Teaching)

Implementation
- Do not confuse nevirapine (Viramune) with nelfinavir (Viracept).
- **PO:** May be administered with or without food.
- Shake oral solution prior to administration. Use an oral dosing syringe for amounts <5 mL. Rinse syringe or cup and readminister to ensure patient receives full dose.
- If therapy is interrupted for more than 7 days, restart therapy at 200 mg daily for 14 days, then increase dose to 200 mg twice daily.

Patient/Family Teaching
- Emphasize the importance of taking nevirapine as directed, at evenly spaced times throughout day. Instruct patient to read the *Medication Guide* prior to initiating therapy and with each Rx refill. Do not take more than prescribed amount and do not stop taking without consulting health care professional. Take missed doses as soon as remembered; do not double doses.
- Instruct patient not to share nevirapine with others.
- Advise patient to avoid taking other Rx, OTC, and herbal products without consulting health care professional.
- Inform patient that nevirapine does not cure AIDS or prevent associated or opportunistic infections. Nevirapine does not reduce the risk of transmission of HIV to others through sexual contact or blood contamination. Caution patient to use a condom and avoid sharing needles or donating blood to prevent spreading the AIDS virus to others. Advise patient that the long-term effects of nevirapine are unknown at this time.
- Advise patients taking oral contraceptives to use a nonhormonal method of birth control during nevirapine therapy.
- Instruct patient to notify health care professional immediately if signs and symptoms of hepatitis (flu-like symptoms, tiredness, nausea, lack of appetite, yellow skin or eyes, dark urine, pale stools, pain or sensitivity to touch on right side below ribs), or skin reactions with symptoms (flu-like symptoms, fever, muscle aches, conjunctivitis, blisters, mouth sores, swelling of face, tiredness) occur. Nevirapine should be discontinued immediately.
- Emphasize the importance of regular follow-up exams and blood counts to determine progress and monitor for side effects.

Evaluation/Desired Outcomes
- Delayed progression of AIDS and decreased opportunistic infections in patients with HIV.
- Decrease in viral load and increase in CD4 cell counts.

✦ = Canadian drug name. ▌= Genetic implication.
*CAPITALS indicates life-threatening; underlines indicate most frequent.

niacin (nye-a-sin)
Edur-Acin, Nia-Bid, Niac, Niacels, Niacor, Niaspan, Nicobid, Nico-400, Nicolar, Nicotinex, nicotinic acid, ✦ Novo-Niacin, Slo-Niacin, vitamin B

niacinamide (nye-a-**sin**-a-mide)
nicotinamide

Classification
Therapeutic: lipid-lowering agents, vitamins
Pharmacologic: water soluble vitamins

Pregnancy Category C

Indications
Treatment and prevention of niacin deficiency (pellagra). Adjunctive therapy in certain hyperlipidemias (niacin only).

Action
Required as coenzymes (for lipid metabolism, glycogenolysis, and tissue respiration). Large doses decrease lipoprotein and triglyceride synthesis by inhibiting the release of free fatty acids from adipose tissue and decreasing hepatic lipoprotein synthesis (niacin only). Cause peripheral vasodilation in large doses (niacin only). **Therapeutic Effects:** Decreased blood lipids (niacin only). Supplementation in deficiency states.

Pharmacokinetics
Absorption: Well absorbed following oral administration.
Distribution: Widely distributed following conversion to niacinamide. Enters breast milk.
Metabolism and Excretion: Amounts required for metabolic processes are converted to niacinamide. Large doses of niacin are excreted unchanged in the urine.
Half-life: 45 min.

TIME/ACTION PROFILE (effects on blood lipids)

ROUTE	ONSET	PEAK	DURATION
PO (cholesterol)	several days	unknown	unknown
PO (triglycerides)	several hr	unknown	unknown

Contraindications/Precautions
Contraindicated in: Hypersensitivity to niacin; Some products may contain tartrazine and should be avoided in patients with known hypersensitivity; Alcohol intolerance (Nicotinex only).
Use Cautiously in: Liver disease; Arterial bleeding; History of peptic ulcer disease; Gout; Glaucoma; Diabetes mellitus.

Adverse Reactions/Side Effects
Adverse reactions and side effects refer to doses used to treat hyperlipidemia.
CNS: dizziness, nervousness, panic. **EENT:** blurred vision, loss of central vision, proptosis, toxic amblyopia. **CV:** orthostatic hypotension. **GI:** HEPATOTOXICITY, GI upset, bloating, diarrhea, dry mouth, flatulence, heartburn, hunger pains, nausea, peptic ulceration. **Derm:** flushing of the face and neck, pruritus, burning, dry skin, hyperpigmentation, ↑ sebaceous gland activity, rashes, stinging or tingling of skin. **Metab:** glycosuria, hyperglycemia, hyperuricemia. **MS:** myalgia.

Interactions
Drug-Drug: ↑ risk of myopathy with concurrent use of **HMG-CoA reductase inhibitors**. Additive hypotension with **antihypertensive agents**. Large doses may ↓ uricosuric effects of **probenecid**.

Route/Dosage
PO (Adults and Children): *Dietary supplement*—10–20 mg/day. *Dietary deficiency*—Up to 500 mg/day in divided doses. *Hyperlipidemias–Niacin only*—100–500 mg/day initially; ↑ slowly up to 1–2 g tid (up to 8 g/day).
PO (Children 7–10 yr): *Prevention of deficiency*—13 mg/day.
PO (Children 4–6 yr): *Prevention of deficiency*—12 mg/day.
PO (Children birth–3 yr): *Prevention of deficiency*—5–9 mg/day.

Availability

Niacin (generic available)
Tablets: 25 mg^{OTC}, 50 mg^{OTC}, 100 mg^{OTC}, 125 mg^{OTC}, 250 mg^{OTC}, 400 mg^{OTC}, 500 mg$^{Rx, OTC}$. **Extended-release tablets:** 125 mg$^{Rx, OTC}$, 250 mg$^{Rx, OTC}$, 400 mg^{OTC}, 500 mg$^{Rx, OTC}$, 750 mg$^{Rx, OTC}$, 1000 mg^{OTC}. **Cost:** 500 mg $184.97/90, 750 mg $255.96/90, 1000 mg $331.97/90. **Extended-release capsules:** 125 mg$^{Rx, OTC}$, 250 mg$^{Rx, OTC}$, 300 mg$^{Rx, OTC}$, 400 mg$^{Rx, OTC}$, 500 mg$^{Rx, OTC}$. **Elixir:** 50 mg/5 mL in pints and gallons^{OTC}. *In combination with:* lovastatin (Advicor); simvastatin (Simcor). See Appendix B.

Niacinamide (generic available)
Tablets: 50 mg^{OTC}, 100 mg^{OTC}, 125 mg^{OTC}, 250 mg^{OTC}, 500 mg$^{Rx, OTC}$.

NURSING IMPLICATIONS

Assessment
- **Vitamin Deficiency:** Assess patient for signs of niacin deficiency (*pellagra*—dermatitis, stomatitis, glossitis, anemia, nausea and vomit-

ing, confusion, memory loss, and delirium) prior to and periodically during therapy.
- **Hyperlipidemia:** Obtain a diet history, especially with regard to fat consumption.
- *Lab Test Considerations:* Monitor serum glucose and uric acid levels and hepatic function tests periodically during prolonged high-dose therapy. Notify health care professional if AST, ALT, or LDH becomes elevated. May ↑ prothrombin times and ↓ serum albumin.
- High-dose therapy may cause ↑ serum glucose and uric acid levels.
- When niacin is used as a lipid-lowering agent, serum cholesterol and triglyceride levels should be monitored prior to and periodically during therapy.

Potential Nursing Diagnoses
Imbalanced nutrition: less than body requirements (Indications)
Noncompliance (Patient/Family Teaching)

Implementation
- Because of infrequency of single B-vitamin deficiencies, combinations are commonly administered.
- **PO:** Administer with meals or milk to minimize GI irritation.
- Timed-release tablets and capsules should be swallowed whole, without breaking, crushing, or chewing. Use calibrated measuring device to ensure accurate dose of solution.

Patient/Family Teaching
- Inform patient that cutaneous flushing and a sensation of warmth, especially in the face, neck, and ears; itching or tingling; and headache may occur within the first 2 hr after taking the drug. These effects are usually transient and subside with continued therapy. If flushing is distressing or persistent, aspirin 300 mg given 30 min before each dose or slow upward titration of dose may decrease flushing.
- Advise patient to change positions slowly to minimize orthostatic hypotension.
- Instruct patients taking long-term OTC extended-release niacin to report signs of hepatotoxicity (darkening of urine, light gray–colored stool, loss of appetite, severe stomach pain, yellow eyes or skin) to health care professional.
- Emphasize the importance of follow-up examinations to evaluate progress.
- **Vitamin Deficiency:** Encourage patient to comply with dietary recommendations of health care professional. Explain that the best source of vitamins is a well-balanced diet with foods from the four basic food groups.
- Foods high in niacin include meats, eggs, milk, and dairy products; little is lost during ordinary cooking.
- Patients self-medicating with vitamin supplements should be cautioned not to exceed RDA. The effectiveness of megadoses for treatment of various medical conditions is unproved and may cause side effects.
- **Hyperlipidemia:** Advise patient that this medication should be used in conjunction with dietary restrictions (fat, cholesterol, carbohydrates, alcohol), exercise, and cessation of smoking.

Evaluation/Desired Outcomes
- Prevention and treatment of niacin deficiency.
- Decrease in serum cholesterol and triglyceride levels.

---

niCARdipine (nye-**kar**-di-peen)
Cardene, Cardene SR, Cardene IV

Classification
Therapeutic: antianginals, antihypertensives
Pharmacologic: calcium channel blockers

Pregnancy Category C

Indications
Management of: Hypertension, Angina pectoris, Vasospastic (Prinzmetal's) angina.

Action
Inhibits the transport of calcium into myocardial and vascular smooth muscle cells, resulting in inhibition of excitation-contraction coupling and subsequent contraction. **Therapeutic Effects:** Systemic vasodilation resulting in decreased blood pressure. Coronary vasodilation resulting in decreased frequency and severity of attacks of angina.

Pharmacokinetics
Absorption: Well absorbed following oral administration but extensively metabolized, resulting in ↓ bioavailability.
Distribution: Unknown.
Metabolism and Excretion: Mostly metabolized by the liver; ≤10% excreted unchanged by kidneys.
Half-life: 2–4 hr.

niCARdipine

TIME/ACTION PROFILE (cardiovascular effects)

ROUTE	ONSET	PEAK	DURATION
PO	20 min	0.5–2 hr	8 hr
PO-ER	unknown	unknown	12 hr
IV	within min	45 min	50 hr†

†Following discontinuation

Contraindications/Precautions
Contraindicated in: Hypersensitivity; Sick sinus syndrome; 2nd- or 3rd-degree AV block (unless an artificial pacemaker is in place); SBP <90 mm Hg; Advanced aortic stenosis.
Use Cautiously in: Severe hepatic impairment (dose ↓ recommended); Severe renal impairment (dose ↓ may be necessary); History of serious ventricular arrhythmias or CHF; OB, Lactation, Pedi: Safety not established; Geri: Dose ↓ / slower IV infusion rates recommended due to ↑ risk of hypotension.

Adverse Reactions/Side Effects
CNS: abnormal dreams, anxiety, confusion, dizziness, drowsiness, headache, jitteriness, nervousness, psychiatric disturbances, weakness. **EENT:** blurred vision, disturbed equilibrium, epistaxis, tinnitus. **Resp:** cough, dyspnea, shortness of breath. **CV:** ARRHYTHMIAS, CHF, peripheral edema, bradycardia, chest pain, hypotension, palpitations, syncope, tachycardia. **GI:** ↑ liver function tests, anorexia, constipation, diarrhea, dry mouth, dysgeusia, dyspepsia, nausea, vomiting. **GU:** dysuria, nocturia, polyuria, sexual dysfunction, urinary frequency. **Derm:** dermatitis, erythema multiforme, flushing, ↑ sweating, photosensitivity, pruritus/urticaria, rash. **Endo:** gynecomastia, hyperglycemia. **Hemat:** anemia, leukopenia, thrombocytopenia. **Metab:** weight gain. **MS:** joint stiffness, muscle cramps. **Neuro:** paresthesia, tremor. **Misc:** STEVENS-JOHNSON SYNDROME, gingival hyperplasia.

Interactions
Drug-Drug: Additive hypotension may occur when used concurrently with **fentanyl**, other **antihypertensives**, **nitrates**, acute ingestion of **alcohol**, or **quinidine**. Antihypertensive effects may be ↓ by concurrent use of **NSAIDs**. Concurrent use with **beta blockers**, **digoxin**, **disopyramide**, or **phenytoin** may result in bradycardia, conduction defects, or CHF. **Cimetidine** and **propranolol** may ↓ metabolism and ↑ risk of toxicity. May ↓ the metabolism of and ↑ risk of toxicity from **cyclosporine**, **prazosin**, **quinidine**, or **carbamazepine**.
Drug-Food: Grapefruit and Grapefruit juice ↑ serum levels and effect.

Route/Dosage
PO (Adults): 20 mg 3 times daily, may ↑ q 3 days (range 20–40 mg 3 times daily); or 30 mg twice daily as sustained-release form (up to 60 mg twice daily).
IV (Adults): *To replace PO use* —0.5–2.2 mg/hr continuous infusion. *For acute hypertensive episodes*—5 mg/hr titrated as needed (up to 15 mg/hr).

Availability (generic available)
Capsules: 20 mg, 30 mg. **Sustained-release capsules:** 30 mg, 45 mg, 60 mg. **Injection:** 2.5 mg/mL. **Premixed infusion:** 20 mg/200 mL D5W or 0.9% NaCl, 40 mg/200 mL D5W or 0.9% NaCl.

NURSING IMPLICATIONS
Assessment
- Monitor blood pressure and pulse prior to therapy, during dose titration, and periodically throughout therapy. Monitor ECG periodically during prolonged therapy.
- Monitor intake and output ratios and daily weight. Assess for signs of CHF (peripheral edema, rales/crackles, dyspnea, weight gain, jugular venous distention).
- **Angina:** Assess location, duration, intensity, and precipitating factors of patient's anginal pain.
- ***Lab Test Considerations:*** Total serum calcium concentrations are not affected by calcium channel blockers.
- Monitor serum potassium periodically. Hypokalemia ↑ risk of arrhythmias; should be corrected.
- Monitor renal and hepatic functions periodically during long-term therapy. Several days of therapy may cause ↑ hepatic enzymes, which return to normal upon discontinuation of therapy.

Potential Nursing Diagnoses
Decreased cardiac output (Indications)
Acute pain (Indications)

Implementation
- Do not confuse nicardipine with nifedipine or nimodipine. Do not confuse Cardene (nicardipine) with Cardura (doxazosin), codeine, or Cardizem (diltiazem).
- To transfer from IV nicardipine infusion to oral therapy with other antihypertensive, start oral therapy simultaneously with discontinuation of nicardipine infusion. If transferring to oral nicardipine therapy, administer first dose of a 3-

niCARdipine 917

times-a-day regimen 1 hr prior to discontinuation of infusion.
- Dose adjustments of nicardipine should be made no more frequently than every 3 days.
- **PO:** May be administered without regard to meals. May be administered with meals if GI irritation becomes a problem.
- Do not open, break, crush, or chew sustained-release capsules.

IV Administration

- **Continuous Infusion:** *Diluent:* Dilute each 25-mg ampule with 240 mL of D5W, D5/0.45% NaCl, D5/0.9% NaCl, 0.45% NaCl, or 0.9% NaCl. Infusion is stable for 24 hr at room temperature. *Concentration:* 0.1 mg/mL. *Rate:* Titrate rate according to blood pressure response. Administer through large peripheral veins or central veins to reduce risk of venous thrombosis, phlebitis, local irritation, swelling, extravasation, and vascular impairment. Change infusion site every 12 hours to minimize risk of peripheral venous irritation.
- **Y-Site Compatibility:** amikacin, aminophylline, aztreonam, bivalirudin, butorphanol, calcium gluconate, carboplatin, caspofungin, cefazolin, ceftizoxime, chloramphenicol, cimetidine, cisplatin, clindamycin, cytarabine, daptomycin, dexmedetomidine, diltiazem, dobutamine, docetaxel, dopamine, doxorubicin hydrochloride, enalaprilat, epinephrine, epirubicin, erythromycin, esmolol, famotidine, fenoldopam, fentanyl, gentamicin, hydrocortisone sodium succinate, hydromorphone, labetalol, lidocaine, linezolid, lorazepam, magnesium sulfate, mechlorethamine, methylprednisolone sodium succinate, metronidazole, midazolam, milrinone, morphine, nafcillin, nesiritide, nitroglycerin, nitroprusside, norepinephrine, octreotide, oxaliplatin, oxytocin, palonosetron, penicillin G potassium, potassium chloride, potassium phosphate, quinupristin/dalfopristin, ranitidine, rocuronium, tacrolimus, tirofiban, tobramycin, trimethoprim/sulfamethoxazole, vancomycin, vasopressin, vecuronium, vincristine, voriconazole.
- **Y-Site Incompatibility:** amphotericin B liposome, ampicillin, ampicillin/sulbactam, cefepime, cefoperazone, ertapenem, fluorouracil, furosemide, methotrexate, micafungin, pantoprazole, pemetrexed, thiopental, thiotepa, tigecycline.

Patient/Family Teaching

- Advise patient to take medication exactly as directed, even if feeling well. Take missed doses as soon as possible unless almost time for next dose; do not double doses. May need to be discontinued gradually.
- Instruct patient on technique for monitoring pulse. Instruct patient to contact health care professional if heart rate is <50 bpm.
- Advise patient to avoid grapefruit or grapefruit juice during therapy.
- Caution patient to change positions slowly to minimize orthostatic hypotension.
- May cause drowsiness or dizziness. Advise patient to avoid driving or other activities requiring alertness until response to the medication is known.
- Instruct patient to avoid concurrent use of alcohol or OTC medications, especially cold preparations, without consulting health care professional.
- Advise patient to notify health care professional if irregular heartbeat, dyspnea, swelling of hands and feet, pronounced dizziness, nausea, constipation, or hypotension occurs or if headache is severe or persistent.
- Caution patient to wear protective clothing and to use sunscreen to prevent photosensitivity reactions.
- **Angina:** Instruct patient on concurrent nitrate or beta-blocker therapy to continue taking both medications as directed and to use SL nitroglycerin as needed for anginal attacks.
- Advise patient to contact health care professional if chest pain does not improve, worsens after therapy, or occurs with diaphoresis; if shortness of breath; or if persistent headache occurs.
- Caution patient to discuss exercise restrictions with health care professional prior to exertion.
- **Hypertension:** Encourage patient to comply with other interventions for hypertension (weight reduction, low-sodium diet, smoking cessation, moderation of alcohol consumption, regular exercise, and stress management). Medication controls but does not cure hypertension.
- Instruct patient and family in proper technique for monitoring blood pressure. Advise patient to take blood pressure weekly and to report significant changes to health care professional.

✺ = Canadian drug name. ▮ = Genetic implication.
*CAPITALS indicates life-threatening; underlines indicate most frequent.

Evaluation/Desired Outcomes
- Decrease in blood pressure.
- Decrease in frequency and severity of anginal attacks.
- Decrease in need for nitrate therapy.
- Increase in activity tolerance and sense of well-being.

NICOTINE (nik-o-teen)

nicotine chewing gum
Nicorette, Thrive

nicotine inhaler
Nicotrol Inhaler

nicotine lozenge
Commit

nicotine nasal spray
Nicotrol NS

nicotine transdermal
Nicoderm CQ

Classification
Therapeutic: smoking deterrents

Pregnancy Category D

Indications
Adjunct therapy (with behavior modification) in the management of nicotine withdrawal in patients desiring to give up cigarette smoking.

Action
Provides a source of nicotine during controlled withdrawal from cigarette smoking. **Therapeutic Effects:** Lessened sequelae of nicotine withdrawal (irritability, insomnia, somnolence, headache, and increased appetite).

Pharmacokinetics
Absorption: *Gum, lozenge*—Slowly absorbed from buccal mucosa during chewing/sucking. *Inhaler*—50% of dose is systemically absorbed; most of nicotine released from inhaler is deposited in the mouth; absorption from buccal mucosa is slow,. *Nasal spray*—53% absorbed from nasal mucosa. *Transdermal*—70% of nicotine released from the system is absorbed through the skin.
Distribution: Enter breast milk.
Metabolism and Excretion: Mostly metabolized by the liver. Small amounts are metabolized by kidneys and lungs; 10–20% excreted unchanged by kidneys.
Half-life: 1–2 hr.

TIME/ACTION PROFILE (nicotine blood levels)

ROUTE	ONSET	PEAK	DURATION
gum	rapid	15–30 min	unknown
inhaler	slow	within 15 min	unknown
lozenge	unknown	unknown	unknown
nasal spray	rapid	4–15 min	unknown
transdermal	rapid	2–4 hr	unknown

Contraindications/Precautions
Contraindicated in: Hypersensitivity; Recent history of MI (inhaler or nasal spray); Arrhythmias (inhaler or nasal spray); Severe or worsening angina (inhaler or nasal spray); Severe cardiovascular disease; OB: Effects on fetus unknown; spontaneous abortion has been reported. Encourage behavioral approaches to smoking cessation. Lactation: Excreted in breast milk; weigh risks of nicotine product use against risk of continued smoking. Pedi: Safety not established.

Use Cautiously in: Cardiovascular disease including hypertension; Recent history of MI (gum, lozenge, patch); Arrhythmias (gum, lozenge, patch); Severe or worsening angina (gum, lozenge, patch); Diabetes mellitus; Pheochromocytoma; Peripheral vascular diseases; Hyperthyroidism; Diabetes; Continued smoking; Peptic ulcer disease; Hepatic disease; Bronchospastic lung disease (inhaler or nasal spray); Geri: Begin at lower dosages.

Adverse Reactions/Side Effects
CNS: headache, insomnia, abnormal dreams, dizziness, drowsiness, impaired concentration, nervousness, weakness. **EENT:** sinusitis; *gum*, pharyngitis; *nasal spray*, nasopharyngeal irritation, sneezing, watering eyes, change in smell, earache, epistaxis, eye irritation, hoarseness; *inhaler*, local mouth/throat irritation. **Resp:** *Nasal spray, inhaler*—cough, dyspnea. **CV:** tachycardia, chest pain, hypertension. **GI:** abdominal pain, abnormal taste, constipation, diarrhea, dry mouth, dyspepsia, hiccups, nausea, vomiting; *gum*, belching, ↑ appetite, ↑ salivation, oral injury, sore mouth. **Derm:** *transdermal*—burning at patch site, erythema, pruritus, cutaneous hypersensitivity, rash, sweating. **Endo:** dysmenorrhea. **MS:** arthralgia, back pain, myalgia; *gum*, jaw muscle ache. **Neuro:** paresthesia. **Misc:** allergy.

Interactions
Drug-Drug: Effects of **acetaminophen**, **caffeine**, **imipramine**, **insulin**, **oxazepam**, **pentazocine**, **propranolol**, or other **beta blockers**, **adrenergic antagonists** (**prazosin**, **labetalol**), and **theophylline** may be ↑ during

smoking cessation because of ↓ metabolism; dose ↓ at cessation may be necessary. Doses of adrenergic agonists (e.g., **isoproterenol, phenylephrine**) may need to be ↑ because of lower levels of circulating catecholamines at cessation of smoking. Concurrent treatment with **bupropion** may cause treatment-emergent hypertension.

Route/Dosage

Gum (Adults): If patient smokes < 25 cigarettes/day start with 2 mg gum, if patient smokes ≥ 25 cigarettes/day start with 4 mg gum; Patients should chew one piece of gum every 1–2 hr for 6 wk, then one piece of gum every 2–4 hr for 2 wk, then one piece of gum every 4–8 hr for 2 wk, then discontinue. Should not exceed 24 pieces of gum/day.

Lozenge (Adults): If first cigarette is desired > 30 min after awakening, start with 2 mg lozenge, if first cigarette is desired < 30 min after awakening, start with 4 mg lozenge. Patients should use one lozenge every 1–2 hr for 6 wk, then one lozenge every 2–4 hr for 2 wk, then one lozenge every 4–8 hr for 2 wk, then discontinue. Should not exceed 20 lozenges/day or more than 5 lozenges in 6 hr.

Intranasal (Adults): One spray in each nostril 1–2 times/hr (up to 5 times/hr); may be ↑ up to maximum of 40 times/day (should not exceed 3 mo of therapy).

Inhaln (Adults): Patients are encouraged to use at least 6 cartridges/day for first 3–6 wk, with additional cartridges as necessary (up to 16/day) for 12 wk. Patients are self-titrated to level of nicotine they require (usual usage 6–16 cartridges/day) followed by gradual withdrawal over 6–12 wk (maximum duration of use = 6 mo).

Transdermal (Adults): *Patients smoking >10 cigarettes/day*—Begin with Step 1 (21 mg/day) for 6 wk, followed by Step 2 (14 mg/day) for 2 wk, and then Step 3 (7 mg/day) for 2 wk, then stop (total of 10 wk) (new patch should be applied every 24 hr); *Patients smoking ≤10 cigarettes/day*—Begin with Step 2 (14 mg/day) for 6 wk, followed by Step 3 (7 mg/day) for 2 wk, then stop (total of 8 wk) (new patch should be applied every 24 hr).

Availability (generic available)

Chewing gum (cinnamon, mint, orange, and fruit chill flavors): 2 mg^{OTC}, 4 mg^{OTC}. **Inhalation:** each system contains 168 cartridges, each containing 10 mg of nicotine (deliver 4 mg). **Lozenge (original, mint, cherry, and cappuccino flavors):** 2 mg^{OTC}, 4 mg^{OTC}. **Nasal spray:** 10 mg/mL (0.5 mg/spray) in 10-mL bottles (200 sprays). **Transdermal patch:** 7 mg/day^{OTC}, 14 mg/day^{OTC}, 21 mg/day^{OTC}.

NURSING IMPLICATIONS

Assessment

- Prior to therapy, assess smoking history (number of cigarettes smoked daily, smoking patterns, nicotine content of preferred brand, degree to which patient inhales smoke).
- Assess patient for symptoms of smoking withdrawal (irritability, drowsiness, fatigue, headache, nicotine craving) periodically during nicotine replacement therapy (NRT).
- Evaluate progress in smoking cessation periodically during therapy.
- *Toxicity and Overdose:* Monitor for nausea, vomiting, diarrhea, increased salivation, abdominal pain, headache, dizziness, auditory and visual disturbances, weakness, dyspnea, hypotension, and irregular pulse.

Potential Nursing Diagnoses

Ineffective coping (Indications)

Implementation

- **Gum:** Protect gum from light; exposure to light causes gum to turn brown.
- **Lozenge:** Lozenge should be allowed to dissolve slowly in the mouth; it should not be chewed or swallowed.
- **Transdermal:** Patch can be worn for 16 or 24 hr; the patch can be removed before the patient goes to bed (especially if patient has vivid dreams or sleep disrubances) or can remain on while the patient sleeps (especially if patient craves cigarettes upon awakening).
- **Nasal Spray and Inhaler:** Regular use of the spray or inhaler during the first week of therapy may help patient adjust to irritant effects of the spray.

Patient/Family Teaching

- Explain to patient the necessity of immediate cessation of smoking upon initiation and throughout therapy.
- Encourage patient to participate in a smoking cessation program while using this product.
- Review the patient instruction sheet enclosed in the package.
- Instruct patient in proper method of disposal of unit. Emphasize need to keep out of the reach of children or pets.

✤ = Canadian drug name. ■ = Genetic implication.
*CAPITALS indicates life-threatening; underlines indicate most frequent.

- Nicotine in any form can be harmful to a pregnant woman and/or the fetus. Assist patient in determining risk/benefit of nicotine replacement therapy (NRT) and harm to the fetus versus the likelihood of stopping smoking without NRT.
- Emphasize the importance of regular visits to health care professional to monitor progress of smoking cessation.
- **Gum:** Explain purpose of nicotine gum to patient. The patient should chew 1 piece of gum whenever a craving for nicotine occurs or according to a fixed schedule (every 1–2 hr while awake) as directed. The gum should be chewed slowly until a tingling sensation is felt (about 15 chews). Then, patient should stop chewing and store the gum between the cheek and gums until the tingling sensation disappears (about 1 min). The process of stopping, then resuming chewing should be repeated for approximately 30 min until most of the tingle has disappeared. Rapid, vigorous chewing may result in side effects similar to those of smoking too many cigarettes (headache, dizziness, nausea, increased salivation, heartburn, and hiccups).
- Inform patient that the gum has a slight tobacco/pepper-like taste. Many patients initially find it unpleasant and slightly irritating to the mouth. This usually resolves after several days of therapy.
- Advise patient to carry gum at all times during therapy.
- Advise patient to avoid eating or drinking for 15 min before and during chewing of nicotine gum; these interfere with buccal absorption of nicotine.
- The gum usually can be chewed by denture wearers. Contact dentist if the gum adheres to bridgework.
- Inform patient that they should stop using the gum at the end of 12 wk; if they still feel the need to use the gum after this time period, advise them to contact a health care professional.
- Instruct patient not to swallow gum.
- Dispose of the gum by wrapping in wrapper to prevent ingestion by children and animals. Call the poison control center, emergency department, or health care professional immediately if a child ingests the gum.
- Emphasize the need to discontinue the gum and to inform health care professional if pregnancy occurs.
- **Transdermal:** Instruct patient in application and use of patch. Apply patch at the same time each day. Keep patch in sealed pouch until ready to apply. Apply to clean, dry skin of upper arm or torso free of oil, hair, scars, cuts, burns, or irritation. Press patch firmly in place with palm for 10 sec, making sure there is good contact, especially around the edges. Keep patch in place during showering, bathing, or swimming; replace patches that have fallen off. Wash hands with soap and water after handling patches. Do not trim or cut patch. No more than 1 patch should be worn at a time. Alternate application sites. Dispose of used patches by folding adhesive sides together and replacing in protective pouch or aluminum foil; keep out of reach of children.
- Advise patient that redness, itching, and burning at application site usually subside within 1 hr. Instruct patient to notify health care professional and not apply new patch if signs of allergic reaction (urticaria, generalized rash, hives) or persistent local skin reactions (severe erythema, pruritus, edema) occur.
- May cause drowsiness or dizziness. Caution patient to avoid driving or other activities requiring alertness until response to medication is known.
- Advise patient referred for MRI test to discuss patch with referring health care professional and MRI facility to determine if removal of patch is necessary prior to test and for directions for replacing patch.
- **Nasal Spray:** Instruct patient in proper use of spray. Tilt head back slightly. Do not sniff, swallow, or inhale through nose as spray is being administered. Patients who have successfully stopped smoking should continue to use the same dose for up to 8 wk, after which the spray should be discontinued over the next 4–6 wk.
- Discontinue nasal spray by using ½ dose (1 spray at a time), using the spray less frequently, skipping a dose by not using every hour, or setting a planned stop date for use of the spray.
- Treatment should be discontinued in patients who are unable to stop smoking by the 4th wk of therapy (patient is unlikely to quit on that attempt).
- Patients who fail to stop smoking should be given a therapy holiday before another attempt.
- Instruct patient to replace childproof cap after using and before disposal.
- **Inhalation:** Inhalation regimens should consist of frequent, continuous puffing for 20 minutes.
- Treatment should be discontinued in patients who are unable to stop smoking by the 4th wk of therapy (patient is unlikely to quit on that attempt).

- Patients who fail to stop smoking should be given a therapy holiday before another attempt.
- **Lozenge:** Instruct patient to place lozenge in mouth and allow it to slowly dissolve (20–30 min). Minimize swallowing; advise patient not to chew or swallow lozenge. May cause a warm tingling sensation in mouth. Advise patient to occasionally move lozenge from side to side of mouth until completely dissolved. Instruct patient not to eat or drink 15 min before or while lozenge is in mouth. For best chances of quitting, use at least 9 lozenges/day during 1st 6 wk. Do not use more than 1 lozenge at a time or use continuously one after the another. Lozenge should not be used after 12 wk without consulting health care professional.

Evaluation/Desired Outcomes
- Lessened sequelae of nicotine withdrawal (irritability, insomnia, somnolence, headache, and increased appetite) during smoking cessation.

NIFEdipine (nye-fed-i-peen)
Adalat CC, ✦ Adalat PA, ✦ Adalat XL, Afeditab CR, ✦ Apo-Nifed, Nifedical XL, ✦ Novo-Nifedin, ✦ Nu-Nifed, Procardia, Procardia XL

Classification
Therapeutic: antianginals, antihypertensives
Pharmacologic: calcium channel blockers

Pregnancy Category C

Indications
Management of: Hypertension (extended-release only), Angina pectoris, Vasospastic (Prinzmetal's) angina. **Unlabeled Use:** Prevention of migraine headache. Management of CHF or cardiomyopathy.

Action
Inhibits calcium transport into myocardial and vascular smooth muscle cells, resulting in inhibition of excitation-contraction coupling and subsequent contraction. **Therapeutic Effects:** Systemic vasodilation, resulting in decreased blood pressure. Coronary vasodilation, resulting in decreased frequency and severity of attacks of angina.

Pharmacokinetics
Absorption: Well absorbed after oral administration, but large amounts are rapidly metabolized (primarily by CYP3A4 enzyme system), resulting in ↓ bioavailability (45–70%); bioavailability is ↑ (80%) with long-acting (CC, PA, XL) forms.
Distribution: Unknown.
Protein Binding: 92–98%.
Metabolism and Excretion: Mostly metabolized by the liver.
Half-life: 2–5 hr.

TIME/ACTION PROFILE

ROUTE	ONSET	PEAK	DURATION
PO	20 min	unknown	6–8 hr
PO–PA	unknown	4 hr	12 hr
PO–CC, PA, XL	unknown	6 hr	24 hr

Contraindications/Precautions
Contraindicated in: Hypersensitivity; Sick sinus syndrome; 2nd- or 3rd-degree AV block (unless an artificial pacemaker is in place); Systolic blood pressure <90 mm Hg; Coadministration with grapefruit juice.
Use Cautiously in: Severe hepatic impairment (↓ dose recommended); History of porphyria; Severe renal impairment (↓ dose may be necessary); History of serious ventricular arrhythmias or CHF; OB, Lactation, Pedi: Safety not established; Geri: Short-acting forms appear on Beers list due to ↑ risk of hypotension and constipation (↓ dose recommended); also associated with ↑ incidence of falls.

Adverse Reactions/Side Effects
CNS: headache, abnormal dreams, anxiety, confusion, dizziness, drowsiness, jitteriness, nervousness, psychiatric disturbances, weakness. **EENT:** blurred vision, disturbed equilibrium, epistaxis, tinnitus. **Resp:** cough, dyspnea, shortness of breath. **CV:** ARRHYTHMIAS, CHF, peripheral edema, bradycardia, chest pain, hypotension, palpitations, syncope, tachycardia. **GI:** ↑ liver function tests, anorexia, constipation, diarrhea, dry mouth, dysgeusia, dyspepsia, nausea, vomiting. **GU:** dysuria, nocturia, polyuria, sexual dysfunction, urinary frequency. **Derm:** flushing, dermatitis, erythema multiforme, ↑ sweating, photosensitivity, pruritus/urticaria, rash. **Endo:** gynecomastia, hyperglycemia. **Hemat:** anemia, leukopenia, thrombocytopenia. **Metab:** weight gain. **MS:** joint stiffness, muscle cramps. **Neuro:** paresthesia, tremor. **Misc:** STEVENS-JOHNSON SYNDROME, gingival hyperplasia.

Interactions
Drug-Drug: Additive hypotension may occur when used concurrently with **fentanyl**, other **anti-**

hypertensives, nitrates, acute ingestion of alcohol, or quinidine. Antihypertensive effects may be ↓ by concurrent use of NSAIDs. May ↑ serum levels and risk of toxicity from digoxin. Concurrent use with beta blockers, digoxin, disopyramide, or phenytoin may result in bradycardia, conduction defects, or CHF. Cimetidine and propranolol may ↓ metabolism and ↑ risk of toxicity. May ↓ metabolism of and ↑ risk of toxicity from cyclosporine, prazosin, quinidine, or carbamazepine.

Drug-Food: Grapefruit and grapefruit juice ↑ serum levels and effect.

Route/Dosage
PO (Adults): 10–30 mg 3 times daily (not to exceed 180 mg/day), *or* 10–20 mg twice daily as immediate—release form, *or* 30–90 mg once daily as sustained-release (CC, XL) form (not to exceed 90–120 mg/day).

Availability (generic available)
Capsules: ✤ 5 mg, 10 mg, 20 mg. **Cost:** *Generic*— 10 mg $62.99/90, 20 mg $104.97/90. **Tablets:** ✤ 10 mg. **Extended-release tablets,** (Adalat CC, Afeditab CR, Nifedical XL, Procardia XL): ✤ 10 mg, ✤ 20 mg, 30 mg, 60 mg, 90 mg. **Cost:** *Generic*— 30 mg $94.00/90, 60 mg $164.99/90, 90 mg $174.99/90.

NURSING IMPLICATIONS

Assessment
- Monitor blood pressure and pulse before therapy, during dose titration, and periodically during therapy. Monitor ECG periodically during prolonged therapy.
- Monitor intake and output ratios and daily weight. Assess for signs of CHF (peripheral edema, rales/crackles, dyspnea, weight gain, jugular venous distention).
- **Geri:** Assess fall risk and institute fall prevention strategies.
- Patients receiving digoxin concurrently with nifedipine should have routine tests of serum digoxin levels and be monitored for signs and symptoms of digoxin toxicity.
- **Angina:** Assess location, duration, intensity, and precipitating factors of patient's anginal pain.
- *Lab Test Considerations:* Total serum calcium concentrations are not affected by calcium channel blockers.
- Monitor serum potassium periodically. Hypokalemia increases risk of arrhythmias; should be corrected.
- Monitor renal and hepatic functions periodically during long-term therapy. Several days of therapy may cause increase in hepatic enzymes, which return to normal upon discontinuation of therapy.
- Nifedipine may cause positive ANA and direct Coombs' test results.

Potential Nursing Diagnoses
Decreased cardiac output (Indications)
Acute pain (Indications)

Implementation
- **PO:** May be administered without regard to meals. May be administered with meals if GI irritation becomes a problem.
- Do not open, break, crush, or chew extended-release tablets. Empty tablets that appear in stool are not significant.
- Avoid administration with grapefruit juice.
- Sublingual use is not recommended due to serious adverse drug reactions.

Patient/Family Teaching
- Advise patient to take medication exactly as directed, even if feeling well. Take missed doses as soon as possible unless almost time for next dose; do not double doses. May need to be discontinued gradually.
- Instruct patient on technique for monitoring pulse. Instruct patient to contact health care professional if heart rate is <50 bpm.
- Advise patient to avoid grapefruit or grapefruit juice during therapy.
- Caution patient to change positions slowly to minimize orthostatic hypotension.
- May cause drowsiness or dizziness. Advise patient to avoid driving or other activities requiring alertness until response to the medication is known.
- **Geri:** Teach patients and family about risk for falls and how to reduce risk in the home.
- Instruct patient on importance of maintaining good dental hygiene and seeing dentist frequently for teeth cleaning to prevent tenderness, bleeding, and gingival hyperplasia (gum enlargement).
- Instruct patient to avoid concurrent use of alcohol or OTC medications and natural/herbal products, especially cold preparations, without consulting health care professional.
- Advise patient to notify health care professional if irregular heartbeat, dyspnea, swelling of hands and feet, pronounced dizziness, nausea, constipation, or hypotension occurs or if headache is severe or persistent.
- Caution patient to wear protective clothing and use sunscreen to prevent photosensitivity reactions.

- **Angina:** Instruct patient on concurrent nitrate or beta-blocker therapy to continue taking both medications as directed and use SL nitroglycerin as needed for anginal attacks.
- Inform patient that anginal attacks may occur 30 min after administration because of reflex tachycardia. This is usually temporary and is not an indication for discontinuation.
- Advise patient to contact health care professional if chest pain does not improve, worsens after therapy, or occurs with diaphoresis; if shortness of breath occurs; or if persistent headache occurs.
- Caution patient to discuss exercise restrictions with health care professional before exertion.
- **Hypertension:** Encourage patient to comply with other interventions for hypertension (weight reduction, low-sodium diet, smoking cessation, moderation of alcohol consumption, regular exercise, and stress management). Medication controls but does not cure hypertension.
- Instruct patient and family in proper technique for monitoring blood pressure. Advise patient to take blood pressure weekly and to report significant changes to health care professional.

Evaluation/Desired Outcomes
- Decrease in blood pressure.
- Decrease in frequency and severity of anginal attacks.
- Decrease in need for nitrate therapy.
- Increase in activity tolerance and sense of well-being.

---

nilotinib (ni-lo-ti-nib)
Tasigna

Classification
Therapeutic: antineoplastics
Pharmacologic: enzyme inhibitors, kinase inhibitors

Pregnancy Category D

Indications
Chronic or accelerated phase Philadelphia chromosome positive (Ph+) chronic myelogenous leukemia (CML) which has not responded to other treatment, including imatinib.

Action
Inhibits kinases which may be produced by malignant cell lines. **Therapeutic Effects:** Inhibits production of malignant cells lines with decreased proliferation of leukemic cells.

Pharmacokinetics
Absorption: Well absorbed following oral administration. Blood levels are significantly increased by food.
Distribution: Unknown.
Metabolism and Excretion: Mostly metabolized by the liver; metabolites are not active.
Half-life: 17 hr.

TIME/ACTION PROFILE (blood levels)

ROUTE	ONSET	PEAK	DURATION
PO	unknown	3 hr	12 hr

Contraindications/Precautions
Contraindicated in: Hypokalemia or hypomagnesemia; Long QT syndrome; Concurrent use of medications known to prolong QT interval; Concurrent use of strong inhibitors of the CYP3A4 enzyme system (↑ risk of toxicity); Concurrent use of strong inducers of the CYP3A4 enzyme system (may ↓ effectiveness); Concurrent grapefruit juice (may ↑ risk of toxicity); Galactose intolerance, severe lactase deficiency or glucose-galactose malabsorption (capsules contain lactose); OB, Lactation: Pregnancy or lactation.
Use Cautiously in: Concurrent use of other drugs that prolong QT interval; Electrolyte abnormalities; correct prior to administration to ↓ risk of arrhythmias; Hepatic impairment (↓ dose required for Grade 3 elevated bilirubin, transaminases or lipase); OB: Women with child-bearing potential (effective contraception required); Pedi: Safety not established.

Adverse Reactions/Side Effects
CNS: fatigue, headache, dizziness. **EENT:** vertigo. **CV:** ARRHYTHMIAS, hypertension, palpitations, QT prolongation. **GI:** constipation, diarrhea, nausea, vomiting, abdominal discomfort, anorexia, dyspepsia, flatulence, hepatotoxicity. **Derm:** pruritus, rash, alopecia, flushing. **F and E:** hyperkalemia, hypocalcemia, hypokalemia, hyponatremia, hypophosphatemia. **Hemat:** MYELOSUPRESSION. **Metab:** ↑ lipase, hyperglycemia. **MS:** musculoskeletal pain. **Neuro:** paresthesia. **Misc:** fever, night sweats.

Interactions
Drug-Drug: Strong **inhibitors of the CYP3A4 enzyme system** including **ketoconazole**, **itraconaole**, **voriconazole**, **clarithromycin**, **telithromycin**, **atazanavir**, **indinavir**, **nelfinavir**,

indinavir, **ritonavir**, **saquinavir**, and **nefazodone** may result in ↑ blood levels and toxicity and should be avoided; if concurrent use in necessary, dose ↓ by 50% (400 mg once daily) may be required. Strong **inducers of the CYP3A4 enzyme system** including **carbamazepine**, **dexamethasone**, **phenobarbital**, **phenytoin**, **rifabutin**, **rifampin**, and **rifapentin** may ↓ blood levels and effectiveness and should be avoided if possible; if required, dose ↑ may be necessary. Nilotinib inhibits the following enzyme systems: **CYP3A4**, **CYP2C8**, **CYP2C9**, and **CYP2D6**; concurrent use of drugs metabolized by these systems may result in toxicity of these agents. Nilotinib induces the following enzyme systems: **CYP2D6**, **CYP2C8**, **CYP2C9**; concurrent use of drugs metabolized by these systems may result ↓ therapeutic effectiveness of these agents. Concurrent use of other **drugs that prolong QT interval**; may ↑ risk of serious arrhythmias; avoid concomitant use.

Drug-Natural Products: St. John's wort may ↓ levels and effectiveness; avoid concurrent use.
Drug-Food: Grapefruit juice may ↑ blood levels and should be avoided.

Route/Dosage
PO (Adults): 400 mg twice daily; adjustment may be required for toxicity and/or drug interactions.

Availability
Capsules: 200 mg.

NURSING IMPLICATIONS

Assessment
- Monitor ECG to assess the QTc interval at baseline, 7 days after initiation of therapy, and periodically thereafter. For ECGs with QTc >480 msec, withhold nilotinib and check serum potassium and magnesium. If below lower limit of normal, correct to normal with supplements. Review concommitant medications for effects on electrolytes. If QTc returns to <450 msec and within 20 msec of baseline within 2 wk, return ot prior dose. If QTc is <480 msec and >450 msec after 2 wk, reduce nilotinib dose to 400 mg once daily. Following dose reduction to 400 mg once daily, if QTc return to >480 msec, discontinue nilotinib. Repeat ECG approximately 7 days after any dose adjustment.
- Monitor for myelosuppression. Assess for bleeding (bleeding gums, bruising, petechiae, blood in stools, urine, emesis) and avoid IM injections and taking rectal temperatures if platelet count is low. Apply pressure to venipuncture sites for at least 10 min. Assess for signs of infection during neutropenia. Anemia may occur. Monitor for fatigue, dyspnea, and othrostatic hypotension.
- **Lab Test Considerations:** Monitor serum electrolytes prior to and periodically during therapy. May cause hypokalemia, hypomagnesemia, hypophosphatemia, hyperkalemia, hypocalcemia, hyperglycemia, and hyponatremia.
- Monitor CBC every 2 wk for first 2 mo and monthly thereafter or as indicated. May cause Grade 3/4 thrombocytopenia, neutropenia, and anemia. If ANC is $<1.0 \times 10^9$/L and/or platelet counts $<50 \times 10^9$/L, stop nilotinib and monitor blood counts. Resume within 2 wk at prior dose if ANC $>1.0 \times 10^9$/L and platelets $>50 \times 10^9$/L. If blood counts remain low for >2 wk, reduce dose to 400 mg once daily. Myelosuppression is generally reversible.
- May cause ↑ serum lipase or amylase. If ↑ to ≥Grade 3, withhold nilotinib and monitor serum levels. Resume treatment at 400 mg once daily if serum lipase or amylase return to ≤Grade 1.
- May cause ↑ serum bilirubin. If ↑ to ≥Grade 3, withhold nilotinib and monitor bilirubin. Resume treatment at 400 mg once daily if serum lipase or amylase return to ≤Grade 1.
- May cause ↑ serum hepatic tranaminases. If ↑ to ≥Grade 3, withhold nilotinib and monitor serum ALT, AST, and alkaline phosphatase. Resume treatment at 400 mg once daily if serum lipase or amylase return to ≤Grade 1.

Potential Nursing Diagnoses
Deficient knowledge, related to medication regimen (Patient/Family Teaching)

Implementation
- Correct hypokalemia and hypomagnesemia prior to beginning therapy.
- **PO:** Administer twice daily at 12-hr intervals on an empty stomach, at least 2 hr before and 1 hr after food. Capsule should be swallowed whole with water; do not open capsule.

Patient/Family Teaching
- Instruct patient to take nilotinib as directed, approximately 12 hr apart. If a dose is missed, skip dose and resume taking next prescribed dose. Advise patients to avoid grapefruit products during therapy. Nilotinib is a long-term treatment; do not stop medication or change dose without consulting health care professional. Advise patient to read the *Medication Guide* before starting and with each Rx refill.
- May cause dizziness. Caution patient to avoid driving or other activities requiring alertness until response to medication is known.

- Advise patient to consult health care professional before taking any Rx, OTC, herbal, or vitamin products, especially St. John's wort, during therapy.
- Instruct patient to notify health care professional promptly if fever; chills; cough; hoarseness; sore throat; signs of infection; lower back or side pain; painful or difficulty urination; bleeding gums; bruising; petechiae; blood in stools, urine, or emesis; increased fatigue; dyspnea; or orthostatic hypotension occurs. Caution patient to avoid crowds and persons with known infections. Instruct patients to use a soft toothbrush and electric razor and to avoid falls. Caution patient not to drink alcoholic beverages or take medication containing aspirin or NSAIDs; may precipitate bleeding.
- Instruct patient not to receive any vaccinations without advice of health care professional.
- Discuss the possibility of hair loss with patient. Explore methods of coping. Regrowth usually occurs 2–3 mo after discontinuation of therapy.
- Advise women of childbearing potential to use effective contraception during therapy.

Evaluation/Desired Outcomes
- Decrease in production of leukemic cells.

---

nimodipine (nye-moe-di-peen)

Classification
Therapeutic: subarachnoid hemorrhage therapy agents
Pharmacologic: calcium channel blockers

Pregnancy Category C

Indications
Management of subarachnoid hemorrhage.

Action
Inhibits the transport of calcium into vascular smooth muscle cells, resulting in inhibition of excitation-contraction coupling and subsequent contraction. Potent peripheral vasodilator. **Therapeutic Effects:** Prevention of vascular spasm after subarachnoid hemorrhage, resulting in decreased neurologic impairment.

Pharmacokinetics
Absorption: Well absorbed following oral administration but extensively metabolized, resulting in ↓ bioavailability.
Distribution: Crosses the blood-brain barrier; remainder of distribution unknown.
Protein Binding: >95%.
Metabolism and Excretion: Mostly metabolized by the liver; ≤10% excreted unchanged by kidneys.
Half-life: 1–2 hr.

TIME/ACTION PROFILE (vasodilation)

ROUTE	ONSET	PEAK	DURATION
PO	unknown	1 hr	4 hr

Contraindications/Precautions
Contraindicated in: Hypersensitivity; Sick sinus syndrome; 2nd- or 3rd-degree AV block (unless a pacemaker is present); Systolic BP <90 mm Hg.
Use Cautiously in: Severe hepatic impairment (dose ↓ recommended); Severe renal impairment; History of serious ventricular arrhythmias or CHF; OB, Lactation, Pedi: Safety not established; Geri: Dose ↓ recommended due to ↑ risk of hypotension.

Adverse Reactions/Side Effects
CNS: abnormal dreams, anxiety, confusion, dizziness, drowsiness, headache, nervousness, psychiatric disturbances, weakness. **EENT:** blurred vision, disturbed equilibrium, epistaxis, tinnitus. **Resp:** cough, dyspnea. **CV:** ARRHYTHMIAS, CHF, bradycardia, chest pain, hypotension, palpitations, peripheral edema, syncope, tachycardia. **GI:** ↑ liver enzymes, anorexia, constipation, diarrhea, dry mouth, dysgeusia, dyspepsia, nausea, vomiting. **GU:** dysuria, nocturia, polyuria, sexual dysfunction, urinary frequency. **Derm:** dermatitis, erythema multiforme, flushing, increased sweating, photosensitivity, pruritus/urticaria, rash. **Endo:** gynecomastia, hyperglycemia. **Hemat:** anemia, leukopenia, thrombocytopenia. **Metab:** weight gain. **MS:** joint stiffness, muscle cramps. **Neuro:** paresthesia, tremor. **Misc:** STEVENS-JOHNSON SYNDROME, gingival hyperplasia.

Interactions
Drug-Drug: Additive hypotension may occur when used concurrently with **fentanyl**, other **antihypertensives**, **nitrates**, acute ingestion of **alcohol**, or **quinidine**. Concurrent use with **beta blockers**, **digoxin**, **disopyramide**, or **phenytoin** may result in bradycardia, conduction defects, or CHF.
Drug-Natural Products: **Grapefruit** and **grapefruit juice** ↑ serum levels and effect.

Route/Dosage
PO (Adults): 60 mg q 4 hr for 21 days; therapy should be started within 96 hr of subarachnoid hemorrhage.

Hepatic Impairment
PO (Adults): 30 mg q 4 hr for 21 days; therapy should be started within 96 hr of subarachnoid hemorrhage.

Availability (generic available)
Capsules: 30 mg.

NURSING IMPLICATIONS
Assessment
- Assess patient's neurologic status (level of consciousness, movement) prior to and periodically following administration.
- Monitor blood pressure and pulse prior to therapy and periodically during therapy.
- Monitor intake and output ratios and daily weight. Assess for signs of CHF (peripheral edema, rales/crackles, dyspnea, weight gain, jugular venous distention).
- **Lab Test Considerations:** Total serum calcium concentrations are not affected by calcium channel blockers.
- Monitor serum potassium periodically. Hypokalemia ↑ risk of arrhythmias; should be corrected.
- Monitor renal and hepatic functions periodically. Several days of therapy may cause ↑ hepatic enzymes, which return to normal upon discontinuation of therapy.
- May occasionally cause ↓ platelet count.

Potential Nursing Diagnoses
Ineffective tissue perfusion (Indications)

Implementation
- Do not confuse nimodipine with nicardipine or nifedipine.
- Begin administration within 96 hr of subarachnoid hemorrhage and continue every 4 hr for 21 consecutive days.
- **PO:** If patient is unable to swallow capsule, make a hole in both ends of the capsule with a sterile 18-gauge needle and extract the contents into a syringe. Empty contents into water or nasogastric tube and flush with 30 mL normal saline.

Patient/Family Teaching
- Advise patient to take medication as directed, even if feeling well. Take missed doses as soon as possible unless almost time for next dose; do not double doses. May need to be discontinued gradually.
- Advise patient to avoid grapefruit or grapefruit juice during therapy.
- Caution patient to change positions slowly to minimize orthostatic hypotension.
- May cause drowsiness or dizziness. Advise patient to avoid driving or other activities requiring alertness until response to the medication is known.
- Instruct patient to avoid concurrent use of alcohol or OTC medications, especially cold preparations, without consulting health care professional.
- Advise patient to notify health care professional if irregular heartbeats, dyspnea, swelling of hands and feet, pronounced dizziness, nausea, constipation, or hypotension occurs or if headache is severe or persistent.
- Caution patient to wear protective clothing and use sunscreen to prevent photosensitivity reactions.

Evaluation/Desired Outcomes
- Improvement in neurologic deficits due to vasospasm following subarachnoid hemorrhage.

---

nisoldipine (nye-**sole**-di-peen)
Sular

Classification
Therapeutic: antihypertensives
Pharmacologic: calcium channel blockers

Pregnancy Category C

Indications
Management of hypertension.

Action
Inhibits the transport of calcium into vascular smooth muscle cells, resulting in inhibition of vasoconstriction and dilation of arterioles. **Therapeutic Effects:** Systemic vasodilation, resulting in decreased blood pressure.

Pharmacokinetics
Absorption: Well absorbed (87%) following oral administration but rapidly and extensively metabolized in the gut wall, resulting in 5% bioavailability.
Distribution: Unknown.
Metabolism and Excretion: Highly metabolized CYP3A4 enzyme system.
Half-life: 7–12 hr.

nisoldipine

TIME/ACTION PROFILE (antihypertensive effects)

ROUTE	ONSET	PEAK	DURATION
PO	unknown	6–12 hr	24 hr

Contraindications/Precautions
Contraindicated in: Hypersensitivity; Cross-sensitivity with calcium channel blockers may occur; Concurrent phenytoin use.
Use Cautiously in: CHF/left ventricular dysfunction; Hepatic impairment (dose ↓ may be necessary); Coronary artery disease (may precipitate angina); OB, Lactation, Pedi: Safety not established; Geri: Dose ↓ may be necessary due to age-related ↓ in hepatic, renal or cardiac function.

Adverse Reactions/Side Effects
CNS: headache, dizziness. **EENT:** pharyngitis, sinusitis. **CV:** peripheral edema, chest pain, hypotension, palpitations. **GI:** nausea. **Derm:** rash. **Endo:** gynecomastia.

Interactions
Drug-Drug: Additive hypotension may occur with other **antihypertensives**, acute ingestion of **alcohol**, or **nitrates**. Antihypertensive effects may be decreased by concurrent use of **NSAIDs**. **Phenytoin** or **other CYP3A4 inducers** ↓ blood levels and effectiveness (avoid concurrent use).
Drug-Food: Grapefruit and **grapefruit juice** ↑ serum levels and effect. Blood levels are ↑ by concurrent ingestion of a **high-fat meal** and should be avoided.

Route/Dosage
PO (Adults): *Extended-release tablets*—20 mg/day as a single dose initially; may be ↑ by 10 mg/day q 7 days, up to 60 mg/day (usual range 20–40 mg/day); *Geomatric extended-release tablets*—17 mg/day as a single dose initially; may be ↑ by 8.5 mg/day q 7 days, up to 34 mg/day (usual range 8.5–34 mg/day).

Hepatic Impairment
PO (Adults): *Geomatric extended-release tablets*—Initial dose should not exceed 8.5 mg/day.

Availability (generic available)
Extended-release tablets: 20 mg, 30 mg, 40 mg. **Cost:** 10 mg $179.98/90, 20 mg $225.97/90, 30 mg $239.99/90, 40 mg $240.32/90. **Geomatrix extended-release tablets:** 8.5 mg, 17 mg, 25.5 mg, 34 mg.

NURSING IMPLICATIONS

Assessment
- Monitor blood pressure and pulse prior to therapy, during dosage titration, and periodically throughout therapy. Monitor ECG periodically during prolonged therapy.
- Monitor intake and output ratios and daily weight. Assess for signs of CHF (peripheral edema, rales/crackles, dyspnea, weight gain, jugular venous distention).
- *Lab Test Considerations:* Total serum calcium concentrations are not affected by calcium channel blockers.

Potential Nursing Diagnoses
Decreased cardiac output (Indications)

Implementation
- **PO:** Avoid administration within 1 hr of high-fat meals or grapefruit products.
- Do not break, crush, or chew tablets.

Patient/Family Teaching
- Advise patient to take medication exactly as directed, even if feeling well. If a dose is missed, take as soon as possible unless almost time for next dose; do not double doses. May need to be discontinued gradually.
- Advise patient to avoid grapefruit or grapefruit juice during therapy.
- Encourage patient to comply with other interventions for hypertension (weight reduction, low-sodium diet, smoking cessation, moderation of alcohol consumption, regular exercise, and stress management). Medication controls but does not cure hypertension.
- Instruct patient and family in proper technique for monitoring blood pressure. Advise patient to take blood pressure weekly and to report significant changes to health care professional.
- Caution patient to change positions slowly to minimize orthostatic hypotension.
- May cause dizziness. Advise patient to avoid driving or other activities requiring alertness until response to the medication is known.
- Instruct patient to avoid concurrent use of alcohol or OTC medications, especially cold preparations, without consulting health care professional.
- Advise patient to notify health care professional if irregular heartbeat, dyspnea, swelling of hands and feet, pronounced dizziness, nausea, constipation, or hypotension occurs or if headache is severe or persistent.

Evaluation/Desired Outcomes
- Decrease in blood pressure.

---

nitrofurantoin
(nye-troe-fyoor-**an**-toyn)
✦ Apo-Nitrofurantoin, Furadantin, Macrobid, Macrodantin

Classification
Therapeutic: anti-infectives

Pregnancy Category B

Indications
Prevention and treatment of urinary tract infections caused by susceptible organisms; not effective in systemic bacterial infections.

Action
Interferes with bacterial enzymes. **Therapeutic Effects:** Bactericidal or bacteriostatic action against susceptible organisms. **Spectrum:** Many gram-negative and some gram-positive organisms, specifically: *Citrobacter, Corynebacterium, Enterobacter, Escherichia coli, Klebsiella, Neisseria, Salmonella, Shigella, Staphylococcus aureus, Staphylococcus epidermidis, Enterococcus.*

Pharmacokinetics
Absorption: Readily absorbed after oral administration. Absorption is slower but more complete with macrocrystals (Macrodantin).
Distribution: Crosses placenta; enters breast milk.
Protein Binding: 40%.
Metabolism and Excretion: Partially metabolized by the liver; 30–50% excreted unchanged by the kidneys.
Half-life: 20 min (↑ in renal impairment).

TIME/ACTION PROFILE (urine levels)

ROUTE	ONSET	PEAK	DURATION
PO	unknown	30 min	6–12 hr

Contraindications/Precautions
Contraindicated in: Hypersensitivity; Hypersensitivity to parabens (suspension); Oliguria, anuria, or significant renal impairment (CCr <60 mL/min); History of cholestatic jaundice or hepatic impairment with previous use of nitrofurantoin; Pregnancy near term and infants <1 mo (↑ risk of hemolytic anemia).

Use Cautiously in: Glucose–6–phosphate dehydrogenase (G6PD) deficiency (↑ risk of hemolytic anemia, especially in Blacks and Mediterranean and Near-Eastern ethnic groups); Patients with diabetes or debilitated patients (neuropathy may be more common); OB: Safety not established but has been used safely in pregnant women. Lactation: May cause hemolysis in infants with G6PD deficiency who are breastfed; Geri: Appears on Beers list; ↑ risk for renal, hepatic, and pulmonary reactions.

Adverse Reactions/Side Effects
CNS: dizziness, drowsiness, headache. **EENT:** nystagmus. **Resp:** PNEUMONITIS, PULMONARY FIBROSIS. **CV:** chest pain. **GI:** HEPATOTOXICITY, PSEUDOMEMBRANOUS COLITIS, anorexia, nausea, vomiting, abdominal pain, diarrhea. **GU:** rust/brown discoloration of urine. **Derm:** photosensitivity. **Hemat:** blood dyscrasias, hemolytic anemia. **Neuro:** peripheral neuropathy. **Misc:** hypersensitivity reactions.

Interactions
Drug-Drug: Probenecid and **sulfinpyrazone** prevent high urinary concentrations; may ↓ effectiveness. **Antacids** may ↓ absorption. ↑ risk of neurotoxicity with **neurotoxic drugs**. ↑ risk of hepatotoxicity with **hepatotoxic drugs**. ↑ risk of pneumonitis with **drugs having pulmonary toxicity**.

Route/Dosage
PO (Adults): *Treatment of active infection*—50–100 mg q 6–8 hr *or* 100 mg q 12 hr as extended-release product. *Chronic suppression*—50–100 mg single evening dose.

PO (Children >1 mo): *Treatment of active infection*—5–7 mg/kg/day divided q 6 hr; maximum dose: 400 mg/day. *Chronic suppression*—1–2 mg/kg/day as a single dose at bedtime; maximum dose: 100 mg/day (unlabeled).

Availability (generic available)
Tablets: 50 mg, 100 mg. **Oral suspension:** 25 mg/5 mL. **Capsules:** 25 mg, 50 mg, 100 mg. **Extended-release capsules:** 100 mg.

NURSING IMPLICATIONS

Assessment
- Assess for signs and symptoms of urinary tract infection (frequency, urgency, pain, and burning on urination; fever; cloudy or foul-smelling urine) before and periodically during therapy.
- Obtain specimens for culture and sensitivity before and during drug administration.
- Monitor intake and output ratios. Report significant discrepancies in totals.
- Monitor bowel function. Diarrhea, abdominal cramping, fever, and bloody stools should be reported to health care professional promptly as a sign of pseudomembranous colitis. May

begin up to several weeks following cessation of therapy.
* Assess for signs and symptoms of pulmonary reactions periodically during therapy. Acute reactions (fever, chills, cough, chest pain, dyspnea, pulmonary infiltration with consolidation or pleural effusion on x-ray, eosinophilia) usually occur within first week of treatment and resolve when therapy is discontinued. Chronic reactions (malaise, dyspnea on exertion, cough, altered pulmonary function) may indicate pneumonitis or pulmonary fibrosis and are more common in patients taking nitrofurantoin for 6 mo or longer.
* **Lab Test Considerations:** Monitor CBC routinely with patients on prolonged therapy.
* Monitor liver function tests periodically during therapy. May cause ↑ serum glucose, bilirubin, alkaline phosphatase, BUN, and creatinine. If hepatotoxicity occurs, discontinue therapy.
* Monitor renal function periodically during therapy.

Potential Nursing Diagnoses
Risk for infection (Indications)

Implementation
* **PO:** Administer with food or milk to minimize GI irritation, to delay and increase absorption, to increase peak concentration, and to prolong duration of therapeutic concentration in the urine.
* Do not crush tablets or open capsules.
* Administer liquid preparations with calibrated measuring device. Shake well before administration. Oral suspension may be mixed with water, milk, fruit juices, or infant formula. Rinse mouth with water after administration of oral suspension to avoid staining teeth.

Patient/Family Teaching
* Instruct patient to take medication around the clock, as directed. Take missed doses as soon as remembered and space next dose 2–4 hr apart. Do not skip or double up on missed doses.
* May cause dizziness or drowsiness. Caution patient to avoid driving or other activities requiring alertness until response to medication is known.
* Inform patient that medication may cause a rust-yellow to brown discoloration of urine, which is not significant.
* Advise patient to notify health care professional if fever, chills, cough, chest pain, dyspnea, skin rash, numbness or tingling of the fingers or toes, or intolerable GI upset occurs. Signs of superinfection (milky, foul-smelling urine; perineal irritation; dysuria) should also be reported.
* Instruct patient to notify health care professional if fever and diarrhea develop, especially if stool contains blood, pus, or mucus. Advise patient not to treat diarrhea without consulting health care professional.
* Instruct patient to consult health care professional if no improvement is seen within a few days after initiation of therapy.

Evaluation/Desired Outcomes
* Resolution of the signs and symptoms of infection. Therapy should be continued for a minimum of 7 days and for at least 3 days after the urine has become sterile.
* Decrease in the frequency of infections in chronic suppressive therapy.

---

nitroglycerin
(nye-tro-**gli**-ser-in)

extended-release capsules
Nitro-Time, ✽ Nitrogard SR

intravenous
Nitro-Bid IV, Tridil

translingual spray
Nitrolingual, Nitromist

ointment
Nitro-Bid

sublingual
Nitrostat, NitroQuick

transdermal system
Minitran, Nitrek, Nitro-Dur

Classification
Therapeutic: antianginals
Pharmacologic: nitrates

Pregnancy Category C

Indications
Acute (**translingual and SL**) and long-term prophylatic (**oral, transdermal**) management of angina pectoris. **PO:** Adjunct treatment of CHF. **IV:** Adjunct treatment of acute MI. Production of controlled hypotension during surgical procedures. Treatment of CHF associated with acute MI.

✽ = Canadian drug name. ▮ = Genetic implication.
*CAPITALS indicates life-threatening; underlines indicate most frequent.

nitroglycerin

Action
Increases coronary blood flow by dilating coronary arteries and improving collateral flow to ischemic regions. Produces vasodilation (venous greater than arterial). Decreases left ventricular end-diastolic pressure and left ventricular end-diastolic volume (preload). Reduces myocardial oxygen consumption. **Therapeutic Effects:** Relief or prevention of anginal attacks. Increased cardiac output. Reduction of blood pressure.

Pharmacokinetics
Absorption: Well absorbed after oral, buccal, and sublingual administration. Also absorbed through skin. Orally administered nitroglycerin is rapidly metabolized, leading to decreased bioavailability.
Distribution: Unknown.
Metabolism and Excretion: Undergoes rapid and almost complete metabolism by the liver; also metabolized by enzymes in bloodstream.
Half-life: 1–4 min.

TIME/ACTION PROFILE (cardiovascular effects)

ROUTE	ONSET	PEAK	DURATION
SL	1–3 min	unknown	30–60 min
PO-ER	40–60 min	unknown	8–12 hr
TD-Oint	20–60 min	unknown	4–8 hr
TD-Patch	40–60 min	unknown	8–24 hr
IV	immediate	unknown	several min

Contraindications/Precautions
Contraindicated in: Hypersensitivity; Severe anemia; Pericardial tamponade; Constrictive pericarditis; Alcohol intolerance (large IV doses only); Concurrent use of PDE-5 inhibitor (sildenafil, tadalafil, vardenafil).
Use Cautiously in: Head trauma or cerebral hemorrhage; Glaucoma; Hypertrophic cardiomyopathy; Severe liver impairment; Malabsorption or hypermotility (PO); Hypovolemia (IV); Normal or decreased pulmonary capillary wedge pressure (IV); Cardioversion (remove transdermal patch before procedure); OB: May compromise maternal/fetal circulation; Lactation, Pedi: Safety not established.

Adverse Reactions/Side Effects
CNS: dizziness, headache, apprehension, restlessness, weakness. **EENT:** blurred vision. **CV:** hypotension, tachycardia, syncope. **GI:** abdominal pain, nausea, vomiting. **Derm:** contact dermatitis (transdermal or ointment). **Misc:** alcohol intoxication (large IV doses only), cross-tolerance, flushing, tolerance.

Interactions
Drug-Drug: Concurrent use of nitrates in any form with **sildenafil**, **tadalafil**, and **vardenafil** ↑ risk of serious and potentially fatal hypotension; concurrent use is contraindicated. Additive hypotension with **antihypertensives**, acute ingestion of **alcohol**, **beta blockers**, **calcium channel blockers**, **haloperidol**, or **phenothiazines**. Agents having anticholinergic properties (**tricyclic antidepressants**, **antihistamines**, **phenothiazines**) may ↓ absorption of lingual, or sublingual nitroglycerin.

Route/Dosage
SL (Adults): 0.3–0.6 mg; may repeat q 5 min for 2 additional doses for acute attack.
Translingual Spray (Adults): 1–2 sprays; may be repeated q 5 min for 2 additional doses for acute attack. Both may also be used prophylactically 5–10 min before activities that may precipitate an acute attack.
PO (Adults): 2.5–9 mg q 8–12 hr.
IV (Adults): 5 mcg/min; increase by 5 mcg/min q 3–5 min to 20 mcg/min; if no response, increase by 10–20 mcg/min q 3–5 min (dosing determined by hemodynamic parameters; max: 200 mcg/min).
Transdermal (Adults): *Ointment*—1–2 in. q 6–8 hr. *Transdermal patch*—0.2–0.4 mg/hr initially; may titrate up to 0.4–0.8 mg/hr. Patch should be worn 12–14 hr/day and then taken off for 10–12 hr/day.

Availability (generic available)
Extended-release capsules: 2.5 mg, 6.5 mg, 9 mg. **Sublingual tablets:** 0.3 mg, 0.4 mg, 0.6 mg. **Cost:** *NitroQuick*—0.3 mg $6.82/100, 0.4 mg $6.82/100, 0.6 mg $6.82/100; *Nitrostat*—0.3 mg $9.09/100, 0.4 mg $9.09/100, 0.6 mg $9.09/100. **Translingual spray (Nitrolingual):** 400 mcg/spray in 4.9–g canister (60 doses) or 12-g (200 doses) bottle, NitroMist 400 mcg/spray in 8.5 g canister (230 doses). **Transdermal systems:** 0.1 mg/hr, 0.2 mg/hr, 0.3 mg/hr, 0.4 mg/hr, 0.6 mg/hr, 0.8 mg/hr. **Transdermal ointment:** 2%. **Injection:** 5 mg/mL. **Premixed solution:** 25 mg/250 mL, 50 mg/250 mL, 50 mg/500 mL, 100 mg/250 mL, 200 mg/500 mL.

NURSING IMPLICATIONS

Assessment
- Assess location, duration, intensity, and precipitating factors of patient's anginal pain.
- Monitor blood pressure and pulse before and after administration. Patients receiving IV nitroglycerin require continuous ECG and blood

nitroglycerin

pressure monitoring. Additional hemodynamic parameters may be monitored.
- **Lab Test Considerations:** May cause ↑ urine catecholamine and urine vanillylmandelic acid concentrations.
- Excessive doses may cause ↑ methemoglobin concentrations.
- May cause falsely ↑ serum cholesterol levels.

Potential Nursing Diagnoses
Acute pain (Indications)
Ineffective tissue perfusion (Indications)

Implementation
- **PO:** Administer dose 1 hr before or 2 hr after meals with a full glass of water for faster absorption. Sustained-release preparations should be swallowed whole; do not break, crush, or chew.
- **SL:** Tablet should be held under tongue until dissolved. Avoid eating, drinking, or smoking until tablet is dissolved.
- **Translingual spray:** Spray *Nitrolingual* under tongue. Spray *Nitromist* on or under tongue.

IV Administration
- **IV:** Doses must be diluted and administered as an infusion. Standard infusion sets made of polyvinyl chloride (PVC) plastic may absorb up to 80% of the nitroglycerin in solution. Use glass bottles only and special tubing provided by manufacturer.
- **Continuous Infusion:** *Diluent:* Vials must be diluted in D5W or 0.9% NaCl. Premixed infusions already diluted in D5W and are ready to be administered (no further dilution needed). Admixed solutions stable for 48 hr at room temperature or 7 days if refrigerated. Stability of premixed solutions based on manufacturer's expiration date. *Concentration:* Should not exceed 400 mcg/mL. *Rate:* See Route/Dosage section. Administer via infusion pump to ensure accurate rate. Titrate rate according to patient response.
- **Y-Site Compatibility:** acyclovir, alfentanil, amikacin, aminophylline, amiodarone, amphotericin B cholesteryl, amphotericin B liposome, argatroban, ascorbic acid, atropine, azathioprine, aztreonam, benztropine, bivalirudin, bumetanide, buprenorphine, butorphanol, calcium chloride, calcium gluconate, carboplatin, caspofungin, cefazolin, cefoperazone, cefotaxime, cefotetan, cefoxitin, ceftazidime, ceftizoxime, ceftriaxone, cefuroxime, chloramphenicol, chlorpromazine, cimetidine, cisatracurium, cisplatin, clindamycin, clonidine, cyanocobalamin, cyclophosphamide, cyclosporine, cytarabine, dactinomycin, dexamethasone sodium phosphate, dexmedetomidine, digoxin, diltiazem, diphenhydramine, dobutamine, docetaxel, dopamine, doxorubicin, doxycycline, drotrecogin, enalaprilat, ephedrine, epinephrine, epirubicin, epoetin alfa, eptifibatide, ertapenem, erythromycin, esmolol, etoposide, etoposide phosphate, famotidine, fenoldopam, fentanyl, fluconazole, fludarabine, fluorouracil, folic acid, ganciclovir, gemcitabine, gentamicin, glycopyrrolate, granisetron, heparin, hydrocortisone sodium succinate, hydromorphone, ifosfamide, imipenem-cilastatin, indomethacin, insulin, isoproterenol, ketorolac, labetalol, lidocaine, linezolid, lorazepam, magnesium sulfate, mannitol, mechlorethamine, meperidine, metaraminol, methicillin, methotrexate, methoxamine, methyldopa, methylprednisolone, metoclopramide, metoprolol, metronidazole, micafungin, miconazole, midazolam, milrinone, minocycline, mitoxantrone, morphine, moxalactam, nafcillin, nalbuphine, naloxone, nesiritide, nicardipine, nitroprusside, norepinephrine, octreotide, ondansetron, oxacillin, oxaliplatin, oxytocin, paclitaxel, palonosetron, pancuronium, pantoprazole, papaverine, pemetrexed, penicillin G sodium, pentamidine, pentazocine, pentobarbital, phenobarbital, phentolamine, phenylephrine, phytonadione, piperacillin/tazobactam, potassium chloride, procainamide, prochlorperazine, promethazine, propofol, propranolol, protamine, pyridoxime, quinapristin-dalfopristin, ranitidine, remifentanil, ritodrine, rocuronium, sodium bicarbonate, streptokinase, succinylcholine, sufentanil, tacrolimus, teniposide, theophylline, thiamine, thiopental, ticarcillin/clavulanate, tigecycline, tirofiban, tobramycin, tolazoline, trimethophan, urokinase, vasopressin, vecuronium, verapamil, vincristine, vinorelbine, voriconazole, warfarin.
- **Y-Site Incompatibility:** alteplase, dantrolene, daptomycin, diazepam, diazoxide, lansoprazole, levofloxacin, phenytoin, trimethoprim/sulfamethoxazole.
- **Additive Incompatibility:** Manufacturer recommends that nitroglycerin not be admixed with other medications.

🍁 = Canadian drug name. ❊ = Genetic implication.
*CAPITALS indicates life-threatening; underlines indicate most frequent.

- **Topical:** Sites of topical application should be rotated to prevent skin irritation. Remove patch or ointment from previous site before application.
- Doses may be increased to the highest dose that does not cause symptomatic hypotension.
- Apply ointment by using dose-measuring application papers supplied with ointment. Squeeze ointment onto measuring scale printed on paper. Use paper to spread ointment onto nonhairy area of skin (chest, abdomen, thighs; avoid distal extremities) in a thin, even layer, covering a 2–3-in. area. Do not allow ointment to come in contact with hands. Do not massage or rub in ointment; this will increase absorption and interfere with sustained action. Apply occlusive dressing if ordered.
- Transdermal patches may be applied to any hairless site (avoid distal extremities or areas with cuts or calluses). Apply firm pressure over patch to ensure contact with skin, especially around edges. Apply a new dose unit if the first one becomes loose or falls off. Units are waterproof and not affected by showering or bathing. Do not cut or trim system to adjust dosage. Do not alternate between brands of transdermal products; dose may not be equivalent. Remove patches before MRI, cardioversion or defibrillation to prevent patient burns. Patch may be worn for 12–14 hr and removed for 10–12 hr at night to prevent development of tolerance.

Patient/Family Teaching
- Instruct patient to take medication as directed, even if feeling better. Take missed doses as soon as remembered unless next dose is scheduled within 2 hr (6 hr with extended-release preparations). Do not double doses. Do not discontinue abruptly; gradual dose reduction may be necessary to prevent rebound angina.
- Caution patient to change positions slowly to minimize orthostatic hypotension. First dose should be taken while in a sitting or reclining position, especially in geriatric patients.
- Advise patient to avoid concurrent use of alcohol with this medication. Patient should also consult health care professional before taking OTC medications while taking nitroglycerin.
- Inform patient that headache is a common side effect that should decrease with continuing therapy. Aspirin or acetaminophen may be ordered to treat headache. Notify health care professional if headache is persistent or severe.
- Advise patient to notify health care professional if dry mouth or blurred vision occurs.
- **Acute Anginal Attacks:** Advise patient to sit down and use medication at first sign of attack. Relief usually occurs within 5 min. Dose may be repeated if pain is not relieved in 5–10 min. Call health care professional or go to nearest emergency room if anginal pain is not relieved by 3 tablets in 15 min.
- **SL:** Inform patient that tablets should be kept in original glass container or in specially made metal containers, with cotton removed to prevent absorption. Tablets lose potency in containers made of plastic or cardboard or when mixed with other capsules or tablets. Exposure to air, heat, and moisture also causes loss of potency. Instruct patient not to open bottle frequently, handle tablets, or keep bottle of tablets next to body (i.e., shirt pocket) or in automobile glove compartment. Advise patient that tablets should be replaced 6 mo after opening to maintain potency.
- **Lingual Spray:** Instruct patient to lift tongue and spray dose under tongue (*Nitrolingual, NitroMist*) or on tongue (*NitroMist*).

Evaluation/Desired Outcomes
- Decrease in frequency and severity of anginal attacks.
- Increase in activity tolerance. During long-term therapy, tolerance may be minimized by intermittent administration in 12–14 hr or 10–12 hr off intervals.
- Controlled hypotension during surgical procedures.
- Treatment of CHF associated with acute MI.

HIGH ALERT

nitroprusside
(nye-troe-**pruss**-ide)
Nitropress

Classification
Therapeutic: antihypertensives
Pharmacologic: vasodilators

Pregnancy Category C

Indications
Hypertensive crises. Controlled hypotension during anesthesia. Cardiac pump failure or cardiogenic shock (alone or with dopamine).

Action
Produces peripheral vasodilation by a direct action on venous and arteriolar smooth muscle.
Therapeutic Effects: Rapid lowering of blood pressure. Decreased cardiac preload and afterload.

Pharmacokinetics
Absorption: IV administration results in complete bioavailability.
Distribution: Unknown.
Metabolism and Excretion: Rapidly metabolized in RBCs and tissues to cyanide and subsequently by the liver to thiocyanate.
Half-life: 2 min.

TIME/ACTION PROFILE (hypotensive effect)

ROUTE	ONSET	PEAK	DURATION
IV	immediate	rapid	1–10 min

Contraindications/Precautions
Contraindicated in: Hypersensitivity; ↓ cerebral perfusion.
Use Cautiously in: Renal disease (↑ risk of thiocyanate accumulation); Hepatic disease (↑ risk of cyanide accumulation); Hypothyroidism; Hyponatremia; Vitamin B deficiency; OB, Lactation: Safety not established; Geri: May have ↑ sensitivity to drug effects.

Adverse Reactions/Side Effects
CNS: dizziness, headache, restlessness. **EENT:** blurred vision, tinnitus. **CV:** dyspnea, hypotension, palpitations. **GI:** abdominal pain, nausea, vomiting. **F and E:** acidosis. **Local:** phlebitis at IV site. **Misc:** CYANIDE TOXICITY, thiocyanate toxicity.

Interactions
Drug-Drug: ↑ hypotensive effect with **ganglionic blocking agents**, **general anesthetics**, and other **antihypertensives**. **Estrogens** and **sympathomimetics** may ↓ the response to nitroprusside.

Route/Dosage
IV (Adults and Children): 0.3 mcg/kg/min initially; may be ↑ as needed up to 10 mcg/kg/min (usual dose is 3 mcg/kg/min; not to exceed 10 min of therapy at 10 mcg/kg/min infusion rate).

Availability (generic available)
Injection: 25 mg/mL.

NURSING IMPLICATIONS

Assessment
- Monitor blood pressure, heart rate, and ECG frequently throughout therapy; continuous monitoring is preferred. Consult physician for parameters. Monitor for rebound hypertension following discontinuation of nitroprusside.
- Pulmonary capillary wedge pressure (PCWP) may be monitored in patients with MI or CHF.
- *Lab Test Considerations:* May cause ↓ bicarbonate concentrations, Pco_2, and pH.
- May cause ↑ lactate concentrations.
- May cause ↑ serum cyanide and thiocyanate concentrations.
- Monitor serum methemoglobin concentrations in patients receiving >10 mg/kg and exhibiting signs of impaired oxygen delivery despite adequate cardiac output and arterial Pco_2 (blood is chocolate brown without change on exposure to air). Treatment of methemoglobinemia is 1–2 mg/kg of methylene blue IV administered over several minutes.
- *Toxicity and Overdose:* If severe hypotension occurs, drug effects are quickly reversed, within 1–10 min, by decreasing rate or temporarily discontinuing infusion. May place patient in Trendelenburg position to maximize venous return.
- Monitor plasma thiocyanate levels daily in patients receiving prolonged infusions at a rate >3 mcg/kg/min or 1 mcg/kg/min in patients with anuria. Thiocyanate levels should not exceed 1 millimole/liter.
- Signs and symptoms of thiocyanate toxicity include tinnitus, toxic psychoses, hyperreflexia, confusion, weakness, seizures, and coma.
- Cyanide toxicity may manifest as lactic acidosis, hypoxemia, tachycardia, altered consciousness, seizures, and characteristic breath odor similar to almonds.
- Acute treatment of cyanide toxicity includes 4–6 mg/kg of *sodium nitrite* (as a 3% solution) over 2–4 min. This acts as a buffer for cyanide by converting 10% of hemoglobin to methemoglobin. If administration of sodium nitrite is delayed, inhalation of crushed ampule (vaporole, aspirole) of *amyl nitrite* for 15–30 sec of every minute should be started until sodium nitrite is running. Following completion of sodium nitrite infusion, administer *sodium thiosulfate* 150–200 mcg/kg (available as 25% and 50% solutions). This will convert cyanide to thiocyanate, which may then be eliminated. If required, entire regimen may be repeated in 2 hr at 50% of the initial doses.

Potential Nursing Diagnoses
Ineffective tissue perfusion (Indications)

Implementation
- If infusion of 10 mcg/kg/min for 10 min does not produce adequate reduction in blood pres-

sure, manufacturer recommends nitroprusside be discontinued.
- May be administered in left ventricular CHF concurrently with an inotropic agent (dopamine, dobutamine) when effective doses of nitroprusside restore pump function and cause excessive hypotension.

IV Administration
- **Continuous Infusion:** *Diluent:* Dilute 50 mg of nitroprusside in 250–1000 mL of D5W. Wrap infusion in aluminum foil to protect from light; administration set tubing need not be covered. Amber plastic bags do not offer sufficient protection from light; wrap must be opaque. Freshly prepared solution has a slight brownish tint; discard if solution is dark brown, orange, blue, green, or dark red. Solution must be used within 24 hr of preparation. *Concentration:* 50–200 mcg/mL. *Rate:* Based on patient's weight (see Route/Dosage section). Administer via infusion pump to ensure accurate dosage rate.
- **Y-Site Compatibility:** amikacin, aminophylline, argatroban, atropine, aztreonam, bivalirudin, bumetanide, calcium chloride, calcium gluconate, cefazolin, cefotaxime, cefoxitin, ceftizoxime, ceftriaxone, cefuroxime, chloramphenicol, cimetidine, clindamycin, cyclosporine, daptomycin, dexamethasone sodium phosphate, digoxin, diltiazem, dopamine, doxycycline, enalaprilat, epinephrine, ertapenem, esmolol, famotidine, fenoldopam, fentanyl, fluconazole, furosemide, ganciclovir, gentamicin, granisetron, heparin, hydrocortisone sodium succinate, hydromorphone, insulin, isoproterenol, ketorolac, labetalol, lidocaine, linezolid, lorazepam, magnesium sulfate, meperidine, methylprednisolone sodium succinate, metoclopramide, metoprolol, metronidazole, micafungin, midazolam, milrinone, morphine, nafcillin, nesiritide, nicardipine, nitroglycerin, norepinephrine, ondansetron, palonosetron, pancuronium, pantoprazole, penicillin G potassium, phenylephrine, phytonadione, piperacillin/tazobactam, potassium chloride, potassium phosphate, procainamide, propofol, propranolol, protamine, ranitidine, sodium bicarbonate, tacrolimus, ticarcillin/clavulanate, tirofiban, tobramycin, vancomycin, vasopressin, verapamil.
- **Y-Site Incompatibility:** acyclovir, ampicillin, caspofungin, ceftazidime, diazepam, diphenhydramine, erythromycin, hydralazine, hydroxyzine, levofloxacin, phenytoin, prochlorperazine, promethazine, quinupristin/dalfopristin, trimethoprim/sulfamethoxazole, voriconazole.

Patient/Family Teaching
- Advise patient to report the onset of tinnitus, dyspnea, dizziness, headache, or blurred vision immediately.

Evaluation/Desired Outcomes
- Decrease in blood pressure without the appearance of side effects.
- Treatment of cardiac pump failure or cardiogenic shock.

---

nizatidine, See HISTAMINE H$_2$ ANTAGONISTS.

HIGH ALERT

norepinephrine
(**nor**-ep-i-nef-rin)
Levophed

Classification
Therapeutic: vasopressors

Pregnancy Category C

Indications
Produces vasoconstriction and myocardial stimulation, which may be required after adequate fluid replacement in the treatment of severe hypotension and shock.

Action
Stimulates alpha-adrenergic receptors located mainly in blood vessels, causing constriction of both capacitance and resistance vessels. Also has minor beta-adrenergic activity (myocardial stimulation). **Therapeutic Effects:** Increased blood pressure. Increased cardiac output.

Pharmacokinetics
Absorption: IV administration results in complete bioavailability.
Distribution: Concentrates in sympathetic nervous tissue. Does not cross the blood-brain barrier but readily crosses the placenta.
Metabolism and Excretion: Taken up and metabolized rapidly by sympathetic nerve endings.
Half-life: Unknown.

TIME/ACTION PROFILE (effects on blood pressure)

ROUTE	ONSET	PEAK	DURATION
IV	immediate	rapid	1–2 min

Contraindications/Precautions
Contraindicated in: Vascular, mesenteric, or peripheral thrombosis; OB: ↓ uterine blood flow; Hypoxia; Hypercarbia; Hypotension secondary to hypovolemia (without appropriate volume replacement); Hypersensitivity to bisulfites.
Use Cautiously in: Hypertension; Concurrent use of MAO inhibitors, tricyclic antidepressants, or cyclopropane or halothane anesthetics; Hyperthyroidism; Cardiovascular disease; Lactation: Safety not established.

Adverse Reactions/Side Effects
CNS: anxiety, dizziness, headache, insomnia, restlessness, tremor, weakness. **Resp:** dyspnea. **CV:** arrhythmias, bradycardia, chest pain, hypertension. **GU:** decreased urine output, renal failure. **Endo:** hyperglycemia. **F and E:** metabolic acidosis. **Local:** phlebitis at IV site. **Misc:** fever.

Interactions
Drug-Drug: Use with **cyclopropane** or **halothane anesthesia**, **cardiac glycosides**, **doxapram**, or local use of **cocaine** may result in ↑ myocardial irritability. Use with **MAO inhibitors**, **methyldopa**, **doxapram**, or **tricyclic antidepressants** may result in severe hypertension. **Alpha-adrenergic blockers** can prevent pressor response. **Beta blockers** may exaggerate hypertension or block cardiac stimulation. Concurrent use with **ergot alkaloids** (**ergotamine**, **ergonovine**, **methylergonovine**, or **oxytocin**) may result in enhanced vasoconstriction and hypertension.

Route/Dosage
IV (Adults): 0.5–1 mcg/min initially, followed by maintenance infusion of 2–12 mcg/min titrated by blood pressure response (average rate 2–4 mcg/min, up to 30 mcg/min for refractory shock have been used).
IV (Children): 0.1 mcg/kg/min initially; may be followed by infusion titrated to blood pressure response, up to 1 mcg/kg/min.

Availability
Injection: 1 mg/mL in 4-mL ampules.

NURSING IMPLICATIONS

Assessment
- Monitor blood pressure every 2–3 min until stabilized and every 5 min thereafter. Systolic blood pressure is usually maintained at 80–100 mm Hg or 30–40 mm Hg below the previously existing systolic pressure in previously hypertensive patients. Consult physician for parameters. Continue to monitor blood pressure frequently for hypotension following discontinuation of norepinephrine.
- ECG should be monitored continuously. CVP, intra-arterial pressure, pulmonary artery diastolic pressure, pulmonary capillary wedge pressure (PCWP), and cardiac output may also be monitored.
- Monitor urine output and notify health care professional if it decreases to <30 mL/hr.
- Assess IV site frequently throughout infusion. A large vein should be used to minimize risk of extravasation, which may cause tissue necrosis. Phentolamine 5–10 mg may be added to each liter of solution to prevent sloughing of tissue in extravasation. If extravasation occurs, the site should be infiltrated promptly with 10–15 mL of 0.9% NaCl solution containing 5–10 mg of phentolamine to prevent necrosis and sloughing. If prolonged therapy is required or if blanching along the course of the vein occurs, change injection sites to provide relief from vasoconstriction.
- *Toxicity and Overdose:* If overdose occurs, discontinue norepinephrine and administer fluid and electrolyte replacement therapy. An alpha-adrenergic blocking agent (phentolamine 5–10 mg) may be administered intravenously to treat hypertension.

Potential Nursing Diagnoses
Decreased cardiac output (Indications)
Ineffective tissue perfusion (Indications)

Implementation
- *High Alert:* Vasoactive medications are inherently dangerous. Have second practitioner independently check original order, dose calculations, and infusion pump programming. Establish maximum dose limits. Norepinephrine overdose can result in severe peripheral vasoconstriction with resultant ischemia and necrosis of peripheral tissue. Assess peripheral circulation frequently.
- Volume depletion should be corrected, if possible, prior to initiation of norepinephrine.
- Heparin may be added to each 500 mL of solution to prevent thrombosis in the infused vein, perivenous reactions, and necrosis in patients with severe hypotension following MI.
- Norepinephrine may deplete plasma volume and cause ischemia of vital organs, resulting in hypotension when discontinued, if used for

prolonged periods. Prolonged or large doses may also decrease cardiac output.
- Infusion should be discontinued gradually, upon adequate tissue perfusion and maintenance of blood pressure, to prevent hypotension. Do not resume therapy unless blood pressure falls to 70–80 mm Hg.

IV Administration

- **Continuous Infusion:** *Diluent:* Dilute 4 mg in 1000 mL of D5W or D5/0.9% NaCl. Do not dilute in 0.9% NaCl without dextrose. *Concentration:* 4 mcg/mL Do not use discolored solutions (pink, yellow, brown) or those containing a precipitate. *Rate:* Titrate infusion rate according to patient response, using slowest possible rate to correct hypotension. Administer via infusion pump to ensure accurate dosage.
- **Y-Site Compatibility:** alfentanil, amikacin, amiodarone, anidulafungin, argatroban, ascorbic acid, atracurium, atropine, benztropine, bivalirudin, bumetanide, buprenorphine, butorphanol, calcium chloride, calcium gluconate, carboplatin, caspofungin, cefazolin, cefonicid, cefoperazone, cefotaxime, cefotetan, cefoxitin, ceftazidime, ceftizoxime, ceftriaxone, cefuroxime, chloramphenicol, chrlopromazine, cimetidine, cisatracurium, cisplatin, clindamycin, cyanocobalamin, cyclophosphamide, cyclosporine, cytarabine, daptomycin, dexamethasone, digoxin, diltiazem, diphenhydramine, dobutamine, docetaxel, dopamine, doripenem, doxycycline, enalaprilat, ephedrine, epinephrine, epirubicin, epoetin alfa, ertapenem, erythromycin, esmolol, etoposide, etoposide phosphate, famotidine, fenoldopam, fentanyl, fluconazole, fludarabine, gemcitabine, gentamicin, glycopyrrolate, granisetron, heparin, hetastarch, hydrocortisone sodium succinate, hydromorphone, ifosfamide, imipenem/cilastatin, isoproterenol, ketorolac, labetalol, lidocaine, linezolid, lorazepam, magnesium sulfate, mannitol, mechlorethamine, meperidine, meropenem, metaraminol, methotrexate, methoxamine, methyldopa, methylprednisolone, metoclopramide, metoprolol, metronidazole, micafungin, miconazole, midazolam, milrinone, mitoxantrone, morphine, multivitamins, mycophenolate, nafcillin, nalbuphine, naloxone, nicardipine, nitroglycerin, nitroprusside, octreotide, ondansetron, oxacillin, oxaliplatin, oxytocin, paclitaxel, palonosetron, papaverine, pemetrexed, penicillin G, pentamidine, pentazocine, phentolamine, phenylephrine, phytonadione, piperacillin/tazobactam, potassium chloride, procainamide, prochlorperazine, promethazine, propofol, propranolol, protamine, pyridoxime, ranitidine, remifentanil, streoptokinase, succinylcholine, sufentanil, tacrolimus, teniposide, theophylline, thiamine, thiotepa, ticarcillin/clavulanate, tigecycline, tirofiban, tobramycin, tolazoline, trimetaphan, urokinase, vancomycin, vasorpessin, vecuronium, verapamil, vincristine, vinorelbine, vitamin B complex with C, voriconazole.
- **Y-Site Incompatibility:** aminophylline, amphotericin B colloidal, azathioprine, dantrolene, diazepam, diazoxide, drotrecogin, folic acid, ganciclovir, indomethacin, pentobarbital, phenobarbital, phenytoin, sodium bicarbonate, thiopental, trimethoprim/sulfamethoxazole.

Patient/Family Teaching
- Instruct patient to report headache, dizziness, dyspnea, chest pain, or pain at infusion site promptly.

Evaluation/Desired Outcomes
- Increase in blood pressure to normal range.
- Increased tissue perfusion.

---

norethindrone, See CONTRACEPTIVES, HORMONAL.

---

norethindrone/ethinyl acetate, See CONTRACEPTIVES, HORMONAL.

---

nortriptyline (nor-trip-ti-leen)
Aventyl, Pamelor

Classification
Therapeutic: antidepressants
Pharmacologic: tricyclic antidepressants

Pregnancy Category D

Indications
Various forms of depression. **Unlabeled Use:** Management of chronic neurogenic pain.

Action
Potentiates the effect of serotonin and norepinephrine. Has significant anticholinergic properties. **Therapeutic Effects:** Antidepressant action that develops slowly over several weeks.

Pharmacokinetics
Absorption: Well absorbed after oral administration.
Distribution: Widely distributed. Enters breast milk in small amounts; probably crosses the placenta.

Protein Binding: 92%.
Metabolism and Excretion: Extensively metabolized by the liver, much of it on its first pass. Some is converted to active compounds. Undergoes enterohepatic recirculation and secretion into gastric juices.
Half-life: 18–28 hr.

TIME/ACTION PROFILE (antidepressant effect)

ROUTE	ONSET	PEAK	DURATION
PO	2–3 wk	6 wk	unknown

Contraindications/Precautions
Contraindicated in: Hypersensitivity; Angle-closure glaucoma; Alcohol intolerance (solution only).
Use Cautiously in: Pre-existing cardiovascular disease; History of seizures; Asthma; May ↑ risk of suicide attempt/ideation especially during early treatment or dose adjustment; risk may be greater in children and adolescents; OB: Use only if clearly needed and maternal benefits outweigh risk to fetus; Lactation: May result in sedation in infant; discontinue drug or bottle-feed; Pedi: Safety not established; Geri: More susceptible to adverse reactions; dose reduction recommended). Pre-existing cardiovascular disease. Geriatric men with prostatic hyperplasia may be more susceptible to urinary retention.

Adverse Reactions/Side Effects
CNS: drowsiness, fatigue, lethargy, agitation, confusion, extrapyramidal reactions, hallucinations, headache, insomnia. **EENT:** blurred vision, dry eyes, dry mouth. **CV:** ARRHYTHMIAS, hypotension, ECG changes. **GI:** constipation, nausea, paralytic ileus, unpleasant taste, weight gain. **GU:** urinary retention. **Derm:** photosensitivity. **Endo:** gynecomastia. **Hemat:** blood dyscrasias.

Interactions
Drug-Drug: May cause hypertension, hyperpyrexia, seizures, and death when used with **MAO inhibitors** (avoid concurrent use—discontinue 2 wk before starting nortriptyline). May prevent the therapeutic response to most **antihypertensives**. Hypertensive crisis may occur with **clonidine**. ↑ CNS depression with other **CNS depressants**, including **alcohol, antihistamines, opioids,** and **sedative/hypnotics**. Adrenergic effects may be ↑ with other **adrenergic agents,** including **vasoconstrictors** and **decongestants**. ↑ anticholinergic effects with other **drugs possessing anticholinergic properties,** including **antihistamines, antidepressants, atropine, haloperidol, phenothiazines, quinidine,** and **disopyramide**. **Cimetidine, fluoxetine,** or **hormonal contraceptives** ↑ blood levels and risk of toxicity. ↑ risk of agranulocytosis with **antithyroid agents**.
Drug-Natural Products: Concomitant use of **kava-kava, valerian,** or **chamomile** can ↑ CNS depression. **St. John's wort** may ↓ serum concentrations and efficacy. ↑ anticholinergic effects with **jimson weed** and **scopolia**.

Route/Dosage
PO (Adults): 25 mg 3–4 times daily, up to 150 mg/day.
PO (Geriatric Patients or Adolescents): 30–50 mg/day in divided doses or as a single dose.

Availability (generic available)
Capsules: 10 mg, 25 mg, 50 mg, 75 mg. **Oral solution:** 10 mg/5 mL.

NURSING IMPLICATIONS
Assessment
- Monitor mental status (orientation, mood, behavior). Assess for suicidal tendencies, especially during early therapy. Restrict amount of drug available to patient.
- Assess weight and BMI initially and throughout treatment.
- Monitor blood pressure and pulse rate before and during initial therapy. Report significant decreases in blood pressure or a sudden increase in pulse rate.
- Monitor baseline and periodic ECGs in geriatric patients or patients with heart disease. May cause prolonged PR and QT intervals and may flatten T waves.
- For overweight/obese individuals, monitor FBS and cholesterol levels.
- **Pain:** Assess type, location, and severity of pain before and periodically during therapy. Use pain scale to monitor effectiveness of medication.
- *Lab Test Considerations:* Assess leukocyte and differential blood counts, liver function, and serum glucose periodically. May cause ↑ serum bilirubin and alkaline phosphatase. May cause bone marrow depression. Serum glucose may be ↑ or ↓.
- Serum levels may be monitored in patients who fail to respond to usual therapeutic dose. Therapeutic plasma concentration range is 50–150 ng/mL.

- May cause alterations in blood glucose levels.
- ***Toxicity and Overdose:*** Symptoms of acute overdose include disturbed concentration, confusion, restlessness, agitation, seizures, drowsiness, mydriasis, arrhythmias, fever, hallucinations, vomiting, and dyspnea.
- Treatment of overdose includes gastric lavage, activated charcoal, and a stimulant cathartic. Maintain respiratory and cardiac function (monitor ECG for at least 5 days) and temperature. Medications may include digoxin for CHF, antiarrhythmics, and anticonvulsants.

Potential Nursing Diagnoses
Ineffective coping (Indications)
Risk for injury (Side Effects)
Chronic pain (Indications)
Sexual dysfunction (Side Effects)

Implementation
- Do not confuse nortriptyline with desipramine.
- Taper to avoid withdrawal effects. Reduce dose 50% for 3 days, then by 50% for 3 more days, then discontinue.
- **PO:** Administer medication with meals to minimize gastric irritation.
- May be given as a single dose at bedtime to minimize sedation during the day. Dose increases should be made at bedtime because of sedation.

Patient/Family Teaching
- Instruct patient to take medication as directed. Take missed doses as soon as possible unless almost time for next dose; if regimen is a single dose at bedtime, do not take in the morning because of side effects. Advise patient that drug effects may not be noticed for at least 2 wk. Abrupt discontinuation may cause nausea, vomiting, diarrhea, headache, trouble sleeping with vivid dreams, and irritability.
- May cause drowsiness and blurred vision. Caution patient to avoid driving and other activities requiring alertness until response to drug is known.
- Instruct patient to notify health care professional if visual changes occur. Inform patient that periodic glaucoma testing may be required during long-term therapy.
- Caution patient to make position changes slowly to minimize orthostatic hypotension. (This side effect is less pronounced with this medication than with other tricyclic antidepressants.).
- Advise patient to avoid alcohol or other CNS depressant drugs during therapy and for at least 3–7 days after therapy has been discontinued.
- Instruct patient to notify health care professional if urinary retention occurs or if dry mouth or constipation persists. Sugarless candy or gum may diminish dry mouth, and an increase in fluid intake or bulk may prevent constipation. If symptoms persist, dose reduction or discontinuation may be necessary. Consult health care professional if dry mouth persists for more than 2 wk.
- Caution patient to use sunscreen and protective clothing to prevent photosensitivity reactions.
- Alert patient that urine may turn blue-green in color.
- Inform patient of need to monitor dietary intake. Increase in appetite may lead to undesired weight gain. Refer as appropriate for nutritional, weight, or medical management.
- May have teratogenic effects. Instruct patient to notify health care professional immediately if pregnancy is planned or suspected.
- Advise patient to notify health care professional of medication regimen before treatment or surgery.
- Therapy for depression is usually prolonged. Emphasize the importance of follow-up exams and participation in prescribed psychotherapy to improve coping skills.
- Refer to local support group.

Evaluation/Desired Outcomes
- Increased sense of well-being.
- Renewed interest in surroundings.
- Increased appetite.
- Improved energy level.
- Improved sleep.
- Decrease in severity of chronic neurogenic pain. Patients may require 2–6 wk of therapy before full therapeutic effects of medication are seen.

NPH insulin (isophane insulin suspension), See INSULINS (intermediate-acting).

NPH/regular insulin mixtures, See INSULIN (mixtures).

nystatin (nye-stat-in)
Mycostatin, ✤Nadostine, Nilstat, ✤PMS-Nystatin

nystatin **939**

Classification
Therapeutic: antifungals (topical/local)

Pregnancy Category B

For other nystatin dosage forms, see antifungals (topical) and antifungals (vaginal).

Indications
Lozenges, oral suspension: Local treatment of oropharyngeal candidiasis. Treatment of intestinal candidiasis.

Action
Binds to fungal cell membrane, allowing leakage of cellular contents. **Therapeutic Effects:** Fungistatic or fungicidal action. **Spectrum:** Active against most pathogenic *Candida* species, including *C. albicans*.

Pharmacokinetics
Absorption: Poorly absorbed; action is primarily local.
Distribution: Unknown.
Metabolism and Excretion: Excreted unchanged in the feces after oral administration.
Half-life: Unknown.

TIME/ACTION PROFILE (antifungal effects)

ROUTE	ONSET	PEAK	DURATION
Top	rapid	unknown	2 hr†

†Maintenance of saliva levels required to inhibit growth of Candida species after oral dissolution of 2 lozenges

Contraindications/Precautions
Contraindicated in: Hypersensitivity; Some products may contain ethyl alcohol or benzyl alcohol—avoid use in patients who may be hypersensitive to or intolerant of these additives.
Use Cautiously in: Denture wearers (dentures require soaking in nystatin suspension); Pedi: Lozenges, pastilles, or troches may pose a choking risk for children <5 yr.

Adverse Reactions/Side Effects
GI: diarrhea, nausea, stomach pain (large doses), vomiting. **Derm:** contact dermatitis, Stevens-Johnson syndrome.

Interactions
Drug-Drug: None significant.

Route/Dosage
PO (Adults and Children): 400,000–600,000 units 4 times daily as oral suspension or 200,000–400,000 units 4–5 times daily as pastilles (lozenges).

PO (Infants): 200,000 units 4 times daily or 100,000 units to each side of the mouth 4 times daily.
PO (Neonates, Premature, and Low Birth Weight): 100,000 units 4 times daily or 50,000 units to each side of the mouth 4 times a day.

Availability (generic available)
Oral suspension: 100,000 units/mL. **Oral pastilles (lozenges, troches):** 200,000 units/troche. **Powder for oral suspension:** ⅛ tsp = 500,000 unitss. **Oral tablets:** 500,000 units.

NURSING IMPLICATIONS

Assessment
- Inspect oral mucous membranes before and frequently throughout therapy. Increased irritation of mucous membranes may indicate need to discontinue medication.

Potential Nursing Diagnoses
Risk for impaired skin integrity (Indications)
Risk for infection (Indications)

Implementation
- **PO:** Suspension should be administered by placing ½ of dose in each side of mouth. Patient should hold suspension in mouth or swish throughout mouth for several minutes before swallowing, then gargle and swallow. Use calibrated measuring device for liquid doses. Shake well before administration. Pedi: For neonates and infants, paint suspension into recesses of the mouth.
- To prepare oral solution from powder, add ⅛ tsp (approximately 500,000 units) to 120 mL of water and stir well. Prepare immediately before use; contains no preservatives.
- Lozenges (pastilles) should be allowed to dissolve slowly and completely in mouth; do not chew or swallow whole. Nystatin vaginal tablets can be administered orally for treatment of oral candidiasis.

Patient/Family Teaching
- Instruct patient to take medication as directed. If a dose is missed, take as soon as remembered but not if almost time for next dose. Do not double doses. Therapy should be continued for at least 2 days after symptoms subside.
- Pedi: Instruct parents or caregivers of infants and children on correct dose and administration. Remind them to use only the measuring devise dispensed with the product.

- Advise patient to report increased irritation of mucous membranes or lack of therapeutic response to health care professional.

Evaluation/Desired Outcomes
- Decrease in stomatitis.
- To prevent relapse after oral therapy, therapy should be continued for 48 hr after symptoms have disappeared and cultures are negative.
- Therapy for a period of 2 wk is usually sufficient, but more prolonged therapy may be necessary.

nystatin, See ANTIFUNGALS (TOPICAL).

nystatin, See ANTIFUNGALS (VAGINAL).

octreotide (ok-tree-oh-tide)
Sandostatin, Sandostatin LAR

Classification
Therapeutic: antidiarrheals, hormones

Pregnancy Category B

Indications
Treatment of severe diarrhea and flushing episodes in patients with GI endocrine tumors, including metastatic carcinoid tumors and vasoactive intestinal peptide tumors (VIPomas). Treatment of acromegaly. **Unlabeled Use:** Management of diarrhea in AIDS patients, patients with fistulas, chemotherapy-induced diarrhea, and graft- vs. host–disease-induced diarrhea. Treatment of hyperinsulinemic hypoglycemia of infancy. Management of postoperative chylothorax.

Action
Suppresses secretion of serotonin and gastroenterohepatic peptides. Increases absorption of fluid and electrolytes from the GI tract and increases transit time. Decreases levels of serotonin metabolites. Also suppresses growth hormone, insulin, and glucagon. **Therapeutic Effects:** Control of severe flushing and diarrhea associated with GI endocrine tumors.

Pharmacokinetics
Absorption: Well absorbed following subcut administration and IM administration of depot form.
Distribution: Unknown.
Protein Binding: 65%.
Metabolism and Excretion: Extensive hepatic metabolism; 32% excreted unchanged in urine.
Half-life: 1.5 hr.

TIME/ACTION PROFILE (control of symptoms)

ROUTE	ONSET	PEAK	DURATION
Subcut, IV	unknown	unknown	up to 12 hr
IM (LAR)	unknown	2 wk	up to 4 wk

Contraindications/Precautions
Contraindicated in: Hypersensitivity.
Use Cautiously in: Gallbladder disease (↑ risk of stone formation); Renal impairment (dose ↓ may be necessary); Hyperglycemia or hypoglycemia (changes in blood glucose may occur); Fat malabsorption (may be aggravated); OB, Lactation: Safety not established.

Adverse Reactions/Side Effects
CNS: dizziness, drowsiness, fatigue, headache, weakness. **EENT:** visual disturbances. **CV:** bradycardia, edema, orthostatic hypotension, palpitations. **GI:** ILEUS, abdominal pain, cholelithiasis, diarrhea, fat malabsorption, nausea, vomiting. **Derm:** flushing. **Endo:** hyperglycemia, hypoglycemia, hypothyroidism. **Local:** injection-site pain.

Interactions
Drug-Drug: May alter requirements for **insulin** or **oral hypoglycemic agents**. May ↓ blood levels of **cyclosporine**. May ↑ levels of QTc-prolonging agents.

Route/Dosage
Carcinoid Tumors
Subcut, IV (Adults): *Sandostatin*—100–600 mcg/day in 2–4 divided doses during first 2 wk of therapy (range 50–1500 mcg/day).
IM (Adults): *Sandostatin LAR*—20 mg q 4 wk for 2 mo; dose may be further adjusted.

VIPomas
Subcut, IV (Adults): *Sandostatin*—200–300 mcg/day in 2–4 divided doses during first 2 wk of therapy (range 150–750 mcg/day).
IM (Adults): *Sandostatin LAR*—20 mg q 2 wk for 2 mo; dose may be further adjusted.

Suppression of Growth Hormone (Acromegaly)
Subcut, IV (Adults): *Sandostatin*—50–100 mcg 3 times daily; titrate to achieve growth hormone levels <5 ng/mL or IGF-I levels <1.9 units/mL (males) or <2.2 units/mL (females) (usual effective dose = 100–200 mcg 3 times daily.
IM (Adults): *Sandostatin LAR*—20 mg q 4 wk for 3 mo, then adjusted on the basis of growth hormone levels.

Antidiarrheal
Subcut, IV (Adults): *AIDS-related*-100–1800 mcg/day (unlabeled).
Subcut, IV (Children): 1–10 mcg/kg q 12 hr or 1 mcg/kg IV bolus followed by a continuous infusion of 1 mcg/kg/hr.

Persistent Hyperinsulinemic Hypoglycemia of Infancy
IV (Infants): Initially 2–10 mcg/kg/day divided q 12 hr up to 40 mcg/kg/day divided q 6–8 hr.

Chylothorax
Subcut (Adults): 50–100 mcg q 8 hr.
Subcut (Children): 40 mcg/kg/day.

IV (Children): 0.3–10 mcg/kg/hr continuous infusion.

Availability (generic available)
Injection: 0.05 mg/mL, 0.1 mg/mL, 0.2 mg/mL, 0.5 mg/mL, 1 mg/mL. **Depot injection:** 10 mg, 20 mg, 30 mg.

NURSING IMPLICATIONS
Assessment
- Assess frequency and consistency of stools and bowel sounds throughout therapy.
- Monitor pulse and blood pressure prior to and periodically during therapy.
- Assess patient's fluid and electrolyte balance and skin turgor for dehydration.
- Monitor diabetic patients for signs of hypoglycemia. May require reduction in requirements for insulin and sulfonylureas and treatment with diazoxide.
- Assess for gallbladder disease; assess for pain and monitor ultrasound examinations of gallbladder and bile ducts prior to and periodically during prolonged therapy.
- *Lab Test Considerations:* Monitor 5-HIAA (urinary 5-hydroxyindoleacetic acid), plasma serotonin, and plasma substance P in patients with carcinoid; plasma vasoactive intestinal peptide (VIP) in patients with VIPoma; and free T_4 and serum glucose concentrations prior to and periodically during therapy in all patients taking octreotide.
- Monitor quantitative 72-hr fecal fat and serum carotene determinations periodically for possible drug-induced aggravations of fat malabsorption.
- May cause a slight ↑ in liver enzymes.
- May cause ↓ serum thyroxine (T_4) concentrations.

Potential Nursing Diagnoses
Diarrhea (Indications)

Implementation
- Do not use solution that is discolored or contains particulate matter. Ampules should be refrigerated but may be stored at room temperature for the days they will be used. Discard unused solution.
- **Subcut:** Administer the smallest volume needed to achieve required dose to prevent pain at injection site. Rotate injection sites; avoid multiple injections in same site within short periods of time. Preferred injection sites are the hip, thigh, or abdomen.
- Administer injections between meals and at bedtime to avoid GI side effects.
- Allow medication to reach room temperature prior to injection to minimize local reactions at injection site.
- **IM:** Mix IM solution by adding diluent included in kit. Administer immediately after mixing into the gluteal muscle. Avoid using deltoid site due to pain of injection.
- Patients with carcinoid tumors and VIPomas should continue to receive subcut dose for 2 wk following switch to IM depot form to maintain therapeutic level.

IV Administration
- **Direct IV:** *Diluent:* May be administered undiluted. *Rate:* Administer over 3 min.
- **Intermittent Infusion:** *Diluent:* Dilute in 50–200 mL of 0.9% NaCl or D5W. *Concentration:* 1.5–250 mcg/mL. *Rate:* Infuse over 15–30 min.
- **Y-Site Compatibility:** acyclovir, alfentanyl, allopurinol, amifostine, amikacin, aminocaproic acid, aminophylline, amiodarone, amphotericin B colloidal, amphotericin B lipid complex, amphotericin B liposome, ampicillin, ampicillin/sulbactam, anidulafungin, argatroban, atenolol, atracurium, azithromycin, aztreoman, bivalirudin, bleomycin, bumetanide, buprenorphine, busulfan, butorphanol, calcium chloride, calcium gluconate, capreomycin, carboplatin, carmustine, caspofungin, cefazolin, cefepime, cefotaxime, cefotetan, cefoxitin, ceftazidime, ceftizoxime, ceftriaxone, cefuroxime, chloramphenicol, chlorpromazine, cimetidine, ciprofloxacin, cisatracurium, cisplatin, clindamycin, cyclosporine, cytarabine, dacarbazine, dactinomycin, dantrolene, daptomycin, daunorubicin hydrochloride, daunorubicin liposome, dexamethasone sodium phosphate, dexmeditomidine, dexrazoxane, digoxin, diltiazem, diphenhydramine, dobutamine, docetaxel, dolasetron, dopamine, doxorubicin hydrochloride, doxorubicin liposome, doxycycline, droperidol, enalaprilat, ephedrine, epinephrine, epirubicin, eptifibitide, ertapenem, erythromycin, esmolol, etoposide, etoposide phosphate, famotidine, fenoldopam, fentanyl, fluconazole, fludarabine, fluorouracil, foscarnet, fosphenytoin, furosemide, galium nitrate, ganciclovir, gemcitabine, gentamicin, glycopyrrolate, granisetron, haloperidol, heparin, hydralazine, hydrocortisone, hydromorphone, idarubicin, ifosfamide, imipenem/cilastatin, insulin, irinotecan, isoproterenol, ketorolac, labetalol, lansoprazole, leucovorin, levofloxacin, lidocaine, linezolid, lorazepam, magnesium hydroxice, mannitol, mechlorethamine, mel-

phalan, meperidine, meropenem, mesna, methylprednisolone, methotrexate, methyldopate, metoclopramide, metoprolol, metronidazole, midazolam, milrinone, minocycline, mitomycin, mitoxantrone, mivacurium, morphine, mycophenolate, nafcillin, nalbuphine, naloxone, nesiritide, nicardipine, nitroglycerin, nitroprusside, norepinephrine, ondansetron, oxaliplatin, paclitaxel, palonosetron, pamidronate, pancuronium, pemetrexed, pentamidine, pentazocine, pentobarbital, phenobarbital, phentolamine, phenylephrine, piperacillin/tazobactam, potassium acetate, potassium chloride, potassium phosphates, procainamide, prochlorperazine, promethazine, propranolol, quinapristin/dalfopristin, ranitidine, remifentanil, rocuronium, sodium acetate, sodium bicarbonate, sodium phosphates, streptozocin, succinylcholine, sufentanil, tacrolimus, teniposide, thiopental, thiotepa, ticarcillin/clavulanate, tigecycline, tirofiban, tobramycin, topotecan, trimethoprim/sulfamethoxazole, vancomycin, vasopressin, vecuronium, verapamil, vinblastine, vincristine, vinorelbine, voriconazole, zidovudine, zolendronic acid.

- **Y-Site Incompatibility:** dantrolene, diazepam, micafungin, phenytoin.

Patient/Family Teaching
- May cause dizziness, drowsiness, or visual disturbances. Caution patient to avoid driving or other activities requiring alertness until response to medication is known.
- Advise patient to change positions slowly to minimize orthostatic hypotension.
- **Home Care Issues:** Instruct patients administering octreotide at home on correct technique for injection, storage, and disposal of equipment.
- Instruct patient to administer octreotide exactly as directed. If a dose is missed, administer as soon as possible, then return to regular schedule. Do not double doses.

Evaluation/Desired Outcomes
- Decrease in severity of diarrhea and improvement of electrolyte imbalances in patients with carcinoid or VIP-secreting tumors.
- Relief of symptoms and suppressed tumor growth in patients with pituitary tumors associated with acromegaly.
- Management of diarrhea in patients with AIDS.

olanzapine (oh-lan-za-peen)
Zyprexa, Zyprexa Zydis

Classification
Therapeutic: antipsychotics, mood stabilizers
Pharmacologic: thienobenzodiazepines

Pregnancy Category C

Indications
Acute and maintenance treatment of schizophrenia. Acute treatment of manic episodes associated with bipolar I disorder (may be used alone or with lithium or valproate). Maintenance therapy of bipolar I disorder. Acute agitation due to schizophrenia or bipolar I mania (IM). Depressive episodes associated with bipolar I disorder (when used with fluoxetine). Treatment-resistant depression (when used with fluoxetine). **Unlabeled Use:** Management of anorexia nervosa. Treatment of nausea and vomiting related to highly emetogenic chemotherapy.

Action
Antagonizes dopamine and serotonin type 2 in the CNS. Also has anticholinergic, antihistaminic, and anti–alpha$_1$-adrenergic effects. **Therapeutic Effects:** Decreased manifestations of psychoses.

Pharmacokinetics
Absorption: Well absorbed but rapidly metabolized by first-pass effect, resulting in 60% bioavailability. Conventional tablets and orally disintegrating tablets (Zydis) are bioequivalent. IM administration results in significantly higher blood levels (5 times that of oral).
Distribution: Extensively distributed.
Protein Binding: 93%.
Metabolism and Excretion: Highly metabolized (mostly by the hepatic P450 CYP 1A2 system); 7% excreted unchanged in urine.
Half-life: 21–54 hr.

TIME/ACTION PROFILE (antipsychotic effects)

ROUTE	ONSET	PEAK*	DURATION
PO	unknown	6 hr	unknown
IM	rapid	15–45 min	2–4 hr

*Blood levels

Contraindications/Precautions
Contraindicated in: Hypersensitivity; Lactation: Discontinue drug or bottle feed; **Orally disintegrating tablets only:** Phenylketonuria (orally disintegrating tablets contain aspartame).

Use Cautiously in: Patients with hepatic impairment; Patients at risk for aspiration; Cardiovascular or cerebrovascular disease; History of seizures; History of attempted suicide; Diabetes or risk factors for diabetes (may worsen glucose control); Prostatic hyperplasia; Angle-closure glaucoma; History of paralytic ileus; Dysphagia and aspiration have been associated with antipsychotic drug use; use with caution in patients at risk for aspiration; OB, Pedi: Safety not established; Geri: Geriatric patients (may require ↓ doses; ↑ risk of mortality in elderly patients treated for dementia-related psychosis).

Adverse Reactions/Side Effects

CNS: NEUROLEPTIC MALIGNANT SYNDROME, SEIZURES, SUICIDAL THOUGHTS, agitation, dizziness, headache, restlessness, sedation, weakness, dystonia, insomnia, mood changes, personality disorder, speech impairment, tardive dyskinesia. **EENT:** amblyopia, rhinitis, ↑ salivation, pharyngitis. **Resp:** cough, dyspnea. **CV:** orthostatic hypotension, tachycardia, chest pain. **GI:** constipation, dry mouth, abdominal pain, ↑ appetite, weight loss or gain, nausea, ↑ thirst. **GU:** ↓ libido, urinary incontinence. **Hemat:** AGRANULOCYTOSIS, leukopenia, neutropenia. **Derm:** photosensitivity. **Endo:** amenorrhea, galactorrhea, gynecomastia, hyperglycemia, goiter. **Metab:** dyslipidemia. **MS:** hypertonia, joint pain. **Neuro:** tremor. **Misc:** fever, flu-like syndrome.

Interactions

Drug-Drug: Effects may be ↓ by concurrent **carbamazepine**, **omeprazole**, or **rifampin**. ↑ hypotension may occur with **antihypertensives**. ↑ CNS depression may occur with concurrent use of **alcohol** or other **CNS depressants**. May antagonize the effects of **levodopa** or other **dopamine agonists**. Nicotine can ↓ olanzapine levels.

Route/Dosage

PO (Adults —Most Patients): *Schizophrenia*—5–10 mg/day initially; may ↑ at weekly intervals by 5 mg/day (not to exceed 20 mg/day). *Bipolar I mania*—10–15 mg/day initially (use 10 mg/day when used with lithium or valproate); may ↑ every 24 hr by 5 mg/day (not to exceed 20 mg/day); *Depressive episodes associated with bipolar I disorder*—5 mg/day with fluoxetine 20 mg/day (both given in evening); may ↑ fluoxetine dose up to 50 mg/day and olanzapine dose up to 12.5 mg/day; *Treatment-resistant depression*—5 mg/day with fluoxetine 20 mg/day (both given in evening); may ↑ fluoxetine dose up to 50 mg/day and olanzapine dose up to 20 mg/day.

PO (Adults —Debilitated or Nonsmoking Female Patients ≥65 yr): Initiate therapy at 5 mg/day.
IM (Adults): *Acute agitation*—5–10 mg, may repeat in 2 hr, then 4 hr later.
IM (Adults >65 yr): Initiate therapy with 5 mg.

Availability

Tablets: 2.5 mg, 5 mg, 7.5 mg, 10 mg, 15 mg, 20 mg. **Cost:** 2.5 mg $556.93/90, 5 mg $645.82/90, 7.5 mg $805.91/90, 10 mg $1,007.96/90, 15 mg $1,475.96/90, 20 mg $1,860.77/90. **Orally disintegrating tablets (Zydis):** 5 mg, 10 mg, 15 mg, 20 mg. **Cost:** 5 mg $765.95/90, 10 mg $1,139.83/90, 15 mg $1,648.53/90, 20 mg $2,163.23/90. **Powder for injection:** 10 mg/vial. *In combination with:* fluoxetine (Symbyax; see Appendix B).

NURSING IMPLICATIONS

Assessment

- Assess mental status (orientation, mood, behavior) before and periodically during therapy. Monitor closely for notable changes in behavior that could indicate the emergence or worsening of suicidal thoughts or behavior or depression.
- Monitor blood pressure (sitting, standing, lying), ECG, pulse, and respiratory rate before and frequently during dose adjustment.
- Assess weight and BMI initially and throughout therapy.
- Assess fasting blood glucose and cholesterol levels initially and throughout therapy.
- Observe patient carefully when administering medication to ensure that medication is taken and not hoarded or cheeked.
- Assess fluid intake and bowel function. Increased bulk and fluids in the diet may help minimize constipation.
- Monitor patient for onset of akathisia (restlessness or desire to keep moving) and extrapyramidal side effects (*parkinsonian*—difficulty speaking or swallowing, loss of balance control, pill rolling of hands, mask-like face, shuffling gait, rigidity, tremors; and *dystonic*—muscle spasms, twisting motions, twitching, inability to move eyes, weakness of arms or legs) every 2 mo during therapy and 8–12 wk after therapy has been discontinued. Report these symptoms if they occur, as reduction in dose or discontinuation of medication may be necessary. Trihexyphenidyl or benztropine may be used to control symptoms.
- Monitor for tardive dyskinesia (uncontrolled rhythmic movement of mouth, face, and ex-

olanzapine

tremities; lip smacking or puckering; puffing of cheeks; uncontrolled chewing; rapid or worm-like movements of tongue, excessive blinking of eyes). Report immediately; may be irreversible.
- Monitor for development of neuroleptic malignant syndrome (fever, respiratory distress, tachycardia, seizures, diaphoresis, hypertension or hypotension, pallor, tiredness, severe muscle stiffness, loss of bladder control). Notify health care professional immediately if these symptoms occur.
- Monitor for symptoms related to hyperprolactinemia (menstrual abnormalities, galactorrhea, sexual dysfunction).
- *Lab Test Considerations:* Evaluate CBC, liver function tests, and ocular examinations periodically during therapy. May cause ↓ platelets. May cause ↑ bilirubin, AST, ALT, GGT, CPK, and alkaline phosphatase.
- Monitor blood glucose prior to and periodically during therapy.
- Monitor serum prolactin prior to and periodically during therapy. May cause ↑ serum prolactin levels.
- Monitor CBC frequently during initial months of therapy in patients with pre-existing or history of low WBC. May cause leukopenia, neutropenia, or agranulocytosis. Discontinue therapy if this occurs.

Potential Nursing Diagnoses
Disturbed thought process (Indications)
Impaired oral mucous membrane (Side Effects)
Sexual dysfunction (Side Effects)

Implementation
- Do not confuse Zyprexa (olanzapine) with Celexa (citalopram) or Zyrtec (cetirizine).
- **PO:** May be administered without regard to meals.
- For orally disintegrating tablets, peel back foil on blister, do not push tablet through foil. Using dry hands, remove from foil and place entire tablet in mouth. Tablet will disintegrate with or without liquid.
- **IM:** Reconstitute with 2.1 mL of sterile water for injection for a concentration of 5 mg/mL. Solution should be clear and yellow; do not administer solutions that are discolored or contain particulate matter. Inject slowly, deep into muscle. Do not administer IV or subcutaneously. Administer within 1 hr of reconstitution. Discard unused solution.

Patient/Family Teaching
- Advise patient to take medication as directed and not to skip doses or double up on missed doses. May need to discontinue gradually.
- Inform patient of possibility of extrapyramidal symptoms and tardive dyskinesia. Instruct patient to report these symptoms immediately to health care professional.
- Advise patient to change positions slowly to minimize orthostatic hypotension.
- Medication may cause drowsiness. Caution patient to avoid driving or other activities requiring alertness until response to the medication is known.
- Advise patient and family to notify health care professional if thoughts about suicide or dying, attempts to commit suicide; new or worse depression; new or worse anxiety; feeling very agitated or restless; panic attacks; trouble sleeping; new or worse irritability; acting aggressive; being angry or violent; acting on dangerous impulses; an extreme increase in activity and talking, other unusual changes in behavior or mood occur.
- Caution patient to avoid taking alcohol and to notify health care professional prior to taking other Rx, OTC, or herbal products concurrently with this medication.
- Advise patient to use sunscreen and protective clothing when exposed to the sun. Extremes of temperature (exercise, hot weather, hot baths or showers) should also be avoided; this drug impairs body temperature regulation.
- Instruct patient to use saliva substitute, frequent mouth rinses, good oral hygiene, and sugarless gum or candy to minimize dry mouth. Consult dentist if dry mouth continues for >2 wk.
- Advise patient to notify health care professional of medication regimen before treatment or surgery.
- Instruct patient to notify health care professional promptly if sore throat, fever, unusual bleeding or bruising, rash, weakness, tremors, visual disturbances, dark-colored urine, clay-colored stools, menstrual abnormalities, galactorrhea or sexual dysfunction occur.
- Advise patient to notify health care professional if pregnancy is planned or suspected, or if breastfeeding or planning to breastfeed.
- Emphasize the importance of routine follow-up exams and continued participation in psychotherapy.

✱ = Canadian drug name. ❄ = Genetic implication.
*CAPITALS indicates life-threatening; underlines indicate most frequent.

Evaluation/Desired Outcomes
- Decrease in excitable, manic behavior.
- Decrease in positive symptoms (delusions, hallucinations) of schizophrenia.
- Decrease in negative symptoms (social withdrawal, flat, blunted affect) of schizophrenia.
- Increased sense of well-being.
- Decreased agitation.

---

olmesartan, See ANGIOTENSIN II RECEPTOR ANTAGONISTS.

---

olopatadine (nasal spray)
(o-lo-**pa**-ta-deen)
Patanase

Classification
Therapeutic: allergy, cold, and cough remedies
Pharmacologic: antihistamines

Pregnancy Category C

Indications
Relief of symptoms of allergic rhinitis.

Action
Antagonizes the effects of histamine at histamine$_1$ receptor sites; does not bind to or inactivate histamine. **Therapeutic Effects:** Decreased symptoms of histamine excess including rhinorrhea, sneezing, and nasal itching.

Pharmacokinetics
Absorption: 57% absorbed from nasal mucosa.
Distribution: Unknown.
Metabolism and Excretion: Minimal metabolism; 70% eliminated in urine mostly as unchanged drug; 17% fecal elimination.
Half-life: 8–12 hr.

TIME/ACTION PROFILE

ROUTE	ONSET	PEAK	DURATION
Nasal	rapid	unknown	12 hr

Contraindications/Precautions
Contraindicated in: None noted.
Use Cautiously in: Nasal pathology other than allergic rhinitis; Geri: Dose cautiously in elderly patients; consider age-related decrease in organ function and concurrent medications; Lactation, OB: Use in pregnancy or lactation only when maternal benefit outweighs fetal risk; Pedi: Safe use in children <12 yr not established.

Adverse Reactions/Side Effects
CNS: drowsiness, headache. **EENT:** epistaxis, nasal perforation, nasal ulcerations, pharyngolaryngeal pain, postnasal drip. **GI:** bitter taste. **Resp:** cough.

Interactions
Drug-Drug: ↑ CNS depression may occur with **alcohol**; avoid concurrent use.

Route/Dosage
Intranasal (Adults and Children ≥ 12 yr): 2 sprays in each nostril twice daily.

Availability
Nasal spray: 665 mcg/100 microliter (0.6%) spray in 30.5-g bottle (provides 240 metered sprays).

NURSING IMPLICATIONS

Assessment
- Assess for symptoms of seasonal allergic rhinitis (sneezing, runny nose, nasal itching) prior to and during therapy.

Potential Nursing Diagnoses
Ineffective airway clearance (Indications)

Implementation
- Administer 2 sprays per nostril twice daily.

Patient/Family Teaching
- Instruct patient to prime nasal spray by releasing 5 sprays or spraying until a fine mist appears before initial use. If unit has not been used within 7 days, re-prime with 2 sprays.
- May cause drowsiness. Advise patient to avoid driving or other activities that require alertness until response to medication is known.
- Instruct patient to avoid concurrent use of alcohol or other CNS depressants.

Evaluation/Desired Outcomes
- Relief of symptoms of seasonal allergic rhinitis.

---

olsalazine (ole-**sal**-a-zeen)
Dipentum

Classification
Therapeutic: gastrointestinal anti-inflammatories

Pregnancy Category C

Indications
Ulcerative colitis (when patients cannot tolerate sulfasalazine).

Action
Locally acting anti-inflammatory action in the colon, where activity is probably due to inhibition of

olsalazine **947**

prostaglandin synthesis. **Therapeutic Effects:** Reduction in the symptoms of inflammatory bowel disease.

Pharmacokinetics
Absorption: Acts locally in colon, where 98–99% is converted to mesalamine (5-aminosalicylic acid).
Distribution: Action is primarily local and remains in the colon.
Metabolism and Excretion: 2% absorbed into systemic circulation is rapidly metabolized; mostly eliminated as mesalamine in the feces.
Half-life: 0.9 hr.

TIME/ACTION PROFILE (levels)

ROUTE	ONSET	PEAK	DURATION
PO	unknown	1 hr; 4–8 hr	12 hr

Contraindications/Precautions
Contraindicated in: Hypersensitivity reactions to salicylates; Cross-sensitivity with furosemide, sulfonylurea hypoglycemic agents, or carbonic anhydrase inhibitors may exist; Glucose-6–phosphate dehydrogenase (G6PD) deficiency; Urinary tract or intestinal obstruction; Porphyria; Lactation: Lactation; Pedi: Children <2 yr (safety not established).
Use Cautiously in: Severe hepatic or renal impairment; Renal impairment (↑ risk of renal tubular damage); OB: Pregnancy; Geri: Consider ↓ body mass, hepatic/renal/cardiac function, intercurrent illness and drug therapies.

Adverse Reactions/Side Effects
CNS: ataxia, confusion, dizziness, drowsiness, headache, mental depression, psychosis, restlessness. **GI:** diarrhea, abdominal pain, anorexia, exacerbation of colitis, drug-induced hepatitis, nausea, vomiting. **Derm:** itching, rash. **Hemat:** blood dyscrasias.

Interactions
Drug-Drug: ↑ risk of bleeding after neuraxial anesthesia with **low molecular weight heparins** and **heparinoids**; discontinue olsalazine before initiation of therapy or monitor closely if discontinuation not possible. May ↓ metabolism, and ↑ effects/toxicity of **mercaptopurine** or **thioguanine** with and ↑ risk of myelosuppression (use lowest possible dose and monitor closely). ↑ risk of developing Reye's syndrome; avoid olsalazine during 6 wk after **varicella vaccine**.

Route/Dosage
PO (Adults): 500 mg twice daily.

Availability
Capsules: 250 mg.

NURSING IMPLICATIONS
Assessment
- Assess patient for allergy to sulfonamides and salicylates. Patients allergic to sulfasalazine may take mesalamine or olsalazine without difficulty, but therapy should be discontinued if rash or fever occur.
- Monitor intake and output ratios. Fluid intake should be sufficient to maintain a urine output of at least 1200–1500 mL daily to prevent crystalluria and stone formation.
- **Inflammatory Bowel Disease:** Assess abdominal pain and frequency, quantity, and consistency of stools at the beginning of and throughout therapy.
- *Lab Test Considerations:* Monitor urinalysis, BUN, and serum creatinine prior to and periodically during therapy.
- Olsalazine may cause ↑ AST and ALT levels.
- *Lab Test Considerations:* Monitor CBC prior to and every 3–6 mo during prolonged therapy. Discontinue olsalazine if blood dyscrasias occur.

Potential Nursing Diagnoses
Acute pain (Indications)
Diarrhea (Indications)

Implementation
- **PO:** Administer with food in evenly divided doses every 12 hr.

Patient/Family Teaching
- Instruct patient to take medication as directed, even if feeling better. Take missed doses as soon as remembered unless almost time for next dose.
- May cause dizziness. Caution patient to avoid driving or other activities that require alertness until response to medication is known.
- Advise patient to notify health care professional if skin rash, sore throat, fever, mouth sores, unusual bleeding or bruising, wheezing, fever, or hives occurs.
- Instruct patient to notify health care professional if symptoms do not improve after 1–2 mo of therapy.
- Instruct patient to notify health care professional if symptoms worsen or do not improve.

= Canadian drug name. = Genetic implication.
*CAPITALS indicates life-threatening; underlines indicate most frequent.

If symptoms of acute intolerance (cramping, acute abdominal pain, bloody diarrhea, fever, headache, rash) occur, discontinue therapy and notify health care professional immediately.
- Inform patient that proctoscopy and sigmoidoscopy may be required periodically during treatment to determine response.

Evaluation/Desired Outcomes
- Decrease in diarrhea and abdominal pain.
- Return to normal bowel pattern in patients with inflammatory bowel disease. Effects may be seen within 3–21 days. The usual course of therapy is 3–6 wk.
- Maintenance of remission in patients with inflammatory bowel disease.
- Decrease in pain and inflammation, and increase in mobility in patients with rheumatoid arthritis.

---

omalizumab (o-ma-liz-u-mab)
Xolair

Classification
Therapeutic: antiasthmatics
Pharmacologic: monoclonal antibodies

Pregnancy Category B

Indications
Moderate to severe asthma not controlled by inhaled corticosteroids.

Action
Inhibits binding of IgE to receptors on mast cells and eosinophils; preventing the release of mediators of the allergic response. Also decreases amount of IgE receptors on basophils. **Therapeutic Effects:** Decreased incidence of exacerbations of asthma.

Pharmacokinetics
Absorption: 62% absorbed slowly from subcut sites.
Distribution: Enters breast milk.
Metabolism and Excretion: Degraded similarly to IgG via binding degradation, reticuloendothelial system and the liver.
Half-life: 26 days.

TIME/ACTION PROFILE (effects on IgE levels)

ROUTE	ONSET	PEAK	DURATION
Subcut	within 1 hr	unknown	up to 1 yr

Contraindications/Precautions
Contraindicated in: Hypersensitivity; Acute bronchospasm.

Use Cautiously in: Chronic use of inhaled corticosteroids; OB: Use in pregnancy only if clearly needed; enroll pregnant women with at least one exposure to omalizumab in the Xolair Pregnancy Exposure Registry (1-866-496-5247); Lactation: Safety not established; Pedi: Children <12 yr (safety not established).

Adverse Reactions/Side Effects
Local: injection site reactions. **Misc:** allergic reactions including ANAPHYLAXIS, ↑ risk of malignancy.

Interactions
Drug-Drug: None noted.

Route/Dosage
Subcut (Adults and Children >12 yr): 150–375 mg every 2–4 wk (determined by pretreatment serum IgE level and body weight).

Availability
Powder for injection: 150 mg/vial.

NURSING IMPLICATIONS
Assessment
- Assess lung sounds and respiratory function prior to and periodically during therapy.
- Assess allergy symptoms (rhinitis, conjunctivitis, hives) before and periodically throughout therapy.
- Assess for allergic reactions (urticaria, tongue and/or throat edema) within 2 hr of first or subsequent injections. Observe patient following injection. Epinephrine, diphenhydramine, and corticosteroids should be available in case of anaphylaxis.
- Monitor for injection site reactions (bruising, redness, warmth, burning, stinging, itching, hives, pain, induration, mass, inflammation). Usually occur within 1 hr of injection, last <8 days, and decrease in frequency with subsequent dosing.
- *Lab Test Considerations:* Serum IgE levels will ↑ following administration and may persist for up to 1 year following discontinuation. Serum total IgE levels obtained <1 year following discontinuation may not reflect steady state free IgE levels and should not be used to reassess the dosing regimen.

Potential Nursing Diagnoses
Ineffective airway clearance

Implementation
- Doses of inhaled corticosteroids may be gradually decreased with supervision of health care professional; do not discontinue abruptly.

omega-3-acid ethyl esters **949**

- **Subcut:** To reconstitute draw 1.4 mL of sterile water for injection into a 3-cc syringe with a 1-inch 18-gauge needle. With the vial upright on a flat surface, inject the sterile water into vial. Keep vial upright and gently swirl for approximately 1 min to evenly wet powder. Do not shake. Lyophilized omalizumab takes 15–20 min to dissolve. Gently swirl vial for 5–10 seconds every 5 min to dissolve any remaining particles. Solution should be clear or slightly opalescent and may have small bubbles or foam around edge of vial. Do not use if particles are visible or if contents do not dissolve completely within 40 min. Invert vial for 15 seconds to allow solution to drain toward stopper. Solution may be somewhat viscous. In order to obtain full 1.2 mL dose, all of solution must be withdrawn from the vial using a new 3-cc syringe with an 18-gauge needle, before expelling any air or excess solution from syringe. Administer within 8 hr if refrigerated or within 4 hr if stored at room temperature. Discard unused solution.
- Replace the 18-gauge needle with a 25-gauge needle for subcut injection. Because solution is slightly viscous, injection may take 5–10 seconds to administer. Divide doses >150 mg into 2 injection sites.

Patient/Family Teaching

- Explain purpose of medication to patient. Inform patient that they may not see immediate results from omalizumab therapy.
- Instruct patient not to discontinue or reduce other asthma medications, especially inhaled corticosteroids, without consulting health care professional.

Evaluation/Desired Outcomes

- Decreased incidence of exacerbations of asthma.

---

omega-3-acid ethyl esters
(oh**me**-ga three **as**-id eth-il **es**-ters)
Lovaza

Classification
Therapeutic: lipid-lowering agents
Pharmacologic: fatty acids

Pregnancy Category C

Indications
Hypertriglyceridemia (triglycerides ≥500 mmg/dL) in adults; used with specific diet.

Action
Inhibits synthesis of triglycerides. **Therapeutic Effects:** Lowering of triglycerides.

Pharmacokinetics
Absorption: Well absorbed.
Distribution: Unknown.
Metabolism and Excretion: Incorporated into phospholipids.
Half-life: Unknown.

TIME/ACTION PROFILE (lowering of triglycerides)

ROUTE	ONSET	PEAK	DURATION
PO	unknown	2 mo	unknown

Contraindications/Precautions
Contraindicated in: Hypersensitivity.
Use Cautiously in: Allery/hypersensitivity to fish; OB, Lactation: Pregnancy or lactation; Pedi: Children (safety not established).

Adverse Reactions/Side Effects
GI: altered taste, eructation. **Derm:** rash.

Interactions
Drug-Drug: May ↑ risk of bleeding with **aspirin** or **warfarin**.

Route/Dosage
PO (Adults): 4 g/day; may be given as a single dose or 2 g twice daily.

Availability
Gelatin capsules (oil-filled): 1 g.

NURSING IMPLICATIONS

Assessment
- Obtain a diet history, especially with regard to fat consumption.
- *Lab Test Considerations:* Monitor serum triglyceride levels prior to and periodically during therapy.
- Monitor serum ALT periodically during therapy. May cause ↑ serum ALT without concurrent ↑ in AST levels.
- Monitor serum LDL cholesterol levels periodically during therapy. May cause ↑ in serum LDL levels.

Potential Nursing Diagnoses
Noncompliance (Patient/Family Teaching)

✱ = Canadian drug name. ❋ = Genetic implication.
*CAPITALS indicates life-threatening; underlines indicate most frequent.

Implementation
- An appropriate lipid-lowering diet should be followed before therapy and should continue during therapy.
- **PO:** May be taken as a single 4-g dose or as 2 g twice daily. May be administered with meals.

Patient/Family Teaching
- Instruct patient to take medication as directed, not to skip doses or double up on missed doses. Medication helps control but does not cure elevated serum triglyceride levels.
- Advise patient that this medication should be used in conjunction with diet restrictions (fat, cholesterol, carbohydrates, alcohol), exercise, weight loss in overweight patients, and control of medical problems (such as diabetes mellitus and hypothyroidism) that may contribute to hypertriglyceridemia.
- Emphasize the importance of follow-up exams to determine effectiveness.

Evaluation/Desired Outcomes
- Lowering of serum triglyceride levels. Patients who do not have an adequate response after 2 mo of treatment should be withdrawn from therapy.

---

omeprazole (o-mep-ra-zole)
✦ Losec, Prilosec, Prilosec OTC

Classification
Therapeutic: antiulcer agents
Pharmacologic: proton-pump inhibitors

Pregnancy Category C

Indications
GERD/maintenance of healing in erosive esophagitis. Duodenal ulcers (with or without anti-infectives for *Helicobacter pylori*). Short-term treatment of active benign gastric ulcer. Pathologic hypersecretory conditions, including Zollinger-Ellison syndrome. Reduction of risk of GI bleeding in critically ill patients. **OTC:** Heartburn occurring ≥twice/wk.

Action
Binds to an enzyme on gastric parietal cells in the presence of acidic gastric pH, preventing the final transport of hydrogen ions into the gastric lumen. **Therapeutic Effects:** Diminished accumulation of acid in the gastric lumen with lessened gastroesophageal reflux. Healing of duodenal ulcers.

Pharmacokinetics
Absorption: Rapidly absorbed following oral administration; immediate release formulation contains bicarbonate to prevent acid degradation. **Distribution:** Good distribution into gastric parietal cells.
Protein Binding: 95%.
Metabolism and Excretion: Extensively metabolized by the liver.
Half-life: 0.5–1 hr (↑ in liver disease to 3 hr).

TIME/ACTION PROFILE (antisecretory effects)

ROUTE	ONSET	PEAK	DURATION
PO-delayed release	within 1 hr	within 2 hr	72–96 hr

Contraindications/Precautions
Contraindicated in: Hypersensitivity; Lactation: Discontinue omeprazole or discontinue breastfeeding.
Use Cautiously in: Liver disease (dose ↓ may be necessary); OB, Lactation, Pedi: Safety not established in pregnant or breastfeeding women, or children <1 yr; Geri: ↑ risk of hip fractures in patients using high doses for >1 year.

Adverse Reactions/Side Effects
CNS: dizziness, drowsiness, fatigue, headache, weakness. **CV:** chest pain. **GI:** abdominal pain, acid regurgitation, constipation, diarrhea, flatulence, nausea, vomiting. **Derm:** itching, rash. **Misc:** allergic reactions.

Interactions
Drug-Drug: Omeprazole is metabolized by the CYP450 enzyme system and may compete with other agents metabolized by this system. ↓ metabolism and may ↑ effects of **antifungal agents, diazepam, digoxin, flurazepam, triazolam, cyclosporine, phenytoin, saquinavir, tacrolimus,** and **warfarin.** May ↓ absorption of drugs requiring acid pH, including **ketoconazole, itraconazole, ampicillin, iron salts,** and **digoxin.** Has been used safely with **antacids.** May significantly ↓ effects of **atazanavir** and **nelfinavir** (concurrent use not recommended). May ↑ risk of bleeding with **warfarin** (monitor INR/PT). May ↓ the antiplatelet effects of **clopidogrel.**

Route/Dosage
PO (Adults): *GERD/erosive esophagitis*—20 mg once daily. *Duodenal ulcers associated with H. pylori*—40 mg once daily in the morning with clarithromycin for 2 wk, then 20 mg once daily for 2 wk *or* 20 mg twice daily with clarithromycin 500 mg twice daily and amoxicillin 1000 mg twice daily for 10 days (if ulcer is present at beginning of therapy, continue omeprazole 20 mg daily for 18 more days); has also been used with clarithromycin and metronidazole. *Gastric ulcer*—40 mg

once daily for 4–6 wk. *Reduction of the risk of GI bleeding in critically ill patients*—40 mg initially, then another 40 mg 6–8 hr later, followed by 40 mg once daily for up to 14 days. *Gastric hypersecretory conditions*—60 mg once daily initially; may be increased up to 120 mg 3 times daily (doses >80 mg/day should be given in divided doses); *OTC*—20 mg once daily for up to 14 days.
PO (Children 1–16 yr and 5–9 kg): *GERD/erosive esophagitis*—5 mg once daily.
PO (Children 1–16 yr and 10–19 kg): *GERD/erosive esophagitis*—10 mg once daily.
PO (Children 1–16 yr and ≥20 kg): *GERD/erosive esophagitis*—20 mg once daily.

Availability (generic available)
Delayed-release capsules: 10 mg, 20 mg[Rx, OTC], 40 mg. **Delayed-release powder for oral suspension (peach-mint):** 2.5 mg/packet, 10 mg/packet. *In combination with:* metronidazole and clarithromycin in a compliance package (Losec 1-2-3 M); with amoxicillin and clarithromycin in a compliance package (Losec 1-2-3-A) (both in Canada only); with sodium bicarbonate (Zegerid; see Appendix B).

NURSING IMPLICATIONS

Assessment
- Assess patient routinely for epigastric or abdominal pain and frank or occult blood in the stool, emesis, or gastric aspirate.
- *Lab Test Considerations:* Monitor CBC with differential periodically during therapy.
- May cause ↑ AST, ALT, alkaline phosphatase, and bilirubin.
- May cause serum gastrin concentrations to ↑ during first 1–2 wk of therapy. Levels return to normal after discontinuation of omeprazole.
- Monitor INR and prothrombin time in patients taking warfarin.

Potential Nursing Diagnoses
Acute pain (Indications)

Implementation
- Do not confuse Prilosec (omeprazole) with Prinivil (lisinopril).
- **PO:** Administer doses before meals, preferably in the morning. Capsules should be swallowed whole; do not crush or chew. Capsules may be opened and sprinkled on cool applesauce, entire mixture should be ingested immediately and followed by a drink of water. Do not store for future use.
- *Powder for oral suspension:* Administer on empty stomach, as least 1 hr before a meal. For patients with nasogastric or enteral feeding, suspend feeding for 3 hr before and 1 hr after administration. Empty packet contents into a small cup containing 1–2 tablespoons of water. **Do not use other liquids or foods.** If administered through a nasogastric tube, suspend in 20 mL of water. Stir well and drink immediately. Refill cup with water and drink again.
- May be administered concurrently with antacids.

Patient/Family Teaching
- Instruct patient to take medication as directed for the full course of therapy, even if feeling better. Take missed doses as soon as remembered but not if almost time for next dose. Do not double doses.
- May cause occasional drowsiness or dizziness. Caution patient to avoid driving or other activities requiring alertness until response to medication is known.
- Advise patient to consult health care professional before taking any Rx, OTC, or herbal products with omeprazole.
- Advise patient to avoid alcohol, products containing aspirin or NSAIDs, and foods that may cause an increase in GI irritation.
- Advise patient to report onset of black, tarry stools; diarrhea; abdominal pain; or persistent headache to health care professional promptly.

Evaluation/Desired Outcomes
- Decrease in abdominal pain or prevention of gastric irritation and bleeding. Healing of duodenal ulcers can be seen on x-ray examination or endoscopy.
- Decrease in symptoms of GERD and erosive esophagitis. Therapy is continued for 4–8 wk after initial episode.

---

ondansetron (on-dan-se-tron)
Zofran, Zofran ODT

Classification
Therapeutic: antiemetics
Pharmacologic: 5-HT₃ antagonists

Pregnancy Category B

Indications
Prevention of nausea and vomiting associated with chemotherapy or radiation therapy. **IM, IV:** Pre-

ondansetron

vention and treatment of postoperative nausea and vomiting.

Action
Blocks the effects of serotonin at $5\text{-}HT_3$–receptor sites (selective antagonist) located in vagal nerve terminals and the chemoreceptor trigger zone in the CNS. **Therapeutic Effects:** Decreased incidence and severity of nausea and vomiting following chemotherapy or surgery.

Pharmacokinetics
Absorption: IV administration results in complete bioavailability; 100% absorbed following oral administration.
Distribution: Unknown.
Metabolism and Excretion: Extensively metabolized by the liver; 5% excreted unchanged by the kidneys.
Half-life: *Adults:* 3.5–5.5 hr; *Children 5 mo–12 yrs:* 2.9 hr.

TIME/ACTION PROFILE (antiemetic effect)

ROUTE	ONSET	PEAK	DURATION
PO, IV	rapid	15–30 min	4 hr–8 hr
IM	rapid	40 min	unknown

Contraindications/Precautions
Contraindicated in: Hypersensitivity; Orally disintegrating tablets contain aspartame and should not be used in patients with phenylketonuria.
Use Cautiously in: Liver impairment (daily dose not to exceed 8 mg); Abdominal surgery (may mask ileus); OB, Lactation, Pedi: Pregnancy, lactation, or children ≤3 yr (safety not established).

Adverse Reactions/Side Effects
CNS: headache, dizziness, drowsiness, fatigue, weakness. **GI:** constipation, diarrhea, abdominal pain, dry mouth, ↑ liver enzymes. **Neuro:** extrapyramidal reactions.

Interactions
Drug-Drug: May be affected by **drugs altering the activity of liver enzymes**.

Route/Dosage
PO (Adults and Children >11 yr): *Prevention of chemotherapy-induced nausea/vomiting*—8 mg 30 min prior to chemotherapy and repeated 8 hr later; 8 mg q 12 hr may be given for 1–2 days following chemotherapy. *Prevention of radiation-induced nausea/vomiting*—8 mg 1–2 hr prior to radiation; may be repeated q 8 hr, depending on type, location, and extent of radiation. *Prevention of postoperative nausea/vomiting*—16 mg 1 hr before induction of anesthesia.
PO (Children 4–11 yr): *Prevention of chemotherapy-induced nausea/vomiting*—4 mg 30 min prior to chemotherapy and repeated 4 and 8 hr later; 4 mg q 8 hr may be given for 1–2 days following chemotherapy.
IV (Adults): *Prevention of chemotherapy-induced nausea/vomiting*—0.15 mg/kg 15–30 min prior to chemotherapy, repeated 4 and 8 hr later, or 32-mg single dose 30 min prior to chemotherapy (lower doses have been used).
IM, IV (Adults): *Prevention of postoperative nausea/vomiting*—4 mg before induction of anesthesia or postoperatively.
IV (Children 6 mo–18 yr): *Prevention of chemotherapy-induced nausea/vomiting*—0.15 mg/kg 15–30 min prior to chemotherapy, repeated 4 and 8 hr later.
IV (Children 2–12 yr and ≤40 kg): *Prevention of postoperative nausea/vomiting*—0.1 mg/kg.
IV (Children >40 kg): *Prevention of postoperative nausea/vomiting*—4 mg.

Hepatic Impairment
PO, IM, IV (Adults): Not to exceed 8 mg/day.

Availability (generic available)
Orally disintegrating tablets (contain aspartame) (strawberry flavor): 4 mg, 8 mg. **Cost:** *Generic*—4 mg $549.00/30. **Tablets:** 4 mg, 8 mg, 24 mg. **Cost:** *Generic*—4 mg $569.99/30, 8 mg $1,048.95/30. **Oral solution (strawberry flavor):** 4 mg/5 mL. **Solution for injection:** 2 mg/mL. **Premixed infusion:** 32 mg/50 mL D5W.

NURSING IMPLICATIONS

Assessment
- Assess patient for nausea, vomiting, abdominal distention, and bowel sounds prior to and following administration.
- Assess patient for extrapyramidal effects (involuntary movements, facial grimacing, rigidity, shuffling walk, trembling of hands) periodically during therapy.
- *Lab Test Considerations:* May cause transient ↑ in serum bilirubin, AST, and ALT levels.

Potential Nursing Diagnoses
Imbalanced nutrition: less than body requirements (Indications)
Diarrhea (Side Effects)
Constipation (Side Effects)

Implementation
- Do not confuse Zofran (ondansetron) with Zosyn (piperacillin/tazobactam).
- First dose is administered prior to emetogenic event.

- **PO:** For orally disintegrating tablets, do not attempt to push through foil backing; with dry hands, peel back backing and remove tablet. Immediately place tablet on tongue; tablet will dissolve in seconds, then swallow with saliva. Administration of liquid is not necessary.

IV Administration

- **Direct IV:** Administer undiluted (2 mg/mL) immediately before induction of anesthesia or postoperatively if nausea and vomiting occur shortly after surgery. *Rate:* Administer over at least 30 sec and preferably over 2–5 min.
- **Intermittent Infusion:** *Diluent:* Dilute doses for prevention of nausea and vomiting associated with chemotherapy in 50 mL of D5W, 0.9% NaCl, D5/0.9% NaCl, D5/0.45% NaCl. Solution is clear and colorless. Stable for 7 days at room temperature following dilution. *Concentration:* 1 mg/mL. *Rate:* Administer each dose over 15 min.
- **Syringe Compatibility:** alfentanil, atropine, fentanyl, glycopyrrolate, meperidine, metoclopramide, midazolam, morphine, naloxone, neostigmine, propofol.
- **Syringe Incompatibility:** droperidol.
- **Y-Site Compatibility:** aldesleukin, amifostine, amikacin, azithromycin, aztreonam, bleomycin, carboplatin, carmustine, cefazolin, cefotaxime, cefoxitin, ceftazidime, ceftizoxime, cefuroxime, chlorpromazine, cimetidine, cisatracurium, cisplatin, cladribine, clindamycin, cyclophosphamide, cytarabine, dacarbazine, dactinomycin, daunorubicin, dexamethasone sodium phosphate, dexmedetomidine, diphenhydramine, docetaxel, dopamine, doxorubicin, doxorubicin liposome, doxycycline, droperidol, etoposide, etoposide phosphate, famotidine, fenoldopam, filgrastim, floxuridine, fluconazole, fludarabine, gemcitabine, gentamicin, haloperidol, heparin, hydrocortisone sodium succinate, hydrocortisone sodium phosphate, hydromorphone, ifosfamide, imipenem/cilastatin, linezolid, magnesium sulfate, mannitol, mechlorethamine, melphalan, meperidine, mesna, methotrexate, metoclopramide, mitomycin, mitoxantrone, morphine, oxaliplatin, paclitaxel, pentostatin, piperacillin/tazobactam, potassium chloride, promethazine, prochlorperazine edisylate, ranitidine, remifentanil, sodium acetate, streptozocin, teniposide, thiotepa, ticarcillin/clavulanate, topotecan, vancomycin, vinblastine, vincristine, vinorelbine, zidovudine.
- **Y-Site Incompatibility:** acyclovir, allopurinol, aminophylline, amphotericin B, amphotericin B cholesteryl sulfate, ampicillin, ampicillin/sulbactam, amsacrine, cefepime, cefoperazone, furosemide, ganciclovir, lansoprazole, lorazepam, methylprednisolone sodium succinate, pemetrexed, sargramostim, sodium bicarbonate.

Patient/Family Teaching

- Instruct patient to take ondansetron as directed.
- Advise patient to notify health care professional immediately if involuntary movement of eyes, face, or limbs occurs.

Evaluation/Desired Outcomes

- Prevention of nausea and vomiting associated with initial and repeat courses of emetogenic cancer chemotherapy.
- Prevention of postoperative nausea and vomiting.
- Prevention of nausea and vomiting due to radiation therapy.

---

oprelvekin (o-**prell**-ve-kin)
Neumega

Classification
Therapeutic: colony-stimulating factors
Pharmacologic: interleukins, thrombopoetic growth factors

Pregnancy Category C

Indications

Prevention of severe thrombocytopenia and reduction of the need for platelet transfusions following myelosuppressive chemotherapy in patients with nonmyeloid malignancies at risk for thrombocytopenia.

Action

Stimulates production of megakaryocytes and platelets. **Therapeutic Effects:** Increased platelet count.

Pharmacokinetics

Absorption: >80% absorbed following subcut administration.
Distribution: Unknown.
Metabolism and Excretion: Appears to be mostly metabolized, with metabolites eliminated by kidneys.
Half-life: 6.9 hr.

orlistat

TIME/ACTION PROFILE (↑ in platelet count)

ROUTE	ONSET	PEAK	DURATION
Subcut	5–9 days	unknown	7–14 days†

†Counts continue to rise for 7 days following discontinuation and then return to baseline by 14 days

Contraindications/Precautions
Contraindicated in: Hypersensitivity; Lactation: Lactation.
Use Cautiously in: Any condition in which sodium and water retention would pose problems (CHF, renal disease); Pre-existing pericardial effusion or ascites (may be exacerbated); History of atrial arrhythmias (especially if receiving cardiac medications or previous doxorubicin therapy); Pre-existing papilledema or tumors of the CNS; OB, Pedi: Safety not established.

Adverse Reactions/Side Effects
These effects occurred in patients who had recently received myelosuppressive chemotherapy. **CNS:** dizziness, headache, insomnia, nervousness, weakness. **EENT:** conjunctival hemorrhage, blurred vision, changes in visual acuity, blindness, papilledema, pharyngitis, rhinitis. **Resp:** cough, dyspnea, pleural effusions. **CV:** VENTRICULAR ARRHYTHMIAS, atrial fibrillation, edema, palpitations, syncope, tachycardia, vasodilation, ventricular arrhythmias. **GI:** anorexia, constipation, diarrhea, dyspepsia, mucositis, nausea, oral moniliasis, vomiting, abdominal pain. **Derm:** alopecia, ecchymoses, rash. **F and E:** sodium and water retention. **Local:** injection site reactions. **MS:** bone pain, myalgia. **Misc:** chills, fever, infection, pain.

Interactions
Drug-Drug: None significant.

Route/Dosage
Subcut (Adults): 50 mcg/kg once daily for 10–21 days.

Availability
Powder for injection: 5 mg/vial.

NURSING IMPLICATIONS
Assessment
- Assess patient for signs of fluid retention (dyspnea on exertion, peripheral edema) during therapy. Fluid retention is a common side effect that usually resolves within several days following discontinuation of oprelvekin.
- *Lab Test Considerations:* Monitor platelet count prior to and periodically during therapy, especially at expected nadir. Therapy is continued until postnadir platelet count is ≥50,000 cells/mL.
- CBC should be monitored prior to and at regular intervals during therapy. Decrease in hemoglobin concentration, hematocrit, and RBC count may occur because of increased plasma volume (dilutional anemia); usually begins within 3–5 days of therapy and is reversible within a week of discontinuation of therapy.
- Monitor electrolyte concentrations in patients receiving chronic diuretic therapy. Hypokalemia may be fatal.
- May cause an ↑ in plasma fibrinogen.

Potential Nursing Diagnoses
Excess fluid volume (Side Effects)

Implementation
- Therapy should be started within 6–24 hr after completion of chemotherapy and continued for 10–21 days.
- Treatment should be discontinued at least 2 days prior to next planned chemotherapy cycle.
- **Subcut:** Reconstitute with 1 mL of sterile water for injection without preservatives for a concentration of 5 mg/mL. Direct diluent to sides of vial and swirl gently. Solution is clear and colorless. Do not administer solutions that are discolored or contain particulate matter. Do not shake or agitate vigorously. Do not freeze. Do not reuse vials. Administer within 3 hr of reconstitution as a single injection in abdomen, hip, thigh, or upper arm.

Patient/Family Teaching
- Instruct patient in proper technique for preparation and administration of medication. Provide a puncture-resistant container for disposal of needles.
- May cause transient blurred vision or dizziness. Caution patient to avoid driving or other activities requiring alertness until response to medication is known.
- Advise patient to notify health care professional if pregnancy is planned or suspected.
- Inform patient of side effects and advise patient to notify health care professional if chest pain, shortness of breath, fatigue, blurred vision, or irregular heartbeat persists.

Evaluation/Desired Outcomes
- Increase in postnadir platelet count to ≥50,000 cells/mL.

orlistat (or-li-stat)
Alli, Xenical

orlistat

Classification
Therapeutic: weight control agents
Pharmacologic: lipase inhibitors

Pregnancy Category B

Indications
Obesity management (weight loss and maintenance) when used in conjunction with a reduced-calorie diet in patients with an initial BMI ≥ 30 kg/m^2 or ≥ 27 kg/m^2 in the presence of additional risk factors (diabetes, hypertension, hyperlipidemia). Reduces the risk of weight regain after prior loss. May delay onset of type 2 diabetes in prediabetic patients.

Action
Decreases the absorption of dietary fat by reversibly inhibiting enzymes (lipases), which are necessary for the breakdown and subsequent absorption of fat. **Therapeutic Effects:** Weight loss and maintenance in obese patients. Delayed onset of type 2 diabetes.

Pharmacokinetics
Absorption: Minimal systemic absorption.
Distribution: Action is local, within the GI tract.
Protein Binding: Minimally absorbed drug is >99% bound to plasma proteins.
Metabolism and Excretion: Major route is fecal elimination of unabsorbed drug.
Half-life: 1–2 hr.

TIME/ACTION PROFILE (effects on fecal fat)

ROUTE	ONSET	PEAK	DURATION
PO	24–48 hr	unknown	48–72 hr†

†Following discontinuation

Contraindications/Precautions
Contraindicated in: Hypersensitivity; Chronic malabsorption syndrome or cholestasis; OB, Lactation: Effects of orlistat on developing fetus or breastfeeding infant are unknown.
Use Cautiously in: Pedi: Safety not established for children < 12.

Adverse Reactions/Side Effects
With initial use; incidence decreases with prolonged use.
GI: HEPATOTOXICITY, fecal urgency, flatus with discharge, increased defecation, oily evacuation, oily spotting, fecal incontinence.

Interactions
Drug-Drug: ↓ absorption of some **fat-soluble vitamins**, **beta-carotene**, and **levothyroxine** (separate orlistat and levothyroxine by ≥ 4 hr).

Route/Dosage
PO (Adults and adolescents ≥ 12 yr): 60–120 mg 3 times daily with each meal containing fat.

Availability
Capsules: 60 mg^{OTC}, 120 mg.

NURSING IMPLICATIONS

Assessment
- Monitor patients for weight loss and adjust concurrent medications (antihypertensives, antidiabetics, lipid-lowering agents) as needed.

Potential Nursing Diagnoses
Disturbed body image (Indications)
Imbalanced nutrition: more than body requirements (Indications)

Implementation
- **PO:** Administer one capsule 3 times daily with or up to 1 hour after a meal. If a meal is missed or contains no fat, dose of orlistat can be omitted.
- A supplemental multivitamin containing vitamins A, D, E, K, and beta-carotene should be taken daily, at least 2 hr before or after orlistat dose.
- Psyllium 6 g with each dose or 12 g at bedtime may decrease GI side effects.

Patient/Family Teaching
- Instruct patient to take orlistat with meals as directed. If a meal is missed or contains no fat, orlistat dose can be omitted. Do not take more than recommended dose; does not improve benefit.
- Instruct patient to adhere to a reduced-calorie diet. Daily intake of fat should be distributed over three main meals. Meals should contain no more than 30% fat. Taking orlistat with a meal high in fat may increase the GI side effects.
- Advise patient that regular physical activity, approved by a health care professional, should be used in conjunction with orlistat and diet.
- Inform patient of common GI side effects (oily spotting, gas with discharge, urgent need to go to the bathroom, oily or fatty stools, an oily discharge, increased number of bowel movements, inability to control bowel movements). Oil in bowel movement may be clear or have orange or brown colorations. GI side effects usually occur in first weeks of treatment and are more increased following a meal high in

fat. May lessen or disappear, or may continue for 6 mo or longer.
- Advise patient to notify health care professional if signs and symptoms of hepatotoxicity (weakness, fatigue, fever, jaundice, brown urine, abdominal pain, nausea, vomiting, light-colored stools, itching, loss of appetite) occur.
- Advise patient to notify health care professional prior to taking other Rx, OTC, or herbal products.
- Advise patient to notify health care professional if pregnancy is planned or suspected.

Evaluation/Desired Outcomes
- Slow, consistent weight loss when combined with a reduced-calorie diet.
- Delayed onset of type 2 diabetes.

---

oseltamivir (o-sel-tam-i-vir)
Tamiflu

Classification
Therapeutic: antivirals
Pharmacologic: neuramidase inhibitors

Pregnancy Category C

Indications
Treatment of uncomplicated acute illness due to influenza infection in adults and children ≥1 yr who have had symptoms for ≤2 days. Prevention of influenza in patients ≥1 yr.

Action
Inhibits the enzyme neuraminidase, which may alter virus particle aggregation and release. **Therapeutic Effects:** Reduced duration or prevention of flu-related symptoms.

Pharmacokinetics
Absorption: Rapidly absorbed from the GI tract and converted by the liver to the active form, oseltamivir carboxylate. 75% reaches systemic circulation as the active drug.
Distribution: Unknown.
Metabolism and Excretion: Rapidly metabolized by the liver to oseltamivir carboxylate, the active drug. >99% excreted unchanged in urine.
Half-life: Oseltamivir carboxylate—6–10 hr.

TIME/ACTION PROFILE (blood levels)

ROUTE	ONSET	PEAK	DURATION
PO	unknown	unknown	12 hr

Contraindications/Precautions
Contraindicated in: Hypersensitivity; Pedi: Children <1 yr.

Use Cautiously in: Pedi: Children ≥1 yr (may be at ↑ risk for neuropsychiatric events); OB, Lactation: Safety not established; use only if potential benefits outweigh possible risks.

Adverse Reactions/Side Effects
CNS: SEIZURES, abnormal behavior, agitation, confusion, delirium, hallucinations, insomnia, nightmares, vertigo. **Resp:** bronchitis. **GI:** nausea, vomiting.

Interactions
Drug-Drug: None significant.

Route/Dosage
Treatment of Influenza
PO (Adults and Children > 40kg): 75 mg twice daily for 5 days.
PO (Children 23–40 kg): 60 mg twice daily.
PO (Children 15–23 kg): 45 mg twice daily.
PO (Children ≤ 15 kg and ≥ 1 yr): 30 mg twice daily.

Renal Impairment
PO (Adults): *CCr < 30 mL/min*—75 mg once daily for 5 days.

Influenza Prevention
PO (Adults and Children ≥ 13 yrs): 75 mg once daily for at least 10 days.
PO (Children >40 kg): 75 mg once daily for 10 days.
PO (Children 23–40 kg): 60 mg once daily for 10 days.
PO (Children 15–23 kg): 45 mg once daily for 10 days.
PO (Children ≤15 kg and ≥1 yr): 30 mg once daily.

Renal Impairment
PO (Adults and Children ≥ 13 yrs): *CCr 10–30 mL/min*—75 mg every other day *or* 30 mg every day.

Availability
Capsules: 30 mg, 45 mg, 75 mg. **Cost:** 75 mg $84.99/10. **Oral suspension (tutti-frutti flavor):** 12 mg/mL.

NURSING IMPLICATIONS

Assessment
- Monitor influenza symptoms (sudden onset of fever, cough, headache, fatigue, muscular weakness, sore throat). Additional supportive treatment may be indicated to treat symptoms.

Potential Nursing Diagnoses
Risk for infection (Indications)

Implementation
- Treatment with oseltamivir should be started as soon as possible from the first sign of flu symptoms.
- Consider available information on influenza drug susceptibility patterns and treatment effects before using oseltamivir for prophylaxis.
- **PO:** May be administered with food or milk to minimize GI irritation.
- To prepare oral solution, tap closed bottle to loosen powder. Add total amount of water for constitution and shake closed bottle for 15 seconds. Remove childproof cap and push bottle adaptor into neck of bottle. Close bottle with childproof top tightly, assuring proper seating of bottle adaptor and childproof status. Shake well before use. Use within 10 days of constitution. If oral suspension is not available, capsules can be opened and mixed with sweetened liquids, such as regular or sugar-free chocolate syrup.
- Dosing errors have occurred due to oseltamivir dosing in mg and solution in mL. Make sure units of measure on prescription instructions match dosing device provided with the drug.

Patient/Family Teaching
- Instruct patient to take oseltamivir as soon as influenza symptoms appear and to continue to take it as directed, for the full course of therapy, even if feeling better. Take missed doses as soon as remembered unless within 2 hr of next dose. Do not double doses.
- Caution patient that oseltamivir should not be shared with anyone, even if they have the same symptoms.
- Advise patient that oseltamivir is not a substitute for a flu shot. Patients should receive annual flu shot according to immunization guidelines.
- Advise patients to report behavioral changes (hallucinations, delirium, and abnormal behavior) to health care professional immediately.
- Advise patient to consult health care professional before taking other medications concurrently with oseltamivir.

Evaluation/Desired Outcomes
- Reduced duration or prevention of flu-related symptoms.

---

oxacillin, See PENICILLINS, PENICILLINASE RESISTANT.

---

oxaliplatin (ox-a-li-pla-tin)
Eloxatin

Classification
Therapeutic: antineoplastics
Pharmacologic: alkylating agents

Pregnancy Category D

Indications
Used in combination with 5–fluorouracil and leucovorin in the treatment of advanced or metastatic colon or rectal cancer. **Unlabeled Use:** Treatment of ovarian cancer that has progressed despite treatment with other agents.

Action
Inhibits DNA replication and transcription by incorporating platinum into normal cross-linking (cell-cycle nonspecific). **Therapeutic Effects:** Death of rapidly replicating cells, particularly malignant ones.

Pharmacokinetics
Absorption: IV administration results in complete bioavailability.
Distribution: Extensive tissue distribution.
Protein Binding: >90% (platinum).
Metabolism and Excretion: Undergoes rapid and extensive nonenzymatic biotransformation; excreted mostly by the kidneys.
Half-life: 391 hours.

TIME/ACTION PROFILE

ROUTE	ONSET	PEAK	DURATION
IV	unknown	unknown	unknown

Contraindications/Precautions
Contraindicated in: Hypersensitivity; Hypersensitivity to other platinum compounds; OB, Lactation: Pregnancy or lactation.
Use Cautiously in: Renal impairment; Geri: ↑ risk of adverse reactions; Pedi: Safety not established.

Adverse Reactions/Side Effects
Adverse reactions are noted for the combination of oxaliplatin, 5–FU and leucovorin.
CNS: fatigue. **CV:** chest pain, edema, thromboembolism. **EENT:** visual abnormalities. **Resp:** PULMONARY FIBROSIS, coughing, dyspnea. **GI:** diar-

rhea, nausea, vomiting, abdominal pain, anorexia, gastroesophageal reflux, stomatitis. **F and E:** dehydration, hypokalemia. **Hemat:** leukopenia, NEUTROPENIA, THROMBOCYTOPENIA, anemia. **Local:** injection site reactions. **MS:** back pain. **Neuro:** neurotoxicity. **Misc:** ANAPHYLAXIS/ANAPHYLACTOID REACTIONS, fever.

Interactions
Drug-Drug: Concurrent use of **nephrotoxic agents** may ↑ toxicity.

Route/Dosage
IV (Adults): *Day 1* — 85 mg/m^2 with leucovorin 200 mg/m^2 at the same time over 2 hr, followed by 5–fluorouracil 400 mg/m^2 bolus over 2–4 min, then 5–fluorouracil 600 mg/m^2 as a 22 hr infusion. *Day 2* — leucovorin 200 mg/m^2 over 2 hr, followed by 5–fluorouracil 400 mg/m^2 bolus over 2–4 min, then 5–fluorouracil 600 mg/m^2 as a 22 hr infusion. Cycle is repeated every 2 wk. Dosage reduction/alteration may be required for neurotoxicity or other serious adverse effects.

Availability (generic available)
Solution for injection: 5 mg/mL.

NURSING IMPLICATIONS

Assessment
- Assess for peripheral sensory neuropathy. *Acute onset* occurs within hr to 1–2 days of dosing, resolves within 14 days, and frequently recurs with further dosing (transient paresthesia, dysesthesia and hypothesia of hands, feet, perioral area, or throat). Symptoms may be precipitated or exacerbated by exposure to cold or cold objects. May also cause jaw spasm, abnormal tongue sensation, dysarthria, eye pain, and a feeling of chest pressure. *Persistent* (>14 days) causes paresthesias, dysesthesias, and hypoesthesias, but may also include deficits in proprioception that may interfere with daily activities (walking, writing, swallowing). Persistent neuropathy may occur without prior acute neuropathy and may improve upon discontinuation of oxaliplatin.
- Assess for signs of pulmonary fibrosis (nonproductive cough, dyspnea, crackles, radiological; infiltrates). May be fatal. Discontinue oxaliplatin if pulmonary fibrosis occurs.
- Monitor for signs of anaphylaxis (rash, hives, swelling or lips or tongue, sudden cough). Epinephrine, corticosteroids, and antihistamines should be readily available.
- *Lab Test Considerations:* Monitor WBC with differential, hemoglobin, platelet count, and blood chemistries (ALT, AST, bilirubin, and creatinine) before each oxaliplatin cycle.

Potential Nursing Diagnoses
Nausea (Adverse Reactions)

Implementation
- Extravasation may result in local pain and inflammation that may be severe and lead to necrosis.
- Premedicate patient with antiemetics with or without dexamethasone. Prehydration is not required.

IV Administration
- **Intermittent Infusion:** Protect concentrated solution from light; do not freeze. *Diluent:* Must be further diluted with 250–500 mL of D5W. **Do not use 0.9% NaCl or any other chloride-containing solution for final solution.** Do not use aluminum needles or administration sets containing aluminum parts; aluminum may cause degradation of platinum compounds. May be stored in refrigerator for 24 hr or 6 hr at room temperature. Diluted solution is not light-sensitive. Do not administer solutions that are discolored or contain particulate matter. *Concentration:* 0.2–0.6 mg/mL. *Rate:* Administer oxaliplatin simultaneously with leucovorin in separate bags via Y-line over 120 min. Prolonging infusion time to 6 hr may decrease acute toxicities. Infusion times for fluorouracil and leucovorin do not need to change.
- **Y-Site Compatibility:** alfentanil, amifostine, amikacin, aminocaproic acid, amiodarone, amphotericin B colloid, amphotericin B liposome, ampicillin, ampicillin/sulbactam, anidulafungin, atracurium, azithromycin, aztreonam, bivalirudin, bleomycin, bumetanide, buprenorphine, butorphanol, calcium chloride, calcium gluconate, carboplatin, caspofungin, cefotetan, cefoxitin, ceftazidime, ceftizoxime, ceftriaxone, cefuroxime, chloramphenicol, cimetidine, ciprofloxacin, cisatracurium, cisplatin, clindamycin, cyclophosphamide, cyclosporine, cytarabine, dacarbazine, dactinomycin, daptomycin, daunorubicin, dexamethasone sodium phosphate, dexmeditomidine, dexrazoxane, digoxin, diltiazem, diphenhydramine, dobutamine, docetaxel, dolasetron, dopamine, doxacurium, doxorubicin, doxycycline, droperidol, enalaprilat, ephedrine, epinephrine, epirubicin, ertapenem, erythromycin, esmolol, etoposide, etoposide phosphate, famotidine, fenoldopam, fentanyl, fluconazole, fludarabine, foscarnet, fosphenytoin, furosemide, gemcita-

bine, gentamicin, glycopyrrolate, granisetron, haloperidol, heparin, hetastarch, hydralazine, hydrocortisone, hydromorphone, idarubicin, ifosfamide, imipenem/cilastatin, inamrinone, insulin, irinotecan, isoproterenol, ketorolac, labetalol, leucovorin, levofloxacin, levorphanol, lidocaine, linezolid, lorazepam, magnesium sulfate, mannitol, meperidine, meropenem, mesna, metaraminol, methyldopate, methylprednisolone sodium succinate, metoclopramide, metoprolol, metronidazole, midazolam, milrinone, mitoxantrone, morphine, nafcillin, nalbuphine, naloxone, nesiritide, nicardipine, nitroglycerin, nitroprusside, norepinephrine, octreotide, ondansetron, paclitaxel, palonosetron, pancuronium, pemetrexed, pentamidine, pentazocine, phentolamine, phenylephrine, potassium chloride, potassium phosphates, procainamide, prochlorperazine, promethazine, propranolol, quinupristin/dalfopristin, ranitidine, rocuronium, sodium acetate, sodium phosphates, succinylcholine, sufentanil, tacrolimus, teniposide, theophylline, thiotepa, ticarcillin/clavulanate, tigecycline, tirofiban, tobramycin, tolazoline, topotecan, trimethobenzamide, trimethoprim/sulfamethoxazole, vancomycin, vasopressin, vecuronium, verapamil, vinblastine, vincristine, vinorelbine, voriconazole, zidovudine.

- **Y-Site Incompatibility:** cefepime, cefoperazone, dantrolene, diazepam. Alkaline solutions, chloride-containing solutions. Infusion line should be flushed with D5W prior to administration of other solutions or medications.

Patient/Family Teaching

- Inform patients and caregivers of potential for peripheral neuropathy and potentiation by exposure to cold or cold objects. Advise patient to avoid cold drinks, use of ice in drinks or as ice packs, and to cover exposed skin prior to exposure to cold temperature or cold objects. Caution patients to cover themselves with a blanket during infusion, do not breathe deeply when exposed to cold air, wear warm clothing, and cover mouth and nose with a scarf or pull-down ski cap to warm the air that goes to their lungs, do not take things from the freezer or refrigerator without wearing gloves, drink fluids warm or at room temperature, always drink through a straw, do not use ice chips for nausea, be aware that most metals (car doors, mailbox) are cold; wear gloves to touch, do not run air conditioning at high levels in house or car, if hands get cold wash them with warm water. Advise health care professional of how you did since last treatment before next infusion.
- Instruct patient to notify health care professional immediately if signs of low blood cell counts (fever, persistent diarrhea, infection) or if persistent vomiting, signs of dehydration, cough or breathing difficulty, thirst, dry mouth, dizziness, decreased urination or signs of allergic reactions occur.

Evaluation/Desired Outcomes

- Decrease in size and spread of malignancies.

---

oxaprozin (ox-a-**proe**-zin)
Daypro

Classification
Therapeutic: antirheumatics, nonsteroidal anti-inflammatory agents

Pregnancy Category C (first and second trimester), D (third trimester)

Indications
Osteoarthritis. Rheumatoid arthritis. Juvenile rheumatoid arthritis.

Action
Inhibits prostaglandin synthesis. **Therapeutic Effects:** Suppression of pain and inflammation.

Pharmacokinetics
Absorption: Well absorbed following oral administration (80%); 35% is rapidly converted to an active metabolite.
Distribution: Unknown.
Protein Binding: 99.9%.
Metabolism and Excretion: The active metabolite is metabolized by the liver to inactive compounds.
Half-life: 42–50 hr.

TIME/ACTION PROFILE (antirheumatic action)

ROUTE	ONSET	PEAK	DURATION
PO	within 7 days	unknown	unknown

Contraindications/Precautions
Contraindicated in: Hypersensitivity; Cross-sensitivity may exist with other NSAIDs, including aspirin; Active GI bleeding or ulcer disease; Peri-operative pain from coronary artery bypass graft (CABG) surgery; Lactation: Lactation.
Use Cautiously in: Cardiovascular disease or risk factors for cardiovascular disease (may ↑

risk of serious cardiovascular thrombotic events, myocardial infarction, and stroke, especially with prolonged use); Severe hepatic disease; Renal impairment (lower initial dose may be necessary); History of ulcer disease; OB: May cause premature closure of the ductus arteriosus; not recommended for use in the second half of pregnancy; Pedi: Children <6 yr (safety not established); Geri: Appears on Beers list; at ↑ risk of GI bleeding; may require ↓ dose due to age-related ↓ in renal function.

Adverse Reactions/Side Effects
CNS: agitation, anxiety, confusion, depression, dizziness, drowsiness, fatigue, headache, insomnia, malaise, weakness. **EENT:** abnormal vision, tinnitus. **Resp:** dyspnea, hypersensitivity pneumonitis. **CV:** edema, vasculitis. **GI:** GI BLEEDING, abdominal pain, diarrhea, dyspepsia, ↑ liver enzymes, anorexia, cholestatic jaundice, constipation, dry mouth, duodenal ulcer, flatulence, gastritis, increased appetite, nausea, stomatitis, vomiting. **GU:** albuminuria, azotemia, interstitial nephritis. **Derm:** EXFOLIATIVE DERMATITIS, STEVENS-JOHNSON SYNDROME, TOXIC EPIDERMAL NECROLYSIS, ↑ sweating, photosensitivity, pruritus, rash. **Hemat:** prolonged bleeding time. **Metab:** weight gain. **Neuro:** paresthesia, tremor. **Misc:** allergic reactions including ANAPHYLAXIS, ANGIONEUROTIC EDEMA.

Interactions
Drug-Drug: ↑ adverse GI effects and toxicity with **aspirin**, other **NSAIDs**, **potassium supplements**, **corticosteroids**, or **alcohol**. Chronic use with **acetaminophen** may ↑ risk of adverse renal reactions. May ↓ effectiveness of **diuretics** or **antihypertensive** therapy. May ↑ hypoglycemic effects of **insulin** or **oral hypoglycemic agents**. ↑ risk of toxicity from **methotrexate**. ↑ risk of bleeding with **cefotetan, cefoperazone, thrombolytic agents, anticoagulants, ticlopidine, clopidogrel, eptifibatide,** or **tirofiban**. ↑ risk of adverse hematologic reactions with **antineoplastics** or **radiation therapy**.
Drug-Natural Products: ↑ anticoagulant effect and bleeding risk with **arnica, chamomile, clove, feverfew, garlic, ginger, ginkgo, Panax ginseng**, and others.

Route/Dosage
Osteoarthritis or Rheumatoid Arthritis
PO (Adults): 1200 mg once daily; onset may be more rapid with an initial 1800-mg dose. Patients with low body weight, mild disease, or renal impairment may be started at 600 mg/day (not to exceed 1800 mg/day or 26 mg/kg/day). Daily doses >1200 mg should be given in 2–3 divided doses. Consideration should be given to decreasing dose to lowest effective amount.

Juvenile Rheumatoid Arthritis
PO (Children 6–16 yr): ≥55 kg-1200 mg once daily; *32–54 kg*-900 mg once daily; *22–31 kg*-600 mg once daily.

Availability (generic available)
Tablets: 600 mg.

NURSING IMPLICATIONS
Assessment
- Patients who have asthma, aspirin-induced allergy, and nasal polyps are at increased risk for developing hypersensitivity reactions. Monitor for rhinitis, asthma, and urticaria.
- Assess pain and range of motion prior to and periodically during therapy.
- **Lab Test Considerations:** May cause prolonged bleeding time, which may persist for up to 2 wk following discontinuation of therapy.
- Evaluate BUN, serum creatinine, CBC, and liver function tests periodically in patients receiving prolonged therapy. Serum potassium, BUN, serum creatinine, alkaline phosphatase, LDH, AST, and ALT tests may show ↑ levels. Blood glucose, hemoglobin, and hematocrit concentrations, leukocyte and platelet counts, and CCr may be ↓.

Potential Nursing Diagnoses
Acute pain (Indications)

Implementation
- Administration in higher than recommended doses does not provide increased effectiveness but may cause increased side effects. Use lowest effective dose for shortest period of time.
- **PO:** Administer with food or antacids to decrease GI irritation.

Patient/Family Teaching
- Advise patient to take oxaprozin with a full glass of water and to remain in an upright position for 15–30 min after administration.
- Instruct patient to take medication as directed. Take missed doses as soon as remembered but not if almost time for the next dose. Do not double doses.
- May cause drowsiness and dizziness. Advise patient to avoid driving or other activities requiring alertness until response to the medication is known.
- Caution patient to avoid the concurrent use of alcohol, aspirin, acetaminophen, and other

oxazepam **961**

OTC or herbal products without consulting health care professional.
- Advise patient to notify health care professional of medication regimen prior to treatment or surgery. Oxaprozin should be discontinued 2 wk prior to surgery.
- Caution patient to use sunscreen and protective clothing to prevent photosensitivity reactions.
- Advise patient to consult health care professional if rash, itching, visual disturbances, tinnitus, weight gain, edema, black stools, persistent headache, or influenza-like syndrome (chills, fever, muscle aches, pain) occurs.

Evaluation/Desired Outcomes
- Decreased pain and improved joint mobility. Maximum effectiveness may require 2 wk or more of continuous therapy. Patients who do not respond to one NSAID may respond to another.

---

oxazepam (ox-az-e-pam)
♣Apo-Oxazepam, ♣Novoxapam, Serax

Classification
Therapeutic: antianxiety agents, sedative/hypnotics
Pharmacologic: benzodiazepines

Schedule IV

Pregnancy Category D

Indications
Management of anxiety, anxiety associated with depression. Symptomatic treatment of alcohol withdrawal.

Action
Depresses the CNS, probably by potentiating GABA, an inhibitory neurotransmitter. **Therapeutic Effects:** Decreased anxiety. Diminished symptoms of alcohol withdrawal.

Pharmacokinetics
Absorption: Well absorbed following oral administration. Absorption is slower than with other benzodiazepines.
Distribution: Widely distributed. Crosses the blood-brain barrier. May cross the placenta and enter breast milk.
Metabolism and Excretion: Metabolized by the liver to inactive compounds.
Protein Binding: 97%.

Half-life: 5–15 hr.

TIME/ACTION PROFILE (sedation)

ROUTE	ONSET	PEAK	DURATION
PO	45–90 min	unknown	6–12 hr

Contraindications/Precautions
Contraindicated in: Hypersensitivity; Cross-sensitivity with other benzodiazepines may exist; Comatose patients or those with pre-existing CNS depression; Uncontrolled severe pain; Angle-closure glaucoma; Some products contain tartrazine and should be avoided in patients with known intolerance; OB, Lactation: Pregnancy or lactation.
Use Cautiously in: Hepatic dysfunction (may be preferred over some benzodiazepines due to short half-life); History of suicide attempt or drug abuse; Debilitated patients (initial dosage ↓ recommended); Severe chronic obstructive pulmonary disease; Myasthenia gravis; Pedi: Children <6 yr (safety not established) for children <6 yr.; Geri: Appears on Beers list (associated with ↑ risk of falls; ↓ dose required); ↑ sensitivity to benzodiazepines.

Adverse Reactions/Side Effects
CNS: <u>dizziness</u>, <u>drowsiness</u>, confusion, hangover, headache, impaired memory, mental depression, paradoxical excitation, slurred speech. **EENT:** blurred vision. **Resp:** respiratory depression. **CV:** tachycardia. **GI:** constipation, diarrhea, drug-induced hepatitis, nausea, vomiting, weight gain (unusual). **GU:** urinary problems. **Derm:** rashes. **Hemat:** leukopenia. **Misc:** physical dependence, psychological dependence, tolerance.

Interactions
Drug-Drug: Additive CNS depression with other CNS depressants, including **alcohol**, **antihistamines**, **antidepressants**, **opioid analgesics**, and other **sedative/hypnotics** (including other **benzodiazepines**). May ↓ the therapeutic effectiveness of **levodopa**. **Hormonal contraceptives** or **phenytoin** may ↓ effectiveness. **Theophylline** may ↓ sedative effects.
Drug-Natural Products: Concomitant use of **kava-kava**, **valerian**, **skullcap**, **chamomile**, or **hops** can ↑ CNS depression.

Route/Dosage
PO (Adults): *Antianxiety agent*—10–30 mg 3–4 times daily. *Sedative/hypnotic/management of alcohol withdrawal*—15–30 mg 3–4 times daily.

♣ = Canadian drug name. 🧬 = Genetic implication.
*CAPITALS indicates life-threatening; <u>underlines</u> indicate most frequent.

PO (Geriatric Patients): 5 mg 1–2 times daily initially or 10 mg 3 times daily; may be ↑ as needed.

Availability (generic available)
Capsules: 10 mg, 15 mg, 30 mg. **Tablets:** ✢ 10 mg, 15 mg, ✢ 30 mg.

NURSING IMPLICATIONS
Assessment
- Assess patient for anxiety and orientation, mood and behavior.
- Assess level of sedation (ataxia, dizziness, slurred speech) periodically throughout therapy.
- Assess regularly for continued need for treatment.
- Prolonged high-dose therapy may lead to psychological or physical dependence. Restrict the amount of drug available to patient.
- Geri: Assess CNS effects and risk of falls. Institute falls prevention strategies.
- **Lab Test Considerations:** Monitor CBC and liver function tests periodically during prolonged therapy.
- May cause decreased thyroidal uptake of sodium iodide ^{123}I and ^{131}I.

Potential Nursing Diagnoses
Anxiety (Indications)
Ineffective coping (Indications)
Risk for injury (Side Effects)

Implementation
- Medication should be tapered at the completion of therapy (taper by 0.5 mg q 3 days). Sudden cessation of medication may lead to withdrawal (insomnia, irritability, nervousness, tremors).
- **PO:** Administer with food if GI irritation becomes a problem.

Patient/Family Teaching
- Instruct patient to take oxazepam exactly as directed. Missed doses should be taken within 1 hr; if remembered later, omit and return to regular dosing schedule. Do not double or increase doses. If dose is less effective after a few weeks, notify health care professional.
- Inform patient that oxazepam is usually prescribed for short-term use. Encourage patient to participate in psychotherapy to address source of anxiety and improve coping skills. Teach other methods to decrease anxiety, such as increased exercise, support group, relaxation techniques.
- Encourage patient to participate in psychotherapy to address source of anxiety and improve coping skills.
- Teach other methods to decrease anxiety, such as increased exercise, support group, relaxation techniques.
- May cause drowsiness or dizziness. Caution patient to avoid driving or other activities requiring alertness until response to medication is known.
- Advise patient to avoid the use of alcohol and to consult health care professional prior to the use of OTC preparations that contain antihistamines or alcohol.
- Advise patient to inform health care professional if pregnancy is planned or suspected.
- Advise patient to notify health care professional of medication regimen prior to treatment or surgery.
- Emphasize the importance of follow-up exams to monitor effectiveness of medication.
- Geri: Instruct patient and family how to reduce falls risk at home.

Evaluation/Desired Outcomes
- Decreased sense of anxiety.
- Increased ability to cope.
- Prevention or relief of acute agitation, tremor, and hallucinations during alcohol withdrawal.

---

oxcarbazepine
(ox-kar-**baz**-e-peen)
Trileptal

Classification
Therapeutic: anticonvulsants
Pharmacologic: carbamazepine analogues

Pregnancy Category C

Indications
Monotherapy or adjunctive therapy of partial seizures in adults and children 4 yr and older with epilepsy. Adjunctive therapy in patients 2–16 yr with epilepsy. **Unlabeled Use:** Management of trigeminal neuralgia.

Action
Blocks sodium channels in neural membranes, stabilizing hyperexcitable states, inhibiting repetitive neuronal firing, and decreasing propagation of synaptic impulses. **Therapeutic Effects:** Decreased incidence of seizures.

Pharmacokinetics
Absorption: Rapidly absorbed after oral administration and rapidly converted to the active 10-hydroxy metabolite (MHD).

Distribution: Enters breast milk in significant amounts.
Metabolism and Excretion: Extensively converted to MHD, which is then primarily excreted by the kidneys.
Half-life: *Oxcarbazepine*—2 hr; *MHD*—9 hr.

TIME/ACTION PROFILE (blood levels)

ROUTE	ONSET	PEAK	DURATION
PO 12 hr	PO	rapid	4.5 hr†

†Steady-state levels of MHD are reached after 2–3 days during twice-daily dosing

Contraindications/Precautions
Contraindicated in: Hypersensitivity; cross-sensitivity with carbamazepine may occur; Lactation: Lactation.
Use Cautiously in: All patients (may ↑ risk of suicidal thoughts/behaviors); Renal impairment (dose ↓ recommended if CCr <30 mL/min); OB: May be teratogenic; use only if potential benefit justifies potential risk to the fetus; Pedi: Children <4 yr (safety not established).

Adverse Reactions/Side Effects
CNS: SUICIDAL THOUGHTS, dizziness/vertigo, drowsiness/fatigue, headache, cognitive symptoms. **EENT:** abnormal vision, diplopia, nystagmus. **GI:** abdominal pain, dyspepsia, nausea, vomiting, thirst. **Derm:** acne, rash, urticaria. **F and E:** hyponatremia. **Neuro:** ataxia, gait disturbances, tremor. **Misc:** allergic reactions, hypersensitivity reactions including STEVENS-JOHNSON SYNDROME and MULTIORGAN REACTIONS, lymphadenopathy.

Interactions
Drug-Drug: May inhibit the CYP 2C19 enzyme system and would be expected to alter the effects of other drugs that are metabolized by this system. Oxcarbazepine and MHD induce the P450 3A4/5 enzyme systems and would be expected to alter the effects of other drugs that are metabolized by this system. This may result in ↓ levels and effectiveness of **hormonal contraceptives, felodipine, isradipine, nicardipine, nifedipine,** and **nimodipine**. In addition, oxcarbazepine itself is metabolized by cytochrome P450 system and other **drugs that alter the activity of this system**. ↑ CNS depression may occur with other CNS depressants, including **alcohol, antihistamines, antidepressants, sedative/hypnotics,** and **opioids**. **Carbamazepine, phenobarbital, phenytoin, valproic acid,** and **verapamil** ↓

levels. May ↑ serum levels and effects of **phenytoin** (dose ↓ of phenytoin may be required).

Route/Dosage
(Tablets and oral suspension can be interchanged at equal doses.)
PO (Adults): *Adjunctive therapy*—300 mg twice daily, may be ↑ by up to 600 mg/day at weekly intervals up to 1200 mg/day (up to 2400 mg/day may be needed); *Conversion to monotherapy*—300 mg twice daily; may be ↑ by 600 mg/day at weekly intervals, whereas other antiepileptic drugs are tapered over 3–6 wk; dose of oxcarbazepine should be ↑ up to 2400 mg/day over a period of 2–4 wk; *Initiation of monotherapy*—300 mg twice daily, ↑ by 300 mg/day every third day, up to 1200 mg/day. Maximum maintenance dose should be achieved over 2–4 wk.

PO (Children 2–16 yr): *Adjunctive therapy*—4–5 mg/kg twice daily (up to 600 mg/day), ↑ over 2 wk to achieve 900 mg/day in patients 20–29 kg, 1200 mg/day in patients 29.1–39 kg and 1800 mg/day in patients >39 kg (range 6–51 mg/kg/day). In patients <20 kg, initial dose of 16–20 mg/kg/day may be used not to exceed 60 mg/kg/day. *Conversion to monotherapy*—8–10 mg/kg/day given twice daily; may be ↑ by 10 mg/kg/day at weekly intervals, whereas other antiepileptic drugs are tapered over 3–6 wk; dose of oxcarbazepine should be ↑ up to 600–900 mg/day in patients ≤20 kg, 900–1200 mg/day in patients 25–30 kg, 900–1500 mg/day in patients 35–40 kg. 1200–1500 mg/day in patients 45 kg, 1200–1800 mg/day in patients 50–55 kg, 1200–2100 mg/day in patients 60–65 kg, and 1500–2100 mg/day in patients 70 kg. Maximum maintenance dose should be achieved over 2–4 wk.

Renal Impairment
PO (Adults): *CCr <30 mL/min*—Initiate therapy at 300 mg/day and ↑ slowly to achieve desired response.

Availability (generic available)
Tablets: 150 mg, 300 mg, 600 mg. **Cost:** *Generic*—150 mg $53.79/100, 300 mg $375.97/180, 600 mg $742.97/180, 150 mg $96.21/100, 300 mg $175.70/100, 600 mg $322.94/100. **Oral suspension:** 300 mg/5 mL. **Cost:** $155.23/250 mL.

✱ = Canadian drug name. ≡ = Genetic implication.
*CAPITALS indicates life-threatening; underlines indicate most frequent.

NURSING IMPLICATIONS
Assessment
- Monitor closely for notable changes in behavior that could indicate the emergence or worsening of suicidal thoughts or behavior or depression.
- **Seizures:** Assess frequency, location, duration, and characteristics of seizure activity. Hyponatremia may increase frequency and severity of seizures.
- Monitor patient for CNS changes. May manifest as cognitive symptoms (psychomotor slowing, difficulty with concentration, speech or language problems), somnolence or fatigue, or coordination abnormalities (ataxia, gait disturbances).
- *Lab Test Considerations:* Monitor ECG and serum electrolytes before and periodically during therapy. May cause hyponatremia. Usually occurs during the first 3 mo of therapy. May require dose reduction, fluid restriction, or discontinuation of therapy. Sodium levels return to normal within a few days of discontinuation.

Potential Nursing Diagnoses
Risk for injury (Indications, Side Effects)

Implementation
- Implement seizure precautions as indicated.
- **PO:** Administer twice daily with or without food.
- Shake oral suspension well and prepare dose immediately after. Withdraw using oral dosing syringe supplied by manufacturer. May be mixed in a small glass of water just prior to administration or swallowed directly from syringe. Rinse syringe with warm water and allow to dry.

Patient/Family Teaching
- Instruct patient to take oxcarbazepine in equally spaced doses, as directed. Take missed doses as soon as possible but not just before next dose; do not double dose. Notify health care professional if more than 1 dose is missed. Medication should be gradually discontinued to prevent seizures. Instruct patient to read the *Medication Guide* before starting and with each Rx refill, changes may occur.
- May cause dizziness, drowsiness, or CNS changes. Advise patients to avoid driving or other activities requiring alertness until response to medication is known. Do not resume driving until physician gives clearance based on control of seizure disorder.
- Advise patient not to take alcohol or other CNS depressants concurrently with this medication.
- Advise patient and family to notify health care professional if thoughts about suicide or dying, attempts to commit suicide; new or worse depression; new or worse anxiety; feeling very agitated or restless; panic attacks; trouble sleeping; new or worse irritability; acting aggressive; being angry or violent; acting on dangerous impulses; an extreme increase in activity and talking, other unusual changes in behavior or mood occur.
- Advise female patients to use an additional nonhormonal method of contraception during therapy and until next menstrual period. Instruct patient to notify health care professional if pregnancy is planned or suspected.
- Instruct patient to notify health care professional of medication regimen before treatment or surgery.
- Advise patients to carry identification describing disease and medication regimen at all times.

Evaluation/Desired Outcomes
- Absence or reduction of seizure activity.

---

oxiconazole, See ANTIFUNGALS (TOPICAL).

OXYBUTYNIN (ox-i-byoo-ti-nin)
oxybutynin (oral)
Ditropan, Ditropan XL

oxybutynin (gel)
Gelnique

oxybutynin (transdermal system)
Oxytrol

Classification
Therapeutic: urinary tract antispasmodics
Pharmacologic: anticholinergics

Pregnancy Category B

Indications
Urinary symptoms that may be associated with neurogenic bladder including: Frequent urination, Urgency, Nocturia, Urge incontinence. Overactive bladder with symptoms of urge incontinence, urgency, and frequency.

Action
Inhibits the action of acetylcholine at postganglionic receptors. Has direct spasmolytic action on smooth muscle, including smooth muscle lining the GU tract, without affecting vascular smooth

OXYBUTYNIN

muscle. **Therapeutic Effects:** Increased bladder capacity. Delayed desire to void. Decreased urge incontinence, urinary urgency, and frequency and decreased number of urinary accidents associated with overactive bladder.

Pharmacokinetics
Absorption: Rapidly absorbed following oral administration, but undergoes extensive first-pass metabolism; XL tablets provide extended release. Transdermal absorption occurs by passive diffusion through intact skin and bypasses the first-pass effect.
Distribution: Widely distributed.
Metabolism and Excretion: Extensively metabolized by the liver (CYP3A4 enzyme system); one metabolite is pharmacologically active; metabolites are renally excreted with negligible (<0.1%) excretion of unchanged drug.
Half-life: 7–8 hr (oral and patch); 64 hr (gel).

TIME/ACTION PROFILE (urinary spasmolytic effect)

ROUTE	ONSET	PEAK	DURATION
PO	30–60 min	3–6 hr	6–10 hr (up to 24 hr with XL tablet)
TD-patch	within 24 hr	36 hr	3–4 days
TD-gel	unknown	unknown	24 hr

Contraindications/Precautions
Contraindicated in: Hypersensitivity; Uncontrolled angle-closure glaucoma; Intestinal obstruction or atony; Urinary retention.
Use Cautiously in: Hepatic/renal impairment; Bladder outflow obstruction; Ulcerative colitis; Benign prostatic hyperplasia; Cardiovascular disease; Reflux esophagitis or gastrointestinal obstructive disorders; Patients with dementia receiving acetylcholinesterase inhibitors; Myasthenia gravis; OB, Lactation: Pregnancy or lactation; Pedi: Oral: Safety not established in children <5 yr; Patch and gel: Safety not established in children <18 yr; Geri: Appears on Beers list. Poorly tolerated due to anticholinergic effects. Initiate treatment at lower doses.

Adverse Reactions/Side Effects
CNS: dizziness, drowsiness, agitation, confusion, hallucinations, headache. **EENT:** blurred vision. **CV:** tachycardia. **GI:** constipation, dry mouth, nausea, abdominal pain, diarrhea. **GU:** urinary retention. **Derm:** ↓ sweating, *transdermal only:* application site reactions, pruritus. **Metab:** hyperthermia.

Interactions
Drug-Drug: ↑ anticholinergic effects with other **agents having anticholinergic properties**, including **amantadine, antidepressants, phenothiazines, disopyramide,** and **haloperidol**. Additive CNS depression with other **CNS depressants**, including **alcohol, antihistamines, antidepressants, opioids,** and **sedative/hypnotics. Ketoconazole, itraconazole, erythromycin,** and **clarithromycin** may ↑ effects.

Route/Dosage
PO (Adults): *Immediate-release tablets*—5 mg 2–3 times daily (not to exceed 5 mg 4 times daily) (may start with 2.5 mg 2–3 times daily in elderly). *Extended-release tablets*—5–10 mg once daily; may ↑, as needed, (in 5-mg increments) up to maximum dose of 30 mg/day.
PO (Children >5 yr): *Immediate-release tablets*—5 mg 2–3 times daily (not to exceed 15 mg/day). *Extended-release tablets (children ≥6 yr)*—5 mg once daily; may ↑, as needed, (in 5-mg increments) up to maximum dose of 20 mg/day.
PO (Children 1–5 yr): 0.2 mg/kg/dose 2–3 times daily.
Transdermal (Adults): *Patch*—Apply one 3.9 mg system twice weekly (every 3–4 days); *Gel*—Apply contents of one sachet (100 mg/g) once daily.

Availability (generic available)
Tablets: 5 mg. **Cost:** *Generic*—$29.97/180. **Extended-release tablets:** 5 mg, 10 mg, 15 mg. **Cost:** *Generic*—5 mg $260.98/90, 10 mg $262.80/90, 15 mg $269.99/90. **Syrup:** 5 mg/5 mL. **Cost:** *Generic*—$35.95/480 mL. **Gel:** 1 g unit dose (sachet) contains 100 mg/g (10%).
Transdermal system: 3.9 mg/day system. **Cost:** $106.50/8 patches.

NURSING IMPLICATIONS

Assessment
- Monitor voiding pattern and intake and output ratios, and assess abdomen for bladder distention prior to and periodically during therapy. Catheterization may be used to assess postvoid residual. Cystometry is usually performed to diagnose type of bladder dysfunction prior to prescription of oxybutynin.
- Geri: Assess geriatric patients for anticholinergic effects (sedation and weakness).

Potential Nursing Diagnoses
Impaired urinary elimination (Indications)
Acute pain (Indications)

Implementation
- Do not confuse Ditropan (oxybutynin) with diazepam.
- **PO:** Immediate release tabs should be administered on an empty stomach; XL tablets may be given with or without food. XL tablets should be swallowed whole; do not break, crush, or chew.
- **Transdermal patch:** Apply patch on same two days each week (Sunday/Wednesday, Monday/Thursday) to hip, abdomen, or buttock in an area that is clean, dry, and without irritation. Patch should be worn continuously.
- **Transdermal gel:** Apply clear, colorless gel once daily to intact skin on abdomen (avoid area around navel), upper arms/shoulders, or thighs until dry. Rotate sites; do not use same site on consecutive days.

Patient/Family Teaching
- Instruct patient to take oxybutinin as directed. Take missed doses as soon as remembered unless almost time for next dose. Advise patient to read *Information for the Patient* prior to beginning therapy and with each Rx refill in case of new information.
- May cause drowsiness or blurred vision. Advise patient to avoid driving and other activities requiring alertness until response to medication is known.
- Advise patient to avoid concurrent use of alcohol and other CNS depressants while taking this medication.
- Instruct patient that frequent rinsing of mouth, good oral hygiene, and sugarless gum or candy may decrease dry mouth. Health care professional should be notified if mouth dryness persists >2 wk.
- Inform patient that oxybutynin decreases the body's ability to perspire. Avoid strenuous activity in a warm environment because overheating may occur.
- Advise patient to notify health care professional if urinary retention occurs or if constipation persists. Discuss methods of preventing constipation, such as increasing dietary bulk, increasing fluid intake, and increasing mobility.
- Instruct patient to consult health care professional before taking any other Rx, OTC, or herbal products.
- Advise patient to notify health care professional if pregnancy is planned or suspected or if breastfeeding.
- Discuss need for continued medical follow-up. Periodic cystometry may be used to evaluate effectiveness. Ophthalmic exams should be performed periodically to detect glaucoma, especially in patients over 40 yr of age.
- **Transdermal patch:** Instruct patient on correct application and disposal of patch. Open pouch by tearing along arrows; apply immediately. Apply ½ patch to skin by removing ½ protective cover and applying firmly to skin. Apply second half by bending in half and rolling patch onto skin while removing protective liner. Press patch firmly in place.
- Remove slowly; fold in half, sticky sides together, and discard. Wash site with mild soap and water or a small amount of baby oil.
- Advise patient referred for MRI to remove patch prior to test and give directions for replacing patch.
- **Transdermal gel:** Instruct patient on correct application of oxybutynin gel. Do not apply to recently shaved skin, skin with rashes, or areas treated with lotions, oils, or powders; may be used with sunscreen. Wash area with mild soap and water and dry completely before applying. Tear packet open just before use and squeeze entire contents into hand or directly onto application site. Amount of gel will be size of a nickel on the skin. Gently rub into skin until dry. Wash hands immediately following application. Avoid application near open fire or when smoking; medication is flammable. Do not shower, bathe, swim, exercise, or immerse the application site in water within 1 hr after application. Cover application site with clothing if close skin-to-skin contact at application site is anticipated.

Evaluation/Desired Outcomes
- Relief of bladder spasm and associated symptoms (frequency, urgency, nocturia, and incontinence) in patients with a neurogenic or overactive bladder.

HIGH ALERT

oxycodone (ox-i-koe-done)
Endocodone, M-Oxy, Oxycontin, Oxy-FAST, OxyIR, Percolone, Roxicodone, ♣ Supeudol

oxycodone/acetaminophen†
Endocet, Magnacet, Oxycet, Percocet, Primalev, Roxicet, Roxilox, Tylox

oxycodone/aspirin†
Endodan, ♣ Oxycodan, Percodan

oxycodone/ibuprofen

Combunox

Classification
Therapeutic: opioid analgesics
Pharmacologic: opioid agonists, opioid agonists/nonopioid analgesic combinations

Schedule II

Pregnancy Category C (oxycodone alone or with acetaminophen or ibuprofen), D (with aspirin)

†See also acetaminophen, ibuprofen, and salicylates monographs

Indications
Moderate to severe pain.

Action
Binds to opiate receptors in the CNS. Alter the perception of and response to painful stimuli, while producing generalized CNS depression. **Therapeutic Effects:** Decreased pain.

Pharmacokinetics
Absorption: Well absorbed from the GI tract.
Distribution: Widely distributed. Crosses the placenta; enters breast milk.
Metabolism and Excretion: Mostly metabolized by the liver.
Half-life: 2–3 hr.

TIME/ACTION PROFILE (analgesic effects)

ROUTE	ONSET	PEAK	DURATION
PO	10–15 min	60–90 min	3–6 hr
PO-CR	10–15 min	3 hr	12 hr

Contraindications/Precautions
Contraindicated in: Hypersensitivity to oxycodone (cross-sensitivity may exist to other opioids); Hypersensitivity to acetaminophen/aspirin/ibuprofen (for combination products); Aspirin- and ibuprofen-containing products should be avoided in patients with bleeding disorders or thrombocytopenia; Acetaminophen-containing products should be avoided in patients with severe hepatic or renal disease; Ibuprofen-containing products should be avoided in patients undergoing coronary artery bypass graft surgery; OB, Lactation: Avoid chronic use; Some products contain alcohol or bisulfites and should be avoided in patients with known intolerance or hypersensitivity.
Use Cautiously in: Head trauma; ↑ intracranial pressure; Severe renal, hepatic, or pulmonary disease; Cardiovascular disease (ibuprofen-containing products only); History of peptic ulcer disease (ibuprofen-containing products only); Hypothyroidism; Adrenal insufficiency; Alcoholism; Geri: Geriatric or debilitated patients (initial dose ↓ recommended); Undiagnosed abdominal pain; Prostatic hyperplasia.

Adverse Reactions/Side Effects
Noted for oxycodone only; see acetaminophen/aspirin/ibuprofen monographs for specific information on individual components.
CNS: confusion, sedation, dizziness, dysphoria, euphoria, floating feeling, hallucinations, headache, unusual dreams. **EENT:** blurred vision, diplopia, miosis. **Resp:** RESPIRATORY DEPRESSION. **CV:** orthostatic hypotension. **GI:** constipation, dry mouth, nausea, vomiting. **GU:** urinary retention. **Derm:** flushing, sweating. **Misc:** physical dependence, psychological dependence, tolerance.

Interactions
Drug-Drug: Use with caution in patients receiving **MAO inhibitors** (may result in unpredictable reactions— ↓ initial dose of oxycodone to 25% of usual dose). ↑ CNS depression with **alcohol**, **antihistamines**, and **sedative/hypnotics**. Administration of **partial-antagonist opioid analgesics** may precipitate withdrawal in physically dependent patients. **Nalbuphine**, **buprenorphine**, or **pentazocine** may ↓ analgesia.
Drug-Natural Products: Concomitant use of **kava-kava**, **valerian**, or **chamomile** can ↑ CNS depression.

Route/Dosage
Larger doses may be required during chronic therapy. Consider cumulative effects of additional acetaminophen/aspirin/ibuprofen; if toxic levels are exceeded, change to pure oxycodone product.
PO (Adults ≥50 kg): 5–10 mg q 3–4 hr initially, as needed. Controlled-release tablets (Oxycontin) may be given q 12 hr after careful consideration as to dose, indication, and previous analgesic use/abuse history; if using combination products, acetaminophen or aspirin dose should not exceed 4 g/day and should not exceed 4 tablets/day of ibuprofen-containing products.

PO (Adults <50 kg or Children 6–12 yr): 1.25 mg every 6 hr as needed or 0.2 mg/kg q 3–4 hr initially, as needed.

PO (Children >12): 2.5 mg every 6 hr as needed.

Rect (Adults): 10–40 mg 3–4 times daily initially, as needed.

✣ = Canadian drug name. = Genetic implication.
*CAPITALS indicates life-threatening; underlines indicate most frequent.

Availability (generic available)

Oxycodone
Tablets (Percolone, Roxicodone): 5 mg, 15 mg, 30 mg. **Cost:** *Generic*— 5 mg $24.99/30, 15 mg $26.99/30, 30 mg $36.99/30. **Immediate-release capsules (OxyIR):** 5 mg. **Cost:** *Generic*— $13.99/30. **Controlled-release tablets (Oxycontin):** 10 mg, 20 mg, 40 mg, 80 mg. **Cost:** *Generic*— 10 mg $43.99/30, 20 mg $79.99/30, 40 mg $139.99/30, 80 mg $250.01/30. **Oral solution (Roxicodone) (burgundy cherry):** 5 mg/5 mL in 500-mL bottle. **Concentrated oral solution (Roxicodone Intensol, OxyFAST):** 20 mg/mL in 30-mL bottle with dropper. **Cost:** *Generic*— $33.99/30 mL. **Suppositories:** ✣ 10 mg, ✣ 20 mg.

Oxycodone/Acetaminophen
Tablets: 2.5 mg oxycodone with 300 mg acetaminophen (Primalev), 2.5 mg oxycodone with 325 mg acetaminophen (Percocet), 2.5 mg oxycodone with 400 mg acetaminophen (Magnacet), 5 mg oxycodone with 300 mg acetaminophen (Primalev), 5 mg oxycodone with 325 mg acetaminophen (Endocet, Oxycet, Percocet, Roxicet), 5 mg oxycodone with 400 mg acetaminophen (Magnacet), 7.5 mg oxycodone with 300 mg acetaminophen (Primalev), 7.5 mg oxycodone with 325 mg acetaminophen (Endocet, Percocet), 7.5 mg oxycodone with 400 mg acetaminophen (Magnacet), 7.5 mg oxycodone with 500 mg acetaminophen (Endocet), 10 mg oxycodone with 300 mg acetaminophen (Primalev), 10 mg oxycodone with 325 mg acetaminophen (Endocet, Percocet), 10 mg oxycodone with 400 mg acetaminophen (Magnacet), 10 mg oxycodone with 650 mg acetaminophen (Endocet, Percocet). **Cost:** *Generic*— 5/325 mg $16.99/30, 7.5/325 mg $47.99/30, 10/325 mg $60.99/30, 10/650 mg $49.99/30. **Capsules (Roxilox, Tylox):** 5 mg oxycodone with 500 mg acetaminophen. **Cost:** *Generic*— $23.99/30. **Caplets (Roxicet 5/500):** 5 mg oxycodone with 500 mg acetaminophen. **Oral solution (Roxicet) (mint):** 5 mg oxycodone with 325 mg acetaminophen/5 mL. **Cost:** $43.43/500 mL.

Oxycodone/Aspirin
Tablets: 4.88 mg oxycodone with 325 mg aspirin.

Oxycodone/Ibuprofen
Tablets: 5 mg oxycodone with 400 mg ibuprofen.

NURSING IMPLICATIONS

Assessment
- Assess type, location, and intensity of pain prior to and 1 hr (peak) after administration. When titrating opioid doses, increases of 25–50% should be administered until there is a 50% reduction in the patient's pain rating on a numerical or visual analogue scale or the patient reports satisfactory pain relief. A repeat dose can be safely administered at the time of the peak if previous dose is ineffective and side effects are minimal.
- Patients taking controlled-release tablets may require additional short-acting opioid doses for breakthrough pain. Doses should be equivalent to 10–20% of 24 hr total and given every 2 hr as needed.
- An equianalgesic chart (see Appendix K) should be used when changing routes or when changing from one opioid to another.
- Assess blood pressure, pulse, and respirations before and periodically during administration. If respiratory rate is <10/min, assess level of sedation. Physical stimulation may be sufficient to prevent significant hypoventilation. Dose may need to be decreased by 25–50%. Initial drowsiness will diminish with continued use.
- Prolonged use may lead to physical and psychological dependence and tolerance. This should not prevent patient from receiving adequate analgesia. Most patients who receive oxycodone for pain do not develop psychological dependence. Progressively higher doses may be required to relieve pain with long-term therapy.
- Assess bowel function routinely. Prevention of constipation should be instituted with increased intake of fluids and bulk, and laxatives to minimize constipating effects. Stimulant laxatives should be administered routinely if opioid use exceeds 2–3 days, unless contraindicated.
- *Lab Test Considerations:* May ↑ plasma amylase and lipase levels.
- *Toxicity and Overdose:* If an opioid antagonist is required to reverse respiratory depression or coma, naloxone (Narcan) is the antidote. Dilute the 0.4-mg ampule of naloxone in 10 mL of 0.9% NaCl and administer 0.5 mL (0.02 mg) by direct IV push every 2 min. For children and patients weighing <40 kg, dilute 0.1 mg of naloxone in 10 mL of 0.9% NaCl for a concentration of 10 mcg/mL and administer 0.5 mcg/kg every 2 min. Titrate dose to avoid withdrawal, seizures, and severe pain.

Potential Nursing Diagnoses
Acute pain (Indications)
Disturbed sensory perception (visual, auditory) (Side Effects)
Risk for injury (Side Effects)

Implementation
- **_High Alert:_** Accidental overdosage of opioid analgesics has resulted in fatalities. Before administering, clarify all ambiguous orders; have second practitioner independently check original order and dose calculations. Do not confuse oxycodone with OxyContin.
- Regularly administered doses may be more effective than prn administration. Analgesic is more effective if given before pain becomes severe.
- Coadministration with nonopioid analgesics may have additive analgesic effects and may permit lower doses. Medication should be discontinued gradually after long-term use to prevent withdrawal symptoms.
- **PO:** May be administered with food or milk to minimize GI irritation.
- Administer solution with properly calibrated measuring device.
- Controlled-release tablets should be swallowed whole; do not crush, break, or chew. Taking broken, chewed, or crushed controlled-release tablets leads to rapid release and absorption of a potentially fatal dose of oxycodone.
- **Controlled Release:** Dose should be based on 24-hr opioid requirement determined with short-acting opioids then converted to controlled-release form.

Patient/Family Teaching
- Instruct patient on how and when to ask for and take pain medication. Caution patient not to increase the dose of controlled-release oxycodone without consulting health care professional.
- Caution patient that controlled-release oxycodone is a potential drug of abuse. Medication should be protected from theft and never given to anyone other than the individual for whom it was prescribed.
- May cause drowsiness or dizziness. Advise patient to call for assistance when ambulating or smoking. Caution patient to avoid driving and other activities requiring alertness until response to medication is known.
- Advise patients taking *Oxycontin* tablets that empty matrix tablets may appear in stool.
- Advise patient to make position changes slowly to minimize orthostatic hypotension.
- Advise patient to avoid concurrent use of alcohol or other CNS depressants with this medication.
- Encourage patient to turn, cough, and breathe deeply every 2 hr to prevent atelectasis.

Evaluation/Desired Outcomes
- Decrease in severity of pain without a significant alteration in level of consciousness or respiratory status.

HIGH ALERT

oxymorphone (ox-i-mor-fone)
Opana, Opana ER

Classification
Therapeutic: opioid analgesics
Pharmacologic: opioid agonists

Schedule II

Pregnancy Category C

Indications
Management of moderate to severe pain. Extended-release tablets should only be used in patients who require continuous 24-hr management of chronic pain. Supplement in balanced anesthesia.

Action
Binds to opiate receptors in the CNS. Alters the perception of and response to painful stimuli, while producing generalized CNS depression. **Therapeutic Effects:** Decrease in pain.

Pharmacokinetics
Absorption: 10% absorbed following oral administration. Food and alcohol significantly ↑ absorption (38%). Well absorbed following IM, subcut or rectal administration.
Distribution: Widely distributed; crosses placenta, enters breast milk.
Metabolism and Excretion: Mostly metabolized by the liver; at least 2 metabolites are pharmacologically active, <1% excreted unchanged in urine.
Half-life: 2.6–4 hr.

✦ = Canadian drug name. ☒ = Genetic implication.
*CAPITALS indicates life-threatening; underlines indicate most frequent.

oxymorphone

TIME/ACTION PROFILE (analgesic effects)

ROUTE	ONSET	PEAK	DURATION
PO	unknown	unknown	4–6 hr
PO ER	unknown	unknown	12 hr
IM	10–15 min	30–90 min	3–6 hr
IV	5–10 min	15–30 min	3–6 hr
Subcut	10–20 min	unknown	3–4 hr

Contraindications/Precautions

Contraindicated in: Hypersensitivity; Concurrent alcohol; Moderate/severe hepatic impairment; Respiratory depression (unless monitoring and resuscitative equipment are readily available); Known/suspected paralytic ileus.

Use Cautiously in: Acute alcoholism or delirium tremens or other toxic psychoses; Mild hepatic impairment; Head injury/ ↑ intracranial pressure (may obscure neurologic signs and further ↑ pressure); Volume depletion or drugs that may cause hypotension including diuretics and phenothiazines (↑ risk of severe hypotension); Circulatory shock (may ↑ risk of severe hypotension); Adrenocortical insufficiency; Hypothyroidism; Prostatic hypertrophy or ureteral stricture; Severe pulmonary or renal impairment; Biliary tract disease or pancreatitis; OB: Use only in pregnancy if maternal benefit outweighs fetal risk; Lactation: Lactation; Geri: Blood levels are ↑ ; dose accordingly.

Exercise Extreme Caution in: Conditions association with hypoxia, hypercapnea, ↓ respiratory reserve (including asthma, COPD, cor pulmonale, morbid obesity, sleep apnea, myxedema, kyphoscoliosis, CNS depression and coma).

Adverse Reactions/Side Effects

CNS: confusion, sedation, dizziness, dysphoria, euphoria, floating feeling, hallucinations, headache, unusual dreams. **EENT:** blurred vision, diplopia, miosis. **Resp:** RESPIRATORY DEPRESSION. **CV:** orthostatic hypotension. **GI:** constipation, dry mouth, nausea, vomiting. **GU:** urinary retention. **Derm:** flushing, sweating. **Misc:** physical dependence, psychological dependence, tolerance.

Interactions

Drug-Drug: Use with caution in patients receiving **MAO inhibitors** (may result in unpredictable reactions— ↓ initial dose of oxymorphone to 25% of usual dose). ↑ risk of CNS depression, hypotension and respiratory depression with **alcohol**, other **opioids** or **CNS depressants** including **sedatives**, **hypnotics**, **general anesthetics**, **phenothiazines**, **tranquilizers**, **skeletal muscle relaxants**, or **sedating antihistamines**; may initiate therapy with ⅓ to ½ usual starting dose. **Drugs that may cause volume depletion or hypotension** including **diuretics**, **phenothiazines** may ↑ risk of severe hypotension. Administration of **partial-antagonist opioid analgesics** may precipitate withdrawal in physically dependent patients. **Nalbuphine, buprenorphine,** or **pentazocine** ↓ analgesia.

Drug-Natural Products: Concomitant use of **kava-kava, valerian,** or **chamomile** can ↑ CNS depression.

Route/Dosage

Larger doses may be required during chronic therapy.

PO (Adults): *Opioid-naive patients*—10–20 mg every 4–6 hr, some patients may require initial dose of 5 mg, not to exceed 20 mg. Once optimal analgesia is obtained, chronic pain patients may be converted to an equivalent 24-hour dose given as extended release tablets every 12 hr.

Subcut, IM (Adults): 1–1.5 mg q 3–6 hr as needed. *Analgesia during labor*—0.5–1 mg.

IV (Adults): 0.5 mg q 3–6 hr as needed; increase as needed.

Availability

Tablets (Opana): 5 mg, 10 mg. **Extended-release tablets (Opana ER):** 5 mg, 7.5 mg, 10 mg, 15 mg, 20 mg, 30 mg, 40 mg. **Solution for injection:** 1 mg/mL.

NURSING IMPLICATIONS

Assessment

- Assess type, location, and intensity of pain prior to and 1 hr following IM and 15–30 min (peak) following IV administration. When titrating opioid doses, increases of 25–50% should be administered until there is either a 50% reduction in the patient's pain rating on a numerical or visual analogue scale or the patient reports satisfactory pain relief. A repeat dose can be safely administered at the time of the peak if previous dose is ineffective and side effects are minimal.
- Patients taking controlled-release tablets should also be given supplemental short-acting opioid doses for breakthrough pain.
- An equianalgesic chart (see Appendix K) should be used when changing routes or when changing from one opioid to another.
- Assess blood pressure, pulse, and respirations before and periodically during administration. If respiratory rate is <10/min, assess level of sedation. Physical stimulation may be sufficient to prevent significant hypoventilation. Dose may need to be decreased by 25–50%. Initial drowsiness will diminish with continued use.

- Prolonged use may lead to physical and psychological dependence and tolerance. This should not prevent patient from receiving adequate analgesia. Most patients who receive oxymorphone for pain do not develop psychological dependence. Progressively higher doses may be required to relieve pain with long-term therapy.
- Assess bowel function routinely. Prevention of constipation should be instituted with increased intake of fluids and bulk, and laxatives. Stimulant laxatives should be administered routinely if opioid use exceeds 2–3 days, unless contraindicated.
- *Lab Test Considerations:* May ↑ plasma amylase and lipase levels.
- ***Toxicity and Overdose:*** If an opioid antagonist is required to reverse respiratory depression or coma, naloxone (Narcan) is the antidote. Dilute the 0.4-mg ampule of naloxone in 10 mL of 0.9% NaCl and administer 0.5 mL (0.02 mg) by direct IV push every 2 min. For children and patients weighing <40 kg, dilute 0.1 mg of naloxone in 10 mL of 0.9% NaCl for a concentration of 10 mcg/mL and administer 0.5 mcg/kg every 2 min. Titrate dose to avoid withdrawal, seizures, and severe pain.

Potential Nursing Diagnoses
Acute pain (Indications)
Disturbed sensory perception (visual, auditory) (Side Effects)
Risk for injury (Side Effects)

Implementation
- *High Alert:* Accidental overdose of opioid analgesics has resulted in fatalities. Before administering, clarify all ambiguous orders; have second practitioner independently check original order, dose calculations, and infusion pump settings.
- Explain therapeutic value of medication prior to administration to enhance the analgesic effect.
- Regularly administered doses may be more effective than prn administration. Analgesic is more effective if given before pain becomes severe.
- Coadministration with nonopioid analgesics may have additive analgesic effects and may permit lower doses.
- Medication should be discontinued gradually after long-term use to prevent withdrawal symptoms.
- **PO:** Administer at least 1 hr prior to or 2 hr after eating.
- Controlled-release tablets should be swallowed whole; do not break, crush, or chew.
- **Controlled Release:** Patients should be titrated to mild to no pain with the regular use of no more than 2 doses of supplemental analgesia (rescue) per 24 hr. Dose should be based on 24-hr opioid requirement determined with short-acting opioids then converted to controlled-release form.
- If patient is opioid-naive, start with 5 mg every 12 hr, then titrate in increments of 5–10 mg every 12 hr every 3–7 days to a level that provides adequate analgesia with minimal side effects.
- If converting from *Opana* to *Opana ER*, administer half the patient's total daily dose of *Opana* as *Opana ER* every 12 hr.
- If converting from parenteral oxymorphone, administer 10 times the patient's total daily parenteral oxymorphone dose as *Opana ER* in two equally divided doses every 12 hr.
- If converting from other opioids, 10 mg of oral oxymorphone is equianalgesic to hydrocodone 20 mg, oxycodone 20 mg, methadone 20 mg, and morphine 30 mg orally.

IV Administration
- **Direct IV:** Administer undiluted. *Concentration:* 1 mg/mL. *Rate:* Give over 2–3 min.
- **Syringe Compatibility:** glycopyrrolate, hydroxyzine, ranitidine.

Patient/Family Teaching
- Instruct patient on how and when to ask for pain medication.
- Instruct patient to take oxymorphone as directed and not to adjust dose without consulting health care professional. Take missed doses as soon as possible if on chronic therapy. If almost time for next dose, skip dose and return to regular schedule. Do not double doses unless advised by health care professional. Do not stop taking oxymorphone abruptly, may cause withdrawal symptoms. Discontinue gradually under supervision of health care professional. Caution patient to keep medication out of reach of children and pets.
- Caution patient not to share this medication; may cause harm or death and is against the law.

- Medication may cause drowsiness or dizziness. Advise patient to call for assistance when ambulating or smoking. Caution patient to avoid driving and other activities requiring alertness until response to medication is known.
- Advise patient to make position changes slowly to minimize orthostatic hypotension.
- Advise patient to avoid concurrent use of alcohol or other CNS depressants with this medication.
- Caution patient not to take any new Rx, OTC, or herbal products without notifying health care professional.
- Encourage patient to turn, cough, and breathe deeply every 2 hr to prevent atelectasis.
- OB: Advise patient to notify health care professional if pregnancy is planned or suspected.

Evaluation/Desired Outcomes
- Decrease in severity of pain without a significant alteration in level of consciousness or respiratory status.

HIGH ALERT

oxytocin (ox-i-toe-sin)
Pitocin, ✤ Syntocinon

Classification
Therapeutic: hormones
Pharmacologic: oxytocics

Pregnancy Category X

Indications
IV: Induction of labor at term. **IV:** Facilitation of threatened abortion. **IV, IM:** Postpartum control of bleeding after expulsion of the placenta.

Action
Stimulates uterine smooth muscle, producing uterine contractions similar to those in spontaneous labor. Has vasopressor and antidiuretic effects. **Therapeutic Effects:** Induction of labor. Control of postpartum bleeding.

Pharmacokinetics
Absorption: IV administration results in 100% bioavailability.
Distribution: Widely distributed in extracellular fluid. Small amounts reach fetal circulation.
Metabolism and Excretion: Rapidly metabolized by liver and kidneys.
Half-life: 3–9 min.

TIME/ACTION PROFILE (reduction in uterine contractions)

ROUTE	ONSET	PEAK	DURATION
IV	immediate	unknown	1 hr
IM	3–5 min	unknown	30–60 min

Contraindications/Precautions
Contraindicated in: Hypersensitivity; Anticipated nonvaginal delivery.
Use Cautiously in: OB: First and second stages of labor; slow infusion over 24 hr has caused water intoxication with seizure and coma or maternal death due to oxytocin's antidiuretic effect.

Adverse Reactions/Side Effects
Maternal adverse reactions are noted for IV use only.
CNS: *maternal*—COMA, SEIZURES; *fetal*, INTRACRANIAL HEMORRHAGE. **Resp:** *fetal*—ASPHYXIA, hypoxia. **CV:** *maternal*—hypotension; *fetal*, arrhythmias. **F and E:** *maternal*—hypochloremia, hyponatremia, water intoxication. **Misc:** *maternal*— ↑ uterine motility, painful contractions, abruptio placentae, ↓ uterine blood flow, hypersensitivity.

Interactions
Drug-Drug: Severe hypertension may occur if oxytocin follows administration of **vasopressors**. Concurrent use with **cyclopropane** anesthesia may result in excessive hypotension.

Route/Dosage
Induction/Stimulation of Labor
IV (Adults): 0.5–2 milliunits/min; ↑ by 1–2 milliunits/min q 15–60 min until pattern established (usually 5–6 milliunits/min; maximum 20 milliunits/min), then ↓ dose.

Postpartum Hemorrhage
IV (Adults): 10 units infused at 20–40 milliunits/min.
IM (Adults): 10 units after delivery of placenta.

Incomplete/Inevitable Abortion
IV (Adults): 10 units at a rate of 20–40 milliunits/min.

Availability (generic available)
Solution for injection: 10 units/mL.

NURSING IMPLICATIONS

Assessment
- Fetal maturity, presentation, and pelvic adequacy should be assessed prior to administration of oxytocin for induction of labor.
- Assess character, frequency, and duration of uterine contractions; resting uterine tone; and

fetal heart rate frequently throughout administration. If contractions occur <2 min apart and are >50–65 mm Hg on monitor, if they last 60–90 sec or longer, or if a significant change in fetal heart rate develops, stop infusion and turn patient on her left side to prevent fetal anoxia. Notify health care professional immediately.
- Monitor maternal blood pressure and pulse frequently and fetal heart rate continuously throughout administration.
- This drug occasionally causes water intoxication. Monitor patient for signs and symptoms (drowsiness, listlessness, confusion, headache, anuria) and notify physician or other health care professional if they occur.
- *Lab Test Considerations:* Monitor maternal electrolytes. Water retention may result in hypochloremia or hyponatremia.

Potential Nursing Diagnoses
Deficient knowledge, related to medication regimen (Patient/Family Teaching)

Implementation
- Do not confuse Pitocin (oxytocin) with Pitressin (vasopressin).
- Do not administer oxytocin simultaneously by more than one route.

IV Administration

- **Continuous Infusion:** Rotate infusion container to ensure thorough mixing. Store solution in refrigerator, but do not freeze.
- Infuse via infusion pump for accurate dose. Oxytocin should be connected via Y-site injection to an IV of 0.9% NaCl for use during adverse reactions.
- Magnesium sulfate should be available if needed for relaxation of the myometrium.

- **Induction of Labor:** *Diluent:* Dilute 1 mL (10 units) in 1 L of compatible infusion fluid (0.9% NaCl, D5W, or LR). *Concentration:* 10 milliunits/mL. *Rate:* Begin infusion at 0.5–2 milliunits/min (0.05–0.2 mL); increase in increments of 1–2 milliunits/min at 15–30-min intervals until contractions simulate normal labor.
- **Postpartum Bleeding:** *Diluent:* For control of postpartum bleeding, dilute 1–4 mL (10–40 units) in 1 L of compatible infusion fluid. *Concentration:* 10–40 milliunits/mL. *Rate:* Begin infusion at a rate of 20–40 milliunits/min to control uterine atony. Adjust rate as indicated.
- **Incomplete or Inevitable Abortion:** *Diluent:* For incomplete or inevitable abortion, dilute 1 mL (10 units) in 500 mL of 0.9% NaCl or D5W. *Concentration:* 20 milliunits/mL. *Rate:* Infuse at a rate of 20–40 milliunits/min.
- **Y-Site Compatibility:** heparin, hydrocortisone sodium succinate, insulin, meperidine, morphine, potassium chloride, vitamin B complex with C, warfarin, zidovudine.
- **Solution Compatibility:** dextrose/Ringer's or lactated Ringer's combinations, dextrose/saline combinations, Ringer's or lactated Ringer's injection, D5W, D10W, 0.45% NaCl, 0.9% NaCl.

Patient/Family Teaching
- Advise patient to expect contractions similar to menstrual cramps after administration has started.

Evaluation/Desired Outcomes
- Onset of effective contractions.
- Increase in uterine tone.
- Reduction in postpartum bleeding.

paclitaxel (pak-li-tax-el)
Onxol, Taxol

paclitaxel protein-bound particles (albumin-bound)
Abraxane

Classification
Therapeutic: antineoplastics
Pharmacologic: taxoids

Pregnancy Category D

Indications
Paclitaxel: Advanced ovarian cancer (with cisplatin). Non-small cell lung cancer when potentially curative surgery and/or radiation therapy is not an option. Metastatic breast cancer unresponsive to other therapy. Node-positive breast cancer when administered sequentially to standard combination chemotherapy that includes doxorubicin. Treatment of AIDS-related Kaposi's sarcoma. **Paclitaxel (albumin-bound):** Metastatic breast cancer after treatment failure or relapse where therapy included an anthracycline.

Action
Interferes with the normal cellular microtubule function that is required for interphase and mitosis. **Therapeutic Effects:** Death of rapidly replicating cells, particularly malignant ones.

Pharmacokinetics
Absorption: IV administration results in complete bioavailability.
Distribution: Cross the placenta.
Protein Binding: 89–98%.
Metabolism and Excretion: Highly metabolized by the liver, <10% excreted unchanged in urine.
Half-life: *Paclitaxel*—13–52 hr; *Paclitaxel protein-bound particles (albumin-bound)*—27 hr.

TIME/ACTION PROFILE (effect on WBCs)

ROUTE	ONSET	PEAK	DURATION
IV	unknown	11 days	3 wk

Contraindications/Precautions
Contraindicated in: Hypersensitivity to paclitaxel or to castor oil (non-protein-bound vehicle contains polyoxyethylated castor oil); Known alcohol intolerance; OB, Lactation: Pregnancy or lactation; ANC ≤1500/mm³ in patients with ovarian, lung, or breast cancer; ANC ≤1000/mm³ in patients with AIDS-related Kaposi's sarcoma.
Use Cautiously in: Moderate or severe hepatic impairment; Geri: ↑ risk of neuropathy, myelosuppression, and cardiovascular events; OB: Childbearing potential; Active infection; Decreased bone marrow reserve; Pedi: Safety and effectiveness not established.

Adverse Reactions/Side Effects
CV: ECG changes, hypotension, bradycardia. **GI:** abnormal liver function tests, diarrhea, mucositis, nausea, vomiting. **Derm:** alopecia. **Hemat:** anemia, neutropenia, thrombocytopenia. **MS:** arthralgia, myalgia. **Neuro:** peripheral neuropathy. **Resp:** cough, dyspnea. **Local:** injection site reactions. **Misc:** hypersensitivity reactions including ANAPHYLAXIS and STEVENS-JOHNSON SYNDROME, TOXIC EPIDERMAL NECROLYSIS.

Interactions
Drug-Drug: **Ketoconazole**, **verapamil**, **quinidine**, **cyclosporine**, **diazepam**, **dexamethasone**, **teniposide**, **etoposide**, or **vincristine** may ↓ metabolism and ↑ risk of serious toxicity; concurrent use should be undertaken with caution. ↑ risk of myelosuppression with other **antineoplastics** or **radiation therapy**. Myelosuppression ↑ when given after **cisplatin**. May ↑ levels and toxicity of **doxorubicin**. May ↓ antibody response to and ↑ risk of adverse reactions from **live-virus vaccines**.

Route/Dosage
Many other regimens are used.

Paclitaxel
Ovarian Cancer
IV (Adults): *Previously untreated patients*—175 mg/m² over 3 hr every 3 wk, or 135 mg/m² over 24 hr every 3 wk, followed by cisplatin; *Previously treated patients*—135 mg/m² or 175 mg/m² over 3 hr every 3 wk.

Breast Cancer
IV (Adults): *Adjuvant treatment of node-positive breast cancer*—175 mg/m² over 3 hr every 3 wk for 4 courses administered sequentially to doxorubicin-containing combination chemotherapy; *Failure of initial therapy for metastatic disease or relapse within 6 mo of adjuvant therapy*—175 mg/m² over 3 hr every 3 wk.

Non-Small Cell Lung Cancer
IV (Adults): 135 mg/m^2 over 24 hr every 3 wk, followed by cisplatin.

AIDS-Related Kaposi's Sarcoma
IV (Adults): 135 mg/m^2 over 3 hr every 3 wk or 100 mg/m^2 over 3 hr every 2 wk (dose reduction/adjustment may be necessary in patients with advanced HIV infection).

Paclitaxel Protein-Bound Particles (albumin-bound)
IV (Adults): 260 mg/m^2 over 30 min every 3 wk.

Hepatic Impairment
IV (Adults): *Moderate hepatic impairment (AST levels <10× ULN and bilirubin levels 1.26–2× ULN)* — 200 mg/m^2 over 30 min every 3 wk; *Severe hepatic impairment (AST levels <10× ULN and bilirubin levels 2.01–5× ULN)* — 130 mg/m^2 over 30 min every 3 wk; dose may be ↑ to 200 mg/m^2 for subsequent courses based on individual tolerance; *Severe hepatic impairment (AST levels >10× ULN or bilirubin levels >5× ULN)* — Avoid use.

Availability

Paclitaxel (generic available)
Solution for injection: 6 mg/mL.

Paclitaxel Protein-Bound Particles (albumin-bound)
Powder for injection: 100 mg/vial.

NURSING IMPLICATIONS

Assessment
- Monitor vital signs frequently, especially during first hr of the infusion.
- Monitor cardiovascular status especially during first 3 hr of infusion. Hypotension and bradycardia are common but usually do not require treatment. Continuous ECG monitoring is recommended only for patients with serious underlying conduction abnormalities.
- Monitor for bone marrow depression. Assess for bleeding (bleeding gums, bruising, petechiae, guaiac stools, urine, and emesis) and avoid IM injections and taking rectal temperatures if platelet count is low. Apply pressure to venipuncture sites for 10 min. Assess for signs of infection during neutropenia. Anemia may occur. Monitor for dyspnea and orthostatic hypotension. Granulocyte-colony stimulating factor (G-CSF) may be used if necessary.
- Assess for development of peripheral neuropathy. If severe symptoms occur, subsequent dose should be reduced by 20%.
- Monitor intake and output, appetite, and nutritional intake. Paclitaxel causes nausea and vomiting in 50% of patients. Prophylactic antiemetics may be used. Adjust diet as tolerated to help maintain fluid and electrolyte balance and nutritional status.
- Assess patient for arthralgia and myalgia, which usually begin 2–3 days after therapy and resolve within 5 days. Pain is usually relieved by nonopioid analgesics but may be severe enough to require treatment with opioid analgesics.
- **Paclitaxel:** Monitor for hypersensitivity reactions continuously during the first 30 min and frequently thereafter. These occur frequently (19%), usually during the first 10 min of paclitaxel infusion, after the first or second dose. Pretreatment is recommended for **all** patients and should include dexamethasone 20 mg PO (10 mg for patients with advanced HIV disease) 12 and 6 hours prior to paclitaxel, diphenhydramine 50 mg IV 30–60 min prior to paclitaxel, and cimetidine 300 mg or ranitidine 50 mg IV 30–60 min prior to paclitaxel. Most common manifestations are dyspnea, flushing, tachycardia, rash, hypotension, and chest pain. If these occur, stop infusion and notify health care professional. Treatment may include bronchodilators, epinephrine, antihistamines, and corticosteroids. Keep these agents and resuscitative equipment close by in the event of an anaphylactic reaction. Other manifestations of hypersensitivity reactions include flushing and rash.
- No premedication for hypersensitivity is required for paclitaxel protein-bound (albumin-bound).
- ***Lab Test Considerations:*** Monitor CBC and differential prior to and periodically during therapy. The nadir of leukopenia occurs in 11 days, with recovery by days 15–21. Notify health care professional if the leukocyte count is <1500/mm^3 (1000/mm^3 in AIDS-related Kaposi's sarcoma) or if the platelet count is <100,000/mm^3. Subsequent doses are usually held until leukocyte count is >1500/mm^3 (1000/mm^3 in AIDS-related Kaposi's sarcoma) and platelet count is >100,000/mm^3.
- Monitor liver function studies (AST, ALT, LDH, bilirubin) prior to and periodically during therapy to detect hepatotoxicity.

Potential Nursing Diagnoses
Risk for infection (Adverse Reactions)
Risk for injury (Adverse Reactions)

Implementation
- Do not confuse Taxol (paclitaxel) with Taxotere (docetaxel). Do not confuse paclitaxel with Paxil (paroxetine).

Paclitaxel

IV Administration

- **Continuous Infusion:** Paclitaxel must be diluted prior to injection. ***Diluent:*** Dilute contents of 5-mL (30-mg) vials with the following diluents: 0.9% NaCl, D5W, D5/0.9% NaCl, or dextrose in Ringer's solution. ***Concentration:*** 0.3–1.2 mg/mL. Although haziness in the solution is normal, inspect for particulate matter or discoloration before use. Use an in-line filter of not >0.22-micron pore size. Solutions are stable for 27 hr at room temperature and lighting. Do not use PVC containers or administration sets. ***Rate:*** Dose for *breast cancer or AIDS-related Kaposi's sarcoma* is administered over 3 hr. Dose for *ovarian cancer* is administered as a 24-hr infusion.

- **Y-Site Compatibility:** acyclovir, alfentanyl, allopurinol, amifostine, amikacin, aminophylline, ampicillin, ampicillin/sulbactam, anidulafungin, atracurium, aztreonam, bivalirudin, bleomycin, bumetanice, buprenorphine, butorphanol, calcium chloride, calcium gluconate, carboplatin, carmustine, caspofungin, cefazolin, cefepime, cefoperazone, cefotaxime, cefotetan, cefoxitin, ceftazidime, ceftizoxime, ceftriaxone, cefuroxime, chloramphenicol, cimetidine, ciprofloxacin, cisatracurium, cisplatin, cladribine, clindamycin, cyclophosphamide, cyclosporine, cytarabine, dacarbazine, dactinomycin, dantrolene, daptomycin, daunorubicin hydrochloride, dexamethasone sodium phosphate, dexrazoxane, diltiazem, diphenhydramine, dobutamine, dopamine, doripenem, doxorubicin hydrochloride, droperidol, enalaprilat, ephedrine, epinephrine, epirubicin, ertapenem, erythromycin, esmolol, etoposide, etoposide phosphate, famotidine, fenoldopam, fentanyl, floxuridine, fluconazole, fludarabine, fluorouracil, foscarnet, fosphenytoin, furosemide, ganciclovir, gemcitabine, gentamicin, glycopyrrolate, granisetron, haloperidol, heparin, hetastarch, hydralazine, hydrocortisone, hydromorphone, ifosfamide, imipenem/cilastatin, inamrinone, insulin, irinotecan, isoproterenol, ketorolac, leucovorin, levofloxacin, levorphanol, lidocaine, linezolid, lorazepam, magnesium sulfate, mannitol, meperidine, meropenem, mesna, metaraminol, methohexital, methotrexate, methyldopate, metoclopramide, metoprolol, metronidazole, midazolam, milrinone, mitomycin, morphine, nafcillin, nalbuphine, naloxone, nesiritide, nitroglycerin, nitroprusside, norepinephrine, octreotide, ondansetron, oxaliplatin, palonosetron, pancuronium, pantoprazole, pemetrexed, pentamidine, pentazocine, pentobarbital, pentostatin, phenobarbital, phentolamine, phenylephrine, piperacillin/tazobactam, potassium chloride, procainamide, prochlorperazine edisylate, promethazine, propofol, quinupriatin/dalfopriatin, ranitidine, remifentanil, rituximab, sodium acetate, sodium bicarbonate, sodium phosphates, streptozocin, succinylcholine, sufentanil, tacrolimus, teniposide, theophylline, thiopental, thiotepa, ticarcillin/clavulanate, tigecycline, tirofiban, tobramycin, tolazoline, topotecan, trastuzumab, trimethobenzamide, trimethoprim/sulfamethoxazole, vancomycin, vasopressin, vecuronium, verapamil, vinblastine, vincristine, vinorelbine, voriconazole, zidovudine.

- **Y-Site Incompatibility:** amiodarone, amphotericin B cholesteryl, amphotericin B colloidal, amphotericin B liposome, chlorpromazine, diazepam, digoxin, doxorubicin liposome, hydroxyzine, idarubicin, indomethacin, labetalol, methylprednisolone sodium succinate, mitoxantrone, phenytoin, propranolol.

Paclitaxel Protein-Bound Particles (albumin-bound)

IV Administration

- **Intermittent Infusion:** Reconstitute by slowly adding 20 mL to each vial over at least 1 min for a concentration of 5 mg/mL. Direct solution to inside wall of vial to prevent foaming. Allow vial to sit for at least 5 min to ensure proper wetting of cake/powder. Gently swirl or invert vial for at least 2 min until powder is completely dissolved; avoid foaming. If foaming or clumping occurs, allow vial to stand for 15 min until foaming dissolves. Solution should be milky and homogenous without visible particles. If particles or settling are visible, gently invert vial to resuspend. Inject appropriate amount into sterile PVC IV bag. Do not use an in-line filter during administration. Do not administer solutions that are discolored or contain particulate matter. Reconstituted solution should be administered immediately but is stable for 8 hr if refrigerated. Discard unused portion. *Rate:* Administer over no more than 30 min. Monitor infusion site closely for infiltration.

Patient/Family Teaching
- Instruct patient to notify health care professional promptly if fever; chills; cough; hoarseness; sore throat; signs of infection; lower back or side pain; painful or difficult urination; bleeding gums; bruising; petechiae; blood in stools, urine, or emesis; dyspnea; or orthostatic hypotension occurs. Caution patient to avoid crowds and persons with known infections. Instruct patient to use soft toothbrush and electric razor and to avoid falls. Caution patient not to drink alcoholic beverages or to take medication containing aspirin or NSAIDs; may precipitate gastric bleeding.
- Instruct patient to notify health care professional if abdominal pain, yellow skin, weakness, paresthesia, gait disturbances, or joint or muscle aches occur.
- Instruct patient to inspect oral mucosa for redness and ulceration. If mouth sores occur, advise patient to use sponge brush and rinse mouth with water after eating and drinking. Stomatitis usually resolves in 5–7 days.
- Discuss with patient the possibility of hair loss. Complete hair loss usually occurs between days 14 and 21 and is reversible after discontinuation of therapy. Explore coping strategies.
- Advise patient to use a nonhormonal method of contraception. Advise male patients not to father a child while receiving paclitaxel.
- Instruct patient not to receive any vaccinations without advice of health care professional.
- Emphasize the need for periodic lab tests to monitor for side effects.

Evaluation/Desired Outcomes
- Decrease in size or spread of malignancy.

---

palifermin (pa-liff-er-min)
Kepivance

Classification
Therapeutic: cytoprotective agents
Pharmacologic: keratinocyte growth factors (rDNA)

Pregnancy Category C

Indications
To decrease incidence/duration of severe oral mucositis associated with myelotoxic therapy requiring stem cell support for hematologic malignancies.

Action
Enhances proliferation of epithelial cells. **Therapeutic Effects:** Decreased incidence/duration of mucositis.

Pharmacokinetics
Absorption: IV administration results in complete bioavailability.
Distribution: Distributes into extravascular space.
Metabolism and Excretion: Unknown.
Half-life: 4.5 hr.

TIME/ACTION PROFILE (levels)

ROUTE	ONSET	PEAK	DURATION
IV	unknown	end of dose	unknown

Contraindications/Precautions
Contraindicated in: Hypersensitivity to palifermin or other *E. coli*-derived proteins.
Use Cautiously in: OB: Use only if maternal benefit outweighs fetal risk; Lactation: Pedi: Safety not established.

Adverse Reactions/Side Effects
Derm: skin toxicity. **GI:** oral toxicity. **Metab:** ↑ amylase, ↑ lipase. **MS:** arthralgia. **Neuro:** dysesthesia.

Interactions
Drug-Drug: Binds to and inactivates **heparin** (flush tubing between use). Administration within 24 hr after **myelotoxic therapy (chemotherapy/radiation)** ↑ severity and duration of mucositis.

Route/Dosage
IV (Adults): 60 mcg/kg/day for 3 days before and 3 days after myelotoxic therapy.

Availability
Powder for injection: 6.25 mg/vial.

NURSING IMPLICATIONS

Assessment
- Assess level of oral mucositis prior to and periodically during therapy.
- *Lab Test Considerations:* May cause ↑ serum lipase and amylase; usually reversible.
- May cause proteinuria.

Potential Nursing Diagnoses
Acute pain (Indications)
Impaired oral mucous membrane (Indications)

Implementation
- Do not administer palifermin within 24 hr before, during infusion, or 24 hr after infusion of myelotoxic chemotherapy.

- Administer doses for 3 consecutive days before (third dose 24–48 hr prior to chemotherapy) and 3 consecutive days after myelotoxic chemotherapy (fourth dose on same days as hematopoietic stem cells infusion and at least 4 days after most recent palifermin administration) for a total of 6 doses.

IV Administration

- **Direct IV:** *Diluent:* Reconstitute palifermin powder by slowly injecting 1.2 mL of sterile water for injection aseptically. *Concentration:* 5 mg/mL. Swirl gently; do not shake or vigorously agitate. Solution should be clear and colorless; do not administer solution that is discolored or contains particulate matter. Dissolution usually takes less than 3 minutes. Administer immediately after reconstitution or refrigerate and administer within 24 hr. Do not freeze. Allow to reach room temperature for up to 1 hr. Protect from light. Discard palifermin after expiration date or if left at room temperature for more than 1 hr. *Rate:* Administer via bolus injection. Do not use a filter.
- **Y-Site Incompatibility:** heparin. If heparin solution is used to maintain IV line, flush with 0.9% NaCl prior to and after use of palifermin.

Patient/Family Teaching

- Inform patient of evidence of tumor growth and stimulation in cell culture and animal models.
- Advise patient to notify health care professional if rash, erythema, edema, pruritus, oral/perioral dysesthesia (tongue discoloration, tongue thickening, alteration of taste) occur.

Evaluation/Desired Outcomes

- Decrease in incidence and duration of oral mucositis in patients receiving myelotoxic therapy requiring hematopoietic stem cell support.

---

paliperidone (pa-li-**per**-i-done)
Invega, Invega Sustenna

Classification
Therapeutic: antipsychotics
Pharmacologic: benzisoxazoles

Pregnancy Category C

Indications
PO, IM: Acute and maintenance treatment of schizophrenia. **PO:** Acute treatment of schizoaffective disorder (as monotherapy or as adjunct to mood stabilizers and/or antidepressants).

Action
May act by antagonizing dopamine and serotonin in the CNS. Paliperidone is the active metabolite of risperidone. **Therapeutic Effects:** Decreased manifestations of schizophrenia. Decreased manifestations of schizoaffective disorder.

Pharmacokinetics
Absorption: 28% absorbed following oral administration, food ↑ absorption; slowly absorbed after IM administration (concentrations higher and more rapidly achieved with administration into deltoid muscle).
Distribution: Unknown.
Metabolism and Excretion: 59% excreted unchanged in urine; 32% excreted in urine as metabolites.
Half-life: 23 hr (PO); 25–49 days (IM).

TIME/ACTION PROFILE (blood levels)

ROUTE	ONSET	PEAK	DURATION
PO	unknown	24 hr	24 hr
IM	unknown	13 days	1 mo

Contraindications/Precautions
Contraindicated in: Hypersensitivity to paliperidone or risperidone; Concurrent use of drugs known to cause QTc prolongation (including quinidine, procainamide, sotalol, amiodarone, chlorpromazine, thioridazine, moxifloxacin); History of congenital QTc prolongation or other cardiac arrhythmias; Bradycardia, hypokalemia, hypomagnesemia (↑ risk of QTc prolongation); Pre-existing severe GI narrowing (due to nature of tablet formulation); CCr < 50 mL/min (for IM); Lactation: Discontinue drug or bottle feed.
Use Cautiously in: Patients with Parkinson's Disease or dementia with Lewy Bodies (↑ sensitivity to effects of antipsychotics); History of suicide attempt; Patients at risk for aspiration pneumonia; History of seizures; Conditions which may ↑ body temperature (strenuous exercise, exposure to extreme heat, concurrent anticholinergics or risk of dehydration); ↓ GI transit time (may ↑ blood levels); May mask symptoms of some drug overdoses, intestinal obstruction, Reye's Syndrome or brain tumor (due to antiemetic effect); Diabetes mellitus; Severe hepatic impairment; Renal impairment (dose ↓ recommended if CCr <80 mL/min); OB: Safety not established; use only if maternal benefit outweighs fetal risk; Pedi: Safety not established; Geri: ↑ risk of mortality in elderly patients treated for dementia-related psychosis; consider age-related ↓ in renal function.

Adverse Reactions/Side Effects

CNS: NEUROLEPTIC MALIGNANT SYNDROME, SUICIDAL THOUGHTS, drowsiness, headache, anxiety, confusion, dizziness, extrapyramidal disorders (dose related), fatigue, Parkinsonism (dose related), syncope, tardive dyskinesia, weakness. **EENT:** blurred vision. **Resp:** dyspnea, cough. **CV:** palpitations, tachycardia (dose related), bradycardia, orthostatic hypotension, ↑ QTc interval. **GI:** abdominal pain, dry mouth, dyspepsia, nausea, swollen tongue. **GU:** impotence, priapism. **Endo:** amenorrhea, galactorrhea, gynecomastia, hyperglycemia. **Hemat:** AGRANULOCYTOSIS, leukopenia, neutropenia. **MS:** back pain, dystonia (dose related). **Neuro:** akithisia, dyskinesia, tremor (dose related). **Misc:** fever.

Interactions

Drug-Drug: ↑ risk of CNS depression with other **CNS depressants** including **alcohol**, **antihistamines**, **sedative/hypnotics**, or **opioid analgesics**. May antagonize the effects of **levodopa** or other **dopamine agonists**. ↑ risk of orthostatic hypotension with **antihypertensives**, **nitrates**, or other **agents that lower blood pressure**. **Carbamazepine** may ↓ levels/effects.

Route/Dosage

Schizophrenia

PO (Adults): 6 mg/day; may titrate by 3 mg/day at intervals of at least 5 days (range 3–12 mg/day).
IM (Adults): 234 mg initially, then 156 mg one week later; continue with monthly maintenance dose of 117 mg (range of 39–234 mg based on efficacy and/or tolerability).

Renal Impairment

PO (Adults): *CCr 50–79 mL/min*—3 mg/day initially; dose may be ↑ to maximum of 6 mg/day; *CCr 10–<50 mL/min*—1.5 mg/day initially; dose may be ↑ to maximum of 3 mg/day.

Renal Impairment

IM (Adults): *CCr 50–79 mL/min*—156 mg initially, then 117 mg one week later; continue with monthly maintenance dose of 78 mg; *CCr <50 mL/min*—Contraindicated.

Schizoaffective Disorder

PO (Adults): 6 mg/day; may titrate by 3 mg/day at intervals of at least 4 days (range 3–12 mg/day).

Renal Impairment

PO (Adults): *CCr 50–79 mL/min*—3 mg/day initially; dose may be ↑ to maximum of 6 mg/day; *CCr 10–<50 mL/min*—1.5 mg/day initially; dose may be ↑ to maximum of 3 mg/day.

Availability

Extended-release tablets (Invega): 1.5 mg, 3 mg, 6 mg, 9 mg. **Intramuscular injection (Invega Sustenna):** 39 mg, 78 mg, 117 mg, 156 mg, 234 mg.

NURSING IMPLICATIONS

Assessment

- Monitor patient's mental status (orientation, mood, behavior) before and periodically during therapy. Monitor closely for notable changes in behavior that could indicate the emergence or worsening of suicidal thoughts or behavior or depression, especially during early therapy. Restrict amount of drug available to patient.
- Assess weight and BMI initially and throughout therapy.
- Monitor blood pressure (sitting, standing, lying down) and pulse before and periodically during therapy. May cause prolonged QT interval, tachycardia, and orthostatic hypotension.
- Observe patient when administering medication to ensure that medication is actually swallowed and not hoarded or cheeked.
- Monitor patient for onset of extrapyramidal side effects (*akathisia*—restlessness; *dystonia*—muscle spasms and twisting motions; or *pseudoparkinsonism*—mask-like face, rigidity, tremors, drooling, shuffling gait, dysphagia). Report these symptoms; reduction of dose or discontinuation of medication may be necessary.
- Monitor for tardive dyskinesia (involuntary rhythmic movement of mouth, face, and extremities). Report immediately; may be irreversible.
- Monitor for development of neuroleptic malignant syndrome (fever, respiratory distress, tachycardia, seizures, diaphoresis, hypertension or hypotension, pallor, tiredness). Discontinue paliperidone and notify health care professional immediately if these symptoms occur.
- Monitor for symptoms related to hyperprolactinemia (menstrual abnormalities, galactorrhea, sexual dysfunction).
- **Lab Test Considerations:** Monitor fasting blood glucose and cholesterol levels before and periodically during therapy.
- Monitor serum prolactin prior to and periodically during therapy. May cause ↑ serum prolactin levels.

- Monitor CBC frequently during initial months of therapy in patients with pre-existing or history of low WBC. May cause leukopenia, neutropenia, or agranulocytosis. Discontinue therapy if this occurs.

Potential Nursing Diagnoses
Risk for self-directed violence (Indications)
Impaired oral mucous membrane (Side Effects)
Disturbed sensory perception : (specify: visual, auditory, kinesthetic, gustatory, tactile, olfactory) (Indications)

Implementation
- **PO:** Administer once daily in the morning without regard to food. Tablets should be swallowed whole; do not crush, break or chew.
- **IM:** Administer initial and second doses in deltoid using a 1 ½-inch, 22G needle for patients ≥90 kg (≥200 lb) or 1-inch 23G needle for patients <90 kg (<200 lb). Monthly maintenance doses can be administered in either deltoid or gluteal sites. For gluteal injection, use 1 ½-inch, 22G needle regardless of patient weight. To avoid missed dose, may give second dose 2 days before or after the one-week timepoint. Monthly doses may be given up to 7 days before or after the monthly timepoint. *After 1st month, if missed dose is within 6 wk of scheduled dose,* administer previous dose as soon as possible. *If >6 wk and <6 mo of scheduled dose,* resume with previous dose by administering dose in deltoid as soon as possible, a second dose in deltoid in 1 wk, followed by monthly doses in deltoid or gluteal sites. *If >6 mo since scheduled dose,* administer using initial dosing schedule.

Patient/Family Teaching
- Instruct patient to take medication as directed. Advise patient that appearance of tablets in stool is normal and not of concern.
- Inform patient of the possibility of extrapyramidal symptoms. Instruct patient to report these symptoms immediately to health care professional.
- Advise patient to change positions slowly to minimize orthostatic hypotension.
- May cause drowsiness. Caution patient to avoid driving or other activities requiring alertness until response to medication is known.
- Advise patient and family to notify health care professional if thoughts about suicide or dying, attempts to commit suicide; new or worse depression; new or worse anxiety; feeling very agitated or restless; panic attacks; trouble sleeping; new or worse irritability; acting aggressive; being angry or violent; acting on dangerous impulses; an extreme increase in activity and talking, other unusual changes in behavior or mood occur.
- Advise patient that extremes in temperature should also be avoided; this drug impairs body temperature regulation.
- Caution patient to avoid concurrent use of alcohol, other CNS depressants, and Rx, OTC, or herbal products without consulting health care professional.
- Advise patient to seek nutritional, weight, or medical management as needed for weight gain or cholesterol elevation.
- Advise female patients to notify health care professional if pregnancy is planned or suspected, or if breastfeeding or planning to breastfeed.
- Advise patient to notify health care professional of medication regimen before treatment or surgery.
- Instruct patient to notify health care professional promptly if sore throat, fever, unusual bleeding or bruising, rash, tremors, menstrual abnormalities, galactorrhea, or sexual dysfunction occur.
- Emphasize the importance of routine follow-up exams to monitor side effects and continued participation in psychotherapy to improve coping skills.

Evaluation/Desired Outcomes
- Decrease in excited, manic behavior.
- Decrease in positive symptoms (delusions, hallucinations) of schizophrenia.
- Decrease in negative symptoms (social withdrawal, flat, blunted affect) of schizophrenia.

---

palonosetron
(pa-lone-**o**-se-tron)
Aloxi

Classification
Therapeutic: antiemetics
Pharmacologic: 5-HT$_3$ antagonists

Pregnancy Category B

Indications
Prevention of acute and delayed nausea and vomiting caused by initial or repeat courses of moderate or highly emetogenic chemotherapy (intravenous). Prevention of acute nausea and vomiting

caused by initial or repeat courses of moderately emetogenic chemotherapy (oral). Prevention of postoperative nausea and vomiting (PONV) for up to 24 hr after surgery (intravenous).

Action
Blocks the effects of serotonin at receptor sites (selective antagonist) located in vagal nerve terminals and in the chemoreceptor trigger zones in the CNS. **Therapeutic Effects:** Decreased incidence and severity of nausea and vomiting following emetogenic chemotherapy or surgery.

Pharmacokinetics
Absorption: IV administration results in complete bioavailability; oral bioavailability = 97%.
Distribution: Unknown.
Metabolism and Excretion: 50% metabolized; 40% excreted unchanged in urine.
Half-life: 40 hr.

TIME/ACTION PROFILE

ROUTE	ONSET	PEAK	DURATION
IV	within 30 min	unknown	7 days
PO	within 1 hr	unknown	7 days

Contraindications/Precautions
Contraindicated in: Hypersensitivity; cross sensitivity with other 5-HT$_3$ antagonists may occur; Lactation: Lactation.
Use Cautiously in: OB, Pedi: Safety not established.

Adverse Reactions/Side Effects
CNS: dizziness, headache. **GI:** constipation, diarrhea.

Interactions
Drug-Drug: None significant.

Route/Dosage
IV (Adults): *Prevention of chemotherapy-induced nausea/vomiting*—0.25 mg 30 min before start of chemotherapy; *Prevention of PONV*—0.075 mg given immediately before induction of anesthesia.

PO (Adults): 0.5 mg 1 hr before start of chemotherapy.

Availability
Solution for IV injection: 0.05 mg/mL. **Capsules:** 0.5 mg.

NURSING IMPLICATIONS

Assessment
- Assess patient for nausea, vomiting, abdominal distention, and bowel sounds prior to and following administration.

- **Lab Test Considerations:** May cause transient ↑ in serum bilirubin, AST, and ALT levels.

Potential Nursing Diagnoses
Imbalanced nutrition: less than body requirements (Indications)
Diarrhea (Side Effects)
Constipation (Side Effects)

Implementation
- First dose is administered prior to emetogenic event.
- Repeated dose within a 7 day period is not recommended.
- PO: May be administered with or without food 1 hr prior to the start of chemotherapy.

IV Administration
- **Direct IV:** Administer dose undiluted 30 min prior to chemotherapy or immediately prior to the induction of anesthesia. Flush line prior to and after administration with 0.9% NaCl. Do not administer solutions that are discolored or contain particulate matter. ***Concentration:*** 0.05 mg/mL. ***Rate:*** Administer over 30 seconds for chemotherapy and over 10 seconds for postoperative nausea and vomiting.
- **Syringe Compatibility:** dexamethasone.
- **Y-Site Compatibility:** alfentanil, amifostine, amikacin, aminocaproic acid, aminophylline, amiodarone, amphotericin B liposome, ampicillin, ampicillin/sulbactam, atracurium, atropine, azithromycin, aztreonam, bivalirudin, bleomycin, bretylium, bumetanide, buprenorphine, busulfan, butorphanol, calcium acetate, calcium chloride, calcium gluconate, carboplatin, carmustine, caspofungin, cefazolin, cefepime, cefotaxime, cefotetan, cefoxitin, ceftazidime, ceftizoxime, ceftriaxone, cefuroxime, chloramphenicol, chlorpromazine, cimetidine, ciprofloxacin, cisatracurium, cisplatin, clindamycin, cyclophosphamide, cyclosporine, cytarabine, dacarbazine, dactinomycin, dantrolene, daptomycin, daunorubicin, dexamethasone sodium phosphate, dexmedetomidine, dexrazoxane, digoxin, diltiazem, diphenhydramine, dobutamine, docetaxel, dopamine, doxacurium, doxorubicin hydrochloride, droperidol, enalaprilat, ephedrine, epinephrine, epirubicin, eptifibitide, erythromycin, esmolol, etoposide, etoposide phosphate, famotidine, fenoldopam, fentanyl, fluconazole, fludarabine, fluorouracil, foscarnet, fosphenytoin, furosemide, gemcitabine, gentamicin, glycopyrrolate, haloperidol, heparin, hydralazine, hydrocortisone, hydromorphone, idarubicin, ifosfamide, inamrinone,

insulin, irinotecan, isoproterenol, ketorolac, labetalol, leucovorin, levofloxacin, lidocaine, linezolid, lorazepam, magnesium sulfate, mannitol, mechlorethamine, melphalan, meperidine, meropenem, mesna, metaraminol, methotrexate, methyldopate, metoclopramide, metoprolol, metronidazole, midazolam, milrinone, mitomycin, mitoxantrone, mivacurium, morphine, nalbuphine, naloxone, neostigmine, nesiritide, nicardipine, nitroglycerin, nitroprusside, norepinephrine, octreotide, oxaliplatin, oxytocin, paclitaxel, pamidronate, pancuronium, pentazocine, phenobarbital, phentolamine, phenylephrine, piperacillin/tazobactam, potassium acetate, potassium chloride, potassium phosphates, procainamide, prochlorperazine, promethazine, propranolol, quinupristin/dalfopristin, ranitidine, remifentanil, rocuronium, sodium acetate, sodium bicarbonate, sodium phosphates, streptozocin, succinylcholine, sufentanil, tacrolimus, teniposide, theophylline, thiotepa, ticarcillin/clavulanate, tigecycline, tirofiban, tobramycin, topotecan, trimethobenzamide, trimethoprim/sulfamethoxazole, vancomycin, vasopressin, vecuronium, verapamil, vinblastine, vincristine, vinorelbine, zidovudine.

- **Y-Site Incompatibility:** acyclovir, allopurinol, amphotericin B colloidal, diazepam, doxycycline, ganciclovir, imipenem/cilastatin, methylprednisolone, minocycline, nafcillin, pantoprazole, pentamidine, pentobarbital, phenytoin, thiopental.

Patient/Family Teaching
- Inform patient of purpose of medication.
- Advise patient to notify health care professional if nausea or vomiting occur.

Evaluation/Desired Outcomes
- Prevention of nausea and vomiting associated with initial and repeat courses of emetogenic cancer chemotherapy or surgery.

---

pamidronate (pa-mid-roe-nate)
Aredia

Classification
Therapeutic: bone resorption inhibitors
Pharmacologic: biphosphonates, hypocalcemics

Pregnancy Category D

Indications
Moderate to severe hypercalcemia associated with malignancy. Osteolytic bone lesions associated with multiple myeloma or breast cancer. Moderate to severe Paget's disease.

Action
Inhibits resorption of bone. **Therapeutic Effects:** Decreased serum calcium. Decreased skeletal destruction in multiple myeloma or breast cancer. Decreased skeletal complications in Paget's disease.

Pharmacokinetics
Absorption: IV administration results in complete bioavailability.
Distribution: Rapidly absorbed by bone. Reaches high concentrations in bone, liver, spleen, teeth, and tracheal cartilage. Approximately 50% of a dose is retained by bone and then slowly released.
Metabolism and Excretion: 50% is excreted unchanged in the urine.
Half-life: Elimination half-life from plasma is biphasic—1st phase 1.6 hr, 2nd phase 27.2 hr. Elimination half-life from bone is 300 days.

TIME/ACTION PROFILE (effect on serum calcium)

ROUTE	ONSET	PEAK	DURATION
IV	24 hr	7 days	unknown

Contraindications/Precautions
Contraindicated in: Hypersensitivity to pamidronate, other biphosphonates, or mannitol; OB, Lactation: Pregnancy or lactation.
Use Cautiously in: Underlying cardiovascular disease, especially CHF (initiate saline hydration cautiously); Concurrent dental surgery (may ↑ risk of jaw osteonecrosis); History of thyroid surgery (may be at ↑ risk for hypocalcemia); Renal impairment (dose ↓ recommended); Pedi: Safety not established.

Adverse Reactions/Side Effects
CNS: fatigue. **EENT:** conjunctivitis, blurred vision, eye pain/inflammation, rhinitis. **Resp:** rales. **CV:** arrhythmias, hypertension, syncope, tachycardia. **GI:** nausea, abdominal pain, anorexia, constipation, vomiting. **F and E:** hypocalcemia, hypokalemia, hypomagnesemia, hypophosphatemia, fluid overload. **GU:** nephrotoxicity. **Hemat:** leukopenia, anemia. **Local:** phlebitis at injection site. **Metab:** hypothyroidism. **MS:** muscle

stiffness, musculoskeletal pain, osteonecrosis (primarily of jaw). **Misc:** fever, generalized pain.

Interactions
Drug-Drug: Hypokalemia and hypomagnesemia may ↑ risk of **digoxin** toxicity. **Calcium** and **vitamin D** will antagonize the beneficial effects of pamidronate. Concurrent use of **thalidomide** may ↑ risk of renal dysfunction.

Route/Dosage
Single doses should not exceed 90 mg.

Hypercalcemia of Malignancy
IV (Adults): *Moderate hypercalcemia*—30–90 mg; may be repeated after 7 days.

Osteolytic Lesions from Multiple Myeloma
IV (Adults): 90 mg monthly.

Osteolytic Lesions from Metastatic Breast Cancer
IV (Adults): 90 mg q 3–4 wk.

Paget's Disease
IV (Adults): 90–180 mg/treatment; may be given as 30 mg daily for 3 days up to 30 mg/wk for 6 wk. Single doses of 60–90 mg may also be effective.

Availability (generic available)
Powder for injection: 30 mg/vial, 90 mg/vial.

NURSING IMPLICATIONS

Assessment
- Monitor intake/output ratios and blood pressure frequently during therapy. Assess for signs of fluid overload (edema, rales/crackles).
- Monitor symptoms of hypercalcemia (nausea, vomiting, anorexia, weakness, constipation, thirst, and cardiac arrhythmias).
- Observe for evidence of hypocalcemia (paresthesia, muscle twitching, laryngospasm, and Chvostek's or Trousseau's sign). Protect symptomatic patients by elevating and padding side rails; keep bed in low position.
- Monitor IV site for phlebitis (pain, redness, swelling). Symptomatic treatment should be used if this occurs.
- Assess for bone pain. Treatment with nonopioid or opioid analgesics may be necessary.
- *Lab Test Considerations:* Assess serum creatinine prior to each treatment. Withhold dose if renal function has deteriorated in patients treated for bone metastases.
- Monitor serum electrolytes (including calcium, phosphate, potassium, and magnesium), hemoglobin, and creatinine closely. Monitor CBC and platelet count during the first 2 wk of therapy. May cause hyperkalemia or hypokalemia, hypernatremia, and hematuria.
- Monitor renal function periodically during therapy.

Potential Nursing Diagnoses
Acute pain (Indications, Side Effects)
Risk for injury (Indications)

Implementation
- Initiate a vigorous saline hydration, maintaining a urine output of 2000 mL/24 hr, concurrently with pamidronate therapy. Patients should be adequately hydrated, but avoid overhydration. Use caution in patients with underlying cardiovascular disease, especially CHF. Do not use diuretics prior to treatment of hypovolemia.
- Patients with severe hypercalcemia should be started at the 90-mg dose.

IV Administration

- **IV:** Reconstitute by adding 10 mL of sterile water for injection to each vial. *Concentration:* 30 mg/10 mL or 90 mg/10 mL. Allow drug to dissolve before withdrawing. Solution is stable for 24 hr if refrigerated.
- **Hypercalcemia:** *Diluent:* Dilute further in 1000 mL of 0.45% NaCl, 0.9% NaCl, or D5W. Solution is stable for 24 hr at room temperature. *Rate:* Administer 60-mg infusion over at least 4 hr and 90-mg infusion over 24 hr.
- **Multiple Myeloma:** *Diluent:* Dilute reconstituted solution in 500 mL of 0.45% NaCl, 0.9% NaCl, or D5W. *Rate:* Administer over 4 hr.
- **Paget's Disease:** Dilute reconstituted solution in 500 mL of 0.45% NaCl, 0.9% NaCl, or D5W.
- *Rate:* Administer over 4 hr.
- **Y-Site Compatibility:** bivalirudin, daptomycin, ertapenem, nesiritide, octreotide, oxytocin, palonosetron, pemetrexed, teniposide, thiotepa, tigecycline, tirofiban, voriconazole.
- **Y-Site Incompatibility:** caspofungin.
- **Additive Incompatibility:** Calcium-containing solutions, such as Ringer's solution.

Patient/Family Teaching
- Advise patient to report signs of hypercalcemic relapse (bone pain, anorexia, nausea, vomiting, thirst, lethargy) or eye problems (pain, inflammation, blurred vision, conjunctivitis) to health care professional promptly.
- Advise patient to notify nurse of pain at the infusion site.

- Encourage patient to comply with dietary recommendations. Diet should contain adequate amounts of calcium and vitamin D.
- Advise patient to notify health care professional if bone pain is severe or persistent.
- Advise patient to inform health care professional of pamidronate therapy prior to dental surgery.
- Emphasize the need for keeping follow-up exams to monitor progress, even after medication is discontinued, to detect relapse.

Evaluation/Desired Outcomes
- Lowered serum calcium levels.
- Decreased pain from lytic lesions.

pancrelipase (pan-kre-li-pase)
Creon, Enzymase-16, Ilozyme, Pancrease MT 4, Pancrease MT 10, Pancrease MT 16, Pancrease MT 20, Pancrebarb MS-8, Ultrase MT 12, Ultrase MT 20, Viokase, Zenpep

Classification
Therapeutic: digestive agent
Pharmacologic: pancreatic enzymes

Pregnancy Category C

Indications
Pancreatic insufficiency associated with: Chronic pancreatitis, Pancreatectomy, Cystic fibrosis, GI bypass surgery, Ductal obstruction secondary to tumor.

Action
Contains lipolytic, amylolytic, and proteolytic activity. **Therapeutic Effects:** Increased digestion of fats, carbohydrates, and proteins in the GI tract.

Pharmacokinetics
Absorption: Unknown.
Distribution: Unknown.
Metabolism and Excretion: Unknown.
Half-life: Unknown.

TIME/ACTION PROFILE (digestant effects)

ROUTE	ONSET	PEAK	DURATION
PO	rapid	unknown	unknown

Contraindications/Precautions
Contraindicated in: Hypersensitivity to hog proteins.
Use Cautiously in: OB, Lactation: Safety not established.

Adverse Reactions/Side Effects
EENT: nasal stuffiness. **Resp:** dyspnea, shortness of breath, wheezing. **GI:** abdominal pain (high doses only), diarrhea, nausea, stomach cramps, oral irritation. **GU:** hematuria. **Derm:** hives, rash. **Metab:** hyperuricemia. **Misc:** allergic reactions.

Interactions
Drug-Drug: Antacids (**calcium carbonate** or **magnesium hydroxide**) may ↓ effectiveness of pancrelipase. May ↓ the absorption of concurrently administered **iron supplements**.
Drug-Food: Alkaline foods destroy coating on enteric-coated products.

Route/Dosage
PO (Adults): 1–3 capsule(s) before or with meals; dose may be increased as needed (up to 8 capsules may be needed), *or* 1–2 delayed-release capsule(s), *or* 0.7 g powder.
PO (Children): 1–3 capsule(s) before or with meals; dose may be increased as needed, *or* 1–2 delayed-release capsule(s), *or* 0.7 g powder.

Availability (generic available)
Capsules: 8000 units lipase/30,000 units protease and amylase. **Delayed-release capsules:** 4000 units lipase/12,000 units protease and amylase, 4000 units lipase/25,000 units protease/25,000 units amylase, 4500 units lipase/25,000 units protease/20,000 units amylase, 5000 units lipase/17,000 units protease/27,000 units amylase, 6000 units lipase/19,000 units protease/30,000 units amylase, 8000 units lipase/45,000 units protease/40,000 units amylase, ❋ 8000 units lipase/30,000 units protease and amylase, 10,000 units lipase/30,000 units protease and amylase, 10000 units lipase/34,000 units protease/55,000 units amylase, 12,000 units lipase/39,000 units protease and amylase, 12,000 units lipase/38,000 units protease/60,000 units amylase, 15,000 units lipase/51,000 units protease/82,000 units amylase, 16,000 units lipase/48,000 units protease and amylase, 16,000 units lipase/52,000 units protease and amylase, 20,000 units lipase/44,000 units protease/56,000 units amylase, ❋ 20,000 units lipase/55,000 units protease and amylase, 20,000 units lipase/65,000 units protease and amylase, 20,000 units lipase/68,000 units protease/109,000 units amylase, 24,000 units lipase/76,000 units protease/120,000 units amylase. **Powder:** 16,800 units lipase/70,000 units protease and amylase.

❋ = Canadian drug name. ❋ = Genetic implication.
*CAPITALS indicates life-threatening; underlines indicate most frequent.

NURSING IMPLICATIONS
Assessment
- Assess patient's nutritional status (height, weight, skin-fold thickness, arm muscle circumference, and lab values) prior to and periodically throughout therapy.
- Monitor stools for high fat content (steatorrhea). Stools will be foul-smelling and frothy.
- Assess patient for allergy to pork; sensitivity to pancrelipase may exist.
- *Lab Test Considerations:* May cause ↑ serum and urine uric acid concentrations.

Potential Nursing Diagnoses
Imbalanced nutrition: less than body requirements (Indications)

Implementation
- **PO:** Administer immediately before or with meals and snacks.
- Swallow capsules whole. If unable to swallow, capsules may be opened and sprinkled on foods. Capsules filled with enteric-coated beads should not be chewed (sprinkle on soft, acidic foods that can be swallowed without chewing, such as applesauce or Jell-O).
- Pancrelipase is destroyed by acid. Concurrent sodium bicarbonate or aluminum-containing antacids may be used with nonenteric-coated preparations to neutralize gastric pH. Enteric-coated beads are designed to withstand the acid pH of the stomach. These medications should not be chewed or mixed with alkaline foods prior to ingestion or coating will be destroyed.
- Do not mix *Zenpep* capsule contents directly into formula or breast milk prior to administration. Administer with applesauce, bananas, or pears (commercially prepared) and follow with breast milk or formula. *Zenpep* product is not interchangeable with other pancrealipase products.

Patient/Family Teaching
- Encourage patients to comply with diet recommendations of health care professional (generally high-calorie, high-protein, low-fat). Dose should be adjusted for fat content of diet. Usually 300 mg of pancrelipase is necessary to digest every 17 g of dietary fat. If a dose is missed, it should be omitted.
- Instruct patient not to chew tablets and to swallow them quickly with plenty of liquid to prevent mouth and throat irritation. Patient should be sitting upright to enhance swallowing. Eating immediately after taking medication helps further ensure that the medication is swallowed and does not remain in contact with mouth and esophagus for a prolonged period. Patient should avoid sniffing powdered contents of capsules, as sensitization of nose and throat may occur (nasal stuffiness or respiratory distress).
- Instruct patient to notify health care professional if joint pain, swelling of legs, gastric distress, or rash occurs.
- Advise female patients to notify health care professional if pregnancy is planned or suspected.

Evaluation/Desired Outcomes
- Improved nutritional status in patients with pancreatic insufficiency.
- Normalization of stools in patients with steatorrhea.

HIGH ALERT

pancuronium
(pan-cure-**oh**-nee-yum)

Classification
Therapeutic: neuromuscular blocking agents—nondepolarizing

Pregnancy Category C

Indications
Induction of skeletal muscle paralysis and facilitation of intubation after induction of anesthesia in surgical procedures. Facilitation of compliance during mechanical ventilation.

Action
Prevents neuromuscular transmission by blocking the effect of acetylcholine at the myoneural junction. Has no analgesic or anxiolytic properties.
Therapeutic Effects: Skeletal muscle paralysis.

Pharmacokinetics
Absorption: Following IV administration, absorption is essentially complete.
Distribution: Rapidly distributes into extracellular fluid; small amounts cross the placenta.
Metabolism and Excretion: Excreted mostly unchanged by the kidneys; small amounts are eliminated in bile.
Half-life: 2 hr.

TIME/ACTION PROFILE (neuromuscular blockade)

ROUTE	ONSET	PEAK	DURATION
IV	30–45 sec	3–4.5 min	40–60 min

Contraindications/Precautions
Contraindicated in: Hypersensitivity; Hypersensitivity to bromides; Lactation: Lactation.

Use Cautiously in: Patients with underlying cardiovascular disease (↑ risk of arrhythmias); Dehydration or electrolyte abnormalities (should be corrected); Situations in which histamine release would be problematic; Fractures or muscle spasm; Patients with impaired renal function (↓ elimination); Hyperthermia (↑ duration/intensity of paralysis); Patients with significant hepatic impairment (altered response); Shock; Extensive burns (may be more resistant to effects); Low plasma pseudocholinesterase levels (may be seen in association with anemia, dehydration, cholinesterase inhibitors/insecticides, severe liver disease, pregnancy, or hereditary predisposition); Obese patients; OB: Safety not established; may be used during caesarian section; Pedi: Contains benzyl alcohol which can cause potentially fatal gasping syndrome in neonates; Geri: Age-related ↓ in renal function may result in prolonged effects.
Exercise Extreme Caution in: Patients with neuromuscular diseases such as myasthenia gravis (small test dose may be used to assess response).

Adverse Reactions/Side Effects
Resp: bronchospasm. **CV:** hypertension, tachycardia. **GI:** excessive salivation. **Derm:** rash. **Misc:** allergic reactions including ANAPHYLAXIS.

Interactions
Drug-Drug: Intensity and duration of paralysis may be prolonged by pretreatment with **succinylcholine**, **general anesthesia** (inhalation), **aminoglycosides**, **vancomycin**, **tetracyclines**, **polymyxin B**, **colistin**, **cyclosporine**, **calcium channel blockers**, **clindamycin**, **lidocaine**, and other **local anesthetics**, **lithium**, **quinidine**, **procainamide**, **beta blockers**, **potassium-losing diuretics**, or **magnesium**. **Inhalation anesthetics** including **enflurane**, **isoflurane**, **halothane**, **desflurane**, **sevoflurane** may enhance effects. Higher infusion rates may be required and duration of action may be shortened in patients receiving long-term **carbamazepine**, **steroids (chronic)**, **azathioprine** or **phenytoin**.

Route/Dosage
IV (Adults and Children >12 yr): 0.15 mg/kg initially; incremental doses of 0.15 mg/kg may be given q 20–60 min as needed to maintain paralysis or as a continuous infusion of 0.02–0.04 mg/kg/hr or 0.4–0.6 mcg/kg/min. .
IV (Children > 1 yr): 0.15 mg/kg q 30–60 min as needed or as a continuous infusion of 0.03–0.1 mg/kg/hr or 0.5–1.7 mcg/kg/min.
IV (Neonates and Infants): 0.1 mg/kg q 30–60 min as needed or as a continuous infusion of 0.02–0.04 mg/kg/hr or 0.4–0.6 mcg/kg/min.

Availability (generic available)
Injection: 1 mg/mL, 2 mg/mL.

NURSING IMPLICATIONS

Assessment
- Assess respiratory status continuously throughout therapy with neuromuscular blocking agents. These medications should be used only to facilitate intubation or in patients already intubated.
- Neuromuscular response should be monitored with a peripheral nerve stimulator intraoperatively. Paralysis is initially selective and usually occurs sequentially in the following muscles: levator muscles of eyelids, muscles of mastication, limb muscles, abdominal muscles, muscles of the glottis, intercostal muscles, and the diaphragm. Recovery of muscle function usually occurs in reverse order.
- Monitor ECG, heart rate, and blood pressure throughout administration.
- Observe the patient for residual muscle weakness and respiratory distress during the recovery period.
- Monitor infusion site frequently. If signs of tissue irritation or extravasation occur, discontinue and restart in another vein.
- ***Toxicity and Overdose:*** If overdose occurs, use peripheral nerve stimulator to determine the degree of neuromuscular blockade. Maintain airway patency and ventilation until recovery of normal respirations occurs.
- Administration of anticholinesterase agents (neostigmine, pyridostigmine) may be used to antagonize the action of neuromuscular blocking agents once the patient has demonstrated some spontaneous recovery from neuromuscular block. Atropine is usually administered prior to or concurrently with anticholinesterase agents to counteract the muscarinic effects.
- Administration of fluids and vasopressors may be necessary to treat severe hypotension or shock.

Potential Nursing Diagnoses
Ineffective breathing pattern (Indications)
Impaired verbal communication (Side Effects)
Fear (Side Effects)

Implementation

- **High Alert:** Unintended administration of a neuromuscular blocking agent instead of administration of the intended medication or administration of a neuromuscular blocking agent in the absence of ventilatory support has resulted in serious harm or death. Confusing similarities in packaging and insufficiently controlled access to these medications are often implicated in these medication errors. Store these products in a separate, locked container.
- Dose is titrated to patient response.
- Neuromuscular blocking agents have *no* effect on consciousness or pain threshold. Adequate anesthesia/analgesia should *always* be used when neuromuscular blocking agents are used as an adjunct to surgical procedures or when painful procedures are performed. Benzodiazepines and/or analgesics should be administered concurrently when prolonged neuromuscular blocker therapy is used for ventilator patients, because patient is awake and able to feel all sensations.
- If eyes remain open throughout prolonged administration, protect corneas with artificial tears.
- Store pancuronium in refrigerator. To prevent absorption by plastic, pancuronium should not be stored in plastic syringes. May be administered in plastic syringes.
- Most neuromuscular blocking agents are incompatible with barbiturates and sodium bicarbonate. Do not admix.

IV Administration

- **Direct IV:** *Diluent:* May be administered undiluted. *Concentration:* 1 mg/mL (10-mL vial); 2 mg/mL (2-mL or 5-mL vial). *Rate:* Administer over 1–2 min.
- **Intermittent Infusion:** *Diluent:* Add 100 mg of pancuroniuum to 250 mL of D5W, 0.9% NaCl, D5/0.9% NaCl, or LR. *Concentration:* 0.4 mg/mL. *Rate:* Based on patient's weight (see Route/Dosage section).
- **Y-Site Compatibility:** aminophylline, cefazolin, cefuroxime, cimetidine, daptomycin, diltiazem, dobutamine, dopamine, epinephrine, ertapenem, esmolol, etomidate, fenoldopam, fentanyl, fluconazole, gentamicin, granisetron, heparin, hydrocortisone sodium succinate, hydromorphone, isoproterenol, levofloxacin, linezolid, lorazepam, midazolam, morphine, nitroglycerin, nitroprusside, palonosetron, piperacillin/tazobactam, quinupristin/dalfopristin, ranitidine, trimethoprim/sulfamethoxazole, tacrolimus, tirofiban, vancomycin, voriconazole.
- **Y-Site Incompatibility:** caspofungin, diazepam, pantoprazole, thiopental.

Patient/Family Teaching

- Explain all procedures to patient receiving neuromuscular blocker therapy without general anesthesia, because consciousness is not affected by neuromuscular blocking agents alone.
- Reassure patient that communication abilities will return as the medication wears off.

Evaluation/Desired Outcomes

- Adequate suppression of the twitch response when tested with peripheral nerve stimulation and subsequent muscle paralysis.
- Improved compliance during mechanical ventilation.

---

panitumumab
(pan-i-**tu**-mu-mab)
Vectibix

Classification
Therapeutic: antineoplastics
Pharmacologic: monoclonal antibodies

Pregnancy Category C

Indications
Treatment of metastatic colorectal cancer that expresses EGFR (epidermal growth factor receptor) and has failed conventional treatments (to be used as monotherapy).

Action
Binds to EGFR resulting in inactivation of kinases that regulate proliferation and transformation.
Therapeutic Effects: Decreased progression of colorectal cancer.

Pharmacokinetics
Absorption: IV administration results in complete bioavailability.
Distribution: Monoclonal antibodies cross the placenta and enter breast milk.
Metabolism and Excretion: Unknown.
Half-life: 7.5 days.

TIME/ACTION PROFILE

ROUTE	ONSET	PEAK	DURATION
IV	unknown	end of infusion	unknown

Contraindications/Precautions
Contraindicated in: Concurrent leucovorin; Patients whose tumors have KRAS mutations in

panitumumab

codon 12 or 13 (not effective); OB, Lactation: Pregnancy or lactation.
Use Cautiously in: Pedi: Safety not established.

Adverse Reactions/Side Effects
CNS: <u>fatigue</u>. **EENT:** OCULAR TOXICITY, eyelash growth. **Resp:** PULMONARY FIBROSIS, <u>cough</u>. **GI:** <u>abdominal pain</u>, <u>constipation</u>, <u>diarrhea</u>, <u>nausea</u>, vomiting, stomatitis. **Derm:** DERMATOLOGIC TOXICITY, <u>paromychia</u>, photosensitivity. **F and E:** <u>edema</u>, hypocalcemia, <u>hypomagnesemia</u>. **Misc:** INFUSION REACTIONS.

Interactions
Drug-Drug: None noted.

Route/Dosage
IV (Adults): 6 mg/kg as a 60-min infusion every 14 days; ↓ infusion rates and dose modifications are recommended for infusion reactions and other serious toxicities.

Availability
Solution for IV administration (requires dilution): 20 mg/mL in 5-mL vials (100 mg/vial).

NURSING IMPLICATIONS

Assessment
- Assess for dermatologic toxicity (dermatitis acneiform, pruritus, erythema, rash, skin exfoliation, paronychia, dry skin, skin fissures). If severe, may lead to infection (sepsis, septic death, abscesses requiring incision and drainage). With severe reactions, withhold panitumumab and monitor for inflammatory or infectious sequelae.
- Monitor for severe infusion reactions (anaphylactic reaction, bronchospasm, fever, chills, hypotension). If severe reaction occurs, stop panitumumab; may require permanent discontinuation.
- Assess for pulmonary fibrosis (cough, wheezing, exertional dyspnea, interstitial lung disease, pneumonitis, lung infiltrates). Permanently discontinue panitumumab if these signs occur.
- Monitor for diarrhea during therapy.
- ***Lab Test Considerations:*** Monitor electrolyte levels periodically during and for 8 wk after completion of therapy. May cause hypomagnesemia and hypocalcemia.

Potential Nursing Diagnoses
Risk for impaired skin integrity (Adverse Reactions)
Impaired gas exchange (Adverse Reactions)

Implementation

IV Administration

- **Intermittent Infusion:** ***Diluent:*** Withdraw necessary amount of panitumumab. Dilute to a volume of 100 mL with 0.9% NaCl; dilute doses >1000 mg with 150 mL. ***Concentration:*** 10 mg/mL. Mix by inverting gently; do not shake. Administer via infusion pump using a low-protein binding 0.2 mcg or 0.22 mcg in-line filter. Solution is colorless and may contain a small amount of visible translucent to white, amorphous, proteinaceous particles. Do not administer solutions that are discolored or contain particulate matter. Store in refrigerator; do not freeze. Use diluted solution within 6 hr of preparation if stored at room temperature or within 24 hr if refrigerated. ***Rate:*** Administer over 60 min every 14 days. Administer doses >1000 mg over 90 min.
- If mild to moderate infusion reaction (Grade 1 or 2) occurs decrease infusion rate by 50%. If severe reaction (Grade 3 or 4) occurs, immediately and permanently discontinue panitumumab.
- If severe dermatologic toxicities (Grade 3 or higher) or those considered intolerable occur, withhold panitumumab. If toxicity does not improve to ≤ grade 2 within 1 mo, discontinue permanently. If toxicity improves to ≤ grade 2 and patient improves symptomatically after withholding no more than 2 doses, resume therapy at 50% dose. If toxicities recur, permanently discontinue panitumumab. If toxicities do not recur, increase subsequent doses in 25% increments of the original dose until recommended dose of 6 mg/kg is reached.
- **Y-Site Incompatibility:** Flush line before and after administration with 0.9% NaCl. Do not mix with other medications or solutions.

Patient/Family Teaching
- May cause photosensitivity. Caution patient to wear sunscreen and hats and to limit sun exposure.
- Advise patient that panitumumab may cause fertility impairment and may have teratogenic effects. Caution women of childbearing yr to use contraception during and for at least 6 mo after the last dose and not to breastfeed during and for at least 2 mo after the last dose of panitumumab.

- Inform patient of potential for dermatologic toxicity, infusion reactions, pulmonary fibrosis, and impairment of fertility. Advise patient to notify health care professional if skin or ocular changes or dyspnea occur. Advise patient that periodic electrolyte monitoring is required.

Evaluation/Desired Outcomes
- Decreased progression of colorectal cancer.

---

pantoprazole
(pan-**toe**-pra-zole)
◆ Pantoloc, Protonix, Protonix IV

Classification
Therapeutic: antiulcer agents
Pharmacologic: proton-pump inhibitors

Pregnancy Category B

Indications
Erosive esophagitis associated with GERD. Decrease relapse rates of daytime and nighttime heartburn symptoms on patients with GERD. Pathologic gastric hypersecretory conditions. **Unlabeled Use:** Adjunctive treatment of duodenal ulcers associated with *Helicobacter pylori*.

Action
Binds to an enzyme in the presence of acidic gastric pH, preventing the final transport of hydrogen ions into the gastric lumen. **Therapeutic Effects:** Diminished accumulation of acid in the gastric lumen, with lessened acid reflux. Healing of duodenal ulcers and esophagitis. Decreased acid secretion in hypersecretory conditions.

Pharmacokinetics
Absorption: Tablet is enteric-coated; absorption occurs only after tablet leaves the stomach.
Distribution: Unknown.
Protein Binding: 98%.
Metabolism and Excretion: Mostly metabolized by the liver via the cytochrome P450 (CYP) system (primarily CYP2C19 isoenzyme, but also the CYP3A4 isoenzyme) (the CYP2C19 enzyme system exhibits genetic polymorphism; 15–20% of Asian patients and 3–5% of Caucasian and Black patients may be poor metabolizers and may have significantly ↑ pantoprazole concentrations and an ↑ risk of adverse effects); inactive metabolites are excreted in urine (71%) and feces (18%).
Half-life: 1 hr.

TIME/ACTION PROFILE (effect on acid secretion)

ROUTE	ONSET†	PEAK	DURATION†
PO	2.5 hr	unknown	1 wk
IV	15–30 min	2 hr	unknown

†Onset = 51% inhibition; duration = return to normal following discontinuation

Contraindications/Precautions
Contraindicated in: Hypersensitivity; OB: Should be used during pregnancy only if clearly needed. Lactation: Discontinue breastfeeding due to potential for serious adverse reactions in infants.
Use Cautiously in: Pedi: Safety not established.

Adverse Reactions/Side Effects
CNS: headache. **GI:** abdominal pain, diarrhea, eructation, flatulence. **Endo:** hyperglycemia.

Interactions
Drug-Drug: May ↓ absorption of drugs requiring acid pH, including **ketoconazole**, **itraconazole**, **atazanavir**, **ampicillin esters**, and **iron salts**. May ↑ risk of bleeding with **warfarin** (monitor INR/PT). May ↓ the antiplatelet effects of **clopidogrel**.

Route/Dosage
PO (Adults): *GERD*—40 mg once daily; *Gastric hypersecretory conditions*—40 mg twice daily, up to 120 mg twice daily.
PO (Children): 0.5–1 mg/kg/day.
IV (Adults): *GERD*—40 mg once daily for 7–10 days. *Gastric hypersecretory conditions*—80 mg q 12 hr (up to 240 mg/day).

Availability (generic available)
Delayed-release tablets: 20 mg, 40 mg. **Cost:** 20 mg $353.61/90, 40 mg $351.97/90. **Powder for injection:** 40 mg/vial.

NURSING IMPLICATIONS

Assessment
- Assess patient routinely for epigastric or abdominal pain and for frank or occult blood in stool, emesis, or gastric aspirate.
- *Lab Test Considerations:* May cause abnormal liver function tests, including ↑ AST, ALT, alkaline phosphatase, and bilirubin.

Potential Nursing Diagnoses
Acute pain (Indications)

Implementation
- Patients receiving pantoprazole IV should be converted to PO dosing as soon as possible.
- **PO:** May be administered with or without food. Do not break, crush, or chew tablets.

pantoprazole 991

- Antacids may be used concurrently.

IV Administration

- **IV:** Reconstitute each vial with 10 mL of 0.9% NaCl. Reconstituted solution is stable for 6 hr at room temperature.
- **Direct IV:** *Diluent:* Administer undiluted. *Concentration:* 4 mg/mL. *Rate:* Administer over at least 2 min.
- **Intermittent Infusion:** *Diluent:* Dilute further with D5W, 0.9% NaCl, or LR. *Concentration:* 0.4–0.8 mg/mL. Diluted solution is stable for 24 hr at room temperature. *Rate:* Administer over 15 min at a rate of <3 mg/min.
- **Y-Site Compatibility:** acyclovir, allopurinol, amifostine, amikacin, animocaproic acid, aminophylline, amphotericin B liposome, ampicillin, amipcillin/sulbactam, anidulafungin, azithromycin, bleomycin, calcium gluconate, carboplatin, carmustine, cefazolin, cefoxitin, ceftazidime, ceftizoxime, ceftriaxone, cefuroxime, clindamycin, cyclophosphamide, cyclosporine, cytarabine, digoxin, dimenhydrinate, docetaxel, dopamine, doripenem, doxycycline, enalaprilat, epinephrine, ertapenem, fluorouracil, foscarnet, fosphenytoin, furosemide, ganciclovir, gentamicin, granisetron, heparin, hetastarch, hydrocortisone, hydromorphone, imipenem/cilastatin, inamrinone, insulin, irinotecan, isoproterenol, magnesium sulfate, mannitol, mesna, methohexital, methyldopate, metoclopramide, nafcillin, nitroglycerin, nitroprusside, ofloxacin, oxytocin, paclitaxel, pentazocine, pentobarbital, phenobarbital, phentolamine, phenylephrine, piperacillin/tazobactam, potassium chloride, procainamide, rifampin, sodium bicarbonate, succinylcholine, sufentanil, tacrolimus, teniposide, theophylline, thiopental, ticarcillin/clavulanate, tigecycline, tirofiban, tobramycin, trimethoprim/sulfamethoxazole, vasopressin, zidovudine.
- **Y-Site Incompatibility:** alfentanil, amphotericin B colloidal, atracurium, aztreonam, buprenorphine, butorphanol, calcium acetate, calcium chloride, cefoeprazone, cefotaxime, cefotetan, chloramphenicol, chlorpromazine, cimetidine, ciprofloxacin, cisatracurium, cisplatin, dacarbazine, dactinomycin, dantrolene, daptomycin, daunorubicin hydrochloride, dexamethasone, dexmedetomidine, dexrazoxane, diazepam, diltiazem, diphenhydramine, dobutamine, dolasetron, doxacurium, doxorubicin hydrochloride, droperidol, ephedrine, epirubicin, esmolol, etoposide, etoposide phosphate, famotidine, fenoldopam, fentanyl, fluconazole, fludarabine, gemcitabine, glycopyrrolate, haloperidol, hydralazine, hydroxyzine, idarubicin, ifosfamide, ketorolac, labetalol, leucovorin, levofloxacin, levorphanol, lidocaine, linezolid, lorazepam, mechlorethamine, melphalan, meperidine, methotrexate, methylprednisolone, metoprolol, metronidazole, midazolam, milrinone, mitomycin, mitoxantrone, mivacurium, nalbuphine, naloxone, nesiritide, nicardipine, ondansetron, palonosetron, pancuronium, pemetrexed, pentamidine, phenytoin, potassium phosphates, prochlorperazine, promethazine, propranolol, quinupristin/dalfopristin, ranitidine, remifentanil, rocuronium, sodium acetate, sodium phosphates, streptozocin, thiotepa, tolazoline, topotecan, trimethobenzamide, vancomycin, vecuronium, verapamil, vinblastine, vincristine, vinorelbine, voriconazole, solutions containing zinc.

Patient/Family Teaching

- Instruct patient to take medication as directed for the full course of therapy, even if feeling better.
- Advise patient to avoid alcohol, products containing aspirin or NSAIDs, and foods that may cause an increase in GI irritation.
- Advise patient to report onset of black, tarry stools; diarrhea; or abdominal pain to health care professional promptly.
- Advise female patients to notify health care professional if pregnancy is planned or suspected or if breastfeeding.
- Instruct patient to consult health care professional prior to taking other Rx, OTC, or herbal products.

Evaluation/Desired Outcomes

- Decrease in abdominal pain heartburn, gastric irritation and bleeding in patients with GERD; may require up to 4 wk of therapy.
- Healing in patients with erosive esophagitis. Therapy is continued for up to 8 wk.

---

paricalcitol, See **VITAMIN D COMPOUNDS.**

✦ = Canadian drug name. ■ = Genetic implication.
*CAPITALS indicates life-threatening; underlines indicate most frequent.

paroxetine hydrochloride
(par-**ox**-e-teen)
Paxil, Paxil CR

paroxetine mesylate
Pexeva

Classification
Therapeutic: antianxiety agents, antidepressants
Pharmacologic: selective serotonin reuptake inhibitors (SSRIs)

Pregnancy Category D

Indications
Paxil, Paxil CR, Pexeva: Major depressive disorder, panic disorder. **Paxil, Pexeva:** Obsessive compulsive disorder (OCD), generalized anxiety disorder (GAD). **Paxil, Paxil CR:** Social anxiety disorder. **Paxil:** Post-traumatic stress disorder (PTSD). **Paxil CR:** Premenstrual dysphoric disorder (PMDD).

Action
Inhibits neuronal reuptake of serotonin in the CNS, thus potentiating the activity of serotonin; has little effect on norepinephrine or dopamine.
Therapeutic Effects: Antidepressant action. Decreased frequency of panic attacks, OCD, or anxiety. Improvement in manifestations of post-traumatic stress disorder. Decreased dysphoria prior to menses.

Pharmacokinetics
Absorption: Completely absorbed following oral administration. Controlled-release tablets are enteric-coated and control medication release over 4–5 hr.
Distribution: Widely distributed throughout body fluids and tissues, including the CNS; cross the placenta and enter breast milk.
Protein Binding: 95%.
Metabolism and Excretion: Highly metabolized by the liver (partly by P450 2D6 enzyme system); 2% excreted unchanged in urine.
Half-life: 21 hr.

TIME/ACTION PROFILE (antidepressant action)

ROUTE	ONSET	PEAK	DURATION
PO	1–4 wk	unknown	unknown

Contraindications/Precautions
Contraindicated in: Hypersensitivity; Concurrent MAO inhibitor, thioridazine, or pimozide therapy.

Use Cautiously in: Risk of suicide (may ↑ risk of suicide attempt/ideation especially during early treatment or dose adjustment); History of seizures; History of bipolar disorder; OB: Use during the first trimester may be associated with an increased risk of cardiac malformations—consider fetal risk/maternal benefit; use during third trimester may result in neonatal serotonin syndrome requiring prolonged hospitalization, respiratory and nutritional support; Lactation: Safety not established; discontinue drug or bottle feed; Pedi: May ↑ risk of suicide attempt/ideation especially during early treatment or dose adjustment; may be greater in children and adolescents (safety in children/adolescents not established); Geri: Severe renal hepatic impairment; geriatric or debilitated patients (daily dose should not exceed 40 mg); history of mania/risk of suicide.

Adverse Reactions/Side Effects
CNS: NEUROLEPTIC MALIGNANT SYNDROME, SUICIDAL THOUGHTS, anxiety, dizziness, drowsiness, headache, insomnia, weakness, agitation, amnesia, confusion, emotional lability, hangover, impaired concentration, malaise, mental depression, syncope. **EENT:** blurred vision, rhinitis. **Resp:** cough, pharyngitis, respiratory disorders, yawning. **CV:** chest pain, edema, hypertension, palpitations, postural hypotension, tachycardia, vasodilation. **GI:** constipation, diarrhea, dry mouth, nausea, abdominal pain, decreased appetite, dyspepsia, flatulence, increased appetite, taste disturbances, vomiting. **GU:** ejaculatory disturbance, decreased libido, genital disorders, urinary disorders, urinary frequency. **Derm:** sweating, photosensitivity, pruritus, rash. **Metab:** weight gain, weight loss. **MS:** back pain, myalgia, myopathy. **Neuro:** paresthesia, tremor. **Misc:** SEROTONIN SYNDROME, chills, fever.

Interactions
Drug-Drug: Serious, potentially fatal reactions (hyperthermia, rigidity, myoclonus, autonomic instability, with fluctuating vital signs and extreme agitation, which may proceed to delirium and coma) may occur with concurrent **MAO inhibitor** therapy. MAO inhibitors should be stopped at least 14 days prior to paroxetine therapy. Paroxetine should be stopped at least 14 days prior to MAO inhibitor therapy. May ↓ metabolism and ↑ effects of certain **drugs that are metabolized by the liver**, including other **antidepressants, phenothiazines, class IC antiarrhythmics, risperidone, atomoxetine, theophylline, procyclidine,** and **quinidine**. Concurrent use should be undertaken with caution. Concurrent use with **pimozide** or **thiorida-**

paroxetine hydrochloride 993

zine may ↑ risk of QT interval prolongation and torsades de pointes. Concurrent use is contraindicated. **Cimetidine** ↑ blood levels. **Phenobarbital** and **phenytoin** may ↓ effectiveness. Concurrent use with **alcohol** is not recommended. May ↓ the effectiveness of **digoxin** and **tamoxifen**. May ↑ risk of bleeding with **warfarin**, **aspirin**, or **NSAIDS**. Concurrent use with **5-HT₁ agonists** (**frovatriptan**, **naratriptan**, **rizatriptan**, **sumatriptan**, **zolmitriptan**), **linezolid**, **lithium**, or **tramadol** may result in ↑ serotonin levels and lead to serotonin syndrome.

Drug-Natural Products: ↑ risk of serotonergic side effects including serotonin syndrome with **St. John's wort, SAMe**, and **tryptophan**.

Route/Dosage
Depression
PO (Adults): 20 mg as a single dose in the morning; may be ↑ by 10 mg/day at weekly intervals (not to exceed 50 mg/day). *Controlled-release tablets*— 25 mg once daily initially. May ↑ at weekly intervals by 12.5 mg (not to exceed 62.5 mg/day).

PO (Geriatric Patients or Debilitated Patients): 10 mg/day initially; may be slowly ↑ (not to exceed 40 mg/day). *Controlled-release tablets*— 12.5 mg once daily initially; may be slowly ↑ (not to exceed 50 mg/day).

Obsessive-Compulsive Disorder
PO (Adults): 20 mg/day initially; ↑ by 10 mg/day at weekly intervals up to 40 mg (not to exceed 60 mg/day).

Panic Disorder
PO (Adults): 10 mg/day initially; ↑ by 10 mg/day at weekly intervals up to 40 mg (not to exceed 60 mg/day). *Controlled-release tablets*— 12.5 mg/day initially; ↑ by 12.5 mg/day at weekly intervals (not to exceed 75 mg/day).

Social Anxiety Disorder
PO (Adults): 20 mg/day. *Controlled-release tablets*— 12.5 mg/day initially; may ↑ by 12.5 mg/day weekly intervals (not to exceed 37.5 mg/day).

Generalized anxiety disorder
PO (Adults): 20 mg once daily initially; ↑ by 10 mg/day at weekly intervals (not to exceed 50 mg/day).

Post-traumatic Stress Disorder
PO (Adults): 20 mg/day initially; may be ↑ by 10 mg/day at weekly intervals (not to exceed 50 mg/day).

Premenstrual Dysphoric Disorder
PO (Adults): *Controlled-release tablets*— 12.5 mg once daily throughout menstrual cycle or during luteal phase of menstrual cycle only; may be ↑ to 25 mg/day after one week.

Hepatic Impairment
PO (Adults): *Severe hepatic impairment*— 10 mg/day initially; may be slowly ↑ (not to exceed 40 mg/day). *Controlled-release tablets*— 12.5 mg once daily initially; may be slowly ↑ (not to exceed 50 mg/day).

Renal Impairment
PO (Adults): *Severe renal impairment*— 10 mg/day initially; may be slowly ↑ (not to exceed 40 mg/day). *Controlled-release tablets*— 12.5 mg once daily initially; may be slowly ↑ increased (not to exceed 50 mg/day).

Availability (generic available)
Paroxetine hydrochloride tablets: 10 mg, 20 mg, 30 mg, 40 mg. **Cost:** *Generic*— 10 mg $89.96/90, 20 mg $28.99/90, 30 mg $101.97/90, 40 mg $110.96/90. **Paroxetine hydrochloride controlled-release tablets:** 12.5 mg, 25 mg, 37.5 mg. **Cost:** 12.5 mg $297.99/90, 25 mg $303.95/90, 37.5 mg $317.99/90. **Paroxetine hydrochloride oral suspension (orange flavor):** 10 mg/5 mL. **Cost:** $166.90/250 mL. **Paroxetine mesylate tablets:** 10 mg, 20 mg, 30 mg, 40 mg. **Cost:** 20 mg $352.95/90, 30 mg $256.21/90, 40 mg $383.97/90.

NURSING IMPLICATIONS

Assessment
- Monitor appetite and nutritional intake. Weigh weekly. Notify health care professional of continued weight loss. Adjust diet as tolerated to support nutritional status.
- **Depression:** Monitor mental status (orientation, mood, behavior). Inform health care professional if patient demonstrates significant increase in anxiety, nervousness, or insomnia.
- Assess for suicidal tendencies, especially during early therapy. Restrict amount of drug available to patient. Risk may be increased in children, adolescents, and adults ≤24 yr.
- Assess for serotonin syndrome (mental changes [agitation, hallucinations, coma], autonomic instability [tachycardia, labile blood pressure, hyperthermia], neuromuscular aberations [hyper reflexia, incoordination], and/or GI symptoms [nausea, vomiting, diarrhea]),

especially in patients taking other serotonergic drugs (SSRIs, SNRIs, triptans).
- **OCD:** Assess patient for frequency of obsessive-compulsive behaviors. Note degree to which these thoughts and behaviors interfere with daily functioning.
- **Panic Attacks:** Assess frequency and severity of panic attacks.
- **Social Anxiety Disorder:** Assess frequency and severity of episodes of anxiety.
- **Post-traumatic Stress Disorder:** Assess manifestations of post-traumatic stress disorder periodically during therapy.
- **Premenstrual Dysphoria:** Assess symptoms of premenstrual distress prior to and during therapy.
- *Lab Test Considerations:* Monitor CBC and differential periodically during therapy. Report leukopenia or anemia.

Potential Nursing Diagnoses
Ineffective coping (Indications)
Risk for injury (Side Effects)

Implementation
- Do not confuse paroxetine (Paxil) with paclitaxel (Taxol).
- Paroxetine mesylate (Pexeva) cannot be substituted with paroxetine (Paxil or Paxil CR) or generic paroxetine.
- Periodically reassess dose and continued need for therapy.
- **PO:** Administer as a single dose in the morning. May administer with food to minimize GI irritation.
- Tablets should be swallowed whole. Do not crush, break, or chew.
- Taper to avoid potential withdrawal reactions.

Patient/Family Teaching
- Instruct patient to take paroxetine as directed. Take missed doses as soon as possible and return to regular dosing schedule. Do not double doses. Caution patient to consult health care professional before discontinuing paroxetine. Daily doses should be decreased slowly. Abrupt withdrawal may cause dizziness, sensory disturbances, agitation, anxiety, nausea, and sweating.
- May cause drowsiness or dizziness. Caution patient to avoid driving and other activities requiring alertness until response to the drug is known.
- Advise patient, family and caregivers to look for suicidality, especially during early therapy or dose changes. Notify health care professional immediately if thoughts about suicide or dying, attempts to commit suicide, new or worse depression or anxiety, agitation or restlessness, panic attacks, insomnia, new or worse irritability, aggressiveness, acting on dangerous impulses, mania, or other changes in mood or behavior or if symptoms of serotonin syndrome occur.
- Advise patient to avoid alcohol or other CNS-depressant drugs during therapy and to consult with health care professional before taking other medications or herbal products with paroxetine.
- Inform patient that frequent mouth rinses, good oral hygiene, and sugarless gum or candy may minimize dry mouth. Saliva substitute may be used. Consult dentist if dry mouth persists for more than 2 wk.
- Instruct female patient to inform health care professional if pregnancy is planned or suspected or if she is breastfeeding.
- Advise patient to notify health care professional if headache, weakness, nausea, anorexia, anxiety, or insomnia persists.
- Emphasize the importance of follow-up exams to monitor progress. Encourage patient participation in psychotherapy to improve coping skills.
- Refer patient to local support group.

Evaluation/Desired Outcomes
- Increased sense of well-being.
- Renewed interest in surroundings. May require 1–4 wk of therapy to obtain antidepressant effects.
- Decrease in obsessive-compulsive behaviors.
- Decrease in frequency and severity of panic attacks.
- Decrease in frequency and severity of episodes of anxiety.
- Improvement in manifestations of post-traumatic stress disorder.
- Decreased dysphoria prior to menses.

---

pazopanib (paz-oh-pi-nab)
Votrient

Classification
Therapeutic: antineoplastics
Pharmacologic: kinase inhibitors

Pregnancy Category D

Indications
Treatment of advanced renal cell carcinoma.

Action
Acts as a tyrosine kinase inhibitor of several vascular endothelial growth factor receptors

pazopanib

(VEGFRs), platelet-derived growth factor receptor, fibroblast growth factor receptor, cytokine receptor, interleukin-2 receptor inducible T-cell kinase, leukocyte-specific protein tyrosine kinase, and transmembrane glycoprotein receptor tyrosine kinase. Overall effect is decreased angiogenesis in tumors. **Therapeutic Effects:** Decreased growth and spread of renal cell carcinoma.

Pharmacokinetics

Absorption: Well absorbed following oral administration; crushing tablet and ingesting food ↑ absorption.
Distribution: unknown.
Protein Binding: >99%.
Metabolism and Excretion: Mostly metabolized by the liver (primarily by the CYP3A4 enzyme system, minor amounts by CYP1A2 and CYP2C8) followed by elimination in feces; <4% excreted by the kidneys.
Half-life: 30.9 hr.

TIME/ACTION PROFILE (blood levels)

ROUTE	ONSET	PEAK	DURATION
PO	PO	2–4 hr	24 hr

Contraindications/Precautions

Contraindicated in: Severe hepatic impairment; History of hemoptysis, cerebral or GI bleeding in preceding 6 mo; Risk/history of arterial thrombotic events, including MI, angina or ischemic stroke within preceding 6 mo; Concurrent use of strong CYP3A4 inhibitors (if concurrent use is necessary, consider dose reduction of pazopanib); Concurrent use of strong CYP3A4 inducers (may ↓ effectiveness); Concurrent use of drugs that have narrow therapeutic windows and that are metabolized by CYP3A4, CYP2D6, or CYP2C8 enzyme systems (CYP substrates); OB: May cause fetal harm, avoid use during pregnancy; Lactation: Avoid use during breast feeding.
Use Cautiously in: Congenital prolonged QTc interval or concurrent medications/diseases that prolong QTc (may ↑ risk of Torsade de Pointes, a serious arrhythmia); Electrolyte abnormalities (correct prior to use; may ↑ risk of potentially serious arrhythmia); Patients at risk for gastrointestinal perforation/fistula; Surgery; interruption of therapy recommended; Hypertension; control before therapy is initiated; Hypothyroidism (may worsen condition); Concurrent use of inducers of the CYP3A4 enzyme system; consider alternate concurrent medication with little or no enzyme induction potential or avoid pazopanib; Moderate hepatic impairment (dose reduction recommended; Geri: may be more sensitive to drug effects, consider age-related decrease in cardiac, renal, and hepatic function, concurrent disease states and drug therapy; OB: Women with childbearing potential; Pedi: Safe and effective use in children has not been established.

Adverse Reactions/Side Effects

CNS: fatigue, weakness. **CV:** PROLONGED QT INTERVAL, hypertension, altered taste, chest pain, dyspepsia. **GI:** GI PERFORATION/FISTULA, HEPATOTOXICITY, abdominal pain, anorexia, diarrhea, nausea, vomiting. **GU:** proteinuria. **Derm:** alopecia, facial edema, palmar-plantar erythrodysesthesia (hand-foot syndrome), rash, skin depigmentation. **Endo:** hypothyroidism. **Hemat:** BLEEDING, aterial thrombosis. **Metab:** ↑ lipase, weight loss. **Misc:** hair color changes (depigmentation).

Interactions

Drug-Drug: Concurrent use of **strong CYP3A4 inhibitors**, including **ketoconazole**, **ritonavir** and **clarithromycin** may ↑ pazopanib and should be avoided; if required, dose of pazopanib should be decreased to 400 mg daily or more if necessary. Concurrent use of **strong CYP3A4 inducers**, including **rifampin**, may ↓ levels and effectiveness and should be avoided. Concurrent use with **drugs with narrow therapeutic windows that are metabolized by CYP3A4, CYP2D6, or CYP2C8** may ↑ levels of such drugs and the risk of toxicity/adverse reactions is not recommended.

Route/Dosage

PO (Adults): 800 mg once daily; *strong inhibitors or CYP3A4*— 400 mg once daily, further reductions may be necessary.

Hepatic Impairment

PO (Adults): *Moderate hepatic impairment*— 200 mg once daily.

Availability

Tablets: 200 mg, 400 mg.

NURSING IMPLICATIONS

Assessment

- Monitor BP during frequent therapy; may cause hypertension. BP should be well-controlled prior to initiating therapy. If persistent hypertension occurs despite antihypertensive therapy, reduce dose. If hypertension persists and is severe, discontinue therapy.

- Obtain baseline ECG and monitor periodically during therapy. Maintain serum calcium, magnesium, and potassium within normal range during therapy.
- Monitor for signs and symptoms of GI perforation and fistula (abdominal pain, GI bleeding) during therapy.
- **Lab Test Considerations:** Monitor serum liver tests before initiation and at least every 4 wk for first 4 mo or as indicated, then periodically during therapy. *If isolated ALT ↑ between 3 and 8 times the upper limit of normal,* therapy may continue with weekly monitoring of liver function until ALT returns to Grade 1 or baseline. *If isolated ALT ↑ >8 times the upper limit of normal,* stop therapy until ALT returns to Grade 1 or baseline. If benefit outweighs risk, may reintroduce at reduced dose of 400 mg/day with weekly serum liver tests for 8 wk. Following reintroduction, if ALT ↑ >3 times the upper limit of normal recurs, permanently discontinue pazopanib. *If ALT ↑ occurs concurrently with ↑ serum bilirubin >2 times the upper limit of normal,* discontinue pazopanib permanently. Monitor liver function tests until return to baseline. *Patients with only mild indirect hyperbilirubinemia (Gilbert's syndrome) and ↑ ALT >3 times the upper limit of normal should be managed as per recommendations for ↑ ALT.*
- Monitor thyroid function periodically during therapy. May cause hypothyroidism.
- Obtain baseline urinalysis and monitor periodically. May cause proteinuria. Discontinue therapy if Grade 4 proteinuria develops.
- May cause leukopenia, neutropenia, thrombocytopenia, and lymphocytopenia.
- May cause ↑ AST and ↓ serum phosphorous, sodium, and magnesium. May cause ↑ or ↓ serum glucose.

Potential Nursing Diagnoses
Deficient knowledge, related to medication regimen (Patient/Family Teaching)

Implementation
- **PO:** Administer at least 1 hr before or 2 hr after a meal. Swallow tablets whole; do not crush tablets.

Patient/Family Teaching
- Instruct patient to take pazopanib on an empty stomach as dierected. Take missed doses as soon as remembered; if less than 12 hr before next dose, omit dose. Advise patient to read the Medication Guide prior to taking pazopanib and with each Rx refill; new information may be available.
- Advise patient to notify health care professional if yellowing of skin or whites of eyes, unusual darkening of urine, unusual tiredness, or pain in the right upper stomach area occurs.
- Inform patient that diarrhea frequently occurs. Instruct patient on ways to manage diarrhea and to notify health care professional if moderate to severe diarrhea occurs.
- Inform patient that loss of color (depigmentation) of skin or hair may occur during therapy. Explore methods of coping.
- Advise patient to consult health care professional before taking other Rx, OTC, or herbal products.
- Advise female patients to use effective contraception during therapy and to notify health care professional immediately if pregnancy is suspected.

Evaluation/Desired Outcomes
- Decreased growth and spread of renal cell carcinoma.

---

pegaspargase
(peg-ass-**par**-jase)
Oncaspar, PEG-L-asparaginase

Classification
Therapeutic: antineoplastics
Pharmacologic: enzymes

Pregnancy Category C

Indications
Treatment (usually with other agents) of acute lymphoblastic leukemia (ALL) in patients who have had a previous hypersensitivity reaction to native asparaginase.

Action
Consists of L-asparaginase bound to polyethylene glycol (PEG). This compound depletes asparagine, which leukemic cells cannot synthesize. Normal cells are able to produce their own asparagine and are less susceptible to the effects of asparaginase. Binding to PEG renders asparaginase less antigenic and therefore less likely to induce hypersensitivity reactions. **Therapeutic Effects:** Death of leukemic cells.

Pharmacokinetics
Absorption: IV administration results in complete bioavailability.
Distribution: Unknown.

Metabolism and Excretion: Metabolized by serum proteases and in the reticuloendothelial system.
Half-life: 5.7 days (less in patients with previous hypersensitivity to native L-asparaginase).

TIME/ACTION PROFILE (hematologic effects)

ROUTE	ONSET	PEAK	DURATION
IV	rapid	unknown	14 days

Contraindications/Precautions
Contraindicated in: Pancreatitis or history of pancreatitis; History of previous hemorrhagic reaction to asparaginase therapy; Previous hypersensitivity reactions to pegaspargase.
Use Cautiously in: History of previous hypersensitivity reactions to other drugs; Patients with childbearing potential; OB: Lactation: Safety not established.

Adverse Reactions/Side Effects
CNS: SEIZURES, headache, malaise. **GI:** PANCREATITIS, abdominal pain, abnormal liver function tests, anorexia, diarrhea, lip edema, nausea, vomiting. **Derm:** jaundice. **Endo:** hyperglycemia. **F and E:** peripheral edema. **Hemat:** decreased fibrinogen, disseminated intravascular coagulation, hemolytic anemia, increased thromboplastin, leukopenia, pancytopenia, thrombocytopenia. **Local:** injection site hypersensitivity, injection site pain, thrombosis. **MS:** arthralgia, myalgia, pain in extremities. **Neuro:** paresthesia. **Misc:** chills, hypersensitivity reactions, night sweats.

Interactions
Drug-Drug: May alter response to **anticoagulants** or **antiplatelet agents**. May alter the response to other **drugs that are metabolized by the liver**.

Route/Dosage
IM, IV (Adults up to 21 yr, and Children with Body Surface Area ≥0.6 m^2): 2500 IU/m^2 q 14 days (usually in combination with other agents).
IM, IV (Children with Body Surface Area <0.6 m^2): 82.5 IU/kg q 14 days (usually in combination with other agents).

Availability
Injection: 750 IU/mL.

NURSING IMPLICATIONS
Assessment
- Assess patient for previous hypersensitivity reactions to native L-asparaginase. Monitor for hypersensitivity reaction (urticaria, diaphoresis, facial swelling, joint pain, hypotension, bronchospasm). Epinephrine and resuscitation equipment should be readily available. Reaction may occur up to 2 hr after administration.
- Monitor for development of bone marrow depression. Assess for fever, sore throat, and signs of infection. Monitor platelet count throughout therapy. Assess for bleeding (bleeding gums, bruising, petechiae, guaiac test stools, urine, and emesis). Avoid giving IM injections and taking rectal temperatures. Apply pressure to venipuncture sites for 10 min. Anemia may occur. Monitor for increased fatigue, dyspnea, and orthostatic hypotension.
- Monitor patient frequently for signs of pancreatitis (nausea, vomiting, abdominal pain).
- Assess nausea, vomiting, and appetite. Weigh patient weekly. Prophylactic antiemetics may be used prior to administration.
- **Lab Test Considerations:** Monitor CBC prior to and periodically throughout therapy. May alter coagulation studies. Fibrinogen may be decreased; PT and partial thromboplastin time (PTT) may be ↑.
- Monitor serum amylase frequently to detect pancreatitis.
- Monitor blood glucose; may cause hyperglycemia.
- May cause elevated BUN and serum creatinine.
- Hepatotoxicity may be manifested by increased AST, ALT, or bilirubin. Liver function tests usually return to normal after therapy.
- May cause ↓ serum calcium.
- May cause elevated serum and urine uric acid and hyponatremia.

Potential Nursing Diagnoses
Risk for infection (Adverse Reactions)

Implementation
- Do not confuse pegaspargase with asparaginase.
- IM is the preferred route because of a lower incidence of adverse reactions.
- Solutions should be prepared in a biologic cabinet. Wear gloves, gown, and mask while handling medication. Discard equipment in specially designated containers.
- **IM:** Limit single injection volume to 2 mL. If volume of injection is >2 mL, use multiple injection sites.

IV Administration

- **Intermittent Infusion:** *Diluent:* Dilute each dose in 100 mL of 0.9% NaCl or D5W. Do not shake or agitate. Do not use if solution is cloudy or has formed a precipitate.
- Use only 1 dose per vial; do not re-enter the vial. Discard unused portions.
- Keep refrigerated but do not freeze. Freezing destroys activity but does not change the appearance of pegaspargase. *Rate:* Administer over 1–2 hr via Y-site through an infusion that is already running.
- **Additive Incompatibility:** Information unavailable. Do not admix with other medications or solutions.

Patient/Family Teaching

- Inform patient of the possibility of hypersensitivity reactions, including anaphylaxis.
- Advise patient that concurrent use of other medications may increase the risk of bleeding and the toxicity of pegaspargase. Consult health care professional before taking any other medications, including OTC drugs.
- Instruct patient to notify health care professional if abdominal pain, severe nausea and vomiting, jaundice, fever, chills, sore throat, bleeding or bruising, excess thirst or urination, or mouth sores occur. Caution patient to avoid crowds and persons with known infections. Instruct patient to use soft toothbrush, electric razor, and to be especially careful to avoid falls. Patients should also be cautioned not to drink alcoholic beverages or take medications containing aspirin or NSAIDs because these may precipitate gastric bleeding.
- Instruct patient not to receive any vaccinations without advice of health care professional. Advise parents that this may alter child's immunization schedule.
- Emphasize the need for periodic lab tests to monitor for side effects.

Evaluation/Desired Outcomes

- Improvement of hematologic status in patients with leukemia.

---

pegfilgrastim (peg-fil-gra-stim)
Neulasta

Classification
Therapeutic: colony-stimulating factors

Pregnancy Category C

Indications
To decrease the incidence of infection (febrile neutropenia) in patients with nonmyeloid malignancies receiving myelosuppressive antineoplastics associated with a high risk of febrile neutropenia.

Action
Filgrastim is a glycoprotein that binds to and stimulates neutrophils to divide and differentiate. Also activates mature neutrophils. Binding to a polyethylene glycol molecule prolongs its effects.
Therapeutic Effects: Decreased incidence of infection in patients who are neutropenic from chemotherapy.

Pharmacokinetics
Absorption: Well absorbed following subcut administration.
Distribution: Unknown.
Metabolism and Excretion: Unknown.
Half-life: 15–80 hr.

TIME/ACTION PROFILE

ROUTE	ONSET	PEAK	DURATION
Subcut	unknown	unknown	unknown

Contraindications/Precautions
Contraindicated in: Hypersensitivity to filgrastim or *Escherichia coli*-derived proteins.
Use Cautiously in: Patients with sickle cell disease (↑ risk of sickle cell crisis); Concurrent use of lithium; Malignancy with myeloid characteristics; OB, Lactation: Pregnancy or lactation; Pedi: 6 mg fixed dose should not be used in infants, children, and adolescents weighing <45 kg.

Adverse Reactions/Side Effects
Resp: ADULT RESPIRATORY DISTRESS SYNDROME (ARDS). **GI:** SPLENIC RUPTURE. **Hemat:** SICKLE CELL CRISIS, leukocytosis. **MS:** medullary bone pain. **Misc:** allergic reaction including ANAPHYLAXIS.

Interactions
Drug-Drug: Simultaneous use with **antineoplastics** may have adverse effects on rapidly proliferating neutrophils; avoid use for 24 hr before and 24 hr following chemotherapy. **Lithium** may potentiate the release of neutrophils; concurrent use should be undertaken cautiously.

Route/Dosage
Subcut (Adults and Children >45 kg): 6 mg per chemotherapy cycle.

Availability
Solution for injection: 6 mg/0.6 mL in prefilled syringes.

NURSING IMPLICATIONS

Assessment
- Assess patient for bone pain throughout therapy. Pain is usually mild to moderate and controllable with nonopioid analgesics, but may require opioid analgesics.
- Assess patient periodically for signs of ARDS (fever, lung infiltration, respiratory distress). If ARDS occurs, treat condition and discontinue pegfilgrastim and/or withhold until symptoms resolve.
- *Lab Test Considerations:* Obtain CBC and platelet count before chemotherapy. Monitor hematocrit and platelet count regularly.
- May cause elevated LDH, alkaline phosphatase, and uric acid.

Potential Nursing Diagnoses
Risk for infection (Indications)
Acute pain (Side Effects)

Implementation
- Pegfilgrastim should not be administered between 14 and 24 days after administration of cytotoxic chemotherapy.
- Keep patients with sickle cell disease receiving pegfilgrastim well hydrated and monitor for sickle cell crisis.
- **Subcut:** Administer subcut once per chemotherapy cycle. Do not administer solutions that are discolored or contain particulate matter. Do not shake. Store refrigerated; may be allowed to reach room temperature for a maximum of 48 hr, but protect from light.
- Supplied in prefilled syringes. Following administration, activate UltraSafe Needle Guard to prevent needle sticks by placing hands behind needle, grasping guard with one hand, and sliding guard forward until needle is completely covered and guard clicks into place. If audible click is not heard, guard may not be completely activated. Dispose of by placing entire prefilled syringe with guard activated into puncture-proof container.

Patient/Family Teaching
- Advise patient to notify health care professional immediately if signs of allergic reaction (shortness of breath, hives, rash, pruritus, laryngeal edema) or signs of splenic rupture (left upper abdominal or shoulder tip pain) occur.
- Emphasize the importance of compliance with therapy and regular monitoring of blood counts.
- **Home Care Issues:** Instruct patient on correct disposal technique for home administration. Caution patient not to reuse needle, syringe, or drug product. Provide patient with a puncture-proof container for disposal of prefilled syringe.

Evaluation/Desired Outcomes
- Decreased incidence of infection in patients who receive bone marrow–depressing antineoplastics.

---

peginterferon alpha-2a, See INTERFERONS, ALPHA.

---

peginterferon alpha-2b, See INTERFERONS, ALPHA.

---

pemetrexed (pe-me-**trex**-ed)
Alimta

Classification
Therapeutic: antineoplastics
Pharmacologic: antimetabolites, folate antagonists

Pregnancy Category D

Indications
Malignant pleural mesothelioma (with cisplatin) when tumor is unresectable or patient is not a candidate for surgery. Local advanced or metastatic nonsquamous non–small cell lung cancer as initial therapy (with cisplatin), in previously treated patients (as monotherapy), or as maintenance treatment in patients whose disease has not progressed after four cycles of platinum-based chemotherapy.

Action
Disrupts folate dependent metabolic processes involved in thymidine and purine synthesis. Converted intracellularly to polyglutamate form which increases duration of action. **Therapeutic Effects:** Decreases growth and spread of mesothelioma. Improved survival in patients with nonsquamous non-small cell lung cancer.

Pharmacokinetics
Absorption: IV administration results in complete bioavailability.
Distribution: Unknown.

pemetrexed

Metabolism and Excretion: Minimal metabolism; 70–90% excreted unchanged in urine.
Half-life: 3.5 hr (normal renal function).

TIME/ACTION PROFILE (hematologic effects)

ROUTE	ONSET	PEAK	DURATION
IV	unknown	8–15 days	21 days

Contraindications/Precautions
Contraindicated in: Hypersensitivity; CCr <45 mL/min; **OB:** OB, Lactation: Pregnancy, lactation.
Use Cautiously in: Concurrent use of NSAIDs in patients with CCr 45–79 mL/min (avoid those with short half-lives); Third space fluid accumulation (ascites, pleural effusions); consider drainage prior to therapy; Hepatic impairment (dose alteration recommended); Pedi: Safety not established.

Adverse Reactions/Side Effects
Resp: pharyngitis. **CV:** chest pain. **GI:** constipation, nausea, stomatitis, vomiting, anorexia, diarrhea, esophagitis, mouth pain. **Derm:** desquamation, rash. **Hemat:** anemia, leukopenia, thrombocytopenia. **Neuro:** neuropathy. **Misc:** fever, infection.

Interactions
Drug-Drug: NSAIDs, especially those with short half-lives, ↑ blood levels and risk of toxicity; avoid for 2 days before, day of, and 2 days after treatment. **Probenecid** ↑ blood levels. Concurrent use of **nephrotoxic agents** ↑ risk of nephrotoxicity.

Route/Dosage
IV (Adults): *Mesothelioma and non–small cell lung cancer (with cisplatin)* 500—mg/m^2 on day 1 of each 21-day cycle (with cisplatin); concurrent hydration, folic acid, and vitamin B$_{12}$ therapy, and pretreatment with dexamethasone required. *Non–small cell lung cancer (as monotherapy)*—500 mg/m^2 on day 1 of each 21-day cycle (concurrent folic acid, and vitamin B$_{12}$ therapy, and pretreatment with dexamethasone required).

Availability
Lyophilized powder for IV infusion: 500 mg/vial.

NURSING IMPLICATIONS

Assessment
- Monitor for rash during therapy. Pretreatment with dexamethasone 4 mg orally twice daily the day before, the day of, and the day after administration reduces incidence and severity or reaction.
- Monitor for hematologic and GI (mucositis, diarrhea) toxicities. If any Grade 3 or 4 toxicities, except mucositis or diarrhea, requiring hospitalization occur, decrease doses of pemetrexed and cisplatin by 75%. If Grade 3 or 4 mucositis occurs decrease pemetrexed dose by 50% and cisplatin by 100% of previous dose.
- Monitor for bone marrow depression. Assess for bleeding (bleeding gums, bruising, petechiae, guaiac stools, urine, and emesis) and avoid IM injections and taking rectal temperatures if platelet count is low. Apply pressure to venipuncture sites for 10 min. Assess for signs of infection during neutropenia. Anemia may occur; monitor for increased fatigue, dyspnea, and orthostatic hypotension.
- Assess for neurotoxicity during therapy. If Grade 0–1 neurotoxicity occurs, decrease pemetrexed and cisplatin doses by 100% of previous dose. If Grade 2 neurotoxicity occurs, decrease pemetrexed dose by 100% and cisplatin dose by 50% of previous dose. If Grade 3 or 4 neurotoxicity occurs, discontinue therapy.
- *Lab Test Considerations:* Monitor CBC and platelet counts for nadir and recovery, before each dose and on days 8 and 15 of each cycle and chemistry for renal and liver functions periodically. May cause neutropenia, thrombocytopenia, leukopenia, and anemia. A new cycle should not be started unless the ANC is at least 1500 cells/mm^3, platelet count is at least 100,000 cells/mm^3, and creatinine clearance is at least 45 mL/min. If nadir of ANC is less than 500/mm^3 and nadir of platelets are at least 50,000/mm^3 decrease doses of pemetrexed and cisplatin by 75%. If nadir of platelets is less than 50,000/mm^3 regardless of ANC nadir decrease pemetrexed and cisplatin doses by 50%.

Potential Nursing Diagnoses
Risk for injury (Adverse Reactions)

Implementation
- Pemetrexed should be administered under supervision of a physician experienced in the use of chemotherapeutic agents.
- Prepare solution in a biologic cabinet. Wear gloves, gown, and mask while handling medication. Discard equipment in designated containers.
- To reduce toxicity, at least 5 mg of folic acid must be taken daily for 7 days preceding first dose of pemetrexed and should continue during and for 21 days after last dose. Patients must also receive an injection of vitamin B$_{12}$ 1000 mcg during the week preceding first dose of pemetrexed and every 3 cycles thereafter.

Subsequent doses of vitamin B_{12} may be given on same day as pemetrexed.

IV Administration
- **Intermittent Infusion:** Calculate number of pemetrexed 500-mg vials needed; vials contain excess to facilitate delivery. Reconstitute 500 mg with 20 mL of preservative–free 0.9% NaCl. *Concentration:* 25 mg/mL. Swirl gently until powder is completely dissolved. Solution is clear and colorless to yellow or green-yellow. Do not administer if discolored or containing particulate matter. *Diluent:* Dilute further to 100 mL with preservative–free 0.9% NaCl. Solution is stable at room temperature or if refrigerated for up to 24 hr. *Rate:* Administer over 10 min.
- **Y-Site Compatibility:** acyclovir, alfentanil, allopurinol, amifostine, amikacin, aminocaproic acid, aminophylline, amiodarone, amphotericin B liposome, ampicillin, amipicillin/sulbactam, atenolol, atracurium, azithromycin, aztreonam, bivalirudin, bleomycin, bretylium, bumetanide, buprenorphine, butorphanol, carboplatin, carmustine, ceftizoxime, ceftriaxone, cefuroxime, cimetidine, cisatracurium, cisplatin, clindamycin, cyclophosphamide, cyclosporine, cytarabine, dactinomycin, daptomycin, dexamethasone sodium phosphate, dexrazoxane, digoxin, diltiazem, diphenhydramine, docetaxel, dolasetron, dopamine, doxacurium, enalaprilat, ephedrine, epinephrine, eptifibitide, ertapenem, esmolol, etoposide, etoposide phosphate, famotidine, fenoldopam, fentanyl, fluconazole, fludarabine, fluorouracil, foscarnet, fosphenytoin, furosemide, ganciclovir, glycopyrrolate, granisetron, haloperidol, heparin, hydrocortisone sodium succinate, hydromorphone, ifosfamide, imipenem/cilastatin, insulin, isoproterenol, ketorolac, labetalol, leucovorin, levofloxacin, lidocaine, linezolid, lorazepam, magnesium sulfate, mannitol, meperidine, meropenem, mesna, methyldopate, methylprednisolone sodium succinate, metoclopramide, metoprolol, midazolam, milrinone, mitomycin, mivacurium, morphine, moxifloxacin, nafcillin, naloxone, nesiritide, nitroglycerin, norepinephrine, octreotide, oxaliplatin, paclitaxel, pamidronate, pancuronium, pentobarbital, phenobarbital, phentolamine, piperacillin/tazobactam, potassium chloride, potassium phosphates, procainamide, promethazine, propranolol, ranitidine, remifentanil, rocuronium, sodium acetate, sodium bicarbonate, sodium phosphate, succinylcholine, sufentanil, tacrolimus, theophylline, thiopental, thiotepa, ticarcillin/clavulanate, tigecycline, tirofiban, trimethobenzamide, trimethoprim/sulfamethoxazole, vancomycin, vecuronium, verapamil, vinblastine, vincristine, vinorelbine, zidovudine.
- **Y-Site Incompatibility:** amphotericin B colloidal, calcium acetate, calcium chloride, calcium gluconate, caspofungin, cefazolin, cefepime, cefotaxime, cefotetan, cefoxitin, ceftazidime, chloramphenicol, chlorpromazine, ciprofloxacin, dacarbazine, dantrolene, daunorubicin, diazepam, dobutamine, doxorubicin, doxycycline, droperidol, erythromycin, gemcitabine, gentamicin, hydralazine, idarubicin, inamrinone, irinotecan, metronidazole, minocycline, mitoxantrone, nalbuphine, nicardipine, nitroprusside, ondansetron, pantoprazole, pentamidine, pentazocine, phenytoin, prochlorperazine, quinapristin/dalfopristin, tobramycin, topotecan, vasopressin.
- **Additive Incompatibility:** Solutions containing calcium, including Lactated Ringer's and Ringer's solution.

Patient/Family Teaching
- Emphasize the importance of taking prophylactic folic acid and vitamin B_{12} to reduce treatment-related hematologic and GI toxicity.
- Advise patient to avoid becoming pregnant during therapy. If pregnancy is planned or suspected, notify health care professional promptly.

Evaluation/Desired Outcomes
- Decreased growth and spread of mesothelioma or non–small cell lung cancer.

---

penciclovir (pen-sye-kloe-veer)
Denavir

Classification
Therapeutic: antivirals (topical)

Pregnancy Category B

Indications
Recurrent herpes labialis (cold sores).

Action
Inhibits viral DNA synthesis and replication.
Therapeutic Effects: Death of herpes virus. Decreased lesion duration and pain. Active against herpes viruses.

Pharmacokinetics
Absorption: Not absorbed following topical use.
Distribution: Unknown.
Metabolism and Excretion: Converted intracellularly to active triphosphate form; excreted in urine.
Half-life: 2–2.5 hr.

TIME/ACTION PROFILE

ROUTE	ONSET	PEAK	DURATION
Topical	unknown	unknown	unknown

Contraindications/Precautions
Contraindicated in: Hypersensitivity to penciclovir or other components of the formulation.
Use Cautiously in: OB: Lactation: Pedi: Safety not established.

Adverse Reactions/Side Effects
CNS: headache. **Local:** application site reactions.

Interactions
Drug-Drug: None significant.

Route/Dosage
PO (Adults): Apply q 2 hr for 4 days while awake.

Availability
Cream: 1%.

NURSING IMPLICATIONS

Assessment
- Assess lesions prior to and daily during therapy.

Potential Nursing Diagnoses
Risk for impaired skin integrity (Indications)
Risk for infection (Indications, Patient/Family Teaching)
Deficient knowledge, related to medication regimen (Patient/Family Teaching)

Implementation
- Do not confuse Denavir (penciclovir) with indinavir.
- Begin treatment as early as possible, during prodrome or when lesions appear.
- **Topical:** Apply to lesions every 2 hr for 4 days while awake.
- Apply to lips and face only; avoid application to mucous membranes or near the eyes.

Patient/Family Teaching
- Advise patient to apply medication exactly as directed for the full course of therapy. If a dose is missed, apply as soon as possible but not just before next dose is due; do not double doses. Penciclovir should not be used more frequently or longer than prescribed.
- Advise patients that the additional use of OTC creams, lotions, and ointments may delay healing and may cause spreading of lesions.

Evaluation/Desired Outcomes
- More rapid healing of lesions and relief of pain in herpes labialis.

PENICILLINS (pen-i-sill-ins)

penicillin G
Pfizerpen

penicillin V
✤ Apo-Pen VK, ✤ Crystapen, ✤ Novo-Pen-VK, ✤ Nu-Pen-VK, ✤ Penicilline V

procaine penicillin G
Wycillin

benzathine penicillin G
Bicillin L-A, Permapen

Classification
Therapeutic: anti-infectives
Pharmacologic: penicillins

Pregnancy Category B

Indications
Treatment of a wide variety of infections including: Pneumococcal pneumonia, Streptococcal pharyngitis, Syphilis, Gonorrhea strains. Treatment of enterococcal infections (requires the addition of an aminoglycoside). Prevention of rheumatic fever. Should not be used as a single agent to treat anthrax. **Unlabeled Use:** Treatment of Lyme disease. Prevention of recurrent *Streptococal pneumoniae* septicemia in children with sickle-cell disease.

Action
Bind to bacterial cell wall, resulting in cell death. **Therapeutic Effects:** Bactericidal action against susceptible bacteria. **Spectrum:** Active against: Most gram-positive organisms, including many streptococci (*Streptococcus pneumoniae*, group A beta-hemolytic streptococci), staphylococci (non–penicillinase-producing strains) and *Bacillus anthracis*; Some gram-negative organisms, such as *Neisseria meningitidis* and *Neisseria gonorrhoeae* (only penicillin susceptible strains); Some anaerobic bacteria and spirochetes including *Borellia burgdorferi*.

Pharmacokinetics
Absorption: Variably absorbed from the GI tract. *Penicillin V*—resists acid degradation in the GI

tract. *Procaine and benzathine penicillin*—IM absorption is delayed and prolonged and results in sustained therapeutic blood levels.
Distribution: Widely distributed, although CNS penetration is poor in the presence of uninflamed meninges. Cross the placenta and enter breast milk.
Metabolism and Excretion: Minimally metabolized by the liver, excreted mainly unchanged by the kidneys.
Half-life: 30–60 min.

TIME/ACTION PROFILE (blood levels)

ROUTE	ONSET	PEAK	DURATION
Penicillin V PO	rapid	0.5–1 hr	4–6 hr
Penicillin G IM	rapid	0.25–0.5 hr	4–6 hr
Benzathine penicillin IM	delayed	12–24 hr	3 wk
Procaine penicillin IM	delayed	1–4 hr	12 hr
Penicillin G IV	rapid	end of infusion	4–6 hr

Contraindications/Precautions
Contraindicated in: Previous hypersensitivity to penicillins (cross-sensitivity may exist with cephalosporins and other beta-lactams); Hypersensitivity to procaine or benzathine (procaine and benzathine preparations only); Some products may contain tartrazine and should be avoided in patients with known hypersensitivity.
Use Cautiously in: Severe renal insufficiency (dose ↓ recommended); OB: Although safety not established, has been used safely; Lactation: Safety not established; Geri: Consider ↓ body mass, age-related ↓ in renal, hepatic, and cardiac function, comorbidities, and concurrent drug therapy when prescribing and dosing.

Adverse Reactions/Side Effects
CNS: SEIZURES. **GI:** diarrhea, epigastric distress, nausea, vomiting, pseudomembranous colitis. **GU:** interstitial nephritis. **Derm:** rashes, urticaria. **Hemat:** eosinophilia, hemolytic anemia, leukopenia. **Local:** pain at IM site, phlebitis at IV site. **Misc:** allergic reactions including ANAPHYLAXIS and SERUM SICKNESS, superinfection.

Interactions
Drug-Drug: May ↓ effectiveness of oral contraceptive agents. **Probenecid** ↓ renal excretion and ↑ levels therapy may be combined for this purpose). **Neomycin** may ↓ absorption of penicillin V. ↓ elimination of **methotrexate** and ↑ risk of serious toxicity.

Route/Dosage
Penicillin G (aqueous)
IM, IV (Adults): *Most infections*—1–5 million units q 4–6 hr.
IM, IV (Children): 8333–16,667 units/kg q 4 hr; 12,550–25,000 units/kg q 6 hr; up to 250,000 units/kg/day in divided doses, some infections may require up to 300,000 units/kg/day.
IV (Infants >7 days): 25,000 units/kg q 8 hr; *meningitis*—50,000–75,000 units/kg q 6 hr.
IV (Infants <7 days): 25,000 units/kg q 12 hr; *Streptococcus B meningitis*—100,000–150,000 units/kg/day in divided doses.

Penicillin V
PO (Adults and Children ≥12 yr): *Most infections*—125–500 mg q 6–8 hr. *Rheumatic fever prevention*—125–250 mg q 12 hr.
PO (Children <12 yr): *Lyme disease*—12.5 mg/kg q 6 hr (unlabeled); prevention of *Streptococcus pneumoniae* sepsis in children with sickle cell disease—125 mg twice daily.

Benzathine Penicillin G
IM (Adults): *Streptococcal infections/erysipeloid*—1.2 million units single dose. *Primary, secondary, and early latent syphilis*—2.4 million units single dose. *Tertiary and late latent syphilis (not neurosyphilis)*—2.4 million units once weekly for 3 wk. *Prevention of rheumatic fever*—1.2 million units q 3–4 wk.
IM (Children >27 kg): *Streptococcal infections/erysipeloid*—900,000–1.2 million units (single dose). *Primary, secondary, and early latent syphilis*—up to 2.4 million units single dose. *Late latent or latent syphilis of undetermined duration*—50,000 units/kg weekly for 3 wk. *Prevention of rheumatic fever*—1.2 million units q 2–3 wk.
IM (Children <27 kg): *Streptococcal infections/erysipeloid*—300,000–600,000 units single dose. *Primary, secondary, and early latent syphilis*—up to 2.4 million units single dose. *Late latent or latent syphilis of undetermined duration*—50,000 units/kg weekly for 3 wk. *Prevention of rheumatic fever*—1.2 million units q 2–3 wk.

Procaine Penicillin G
IM (Adults): *Moderate or severe infections*—600,000–1.2 million units/day as a single dose or in 2 divided doses. *Neurosyphilis*—2.4 million

units/day with 500 mg probenecid PO 4 times daily for 10–14 days.
IM (Children): *Congenital syphilis*—50,000 units/kg/day for 10–14 days.

Availability

Penicillin G Potassium (generic available)
Powder for injection: 5 million units/vial, 20 million units/vial. **Premixed (frozen) solution for injection:** 1 million units/50 mL, 2 million units/50 mL, 3 million units/50 mL.

Penicillin G Sodium (generic available)
Powder for injection: 5 million units/vial.

Penicillin V Potassium (generic available)
Tablets: 250 mg, 500 mg. **Oral solution:** 125 mg/5 mL, 250 mg/5 mL.

Procaine Penicillin G (generic available)
Suspension for IM injection: 600,000 units/mL.

Benzathine Penicillin G
Suspension for IM injection: 600,000 units/mL.

NURSING IMPLICATIONS

Assessment
- Assess for infection (vital signs; appearance of wound, sputum, urine, and stool; WBC) at beginning of and during therapy.
- Obtain a history to determine previous use of and reactions to penicillins, cephalosporins, or other beta-lactam antibiotics. Persons with a negative history of penicillin sensitivity may still have an allergic response.
- Obtain specimens for culture and sensitivity before initiating therapy. First dose may be given before receiving results.
- Observe patient for signs and symptoms of anaphylaxis (rash, pruritus, laryngeal edema, wheezing). Discontinue drug and notify health care professional immediately if these symptoms occur. Keep epinephrine, an antihistamine, and resuscitation equipment close by in case of an anaphylactic reaction.
- *Lab Test Considerations:* May cause positive direct Coombs' test results.
- Hyperkalemia may develop after large doses of penicillin G potassium.
- Monitor serum sodium concentrations in patient with hypertension or CHF. Hypernatremia may develop after large doses of penicillin sodium.
- May cause ↑ AST, ALT, LDH, and serum alkaline phosphatase concentrations.
- May cause leukopenia and neutropenia, especially with prolonged therapy or hepatic impairment.

Potential Nursing Diagnoses
Risk for infection (Indications, Side Effects)
Noncompliance (Patient/Family Teaching)

Implementation
- Do not confuse penicillin with penicillamine. Do not confuse penicillin G aqueous (potassium or sodium salt) with penicillin G procaine.
- **PO:** Administer around the clock. Penicillin V may be administered without regard for meals.
- Use calibrated measuring device for liquid preparations. Solution is stable for 14 days if refrigerated.
- **IM:** Reconstitute according to manufacturer's directions with sterile water for injection, D5W, or 0.9% NaCl.
- **IM:** Shake medication well before injection. Inject penicillin deep into a well-developed muscle mass at a slow, consistent rate to prevent blockage of the needle. Massage well. Accidental injury near or into a nerve can result in severe pain and dysfunction.
- Penicillin G potassium or sodium may be diluted with lidocaine (without epinephrine) 1% or 2% to minimize pain from IM injection.
- Never give penicillin G benzathine or penicillin G procaine suspensions IV. May cause embolism or toxic reactions.

IV Administration
- **IV:** Change IV sites every 48 hr to prevent phlebitis.
- Administer slowly and observe patient closely for signs of hypersensitivity.
- **Intermittent Infusion:** *Diluent:* Doses of 3 million units or less should be diluted in at least 50 mL of D5W or 0.9% NaCl; doses of more than 3 million units should be diluted with 100 mL. *Concentration:* 100,000–500,000 units/mL (50,000 units/mL in neonates). *Rate:* Infuse over 1–2 hr in adults or 15–30 min in children.
- **Continuous Infusion:** Doses of 10 million units or more may be diluted in 1 or 2 L.
- *Rate:* Infuse over 24 hr.

Penicillin G Potassium
- **Y-Site Compatibility:** acyclovir, amiodarone, cyclophosphamide, diltiazem, enalaprilat, esmolol, fluconazole, foscarnet, heparin, hydro-

morphone, labetalol, magnesium sulfate, meperidine, morphine, nicardipine, perphenazine, potassium chloride, tacrolimus, theophylline, verapamil, vitamin B complex with C.
- **Y-Site Incompatibility:** If aminoglycosides and penicillins must be administered concurrently, administer in separate sites at least 1 hr apart.
- **Additive Incompatibility:** Incompatible with aminoglycosides; do not admix.

Penicillin G Sodium
- **Y-Site Compatibility:** levofloxacin.
- **Y-Site Incompatibility:** If aminoglycosides and penicillins must be administered concurrently, administer in separate sites at least 1 hr apart.
- **Additive Incompatibility:** Incompatible with aminoglycosides; do not admix.

Patient/Family Teaching
- Instruct patient to take medication around the clock and to finish drug completely as directed, even if feeling better. Advise patient that sharing this medication may be dangerous.
- Advise patient to report signs of superinfection (black, furry overgrowth on tongue; vaginal itching or discharge; loose or foul-smelling stools) and allergy.
- Instruct patient to notify health care professional if fever and diarrhea develop, especially if stool contains blood, pus, or mucus. Advise patient not to treat diarrhea without consulting health care professional.
- Instruct patient to notify health care professional if symptoms do not improve.
- Advise patient taking oral contraceptives to use an additional nonhormonal method of contraception during therapy with penicillin and until next menstrual period.
- Patient with an allergy to penicillin should be instructed to always carry an identification card with this information.

Evaluation/Desired Outcomes
- Resolution of signs and symptoms of infection. Length of time for complete resolution depends on the organism and site of infection.

PENICILLINS, PENICILLINASE RESISTANT

dicloxacillin (dye-klox-a-**sill**-in)

nafcillin (naf-**sill**-in)

oxacillin (ox-a-**sill**-in)
Bactocill

Classification
Therapeutic: anti-infectives
Pharmacologic: penicillinase resistant penicillins

Pregnancy Category B

Indications
Treatment of the following infections due to penicillinase-producing staphylococci: Respiratory tract infections, Sinusitis, Skin and skin structure infections. **Dicloxacillin:** Osteomyelitis. **Nafcillin, oxacillin:** Are also used to treat: Bone and joint infections, Urinary tract infections, Endocarditis, Septicemia, Meningitis.

Action
Bind to bacterial cell wall, leading to cell death. Not inactivated by penicillinase enzymes. **Therapeutic Effects:** Bactericidal action. **Spectrum:** Active against most gram-positive aerobic cocci but less so than penicillin. Spectrum is notable for activity against: Penicillinase-producing strains of *Staphylococcus aureus*, *Staphylococcus epidermidis*. Not active against methicillin-resistant staphylococci.

Pharmacokinetics
Absorption: *Dicloxacillin*—Rapidly but incompletely (35–76%) absorbed from the GI tract. *Nafcillin and oxacillin*—Completely absorbed following IV administration; well absorbed from IM sites.

Distribution: Widely distributed; penetration into CSF is minimal, but sufficient in the presence of inflamed meninges; cross the placenta and enter breast milk.

Metabolism and Excretion: *Dicloxacillin*—Some metabolism by the liver (6–10%) and some renal excretion of unchanged drug (60%); small amounts eliminated in the feces via the bile. *Nafcillin, oxacillin*—Partially metabolized by the liver (nafcillin 60%, oxacillin 49%), partially excreted unchanged by the kidneys.

Half-life: *Dicloxacillin*—0.5–1.1 hr (↑ in severe hepatic and renal dysfunction); *nafcillin*—Neonates: 1–5 hr; Children 1 month – 14 yr: 0.75–1.9 hr; Adults: 0.5–1.5 hr (↑ in renal impairment); *oxacillin*—Neonates: 1.6 hr; Children up to 2 yr: 0.9–1.8 hr; Adults: 0.3–0.8 hr (↑ in severe hepatic impairment).

✽ = Canadian drug name. = Genetic implication.
*CAPITALS indicates life-threatening; underlines indicate most frequent.

PENICILLINS, PENICILLINASE RESISTANT

TIME/ACTION PROFILE (blood levels)

ROUTE	ONSET	PEAK	DURATION
Dicloxacillin PO	30 min	30–120 min	6 hr
Nafcillin IM	30 min	60–120 min	4–6 hr
Nafcillin IV	rapid	end of infusion	4–6 hr
Oxacillin IM	rapid	30 min	4–6 hr
Oxacillin IV	rapid	end of infusion	4–6 hr

Contraindications/Precautions

Contraindicated in: Hypersensitivity to penicillins (cross-sensitivity with cephalosporins may exist).

Use Cautiously in: Severe renal or hepatic impairment; OB: Lactation: Safety not established.

Adverse Reactions/Side Effects

CNS: SEIZURES (high doses). **GI:** PSEUDOMEMBRANOUS COLITIS, diarrhea, nausea, vomiting, drug-induced hepatitis. **GU:** interstitial nephritis. **Derm:** rashes, urticaria. **Hemat:** eosinophilia, leukopenia. **Local:** pain at IM sites, phlebitis at IV sites. **Misc:** allergic reactions including ANAPHYLAXIS and SERUM SICKNESS, superinfection.

Interactions

Drug-Drug: Probenecid ↓ renal excretion and ↑ blood levels (treatment may be combined for this purpose). May ↓ effectiveness of **oral contraceptive agents**. May ↓ elimination of **methotrexate** and ↑ risk of serious toxicity.

Route/Dosage

Dicloxacillin

PO (Adults and Children ≥40 kg): 125–250 mg q 6 hr (up to 2 g/day).
PO (Children <40 kg): 6.25–12.5 mg/kg q 6 hr; (up to 12.25 mg/kg q 6 hr has been used for osteomyelitis), maximum: 2 g/day.

Nafcillin

IM (Adults): 500 mg q 4–6 hr.
IM, IV (Children and Infants): 50–200 mg/kg/day divided q 4–6 hr, maximum: 12 g/day.
IM, IV (Neonates 0–4 weeks, < 1200 g): 25 mg/kg q 12 hr.
IM, IV (Neonates 1.2–2 kg): —25 mg/kg q 12 hr for the first 7 days of life, then 25 mg/kg q 8 hr.
IM, IV (Neonates >2 kg): —25 mg/kg q 8 hr for the first 7 days of life, then 25 mg/kg q 6 hr.
IV (Adults): 500–2000 mg q 4–6 hr.

Oxacillin

IM, IV (Adults and Children ≥40 kg): 250–2000 mg q 4–6 hr (up to 12 g/day).
IM, IV (Children <40 kg): 100–200 mg/kg/day divided q 4–6 hr, maximum: 12 g/day.
IM, IV (Neonates < 1200 g): —25 mg/kg q 12 hr.
IM, IV (Neonates ≥2 kg): —25 mg/kg q 8 hr for the first 7 days of life, then 25 mg/kg q 6 hr.
IM, IV (Neonates 1.2–2 kg): —25 mg/kg q 12 hr for the first 7 days of life, then 25 mg/kg q 8 hr.

Availability

Dicloxacillin (generic available)
Capsules: 250 mg, 500 mg. **Oral suspension:** 62.5 mg/5 mL.

Nafcillin (generic available)
Powder for injection: 500 mg/vial, 1 g/vial, 2 g/vial, 10 g/vial.

Oxacillin (generic available)
Powder for injection: 250 mg/vial, 500 mg/vial, 1 g/vial, 2 g/vial, 4 g/vial, 10 g/vial.

NURSING IMPLICATIONS

Assessment

- Assess patient for infection (vital signs; appearance of wound, sputum, urine, and stool; WBC) at beginning of and throughout therapy.
- Obtain a history before initiating therapy to determine previous use of and reactions to penicillins, cephalosporins, or other beta-lactam antibiotics. Persons with a negative history of penicillin sensitivity may still have an allergic response.
- Obtain specimens for culture and sensitivity prior to initiating therapy. First dose may be given before receiving results.
- Observe patient for signs and symptoms of anaphylaxis (rash, pruritus, laryngeal edema, wheezing, abdominal pain). Discontinue the drug and notify the physician or other health care professional immediately if these occur. Keep epinephrine, an antihistamine, and resuscitation equipment close by in the event of an anaphylactic reaction.
- Assess vein for signs of irritation and phlebitis. Change IV site every 48 hr to prevent phlebitis.
- *Lab Test Considerations:* May cause leukopenia and neutropenia, especially with prolonged therapy or hepatic impairment.
- May cause positive direct Coombs' test result.
- May cause ↑ AST, ALT, LDH, and serum alkaline phosphatase concentrations.

Potential Nursing Diagnoses

Risk for infection (Indications, Side Effects)
Noncompliance (Patient/Family Teaching)

Implementation

- **PO:** Administer around the clock on an empty stomach at least 1 hr before or 2 hr after meals. Take with a full glass of water; acidic juices may decrease absorption of penicillins.
- Use calibrated measuring device for liquid preparations. Shake well. Solution is stable for 14 days if refrigerated.

Nafcillin

IV Administration

- **IV, IM:** To reconstitute, add 3.4 mL to each 1-g vial or 6.8 mL to each 2-g vial, for a concentration of 250 mg/mL. Stable for 2–7 days if refrigerated.
- **Direct IV:** *Diluent:* Dilute reconstituted solution with 15–30 mL of sterile water, 0.45% NaCl, or 0.9% NaCl for injection. *Concentration:* 100 mg/mL. *Rate:* Administer over 5–10 min.
- **Intermittent Infusion:** *Diluent:* Dilute with sterile water for injection, 0.9% NaCl, D5W, D10W, D5/0.25% NaCl, D5/0.45% NaCl, D5/0.9% NaCl, D5/LR, Ringer's or LR. Stable for 24 hr at room temperature, 96 hr if refrigerated. *Concentration:* 2–40 mg/mL. *Rate:* Infuse over at least 30–60 min to avoid vein irritation.
- **Y-Site Compatibility:** acyclovir, atropine, cyclophosphamide, diazepam, enalaprilat, esmolol, famotidine, fentanyl, fluconazole, foscarnet, heparin, hydromorphone, magnesium sulfate, morphine, nicardipine, perphenazine, propofol, theophylline, zidovudine.
- **Y-Site Incompatibility:** droperidol, insulin, labetalol, midazolam, nalbuphine, pentazocine, verapamil. If penicillins and aminoglycosides must be administered concurrently, administer at separate sites.

Oxacillin

IV Administration

- **IV, IM:** To reconstitute for IM or IV use, add 1.4 mL of sterile water for injection to each 250-mg vial, 2.7 mL to each 500-mg vial, 5.7 mL to each 1-g vial, 11.5 mL to each 2-g vial, and 23 mL to each 4-g vial, for a concentration of 250 mg/1.5 mL. Stable for 3 days at room temperature or 7 days if refrigerated.
- **Direct IV:** *Diluent:* Further dilute each reconstituted 250-mg or 500-mg vial with 5 mL of sterile water or 0.9% NaCl for injection, 10 mL for each 1-g vial, 20 mL for each 2-g vial, and 40 mL for each 4-g vial. *Concentration:* 100 mg/mL. *Rate:* Administer slowly over 10 min.
- **Intermittent Infusion:** *Diluent:* Dilute with 0.9% NaCl, D5W, D5/0.9% NaCl, or LR. *Concentration:* 0.5–40 mg/mL. *Rate:* May be infused for up to 6 hr.
- **Y-Site Compatibility:** acyclovir, cyclophosphamide, diltiazem, doxapram, famotidine, fluconazole, foscarnet, heparin, hydrocortisone sodium succinate, hydromorphone, labetalol, levofloxacin, magnesium sulfate, meperidine, methotrexate, milrinone, morphine, perphenazine, potassium chloride, tacrolimus, vitamin B complex with C, zidovudine.
- **Y-Site Incompatibility:** sodium bicarbonate, verapamil. If penicillins and aminoglycosides must be administered concurrently, administer at separate sites.

Patient/Family Teaching

- Instruct patient to take medication around the clock and to finish the drug completely as directed, even if feeling better. Missed doses should be taken as soon as remembered. Advise patient that sharing of this medication may be dangerous.
- Advise patient to report signs of superinfection (black, furry overgrowth on the tongue; vaginal itching or discharge; loose or foul-smelling stools) and allergy.
- Instruct patient to notify health care professional if fever and diarrhea develop, especially if stool contains blood, pus, or mucus. Advise patient not to treat diarrhea without consulting health care professional.
- Instruct patient to notify health care professional if symptoms do not improve.

Evaluation/Desired Outcomes

- Resolution of the signs and symptoms of infection. Length of time for complete resolution depends on the organism and site of infection.

---

pentamidine (pen-**tam**-i-deen)
NebuPent, Pentam 300

Classification
Therapeutic: anti-infectives

Pregnancy Category C

Indications

IV: Treatment of *Pneumocystis jirovecii* pneumonia (PCP). **Inhaln:** Prevention of PCP in AIDS

1008 pentamidine

or HIV-positive patients who have had PCP or who have a peripheral CD4 lymphocyte count of ≤200/mm³. **Unlabeled Use: Inhaln:** Treatment of PCP.

Action
Appears to disrupt DNA or RNA synthesis. Also has a direct toxic effect on pancreatic islet cells.
Therapeutic Effects: Death of susceptible organism.

Pharmacokinetics
Absorption: Minimal systemic absorption occurs following inhalation.
Distribution: Widely and extensively distributed but does not cross the blood-brain barrier. Concentrates in liver, kidneys, lungs, and spleen, with prolonged storage in some tissues.
Metabolism and Excretion: 1–30% excreted unchanged by the kidneys. Remainder of metabolic fate unknown.
Half-life: 6.4–9.4 hr (↑ in renal impairment).

TIME/ACTION PROFILE (blood levels)

ROUTE	ONSET	PEAK	DURATION
IV	unknown	end of infusion	24 hr
Inhaln	unknown	unknown	unknown

Contraindications/Precautions
Contraindicated in: History of previous anaphylactic reaction to pentamidine.
Use Cautiously in: Hypotension; Hypertension; Hypoglycemia; Hyperglycemia; Hypocalcemia; Leukopenia; Thrombocytopenia; Anemia; Renal impairment (dose reduction required); Diabetes mellitus; Liver impairment; Cardiovascular disease; Bone marrow depression, previous antineoplastic therapy, or radiation therapy; OB, Lactation: Safety not established during pregnancy; breastfeeding not recommended.

Adverse Reactions/Side Effects
For parenteral form, unless otherwise indicated. **CNS:** anxiety, headache, confusion, dizziness, hallucinations. **EENT:** *inhalation*—burning in throat. **Resp:** *inhalation*—bronchospasm, cough. **CV:** ARRHYTHMIAS, HYPOTENSION. **GI:** PANCREATITIS, abdominal pain, anorexia, drug-induced hepatitis, nausea, unpleasant metallic taste, vomiting. **GU:** nephrotoxicity. **Derm:** pallor, rash. **Endo:** HYPOGLYCEMIA, hyperglycemia. **F and E:** hyperkalemia, hypocalcemia. **Hemat:** anemia, leukopenia, thrombocytopenia. **Local:** *IV*—phlebitis, pruritus, urticaria at IV site; *IM*—sterile abscesses at IM sites. **Misc:** allergic reactions including ANAPHYLAXIS, STEVENS-JOHNSON SYNDROME, chills, fever.

Interactions
Interactions listed for parenteral administration.
Drug-Drug: Concurrent use with **erythromycin IV** may ↑ risk of potentially fatal arrhythmias. Additive nephrotoxicity with other **nephrotoxic agents**, including **aminoglycosides**, **amphotericin B**, and **vancomycin**. Additive bone marrow depression with **antineoplastics** or previous **radiation therapy**. ↑ risk of pancreatitis with **didanosine**. ↑ risk of nephrotoxicity, hypocalcemia, and hypomagnesemia with **foscarnet**.

Route/Dosage
IV (Adults and Children): 4 mg/kg once daily for 14–21 days (longer treatment may be required in AIDS patients; some patients may respond to 3 mg/kg/day).
Inhaln (Adults): *NebuPent*—300 mg q 4 wk, using a Respirgard II jet nebulizer (150 mg q 2 wk has also been used).
Inhaln (Children >5 yr): *NebuPent*—300 mg q 4 wk, using a Respirgard II jet nebulizer (for patients who cannot tolerate trimethoprim/sulfamethoxazole; unlabeled).

Availability (generic available)
Powder for injection: 300 mg. **Solution for aerosol use (NebuPent):** 300 mg.

NURSING IMPLICATIONS

Assessment
- Assess patient for infection (vital signs, sputum, WBC) and monitor respiratory status (rate, character, lung sounds, dyspnea, sputum) at beginning of and throughout therapy.
- Obtain specimens for culture and sensitivity prior to initiating therapy. First dose may be given before receiving results.
- **IV, IM:** Monitor blood pressure frequently during and following IM or IV administration of pentamidine. Patient should be lying down during administration. Sudden, severe hypotension may occur following a single dose. Resuscitation equipment should be immediately available.
- Assess patient for signs of hypoglycemia (anxiety; chills; diaphoresis; cold, pale skin; headache; increased hunger; nausea; nervousness; shakiness) and hyperglycemia (drowsiness; flushed, dry skin; fruit-like breath odor; increased thirst; increased urination; loss of appetite), which may occur up to several months after therapy is discontinued.
- Pulse and ECG should be monitored prior to and periodically during therapy. Fatalities due

to cardiac arrhythmias, tachycardia, and cardiotoxicity have been reported.
- **Inhaln:** A tuberculin skin test, chest x-ray, and sputum culture should be performed prior to administration to rule out tuberculosis.
- **Lab Test Considerations:** *IM, IV*—Monitor blood glucose concentrations prior to, daily during, and for several months following therapy. Severe hypoglycemia and permanent diabetes mellitus have occurred.
- Monitor BUN and serum creatinine prior to and daily during therapy to monitor for nephrotoxicity. Concentrations may be ↑.
- Monitor CBC and platelet count prior to and every 3 days during therapy. Pentamidine may cause leukopenia, anemia, and thrombocytopenia.
- May cause ↑ serum bilirubin, alkaline phosphatase, AST, and ALT concentrations. Monitor liver function tests prior to and every 3 days during therapy.
- Monitor serum calcium and magnesium concentrations prior to and every 3 days during therapy; may cause hypocalcemia and hypomagnesemia.
- May cause ↑ serum potassium concentrations.

Potential Nursing Diagnoses
Risk for infection (Indications, Side Effects)

Implementation
- Pentamidine must be given on a regular schedule for the full course of therapy. Administer missed doses as soon as remembered. If almost time for the next dose, skip the missed dose and return to the regular schedule. Do not double doses.
- **IM:** Dilute 300 mg of pentamidine with 3 mL of sterile water for injection for a concentration of 100 mg/mL. IM administration should be used only for patients with adequate muscle mass and given deep IM via Z-track technique. May cause sterile abscesses.

IV Administration
- **Intermittent Infusion:** *Diluent:* To reconstitute, add 3–5 mL of sterile water for injection or D5W to each 300-mg vial for a concentration of 100, 75, or 60 mg/mL, respectively. Withdraw dose and dilute further in 50–250 mL of D5W. Solution is stable for 48 hr at room temperature. Discard unused portions. *Concentration:* Not to exceed 6 mg/mL for administration. *Rate:* Administer slowly over 1–2 hr.
- **Y-Site Compatibility:** alfentanyl, anidulafungin, atropine, atracurium, benztropine, buprenorphine, calcium gluconate, carboplatin, caspofungin, chlorpromazine, cimetidine, cisplatin, cyanocobalamin, cyclophosphamide, cyclosporine, cytarabine, dactinomycin, daptomycin, dexmedetomidine, diltiazem, diphenhydramine, dobutamine, docetaxel, dopamine, doxacurium, doxycycline, enalaprilat, epinephrine, epirubicin, erythromycin, esmolol, etoposide, etoposide phosphate, famotidine, fenoldopam, fentanyl, fludarabine, gemcitabine, glycopyrrolate, granisetron, hetastarch, hydromorphone, idarubicin, ifosfamide, isoproterenol, labetalol, levofloxacin, lidocaine, lorazepam, mannitol, mechlorethamine, meperidine, metaraminol, methoxamine, metoclopramide, metoprolol, metronidazole, miconazole, midazolam, milrinone, mitoxantrone, multivitamins, naloxone, nesiritide, nitroglycerin, nitroprusside norepinephrine, octreotide, ondansetron, oxaliplatin, oxytocin, paclitaxel, pancuronium, papaverine, pentazocine, phentolamine, phytonadione, procainamide, promethazine, propranolol, pyridoxime, quinupristin/dalfopristin, ranitidine, rituximab, rocuronium, sodium acetate, succinylcholine, sufentanil, tacrolimus, teniposide, theophylline, thiamine, thiotepa, tigecycline, tolazoline, trastuzumab, trimetaphan, urokinase, vancomycin, vasopressin, verapamil, vincristine, vinorelbine, voriconazole, zidovudine.
- **Y-Site Incompatibility:** acyclovir, aldesleukin, amikacin, aminophylline, amphotericin B colloidal, amphotericin B liposome, ampicillin, ampicillin/sulbactam, ascorbic acid, azathioprine, azotreonam, bivalirudin, bumetanide, butorphanol, cefazolin, cefonicid, cefoperazone, cefotaxime, cefotetan, cefoxitin, ceftazidime, ceftriaxone, cefuroxime, chloramphenicol, clindamycin, dantrolene, dexamethasone, diazepam, diazoxide, digoxin, doxorubicin, ephedrine, epoetin alfa, eftifibatide, ertapenem, fluorouracil, folic acid, foscarnet, furosemide, gentamicin, heparin, hydrocortisone, inamrinone, indomethacin, insulin, ketorolac, linezolid, magnesium sulfate, methotrexate, methyldopate, methylprednisolone, morphine, nafcillin, nalbuphine, oxacillin, palonosetron, pantoprazole, pemetrexed, penicillin G, pentobarbital, phenobarbital, phenylephrine, phe-

nytoin, piperacillin/tazobactam, potassium chloride, prochlorperazine, protamine, sodium bicarbonate, streptokinase, ticarcillin/clavulanate, tobramycin, trimethoprim/sulfamethoxazole, vecuronium.
- **Inhaln:** If using inhalation bronchodilator, administer bronchodilator 5–10 min prior to pentamidine administration.
- Administer in a well-ventilated area.
- Administration with patient in supine or recumbent position appears to provide a more uniform distribution of pentamidine.
- *NebuPent* Dilute 300 or 600 mg (for prophylaxis or treatment, respectively) in 6 mL of sterile water for injection. Place reconstituted solution into Respirgard II nebulizer. Do not dilute with 0.9% NaCl or admix with other medications, as solution will form a precipitate. Do not use Respirgard II nebulizer for other medications.
- Administer inhalation dose through nebulizer until chamber is empty, approximately 30–45 min.
- Administer with the flow rate of the nebulizer at the midflow mark (5–7 L/min) over approximately 15 min until the chamber is empty.

Patient/Family Teaching
- Inform patient of the importance of completing the full course of pentamidine therapy, even if feeling better.
- **IV:** Instruct patient to notify health care professional promptly if fever; sore throat; signs of infection; bleeding of gums; unusual bruising; petechiae; or blood in stool, urine, or emesis occurs. Caution patient to avoid crowds and persons with known infections. Instruct patient to use soft toothbrush and electric razor and to avoid falls. Patient should not be given IM injections or rectal thermometers. Patient should be cautioned not to drink alcoholic beverages or take medication containing aspirin or NSAIDs, as these may precipitate gastric bleeding.
- Caution patient to make position changes slowly to minimize orthostatic hypotension.
- **Inhaln:** Advise patient that an unpleasant metallic taste may occur with pentamidine administration but is not significant.
- Inform patients who continue to smoke that bronchospasm and coughing during therapy are more likely.

Evaluation/Desired Outcomes
- Prevention or resolution of the signs and symptoms of PCP in HIV-positive patients.

HIGH ALERT

pentazocine (pen-taz-oh-seen)
Talwin, Talwin NX

Classification
Therapeutic: opioid analgesics
Pharmacologic: opioid agonists/antagonists

Schedule IV

Pregnancy Category C

Indications
Moderate to severe pain. Also used for: Analgesia during labor, Sedation prior to surgery, Supplemention in balanced anesthesia.

Action
Binds to opiate receptors in the CNS. Alters perception of and response to painful stimuli, while producing generalized CNS depression. Has partial antagonist properties, which may result in opioid withdrawal in physically dependent patients. **Therapeutic Effects:** Decrease in moderate to severe pain.

Pharmacokinetics
Absorption: Well absorbed following oral, IM, and subcut administration. Small amount (0.5 mg) of naloxone in tablets included to prevent parenteral abuse.
Distribution: Widely distributed. Crosses the placenta.
Metabolism and Excretion: Mostly metabolized by the liver. Small amounts excreted unchanged by the kidneys.
Half-life: 2–3 hr.

TIME/ACTION PROFILE (analgesia)

ROUTE	ONSET	PEAK	DURATION
PO	15–30 min	60–90 min	3 hr
IM, subcut	15–20 min	30–60 min	2–3 hr
IV	2–3 min	15–30 min	2–3 hr

Contraindications/Precautions
Contraindicated in: Hypersensitivity; Patients who are physically dependent on opioids (may precipitate withdrawal).
Use Cautiously in: Head trauma; History of drug abuse; ↑ intracranial pressure; Severe renal, hepatic, or pulmonary disease; Hypothyroidism; Adrenal insufficiency; Alcoholism; Debilitated patients or patients with severe liver impairment (dose ↓ recommended); Undiagnosed abdominal pain; Prostatic hyperplasia; Patients who have recently received opioid agonists; OB: Has been used during labor but may cause respiratory depression in the newborn; Lactation: Pedi: Safety

pentazocine **1011**

not established; **Geri:** Appears on Beers list and is associated with ↑ risk of falls. More susceptible to adverse CNS effects; dose ↓ recommended.

Adverse Reactions/Side Effects
CNS: <u>dizziness</u>, euphoria, hallucinations, <u>headache</u>, <u>sedation</u>, confusion, dysphoria, floating feeling, unusual dreams. **EENT:** blurred vision, diplopia, miosis (high doses). **Resp:** respiratory depression. **CV:** hypertension, hypotension, palpitations. **GI:** <u>nausea</u>, constipation, dry mouth, ileus, vomiting. **GU:** urinary retention. **Derm:** clammy feeling, sweating. **Local:** severe tissue damage at subcut sites. **Misc:** physical dependence, psychological dependence, tolerance.

Interactions
Drug-Drug: Use with caution in patients receiving **MAO inhibitors** (may result in unpredictable reactions— ↓ initial dose of pentazocine to 25% of usual dose). Additive CNS depression with **alcohol**, **antihistamines**, and **sedative/hypnotics**. May precipitate withdrawal in patients who are physically dependent on **opioid analgesic agonists**. May ↓ analgesic effects of other **opioids**.
Drug-Natural Products: Concomitant use of **kava-kava**, **valerian**, or **chamomile** can ↑ CNS depression.

Route/Dosage
PO (Adults): 50–100 mg q 3–4 hr (not to exceed 600 mg/day).
Subcut, IV, IM (Adults): 30 mg q 3–4 hr (not to exceed 30 mg/dose IV or 60 mg/dose IM or subcut; not to exceed 360 mg/day subcut, IV, or IM). *Obstetrical use*— 20 mg IV or 30 mg IM when contractions become regular, may repeat q 2–3 hr for 2–3 doses.

Availability
Tablets: 50 mg (with 0.5 mg naloxone), ✺ 50 mg. **Injection:** 30 mg/mL. *In combination with:* acetaminophen (Talacen). See Appendix B.

NURSING IMPLICATIONS

Assessment
- Assess type, location, and intensity of pain prior to and 1 hr following PO, subcut, or IM and 15–30 min (peak) following IV administration. When titrating opioid doses, increases of 25–50% should be administered until there is either a 50% reduction in the patient's pain rating on a numeric or visual analogue scale or the patient reports satisfactory pain relief. A repeat dose can be safely administered at the time of the peak if previous dose is ineffective and side effects are minimal. Patients requiring doses higher than 100 mg should be converted to an opioid agonist. Pentazocine is not recommended for prolonged use or as first-line therapy for acute or cancer pain.
- An equianalgesic chart (see Appendix K) should be used when changing routes or when changing from one opioid to another.
- Assess blood pressure, pulse, and respirations before and periodically during administration. If respiratory rate is <10/min, assess level of sedation. Physical stimulation may be sufficient to prevent significant hypoventilation. Dose may need to be decreased by 25–50%. Pentazocine produces respiratory depression, but this does not markedly increase with increased doses.
- Assess prior analgesic history. Antagonistic properties may induce withdrawal symptoms (vomiting, restlessness, abdominal cramps, and increased blood pressure and temperature) in patients physically dependent on opioids.
- Although this drug has a low potential for dependence, prolonged use may lead to physical and psychological dependence and tolerance. This should not prevent patient from receiving adequate analgesia. Most patients receiving pentazocine for pain do not develop psychological dependence. If tolerance develops, changing to an opioid agonist may be required to relieve pain.
- **Geri:** Assess falls risk and implement prevention strategies. Assess for adverse CNS effects.
- *Lab Test Considerations:* May cause ↑ serum amylase and lipase levels.
- *Toxicity and Overdose:* If an opioid antagonist is required to reverse respiratory depression or coma, naloxone (Narcan) is the antidote. Dilute the 0.4-mg ampule of naloxone in 10 mL of 0.9% NaCl and administer 0.5 mL (0.02 mg) by direct IV push every 2 min. For patients weighing <40 kg, dilute 0.1 mg of naloxone in 10 mL of 0.9% NaCl for a concentration of 10 mcg/mL and administer 0.5 mcg/kg every 2 min. Titrate dose to avoid withdrawal, seizures, and severe pain.

Potential Nursing Diagnoses
Acute pain (Indications)
Risk for injury (Side Effects)

✺ = Canadian drug name.   ❀ = Genetic implication.
*CAPITALS indicates life-threatening; <u>underlines</u> indicate most frequent.

Disturbed sensory perception (visual, auditory) (Side Effects)

Implementation
- **High Alert:** Accidental overdose of opioid analgesics has resulted in fatalities. Before administering, clarify all ambiguous orders; have second practitioner independently check original order and dose calculations.
- Explain therapeutic value of medication prior to administration to enhance the analgesic effect.
- Regularly administered doses may be more effective than prn administration. Analgesic is more effective if administered before pain becomes severe.
- Coadministration with nonopioid analgesics may have additive effects and may permit lower opioid doses.
- **PO:** Talwin NX contains 0.5 mg of naloxone, which has no pharmacologic activity when administered orally. If the product is abused by injection, naloxone antagonizes pentazocine. Parenteral use of oral pentazocine may lead to severe, potentially fatal reactions (pulmonary emboli, vascular occlusion, ulceration and abscess, and withdrawal symptoms in opioid-dependent individuals).
- **IM, Subcut:** Administer IM injections deep into well-developed muscle. Rotate sites of injections. Subcut route may cause tissue damage with repeated injections.

IV Administration
- **Direct IV:** *Diluent:* Manufacturer recommends diluting each 5 mg with at least 1 mL of sterile water for injection. *Concentration:* 5 mg/mL. *Rate:* Administer slowly, each 5 mg over at least 1 min.
- **Syringe Compatibility:** atropine, chlorpromazine, cimetidine, dimenhydrinate, diphenhydramine, droperidol, hydroxyzine, metoclopramide, perphenazine, prochlorperazine edisylate, promazine, promethazine, ranitidine, scopolamine.
- **Syringe Incompatibility:** glycopyrrolate, heparin, pentobarbital.
- **Y-Site Compatibility:** heparin, hydrocortisone sodium succinate, potassium chloride, vitamin B complex with C.
- **Y-Site Incompatibility:** nafcillin.

Patient/Family Teaching
- Instruct patient on how and when to ask for pain medication.
- Medication may cause drowsiness, dizziness, or hallucinations, particularly in geriatric patients. Advise patient to call for assistance when ambulating and to avoid driving or other activities requiring alertness until response to medication is known. Institute fall prevention strategies and teach patient or family how to prevent falls at home.
- Caution patient to change positions slowly to minimize orthostatic hypotension.
- Advise patient to avoid concurrent use of alcohol and other CNS depressants.
- Encourage patient to turn, cough, and breathe deeply every 2 hr to prevent atelectasis.
- Advise patient that frequent mouth rinses, good oral hygiene, and sugarless gum or candy may decrease dry mouth.

Evaluation/Desired Outcomes
- Decrease in severity of pain without a significant alteration in level of consciousness or respiratory status.

---

perindopril, See ANGIOTENSIN-CONVERTING ENZYME (ACE) INHIBITORS.

---

permethrin (per-meth-rin)
Acticin, Elimite, Nix

Classification
Therapeutic: pediculocides

Pregnancy Category B

Indications
1% lotion: Eradication of *Pediculus humanus capitis* (head lice and their eggs): Prevention of infestation of head lice during epidemics. **5% cream:** Eradication of *Sarcoptes scabiei* (scabies).

Action
Causes repolarization and paralysis in lice by disrupting sodium transport in normal nerve cells.
Therapeutic Effects: Death of parasites.

Pharmacokinetics
Absorption: Small amounts (<2%) systemically absorbed. Remains on hair for 10 days.
Distribution: Unknown.
Metabolism and Excretion: Rapidly inactivated by enzymes.
Half-life: Unknown.

TIME/ACTION PROFILE (pediculocidal action)

ROUTE	ONSET	PEAK	DURATION
Topical	10 min	unknown	14 days

Contraindications/Precautions
Contraindicated in: Hypersensitivity to permethrin, pyrethrins (insecticides or veterinary pesticides), chrysanthemums, or isopropyl alcohol; Lactation: Lactation.
Use Cautiously in: OB: Use only if clearly needed; Pedi: Children <2 yr (1% lotion); Children <2 mo (5% cream).

Adverse Reactions/Side Effects
Derm: burning, itching, rash, redness, stinging, swelling. **Neuro:** numbness, tingling.

Interactions
Drug-Drug: No significant interactions.

Route/Dosage
Head Lice (Treatment and Prevention)
Topical (Adults and Children >2 yr): 1% lotion applied to the hair, left on for 10 min, then rinsed, for 1 application.

Scabies
Topical (Adults and Children): Massage 5% cream into all skin surfaces. Leave on for 8–14 hr, then wash off.
Topical (Infants >2 mo): Massage 5% cream into hairline, scalp, neck, temple, and forehead. Leave on for 8–14 hr, then wash off.

Availability (generic available)
Liquid cream rinse (lotion): 1%^{OTC}. **Cream:** 5%.

NURSING IMPLICATIONS

Assessment
- **Head Lice:** Assess scalp for presence of lice and their ova (nits) prior to and 1 wk after application of permethrin.
- **Scabies:** Assess skin for scabies prior to and following therapy.

Potential Nursing Diagnoses
Impaired home maintenance (Indications)
Bathing/hygiene self-care deficit (Indications)

Implementation
- **Topical:** For topical application only.

Patient/Family Teaching
- Instruct patient to notify health care professional if scalp itching, numbness, redness, or rash occurs.
- Instruct patient to avoid getting Elimite cream in eyes. If this occurs, eyes should be flushed thoroughly with water. Health care professional should be contacted if eye irritation persists.
- Advise patient that others residing in the home should also be checked for lice.
- Instruct patient on methods of preventing reinfestation. All clothes, including outdoor apparel and household linens, should be machine-washed using very hot water and dried for at least 20 min in a hot dryer. Dry-clean nonwashable clothes. Brushes and combs should be soaked in hot (130°F), soapy water for 5–10 min. Remind patient that brushes and combs should not be shared. Wigs and hairpieces should be shampooed. Rugs and upholstered furniture should be vacuumed. Toys should be washed in hot, soapy water. Items that cannot be washed should be sealed in a plastic bag for 2 wk.
- If patient is a child, instruct parents to notify school nurse or day care center so that classmates and playmates can be checked.
- **Head Lice:** Instruct patient to wash hair with regular shampoo, rinse, and towel dry. Each container holds enough medication for one treatment. Shake the container well. Thoroughly wet scalp and hair with the lotion. The patient should use as much of the solution as needed to coat entire head of hair, then discard remainder of solution. Allow lotion to remain on hair for 10 min, then thoroughly rinse hair and towel dry with a clean towel. Comb hair with a fine-toothed comb to remove dead lice and eggs (not necessary but may be desired for cosmetic effects). Products are available for removal of nits (Rid Lice Egg Loosener Gel®Step 2). Schools usually require children to be nit-free prior to returning to school.
- Explain to patient that permethrin will protect from reinfestation for 2 wk. These effects continue even when the patient resumes regular shampooing.
- **Scabies:** Instruct patient to massage thoroughly into the skin from head to soles of feet. Treat infants on the hairline, neck, scalp, temple, and forehead. Remove the cream by washing after 8–14 hr. Usually 30 g (½ tube) is sufficient for adults. One application is curative.

Evaluation/Desired Outcomes
- The absence of lice and eggs 1 wk after therapy. A second application is indicated if lice are detected at this time.
- Prevention of infestation of head lice during epidemics.
- Eradication of scabies following one application.

- If resistance to permethrin develops, malathion may be used.

phenazopyridine
(fen-az-oh-**peer**-i-deen)
Azo-Standard, Baridium, ♣ Phenazo, Prodium, Pyridium, Pyridium Plus, UTI Relief

Classification
Therapeutic: nonopioid analgesics
Pharmacologic: urinary tract analgesics

Pregnancy Category B

Indications
Provides relief from the following urinary tract symptoms, which may occur in association with infection or following urologic procedures: Pain, Itching, Burning, Urgency, Frequency.

Action
Acts locally on the urinary tract mucosa to produce analgesic or local anesthetic effects. Has no antimicrobial activity. **Therapeutic Effects:** Diminished urinary tract discomfort.

Pharmacokinetics
Absorption: Appears to be well absorbed following oral administration.
Distribution: Unknown. Small amounts cross the placenta.
Metabolism and Excretion: Rapidly excreted unchanged in the urine.
Half-life: Unknown.

TIME/ACTION PROFILE (urinary analgesia)

ROUTE	ONSET	PEAK	DURATION
PO	unknown	5–6 hr	6–8 hr

Contraindications/Precautions
Contraindicated in: Hypersensitivity; Glomerulonephritis; Severe hepatitis, uremia, or renal failure; Renal insufficiency; Glucose-6–phosphate dehydrogenase (G6PD) deficiency.
Use Cautiously in: Hepatitis; OB: Lactation: Safety not established.

Adverse Reactions/Side Effects
CNS: headache, vertigo. **GI:** hepatotoxicity, nausea. **GU:** bright-orange urine, renal failure. **Derm:** rash. **Hemat:** hemolytic anemia, methemoglobinemia.

Interactions
Drug-Drug: None significant.

Route/Dosage
PO (Adults): 200 mg 3 times daily for 2 days.
PO (Children): 4 mg/kg 3 times daily for 2 days.

Availability (generic available)
Tablets: 95 mg^{OTC}, 100 mg, ♣ 100 mg^{OTC}, ♣ 200 mg^{OTC}, 200 mg.

NURSING IMPLICATIONS
Assessment
- Assess patient for urgency, frequency, and pain on urination prior to and throughout therapy.
- *Lab Test Considerations:* Renal function should be monitored periodically during course of therapy.
- Interferes with urine tests based on color reactions (glucose, ketones, bilirubin, steroids, protein).

Potential Nursing Diagnoses
Acute pain (Indications)
Impaired urinary elimination (Indications)

Implementation
- Medication should be discontinued after pain or discomfort is relieved (usually 2 days for treatment of urinary tract infection). Concurrent antibiotic therapy should continue for full prescribed duration.
- **PO:** Administer medication with or following meals to decrease GI irritation. Do not crush, break, or chew tablet.

Patient/Family Teaching
- Instruct patient to take medication exactly as directed. If a dose is missed, take as soon as remembered unless almost time for next dose.
- Advise patient that while phenazopyridine administration is stopped once pain or discomfort is relieved, concurrent antibiotic therapy must be continued for full duration of therapy. Do not save unused portion of phenazopyridine without consulting health care professional.
- Inform patient that drug causes reddish-orange discoloration of urine that may stain clothing or bedding. Sanitary napkin may be worn to avoid clothing stains. May also cause staining of soft contact lenses.
- Instruct patient to notify health care professional if rash, skin discoloration, or unusual tiredness occurs.

Evaluation/Desired Outcomes
- Decrease in pain and burning on urination.

phenelzine, See MONOAMINE OXIDASE (MAO) INHIBITORS.

phenobarbital
(fee-noe-**bar**-bi-tal)
✦Ancalixir, Luminal, Solfoton

Classification
Therapeutic: anticonvulsants, sedative/hypnotics
Pharmacologic: barbiturates

Schedule IV

Pregnancy Category D

Indications
Anticonvulsant in tonic-clonic (grand mal), partial, and febrile seizures in children. Preoperative sedative and in other situations in which sedation may be required. Hypnotic (short-term). **Unlabeled Use:** Prevention/treatment of hyperbilirubinemia in neonates.

Action
Produces all levels of CNS depression. Depresses the sensory cortex, decreases motor activity, and alters cerebellar function. Inhibits transmission in the nervous system and raises the seizure threshold. Capable of inducing (speeding up) enzymes in the liver that metabolize drugs, bilirubin, and other compounds. **Therapeutic Effects:** Anticonvulsant activity. Sedation.

Pharmacokinetics
Absorption: Absorption is slow but relatively complete (70–90%).
Distribution: Unknown.
Metabolism and Excretion: 75% metabolized by the liver, 25% excreted unchanged by the kidneys.
Half-life: Neonates: 1.8–8.3 days; Infants: 0.8–5.5 days; Children: 1.5–3 days; Adults: 2–6 days.

TIME/ACTION PROFILE (sedation†)

ROUTE	ONSET	PEAK	DURATION
PO	30–60 min	unknown	>6 hr
IM, subcut	10–30 min	unknown	4–6 hr
IV	5 min	30 min	4–6 hr

†Full anticonvulsant effects occur after 2–3 wk of chronic dosing unless a loading dose has been used

Contraindications/Precautions
Contraindicated in: Hypersensitivity; Comatose patients or those with pre-existing CNS depression; Severe respiratory disease with dyspnea or obstruction; Uncontrolled severe pain; Known alcohol intolerance (elixir only); Lactation: Discontinue drug or bottle feed.

Use Cautiously in: Hepatic dysfunction; Severe renal impairment; History of suicide attempt or drug abuse; Hypnotic use should be short-term. Chronic use may lead to dependence; OB: Chronic use during pregnancy results in drug dependency in the infant; may result in coagulation defects and fetal malformation; acute use at term may result in respiratory depression in the newborn; Geri: Iinitial dose reduction recommended; Hypnotic use should be short-term. Chronic use may lead to dependence.

Adverse Reactions/Side Effects
CNS: hangover, delirium, depression, drowsiness, excitation, lethargy, vertigo. **Resp:** respiratory depression; *IV*, LARYNGOSPASM, bronchospasm. **CV:** *IV*—hypotension. **GI:** constipation, diarrhea, nausea, vomiting. **Derm:** photosensitivity, rashes, urticaria. **Local:** phlebitis at IV site. **MS:** arthralgia, myalgia, neuralgia. **Misc:** hypersensitivity reactions including ANGIOEDEMA and SERUM SICKNESS, physical dependence, psychological dependence.

Interactions
Drug-Drug: Additive CNS depression with other **CNS depressants**, including **alcohol**, **antihistamines**, **opioid analgesics**, and other **sedative/hypnotics**. May induce hepatic enzymes that metabolize other drugs, ↓ their effectiveness, including **hormonal contraceptives**, **warfarin**, **chloramphenicol**, **cyclosporine**, **dacarbazine**, **corticosteroids**, **tricyclic antidepressants**, **felodipine**, **clonazepam**, **carbamazepine**, **verapamil**, **theophylline**, **metronidazole**, and **quinidine**. May ↑ risk of hepatic toxicity of **acetaminophen**. **MAO inhibitors**, **valproic acid**, or **divalproex** may ↓ metabolism of phenobarbital, ↑ sedation. **Rifampin** may ↑ metabolism of and ↓ effects of phenobarbital. May ↑ risk of hematologic toxicity with **cyclophosphamide**.
Drug-Natural Products: Concomitant use of **kava-kava**, **valerian,**, **chamomile**, or **hops** can ↑ CNS depression. **St. John's wort** may ↓ effects.

Route/Dosage

Status Epilepticus
IV (Adults and Children >1 month): 15–18 mg/kg in a single or divided dose, maximum loading dose 20 mg/kg.
IV (Neonates): 15–20 mg/kg in a single or divided dose.

✦ = Canadian drug name. ▆ = Genetic implication.
*CAPITALS indicates life-threatening; underlines indicate most frequent.

Maintenance Anticonvulsant
IV, PO (Adults and Children > 12 yr): 1–3 mg/kg/day as a single dose or 2 divided doses.
IV, PO (Children 5–12 yr): 4–6 mg/kg/day in 1–2 divided doses.
IV, PO (Children 1–5 yr): 6–8 mg/kg/day in 1–2 divided doses.
IV, PO (Infants): 5–6 mg/kg/day in 1–2 divided doses.
IV, PO (Neonates): 3–4 mg/kg/day once daily, may need to increase up to 5 mg/kg/day by 2nd week of therapy.

Sedation
PO, IM (Adults): 30–120 mg/day in 2–3 divided doses. *Preoperative sedation*—100–200 mg IM 1–1.5 hours before the procedure.
PO (Children): 2 mg/kg 3 times daily. *Preoperative sedation*—1–3 mg/kg PO/IM/IV 1–1.5 hours before the procedure.

Hypnotic
PO, Subcut, IV, IM (Adults): 100–320 mg at bedtime.
IV, IM, Subcut (Children): 3–5 mg/kg at bedtime.

Hyperbilirubinemia
PO (Adults): 90–180 mg/day in 2–3 divided doses.
PO (Children <12 yr): 3–8 mg/kg/day in 2–3 divided doses, doses up to 12 mg/kg/day have been used.

Availability (generic available)
Tablets: 8 mg, 15 mg, 30 mg, 60 mg, 100 mg. **Capsules:** 15 mg. **Elixir:** 20 mg/5 mL. **Injection:** 30 mg/mL in 1-mL prefilled syringes, 60 mg/mL in 1-mL prefilled syringes, 65 mg/mL in 1-mL vials, 130 mg/mL in 1-mL prefilled syringes, 1-mL vials, and 1-mL ampules. ***In combination with:*** phenytoin. See Appendix B.

NURSING IMPLICATIONS

Assessment
- Monitor respiratory status, pulse, and blood pressure frequently in patients receiving phenobarbital IV. Equipment for resuscitation and artificial ventilation should be readily available. Respiratory depression is dose-dependent.
- Prolonged therapy may lead to psychological or physical dependence. Restrict amount of drug available to patient, especially if depressed, suicidal, or with a history of addiction.
- Geri: Elderly patients may react to phenobarbital with marked excitement, depression, and confusion. Monitor for these adverse reactions.
- **Seizures:** Assess location, duration, and characteristics of seizure activity.
- **Sedation:** Assess level of consciousness and anxiety when used as a preoperative sedative.
- Assess postoperative patients for pain with a pain scale. Phenobarbital may increase sensitivity to painful stimuli.
- ***Lab Test Considerations:*** Patients on prolonged therapy should have hepatic and renal function and CBC evaluated periodically.
- Monitor serum folate concentrations periodically during therapy because of increased folate requirements of patients on long-term anticonvulsant therapy with phenobarbital.
- May cause ↓ serum bilirubin concentrations in neonates, in patients with congenital nonhemolytic unconjugated hyperbilirubinemia, and in epileptics.
- ***Toxicity and Overdose:*** Serum phenobarbital levels may be monitored when used as an anticonvulsant. Therapeutic blood levels are 10–40 mcg/mL. Symptoms of toxicity include confusion, drowsiness, dyspnea, slurred speech, and staggering.

Potential Nursing Diagnoses
Risk for injury (Indications, Side Effects)
Acute confusion (Side Effects)

Implementation
- Do not confuse phenobarbital with pentobarbital.
- Supervise ambulation and transfer of patients following administration. Two side rails should be raised and call bell within reach at all times. Keep bed in low position. Institute seizure and fall precautions.
- When changing from phenobarbital to another anticonvulsant, gradually decrease phenobarbital dose while concurrently increasing dose of replacement medication to maintain anticonvulsant effects.
- **PO:** Tablets may be crushed and mixed with food or fluids (do not administer dry) for patients with difficulty swallowing. Oral solution may be taken undiluted or mixed with water, milk, or fruit juice. Use calibrated measuring device for accurate measurement of liquid doses.
- **IM:** Injections should be given deep into the gluteal muscle to minimize tissue irritation. Do not inject >5 mL into any one site, because of tissue irritation.

IV Administration
- **IV:** Doses may require 15–30 min to reach peak concentrations in the brain. Administer

minimal dose and wait for effectiveness before administering 2nd dose to prevent cumulative barbiturate-induced depression.
- **Direct IV:** *Diluent:* Reconstitute sterile powder for IV dose with a minimum of 3 mL of sterile water for injection. Dilute further with 10 mL of sterile water. Do not use solution that is not absolutely clear within 5 min after reconstitution or that contains a precipitate. Discard powder or solution that has been exposed to air for longer than 30 min.
- Solution is highly alkaline; avoid extravasation, which may cause tissue damage and necrosis. If extravasation occurs, injection of 5% procaine solution into affected area and application of moist heat may be ordered. *Concentration:* 130 mg/mL (undiluted). *Rate:* Do not inject IV faster than 1 mg/kg/min with a maximum of 30 mg over 1 min in infants and children and 60 mg over 1 min in adults. Titrate slowly for desired response. Rapid administration may result in respiratory depression.
- **Y-Site Compatibility:** doxapram, enalaprilat, fentanyl, fosphenytoin, levofloxacin, linezolid, meropenem, methadone, morphine, propofol, sufentanil.
- **Y-Site Incompatibility:** amphotericin B cholesteryl sulfate complex, lansoprazole.

Patient/Family Teaching
- Advise patient to take medication as directed. Take missed doses as soon as remembered if not almost time for next dose; do not double doses.
- Advise patients on prolonged therapy not to discontinue medication without consulting health care professional. Abrupt withdrawal may precipitate seizures or status epilepticus.
- Medication may cause daytime drowsiness. Caution patient to avoid driving and other activities requiring alertness until response to medication is known. Do not resume driving until physician gives clearance based on control of seizure disorder.
- Caution patient to avoid taking alcohol or other CNS depressants concurrently with this medication.
- Advise female patients using oral contraceptives to use an additional nonhormonal contraceptive during therapy and until next menstrual period. Instruct patient to contact health care professional immediately if pregnancy is planned or suspected.
- Advise patient to notify health care professional if fever, sore throat, mouth sores, unusual bleeding or bruising, nosebleeds, or petechiae occur.
- Teach sleep hygiene techniques (dark room, quiet, bedtime ritual, limit daytime napping, avoid nicotine and caffeine).
- Pedi: Advise parents or caregivers that child may experience irritability, hyperactivity, and/or sleep disturbances, which may diminish in a few days to a few weeks or may persist until drug is stopped. An alternative medication can be considered. Instruct parents to monitor for skin rash occurring 7-20 days after treatment begins and to contact a health care provider if rash occurs. Teach family about symptoms of toxicity (staggering, drowsiness, slurred speech).

Evaluation/Desired Outcomes
- Decrease or cessation of seizure activity without excessive sedation. Several weeks may be required to achieve maximum anticonvulsant effects.
- Preoperative sedation.
- Improvement in sleep patterns.
- Decrease in serum bilirubin levels.

---

phentermine (fen-ter-meen)
Adipex-P, Banobese, Fastin, Ionamin, Obi-Nix, OBY-CAP, Phentercot, Phentride, T-Diet, Teramine, Zantryl

Classification
Therapeutic: weight control agents
Pharmacologic: appetite suppressants

Schedule IV

Pregnancy Category UK

Indications
Short-term treatment of obesity in conjunction with other interventions (dietary restriction, exercise); used to produce and maintain weight loss in patients with a BMI ≥ 30 kg/m^2 or ≥ 27 kg/m^2 in the presence of other risk factors (diabetes, hypertension, hyperlipidemia).

Action
Decreases hunger by altering the chemical control of nerve impulse transmission in the appetite control center of the hypothalamus. **Therapeutic Effects:** Appetite suppression with resultant weight loss.

Pharmacokinetics
Absorption: Unknown.
Distribution: Unknown.
Metabolism and Excretion: Metabolized by the liver.
Half-life: 19–24 hr.

TIME/ACTION PROFILE (appetite suppression)

ROUTE	ONSET	PEAK	DURATION
PO-hydro-chloride	unknown	unknown	4 hr†
PO-resin complex	unknown	unknown	12–14 hr

†For 8-mg tablets, increase to 12–14 hr for 30-mg capsules or 37.5-mg tablets

Contraindications/Precautions
Contraindicated in: Hypersensitivity or known intolerance to sympathomimetic amines; Cardiovascular disease; Hyperthyroidism; Moderate to severe hypertension; History of drug abuse; Agitation; Glaucoma; Concurrent or recent (within 14 days) MAO inhibitor therapy; Concurrent SSRI antidepressants.
Use Cautiously in: Mild hypertension; Diabetes mellitus; Pregnancy, lactation, or children <12 yr (safety not established).

Adverse Reactions/Side Effects
CNS: CNS stimulation, confusion, dizziness, dysphoria, euphoria, headache, insomnia, mental depression, restlessness. **EENT:** blurred vision. **CV:** hypertension, palpitations, tachycardia. **GI:** constipation, diarrhea, dry mouth, nausea, unpleasant taste, vomiting. **GU:** changes in libido, erectile dysfunction.

Interactions
Drug-Drug: Concurrent use with **MAO inhibitors** may result in hypertensive crisis (do not use within 14 days of MAO inhibitors). Increased risk of adverse CNS events with **alcohol**. Concurrent use with **SSRI antidepressants** is not recommended. May decrease **insulin** requirements in diabetic patients.

Route/Dosage
PO (Adults): *Phentermine hydrochloride tablets or capsules*—8 mg 3 times daily or 15–37.5 mg once daily; *Phentermine resin complex capsules*—15–30 mg once daily.

Availability (generic available)
Phentermine hydrochloride tablets: 8 mg, 37.5 mg. **Phentermine hydrochloride capsules:** 15 mg, 18.75 mg, 30 mg, 37.5 mg. **Phentermine resin complex capsules:** 15 mg, 30 mg.

NURSING IMPLICATIONS

Assessment
- Monitor patients for weight loss and adjust concurrent medications (antihypertensives, antidiabetics, lipid-lowering agents) as needed.

Potential Nursing Diagnoses
Disturbed body image (Indications)
Imbalanced nutrition: more than body requirements (Indications)
Deficient knowledge, related to medication regimen (Patient/Family Teaching)

Implementation
- **PO:** Administer 30 min before meals or as a single dose before breakfast or 10–14 hr before retiring.

Patient/Family Teaching
- Instruct patient to take medication as directed and not to exceed dose recommended. Medication may need to be discontinued gradually.
- May cause drowsiness. Advise patient to avoid driving or other activities requiring alertness until response to medication is known.
- Caution patient to avoid using alcohol or other CNS depressants with this medication.
- Advise patient to notify health care professional immediately if chest pain, decreased exercise tolerance, fainting, or swelling of the feet or lower legs occurs.

Evaluation/Desired Outcomes
- Gradual weight loss.

---

phentolamine
(fen-**tole**-a-meen)
Oraverse, Regitine, ✦ Rogitine

Classification
Therapeutic: agents for pheochromocytoma
Pharmacologic: alpha-adrenergic blockers

Pregnancy Category C

Indications
IV: Control of blood pressure during surgical removal of a pheochromocytoma. **IV, Infiltration:** Prevention and treatment of dermal necrosis and sloughing following extravasation of norepinephrine, phenylephrine, or dopamine. **Local:** Reversal of soft-tissue anesthesia (of lip and tongue) resulting from an intraoral submucosal injection of a local anesthetic containing a vasoconstrictor. **Unlabeled Use: IM, IV:** Treatment of hypertension associated with pheochromocytoma or adrenergic (sympathetic) excess, such as administration of phenylephrine, tyramine-containing foods in

phentolamine 1019

patients on MAO inhibitor therapy, or clonidine withdrawal.

Action
Produces incomplete and short-lived blockade of alpha-adrenergic receptors located primarily in smooth muscle and exocrine glands. Induces hypotension by direct relaxation of vascular smooth muscle and by alpha blockade. Increases blood flow to submucosal tissue through blockade of alpha receptors. **Therapeutic Effects:** Reduction of blood pressure in situations in which hypertension is due to adrenergic (sympathetic) excess. When infiltrated locally, reverses vasoconstriction caused by norepinephrine or dopamine. Reverses local anesthetic effects (restores normal lip and tongue sensation).

Pharmacokinetics
Absorption: Well absorbed following IM administration; completely available after local injection.
Distribution: Unknown.
Metabolism and Excretion: 10% excreted unchanged by kidneys.
Half-life: 19 min (IV); 2–3 hr (local injection).

TIME/ACTION PROFILE (alpha-adrenergic blockade)

ROUTE	ONSET	PEAK	DURATION
IM	unknown	20 min	30–45 min
IV	immediate	2 min	15–30 min
Local	rapid	10–20 min	unknown

Contraindications/Precautions
Contraindicated in: Hypersensitivity; Coronary or cerebral arteriosclerosis; Renal impairment.
Use Cautiously in: Peptic ulcer disease; OB, Lactation: Safety not established; Pedi: Children <6 yr or <15 kg (Oraverse) (safety not established); Geri: More susceptible to hypotensive effects; ↓ dose recommended.

Adverse Reactions/Side Effects
With parenteral use.
CNS: CEREBROVASCULAR SPASM, dizziness, weakness. **EENT:** nasal stuffiness. **CV:** HYPOTENSION, MI, angina, arrhythmias, tachycardia. **GI:** abdominal pain, diarrhea, nausea, vomiting, aggravation of peptic ulcer. **Derm:** flushing. **Local:** injection site pain (local).

Interactions
Drug-Drug: Antagonizes the effects of **alpha-adrenergic stimulants**. May ↓ pressor response to **ephedrine** or **phenylephrine**. Severe hypotension may occur with concurrent use of **epinephrine** or **methoxamine**. Use with **guanadrel** may result in exaggerated hypotension and bradycardia. ↓ peripheral vasoconstriction from high doses of **dopamine**.

Route/Dosage

Hypertension Associated with Pheochromocytoma—Before/During Surgery
IV (Adults): 5 mg given 1–2 hr preop, repeated as necessary. May be infused at a rate of 0.5–1 mg/min during surgery.
IV, IM (Children): 1 mg or 0.1 mg/kg (3 mg/m^2) given 1–2 hr preop, repeated IV as necessary during surgery.

Prevention of Dermal Necrosis during Infusion of Norepinephrine, Phenylephrine, or Dopamine
IV (Adults): Add 10 mg phentolamine to every 1000 mL of fluid containing norepinephrine.

Treatment of Dermal Necrosis Following Extravasation of Norepinephrine, Phenylephrine, or Dopamine
Infiltrate (Adults): 5–10 mg.
Infiltrate (Children): 0.1–0.2 mg/kg (up to 10 mg).

Reversal of Intraoral Submucosal Anesthesia Following Dental Procedures (Oraverse)
Infiltrate or Block Injection (Adults and Children ≥6 yr and >30 kg): Dose administered is based on number of cartridges of local anesthetic with vasoconstrictor administered: *½ cartridge local anesthetic*—0.2 mg phentolamine (½ cartridge); *1 cartridge local anesthetic*—0.4 mg phentolamine (1 cartridge); *2 cartridges local anesthetic*—0.8 mg phentolamine (2 cartridges).

Infiltrate or Block Injection (Children ≥6 yr and 15–30 kg): Do not exceed dose of 0.2 mg (½ cartridge).

Availability (generic available)
Powder for injection: 5 mg/vial. **Injection for local infiltration/block injection:** 0.4 mg/cartridge.

NURSING IMPLICATIONS

Assessment
- Monitor blood pressure, pulse, and ECG every 2 min until stable during IV administration. If

hypotensive crisis occurs, epinephrine is contraindicated and may cause paradoxic further decrease in blood pressure; norepinephrine may be used.

Potential Nursing Diagnoses
Ineffective tissue perfusion (Indications)
Risk for injury (Indications)

Implementation
- Patient should remain supine throughout parenteral administration.

IV Administration
- **IV:** *Diluent:* Reconstitute each 5 mg with 1 mL of sterile water for injection or 0.9% NaCl. Discard unused solution. *Concentration:* 5 mg/mL. *Rate:* Inject each 5 mg over 1 min.
- **Continuous Infusion:** Dilute 5–10 mg in 500 mL of D5W.
- *Rate:* Titrate infusion rate according to patient response.
- May also add 10 mg to every 1000 mL of fluid containing norepinephrine for prevention of dermal necrosis and sloughing. Does not affect pressor effect of norepinephrine.
- **Syringe Compatibility:** papaverine.
- **Y-Site Compatibility:** alfentanil, amikacin, aminophylline, amiodarone, ascorbic acid, atropine, aztreonam, benztropine, bumetanide, buprenorphine, butorphanol, calcium chloride, calcium gluconate, ceftazidime, ceftriaxone, chlorpromazine, cimetidine, cyanocobalamin, cyclosporine, dactinomycin, daptomycin, digoxin, diltiazem, diphenhydramine, dobutamine, docetaxel, dobutamine, docetaxel, dopamine, doxycycline, enalaprilat, epinephrine, epoetin, ertapenem, erythromycin, esmolol, etoposide phosphate, famotidine, fenoldopam, fentanyl, fluconazole, fludarabine, folic acid, gemcitabine, gentamicin, glycopyrrolate, granisetron, heparin, hydrocortisone sodium succinate, imipenem-cilastatin, isoproterenol, labetalol, lidocaine, linezolid, lorazepam, magnesium sulfate, mannitol, mechlorethamine, meperidine, metaraminol, methoxamine, methyldopa, metoclopramide, metoprolol, metronidazole, midazolam, minocycline, mitoxantrone, morphine, multivitamin injection, nafcillin, naloxone, nesiritide, nitroglycerin, nitroprusside, norepinephrine, octreotide, ondansetron, oxaliplatin, oxytocin, paclitaxel, palonosetron, pantoprazole, pemetrexed, pentamidine, pentazocine, phenylephrine, phytonadione, piperacillin/tazobactam, potassium chloride, procainamide, prochlorperazine, promethazine, propranolol, protamine, pyridoxine, quinidine, ranitidine, sodium bicarbonate, streptokinase, succinylcholine, sufentanil, tacrolimus, teniposide, theophylline, thiamine, thiotepa, ticarcillin/clavulanate, tirofiban, tobramycin, tolazoline, trimethophan, vancomycin, vasopressin, verapamil, vinorelbine, voriconazole.
- **Y-Site Incompatibility:** amphotericin B colloidal, cefazolin, cefoperazone, cefotetan, cefoxitin, cefuroxime, chloramphenicol, clindamycin, dantrolene, dexamethasone, diazepam, diazoxide, furosemide, ganciclovir, insulin, ketorolac, moxalactam, penicillin G, pentobarbital, phenobarbital, phenytoin, trimethoprim/sulfamethoxazole.
- **Additive Compatibility:** dobutamine, norepinephrine.
- **Infiltration:** Dilute 5–10 mg of phentolamine in 10 mL of 0.9% NaCl. For children, use 0.1–0.2 mg/kg up to a maximum of 10 mg. Infiltrate site of extravasation promptly. Must be given within 12 hr of extravasation to be effective.

Patient/Family Teaching
- Advise patient to change positions slowly to minimize orthostatic hypotension.
- Instruct patient to notify health care professional if chest pain occurs during IV infusion.

Evaluation/Desired Outcomes
- Decrease in blood pressure.
- Prevention of dermal necrosis and sloughing in extravasation of norepinephrine, dopamine, and phenylephrine.
- Restoration of normal lip and tongue sensation following local anesthesia.

---

phenytoin (fen-i-toyn)
Dilantin, Phenytek

Classification
Therapeutic: antiarrhythmics (group IB), anticonvulsants
Pharmacologic: hydantoins

Pregnancy Category D

Indications
Treatment/prevention of tonic-clonic (grand mal) seizures and complex partial seizures. **Unlabeled Use:** As an antiarrhythmic, particularly for ventricular arrhythmias associated with digoxin toxicity, prolonged QT interval, and surgical repair of congenital heart diseases in children. Management of neuropathic pain, including trigeminal neuralgia.

phenytoin 1021

Action
Limits seizure propagation by altering ion transport. May also decrease synaptic transmission. Antiarrhythmic properties as a result of shortening the action potential and decreasing automaticity. **Therapeutic Effects:** Diminished seizure activity. Termination of ventricular arrhythmias.

Pharmacokinetics
Absorption: Absorbed slowly from the GI tract. Bioavailability differs among products; the Dilantin and Phenytek preparations are considered to be "extended" products. Other products are considered to be prompt release.

Distribution: Distributes into CSF and other body tissues and fluids. Enters breast milk; crosses the placenta, achieving similar maternal/fetal levels. Preferentially distributes into fatty tissue.

Protein Binding: Adults 90–95%; decreased protein binding in neonates (up to 20% free fraction available), infants (up to 15% free), and patients with hyperbilirubinemia, hypoalbuminemia, severe renal dysfunction or uremia.

Metabolism and Excretion: Mostly metabolized by the liver; minimal amounts excreted in the urine.

Half-life: 22 hr (range 7–42 hr).

TIME/ACTION PROFILE (anticonvulsant effect)

ROUTE	ONSET	PEAK	DURATION
PO	2–24 hr (1 wk)*	1.5–3 hr	6–12 hr
PO-ER	2–24 hr (1 wk)	4–12 hr	12–36 hr
IV	0.5–1 hr (1 wk)	rapid	12–24 hr

*( ) = time required for onset of action without a loading dose

Contraindications/Precautions
Contraindicated in: Hypersensitivity; Hypersensitivity to propylene glycol (phenytoin injection only); Alcohol intolerance (phenytoin injection and liquid only); Sinus bradycardia, sinoatrial block, 2nd- or 3rd-degree heart block, or Stokes-Adams syndrome (phenytoin injection only).

Use Cautiously in: All patients (may ↑ risk of suicidal thoughts/behaviors); Hepatic or renal disease (↑ risk of adverse reactions; dose reduction recommended for hepatic impairment); Patients with severe cardiac or respiratory disease (use of IV phenytoin may result in an ↑ risk of serious adverse reactions); OB: Safety not established; may result in fetal hydantoin syndrome if used chronically or hemorrhage in the newborn if used at term; use with extreme caution; Lactation: Safety not established; Pedi: Suspension contains sodium benzoate, a metabolite of benzyl alcohol that can cause potentially fatal gasping syndrome in neonates; Geri: Use of IV phenytoin may result in an ↑ risk of serious adverse reactions.

Exercise Extreme Caution in: Patients positive for HLA-B*1502 allele (unless exceptional circumstances exist where benefits clearly outweigh the risks).

Adverse Reactions/Side Effects
Most listed are for chronic use of phenytoin. **CNS:** SUICIDAL THOUGHTS, ataxia, agitation, confusion, dizziness, drowsiness, dysarthria, dyskinesia, extrapyramidal syndrome, headache, insomnia, weakness. **EENT:** diplopia, nystagmus. **CV:** hypotension (↑ with IV phenytoin), tachycardia. **GI:** gingival hyperplasia, nausea, constipation, drug-induced hepatitis, vomiting. **Derm:** hypertrichosis, rash, exfoliative dermatitis, pruritus, purple glove syndrome. **Hemat:** AGRANULOCYTOSIS, APLASTIC ANEMIA, leukopenia, megaloblastic anemia, thrombocytopenia. **MS:** osteomalacia, osteoporosis. **Misc:** allergic reactions including STEVENS-JOHNSON SYNDROME, fever, lymphadenopathy.

Interactions
Drug-Drug: Disulfiram, acute ingestion of **alcohol**, **amiodarone**, **ethosuximide**, **isoniazid**, **chloramphenicol**, **sulfonamides**, **fluoxetine**, **gabapentin**, **H2 antagonists**, **benzodiazepines**, **omeprazole**, **ketoconazole**, **fluconazole**, **estrogens**, **succinamides**, **halothane**, **methylphenidate**, **phenothiazines**, **salicylates**, **ticlopidine**, **tolbutamide**, **topiramate**, **trazodone**, **felbamate**, and **cimetidine** may ↑ phenytoin blood levels. **Barbiturates**, **carbamazepine**, **reserpine**, and chronic ingestion of **alcohol** may ↓ phenytoin blood levels. Phenytoin may ↓ the effects of **amiodarone**, **benzodiazepines**, **carbamazepine**, **chloramphenicol**, **corticosteroids**, **disopyramide**, **warfarin**, **felbamate**, **doxycycline**, **lamotrigine**, **oral contraceptives**, **paroxetine**, **propafenone**, **rifampin**, **ritonavir**, **quinidine**, **tacrolimus**, **theophylline**, **topiramate**, **tricyclic antidepressants**, **zonisamide**, **methadone**, **cyclosporine**, and **estrogens**. IV phenytoin and **dopamine** may cause additive hypotension. Additive CNS depression with other

CNS depressants, including **alcohol**, **antihistamines**, **antidepressants**, **opioids**, and **sedative/hypnotics**. **Antacids** may ↓ absorption of orally administered phenytoin. ↑ systemic clearance of antileukemic drugs **teniposide** and **methotrexate** which has been associated with a worse event free survival, phenytoin use is not recommended in children undergoing chemotherapy for acute lymphocytic leukemia. **Calcium** and **sucralfate** ↓ phenytoin absorption.
Drug-Food: Phenytoin may ↓ absorption of **folic acid**. Concurrent administration of **enteral tube feedings** may ↓ phenytoin absorption.

Route/Dosage
IM administration is not recommended due to erratic absorption and pain on injection.

Anticonvulsant
PO (Adults): Loading dose of 15–20 mg/kg as extended capsules in 3 divided doses given every 2–4 hr; maintenance dose 5–6 mg/kg/day given in 1–3 divided doses; usual dosing range = 200–1200 mg/day.
PO (Children 10–16 yr): 6–7 mg/kg/day in 2–3 divided doses.
PO (Children 7–9 yr): 7–8 mg/kg/day in 2–3 divided doses.
PO (Children 4–6 yr): 7.5–9 mg/kg/day in 2–3 divided doses.
PO (Children 0.5–3 yr): 8–10 mg/kg/day in 2–3 divided doses.
PO (Neonates up to 6 mo): 5–8 mg/kg/day in 2 divided doses, may require q 8 hr dosing.
IV (Adults): *Status epilepticus loading dose*—15–20 mg/kg. Rate not to exceed 25–50 mg/min. *Maintenance dose*—same as PO dosing above.
IV (Children): *Status epilepticus loading dose*—15–20 mg/kg at 1–3 mg/kg/min. *Maintenance dose*—same as PO dosing above.

Antiarrhythmic
IV (Adults): 50–100 mg q 10–15 min until arrhythmia is abolished, or a total of 15 mg/kg has been given, or toxicity occurs.
PO (Adults): Loading dose: 250 mg QID for 1 day, then 250 mg BID for 2 days, then maintenance at 300–400 mg/day in divided doses 1–4 times/day.
IV (Children): 1.25 mg/kg q 5 min, may repeat up to total loading dose of 15 mg/kg. *Maintenance dose*—5–10 mg/kg/day in 2–3 divided doses IV or PO.

Availability (generic available)
Chewable tablets: 50 mg. **Cost:** $41.99/90.
Oral suspension: 125 mg/5 mL. **Cost:** *Generic*—$28.99/237 mL. **Extended-release capsules:** 30 mg, 100 mg, 200 mg, 300 mg. **Cost:** *Dilantin*—30 mg $34.99/90; *Phenytek*—200 mg $65.97/90, 300 mg $95.27/90; *Generic*—100 mg $23.18/90. **Injection:** 50 mg/mL.

NURSING IMPLICATIONS
Assessment
- Monitor closely for notable changes in behavior that could indicate the emergence or worsening of suicidal thoughts or behavior or depression.
- Assess oral hygiene. Vigorous cleaning beginning within 10 days of initiation of phenytoin therapy may help control gingival hyperplasia.
- Assess patient for phenytoin hypersensitivity syndrome (fever, skin rash, lymphadenopathy). Rash usually occurs within the first 2 wk of therapy. Hypersensitivity syndrome usually occurs at 3–8 wk but may occur up to 12 wk after initiation of therapy. May lead to renal failure, rhabdomyolysis, or hepatic necrosis; may be fatal.
- Observe patient for development of rash. Discontinue phenytoin at the first sign of skin reactions. Serious adverse reactions such as exfoliative, purpuric, or bullous rashes or the development of lupus erythematosus, Stevens-Johnson syndrome, or toxic epidermal necrolysis preclude further use of phenytoin or fosphenytoin. Stevens-Johnson syndrome and toxic epidermal necrolysis are significantly more common in patients with a particular human leukocyte antigen (HLA) allele, HLA-B*1502 (occurs almost exclusively in patients with Asian ancestry, including Han Chinese, Filipinos, Malaysians, South Asian Indians, and Thais). Avoid using phenytoin or fosphenytoin as alternatives to carbamazepine for patients who test positive. If less serious skin eruptions (measles-like or scarlatiniform) occur, phenytoin may be resumed after complete clearing of the rash. If rash reappears, further use of fosphenytoin or phenytoin should be avoided.
- **Seizures:** Assess location, duration, frequency, and characteristics of seizure activity. EEG may be monitored periodically throughout therapy.
- Monitor blood pressure, ECG, and respiratory function continuously during administration of IV phenytoin and throughout period when peak serum phenytoin levels occur (15–30 min after administration).

- **Arrhythmias:** Monitor ECG continuously during treatment of arrhythmias.
- *Lab Test Considerations:* Monitor CBC, serum calcium, albumin, and hepatic function tests prior to and monthly for the first several months, then periodically during therapy.
- May cause ↑ serum alkaline phosphatase, GGT, and glucose levels.
- Monitor serum folate concentrations periodically during prolonged therapy.
- *Toxicity and Overdose:* Monitor serum phenytoin levels routinely. Therapeutic blood levels are 10–20 mcg/mL (8–15 mcg/mL in neonates) in patients with normal serum albumin and renal function. In patients with altered protein binding (neonates, patients with renal failure, hypoalbuminemia, acute trauma), free phenytoin serum concentrations should be monitored. Therapeutic serum free phenytoin levels are 1–2 mcg/mL.
- Progressive signs and symptoms of phenytoin toxicity include nystagmus, ataxia, confusion, nausea, slurred speech, and dizziness.

Potential Nursing Diagnoses
Risk for injury (Indications)
Impaired oral mucous membrane (Side Effects)

Implementation
- Implement seizure precautions.
- When transferring from phenytoin to another anticonvulsant, dosage adjustments are made gradually over several weeks.
- When substituting *fosphenytoin* for oral *phenytoin* therapy, the same total daily dose may be given as a single dose. Unlike parenteral phenytoin, fosphenytoin may be given safely by the IM route.
- **PO:** Administer with or immediately after meals to minimize GI irritation. Shake liquid preparations well before pouring. Use a calibrated measuring device for accurate dose. Chewable tablets must be crushed or chewed well before swallowing. Capsules may be opened and mixed with food or fluids for patients with difficulty swallowing. To prevent direct contact of alkaline drug with mucosa, have patient swallow a liquid first, follow with mixture of medication, then follow with a full glass of water or milk or with food.
- If patient is receiving enteral tube feedings, 2 hr should elapse between feeding and phenytoin administration. If phenytoin is administered via nasogastric tube, flush tube with 2–4 oz water before and after administration.
- Do not interchange chewable phenytoin tablets with phenytoin sodium capsules, because they are not bioequivalent.
- Capsules labeled "extended" may be used for once-a-day dose; those labeled "prompt" may result in toxic serum levels if used for once-a-day dose.

IV Administration
- **IV:** Slight yellow color will not alter solution potency. If refrigerated, may form precipitate, which dissolves after warming to room temperature. Discard solution that is not clear.
- To prevent precipitation and minimize local venous irritation, follow infusion with 0.9% NaCl through the same needle or catheter. Avoid extravasation; phenytoin is caustic to tissues; may lead to purple glove syndrome. Monitor infusion site closely.
- **Direct IV:** Administer undiluted. *Rate:* Administer at a rate not to exceed 50 mg over 1 min in adults or 1–3 mg/kg/min in neonates. Rapid administration may result in severe hypotension, cardiovascular collapse, or CNS depression.
- **Intermittent Infusion:** *Diluent:* Administer by mixing with no more than 50 mL of 0.9% NaCl. *Concentration:* 1–10 mg/mL. Administer immediately following admixture. Use tubing with a 0.45- to 0.22-micron in-line filter. *Rate:* Complete infusion within 1 hr at a rate not to exceed 50 mg/min. In patients who may develop hypotension, patients with cardiovascular disease, or geriatric patients maximum rate of 25 mg/min [may be as low as 5–10 mg/min]. Maximum rate in neonates is 1–3 mg/kg/min. Monitor cardiac function and blood pressure throughout infusion.
- **Y-Site Compatibility:** cisplatin, foscarnet, tacrolimus.
- **Y-Site Incompatibility:** acyclovir, alfentanil, amikacin, aminophylline, amphotericin B cholesteryl, amphotericin B colloidal, amphotericin B liposome, ampicillin, ampicillin/sulbactam, ascorbic acid, atracurium, atropine, azathioprine, aztreonam, benztropine, bivalirudin, bumetanide, buprenorphine, butorphanol, calcium chloride, calcium gluconate, carboplatin, caspofungin, cefamandole, cefazolin, cefepime, cefmetazole, cefonocid, cefoperazone, cefotaxime, cefotetan, cefoxitin, ceftazidime,

ceftizoxime, ceftriaxone, cefuroxime, chloramphenicol, chlorpormazine, cimetidine, ciprofloxacin, clindamycin, cyanocobalamine, cyclophosphamide, cyclosporine, cytarabine, dactinomycin, dantrolene, daptomycin, dexamethasone, dexmeditomidine, diltiazem, diazoxide, digoxin, diltiazem, diphenhydramine, dobutamine, docetaxel, dopamine, doxacurium, doxorubicin hydrochloride, doxycycline, enalaprilat, ephedrine, epinephrine, epirubicin, epoetin, ertapenem, erythromycin, etoposide, etoposide phosphate, fenoldopam, fentanyl, fludarabine, fluorouracil, folic acid, furosemide, ganciclovir, gemcitabine, gentamicin, glycopyrrolate, granisetron, haloperidol, heparin, hetastarch, hydralazine, hydrocortisone sodium succinate, hydromorphone, hydroxyzine, ifosfamide, imipenem/cilastatin, inamrinone, indomethacin, insulin, isoproterenol, ketorolac, labetalol, levofloxacin, lidocaine, linezolid, lorazepam, magnesium sulfate, mannitol, mechlorethamine, meperidine, metaraminol, methadone, methotrexate, methoxamine, methyldopate, methylprednisolone, metoclopramide, mezlocillin, micafungin, miconazole, midazolam, milrinone, mitoxantrone, morphine, multivitamin infusion, nafcillin, nalbuphine, naloxone, nesiritide, netilmicin, nitroglycerin, nitroprusside, norepinpehrine, octreotide, ondansetron, oxacillin, oxytocin, paclitaxel, palonosetron, pantoprazole, papaverine, pemetrexed, penicillin G, pentamidine, pentazocine, pentobarbital, phenobarbital, phentolamine, phenylephrine, phytonadione, piperacillin/tazobactam, potassium chloride, procainamide, prochlorperazine, promethazine, propofol, propranolol, protamine, pyridoxime, quinapristin/dalfopristin, ranitidine, ritodrine, rocuronium, sodium acetate, sodium bicarbonate, streptokinase, succinylcholine, sufentanil, teniposide, theophylline, thiamine, thiotepa, ticarcillin/clavulanate, tigecycline, tirofiban, tobramycin, tolazoline, trimethaphan, trimethoprim/sulfamethoxazole, urokinase, vancomycin, vasopressin, vecuronium, verapamil, vincristine, vinorelbine, vitamin B complex with C, voriconazole.

- **Additive Incompatibility:** Do not admix with other solutions or medications, especially dextrose, because precipitation will occur.

Patient/Family Teaching

- Instruct patient to take medication as directed, at the same time each day. If a dose is missed from a once-a-day schedule, take as soon as possible and return to regular dosing schedule. If taking several doses a day, take missed dose as soon as possible within 4 hr of next scheduled dose; do not double doses. Consult health care professional if doses are missed for 2 consecutive days. Abrupt withdrawal may lead to status epilepticus.
- May cause drowsiness or dizziness. Caution patient to avoid driving or other activities requiring alertness until response to medication is known. Do not resume driving until physician gives clearance based on control of seizure disorder.
- Caution patient to avoid taking alcohol, OTC medications, or herbal medications concurrently with phenytoin without consulting health care professional.
- Instruct patient on importance of maintaining good dental hygiene and seeing dentist frequently for teeth cleaning to prevent tenderness, bleeding, and gingival hyperplasia. Institution of oral hygiene program within 10 days of initiation of phenytoin therapy may minimize growth rate and severity of gingival enlargement. Patients under 23 yr of age and those taking doses >500 mg/day are at increased risk for gingival hyperplasia.
- Advise patient that brands of phenytoin may not be equivalent. Check with health care professional if brand or dose form is changed.
- Advise diabetic patients to monitor blood glucose carefully and to notify health care professional of significant changes.
- Instruct patient to notify health care professional of medication regimen prior to treatment or surgery.
- Advise patient not to take phenytoin within 2–3 hr of antacids.
- Advise female patients to use an additional non-hormonal method of contraception during therapy. Instruct patient to notify health care professional if pregnancy is planned or suspected.
- Advise patient to carry identification describing disease process and medication regimen at all times.
- Instruct patients that behavioral changes, skin rash, fever, sore throat, mouth ulcers, easy bruising, petechiae, unusual bleeding, abdominal pain, chills, pale stools, dark urine, jaundice, severe nausea or vomiting, drowsiness, slurred speech, unsteady gait. swollen glands,or persistent headache should be reported to health care professional immediately. Advise patient and family to notify health care professional if thoughts about suicide or dying,

attempts to commit suicide; new or worse depression; new or worse anxiety; feeling very agitated or restless; panic attacks; trouble sleeping; new or worse irritability; acting aggressive; being angry or violent; acting on dangerous impulses; an extreme increase in activity and talking, other unusual changes in behavior or mood occur.
- Emphasize the importance of routine exams to monitor progress. Patient should have routine physical exams, especially monitoring skin and lymph nodes, and EEG testing.

Evaluation/Desired Outcomes
- Decrease or cessation of seizures without excessive sedation.
- Suppression of arrhythmias.
- Relief of neuropathic pain.

phosphate/biphosphate
(foss-fate/bye-foss-fate)
Fleet Enema, OsmoPrep, Visicol

Classification
Therapeutic: laxatives (saline)

Pregnancy Category C

Indications
Intermittent treatment of chronic constipation. **Visicol and OsmoPrep:** Cleansing of the bowel as a preparation for colonoscopy in adults 18 yr of age or older.

Action
Osmotically active in the lumen of the GI tract. Produces laxative effect by causing water retention and stimulation of peristalsis. Stimulates motility and inhibits fluid and electrolyte absorption from the small intestine. **Therapeutic Effects:** Relief of constipation. Emptying of the bowel.

Pharmacokinetics
Absorption: 1–20% of rectally administered sodium and phosphate may be absorbed; some absorption follows oral administration.
Distribution: Unknown.
Metabolism and Excretion: Excreted by the kidneys.
Half-life: Unknown.

TIME/ACTION PROFILE (laxative effect)

ROUTE	ONSET	PEAK	DURATION
PO	0.5–3 hr	unknown	unknown
Rect	2–5 min	unknown	unknown

Contraindications/Precautions
Contraindicated in: Hypersensitivity; Abdominal pain, nausea, or vomiting, especially when associated with fever or other signs of an acute abdomen; Severe renal or cardiovascular disease; Intestinal obstruction; OB: Not recommended for use at term; *Visicol and OsmoPrep*—CHF, ascites, unstable angina, acute colitis, toxic megacolon, or hypomotility syndrome; Pedi: Children <2 yr.

Use Cautiously in: Excessive or chronic use (may lead to dependence); Renal or cardiovascular disease, dehydration or concurrent use of diuretics or other drugs known to alter electrolytes (correct abnormalities prior to administration); Dehydration, renal dysfunction, bowel obstruction, active colitis, or concurrent use of diuretics, ACE inhibitors, ARBs, or NSAIDs (↑ risk of acute phosphate nephropathy); OB: May cause sodium retention and edema; Geri: May be more sensitive to effects; *Visicol*—use cautiously within 3 mo of MI or cardiac surgery or in patients with acute exacerbations of inflammatory bowel disease.

Adverse Reactions/Side Effects
CNS: *Visicol*—dizziness, headache. **CV:** AR-RHYTHMIAS. **GI:** cramping, nausea, colonic aphtous ulcerations; *Visicol and OsmoPrep*, abdominal bloating, abdominal pain, vomiting. **F and E:** hyperphosphatemia, hypocalcemia, hypokalemia, sodium retention. **GU:** renal dysfunction.

Interactions
Drug-Drug: *Visicol and OsmoPrep*—Concurrently administered oral medications may not be absorbed due to rapid peristalsis and diarrhea.

Route/Dosage
Each Fleet Enema contains 4.4 g sodium/118 mL.
PO (Adults: *Visicol*—evening before colonoscopy: 3 tablets every 15 min (with at least 8 oz of water), last dose will be 2 tablets (total of 20 tablets); on morning of colonoscopy starting 3–5 hr before procedure, 3 tablets every 15 min (with at least 8 oz of clear liquids), last dose will be 2 tablets (total of 20 tablets); should not be repeated in less than 7 days; *OsmoPrep*—evening before colonoscopy: 4 tablets every 15 min (with at least 8 oz of water) for a total of 20 tablets; on morning of colonoscopy starting 3–5 hr before procedure, 4 tablets every 15 min (with at least 8 oz of clear liquids), for a total of 12 tablets; should not be repeated in less than 7 days.
Rect (Adults and Children >12 yr): 118 mL Fleet Enema.

phytonadione

Rect (Children >2 yr): ½ of the adult dose.

Availability (generic available)
Enema: 7 g sodium phosphate and 19 g sodium biphosphate/118 mL in 67.5- and 133-mL containers. **Tablets (Visicol):** 1.5 g. **Tablets (OsmoPrep):** 1.5 g.

NURSING IMPLICATIONS

Assessment
- Assess patient for fever, abdominal distention, presence of bowel sounds, and usual pattern of bowel function.
- Assess color, consistency, and amount of stool produced.
- May rarely cause arrhythmias. Monitor patients with underlying cardiovascular disease, renal disease, bowel perforation, misuse or overdose.
- **Lab Test Considerations:** May cause increased serum sodium and phosphorus levels, decreased serum calcium and potassium levels, and acidosis. Electrolyte changes are transient, self-limiting, do not require treatment and are not usually associated with adverse clinical events.

Potential Nursing Diagnoses
Constipation (Indications)

Implementation
- Do not administer at bedtime or late in the day.
- **PO:** Administer on an empty stomach for more rapid results. Mix dose in at least ½ glass cold water. May be followed by carbonated beverage or fruit juice to improve flavor.
- See Route and Dose section for dosing of *Visicol* and *OsmoPrep*. Undigested *Visicol* tablets may appear in the stool or be visualized during colonoscopy.
- **Rect:** Position patient on left side with knee slightly flexed. Insert prelubricated tip about 2 inches into rectum, aiming toward the umbilicus. Gently squeeze bottle until empty. Discontinue if resistance is met, because perforation may occur if contents are forced into rectum.

Patient/Family Teaching
- Advise patient that laxatives should be used only for short-term therapy. Long-term therapy may cause electrolyte imbalance and dependence.
- Caution patient on sodium restriction that this product has a high sodium content.
- Advise patient not to take oral form of this medication within 2 hr of other medications.
- Encourage patient to use other forms of bowel regulation, such as increasing bulk in the diet, fluid intake, and mobility. Normal bowel habits may vary from 3 times/day to 3 times/wk.
- Advise patient to notify health care professional if unrelieved constipation, rectal bleeding, or symptoms of electrolyte imbalance (muscle cramps or pain, weakness, dizziness, and so forth) occur.

Evaluation/Desired Outcomes
- Soft, formed bowel movement.
- Evacuation of the bowel.

---

phytonadione
(fye-toe-na-**dye**-one)
Mephyton, vitamin K

Classification
Therapeutic: antidotes, vitamins
Pharmacologic: fat-soluble vitamins

Pregnancy Category C

Indications
Prevention and treatment of hypoprothrombinemia, which may be associated with: Excessive doses of oral anticoagulants, Salicylates, Certain anti-infective agents, Nutritional deficiencies, Prolonged total parenteral nutrition. Prevention of hemorrhagic disease of the newborn.

Action
Required for hepatic synthesis of blood coagulation factors II (prothrombin), VII, IX, and X.
Therapeutic Effects: Prevention of bleeding due to hypoprothrombinemia.

Pharmacokinetics
Absorption: Well absorbed following oral or subcut administration. Oral absorption requires presence of bile salts. Some vitamin K is produced by bacteria in the GI tract.
Distribution: Crosses the placenta; does not enter breast milk.
Metabolism and Excretion: Rapidly metabolized by the liver.
Half-life: Unknown.

TIME/ACTION PROFILE

ROUTE	ONSET	PEAK†	DURATION‡
PO	6–12 hr	unknown	unknown
Subcut	1–2 hr	3–6 hr	12–14 hr
IV	1–2 hr	3–6 hr	12 hr

†Control of hemorrhage
‡Normal PT achieved

Contraindications/Precautions
Contraindicated in: Hypersensitivity; Hypersensitivity or intolerance to benzyl alcohol (injection only).

Use Cautiously in: Impaired liver function.
Exercise Extreme Caution in: Severe life-threatening reactions have occurred following IV administration, use other routes unless risk is justified.

Adverse Reactions/Side Effects
GI: gastric upset, unusual taste. **Derm:** flushing, rash, urticaria. **Hemat:** hemolytic anemia. **Local:** erythema, pain at injection site, swelling. **Misc:** allergic reactions, hyperbilirubinemia (large doses in very premature infants), kernicterus.

Interactions
Drug-Drug: Large doses will counteract the effect of **warfarin**. Large doses of **salicylates** or broad-spectrum **anti-infectives** may ↑ vitamin K requirements. **Bile acid sequestrants**, **mineral oil**, and **sucralfate** may ↓ vitamin K absorption from the GI tract.

Route/Dosage
IV use of phytonadione should be reserved for patients with serious or life-threatening bleeding and elevated INR. Oral route is preferred in patients with elevated INRs and no serious or life-threatening bleeding. IM route should generally be avoided because of risk of hematoma formation.

Treatment of Hypoprothrombinemia due to Vitamin K Deficiency (from factors other than warfarin)
Subcut, IV (Adults): 10 mg.
PO (Adults): 2.5–25 mg/day.
Subcut, IV (Children >1 month): 1–2 mg single dose.
PO (Children >1 month): 2.5–5 mg/day.

Vitamin K Deficiency (Supratherapeutic INR) Secondary to Warfarin
PO (Adults): *INR ≥5 and <9 (no significant bleeding)*—Hold warfarin and give 1–2.5 mg vitamin K; if more rapid reversal required, given ≤5 mg vitamin K; *INR >9 (no significant bleeding)*—Hold warfarin and give 2.5–5 mg vitamin K.
IV (Adults): *Elevated INR with serious or life-threatening bleeding*—10 mg slow infusion.

Prevention of Hypoprothrombinemia during Total Parenteral Nutrition
IV (Adults): 5–10 mg once weekly.
IV (Children): 2–5 mg once weekly.

Prevention of Hemorrhagic Disease of Newborn
IM (Neonates): 0.5–1 mg, within 1 hr of birth, may repeat in 6–8 hr if needed. May be repeated in 2–3 wk if mother received previous anticonvulsant/anticoagulant/anti-infective/antitubercular therapy. 1–5 mg may be given IM to mother 12–24 hr before delivery.

Treatment of Hemorrhagic Disease of Newborn
IM, Subcut (Neonates): 1–2 mg/day.

Availability (generic available)
Tablets: 5 mg. **Injection:** 2 mg/mL, 10 mg/mL.

NURSING IMPLICATIONS

Assessment
- Monitor for frank and occult bleeding (guaiac stools, Hematest urine, and emesis). Monitor pulse and blood pressure frequently; notify physician immediately if symptoms of internal bleeding or hypovolemic shock develop. Inform all personnel of patient's bleeding tendency to prevent further trauma. Apply pressure to all venipuncture sites for at least 5 min; avoid unnecessary IM injections.
- **Pedi:** Monitor for side effects and adverse reactions. Children may be especially sensitive to the effects and side effects of vitamin K. Neonates, especially premature neonates, may be more sensitive than older children.
- ***Lab Test Considerations:*** Monitor prothrombin time (PT) prior to and throughout vitamin K therapy to determine response to and need for further therapy.

Potential Nursing Diagnoses
Imbalanced nutrition: less than body requirements (Indications)
Ineffective tissue perfusion (Indications)

Implementation
- The parenteral route is preferred for phytonadione therapy but, because of severe, potentially fatal hypersensitivity reactions, IV vitamin K is not recommended.
- Administration of whole blood or plasma may also be required in severe bleeding because of the delayed onset of this medication.
- Phytonadione is an antidote for warfarin overdose but does not counteract the anticoagulant activity of heparin.

1028 pilocarpine (oral)

IV Administration

- **Intermittent Infusion:** *Diluent:* Dilute in 0.9% NaCl, D5W, or D5/0.9% NaCl. *Rate:* Administer over 30–60 min. Rate should not exceed 1 mg/min.
- **Y-Site Compatibility:** alfentanil, amikacin, aminophylline, ascorbic acid, atracurium, atropine, azathioprine, aztreonam, bumetanide, buprenorphine, butorphanol, calcium chloride, calcium gluconate, cefazolin, cefonocid, cefoperazone, cefotaxime, cefotetan, cefoxitin, ceftazidime, ceftizoxime, ceftriaxone, cefuroxime, chloramphenicol, chlorpromazine, cimetidine, clindamycin, cyanocobalamin, cyclosporine, dexamethasone sodium phosphate, digoxin, diphenhydramine, dopamine, doxycycline, enalaprilat, ephedrine, epinephrine, epoetin alfa, erythromycin, esmolol, famotidine, fentanyl, fluconazole, folic acid, furosemide, ganciclovir, gentamicin, glycopyrronate, heparin, hydrocortisone sodium succinate, imipenem/cilastatin, indomethacin, insulin, isoproterenol, ketorolac, labetalol, lidocaine, mannitol, meperidine, metaraminol, methoxamine, methyldopa, metoclopramide, metoprolol, metronidazole, midazolam, morphine, multivitamins, nafcillin, nalbuphine, naloxone, nitroglycerin, nitroprusside, norepinephrine, ondansetron, oxacillin, oxytocin, papaverine, penicillin G potassium, pentamidine, pentazocine, pentobarbital, phenobarbital, phentolamine, phenylephrine, potassium chloride, procainamide, prochlorperazine, propranolol, pyridoxime, ranitidine, sodium bicarbonate, streptokinase, succinylcholine, sufentanil, theophylline, thiamine, ticarcillin/clavulanate, tobramycin, tolazoline, trimethaphan, urokinase, vancomycin, vasopressin, verapamil, vitamin B with C.
- **Y-Site Incompatibility:** dantrolene, diazepam, diazoxide, magnesium sulfate, phenytoin, trimethoprim/sulfamethoxazole.

Patient/Family Teaching

- Instruct patient to take phytonadione as directed. Take missed doses as soon as remembered unless almost time for next dose. Notify health care professional of missed doses.
- Cooking does not destroy substantial amounts of vitamin K. Patient should not drastically alter diet while taking vitamin K. See Appendix M for foods high in vitamin K.
- Caution patient to avoid IM injections and activities leading to injury. Use a soft toothbrush, do not floss, and shave with an electric razor until coagulation defect is corrected.
- Advise patient to report any symptoms of unusual bleeding or bruising (bleeding gums; nosebleed; black, tarry stools; hematuria; excessive menstrual flow).
- Patients receiving vitamin K therapy should be cautioned not to take other Rx, OTC, or herbal products without advice of health care professional.
- Advise patient to inform health care professional of medication regimen prior to treatment or surgery.
- Advise patient to carry identification at all times describing disease process.
- Emphasize the importance of frequent lab tests to monitor coagulation factors.

Evaluation/Desired Outcomes

- Prevention of spontaneous bleeding or cessation of bleeding in patients with hypoprothrombinemia secondary to impaired intestinal absorption or oral anticoagulant, salicylate, or anti-infective therapy.
- Prevention of hemorrhagic disease in the newborn.

---

pilocarpine (oral)†
(pye-loe-**kar**-peen)
Salagen

Classification
Therapeutic: none assigned
Pharmacologic: cholinergics

Pregnancy Category C

†For ophthalmic use of pilocarpine, see Appendix C

Indications
Management of xerostomia, which may occur as a consequence of radiation therapy for cancer of the head and neck. Treatment of dry mouth in patients with Sjögren's syndrome.

Action
Stimulates cholinergic receptors, resulting in primarily muscarinic action, including stimulation of exocrine glands. Other effects include: Increased sweating, gastric secretions, Increased bronchial secretions, Increased tone and motility of the urinary tract, gallbladder, and biliary duct smooth muscle. **Therapeutic Effects:** Increased salivary gland secretion.

Pharmacokinetics
Absorption: Well absorbed after oral administration.
Distribution: Unknown.

Metabolism and Excretion: Inactivated at neuronal synapses and in plasma. Some unchanged pilocarpine and metabolites are excreted in urine.
Half-life: *After 5-mg dose for 2 days*—0.8 hr; *after 10-mg dose for 2 days*—1.3 hr.

TIME/ACTION PROFILE

ROUTE	ONSET	PEAK	DURATION
PO	20 min	1 hr	3–5 hr

Contraindications/Precautions
Contraindicated in: Hypersensitivity; Uncontrolled asthma; Angle-closure glaucoma; Iritis.
Use Cautiously in: History of pulmonary disease (asthma, bronchitis, or chronic obstructive pulmonary disease); Biliary tract disease or cholelithiasis; Cardiovascular disease; Retinal disease; Nephrolithiasis; History of psychiatric or cognitive disorders; OB: Pregnancy, lactation, or children (safety not established).

Adverse Reactions/Side Effects
CNS: dizziness, headache, weakness. **EENT:** amblyopia, epistaxis, rhinitis. **CV:** edema, hypertension, tachycardia. **GI:** <u>nausea</u>, <u>vomiting</u>, dyspepsia, dysphagia. **GU:** urinary frequency. **Derm:** <u>flushing</u>, <u>sweating</u>. **Neuro:** tremors. **Misc:** chills, voice change.

Interactions
Drug-Drug: Concurrent use of **anticholinergics** will ↓ the effectiveness of pilocarpine. Concurrent use of **bethanechol** or **ophthalmic cholinergics** may result in ↑ cholinergic effects. Concurrent use with **beta blockers** may ↑ the risk of adverse cardiovascular reactions (conduction disturbances).

Route/Dosage
Head and Neck Cancer Patients
PO (Adults): 5 mg three times daily initially, then titrated to need/response, usual range 15–30 mg/day (no single should exceed 10 mg).

Patients with Sjögren's Syndrome
PO (Adults): 5 mg four times daily.

Availability
Tablets: 5 mg, 7.5 mg.

NURSING IMPLICATIONS
Assessment
- Assess oral mucosa for dryness and ulceration periodically during therapy.

Potential Nursing Diagnoses
Impaired oral mucous membrane (Indications)

Implementation
- **PO:** Use lowest dose that is tolerated and effective for maintenance.

Patient/Family Teaching
- Instruct patient to take medication as directed.
- Caution patient that pilocarpine may cause visual changes, especially at night; avoid driving or other activities requiring alertness until effects of medication are known.
- Advise patient to drink adequate daily fluids (1500–2000 mL/day), especially if sweating occurs. Less than adequate fluid intake may lead to dehydration.

Evaluation/Desired Outcomes
- Increased salivary gland secretion in patients with xerostomia.
- Decrease in dry mouth in patients with Sjögren's syndrome. Full effects in cancer patients may not be seen for up to 12 weeks or 6 weeks in patients with Sjögren's syndrome.

---

pimecrolimus
(pi-me-**cro**-li-mus)
Elidel

Classification
Therapeutic: immunosuppressants (topical)

Indications
Short-term and intermittent long-term management of mild to moderate atopic dermatitis unresponsive to or in patients intolerant of conventional treatment.

Action
Inhibits T-cell and mast cell activation by interfering with production of inflammatory cytokines.
Therapeutic Effects: Decreased severity of atopic dermatatis.

Pharmacokinetics
Absorption: Minimally absorbed through intact skin.
Distribution: Local distribution after topical administration.
Metabolism and Excretion: Systemic metabolism and excretion is negligible with local application.
Half-life: Not applicable.

pioglitazone

TIME/ACTION PROFILE (improvement in symptoms)

ROUTE	ONSET	PEAK	DURATION
topical	within 6 days	unknown	unknown

Contraindications/Precautions
Contraindicated in: Hypersensitivity; Should not be applied to areas of active cutaneous viral infections (increased risk of dissemination); Concurrent use of occlusive dressings; Netherton's syndrome (increased absorption of pimecrolimus); Lactation: Discontinue breastfeeding.
Use Cautiously in: Possible risk of cancer. Do not use as first-line therapy; Clinical infection at treatment site (infection should be treated/cleared prior to use); Skin papillomas (warts); allow treatment/resolution prior to use; Natural/artificial sunlight (minimize exposure); OB: Use only if clearly needed; Pedi: Use only if other treatments have failed; safety not established in children <2 yr.

Adverse Reactions/Side Effects
Local: burning. **Misc:** increased risk of lymphoma/skin cancer.

Interactions
Drug-Drug: None significant as systemic absorption is negligible.

Route/Dosage
Topical (Adults and Children ≥2 yr): Apply thin film twice daily; rub in gently and completely.

Availability
Cream: 1% in 30-g, 60-g, and 100-g tubes. **Cost:** $75.99/30 g, $141.58/60 g, $220.98/100 g.

NURSING IMPLICATIONS

Assessment
- Assess skin lesions prior to and periodically during therapy. Discontinue therapy after signs and symptoms of atopic dermatitis have resolved. Resume treatment at the first signs and symptoms of recurrence.

Potential Nursing Diagnoses
Impaired skin integrity (Indications)

Implementation
- **Topical:** Apply a thin layer to affected area twice daily and rub in gently and completely. May be used on all skin areas including head, neck, and intertriginous areas. Do not use with occlusive dressings.

Patient/Family Teaching
- Instruct patient on correct technique for application. Apply only as directed to external areas. Wash hands following application, unless hands are areas of application.
- Caution patient to avoid exposure to natural or artificial sunlight, including tanning beds, while using cream.
- Advise patient that pimecrolimus may cause skin burning. This occurs most commonly during first few days of application, is of mild to moderate severity, and improves within 5 days or as atopic dermatitis resolves.
- Advise patient to notify health care provider if no improvement is seen following 6 wk of treatment or at any time if condition worsens.

Evaluation/Desired Outcomes
- Resolution of signs and symptoms of atopic dermatitis.

---

pioglitazone (pi-o-glit-a-zone)
Actos

Classification
Therapeutic: antidiabetics (oral)
Pharmacologic: thiazolidinediones

Pregnancy Category C

Indications
Type 2 diabetes mellitus (with diet and exercise); may be used with metformin, sulfonylureas, or insulin.

Action
Improves sensitivity to insulin by acting as an agonist at receptor sites involved in insulin responsiveness and subsequent glucose production and utilization. Requires insulin for activity. **Therapeutic Effects:** Decreased insulin resistance, resulting in glycemic control without hypoglycemia.

Pharmacokinetics
Absorption: Well absorbed following oral administration.
Distribution: Unknown.
Protein Binding: >99% bound to plasma proteins. Active metabolites are also highly (>99%) bound.
Metabolism and Excretion: Extensively metabolized by the liver; at least two metabolites have pharmacologic activity. Minimal renal excretion of unchanged drug.
Half-life: *Pioglitazone*—3–7 hr; *total pioglitazone (pioglitazone plus metabolites)*—16–24 hr.

pioglitazone

TIME/ACTION PROFILE (effects on blood glucose)

ROUTE	ONSET	PEAK	DURATION
PO	30 min	2–4 hr	24 hr

Contraindications/Precautions
Contraindicated in: Hypersensitivity; Type 1 diabetes; Diabetic ketoacidosis; Clinical evidence of active liver disease or ↑ ALT (>2.5 times upper limit of normal); OB, Lactation: Insulin should be used to control blood glucose levels; Pedi: Children.

Use Cautiously in: Edema; CHF (avoid use in moderate to severe CHF); Hepatic impairment; Women (may ↑ distal upper and lower limb fractures); Women with childbearing potential (may restore ovulation and ↑ risk of pregnancy).

Adverse Reactions/Side Effects
CV: CHF, edema. **EENT:** macular edema. **GI:** hepatitis, ↑ liver enzymes. **Hemat:** anemia. **Misc:** fractures (arm, hand, foot) in female patients.

Interactions
Drug-Drug: May ↓ efficacy of **hormonal contraceptives**. Pioglitazone is metabolized by the **CYP450 3A4** enzyme system. Concurrent use of drugs that alter the activity of this system may result in drug-drug interactions. **Ketoconazole** may ↑ effects of pioglitazone. Concurrent use with **insulin** may ↑ risk of CHF (consider predisposing factors).

Drug-Natural Products: Glucosamine may worsen blood glucose control. **Chromium**, and **coenzyme Q-10** may produce ↑ hypoglycemic effects.

Route/Dosage
PO (Adults): 15–30 mg once daily, may be ↑ to 45 mg/day if needed. Doses >30 mg have not been evaluated in combination with insulin and other antidiabetics.

Availability
Tablets: 15 mg, 30 mg, 45 mg. **Cost:** 15 mg $329.97/90, 30 mg $505.97/90, 45 mg $549.97/90. *In combination with:* Metformin (Actoplus Met, Actoplus Met XR), glimepride (Duetact); see Appendix B.

NURSING IMPLICATIONS

Assessment
- Observe patient taking concurrent insulin for signs and symptoms of hypoglycemic reactions (sweating, hunger, weakness, dizziness, tremor, tachycardia, anxiety).
- Assess for signs and symptoms of heart failure (edema, dyspnea, rapid weight gain, unusual tiredness).
- *Lab Test Considerations:* Monitor serum glucose and Hb A_{1c} periodically during therapy to evaluate effectiveness.
- Monitor CBC with differential periodically during therapy. May cause ↓ in hemoglobin and hematocrit, usually during the first 4–12 wk of therapy; then levels stabilize.
- Monitor serum ALT levels before starting therapy and periodically thereafter or if jaundice or symptoms of hepatic dysfunction occur. Pioglitazone should not be started in patients with active liver disease or ALT levels >2.5 times the upper limit of normal. Patients with mild ALT ↑ should have more frequent monitoring. If ALT ↑ to >3 times the upper limit of normal, recheck ALT promptly. Discontinue pioglitazone if ALT remains >3 times normal.
- May cause transient ↑ in CPK levels.

Potential Nursing Diagnoses
Imbalanced nutrition: more than body requirements (Indications)
Noncompliance (Patient/Family Teaching)

Implementation
- Patients stabilized on a diabetic regimen who are exposed to stress, fever, trauma, infection, or surgery may require administration of insulin.
- **PO:** May be administered with or without meals.

Patient/Family Teaching
- Instruct patient to take medication as directed. If dose for 1 day is missed, do not double dose the next day.
- Explain to patient that this medication controls hyperglycemia but does not cure diabetes. Therapy is long-term.
- Review signs of hypoglycemia and hyperglycemia with patient. If hypoglycemia occurs, advise patient to take a glass of orange juice or 2–3 tsp of sugar, honey, or corn syrup dissolved in water and notify health care professional.
- Encourage patient to follow prescribed diet, medication, and exercise regimen to prevent hypoglycemic or hyperglycemic episodes.
- Instruct patient in proper testing of serum glucose and ketones. These tests should be closely

monitored during periods of stress or illness, and health care professional should be notified if significant changes occur.
- Advise patient to notify health care professional immediately if signs of hepatic dysfunction (nausea, vomiting, abdominal pain, fatigue, anorexia, dark urine, jaundice) or CHF (edema, shortness of breath, rapid weight gain, tiredness) occur.
- Insulin is the preferred method of controlling blood glucose during pregnancy. Counsel female patients that higher doses of oral contraceptives or a form of contraception other than oral contraceptives may be required and to notify health care professional promptly if pregnancy is planned or suspected.
- Advise patient to inform health care professional of medication regimen before treatment or surgery.
- Advise patient to carry a form of sugar (sugar packets, candy) and identification describing disease process and medication regimen at all times.
- Emphasize the importance of routine follow-up exams.

Evaluation/Desired Outcomes
- Control of blood glucose levels.

---

piperacillin/tazobactam
(pi-**per**-a-sill-in/tay-zoe-**bak**-tam)
Zosyn

Classification
Therapeutic: anti-infectives
Pharmacologic: extended spectrum penicillins

Pregnancy Category B

Indications
Appendicitis and peritonitis. Skin and skin structure infections. Gynecologic infections. Community-acquired and nosocomial pneumonia caused by piperacillin-resistant, beta-lactamase–producing bacteria.

Action
Piperacillin: Binds to bacterial cell wall membrane, causing cell death. Spectrum is extended compared with other penicillins. **Tazobactam:** Inhibits beta-lactamase, an enzyme that can destroy penicillins. **Therapeutic Effects:** Death of susceptible bacteria. **Spectrum:** Active against piperacillin-resistant, beta-lactamase–producing: *Bacteroides fragilis, E. coli, Acinetobacter baumannii, Klebsiella pneumoniae, Pseudomonas aeruginosa, Staphylococcus aureus, Haemophilus influenzae.*

Pharmacokinetics
Absorption: Piperacillin is well absorbed (80%) from IM sites.
Distribution: Widely distributed. Enter CSF well only when meninges are inflamed. Crosses the placenta and enters breast milk in low concentrations.
Metabolism and Excretion: Piperacillin (68%) and tazobactam (80%) are mostly excreted unchanged by the kidneys.
Half-life: Adults: 0.7–1.2 hr; Children 6 mo–12 yr: 0.7–0.9 hr; Infants 2–5 mo: 1.4 hr.

TIME/ACTION PROFILE (piperacillin blood levels)

ROUTE	ONSET	PEAK	DURATION
IV	rapid	end of infusion	4–6 hr

Contraindications/Precautions
Contraindicated in: Hypersensitivity to penicillins, beta-lactams, cephalosporins, or tazobactam (cross-sensitivity may occur).
Use Cautiously in: Renal impairment (dosage reduction or increased interval recommended if CCr <40 mL/min); Sodium restriction; OB: Lactation: Safety not established.

Adverse Reactions/Side Effects
CNS: SEIZURES (higher doses), confusion, dizziness, headache, insomnia, lethargy. **GI:** PSEUDOMEMBRANOUS COLITIS, diarrhea, constipation, drug-induced hepatitis, nausea, vomiting. **GU:** interstitial nephritis. **Derm:** rashes (↑ in cystic fibrosis patients), urticaria. **Hemat:** bleeding, leukopenia, neutropenia, thrombocytopenia. **Local:** pain, phlebitis at IV site. **Misc:** hypersensitivity reactions, including ANAPHYLAXIS and SERUM SICKNESS, fever (↑ in cystic fibrosis patients), superinfection.

Interactions
Drug-Drug: Probenecid ↓ renal excretion and ↑ blood levels. May alter excretion of **lithium**. **Potassium-losing diuretics, corticosteroids,** or **amphotericin B** may ↑ risk of hypokalemia. ↑ risk of hepatotoxicity with other **hepatotoxic agents**. May ↓ levels/effects of **aminoglycosides** in patients with renal impairment. May ↑ levels and risk of toxicity from **methotrexate**.

Route/Dosage
Contains 2.79 mEq (64 mg) sodium/g of piperacillin; adult doses below expressed as combined piperacillin/tazobactam content.

piperacillin/tazobactam

IV (Adults): *Most infections*—3.375 g q 6 hr. *Nosocomial pneumonia*—4.5 g q 6 hr.
IV (Adults): *Nosocomial pneumonia*—4.5 g q 6 hr.
IV (Adults and Children >40 kg): *Appendicitis and/or peritonitis*—3.375 g q 6 hr.
IV (Children ≥9 mo and ≤40 kg): *Appendicitis and/or peritonitis*—300 mg piperacillin component/kg/day divided q 8 hr.
IV (Infants 2–9 mo): *Appendicitis and/or peritonitis*—240 mg piperacillin component/kg/day divided q 8 hr.
IV (Infants and Children ≥6 mo): 240–400 mg/piperacillin component/kg/day divided q 6–8 hr (higher end of dosing range for serious pseudomonal infections); Max dose: 16 g piperacillin/day.
IV (Infants <6 mo): 150–300 mg/piperacillin component/kg/day divided q 6–8 hr.

Renal Impairment
IV (Adults): *CCr 20–40 mL/min*—2.25 g q 6 hr (3.375 g q 6 hr for nosocomial pneumonia); *CCr <20 mL/min*—2.25 g q 8 hr (2.25 g q 6 hr for nosocomial pneumonia); *Hemodialysis*—2.25 g q 12 h (2.25 g q 8 hr for nosocomial pneumonia).

Availability (generic available)
Powder for injection: 2-g piperacillin/0.25-g tazobactam vials and 50-mL premixed frozen containers, 3-g piperacillin/0.375-g tazobactam vials and 50-mL premixed frozen containers, 4-g piperacillin/0.5-g tazobactam vials and 50-mL premixed frozen containers, 36– piperacillin/4.5-g tazobactam bulk vials.

NURSING IMPLICATIONS

Assessment
- Assess patient for infection (vital signs; appearance of wound, sputum, urine, and stool; WBC) at beginning of and during therapy.
- Obtain a history before initiating therapy to determine previous use of and reactions to penicillins or cephalosporins. Persons with a negative history of penicillin sensitivity may still have an allergic response.
- Obtain specimens for culture and sensitivity prior to initiating therapy. First dose may be given before receiving results.
- Observe patient for signs and symptoms of anaphylaxis (rash, pruritus, laryngeal edema, wheezing). Discontinue the drug and notify health care professional immediately if these occur. Keep epinephrine, an antihistamine, and resuscitation equipment close by in the event of an anaphylactic reaction.
- Monitor bowel function. Diarrhea, abdominal cramping, fever, and bloody stools should be reported to health care professional promptly as a sign of pseudomembranous colitis. May begin up to several weeks following cessation of therapy.
- *Lab Test Considerations:* Evaluate renal and hepatic function, CBC, serum potassium, and bleeding times prior to and routinely during therapy.
- May cause positive direct Coombs' test result.
- May cause ↑ BUN, creatinine, AST, ALT, serum bilirubin, alkaline phosphatase, and LDH.
- May cause leukopenia and neutropenia, especially with prolonged therapy or hepatic impairment.
- May cause prolonged prothrombin and partial thromboplastin time.
- May cause ↓ hemoglobin and hematocrit and thrombocytopenia, eosinophilia, leukopenia, and neutropenia. It also may cause proteinuria; hematuria; pyuria; hyperglycemia; ↓ total protein or albumin; and abnormalities in sodium, potassium, and calcium levels.

Potential Nursing Diagnoses
Risk for infection (Indications, Side Effects)
Deficient knowledge, related to medication regimen (Patient/Family Teaching)

Implementation
- Do not confuse Zosyn (piperacillin/tazobactam) with Zofran (ondansetron).

IV Administration

- **Intermittent Infusion:** Reconstitute each 1 g of piperacillin with at least 5 mL of 0.9% NaCl, sterile water for injection, or D5W. ***Diluent:*** Dilute further in 50–100 mL of 0.9% NaCl, D5W, D5/0.9% NaCl, or LR. Reconstituted vials stable for 24 hr at room temperature or 48 hr if refrigerated. Infusion stable for 24 hr at room temperature or 7 days if refrigerated. ***Rate:*** Infuse over 30 min.
- **Y-Site Compatibility:** alfentanil, allopurinol, amifostine, amikacin, aminophylline, amphotericin B liposome, anidulafungin, aztreonam, bivalirudin, bleomycin, bumetanide, buprenorphine, busulfan, butorphanol, calcium acetate, calcium chloride, calcium gluconate, carboplatin, carmustine, cefepime, chloramphenicol, cimetidine, clindamycin, cyclophosphamide,

cyclosporine, cytarabine, dactinomycin, daptomycin, dexamethasone, dexmedetomidine, dexrazoxane, diazepam, digoxin, diphenhydramine, docetaxel, dopamine, doxacurium, enalaprilat, ephedrine, epinephrine, erythromycin, esmolol, etoposide, etoposide phosphate, fenoldopam, fentanyl, floxuridine, fluconazole, fludarabine, fluorouracil, foscarnet, fosphenytoin, furosemide, granisetron, heparin, hetastarch, hydrocortisone, hydromorphone, ifosfamide, isoproterenol, ketorolac, leucovorin, lidocaine, linezolid, lorazepam, magnesium sulfate, mannitol, mechlorethamine, melphalan, meperidine, mesna, metaraminol, methotrexate, methylprednisolone, metoclopramide, metoprolol, metronidazole, milrinone, morphine, naloxone, nitroglycerin, nitroprusside, norepinephrine, octreotide, ondansetron, oxytocin, paclitaxel, palonosetron, pancuronium, pantoprazole, pemetrexed, pentobarbital, phenobarbital, phentolamine, phenylephrine, plicamycin, potassium chloride, potassium phosphates, procainamide, ranitidine, remifentanil, rituximab, sargramostim, sodium acetate, sodium bicarbonate, sodium phosphates, succinylcholine, sufentanil, tacrolimus, teniposide, theophylline, thiotepa, tigecycline, tirofiban, trimethobenzamide, trimethoprim/sulfamethoxazole, vasopressin, vinblastine, vincristine, voriconazole, zidovudine.

- **Y-Site Incompatibility:** acyclovir, amiodarone, amphotericin B cholesteryl, amphotericin B colloidal, azithromycin, caspofungin, chlorpromazine, ciprofloxacin, cisplatin, codeine, dacarbazine, dantrolene, daunorubicin, diltiazem, dobutamine, doxorubicin, doxorubicin liposome, doxycycline, droperidol, drotrecogin, epirubicin, famotidine, ganciclovir, gemcitabine, glycopyrrolate, haloperidol, hydralazine, hydroxyzine, idarubicin, inamrinone, insulin, labetalol, levofloxacin, methyldopate, midazolam, mitomycin, mitoxantrone, nalbuphine, nesiritide, pentamidine, pentazocine, phenytoin, prochlorperazine, promethazine, propranolol, quinupristin/dalfopristin, rocuronium, streptozocin, thiopental, tobramycin, tranexamic acid, trastuzumab, vecuronium, verapamil, vinorelbine.

Patient/Family Teaching
- Advise patient to report signs of superinfection (black furry overgrowth on tongue, vaginal itching or discharge, loose or foul-smelling stools) and allergy.
- Caution patient to notify health care professional if fever and diarrhea occur, especially if stool contains blood, pus, or mucus. Advise patient not to treat diarrhea without consulting health care professional. May occur up to several weeks after discontinuation of medication.

Evaluation/Desired Outcomes
- Resolution of the signs and symptoms of infection. Length of time for complete resolution depends on the organism and site of infection.

---

piroxicam (peer-ox-i-kam)
✤ Apo-Piroxicam, Feldene,
✤ Novo-Pirocam, ✤ Nu-Pirox,
✤ PMS-Piroxicam

Classification
Therapeutic: antirheumatics, nonsteroidal anti-inflammatory agents

Pregnancy Category C

Indications
Management of inflammatory disorders, including: Rheumatoid arthritis, Osteoarthritis. **Unlabeled Use:** Management of dysmenorrhea.

Action
Inhibits prostaglandin synthesis. **Therapeutic Effects:** Suppression of pain and inflammation.

Pharmacokinetics
Absorption: Well absorbed from the GI tract.
Distribution: Unknown. Enters breast milk in small amounts.
Metabolism and Excretion: Mostly metabolized by the liver. Minimal amounts excreted unchanged by the kidneys.
Half-life: 50 hr.

TIME/ACTION PROFILE

ROUTE	ONSET	PEAK	DURATION
PO (analgesic effect)	1 hr	unknown	48–72 hr
PO (anti-inflammatory effect)	7–12 days	2–3 wk†	unknown

†May take up to 12 wk

Contraindications/Precautions
Contraindicated in: Hypersensitivity; Cross-sensitivity may exist with other NSAIDs, including aspirin; Active GI bleeding or ulcer disease; Peri-operative pain from coronary artery bypass graft (CABG) surgery; Lactation: Lactation.

Use Cautiously in: Cardiovascular disease or risk factors for cardiovascular disease (may ↑ risk of serious cardiovascular thrombotic events, myocardial infarction, and stroke, especially with

piroxicam 1035

prolonged use); Severe hepatic disease; History of ulcer disease; Renal impairment (dosage reduction recommended); OB: Avoid use during 2nd half of pregnancy; Pedi: Safety not established; Geri: Appears on Beers list; ↑ risk for GI bleeding, edema and renal failure.

Adverse Reactions/Side Effects
CNS: drowsiness, headache, dizziness. **EENT:** blurred vision, tinnitus. **CV:** edema. **GI:** DRUG-INDUCED HEPATITIS, GI BLEEDING, discomfort, dyspepsia, nausea, vomiting, anorexia, constipation, diarrhea, flatulence. **GU:** renal failure. **Derm:** EXFOLIATIVE DERMATITIS, STEVENS-JOHNSON SYNDROME, TOXIC EPIDERMAL NECROLYSIS, rashes. **Hemat:** blood dyscrasias, prolonged bleeding time. **Misc:** allergic reactions including ANAPHYLAXIS.

Interactions
Drug-Drug: Concurrent use with **aspirin** ↓ levels and may ↓ effectiveness. ↑ risk of bleeding with **anticoagulants, cefoperazone, cefotetan, heparin, ticlopidine, clopidogrel, eptifibatide, tirofiban, thrombolytic agents, valproic acid.** ↑ adverse GI side effects with **aspirin, corticosteroids,** and other **NSAIDs. Probenecid** ↑ levels and may ↑ toxicity. May ↓ response to **antihypertensives** or **diuretics.** May ↑ serum levels and risk of toxicity from **lithium**. May ↑ risk of hypoglycemia from **insulin** or **oral hypoglycemic agents**. ↑ risk of adverse renal effects with **cyclosporine** or chronic use of **acetaminophen**. May ↑ risk of hematologic toxicity from **antineoplastics** or **radiation therapy**.

Drug-Natural Products: ↑ bleeding risk with **arnica, chamomile, clove, dong quai, fenugreek, feverfew, garlic, ginger, ginkgo,** and **Panax ginseng.**

Route/Dosage
PO (Adults): *Anti-inflammatory*—10–20 mg/day; may be given as single dose or 2 divided doses. *Antidysmenorrheal*—40 mg initially, then 20 mg/day.

PO (Geriatric Patients): 10 mg/day initially.

Availability (generic available)
Capsules: 10 mg, 20 mg. **Suppositories:** ✦ 10 mg, ✦ 20 mg.

NURSING IMPLICATIONS

Assessment
- Patients who have asthma, aspirin-induced allergy, and nasal polyps are at increased risk for developing hypersensitivity reactions. Monitor for rhinitis, asthma, and urticaria.
- **Arthritis:** Assess pain and range of motion prior to and 1–2 hr following administration.
- ***Lab Test Considerations:*** Bleeding time may be prolonged for up to 2 wk following discontinuation of therapy.
- May cause ↓ hemoglobin, hematocrit, leukocyte, and platelet counts.
- Monitor liver function tests periodically during therapy. May cause ↑ serum alkaline phosphatase, LDH, AST, and ALT concentrations.
- Monitor BUN, serum creatinine, and electrolytes periodically during therapy. May cause ↑ BUN, serum creatinine, and electrolyte concentrations and ↓ urine electrolyte concentrations.

Potential Nursing Diagnoses
Acute pain (Indications)
Impaired physical mobility (Indications)

Implementation
- Administration in higher than recommended doses does not provide increased effectiveness but may cause increased side effects, especially in geriatric patients. Use lowest effective dose for shortest period of time.
- **PO:** Administer after meals or with food or an antacid containing aluminum or magnesium to minimize gastric irritation.
- Administer as soon as possible after the onset of menses. Prophylactic use has not been proved effective.

Patient/Family Teaching
- Advise patient to take this medication with a full glass of water and to remain in an upright position for 15–30 min after administration.
- Instruct patient to take medication as directed. Take missed doses as soon as remembered but not if almost time for the next dose. Do not double doses.
- May cause drowsiness or dizziness. Advise patient to avoid driving or other activities requiring alertness until response to the medication is known.
- Caution patient to avoid the concurrent use of alcohol, aspirin, acetaminophen, or other OTC or herbal products without consulting health care professional.
- Advise patient to inform health care professional of medication regimen prior to treatment or surgery.

✦ = Canadian drug name. ❚ = Genetic implication.
*CAPITALS indicates life-threatening; underlines indicate most frequent.

- Caution patient to use sunscreen and protective clothing to prevent photosensitivity reaction (rare).
- Advise patient to consult health care professional if rash, itching, visual disturbances, tinnitus, weight gain, edema, black stools, persistent headache, or influenza-like syndrome (chills, fever, muscle aches, pain) occurs.

Evaluation/Desired Outcomes
- Decreased pain and improved joint mobility. Partial arthritic relief is usually seen within 2 wk, but maximum effectiveness may require up to 12 wk of continuous therapy. Patients who do not respond to one NSAID may respond to another.

---

pitavastatin, See HMG-CoA REDUCTASE INHIBITORS (statins).

---

polyethylene glycol
(po-lee-**eth**-e-leen **glye**-kole)
GlycoLax, MiraLax

Classification
Therapeutic: laxatives
Pharmacologic: osmotics

Pregnancy Category C

Indications
Treatment of occasional constipation.

Action
Polyethylene glycol (PEG) in solution acts as an osmotic agent, drawing water into the lumen of the GI tract. **Therapeutic Effects:** Evacuation of the GI tract without water or electrolyte imbalance.

Pharmacokinetics
Absorption: Nonabsorbable.
Distribution: Unknown.
Metabolism and Excretion: Excreted in fecal contents.
Half-life: Unknown.

TIME/ACTION PROFILE (bowel movement)

ROUTE	ONSET	PEAK	DURATION
PO	unknown	2–4 days	unknown

Contraindications/Precautions
Contraindicated in: GI obstruction; Gastric retention; Toxic colitis; Megacolon.
Use Cautiously in: Abdominal pain of uncertain cause, particularly if accompanied by fever; OB: Pedi: Safety not established.

Adverse Reactions/Side Effects
GI: abdominal bloating, cramping, flatulence, nausea.

Interactions
Drug-Drug: None significant.

Route/Dosage
PO (Adults): 17 g (heaping tablespoon) in 8 oz of water; may be used for up to 2 wk.

Availability (generic available)
Powder: 14-oz, 24-oz, and 26-oz containers.

NURSING IMPLICATIONS

Assessment
- Assess patient for abdominal distention, presence of bowel sounds, and usual pattern of bowel function.
- Assess color, consistency, and amount of stool produced.

Potential Nursing Diagnoses
Constipation (Indications)
Diarrhea (Side Effects)

Implementation
- **PO:** Dissolve powder in 8 oz of water prior to administration.

Patient/Family Teaching
- Inform patient that 2–4 days may be required to produce a bowel movement. PEG should not be used for more than 2 wk. Prolonged, frequent, or excessive use may result in electrolyte imbalance and laxative dependence.
- Advise patient to notify health care professional if unusual cramps, bloating, or diarrhea occurs.

Evaluation/Desired Outcomes
- A soft, formed bowel movement.

---

polyethylene glycol/ electrolyte
(po-lee-**eth**-e-leen **glye**-kole/e-**lek**-troe-lite)
Colyte, GoLYTELY, ✽Klean-Prep, MoviPrep, NuLytely, TriLyte

Classification
Therapeutic: laxatives
Pharmacologic: osmotics

Pregnancy Category C

Indications
Bowel cleansing in preparation for GI examination. **Unlabeled Use:** Treatment of acute iron overdose in children.

Action
Polyethylene glycol (PEG) in solution acts as an osmotic agent, drawing water into the lumen of the GI tract. **Therapeutic Effects:** Evacuation of the GI tract without water or electrolyte imbalance.

Pharmacokinetics
Absorption: Ions in the solution are nonabsorbable.
Distribution: Unknown.
Metabolism and Excretion: Solution is excreted in fecal contents.
Half-life: Unknown.

TIME/ACTION PROFILE

ROUTE	ONSET	PEAK	DURATION
PO	1 hr	unknown	4 hr

Contraindications/Precautions
Contraindicated in: GI obstruction; Gastric retention; Toxic colitis; Megacolon.
Use Cautiously in: Patients with absent or diminished gag reflex; Unconscious or semicomatose states, in which administration is via NG tube; History of ulcerative colitis (increased risk of hypoglycemia, dehydration, and hypokalemia); Barium enema using double-contrast technique (may not allow proper barium coating of mucosa); Abdominal pain of uncertain cause, particularly if accompanied by fever; Geri: May be more sensitive to effects; Pedi: Children (safety not established; children <2 yr more prone to hypoglycemia, dehydration, and hypokalemia).

Adverse Reactions/Side Effects
GI: <u>abdominal fullness</u>, diarrhea, bloating, cramps, nausea, vomiting. **Misc:** allergic reactions (rare).

Interactions
Drug-Drug: Interferes with the absorption of **orally administered medications** by decreasing transit time (do not administer within 1 hr of start of therapy).

Route/Dosage
PO (Adults): 240 mL q 10 min (up to 4 L) until fecal discharge appears clear and has no solid material; may be given through NG tube at 20–30 mL/min (up to 4 L).
PO (Children ≥6 mo): 25 mL/kg/hr until fecal discharge is clear and has no solid material; may also be given through an NG tube (unlabeled).

Availability (generic available)
Powder for oral solution (regular, pineapple, citrus berry, lemon lime, orange, cherry flavor): CoLyte, NuLytely, TriLyte—powder in bottles for reconstitution, GoLYTELY—powder in packets and bottles for reconstitution, MoviPrep—powder in pouches for reconstitution.

NURSING IMPLICATIONS

Assessment
- Assess color, consistency, and amount of stool produced.
- Monitor semiconscious or unconscious patients closely for regurgitation when administering via NG tube.

Potential Nursing Diagnoses
Diarrhea (Side Effects)

Implementation
- Do not add extra flavorings or additional ingredients to solution prior to administration.
- Patient avoid solid food within 1–2 hr of administration, but should be adequately hydrated prior to, during, and after administration.
- Patient should be allowed only clear liquids after administration.
- May be administered on the morning of the examination as long as time is allotted to drink solution (3 hr) and evacuate bowel (1 additional hr). For barium enema, administer solution early evening (6 PM) prior to exam to allow proper mucosal coating by barium.
- **PO:** Solution may be reconstituted with tap water. Shake vigorously until powder is dissolved.
- May be administered via NG tube at a rate of 20–30 mL/min.

Patient/Family Teaching
- Instruct patient to drink 240 mL every 10 min until 4 L have been consumed or fecal discharge is clear and free of solid matter. Rapidly drinking each 240 mL is preferred over drinking small amounts continuously.

Evaluation/Desired Outcomes
- Diarrhea, which cleanses the bowel within 4 hr. The first bowel movement usually occurs within 1 hr of administration.

---

posaconazole
(po-sa-**kon**-a-zole)
Noxafil

✚ = Canadian drug name. 🧬 = Genetic implication.
*CAPITALS indicates life-threatening; <u>underlines</u> indicate most frequent.

posaconazole

Classification
Therapeutic: antifungals
Pharmacologic: triazoles

Pregnancy Category C

Indications
Prevention of invasive aspergillus and candida infections in severely immunocompromised patients. Treatment of orpharyngeal candidiasis (including candidiasis unresponsive to itraconazole or fluconazole).

Action
Blocks ergosterol synthesis, a major component of fungal plasma membrane. **Therapeutic Effects:** Fungistatic/fungicidal action against susceptible fungi.

Pharmacokinetics
Absorption: Well absorbed following oral administration; absorption is optimized by food.
Distribution: Extensive extravascular distribution and penetration into body tissues.
Protein Binding: >98%.
Metabolism and Excretion: Some metabolism via UDP glucuronidation; 66% eliminated unchanged in feces, 13% in urine (mostly as metabolites).
Half-life: 35 hr.

TIME/ACTION PROFILE (blood levels)

ROUTE	ONSET	PEAK	DURATION
PO	unknown	3–5 hr	8 hr

Contraindications/Precautions
Contraindicated in: Hypersensitivity; Concurrent use of pimozide or quinidine (↑ risk of serious arrhythmias); Concurrent use of ergot alkaloids (↑ risk of ergotism); Concurrent use of sirolimus (↑ risk of sirolimus toxicity).
Use Cautiously in: History of/predisposition to QTc prolongation including congenital QTc prolongation, concurrent medications that prolong QTc, high cumulative anthracycline history or electrolyte abnormalities (hypokalemia, hypomagnesemia); correct pre-existing abnormalities prior to administration; Hypersensitivity to other azole antifungals; Severe diarrhea, vomiting, or renal impairment (monitor for breakthrough fungal infections); OB, Lactation: Use only if maternal benefit outweighs risk to child; Pedi: Children <13 yr (safety not established).

Adverse Reactions/Side Effects
GI: HEPATOCELLULAR DAMAGE, diarrhea, nausea, vomiting. **Endo:** adrenal insufficiency. **Metab:** ALLERGIC REACTIONS.

Interactions
Drug-Drug: Posaconazole inhibits the CYP3A4 enzyme systems and should be expected to interact with other drugs affected by this system. **Rifabutin**, **phenytoin**, **cimetidine**, and **efavirenz** ↓ levels and may ↓ antifungal effectiveness; avoid concurrent use. ↑ **cyclosporine**, **sirolimus**, and **tacrolimus** levels and risk of toxicity; use with sirolimus contraindicated; for cyclosporine and tacrolimus, ↓ dose initially and monitor levels frequently. **Esomeprazole** and **metoclopramide** may ↓ levels and may ↓ antifungal effectiveness. ↑ **rifabutin** levels; avoid concurrent use. May ↑ **digoxin** levels; monitor levels frequently. ↑ **phenytoin**, **midazolam**, **ritonavir**, and **atazanavir** levels; monitor for excess clinical effect. ↑ levels and risk of toxicity from **ergot alkaloids**, including **ergotamine** and **dihydroergotamine**; concurrent administration is contraindicated. ↑ levels and risk of neurotoxicity of **vinca alkaloids**, including **vincristine** and **vinblastine**; consider dose adjustment. ↑ levels and risk of toxicity of **HMG CoA reductase inhibitors (statins)**; consider ↓ statin dose. May ↑ levels and risk of adverse cardiovascular reactions to **calcium channel blockers**; consider dosage reduction.

Route/Dosage
PO (Adults and Children ≥13 yr): *Prophylaxis of invasive fungal infections*—200 mg 3 times daily.

PO (Adults): *Oropharyngeal candidiasis*—100 mg 2 times daily for 1 day, then 100 mg daily for 13 days; *Refractory oropharyngeal candidiasis*—400 mg 2 times daily.

Availability
Oral suspension (cherry): 40 mg/mL.

NURSING IMPLICATIONS

Assessment
- Assess for signs and symptoms of fungal infection.
- **Lab Test Considerations:** Monitor liver function tests prior to and periodically during therapy. May cause ↑ ALT, ↑ AST, ↑ alkaline phosphatase and ↑ total bilirubin levels; generally reversible on discontinuation. Discontinue posaconazole if clinical signs and symptoms of liver disease develop.

Potential Nursing Diagnoses
Risk for infection (Indications)

Implementation
- **PO:** Shake suspension well before use. Administer with a full meal, liquid nutritional supple-

ment or an acidic carbonated beverage (ginger ale) to enhance absorption. Rinse spoon for administration with water after each use. Alternative therapy or close monitoring for breakthrough fungal infections should be considered for patients unable to eat a full meal or tolerate a nutritional supplement.

Patient/Family Teaching
- Instruct patient to take posaconazole during or immediately (within 20 min) following a full meal or liquid nutritional supplement in order to enhance absorption. Take missed doses as soon as remembered. Instruct patient to read the *Patient Information* before taking posaconazole and with each Rx refill; may be new information.
- Advise patient to notify health care professional if severe diarrhea or vomiting occur; may decrease posaconazole blood levels and allow breakthrough fungal infections.
- Instruct patient to consult health care professional prior to taking Rx, OTC, or herbal products during posaconazole therapy.
- Advise patient to notify health care professional if pregnancy is planned or suspected or if breastfeeding.

Evaluation/Desired Outcomes
- Resolution of clinical and laboratory indications of fungal infections. Duration of therapy is based on recovery from infection or neutropenia or immunosuppression.

---

potassium and sodium phosphates
(po-**tas**-e-um/**soe**-dee-yum **foss**-fates)
K-Phos M.F, K-Phos Neutral, K-Phos No. 2, Neutra-Phos, Uro-KP Neutral

Classification
Therapeutic: antiurolithics, mineral and electrolyte replacements/supplements

Pregnancy Category C

Indications
Treatment and prevention of phosphate depletion in patients who are unable to ingest adequate dietary phosphate. Adjunct therapy of urinary tract infections with methenamine hippurate or mandelate. Prevention of calcium urinary stones. Phosphate salts of potassium may be used in hypokalemic patients with metabolic acidosis or coexisting phosphorus deficiency.

Action
Phosphate is present in bone and is involved in energy transfer and carbohydrate metabolism. Serves as a buffer for the excretion of hydrogen ions by the kidneys. Dibasic potassium phosphate is converted in renal tubule to monobasic salt, resulting in urinary acidification, which is required for methenamine hippurate or mandelate to be active as urinary anti-infectives. Acidification of urine increases solubility of calcium, decreasing calcium stone formation. **Therapeutic Effects:** Replacement of phosphorus in deficiency states. Urinary acidification. Increased efficacy of methenamine. Decreased formation of calcium urinary tract stones.

Pharmacokinetics
Absorption: Well absorbed following oral administration. Vitamin D promotes GI absorption of phosphates.
Distribution: Phosphates enter extracellular fluids and are then actively transported to sites of action.
Metabolism and Excretion: Excreted mainly (>90%) by the kidneys.
Half-life: Unknown.

TIME/ACTION PROFILE (effects on serum phosphate levels)

ROUTE	ONSET	PEAK	DURATION
PO	unknown	unknown	unknown

Contraindications/Precautions
Contraindicated in: Hyperkalemia (potassium salts); Hyperphosphatemia; Hypocalcemia; Severe renal impairment; Untreated Addison's disease (potassium salts).
Use Cautiously in: Hyperparathyroidism; Cardiac disease; Hypernatremia (sodium phosphate only); Hypertension (sodium phosphate only); Renal impairment.

Adverse Reactions/Side Effects
Related to hyperphosphatemia, unless otherwise indicated.
CNS: confusion, dizziness, headache, weakness.
CV: ARRHYTHMIAS, CARDIAC ARREST, bradycardia, ECG changes (absent P waves, widening of the QRS complex with biphasic curve, peaked T waves), edema. **GI:** diarrhea, abdominal pain, nausea, vomiting. **F and E:** hyperkalemia, hypernatremia, hyperphosphatemia, hypocalcemia, hy-

pomagnesemia. **MS:** *hypocalcemia, hyperkalemia*—muscle cramps. **Neuro:** flaccid paralysis, heaviness of legs, paresthesias, tremors.

Interactions
Drug-Drug: Concurrent use of **potassium-sparing**, **diuretics**, **ACE inhibitors**, or **angiotensin II receptor blockers** with potassium phosphates may result in hyperkalemia. Concurrent use of **corticosteroids** with sodium phosphate may result in hypernatremia. Concurrent administration of **calcium-, magnesium-,** or **aluminum-containing compounds** ↓ absorption of phosphates by formation of insoluble complexes. **Vitamin D** enhances the absorption of phosphates.
Drug-Food: Oxalates (in spinach and rhubarb) and **phytates** (in bran and whole grains) may ↓ absorption of phosphates by binding them in the GI tract.

Route/Dosage

Phosphorous Supplementation
PO (Adults and Children >4 yr): 250–500 mg (8–16 mmol) phosphorus (1–2 packets) 4 times daily.
PO (Children <4 yr): 250 mg (8 mmol) phosphorus (1 packet) 4 times daily.

Urinary Acidification
PO (Adults): 2 tablets 4 times/day.

Maintenance Phosphorus
PO (Adults): 50–150 mmol/day in divided doses.
PO (Children): 2–3 mmol/kg/day in divided doses.

Availability

Potassium and Sodium Phosphates
Tablets (K-Phos MF): elemental phosphorus 125.6 mg (4 mmol), sodium 67 mg (2.9 mEq), and potassium 44.5 mg (1.1 mEq). **Tablets (K-Phos Neutral):** elemental phosphorus 250 mg (8 mmol), sodium 298 mg (13 mEq), and potassium 45 mg (1.1 mEq). **Tablets (K-Phos No.2):** elemental phosphorus 250 mg (8 mmol), sodium 134 mg (5.8 mEq), and potassium 88 mg (2.3 mEq). **Tablets (Uro-KP Neutral):** elemental phosphorus 258 mg, sodium 262.4 mg (10.8 mEq), and potassium 49.4 mg (1.3 mEq). **Powder for oral solution (Neutra-Phos):** elemental phosphorus 250 mg (8 mmol), sodium 164 mg (7.1 mEq), and potassium 278 mg (7.1 mEq)/packet.

NURSING IMPLICATIONS

Assessment
- Assess patient for signs and symptoms of hypokalemia (weakness, fatigue, arrhythmias, presence of U waves on ECG, polyuria, polydipsia) and hypophosphatemia (anorexia, weakness, decreased reflexes, bone pain, confusion, blood dyscrasias) throughout therapy.
- Monitor intake and output ratios and daily weight. Report significant discrepancies.
- ● *Lab Test Considerations:* Monitor serum phosphate, potassium, sodium, and calcium levels prior to and periodically throughout therapy. Increased phosphate may cause hypocalcemia.
- Monitor renal function studies prior to and periodically throughout therapy.
- Monitor urinary pH in patients receiving potassium and sodium phosphate as a urinary acidifier.

Potential Nursing Diagnoses
Imbalanced nutrition: less than body requirements (Indications)

Implementation
- **PO:** Tablets should be dissolved in a full glass of water. Allow mixture to stand for 2–5 min to ensure it is fully dissolved. Solutions prepared by pharmacy should not be further diluted.
- Medication should be administered after meals to minimize gastric irritation and laxative effect.
- Do not administer simultaneously with antacids containing aluminum, magnesium, or calcium.

Patient/Family Teaching
- Explain to the patient the purpose of the medication and the need to take as directed. Take missed doses as soon as remembered unless within 1 or 2 hr of the next dose. Explain that the tablets should not be swallowed whole. Tablets should be dissolved in water.
- Instruct patients in low-sodium diet (see Appendix M).
- Advise patient of the importance of maintaining a high fluid intake (drinking at least one 8-oz glass of water each hr) to prevent kidney stones.
- Instruct the patient to promptly report diarrhea, weakness, fatigue, muscle cramps, unexplained weight gain, swelling of lower extremities, shortness of breath, unusual thirst, or tremors.

Evaluation/Desired Outcomes
- Prevention and correction of serum phosphate and potassium deficiencies.

POTASSIUM SUPPLEMENTS 1041

- Maintenance of acid urine.
- Decreased urine calcium, which prevents formation of renal calculi.

potassium iodide, See IODINE, IODIDE.

HIGH ALERT

POTASSIUM SUPPLEMENTS
(poe-**tass**-ee-um)

potassium acetate

potassium bicarbonate
K+Care ET, K-Electrolyte, K-Ide, Klor-Con/EF, K-Lyte, K-Vescent

potassium bicarbonate/potassium chloride
K-Lyte/Cl, ✤Neo-K, ✤Potassium Sandoz

potassium bicarbonate/potassium citrate
Effer-K, K-Lyte DS

potassium chloride
✤Apo-K, Cena-K, Gen-K, K+ Care, K+ 10, ✤Kalium Durules, Kaochlor, Kaochlor S-F, Kaon-Cl, Kay Ciel, KCl, K-Dur, K-Lease, ✤K-Long, K-Lor, Klor-Con, Klorvess Liquid, Klotrix, K-Lyte/Cl Powder, K-Med, K-Norm, K-Sol, K-Tab, Micro-K, Micro-K ExtenCaps, Micro-LS, Potasalan, Roychlor, Rum-K, Slow-K, Ten-K

potassium chloride/potassium bicarbonate/potassium citrate
Kaochlor Eff

potassium gluconate
Kaon, Kaylixir, K-G Elixir, ✤Potassium-Rougier

potassium gluconate/potassium chloride
Kolyum

potassium gluconate/potassium citrate
Twin-K

trikates (potassium acetate/potassium bicarbonate/potassium citrate)
Tri-K

Classification
Therapeutic: mineral and electrolyte replacements/supplements

Pregnancy Category C

Indications
PO, IV: Treatment/prevention of potassium depletion. **IV:** Arrhythmias due to digoxin toxicity.

Action
Maintain acid-base balance, isotonicity, and electrophysiologic balance of the cell. Activator in many enzymatic reactions; essential to transmission of nerve impulses; contraction of cardiac, skeletal, and smooth muscle; gastric secretion; renal function; tissue synthesis; and carbohydrate metabolism. **Therapeutic Effects:** Replacement. Prevention of deficiency.

Pharmacokinetics
Absorption: Well absorbed following oral administration.
Distribution: Enters extracellular fluid; then actively transported into cells.
Metabolism and Excretion: Excreted by the kidneys.
Half-life: Unknown.

TIME/ACTION PROFILE (increase in serum potassium levels)

ROUTE	ONSET	PEAK	DURATION
PO	unknown	1–2 hr	unknown
IV	rapid	end of infusion	unknown

Contraindications/Precautions
Contraindicated in: Hyperkalemia; Severe renal impairment; Untreated Addison's disease; Severe tissue trauma; Hyperkalemic familial periodic paralysis; Some products may contain tartrazine (FDC yellow dye #5) or alcohol; avoid using in patients with known hypersensitivity or intolerance; Potassium acetate injection contains aluminum, which may become toxic with prolonged use to high risk groups (renal impairment, premature neonates).
Use Cautiously in: Cardiac disease; Renal impairment; Diabetes mellitus (liquids may contain sugar); Hypomagnesemia (may make correction

P

✤ = Canadian drug name. ▌ = Genetic implication.
*CAPITALS indicates life-threatening; underlines indicate most frequent.

of hypokalemia more difficult); GI hypomotility including dysphagia or esophageal compression from left atrial enlargement (tablets, capsules); Patients receiving potassium-sparing drugs.

Adverse Reactions/Side Effects
CNS: confusion, restlessness, weakness. **CV:** ARRHYTHMIAS, ECG changes. **GI:** abdominal pain, diarrhea, flatulence, nausea, vomiting; *tablets, capsules only*, GI ulceration, stenotic lesions. **Local:** irritation at IV site. **Neuro:** paralysis, paresthesia.

Interactions
Drug-Drug: Use with **potassium-sparing diuretics** or **ACE inhibitors** or **angiotensin II receptor antagonists** may lead to hyperkalemia. **Anticholinergics** may ↑ GI mucosal lesions in patients taking wax-matrix potassium chloride preparations.

Route/Dosage
Expressed as mEq of potassium. Potassium acetate contains 10.2 mEq/g; potassium bicarbonate contains 10 mEq potassium/g; potassium chloride contains 13.4 mEq potassium/g; potassium gluconate contains 4.3 mEq/g.

Normal Daily Requirements
PO, IV (Adults): 40–80 mEq/day.
PO, IV (Children): 2–3 mEq/kg/day.
PO, IV (Neonates): 2–6 mEq/kg/day.

Prevention of Hypokalemia during Diuretic Therapy
PO (Adults): 20–40 mEq/day in 1–2 divided doses; single dose should not exceed 20 mEq.
PO (Neonates, Infants, and Children): 1–2 mEq/kg/day in 1–2 divided doses.

Treatment of Hypokalemia
PO (Adults): 40–100 mEq/day in divided doses.
PO (Neonates, Infants, and Children): 2–5 mEq/kg/day in divided doses.
IV (Adults): *Serum potassium >2.5 mEq/L—* Up to 20 mEq/day as an infusion (not to exceed 10 mEq/hr) or a concentration of 40 mEq/L via peripheral line (up to 100 mEq/L have been used via central line [unlabeled]). *Serum potassium <2 mEq/L with symptoms—* Up to 40 mEq/day as an infusion (rate should generally not exceed 20 mEq/hr).
IV (Neonates, Infants, and Children): 0.5–1 mEq/kg/dose (maximum 30 mEq/dose) as an infusion to infuse at 0.3–0.5 mEq/kg/hr (maximum infusion rate 1 mEq/kg/hr).

Availability

Potassium Acetate (generic available)
Concentrate for injection (contains aluminum): 2 mEq/mL in 20-, 50-, and 100-mL vials, 4 mEq/mL in 50-mL vials.

Potassium Bicarbonate
Tablets for effervescent oral solution: 25 mEq.

Potassium Bicarbonate/Potassium Chloride
Packets for effervescent oral solution: 20 mEq/2.8-g packet. **Tablets for effervescent oral solution:** ✦ 12 mEq, 20 mEq, 25 mEq, 50 mEq.

Potassium Bicarbonate/Potassium Citrate
Tablets for effervescent oral solution: 25 mEq, 50 mEq. **Cost:** 25 mEq $122.98/90, 50 mEq $213.97/90.

Potassium Chloride (generic available)
Extended-release tablets: 8 mEq, 10 mEq, 20 mEq. **Cost:** *Generic—* 10 mEq $22.49/90, 20 mEq $32.97/90. **Extended-release capsules:** 8 mEq, 10 mEq. **Cost:** *Generic—* 10 mEq $24.74/90. **Oral solution:** 20 mEq/15 mL, 40 mEq/15 mL. **Cost:** *Generic—* 20 mEq/15 mL $8.99/473 mL, 40 mEq/15 mL $19.97/480 mL. **Powder/packets for oral solution:** 20-mEq/1.5-g packet, 25-mEq/1.8-g packet. **Packets for oral suspension:** 20-mEq/1.5-g packet. **Concentrate for injection:** 0.1 mEq/mL in 10-mEq ampules and vials, 0.2 mEq/mL in 10- and 20-mEq ampules and vials, 0.3 mEq/mL in 30-mEq ampules and vials, 0.4 mEq/mL in 20- and 40-mEq ampules and vials, 1.5 mEq/mL, 2 mEq/mL, 3 mEq/mL. **Solution for IV infusion:** 10 mEq/L in various dextrose and saline solutions in 250-, 500-, and 100-mL containers, 20 mEq/L in dextrose/saline/LRs in 250-, 500-, and 100-mL containers, 30 mEq/L in various dextrose and saline solutions in 250-, 500-, and 100-mL containers, 40 mEq/L in various dextrose and saline solutions in 250-, 500-, and 100-mL containers.

Potassium Chloride/Potassium Bicarbonate/Potassium Citrate
Tablets for effervescent oral solution: 20 mEq.

Potassium Gluconate (generic available)
Tablets: 2 mEq, 5 mEq. **Elixir:** 20 mEq/15 mL.

Potassium Gluconate/Potassium Chloride
Oral solution: 20 mEq/15 mL. **Powder for oral solution:** 20 mEq/5-g packet.

POTASSIUM SUPPLEMENTS 1043

Potassium Gluconate/Potassium Citrate
Oral solution: 20 mEq/15 mL.

Trikates (Potassium Acetate/Potassium Bicarbonate/Potassium Citrate)
Oral solution: 15 mEq/5 mL.

NURSING IMPLICATIONS
Assessment
- Assess for signs and symptoms of hypokalemia (weakness, fatigue, U wave on ECG, arrhythmias, polyuria, polydipsia) and hyperkalemia (see Toxicity and Overdose).
- Monitor pulse, blood pressure, and ECG periodically during IV therapy.
- **Lab Test Considerations:** Monitor serum potassium before and periodically during therapy. Monitor renal function, serum bicarbonate, and pH. Determine serum magnesium level if patient has refractory hypokalemia; hypomagnesemia should be corrected to facilitate effectiveness of potassium replacement. Monitor serum chloride because hypochloremia may occur if replacing potassium without concurrent chloride.
- ***Toxicity and Overdose:*** Symptoms of toxicity are those of hyperkalemia (slow, irregular heartbeat; fatigue; muscle weakness; paresthesia; confusion; dyspnea; peaked T waves; depressed ST segments; prolonged QT segments; widened QRS complexes; loss of P waves; and cardiac arrhythmias).
- Treatment includes discontinuation of potassium, administration of sodium bicarbonate to correct acidosis, dextrose and insulin to facilitate passage of potassium into cells, calcium salts to reverse ECG effects (in patients who are not receiving digoxin), sodium polystyrene used as an exchange resin, and/or dialysis for patient with impaired renal function.

Potential Nursing Diagnoses
Imbalanced nutrition: less than body requirements (Indications)

Implementation
- ***High Alert:*** Medication errors involving too rapid infusion or bolus IV administration of potassium chloride have resulted in fatalities. See IV administration guidelines below.
- Do not confuse K-Dur with Imdur (isosorbide mononitrate). Do not confuse Micro-K with micronase (glyburide).
- For most purposes, potassium chloride should be used, except for renal tubular acidoses (hyperchloremic acidosis), in which other salts are more appropriate (potassium bicarbonate, potassium citrate, or potassium gluconate).
- If hypokalemia is secondary to diuretic therapy, consideration should be given to decreasing the dose of diuretic, unless there is a history of significant arrhythmias or concurrent digitalis glycoside therapy.
- **PO:** Administer with or after meals to decrease GI irritation.
- Use of tablets and capsules should be reserved for patients who cannot tolerate liquid preparations.
- Dissolve effervescent tablets in 3–8 oz of cold water. Ensure that effervescent tablet is fully dissolved. Powders and solutions should be diluted in 3–8 oz of cold water or juice (do not use tomato juice if patient is on sodium restriction). Instruct patient to drink slowly over 5–10 min.
- Tablets and capsules should be taken with a meal and full glass of water. Do not chew or crush enteric-coated or extended-release tablets or capsules. Micro-K ExtenCaps capsules can be opened and sprinkled on soft food (pudding, applesauce) and swallowed immediately with a glass of cool water or juice.
- **IV:** Assess for extravasation; severe pain and tissue necrosis may occur. ***High Alert:*** Never administer potassium IV push or bolus.

Potassium Acetate
- **Continuous Infusion:** ***High Alert:*** Do not administer undiluted. Each single dose *must* be diluted and thoroughly mixed in 100–1000 mL of dextrose, saline, Ringer's or LR, dextrose/saline, dextrose/Ringer's, or LR combinations. Usually limited to 80 mEq/L via peripheral line (200 mEq/L via central line).
- ***Rate: High Alert:*** Infuse slowly, at a rate up to 10 mEq/hr in adults or 0.5 mEq/kg/hr in children on general care areas. Check hospital policy for maximum infusion rates (maximum rate in monitored setting 40 mEq/hr in adults or 1 mEq/kg/hr in children).
- **Y-Site Compatibility:** ciprofloxacin.

Potassium Chloride
- **Continuous Infusion:** ***High Alert:*** Do not administer concentrations of ≥1.5 mEq/mL undiluted; fatalities have occurred. Concentrated products have black caps on vials or black stripes above constriction on ampules and are labeled with a warning about dilution

requirement. Each single dose must be diluted and thoroughly mixed in 100–1000 mL of IV solution. Usually limited to 80 mEq/L via peripheral line (200 mEq/L via central line).

- Concentrations of 0.1 and 0.4 mEq/mL are intended for administration via calibrated infusion device and do not require dilution.
- ***Rate: High Alert:*** Infuse slowly, at a rate up to 10 mEq/hr in adults or 0.5 mEq/kg/hr in children in general care areas. Check hospital policy for maximum infusion rates (maximum rate in monitored setting 40 mEq/hr in adults or 1 mEq/kg/hr in children). Use an infusion pump.
- **Solution Compatibility:** May be diluted in dextrose, saline, Ringer's solution, LR, dextrose/saline, dextrose/Ringer's solution, and dextrose/LR combinations. Commercially available premixed with many of the above IV solutions.
- **Y-Site Compatibility:** acyclovir, allopurinol, amifostine, aminophylline, amiodarone, ampicillin, atropine, aztreonam, betamethasone, bivalirudin, calcium gluconate, chlordiazepoxide, chlorpromazine, ciprofloxacin, cisatracurium, cladribine, cyanocobalamin, dexamethasone sodium phosphate, dexmedetomidine, digoxin, diltiazem, diphenhydramine, dobutamine, docetaxel, dopamine, doxorubicin liposome, droperidol, drotrecogin, edrophonium, enalaprilat, epinephrine, ertapenem, esmolol, conjugated estrogens, ethacrynate sodium, etoposide phosphate, famotidine, fenoldopam, fentanyl, filgrastim, fludarabine, fluorouracil, furosemide, gemcitabine, granisetron, heparin, hydralazine, idarubicin, inamrinone, indomethacin, insulin, isoproterenol, kanamycin, labetalol, lidocaine, linezolid, lorazepam, magnesium sulfate, melphalan, menadiol, meperidine, meropenem, methoxamine, methylergonovine, midazolam, milrinone, morphine, neostigmine, nicardipine, nitroprusside, norepinephrine, ondansetron, oxacillin, oxaliplatin, oxytocin, paclitaxel, pantoprazole, pemetrexed, penicillin G potassium, pentazocine, phytonadione, piperacillin/tazobactam, procainamide, prochlorperazine, propofol, propranolol, pyridostigmine, quinupristin/dalfopristin, remifentanil, sargramostim, scopolamine, sodium bicarbonate, succinylcholine, tacrolimus, teniposide, theophylline, thiotepa, tirofiban, vinorelbine, warfarin, zidovudine.
- **Y-Site Incompatibility:** amphotericin B cholesteryl sulfate complex, azithromycin, diazepam, ergotamine tartrate, lansoprazole, phenytoin.
- **Additive Compatibility:** calcium gluconate, cimetidine, dobutamine, dopamine, furosemide, heparin, hydrocortisone, hydromorphone, lidocaine, ranitidine, sodium bicarbonate, vitamin B complex with C.

Patient/Family Teaching

- Explain to patient purpose of the medication and the need to take as directed, especially when concurrent digoxin or diuretics are taken. Take missed doses as soon as remembered within 2 hr; if not, return to regular dose schedule. Do not double dose.
- Emphasize correct method of administration. GI irritation or ulceration may result from chewing enteric-coated tablets or insufficient dilution of liquid or powder forms.
- Some extended-release tablets are contained in a wax matrix that may be expelled in the stool. This occurrence is not significant.
- Instruct patient to avoid salt substitutes or low-salt milk or food unless approved by health care professional. Patient should be advised to read all labels to prevent excess potassium intake.
- Advise patient regarding sources of dietary potassium (see Appendix M). Encourage compliance with recommended diet.
- Instruct patient to report dark, tarry, or bloody stools; weakness; unusual fatigue; or tingling of extremities. Notify health care professional if nausea, vomiting, diarrhea, or stomach discomfort persists. Dosage may require adjustment.
- Emphasize the importance of regular follow-up exams to monitor serum levels and progress.

Evaluation/Desired Outcomes

- Prevention and correction of serum potassium depletion.
- Cessation of arrhythmias caused by digoxin toxicity.

---

pramipexole (pra-mi-**pex**-ole)
Mirapex

Classification
Therapeutic: antiparkinson agents
Pharmacologic: dopamine agonists

Pregnancy Category C

Indications

Management of Parkinson's disease. Restless leg syndrome.

Action
Stimulates dopamine receptors in the striatum of the brain. **Therapeutic Effects:** Decreased tremor and rigidity in Parkinson's disease. Decreased leg restlessness.

Pharmacokinetics
Absorption: >90% absorbed following oral administration.
Distribution: Widely distributed.
Metabolism and Excretion: 90% excreted unchanged in urine.
Half-life: 8 hr (↑ in geriatric patients and patients with renal impairment).

TIME/ACTION PROFILE (blood levels)

ROUTE	ONSET	PEAK	DURATION
PO	unknown	2 hr	8 hr

Contraindications/Precautions
Contraindicated in: Hypersensitivity.
Use Cautiously in: Renal impairment (↑ dosing interval recommended if CCr <60 mL/min); OB, Lactation: Pedi: Safety not established; Geri: ↑ risk of hallucinations.

Adverse Reactions/Side Effects
CNS: SLEEP ATTACKS, amnesia, dizziness, drowsiness, hallucinations, weakness, abnormal dreams, confusion, dyskinesia, extrapyramidal syndrome, headache, insomnia, urges (gambling, sexual). **CV:** postural hypotension. **Derm:** melanoma. **GI:** constipation, dry mouth, dyspepsia, nausea, tooth disease. **GU:** urinary frequency. **MS:** leg cramps. **Neuro:** hypertonia, unsteadiness/falling.

Interactions
Drug-Drug: Concurrent **levodopa** ↑ risk of hallucinations and dyskinesia. Effectiveness may be ↑ by **cimetidine**. Effectiveness may be ↓ by **dopamine antagonists**, including **butyrophenones**, **metoclopramide**, **phenothiazines**, or **thioxanthenes**.

Route/Dosage
PO (Adults): *Parkinson's disease*—0.125 mg 3 times daily initially; may be ↑ q 5–7 days (range 1.5–4.5 mg/day in 3 divided doses). *Restless Lag Syndrome*—0.125 mg daily 1–3 hr before bedtime. May be ↑ at 4–7 day intervals to 0.25 mg daily, then up to 0.5 mg daily.

Renal Impairment
PO (Adults): *Parkinson's disease*—*CCr 35–59 mL/min*—0.125 mg twice daily initially, may be ↑ q 5–7 days up to 1.5 mg twice daily; *CCr 15–34 mL/min*—0.125 mg daily initially, may be ↑ q 5–7 days up to 1.5 mg daily. *Restless Leg Syndrome*—0.125 mg daily 1–3 hr before bedtime. May be ↑ at 14-day intervals to 0.25 mg daily, then up to 0.5 mg daily.

Availability (generic available)
Tablets: 0.125 mg, 0.25 mg, 0.5 mg, 0.75 mg, 1 mg, 1.5 mg. **Cost:** 0.125 mg $517.05/270, 0.25 mg $491.97/270, 0.5 mg $605.96/270, 1 mg $574.97/270, 1.5 mg $605.96/270.

NURSING IMPLICATIONS

Assessment
- Assess patient for confusion or hallucinations. Notify health care professional if these occur.
- Monitor ECG and blood pressure frequently during dosage adjustment and periodically throughout therapy.
- Assess patient for drowsiness and sleep attacks. Drowsiness is a common side effect of pramipexole, but sleep attacks or episodes of falling asleep during activities that require active participation may occur without warning. Assess patient for concomitant medications that have sedating effects or may increase serum pramipexole levels (see Interactions). May require discontinuation of therapy.
- **Parkinson's Disease:** Assess patient for signs and symptoms of Parkinson's disease (tremor, muscle weakness and rigidity, ataxia) before and throughout therapy.
- **Restless Leg Syndrome:** Assess sleep patterns and frequency of restless leg disturbances.

Potential Nursing Diagnoses
Impaired physical mobility (Indications)
Risk for injury (Indications, Side Effects)

Implementation
- An attempt to reduce the dose of levodopa/carbidopa may be made cautiously during pramipexole therapy.
- **PO:** Administer with meals to minimize nausea; usually resolves with continued therapy.

Patient/Family Teaching
- Instruct patient to take medication as directed. Take missed doses as soon as remembered if it is not almost time for next dose. Do not double doses. Consult health care professional before reducing dose or discontinuing medication. Advise patient to read the *Patient Information*

sheet before taking and with each Rx refill, changes may occur.
- May cause drowsiness and unexpected episodes of falling asleep. Caution patient to avoid driving or other activities requiring alertness until response to medication is known. Advise patient to notify health care professional if episodes of falling asleep occur.
- Advise patient to change position slowly to minimize orthostatic hypotension. May occur more frequently during initial therapy.
- Instruct patient to consult health care professional before taking any other Rx, OTC, or herbal products with pramipexole.
- Advise patient to have periodic skin exams to check for lesions that may be melanoma.
- Advise patient to notify health care professional if new or increased gambling, sexual, or other intense urges occur.
- Advise female patient to notify health care professional if pregnancy is planned or suspected or if breastfeeding or planning to breastfeed.

Evaluation/Desired Outcomes
- Decreased tremor and rigidity in Parkinson's disease.
- Decrease in restless legs and improved sleep.

HIGH ALERT

pramlintide (pram-lin-tide)
Symlin

Classification
Therapeutic: antidiabetics
Pharmacologic: hormones

Pregnancy Category C

Indications
Used with mealtime insulin in the management of diabetics whose blood sugar cannot be controlled by optimal insulin therapy; can be used with other agents (sulfonylureas, metformin).

Action
Acts as a synthetic analogue of amylin, an endogenous pancreatic hormone that helps to control postprandial hyperglycemia; effects include slowed gastric emptying, suppression of glucagon secretion and regulation of food intake. **Therapeutic Effects:** Improved control of postprandial hyperglycemia.

Pharmacokinetics
Absorption: 30–40% absorbed following subcutaneous administration.
Distribution: Does not appear to significantly cross the placenta.
Metabolism and Excretion: Metabolized by the kidneys; major metabolite has pharmacologic properties similar to the parent compound.
Half-life: 48 min.

TIME/ACTION PROFILE (effect on blood sugar*)

ROUTE	ONSET	PEAK	DURATION
Subcut	rapid	20 min	3 hr

*Blood level

Contraindications/Precautions
Contraindicated in: Hypersensitivty; Inability to identify hypoglycemia; Gastroparesis or need for medications to stimulate gastric motility; Poor compliance with current insulin regimen or self-monitoring; HbA1c >9%; Recurring severe hypoglycemia within the last 6 mo, requiring treatment; OB: Insulin is the drug of choice for blood glucose control during pregnancy; Pedi: Safety not established.
Use Cautiously in: Lactation: Lactation.

Adverse Reactions/Side Effects
Noted for concurrent use with insulin.
CNS: dizziness, fatigue, headache. **Resp:** cough. **GI:** nausea, abdominal pain, anorexia, vomiting. **Endo:** HYPOGLYCEMIA. **Derm:** local allergy. **MS:** arthralgia. **Misc:** injection site reactions, systemic allergic reactions.

Interactions
Drug-Drug: ↑ likelihood of hypoglycemia with short-acting **insulin**; ↓ dose of short-acting premeal insulin by 50%. Avoid concurrent use with other agents that ↓ GI motility, including **atropine** and other **anticholinergics**. Avoid concurrent use with other agents that ↓ GI absorption of nutrients, including α-glucosidase inhibitors including **acarbose** and **miglitol**. May delay oral absorption of concurrently administered drugs; if prompt absorption is desired, administer 1 hr before or 2 hr after pramlintide.

Route/Dosage

Insulin-using Type 2 Diabetes
Subcut (Adults): 60 mcg, immediately prior to major meals initially, if no significant nausea occurs, dose may be ↑ to 120 mcg.

Type 1 Diabetes
Subcut (Adults): 15 mcg, immediately prior to major meals initially, if no significant nausea occurs, dose may be ↑ by 15 mcg every 3 days up to 60 mcg.

Availability
Pen-injector: 1000 mcg/mL. **Solution for injection:** 600 mcg/mL.

NURSING IMPLICATIONS
Assessment
- Assess hemoglobin A1c, recent blood glucose monitoring data, history of insulin-induced hypoglycemia, current insulin regimen, and body weight prior to initiation of therapy.
- Assess for signs and symptoms of hypoglycemia (hunger, headache, sweating, tremor, irritability, difficulty concentrating, loss of consciousness, coma, seizure), occurs within 3 hr of injection. Pramlintide alone does not cause hypoglycemia, may increase risk when administered with insulin.
- *Lab Test Considerations:* Monitor blood glucose frequently, including pre- and post-meals and at bedtime.

Potential Nursing Diagnoses
Noncompliance (Patient/Family Teaching)

Implementation
- *High Alert:* Dose errors are a potential problem with administration of pramlintide. Pramlintide is available in a concentration of 0.6 mg/mL, dosing is in mcg, and insulin syringe for administration is in units. Carefully review dosing and conversion table prior to administration.
- Administer pramlintide and insulin as separate injections; do not mix.
- Adjust insulin doses to optimize glycemic control once target dose of pramlintide is achieved and nausea has subsided.
- **Subcut:** Administer immediately prior to major meals ≥250 kcal or containing ≥30 g of carbohydrate. Reduce preprandial rapid-acting, short-acting, and fixed-mix insulin doses by 50%. Use a U-100 syringe (preferably a 0.3 mL size) for optimal accuracy. Administer into abdomen or thigh, rotating injection sites. Do not administer solutions that are cloudy. Store unopened vials in refrigerator. Opened vials may be refrigerated or kept at room temperature for up to 28 days.

Patient/Family Teaching
- Instruct patient in proper use of pramlintide (injection technique, timing of doses, storage, and disposal of equipment). Make sure patient understands dosing and preparation of correct dose. Emphasize importance of adherence to meal planning, physical activity, recognition and management of hypoglycemia and hyperglycemia, and assessment of diabetes complications. Advise patient to read the *Medication Guide* before use and with each refill for new information.
- Review with patient how to handle illness or stress, inadequate or omitted insulin dose, inadvertent administration of increased dose of insulin or pramlintide, inadequate food intake or missed meals. If a dose is missed, wait until the next meal and take usual dose; do not give an additional injection.
- Instruct patient to contact health care professional at least once a week until target dose of pramlintide is achieved, pramlintide is well-tolerated, and blood glucose concentrations are stable.
- May cause difficulty concentrating. Caution patient to avoid driving or other activities requiring alertness until response to medication is known.
- Inform patient that signs of local allergy (redness, swelling, itching at site of injection) usually resolve within a few days to a few weeks; may be related to pramlintide, irritants in skin cleansing agent or improper injection technique.
- Advise patient to contact health care professional if recurrent nausea or hypoglycemia occur; may lead to increased risk of severe hypoglycemia. Discontinue pramlintide therapy if recurrent unexplained hypoglycemia requiring medical assistance, persistent clinically significant nausea, or noncompliance with self-monitoring of blood glucose concentrations, insulin dose adjustments, or scheduled health care professional contacts or recommended clinic visits occur.
- Advise patient to contact health care professional before taking other Rx, OTC, vitamins, or herbal products with pramlintide and to avoid concurrent alcohol use.
- Advise female patients to notify health care professional if pregnancy is planned or suspected or if breastfeeding.

Evaluation/Desired Outcomes
- Reduction in postprandial glucose concentrations.

prasugrel (pra-soo-grel)
Effient

Classification
Therapeutic: antiplatelet agents
Pharmacologic: thienopyridines

Pregnancy Category B

Indications
Reduction of thrombotic cardiovascular events (including stent thrombosis) in patients with acute coronary syndrome who will be managed with PCI including patients with unstable angina or non-ST-elevation myocardial infarction (NSTEMI). Reduction of thrombotic cardiovascular events (including stent thrombosis) in patients with STEMI when managed with either primary/delayed PCI.

Action
Acts by irreversibly binding its active metabolite to the $P2Y_{12}$ class of ADP receptors on platelets; inhibiting platelet activation and aggregation. **Therapeutic Effects:** Decreased thrombotic events including cardiovascular death, nonfatal myocardial infarction (MI) and nonfatal stroke.

Pharmacokinetics
Absorption: Well absorbed following oral administration (79%), then rapidly converted to an active metabolite.
Distribution: Unknown.
Protein Binding: *Active metabolite*—98%.
Metabolism and Excretion: Active metabolite is metabolized to two inactive compounds; 68% excreted in the urine and 27% in feces as inactive metabolites.
Half-life: *Active metabolite*—7 hr (range 2–15 hr).

TIME/ACTION PROFILE (effect on platelet function)

ROUTE	ONSET	PEAK	DURATION
PO	within 1 hr	2 hr	5–9 days†

† Following discontinuation.

Contraindications/Precautions
Contraindicated in: Hypersensitivity; Active pathological bleeding; History of transient ischemic attack or stroke.
Use Cautiously in: Patients about to undergo coronary artery bypass grafting (CABG) (↑ risk of bleeding; discontinue at least 7 days prior to surgery); Premature discontinuation (↑ risk of stent thrombosis, MI, and death); Body weight <60 kg, propensity to bleed, severe hepatic impairment, concurrent use of medications that increase the risk of bleeding (↑ risk of bleeding); Hypotension in the setting of recent coronary angiography, PCI, CABG, or other surgical procedure (suspect bleeding but do not discontinue prasugrel); Geri: Use in patients ≥75 yr of age generally not recommended (↑ risk of fatal/intracranial bleeding and questionable benefit, except in high-risk patients such as diabetes or prior MI); OB: Use during pregnancy only if potential benefit to mother justifies potential risk to fetus; Lactation: Use during nursing only if potential benefit to the mother justifies potential risk to nursing infant; Pedi: Safe and effective use in children has not been established.

Adverse Reactions/Side Effects
CNS: dizziness, fatigue, headache. **Resp:** cough, dyspnea. **CV:** atrial fibrillation, bradycardia, hypertension, hypotension, peripheral edema. **GI:** diarrhea, nausea. **Derm:** rash. **Hemat:** BLEEDING, THROMBOTIC THROMBOCYTOPENIC PURPURA, leukopenia. **Metab:** hyperlipidemia/hypercholesterolemia. **MS:** back pain, extremity pain. **Misc:** fever, non-cardiac chest pain.

Interactions
Drug-Drug: ↑ risk of bleeding with **warfarin**, **NSAIDs**.

Route/Dosage
Aspirin 75–325 mg/daily should be taken concurrently.
PO (Adults ≥60 kg): 60 mg initially as a loading dose, then 10 mg once daily.
PO (Adults < 60 kg): Consider maintenance dose of 5 mg once daily.

Availability
Tablets: 5 mg, 10 mg.

NURSING IMPLICATIONS

Assessment
- Assess patient for symptoms of stroke, peripheral vascular disease, or MI periodically during therapy.
- Monitor patient for signs of thrombotic thrombocytic purpura (thrombocytopenia, microangiopathic hemolytic anemia, neurologic findings, renal dysfunction, fever). May rarely occur, even after short exposure (<2 wk). Requires prompt treatment.
- *Lab Test Considerations:* Monitor bleeding time during therapy. Prolonged bleeding time, which is time- and dose-dependent, is expected.

- Monitor CBC with differential and platelet count periodically during therapy. Thrombocytopenia and anemia may rarely occur.

Potential Nursing Diagnoses
Risk for injury (Indications, Side Effects)

Implementation
- Discontinue prasugrel 7 days before planned surgical procedures.
- Patients should take aspirin 75–325 mg daily with prasugrel.
- **PO:** Administer once daily without regard to food.

Patient/Family Teaching
- Instruct patient to take medication as directed. Take missed doses as soon as possible unless almost time for next dose; do not double doses. Do not discontinue without consulting health care professional. Advise patient to read *Medication Guide* before taking and with each Rx refill; new information may be available.
- Advise patient to notify health care professional promptly if fever, weakness, skin paleness, purple skin patches, yellowing of skin or eyes, chills, sore throat, neurological changes, or unusual bleeding or bruising occurs.
- Advise patient to notify health care professional of medication regimen prior to treatment or surgery.
- Instruct patient to avoid taking other Rx, OTC, or herbal products, especially those containing NSAIDs without consulting health care professional.

Evaluation/Desired Outcomes
- Prevention of stroke, MI, and vascular death in patients at risk.

---

pravastatin, See HMG-CoA REDUCTASE INHIBITORS (statins).

---

prazosin (pra-zoe-sin)
Minipress

Classification
Therapeutic: antihypertensives
Pharmacologic: peripherally acting antiadrenergics

Pregnancy Category C

Indications
Mild to moderate hypertension. **Unlabeled Use:** Management of urinary outflow obstruction in patients with benign prostatic hyperplasia.

Action
Dilates both arteries and veins by blocking postsynaptic alpha$_1$-adrenergic receptors. Decreases contractions in smooth muscle of prostatic capsule. **Therapeutic Effects:** Lowering of blood pressure. Decreased cardiac preload and afterload. Decreased symptoms of prostatic hyperplasia (urinary urgency, urinary hesitancy, nocturia).

Pharmacokinetics
Absorption: 60% absorbed following oral administration.
Distribution: Widely distributed.
Protein Binding: 97%.
Metabolism and Excretion: Extensively metabolized by the liver. Minimal (5–10%) renal excretion of unchanged drug.
Half-life: 2–3 hr.

TIME/ACTION PROFILE (antihypertensive effects)

ROUTE	ONSET	PEAK	DURATION
PO	2 hr	2–4 hr†	10 hr

†Following single dose; maximal antihypertensive effects occur after 3–4 wk of chronic dosing

Contraindications/Precautions
Contraindicated in: Hypersensitivity.
Use Cautiously in: Renal insufficiency (↑ sensitivity to effects; dose reduction may be required); OB, Lactation: Pedi: Safety not established; Angina pectoris; When adding diuretics (↓ dose of prazosin); Patients undergoing cataract surgery (↑ risk of intraoperative floppy iris syndrome).

Adverse Reactions/Side Effects
CNS: dizziness, headache, weakness, drowsiness, mental depression, syncope. **EENT:** blurred vision, intraoperative floppy iris syndrome. **CV:** first-dose orthostatic hypotension, palpitations, angina, edema. **GI:** abdominal cramps, diarrhea, dry mouth, nausea, vomiting. **GU:** erectile dysfunction, priapism.

Interactions
Drug-Drug: Additive hypotension with acute ingestion of **alcohol**, other **antihypertensives**, or **nitrates**. Antihypertensive effects may be ↓ by **NSAIDs**.

Route/Dosage
Hypertension
PO (Adults): 1 mg 2–3 times daily (give first dose at bedtime) for initial 3 days of therapy, then ↑ gradually to maintenance dose of 6–15 mg/day in 2–3 divided doses (not to exceed 20–40 mg/day).
PO (Children): 50–400 mcg (0.05–0.4 mg)/kg/day in 2–3 divided doses (not to exceed 7 mg/dose or 15 mg/day).

Benign Prostatic Hyperplasia
PO (Adults): 1–5 mg twice daily.

Availability (generic available)
Capsules: 1 mg, 2 mg, 5 mg. **Cost:** *Generic*—1 mg $35.96/180, 2 mg $43.00/180, 5 mg $93.98/180. **Tablets:** ✱ 1 mg, ✱ 2 mg, ✱ 5 mg.

NURSING IMPLICATIONS
Assessment
- Assess for first-dose orthostatic reaction (dizziness, weakness) and syncope. May occur 30 min–2 hr after initial dose and occasionally thereafter. Incidence may be dose related. Volume-depleted or sodium-restricted patients may be more sensitive. Observe patient closely during this period; take precautions to prevent injury. First dose may be given at bedtime to minimize this reaction.
- Monitor intake and output ratios and daily weight; assess for edema daily, especially at beginning of therapy.
- **Hypertension:** Monitor blood pressure and pulse frequently during initial dosage adjustment and periodically throughout therapy. Report significant changes.
- Monitor frequency of prescription refills to determine adherence.
- **Benign Prostatic Hyperplasia:** Assess patient for symptoms of prostatic hyperplasia (urinary hesitancy, feeling of incomplete bladder emptying, interruption of urinary stream, impairment of size and force of urinary stream, terminal urinary dribbling, straining to start flow, dysuria, urgency) before and periodically during therapy.
- Rule out prostatic carcinoma before therapy; symptoms are similar.

Potential Nursing Diagnoses
Risk for injury (Side Effects)
Noncompliance (Patient/Family Teaching)

Implementation
- May be used in combination with diuretics or beta blockers to minimize sodium and water retention. If these are added to prazosin therapy, reduce dose of prazosin initially and titrate to effect.
- **PO:** Administer daily dose at bedtime. If necessary, dose may be increased to twice daily.

Patient/Family Teaching
- Instruct patient to take medication at the same time each day. Take missed doses as soon as remembered. If not remembered until next day, omit; do not double doses.
- Advise patient to weigh self twice weekly and assess feet and ankles for fluid retention.
- May cause dizziness or drowsiness. Advise patient to avoid driving or other activities requiring alertness until response to the medication is known.
- Caution patient to avoid sudden changes in position to decrease orthostatic hypotension. Alcohol, CNS depressants, standing for long periods, hot showers, and exercising in hot weather should be avoided because of enhanced orthostatic effects.
- Advise patient to consult health care professional before taking any cough, cold, or allergy remedies.
- Instruct patient to notify health care professional of medication regimen before any surgery.
- Advise patient to notify health care professional if frequent dizziness, fainting, or swelling of feet or lower legs occurs.
- Emphasize the importance of follow-up exams to evaluate effectiveness of medication.
- **Hypertension:** Emphasize the importance of continuing to take this medication as directed, even if feeling well. Medication controls but does not cure hypertension.
- Encourage patient to comply with additional interventions for hypertension (weight reduction, low-sodium diet, smoking cessation, moderation of alcohol consumption, regular exercise, and stress management).
- Instruct patient and family on proper technique for blood pressure monitoring. Advise them to check blood pressure at least weekly and to report significant changes.

Evaluation/Desired Outcomes
- Decrease in blood pressure without appearance of side effects.
- Decrease in symptoms of prostatic hyperplasia.

prednicarbate, See CORTICOSTEROIDS (TOPICAL/LOCAL).

predniSOLONE, See **CORTICOSTEROIDS (SYSTEMIC).**

predniSONE, See **CORTICOSTEROIDS (SYSTEMIC).**

pregabalin (pre-**gab**-a-lin)
Lyrica

Classification
Therapeutic: analgesics, anticonvulsants
Pharmacologic: gamma aminobutyric acid (GABA) analogues, nonopioid analgesics

Schedule V

Pregnancy Category C

Indications
Pain due to: diabetic peripheral neuropathy, postherpetic neuralgia, fibromyalgia. Adjunctive therapy of partial-onset seizures in adults.

Action
Binds to calcium channels in CNS tissues which regulate neurotransmitter release. Does not bind to opioid receptors. **Therapeutic Effects:** Decreased neuropathic or post-herpetic pain. Decreased partial-onset seizures.

Pharmacokinetics
Absorption: Well absorbed (90%) following oral administration.
Distribution: Probably crosses the blood-brain barrier.
Metabolism and Excretion: Minimally metabolized, 90% excreted unchanged in urine.
Half-life: 6 hr.

TIME/ACTION PROFILE (↓ post–herpetic pain)

ROUTE	ONSET	PEAK	DURATION
PO	unknown	2–4 wk	unknown

Contraindications/Precautions
Contraindicated in: Myopathy (known/suspected); Lactation: Lactation.
Use Cautiously in: All patients (may ↑ risk of suicidal thoughts/behaviors); Renal impairment (dose alteration recommended for CCr <60 mL/min); CHF; History of drug dependence/drug-seeking behavior; OB: Use only if maternal benefit outweighs fetal risk; may ↑ risk of male-mediated teratogenicity; Pedi: Safety not established; Geri: Consider age-related ↓ in renal function when determining dose.

Adverse Reactions/Side Effects
CNS: SUICIDAL THOUGHTS, dizziness, drowsiness, impaired attention/concentration/thinking. **CV:** edema. **EENT:** blurred vision. **GI:** dry mouth, abdominal pain, constipation, ↑ appetite, vomiting. **Hemat:** ↓ platelet count. **Metab:** weight gain. **Misc:** allergic reactions, fever.

Interactions
Drug-Drug: Concurrent use with **thiazolidinediones (pioglitazone, rosiglitazone)** may ↑ risk of fluid retention. ↑ risk of CNS depression with other **CNS depressants** including **opioids, alcohol, benzodiazepines,** or other **sedatives/hypnotics**.

Route/Dosage
PO (Adults): *Diabetic neuropathic pain*—50 mg three times daily, ↑ over 7 days up to 100 mg 3 times daily; *Partial onset seizures*—150 mg/day initially in 2–3 divided doses, may be gradually ↑ to 600 mg/day; *Post-herpetic neuralgia*—75 mg twice daily or 50 mg 3 times daily initially, may be ↑ over 7 days to 300 mg/day in 2–3 divided doses, after 2–4 wk may be ↑ to 600 mg/day in 2–3 divided doses; *Fibromyalgia*—75 mg twice daily initially, may be ↑ to 150 mg twice daily within 1 wk based on efficacy and tolerability. May be ↑ to 225 twice daily.

Renal Impairment
PO (Adults): *CCr 30–60 mL/min*—75–300 mg/day in 2–3 divided doses; *CCr 15–30 mL/min*—25–150 mg/day in 1–2 divided doses; *CCr <15 mL/min*—25–75 mg/day as a single daily dose.

Availability
Capsules: 25 mg, 50 mg, 75 mg, 100 mg, 150 mg, 200 mg, 225 mg, 300 mg. **Cost:** 25 mg $335.95/180, 50 mg $335.95/180, 75 mg $335.95/180, 100 mg $335.95/180, 150 mg $335.95/180, 200 mg $343.94/180, 225 mg $337.01/180, 300 mg $351.92/180.

NURSING IMPLICATIONS

Assessment
- Monitor closely for notable changes in behavior that could indicate the emergence or worsening of suicidal thoughts or behavior or depression.

procainamide

- **Diabetic Peripheral Neuropathy, Postherpetic Neuralgia, and Fibromylagia:** Assess location, characteristics, and intensity of pain periodically during therapy.
- **Seizures:** Assess location, duration, and characteristics of seizure activity.
- *Lab Test Considerations:* May cause ↑ creatine kinase levels.
- May cause ↓ platelet count.

Potential Nursing Diagnoses
Risk for injury (Adverse Reactions)

Implementation
- Pregabalin should be discontinued gradually over at least 1 wk. Abrupt discontinuation may cause insomnia, nausea, headache, and diarrhea when used for pain and may cause increase in seizure frequency when treating seizures.
- **PO:** May be administered without regard to meals.

Patient/Family Teaching
- Instruct patient to take medication as directed. Do not discontinue abruptly; may cause insomnia, nausea, headache, or diarrhea or increase in frequency of seizures. Advise patient to read the *Patient Information Leaflet* prior to taking pregabalin.
- May cause dizziness, drowsiness, and blurred vision. Caution patient to avoid driving or activities requiring alertness until response to medication is known. Advise patient to notify health care professional if changes in vision occur. Seizure patients should not resume driving until physician gives clearance based on control of seizure disorder.
- Instruct patient to promptly report unexplained muscle pain, tenderness, or weakness, especially if accompanied by malaise or fever. Discontinue therapy if myopathy is diagnosed or suspected or if markedly elevated creatine kinase levels occur.
- Advise patient and family to notify health care professional if thoughts about suicide or dying, attempts to commit suicide; new or worse depression; new or worse anxiety; feeling very agitated or restless; panic attacks; trouble sleeping; new or worse irritability; acting aggressive; being angry or violent; acting on dangerous impulses; an extreme increase in activity and talking, other unusual changes in behavior or mood occur.
- Inform patient that pregabalin may cause edema and weight gain.
- Caution patient to avoid alcohol or other CNS depressants with pregabalin.
- Advise female patient to notify health care professional if pregnancy is planned or suspected or if breastfeeding. Inform male patients who plan to father a child of the potential risk of male-mediated teratogenicity.
- Instruct patient to notify health care professional of medication regimen before treatment or surgery.
- Advise patient to carry identification describing disease process and medication regimen at all times.

Evaluation/Desired Outcomes
- Decrease in intensity of chronic pain.
- Decrease in the frequency or cessation of seizures.

---

procainamide
(proe-**kane**-ah-mide)

Classification
Therapeutic: antiarrhythmics (class IA)

Pregnancy Category C

Indications
Treatment of a wide variety of ventricular and atrial arrhythmias, including: Atrial premature contractions, Premature ventricular contractions, Ventricular tachycardia, Paroxysmal atrial tachycardia. Maintenance of normal sinus rhythm after conversion from atrial fibrillation or flutter.

Action
Decreases myocardial excitability. Slows conduction velocity. May depress myocardial contractility. **Therapeutic Effects:** Suppression of arrhythmias.

Pharmacokinetics
Absorption: Well absorbed (75–90%) following IM administration.
Distribution: Rapidly and widely distributed.
Metabolism and Excretion: Converted by the liver to *N*-acetylprocainamide (NAPA), an active antiarrhythmic compound. Remainder (40–70%) excreted unchanged by the kidneys.
Half-life: 2.5–4.7 hr (NAPA—7 hr); prolonged in renal impairment.

TIME/ACTION PROFILE (antiarrhythmic effects)

ROUTE	ONSET	PEAK	DURATION
IV	immediate	25–60 min	3–4 hr
IM	10–30 min	15–60 min	3–4 hr

Contraindications/Precautions
Contraindicated in: Hypersensitivity; AV block; Myasthenia gravis; Hypersensitivity to tartrazine

procainamide **1053**

(FDC yellow dye #5; present in some oral products).
Use Cautiously in: MI or cardiac glycoside toxicity; Geri: CHF, renal or hepatic insufficiency, geriatric patients (dose reduction or increased dosing intervals recommended); OB, Lactation: Pedi: Safety not established.

Adverse Reactions/Side Effects
CNS: SEIZURES, confusion, dizziness. **CV:** ASYSTOLE, HEART BLOCK, VENTRICULAR ARRHYTHMIAS, hypotension. **GI:** diarrhea, anorexia, bitter taste, nausea, vomiting. **Derm:** rashes. **Hemat:** AGRANULOCYTOSIS, eosinophilia, leukopenia, thrombocytopenia. **Misc:** chills, drug-induced systemic lupus syndrome, fever.

Interactions
Drug-Drug: May have additive or antagonistic effects with other **antiarrhythmics**. Additive neurologic toxicity (confusion, seizures) with **lidocaine**. **Antihypertensives** and **nitrates** may potentiate hypotensive effect. Potentiates **neuromuscular blocking agents**. May partially antagonize the therapeutic effects of **anticholinesterase agents** in myasthenia gravis. ↑ risk of arrhythmias with **pimozide**. Additive anticholinergic effects with other **drugs possessing anticholinergic properties**, including **antihistamines**, **antidepressants**, **atropine**, **haloperidol**, and **phenothiazines**. Effects of procainamide may be ↑ by **cimetidine**, **quinidine**, or **trimethoprim**.

Route/Dosage
IM (Adults): 50 mg/kg/day in divided doses q 3–6 hr.

IV (Adults): 100 mg q 5 min until arrhythmia is abolished or 1000 mg have been given; wait at least 10 min until further dosing *or* loading infusion of 500–600 mg over 30–60 min followed by maintenance infusion of 1–4 mg/min.

Availability (generic available)
Injection: 100 mg/mL, 500 mg/mL.

NURSING IMPLICATIONS

Assessment
- Monitor ECG, pulse, and blood pressure continuously throughout IV administration. Parameters should be monitored periodically during oral administration. IV administration is usually discontinued if any of the following occur: arrhythmia is resolved, QRS complex widens by 50%, PR interval is prolonged, blood pressure drops >15 mm Hg, or toxic side effects develop. Patient should remain supine throughout IV administration to minimize hypotension.
- **Lab Test Considerations:** Monitor CBC every 2 wk during the first 3 mo of therapy. May cause ↓ leukocyte, neutrophil, and platelet counts. Therapy may be discontinued if leukopenia occurs. Blood counts usually return to normal within 1 mo of discontinuation of therapy.
- Monitor ANA periodically during prolonged therapy or if symptoms of lupus-like reaction occur. Therapy is discontinued if a steady increase in ANA titer occurs.
- May cause ↑ AST, ALT, alkaline phosphatase, LDH, bilirubin, and a positive Coombs' test result.
- ***Toxicity and Overdose:*** Serum procainamide and *N*-acetylprocainamide levels may be monitored periodically during dosage adjustment. Therapeutic blood level of procainamide is 4–8 mcg/mL.
- Toxicity may occur with procainamide blood levels of 8–16 mcg/mL or greater.
- Signs of toxicity include confusion, dizziness, drowsiness, decreased urination, nausea, vomiting, and tachyarrhythmias.

Potential Nursing Diagnoses
Decreased cardiac output (Indications)

Implementation
- **IM:** Used only when IV route is not feasible.

IV Administration

- **Direct IV:** (only to be used for life-threatening arrhythmias). ***Diluent:*** Dilute each 100 mg of procainamide with 10 mL of 0.9% NaCl. ***Rate:*** Not to exceed 25 mg/min. Rapid administration may cause ventricular fibrillation or asystole.
- **Intermittent Infusion (preferred route of administration):** ***Diluent:*** Add 2 g of procainamide to 250 mL of 0.9% NaCl. ***Concentration:*** 8 mg/mL. ***Rate:*** Administer initial infusion over 30–60 min. Administer maintenance infusion at rate of 1–4 mg/min to maintain control of arrhythmia.
- **Y-Site Compatibility:** alfentanil, amikacin, aminophylline, amiodarone, amphotericin B liposome, anidulafungin, ascorbic acid, atracurium, atropine, azathioprine, aztreonam, benztropine, bivalirudin, bleomycin, bumetanide, buprenorphine, butorphanol, calcium chloride, calcium gluconate, caspofungin, cefazo-

✻ = Canadian drug name. = Genetic implication.
*CAPITALS indicates life-threatening; underlines indicate most frequent.

lin, cefotaxime, cefoxitin, ceftazidime, ceftriaxone, cefuroxime, chlorpromazine, cimetidine, cisatracurium, cisplatin, clindamycin, cyanocobalamin, cyclophosphamide, cyclosporine, cytarabine, dactinomycin, daptomycin, dexamethasone, dexmedetomidine, digoxin, diphenhydramine, dobutamine, docetaxel, dopamine, doxacurium doxorubicin, doxycycline, enalaprilat, ephedrine, epinephrine, epirubicin, epoetin alfa, eptifibatide, ertapenem, erythromycin, esmolol, etoposide, etoposide phosphate, famotidine, fenoldopam, fentanyl, fluconazole, fludarabine, fluorouracil, folic acid, furosemide, gemcitabine, gentamicin, glycopyrrolate, granisetron, heparin, hetastarch, hydrocortisone, hydromorphone, idarubicin, ifosfamide, indomethacin, insulin, isoproterenol, ketorolac, labetalol, lidocaine, linezolid, lorazepam, magnesium sulfate, mannitol, mechlorethamine, meperidine, metaraminol, methotrexate, methoxamine, methyldopate, methylprednisolone, metoclopramide, metoprolol, midazolam, mitoxantrone, morphine, multivitamins, nafcillin, nalbuphine, naloxone, nitroglycerin, nitroprusside, norepinephrine, octreotide, ondansetron, oxacillin, oxaliplatin, oxytocin, paclitaxel, palonosetron, pancuronium, pantoprazole, papaverine, penicillin G, pentamidine, pentazocine, pentobarbital, phenobarbital, phentolamine, phenylephrine, phytonadione, piperacillin/tazobactam, potassium chloride, prochlorperazine, promethazine, propranolol, protamine, pyridoxime, quinupristin/dalfopristin, ranitidine, remifentanil, rocuronium, sodium bicarbonate, streptokinase, succinylcholine, sufentanil, tacrolimus, teniposide, theophylline, thiamine, thioptepa, ticarcillin/clavulanate, tigecycline, tirofiban, tobramycin, tolazoline, trimetaphan, urokinase, vancomycin, vasopressin, vecuronium, verapamil, vincristine, vinorelbine, vitamin B complex with C, voriconazole.
- **Y-Site Incompatibility:** acyclovir, azathioprine, carboplatin, ceftizoxime, chloramphenicol, dantrolene, diazepam, diazoxide, ganciclovir, hydralazine, metronidazole, milrinone, phenytointrimethoprim/sulfamethoxazole.

Patient/Family Teaching
- May cause dizziness. Caution patient to request assistance with ambulation until response to medication is known.
- Advise patient to notify health care professional immediately if signs of drug-induced lupus syndrome (fever, chills, joint pain or swelling, pain with breathing, skin rash), leukopenia (sore throat, mouth, or gums), or thrombocytopenia (unusual bleeding or bruising) occur. Medication may be discontinued if these occur.
- Advise patient to carry identification at all times describing disease process and medication regimen.
- Emphasize the importance of routine follow-up exams to monitor progress.

Evaluation/Desired Outcomes
- Resolution of cardiac arrhythmias without detrimental side effects.

procaine penicillin G, See **PENICILLINS.**

procarbazine
(proe-**kar**-ba-zeen)
Matulane, ✤ Natulan

Classification
Therapeutic: antineoplastics
Pharmacologic: alkylating agents

Pregnancy Category D

Indications
Hodgkin's disease (with other treatment modalities). **Unlabeled Use:** Other lymphomas. Brain and lung tumors. Multiple myeloma. Malignant melanoma. Polycythemia vera.

Action
Appears to inhibit DNA, RNA, and protein synthesis (cell-cycle S-phase–specific). **Therapeutic Effects:** Death of rapidly replicating cells, particularly malignant ones.

Pharmacokinetics
Absorption: Well absorbed following oral administration.
Distribution: Widely distributed; crosses the blood-brain barrier.
Metabolism and Excretion: Metabolized by the liver; <5% excreted unchanged by the kidneys; some respiratory elimination as methane and carbon dioxide.
Half-life: 1 hr.

TIME/ACTION PROFILE (effects on blood counts)

ROUTE	ONSET	PEAK	DURATION
PO	14 days	2–8 wk	28 days or more (up to 6 wk)

Contraindications/Precautions
Contraindicated in: Hypersensitivity; Alcoholism; Severe renal or liver impairment; Pheochromocytoma; CHF; OB, Lactation: Pregnancy or lactation.
Use Cautiously in: Infection; ↓ bone marrow reserve; Headache; Psychiatric illness; Liver impairment; Cardiovascular disease; OB: Women with childbearing potential should be advised to avoid pregnancy; Pedi: Very close clinical monitoring required due to potential for toxicity.

Adverse Reactions/Side Effects
CNS: SEIZURES, confusion, dizziness, drowsiness, hallucinations, headache, mania, mental depression, nightmares, psychosis, syncope, tremor. **EENT:** nystagmus, photophobia, retinal hemorrhage. **Resp:** cough, pleural effusions. **CV:** edema, hypotension, tachycardia. **GI:** nausea, vomiting, anorexia, diarrhea, dry mouth, dysphagia, hepatic dysfunction, stomatitis. **GU:** gonadal suppression. **Derm:** alopecia, photosensitivity, pruritus, rashes. **Endo:** gynecomastia. **Hemat:** anemia, leukopenia, thrombocytopenia. **Neuro:** neuropathy, paresthesia. **Misc:** ascites, secondary malignancy.

Interactions
Drug-Drug: Concurrent use with **sympathomimetics** including **methylphenidate** may produce life-threatening hypertension (avoid concurrent use during and for 14 days following procarbazine). Deep coma and death may result from concurrent use of **opioid analgesics**; avoid **meperidine**. Use small incremental doses of other agents and titrate to effect. ↑ bone marrow depression may occur with other **antineoplastics** or **radiation therapy**. Seizures and hyperpyrexia may occur with concurrent use of **MAO inhibitors**, **tricyclic antidepressants**, **SSRI antidepressants** (should not be used within 5 wk of **fluoxetine**), or **carbamazepine**. May ↓ serum **digoxin** levels. Concurrent use with **levodopa** may result in flushing and hypertension. ↑ CNS depression with other **CNS depressants**, including **alcohol**, **antidepressants**, **antihistamines**, **opioid analgesics**, **phenothiazines**, and **sedative/hypnotics**. Disulfiram-like reaction may occur with **alcohol**. **Cigarette smoking** may ↑ the risk of secondary lung cancer.
Drug-Food: Ingestion of foods high in **tyramine** content (see Appendix M) may result in hypertension. Ingestion of foods high in **caffeine** content may result in arrhythmias.

Route/Dosage
PO (Adults): 2–4 mg/kg/day as a single dose or in divided doses for 1 wk, then 4–6 mg/kg/day until response is obtained; then maintenance dose of 1–2 mg/kg/day. Dosage should be rounded off to the nearest 50 mg.
PO (Children): 50 mg/m^2/day for 7 days, then 100 mg/m^2/day, maintenance dose of 50 mg/m^2/day.

Availability
Capsules: 50 mg.

NURSING IMPLICATIONS
Assessment
- Monitor blood pressure, pulse, and respiratory rate periodically during therapy. Report significant changes to health care professional.
- Assess nutritional status (appetite, intake and output ratios, weight, frequency and amount of emesis). Anorexia and weight loss can be decreased by feeding light, frequent meals. Nausea and vomiting can be minimized by administering an antiemetic at least 1 hr prior to receiving medication. Phenothiazine antiemetics should be avoided.
- Monitor for bone marrow depression. Assess for bleeding (bleeding gums, bruising, petechiae, guaiac stools, urine, and emesis) and avoid IM injections and taking rectal temperatures if platelet count is low. Apply pressure to venipuncture sites for 10 min. Assess for signs of infection during neutropenia. Anemia may occur. Monitor for increased fatigue, dyspnea, and orthostatic hypotension.
- Concurrent ingestion of tyramine-rich foods and many medications may result in life-threatening hypertensive crisis. Signs and symptoms of hypertensive crisis include chest pain, severe headache, nausea and vomiting, photosensitivity, and enlarged pupils. Treatment includes IV phentolamine.
- Procarbazine should be discontinued until side effects clear and then resumed at a lower dose if leukopenia, thrombocytopenia, hypersensitivity reaction, stomatitis (first small ulceration or persistent soreness), diarrhea, hemorrhage, or bleeding tendencies occur.
- *Lab Test Considerations:* Monitor hemoglobin, hematocrit, WBC, differential, reticulocytes, and platelet count prior to and every 3–4 days during therapy. Notify physician if WBC <4000/mm^3 or platelet count <100,000/mm^3.

Therapy should be discontinued and resumed at a lower dose when counts improve. The nadir of leukopenia and thrombocytopenia occurs in approximately 2–8 wk, and recovery usually occurs in about 6 wk. Anemia also may occur.
- Assess hepatic and renal function prior to therapy. Monitor urinalysis, AST, ALT, alkaline phosphatase, and BUN at least weekly during therapy.
- Closely monitor serum glucose in diabetic patients. Oral hypoglycemics or insulin dosage may need to be reduced, because hypoglycemic effects are enhanced.
- Bone marrow aspiration studies are recommended prior to initiation of therapy and at time of maximum hematologic response to ensure adequate bone marrow reserve.

Potential Nursing Diagnoses
Risk for infection (Adverse Reactions)
Imbalanced nutrition: less than body requirements (Adverse Reactions)

Implementation
- **PO:** Administer with food or fluids if GI irritation occurs. Confer with pharmacist regarding opening of capsules if patient has difficulty swallowing.

Patient/Family Teaching
- Emphasize the need to take medication as directed. Take missed doses as soon as remembered within a few hours but not if several hours have passed or if almost time for next dose. Health care professional should be consulted if vomiting occurs shortly after a dose is taken.
- Instruct patient to notify health care professional promptly if signs of infection (fever, sore throat, chills, cough, thickened bronchial secretions, hoarseness, pain in lower back or side, difficult or painful urination); bleeding gums; bruising; petechiae; or blood in stool, urine, or emesis occurs. Caution patient to avoid crowds and persons with known infections. Instruct patient to use soft toothbrush and electric razor and to avoid falls. Patient should not receive IM injections or rectal temperatures. Caution patient not to drink alcoholic beverages or take medication containing aspirin or NSAIDs; may precipitate gastric bleeding.
- Caution patient to avoid alcohol, caffeinated beverages, CNS depressants, OTC drugs, and foods or beverages containing tyramine (see Appendix M for foods included) during therapy and for at least 2 wk after therapy has been discontinued, because they may precipitate a hypertensive crisis.
- Advise patient that an additional interaction of alcohol with procarbazine is a disulfiram-like reaction (flushing, nausea, vomiting, headache, abdominal cramps).
- Instruct patient to inspect oral mucosa for erythema and ulceration. If ulceration occurs, advise patient to notify health care professional and to use sponge brush and rinse mouth with water after eating and drinking. Topical agents may be used if mouth pain interferes with eating. Stomatitis pain may require treatment with opioid analgesics.
- May cause drowsiness or dizziness. Caution patient to avoid driving or other activities that require alertness until response to medication is known.
- Advise patient that this medication may have teratogenic effects. Contraception should be practiced during therapy and for at least 4 mo after therapy is concluded.
- Discuss the possibility of hair loss with patient. Explore methods of coping.
- Caution patient to use sunscreen and protective clothing to prevent photosensitivity reactions.
- Instruct patient not to receive any vaccinations without advice of health care professional.
- Advise patient to notify health care professional of medication regimen prior to treatment or surgery. This therapy usually should be withdrawn at least 2 wk prior to surgery.
- Instruct patient to inform health care professional if muscle or joint pain, nausea, vomiting, sweating, tiredness, weakness, constipation, headache, difficulty swallowing, or loss of appetite becomes pronounced.
- Advise patient to carry identification describing medication regimen at all times.
- Emphasize the need for periodic lab tests to monitor for side effects.

Evaluation/Desired Outcomes
- Decrease in size and spread of malignant tissue in Hodgkin's disease.

---

prochlorperazine
(proe-klor-**pair**-a-zeen)
Compro, ✤ Stemetil

Classification
Therapeutic: antiemetics, antipsychotics
Pharmacologic: phenothiazines

Pregnancy Category C

Indications
Management of nausea and vomiting. Treatment of psychoses. Treatment of anxiety.

Action
Alters the effects of dopamine in the CNS. Possesses significant anticholinergic and alpha-adrenergic blocking activity. Depresses the chemoreceptor trigger zone (CTZ) in the CNS.
Therapeutic Effects: Diminished nausea and vomiting. Diminished signs and symptoms of psychoses or anxiety.

Pharmacokinetics
Absorption: Absorption from tablet is variable; may be better with oral liquid formulations. Well absorbed after IM administration.
Distribution: Widely distributed, high concentrations in the CNS. Crosses the placenta and probably enters breast milk.
Protein Binding: ≥90%.
Metabolism and Excretion: Highly metabolized by the liver and GI mucosa. Converted to some compounds with antipsychotic activity.
Half-life: Unknown.

TIME/ACTION PROFILE (antiemetic effect)

ROUTE	ONSET	PEAK	DURATION
PO	30–40 min	unknown	3–4 hr
Rect	60 min	unknown	3–4 hr
IM	10–20 min	10–30 min	3–4 hr
IV	rapid (min)	10–30 min	3–4 hr

Contraindications/Precautions
Contraindicated in: Hypersensitivity; Cross-sensitivity with other phenothiazines may exist; Angle-closure glaucoma; Bone marrow depression; Severe liver or cardiovascular disease; Hypersensitivity to bisulfites or benzyl alcohol (some parenteral products); Pedi: Children <2 yr or <9.1 kg.
Use Cautiously in: Diabetes mellitus; Respiratory disease; Prostatic hypertrophy; CNS tumors; Epilepsy; Intestinal obstruction; OB, Lactation: Safety not established; Geri: Dose ↓ recommended; ↑ risk of mortality in elderly patients treated for dementia-related psychosis.

Adverse Reactions/Side Effects
CNS: NEUROLEPTIC MALIGNANT SYNDROME, extrapyramidal reactions, sedation, tardive dyskinesia. **EENT:** blurred vision, dry eyes, lens opacities. **CV:** ECG changes, hypotension, tachycardia. **GI:** constipation, dry mouth, anorexia, drug-induced hepatitis, ileus. **GU:** pink or reddish-brown discoloration of urine, urinary retention. **Derm:** photosensitivity, pigment changes, rashes. **Endo:** galactorrhea. **Hemat:** AGRANULOCYTOSIS, leukopenia. **Metab:** hyperthermia. **Misc:** allergic reactions.

Interactions
Drug-Drug: Additive hypotension with **antihypertensives**, **nitrates**, or acute ingestion of **alcohol**. Additive CNS depression with other **CNS depressants**, including **alcohol**, **antidepressants**, **antihistamines**, **opioid analgesics**, **sedative/hypnotics**, or **general anesthetics**. Additive anticholinergic effects with other **drugs possessing anticholinergic properties**, including **antihistamines**, some **antidepressants**, **atropine**, **haloperidol**, and other **phenothiazines**. **Lithium** ↑ risk of extrapyramidal reactions. May mask early signs of **lithium** toxicity. ↑ risk of agranulocytosis with **antithyroid agents**. ↓ beneficial effects of **levodopa**. **Antacids** may ↓ absorption.
Drug-Natural Products: Concomitant use of **kava-kava**, **valerian**, **chamomile**, or **hops** can ↑ CNS depression. ↑ anticholinergic effects with **angel's trumpet**, **jimson weed**, and **scopolia**.

Route/Dosage
Pediatric dose should not exceed 10 mg on the 1st day and then should not exceed 20 mg/day in children 2–5 yr or 25 mg/day in children 6–12 yr.

Antiemetic
PO (Adults and Children ≥12 yr): 5–10 mg 3–4 times daily (not to exceed 40 mg/day).
PO (Children 18–39 kg): 2.5 mg 3 times daily or 5 mg twice daily (not to exceed 15 mg/day).
PO (Children 14–17 kg): 2.5 mg 2–3 times daily (not to exceed 10 mg/day).
PO (Children 9–13 kg): 2.5 mg 1–2 times daily (not to exceed 7.5 mg/day).
IM (Adults and Children ≥12 yr): 5–10 mg q 3–4 hr as needed. *Nausea/vomiting associated with surgery*—5–10 mg; may be repeated once.
IM (Children 2–12 yr): 132 mcg (0.132 mg)/kg; usually only 1 dose is required.
IV (Adults and Children ≥12 yr): 2.5–10 mg (not to exceed 40 mg/day). *Nausea/vomiting associated with surgery*—5–10 mg; may be repeated once.
Rect (Adults): 25 mg twice daily.

Rect (Children 18–39 kg): 2.5 mg 3 times daily or 5 mg twice daily (not to exceed 15 mg/day).
Rect (Children 14–17 kg): 2.5 mg 2–3 times daily (not to exceed 10 mg/day).
Rect (Children 9–13 kg): 2.5 mg 1–2 times daily (not to exceed 7.5 mg/day).

Antipsychotic
PO (Adults and Children ≥12 yr): 5–10 mg 3–4 times daily; may be increased q 2–3 days (up to 150 mg/day).
PO (Children 2–12 yr): 2.5 mg 2–3 times daily.
IM (Adults): 10–20 mg q 2–4 hr for up to 4 doses, then 10–20 mg q 4–6 hr (up to 200 mg/day).
IM (Children 2–12 yr): 132 mcg (0.132 mg)/kg (not to exceed 10 mg/dose).
IV (Adults and Children ≥12 yr): 2.5–10 mg (up to 40 mg/day).
Rect (Adults): 10 mg 3–4 times daily; may be increased by 5–10 mg q 2–3 days as needed.

Antianxiety
PO (Adults and Children ≥12 yr): 5 mg 3–4 times daily (not to exceed 20 mg/day or longer than 12 wk).
IM (Adults and Children ≥12 yr): 5–10 mg q 3–4 hr as needed (up to 40 mg/day).
IM (Children 2–12 yr): 132 mcg (0.132 mg)/kg.
IV (Adults): 2.5–10 mg (up to 40 mg/day).

Availability (generic available)
Tablets: 5 mg, 10 mg. **Syrup (fruit flavor):** ✱5 mg/5 mL (mesylate). **Solution for injection:** 5 mg/mL (edisylate), ✱5 mg/mL (mesylate). **Suppositories:** 25 mg.

NURSING IMPLICATIONS

Assessment
- Monitor blood pressure (sitting, standing, lying down), ECG, pulse, and respiratory rate before and frequently during the period of dosage adjustment. May cause Q-wave and T-wave changes in ECG.
- Assess patient for level of sedation after administration.
- Monitor patient for onset of akathisia (restlessness or desire to keep moving) and extrapyramidal side effects (*parkinsonian*—difficulty speaking or swallowing, loss of balance control, pill rolling, mask-like face, shuffling gait, rigidity, tremors; and *dystonic*—muscle spasms, twisting motions, twitching, inability to move eyes, weakness of arms or legs) every 2 mo during therapy and 8–12 wk after therapy has been discontinued. Report these symptoms; reduction in dosage or discontinuation may be necessary. Trihexyphenidyl or diphenhydramine may be used to control these symptoms.
- Monitor for tardive dyskinesia (uncontrolled rhythmic movement of mouth, face, and extremities; lip smacking or puckering; puffing of cheeks; uncontrolled chewing; rapid or worm-like movements of tongue). Report immediately; may be irreversible.
- Monitor for development of neuroleptic malignant syndrome (fever, respiratory distress, tachycardia, seizures, diaphoresis, hypertension or hypotension, pallor, tiredness, severe muscle stiffness, loss of bladder control). Notify health care professional immediately if these symptoms occur.
- **Antiemetic:** Assess patient for nausea and vomiting before and 30–60 min after administration.
- **Antipsychotic:** Monitor patient's mental status (orientation to reality and behavior) before and periodically during therapy.
- Observe patient carefully when administering oral medication to ensure that medication is actually taken and not hoarded.
- Assess fluid intake and bowel function. Increased bulk and fluids in the diet may help minimize constipation.
- **Anxiety:** Assess degree and manifestations of anxiety and mental status before and periodically during therapy.
- *Lab Test Considerations:* CBC and liver function tests should be evaluated periodically during therapy. May cause blood dyscrasias, especially between wk 4 and 10 of therapy. Hepatotoxicity is more likely to occur between wk 2 and 4 of therapy. May recur if medication is restarted. Liver function abnormalities may require discontinuation of therapy.
- May cause false-positive or false-negative pregnancy test results and false-positive urine bilirubin test results.
- May cause ↑ serum prolactin levels.

Potential Nursing Diagnoses
Deficient fluid volume (Indications)
Disturbed thought process (Indications)

Implementation
- Do not confuse prochlorperazine with chlorpromazine.
- To prevent contact dermatitis, avoid getting solution on hands.

prochlorperazine

- Phenothiazines should be discontinued 48 hr before and not resumed for 24 hr after myelography; they lower seizure threshold.
- **PO:** Administer with food, milk, or a full glass of water to minimize gastric irritation.
- **IM:** Do not inject subcut. Inject slowly, deep into well-developed muscle. Keep patient recumbent for at least 30 min after injection to minimize hypotensive effects. Slight yellow color will not alter potency. Do not administer solution that is markedly discolored or that contains a precipitate.

IV Administration

- **Direct IV:** *Concentration:* Dilute to a concentration of 1 mg/mL. *Rate:* Administer at a rate of 1 mg/min; not to exceed 5 mg/min.
- **Intermittent Infusion:** *Diluent:* Dilute 20 mg in up to 1 L dextrose, saline, Ringer's or LR, dextrose/saline, dextrose/Ringer's, or lactated Ringer's combinations.
- **Continuous Infusion:** Has been used as infusion with 20 mg/L of compatible solution.
- **Syringe Incompatibility:** Manufacturer does not recommend mixing prochlorperazine with other medications in syringe.
- **Y-Site Compatibility:** amsarcine, calcium gluconate, cisatracurium, cisplatin, cladribine, cyclophosphamide, cytarabine, dexmedetomidine, doxorubicin, doxorubicin liposome, fluconazole, granisetron, heparin, hydrocortisone sodium succinate, linezolid, melphalan, methotrexate, ondansetron, oxaliplatin, paclitaxel, potassium chloride, propofol, remifentanil, sargramostim, sufentanil, teniposide, thiotepa, topotecan, vinorelbine, vitamin B complex with C.
- **Y-Site Incompatibility:** aldesleukin, allopurinol, amifostine, amphotericin B cholesteryl, amifostine, aztreonam, bivalirudin, cefepime, etoposide phosphate, fenoldopam, filgrastim, fludarabine, foscarnet, gemcitabine, pemetrexed, piperacillin/tazobactam.

Patient/Family Teaching

- Instruct patient to take medication as directed, not to skip doses or double up on missed doses. Take missed doses as soon as remembered unless almost time for next dose. If more than 2 doses are scheduled each day, missed dose should be taken within about 1 hr of the ordered time. Abrupt withdrawal may lead to gastritis, nausea, vomiting, dizziness, headache, tachycardia, and insomnia.
- Inform patient of possibility of extrapyramidal symptoms and tardive dyskinesia. Instruct patient to report these symptoms immediately to health care professional.
- Advise patient to change positions slowly to minimize orthostatic hypotension.
- May cause drowsiness. Caution patient to avoid driving or other activities requiring alertness until response to medication is known.
- Caution patient to avoid taking alcohol or other CNS depressants concurrently with this medication.
- Advise patient to use sunscreen and protective clothing when exposed to the sun to prevent photosensitivity reactions. Extremes in temperature should also be avoided, because this drug impairs body temperature regulation.
- Instruct patient to use frequent mouth rinses, good oral hygiene, and sugarless gum or candy to minimize dry mouth. Consult health care professional if dry mouth continues for >2 wk.
- Advise patient not to take prochlorperazine within 2 hr of antacids or antidiarrheal medication.
- Advise patient that increasing bulk and fluids in the diet and exercise may help minimize the constipating effects of this medication.
- Inform patient that this medication may turn urine pink to reddish-brown.
- Advise patient to notify health care professional of medication regimen before treatment or surgery.
- Instruct patient to notify health care professional promptly if sore throat, fever, unusual bleeding or bruising, skin rashes, weakness, tremors, visual disturbances, dark-colored urine, or clay-colored stools are noted.
- Emphasize the importance of routine follow-up exams to monitor response to medication and detect side effects. Periodic ocular exams are indicated. Encourage continued participation in psychotherapy as ordered by health care professional.

Evaluation/Desired Outcomes

- Relief of nausea and vomiting.
- Decrease in excitable, paranoic, or withdrawn behavior when used as an antipsychotic.
- Decrease in feelings of anxiety.

progesterone
(proe-**jess**-te-rone)
Crinone, Endometrin, Prochieve, Prometrium

Classification
Therapeutic: hormones
Pharmacologic: progestins

Pregnancy Category D

Indications
Secondary amenorrhea and abnormal uterine bleeding due to hormonal imbalance. **Prometrium:** Prevention of cell overgrowth in the uterine lining in postmenopausal women who have not had a hysterectomy (with estrogen). Part of assisted reproductive technology (ART) in the management of infertility (4% and 8% vaginal gel). **Endometrin:** Support of embryo implantation and early pregnancy. **Unlabeled Use:** Corpus luteum dysfunction.

Action
Produces: Secretory changes in the endometrium, Increase in basal body temperature, Histologic changes in vaginal epithelium, Relaxation of uterine smooth muscle, Mammary alveolar tissue growth, Pituitary inhibition, Withdrawal bleeding in the presence of estrogen. **Therapeutic Effects:** Restoration of hormonal balance with control of uterine bleeding. Successful outcome in assisted reproduction.

Pharmacokinetics
Absorption: Micronization increases oral and vaginal absorption.
Distribution: Enters breast milk.
Protein Binding: ≥90%.
Metabolism and Excretion: Metabolized by the liver; 50–60% eliminated by kidneys; 10% eliminated in feces.
Half-life: Several minutes.

TIME/ACTION PROFILE (blood levels)

ROUTE	ONSET	PEAK	DURATION
PO	unknown	2–4 hr	unknown
Vaginal	unknown	34.8–55 hr	unknown
IM	unknown	19.6–28 hr	unknown

Contraindications/Precautions
Contraindicated in: Hypersensitivity; Hypersensitivity to parabens or sesame oil (IM suspension only); Thromboembolic disease; Cerebrovascular disease; Severe liver disease; Breast or genital cancer; Porphyria; Missed abortion; OB: Contraindicated except in corpus luteum dysfunction.

Use Cautiously in: History of liver disease; Renal disease; Cardiovascular disease; Seizure disorders; Mental depression.

Adverse Reactions/Side Effects
CNS: depression. **EENT:** retinal thrombosis. **CV:** PULMONARY EMBOLISM, THROMBOEMBOLISM, thrombophlebitis. **GI:** gingival bleeding, hepatitis. **GU:** cervical erosions. **Derm:** chloasma, melasma, rashes. **Endo:** amenorrhea, breakthrough bleeding, breast tenderness, changes in menstrual flow, galactorrhea, spotting. **F and E:** edema. **Local:** irritation or pain at IM injection site. **Misc:** allergic reactions including ANAPHYLAXIS and ANGIOEDEMA, weight gain, weight loss.

Interactions
Drug-Drug: May ↓ effectiveness of **bromocriptine** when used concurrently for galactorrhea and amenorrhea.

Route/Dosage
PO (Adults): *Secondary amenorrhea*—400 mg once daily in the evening for 10 days; *prevention of postmenopausal estrogen-induced endometrial hyperplasia*—200 mg once daily at bedtime for 14 days on days 8–21 of a 28-day cycle or on days 12–25 of a 30-day cycle; if patient currently receives ≥1.25 mg/day of estrogen, then a daily of dose of 300 mg of progesterone as 100 mg 2 hr after breakfast and 200 mg at bedtime is used; further adjustments may be required.

Vag (Adults): *Secondary amenorrhea*—45 mg (1 applicatorful of 4% gel) once every other day for up to 6 doses, may be increased to 90 mg (1 applicatorful of 8% gel) once every other day for up to 6 doses; *Corpus luteum insufficiency or assisted reproduction technology*—For luteal phase support: 90 mg (1 applicatorful of 8% gel) once daily; for *in vitro* fertilization: 90 mg (1 applicatorful of 8% gel) once daily beginning within 24 hr of embryo transfer and continued through day 30 post-transfer (if pregnancy occurs, treatment may be continued for up to 10–12 wk); *partial or complete ovarian failure*—90 mg (1 applicatorful of 8% gel) twice daily while undergoing donor oocyte transfer (if pregnancy occurs, treatment may be continued for up to 10–12 wk) *Support of embryo implantation and early pregnancy*—100 mg insert 2 or 3 times daily for up to 10 wk.

IM (Adults): *Secondary amenorrhea*—100–150 mg (single dose) or 5–10 mg daily for 6–8 days given 8–10 days before expected menstrual period. *Dysfunctional uterine bleeding*—5–10 mg daily for 6 days. *Corpus luteum insufficiency*—12.5 mg/day at onset of ovulation for 2

promethazine

wk; may continue until 11th wk of gestation (unlabeled).

Availability (generic available)
Micronized capsules (Prometrium): 100 mg, 200 mg. **Cost:** 100 mg $48.99/30, 200 mg $85.99/30. **Bioadhesive vaginal gel (Crinone, Prochieve):** 4%, 8%. **Vaginal tablets (Endometrin):** 100 mg. **Injection:** 50 mg/mL in 10-mL vials.

NURSING IMPLICATIONS

Assessment
- Blood pressure be monitored periodically during therapy.
- Monitor intake and output ratios and weekly weight. Report significant discrepancies or steady weight gain.
- **Amenorrhea:** Assess patient's usual menstrual history. Administration of drug usually begins 8–10 days before anticipated menstruation. Withdrawal bleeding usually occurs 48–72 hr after course of therapy. Therapy should be discontinued if menses occur during injection series.
- **Dysfunctional Bleeding:** Monitor pattern and amount of vaginal bleeding (pad count). Bleeding should end by sixth day of therapy. Therapy should be discontinued if menses occur during injection series.
- *Lab Test Considerations:* Monitor hepatic function before and periodically during therapy.
- May cause ↑ plasma amino acid and alkaline phosphatase levels.
- May ↓ pregnanediol excretion concentrations.
- May cause ↑ serum concentrations of LDL and ↓ concentrations of HDL.
- High doses may ↑ sodium and chloride excretion.
- May alter thyroid function test results.

Potential Nursing Diagnoses
Sexual dysfunction (Indications)

Implementation
- **IM:** Shake vial before preparing IM dose. Administer deep IM. Rotate sites.
- **Vag:** Vaginal gel and insert are administered with disposable applicator provided by manufacturer.
- If dose increase is required from 4% gel to 8% gel, doubling the volume of the 4% gel will not accomplish dose increase; changing to 8% gel is required.

Patient/Family Teaching
- Advise patient to report signs and symptoms of fluid retention (swelling of ankles and feet, weight gain), thromboembolic disorders (pain, swelling, tenderness in extremities, headache, chest pain, blurred vision), mental depression, or hepatic dysfunction (yellowed skin or eyes, pruritus, dark urine, light-colored stools) to health care professional.
- Instruct patient to notify health care professional if change in vaginal bleeding pattern or spotting occurs.
- Instruct patient to stop taking medication and notify health care professional if pregnancy is suspected.
- Caution patient to use sunscreen and protective clothing to prevent photosensitivity reactions.
- Advise patient to notify health care professional of medication regimen before treatment or surgery.
- Emphasize the importance of routine follow-up physical exams, including blood pressure; breast, abdomen, and pelvic examinations; and Pap smears.
- **Vag:** Instruct patient not to use vaginal gel concurrently with other vaginal agents. If these agents must be used concurrently, administer at least 6 hr before or after vaginal gel.

Evaluation/Desired Outcomes
- Development of normal cyclic menses.
- Successful outcome in assisted reproduction.

HIGH ALERT

promethazine
(proe-**meth**-a-zeen)
✽ Histantil, Promethacon

Classification
Therapeutic: antiemetics, antihistamines, sedative/hypnotics
Pharmacologic: phenothiazines

Pregnancy Category C

Indications
Treatment of various allergic conditions and motion sickness. Preoperative sedation. Treatment and prevention of nausea and vomiting. Adjunct to anesthesia and analgesia.

✽ = Canadian drug name. ▓ = Genetic implication.
*CAPITALS indicates life-threatening; underlines indicate most frequent.

promethazine

Action
Blocks the effects of histamine. Has inhibitory effect on the chemoreceptor trigger zone in the medulla, resulting in antiemetic properties. Alters the effects of dopamine in the CNS. Possesses significant anticholinergic activity. Produces CNS depression by indirectly decreased stimulation of the CNS reticular system. **Therapeutic Effects:** Relief of symptoms of histamine excess usually seen in allergic conditions. Diminished nausea or vomiting. Sedation.

Pharmacokinetics
Absorption: Well absorbed after oral (88%) and IM administration; rectal administration may be less reliable.
Distribution: Widely distributed; crosses the blood-brain barrier and the placenta.
Protein Binding: 65–90%.
Metabolism and Excretion: Metabolized by the liver.
Half-life: 9–16 hr.

TIME/ACTION PROFILE (noted as antihistaminic effects; sedative effects last 2–8 hr)

ROUTE	ONSET	PEAK	DURATION
PO, IM	20 min	unknown	4–12 hr
Rectal	20 min	unknown	4–12 hr
IV	3–5 min	unknown	4–12 hr

Contraindications/Precautions
Contraindicated in: Hypersensitivity; Comatose patients; Prostatic hypertrophy; Bladder neck obstruction; Some products contain alcohol or bisulfites and should be avoided in patients with known intolerance; Angle-closure glaucoma; Pedi: May cause fatal respiratory depression in children <2 yr.
Use Cautiously in: IV administration may cause severe injury to tissue; Hypertension; Cardiovascular disease; Impaired liver function; Prostatic hypertrophy; Glaucoma; Asthma; Sleep apnea; Epilepsy; Underlying bone marrow depression; Pedi: For children >2 yr, use lowest effective dose, avoid concurrent respiratory depressants; OB: Has been used safely during labor; avoid chronic use during pregnancy; Lactation: Safety not established; may cause drowsiness in infant; Geri: Appears on Beers list. Sensitive to anticholinergic effects and have ↑ risk for side effects.

Adverse Reactions/Side Effects
CNS: NEUROLEPTIC MALIGNANT SYNDROME, confusion, disorientation, sedation, dizziness, extrapyramidal reactions, fatigue, insomnia, nervousness. **EENT:** blurred vision, diplopia, tinnitus. **CV:** bradycardia, hypertension, hypotension, tachycardia. **GI:** constipation, drug-induced hepatitis, dry mouth. **Derm:** photosensitivity, severe tissue necrosis upon infiltration at IV site, rashes. **Hemat:** blood dyscrasias.

Interactions
Drug-Drug: Additive CNS depression with other **CNS depressants**, including **alcohol**, other **antihistamines**, **opioid analgesics**, and other **sedative/hypnotics**. Neuroleptic malignant syndrome can occur when used concurrently with **antipsychotics**. Additive anticholinergic effects with other **drugs possessing anticholinergic properties**, including other **antihistamines**, **antidepressants**, **atropine**, **haloperidol**, other **phenothiazines**, **quinidine**, and **disopyramide**. May precipitate seizures when used with **drugs that lower seizure threshold**. Concurrent use with **MAO inhibitors** may result in ↑ sedation and anticholinergic side effects.

Route/Dosage
Antihistamine
PO (Adults): 6.25–12.5 mg 3 times/day and 25 mg at bedtime.
PO (Children ≥2 yr): 0.1 mg/kg/dose (not to exceed 12.5 mg) q 6 hr during the day and 0.5 mg/kg/dose (not to exceed 25 mg) at bedtime.
IM, IV, Rect (Adults): 25 mg; may repeat in 2 hr.
Rect (Children ≥2 yr): 0.125 mg/kg q 4–6 hr *or* 0.5 mg/kg at bedtime.

Antivertigo (Motion Sickness)
PO (Adults): 25 mg 30–60 min before departure; may be repeated in 8–12 hr.
PO, Rect (Children ≥2 yr): 0.5 mg/kg (not to exceed 25 mg) 30–60 min before departure; may be given q 12 hr as needed.

Sedation
PO, Rect, IM, IV (Adults): 25–50 mg; may repeat q 4–6 hr if needed.
PO, Rect, IM (Children >2 yr): 0.5–1 mg/kg (not to exceed 50 mg) q 6 hr as needed.

Sedation during Labor
IM, IV (Adults): 50 mg in early labor; when labor is established, additional doses of 25–75 mg may be given 1–2 times at 4-hr intervals (should not exceed 100 mg/24 hr).

Antiemetic
PO, Rect, IM, IV (Adults): 12.5–25 mg q 4 hr as needed; initial PO dose should be 25 mg.
PO, Rect, IM, IV (Children ≥2 yr): 0.25–1 mg/kg (not to exceed 25 mg) q 4–6 hr.

promethazine **1063**

Availability (generic available)
Tablets: 12.5 mg, 25 mg, ✱ 25 mg^OTC, 50 mg, ✱ 50 mg^OTC. **Syrup (cherry flavor):** 6.25 mg/5 mL, ✱ 10 mg/5 mL^OTC. **Injection:** 25 mg/mL, 50 mg/mL. **Suppositories:** 12.5 mg, 25 mg, 50 mg. *In combination with:* codeine, dextromethorphan, and/or phenylephrine in a variety of cough and cold preparations.

NURSING IMPLICATIONS

Assessment
- Monitor blood pressure, pulse, and respiratory rate frequently in patients receiving IV doses.
- Assess level of sedation after administration. Risk of sedation and respiratory depression are increased when administered concurrently with other drugs that cause CNS depression.
- Monitor patient for onset of extrapyramidal side effects (*akathisia*—restlessness; *dystonia*—muscle spasms and twisting motions; *pseudoparkinsonism*—mask-like face, rigidity, tremors, drooling, shuffling gait, dysphagia). Notify health care professional if these symptoms occur.
- Geri: Assess for adverse anticholinergic effects (delirium, acute confusion, dizziness, dry mouth, blurred vision, urinary retention, constipation, tachycardia).
- **Allergy:** Assess allergy symptoms (rhinitis, conjunctivitis, hives) before and periodically throughout course of therapy.
- **Antiemetic:** Assess patient for nausea and vomiting before and after administration.
- **IV:** *High Alert:* If administered IV, assess for burning and pain at IV site; may cause severe tissue injury. Avoid IV administration, if possible. If pain occurs, discontinue administration immediately.
- *Lab Test Considerations:* May cause false-positive or false-negative pregnancy test results.
- Evaluate CBC periodically during chronic therapy; blood dyscrasias may occur.
- May cause ↑ serum glucose.
- May cause false-negative results in skin tests using allergen extracts. Promethazine should be discontinued 72 hr before the test.

Potential Nursing Diagnoses
Deficient fluid volume (Indications)
Risk for injury (Side Effects)

Implementation
- When administering promethazine concurrently with opioid analgesics, supervise ambulation closely to prevent injury from increased sedation.
- **PO:** Administer with food, water, or milk to minimize GI irritation. Tablets may be crushed and mixed with food or fluids for patients with difficulty swallowing.
- **IM:** Administer deep into well-developed muscle. Subcut or inadvertent intra-arterial administration may cause severe tissue necrosis.

IV Administration
- **Direct IV:** *Diluent:* Dilute with 0.9% NaCl or D5W. *Concentration:* Doses should not exceed a concentration of 25 mg/mL. Administer through a large-bore vein through a running IV line into the most distal port. Slight yellow color does not alter potency. Do not use if precipitate is present. *Rate:* Administer each 25 mg slowly, over at least 10–15 min (maximum rate = 25 mg/min). Rapid administration may produce a transient fall in blood pressure.
- **Syringe Compatibility:** butorphanol, cimetidine, dihydroergotamine, droperidol, fentanyl, glycopyrrolate, hydromorphone, metoclopramide, midazolam, pentazocine, ranitidine, scopolamine.
- **Syringe Incompatibility:** heparin, ketorolac, pentobarbital, phenobarbital, phenytoin, thiopental.
- **Y-Site Compatibility:** alfentanil, amifostine, amikacin, amsacrine, anidulafungin, ascorbic acid, atracurium, atropine, benztropine, bivalirudin, bumetanide, buprenorphine, butorphanol, calcium chloride, calcium gluconate, carboplatin, caspofungin, cimetidine, ciprofloxacin, cisatracurium, cisplatin, cladribine, codeine, cyclophosphamide, cyclosporine, cytarabine, dactinomycin, daptomycin, dexmedetomidine, digoxin, diltiazem, diphenhydramine, dobutamine, docetaxel, dopamine, doxacurium, doxorubicin, enalaprilat, ephedrine, epinephrine, epirubicin, epoetin alfa, eftifibatide, erythromycin, esmolol, etoposide, etoposide phosphate, famotidine, fenoldopam, fentanyl, filgrastim, fluconazole, fludarabine, gemcitabine, gentamycin, glycopyrrolate, granisetron, hetastarch, hydromorphone, ifosfamide, insulin, isoproterenol, labetalol, levofloxacin, lidocaine, linezolid, lorazepam, magnesium sulfate, mannitol, mechlorethamine, melphalan, meperidine, metaraminol, methoxamine, methyldopate, metoclopramide, metoprolol, metronidazole, midazolam, milri-

✱ = Canadian drug name. ≡ = Genetic implication.
*CAPITALS indicates life-threatening; underlines indicate most frequent.

none, mitoxantrone, morphine, nalbuphine, naloxone, nitroglycerin, norepinephrine, octreotide, ondansetron, oxaliplatin, oxytocin, paclitaxel, palonosetron, pancuronium, pemetrexed, pentamidine, pentazocine, phentolamine, phenylephrine, procainamide, prochlorperazine, propranolol, protamine, pyridoxime, quinupristin/dalfopristin, ranitidine, remifentanil, rituximab, rocuronium, sargramostim, sodium acetate, succinylcholine, sufentanil, tacrolimus, teniposide, theophylline, thiamine, thiotepa, tigecycline, tirofiban, tobramycin, tolazoline, trastuzumab, trimetaphan, vancomycin, vasopressin, vecuronium, verapamil, vincristine, vinorelbine, voriconazole.

- **Y-Site Incompatibility:** acyclovir, aldesleukin, allopurinol, aminophylline, amphotericin B cholesteryl, amphotericin B colloidal, amphotericin B liposome, ampicillin, ampicillin/sulbactam, azathioprine, cefazolin, cefepime, cefonocid, cefoperazone, cefotaxime, cefotetan, cefoxitin, ceftazidime, ceftizoxime, ceftriaxone, cefuroxime, chloramphenicol, clindamycin, dantrolene, dexamethasone, diazepam, diazoxide, doxorubicin liposome, ertapenem, fluorouracil, folic acid, foscarnet, furosemide, ganciclovir, inamrinone, indomethacin, ketorolac, methylprednisolone, nafcillin, nitroprusside, oxacillin, pantoprazole, penicillin G, pentobarbital, phenobarbital, phenytoin, piperacillin/tazobactam, sodium bicarbonate, streptokinase, ticarcillin/clavulanate, trimethoprim/sulfamethoxazole, urokinase.

Patient/Family Teaching
- Review dose schedule with patient. If medication is ordered regularly and a dose is missed, take as soon as remembered unless time for next dose. Pedi: Caution caregivers to use only the measuring device accompanying the liquid medication and not to use household measuring devices..
- May cause drowsiness. Caution patient to avoid driving or other activities requiring alertness until response to medication is known.
- Advise patient that frequent mouth rinses, good oral hygiene, and sugarless gum or candy may decrease dry mouth. Health care professional should be notified if dry mouth persists >2 wk.
- Caution patient to use sunscreen and protective clothing to prevent photosensitivity reactions.
- Advise patient to change positions slowly to minimize orthostatic hypotension. Geri: Geriatric patients are at increased risk.
- Caution patient to avoid concurrent use of alcohol and other CNS depressants with this medication.
- Instruct patient to notify health care professional if sore throat, fever, jaundice, or uncontrolled movements are noted.
- Geri: Teach patient and family about anticholinergic effects and to contact a health care professional if such effects persist.
- **Motion Sickness:** When used as prophylaxis for motion sickness, advise patient to take medication at least 30 min and preferably 1–2 hr before exposure to conditions that may cause motion sickness.

Evaluation/Desired Outcomes
- Relief from allergic symptoms.
- Prevention of motion sickness.
- Sedation.
- Relief from nausea and vomiting.

---

propafenone
(proe-**paff**-e-nown)
Rythmol, Rythmol SR

Classification
Therapeutic: antiarrhythmics (class IC)

Pregnancy Category C

Indications
Treatment of life-threatening ventricular arrhythmias, including ventricular tachycardia (immediate-release only). Prolongs the time to recurrence of symptomatic paroxysmal atrial arrhythmias, including paroxysmal atrial fibrillation/flutter (PAF) and paroxysmal supraventricular tachycardia (PSVT). **Unlabeled Use:** Single dose treatment for atrial fibrillation.

Action
Slows conduction in cardiac tissue by altering transport of ions across cell membranes. **Therapeutic Effects:** Suppression of ventricular arrhythmias.

Pharmacokinetics
Absorption: Although well absorbed following oral administration, undergoes rapid hepatic metabolism (bioavailability 3–11%).
Distribution: Widely distributed; crosses the placenta.
Metabolism and Excretion: Extensively metabolized by the liver (CYP1A2, CYP2D6, and CYP3A4 enzyme systems), some metabolites have antiarrhythmic activity. >90% of patients are considered extensive metabolizers. Others metabolize propafenone more slowly.

Half-life: 2–10 hr in extensive metabolizers, 10–32 hr in slow metabolizers.

TIME/ACTION PROFILE (antiarrhythmic effects)

ROUTE	ONSET	PEAK	DURATION
PO	hr–days	4–5 days†	hr

†Chronic dosing

Contraindications/Precautions
Contraindicated in: Hypersensitivity; Cardiogenic shock; Conduction disorders including sick sinus syndrome and AV block (without a pacemaker); Bradycardia; Severe hypotension; Concurrent quinidine or amiodarone; Nonallergic bronchospasm; Electrolyte disturbances; Uncontrolled CHF.

Use Cautiously in: Severe hepatic or renal impairment (dose ↓ may be necessary); Geri: Lower doses may be necessary due to age-related ↓ in renal/hepatic/cardiovascular function, concurrent chronic illnesses and medications; OB, Lactation: Pedi: Safety not established.

Adverse Reactions/Side Effects
CNS: dizziness, shaking, weakness. **EENT:** blurred vision. **CV:** SUPRAVENTRICULAR ARRHYTHMIA, VENTRICULAR ARRHYTHMIAS, conduction disturbances, angina, bradycardia, hypotension. **GI:** altered taste, constipation, nausea, vomiting, diarrhea, dry mouth. **Derm:** rash. **MS:** joint pain.

Interactions
Drug-Drug: Any **inhibitors of the CYP1A2, CYP2D6, or CYP3A4 enzyme systems** may ↑ levels, including **desipramine**, **paroxetine**, **ritonavir**, **sertraline**, **ketoconazole**, **saquinavir**, **erythromycin** (blood level monitoring recommended). **Quinidine** is a strong inhibitor of CYP2D6 and significantly ↑ levels of propafenone; concurrent use is not recommended. Propafenone is also an inhibitor of CYP2D6 and may ↑ levels of **desipramine**, **imipramine**, **haloperidol**, and **venlafaxine**. Significantly ↑ serum **digoxin** levels (blood level monitoring recommended, ↓ dose may be required). ↑ blood levels of **metoprolol** and **propranolol** (↓ dose may be required). Concurrent use of **local anesthetics** may ↑ risk of CNS adverse reactions. ↑ effects of **warfarin** (↓ warfarin dose if necessary, monitor INR). Concurrent use with **amiodarone** can adversely effect conduction/repolarization and should be avoided. May ↑ risk of CNS adverse reactions with **lidocaine**. May ↑ cyclosporine trough blood levels and risk of nephrotoxicity. **Rifampin** may ↓ serum levels and effectiveness. **Cimetidine** may ↑ serum levels.

Drug-Food: Grapefruit juice may ↑ levels.

Route/Dosage
PO (Adults): 150 mg q 8 hr; may be gradually ↑ at 3–4-day intervals as required up to 300 mg q 8–12 hr. *Single dose treatment of atrial fibrillation (unlabeled)*—450 or 600 mg; *Sustained release*—225 mg q 12 hr; may be gradually ↑ at a minimum of 5-day intervals as required to 325 mg q 12 hr; if further ↑ is needed, may ↑ to 425 mg q 12 hr.

Availability (generic available)
Tablets: 150 mg, 225 mg, 300 mg. Cost: *Generic*—150 mg $316.95/270, 225 mg $355.00/270, 300 mg $593.95/270. **Sustained-release capsules:** 225 mg, 325 mg, 425 mg.

NURSING IMPLICATIONS

Assessment
- Monitor ECG or use Holter monitor prior to and periodically during therapy. May cause PR and QT prolongation.
- Monitor blood pressure and pulse periodically during therapy.
- Monitor intake and output ratios and daily weight. Assess patients for signs of CHF (peripheral edema, rales/crackles, dyspnea, weight gain, jugular venous distention). May require reduction or discontinuation of therapy.
- *Lab Test Considerations:* May cause ↑ ANA titer, which is usually asymptomatic and reversible.
- Monitor prothrombin level in patients taking warfarin; may ↑ effects of warfarin.
- *Toxicity and Overdose:* Signs of toxicity include hypotension, excessive drowsiness, and decreased or abnormal heart rate. Notify health care professional if these signs occur.

Potential Nursing Diagnoses
Decreased cardiac output (Indications)

Implementation
- **PO:** Propafenone therapy should be initiated in a hospital with facilities for cardiac rhythm monitoring. Most serious proarrhythmic effects are seen in the first 2 wk of therapy.
- Swallow sustained-release capsules whole; do not open, crush or chew.

- Previous antiarrhythmic therapy should be withdrawn 2–5 half-lives before starting propafenone.
- Dose adjustments should be at least 3–4 days apart because of the long half-life of propafenone.
- Correct pre-existing hypokalemia or hyperkalemia prior to instituting therapy.

Patient/Family Teaching
- Instruct patient to take medication around the clock as directed, even if feeling better. Take missed doses as soon as remembered if within 4 hr; omit if remembered later. Gradual dosage reduction may be necessary.
- May cause dizziness. Caution patient to avoid driving and other activities requiring alertness until response to medication is known.
- Advise patient to notify health care professional of medication regimen prior to treatment or surgery.
- Instruct patient to notify health care professional if fever, sore throat, chills, or unusual bleeding or bruising occurs or if chest pain, shortness of breath, diaphoresis, palpitations, or visual changes become bothersome.
- Advise patient to carry identification describing disease process and medication regimen at all times.
- Emphasize the importance of follow-up exams to monitor progress.

Evaluation/Desired Outcomes
- Decrease in frequency of ventricular arrhythmias.
- Prolonged time to recurrence of symptomatic paroxysmal atrial arrhythmias, including paroxysmal atrial fibrillation/flutter and PSVT.

HIGH ALERT

propofol (proe-poe-fol)
Diprivan

Classification
Therapeutic: general anesthetics

Pregnancy Category B

Indications
Induction of general anesthesia in children >3 yr and adults. Maintenance of balanced anesthesia when used with other agents in children >2 mo and adults. Initiation and maintenance of monitored anesthesia care (MAC). Sedation of intubated, mechanically ventilated patients in intensive care units (ICUs).

Action
Short-acting hypnotic. Mechanism of action is unknown. Produces amnesia. Has no analgesic properties. **Therapeutic Effects:** Induction and maintenance of anesthesia.

Pharmacokinetics
Absorption: Administered IV only, resulting in complete absorption.
Distribution: Rapidly and widely distributed. Crosses the blood-brain barrier well; rapidly redistributed to other tissues. Crosses the placenta and enters breast milk.
Protein Binding: 95–99%.
Metabolism and Excretion: Rapidly metabolized by the liver.
Half-life: 3–12 hr (blood-brain equilibration half-life 2.9 min).

TIME/ACTION PROFILE (loss of consciousness)

ROUTE	ONSET	PEAK	DURATION†
IV	40 sec	unknown	3–5 min

†Time to recovery is 8 min (up to 19 min if opioid analgesics have been used)

Contraindications/Precautions
Contraindicated in: Hypersensitivity to propofol, soybean oil, egg lecithin, or glycerol; OB: Crosses placenta; may cause neonatal depression; Lactation: Enters breast milk; effects on newborn unknown.
Use Cautiously in: Cardiovascular disease; Lipid disorders (emulsion may have detrimental effect); ↑ intracranial pressure; Cerebrovascular disorders; Hypovolemic patients (lower induction and maintenance dosage reduction recommended); Pedi: Not recommended for induction of anesthesia in children <3 yr, or for maintenance of anesthesia in infants <2 mo; not for ICU or pre-procedure sedation; Geri: Lower induction and maintenance dose reduction recommended.

Adverse Reactions/Side Effects
CNS: dizziness, headache. **Resp:** APNEA, cough. **CV:** bradycardia, hypotension, hypertension. **GI:** abdominal cramping, hiccups, nausea, vomiting. **Derm:** flushing. **Local:** burning, pain, stinging, coldness, numbness, tingling at IV site. **MS:** involuntary muscle movements, perioperative myoclonia. **GU:** discoloration of urine (green). **Misc:** PROPOFOL INFUSION SYNDROME, fever.

Interactions
Drug-Drug: Additive CNS and respiratory depression with **alcohol**, **antihistamines**, **opioid analgesics**, and **sedative/hypnotics** (dose ↓

may be required). **Theophylline** may antagonize the CNS effects of propofol. Propofol may ↑ levels of **alfentanil**. Cardiorespiratory instability can occur when used with **acetazolamide**. Serious bradycardia can occur with concurrent use of **fentanyl** in children. ↑ risk of hypertriglyceridemia with **intravenous fat emulsion**.

Route/Dosage

General Anesthesia
IV (Adults <55 yr): *Induction*—40 mg q 10 sec until induction achieved (2–2.5 mg/kg total). *Maintenance*—100–200 mcg/kg/min. Rates of 150–200 mcg/kg/min are usually required during first 10–15 min after induction, then ↓ by 30–50% during first 30 min of maintenance. Rates of 50–100 mcg/kg/min are associated with optimal recovery time. May also be given intermittently in increments of 25–50 mg.
IV (Geriatric Patients, Cardiac patients, Debilitated Patients, or Hypovolemic Patients): *Induction*—20 mg q 10 sec until induction achieved (1–1.5 mg/kg total). *Maintenance*—50–100 mcg/kg/min (dose in cardiac anesthesia ranges from 50–150 mcg/kg/min depending on concurrent use of opioid).
IV (Adults Undergoing Neurosurgical Procedures): *Induction*—20 mg q 10 sec until induction achieved (1–2 mg/kg total). *Maintenance*—100–200 mcg/kg/min.
IV (Children ≥3 yr–16 yr): *Induction*—2.5–3.5 mg/kg, use lower dose for children ASA III or IV.
IV (Children 2 mo–16 yr): *Maintenance*—125–300 mcg/kg/min (following first 30 min of maintenance, rate should be ↓ if possible), younger children may require larger infusion rates compared to older children.

Monitored Anesthesia Care (MAC) Sedation
IV (Adults <55 yr): *Initiation*—100–150 mcg/kg/min infusion *or* 0.5 mg/kg as slow injection. *Maintenance*—25–75 mcg/kg/min infusion or incremental boluses of 10–20 mg.
IV (Geriatric Patients, Debilitated Patients, or ASA III/IV Patients): *Initiation*—Use slower infusion or injection rates. *Maintenance*—20% less than the usual adult infusion dose; rapid/repeated bolus dosing should be avoided.

ICU Sedation
IV (Adults): 5 mcg/kg/min for a minimum of 5 min. Additional increments of 5–10 mcg/kg/min over 5–10 min may be given until desired response is obtained. (Range 5–50 mcg/kg/min.) Dose should be reassessed every 24 hr.

Availability (generic available)
Injection: 10 mg/mL.

NURSING IMPLICATIONS

Assessment
- Assess respiratory status, pulse, and blood pressure continuously throughout propofol therapy. Frequently causes apnea lasting ≥60 sec. Maintain patent airway and adequate ventilation. Propofol should be used only by individuals experienced in endotracheal intubation, and equipment for this procedure should be readily available.
- Assess level of sedation and level of consciousness throughout and following administration.
- When using for ICU sedation, wake-up and assessment of CNS function should be done daily during maintenance to determine minimum dose required for sedation. Maintain a light level of sedation during these assessments; do not discontinue. Abrupt discontinuation may cause rapid awakening with anxiety, agitation, and resistance to mechanical ventilation.
- Monitor for propofol infusion syndrome (severe metabolic acidosis, hyperkalemia, lipemia, rhabdomyolysis, hepatomegaly, cardiac and renal failure). Most frequent with prolonged, high-dose infusions (>5 mg/kg/hr for >48 hr) but has also been reported following large-dose, short-term infusions during surgical anesthesia. If prolonged sedation or increasing dose is required, or metabolic acidosis occurs, consider alternative means of sedation.
- ***Toxicity and Overdose:*** If overdose occurs, monitor pulse, respiration, and blood pressure continuously. Maintain patent airway and assist ventilation as needed. If hypotension occurs, treatment includes IV fluids, repositioning, and vasopressors.

Potential Nursing Diagnoses
Ineffective breathing pattern (Adverse Reactions)
Risk for injury (Side Effects)

Implementation
- Do not confuse Diprivan (propofol) with Diflucan (fluconazole).

✦ = Canadian drug name. = Genetic implication.
*CAPITALS indicates life-threatening; underlines indicate most frequent.

- Dose is titrated to patient response.
- Propofol has no effect on the pain threshold. Adequate analgesia should *always* be used when propofol is used as an adjunct to surgical procedures.

IV Administration

- **Direct IV:** *Diluent:* Usually administered undiluted. If dilution is necessary, use only D5W. Shake well before use. Solution is opaque, making detection of contaminants difficult. Do not use if separation of the emulsion is evident. Contains no preservatives; maintain sterile technique and administer immediately after preparation. *Concentration:* Undiluted: 10 mg/mL. If dilution is necessary, dilute to concentration ≥2 mg/mL.
- Discard unused portions and IV lines at the end of anesthetic procedure or within 6 hr. For ICU sedation, discard after 12 hr if administered directly from vial or after 6 hr if transferred to a syringe or other container. Do not administer via filter <5–micron pore size.
- Aseptic technique is essential. Solution is capable of rapid growth of bacterial contaminants. Infections and subsequent deaths have been reported. *Rate:* Administer over 3–5 min. Titrate to desired level of sedation. Frequently causes pain, burning, and stinging at injection site; use larger veins of the forearm, antecubital fossa, or a dedicated IV catheter. Lidocaine 10–20 mg IV may be administered prior to injection to minimize pain. Pedi: Induction doses may be administered over 20–30 seconds.
- **Intermittent/Continuous Infusion:** *Diluent:* Administer undiluted. Allow 3 to 5 minutes between dose adjustments to allow for and assess the clinical effects. *Concentration:* 10 mg/mL. *Rate:* Based on patient's weight (see Route/Dosage section).
- **Solution Compatibility:** D5W, LR, D5/LR, D5/0.45% NaCl, D5/0.2% NaCl.
- **Y-Site Compatibility:** acyclovir, alfentanil, aminophylline, ampicillin, aztreonam, bumetanide, buprenorphine, butorphanol, calcium gluconate, carboplatin, cefazolin, cefepime, cefotaxime, cefoxitin, ceftizoxime, ceftriaxone, cefuroxime, chlorpromazine, cimetidine, cisplatin, clindamycin, cyclophosphamide, cyclosporine, cytarabine, dexamethasone, dexmedetomidine, diphenhydramine, dobutamine, dopamine, doxycycline, droperidol, enalaprilat, epinephrine, esmolol, famotidine, fenoldopam, fentanyl, fluconazole, fluorouracil, furosemide, ganciclovir, glycopyrrolate, granisetron, haloperidol, heparin, hydrocortisone sodium succinate, hydromorphone, ifosfamide, imipenem/cilastatin, inamrinone, insulin, isoproterenol, ketamine, labetalol, levorphanol, lidocaine, lorazepam, magnesium sulfate, mannitol, meperidine, milrinone, nafcillin, nalbuphine, naloxone, nitroglycerin, nitroprusside, norepinephrine, paclitaxel, pentobarbital, phenobarbital, potassium chloride, prochlorperazine, propranolol, ranitidine, scopolamine, sodium bicarbonate, succinylcholine, sufentanil, thiopental, ticarcillin/clavulanate, vecuronium.
- **Y-Site Incompatibility:** amikacin, amphotericin B, calcium chloride, ciprofloxacin, diazepam, digoxin, doxorubicin, gentamicin, levofloxacin, methotrexate, methylprednisolone sodium succinate, metoclopramide, mitoxantrone, phenytoin, tobramycin, verapamil.

Patient/Family Teaching

- Inform patient that this medication will decrease mental recall of the procedure.
- May cause drowsiness or dizziness. Advise patient to request assistance prior to ambulation and transfer and to avoid driving or other activities requiring alertness for 24 hr following administration.
- Advise patient to avoid alcohol or other CNS depressants without the advice of a health care professional for 24 hr following administration.

Evaluation/Desired Outcomes

- Induction and maintenance of anesthesia.
- Amnesia.
- Sedation in mechanically ventilated patients in an intensive care setting.

PROPOXYPHENE

propoxyphene hydrochloride
(pro-**pox**-i-feen hye-droe-**klor**-ide)
✦ 642 Tab, Darvon

propoxyphene hydrochloride/ acetaminophen

propoxyphene napsylate
(pro-**pox**-i-feen **nap**-si-late)
Darvon N

propoxyphene napsylate/ acetaminophen
Darvocet A500, Darvocet-N 50, Darvocet-N 100

PROPOXYPHENE

Classification
Therapeutic: opioid analgesics
Pharmacologic: opioid agonists, opioid agonists/nonopioid analgesic combinations

Pregnancy Category C
See also Acetaminophen monograph

Indications
Mild to moderate pain.

Action
Binds to opiate receptors in the CNS. Alters the perception of and response to painful stimuli, while producing generalized CNS depression.
Therapeutic Effects: Decrease in mild to moderate pain.

Pharmacokinetics
Absorption: Well absorbed following oral administration. Napsylate salt is more slowly absorbed.
Distribution: Widely distributed. Probably crosses the placenta. Enters breast milk in small amounts.
Metabolism and Excretion: Mostly metabolized by the liver. Some conversion to norpropoxyphene, a toxic metabolite. This metabolite accumulates in elderly patients and patients with decreased renal function.
Half-life: 6–12 hr.

TIME/ACTION PROFILE (analgesic effect)

ROUTE	ONSET	PEAK	DURATION
PO	15–60 min	2–3 hr	4–6 hr

Contraindications/Precautions
Contraindicated in: Hypersensitivity; History of suicidal ideation; OB, Lactation: Pedi: Safety not established.
Use Cautiously in: Head trauma; ↑ intracranial pressure; Severe renal, hepatic, or pulmonary disease; Hypothyroidism; Adrenal insufficiency; Alcoholism; Geri: Appears on Beers list. Elderly or debilitated patients require reduced doses; Undiagnosed abdominal pain; Prostatic hyperplasia.

Adverse Reactions/Side Effects
CNS: <u>dizziness</u>, <u>weakness</u>, dysphoria, euphoria, headache, insomnia, paradoxical excitement, sedation. **EENT:** blurred vision. **CV:** hypotension. **GI:** <u>nausea</u>, abdominal pain, constipation, vomiting. **Derm:** rashes. **Misc:** physical dependence, psychological dependence, tolerance.

Interactions
Drug-Drug: Use with extreme caution in patients receiving **MAO inhibitors** (may result in unpredictable, severe, and potentially fatal reactions—decrease initial dose to 25% of usual dose). Use with extreme caution with **alcohol**, **antidepressants**, **sedative/hypnotics**, or **muscle relaxants** (may result in severe CNS depression and possibly death). CYP3A4 inhibitors, including **ritonavir**, **ketoconazole**, **itraconazole**, **clarithromycin**, **nelfinavir**, **nefazodone**, **amiodarone**, **aprepitant**, **diltiazem**, **erythromycin**, **fluconazole**, **fosamprenavir**, or **verapamil** may ↑ propoxyphene levels. CYP3A4 inducers, including **rifampin**, **carbamazepine**, or **phenytoin** may ↑ levels of norpropoxyphene. Smoking ↑ metabolism and may ↓ analgesic effectiveness. Administration of **partial-antagonist opioid analgesics** may precipitate withdrawal in physically dependent patients. **Nalbuphine**, **buprenorphine**, or **pentazocine** may ↓ analgesia.
Drug-Natural Products: Concomitant use of **kava-kava**, **valerian**, or **chamomile** can ↑ CNS depression. St. John's wort may ↓ levels of norpropoxyphene.
Drug-Food: Grapefruit juice may ↑ propoxyphene levels.

Route/Dosage
Consider cumulative effects of additional acetaminophen (should not exceed 4 g acetaminophen/day); if toxic levels are exceeded, change to pure propoxyphene product.
PO (Adults): 65 mg q 4 hr (hydrochloride—Darvon) or 100 mg q 4 hr (napsylate—Darvon-N) as needed (not to exceed 390 mg/day as hydrochloride or 600 mg/day as napsylate). 100 mg propoxyphene napsylate = 65 mg propoxyphene hydrochloride.

Availability (generic available)

Propoxyphene Hydrochloride
Capsules: 65 mg. **Tablets:** ✺ 65 mg.

Propoxyphene Napsylate
Capsules: ✺ 100 mg. **Tablets:** 100 mg.

Propoxyphene Hydrochloride/Acetaminophen
Tablets: propoxyphene 65 mg/acetaminophen 650 mg.

Propoxyphene Napsylate/Acetaminophen
Tablets: propoxyphene 50 mg/acetaminophen 325 mg, propoxyphene 100 mg/acetaminophen

650 mg, propoxyphene 100 mg/acetaminophen 500 mg.

NURSING IMPLICATIONS
Assessment
- Assess type, location, and intensity of pain prior to and 2 hr (peak) following administration. When titrating opioid doses, increases of 25–50% should be administered until there is either a 50% reduction in the patient's pain rating on a numeric or visual analogue scale or the patient reports satisfactory pain relief. A repeat dose can be safely administered at the time of the peak if previous dose is ineffective and side effects are minimal.
- Use an equianalgesic chart (see Appendix K) when changing routes or when changing from one opioid to another.
- Prolonged, high-dose therapy may lead to physical and psychological dependence and tolerance. This should not prevent patient from receiving adequate analgesia. Most patients who receive propoxyphene for pain do not develop psychological dependence. Progressively higher doses or change to a stronger opioid may be required to relieve pain with long-term therapy.
- Assess blood pressure, pulse, and respirations before and periodically during administration. If respiratory rate is <10/min, assess level of sedation. Physical stimulation may be sufficient to prevent significant hypoventilation. Dose may need to be decreased by 25–50%. Initial drowsiness will diminish with continued use.
- Assess bowel function routinely. Prevention of constipation should be instituted with increased intake of fluids and bulk, and laxatives to minimize constipating effects. Stimulant laxatives should be administered routinely if opioid use exceeds 2–3 days, unless contraindicated.
- Geri: Geriatric patients may be more sensitive to CNS effects; monitor closely and assess falls risk.
- *Lab Test Considerations:* May cause ↑ serum amylase and lipase levels.
- May cause ↑ AST, ALT, serum alkaline phosphatase, LDH, and bilirubin concentrations.
- *Toxicity and Overdose:* If an opioid antagonist is required to reverse respiratory depression or coma, naloxone (Narcan) is the antidote. Dilute the 0.4-mg ampule of naloxone in 10 mL of 0.9% NaCl and administer 0.5 mL (0.02 mg) by direct IV push every 2 min. For patients weighing <40 kg, dilute 0.1 mg of naloxone in 10 mL of 0.9% NaCl for a concentration of 10 mcg/mL and administer 0.5 mcg/kg every 2 min. Titrate dose to avoid withdrawal, seizures, and severe pain.

Potential Nursing Diagnoses
Acute pain (Indications)
Disturbed sensory perception (visual, auditory) (Side Effects)
Risk for injury (Side Effects)

Implementation
- Explain therapeutic value of medication prior to administration, to enhance the analgesic effect.
- Regularly administered doses may be more effective than prn administration. Analgesic is more effective if given before pain becomes severe.
- Coadministration with nonopioid analgesics may have additive analgesic effects and may permit lower opioid doses.
- Medication should be discontinued gradually after long-term use to prevent withdrawal symptoms.
- **PO:** Doses may be administered with food or milk to minimize GI irritation.

Patient/Family Teaching
- Advise patient to take medication as directed and not to take more than the recommended amount. Severe and permanent liver damage may result from prolonged use or high doses of acetaminophen. Renal damage may occur with prolonged use of acetaminophen or aspirin. Doses of nonopioid agents should not exceed the maximum recommended daily dose. Instruct patient to read *Medication Guide* before taking and with each Rx refill; new information may be available.
- Instruct patient on how and when to ask for pain medication.
- Caution patient to avoid drinking grapefruit juice during propoxyphene therapy.
- May cause drowsiness or dizziness. Caution patient to avoid driving and other activities requiring alertness until response to the drug is known.
- Geri: Advise geriatric patients of increased risk for CNS effects and potential for falls.
- Advise patient to change positions slowly to minimize orthostatic hypotension.
- Caution patient to avoid concurrent use of alcohol or other CNS depressants with this medication and to notify health care professional before taking other Rx, OTC, or herbal products.
- Encourage patient to turn, cough, and breathe deeply every 2 hr to prevent atelectasis.

- Advise patient that good oral hygiene, frequent mouth rinses, and sugarless gum or candy may decrease dry mouth.

Evaluation/Desired Outcomes
- Decrease in severity of pain without a significant alteration in level of consciousness.

HIGH ALERT

propranolol
(proe-**pran**-oh-lole)

✦Apo-Propranolol, ✦Betachron E-R, Inderal, Inderal LA, InnoPran XL, ✦Novopranol, ✦pms Propranolol

Classification
Therapeutic: antianginals, antiarrhythmics (Class II), antihypertensives, vascular headache suppressants
Pharmacologic: beta blockers

Pregnancy Category C

Indications
Management of hypertension, angina, arrhythmias, hypertrophic cardiomyopathy, thyrotoxicosis, essential tremors, pheochromocytoma. Also used in the prevention and management of MI, and the prevention of vascular headaches. **Unlabeled Use:** Also used to manage alcohol withdrawal, aggressive behavior, antipsychotic-associated akathisia, situational anxiety, and esophageal varices. Post-traumatic stress disorder (PTSD) (Ongoing clinical trials at National Institute for Mental Health [NIMH]).

Action
Blocks stimulation of beta$_1$ (myocardial) and beta$_2$ (pulmonary, vascular, and uterine)-adrenergic receptor sites. **Therapeutic Effects:** Decreased heart rate and blood pressure. Suppression of arrhythmias. Prevention of MI.

Pharmacokinetics
Absorption: Well absorbed but undergoes extensive first-pass hepatic metabolism.
Distribution: Moderate CNS penetration. Crosses the placenta; enters breast milk.
Protein Binding: 93%.
Metabolism and Excretion: Almost completely metabolized by the liver (primarily for CYP2D6 isoenzyme) ▤ (the CYP2D6 enzyme system exhibits its genetic polymorphism; ~7% of population may be poor metabolizers and may have significantly ↑ propranolol concentrations and an ↑ risk of adverse effects).

Half-life: 3.4–6 hr.

TIME/ACTION PROFILE (cardiovascular effects)

ROUTE	ONSET	PEAK	DURATION
PO	30 min	60–90 min†	6–12 hr
PO–ER	unknown	6 hr	24 hr
IV	immediate	1 min	4–6 hr

†Following single dose, full effect not seen until several weeks of therapy

Contraindications/Precautions
Contraindicated in: Uncompensated CHF; Pulmonary edema; Cardiogenic shock; Bradycardia or heart block.
Use Cautiously in: Renal or hepatic impairment; Pulmonary disease (including asthma); Diabetes mellitus (may mask signs of hypoglycemia); Thyrotoxicosis (may mask symptoms); History of severe allergic reactions (may ↑ intensity of response); OB: Crosses the placenta and may cause fetal/neonatal bradycardia, hypotension, hypoglycemia, or respiratory depression. May also ↓ blood supply to the placenta, increase the risk for premature birth or fetal death, and cause intrauterine growth retardation. May ↑ risk of cardiac and pulmonary complications in the infant during the neonatal time frame. Lactation: Appears in breast milk; use formula if propranolol must be taken; Pedi: ↑ risk of hypoglycemia, especially during periods of fasting such as before surgery, during prolonged exertion, or with coexisting renal insufficiency; Geri: ↑ sensitivity to all beta blockers; initial dose reduction and careful titration recommended.

Adverse Reactions/Side Effects
CNS: <u>fatigue</u>, <u>weakness</u>, anxiety, dizziness, drowsiness, insomnia, memory loss, mental depression, mental status changes, nervousness, nightmares. **EENT:** blurred vision, dry eyes, nasal stuffiness. **Resp:** bronchospasm, wheezing. **CV:** ARRHYTHMIAS, BRADYCARDIA, CHF, PULMONARY EDEMA, orthostatic hypotension, peripheral vasoconstriction. **GI:** constipation, diarrhea, nausea. **GU:** <u>erectile dysfunction</u>, ↓ libido. **Derm:** itching, rashes. **Endo:** hyperglycemia, hypoglycemia (↑ in children). **MS:** arthralgia, back pain, muscle cramps. **Neuro:** paresthesia. **Misc:** drug-induced lupus syndrome.

Interactions
Drug-Drug: General anesthesia, IV phenytoin, and verapamil may cause additive myocar-

---

✦ = Canadian drug name. ▤ = Genetic implication.
*CAPITALS indicates life-threatening; underlines indicate most frequent.

propranolol

dial depression. Additive bradycardia may occur with **digoxin**. Additive hypotension may occur with other **antihypertensives**, acute ingestion of **alcohol**, or **nitrates**. Concurrent use with **amphetamines, cocaine, ephedrine, epinephrine, norepinephrine, phenylephrine**, or **pseudoephedrine** may result in unopposed alpha-adrenergic stimulation (excessive hypertension, bradycardia). Concurrent **thyroid** administration may ↓ effectiveness. May alter the effectiveness of **insulin** or **oral hypoglycemics** (dose adjustments may be necessary). May ↓ effectiveness of **beta-adrenergic bronchodilators** and **theophylline**. May ↓ beneficial beta cardiovascular effects of **dopamine** or **dobutamine**. Use cautiously within 14 days of **MAO inhibitor** therapy (may result in hypertension). **Cimetidine** may ↑ blood levels and toxicity. Concurrent **NSAIDs** may ↓ antihypertensive action. **Smoking** ↑ metabolism and ↓ effects; smoking cessation may ↑ effects.

Route/Dosage

PO (Adults): *Antianginal*—80–320 mg/day in 2–4 divided doses or once daily as extended/sustained-release capsules. *Antihypertensive*—40 mg twice daily initially; may be ↑ as needed (usual range 120–240 mg/day; doses up to 1 g/day have been used); *or* 80 mg once daily as extended/sustained-release capsules, ↑ as needed up to 120 mg. *InnoPran XL* dosing form is designed to be given once daily at bedtime. *Antiarrhythmic*—10–30 mg 3–4 times daily. *Prevention of MI*—180–240 mg/day in divided doses. *Hypertrophic cardiomyopathy*—20–40 mg 3–4 times daily. *Adjunct therapy of pheochromocytoma*—20 mg 3 times daily to 40 mg 3–4 times daily concurrently with alpha-blocking therapy, started 3 days before surgery is planned. *Vascular headache prevention*—20 mg 4 times daily *or* 80 mg/day as extended/sustained-release capsules; may be ↑ as needed up to 240 mg/day. *Management of tremor*—40 mg twice daily; may be ↑ up to 120 mg/day (up to 320 mg have been used).

PO (Children): *Antihypertensive/antiarrhythmic*—0.5–1 mg/kg/day in 2–4 divided doses; may be ↑ as needed (usual range for maintenance dose is 2–4 mg/kg/day in 2 divided doses).

IV (Adults): *Antiarrhythmic*—1–3 mg; may be repeated after 2 min and again in 4 hr if needed.

IV (Children): *Antiarrhythmic*—10–100 mcg (0.01–0.1 mg)/kg (up to 1 mg/dose); may be repeated q 6–8 hr if needed.

Availability (generic available)

Oral solution: 4 mg/mL, 8 mg/mL. **Cost:** *Generic*—4 mg/mL $38.54/480 mL. **Tablets:** 10 mg, 20 mg, 40 mg, 60 mg, 80 mg. **Cost:** *Generic*—10 mg $8.99/100, 20 mg $7.99/100, 40 mg $12.22/100, 60 mg $86.65/100, 80 mg $15.59/100. **Sustained-release capsules (Inderal LA):** 60 mg, 80 mg, 120 mg, 160 mg. **Cost:** 60 mg $132.98/90, 80 mg $141.97/90, 120 mg $176.80/90, 120 mg $230.05/90. **Extended-release capsules:** 60 mg, 80 mg, 120 mg, 160 mg. **Cost:** *Generic*—60 mg $99.99/90, 80 mg $141.97/90, 120 mg $176.80/90, 160 mg $230.05/90. **Injection:** 1 mg/mL. *In combination with:* hydrochlorothiazide (Inderide). See Appendix B.

NURSING IMPLICATIONS

Assessment

- Monitor blood pressure and pulse frequently during dose adjustment period and periodically during therapy.
- Abrupt withdrawal of propranolol may precipitate life-threatening arrhythmias, hypertension, or myocardial ischemia. Drug should be tapered over a 2-week period before discontinuation. Assess patient carefully during tapering and after medication is discontinued. Consider that patients taking propranolol for non-cardiac indications may have undiagnosed cardiac disease. Abrupt discontinuation or withdrawal over too-short a period of time (less than 9 days) should be avoided.
- Pedi: Assess pediatric patients for signs and symptoms of hypoglycemia, particularly when oral foods and fluids are restricted.
- Patients receiving **propranolol IV** must have continuous ECG monitoring and may have pulmonary capillary wedge pressure (PCWP) or central venous pressure (CVP) monitoring during and for several hours after administration.
- Assess for orthostatic hypotension when assisting patient up from supine position.
- Monitor intake and output ratios and daily weight. Assess patient routinely for evidence of fluid overload (peripheral edema, dyspnea, rales/crackles, fatigue, weight gain, jugular venous distention).
- **Angina:** Assess frequency and characteristics of anginal attacks periodically during therapy.
- **Vascular Headache Prophylaxis:** Assess frequency, severity, characteristics, and location of vascular headaches periodically during therapy.
- **PTSD:** Assess frequency of symptoms (flashbacks, nightmares, efforts to avoid thoughts or

activities that may trigger memories of the trauma, and hypervigilance) periodically throughout therapy.
- **Lab Test Considerations:** May cause ↑ BUN, serum lipoprotein, potassium, triglyceride, and uric acid levels.
- May cause ↑ ANA titers.
- May cause ↓ or ↑ in blood glucose levels. In labile diabetic patients, hypoglycemia may be accompanied by precipitous ↑ of blood pressure.
- ***Toxicity and Overdose:*** Monitor patients receiving beta blockers for signs of overdose (bradycardia, severe dizziness or fainting, severe drowsiness, dyspnea, bluish fingernails or palms, seizures). Notify health care professional immediately if these signs occur.
- Hypotension may be treated with modified Trendelenburg position and IV fluids unless contraindicated. Vasopressors (epinephrine, norepinephrine, dopamine, dobutamine) may also be used. Hypotension does not respond to beta agonists.
- Glucagon has been used to treat bradycardia and hypotension.

Potential Nursing Diagnoses
Decreased cardiac output (Side Effects)
Noncompliance (Patient/Family Teaching)

Implementation
- **High Alert:** IV vasoactive medications are inherently dangerous. Before administering intravenously, have second practitioner independently check the original order, dose calculations, and infusion pump settings. Also, patient harm or fatalities have occurred when switching from oral to IV *propranolol*; oral and parenteral doses are not interchangeable. IV dose is 1/10 of the oral dose. Change to oral therapy as soon as possible. Do not confuse propranolol with pravachol. Do not confuse Inderal (a brand name of propranolol) with Adderall (an amphetamine/dextroamphetamine combination drug).
- **PO:** Take apical pulse prior to administering. If <50 bpm or if arrhythmia occurs, withhold medication and notify physician or other health care professional.
- Administer with meals or directly after eating to enhance absorption.
- Extended-release capsules should be swallowed whole; do not crush, open, or chew.

Propranolol tablets may be crushed and mixed with food.
- Mix propranolol oral solution with liquid or semisolid food (water, juices, applesauce, puddings). To ensure entire dose is taken, rinse glass with more liquid or have patient consume all of the applesauce or pudding. Do not store after mixing.

IV Administration
- **Direct IV:** ***Diluent:*** Administer undiluted or dilute each 1 mg in 10 mL of D5W for injection. ***Concentration:*** Undiluted: 1 mg/mL. Diluted in 10 mL of D5W: 0.1 mg/mL. ***Rate:*** Administer at 0.5 mg/ min for adults to avoid hypotension and cardiac arrest; do not exceed 1 mg/min. Pedi: Administer over 10 min.
- **Intermittent Infusion:** ***Diluent:*** May be diluted in 50 mL of 0.9% NaCl, D5W, D5/0.45% NaCl, D5/0.9% NaCl, or lactated Ringer's injection. ***Concentration:*** Depends on dose. ***Rate:*** Infuse over 10–15 min.
- **Y-Site Compatibility:** acyclovir, alfentanil, alteplase, amikacin, aminophylline, anidulafungin, ascorbic acid, atracurium, atropine, azathioprine, aztreonam, benztropine, bivalirudin, bumetanide, buprenorphine, butorphanol, calcium chloride, calcium gluconate, carboplatin, caspofungin, cefazolin, cefonocid, cefoperazone, cefotetan, ceftazidime, ceftizoxime, ceftriaxone, cefuroxime, chloramphenicol, chlorpromazine, cimetidine, cisplatin, clindamycin, cyanocobalamin, cyclophosphamide, cyclosporine, cytarabine, dactinomycin, daptomycin, dexamethasone, dexmedetomidine, digoxin, diltiazem, diphenhydramine, dobutamine, docetaxel, dopamine, doxacurium, doxorubicin, doxycycline, enalaprilat, ephedrine, epinephrine, epirubicin, epoetin alfa, eptifibatide, ertapenem, erythromycin, esmolol, etoposide, etoposide phosphate, famotidine, fenoldopam, fentanyl, fluconazole, fludarabine, fluorouracil, folic acid, furosemide, ganciclovir, gemcitabine, gentamicin, glycopyrrolate, granisetron, heparin, hetastarch, hydrocortisone, hydromorphone, idarubicin, ifosfamide, imipenem/cilastatin, inamrinone, isoproterenol, ketorolac, labetalol, levofloxacin, lidocaine, linezolid, lorazepam, magnesium sulfate, mannitol, mechlorethamine, meperidine, metaraminol, methotrexate, methoxamine, methyldopate, methylprednisolone, metoclopramide, metoprolol, metronida-

zole, midazolam, milrinone, mitoxantrone, morphine, multivitamins, nafcillin, nalbuphine, naloxone, nesiritide, nitroglycerin, nitroprusside, norepinephrine, octreotide, ondansetron, oxacillin, oxaliplatin, oxytocin, palonosetron, pancuronium, papaverine, pemetrexed, penicillin G, pentamidine, pentazocine, pentobarbital, phenobarbital, phentolamine, phenylephrine, phytonadione, potassium chloride, procainamide, prochlorperazine, promethazine, propofol, protamine, pyridoxime, quinupristin/dalfopristin, ranitidine, rocuronium, sodium acetate, sodium bicarbonate, streptokinase, succinylcholine, sufentanil, tacrolimus, teniposide, theophylline, thiamine, thiotepa, ticarcillin/clavulanate, tigecycline, tirofiban, tobramycin, tolazoline, trimetaphan, urokinase, vancomycin, vasopressin, vecuronium, verapamil, vincristine, vinorelbine, vitamin B complex with C, voriconazole.
- **Y-Site Incompatibility:** amphotericin B cholesteryl, amphotericin B colloidal, amphotericin B liposome, dantrolene, diazepam, diazoxide, indomethacin, insulin, paclitaxel, pantoprazole, phenytoin, piperacillin/tazobactam, trimethoprim/sulfamethoxazole.

Patient/Family Teaching
- Instruct patient to take medication as directed, at the same time each day, even if feeling well; do not skip or double up on missed doses. Take missed doses as soon as possible up to 4 hr before next dose (8 hr with extended-release propranolol). Inform patient that abrupt withdrawal can cause life-threatening arrhythmias, hypertension, or myocardial ischemia.
- Advise patient to make sure enough medication is available for weekends, holidays, and vacations. A written prescription may be kept in wallet in case of emergency.
- Teach patient and family how to check pulse daily and blood pressure biweekly. Advise patient to hold dose and contact health care professional if pulse is <50 bpm or blood pressure changes significantly.
- May cause drowsiness or dizziness. Caution patients to avoid driving or other activities that require alertness until response to the drug is known.
- Advise patients to change positions slowly to minimize orthostatic hypotension, especially during initiation of therapy or when dose is increased.
- Caution patient that this medication may increase sensitivity to cold.
- Instruct patient to ask a health care professional before taking any OTC medications or herbal products, especially cold preparations, when taking this medication.
- Diabetic patients should closely monitor blood glucose, especially if weakness, malaise, irritability, or fatigue occurs. May mask tachycardia and increased blood pressure as signs of hypoglycemia, but dizziness and sweating may still occur.
- Advise patient to notify health care professional if slow pulse, difficulty breathing, wheezing, cold hands and feet, dizziness, light-headedness, confusion, depression, rash, fever, sore throat, unusual bleeding, or bruising occurs.
- Instruct patient to inform health care professional of medication regimen prior to treatment or surgery.
- Advise patient to carry identification describing disease process and medication regimen at all times.
- **Hypertension:** Reinforce the need to continue additional therapies for hypertension (weight loss, sodium restriction, stress reduction, regular exercise, moderation of alcohol consumption, and smoking cessation). Medication controls but does not cure hypertension.
- **Angina:** Caution patient to avoid overexertion with decrease in chest pain.
- **Vascular Headache Prophylaxis:** Caution patient that sharing this medication may be dangerous.
- **PTSD:** Advise patient that medication may relieve distressing symptoms but that psychotherapy is the primary treatment for the disorder. Refer patient and family to a PTSD support group.

Evaluation/Desired Outcomes
- Decrease in blood pressure.
- Control of arrhythmias without appearance of detrimental side effects.
- Reduction in frequency of anginal attacks.
- Increase in activity tolerance.
- Prevention of MI.
- Prevention of vascular headaches.
- Management of thyrotoxicosis.
- Management of pheochromocytoma.
- Decrease in tremors.
- Management of hypertrophic cardiomyopathy.
- Decrease in symptoms associated with PTSD.

---

propylthiouracil
(proe-pill-thye-oh-**yoor**-a-sill)
✤ Propyl-Thyracil, PTU

propylthiouracil

Classification
Therapeutic: antithyroid agents

Pregnancy Category D

Indications
Palliative treatment of hyperthyroidism. Adjunct in the control of hyperthyroidism in preparation for thyroidectomy or radioactive iodine therapy.

Action
Inhibits the synthesis of thyroid hormones. **Therapeutic Effects:** Decreased signs and symptoms of hyperthyroidism.

Pharmacokinetics
Absorption: Rapidly absorbed from the GI tract.
Distribution: Concentrates in the thyroid gland; crosses the placenta and enters breast milk in low concentrations.
Metabolism and Excretion: Metabolized by the liver.
Half-life: 1–2 hr.

TIME/ACTION PROFILE (effects on clinical thyroid status)

ROUTE	ONSET	PEAK	DURATION
PO	10–21 days†	6–10 wk	wk

†Effects on serum thyroid hormone concentration may occur within 60 min of a single dose

Contraindications/Precautions
Contraindicated in: Hypersensitivity.
Use Cautiously in: ↓ bone marrow reserve; OB: May be used safely; however, fetus may develop thyroid problems; Lactation: Safety not established; Pedi: Children <6 yr (safety not established).

Adverse Reactions/Side Effects
CNS: drowsiness, headache, vertigo. **GI:** HEPATOTOXICITY, nausea, vomiting, diarrhea, loss of taste. **Derm:** rash, skin discoloration, urticaria. **Endo:** hypothyroidism. **Hemat:** AGRANULOCYTOSIS, leukopenia, thrombocytopenia. **MS:** arthralgia. **Misc:** fever, lymphadenopathy, parotitis.

Interactions
Drug-Drug: Additive bone marrow depression with **antineoplastics** or **radiation therapy**. Additive antithyroid effects with **lithium**, **potassium iodide**, or **sodium iodide**. ↑ risk of agranulocytosis with **phenothiazines**.

Route/Dosage
PO (Adults): *Thyrotoxic crisis*—200–400 mg q 4 hr during the first 24 hr. *Hyperthyroidism*—300–900 mg once daily or in 2–4 divided doses initially (up to 1.2 g/day); maintenance dose 50–600 mg/day once daily or in 2–4 divided doses.
PO (Children >10 yr): 50–300 mg/day given once daily or in 2–4 divided doses.
PO (Children 6–10 yr): 50–150 mg/day given once daily or in 2–4 divided doses.

Availability (generic available)
Tablets: 50 mg, ✤ 100 mg.

NURSING IMPLICATIONS

Assessment
- Monitor response of symptoms of hyperthyroidism or thyrotoxicosis (tachycardia, palpitations, nervousness, insomnia, fever, diaphoresis, heat intolerance, tremors, weight loss, diarrhea).
- Assess patient for development of hypothyroidism (intolerance to cold, constipation, dry skin, headache, listlessness, tiredness, or weakness). Dose adjustment may be required.
- Assess patient for skin rash or swelling of cervical lymph nodes. Treatment may be discontinued if this occurs.
- **Lab Test Considerations:** Thyroid function studies should be monitored prior to therapy, monthly during initial therapy, and every 2–3 mo throughout therapy.
- WBC and differential counts should be monitored periodically throughout course of therapy. Agranulocytosis may develop rapidly and usually occurs during first 2 mo. This necessitates discontinuation of therapy.
- May cause increased AST, ALT, LDH, alkaline phosphatase, serum bilirubin, and prothrombin time.

Potential Nursing Diagnoses
Deficient knowledge, related to medication regimen (Patient/Family Teaching)
Noncompliance (Patient/Family Teaching)

Implementation
- Do not confuse propylthiouracil with Purinethol (mercaptopurine).
- Can be compounded by pharmacist into enema or suppository.
- **PO:** Administer at same time in relation to meals every day. Food may either increase or decrease absorption.

Patient/Family Teaching
- Instruct patient to take medication exactly as directed, around the clock. If a dose is missed,

✤ = Canadian drug name. ▤ = Genetic implication.
*CAPITALS indicates life-threatening; underlines indicate most frequent.

take as soon as remembered; take both doses together if almost time for next dose; check with health care professional if more than 1 dose is missed. Consult health care professional prior to discontinuing medication.
- Instruct patient to monitor weight 2–3 times weekly. Report significant changes.
- May cause drowsiness. Caution patient to avoid driving or other activities requiring alertness until response to medication is known.
- Advise patient to consult health care professional regarding dietary sources of iodine (iodized salt, shellfish).
- Advise patient to report sore throat, fever, chills, headache, malaise, weakness, yellowing of eyes or skin, unusual bleeding or bruising, symptoms of hyperthyroidism or hypothyroidism, or rash to health care professional promptly.
- Instruct patient to consult health care professional before taking any OTC medications containing iodine concurrently with this medication.
- Advise patient to carry identification describing medication regimen at all times and to notify health care professional of medication regimen prior to treatment or surgery.
- Emphasize the importance of routine exams to monitor progress and to check for side effects.

Evaluation/Desired Outcomes
- Decrease in severity of symptoms of hyperthyroidism (lowered pulse rate and weight gain).
- Return of thyroid function studies to normal.
- May be used as short-term adjunctive therapy to prepare patient for thyroidectomy or radiation therapy or may be used in treatment of hyperthyroidism. Treatment of 6 mo to several yr may be necessary, usually averaging 1 yr.

---

protamine sulfate
(proe-ta-meen)

Classification
Therapeutic: antidotes
Pharmacologic: antiheparins

Pregnancy Category C

Indications
Acute management of severe heparin overdosage. Used to neutralize heparin received during dialysis, cardiopulmonary bypass, and other procedures. **Unlabeled Use:** Management of overdose of heparin-like compounds.

Action
A strong base that forms a complex with heparin (an acid). **Therapeutic Effects:** Inactivation of heparin.

Pharmacokinetics
Absorption: Administered IV only, resulting in complete bioavailability.
Distribution: Unknown.
Metabolism and Excretion: Metabolic fate not known. Protamine-heparin complex eventually degrades.
Half-life: Unknown.

TIME/ACTION PROFILE (reversal of heparin effect)

ROUTE	ONSET	PEAK	DURATION
IV	30 sec–1 min	unknown	2 hr†

†Depends on body temperature

Contraindications/Precautions
Contraindicated in: Hypersensitivity to protamine or fish.
Use Cautiously in: Patients who have received previous protamine-containing insulin or vasectomized men (↑ risk of hypersensitivity reactions); OB: Lactation: Pedi: Safety not established.

Adverse Reactions/Side Effects
Resp: dyspnea. **CV:** bradycardia, hypertension, hypotension, pulmonary hypertension. **GI:** nausea, vomiting. **Derm:** flushing, warmth. **Hemat:** bleeding. **MS:** back pain. **Misc:** hypersensitivity reactions, including ANAPHYLAXIS, ANGIOEDEMA, and PULMONARY EDEMA.

Interactions
Drug-Drug: None significant.

Route/Dosage
IV (Adults and Children): *Heparin overdose*—1 mg/100 units of heparin. If given >30 min after heparin, give 0.5 mg/100 units of heparin (not to exceed 100 mg/2 hr). Further doses should be determined by coagulation tests. If heparin was administered subcutaneously, use 1–1.5 mg protamine per 100 units of heparin, give 25–50 mg of the protamine dose slowly followed by a continuous infusion over 8–16 hours. *Enoxaparin overdose*—1 mg/each mg of enoxaparin to be neutralized (unlabeled). *Dalteparin overdose*—1 mg/100 anti-Xa IU of dalteparin. If required, a second dose of 0.5 mg/100 anti-Xa IU of dalteparin may be given 2–4 hr later if laboratory assessment indicates need (unlabeled).

Availability (generic available)
Injection: 10 mg/mL.

NURSING IMPLICATIONS
Assessment
- Assess for bleeding and hemorrhage throughout therapy. Hemorrhage may recur 8–9 hr after therapy because of rebound effects of heparin. Rebound may occur as late as 18 hr after therapy in patients heparinized for cardiopulmonary bypass.
- Assess for allergy to fish (salmon), previous reaction to or use of protamine insulin or protamine sulfate. Vasectomized and infertile men also have higher risk of hypersensitivity reaction.
- Observe patient for signs and symptoms of hypersensitivity reaction (hives, edema, coughing, wheezing). Keep epinephrine, an antihistamine, and resuscitative equipment close by in the event of anaphylaxis.
- Assess for hypovolemia before initiation of therapy. Failure to correct hypovolemia may result in cardiovascular collapse from peripheral vasodilating effects of protamine sulfate.
- *Lab Test Considerations:* Monitor clotting factors, activated clotting time (ACT), activated partial thromboplastin time (aPTT), and thrombin time (TT) 5–15 min after therapy and again as necessary.

Potential Nursing Diagnoses
Risk for injury (Indications)
Ineffective tissue perfusion (Indications)

Implementation
- Discontinue heparin infusion. In milder cases, overdosage may be treated by heparin withdrawal alone.
- In severe cases, fresh frozen plasma or whole blood may also be required to control bleeding.
- Dose varies with type of heparin, route of heparin therapy, and amount of time elapsed since discontinuation of heparin.
- Do not administer >100 mg in 2 hr without rechecking clotting studies, as protamine sulfate has its own anticoagulant properties.

IV Administration
- **Direct IV:** *Diluent:* May be administered undiluted. If further dilution is desired, D5W or 0.9% NaCl may be used. *Concentration:* 10 mg/mL. *Rate:* Administer by slow IV push over 1–3 min. Rapid infusion rate may result in hypotension, bradycardia, flushing, or feeling of warmth. If these symptoms occur, stop infusion and notify physician. No more than 50 mg should be administered within a 10–min period.
- **Y-Site Compatibility:** amikacin, aminophylline, atropine, aztreonam, bumetanide, calcium chloride, calcium gluconate, cimetidine, clindamycin, cyclosporine, digoxin, diphenhydramine, doxycycline, enalaprilat, epinephrine, erythromycin, esmolol, famotidine, fentanyl, fluconazole, ganciclovir, gentamicin, hydroxyzine, imipenem/cilastatin, isoproterenol, labetalol, lidocaine, meperidine, metoclopramide, metoprolol, metronidazole, midazolam, morphine, nitroglycerin, nitroprusside, norepinephrine, ondansetron, phenylephrine, potassium chloride, procainamide, prochlorperazine, promethazine, propranolol, ranitidine, sodium bicarbonate, tobramycin, vancomycin, verapamil.
- **Y-Site Incompatibility:** ampicillin, ampicillin/sulbactam, cefazolin, cefotaxime, cefoxitin, ceftazidime, cefuroxime, chloramphenicol, dexamethasone sodium phosphate, diazepam, furosemide, hydrocortisone sodium succinate, insulin, ketorolac, methylprednisolone sodium succinate, nafcillin, penicillin G potassium, phenytoin, ticarcillin/clavulanate, trimethoprim/sulfamethoxazole.

Patient/Family Teaching
- Explain purpose of the medication to patient. Instruct patient to report recurrent bleeding immediately.
- Advise patient to avoid activities that may result in bleeding (shaving, brushing teeth, receiving injections or rectal temperatures, or ambulating) until risk of hemorrhage has passed.

Evaluation/Desired Outcomes
- Control of bleeding.
- Normalization of clotting factors in heparinized patients.

---

pseudoephedrine
(soo-doe-e-**fed**-rin)
✤ Balminil Decongestant Syrup, Cenafed, Congestaid, Decofed, Dimetapp Maximum Strength 12–Hour Non-Drowsy Extentabs, Dimetapp Decongestant Pediatric, Drixoral 12 Hour Non-Drowsy Formula, Efidac 24, ✤ Eltor 120, Genafed, Halofed, Kid Kare, Medi-First Sinus Decongestant,

---

✤ = Canadian drug name. ☗ = Genetic implication.
*CAPITALS indicates life-threatening; underlines indicate most frequent.

pseudoephedrine

PediaCare Infants' Decongestant Drops, Pediatric Nasal Decongestant, Simply Stuffy, Sinustop, ✤ Robidrine, Silfedrine, Sudafed, Sudafed Childrens's Non-Drowsy, Sudafed 12 Hour, Sudafed Non-Drowsy Maximum Strength, Sudodrin, Triaminic Allergy Congestion Softchews, Unifed

Classification
Therapeutic: allergy, cold, and cough remedies, nasal drying agents/decongestants
Pharmacologic: adrenergics

Pregnancy Category B

Indications
Symptomatic management of nasal congestion associated with acute viral upper respiratory tract infections. Used in combination with antihistamines in the management of allergic conditions. Used to open obstructed eustachian tubes in chronic otic inflammation or infection.

Action
Stimulates alpha- and beta-adrenergic receptors. Produces vasoconstriction in the respiratory tract mucosa (alpha-adrenergic stimulation) and possibly bronchodilation ($beta_2$-adrenergic stimulation). **Therapeutic Effects:** Reduction of nasal congestion, hyperemia, and swelling in nasal passages.

Pharmacokinetics
Absorption: Well absorbed after oral administration.
Distribution: Appears to enter the CSF; probably crosses the placenta and enters breast milk.
Metabolism and Excretion: Partially metabolized by the liver. 55–75% excreted unchanged by the kidneys (depends on urine pH).
Half-life: Children: 3.1 hr; Adults: 9–16 hr (depends on urine pH).

TIME/ACTION PROFILE (decongestant effects)

ROUTE	ONSET	PEAK	DURATION
PO	15–30 min	unknown	4–6 hr
PO-ER	60 min	unknown	12 hr

Contraindications/Precautions
Contraindicated in: Hypersensitivity to sympathomimetic amines; Hypertension; severe coronary artery disease; Concurrent MAO inhibitor therapy; Known alcohol intolerance (some liquid products).
Use Cautiously in: Hyperthyroidism; Diabetes mellitus; Prostatic hyperplasia; Ischemic heart disease; Glaucoma; OB, Lactation: Safety not established; Pedi: Avoid OTC cough and cold products containing this medication in children <4 yr.

Adverse Reactions/Side Effects
CNS: SEIZURES, anxiety, nervousness, dizziness, drowsiness, excitability, fear, hallucinations, headache, insomnia, restlessness, weakness.
Resp: respiratory difficulty. **CV:** CARDIOVASCULAR COLLAPSE, palpitations, hypertension, tachycardia.
GI: anorexia, dry mouth. **GU:** dysuria. **Misc:** diaphoresis.

Interactions
Drug-Drug: Concurrent use with **MAO inhibitors** may cause hypertensive crisis. Additive adrenergic effects with other **adrenergics**. Concurrent use with **beta blockers** may result in hypertension or bradycardia. **Drugs that acidify the urine** may ↓ effectiveness. **Phenothiazines** and **tricyclic antidepressants** potentiate pressor effects. **Drugs that alkalinize the urine (sodium bicarbonate, high-dose antacid therapy)** may intensify effectiveness.
Drug-Food: Foods that acidify the urine may ↓ effectiveness. **Foods that alkalinize the urine** may intensify effectiveness (see lists in Appendix M).

Route/Dosage
PO (Adults and Children >12 yr): 60 mg q 6 hr as needed (not to exceed 240 mg/day) *or* 120 mg extended-release preparation q 12 hr *or* 240 mg extended-release preparation q 24 hr.
PO (Children 6–12 yr): 30 mg q 6 hr as needed (not to exceed 120 mg/day).
PO (Children 4–5 yr): 15 mg q 6 hr (not to exceed 60 mg/day).

Availability (generic available)
Tablets: 30 mg^{OTC}, 60 mg^{OTC}. **Extended-release tablets:** 120 mg^{OTC}. **Controlled-release tablets:** 240 mg^{OTC}. **Capsules:** ✤ 60 mg^{OTC}. **Extended-release capsules:** ✤ 240 mg^{OTC}. **Softgel capsules:** 30 mg^{OTC}. **Liquid (grape and others):** 15 mg/5 mL^{OTC}, 30 mg/5 mL^{OTC}. **Drops (cherry and fruit flavor):** 7.5 mg/0.8 mL ^{OTC}. *In combination with:* antihistamines, acetaminophen, cough suppressants, and expectorants^{OTC}. See Appendix B.

NURSING IMPLICATIONS

Assessment
- Assess congestion (nasal, sinus, eustachian tube) before and periodically during therapy.
- Monitor pulse and blood pressure before beginning therapy and periodically during therapy.

- Assess lung sounds and character of bronchial secretions. Maintain fluid intake of 1500–2000 mL/day to decrease viscosity of secretions.

Potential Nursing Diagnoses
Ineffective airway clearance (Indications)

Implementation
- Administer pseudoephedrine at least 2 hr before bedtime to minimize insomnia.
- **PO:** Extended-release tablets and capsules should be swallowed whole; do not crush, break, or chew. Contents of the capsule can be mixed with jam or jelly and swallowed without chewing for patients with difficulty swallowing.

Patient/Family Teaching
- Instruct patient to take medication as directed and not to take more than recommended. Take missed doses within 1 hr; if remembered later, omit. Do not double doses. Caution parents to avoid OTC cough and cold products while breastfeeding or to children <4 yr.
- Instruct patient to notify health care professional if nervousness, slow or fast heart rate, breathing difficulties, hallucinations, or seizures occur, because these symptoms may indicate overdose.
- Instruct patient to contact health care professional if symptoms do not improve within 7 days or if fever is present.

Evaluation/Desired Outcomes
- Decreased nasal, sinus, or eustachian tube congestion.

---

psyllium (sill-i-yum)
Alramucil, Cillium, Effer-Syllium, Fiberall, Fibrepur, Hydrocil, ✤Karacil, Konsyl, Metamucil, Modane Bulk, Mylanta Natural Fiber Supplement, Naturacil Caramels, ✤Natural Source Fibre Laxative, Perdiem, ✤Prodiem, Pro-Lax, Reguloid Natural, Serutan, Siblin, Syllact, Vitalax, V-Lax

Classification
Therapeutic: laxatives
Pharmacologic: bulk-forming agents

Pregnancy Category UK

Indications
Management of simple or chronic constipation, particularly if associated with a low-fiber diet. Useful in situations in which straining should be avoided (after MI, rectal surgery, prolonged bed rest). Used in the management of chronic watery diarrhea.

Action
Combines with water in the intestinal contents to form an emollient gel or viscous solution that promotes peristalsis and reduces transit time. **Therapeutic Effects:** Relief and prevention of constipation.

Pharmacokinetics
Absorption: Not absorbed from the GI tract.
Distribution: No distribution occurs.
Metabolism and Excretion: Excreted in feces.
Half-life: Unknown.

TIME/ACTION PROFILE (laxative effect)

ROUTE	ONSET	PEAK	DURATION
PO	12–24 hr	2–3 days	unknown

Contraindications/Precautions
Contraindicated in: Hypersensitivity; Abdominal pain, nausea, or vomiting (especially when associated with fever); Serious adhesions; Dysphagia.
Use Cautiously in: Some dosage forms contain sugar, aspartame, or excessive sodium and should be avoided in patients on restricted diets; OB: Lactation: Has been used safely.

Adverse Reactions/Side Effects
Resp: bronchospasm. **GI:** cramps, intestinal or esophageal obstruction, nausea, vomiting.

Interactions
Drug-Drug: May ↓ absorption of **warfarin, salicylates**, or **digoxin**.

Route/Dosage
PO (Adults): 1–2 tsp/packet/wafer (3–6 g psyllium) in or with a full glass of liquid 2–3 times daily. Up to 30 g daily in divided doses.
PO (Children >6 yr): 1 tsp/packet/wafer (1.5–3 g psyllium) in or with 4–8 oz glass of liquid 2–3 times daily. Up to 15 g daily in divided doses.

Availability (generic available)
Powder: 3.3–3.5 g/dose or packet[OTC]. **Effervescent powder:** 3–3.5 g/dose or packet[OTC]. **Granules:** 2.5 g/dose[OTC]. **Wafers:** 3.4 g/dose[OTC].

✤ = Canadian drug name. ▮ = Genetic implication.
*CAPITALS indicates life-threatening; underlines indicate most frequent.

NURSING IMPLICATIONS
Assessment
- Assess patient for abdominal distention, presence of bowel sounds, and usual pattern of bowel function.
- Assess color, consistency, and amount of stool produced.
- *Lab Test Considerations:* May cause elevated blood glucose levels with prolonged use of preparations containing sugar.

Potential Nursing Diagnoses
Constipation (Indications)

Implementation
- Packets are not standardized for volume, but each contains 3–3.5 g of psyllium.
- **PO:** Administer with a full glass of water or juice, followed by an additional glass of liquid. Solution should be taken immediately after mixing; it will congeal. Do not administer without sufficient fluid and do not chew granules.

Patient/Family Teaching
- Encourage patient to use other forms of bowel regulation, such as increasing bulk in the diet, increasing fluid intake, and increasing mobility. Normal bowel habits are individualized and may vary from 3 times/day to 3 times/wk.
- May be used for long-term management of chronic constipation.
- Instruct patients with cardiac disease to avoid straining during bowel movements (Valsalva maneuver).
- Advise patient not to use laxatives when abdominal pain, nausea, vomiting, or fever is present.

Evaluation/Desired Outcomes
- A soft, formed bowel movement, usually within 12–24 hr. May require 3 days of therapy for results.

---

pyrazinamide
(peer-a-**zin**-a-mide)
✤ PMS Pyrazinamide, ✤ Tebrazid

Classification
Therapeutic: antituberculars

Pregnancy Category C

Indications
Used in combination with other agents in the treatment of active tuberculosis.

Action
Mechanism not known. **Therapeutic Effects:** Bacteriostatic action against susceptible mycobacteria. **Spectrum:** Active against mycobacteria only.

Pharmacokinetics
Absorption: Well absorbed after oral administration.
Distribution: Widely distributed. Reaches high concentrations in the CNS (same as plasma). Excreted in breast milk.
Metabolism and Excretion: Mostly metabolized by the liver. Metabolite (pyrazinoic acid) has antimycobacterial activity; 3–4% excreted unchanged by the kidneys.
Half-life: *Pyrazinamide*—9.5 hr. *Pyrazinoic acid*—12 hr. Both are prolonged in renal impairment.

TIME/ACTION PROFILE (blood levels)

ROUTE	ONSET	PEAK	DURATION
PO	unknown	1–2 hr (4–5 hr†)	24 hr

†For pyrazinoic acid

Contraindications/Precautions
Contraindicated in: Hypersensitivity; Cross-sensitivity with ethionamide, isoniazid, niacin, or nicotinic acid may exist; Severe liver impairment.
Use Cautiously in: Gout; Diabetes mellitus; Acute intermittent porphyria; OB: Safety not established.

Adverse Reactions/Side Effects
GI: HEPATOTOXICITY, anorexia, diarrhea, nausea, vomiting. **GU:** dysuria. **Derm:** acne, itching, photosensitivity, skin rash. **Hemat:** anemia, thrombocytopenia. **Metab:** hyperuricemia. **MS:** arthralgia, gouty arthritis.

Interactions
Drug-Drug: Concurrent use with **rifampin** may result in life-threatening hepatoxicity and should be avoided. May ↓ blood levels and effectiveness of **cyclosporine**. May ↓ effectiveness of **antigout agents**.

Route/Dosage
PO (Adults and Children): 15–30 mg/kg/day as a single dose. Up to 60 mg/kg/day has been used in isoniazid-resistant tuberculosis (not to exceed 2 g/day as a single dose or 3 g/day in divided doses). May also be given as 50–70 mg/kg 2–3 times weekly (not to exceed 2 g/dose on daily regimen, 3 g/dose for 3-times-weekly regimen, or 4 g/dose for twice-weekly regimen). *Patients with HIV*—20–30 mg/kg/day for first 2 mo of therapy; further dosing depends on regimen employed.

Availability (generic available)
Tablets: 500 mg. *In combination with:* rifampin and isoniazid (Rifater). See Appendix B.

NURSING IMPLICATIONS
Assessment
- Perform mycobacterial studies and susceptibility tests before and periodically during therapy to detect possible resistance.
- **Lab Test Considerations:** Evaluate hepatic function before and every 2–4 wk during therapy. Increased AST and ALT may not be predictive of clinical hepatitis and may return to normal levels during treatment. Patients with impaired liver function should receive pyrazinamide therapy only if crucial to treatment.
- Monitor serum uric acid concentrations during therapy. May cause ↑ resulting in precipitation of acute gout.
- May interfere with urine ketone determinations.

Potential Nursing Diagnoses
Risk for infection (Indications)
Noncompliance (Patient/Family Teaching)

Implementation
- **PO:** May be given concurrently with isoniazid.

Patient/Family Teaching
- Advise patient to take medication as directed and not to skip doses or double up on missed doses. Take missed doses as soon as remembered unless almost time for next dose. Emphasize the importance of continuing therapy even after symptoms have subsided. Length of therapy depends on regimen being used and underlying disease states.
- Inform diabetic patients that pyrazinamide may interfere with urine ketone measurements.
- Advise patients to notify health care professional if no improvement is noticed after 2–3 wk of therapy or if fever, anorexia, malaise, nausea, vomiting, darkened urine, yellowish discoloration of the skin and eyes, pain, or swelling of the joints occurs.
- Advise patients to use sunscreen and protective clothing to prevent photosensitivity reactions.
- Emphasize the importance of regular follow-up exams to monitor progress and check for side effects.

Evaluation/Desired Outcomes
- Resolution of signs and symptoms of tuberculosis.
- Negative sputum cultures.

---

pyridostigmine
(peer-id-oh-**stig**-meen)
Mestinon, ✻Mestinon SR, Mestinon Timespan, Regonol

Classification
Therapeutic: antimyasthenics
Pharmacologic: cholinergics

Pregnancy Category C

Indications
Used to increase muscle strength in the symptomatic treatment of myasthenia gravis. Reversal of nondepolarizing neuromuscular blocking agents. Prophylaxis of lethal effects of poisoning with the nerve agent soman.

Action
Inhibits the breakdown of acetylcholine and prolongs its effects (anticholinesterase). Effects include: Miosis, Increased intestinal and skeletal muscle tone, Bronchial and ureteral constriction, Bradycardia, Increased salivation, Lacrimation, Sweating. **Therapeutic Effects:** Improved muscular function in patients with myasthenia gravis. Reversal of paralysis from nondepolarizing neuromuscular blocking agents. Prevention of Soman nerve gas toxicity.

Pharmacokinetics
Absorption: Poorly absorbed after oral administration, necessitating large oral doses compared with parenteral doses.
Distribution: Appears to cross the placenta.
Metabolism and Excretion: Metabolized by plasma cholinesterases and the liver.
Half-life: *PO*—3.7 hr; *IV*—1.9 hr.

TIME/ACTION PROFILE (cholinergic effects)

ROUTE	ONSET	PEAK	DURATION
PO	30–35 min	unknown	3–6 hr
PO-SR	30–60 min	unknown	6–12 hr
IM	15 min	unknown	2–4 hr
IV	2–5 min	unknown	2–3 hr

Contraindications/Precautions
Contraindicated in: Hypersensitivity to pyridostigmine or bromides; Mechanical obstruction of the GI or GU tract; Known alcohol intolerance (syrup only).
Use Cautiously in: History of asthma; Ulcer disease; Cardiovascular disease; Epilepsy; Hyperthyroidism; OB: May cause uterine irritability after IV administration near term; 20% of newborns dis-

pyridostigmine

play transient muscle weakness; Lactation: Pedi: Safety not established.

Adverse Reactions/Side Effects
CNS: SEIZURES, dizziness, weakness. **EENT:** lacrimation, miosis. **Resp:** bronchospasm, excessive secretions. **CV:** bradycardia, hypotension. **GI:** abdominal cramps, diarrhea, excessive salivation, nausea, vomiting. **Derm:** sweating, rashes.

Interactions
Drug-Drug: Cholinergic effects may be antagonized by other **drugs possessing anticholinergic properties**, including **antihistamines, antidepressants, atropine, haloperidol, phenothiazines, procainamide, quinidine**, or **disopyramide**. Prolongs the action of **depolarizing muscle-relaxing agents** and **cholinesterase inhibitors (succinylcholine, decamethonium)**. ↑ toxicity with other **cholinesterase inhibitors**, including **echothiophate**.

Route/Dosage
Myasthenia Gravis
PO (Adults): *Tablets/syrup*—30–60 mg q 3–4 hr initially; then adjusted as required; usual maintenance dose is 600 mg/day in divided doses (range 60–1500 mg/day). *Extended-release tablets*—180–540 mg 1–2 times daily (dosing interval should be at least 6 hr; may be associated with increased risk of cholinergic crisis; concurrent immediate-release products may be required).
PO (Children): 7 mg/kg (200 mg/m^2)/day in 5–6 divided doses.
IM, IV (Adults): 2 mg ($\frac{1}{30}$ of oral dose); may be repeated q 2–3 hr. *During labor/delivery*—1 mg before second stage of labor is complete.
IM (Neonates Born to Myasthenic Mothers): 50–150 mcg/kg q 4–6 hr.

Antidote for Nondepolarizing Neuromuscular Blocking Agents
IV (Adults): 10–20 mg; pretreat with 0.6–1.2 mg atropine IV.

Prevention of Soman Nerve Gas Effects
PO (Adults): 30 mg every 8 hr before exposure, stopped on exposure to gas.

Availability (generic available)
Tablets: 60 mg. **Extended-release tablets:** 180 mg. **Syrup:** 60 mg/5 mL. **Injection:** 5 mg/mL.

NURSING IMPLICATIONS
Assessment
- Assess pulse, respiratory rate, and blood pressure before administration. Report significant changes in heart rate.
- **Myasthenia Gravis:** Assess neuromuscular status, including vital capacity, ptosis, diplopia, chewing, swallowing, hand grasp, and gait before administering and at peak effect. Patients with myasthenia gravis may be advised to keep a daily record of their condition and the effects of this medication.
- Assess patient for overdose, underdose, or resistance. Both have similar symptoms (muscle weakness, dyspnea, dysphagia), but symptoms of overdosage usually occur within 1 hr of administration, whereas symptoms of underdose occur ≥3 hr after administration. Overdose (cholinergic crisis) symptoms may also include increased respiratory secretions and saliva, bradycardia, nausea, vomiting, cramping, diarrhea, and diaphoresis. A Tensilon test (edrophonium chloride) may be used to differentiate between overdosage and underdosage.
- **Antidote to Nondepolarizing Neuromuscular Blocking Agents:** Monitor reversal of effect of neuromuscular blocking agents with a peripheral nerve stimulator. Recovery usually occurs consecutively in the following muscles: diaphragm, intercostal muscles, muscles of the glottis, abdominal muscles, limb muscles, muscles of mastication, and levator muscles of eyelids. Closely observe patient for residual muscle weakness and respiratory distress throughout the recovery period. Maintain airway patency and ventilation until recovery of normal respirations occurs.
- ***Toxicity and Overdose:*** Atropine is the antidote.

Potential Nursing Diagnoses
Impaired physical mobility (Indications)
Ineffective breathing pattern (Indications)

Implementation
- For patients who have difficulty chewing, pyridostigmine may be administered 30 min before meals.
- Oral dose is not interchangeable with IV dose. Parenteral form is 30 times more potent.
- When used as an antidote to nondepolarizing neuromuscular blocking agents, atropine may be ordered before or currently with large doses of pyridostigmine to prevent or to treat bradycardia and other side effects.

- **PO:** Administer with food or milk to minimize side effects. Extended-release tablets should be swallowed whole; do not crush, break, or chew. Regular tablets or syrup may be administered with extended-release tablets for optimum control of symptoms. Mottled appearance of sustained-release tablet does not affect potency.

IV Administration

- **Direct IV:** Administer undiluted. Do not add to IV solutions. May be given through Y-site of infusion of D5W, 0.9% NaCl, LR, D5/Ringer's solution, or D5/LR. *Concentration:* 5 mg/mL. *Rate:* For myasthenia gravis, administer each 0.5 mg over 1 min. For reversal of nondepolarizing neuromuscular blocking agents, administer each 5 mg over 1 min.
- **Syringe Compatibility:** glycopyrrolate.
- **Y-Site Compatibility:** heparin, hydrocortisone sodium succinate, potassium chloride, vitamin B complex with C.

Patient/Family Teaching

- Instruct patient to take medication as directed. Do not skip or double up on missed doses. Patients with a history of dysphagia should have a nonelectric or battery-operated back-up alarm clock to remind them of exact dose time. Patients with dysphagia may not be able to swallow medication if the dose is not taken exactly on time. Taking dose late may result in myasthenic crisis. Taking dose early may result in cholinergic crisis. Patients with myasthenia gravis must continue this regimen as a life-long therapy.
- Advise patient to carry identification describing disease and medication regimen at all times.
- Instruct patient to space activities to avoid fatigue.

Evaluation/Desired Outcomes

- Relief of ptosis and diplopia; improved chewing, swallowing, extremity strength, and breathing without the appearance of cholinergic symptoms.
- Reversal of nondepolarizing neuromuscular blocking agents in general anesthesia.
- Prevention of Soman nerve gas toxicity.

---

pyridoxine (peer-i-**dox**-een)
Beesix, Doxine, Nestrex, Pyri, Rodex, Vitabee 6, vitamin B_6

---

pyridoxine 1083

Classification
Therapeutic: vitamins
Pharmacologic: water soluble vitamins

Pregnancy Category A

Indications
Treatment and prevention of pyridoxine deficiency (may be associated with poor nutritional status or chronic debilitating illnesses). Treatment of pyridoxine-dependent seizures in infants. Treatment and prevention of neuropathy, which may develop from isoniazid, penicillamine, or hydralazine therapy. Management of isoniazid overdose >10 g.

Action
Required for amino acid, carbohydrate, and lipid metabolism. Used in the transport of amino acids, formation of neurotransmitters, and synthesis of heme. **Therapeutic Effects:** Prevention of pyridoxine deficiency. Prevention or reversal of neuropathy associated with hydralazine, penicillamine, or isoniazid therapy.

Pharmacokinetics
Absorption: Well absorbed from the GI tract.
Distribution: Stored in liver, muscle, and brain. Crosses the placenta and enters breast milk.
Metabolism and Excretion: Converted in RBCs to pyridoxal phosphate and another active metabolite. Amounts in excess of requirements are excreted unchanged by the kidneys.
Half-life: 15–20 days.

TIME/ACTION PROFILE

ROUTE	ONSET	PEAK	DURATION
PO, IM, IV	unknown	unknown	unknown

Contraindications/Precautions
Contraindicated in: Hypersensitivity to pyridoxine or any component.
Use Cautiously in: Parkinson's disease (treatment with levodopa only); OB: Chronic ingestion of large doses may produce pyridoxine-dependency syndrome in newborn.

Adverse Reactions/Side Effects
Adverse reactions listed are seen with excessive doses only.
Neuro: sensory neuropathy, paresthesia. **Misc:** pyridoxine-dependency syndrome.

Interactions
Drug-Drug: Interferes with the therapeutic response to **levodopa** when used without carbi-

---

✤ = Canadian drug name. 🧬 = Genetic implication.
*CAPITALS indicates life-threatening; underlines indicate most frequent.

pyridoxine

dopa. Requirements are increased by **isoniazid**, **hydralazine**, **chloramphenicol**, **penicillamine**, **estrogens**, and **immunosuppressants**. Decreases serum levels of **phenobarbital** and **phenytoin**.

Route/Dosage

Prevention of Deficiency (Recommended Daily Allowance)

PO (Adults and Children >14 yr): 1.2–1.7 mg/day (larger doses required with cycloserine, ethionamide, hydralazine, immunosuppressants, isoniazid, penicillamine, and estrogen-containing oral contraceptives).
PO (Children 9–13 yr): 1 mg/day (larger doses required with cycloserine, ethionamide, hydralazine, immunosuppressants, isoniazid, and penicillamine).
PO (Children 1–8 yr): 0.5–0.6 mg/day (larger doses required with cycloserine, ethionamide, hydralazine, immunosuppressants, isoniazid, and penicillamine).
PO (Infants 6–12 mo): 0.3 mg/day.
PO (Infants < 6 mo): 0.1 mg/day.

Treatment of Deficiency

PO (Adults): 2.5–10 mg/day until clinical signs are corrected, then 2–5 mg/day.
PO (Children): 5–25 mg/day for 3 weeks, then 1.5–2.5 mg/day.

Pyridoxine-Dependent Seizures

PO, IM, IV (Neonates and Infants): 10–100 mg initially then 50—100 mg/day orally.

Drug-Induced Neuritis

PO (Adults): Treatment—100–300 mg/day; Prophylaxis—25–100 mg/day.
PO (Children): Treatment—10–50 mg/day; Prophylaxis—1–2 mg/kg/day.

Isoniazid Overdose (>10 g)

IM, IV (Adults and Children): Amount in mg equal to amount of isoniazid ingested given as 1–4 g IV, then 1 g IM q 30 min.

Availability (generic available)

Tablets: 20 mg^{OTC}, 25 mg^{OTC}, 50 mg^{OTC}, 100 mg^{OTC}, 250 mg^{OTC}, 500 mg^{OTC}. **Extended-release tablets:** 100 mg^{OTC}, 200 mg^{OTC}, 500 mg^{OTC}. **Extended-release capsules:** 150 mg^{OTC}. **Injection:** 100 mg/mL in 10- and 30-mL vials. *In combination with:* vitamins, minerals, and trace elements in a variety of multivitamin preparations^{OTC}.

NURSING IMPLICATIONS

Assessment

- Assess patient for signs of vitamin B$_6$ deficiency (anemia, dermatitis, cheilosis, irritability, seizures, nausea, and vomiting) before and periodically throughout therapy. Institute seizure precautions in pyridoxine-dependent infants.
- ***Lab Test Considerations:*** May cause false elevations in urobilinogen concentrations.

Potential Nursing Diagnoses

Imbalanced nutrition: less than body requirements (Indications)

Implementation

- Because of infrequency of single B-vitamin deficiencies, combinations are commonly administered.
- Administration of parenteral vitamin B$_6$ is limited to patients who are NPO or who have nausea and vomiting or malabsorption syndromes.
- Protect parenteral solution from light; decomposition will occur.
- **PO:** Extended-release capsules and tablets should be swallowed whole, without crushing, breaking, or chewing. For patients unable to swallow capsule, contents of capsules may be mixed with jam or jelly.
- **IM:** Rotate sites; burning or stinging at site may occur.
- **IV:** May be administered slowly by direct IV or as infusion in standard IV solutions. Monitor respiratory rate, heart rate, and blood pressure when administering large IV doses.
- Pyridoxine-dependent seizures should cease within 2–3 min of IV administration.
- ***Rate:*** Infusion rates of 15–30 min and up to 3 hr have been used.
- **Additive Incompatibility:** alkaline solutions, riboflavin.

Patient/Family Teaching

- Instruct patient to take medication as directed. If a dose is missed, it may be omitted because an extended period of time is required to become deficient in vitamin B$_6$.
- Encourage patient to comply with diet recommended by health care professional. Explain that the best source of vitamins is a well-balanced diet with foods from the four basic food groups. Foods high in vitamin B$_6$ include bananas, whole-grain cereals, potatoes, lima beans, and meats.
- Patients self-medicating with vitamin supplements should be cautioned not to exceed RDA. The effectiveness of megadoses for treatment of various medical conditions is unproved and

may cause side effects, such as unsteady gait, numbness in feet, and difficulty with hand co-ordination.
• Emphasize the importance of follow-up exams to evaluate progress.

Evaluation/Desired Outcomes
• Decrease in the symptoms of vitamin B_6 deficiency.

pyrimethamine
(peer-i-**meth**-a-meen)
Daraprim

Classification
Therapeutic: antimalarials, antiprotozoals

Pregnancy Category C

Indications
Used in combination with other antimalarials in the treatment of chloroquine-resistant malaria. Used in combination with a sulfonamide in the treatment of toxoplasmosis. **Unlabeled Use:** Used in combination with other agents (sulfonamides, dapsone) in the treatment of *Pneumocystis jirovecii* pneumonia.

Action
Binds to an enzyme in the protozoa, which results in depletion of folic acid. **Therapeutic Effects:** Death and arrested growth of susceptible organisms (protozoa).

Pharmacokinetics
Absorption: Well absorbed after oral administration.
Distribution: Widely distributed with high concentrations achieved in blood cells, kidneys, lungs, liver, and spleen. Some enters CSF (13–26% of serum levels). Crosses the placenta and enters breast milk.
Metabolism and Excretion: Mostly metabolized by the liver. 20–30% excreted unchanged by the kidneys.
Half-life: 4 days (shortened in patients with AIDS).

TIME/ACTION PROFILE (blood levels)

ROUTE	ONSET	PEAK	DURATION
PO	unknown	3 hr	2 wk†

†Suppressive levels

Contraindications/Precautions
Contraindicated in: Hypersensitivity; OB: First 14–16 wk of pregnancy; Megaloblastic anemia caused by folate deficiency; Concurrent folate antagonist therapy (because of risk of megaloblastic anemia); Tablets contain lactose and potato starch and should be avoided in patients with known hypersensitivity/intolerance.
Use Cautiously in: History of seizures (high doses); Underlying anemia or bone marrow depression; Impaired liver function; G6PD deficiency; OB: Pregnancy >16 wk (may require concurrent leucovorin); Lactation: Large doses to mother may cause folic acid deficiency in infant.

Adverse Reactions/Side Effects
CNS: SEIZURES (high doses), headache, insomnia, light-headedness, malaise, mental depression. **Resp:** dry throat, pulmonary eosinophilia. **CV:** ARRHYTHMIAS (large doses). **GI:** atrophic glossitis (high doses), anorexia, diarrhea, nausea. **GU:** hematuria. **Derm:** abnormal pigmentation, dermatitis. **Hemat:** megaloblastic anemia (high doses), pancytopenia, thrombocytopenia. **Misc:** fever.

Interactions
Drug-Drug: ↑ risk of bone marrow depression with other **bone marrow depressants**, including **antineoplastics**, **proguanil**, or **radiation therapy**. ↑ risk of megaloblastic anemia with folate antagonists (**methotrexate**); concurrent use should be avoided.

Route/Dosage

Treatment of Malaria
PO (Adults and Children >10 yr): 50 mg/day for 2 days, then 25 mg once weekly in combination with other agents.
PO (Children 4–10 yr): 25 mg daily for 2 days, then 12.5 mg once weekly in combination with other agents.

Toxoplasmosis
PO (Adults): 50–200 mg/day for 1–2 days, followed by 25–50 mg/day for 2–6 wk; given with a sulfonamide.
PO (Children): 1 mg/kg/day for 1–3 days, then 0.5 mg/kg/day for 4–6 wk; given with a sulfonamide.

Toxoplasmosis in AIDS Patients
PO (Adults): 100–200 mg/day for 1–2 days, followed by 50–100 mg/day for 3–6 wk, then 25–50 mg/day for life; given with clindamycin or sulfadiazine.

pyrimethamine

Availability
Tablets: 25 mg. *In combination with:* sulfadoxine (Fansidar). See Appendix B.

NURSING IMPLICATIONS

Assessment
- Assess patient for improvement in signs and symptoms of infection daily during therapy.
- *Lab Test Considerations:* Monitor CBC and platelet count periodically during therapy; semiweekly in patients with toxoplasmosis. May cause ↓ WBC and platelet counts.

Potential Nursing Diagnoses
Risk for infection (Indications)

Implementation
- Leucovorin may be administered concurrently to prevent folic acid deficiency and restore normal hematopoiesis.
- **PO:** Administer with milk or meals to minimize GI distress.
- Tablets may be crushed and mixed with saline or with other vehicles by pharmacist for patients with difficulty swallowing.

Patient/Family Teaching
- Instruct patient to take medication as directed on a regular schedule and continue full course of therapy, even if feeling better. Take missed doses as soon as remembered unless almost time for next dose; do not double doses.
- Advise patient to notify health care professional promptly if sore throat, pallor, purpura, or glossitis occurs. Instruct patient to stop taking pyrimethamine and notify health care professional immediately at the first sign of a skin rash or if no improvement is seen within a few days.
- Emphasize the importance of lab tests at scheduled intervals, especially in patients taking high doses. Tests should not be delayed or missed.

Evaluation/Desired Outcomes
- Improvement in the signs and symptoms of malaria.
- Improvement in signs and symptoms of toxoplasmosis.

quetiapine (kwet-**eye**-a-peen)
Seroquel, Seroquel XR

Classification
Therapeutic: antipsychotics, mood stabilizers

Pregnancy Category C

Indications
Schizophrenia. Depressive episodes with bipolar disorder. Acute manic episodes associated with bipolar I disorder (as monotherapy or with lithium or divalproex). Maintenance treatment of bipolar I disorder (with lithium or divalproex).

Action
Probably acts by serving as an antagonist of dopamine and serotonin. Also antagonizes histamine H_1 receptors and alpha$_1$-adrenergic receptors. **Therapeutic Effects:** Decreased manifestations of psychoses, depression, or acute mania.

Pharmacokinetics
Absorption: Well absorbed after oral administration.
Distribution: Widely distributed.
Metabolism and Excretion: Extensively metabolized by the liver (mostly by P450 CYP3A4 enzyme system); <1% excreted unchanged in the urine.
Half-life: 6 hr.

TIME/ACTION PROFILE (antipsychotic effects)

ROUTE	ONSET	PEAK	DURATION
PO	unknown	unknown	8–12 hr
PO-XR	unknown	unknown	unknown

Contraindications/Precautions
Contraindicated in: Hypersensitivity; Lactation: Lactation.
Use Cautiously in: Cardiovascular disease, cerebrovascular disease, dehydration or hypovolemia (↑ risk of hypotension); History of seizures, Alzheimer's dementia; Diabetes (may ↑ risk of hyperglycemia); Patients at risk for aspiration pneumonia; Hepatic impairment (dose ↓ may be necessary); Hypothyroidism (may be exacerbated); History of suicide attempt; OB: Safety not established; Pedi: May ↑ risk of suicide attempt/ideation especially during early treatment or dose adjustment; risk may be greater in children or adolescents; Geri: May require ↓ doses; ↑ risk of mortality in elderly patients treated for dementia-related psychosis.

Adverse Reactions/Side Effects
CNS: NEUROLEPTIC MALIGNANT SYNDROME, SEIZURES, dizziness, cognitive impairment, extrapyramidal symptoms, sedation, tardive dyskinesia. **EENT:** ear pain, rhinitis, pharyngitis. **Resp:** cough, dyspnea. **CV:** palpitations, peripheral edema, postural hypotension. **GI:** anorexia, constipation, dry mouth, dyspepsia. **Derm:** sweating. **Hemat:** leukopenia. **Metab:** weight gain, hyperglycemia. **Misc:** flu-like syndrome.

Interactions
Drug-Drug: ↑ CNS depression may occur with **alcohol**, **antihistamines**, **opioid analgesics**, and **sedative/hypnotics**. ↑ risk of hypotension with acute ingestion of **alcohol** or **antihypertensives**. **Phenytoin** and **thioridazine** ↑ clearance and ↓ effectiveness of quetiapine (dose change may be necessary); similar effects may occur with **carbamazepine**, **barbiturates**, **rifampin**, or **corticosteroids**. Effects may be ↑ by **ketoconazole**, **itraconazole**, **fluconazole**, **protease inhibitors** or **erythromycin**, as well as by other **agents that inhibit the cytochrome P450 CYP3A4 enzyme**.

Route/Dosage
PO (Adults): *Schizophrenia*—25 mg twice daily initially, ↑ by 25–50 mg 2–3 times daily over 3 days, up to 300–400 mg/day in 2–3 divided doses by the 4th day (not to exceed 800 mg/day); or 300 mg once daily as extended-release tablets, ↑ by 300 mg/day, up to 400–800 mg/day (not to exceed 800 mg/day). Elderly patients or patients with hepatic impairment should be started on immediate-release product and converted to extended-release product once effective dose is reached. *Bipolar Mania*—Immediate-release: 50 mg twice daily on day 1, ↑ dose by 100 mg/day up to 200 mg twice daily on day 4, then may ↑ in ≤200 mg/day increments up to 400 mg twice daily on day 6 if required; Extended-release: 300 mg once daily on Day 1, then 600 mg once daily on Day 2, then 400–800 mg once daily starting on Day 3. *Bipolar Depression*—Immediate-release or extended-release: 50 mg once daily at bedtime on Day 1, then 100 mg daily at bedtime on Day 2, then 200 mg daily at bedtime on Day 3, then 300 mg daily at bedtime thereafter. *Bipolar Maintenance*—Continue at the dose required to maintain symptom remission (usual dosage: 400–800 mg/day given as once daily dose [extended-release] or in two divided doses [immediate-release]).

quetiapine

Availability
Tablets: 25 mg, 50 mg, 100 mg, 200 mg, 300 mg, 400 mg. **Cost:** 25 mg $360.95/180, 50 mg $604.78/180, 100 mg $610.97/180, 200 mg $1,142.96/180, 300 mg $1,579.93/180, 400 mg $1,787.40/180. **Extended-release Tablets:** 50 mg, 150 mg, 200 mg, 300 mg, 400 mg. **Cost:** 200 mg $395.00/60, 300 mg $510.00/60, 400 mg $595.00/60.

NURSING IMPLICATIONS

Assessment
- Monitor mental status (mood, orientation, behavior) before and periodically during therapy.
- Assess for suicidal tendencies, especially during early therapy. Restrict amount of drug available to patient. Risk may be increased in children, adolescents, and adults ≤24 yr.
- Assess weight and BMI initially and throughout therapy.
- Monitor blood pressure (sitting, standing, lying) and pulse before and frequently during initial dose titration. If hypotension occurs during dose titration, return to the previous dose.
- Observe patient carefully when administering to ensure medication is swallowed and not hoarded or cheeked.
- Monitor for onset of extrapyramidal side effects (*akathisia*—restlessness; *dystonia*—muscle spasms and twisting motions; or *pseudoparkinsonism*—mask-like faces, rigidity, tremors, drooling, shuffling gait, dysphagia). Report these symptoms; reduction of dose or discontinuation may be necessary. Trihexyphenidyl or benztropine may be used to control these symptoms.
- Monitor for tardive dyskinesia (involuntary rhythmic movement of mouth, face, and extremities). Report immediately; may be irreversible.
- Monitor for development of neuroleptic malignant syndrome (fever, respiratory distress, tachycardia, seizures, diaphoresis, hypertension or hypotension, pallor, tiredness). Notify health care professional immediately if these symptoms occur.
- **Lab Test Considerations:** May cause asymptomatic ↑ in AST and ALT.
- May also cause anemia, thrombocytopenia, leukocytosis, and leukopenia.
- May cause ↑ total cholesterol and triglycerides.
- Obtain fasting blood glucose and cholesterol levels initially and throughout therapy.

Potential Nursing Diagnoses
Risk for self-directed violence (Indications)
Disturbed thought process (Indications)
Imbalanced nutrition: risk for more than body requirements (Side Effects)

Implementation
- If therapy is reinstituted after an interval of ≥1 wk off, follow initial titration schedule.
- **PO:** May be administered without regard to food. Extended-release tablets should be swallowed whole, do not break, crush, or chew.

Patient/Family Teaching
- Instruct patient to take medication as directed.
- Inform patient of the possibility of extrapyramidal symptoms. Instruct patient to report symptoms immediately to health care professional.
- Advise patient to change positions slowly to minimize orthostatic hypotension.
- May cause drowsiness. Caution patient to avoid driving or other activities requiring alertness until response to medication is known.
- Advise patient to avoid extremes in temperature; this drug impairs body temperature regulation.
- Caution patient to avoid concurrent use of alcohol, other CNS depressants, and OTC or herbal medications without consulting health care professional.
- Advise female patients to notify health care professional if pregnancy is planned or suspected or if they are breastfeeding or planning to breastfeed.
- Advise patient and family to notify health care professional if thoughts about suicide or dying, attempts to commit suicide; new or worse depression; new or worse anxiety; feeling very agitated or restless; panic attacks; trouble sleeping; new or worse irritability; acting aggressive; being angry or violent; acting on dangerous impulses; an extreme increase in activity and talking, other unusual changes in behavior or mood occur.
- Refer patient for nutritional, weight or medical management of dyslipidemia as indicated.
- Advise patient to notify health care professional of medication regimen before treatment or surgery.
- Instruct patient to notify health care professional promptly of sore throat, fever, unusual bleeding or bruising, or rash.
- Emphasize importance of routine follow-up exams to monitor side effects and continued participation in psychotherapy as indicated to improve coping skills. Ophthalmologic exams

should be performed before and every 6 months during therapy.

Evaluation/Desired Outcomes
- Decrease in excited, manic, behavior.
- Decrease in signs of depression in patients with bipolar disorder.
- Decrease in manic episodes in patients with bipolar I disorder.
- Decrease in positive symptoms (delusions, hallucinations) of schizophrenia.
- Decrease in negative symptoms (social withdrawal, flat, blunt affect) of schizophrenia.

---

quinapril, See ANGIOTENSIN-CONVERTING ENZYME (ACE) INHIBITORS.

QUINIDINE (kwin-i-deen)
quinidine gluconate
✦ Apo-Quin-G
quinidine sulfate
✦ Apo-Quinidine

Classification
Therapeutic: antiarrhythmics (class IA)

Pregnancy Category C

Indications
Restoration and maintenance of sinus rhythm in patients with atrial fibrillation or flutter. Prevention of recurrent ventricular arrhythmias. Treatment of malaria.

Action
Decrease myocardial excitability. Slow conduction velocity. **Therapeutic Effects:** Suppression of arrhythmias.

Pharmacokinetics
Absorption: Bioavailability of oral formulations is 70–80%. Extended-release preparations are absorbed slowly following oral administration.
Distribution: Widely distributed. Cross the placenta; enter breast milk.
Metabolism and Excretion: Metabolized by the liver; 5–20% excreted unchanged by the kidneys.
Half-life: 6–8 hr (increased in CHF or severe liver impairment).

TIME/ACTION PROFILE (antiarrhythmic effects)

ROUTE	ONSET	PEAK	DURATION
PO (sulfate)	30 min	1–1.5 hr	6–8 hr
PO (sulfate-ER)	unknown	4 hr	8–12 hr
PO (gluconate)	unknown	3–4 hr	6–8 hr
IV	1–5 min	rapid	6–8 hr

Contraindications/Precautions
Contraindicated in: Hypersensitivity; Conduction defects (in the absence of a pacemaker); Myasthenia gravis.
Use Cautiously in: CHF (dose reduction recommended); Severe liver disease (dose reduction recommended); Hypokalemia or hypomagnesemia (↑ risk of torsades de pointes); Bradycardia (↑ risk of torsades de pointes); Renal impairment; OB, Lactation: Pedi: Safety not established; extended-release preparations should not be used in children.

Adverse Reactions/Side Effects
CNS: dizziness, confusion, fatigue, headache, syncope, vertigo. **EENT:** blurred vision, diplopia, mydriasis, photophobia, tinnitus. **CV:** HYPOTENSION, TORSADES DE POINTES, arrhythmias, palpitations, tachycardia. **GI:** anorexia, abdominal cramping, diarrhea, nausea, vomiting, drug-induced hepatitis. **Derm:** rash. **Hemat:** AGRANULOCYTOSIS, hemolytic anemia, thrombocytopenia. **Neuro:** ataxia, tremor. **Misc:** fever.

Interactions
Drug-Drug: May ↑ risk of QT interval prolongation when used with **tricyclic antidepressants, erythromycin, clarithromycin, haloperidol, sotalol,** or **fluoroquinolones.** ↑ serum **digoxin** levels and may cause toxicity (dose reduction recommended). **Phenytoin, phenobarbital, carbamazepine,** or **rifampin** may ↑ metabolism and ↓ effectiveness. **Cimetidine, diltiazem, verapamil, amiodarone, ketoconazole, itraconazole,** and **protease inhibitors** ↓ metabolism and may ↑ blood levels. Excretion is delayed and effects ↑ by drugs that alkalinize the urine, including **carbonic anhydrase inhibitors, thiazide diuretics,** and **sodium bicarbonate.** Potentiates the effects of **neuromuscular blocking agents** and **warfarin.** Additive hypotension with **antihypertensives, nitrates,** and acute ingestion of **alcohol.** May increase **procainamide, haloper-**

idol, **mexiletine**, or **tricyclic antidepressant** levels and risk of toxicity. May antagonize **anticholinesterase therapy** in patients with myasthenia gravis. Additive anticholinergic effects may occur with **agents having anticholinergic properties** (including **antihistamines**, **tricyclic antidepressants**).

Drug-Food: **Grapefruit juice** ↑ serum levels and effect (avoid concurrent use). **Foods that alkalinize the urine** (see Appendix M) may ↑ serum quinidine levels and the risk of toxicity.

Route/Dosage

Quinidine Gluconate (62% Quinidine)
PO (Adults): 324–972 mg q 8–12 hr.
IV (Adults): 200–400 mg given at a rate ≤10 mg/min until arrhythmia is suppressed, QRS complex widens, bradycardia or hypotension occurs.

Quinidine Sulfate (83% Quinidine)
PO (Adults): *Atrial/ventricular arrhythmias*— 200–400 mg q 4–6 hr; may be ↑ to achieve therapeutic response (not to exceed 3–4 g/day).
PO (Children): 6 mg/kg 4–5 times daily.

Availability (generic available)

Quinidine Gluconate
Extended-release tablets: 324 mg. **Solution for Injection:** 80 mg/mL in 10-mL vials.

Quinidine Sulfate
Tablets: 200 mg, 300 mg. **Extended-release tablets:** 300 mg.

NURSING IMPLICATIONS

Assessment
- Monitor ECG, pulse, and blood pressure continuously throughout IV administration and periodically during oral administration. IV administration is usually discontinued if any of the following occur: arrhythmia is resolved, QRS complex widens by 50%, PR or QT intervals are prolonged, or frequent ventricular ectopic beats or tachycardia, bradycardia, or hypotension develops. Patient should remain supine throughout IV administration to minimize hypotension.
- *Lab Test Considerations:* Monitor hepatic and renal function, CBC, and serum potassium and magnesium levels periodically during prolonged therapy.
- *Toxicity and Overdose:* Serum quinidine levels may be monitored periodically during dose adjustment. Therapeutic serum concentrations are 2–6 mcg/mL. Toxic effects usually occur at concentrations >8 mcg/mL.
- Signs and symptoms of toxicity or cinchonism include tinnitus, hearing loss, visual disturbances, headache, nausea, and dizziness. These may occur after a single dose.
- Cardiac signs of toxicity include QRS widening, cardiac asystole, ventricular ectopic beats, idioventricular rhythms (ventricular tachycardia, ventricular fibrillation), paradoxical tachycardia, and torsades de pointes.

Potential Nursing Diagnoses
Decreased cardiac output (Indications)

Implementation
- Do not confuse quinidine with quinine.
- **PO:** Administer with a full glass of water on an empty stomach either 1 hr before or 2 hr after meals for faster absorption. If GI irritation becomes a problem, may be administered with or immediately after meals. Extended-release preparations should be swallowed whole; do not break, crush, or chew.

IV Administration
- **IV:** Use only clear, colorless solution.
- **Intermittent Infusion:** *Diluent:* Dilute 800 mg of quinidine gluconate (10 mL) in 50 mL of D5W. Infusion is stable for 24 hr at room temperature or 48 hr if refrigerated. *Concentration:* 16 mg/mL. *Rate:* Administer quinidine gluconate at a rate not to exceed 0.25 mg/kg/min. Administer via infusion pump to ensure accurate dose. Rapid administration may cause peripheral vascular collapse and severe hypotension.
- **Y-Site Compatibility:** amikacin, atropine, bumetanide, calcium gluconate, caspofungin, cimetidine, cyclosporine, digoxin, diltiazem, diphenhydramine, dobutamine, dopamine, doxycycline, enalaprilat, epinephrine, erythromycin, esmolol, famotidine, fenoldopam, fentanyl, fluconazole, gentamicin, granisetron, hydromorphone, imipenem, isoproterenol, labetalol, lidocaine, linezolid, lorazepam, meperidine, metoclopramide, metoprolol, milrinone, morphine, nesiritide, nitroglycerin, norepinephrine, ondansetron, palonosetron, phenylephrine, phytonadione, potassium chloride, procainamide, prochlorperazine, promethazine, propranolol, protamine, ranitidine, succinylcholine, tacrolimus, tirofiban, tobramycin, vancomycin, vasopressin, verapamil, voriconazole.
- **Y-Site Incompatibility:** acyclovir, aminophylline, ampicillin, ampicillin/sulbactam, aztreonam, cefazolin, cefotaxime, cefoxitin, ceftazidime, ceftizoxime, ceftriaxone, cefuroxime,

chloramphenicol, clindamycin, daptomycin, dexamethasone, ertapenem, furosemide, ganciclovir, hydrocortisone sodium succinate, insulin, ketorolac, methylprednisolone sodium succinate, metronidazole, nafcillin, nitroprusside, pantoprazole, penicillin G potassium, phenytoin, piperacillin/tazobacatam, sodium bicarbonate, sulfamethoxazole/trimethoprim, ticarcillin/clavulanate.

Patient/Family Teaching

- Instruct patient to take medication around the clock, exactly as directed, even if feeling well. Take missed doses as soon as remembered if within 2 hr; if remembered later, omit. Do not double doses.
- Instruct patient or family member on how to take pulse. Advise patient to report changes in pulse rate or rhythm to health care professional.
- May cause dizziness or blurred vision. Caution patient to avoid driving or other activities requiring alertness until response to medication is known.
- Inform patient that quinidine may cause increased sensitivity to light. Dark glasses may minimize this effect.
- Advise patient to inform health care professional of medication regimen prior to treatment or surgery.
- Instruct patient not to take Rx, OTC, or herbal products with quinidine without consulting health care professional.
- Advise patient to consult health care professional if symptoms of cinchonism, rash, or dyspnea occur or if diarrhea is severe or persistent.
- Advise patient to carry identification at all times describing disease process and medication regimen.
- Emphasize the importance of routine follow-up exams to monitor progress.

Evaluation/Desired Outcomes

- Decrease or cessation of cardiac arrhythmia.
- Resolution of malarial infection.

---

quinine (kwi-nine)
Qualaquin

Classification
Therapeutic: antimalarials

Pregnancy Category C

---

quinine 1091

Indications
Chloroquine-resistant falciparum malaria (alone or with pyrimethamine and a sulfonamide or with a tetracycline; has also been used with clindamycin and mefloquine depending on origin of illness). **Unlabeled Use:** Leg cramps (not recommended due to cardiac side effects).

Action
Disrupts metabolism of the erythrocytic phase of *Plasmodium falciparum*. Increases the refractory period of skeletal muscle, increases the distribution of calcium within muscle fibers, decreases the excitability of motor end-plate regions, resulting in decreased response to repetitive nerve stimulation and acetylcholine. **Therapeutic Effects:** Death of *P. falciparum*.

Pharmacokinetics
Absorption: Rapidly and almost completely (80%) absorbed following oral administration.
Distribution: Varies with condition and patient; does not enter CSF well. Crosses the placenta and enters breast milk.
Protein Binding: >90% in patients with cerebral malaria, pregnant women, and children; 85–90% in patients with uncomplicated malaria; 70% in healthy adults.
Metabolism and Excretion: >80% metabolized by the liver; metabolites have less activity than quinine; metabolites excreted in urine. 20% excreted unchanged in urine. Excretion ↑ in acidic urine.
Half-life: 11 hr (↑ in patients with malaria).

TIME/ACTION PROFILE (antimalarial blood levels)

ROUTE	ONSET	PEAK	DURATION
PO	unknown	3.2–5.9 hr	8 hr

Contraindications/Precautions
Contraindicated in: Hypersensitivity to quinine, quinidine, or mefloquine; History of previous serious adverse reaction to quinine including thrombotic thrombocytopenic purpura, thrombocytopenia, acute intravascular hemolysis, hemoglobinuria, or hemoglobinemia; QTc prolongation or conditions predisposing to QTc prolongation including hypokalemia and bradycardia; Concurrent use of Class IA or Class III antiarrhythmics, mefloquine, pimozide, or macrolide anti-infectives (↑ risk of arrhythmias); G6PD deficiency; Myasthenia gravis; Optic neuritis; OB: Use only if potential maternal benefit outweighs

---

✦ = Canadian drug name. ■ = Genetic implication.
*CAPITALS indicates life-threatening; underlines indicate most frequent.

fetal risk; consider alternative therapies; Lactation: Discontinue drug or breastfeeding; Geri: Avoid if possible (↑ risk of arrhythmias).
Use Cautiously in: Recurrent or interrupted malaria therapy; History of arrhythmias, especially QTc prolongation; Atrial fibrillation/flutter (may cause paradoxical ↑ in ventricular response); Hypoglycemia; History of thrombocytopenic purpura; Pedi: Safety not established for children <16 yr.

Adverse Reactions/Side Effects
CV: CARDIAC ARRHYTHMIAS. **GI:** abdominal cramps/pain, diarrhea, nausea, vomiting, hepatotoxicity. **Derm:** rash. **Endo:** hypoglycemia (↑ in pregnancy). **Hemat:** bleeding, blood dyscrasias, thrombotic thrombocytopenic pupura, thrombocytopenia. **Misc:** cinchonism, hypersensitivity reactions including fever and ANAPHYLAXIS, HEMOLYTIC UREMIC SYNDROME, STEVENS-JOHNSON SYNDROME.

Interactions
Drug-Drug: Concurrent use of Class IA antiarrhythmics (**quinidine**, **procainamide**, **disopyramide**, Class III antiarrhythmics, mefloquine, pimozide, or macrolide anti-infectives ↑ risk of arrhythmias and should be avoided. **Antacids** ↓ absorption. **Cimetidine** ↓ metabolism and may ↑ effects. **Rifampin** and **rifabutin** ↑ metabolism and may ↓ effects; concurrent use with rifampin should be avoided. May ↑ effects of **neuromuscular blocking agents**. May ↑ **digoxin** levels; dose adjustments may be necessary. May ↑ risk of hemolytic, ototoxic, or neurotoxic reactions when used concurrently with **agents sharing these toxicities**. Concurrent use with **quinidine** may ↑ risk of adverse cardiovascular reactions. May ↑ risk of bleeding with **warfarin**. Concurrent use with **mefloquine** ↑ risk of seizures and adverse cardiovascular reactions. **Urinary alkalinizers** including **acetazolamide** and **sodium bicarbonate** may ↑ blood levels. Quinine inhibits the CYP3A4 and CYP2D6 enzyme systems and can ↑ levels of **carbamazepine**, **phenobarbital**, **phenytoin**, **atorvastatin**, **simvastatin**, **lovastatin**, **dextromethorphan**, **metoprolol**, **flecainide**, and **paroxetine**. **Carbamazepine**, **phenobarbital**, and **phenytoin** induce metabolism and ↓ levels of quinine; frequent monitoring recommended.

Route/Dosage
PO (Adults): *Malaria*—648 mg every 8 hr for 7 days.

Renal Impairment
PO (Adults): *Severe chronic renal failure*—648 mg initially, then 324 mg every 12 hr for 7 days.

Availability
Capsules: 325 mg. **Tablets:** 324 mg.

NURSING IMPLICATIONS

Assessment
- **Malaria:** Assess patient for improvement in signs and symptoms of condition daily during therapy.
- *Lab Test Considerations:* May cause ↑ urinary 17-ketogenic steroids when metyrapone or Zimmerman method is used.
- *Toxicity and Overdose:* Plasma quinine levels of >10 mcg/mL may cause tinnitus and impaired hearing.
- Signs of toxicity or cinchonism include tinnitus, headache, nausea, and slightly disturbed vision; usually disappear rapidly upon discontinuing quinine.

Potential Nursing Diagnoses
Risk for infection (Indications)

Implementation
- **PO:** Administer with or after meals to minimize GI distress. Aluminum-containing antacids will decrease and delay absorption; avoid concurrent use.

Patient/Family Teaching
- Instruct patient to take medication as directed and continue full course of therapy, even if feeling better. Take missed doses as soon as remembered, unless almost time for the next dose. If more than 4 hr has elapsed since missed dose, wait and take the next dose as scheduled. Do not double doses or take more than recommended. Advise patient to read the *Patient Information* leaflet prior to starting therapy and with each Rx refill.
- Review methods of minimizing exposure to mosquitoes with patients receiving quinine (use insect repellent, wear long-sleeved shirt and long trousers, use screen or netting).
- Quinine may cause visual changes. Caution patient to avoid driving or other activities requiring alertness until response to medication is known.
- May cause diarrhea, nausea, stomach cramps or pain, vomiting, or ringing in the ears. Advise patient to notify health care professional promptly if these become pronounced.
- Advise patient to stop quinine and notify health care professional of any evidence of allergy

(flushing, itching, rash, fever, facial swelling, stomach pain, difficult breathing, ringing in the ears, visual problems).
- Instruct patient to consult health care professional before taking any Rx, OTC, or herbal products with quinine.
- Advise patient to notify health care professional if pregnancy is planned or suspected or if breastfeeding.

Evaluation/Desired Outcomes
- Prevention of or improvement in signs and symptoms of malaria.

---

quinupristin/dalfopristin
(kwin-oo-**pris**-tin/dal-foe-**pris**-tin)
Synercid

Classification
Therapeutic: anti-infectives
Pharmacologic: streptogramins

Pregnancy Category B

Indications
Treatment of serious or life-threatening infections associated with vancomycin-resistant *Enterococcus faecium* (VREF). Complicated skin/skin structure infections caused by *Staphylococcus aureus* (methicillin, susceptible) or *Streptococcus pyogenes*.

Action
Quinupristin inhibits the late phase of protein synthesis at the level of the bacterial ribosome; dalfopristin inhibits the early phase. **Therapeutic Effects:** Bacteriostatic effect against susceptible organisms. **Spectrum:** Active against vancomycin-resistant and multidrug-resistant strains of *E. faecium*, *S. aureus* (methicillin-susceptible), and *S. pyogenes*. Not active against *E. faecalis*.

Pharmacokinetics
Absorption: IV administration results in complete bioavailability.
Distribution: Unknown.
Protein Binding: Moderate.
Metabolism and Excretion: Both are converted to compounds with additional anti-infective activity; parent drugs and metabolites are mostly excreted in feces (75–77%); 15% of quinupristin and 17% of dalfopristin excreted in urine.
Half-life: *Quinupristin*—0.85 hr; *dalfopristin*—0.7 hr.

TIME/ACTION PROFILE

ROUTE	ONSET	PEAK	DURATION
IV	rapid	end of infusion	8–12 hr

Contraindications/Precautions
Contraindicated in: Hypersensitivity.
Use Cautiously in: Concurrent use of other drugs metabolized by the cytochrome P450 3A4 enzyme system (serious interactions may occur); Hepatic impairment (dose adjustment may be necessary); Patients with a history of GI disease, especially colitis; OB, Lactation: Pedi: Pregnancy, lactation, or children <16 yr (safety not established).

Adverse Reactions/Side Effects
CNS: headache. **CV:** thrombophlebitis. **GI:** PSEUDOMEMBRANOUS COLITIS, diarrhea, nausea, vomiting. **Derm:** pruritus, rash. **Local:** edema/inflammation/pain at infusion site, infusion site reactions. **Misc:** allergic reactions including ANAPHYLAXIS, pain.

Interactions
Drug-Drug: Inhibits the cytochrome P450 3A4 drug metabolizing enzyme system; inhibits metabolism of **cyclosporine**, **midazolam**, and **nifedipine** and ↑ risk of toxicity (careful monitoring required). Similar effects may be expected with concurrent use of **delavirdine**, **nevirapine**, **indinavir**, **ritonavir**, **vinca alkaloids**, **docetaxel**, **paclitaxel**, **diazepam**, **verapamil**, **diltiazem**, **HMG CoA reductase inhibitors**, **tacrolimus**, **methylprednisolone**, **carbamazepine**, **quinidine**, **lidocaine**, and **disopyramide**.

Route/Dosage
IV (Adults): *Vancomycin-resistant E. faecium*—7.5 mg/kg q 8 hr for at least 7 days; *complicated skin/skin structure infections*—7.5 mg/kg q 12 hr for at least 7 days.

Availability
Powder for injection: 500 mg (150 mg quinupristin and 350 mg dalfopristin in 10-mL vials), 600 mg (180 mg quinupristin and 420 mg dalfopristin in 10-mL vials).

NURSING IMPLICATIONS

Assessment
- Assess patient for infection (vital signs; appearance of wound, sputum, urine, and stool; WBC) at beginning of and throughout therapy.

- Obtain specimens for culture and sensitivity before initiating therapy. First dose may be given before receiving results.
- Monitor patient for pain or inflammation at the infusion site frequently throughout infusion. Increasing the volume of diluent from 250 mL to 500 mL or 750 mL or infusing via a peripherally inserted central catheter or central venous catheter may be required.
- Observe patient for signs and symptoms of anaphylaxis (rash, pruritus, laryngeal edema, wheezing). Discontinue drug and notify physician or other health care professional immediately if these problems occur. Keep epinephrine, an antihistamine, and resuscitation equipment close by in case of an anaphylactic reaction.
- Assess patient for myalgia and arthralgia after infusion. May be severe. Reducing dose frequency to every 12 hr may decrease pain. Symptoms usually resolve upon discontinuation of medication.
- **Lab Test Considerations:** May cause ↑ serum total bilirubin concentrations.

Potential Nursing Diagnoses
Risk for infection (Indications, Side Effects)
Diarrhea (Adverse Reactions)

Implementation

IV Administration

- **Intermittent Infusion: *Diluent:*** Reconstitute the 500-mg vial with 5 mL and the 600-mg vial with 6 mL of D5W or sterile water for injection, respectively, for a concentration of 100 mg/mL. Avoid shaking to prevent foam formation. Allow solution to sit until all foam has disappeared. Dilute further with 250 mL of D5W (100 mL can be used for central line administration). May dilute in 500 mL or 750 mL of D5W if severe venous irritation occurs after peripheral administration. Reconstituted vials should be used within 30 min. Infusion is stable for 5 hr at room temperature or 54 hr if refrigerated. *Rate:* Infuse over 60 min. Flush line before and after infusion with D5W.
- **Y-Site Compatibility:** amikacin, amiodarone, anidulafungin, aztreonam, caspofungin, cimetidine, ciprofloxacin, cyclosporine, daptomycin, diltiazem, diphenhydramine, dolasetron, doxycycline, droperidol, enalaprilat, epinephrine, esmolol, fenoldopam, fentanyl, fluconazole, granisetron, haloperidol, hydromorphone, hydroxyzine, isoproterenol, labetalol, levofloxacin, lidocaine, linezolid, lorazepam, meperidine, metoclopramide, metoprolol, midazolam, milrinone, morphine, nicardipine, nitroglycerin, ondansetron, palonosetron, pancuronium, phenylephrine, potassium chloride, procainamide, prochlorperazine, promethazine, propranolol, tacrolimus, tirofiban, tobramycin, verapamil, voriconazole.
- **Y-Site Incompatibility:** acyclovir, aminophylline, ampicillin, ampicillin/sulbacatam, azithromycin, bumetanide, calcium chloride, calcium gluconate, cefazolin, cefepime, cefotaxime, ceftazidime, ceftizoxime, ceftriaxone, cefuroxime, clindamycin, dexamethasone sodium phosphate, diazepam, digoxin, ertapenem, furosemide, ganciclovir, heparin, hydrocortisone sodium succinate, imipenem/cilastatin, insulin, ketorolac, meropenem, methylprednisolone sodium succinate, nitroprusside, pantoprazole, phenytoin, piperacillin/tazobactam, potassium phosphate, ranitidine, sodium bicarbonate, trimethoprim/sulfamethoxazole, ticarcillin/clavulanate.
- **Solution Incompatibility:** 0.9% NaCl.

Patient/Family Teaching
- Instruct patient to notify health care professional if fever and diarrhea develop, especially if stool contains blood, pus, or mucus. Advise patient not to treat diarrhea without consulting health care professional.

Evaluation/Desired Outcomes
- Resolution of signs and symptoms of infection. Length of time for complete resolution depends on the organism and site of infection.

rabeprazole (ra-**bep**-ra-zole)
Aciphex, ♦Pariet

Classification
Therapeutic: antiulcer agents
Pharmacologic: proton-pump inhibitors

Pregnancy Category B

Indications
Gastroesophageal reflux disease (GERD). Duodenal ulcers (including combination therapy with clarithromycin and amoxicillin to erradicate *H. pylori* and prevent recurrence). Pathological hypersecretory conditions, including Zollinger-Ellison syndrome.

Action
Binds to an enzyme in the presence of acidic gastric pH, preventing the final transport of hydrogen ions into the gastric lumen. **Therapeutic Effects:** Diminished accumulation of acid in the gastric lumen, with lessened acid reflux. Healing of duodenal ulcers and esophagitis. Decreased acid secretion in hypersecretory conditions.

Pharmacokinetics
Absorption: Delayed-release tablet is designed to allow rabeprazole, which is not stable in gastric acid, to pass through the stomach intact. Subsequently 52% is absorbed after oral administration.
Distribution: Unknown.
Protein Binding: 96.3%.
Metabolism and Excretion: Mostly metabolized by the liver (hepatic cytochrome P450 3A and 2C19 enzyme systems) ▒ (the CYP2C19 enzyme system exhibits genetic polymorphism; 15–20% of Asian patients and 3–5% of Caucasian and Black patients may be poor metabolizers and may have significantly ↑ rabeprazole concentrations and an ↑ risk of adverse effects); 10% excreted in feces; remainder excreted in urine as inactive metabolites.
Half-life: 1–2 hr.

TIME/ACTION PROFILE (acid suppression)

ROUTE	ONSET	PEAK	DURATION
PO	within 1 hr	unknown	24 hr†

†Suppression continues to increase over the first week of therapy

Contraindications/Precautions
Contraindicated in: Hypersensitivity to rabeprazole or related drugs (benzimidazoles).

Use Cautiously in: Severe hepatic impairment (dose reduction may be necessary); Geri: ↑ risk of hip fractures in patients using high doses for >1 year; OB, Lactation: Pedi: Pregnancy, lactation, or children <12 yr (breastfeeding not recommended; use in pregnancy only if needed; safety not established).

Adverse Reactions/Side Effects
CNS: dizziness, headache, malaise. **GI:** abdominal pain, constipation, diarrhea, nausea. **Derm:** photosensitivity, rash. **MS:** neck pain. **Misc:** allergic reactions, chills, fever.

Interactions
Drug-Drug: Rabeprazole is metabolized by the CYP450 enzyme system and may interact with other drugs metabolized by this sytem. May ↓ absorption of drugs requiring acid pH, including **ketoconazole**, **itraconazole**, **atazanavirampicillin esters**, and **iron salts**. May ↑ blood levels of **digoxin**. May ↑ the risk of bleeding with **warfarin** (monitor INR/PT). May ↓ the antiplatelet effects of **clopidogrel**.

Route/Dosage
PO (Adults): *GERD, duodenal ulcers*—20 mg once daily; *prevention of duodenal ulcer recurrence*—20 mg twice daily for 7 days with amoxicillin 1000 mg twice daily for 7 days and clarithromycin 500 mg twice daily for 7 days; *hypersecretory conditions*—60 mg once daily initially, may be adjusted as needed and continued as necessary; doses up to 100 mg daily or 60 mg twice daily have been used.
PO (Children ≥12 yr): *GERD*—20 mg once daily.

Availability
Delayed-release tablets: 20 mg. **Cost:** 20 mg $419.97/90.

NURSING IMPLICATIONS

Assessment
- Assess routinely for epigastric or abdominal pain and frank or occult blood in the stool, emesis, or gastric aspirate.
- **Lab Test Considerations:** Monitor CBC with differential periodically during therapy.

Potential Nursing Diagnoses
Acute pain (Indications)

Implementation
- **PO:** Administer doses before meals, preferably in the morning. Tablets should be swallowed whole; do not break, crush, or chew.

♦ = Canadian drug name. ▒ = Genetic implication.
*CAPITALS indicates life-threatening; underlines indicate most frequent.

Patient/Family Teaching

- Instruct patient to take medication as directed for the full course of therapy, even if feeling better. Take missed doses as soon as remembered but not if almost time for next dose. Do not double doses.
- May cause occasional drowsiness or dizziness. Caution patient to avoid driving or other activities requiring alertness until response to medication is known.
- Advise patient to avoid alcohol, products containing aspirin or NSAIDs, and foods that may cause an increase in GI irritation.
- Caution patients to wear sunscreen and protective clothing to prevent photosensitivity reactions.
- Advise patient to report onset of black, tarry stools; diarrhea; abdominal pain; or persistent headache to health care professional promptly.
- Advise female patients to notify health care professional if pregnancy is planned or suspected or if breastfeeding.
- Instruct patient to consult health care professional prior to taking other Rx, OTC, or herbal products.

Evaluation/Desired Outcomes

- Decrease in abdominal pain or prevention of gastric irritation and bleeding. Healing of duodenal ulcers can be seen on x-ray examination or endoscopy.
- Decrease in symptoms of GERD. Therapy is continued for 4–8 wk after initial episode.

---

raloxifene (ra-**lox**-i-feen)
Evista

Classification
Therapeutic: bone resorption inhibitors
Pharmacologic: selective estrogen receptor modulators

Pregnancy Category X

Indications
Treatment and prevention of osteoporosis in postmenopausal women. Reduction of the risk of breast cancer in postmenopausal women with osteoporosis and those at high risk for invasive breast cancer.

Action
Binds to estrogen receptors, producing estrogen-like effects on bone, resulting in reduced resorption of bone and decreased bone turnover. **Therapeutic Effects:** Prevention of osteoporosis in patients at risk. Decreased risk of breast cancer.

Pharmacokinetics
Absorption: Although well absorbed (>60%), after oral administration, extensive first-pass metabolism results in 2% bioavailability.
Distribution: Highly bound to plasma proteins; remainder of distribution unknown.
Protein Binding: Highly bound to plasma proteins.
Metabolism and Excretion: Extensively metabolized by the liver; undergoes enterohepatic cycling; excreted primarily in feces.
Half-life: 27.7 hr.

TIME/ACTION PROFILE (effects on bone turnover)

ROUTE	ONSET	PEAK	DURATION
PO	unknown	3 mo	unknown

Contraindications/Precautions
Contraindicated in: Hypersensitivity; History of thromboembolic events; OB: Lactation: Not indicated for women with childbearing potential or who are breastfeeding; Pedi: Safety not established.
Use Cautiously in: Potential immobilization (increased risk of thromboembolic events); History of stroke or transient ischemic attack; Atrial fibrillation; Hypertension; Cigarette smoking.

Adverse Reactions/Side Effects
CV: STROKE, deep vein thrombosis, pulmonary embolism, retinal vein thrombosis. **MS:** leg cramps. **Misc:** hot flashes.

Interactions
Drug-Drug: Cholestyramine ↓ absorption (avoid concurrent use). May alter effects of **warfarin** and other **highly protein-bound drugs**. Concurrent systemic **estrogen** therapy is not recommended.

Route/Dosage
PO (Adults): 60 mg once daily.

Availability
Tablets: 60 mg. **Cost:** $269.96/90.

NURSING IMPLICATIONS

Assessment
- Assess patient for bone mineral density with x-ray, serum, and urine bone turnover markers (bone-specific alkaline phosphatase, osteocalcin, and collagen breakdown products) before and periodically during therapy.
- *Lab Test Considerations:* May cause ↑ apolipoprotein A-I and reduced serum total cholesterol, LDL cholesterol, fibrinogen, apolipoprotein B, and lipoprotein.

- May cause ↑ hormone-binding globulin (sex steroid-binding globulin, thyroxine-binding globulin, corticosteroid-binding globulin) with ↑ total hormone concentrations.
- May cause small ↓ in serum total calcium, inorganic phosphate, total protein, and albumin.
- May also cause slight decrease in platelet count.

Potential Nursing Diagnoses
Risk for injury (Indications)

Implementation
- **PO:** May be administered without regard to meals.
- Calcium supplementation should be added to diet if daily intake is inadequate.

Patient/Family Teaching
- Instruct patient to take raloxifene as directed. Discuss the importance of adequate calcium and vitamin D intake or supplementation. Advise patient to discontinue smoking and alcohol consumption.
- Emphasize the importance of regular weight-bearing exercise. Advise patient that raloxifene should be discontinued at least 72 hr before and during prolonged immobilization (recovery from surgery, prolonged bedrest). Instruct patient to avoid prolonged restrictions of movement during travel because of the increased risk of venous thrombosis.
- Advise patient that raloxifene will not reduce hot flashes or flushes associated with estrogen deficiency and may cause hot flashes.
- **OB:** Advise patient that raloxifene may have teratogenic effects. Instruct patient to notify health care provider immediately if pregnancy is planned or suspected.
- Instruct patient to read the patient package insert when initiating therapy and again with each prescription refill.

Evaluation/Desired Outcomes
- Prevention of osteoporosis in postmenopausal women.
- Reduced risk of breast cancer in postmenopausal women with osteoporosis and those at high risk for invasive breast cancer.

---

raltegravir (ral-teg-ra-veer)
Isentress

Classification
Therapeutic: antiretrovirals
Pharmacologic: integrase strand transfer inhibitor (INSTI)

Pregnancy Category C

Indications
HIV-1 infection (with other antiretrovirals) in treatment-experienced or treatment-naïve patients.

Action
Inhibits HIV-1 integrase, which is required for viral replication. **Therapeutic Effects:** Evidence of decreased viral replication and reduced viral load with slowed progression of HIV and its sequelae.

Pharmacokinetics
Absorption: Well absorbed following oral administration.
Distribution: Unknown.
Metabolism and Excretion: Mostly metabolized by the uridine diphosphate glucuronosyltransferase (UGT) A1A enzyme system; 23% excreted in urine as parent drug and metabolite.
Half-life: 9 hr.

TIME/ACTION PROFILE (blood levels)

ROUTE	ONSET	PEAK	DURATION
PO	unknown	3 hr	12 hr

Contraindications/Precautions
Contraindicated in: Lactation: Breast feeding not recommended in HIV-infected patients.
Use Cautiously in: Geri: Choose dose carefully, considering concurrent disease states, drug therapy and age-related ↓ in hepatic and renal function; Concurrent use of medications associated with rhabdomyolysis/myopathy (may ↑ risk); OB: Use in pregnancy only if maternal benefit outweighs fetal risk; Pedi: Safety not established.

Adverse Reactions/Side Effects
CNS: SUICIDAL THOUGHTS, headache, depression, dizziness, fatigue, weakness. **CV:** myocardial infarction. **GI:** diarrhea, abdominal pain, gastritis, hepatitis, vomiting. **GU:** renal failure/impairment. **Hemat:** anemia, neutropenia. **Metab:** lipodystrophy. **Misc:** hypersensitivity reactions, immune reconstitution syndrome, fever.

Interactions
Drug-Drug: Concurrent use with **strong inducers of the UGT A1A enzyme system** including

rifampin may ↓ blood levels and effectiveness. Concurrent use with **strong inhibitors of the UGT A1A enzyme system** including **atazanavir** may ↑ blood levels. ↑ risk of rhabdomyolysis/myopathy **HMG-CoA reductase inhibitors**. **Proton pump inhibitors** may ↑ levels. **Efavirenz**, **etravirine**, and **tipranavir/ritonavir** may ↓ levels.

Route/Dosage
PO (Adults): 400 mg twice daily; ↑ dose to 800 mg twice daily when used with rifampin.

Availability
Tablets: 400 mg.

NURSING IMPLICATIONS
Assessment
- Assess patient for change in severity of HIV symptoms and for symptoms of opportunistic infections during therapy.
- Monitor for anxiety, depression (especially in patients with a history of psychiatric illness), suicidal ideation, and paranoia during therapy.
- *Lab Test Considerations:* Monitor viral load and CD4 counts regularly during therapy.
- May casue ↓ ANC, hemoglobin, and platelet counts.
- May cause ↑ serum glucose, AST, ALT, GGT, total bilirubin, alkaline phosphatase, pancreatic amylase, serum lipase, and creatinine kinase concentrations.

Potential Nursing Diagnoses
Risk for infection (Indications)
Noncompliance (Patient/Family Teaching)

Implementation
- **PO:** May be administered without regard to meals.

Patient/Family Teaching
- Emphasize the importance of taking raltegravir as directed, at evenly spaced times throughout day. Do not take more than prescribed amount and do not stop taking without consulting health care professional. Take missed doses as soon as remembered unless almost time for next dose. Do not double doses. Advise patient to read *Patient Information* sheet before starting therapy and with each prescription renewal in case changes have been made.
- Instruct patient that raltegravir should not be shared with others.
- Advise patient to avoid taking other Rx, OTC, or herbal products without consulting health care professional.
- Inform patient that raltegravir does not cure AIDS or prevent associated or opportunistic infections. Raltegravir does not reduce the risk of transmission of HIV to others through sexual contact or blood contamination. Caution patient to use a condom during sexual contact and to avoid sharing needles or donating blood to prevent spreading the AIDS virus to others. Advise patient that the long-term effects of raltegravir are unknown at this time.
- Advise patient to notify health care professional if they develop any unusual symptoms, if any known symptom persists or worsens, or if depression or suicidal thoughts occur.
- Advise patients to notify health care professional if pregnancy is planned or suspected. Breastfeeding should be avoided during therapy.
- Emphasize the importance of regular follow-up exams and blood counts to determine progress and monitor for side effects.

Evaluation/Desired Outcomes
- Delayed progression of AIDS and decreased opportunistic infections in patients with HIV.
- Decrease in viral load and improvement in CD4 cell counts.

---

ramelteon (ra-mel-tee-on)
Rozerem

Classification
Therapeutic: sedative/hypnotics
Pharmacologic: melatonin receptor agonists

Pregnancy Category C

Indications
Treatment of insomnia characterized by difficult sleep onset.

Action
Activates melatonin receptors, which promotes maintenance of circadian rhythm, a part of the sleep-wake cycle. **Therapeutic Effects:** Easier onset of sleep.

Pharmacokinetics
Absorption: Well absorbed (84%), but bioavailability is low (1.8%) due to extensive first pass liver metabolism. Absorption in increased by a high fat meal.
Distribution: Widely distributed to body tissues.
Metabolism and Excretion: Extensively metabolized by the liver; mainly by CYP1A2 enzyme system. Metabolites are excreted mostly in urine (88%); 4% excreted in feces.
Half-life: 1–2.6 hr.

TIME/ACTION PROFILE (blood levels)

ROUTE	ONSET	PEAK	DURATION
PO	rapid	30–90 min	unknown

Contraindications/Precautions
Contraindicated in: Hypersensitivity; History of angioedema with previous use; Severe hepatic impairment; Concurrent use of fluvoxamine; Lactation: Lactation; Pedi: Safety not established.
Use Cautiously in: Depression or history of suicidal ideation; Moderate hepatic impairment; Concurrent use of CYP3A4 inhibitors, such as ketoconazole; Concurrent use of CYP2C9 inhibitors, such as fluconazole; OB: Use only if maternal benefit outweighs fetal risk.

Adverse Reactions/Side Effects
CNS: abnormal thinking, behavior changes, dizziness, fatigue, hallucinations, headache, insomnia (worsened), sleep—driving. **GI:** nausea. **Endo:** ↑ prolactin levels, ↓ testosterone levels. **Misc:** ANGIOEDEMA.

Interactions
Drug-Drug: Blood levels and effects are ↑ by **fluvoxamine**; concurrent use is contraindicated. Levels and effects may be ↓ by **rifampin**. Concurrent use of CYP3A4 inhibitors, such as **ketoconazole** may ↑ levels and effects; use cautiously. Concurrent use of CYP2C9 inhibitors, such as **fluconazole** may ↑ levels and effects; use cautiously. ↑ risk of excessive CNS depression with other CNS depressants including **alcohol**, **benzodiazepines**, **opioids**, and other **sedative/hypnotics**.

Route/Dosage
PO (Adults): 8 mg within 30 min of going to bed.

Availability
Tablets: 8 mg.

NURSING IMPLICATIONS

Assessment
- Assess sleep patterns before and periodically throughout therapy.

Potential Nursing Diagnoses
Insomnia (Indications)
Risk for injury (Side Effects)

Implementation
- Do not administer with or immediately after a high-fat meal.
- Before administering, reduce external stimuli and provide comfort measures to increase effectiveness of medication.
- **PO:** Administer within 30 min prior to going to bed.

Patient/Family Teaching
- Instruct patient to take ramelteon as directed, within 30 minutes of going to bed and to confine activities to those necessary to prepare for bed. Instruct patient to read the *Medication Guide* before starting and with each Rx refill, changes may occur.
- Causes drowsiness. Caution patient to avoid driving and other activities requiring alertness until response to medication is known.
- Caution patient that complex sleep-related behaviors (sleep-driving, making phone calls, preparing and eating food) may occur while asleep.
- Advise patient to notify health care professional immediately if signs of anaphylaxis (swelling of the tongue or throat, trouble breathing, and nausea and vomiting) or angioedema (severe facial swelling) occur; may occur as early as the first time the product is taken.
- Caution patient to avoid concurrent use of alcohol or other CNS depressants.

Evaluation/Desired Outcomes
- Relief of insomnia.

---

ramipril, See ANGIOTENSIN-CONVERTING ENZYME (ACE) INHIBITORS.

---

ranitidine, See HISTAMINE H₂ ANTAGONISTS.

---

ranolazine (ra-nole-a-zeen)
Ranexa

Classification
Therapeutic: antianginals

Pregnancy Category C

Indications
Chronic angina pectoris.

Action
Does not ↓ blood pressure or heart rate; remainder of mechanism is not known. **Therapeutic Effects:** Decreased frequency of angina.

Pharmacokinetics
Absorption: Highly variable.
Distribution: Unknown.
Metabolism and Excretion: Metabolized in the gut (P-glycoprotein) and by the liver (primarily CYP3A and less by CYP2D6); <5% excreted unchanged in urine and feces.
Half-life: 7 hr.

TIME/ACTION PROFILE (blood levels)

ROUTE	ONSET	PEAK	DURATION
PO	unknown	2–5 hr	12 hr

Contraindications/Precautions
Contraindicated in: Hypersensitivity; Concurrent use of potent inhibitors of CYP3A; Concurrent use of inducers of CYP3A; Hepatic impairment; Lactation: Lactation.
Use Cautiously in: Renal impairment; OB: Use only when potential benefit outweighs risk to fetus; Pedi: Safety not established; Geri: ↑ risk of adverse reactions in patients >75 yr.

Adverse Reactions/Side Effects
CNS: dizziness, headache. **EENT:** tinnitus. **CV:** palpitations, QTc prolongation. **GI:** abdominal pain, constipation, dry mouth, nausea, vomiting.

Interactions
Drug-Drug: **Ketoconazole**, **itraconazole**, **clarithromycin**, **nefazodone**, **nelfinavir**, **ritonavir**, **indinavir**, and **saquinavir** significantly ↑ levels (contraindicated). **Verapamil**, **diltiazem**, **aprepitant**, **erythromycin**, and **fluconazole** ↑ levels (do not exceed ranolazine dose of 500 mg twice daily). **Cyclosporine** may ↑ levels. **Rifampin**, **rifabutin**, **rifapentin**, **phenobarbital**, **phenytoin**, and **carbamazepine** significantly ↓ levels (contraindicated). **Paroxetine** may ↑ levels. ↑ blood levels of **simvastatin** and its active metabolite. May ↓ metabolism and ↑ effects of **tricyclic antidepressants** and **antipsychotics**, dosage adjustments may be necessary. May ↑ **digoxin** levels; dose adjustment may be required.
Drug-Natural Products: **St. John's wort** significantly ↓ levels (contraindicated).
Drug-Food: **Grapefruit juice** ↑ levels (do not exceed ranolazine dose of 500 mg twice daily).

Route/Dosage
PO (Adults): 500 mg twice daily initially, may be ↑ to 1000 mg twice daily.

Availability
Extended-release tablet: 500 mg.

NURSING IMPLICATIONS
Assessment
- Assess location, duration, intensity, and precipitating factors of anginal pain.
- Monitor ECG at baseline and periodically during therapy to evaluate effects on QT interval.
- *Lab Test Considerations:* May cause ↑ serum creatinine. Usually has a rapid onset, but does not progress during therapy and is reversible with discontinuation of ranolazine.
- May cause transient eosinophilia.
- May cause small mean ↓ in hematocrit.

Potential Nursing Diagnoses
Ineffective tissue perfusion (Indications)
Activity intolerance (Indications)

Implementation
- Ranolazine should be used in combination with amlodipine, beta blockers, or nitrates.
- Do not administer with grapefruit juice or grapefruit products.
- **PO:** May be administered without regard to food. Tablets should be swallowed whole; do not break, crush, or chew.

Patient/Family Teaching
- Instruct patient to take ranolazine as directed. If a dose is missed, take the usual dose at the next scheduled time; do not double doses. Explain to patient that ranolazine is used for chronic therapy and will not help an acute anginal episode.
- Advise patient to avoid grapefruit juice and grapefruit products when taking ranolazine.
- May cause dizziness and light-headedness. Caution patient to avoid driving and other activities requiring alertness until response to medication is known.
- Inform patient that ranolazine may cause changes in the ECG. Patient should inform health care professional if they have a personal or family history of QTc prolongation, congenital long QT syndrome, or proarrhythmic conditions such as hypokalemia.
- Advise patient to consult health care professional prior to taking other Rx, OTC, or herbal products.

Evaluation/Desired Outcomes
- Decrease in frequency of angina attacks.

rasagiline (raza-ji-leen)
Azilect

rasagiline

Classification
Therapeutic: antiparkinson agents
Pharmacologic: monoamine oxidase type B inhibitors

Pregnancy Category C

Indications
Parkinson's disease (monotherapy and adjunctive to levodopa).

Action
Irreversibly inactivates monoamine oxidase (MAO) by binding to it at type B (brain sites); inactivation of MAO leads to increased amounts of dopamine available in the CNS. Differs from selegiline by its nonamphetamine characteristics.
Therapeutic Effects: Improvement in symptoms of Parkinson's disease, allowing increase in function.

Pharmacokinetics
Absorption: 36% absorbed following oral administration.
Distribution: Readily crosses the blood-brain barrier.
Metabolism and Excretion: Extensively metabolized by the liver (CYP1A2 enzyme) to an inactive metabolite; less than 1% excreted in urine.
Half-life: 1.3 hr; does not correlate with duration of MAO-B inhibition.

TIME/ACTION PROFILE

ROUTE	ONSET	PEAK	DURATION
PO	rapid	1 hr	40 days*

*Recovery of MAO-B function.

Contraindications/Precautions
Contraindicated in: Hypersensitivity; Concurrent meperidine, tramadol, propoxyphene, methadone, sympathomimetic amines, dextromethorphan, mirtazapine, cyclobenzaprine, cocaine, or St. John's wort; Moderate to severe hepatic impairment; Elective surgery requiring general anesthesia; allow 14 days after discontinuation; Pheochromocytoma.
Use Cautiously in: Mild hepatic impairment (↑ blood levels); OB: Use only if maternal benefit outweighs fetal risk; Lactation: May inhibit lactation; Pedi: Safety not established.

Adverse Reactions/Side Effects
CNS: depression, dizziness, hallucinations, malaise, vertigo. **EENT:** conjunctivitis, rhinitis. **Resp:** asthma. **CV:** chest pain, postural hypotension (may ↑ levodopa-induced hypotension), syncope. **GI:** anorexia, dizziness, dyspepsia, gastroenteritis, vomiting. **GU:** albuminuria, ↓ libido. **Derm:** alopecia, ecchymosis, ↑ melanoma risk, rash. **Endo:** weight loss. **Hemat:** leukopenia. **MS:** arthralgia, arthritis, neck pain. **Neuro:** dyskinesia (may ↑ levodopa-induced dyskinesia), paresthesia. **Misc:** allergic reactions, flu-like syndrome, ↑ fall risk, fever.

Interactions
Drug-Drug: **Ciprofloxacin** and other **inhibitors of the CYP1A2 enzyme** ↑ rasagiline levels; dose adjustment is recommended. **Meperidine** has resulted in life-threatening reactions when used with other MAO inhibitors; wait at least 14 days after discontinuation of rasagiline to initiate meperidine. Similar reactions may occur with **tramadol, methadone, propoxyphene**; concurrent use should be avoided. Concurrent use with **dextromethorphan** may result in psychosis/bizarre behavior and should be avoided. ↑ risk of adverse reactions with **mirtazapine** and **cyclobenzapine**; concurrent use should be avoided. Hypertensive crisis may occur with **sympathomimetic amines** including **amphetamines, cold products**, and some **weight loss products** containing **vasoconstrictors** such as **pseudoephedrine, phenylephrine**, or **ephedrine**; avoid concurrent use. ↑ risk of CNS toxicity with **tricyclic antidepressants, SSRI antidepressants, SNRI antidepressants**, and other **MAO inhibitors**; rasagiline should be discontinued ≥14 days prior to initiation of antidepressants (**fluoxetine** should be discontinued ≥5 weeks prior to rasagiline therapy). Hypertensive crisis may also occur when rasagiline is used with **other MAO inhibitors**; allow at least 14 days between usage.
Drug-Natural Products: Risk of toxicity is ↑ with **St. John's wort**.
Drug-Food: Ingestion of **tyramine-rich foods or beverages** may result in life-threatening hypertensive crisis.

Route/Dosage
PO (Adults): *Monotherapy*—1 mg daily; *adjunct therapy*—0.5 mg daily, may be ↑ to 1 mg daily; *concurrent ciprofloxacin or other CYP1A2 inhibitors*—0.5 mg daily.

Hepatic Impairment
PO (Adults): *Mild hepatic impairment*—1 mg daily; *adjunct therapy*—0.5 mg daily, may be ↑ to 1 mg daily.

Availability
Tablets: 0.5 mg, 1 mg.

NURSING IMPLICATIONS
Assessment
- Assess signs and symptoms of Parkinson's disease (tremor, muscle weakness and rigidity, ataxic gait) prior to and during therapy.
- Monitor blood pressure periodically during therapy.
- Assess skin for melanomas periodically during therapy.
- **Lab Test Considerations:** May cause albuminuria, leukopenia, and abnormal liver function tests.
- ***Toxicity and Overdose:*** Concurrent ingestion of tyramine-rich foods and many medications may result in a life-threatening hypertensive crisis. Signs and symptoms of hypertensive crisis include chest pain, tachycardia or bradycardia, severe headache, neck stiffness or soreness, nausea and vomiting, sweating, photosensitivity, and enlarged pupils.

Potential Nursing Diagnoses
Impaired physical mobility (Indications)
Risk for injury (Indications, Side Effects)

Implementation
- If used in combination with levodopa, a reduction in levodopa dose may be considered based on individual results.
- **PO:** Administer once daily.

Patient/Family Teaching
- Instruct patient to take rasagiline as directed. Missed doses should be omitted and next dose taken at usual time the following day. Do not double doses.
- Caution patient to avoid alcohol, CNS depressants, and foods or beverages containing tyramine (see Appendix M) during and for at least 2 wk after therapy has been discontinued; they may precipitate a hypertensive crisis. Contact health care professional immediately if symptoms of hypertensive crisis develop.
- Instruct patient to consult health care professional before taking any Rx, OTC, or herbal products. Caution patient to avoid use of St. John's Wort and the analgesics meperidine, propoxyphene, tramadol, or methadone during therapy.
- Caution patient to avoid elective surgery requiring general anesthesia, cocaine, or local anesthesia containing sympathomimetic vasoconstrictors within 14 days of discontinuing rasagiline. If surgery is necessary sooner, benzodiazepines, mivacurium, rapacuronium, fentanyl, morphine, and codeine may be used cautiously.
- May cause dizziness or drowsiness. Caution patient to avoid driving and other activities requiring alertness until response to medication is known.
- Caution patient to change positions slowly to minimize orthostatic hypotension. Geriatric patients are at increased risk for this side effect.
- Advise patient to monitor for melanomas frequently and on a regular basis.
- Advise patient to notify health care professional immediately if severe headache, neck stiffness, heart racing, or palpitations, occur.

Evaluation/Desired Outcomes
- Improvement in symptoms of Parkinson's disease, allowing increase in function.

---

rasburicase
(ras-**byoor**-i-case)
Elitek

Classification
Therapeutic: antigout agents, antihyperuricemics
Pharmacologic: enzymes

Pregnancy Category C

Indications
Initial management of increased uric acid levels in children with leukemia, lymphoma, or other malignancies who are being treated with antineoplastics which are expected to produce hyperuricemia.

Action
An enzyme which promotes the conversion of uric acid to allantoin, an inactive, water-soluble compound. Produced by recombinant DNA technology. **Therapeutic Effects:** Decreased sequelae of hyperuricemia (nephropathy, arthropathy).

Pharmacokinetics
Absorption: IV administration results in complete bioavailability.
Distribution: Unknown.
Metabolism and Excretion: Unknown.
Half-life: 18 hr.

TIME/ACTION PROFILE (decrease in uric acid)

ROUTE	ONSET	PEAK	DURATION
IV	rapid	unknown	4–24 hr

Contraindications/Precautions
Contraindicated in: ⚱ G6PD deficiency (↑ risk of severe hemolysis); Previous allergic reaction, hemolysis or methemoglobinemia from rasburicase; Lactation: Lactation.
Use Cautiously in: OB: Pregnancy (use only if clearly needed).

Adverse Reactions/Side Effects
CNS: headache. **Resp:** respiratory distress. **GI:** abdominal pain, constipation, diarrhea, nausea, vomiting, mucositis. **Derm:** rash. **Hemat:** HEMOLYSIS, METHEMOGLOBINEMIA, neutropenia. **Misc:** hypersensitivity reactions including ANAPHYLAXIS, fever, sepsis.

Interactions
Drug-Drug: None known.

Route/Dosage
IV (Children): 0.15 or 0.2 mg/kg daily as a single dose for 5 days.

Availability
Lyophilized powder for reconstitution: 1.5 mg/vial.

NURSING IMPLICATIONS

Assessment
- Monitor patients for signs of allergic reactions and anaphylaxis (chest pain, dyspnea, hypotension, urticaria). If these signs occur, rasburicase should be immediately and permanently discontinued.
- *Lab Test Considerations:* Monitor patients for hemolysis. ⚱ Screen patients at higher risk for G6PD deficiency (patients of African American or Mediterranean ancestry) prior to therapy. If hemolysis occurs, discontinue and do not restart rasburicase.
- Monitor patients for methemoglobinemia. Discontinue rasburicase and do not restart in patients who develop methemoglobinemia.
- May cause spuriously low uric acid levels in blood samples left at room temperature. Collect blood for uric acid levels in pre-chilled tubes containing heparin and immediately immerse and maintain in an ice water bath. Uric acid must be analyzed in plasma. Plasma samples must be assayed within 4 hr of collection.

Potential Nursing Diagnoses
Deficient knowledge, related to medication regimen (Patient/Family Teaching)

Implementation
- Chemotherapy is initiated 4–24 hr after first dose of rasburicase.

IV Administration
- **Intermittent Infusion:** Determine number of vials of rasburicase needed based on patient's weight and dose/kg. Reconstitute in diluent provided. Add 1 mL of diluent provided to each vial and mix by swirling very gently. Do not shake or vortex. Solution should be clear and colorless. Do not use solutions that are discolored or contain particulate matter. *Diluent:* Remove dose from reconstituted vials and inject into infusion bag of 0.9% NaCl for a final total volume of 50 mL. Administer within 24 hr of reconstitution. Store reconstituted or diluted solution in refrigerator for up to 24 hr. *Rate:* Administer over 30 min. Do not administer as a bolus.
- **Y-Site Incompatibility:** Infuse through a separate line. Do not use a filter with infusion. If separate line is not possible, flush line with at least 15 mL of 0.9% NaCl prior to rasburicase infusion.

Patient/Family Teaching
- Inform patient and family of purpose of rasburicase infusion.

Evaluation/Desired Outcomes
- Decrease in plasma uric acid levels in pediatric patients receiving antineoplastics expected to result in tumor lysis and subsequent elevation of plasma uric acid levels.

HIGH ALERT

repaglinide (re-pag-gli-nide)
♣ Gluconorm, Prandin

Classification
Therapeutic: antidiabetics
Pharmacologic: meglitinides

Pregnancy Category C

Indications
Type 2 diabetes mellitus, with diet and exercise; may be used with metformin, rosiglitazone, or pioglitazone.

Action
Stimulates the release of insulin from pancreatic beta cells by closing potassium channels, which results in the opening of calcium channels in beta

cells. This is followed by release of insulin. **Therapeutic Effects:** Lowering of blood glucose levels.

Pharmacokinetics
Absorption: Well absorbed (56%) following oral administration.
Distribution: Unknown.
Protein Binding: >98%.
Metabolism and Excretion: Mostly metabolized by the liver; metabolites are excreted primarily in feces.
Half-life: 1 hr.

TIME/ACTION PROFILE

ROUTE	ONSET	PEAK	DURATION
PO	within 30 min	60–90 min	<4 hr

Contraindications/Precautions
Contraindicated in: Hypersensitivity; Lactation: Lactation; Diabetic ketoacidosis; Type 1 diabetes; Concurrent use of gemfibrozil.
Use Cautiously in: Impaired liver function (longer dosing intervals may be necessary); Severe renal impairment (dose ↓ recommended); Geri: Consider age-related ↓ in renal/hepatic/cardiovascular function; OB, Pedi: Safety not established; insulin recommended to control diabetes during pregnancy.

Adverse Reactions/Side Effects
CV: angina, chest pain. **Endo:** HYPOGLYCEMIA, hyperglycemia.

Interactions
Drug-Drug: Ketoconazole, miconazole, gemfibrozil, itraconazole, and erythromycin may ↓ metabolism and ↑ risk of hypoglycemia; concurrent use with gemfibrozil contraindicated. Effects may also be ↑ by NSAIDs, cyclosporine, hormonal contraceptives, simvastatin, sulfonamides, chloramphenicol, warfarin, probenecid, MAO inhibitors, and beta blockers. Effects may be ↓ by corticosteroids, phenothiazines, thyroid preparations, estrogens, hormonal contraceptives, phenytoin, nicotinic acid, sympathomimetics, isoniazid, and calcium channel blockers. **Drug-Natural Products:** Glucosamine may worsen blood glucose control. Chromium and coenzyme Q-10 may produce ↑ hypoglycemic effects.

Route/Dosage
PO (Adults): 0.5–4 mg taken before meals (not to exceed 16 mg/day).

Renal Impairment
PO (Adults): *Severe renal impairment*—start with 0.5 mg/day and titrate carefully.

Availability
Tablets: 0.5 mg, 1 mg, 2 mg. **Cost:** 0.5 mg $385.64/270, 1 mg $377.70/270, 2 mg $377.97/270. *In combination with:* metformin (PrandiMet); see Appendix B.

NURSING IMPLICATIONS
Assessment
- Observe patient for signs and symptoms of hypoglycemic reactions (abdominal pain, sweating, hunger, weakness, dizziness, headache, tremor, tachycardia, anxiety). Hypoglycemia may be difficult to recognize in geriatric patients and in patients taking beta blockers. Hypoglycemia is more likely to occur with insufficient caloric intake, following intense prolonged exercise, or when alcohol or more than one hypoglycemic agent is used.
- *Lab Test Considerations:* Monitor fasting serum glucose and glycosylated hemoglobin periodically during therapy to evaluate effectiveness.

Potential Nursing Diagnoses
Imbalanced nutrition: more than body requirements (Indications)
Noncompliance (Patient/Family Teaching)

Implementation
- Patients stabilized on a diabetic regimen who are exposed to stress, fever, trauma, infection, or surgery may require administration of insulin. Withhold repaglinide and reinstitute after resolution of acute episode.
- Repaglinide therapy should be temporarily discontinued from patients requiring surgery involving restricted intake of food and fluids.
- There is no fixed dose of repaglinide. Dose is based on periodic monitoring of blood glucose and long-term response is based on glycolysated hemoglobin levels. If adequate response is not achieved, metformin may be added to regimen. If combination therapy is unsuccessful, oral hypoglycemic therapy may need to be discontinued and replaced with insulin.
- When replacing other oral hypoglycemic agents, repaglinide may be started on the day following discontinuation of the other agent. Monitor blood glucose closely. Discontinuation of long-acting oral hypoglycemics may require monitoring for a week or more.
- Short-term repaglinide therapy may be used for patients well controlled with diet experiencing transient loss of control.

- **PO:** Administer up to 30 min before meals. Patients who skip a meal or add an extra meal should skip or add a dose, respectively, for that meal.

Patient/Family Teaching
- Instruct patient to take repaglinide before each meal, exactly as directed.
- Explain to patient that repaglinide helps control hyperglycemia but does not cure diabetes. Therapy is usually long term.
- Encourage patient to follow prescribed diet, medication, and exercise regimen to prevent hyperglycemic or hypoglycemic episodes.
- Review signs of hypoglycemia and hyperglycemia with patient. If hypoglycemia occurs, advise patient to take a glass of orange juice or 2–3 tsp of sugar, honey, or corn syrup dissolved in water, and notify health care professional.
- Instruct patient in proper testing of blood glucose. These tests should be monitored closely during periods of stress or illness and a health care professional notified if significant changes occur.
- Caution patient to avoid taking other Rx, OTC or herbal products, or alcohol during repaglinide therapy without consulting health care professional.
- Insulin is the recommended method of controlling blood glucose during pregnancy. Counsel female patients to use a form of contraception other than oral contraceptives and to notify health care professional promptly if pregnancy is planned or suspected.
- Advise patient to inform health care professional of medication regimen prior to treatment or surgery.
- Advise patient to carry a form of sugar (sugar packets, candy) and identification describing disease process and medication regimen at all times.
- Emphasize the importance of routine follow-up exams and regular testing of blood glucose and glycosylated hemoglobin.

Evaluation/Desired Outcomes
- Control of blood glucose levels without the appearance of hypoglycemic or hyperglycemic episodes.

---

reteplase, See THROMBOLYTIC AGENTS.

Rh$_o$(D) IMMUNE GLOBULIN
(arr aych oh dee im-**yoon** glob-yoo-lin)

Rh$_o$(D) immune globulin standard dose IM
HyperRHO S/D Full Dose, RhoGAM

Rh$_o$(D) immune globulin microdose IM
HyperRHO S/D Mini-Dose, MICRhoGAM, Mini-Gamulin R

Rh$_o$(D) immune globulin IV
WinRho SDF

Rh$_o$(D) immune globulin microdose IM, IV
Rhophylac

Classification
Therapeutic: vaccines/immunizing agents
Pharmacologic: immune globulins

Pregnancy Category C

Indications
IM, IV: Administered to Rh$_o$(D)-negative patients who have been exposed to Rh$_o$(D)-positive blood by: Pregnancy or delivery of a Rh$_o$(D)-positive infant, Abortion of a Rh$_o$(D)-positive fetus, Fetal-maternal hemorrhage due to amniocentesis, other obstetrical manipulative procedure, or intra-abdominal trauma while carrying a Rh$_o$(D)-positive fetus, Transfusion of Rh$_o$(D)-positive blood or blood products to a Rh$_o$(D)-negative patient. **IV:** Management of immune thrombocytopenic purpura (ITP).

Action
Prevent production of anti-Rh$_o$(D) antibodies in Rh$_o$(D)-negative patients who were exposed to Rh$_o$(D)-positive blood. Increase platelet counts in patients with ITP. **Therapeutic Effects:** Prevention of antibody response and hemolytic disease of the newborn (erythroblastosis fetalis) in future pregnancies of women who have conceived a Rh$_o$(D)-positive fetus. Prevention of Rh$_o$(D) sensitization following transfusion accident. Decreased bleeding in patients with ITP.

Pharmacokinetics
Absorption: Completely absorbed with IV administration. Well absorbed from IM sites.
Distribution: Unknown.
Metabolism and Excretion: Unknown.

Rh₀(D) IMMUNE GLOBULIN

Half-life: approximately 25–30 days.

TIME/ACTION PROFILE (blood levels)

ROUTE	ONSET	PEAK	DURATION
IM	rapid	5–10 days	unknown
IV†	unknown	2 hr	unknown

†When given for ITP, platelet counts start to rise in 1–2 days, peak after 5–7 days, and last for 30 days

Contraindications/Precautions
Contraindicated in: Prior hypersensitivity reaction to human immune globulin; Rh₀(D)- or Du-positive patients.
Use Cautiously in: ITP patients with pre-existing anemia (decrease dose if Hgb <10 g/dL). May also cause disseminated intravascular coagulation in ITP patients.

Adverse Reactions/Side Effects
CNS: dizziness, headache. **CV:** hypertension, hypotension. **Derm:** rash. **GI:** diarrhea, nausea, vomiting. **Hemat:** *ITP*—anemia, intravascular hemolysis. **MS:** arthralgia, myalgia. **Local:** pain at injection site. **Misc:** fever.

Interactions
Drug-Drug: May decrease antibody response to some **live-virus vaccines** (**measles**, **mumps**, **rubella**).

Route/Dosage
Rh₀(D) Immune Globulin (for IM use only)

Following Delivery
IM (Adults): *HyperRHO S/D Full Dose, RhoGAM*—1 vial standard dose (300 mcg) within 72 hr of delivery.

Before Delivery
IM (Adults): *HyperRHO S/D Full Dose, RhoGAM*—1 vial standard dose (300 mcg) at 26–28 wk.

Termination of Pregnancy (<13 wk Gestation)
IM (Adults): *HyperRHO S/D Mini-Dose, MICRhoGAM*—1 vial of microdose (50 mcg) within 72 hr.

Termination of Pregnancy (>13 wk Gestation)
IM (Adults): *RhoGAM*—1 vial standard dose (300 mcg) within 72 hr.

Large Fetal-Maternal Hemorrhage (>15 mL)
IM (Adults): *RhoGAM*—20 mcg/mL of Rh₀(D)-positive fetal RBCs.

Transfusion Accident
IM (Adults): *HyperRHO S/D Full Dose, RhoGAM*—(Volume of Rh-positive blood administered × Hct of donor blood)/15 = number of vials of standard dose (300 mcg) preparation (round to next whole number of vials).

Rh₀(D) Immune Globulin IV (for IM or IV Use)

Following Delivery
IM, IV (Adults): *WinRho SDF*—600 IU (120 mcg) within 72 hr of delivery. *Rhophylac*—1500 IU (300 mcg) within 72 hr of delivery.

Prior to Delivery
IM, IV (Adults): *WinRho SDF, Rhophylac*—1500 IU (300 mcg) at 28 wk; if initiated earlier in pregnancy, repeat q 12 wk.

Following Amniocentesis or Chorionic Villus Sampling
IM, IV (Adults): *WinRho SDF (before 34 wk gestation)*—1500 IU (300 mcg) immediately; repeat q 12 wk during pregnancy. *Rhophylac*—1500 IU (300 mcg) within 72 hr of procedure.

Termination of Pregnancy, Amniocentesis, or Any Other Manipulation
IM, IV (Adults): *WinRho SDF*—600 IU (120 mcg) within 72 hr after event.

Large Fetal-Maternal Hemorrhage/Transfusion Accident
IM (Adults): *WinRho SDF*—6000 IU (1200 mcg) q 12 hr until total dose is given (total dose determined by amount of blood loss/hemorrhage).
IV (Adults): 3000 IU (600 mcg) q 8 hr until total dose is given (total dose determined by amount of blood loss/hemorrhage).

Immune Thrombocytopenic Purpura
IV (Adults and Children): *WinRho SDF, Rhophylac*—50 mcg (250 IU)/kg initially (if Hgb <10 g/dL, ↓ dose to 25–40 mcg [125–200 IU]/kg); further dosing/frequency determined by clinical response (range 25–60 mcg [125–300 IU]/kg). Each dose may be given as a single dose or in 2 divided doses on separate days.

Availability
Rh₀(D) Immune Globulin (for IM Use)
Injection: 50 mcg/vial (microdose—MICRhoGAM, HyperRHO S/D Mini-Dose), 300 mcg/vial (standard dose—RhoGAM, HyperRHO S/D Full Dose).

Rh₀(D) Immune Globulin Intravenous (for IM or IV Use)
Injection: 600 IU (120 mcg)/vial, 1500 IU (300 mcg)/vial, 2500 IU (500 mcg)/vial, 5000 IU (1000 mcg)/vial, 15000 IU (3000 mcg)/vial. **Prefilled syringes:** 1500 IU (300 mcg/2 mL).

NURSING IMPLICATIONS
Assessment
- **IV:** Assess vital signs periodically during therapy in patients receiving IV Rh₀(D) immune globulin.
- **ITP:** Monitor patient for signs and symptoms of intravascular hemolysis (IVH) (back pain, shaking chills, fever, hemoglobinuria), anemia, and renal insufficiency. If transfusions are required, use Rh₀(D)-negative packed red blood cells to prevent exacerbation of IVH.
- *Lab Test Considerations: Pregnancy:* Type and crossmatch of mother and newborn's cord blood must be performed to determine need for medication. Mother must be Rh₀(D)-negative and Du-negative. Infant must be Rh₀(D)-positive. If there is doubt regarding infant's blood type or if father is Rh₀(D)-positive, medication should be given.
- An infant born to a woman treated with Rh₀(D) immune globulin antepartum may have a weakly positive direct Coombs' test result on cord or infant blood.
- *ITP:* Monitor platelet counts, RBC counts, hemoglobin, and reticulocyte levels to determine effectiveness of therapy.

Potential Nursing Diagnoses
Deficient knowledge, related to medication regimen (Patient/Family Teaching)

Implementation
- Do not give to infant, to Rh₀(D)-positive individual, or to Rh₀(D)-negative individual previously sensitized to the Rh₀(D) antigen. However, there is no more risk than when given to a woman who is not sensitized. When in doubt, administer Rh₀(D) immune globulin.
- Do not confuse IM and IV formulations. Rh immune globulin for IV administration is labelled 'Rh Immune Globulin Intravenous.' Rh Immune Globulin Intravenous may be given IM; however, Rh Immune Globulin (microdose and standard dose) is for IM use only and cannot be given IV.
- When using prefilled syringes, allow solution to reach room temperature before administration.
- **IM:** Reconstitute Rh₀(D) immune globulin IV for IM use immediately before use with 1.25 mL of 0.9% NaCl. Inject diluent onto inside wall of vial and wet pellet by gently swirling until dissolved. Do not shake.
- Administer into the deltoid muscle. Dose should be given within 3 hr but may be given up to 72 hr after delivery, miscarriage, abortion, or transfusion.

IV Administration
- **Direct IV:** Reconstitute Rh₀(D) immune globulin IV for IV administration immediately before use with 2.5 mL of 0.9% NaCl. Inject diluent onto inside wall of vial and wet pellet by gently swirling until dissolved. Do not shake. *Rate:* Administer over 3–5 min.

Patient/Family Teaching
- **Pregnancy:** Explain to patient that the purpose of this medication is to protect future Rh₀(D)-positive infants.
- **ITP:** Explain purpose of medication to patient.

Evaluation/Desired Outcomes
- Prevention of erythroblastosis fetalis in future Rh₀(D)-positive infants.
- Prevention of Rh₀(D) sensitization following incompatible transfusion.
- Decreased bleeding episodes in patients with ITP.

---

ribavirin (rye-ba-**vye**-rin)
Copegus, Rebetol, Virazole

Classification
Therapeutic: antivirals
Pharmacologic: nucleoside analogues

Pregnancy Category X

Indications
Inhaln: Treatment of severe lower respiratory tract infections caused by the respiratory syncytial virus (RSV) in infants and young children. **PO:** *Rebetol*—with interferon alfa-2b (*Intron A*) or peginterferon alfa-2b (*PegIntron*) in the treatment of chronic hepatitis C in patients who have failed previous therapy. **PO:** *Copegus*—with peginterferon alfa-2a (Pegasys) in the treatment of chronic hepatitis C in patients who have failed previous therapy. **Unlabeled Use:** Early (within

24 hr of symptoms) secondary treatment of influenza A or B in young adults.

Action
Inhibits viral DNA and RNA synthesis and subsequent replication. Must be phosphorylated intracellularly to be active. **Therapeutic Effects: Inhaln:** Virustatic action. **PO:** Decreased progression and sequelae of chronic hepatitis C.

Pharmacokinetics
Absorption: Systemic absorption occurs following nasal and oral inhalation. Rapidly and extensively absorbed following oral administration, but undergoes first-pass hepatic metabolism (64% bioavailability).
Distribution: 70% of inhaled drug is deposited in the respiratory tract. Appears to concentrate in the respiratory tract and red blood cells. Enters breast milk.
Metabolism and Excretion: Eliminated from the respiratory tract by distribution across membranes, macrophages, and ciliary motion. Metabolized primarily by the liver; metabolites are renally excreted.
Half-life: *Inhaln*—9.5 hr (40 days in RBCs); *oral*—43.6 hr (single dose); 12 days (multiple dose).

TIME/ACTION PROFILE (blood levels)

ROUTE	ONSET	PEAK	DURATION
Inhaln	unknown	end of inhaln	unknown
PO	unknown	1.7–3 hr	12 hr

Contraindications/Precautions
Contraindicated in: Hypersensitivity; **Inhalation:** Patients receiving mechanically assisted ventilation; **Oral:** OB, Lactation: Pregnancy or lactation; OB: Male partners of pregnant patients; CCr <50 mL/min; Significant/unstable cardiovascular disease; Hemoglobinopathies; Autoimmune hepatitis or hepatic decompensation before/during treatment (for combined therapy with interferon alfa-2b or peginterferon alfa-2a); Concurrent use of didanosine, stavudine, or zidovudine.
Use Cautiously in: PO: Sarcoidosis (may exacerbate condition); Anemia (dose reduction/discontinuation may be required); Any pre-existing cardiac disease; OB: Patients with childbearing potential.

Adverse Reactions/Side Effects
Inhalation.
CNS: dizziness, faintness. **EENT:** blurred vision, conjunctivitis, erythema of the eyelids, ocular irritation, photosensitivity. **CV:** CARDIAC ARREST, hypotension. **Derm:** rash. **Hemat:** hemolytic anemia (with interferon alpha 2b), reticulocytosis.

Oral (may reflect combination with interferon)
CNS: emotional lability (↑ in children), fatigue (↓ in children), impaired concentration (↓ in children), insomnia (↓ in children), irritability (↓ in children). **EENT:** dry mouth. **Resp:** dyspnea (↓ in children). **GI:** anorexia (↑ in children), dyspepsia (↓ in children), vomiting (↑ in children). **Hemat:** hemolytic anemia. **Derm:** STEVENS-JOHNSON SYNDROME, pruritus (↓ in children). **MS:** arthralgia (↓ in children). **Misc:** fever (↑ in children).

Interactions
Drug-Drug: Oral: May ↓ the antiretroviral action of **stavidine** and **zidovudine**. May ↑ hematologic toxicity of **zidovudine**. May ↑ blood levels and risk of toxicity of **didanosine**. Although used together in the management of hepatitis, concurrent use with **interferon alpha 2b** ↑ risk of hemolytic anemia.

Route/Dosage
Inhaln (Infants and Young Children): 300 mL of 20 mg/mL solution delivered via mist for 12–18 hr/day.

Rebetol (with peginterferon alfa-2b [PegIntron])
PO (Adults >105 kg): 600 mg in the morning, then 800 mg in the evening for 48 wk (viral genotype 1) or 24 wk (viral genotypes 2 and 3).
PO (Adults 86–105 kg): 600 mg in the morning, then 600 mg in the evening for 48 wk (viral genotype 1) or 24 wk (viral genotypes 2 and 3).
PO (Adults 66–85 kg): 400 mg in the morning, then 600 mg in the evening for 48 wk (viral genotype 1) or 24 wk (viral genotypes 2 and 3).
PO (Adults ≤65 kg): 400 mg in the morning, then 400 mg in the evening for 48 wk (viral genotype 1) or 24 wk (viral genotypes 2 and 3).
PO (Children 3–17 yr and >73 kg): 600 mg in the morning and 600 mg in the evening for 48 wk (viral genotype 1) or 24 wk (viral genotypes 2 and 3).
PO (Children 3–17 yr and 60–73 kg): 400 mg in the morning and 600 mg in the evening for 48 wk (viral genotype 1) or 24 wk (viral genotypes 2 and 3).
PO (Children 3–17 yr and 47–59 kg): 400 mg in the morning and 400 mg in the evening for 48 wk (viral genotype 1) or 24 wk (viral genotypes 2 and 3).
PO (Children 3–17 yr and <47 kg): 15 mg/kg/day in 2 divided doses (as oral solution) for 48 wk (viral genotype 1) or 24 wk (viral genotypes 2 and 3).

ribavirin 1109

Rebetol (with interferon alfa-2b [Intron A])
PO (Adults >75 kg): 600 mg in the morning, then 600 mg in the evening for 48 wk (viral genotype 1) or 24 wk (viral genotypes 2 and 3).
PO (Adults ≤75 kg): 400 mg in the morning, then 600 mg in the evening for 48 wk (viral genotype 1) or 24 wk (viral genotypes 2 and 3).
PO (Children >61 kg): Refer to adult dosing.
PO (Children 50–61 kg): 400 mg in the morning and 400 mg in the evening for 48 wk (viral genotype 1) or 24 wk (viral genotypes 2 and 3).
PO (Children 37–49 kg): 200 mg in the morning and 400 mg in the evening for 48 wk (viral genotype 1) or 24 wk (viral genotypes 2 and 3).
PO (Children 25–36 kg): 200 mg in the morning and 200 mg in the evening for 48 wk (viral genotype 1) or 24 wk (viral genotypes 2 and 3).
PO (Children <25 kg): 15 mg/kg/day in 2 divided doses (as oral solution) for 48 wk (viral genotype 1) or 24 wk (viral genotypes 2 and 3).

Copegus—viral genotype 1 or 4 (with peginterferon alfa-2a)
PO (Adults ≥75 kg): 600 mg twice daily for 48 wk.
PO (Adults <75 kg): 500 mg twice daily for 48 wk.

Copegus—viral genotype 2 or 3 (with peginterferon alfa-2a)
PO (Adults): 400 mg twice daily for 24 wk.

Availability
Powder for reconstitution for aerosol use: 6 g/vial. **Capsules (Rebetol):** 200 mg. **Oral solution (Rebetol):** 40 mg/mL. **Tablets (Copegus):** 200 mg, 400 mg, 600 mg. *In combination with:* Rebetrol with interferon alfa-2b (Intron A) as combination therapy for chronic hepatitis C (Rebetron). See Appendix B; *Copegus* is intended for combined therapy with pegylated interferon alfa-2a (*Pegasys*).

NURSING IMPLICATIONS

Assessment
- **RSV:** Assess patient for infection (vital signs, sputum, WBC) at beginning and during therapy.
- Obtain specimens for culture and sensitivity prior to initiating therapy. First dose may be given before receiving results.
- Assess respiratory (lung sounds, quality and rate of respirations) and fluid status prior to and frequently throughout therapy.
- **Chronic Hepatitis C:** Monitor symptoms of hepatitis during therapy.
- Assess patient for signs of depression during therapy. Monitor closely for neuropsychiatric changes, including suicidal thoughts.
- Assess patient for cardiovascular disorders (pulse, blood pressure, chest pain). May cause myocardial infarction.
- Assess for signs of colitis (abdominal pain, bloody diarrhea, fever) and pancreatitis (nausea, vomiting, abdominal pain) during therapy. Discontinue therapy if these occur; may be fatal.
- Assess pulmonary status (lung sounds, respirations) periodically during therapy. May require discontinuation.
- Monitor for hypersensitivity reactions (urticaria, angioedema, bronchoconstriction, anaphylaxis). Discontinue immediately and institute supportive therapy.
- *Lab Test Considerations:* Chronic Hepatitis C: Monitor CBC with differential and platelet count prior to initiation, at week 2, and week 4, and regularly during therapy. If hemoglobin <10 g/dL in patients with no history of cardiac disease or ↓ more than 2 g/dL in any 4 wk treatment period in patients with history of stable cardiac disease, decrease ribavirin dose to 600 mg (200 mg in AM and 400 mg in PM). If hemoglobin <8.5 g/dL in patients with no history of cardiac disease or <12 g/dL despite dose reduction in patients with history of stable cardiac disease, discontinue combination therapy permanently.
- Monitor liver function tests and thyroid stimulating hormone prior to and periodically during therapy.
- Monitor pregnancy tests prior to, monthly during, and for 6 mo following discontinuation of therapy in women of childbearing age. Ribavarin should be started following a negative pregnancy test.
- May cause ↑ serum bilirubin and uric acid levels.

Potential Nursing Diagnoses
Risk for infection (Indications, Side Effects)
Impaired gas exchange (Indications)

✦ = Canadian drug name. 🧬 = Genetic implication.
*CAPITALS indicates life-threatening; underlines indicate most frequent.

Implementation

- **InhaIn:** Infants requiring assisted ventilation should be suctioned every 1–2 hr and pulmonary pressures monitored every 2–4 hr.
- Ribavirin treatment should begin within the first 3 days of RSV infection to be effective.
- Ribavirin aerosol should be administered using the Viratek SPAG model SPAG-2 only. Do not administer via other aerosol-generating devices. Usually administered using an infant oxygen hood attached to the SPAG-2 aerosol generator. Administration by face mask may be used if the oxygen hood cannot be used.
- Reconstitute ribavirin 6-g vial with preservative-free sterile water for injection or inhalation. Transfer to clean, sterilized Erlenmeyer flask of the SPAG-2 reservoir and dilute to a final volume of 300 mL. This recommended concentration (20 mg/mL) in the reservoir provides a concentration of aerosol ribavirin of 190 mcg/liter of air over a 12-hr period. Solution should be discarded and replaced every 24 hr.
- Aerosol treatments should be administered continuously 12–18 hr/day for 3–7 days.
- **PO:** Administer with food. Capsules should be swallowed whole; do not open, crush, or chew.

Patient/Family Teaching

- **RSV:** Explain the purpose and route of treatment to the patient and parents.
- Inform patient and parents that ribavirin may cause blurred vision and photosensitivity.
- **Chronic Hepatitis C:** Instruct patient to take ribavirin at the same time each day for the full course of therapy. Take missed doses as soon as remembered. If total day dose is missed, notify health care professional; do not double doses. Emphasize the importance of routine lab test to monitor for side effects.
- Advise patient to brush teeth twice daily, have regular dental examinations, and rinse mouth thoroughly after vomiting to prevent dental and periodontal disorders.
- Inform patient about teratogenic effects of ribavirin. Instruct women with childbearing potential, and men, to use 2 forms of effective contraception during and for at least 6 mo following conclusion of therapy. Men must use a condom. Avoid breastfeeding during use.
- May cause dizziness, confusion, fatigue, and drowsiness. Caution patient to avoid driving or other activities requiring alertness until response to medication is known.
- Inform patient that ribavirin may not reduce the risk of transmission of HCV to others or prevent cirrhosis, liver failure, or liver cancer.
- Advise patient to consult health care professional before taking any other Rx, OTC, or herbal products.
- Advise patient to stop taking ribavirin and notify health care professional immediately if rash with fever, blisters or sores in mouth, nose, or eyes, or conjunctivitis occurs and to notify health care professional if trouble breathing, hives or swelling, chest pain, severe stomach pain or low back pain, bloody diarrhea or bloody or black stools, bruising or unusual bleeding, change in vision, fever >100.5°F, worsening psoriasis, worsening depression or suicidal thoughts occur.

Evaluation/Desired Outcomes

- Resolution of the signs and symptoms of RSV.
- Decreased progression and sequelae of chronic hepatitis C.

---

rifabutin (riff-a-**byoo**-tin)
Mycobutin

Classification
Therapeutic: agents for atypical mycobacterium

Pregnancy Category B

Indications
Prevention of disseminated *Mycobacterium avium* complex (MAC) disease in patients with advanced HIV infection. **Unlabeled Use:** Treatment of *Helicobacter pylori* ulcer disease which has failed on other regimens (with pantoprazole and amoxicillin).

Action
Appears to inhibit DNA-dependent RNA polymerase in susceptible organisms. **Therapeutic Effects:** Antimycobacterial action against susceptible organisms. **Spectrum:** Active against *M. avium* and most strains of *M. tuberculosis*.

Pharmacokinetics
Absorption: Well absorbed following oral administration (50–85%). Absorption is decreased in HIV-positive patients (20%).
Distribution: Widely distributed to body tissues and fluids.
Metabolism and Excretion: Mostly metabolized by the liver; <5% excreted unchanged by the kidneys.
Half-life: 45 hr.

rifabutin

TIME/ACTION PROFILE (blood levels)

ROUTE	ONSET	PEAK	DURATION
PO	rapid	2–4 hr	24 hr

Contraindications/Precautions
Contraindicated in: Hypersensitivity. Cross-sensitivity with other rifamycins (rifampin) may occur; Active tuberculosis; Concurrent ritonavir or delavirdine.
Use Cautiously in: OB, Lactation: Pedi: Safety not established.

Adverse Reactions/Side Effects
EENT: brown-orange discoloration of tears, ocular disturbances. **Resp:** dyspnea. **CV:** chest pain, chest pressure. **GI:** PSEUDOMEMBRANOUS COLITIS, brown-orange discoloration of saliva, altered taste, drug-induced hepatitis. **GU:** brown-orange discoloration of urine. **Derm:** rash, skin discoloration. **Hemat:** hemolysis, neutropenia, thrombocytopenia. **MS:** arthralgia, myositis. **Misc:** brown-orange discoloration of body fluids, flu-like syndrome.

Interactions
Drug-Drug: Increases metabolism and may decrease the effectiveness of other drugs, including **amprenavir**, **efavirenz**, **indinavir**, **nelfinavir**, **nevirapine**, **saquinavir**, (dosage adjustment may be necessary), **delavirdine**, (concurrent use should be avoided), **corticosteroids**, **disopyramide**, **quinidine**, **opioid analgesics**, **oral hypoglycemic agents**, **warfarin**, **estrogens**, **estrogen-containing contraceptives**, **phenytoin**, **verapamil**, **fluconazole**, **quinidine**, **tocainide**, **theophylline**, **zidovudine**, and **chloramphenicol**. **Ritonavir** increases blood levels of rifabutin (concurrent use is contraindicated), similar effects occur with **efavirenz** and **nevirapine**.

Route/Dosage
PO (Adults): 300 mg once daily. If GI upset occurs, may give as 150 mg twice daily with food. *H. pylori*—300 mg/day (unlabeled).

Availability
Capsules: 150 mg.

NURSING IMPLICATIONS

Assessment
- Monitor patient for signs of active tuberculosis (purified protein derivative [PPD], chest x-ray, sputum culture, blood culture, urine culture, biopsy of suspicious lymph nodes) prior to and throughout therapy. Rifabutin must not be administered to patients with active tuberculosis.
- Monitor bowel function. Diarrhea, abdominal cramping, fever, and bloody stools should be reported to health care professional promptly as a sign of pseudomembranous colitis. May begin up to several weeks following cessation of therapy.
- *Lab Test Considerations:* Monitor CBC periodically during therapy. May cause neutropenia and thrombocytopenia.

Potential Nursing Diagnoses
Risk for infection (Indications)
Noncompliance (Patient/Family Teaching)

Implementation
- Do not confuse rifabutin with rifampin.
- **PO:** May be administered without regard to meals. High-fat meals slow rate but not extent of absorption. May be mixed with foods such as applesauce. If GI upset occurs, administer with food.

Patient/Family Teaching
- Advise patient to take medication as directed. Do not skip doses or double up on missed doses. Emphasize the importance of continuing therapy even if asymptomatic.
- Advise patient to notify health care professional promptly if signs and symptoms of neutropenia (sore throat, fever, signs of infection), thrombocytopenia (unusual bleeding or bruising), or hepatitis (yellow eyes and skin, nausea, vomiting, anorexia, unusual tiredness, weakness) occur.
- Caution patient to avoid the use of alcohol during this therapy, because this may increase the risk of hepatotoxicity.
- Instruct patient to notify health care professional immediately if diarrhea, abdominal cramping, fever, or bloody stools occur and not to treat with antidiarrheals without consulting health care professionals.
- Instruct patient to report symptoms of myositis (myalgia, arthralgia) or uveitis (intraocular inflammation) to health care professional promptly.
- Inform patient that saliva, sputum, sweat, tears, urine, and feces may become red-orange to red-brown and that soft contact lenses may become permanently discolored.
- Advise patient that this medication has teratogenic properties and may decrease the effectiveness of oral contraceptives. Counsel patient

to use a nonhormonal form of contraception throughout therapy.
- Emphasize the importance of regular follow-up exams to monitor progress and to check for side effects.

Evaluation/Desired Outcomes
- Prevention of disseminated MAC in patients with advanced HIV infection.

---

rifampin (rif-am-pin)
Rifadin, Rimactane, ✸ Rofact

Classification
Therapeutic: antituberculars
Pharmacologic: rifamycins

Pregnancy Category C

Indications
Active tuberculosis (with other agents). Elimination of meningococcal carriers. **Unlabeled Use:** Prevention of disease caused by *Haemophilus influenzae* type B in close contacts.

Action
Inhibits RNA synthesis by blocking RNA transcription in susceptible organisms. **Therapeutic Effects:** Bactericidal action against susceptible organisms. **Spectrum:** Broad spectrum notable for activity against: *Mycobacterium* spp, *Staphylococcus aureus*, *H. influenzae*, *Legionella pneumophila*, *Neisseria meningitidis*.

Pharmacokinetics
Absorption: Well absorbed following oral administration.
Distribution: Widely distributed; enters CSF. Crosses placenta; enters breast milk.
Metabolism and Excretion: Mostly metabolized by the liver; 60% eliminated in feces via biliary elimination.
Half-life: 3 hr.

TIME/ACTION PROFILE (blood levels)

ROUTE	ONSET	PEAK	DURATION
PO	rapid	2–4 hr	12–24 hr
IV	rapid	end of infusion	12–24 hr

Contraindications/Precautions
Contraindicated in: Hypersensitivity; Concurrent indinavir, nelfinavir, pyrazinamide, or saquinavir.
Use Cautiously in: History of liver disease; Concurrent use of other hepatotoxic agents; Pregnancy or lactation.

Adverse Reactions/Side Effects
CNS: ataxia, confusion, drowsiness, fatigue, headache, weakness. **EENT:** red discoloration of tears. **GI:** abdominal pain, diarrhea, flatulence, heartburn, nausea, vomiting, drug-induced hepatitis, red discoloration of saliva. **GU:** red discoloration of urine. **Hemat:** hemolytic anemia, thrombocytopenia. **MS:** arthralgia, myalgia. **Misc:** red discoloration of all body fluids, flu-like syndrome.

Interactions
Drug-Drug: ↑ risk of hepatotoxicity with other **hepatotoxic agents**, including **alcohol**, **ketoconazole**, **isoniazid**, **pyrazinamide** (concurrent use with **pyrazinamide** may result in potentially fatal hepatotoxicity and should be avoided). Rifampin significantly ↓ blood levels of **delavirdine**, **indinavir**, **nelfinavir**, and **saquinavir**; concurrent use is contraindicated. Rifampin stimulates liver enzymes, which may ↑ metabolism and ↓ effectiveness of other drugs, including **ritonavir**, **nevirapine**, and **efavirenz** (dose adjustment may be necessary), **corticosteroids**, **disopyramide**, **quinidine**, **opioid analgesics**, **oral hypoglycemic agents**, **warfarin**, **estrogens**, **phenytoin**, **verapamil**, **fluconazole**, **ketoconazole**, **itraconazole**, **quinidine**, **tocainide**, **theophylline**, **chloramphenicol**, and **hormonal contraceptive agents**.

Route/Dosage

Tuberculosis
PO, IV (Adults): 600 mg/day or 10 mg/kg/day (up to 600 mg/day) single dose; may also be given 2–3 times weekly.
PO, IV (Children): 10–20 mg/kg/day single dose (not to exceed 600 mg/day); may also be given 2–3 times weekly.

Asymptomatic Carriers of Meningococcus
PO, IV (Adults): 600 mg q 12 hr for 2 days.
PO, IV (Children ≥1 mo): 10 mg/kg q 12 hr for 2 days.
PO (Infants <1 mo): 5 mg/kg q 12 hr for 2 days.

Prevention of *H. influenzae* Type B Infection
PO (Adults): 600 mg/day for 4 days.
PO (Children): 20 mg/kg/day for 4 days.

Availability (generic available)
Capsules: 150 mg, 300 mg. **Powder for injection:** 600 mg/vial. *In combination with:* isoniazid (IsonaRif, Rifamate); isoniazid and pyrazinamide (Rifater). See Appendix B.

NURSING IMPLICATIONS

Assessment
- Perform mycobacterial studies and susceptibility tests prior to and periodically during therapy to detect possible resistance.
- Assess lung sounds and character and amount of sputum periodically during therapy.
- *Lab Test Considerations:* Evaluate renal function, CBC, and urinalysis periodically and during therapy.
- Monitor hepatic function at least monthly during therapy. May cause ↑ BUN, AST, ALT, and serum alkaline phosphatase, bilirubin, and uric acid concentrations.
- May cause false-positive direct Coombs' test results. May interfere with folic acid and vitamin B assays.
- May interfere with dexamethasone suppression test results; discontinue rifampin 15 days prior to test.
- May interfere with methods for determining serum folate and vitamin B levels and with urine tests based on color reaction.
- May delay hepatic uptake and excretion of sulfobromophthalein (SBP) during SBP uptake and excretion tests; perform test prior to daily dose of rifampin.

Potential Nursing Diagnoses
Risk for infection (Indications)
Noncompliance (Patient/Family Teaching)

Implementation
- Do not confuse rifampin with rifabutin.
- **PO:** Administer medication on an empty stomach at least 1 hr before or 2 hr after meals with a full glass (240 mL) of water. If GI irritation becomes a problem, may be administered with food. Antacids may also be taken 1 hr prior to administration. Capsules may be opened and contents mixed with applesauce or jelly for patients with difficulty swallowing.
- Pharmacist can compound a syrup for patients unable to swallow solids.

IV Administration
- **Intermittent Infusion:** Reconstitute each 600-mg vial with 10 mL of sterile water for injection for a concentration of 60 mg/mL. *Diluent:* Dilute further in 100 mL or 500 mL of D5W or 0.9% NaCl. Reconstituted vials are stable at room temperature for 24 hr. Infusion is stable at room temperature for 4 hr (in D5W) or 24 hr (in 0.9% NaCl). *Concentration:* Final concentration of infusion should not exceed 6 mg/mL. *Rate:* Administer solutions diluted in 100 mL over 30 min and solutions diluted in 500 mL over 3 hr.
- **Y-Site Compatibility:** amiodarone, bumetanide, midazolam, pantoprazole, vancomycin.
- **Y-Site Incompatibility:** diltiazem.

Patient/Family Teaching
- Advise patient to take medication once daily (unless biweekly regimens are used), as directed, and not to skip doses or double up on missed doses. Emphasize the importance of continuing therapy even after symptoms have subsided. Length of therapy for tuberculosis depends on regimen being used and underlying disease states. Patients on short-term prophylactic therapy should also be advised of the importance of compliance with therapy.
- Advise patient to notify health care professional promptly if signs and symptoms of hepatitis (yellow eyes and skin, nausea, vomiting, anorexia, unusual tiredness, weakness) or of thrombocytopenia (unusual bleeding or bruising) occur.
- Caution patient to avoid the use of alcohol during this therapy, because this may increase the risk of hepatotoxicity.
- Instruct patient to report the occurrence of flu-like symptoms (fever, chills, myalgia, headache) promptly.
- Rifampin may occasionally cause drowsiness. Caution patient to avoid driving or other activities requiring alertness until response to medication is known.
- Inform patient that saliva, sputum, sweat, tears, urine, and feces may become red-orange to red-brown and that soft contact lenses may become permanently discolored.
- Advise patient that this medication has teratogenic properties and may decrease the effectiveness of oral contraceptives. Counsel patient to use a nonhormonal form of contraception throughout therapy.
- Emphasize the importance of regular follow-up exams to monitor progress and to check for side effects.

Evaluation/Desired Outcomes
- Decreased fever and night sweats.
- Diminished cough and sputum production.
- Negative sputum cultures.
- Increased appetite.
- Weight gain.

- Reduced fatigue.
- Sense of well-being in patients with tuberculosis.
- Prevention of meningococcal meningitis.
- Prevention of *H. influenzae* type B infection. Prophylactic course is usually short-term.

rifaximin (ri-fax-i-min)
Xifaxan

Classification
Therapeutic: anti-infectives
Pharmacologic: rifamycins

Pregnancy Category C

Indications
Travelers' diarrhea due to noninvasive strains of *Escherichia coli*.

Action
Inhibits bacterial RNA synthesis by binding to bacterial DNA-dependent RNA polymerase. **Therapeutic Effects:** Decreased severity of travelers' diarrhea. **Spectrum:** *Escherichia coli* (enterotoxigenic and enteroaggregative strains).

Pharmacokinetics
Absorption: Poorly absorbed (<0.4%), action is primarily in GI tract.
Distribution: 80–90% concentrated in gut.
Metabolism and Excretion: Almost exclusively excreted unchanged in feces.
Half-life: 6 hr.

TIME/ACTION PROFILE

ROUTE	ONSET	PEAK	DURATION
PO	unknown	unknown	unknown

Contraindications/Precautions
Contraindicated in: Hypersensitivity to rifaximin or other rifamycins; Diarrhea with fever or bloody stools; Diarrhea caused by other infections agents; Lactation: Potential for adverse effects in the infant. Switch to formula for duration of treatment.
Use Cautiously in: OB: Use only if benefit to mother outweighs risk to fetus; Pedi: Safety not established in children <12 yr.

Adverse Reactions/Side Effects
CNS: dizziness. **GI:** PSEUDOMEMBRANOUS COLITIS.

Interactions
Drug-Drug: Although rifaximin induces the CYP 3A4 enzyme system, since it is not absorbed, drug interactions are unlikely.

Route/Dosage
PO (Adults and Children ≥12 yr): 200 mg three times daily for 3 days.

Availability
Tablets: 200 mg.

NURSING IMPLICATIONS

Assessment
- Assess frequency and consistency of stools and bowel sounds prior to and during therapy.
- Assess fluid and electrolyte balance and skin turgor for dehydration.
- *Lab Test Considerations:* May cause lymphocytosis, monocytosis, and neutropenia.

Potential Nursing Diagnoses
Diarrhea (Indications)
Risk for deficient fluid volume (Indications)

Implementation
- **PO:** Administer with or without food, 3 times daily for 3 days.

Patient/Family Teaching
- Instruct patient to take rifaximin as directed and to complete therapy, even if feeling better. Caution patient to stop taking rifaximin if diarrhea symptoms get worse, persist more than 24–48 hr, or are accompanied by fever or blood in the stool. Consult health care professional if these occur.
- May cause dizziness. Caution patient to avoid driving and other activities requiring alertness until response to medication is known.
- Advise female patients to notify health care professional if pregnant or if pregnancy is suspected.

Evaluation/Desired Outcomes
- Decreased severity of travelers' diarrhea.

risedronate (riss-ed-roe-nate)
Actonel

Classification
Therapeutic: bone resorption inhibitors
Pharmacologic: biphosphonates

Pregnancy Category C

Indications
Prevention and treatment of postmenopausal and corticosteroid-induced osteoporosis. Treatment of Paget's disease in men and women. Treatment of osteoporosis in men.

Action
Inhibits bone resorption by binding to bone hydroxyapatite, which inhibits osteoclast activity.

risedronate

Therapeutic Effects: Reversal of the progression of osteoporosis with decreased fractures and other sequelae. Reduced bone turnover and resorption; normalization of serum alkaline phosphatase with reduced complications of Paget's disease.

Pharmacokinetics
Absorption: Rapidly but poorly absorbed following oral administration (0.63% bioavailability).
Distribution: 60% of absorbed dose distributes to bone.
Metabolism and Excretion: 40% of absorbed dose is excreted unchanged by kidneys; unabsorbed drug is excreted in feces.
Half-life: *Initial*—1.5 hr; *terminal*—220 hr (reflects dissociation from bone).

TIME/ACTION PROFILE (effects on serum alkaline phosphatase)

ROUTE	ONSET	PEAK	DURATION
PO	within days	30 days	up to 16 mo

Contraindications/Precautions
Contraindicated in: Hypersensitivity; Hypocalcemia; Lactation: Lactation; Severe renal impairment (CCr <30 mL/min).
Use Cautiously in: History of upper GI disorders; Other disturbances of bone or mineral metabolism (correct abnormalities before initiating therapy); Dietary deficiencies (supplemental vitamin D and calcium may be required); Concurrent dental surgery (may ↑ risk of jaw osteonecrosis); OB, Pedi: Safety not established; use in pregnancy only if potential benefit justifies potential risks.

Adverse Reactions/Side Effects
CNS: weakness. **EENT:** amblyopia, conjunctivitis, dry eyes, eye pain/inflammation, tinnitus. **CV:** chest pain, edema. **GI:** abdominal pain, diarrhea, belching, colitis, constipation, dysphagia, esophagitis, esophageal cancer, esophageal ulcer, gastric ulcer, nausea. **Derm:** rash. **MS:** arthralgia, musculoskeletal pain, osteonecrosis (primarily of jaw). **Misc:** flu-like syndrome.

Interactions
Drug-Drug: Concurrent use with **NSAIDs** or **aspirin** ↑ risk of GI irritation. Absorption is ↓ by **calcium supplements** or **antacids**.
Drug-Food: Food ↓ absorption (administer at least 30 min before breakfast).

Route/Dosage
PO (Adults): *Postmenopausal Osteoporosis*—5 mg daily; *or* 35 mg once weekly; *or* 75 mg taken on two consecutive days for a total of 2 tablets each month; *or* 150 mg once monthly *Osteoporosis in Men*—35 mg once weekly; *Glucocorticoid-induced Osteoporosis*—5 mg daily; *Paget's disease*—30 mg daily for 2 mo; retreatment may be considered after 2 mo off therapy.

Availability
Tablets: 5 mg, 30 mg, 35 mg, 75 mg, 150 mg.
Cost: 5 mg $272.31/90, 30 mg $1,282.24/90, 35 mg $90.97/4, 75 mg $97.47/2. ***In combination with:*** calcium carbonate.

NURSING IMPLICATIONS

Assessment
- **Osteoporosis:** Assess patients via bone density study for low bone mass before and periodically during therapy.
- **Paget's disease:** Assess for symptoms of Paget's disease (bone pain, headache, decreased visual and auditory acuity, increased skull size).
- **Lab Test Considerations:** *Osteoporosis:* Assess serum calcium before and periodically during therapy. Hypocalcemia and vitamin D deficiency should be treated before initiating alendronate therapy. May cause mild, transient ↑ of calcium and phosphate.
- *Paget's disease:* Monitor alkaline phosphatase prior to and periodically during therapy to monitor effectiveness of therapy.

Potential Nursing Diagnoses
Risk for injury (Indications)

Implementation
- **PO:** Administer first thing in the morning with 6–8 oz of plain water, 30 min prior to other medications, beverages, or food. Tablet should be swallowed whole; do not crush, break, or chew.
- Calcium-, magnesium-, or aluminum-containing agents may interfere with absorption of risedronate and should be taken at a different time of day with food.

Patient/Family Teaching
- Instruct patient on the importance of taking as directed, first thing in the morning, 30 min prior to other medications, beverages, or food. Waiting longer than 30 min will improve absorption. Risedronate should be taken with 6–

8 oz of plain water (mineral water, orange juice, coffee, and other beverages decrease absorption). If a dose is missed, skip dose and resume the next morning; do not double doses or take later in the day. Do not discontinue without consulting health care professional.
- Caution patients to remain upright for 30 min following dose to facilitate passage to stomach and minimize risk of esophageal irritation.
- Advise patient to eat a balanced diet and consult health care professional about the need for supplemental calcium and vitamin D (see Appendix M).
- Inform patient that severe musculoskeletal pain may occur within days, months, or yr after starting risendronate. Symptoms my resolve completely after discontinuation or slow or incomplete resolution may occur. Notify health care professional if severe pain occurs.
- Encourage patient to participate in regular exercise and to modify behaviors that increase the risk of osteoporosis (stop smoking, reduce alcohol consumption).
- Advise patient to inform health care professional of risedronate therapy prior to dental surgery.
- Advise female patients to notify health care professional if pregnancy is planned or suspected or if she is nursing.

Evaluation/Desired Outcomes
- Reversal of the progression of osteoporosis with decreased fractures and other sequelae.
- Decrease in serum alkaline phosphatase and the progression of Paget's disease.

---

risperidone (riss-**per**-i-done)
Risperdal, Risperdal M-TAB, Risperdal Consta

Classification
Therapeutic: antipsychotics, mood stabilizers
Pharmacologic: benzisoxazoles

Pregnancy Category C

Indications
Schizophrenia in adults and adolescents age 13–17 yr. Short-term treatment of acute manic or mixed episodes associated with Bipolar I Disorder (oral only) in adults, and children and adolescents aged 10–17 yr, maintenance treatment of Bipolar I Disorder (IM only) in adults only; can be used with lithium or valproate (adults only). Treatment of irritability associated with autistic disorder in children age 5–16 yr.

Action
May act by antagonizing dopamine and serotonin in the CNS. **Therapeutic Effects:** Decreased symptoms of psychoses, bipolar mania, or autism.

Pharmacokinetics
Absorption: 70% after administration of tablets, solution or orally disintegrating tablets. Following IM administration, small initial release of drug, followed by 3–wk lag; the rest of release starts at 3 wk and lasts 4–6 wk.
Distribution: Unknown.
Metabolism and Excretion: Extensively metabolized by the liver. Metabolism is genetically determined; extensive metabolizers (most patients) convert risperidone to 9-hydroxyrisperidone rapidly. Poor metabolizers (6–8% of Whites) convert it more slowly. The 9-hydroxyrisperidone is an antipsychotic compound. Risperidone and its active metabolite are renally eliminated.
Half-life: *Extensive metabolizers*— 3 hr for risperidone, 21 hr for 9-hydroxyrisperidone. *Poor metabolizers*— 20 hr for risperidone and 30 hr for 9-hydroxyrisperidone.

TIME/ACTION PROFILE (clinical effects)

ROUTE	ONSET	PEAK	DURATION
PO	1–2 wk	unknown	up to 6 wk†
IM	3 wk	4–6 wk	up to 6 wk†

†After discontinuation

Contraindications/Precautions
Contraindicated in: Hypersensitivity; Lactation: Discontinue drug or bottle feed.
Use Cautiously in: Debilitated patients, patients with renal or hepatic impairment (initial dose reduction recommended); Underlying cardiovascular disease (↑ risk of arrhythmias and hypotension); History of seizures; History of suicide attempt or drug abuse; Diabetes or risk factors for diabetes (may worsen glucose control); Patients at risk for aspiration; OB, Pedi: Safety not established; Geri: Initial dose ↓ recommended. ↑ risk of mortality in elderly patients treated for dementia-related psychosis.

Adverse Reactions/Side Effects
CNS: NEUROLEPTIC MALIGNANT SYNDROME, SUICIDAL THOUGHTS, aggressive behavior, dizziness, extrapyramidal reactions, headache, ↑ dreams, ↑ sleep duration, insomnia, sedation, fatigue, impaired temperature regulation, nervousness, tardive dyskinesia. **EENT:** pharyngitis, rhinitis, visual disturbances. **Resp:** cough, dyspnea. **CV:** arrhythmias, orthostatic hypotension, tachycardia. **GI:** constipation, diarrhea, dry mouth, nausea, abdominal pain, anorexia, dyspepsia, ↑ saliva-

risperidone **1117**

tion, vomiting, weight gain, weight loss, polydipsia. **GU:** ↓ libido, dysmenorrhea/menorrhagia, difficulty urinating, polyuria. **Derm:** itching/skin rash, dry skin, ↑ pigmentation, sweating, photosensitivity, seborrhea. **Endo:** galactorrhea, hyperglycemia. **Hemat:** AGRANULOCYTOSIS, leukopenia, neutropenia. **MS:** arthralgia, back pain.

Interactions
Drug-Drug: May ↓ the antiparkinsonian effects of **levodopa** or other **dopamine agonists**. **Carbamazepine, phenytoin, rifampin, phenobarbital**, and other **enzyme inducers** ↑ metabolism and may ↓ effectiveness; dose adjustments may be necessary. **Fluoxetine** and paroxetine ↑ blood levels and may ↑ effects; dose adjustments may be necessary. **Clozapine** ↓ metabolism and may ↑ effects of risperidone. ↑ CNS depression may occur with other **CNS depressants**, including **alcohol, antihistamines, sedative/hypnotics**, or **opioid analgesics**.
Drug-Natural Products: Kava, valerian, or chamomile can ↑ CNS depression.

Route/Dosage
Schizophrenia
PO (Adults): 1 mg twice daily, ↑ by 1–2 mg/day no more frequently than every 24 hr to 4–8 mg daily.
PO (Children 13–17 yr): 0.5 mg once daily, ↑ by 0.5–1.0 mg no more frequently than every 24 hr to 3 mg daily. May administer half the daily dose twice daily if drowsiness persists.
IM (Adults): 25 mg every 2 wk; some patients may benefit from a higher dose of 37.5 or 50 mg every 2 wk.

Acute Manic or Mixed Episodes Associated with Bipolar I Disorder
PO (Adults): 2–3 mg/day as a single daily dose, dose may be ↑ at 24–hr intervals by 1 mg (range 1–5 mg/day).
PO (Children 13–17 yr): 0.5 mg once daily, ↑ by 0.5–1 mg no more frequently than every 24 hr to 2.5 mg daily. May administer half the daily dose twice daily if drowsiness persists.
PO (Geriatric Patients or Debilitated Patients): Start with 0.5 mg twice daily; ↑ by 0.5 mg twice daily, up to 1.5 mg twice daily; then ↑ at weekly intervals if necessary. May also be given as a single daily dose after initial titration.

Maintenance Treatment of Bipolar I Disorder
IM (Adults): 25 mg every 2 wk; some patients may benefit from a higher dose of 37.5 or 50 mg every 2 wk.

Irritability Associated with Autistic Disorder
PO (Children 5–16 yr weighing <20 kg): 0.25 mg/day initially. After at least 4 days of therapy, may ↑ to 0.5 mg/day. Dose ↑ in increments of 0.25 mg/day may be considered at 2-wk or longer intervals. May be as a single or divided dose.
PO (Children 5–16 yr weighing >20 kg): 0.5 mg/day initially. After at least 4 days of therapy, may ↑ to 1 mg/day. Dose ↑ in increments of 0.5 mg/day may be considered at 2-wk or longer intervals. May be as a single or divided dose.

Renal Impairment
Hepatic Impairment
PO (Adults): Start with 0.5 mg twice daily; ↑ by 0.5 mg twice daily, up to 1.5 mg twice daily; then ↑ at weekly intervals if necessary. May also be given as a single daily dose after initial titration.

Availability (generic available)
Tablets: 0.25 mg, 0.5 mg, 1 mg, 2 mg, 3 mg, 4 mg. **Cost:** 0.25 mg $605.97/180, 0.5 mg $671.96/180, 1 mg $751.93/180, 2 mg $1,219.95/180, 3 mg $1,489.95/180, 4 mg $1,831.84/180. **Orally disintegrating tablets (Risperdal M-Tabs):** 0.5 mg, 1 mg, 2 mg, 3 mg, 4 mg. **Cost:** 0.5 mg $122.93/28, 1 mg $138.95/28, 2 mg $130.68/28, 3 mg $148.49/28, 4 mg $194.02/28. **Oral solution:** 1 mg/mL. **Cost:** $136.66/30 mL. **Extended-release microspheres for injection (Risperdal Consta):** 12.5 mg/vial kit, 25 mg/vial kit, 37.5 mg/vial kit, 50 mg/vial kit.

NURSING IMPLICATIONS
Assessment
- Monitor patient's mental status (orientation, mood, behavior) before and periodically during therapy. Monitor closely for notable changes in behavior that could indicate the emergence or worsening of suicidal thoughts or behavior or depression.
- Assess weight and BMI initially and throughout therapy.

= Canadian drug name. = Genetic implication.
*CAPITALS indicates life-threatening; underlines indicate most frequent.

risperidone

- Monitor mood changes. Assess for suicidal tendencies, especially during early therapy. Restrict amount of drug available to patient.
- Monitor blood pressure (sitting, standing, lying down) and pulse before and frequently during initial dose titration. May cause prolonged QT interval, tachycardia, and orthostatic hypotension. If hypotension occurs, dose may need to be decreased.
- Observe patient when administering medication to ensure medication is swallowed and not hoarded or cheeked.
- Monitor patient for onset of extrapyramidal side effects (*akathisia*—restlessness; *dystonia*—muscle spasms and twisting motions; or *pseudoparkinsonism*—mask-like face, rigidity, tremors, drooling, shuffling gait, dysphagia). Report these symptoms; reduction of dose or discontinuation may be necessary. Trihexyphenidyl or benztropine may be used to control symptoms.
- Monitor for tardive dyskinesia (involuntary rhythmic movement of mouth, face, and extremities). Report immediately; may be irreversible.
- Monitor for development of neuroleptic malignant syndrome (fever, respiratory distress, tachycardia, seizures, diaphoresis, hypertension or hypotension, pallor, tiredness). Notify health care professional immediately if these symptoms occur.
- *Lab Test Considerations:* May cause ↑ serum prolactin levels.
- May cause ↑ AST and ALT.
- May also cause anemia, thrombocytopenia, leukocytosis, and leukopenia.
- Obtain fasting blood glucose and cholesterol levels initially and periodically during therapy.
- Monitor CBC frequently during initial months of therapy in patients with pre-existing or history of low WBC. May cause leukopenia, neutropenia, or agranulocytosis. Discontinue therapy if this occurs.

Potential Nursing Diagnoses
Risk for self-directed violence (Indications)
Disturbed thought process (Indications)
Risk for injury (Side Effects)

Implementation
- Do not confuse risperidone with reserpine.
- When switching from other antipsychotics, discontinue previous agents when starting risperidone and minimize the period of overlapping antipsychotic agents.
- If therapy is reinstituted after an interval off risperidone, follow initial titration schedule.
- For IM use, establish tolerance with oral dosing before IM use and continue oral dosing for 3 wk following initial IM injection. Do not increase dose more frequently than every 4 wk.
- **PO:** Daily doses can be taken in the morning or evening.
- For orally disintegrating tablets, open blister pack by pealing back foil to expose tablet; do not try to push tablet through foil. Use dry hands to remove tablet from blister and immediately place entire tablet on tongue. Tablets disintegrate in mouth within seconds and can be swallowed with or without liquid. Do not attempt to split or chew tablet. Do not try to store tablets once removed from blister.
- Oral solution can be mixed with water, coffee, orange juice, or low fat milk; do not mix with cola or tea.
- **IM:** Reconstitute with 2 mL of diluent provided by manufacturer. Administer via deep deltoid (1-inch needle) or gluteal (2-inch needle) injection using enclosed safety needle; alternate arms or buttocks with each injection. Allow solution to warm to room temperature prior to injection. Administer immediately after mixed with diluent; shake well to mix suspension. Must be administered within 6 hr of reconstitution. Store dose pack in refrigerator.
- Do not combine dose strengths in a single injection.

Patient/Family Teaching
- Instruct patient to take medication as directed.
- Inform patient of the possibility of extrapyramidal symptoms. Instruct patient to report these symptoms immediately to health care professional.
- Advise patient to change positions slowly to minimize orthostatic hypotension.
- May cause drowsiness. Caution patient to avoid driving or other activities requiring alertness until response to medication is known.
- Advise patient and family to notify health care professional if thoughts about suicide or dying, attempts to commit suicide; new or worse depression; new or worse anxiety; feeling very agitated or restless; panic attacks; trouble sleeping; new or worse irritability; acting aggressive; being angry or violent; acting on dangerous impulses; an extreme increase in activity and talking, other unusual changes in behavior or mood occur.
- Advise patient to use sunscreen and protective clothing when exposed to the sun to prevent photosensitivity reactions. Extremes in temper-

ature should also be avoided; this drug impairs body temperature regulation.
- Caution patient to avoid concurrent use of alcohol, other CNS depressants, and OTC medications or herbal products without consulting health care professional.
- Advise female patients to notify health care professional if pregnancy is planned or suspected, or if breastfeeding or planning to breastfeed.
- Advise patient to notify health care professional of medication regimen before treatment or surgery.
- Instruct patient to notify health care professional promptly if sore throat, fever, unusual bleeding or bruising, rash, or tremors occur.
- Emphasize the importance of routine follow up exams to monitor side effects and continued participation in psychotherapy to improve coping skills.

Evaluation/Desired Outcomes
- Decrease in excited, manic behavior.
- Decrease in positive symptoms (delusions, hallucinations) of schizophrenia.
- Decreased aggression toward others, deliberate self—injury, temper tantrums, and mood changes in children with autism.
- Decrease in negative symptoms (social withdrawal, flat, blunted affects) of schizophrenia.

ritonavir (ri-toe-na-veer)
Norvir

Classification
Therapeutic: antiretrovirals
Pharmacologic: protease inhibitors

Pregnancy Category B

Indications
HIV infection (with other antiretrovirals).

Action
Inhibits the action of HIV protease and prevents the cleavage of viral polyproteins. **Therapeutic Effects:** Increased CD4 cell counts and decreased viral load with subsequent slowed progression of HIV infection and its sequelae.

Pharmacokinetics
Absorption: Appears to be well absorbed after oral administration.
Distribution: Poor CNS penetration.
Protein Binding: 98–99%.
Metabolism and Excretion: Highly metabolized by the liver (by P450 CYP3A and CYP2D6 enzymes); one metabolite has antiretroviral activity; 3.5% excreted unchanged in urine.
Half-life: 3–5 hr.

TIME/ACTION PROFILE (blood levels)

ROUTE	ONSET	PEAK	DURATION
PO	rapid	4 hr*	12 hr

*Nonfasting

Contraindications/Precautions
Contraindicated in: Hypersensitivity; Concurrent use of alfuzosin, amiodarone, dihydroergotamine, ergotamine, ergonovine, flecainide, fluticasone, lovastatin, meperidine, methylergonovine, midazolam, pimozide, propafenone, quinidine, simvastatin, St. John's wort, triazolam, or voriconazole; Hypersensitivity or intolerance to alcohol or castor oil (present in capsules and liquid).

Use Cautiously in: Impaired hepatic function, history of hepatitis; Diabetes mellitus; Hemophilia (↑ risk of bleeding); Structural heart disease, conduction abnormalities, ischemic heart disease or heart failure (↑ risk of heart block); OB, Pedi: Pregnancy or children <12 yr (safety not established); Lactation: Breastfeeding not recommended in HIV-infected patients.

Adverse Reactions/Side Effects
CNS: SEIZURES, abnormal thinking, weakness, dizziness, headache, malaise, somnolence, syncope. **EENT:** pharyngitis, throat irritation. **Resp:** ANGIOEDEMA, bronchospasm. **CV:** heart block, orthostatic hypotension, vasodilation. **GI:** abdominal pain, altered taste, anorexia, diarrhea, nausea, vomiting, constipation, dyspepsia, flatulence. **GU:** renal insufficiency. **Derm:** rash, skin eruptions, sweating, urticaria. **Endo:** hyperglycemia. **F and E:** dehydration. **Metab:** hyperlipidemia. **MS:** ↑ creatine phosphokinase, myalgia. **Neuro:** circumoral paresthesia, peripheral paresthesia. **Misc:** hypersensitivity reactions including STEVENS-JOHNSON SYNDROME and ANAPHYLAXIS, fat redistribution, fever.

Interactions
Drug-Drug: Produces large ↑ in levels and effects of **amiodarone, alfuzosin, flecainide, fluticasone (inhalation), meperidine, pimozidepropafenone,** and **quinidine**; concurrent use should be avoided. Ergot toxicity may occur with concurrent use of **ergonovine, ergotamine methylergonovine,** or **dihydroergotamine**; concurrent use should be avoided. ↑ risk

of rhabdomyolysis with **lovastatin** or **simvastatin**; concurrent use should be avoided. ↑ levels and the risk of excessive sedation and/or respiratory depression from **midazolam** and **triazolam**; concurrent use should be avoided. ↑ levels of **maraviroc**; ↓ maraviroc dose to 150 mg twice daily. ↑ levels of **clarithromycin**; ↓ clarithromycin dose if CCr <60 mL/min. ↑ levels of **rifabutin**; ↓ rifabutin dose to 150 mg every other day or 3 times weekly. May lead to ↓ antifungal effects of **voriconazole**; concurrent use should be avoided. May also ↑ levels and effects of some **opioid analgesics** (**alfentanil, fentanyl, hydrocodone, oxycodone**), **tramadol**; some **NSAIDs** (**diclofenac, ibuprofen, indomethacin**); some **antiarrhythmics** (**disopyramide, lidocaine, mexiletine**); many **antidepressants** (**amitriptyline, clomipramine, desipramine, imipramine, nortriptyline, nefazodone, sertraline, trazodone, fluoxetine, paroxetine, venlafaxine**); some **antiemetics** (**dronabinol, ondansetron**); some **beta blockers** (**metoprolol, pindolol, propranolol, timolol**); many **calcium channel blockers** (**amlodipine, diltiazem, felodipine, isradipine, nicardipine, nifedipine, nimodipine, nisoldipine, verapamil**); some **antineoplastics** (**etoposides, paclitaxel, tamoxifen, vinblastine, vincristine**); some **corticosteroids** (**dexamethasone, prednisone**), most **HMG CoA reductase inhibitors**; some **immunosuppressants** (**cyclosporine, tacrolimus**); some **antipsychotics** (**chlorpromazine, haloperidol, perphenazine, risperidone, thioridazine**); and also **quinidine, saquinavir, methamphetamine**, and **warfarin**. Dosage ↓ may be necessary. ↓ levels and effects of **hormonal contraceptives, zidovudine, bupropion**, and **theophylline**; dose alteration or alternative therapy may be necessary. Levels may be ↑ by **clarithromycin** or **fluoxetine**. ↑ risk of heart block with **beta blockers, verapamil, diltiazem, digoxin**, or **atazanavir**. May ↑ concentrations of phosphodiesterase type 5 inhibitors (PDE5) causing hypotension, visual changes, priapism; ↓ starting doses not to exceed 25 mg within 48 hr for **sildenafil**, 2.5 mg q 72 hr for **vardenafil** and 10 mg q 72 hr for **tadalafil**.
Drug-Natural Products: St. John's wort ↓ levels and may promote resistance; concurrent use not recommended.
Drug-Food: Food ↑ absorption.

Route/Dosage
PO (Adults): 300 mg twice daily for 1 day, then 400 mg twice daily for 3 days, then 500 mg twice daily for 1 day, then 600 mg twice daily as maintenance.
PO (Children): 250 mg/m² twice daily initially; ↑ by 50 mg/m² twice daily q 2–3 days up to 400 mg/m² twice daily (if unable to get up to 400 mg/m² twice daily, additional antiretroviral therapy is required).

Availability
Capsules: 100 mg. **Oral solution:** 80 mg/mL.

NURSING IMPLICATIONS

Assessment
- Assess patient for change in severity of HIV symptoms and for symptoms of opportunistic infections during therapy.
- *Lab Test Considerations:* Monitor viral load and CD4 counts regularly during therapy.
- May cause hyperglycemia.
- May cause ↑ serum AST, ALT, GGT, total bilirubin, CPK, triglycerides, and uric acid concentrations.

Potential Nursing Diagnoses
Risk for infection (Indications)
Noncompliance (Patient/Family Teaching)

Implementation
- Do not confuse with Retrovir (zidovudine).
- **PO:** Administer with a meal or light snack.
- Oral powder may be mixed with chocolate milk, Ensure, or Advera within 1 hr of dosing to improve taste. Capsules should be stored in the refrigerator and protected from light. Use calibrated oral dosing syringe for oral solution. Oral solution does not require refrigeration if used within 30 days and stored below 77°F in the original container. Keep cap tightly closed.
- If nausea occurs on dose of 600 mg twice daily, may titrate by 300 mg twice daily for 1 day, then 400 mg twice daily for 2 days, then 500 mg twice daily for 1 day, then 600 mg twice daily thereafter.
- Patients initiating concurrent therapy with nucleoside analogues may have less GI intolerance by initiating ritonavir for 2 wk and then adding the nucleoside analogue.

Patient/Family Teaching
- Emphasize the importance of taking ritonavir as directed, at evenly spaced times throughout day. Do not take more than prescribed amount and do not stop taking without consulting health care professional. Take missed doses as soon as remembered; do not double doses.
- Instruct patient that ritonavir should not be shared with others.

rituximab **1121**

- Advise patient to avoid taking other Rx, OTC, or herbal products without consulting health care professional.
- Inform patient that ritonavir does not cure AIDS or prevent associated or opportunistic infections. Ritonavir does not reduce the risk of transmission of HIV to others through sexual contact or blood contamination. Caution patient to use a condom during sexual contact and to avoid sharing needles or donating blood to prevent spreading the AIDS virus to others. Advise patient that the long-term effects of ritonavir are unknown at this time.
- Inform patient that ritonavir may cause hyperglycemia. Advise patient to notify health care professional if increased thirst or hunger; unexplained weight loss; increased urination; fatigue; or dry, itchy skin occurs.
- Advise patients taking oral contraceptives to use a nonhormonal method of birth control during ritonavir therapy.
- Inform patient that redistribution and accumulation of body fat may occur, causing central obesity, dorsocervical fat enlargement (buffalo hump), peripheral wasting, breast enlargement, and cushingoid appearance. The cause and long-term effects are not known.
- Emphasize the importance of regular follow-up exams and blood counts to determine progress and monitor for side effects.

Evaluation/Desired Outcomes
- Delayed progression of AIDS and decreased opportunistic infections in patients with HIV.
- Decrease in viral load and improvement in CD4 cell counts.

rituximab (ri-**tux**-i-mab)
Rituxan

Classification
Therapeutic: antineoplastics
Pharmacologic: monoclonal antibodies

Pregnancy Category C

Indications
Treatment of low-grade or follicular, CD20-positive, B-cell non-Hodgkin's lymphoma alone, with, or following treatment with cyclophosphamide, vincristine, and prednisolone (CVP). Moderately-to-severely active rheumatoid arthritis with methotrexate in patients who have had an inadequate response to one of more TNF antagonist therapies.

Action
Binds to the CD20 antigen on the surface of lymphoma cells, preventing the activation process for cell cycle initiation and differentiation. **Therapeutic Effects:** Death of lymphoma cells. Reduced signs and symptoms of rheumatoid arthritis.

Pharmacokinetics
Absorption: IV administration results in complete bioavailability.
Distribution: Binds specifically to CD20 binding sites on lymphoma cells.
Metabolism and Excretion: Unknown.
Half-life: 59.8–174 hr (depending on tumor burden).

TIME/ACTION PROFILE (B-cell depletion)

ROUTE	ONSET	PEAK	DURATION
IV	within 14 days	3–4 wk	6–9 mo†

†Duration of depletion after 4 wk of treatment.

Contraindications/Precautions
Contraindicated in: Hypersensitivity to murine (mouse) proteins; OB: Can pass placental barrier potentially causing fetal B-cell depletion. Give only if clearly needed; Lactation: Potential for immunosuppression in infant. Discontinue nursing.
Use Cautiously in: Pre-existing bone marrow depression; Hepatitis B infection (may reactivate infection during and for several months after treatment); Systemic lupus erythematosus (may cause fatal progressive multifocal leukoencephalopathy); HIV infection (may increase risk of HIV-associated lymphoma); Pedi: Safety not established.

Adverse Reactions/Side Effects
CNS: PROGRESSIVE MULTIFOCAL LEUKOENCEPHALOPATHY, headache. **Resp:** bronchospasm, cough, dyspnea. **CV:** ARRHYTHMIAS, hypotension, peripheral edema. **GI:** abdominal pain, altered taste, dyspepsia. **Derm:** MUCOCUTANEOUS SKIN REACTIONS, flushing, urticaria. **Endo:** hyperglycemia. **F and E:** hypocalcemia. **Hemat:** ANEMIA, NEUTROPENIA, THROMBOCYTOPENIA. **MS:** arthralgia, back pain. **Misc:** allergic reactions including ANAPHYLAXIS and ANGIOEDEMA, infections, INFUSION REACTIONS, TUMOR LYSIS SYNDROME, fever/chills/rigors (infusion related).

Interactions
Drug-Drug: None known.

Route/Dosage
Relapsed or refractory, low-grade or follicular, CD20–positive, B-cell Non-hodgkins lymphoma
IV (Adults): 375 mg/m^2 once weekly for 4–8 doses.

Retreatment Therapy
IV (Adults): 375 mg/m^2 once weekly for 4 doses.

Previously untreated follicular, CD20–positive, B-cell Non-Hodgkins lymphoma
IV (Adults): 375 mg/m^2 given on Day 1 of each cycle of CVP for up to 8 doses.

Previously untreated low-grade, CD20–positive, B-cell Non-Hodgkins lymphoma
IV (Adults): For patients who have not progressed following 6–8 cycles of CVP chemotherapy, 375 mg/m^2 given once weekly for 4 doses given every 6 mo for up to 16 doses.

Diffuse Large B-cell Non-Hodgkins lymphoma
IV (Adults): 375 mg/m^2 given on Day 1 of each cycle of CVP for up to 8 infusions.

Rheumatoid Arthritis
IV (Adults): Two 1000 mg separated by 2 wk.

Availability
Solution for injection (requires dilution): 10 mg/mL in 100-mg and 500-mg vials.

NURSING IMPLICATIONS
Assessment
- Monitor patient for fever, chills/rigors, nausea, urticaria, fatigue, headache, pruritus, bronchospasm, dyspnea, sensation of tongue or throat swelling, rhinitis, vomiting, hypotension, flushing, and pain at disease sites. These infusion-related events occur frequently within 30 min–2 hr of beginning first infusion and may resolve with slowing or discontinuing infusion and treatment with IV saline, diphenhydramine, and acetaminophen. Patients with increased risk (females, patients with pulmonary infiltrates, chronic lymphocytic leukemia, or mantle cell leukemia) may have more severe reactions, which may be fatal. Signs of severe reactions include hypotension, angioedema, hypoxia, or bronchospasm and may require interruption of infusion. May result in pulmonary infiltrates, adult respiratory distress syndrome, MI, ventricular fibrillation, and cardiogenic shock. Monitor closely. Incidence decreases with subsequent infusions.
- Monitor patient for tumor lysis syndrome due to rapid reduction in tumor volume (acute renal failure, hyperkalemia, hypocalcemia, hyperuricemia, or hypophosphatemia) usually occurring 12–24 hr after first infusion. Risks are higher in patients with greater tumor burden; may be fatal. Correct electrolyte abnormalities, monitor renal function and fluid balance, and administer supportive care, including dialysis, as indicated.
- Assess patient for hypersensitivity reactions (hypotension, bronchospasm, angioedema) during administration. May respond to decrease in infusion rate. Premedication with diphenhydramine and acetaminophen is recommended. Treatment includes diphenhydramine, acetaminophen, bronchodilators, or IV saline as indicated. Epinephrine, antihistamines, and corticosteroids should be readily available in the event of a severe reaction. If severe reactions occur, discontinue infusion; may be resumed at 50% of the rate when symptoms have resolved completely.
- Monitor ECG during and immediately after infusion in patients with pre-existing cardiac conditions (arrhythmias, angina) or patients who have developed arrhythmias during previous infusions of rituximab. Life-threatening arrhythmias may occur.
- Assess for signs of progressive multifocal leukoencephalopathy (hemiparesis, apathy, confusion, cognitive deficiencies, and ataxia) periodically during therapy.
- ***Lab Test Considerations:*** Monitor CBC and platelet count regularly during therapy and frequently in patients with blood dyscrasias. May cause anemia, thrombocytopenia, or neutropenia.
- Frequently causes B-cell depletion with an associated ↓ in serum immunoglobulins in a minority of patients; does not appear to cause an increased incidence of infection.

Potential Nursing Diagnoses
Risk for infection (Side Effects)

Implementation
- Transient hypotension may occur during infusion; antihypertensive medications may be held for 12 hr before infusion.
- **Rheumatoid Arthritis:** Administer 100 mg methylprednisolone IV or equivalent 30 min prior to each infusion to minimize infusion reactions.

IV Administration
- **Intermittent Infusion:** ***Diluent:*** Dilute with 0.9% NaCl or D5W. ***Concentration:*** 1–4 mg/

mL. Gently invert bag to mix. Solution is clear and colorless; do not administer solutions that are discolored or contain particulate matter. Discard unused portion remaining in vial. Solution is stable for 12 hr at room temperature and for 24 hr if refrigerated. *Rate:* Do not administer as an IV push or bolus.
- *First infusion:* Administer at an initial rate of 50 mg/hr. If hypersensitivity or infusion-related events do not occur, rate may be escalated in 50 mg/hr increments every 30 min to a maximum of 400 mg/hr.
- *Subsequent infusions:* May be administered at an initial rate of 100 mg/hr and increased by 100-mg/hr increments at 30 min intervals to a maximum of 400 mg/hr.
- **Y-Site Compatibility:** acyclovir, amifostine, amikacin, aminophylline, ampicillin, ampicillin/sulbactam, aztreonan, bleomycin, bumetanide, buprenorphine, busulfan, butorphanol, calcium gluconate, carboplatin, carmustine, cefazolin, cefoperazone, cefotaxime, cefotetan, cefoxitin, ceftazidime, ceftizoxime, ceftriaxone, cefuroxime, chlorproamzine, cimetidine, cisplatin, clindamycin, cyclophosphamide, cytarabine, dactinomycin, daunarubicin hydrochloride, dexamethasone sodium phosphate, dexrazoxane, digoxin, diphenhydramine, dobutamine, docetaxel, dopamine, doxorubicin liposome, doxycycline, droperidol, enalaprilat, etoposide phosphate, famotidine, fentanyl, filgrastim, floxuridine, fluconazole, fludarabine, fluorouracil, ganciclovir, gemcitabine, gentamicin, granisetron, haloperidol, heparin, hydrocortisone, hydromorphone, idarubicin, ifosfamide, imipenem/cilastatin, irinotecan, leucovorin, levorphanol, lorazepam, magnesium sulfate, mannitol, meperidine, mesna, methotrexate, methyprednisolone, metoclopramide, metronidazole, mitomycin, mitoxantrone, morphine, nalbuphine, netilmicin, paclitaxel, pentamidine, piperacillin/tazobactam, plicamycin, potassium chloride, prochlorperazine, promethazine, ranitidine, sargramostim, streptozocin, teniposide, theophylline, thiotepa, ticarcillin/clavulanate, tobramycin, trimethoprim/sulfamethoxazole, trimethobenzamide, vinblastine, vincristine, vinorelbine, zidovudine.
- **Y-Site Incompatibility:** aldesleukin, amphotericin B colloidal, ciprofloxacin, cyclosporine, daunorubicin liposome, doxorubicin hydrochloride, furosemide, levofloxacin, minocycline, ondansetron, quinapristin/dalfopristin, sodium bicarbonate, topotecan, vancomycin.
- **Additive Incompatibility:** Do not admix with other medications.

Patient/Family Teaching
- Inform patient of the purpose of the medication.
- Advise patient to report infusion-related events or symptoms of hypersensitivity reactions immediately.
- Instruct patient to notify health care professional promptly if fever; chills; cough; hoarseness; sore throat; signs of infection; lower back or side pain; painful or difficult urination; bleeding gums; bruising; petechiae; blood in stools, urine, or emesis; increased fatigue; dyspnea; or orthostatic hypotension occurs. Caution patient to avoid crowds and persons with known infections. Instruct patient to use soft toothbrush and electric razor and to avoid falls. Caution patient not to drink alcoholic beverages or take medication containing aspirin or NSAIDs; may precipitate gastric bleeding.
- Instruct patient to use contraception throughout therapy.
- Advise patient to consult health care professional prior to receiving any vaccinations.

Evaluation/Desired Outcomes
- Decrease in spread of malignancy.
- Reduced signs and symptoms of rheumatoid arthritis.

---

rivastigmine (rye-va-**stig**-meen)
Exelon

Classification
Therapeutic: anti-Alzheimer's agents
Pharmacologic: cholinergics (cholinesterase inhibitors)

Pregnancy Category B

Indications
PO: Mild to moderate dementia associated with Alzheimer's disease. **Transdermal:** Treatment of mild to moderate dementia associated with Alzheimer's disease and Parkinson's disease.

Action
Enhances cholinergic function by reversible inhibition of cholinesterase. Does not cure the disease. **Therapeutic Effects:** Decreased dementia (temporary) associated with Alzheimer's disease

and Parkinson's disease. Enhanced cognitive ability.

Pharmacokinetics
Absorption: Well absorbed following oral administration. Transdermal patch is slowly absorbed over 8 hr.
Distribution: Widely distributed.
Metabolism and Excretion: Rapidly and extensively metabolized by the liver; metabolites are excreted by the kidneys.
Half-life: *PO*—1.5 hr; *Transdermal*—24 hr.

TIME/ACTION PROFILE (improvement in dementia)

ROUTE	ONSET	PEAK	DURATION
PO	within 2 wk	up to 12 wk	unknown
Transdermal	unknown	unknown	unknown

Contraindications/Precautions
Contraindicated in: Hypersensitivity to rivastigmine or other carbamates.
Use Cautiously in: History of asthma or obstructive pulmonary disease; History of GI bleeding; Sick sinus syndrome or other supraventricular cardiac conduction abnormalities.
Transdermal: Patients weighing <50 kg; at risk for ↑ adverse reactions; OB, Lactation: Pedi: Safety not established.

Adverse Reactions/Side Effects
CNS: weakness, dizziness, drowsiness, headache, sedation (unusual). **CV:** edema, heart failure, hypotension. **GI:** anorexia, dyspepsia, nausea, vomiting, abdominal pain, diarrhea, flatulence, weight gain (unusual). **Neuro:** tremor. **Misc:** fever, weight loss.

Interactions
Drug-Drug: Nicotine may ↑ metabolism and ↓ levels.

Route/Dosage
PO (Adults): 1.5 mg twice daily initially; after at least 2 wk, dose may be ↑ to 3 mg twice daily. Further increments may be made at 2-wk intervals up to 6 mg twice daily.
Transdermal (Adults): *Initial Dose*—4.6 mg/24-hr transdermal patch intially; may ↑ to 9.5 mg/24-hr transdermal patch after at least 4 wk.

Availability
Capsules: 1.5 mg, 3 mg, 4.5 mg, 6 mg. **Oral Solution:** 2 mg/mL. **Transdermal Patch:** 4.6 mg/24 hr, 9.5 mg/24 hr.

NURSING IMPLICATIONS

Assessment
- Assess cognitive function (memory, attention, reasoning, language, ability to perform simple tasks) periodically throughout therapy.
- Monitor patient for nausea, vomiting, anorexia, and weight loss. Notify health care professional if these side effects occur.

Potential Nursing Diagnoses
Disturbed thought process (Indications)
Impaired environmental interpretation syndrome (Indications)
Imbalanced nutrition: less than body requirements (Side Effects)

Implementation
- Rivastigmine oral solution and capsules may be interchanged at equal doses.
- Patients switching from oral doses of <6 mg to transdermal doses should use 4.6 mg/24 hr patch. Patients taking oral doses of 6 mg–12 mg may be converted directly to 9.5 mg/24 hr patch. Apply patch on the day following the last oral dose.
- **PO:** Administer in the morning and evening with food.
- Oral solution may be administered directly from syringe provided or mixed with a small glass of water, cold fruit juice, or soda. Mixture should be stirred prior to drinking. Ensure patient drinks entire mixture. Oral solution is stable for 4 hours at room temperature when mixed with cold fruit juice or soda. Do not mix with other solutions.
- **Transdermal:** Apply patch to clean, dry, hairless area that will not be rubbed by tight clothing. Upper or lower back is recommended, may also use upper arm or chest. Do not apply to red, irritated or cut skin. Rotate sites to prevent irritation, do not use same site within 14 days. Remove adhesive liner and apply by pressing patch firmly until edges stick well. May be worn during bathing and hot weather. Each 24 hr, remove old patch and discard by folding in half and apply new patch to a new area.

Patient/Family Teaching
- **PO:** Emphasize the importance of taking rivastigmine at regular intervals as directed.
- Explain to patient and caregiver how to use oral dosing syringe provided with oral solution. Remove syringe from protective case and push down and twist child resistant closure to open bottle. Insert syringe into opening in white stopper in bottle. Hold the syringe and pull

plunger to the level corresponding to the prescribed dose. Before removing syringe from bottle, push out larger bubbles (small bubbles will not alter dose) by moving plunger up and down a few times. After large bubbles are gone, move plunger to level of dose. Remove syringe from bottle.
- Caution patient and caregiver that rivastigmine may cause dizziness. Caution patient to avoid driving or other activities requiring alertness until response to medication is known.
- Advise patient and caregiver to notify health care professional if nausea, vomiting, anorexia, or weight loss occur. If adverse effects become intolerable during treatment with *transdermal patch,* instruct patient to discontinue patches for several days and then restart at same or next lower dose level. If treatment is interrupted for more than several days, lowest dose level should be used when restarting and titrate according to Route and Dosage section.
- Advise patient and caregiver to notify health care professional of medication regimen prior to treatment or surgery.
- Inform patient and caregivers that improvement in cognitive functioning may take weeks to months and that the degenerative process is not reversed.
- Advise patient to notify health care professional if pregnancy is planned or suspected or if breastfeeding.
- **Transdermal:** Instruct patient and caregiver on the correct application, rotation, and discarding of patch. Patch should be folded in half and discarded out of reach of children and pets; medication remains in discarded patch. Replace missed doses immediately and apply next patch at usual time. Advise patient and caregiver to avoid contact with eyes and to wash hands after applying patch. Avoid exposure to heat sources (excessive sunlight, saunas, heating pads) for long periods.
- Advise patient referred for MRI test to discuss patch with referring health care professional and MRI facility to determine if removal of patch is necessary prior to test and for directions for replacing patch.

Evaluation/Desired Outcomes
- Temporary improvement in cognitive function (memory, attention, reasoning, language, ability to perform simple tasks) in patients with Alzheimer's disease.
- Improvement in cognitive function and overall functioning in patients with Parkinson's disease.

rizatriptan (riz-a-**trip**-tan)
Maxalt, Maxalt-MLT

Classification
Therapeutic: vascular headache suppressants
Pharmacologic: 5-HT$_1$ agonists

Pregnancy Category C

Indications
Acute treatment of migraine headache.

Action
Acts as an agonist at specific 5-HT$_1$ receptor sites in intracranial blood vessels and sensory trigeminal nerves. **Therapeutic Effects:** Cranial vessel vasoconstriction with associated decrease in release of neuropeptides and resultant decrease in migraine headache.

Pharmacokinetics
Absorption: Completely absorbed after oral administration, but first-pass metabolism results in 45% bioavailability.
Distribution: Unknown.
Metabolism and Excretion: Primarily metabolized by monoamine oxidase-A (MAO-A); minor conversion to an active compound; 14% excreted unchanged in urine.
Half-life: 2–3 hr.

TIME/ACTION PROFILE (blood levels)

ROUTE	ONSET	PEAK	DURATION
PO	30 min	1–1.5 hr	unknown

Contraindications/Precautions
Contraindicated in: Hypersensitivity; Ischemic or vasospastic cardiovascular, cerebrovascular, or peripheral vascular syndromes; History of significant cardiovascular disease; Uncontrolled hypertension; Should not be used within 24 hr of other 5-HT$_1$ agonists or ergot-type compounds (dihydroergotamine); Basilar or hemiplegic migraine; Concurrent MAO-A inhibitor therapy or within 2 wk of discontinuing MAO-A inhibitor therapy; Phenylketonuria (orally disintegrating tablet contains aspartame).
Use Cautiously in: Severe renal impairment, especially in patients on dialysis; Moderate hepatic impairment; OB, Lactation: Pedi: Pregnancy, lac-

tation, or children <18 yr (safety not established).

Exercise Extreme Caution in: Cardiovascular risk factors (hypertension, hypercholesterolemia, cigarette smoking, obesity, diabetes, strong family history, menopausal women or men >40 yr); use only if cardiovascular status has been evaluated and determined to be safe and first dose is administered under supervision.

Adverse Reactions/Side Effects
CNS: dizziness, drowsiness, weakness. **CV:** CORONARY ARTERY VASOSPASM, MI, VENTRICULAR ARRHYTHMIAS, chest pain, myocardial ischemia. **GI:** dry mouth, nausea. **Misc:** hypersensitivity reactions including ANGIOEDEMA, toxic epidermal necrolysis, pain.

Interactions
Drug-Drug: Concurrent use with **MAO-A inhibitors** ↑ levels and adverse reactions (concurrent use or use within 2 wk or MAO inhibitor is contraindicated). Concurrent use with other **5-HT agonists** or **ergot-type compounds (dihydroergotamine)** may result in ↑ vasoactive properties (avoid use within 24 hr of each other). **Propranolol** ↑ levels and risk of adverse reactions (dosage reduction recommended). Concurrent use with **SSRI antidepressants** may result in weakness, hyperreflexia, and incoordination.
Drug-Natural Products: ↑ risk of serotinergic side effects including serotonin syndrome with **St. John's wort** and **SAMe**.

Route/Dosage
PO (Adults): 5–10 mg (use 5-mg dose in patients receiving propranolol); may be repeated in 2 hr; not to exceed 3 doses/24 hr. Dose is same for both types of tablets.

Availability
Tablets: 5 mg, 10 mg. **Cost:** 5 mg $107.44/6, 10 mg $231.99/12. **Orally disintegrating tablets (Maxalt-MLT) (peppermint flavor):** 5 mg, 10 mg. **Cost:** 5 mg $116.58/6, 10 mg $113.99/6.

NURSING IMPLICATIONS

Assessment
- Assess pain location, character, intensity, and duration and associated symptoms (photophobia, phonophobia, nausea, vomiting) during migraine attack.

Potential Nursing Diagnoses
Acute pain (Indications)

Implementation
- **PO:** Tablets should be swallowed whole with liquid.
- Orally disintegrating tablets should be left in the package until use. Remove from the blister pouch. Do not push tablet through the blister; peel open the blister pack with dry hands and place tablet on tongue. Tablet will dissolve rapidly and be swallowed with saliva. No liquid is needed to take the orally disintegrating tablet.

Patient/Family Teaching
- Inform patient that rizatriptan should be used only during a migraine attack. It is meant to be used for relief of migraine attacks but not to prevent or reduce the number of attacks.
- Instruct patient to administer rizatriptan as soon as symptoms of a migraine attack appear, but it may be administered at any time during an attack. If migraine symptoms return, a second dose may be used. Allow at least 2 hr between doses, and do not use more than 30 mg in any 24-hr period.
- If first dose does not relieve headache, additional rizatriptan doses are not likely to be effective; notify health care professional.
- Caution patient not to take rizatriptan within 24 hr of other vascular headache suppressants.
- Advise patient that lying down in a darkened room after rizatriptan administration may further help relieve headache.
- Caution patient not to use rizatriptan if she is pregnant, suspects she is pregnant, plans to become pregnant, or is breastfeeding. Adequate contraception should be used during therapy.
- Advise patient to notify health care professional before next dose of rizatriptan if pain or tightness in the chest occurs during use. If pain is severe or does not subside, notify health care professional immediately. If feelings of tingling, heat, flushing, heaviness, pressure, drowsiness, dizziness, tiredness, or sickness develop, discuss with health care professional at next visit.
- May cause dizziness or drowsiness. Caution patient to avoid driving or other activities requiring alertness until response to medication is known.
- Advise patient to avoid alcohol, which aggravates headaches, during rizatriptan use.

Evaluation/Desired Outcomes
- Relief of migraine attack.

ropinirole (roe-pin-i-role)
Requip, Requip XL

ropinirole 1127

Classification
Therapeutic: antiparkinson agents
Pharmacologic: dopamine agonists

Pregnancy Category C

Indications
Management of signs and symptoms of idiopathic Parkinson's disease. Restless leg syndrome (immediate-release only).

Action
Stimulates dopamine receptors in the brain.
Therapeutic Effects: Decreased tremor and rigidity in Parkinson's disease. Decreased leg restlessness.

Pharmacokinetics
Absorption: 55% absorbed following oral administration.
Distribution: Widely distributed.
Metabolism and Excretion: Extensively metabolized by the liver (by cytochrome P450 CYP1A2 enzyme system); <10% excreted unchanged in urine.
Half-life: 6 hr.

TIME/ACTION PROFILE

ROUTE	ONSET	PEAK	DURATION
PO	unknown	unknown	8 hr

Contraindications/Precautions
Contraindicated in: Hypersensitivity.
Use Cautiously in: Hepatic impairment (slower titration may be required); Severe cardiovascular disease; OB, Lactation: Pedi: Safety not established; may inhibit lactation; Geri: ↑ risk of hallucinations in patients >65 yr.

Adverse Reactions/Side Effects
CNS: SLEEP ATTACKS, dizziness, syncope, confusion, drowsiness, fatigue, hallucinations, headache, dyskinesia, urges (gambling, sexual), weakness. **EENT:** abnormal vision. **CV:** orthostatic hypotension, peripheral edema. **GI:** constipation, dry mouth, dyspepsia, nausea, vomiting. **Derm:** sweating, melanoma.

Interactions
Drug-Drug: Drugs that alter the activity of cytochrome P450 CYP1A2 enzyme system may affect the activity of ropinirole. Effects may be ↑ by **estrogens**. Effects may be ↓ by **phenothiazines**, **butyrophenones**, **thioxanthenes**, or **metoclopramide**. May ↑ effects of **levodopa** (may allow dose reduction of levodopa).

Route/Dosage
PO (Adults): *Parkinson's disease*—Immediate-release: 0.25 mg 3 times daily for 1 wk, then 0.5 mg 3 times daily for 1 wk, then 0.75 mg 3 times daily for 1 wk, then 1 mg 3 times daily for 1 wk; then may ↑ by 1.5 mg/day every wk up to 9 mg/day; then may ↑ by up to 3 mg/day every wk up to 24 mg/day; Extended-release: 2 mg once daily for 1–2 wk; may ↑ by 2 mg/day every wk up to 24 mg/day. *Restless leg syndrome*—0.25 mg once daily initially, 1–3 hr before bedtime. After 2 days, ↑ to 0.5 mg once daily and to 1 mg once daily by the end of first week of dosing, then ↑ by 0.5 mg weekly, up to 4 mg/day as needed/tolerated.

Availability (generic available)
Tablets: 0.25 mg, 0.5 mg, 1 mg, 2 mg, 3 mg, 4 mg, 5 mg. **Cost:** 0.25 mg $569.92/270, 0.5 mg $569.92/270, 1 mg $568.84/270, 2 mg $575.94/270, 3 mg $638.87/270, 4 mg $638.87/270, 5 mg $639.98/270. **Extended-release tablets:** 2 mg, 4 mg, 6 mg, 8 mg, 12 mg.

NURSING IMPLICATIONS

Assessment
- Assess blood pressure periodically during therapy.
- Assess patient for drowsiness and sleep attacks. Drowsiness is a common side effect of ropinirole, but sleep attacks or episodes of falling asleep during activities that require active participation may occur without warning. Assess patient for concomitant medications that have sedating effects or may increase serum ropinirole levels (see Interactions). May require discontinuation of therapy.
- **Parkinson's Disease:** Assess patient for signs and symptoms of Parkinson's disease (tremor, muscle weakness and rigidity, ataxic gait) prior to and during therapy.
- **Restless Leg Syndrome:** Assess sleep patterns and frequency of restless leg disturbances.
- *Lab Test Considerations:* May cause ↑ BUN.

Potential Nursing Diagnoses
Impaired physical mobility (Indications)
Risk for injury (Indications, Side Effects)

Implementation
- **PO:** May be administered with or without food. Administration with food may decrease nausea.

Extended-release tablets should be swallowed whole; do not break, crush, or chew.

Patient/Family Teaching
- Instruct patient to take medication exactly as directed. Missed doses should be taken as soon as possible, but not if almost time for next dose. Do not double doses.
- Caution patient to change positions slowly to minimize orthostatic hypotension.
- May cause drowsiness and unexpected episodes of falling asleep. Caution patient to avoid driving or other activities requiring alertness until response to medication is known. Advise patient to notify health care professional if episodes of falling asleep occur.
- Advise patient to avoid alcohol and other CNS depressants concurrently with ropinirole.
- Advise patient that increasing fluids, sugarless gum or candy, ice, or saliva substitutes may help minimize dry mouth. Consult health care professional if dry mouth continues for >2 wk.
- Advise patient to have periodic skin exams to check for lesions that may be melanoma.
- Advise patient to notify health care professional if new or increased gambling, sexual, or other intense urges occur.

Evaluation/Desired Outcomes
- Decreased tremor and rigidity in Parkinson's disease.
- Decrease in restless legs and improved sleep.

---

ropivacaine, See EPIDURAL LOCAL ANESTHETICS.

---

rosiglitazone
(roe-zi-**glit**-a-zone)
Avandia

Classification
Therapeutic: antidiabetics
Pharmacologic: thiazolidinediones

Pregnancy Category C

Indications
Type 2 diabetes mellitus (with diet and exercise); may be used with metformin, sulfonylureas, or insulin.

Action
Improves sensitivity to insulin by acting as an agonist at receptor sites involved in insulin responsiveness and subsequent glucose production and utilization. Requires insulin for activity. **Therapeutic Effects:** Decreased insulin resistance, resulting in glycemic control without hypoglycemia.

Pharmacokinetics
Absorption: Well absorbed (99%) following oral administration.
Distribution: Unknown.
Protein Binding: 99.8% bound to plasma proteins.
Metabolism and Excretion: Entirely metabolized by the liver.
Half-life: 3.2–3.6 hr (increased in liver disease).

TIME/ACTION PROFILE (effects on blood glucose)

ROUTE	ONSET	PEAK	DURATION
PO	unknown	unknown	12–24 hr

Contraindications/Precautions
Contraindicated in: Hypersensitivity; Diabetic ketoacidosis; Clinical evidence of active liver disease or increased ALT (>2.5 times upper limit of normal); Renal disease or dysfunction (creatinine over 1.5 mg/dL in males or 1.4 mg/dL in females; OB, Lactation: Potential for fetal or infant harm. Insulin monotherapy should be used.; Pedi: Safety and effectiveness not established.
Use Cautiously in: Edema; CHF (avoid use in moderate to severe CHF unless benefits outweigh risks); Concurrent use with insulin (may increase risk of adverse cardiovascular reactions); Hepatic impairment; OB: May restore ovulation and risk of pregnancy in premenopausal women; Geri: Dose reduction and careful titration recommended due to age-related decline in renal function. Avoid maximum dose. Should not be given to patients older than 80 yr.

Adverse Reactions/Side Effects
CV: CHF, edema. **EENT:** new onset and worsening diabetic macular edema. **Derm:** urticaria. **GI:** hepatitis, ↑ liver enzymes. **Hemat:** anemia. **Metab:** lactic acidosis, ↑ total cholesterol, LDL and HDL, weight gain. **Misc:** ANGIOEDEMA (rare), fractures (arm, hand, foot) in female patients.

Interactions
Drug-Drug: Concurrent use with **rifampin** ↓ levels and may ↓ effectiveness. **Gemfibrozil** ↑ levels and may ↑ risk of hypoglycemia (↓ dose of rosiglitazone).
Drug-Natural Products: **Glucosamine** may worsen blood glucose control. **Chromium** and **coenzyme Q-10** may produce additive hypoglycemic effects.

Route/Dosage
PO (Adults): 4 mg as a single dose once daily or 2 mg twice daily; after 8 wk, may be increased if necessary to 8 mg once daily or 4 mg twice daily.

Availability
Tablets: 2 mg, 4 mg, 8 mg. **Cost:** 2 mg $218.99/90, 4 mg $338.96/90, 8 mg $575.95/90. ***In combination with:*** metformin (Avandamet), glimepiride (Avandaryl). See Appendix B.

NURSING IMPLICATIONS
Assessment
- Observe patient taking concurrent insulin for signs and symptoms of hypoglycemia (sweating, hunger, weakness, dizziness, tremor, tachycardia, anxiety).
- Assess patient for edema and signs of CHF (dyspnea, rales/crackles, peripheral edema, weight gain, jugular venous distention). May require discontinuation of rosiglitazone.
- Assess patient for signs of lactic acidosis (malaise, myalgias, respiratory distress, somnolence, nonspecific abdominal distress).
- ***Lab Test Considerations:*** Monitor serum glucose and glycosylated hemoglobin periodically during therapy to evaluate effectiveness.
- Monitor CBC with differential periodically during therapy. May cause ↓ in hemoglobin, hematocrit, and WBC, usually during the first 4–8 wk of therapy; then levels stabilize.
- Monitor AST and ALT prior to initiating therapy and periodically thereafter or if jaundice or symptoms of hepatic dysfunction occur. May cause irreversible ↑ in AST and ALT or hepatic failure (rare). If ALT increases to >3 times the upper limit of normal, recheck ALT promptly. Discontinue rosiglitazone if ALT remains >3 times normal.
- May cause ↑ in total cholesterol, LDL, and HDL and ↓ in free fatty acids.
- Monitor renal function tests prior to initiating therapy and periodically thereafter (BUN, creatinine, creatinine clearance), especially in older adults.

Potential Nursing Diagnoses
Imbalanced nutrition: more than body requirements (Indications)

Implementation
- Patients stabilized on a diabetic regimen who are exposed to stress, fever, trauma, infection, or surgery may require administration of insulin.
- **PO:** May be administered with or without meals.

Patient/Family Teaching
- Instruct patient to take medication as directed. If dose for 1 day is missed, do not double dose the next day.
- Explain to patient that this medication controls hyperglycemia but does not cure diabetes. Therapy is long term.
- Review signs of hypoglycemia and hyperglycemia with patient. If hypoglycemia occurs, advise patient to take a glass of orange juice or 2–3 tsp of sugar, honey, or corn syrup dissolved in water and notify health care professional.
- Encourage patient to follow prescribed diet, medication, and exercise regimen to prevent hypoglycemic or hyperglycemic episodes.
- Instruct patient in proper testing of serum glucose and ketones. These tests should be closely monitored during periods of stress or illness and health care professional notified if significant changes occur.
- Advise patient to notify health care professional immediately if signs of hepatic dysfunction (nausea, vomiting, abdominal pain, fatigue, anorexia, dark urine, jaundice), CHF, or lactic acidosis (malaise, myalgias, respiratory distress, somnolence, nonspecific abdominal distress, hypothermia, hypotension, and bradyarrhythmias) occur.
- Advise patient to inform health care professional of medication regimen prior to treatment, studies using IV contrast, or surgery.
- Advise patient to carry a form of sugar (sugar packets, candy) and identification describing disease process and medication regimen at all times.
- Emphasize the importance of routine follow-up exams.
- OB: Insulin is the preferred method of controlling blood glucose during pregnancy. Counsel female patients that higher doses of oral contraceptives or a form of contraception other than oral contraceptives may be required and to notify health care professional promptly if pregnancy is planned or suspected.

Evaluation/Desired Outcomes
- Control of blood glucose levels.

---

rosuvastatin, See HMG-CoA REDUCTASE INHIBITORS (statins).

SALICYLATES

aspirin (**as**-pir-in)
✦ Apo-ASA, ✦ Apo-ASEN, ✦ Arthrinol, ✦ Arthrisin, ✦ Artria S.R, ASA, ✦ Asaphen, Ascriptin, Aspercin, Aspergum, Aspirtab, ✦ Astrin, Bayer Aspirin, Bufferin, ✦ Coryphen, Easprin, Ecotrin, ✦ Entrophen, Genacote, Halfprin, ✦ Headache Tablets, Healthprin, ✦ Novasen, ✦ PMS-ASA, ✦ Rivasa, St. Joseph Adult Chewable Aspirin, ZORprin

choline salicylate
(**koe**-leen sal-**i**-sil-ate)
Arthropan

choline and magnesium salicylates
(**koe**-leen mag-**neez**-ee-um sal-**i**-sil-ates)
CMT, Tricosal, Trilisate

magnesium salicylate
(mag-**neez**-ee-um sal-**i**-sil-ate)
✦ Doan's Backache Pills, Doan's Regular Strength Tablets, Magan, Mobidin

salsalate (**sal**-sa-late)
Amigesic, Anaflex, Disalcid, Marthritic, Mono-Gesic, Salflex, Salgesic, Salsitab

sodium salicylate
(**soe**-dee-yum sal-**i**-sil-ate)
✦ Dodd's Extra Strength, ✦ Dodd's Pills, ✦ Gin Pain Pills

Classification
Therapeutic: antipyretics, nonopioid analgesics
Pharmacologic: salicylates

Pregnancy Category D (aspirin—first trimester), C (magnesium salicylate, salsalate—first trimester)

Indications
Inflammatory disorders including: Rheumatoid arthritis, Osteoarthritis. Mild to moderate pain. Fever. **Aspirin:** Prophylaxis of transient ischemic attacks and MI.

Action
Produce analgesia and reduce inflammation and fever by inhibiting the production of prostaglandins. **Aspirin Only:** Decreases platelet aggregation. **Therapeutic Effects:** Analgesia. Reduction of inflammation. Reduction of fever. **Aspirin:** Decreased incidence of transient ischemic attacks and MI.

Pharmacokinetics
Absorption: *Aspirin*—Well absorbed from the upper small intestine; absorption from enteric-coated preparations may be unreliable; rectal absorption is slow and variable. *Choline and magnesium salicylates*—Well absorbed after oral administration. *Salsalate*—Splits into 2 molecules of salicylic acid after oral administration; absorbed in the small intestine.
Distribution: All salicylates are rapidly and widely distributed; cross the placenta and enter breast milk.
Metabolism and Excretion: Extensively metabolized by the liver; inactive metabolites excreted by the kidneys. Amount excreted unchanged by the kidneys depends on urine pH; as pH increases, amount excreted unchanged increases from 2–3% up to 80%.
Half-life: 2–3 hr for low doses; up to 15–30 hr with larger doses because of saturation of liver metabolism.

TIME/ACTION PROFILE (analgesia/fever reduction†)

ROUTE	ONSET	PEAK	DURATION
Aspirin–PO	5–30 min	1–3 hr	3–6 hr
Aspirin–PO-ER	5–30 min	2–4 hr	8–12 hr
Aspirin–Rect	1–2 hr	4–5 hr	7 hr
All other salicylates–PO	5–30 min	1–3 hr	3–6 hr

†Antirheumatic effect may take 2–3 wk of chronic dosing

Contraindications/Precautions
Contraindicated in: Hypersensitivity to aspirin, tartrazine (FDC yellow dye #5), or other salicylates; Cross-sensitivity with other NSAIDs may exist (less with nonaspirin salicylates); Bleeding disorders or thrombocytopenia (more important with aspirin); Children or adolescents with viral infections (may increase the risk of Reye's syndrome); **Salsalate:** Peri-operative pain from coronary artery bypass graft (CABG) surgery.
Use Cautiously in: History of GI bleeding or ulcer disease; Chronic alcohol use/abuse; Severe

renal disease (magnesium toxicity may occur with magnesium salicylate); Severe hepatic disease; **Salsalate:** Cardiovascular disease or risk factors for cardiovascular disease (may ↑ risk of serious cardiovascular thrombotic events, myocardial infarction, and stroke, especially with prolonged use); OB: Salicylates may have adverse effects on fetus and mother and, in general, should be avoided during pregnancy, especially during the 3rd trimester; Lactation: Safety not established; Geri: ↑ risk of adverse reactions especially GI bleeding; more sensitive to toxic levels.

Adverse Reactions/Side Effects
EENT: tinnitus. **GI:** GI BLEEDING, dyspepsia, epigastric distress, nausea, abdominal pain, anorexia, hepatotoxicity, vomiting. **Derm:** *salsalate*—EXFOLIATIVE DERMATITIS, STEVENS-JOHNSON SYNDROME, TOXIC EPIDERMAL NECROLYSIS. **Hemat:** *aspirin*—anemia, hemolysis, increased bleeding time. **Misc:** allergic reactions including ANAPHYLAXIS and LARYNGEAL EDEMA.

Interactions
Drug-Drug: Aspirin may ↑ the risk of bleeding with **warfarin**, **heparin**, **heparin-like agents**, **thrombolytic agents**, **ticlopidine**, **clopidogrel**, **abciximab**, **tirofiban**, or **eptifibatide**, although these agents are frequently used safely in combination and in sequence. Ibuprofen may negate the cardioprotective antiplatelet effects of low-dose aspirin. Aspirin may ↑ risk of bleeding with **cefoperazone**, **cefotetan**, and **valproic acid**. May ↑ activity of **penicillins**, **phenytoin**, **methotrexate**, **valproic acid**, **oral hypoglycemic agents**, and **sulfonamides**. May ↓ beneficial effects of **probenecid** or **sulfinpyrazone**. **Corticosteroids** may ↓ serum salicylate levels. **Urinary acidification** ↑ reabsorption and may ↑ serum salicylate levels. **Alkalinization of the urine** or the ingestion of large amounts of **antacids** ↑ excretion and ↓ serum salicylate levels. May blunt the therapeutic response to **diuretics**, and **antihypertensives**. ↑ risk of GI irritation with **NSAIDs**.
Drug-Natural Products: ↑ anticoagulant effect and bleeding risk when using aspirin with **arnica**, **chamomile**, **clove**, **feverfew**, **garlic**, **ginger**, **ginkgo**, **Panax ginseng**, and others.
Drug-Food: Foods capable of **acidifying the urine** (see Appendix M) may ↑ serum salicylate levels.

Route/Dosage
Aspirin
Pain/Fever
PO, Rect (Adults): 325–1000 mg q 4–6 hr (not to exceed 4 g/day). *Extended-release tablets*—650 mg q 8 hr or 800 mg q 12 hr.
PO, Rect (Children 2–11 yr): 10–15 mg/kg q 4–6 hr (not to exceed 4 g/day).

Inflammation
PO (Adults): 2.4 g/day initially; increased to maintenance dose of 3.6–5.4 g/day in divided doses (up to 7.8 g/day for acute rheumatic fever).
PO (Children): 60–100 mg/kg/day in divided doses (up to 130 mg/kg/day for acute rheumatic fever).

Prevention of Transient Ischemic Attacks
PO (Adults): 50–325 mg once daily.

Prevention of Myocardial Infarction
PO (Adults): 80–325 mg once daily.
PO (Children): 3–10 mg/kg once daily (round dose to a convenient amount).

Kawasaki Disease
PO (Children): 80–100 mg/kg/day in 4 divided doses until fever resolves; may be followed by maintenance dose of 3–5 mg/kg/day as a single dose for up to 8 wk.

Choline Salicylate
435 mg of choline salicylate is equivalent to 325 mg of aspirin.
PO (Adults): *Analgesic/antipyretic*—435–669 mg (½–¾ tsp) q 3 hr or 425–870 mg (½–1 tsp) q 4 hr or 870–1305 mg (1–1½ tsp) q 6 hr as needed. *Anti-inflammatory*—4.8–7.2 g/day in divided doses.
PO (Children): *Pain/fever*—2 g/m²/day in 4–6 divided doses. *Inflammation*—107–133 mg/kg/day in 4–6 divided doses (up to 174 mg/kg).

Magnesium Salicylate
PO (Adults): 304 mg q 4 hr or 467 mg q 6 hr.

Choline and Magnesium Salicylates
5 mL of liquid equivalent to 500 mg salicylate or 650 mg of aspirin. Tablet strength expressed in mg of salicylate: 500-mg tablet equivalent to 650 mg of aspirin, 750-mg tablet equivalent to 975 mg of aspirin, 1000-mg tablet equivalent to 1.3 g of aspirin.
PO (Adults): *Anti-inflammatory*—3 g/day of salicylate at bedtime or in 2–3 divided doses (not to exceed 4.5 g/day).
PO (Children >37 kg): 2.25 g of salicylate/day in 2 divided doses.

SALICYLATES

PO (Children <37 kg): 50 mg of salicylate/kg/day in 2 divided doses.

Salsalate
PO (Adults): 1 g 3 times daily initially; further titration may be required.

Sodium Salicylate
PO (Adults): *Pain/fever*—325–650 mg q 4 hr. *Inflammation*—3.6–5.4 g/day in divided doses. **PO (Children):** *Pain/fever*—1.5 g/m²/day in 4–6 divided doses. *Inflammation*—80–100 mg/kg/day in 4–6 divided doses.

Availability
Aspirin (generic available)
Tablets: 81 mg^{OTC}, 162.5 mg^{OTC}, 325 mg^{OTC}, 500 mg^{OTC}, 650 mg^{OTC}, ✢ 975 mg^{OTC}. **Chewable tablets:** ✢ 80 mg^{OTC}, 81 mg^{OTC}. **Chewing gum:** 227 mg^{OTC}. **Dispersible tablets:** 325 mg^{OTC}, 500 mg^{OTC}. **Enteric-coated (delayed-release) tablets:** 80 mg^{OTC}, 165 mg^{OTC}, ✢ 300 mg^{OTC}, 325 mg^{OTC}, 500 mg^{OTC}, ✢ 600 mg^{OTC}, 650 mg^{OTC}, 975 mg^{OTC}. **Extended-release tablets:** ✢ 325 mg^{OTC}, 650 mg^{OTC}, 800 mg. **Delayed-release capsules:** ✢ 325 mg^{OTC}, ✢ 500 mg^{OTC}. **Suppositories:** 60 mg^{OTC}, 120 mg^{OTC}, 125 mg^{OTC}, 130 mg^{OTC}, ✢ 150 mg^{OTC}, ✢ 160 mg^{OTC}, 195 mg^{OTC}, 200 mg^{OTC}, 300 mg^{OTC}, ✢ 320 mg^{OTC}, 325 mg^{OTC}, 600 mg^{OTC}, ✢ 640 mg^{OTC}, 650 mg^{OTC}, 1.2 g^{OTC}. *In combination with:* antihistamines, decongestants, cough suppressants^{OTC}, and opioids. See Appendix B.

Choline Salicylate
Oral solution: 870 mg/5 mL^{OTC}.

Magnesium Salicylate (generic available)
Tablets: 304 mg^{OTC}, 467 mg^{OTC}, 545 mg, 600 mg, 650 mg.

Choline and Magnesium Salicylates (listed as salicylate content)
Tablets: 500 mg, 750 mg, 1000 mg. **Liquid:** 500 mg/5 mL.

Salsalate (generic available)
Tablets: 500 mg, 750 mg. **Cost:** *Disalcid*—500 mg $22.90/20, 750 mg $41.87/30; *generic*—500 mg $32.74/100, 750 mg $41.04/100.

Sodium Salicylate (generic available)
Tablets: 325 mg^{OTC}, 650 mg^{OTC}. **Delayed-release tablets:** 324 mg^{OTC}, 325 mg^{OTC}, 650 mg^{OTC}.

NURSING IMPLICATIONS
Assessment
- Patients who have asthma, allergies, and nasal polyps or who are allergic to tartrazine are at an increased risk for developing hypersensitivity reactions.
- **Pain:** Assess pain and limitation of movement; note type, location, and intensity before and at the peak (see Time/Action Profile) after administration.
- **Fever:** Assess fever and note associated signs (diaphoresis, tachycardia, malaise, chills).
- *Lab Test Considerations:* Monitor hepatic function before antirheumatic therapy and if symptoms of hepatotoxicity occur; more likely in patients, especially children, with rheumatic fever, systemic lupus erythematosus, juvenile arthritis, or pre-existing hepatic disease. May cause ↑ serum AST, ALT, and alkaline phosphatase, especially when plasma concentrations exceed 25 mg/100 mL. May return to normal despite continued use or dose reduction. If severe abnormalities or active liver disease occurs, discontinue and use with caution in future.
- Monitor serum salicylate levels periodically with prolonged high-dose therapy to determine dose, safety, and efficacy, especially in children with Kawasaki disease.
- *Aspirin:* Prolongs bleeding time for 4–7 days and, in large doses, may cause prolonged prothrombin time. Monitor hematocrit periodically in prolonged high-dose therapy to assess for GI blood loss.
- ***Toxicity and Overdose:*** Monitor patient for the onset of tinnitus, headache, hyperventilation, agitation, mental confusion, lethargy, diarrhea, and sweating. If these symptoms appear, withhold medication and notify physician or other health care professional immediately.

Potential Nursing Diagnoses
Acute pain (Indications)
Impaired physical mobility (Indications)

Implementation
- Use lowest effective dose for shortest period of time.
- **PO:** Administer after meals or with food or an antacid to minimize gastric irritation. Food slows but does not alter the total amount absorbed.
- Do not crush or chew enteric-coated tablets. Do not take antacids within 1–2 hr of enteric-

✢ = Canadian drug name. ▇ = Genetic implication.
*CAPITALS indicates life-threatening; underlines indicate most frequent.

coated tablets. Chewable tablets may be chewed, dissolved in liquid, or swallowed whole. Some extended-release tablets may be broken or crumbled but must not be ground up before swallowing. See manufacturer's prescribing information for individual products.

Patient/Family Teaching
- Instruct patient to take salicylates with a full glass of water and to remain in an upright position for 15–30 min after administration.
- Advise patient to report tinnitus; unusual bleeding of gums; bruising; black, tarry stools; or fever lasting longer than 3 days.
- Caution patient to avoid concurrent use of alcohol with this medication to minimize possible gastric irritation; 3 or more glasses of alcohol per day may increase the risk of GI bleeding. Caution patient to avoid taking concurrently with acetaminophen or NSAIDs for more than a few days, unless directed by health care professional to prevent analgesic nephropathy.
- Teach patients on a sodium-restricted diet to avoid effervescent tablets or buffered-aspirin preparations.
- Tablets with an acetic (vinegar-like) odor should be discarded.
- Advise patients on long-term therapy to inform health care professional of medication regimen before surgery. Aspirin may need to be withheld for 1 wk before surgery.
- Pedi: Centers for Disease Control and Prevention warns against giving aspirin to children or adolescents with varicella (chickenpox) or influenza-like or viral illnesses because of a possible association with Reye's syndrome.
- **Transient Ischemic Attacks or MI:** Advise patients receiving aspirin prophylactically to take only prescribed dose. Increasing the dose has not been found to provide additional benefits.

Evaluation/Desired Outcomes
- Relief of mild to moderate discomfort.
- Increased ease of joint movement. May take 2–3 wk for maximum effectiveness.
- Reduction of fever.
- Prevention of transient ischemic attacks.
- Prevention of MI.

---

salmeterol (sal-me-te-role)
Serevent Diskus

Classification
Therapeutic: bronchodilators
Pharmacologic: adrenergics

Pregnancy Category C

Indications
Long-term control of reversible airway obstruction due to asthma and for maintenance treatment of asthma and prevention of bronchospasm. Prevention of exercise-induced asthma. Maintenance treatment to prevent bronchospasm in COPD including chronic bronchitis and emphysema.

Action
Produces accumulation of cyclic adenosine monophosphate (cAMP) at beta$_2$-adrenergic receptors. Relatively specific for beta (pulmonary) receptors. **Therapeutic Effects:** Bronchodilation.

Pharmacokinetics
Absorption: Minimal systemic absorption follows inhalation.
Distribution: Action is primarily local.
Metabolism and Excretion: Unknown.
Half-life: 3–4 hr.

TIME/ACTION PROFILE (bronchodilation)

ROUTE	ONSET	PEAK	DURATION
Inhalation	10–25 min	3–4 hr	12 hr†

†9 hr in adolescents

Contraindications/Precautions
Contraindicated in: Hypersensitivity; Acute attack of asthma (onset of action is delayed).
Use Cautiously in: Cardiovascular disease (including angina and hypertension); Seizure disorders; Diabetes; Glaucoma; Hyperthyroidism; Pheochromocytoma; Excessive use (may lead to tolerance and paradoxical bronchospasm); OB: Use only if potential benefit justifies potential risk to fetus; may inhibit contractions during labor; Lactation: Use only if potential benefit justifies potential risk to infant. Consider discontinuing breast-feeding while on salmeterol; Pedi: Safety not established in children <4 yr (dry powder inhalation may be used in children 4–12 yr; aerosol inhalation may be used in children >12 yr).

Adverse Reactions/Side Effects
CNS: headache, nervousness. **CV:** palpitations, tachycardia. **GI:** abdominal pain, diarrhea, nausea. **MS:** muscle cramps/soreness. **Neuro:** trembling. **Resp:** paradoxical bronchospasm, cough.

Interactions
Drug-Drug: Beta blockers may ↓ therapeutic effects of salmeterol. **MAO inhibitors** and **tricyclic antidepressants** potentiate cardiovascu-

salmeterol 1135

lar effects. ↑ levels and ↑ risk of cardiovascular effects when used with potent CYP3A4 inhibitors (e.g., **ketoconazole**, **itraconazole**, **ritonavir**, **atazanavir**, **clarithromycin**, **indinavir**, **nefazodone**, **nelfinavir**, or **saquinavir**); concurrent use is not recommended.

Drug-Natural Products: Use with caffeine-containing herbs (**cola nut**, **guarana**, **mate**, **tea**, **coffee**) ↑ stimulant effect.

Route/Dosage
Inhaln (Adults and Children ≥4 yr): 50 mcg (one inhalation) twice daily (approximately 12 hr apart). *Exercise-induced bronchospasm*—50 mcg (one inhalation) 30–60 min before exercise.

Availability
Powder for oral inhalation (Serevent Diskus): 50 mcg/blister. *In combination with:* fluticasone (Advair Diskus, see Appendix B).

NURSING IMPLICATIONS

Assessment
- Assess lung sounds, pulse, and blood pressure before administration and periodically during therapy.
- Monitor pulmonary function tests before initiating therapy and periodically during therapy.
- Observe for paradoxical bronchospasm (wheezing, dyspnea, tightness in chest) and hypersensitivity reaction (rash; urticaria; swelling of the face, lips, or eyelids). Frequently occurs with first use of new canister or vial. If condition occurs, withhold medication and notify physician or other health care professional immediately.
- **Lab Test Considerations:** May cause ↑ serum glucose concentrations; occurs rarely with recommended doses and is more pronounced with frequent use of high doses.
- May cause ↓ serum potassium concentrations, which are usually transient and dose related; rarely occurs at recommended doses and is more pronounced with frequent use of high doses.
- ***Toxicity and Overdose:*** Symptoms of overdose include persistent agitation, chest pain or discomfort, decreased blood pressure, dizziness, hyperglycemia, hypokalemia, seizures, tachyarrhythmias, persistent trembling, and vomiting.
- Treatment includes discontinuing salmeterol and other beta-adrenergic agonists and providing symptomatic, supportive therapy. Cardioselective beta blockers are used cautiously because they may induce bronchospasm.

Potential Nursing Diagnoses
Ineffective airway clearance (Indications)

Implementation
- Do not confuse salmeterol with Salbutamol (albuterol).
- **Inhaln:** Once removed from foil overwrap, discard diskus when every blister has been used or 6 wk have passed, whichever comes first.
- Do not use a spacer with powder for inhalation.

Patient/Family Teaching
- Advise patient to take salmeterol as directed. Do not use more than the prescribed dose. If a regularly scheduled dose is missed, use as soon as possible and resume regular schedule. Do not double doses. If symptoms occur before next dose is due, use a rapid-acting inhaled bronchodilator.
- Instruct patient using *powder for inhalation* never to exhale into diskus device and always to hold device in a level horizontal position. Mouthpiece should be kept dry; never wash.
- Caution patient not to use salmeterol to treat acute symptoms. A rapid-acting inhaled beta-adrenergic bronchodilator should be used for relief of acute asthma attacks.
- Advise patients on chronic therapy not to use additional salmeterol to prevent exercise-induced bronchospasm. Patients using salmeterol for prevention of exercise-induced bronchospasm should not use additional doses of salmeterol for 12 hr after prophylactic administration.
- Advise patient to notify health care professional immediately if difficulty in breathing persists after use of salmeterol, if condition worsens, if more inhalations of rapid-acting bronchodilator than usual are needed to relieve an acute attack, or if using 4 or more inhalations of a rapid-acting bronchodilator for 2 or more consecutive days or more than 1 canister in an 8-wk period.
- Salmeterol is often used with inhaled corticosteroids and is not a substitute for corticosteroids or adrenergic bronchodilators. Advise patients using inhalation or systemic corticosteroids to consult health care professional before stopping or reducing therapy.

= Canadian drug name. = Genetic implication.
*CAPITALS indicates life-threatening; underlines indicate most frequent.

- Emphasize the importance of regular follow-up exams to determine progress during therapy.

Evaluation/Desired Outcomes
- Prevention of bronchospasm or reduction of frequency of acute asthma attacks in patients with chronic asthma.
- Prevention of exercise-induced asthma.

---

salsalate, See SALICYLATES.

---

sargramostim
(sar-**gram**-oh-stim)
Leukine, rHu GM-CSF (recombinant human granulocyte/macrophage colony-stimulating factor)

Classification
Therapeutic: colony-stimulating factors
Pharmacologic: biologic response modifiers

Pregnancy Category C

Indications
Acceleration of bone marrow recovery after: Autologous bone marrow transplantation in patients with non-Hodgkin's lymphoma, acute lymphoblastic leukemia, or Hodgkin's disease, Allogenic bone marrow transplantation from HLA-matched donors. Management of bone marrow transplant failure or engraftment delay. After induction chemotherapy for acute myelogenous leukemia (AML) in patients ≥55 yr. Mobilization and after transplant of autologous peripheral blood progenitor cells (PBPCs); increases harvest by leukapheresis.

Action
Consists of a glycoprotein produced by recombinant DNA technique that is capable of binding to and stimulating the production, division, differentiation, and activation of granulocytes and macrophages. **Therapeutic Effects:** Accelerated recovery of bone marrow after autologous bone marrow transplantation, resulting in decreased risk of infection and other complications.

Pharmacokinetics
Absorption: After IV administration, absorption is essentially complete. Well absorbed after subcut administration.
Distribution: Unknown.
Metabolism and Excretion: Unknown.
Half-life: Unknown.

TIME/ACTION PROFILE (noted as effects on blood counts)

ROUTE	ONSET	PEAK	DURATION
Subcut, IV	rapid	unknown	3–7 days

Contraindications/Precautions
Contraindicated in: Presence of ≥10% leukemic myeloid blast cells in bone marrow or peripheral blood; Hypersensitivity to granulocyte macrophage colony-stimulating factor (GM-CSF), yeast products, or additives (mannitol, tromethamine, or sucrose); Pedi: Products containing benzyl alcohol should not be used in newborns.
Use Cautiously in: Pre-existing fluid retention, CHF, or pulmonary infiltrates; Pre-existing cardiac disease; Myeloid malignancies; Previous extensive radiation or chemotherapy (response may be limited); OB: Use only if clearly needed; Lactation, Pedi: Safety not established.

Adverse Reactions/Side Effects
CNS: headache, malaise, weakness. **Resp:** dyspnea. **CV:** pericardial effusion, peripheral edema, transient supraventricular tachycardia. **GI:** diarrhea. **Derm:** itching, rash. **MS:** arthralgia, bone pain, myalgia. **Misc:** chills, fever, first-dose reaction.

Interactions
Drug-Drug: Lithium or **corticosteroids** may potentiate myeloproliferative effects of sargramostim (concurrent use should be undertaken cautiously).

Route/Dosage
After Bone Marrow Transplantation
IV (Adults): 250 mcg/m^2/day for 21 days.

Failure/Delay of Engraftment after Bone Marrow Transplantation
IV (Adults): 250 mcg/m^2/day for 14 days; may be repeated after a 7-day rest between courses; if results are inadequate, a 3rd course at 500 mcg/m^2/day for 14 days may be given after a 7-day rest.

After Chemotherapy for AML
IV (Adults): 250 mcg/m^2/day started around day 11 or 4 days after induction if day 10 bone marrow is hypoplastic with <5% blast cells and continued until absolute neutrophil count (ANC) >1500 cells/mm^3 for 3 consecutive days (not to exceed 42 days); if adverse reactions occur, decrease dose by 50% or temporarily discontinue.

Mobilization of PBPCs
IV, Subcut (Adults): 250 mcg/m^2/day continued throughout collection of PBPCs.

After PBPC Transplantation
IV, Subcut (Adults): 250 mcg/m²/day continued until ANC >1500 cells/mm³ for 3 consecutive days.

Availability
Powder for injection: 250 mcg/vial. **Solution for injection:** 500 mcg/vial.

NURSING IMPLICATIONS
Assessment
- Monitor heart rate, blood pressure, and respiratory status during and immediately after infusion. If dyspnea develops, slow infusion rate by half. Reassess; medication may need to be discontinued. Assess for peripheral edema daily throughout therapy. Capillary leak syndrome (swelling of feet or lower legs, sudden weight gain, dyspnea) and pleural or pericardial effusion may occur, usually at doses >32 mcg/kg/day.
- Monitor for first-dose reaction (flushing, hypotension, syncope, weakness). Does not recur with first dose of each course but may occur with first dose of more than 1 course.
- Assess for fever daily during therapy. Usually mild and dose-related and resolves with discontinuation or administration of antipyretics.
- Assess for arthralgias and myalgias, usually in lower extremities, which tend to occur when granulocyte counts are returning to normal. May also cause mild to moderate bone pain, possibly from bone marrow expansion. Usually occurs over 1–3 days before myeloid recovery and occurs in the sternum, spine, pelvis, and long bones. Treat with analgesics.
- **Lab Test Considerations:** Obtain a CBC with differential and platelet count before chemotherapy and twice weekly during therapy to avoid leukocytosis. Monitor ANC; may increase rapidly. If ANC >20,000/mm³ or 10,000/mm³ after the nadir has occurred or if platelet count >500,000/mm³, interrupt administration and reduce dose by half or discontinue. Excessive blood levels usually return to baseline 3–7 days after discontinuation of therapy. If blast cells appear, sargramostim should be discontinued.
- Monitor renal and hepatic function before and biweekly throughout therapy in patients with renal or hepatic dysfunction. May cause ↑ BUN, creatinine, and hepatic enzymes.
- May cause ↓ serum albumin concentrations.

Potential Nursing Diagnoses
Risk for infection (Indications)

Implementation
- Do not confuse Leukine (sargramostim) with leukeran (chlorambucil) or leucovorin.
- Administer 2–4 hr after bone marrow transplant and no earlier than 24 hr after cytotoxic chemotherapy or 12 hr after last dose of radiotherapy.
- Refrigerate but do not freeze powder, reconstituted solution, or diluted solution. Reconstitute with 1 mL of sterile water without preservatives injected toward side of vial. Swirl gently to avoid foaming. Do not shake. Solution should be clear and colorless. Discard if left at room temperature for >6 hr. Vial is for 1-time use only.
- **Subcut:** Administer reconstituted solution without further dilution.

IV Administration
- **Intermittent Infusion:** *Diluent:* Dilute in 0.9% NaCl. *Concentration:* If final concentration is <10 mcg/mL, add 1 mg human albumin per 1 mL of 0.9% NaCl before addition of sargramostim to prevent absorption of the components of the drug delivery system. Do not administer with an in-line filter. *Rate:* Usually infused over 2–4 hr. Has been administered over 30–60 min, over 5–12 hr, and as a continuous infusion over 24 hr.
- *After bone marrow transplantation or failure of engraftment:* Administer over 2 hr.
- *Chemotherapy for AML:* Administer over 4 hr.
- *Mobilization of PBPCs or PBPC transplant:* Administer as a continuous infusion over 24 hr.
- **Y-Site Compatibility:** amikacin, aminophylline, aztreonam, bleomycin, butorphanol, calcium gluconate, carboplatin, carmustine, cefazolin, cefepime, cefotaxime, cefotetan, ceftizoxime, ceftriaxone, cefuroxime, cimetidine, cisplatin, clindamycin, cyclophosphamide, cyclosporine, cytarabine, dacarbazine, dactinomycin, dexamethasone sodium phosphate, diphenhydramine, dopamine, doxorubicin hydrochloride, doxycycline, droperidol, etoposide, famotidine, fentanyl, floxuridine, fluconazole, fluorouracil, furosemide, gentamicin, granisetron, heparin, idarubicin, ifosfamide, immune globulin, levofloxacin, magnesium sulfate, mannitol, mechlorethamine, meperidine, mesna, methotrexate, metoclopramide, metronidazole, mitoxantrone, pentostatin, pi-

peracillin/tazobactam, potassium chloride, prochlorperazine, promethazine, ranitidine, rituximab, sodium acetate, teniposide, ticarcillin/clavulanate, trastuzumab, trimethoprim/sulfamethoxazole, vinblastine, vincristine, zidovudine.
- **Y-Site Incompatibility:** acyclovir, ampicillin, ampicillin/sulbactam, cefoperazone, chlorpromazine, ganciclovir, haloperidol, hydrocortisone, hydromorphone, hydroxyzine, imipenem/cilastatin, lorazepam, methylprednisolone sodium succinate, mitomycin, morphine, nalbuphine, nesiritide, ondansetron, sodium bicarbonate, tobramycin.
- **Additive Incompatibility:** Do not admix with other medications.

Patient/Family Teaching
- Instruct patient to notify health care professional if dyspnea or palpitations occur.

Evaluation/Desired Outcomes
- Acceleration of bone marrow recovery and decreased incidence of infection in patients after autologous and allogenic bone marrow transplantation, bone marrow transplant failure or engraftment delay, chemotherapy for AML, and PBPC transplantation.

saxagliptin (sax-a-glip-tin)
Onglyza

Classification
Therapeutic: antidiabetics
Pharmacologic: dipeptidyl peptidase-4 inhibitors

Pregnancy Category B

Indications
Adjunct with diet and exercise to improve glycemic control in adults with type 2 diabetes mellitus.

Action
Acts as a competitive inhibitor of dipeptidyl peptidase-4 (DPP4) which slows inactivation of incretin hormones, thereby increasing their concentrations and reducing fasting and postprandial glucose concentrations. **Therapeutic Effects:** Improved control of blood glucose.

Pharmacokinetics
Absorption: Well absorbed following oral administration.
Distribution: Unknown.
Metabolism and Excretion: Metabolized by the liver via the P450 3A4/5 (CYP3A4/5) enzyme system, with conversion to 5–hydroxysaxagliptin, a pharmacologically active metabolite; 24% of saxagliptin is excreted unchanged in urine, 36% of hydroxysaxagliptin is excreted unchanged in urine, 22% is eliminated in feces as unabsorbed drug/metabolites excreted in bile.
Half-life: *Saxagliptin*—2.5 hr; *5–hydroxysaxagliptin*—3.1 hr.

TIME/ACTION PROFILE (DDP-4 inhibition)

ROUTE	ONSET	PEAK	DURATION
PO	unknown	2 hr (4 hr for 5–hydroxy-saxagliptin)†	24 hr

† Blood levels

Contraindications/Precautions
Contraindicated in: Type 1 diabetes; Diabetic ketoacidosis.
Use Cautiously in: Geri: Elderly may be more sensitive to effects; consider age-related decrease in renal function.; OB: use during pregnancy only if clearly needed.; Lactation: Use cautiously during breastfeeding; Pedi: Safe and effective use in children <18 yr has not been established.

Adverse Reactions/Side Effects
CNS: headache. **CV:** peripheral edema (↑ with thiazolidinediones). **GI:** abdominal pain, vomiting. **Hemat:** ↓ lymphocyte count. **Endo:** hypoglycemia (↑ with sulfonylureas). **Misc:** hypersensitivity reactions including urticaria and facial edema.

Interactions
Drug-Drug: Strong **CYP3A4/5 inhibitors**, including **ketoconazole**, **atazanavir**, **clarithromycin**, **indinavir**, **itraconazole**, **nefazodone**, **nelfinavir**, **ritonavir**, **saquinavir**, and **telithromycin** ↑ blood levels; daily dose should not exceed 2.5 mg. ↑ risk of hypoglycemia with **sulfonylureas**.

Route/Dosage
PO (Adults): 2.5–5 mg once daily; *strong P450 3A4/5 (CYP3A4/5) inhibitors*—2.5 mg once daily.

Renal Impairment
PO (Adults): *CCr ≤50 mL/min*—2.5 mg once daily.

Availability
Tablets: 2.5 mg, 5 mg.

NURSING IMPLICATIONS

Assessment
- Observe patient for signs and symptoms of hypoglycemic reactions (abdominal pain, sweating, hunger, weakness, dizziness, headache, tremor, tachycardia, anxiety).
- **Lab Test Considerations:** Monitor hemoglobin A1C prior to and periodically during therapy.
- Monitor renal function prior to and periodically during therapy.
- May cause ↓ absolute lymphocyte count.

Potential Nursing Diagnoses
Imbalanced nutrition: more than body requirements (Indications)
Noncompliance (Patient/Family Teaching)

Implementation
- Patients stabilized on a diabetic regimen who are exposed to stress, fever, trauma, infection, or surgery may require administration of insulin.
- **PO:** May be administered without regard to food.

Patient/Family Teaching
- Instruct patient to take saxagliptin as directed. Take missed doses as soon as remembered, unless it is almost time for next dose; do not double doses. Advise patient to read the Patient Package Insert before starting and with each Rx refill; new information may be available.
- Explain to patient that saxagliptin helps control hyperglycemia but does not cure diabetes. Therapy is usually long term.
- Instruct patient not to share this medication with others, even if they have the same symptoms; it may harm them.
- Encourage patient to follow prescribed diet, medication, and exercise regimen to prevent hyperglycemic or hypoglycemic episodes.
- Review signs of hypoglycemia and hyperglycemia with patient. If hypoglycemia occurs, advise patient to take a glass of orange juice or 2–3 tsp of sugar, honey, or corn syrup dissolved in water, and notify health care professional.
- Instruct patient in proper testing of blood glucose and urine ketones. These tests should be monitored closely during periods of stress or illness and health care professional notified if significant changes occur.
- Advise patient to notify health care professional promptly if swelling of hands, feet, or ankles; rash; hives; or swelling of face, lips, or throat occur.
- Instruct patient to notify health care professional prior to taking any Rx, OTC, and herbal products.
- Advise patient to notify health care professional if pregnancy is planned or suspected or if breastfeeding.

Evaluation/Desired Outcomes
- Improved hemoglobin A1C, fasting plasma glucose and 2-hr post-prandial glucose levels.

---

scopolamine (scoe-**pol**-a-meen)
Scopace, Transderm-Scop, ✥ Transderm-V

Classification
Therapeutic: antiemetics
Pharmacologic: anticholinergics

Pregnancy Category C

Indications
Transdermal: Prevention of motion sickness. Management of nausea and vomiting associated with opioid analgesia or general anesthesia/recovery from anesthesia. **IM, IV, Subcut:** Preoperatively to produce amnesia and to decrease salivation and excessive respiratory secretions. **PO:** Symptomatic treatment of postencephalitis parkinsonism and paralysis agitans. Treatment of spasticity. Inhibits excessive motility and hypertonus of GI tract in irritable colon syndrome, mild dysentery, diverticulitis, and pylorospasm. Prevention of motion sickness.

Action
Inhibits the muscarinic activity of acetylcholine. Corrects the imbalance of acetylcholine and norepinephrine in the CNS, which may be responsible for motion sickness. **Therapeutic Effects:** Reduction of nausea and vomiting. Preoperative amnesia and decreased secretions. Reduction of spasms.

Pharmacokinetics
Absorption: Well absorbed following IM, subcut, and transdermal administration.
Distribution: Crosses the placenta and blood-brain barrier.
Metabolism and Excretion: Mostly metabolized by the liver.

scopolamine

Half-life: 8 hr.

TIME/ACTION PROFILE (antiemetic, sedative properties)

ROUTE	ONSET	PEAK	DURATION
PO, IM, sub-cut	30 min	1 hr	4–6 hr
IV	10 min	1 hr	2–4 hr
Transdermal	4 hr	unknown	72 hr

Contraindications/Precautions
Contraindicated in: Hypersensitivity; Hypersensitivity to bromides (injection only); Angle-closure glaucoma; Acute hemorrhage; Prostatic hyperplasia (oral only); Pyloric obstruction (oral only); Tachycardia secondary to cardiac insufficiency or thyrotoxicosis.
Use Cautiously in: Possible intestinal obstruction; Prostatic hyperplasia; Chronic renal, hepatic, pulmonary, or cardiac disease; OB, Lactation: Safety not established; to minimize exposure to fetus, apply 1 hr prior to cesarean section; Pedi: Geri: ↑ risk of adverse reactions.

Adverse Reactions/Side Effects
CNS: drowsiness, confusion. **EENT:** blurred vision, mydriasis, photophobia. **CV:** tachycardia, palpitations. **GI:** dry mouth, constipation. **GU:** urinary hesitancy, urinary retention. **Derm:** ↓ sweating.

Interactions
Drug-Drug: ↑ anticholinergic effects with **antihistamines, antidepressants, quinidine**, or **disopyramide**. ↑ CNS depression with **alcohol, antidepressants, antihistamines, opioid analgesics**, or **sedative/hypnotics**. May alter the absorption of other **orally administered drugs** by slowing motility of the GI tract. May ↑ GI mucosal lesions in patients taking oral **wax-matrix potassium chloride preparations**.
Drug-Natural Products: ↑ anticholinergic effects with **jimson weed** and **scopolia**.

Route/Dosage
Transdermal (Adults): *Motion sickness*—Apply 1 patch 4 hr prior to travel and then every 3 days (as needed); *Preoperative*—Apply 1 patch the evening before surgery or 1 hr prior to cesarean section (remove 24 hr after surgery).
PO (Adults): 0.4–0.8 mg; may repeat every 8–12 hr as needed (dose may be ↑ in parkinsonism and spastic states); for motion sickness, give at least 1 hr before exposure to motion.
IM, IV, Subcut (Adults): *Antiemetic/anticholinergic*—0.3–0.6 mg; *antisecretory effect*—0.2–0.6 mg; *amnestic effect*—0.32–0.65 mg; *sedation*—0.6 mg 3–4 times daily.

IM, IV, Subcut (Children): *Antiemetic/anticholinergic*—6 mcg/kg or 0.2 mg/m^2.
IM (Children 8–12 yr): *Antisecretory*—0.3 mg.
IM (Children 3–8 yr): *Antisecretory*—0.2 mg.
IM (Children 7 mo–3 yr): *Antisecretory*—0.15 mg.
IM (Children 4–7 mo): *Antisecretory*—0.1 mg.

Availability (generic available)
Transdermal therapeutic system: Transderm-Scop—1.5 mg scopolamine/patch releases 0.5 mg scopolamine over 3 days, ♣Transderm-V—1.5 mg scopolamine/patch releases 1 mg scopolamine over 3 days. **Tablets:** 0.4 mg. **Injection:** 0.3 mg/mL, 0.4 mg/mL.

NURSING IMPLICATIONS

Assessment
- Assess patient for signs of urinary retention periodically during therapy.
- Monitor heart rate periodically during parenteral therapy.
- Assess patient for pain prior to administration. Scopolamine may act as a stimulant in the presence of pain, producing delirium if used without opioid analgesics.
- **Antiemetic:** Assess patient for nausea and vomiting periodically during therapy.

Potential Nursing Diagnoses
Impaired oral mucous membrane (Indications, Side Effects)
Risk for injury (Side Effects)

Implementation
- **PO:** Administer at least 1 hr prior to exposure to travel for motion sickness. Tablets may be crushed or dissolved in water to decrease onset.

IV Administration

- **Direct IV:** *Diluent:* Scopolamine should be diluted with sterile water for injection prior to IV administration. *Concentration:* Dilute dose with an equal volume of diluent. *Rate:* Inject slowly over 2–3 min..
- **Syringe Compatibility:** atropine, butorphanol, chlorpromazine, cimetidine, diphenhydramine, droperidol, fentanyl, glycopyrrolate, hydromorphone, meperidine, metoclopramide, midazolam, morphine, nalbuphine, pentazocine, pentobarbital, perphenazine, prochlorperazine, promethazine, ranitidine, sufentanil, thiopental.

- **Y-Site Compatibility:** fentanyl, heparin, hydrocortisone sodium succinate, hydromorphone, methadone, morphine, potassium chloride, propofol, sufentanil, vitamin B complex with C.

Patient/Family Teaching
- Instruct patient to take medication as directed. Take missed doses as soon as remembered. Do not double doses.
- May cause drowsiness or blurred vision. Caution patient to avoid driving or other activities requiring alertness until response to medication is known.
- Patient should use caution when exercising and in hot weather; overheating may result in heatstroke.
- Advise patient to avoid concurrent use of alcohol and other CNS depressants with this medication.
- Inform patient that frequent mouth rinses, good oral hygiene, and sugarless gum or candy may minimize dry mouth.
- **Transdermal:** Instruct patient on application of transdermal patches. Apply at least 4 hr (US product) before exposure to travel to prevent motion sickness. Wash hands and dry thoroughly before and after application. Apply to hairless, clean, dry area behind ear; avoid areas with cuts or irritation. Apply pressure over system to ensure contact with skin. System is effective for 3 days. If system becomes dislodged, replace with a new system on another site behind the ear. System is waterproof and not affected by bathing or showering.
- Instruct patient to remove patch and notify health care professional immediately if symptoms of acute angle-closure glaucoma (pain or reddening of the eyes with pupil dilation) occur.
- Caution patients engaging in underwater sports of potentially distorting effects of scopolamine.
- For *perioperative nausea and vomiting*, apply patch the night before surgery, or 1 hr prior to Cesarean section to minimize exposure to infant. Keep patch in place for 24 hr, then remove and discard.
- Advise patient referred for MRI test to discuss patch with referring health care professional and MRI facility to determine if removal of patch is necessary prior to test and for directions for replacing patch.

Evaluation/Desired Outcomes
- Decrease in salivation and respiratory secretion preoperatively.
- Postoperative amnesia.
- Prevention of motion sickness.
- Prevention and treatment of opioid- or anesthesia-induced nausea and vomiting.
- Reduction in spasms.
- Reduction in excessive GI motility.

---

selegiline (se-le-ji-leen)
Apo-Selegiline, Carbex, Eldepryl, Gen-Selegiline, Nu-Selegiline, ✦ Novo-Selegiline, SD-Deprenyl, Zelapar

Classification
Therapeutic: antiparkinson agents
Pharmacologic: monoamine oxidase type B inhibitors

Pregnancy Category C

Indications
Management of Parkinson's disease (with levodopa or levodopa/carbidopa) in patients who fail to respond to levodopa/carbidopa alone.

Action
Following conversion by MAO to its active form, selegiline inactivates MAO by irreversibly binding to it at type B (brain) sites. Inactivation of MAO leads to increased amounts of dopamine available in the CNS. **Therapeutic Effects:** Increased response to levodopa/dopamine therapy in Parkinson's disease.

Pharmacokinetics
Absorption: Appears to be well absorbed following oral administration.
Distribution: Widely distributed.
Metabolism and Excretion: Metabolism involves some conversion to amphetamine and methamphetamine. 45% excreted in urine as metabolites.
Half-life: Unknown; orally disintegrating tablets 1.3 hr.

TIME/ACTION PROFILE (onset of beneficial effects in Parkinson's disease)

ROUTE	ONSET	PEAK	DURATION
PO	2–3 days	40–90 min	unknown
Orally disintegrating	5 min	10–15 min	unknown

✦ = Canadian drug name. ▮ = Genetic implication.
*CAPITALS indicates life-threatening; underlines indicate most frequent.

selegiline

Contraindications/Precautions
Contraindicated in: Hypersensitivity; Concurrent meperidine or opioid analgesic therapy (possible fatal reactions); Concurrent use of SSRIs or tricyclic antidepressants.

Use Cautiously in: Doses >10 mg/day (↑ risk of hypertensive reactions with tyramine-containing foods and some medications); History of peptic ulcer disease.

Adverse Reactions/Side Effects
CNS: confusion, dizziness, fainting, hallucinations, insomnia, urges (gambling, sexual), vivid dreams. **Derm:** melanoma. **GI:** nausea, abdominal pain, dry mouth.

Interactions
Drug-Drug: Concurrent use with **meperidine** or other **opioid analgesics** may possibly result in a potentially fatal reaction (excitation, sweating, rigidity, and hypertension; or hypotension and coma). Serotonin syndrome (confusion, agitation, hyperpyrexia, hypertension, seizures) may occur with concurrent use of **nefazodone** or **SSRI antidepressants** (fluoxetine should be discontinued 5 wk prior to selegiline, **venlafaxine** should be discontinued 7 days before selegiline, other agents should be discontinued 2 wk before selegiline). Selegiline should be discontinued 2 wk before **SSRIs** are initiated. Concurrent use with **tricyclic antidepressants** may result in asystole, diaphoresis, hypertension, syncope, behavioral changes, altered consciousness, hyperpyrexia, tremors, muscle rigidity, and seizures (avoid concurrent use; discontinue selegiline 2 wk before initiating tricyclic antidepressant therapy). May initially ↑ risk of side effects of **levodopa/carbidopa** (dose of levodopa/carbidopa may need to be ↓ by 10–30%).
Drug-Food: Doses >10 mg/day may produce hypertensive reactions with **tyramine-containing foods** (see Appendix M).

Route/Dosage
PO (Adults): 5 mg bid, with breakfast and lunch (some patients may require further dividing of doses—2.5 mg 4 times daily).

PO (Adults): *Orally disintegrating tablets*—1.25 mg once daily for at least 6 wk. After 6 wk, may increase to 2.5 mg if effect not achieved and patient is tolerating medication.

Availability (generic available)
Capsules: 5 mg. **Tablets:** 5 mg. **Orally disintegrating tablets:** 1.25 mg.

NURSING IMPLICATIONS

Assessment
- Assess patient for signs and symptoms of Parkinson's disease (tremor, muscle weakness and rigidity, ataxic gait) prior to and during therapy.
- Assess blood pressure periodically during therapy.

Potential Nursing Diagnoses
Impaired physical mobility (Indications)
Risk for injury (Indications, Side Effects)

Implementation
- Do not confuse selegiline with sertraline.
- An attempt to reduce the dose of levodopa/carbidopa by 10–30% may be made after 2–3 days of selegiline therapy.
- **PO:** Administer 5-mg tablet with breakfast and lunch.
- Administer *orally disintegrating tablets* in the morning, before breakfast and without liquid. Remove tablet gently from blister pack with clean, dry hands immediately before administering. Do not attempt to push tablet through backing. Tablet will disintegrate within seconds when placed on tongue. Avoid food or liquid within 5 min of administering orally disintegrating tablets.

Patient/Family Teaching
- Instruct patient to take medication as directed. Take missed doses as soon as possible, but not if late afternoon or evening or almost time for next dose. Do not double doses. Caution patient that taking more than the prescribed dose may increase side effects and place patient at risk for hypertensive crisis if foods containing tyramine are consumed (see Appendix M).
- Advise patients taking selegiline ≥20 mg/day to avoid large amounts of tyramine-containing foods (see Appendix M), alcoholic beverages, large quantities of caffeine-containing beverages, or OTC or herbal cough or cold medications.
- Inform patient and family of the signs and symptoms of MAO inhibitor–induced hypertensive crisis (severe headache, chest pain, nausea, vomiting, photosensitivity, enlarged pupils). Advise patient to notify health care professional immediately if severe headache or any other unusual symptom occurs.
- Caution patient to change positions slowly to minimize orthostatic hypotension.
- Instruct patient to consult health care professional before taking any other Rx, OTC, or herbal products with selegiline.

selegiline transdermal 1143

- Advise patient to have periodic skin exams to check for lesions that may be melanoma.
- Advise patient to notify health care professional if or new or increased gambling, sexual, or other intense urges occur.
- Advise patient that increasing fluids, sugarless gum or candy, ice, or saliva substitutes may help minimize dry mouth. Consult health care professional if dry mouth continues for >2 wk.
- Inform patient that selegiline may cause hallucinations.

Evaluation/Desired Outcomes
- Improved response to levodopa/carbidopa in patients with Parkinson's disease.

---

selegiline transdermal
(se-**le**-ji-leen)
Emsam

Classification
Therapeutic: antidepressants
Pharmacologic: monoamine oxidase type B inhibitors

Pregnancy Category C

Indications
Major depressive disorder.

Action
Following conversion by MAO to its active form, selegiline inactivates MAO by irreversibly binding to it at type B (brain) sites; this results in higher levels of monoamine neurotransmitters in the brain (dopamine, serotonin, norepinephrine). **Therapeutic Effects:** Decreased symptoms of depression.

Pharmacokinetics
Absorption: 25–30% of patch content is transdermally absorbed, blood levels are higher than those following oral administration because there is less first pass hepatic metabolism.
Distribution: Rapidly distributes to all body tissues; crosses the blood brain barrier.
Metabolism and Excretion: Mostly metabolized by the liver, primarily by the CYP2A6, CYP2C9, and CYP3A4/5 enzyme systems. 10% excreted in urine as metabolites, 2% in feces; negligible renal excretion of unchanged drug.
Half-life: 18–25 hr.

TIME/ACTION PROFILE

ROUTE	ONSET	PEAK	DURATION
transdermal	unknown	2 or more wk	2 wk (after discontinuation)

Contraindications/Precautions
Contraindicated in: Hypersensitivity; Pheochromocytoma; Concurrent selective serotonin re-uptake inhibitors (fluoxetine, paroxetine citalopram, escitalopram and others), nonselective serotonin re-uptake inhibitors (venlafaxine, duloxetine), tricyclic antidepressants (amitriptyline, imipramine, and others), carbamazepine, oxcarbazepine, amphetamines, vasoconstrictors (ephedrine, pseudoephedrine), bupropion, meperidine, tramadol, methadone, propoxyphene, dextromethorphan, mirtazapine cyclobenzaprine, other MAO inhibitors (isocarboxazid, phenelzine, tranylcypromine) oral selegiline, sympathomimetic amines, amphetamines, cocaine or local anesthetics with vasoconstrictors; St. John's wort; Alcohol.
Use Cautiously in: Elective surgery within 10 days; benzodiazepines, mivacurium, rapacuronium, fentanyl, morphine and codeine may be used cautiously; May ↑ risk of suicide attempt/ideation especially during early treatment or dose adjustment; risk may be greater in children or adolescents (safe use in children <12 yr not established); History of mania; Dosing at 9 mg/24 hr or 12 mg/24 hr requires dietary modification (avoid foods containing large amounts of tyramine); Geri: May be more susceptible to orthostatic hypotension; OB: Use only if benefit outweighs risk to the fetus; Lactation: Safety not established; Pedi: Safe use in children and adolescents not established.

Adverse Reactions/Side Effects
CNS: insomnia, abnormal thinking, agitation, amnesia, worsening of mania/hypomania. **EENT:** tinnitus. **Resp:** ↑ cough. **CV:** HYPERTENSIVE CRISIS, chest pain, orthostatic hypotension, peripheral edema. **GI:** diarrhea, altered taste, anorexia, constipation, flatulence, gastroenteritis, vomiting. **GU:** dysmenorrhea, metrorrhagia, urinary frequency. **Derm:** application site reactions, acne, ecchymoses, pruritus, sweating. **MS:** mylagia, neck pain, pathologic fracture. **Neuro:** paresthesia.

✱ = Canadian drug name. 🧬 = Genetic implication.
*CAPITALS indicates life-threatening; underlines indicate most frequent.

1144 selegiline transdermal

Interactions
Drug-Drug: Concurrent **selective serotonin re-uptake inhibitors** (**fluoxetine, paroxetine, citalopram, escitalopram** and others), **nonselective serotonin re-uptake inhibitors** (**venlafaxine, duloxetine**), **tricyclic antidepressants** (**amitriptyline, imipramine**, and others), **carbamazepine, oxcarbazepine, amphetamines, vasoconstrictors** (**ephedrine, pseudoephedrine, phenylprolanolamine**), **bupropion, meperidine, tramadol, methadone, propoxyphene, dextromethorphan, mirtazapine, cyclobenzaprine**, other MAO inhibitors (**isocarboxazid, phenelzine, tranylcypromine**) oral **selegiline, sympathomimetic amines, amphetamines, cocaine**, or **local anesthetics with vasoconstrictors**; these may all ↑ risk of hypertensive crisis. (**Fluoxetine** should not be used within 2 wk of initiating therapy).
Drug-Natural Products: St. John's wort may ↑ risk of hypertensive crisis.

Route/Dosage
Transdermal (Adults): 6 mg/24 hr, if necessary, may be increased at 2-wk intervals in increments of 3 mg, up to 12 mg/24 hr.

Availability
Transdermal patch : 6 mg/24 hr, 9 mg/24 hr, 12 mg/24 hr.

NURSING IMPLICATIONS
Assessment
- Assess mental status, mood changes, and anxiety level frequently. Assess for suicidal tendencies, agitation, irritability, and unusual changes in behavior especially during early therapy. Monitor pediatric patients face-to-face weekly during first 4 wk, every other week for 4 wk, at 12 wk, and as clinically indicated during therapy. Restrict amount of drug available to patient.
- Monitor blood pressure and pulse rate before and frequently during therapy. Report significant changes promptly.
- ***Toxicity and Overdose:*** Concurrent ingestion of tyramine-rich foods and many medications may result in a life-threatening hypertensive crisis. Signs and symptoms of hypertensive crisis include chest pain, tachycardia or bradycardia, severe headache, neck stiffness or soreness, nausea and vomiting, sweating, photosensitivity, and enlarged pupils. If hypertensive crisis occurs, discontinue selegiline transdermal and administer phentolamine 5 mg or labetalol 20 mg slowly IV to control hypertension. Manage fever with external cooling. Monitor patient closely until symptoms have stabilized.

Potential Nursing Diagnoses
Ineffective coping (Indications)
Noncompliance (Patient/Family Teaching)

Implementation
- **Transdermal:** Apply system to dry, intact skin on the upper torso such as chest, back, upper thigh, or outer surface of the upper arm once every 24 hr at the same time each day. Avoid areas that are hairy, oily, irritated, broken, scarred, or calloused. Wash area gently with soap and warm water, rinse thoroughly. Allow skin to dry completely before application. Apply immediately after removing from package. Do not alter the system (i.e., cut) in any way before application. Remove liner from adhesive layer and press firmly in place with palm of hand for 30 sec, especially around the edges, to make sure contact is complete. Remove used system and fold so that adhesive edges are together. Only one selegiline patch should be worn at a time. Dispose away from children and pets. Apply new system to a different site. Wash hands thoroughly with soap and water to remove any medicine that may have gotten on them.

Patient/Family Teaching
- Instruct patient to apply patch as directed. Advise patients and caregivers to read the *Medication Guide about Using Antidepressants in Children and Teenagers*. Inform patient that improvement may be noticed after 1 to several weeks of therapy. Advise patient not to discontinue therapy without consulting health care professional.
- Caution patient to avoid alcohol and CNS depressants during and for at least 2 wk after therapy has been discontinued; they may precipitate a hypertensive crisis. Contact health care professional immediately if symptoms of hypertensive crisis develop. Patients taking 9 mg/24 hr or 12 mg/24 hr must avoid foods or beverages containing tyramine (see Appendix M) from the first day of the increased dose through 2 wk after discontinuation of selegiline transdermal therapy.
- Advise patient to avoid exposing application site to external sources of direct heat such as heating pads, electric blankets, heat lamps, saunas, hot tubs, heated water beds, and prolonged direct sunlight.

- May cause dizziness or drowsiness. Caution patient to avoid driving and other activities requiring alertness until response to medication is known.
- Caution patient to change positions slowly to minimize orthostatic hypotension. Geriatric patients are at increased risk for this side effect.
- Advise patient referred for MRI test to discuss patch with referring health care professional and MRI facility to determine if removal of patch is necessary prior to test and for directions for replacing patch.
- Advise patients and caregivers to notify health care professional if severe headache, neck stiffness, heart racing or palpitations, anxiety, agitation, panic attacks, insomnia, irritability, hostility, aggressiveness, impulsivity, akathisia, hypomania, mania, change in behavior, worsening of depression, or suicidal ideation occur, especially during initial therapy or during changes in dose.
- Instruct patient to consult health care professional before taking any Rx, OTC, or herbal products. Caution patient to avoid use of St. John's Wort and the analgesics meperidine, propoxyphene, tramadol, or methadone during therapy.
- Advise patient to notify health care professional of medication regimen before treatment or surgery. If possible, therapy should be discontinued at least 2 wk before surgery.
- Advise patient to notify health care professional if pregnancy is planned or suspected or if breastfeeding.

Evaluation/Desired Outcomes
- Improved mood in depressed patients.
- Decreased anxiety.
- Increased appetite.
- Improved energy level.
- Improved sleep. Evaluate effectiveness of therapy periodically.

---

sennosides (sen-oh-sides)
Black-Draught, Ex-Lax, Ex-Lax Chocolated, Fletchers' Castoria, Maximum Relief Ex-Lax, Sena-Gen, Senexon, Senokot, SenokotXTRA

Classification
Therapeutic: laxatives
Pharmacologic: stimulant laxatives

Pregnancy Category C

Indications
Treatment of constipation, particularly when associated with: Slow transit time, Constipating drugs, Irritable or spastic bowel syndrome, Neurologic constipation.

Action
Active components of senna (sennosides) alter water and electrolyte transport in the large intestine, resulting in accumulation of water and increased peristalsis. **Therapeutic Effects:** Laxative action.

Pharmacokinetics
Absorption: Minimally absorbed following oral administration.
Distribution: Unknown.
Metabolism and Excretion: Unknown.
Half-life: Unknown.

TIME/ACTION PROFILE (laxative effect)

ROUTE	ONSET	PEAK	DURATION
PO	6–12 hr†	unknown	3–4 days

†May take as long as 24 hr

Contraindications/Precautions
Contraindicated in: Hypersensitivity; Abdominal pain of unknown cause, especially if associated with fever; Rectal fissures; Ulcerated hemorrhoids; Known alcohol intolerance (some liquid products).
Use Cautiously in: Chronic use (may lead to laxative dependence); Possible intestinal obstruction; OB, Lactation: Safety not established.

Adverse Reactions/Side Effects
GI: cramping, diarrhea, nausea. **GU:** pink-red or brown-black discoloration of urine. **F and E:** electrolyte abnormalities (chronic use or dependence). **Misc:** laxative dependence.

Interactions
Drug-Drug: May ↓ absorption of other **orally administered drugs** because of ↓ transit time.

Route/Dosage
Larger doses have been used to treat/prevent opioid-induced constipation. Consult labeling of individual OTC products for more speceific dosing information.
PO (Adults and Children >12 yr): 12–50 mg 1–2 times daily.
PO (Children 6–12 yr): 6–25 mg 1–2 times daily.
PO (Children 2–6 yr): 3–12.5 mg 1–2 times daily.

Availability (generic available)
Noted as sennoside content
Tablets: 6 mg^OTC, 8.6 mg^OTC, 15 mg^OTC, 17 mg^OTC, 25 mg^OTC. **Granules:** 15 mg/5 mL^OTC, 20 mg/5 mL^OTC. **Syrup:** 8.8 mg/5 mL^OTC. **Liquid:** 25 mg/15 mL^OTC, 33.3 mg/mL senna concentrate^OTC. *In combination with:* psyllium and docusate^OTC. See Appendix B.

NURSING IMPLICATIONS
Assessment
- Assess patient for abdominal distention, presence of bowel sounds, and usual pattern of bowel function.
- Assess color, consistency, and amount of stool produced.

Potential Nursing Diagnoses
Constipation (Indications)
Diarrhea (Side Effects)

Implementation
- **PO:** Take with a full glass of water. Administer at bedtime for evacuation 6–12 hr later. Administer on an empty stomach for more rapid results.
- Shake oral solution well before administering.
- Granules should be dissolved or mixed in water or other liquid before administration.

Patient/Family Teaching
- Advise patient that laxatives should be used only for short-term therapy. Long-term therapy may cause electrolyte imbalance and dependence.
- Encourage patient to use other forms of bowel regulation, such as increasing bulk in the diet, increasing fluid intake, and increasing mobility. Normal bowel habits are individualized and may vary from 3 times/day to 3 times/wk.
- Inform patient that this medication may cause a change in urine color to pink, red, violet, yellow, or brown.
- Instruct patients with cardiac disease to avoid straining during bowel movements (Valsalva maneuver).
- Advise patient not to use laxatives when abdominal pain, nausea, vomiting, or fever is present.

Evaluation/Desired Outcomes
- A soft, formed bowel movement.

---

sertaconazole
(ser-ta-**kon**-a-zole)
Ertaczo

Classification
Therapeutic: antifungals
Pharmacologic: imidazoles

Indications
Topical treatment of interdigital tinea pedis in immunocompetent patients.

Action
Inhibits synthesis of ergosterol, a component of fungal cell membrane, resulting in cytoplasmic leakage and fungal cell death. **Therapeutic Effects:** Resolution of fungal infection. **Spectrum:** Active against *Trichophyton rubrum*, *Trichophyton mentagrophytes*, *Epidermophyton floccosum*.

Pharmacokinetics
Absorption: Minimal systemic absorption.
Distribution: Unknown.
Metabolism and Excretion: Unknown.
Half-life: Unknown.

TIME/ACTION PROFILE

ROUTE	ONSET	PEAK	DURATION
top	within 2 wk	unknown	unknown

Contraindications/Precautions
Contraindicated in: Hypersensitivity to sertaconazole or other imidazoles.
Use Cautiously in: OB: Use only if clearly needed; Lactation, Pedi: Lactation and children <12 yr (safety not established).

Adverse Reactions/Side Effects
Derm: application site reactions, burning, contact dermatitis, dry skin, tenderness.

Interactions
Drug-Drug: None noted.

Route/Dosage
Topical (Adults and Children >12 yr): Apply twice daily for 4 wk.

Availability
Cream: 2%.

NURSING IMPLICATIONS
Assessment
- Inspect involved areas of skin and mucous membranes before and frequently during therapy. Increased skin irritation may indicate need to discontinue medication.

Potential Nursing Diagnoses
Impaired skin integrity (Indications)
Risk for infection (Indications)

Implementation
- **Topical:** Apply small amount to cover affected areas between the toes and the immediately surrounding healthy skin. Dry affected area well if applied after bathing. Avoid the use of occlusive wrappings or dressings unless directed by health care professional.

Patient/Family Teaching
- Instruct patient to apply medication as directed for full course of therapy, even if symptoms have improved. Emphasize the importance of avoiding the eyes, nose, mouth, and other mucous membranes. Do not use for disorders other than for which it was prescribed.
- Patients with athlete's foot should be taught to wear well-fitting, ventilated shoes and to change shoes and socks at least once a day.
- Advise patient to report increased skin irritation, redness, itching, burning, blistering, swelling, oozing, or lack of response to therapy to health care professional.

Evaluation/Desired Outcomes
- Decrease in skin irritation and resolution of infection. If no clinical improvement is seen in 2 wk, diagnosis should be reviewed. Recurrent fungal infections may be a sign of systemic illness.

---

sertraline (ser-tra-leen)
Zoloft

Classification
Therapeutic: antidepressants
Pharmacologic: selective serotonin reuptake inhibitors (SSRIs)

Pregnancy Category C

Indications
Major depressive disorder. Panic disorder. Obsessive-compulsive disorder (OCD). Post-traumatic stress disorder (PTSD). Social anxiety disorder (social phobia). Premenstrual dysphoric disorder (PMDD). **Unlabeled Use:** Generalized anxiety disorder (GAD).

Action
Inhibits neuronal uptake of serotonin in the CNS, thus potentiating the activity of serotonin. Has little effect on norepinephrine or dopamine. **Therapeutic Effects:** Antidepressant action. Decreased incidence of panic attacks. Decreased obsessive and compulsive behavior. Decreased feelings of intense fear, helplessness, or horror. Decreased social anxiety. Decrease in premenstrual dysphoria.

Pharmacokinetics
Absorption: Appears to be well absorbed after oral administration.
Distribution: Extensively distributed throughout body tissues.
Protein Binding: 98%.
Metabolism and Excretion: Extensively metabolized by the liver; one metabolite has some antidepressant activity; 14% excreted unchanged in feces.
Half-life: 24 hr.

TIME/ACTION PROFILE (antidepressant effect)

ROUTE	ONSET	PEAK	DURATION
PO	within 2–4 wk	unknown	unknown

Contraindications/Precautions
Contraindicated in: Hypersensitivity; Concurrent MAO inhibitor therapy (may result in serious, potentially fatal reactions); Concurrent pimozide; Oral concentrate contains alcohol; avoid in patients with known intolerance.
Use Cautiously in: Severe hepatic or renal impairment; Patients with a history of mania; History of suicide attempt; OB, Lactation: Pregnancy or lactation; Pedi: May ↑ risk of suicide attempt/ideation especially during early treatment or dose adjustment; risk may be greater in children or adolescents.

Adverse Reactions/Side Effects
CNS: NEUROLEPTIC MALIGNANT SYNDROME, SUICIDAL THOUGHTS, dizziness, drowsiness, fatigue, headache, insomnia, agitation, anxiety, confusion, emotional lability, impaired concentration, manic reaction, nervousness, weakness, yawning. **EENT:** pharyngitis, rhinitis, tinnitus, visual abnormalities. **CV:** chest pain, palpitations. **GI:** diarrhea, dry mouth, nausea, abdominal pain, altered taste, anorexia, constipation, dyspepsia, flatulence, ↑ appetite, vomiting. **GU:** sexual dysfunction, menstrual disorders, urinary disorders, urinary frequency. **Derm:** ↑ sweating, hot flashes, rash. **F and E:** hyponatremia. **MS:** back pain, myalgia. **Neuro:** tremor, hypertonia, hypoesthesia, paresthesia, twitching. **Misc:** SEROTONIN SYNDROME, fever, thirst.

Interactions
Drug-Drug: Serious, potentially fatal reactions (hyperthermia, rigidity, myoclonus, autonomic

instability, with fluctuating vital signs and extreme agitation, which may proceed to delirium and coma) may occur with concurrent **MAO inhibitors**. MAO inhibitors should be stopped at least 14 days before sertraline therapy. Sertraline should be stopped at least 14 days before MAO inhibitor therapy. May ↑ **pimozide** levels and the risk of potentially life-threatening cardiovascular reactions. Drugs that affect serotonergic neurotransmitter systems, including **linezolid**, **tramadol**, and **triptans**, ↑ risk of serotonin syndrome. May ↑ sensitivity to **adrenergics** and ↑ the risk of serotonin syndrome. Concurrent use with **alcohol** is not recommended. May ↑ levels/effects of **warfarin, phenytoin, tricyclic antidepressants**, some **benzodiazepines (alprazolam), cloazapine**, or **tolbutamide**. ↑ risk of bleeding with **NSAIDS, aspirin, clopidogrel**, or **warfarin**. **Cimetidine** ↑ blood levels and effects.

Drug-Natural Products: ↑ risk of serotinergic side effects including serotonin syndrome with **St. John's wort** and **SAMe**.

Route/Dosage
Depression/OCD
PO (Adults): 50 mg/day as a single dose in the morning or evening initially; after several weeks may be ↑ at weekly intervals up to 200 mg/day, depending on response.

PO (Children 13–17 yr): *OCD*—50 mg once daily.

PO (Children 6–12 yr): *OCD*—25 mg once daily.

Panic Disorder
PO (Adults): 25 mg/day initially, may ↑ after 1 wk to 50 mg/day.

PTSD
PO (Adults): 25 mg once daily for 7 days, then ↑ to 50 mg once daily; may then be ↑ if needed at intervals of at least 7 days (range 50–200 mg once daily).

Social Anxiety Disorder
PO (Adults): 25 mg once daily initially, then 50 mg once daily; may be ↑ at weekly intervals up to 200 mg/day.

PMDD
PO (Adults): 50 mg/day initially either daily or daily during luteal phase of cycle. Daily dosing may be titrated upward in 50-mg increments at the beginning of a cycle. In luteal phase–only dosing a 50 mg/day titration step for 3 days at the beginning of each luteal phase dosing period should be used (range 50–150 mg/day).

Availability (generic available)
Tablets: 25 mg, 50 mg, 100 mg. **Cost:** *Generic*—25 mg $87.98/90, 50 mg $89.98/90, 100 mg $99.96/90. **Capsules:** ✹ 50 mg, ✹ 100 mg. **Oral concentrate (12% alcohol):** 20 mg/mL in 60-mL bottles. **Cost:** $65.28/60 mL.

NURSING IMPLICATIONS
Assessment
- Assess for suicidal tendencies, especially during early therapy. Restrict amount of drug available to patient. Risk may be increased in children, adolescents, and adults ≤24 yr. After starting therapy, children, adolescents, and young adults should be seen by health care professional at least weekly for 4 wk, every 3 wk for next 4 wk, and on advice of health care professional thereafter.
- Monitor appetite and nutritional intake. Weigh weekly. Notify health care professional of continued weight loss. Adjust diet as tolerated to support nutritional status.
- Assess for serotonin syndrome (mental changes [agitation, hallucinations, coma], autonomic instability [tachycardia, labile blood pressure, hyperthermia], neuromuscular aberrations [hyper-reflexia, incoordination], and/or GI symptoms [nausea, vomiting, diarrhea]), especially in patients taking other serotonergic drugs (SSRIs, SNRIs, triptans).
- **Depression:** Monitor mood changes. Inform health care professional if patient demonstrates significant increase in anxiety, nervousness, or insomnia.
- Assess for suicidal tendencies, especially during early therapy. Restrict amount of drug available to patient.
- **OCD:** Assess patient for frequency of obsessive-compulsive behaviors. Note degree to which these thoughts and behaviors interfere with daily functioning.
- **Panic Attacks:** Assess frequency and severity of panic attacks.
- **PTSD:** Assess patient for feelings of fear, helplessness, and horror. Determine effect on social and occupational functioning.
- **Social Anxiety Disorder:** Assess patient for symptoms of social anxiety disorder (blushing, sweating, trembling, tachycardia during interactions with new people, people in authority, or groups) periodically during therapy.
- **Premenstrual Dysphoric Disorder:** Assess patient for symptoms of premenstrual dys-

phoric disorder (feeling angry, tense, or tired; crying easily, feeling sad or hopeless; arguing with family or friends for no reason; difficulty sleeping or paying attention; feeling out of control or unable to cope; having cramping, bloating, food craving, or breast tenderness) periodically during therapy.

Potential Nursing Diagnoses
Ineffective coping (Indications)
Risk for injury (Side Effects)
Sexual dysfunction (Side Effects)

Implementation
- Do not confuse sertraline with selegiline.
- Periodically reassess dose and continued need for therapy.
- **PO:** Administer as a single dose in the morning or evening.

Patient/Family Teaching
- Instruct patient to take sertraline as directed. Take missed doses as soon as possible and return to regular dosing schedule. Do not double doses.
- May cause drowsiness or dizziness. Caution patient to avoid driving and other activities requiring alertness until response to the drug is known.
- Advise patient, family, and caregivers to look for suicidality, especially during early therapy or dose changes. Notify health care professional immediately if thoughts about suicide or dying, attempts to commit suicide; new or worse depression or anxiety; agitation or restlessness; panic attacks; insomnia; new or worse irritability, aggressiveness, acting on dangerous impulses, mania, or other changes in mood or behavior or if symptoms of serotonin syndrome occur.
- Advise patient to avoid alcohol or other CNS depressant drugs during therapy and to consult with health care professional before taking other medications with sertraline.
- Inform patient that frequent mouth rinses, good oral hygiene, and sugarless gum or candy may minimize dry mouth. If dry mouth persists for more than 2 wk, consult health care professional regarding use of saliva substitute.
- Advise patient to wear sunscreen and protective clothing to prevent photosensitivity reactions.
- Instruct female patient to inform health care professional if pregnancy is planned or suspected or if she is breastfeeding.
- Advise patient to notify health care professional if headache, weakness, nausea, anorexia, anxiety, or insomnia persists.
- Emphasize the importance of follow-up exams to monitor progress. Encourage patient participation in psychotherapy to improve coping skills.

Evaluation/Desired Outcomes
- Increased sense of well-being.
- Renewed interest in surroundings. May require 1–4 wk of therapy to obtain antidepressant effects.
- Decrease in obsessive-compulsive behaviors.
- Decrease in frequency and severity of panic attacks.
- Decrease in symptoms of PTSD.
- Decrease in social anxiety disorder.
- Decrease in symptoms of premenstrual dysphoric disorder.

sevelamer (se-**vel**-a-mer)
Renagel, Renvela

Classification
Therapeutic: electrolyte modifiers
Pharmacologic: phosphate binders

Pregnancy Category C

Indications
Reduction of serum phosphate levels in patients with hyperphosphatemia associated with end-stage renal disease.

Action
A polymer that binds phosphate in the GI tract, preventing its absorption. **Therapeutic Effects:** Decreased serum phosphate levels and reduction in the consequences of hyperphosphatemia (ectopic calcification, secondary hyperparathyroidism with osteitis fibrosa).

Pharmacokinetics
Absorption: Not absorbed; action is local (in GI tract).
Distribution: Unknown.
Metabolism and Excretion: Eliminated in feces.
Half-life: Unknown.

TIME/ACTION PROFILE (decrease in serum phosphate levels)

ROUTE	ONSET	PEAK	DURATION
PO	5 days	2 wk	unknown

✱ = Canadian drug name.   ✣ = Genetic implication.
*CAPITALS indicates life-threatening; underlines indicate most frequent.

Contraindications/Precautions

Contraindicated in: Hypersensitivity; Hypophosphatemia; Bowel obstruction.

Use Cautiously in: Dysphagia, swallowing disorders, severe GI motility disorders, or major GI tract surgery; OB, Lactation: Pedi: Safety not established.

Adverse Reactions/Side Effects

GI: diarrhea, dyspepsia, vomiting, constipation, flatulence, nausea.

Interactions

Drug-Drug: May ↓ absorption of other drugs and ↓ effectiveness, especially **drugs whose efficacy is dependent on tightly controlled blood levels.** ↓ absorption of **ciprofloxacin.**

Route/Dosage

PO (Adults): 800–1600 mg with each meal; may titrate by 800 mg every 2 wk to achieve target serum phosphorus levels.

Availability

Tablets: 400 mg, 800 mg. **Powder for oral suspension:** 800 mg/packet, 2400 mg/packet.

NURSING IMPLICATIONS

Assessment

- Assess patient for GI side effects periodically during therapy.
- *Lab Test Considerations:* Monitor serum phosphorous, calcium, bicarbonate, and chloride levels periodically during therapy.

Potential Nursing Diagnoses

Deficient knowledge, related to medication regimen (Patient/Family Teaching)

Implementation

- Doses of concurrent medications, especially antiarrhythmics, should be spaced at least 1 hr before or 3 hr after sevelamer.
- **PO:** Administer with meals. Do not break, chew, or crush tablets; contents expand in water.
- Place contents of powder packet in a cup and mix thoroughly with at least 1 ounce of water for the 0.8 g dose or 2 ounces of water for the 2.4 g dose packet. Stir mixture vigorously (it does not dissolve) and drink entire preparation within 30 minutes or resuspend the preparation right before drinking.

Patient/Family Teaching

- Instruct patient to take sevelamer with meals as directed and to adhere to prescribed diet.
- Caution patient to space concurrent medications at least 1 hr before or 3 hr after sevelamer.
- Advise patient to notify health care professional if GI effects are severe or prolonged.

Evaluation/Desired Outcomes

- Decrease in serum phosphorous concentration to ≤6 mg/dL. Dose adjustment is based on serum phosphorous concentrations.

---

sibutramine (si-byoo-tra-meen)
Meridia

Classification
Therapeutic: weight control agents
Pharmacologic: appetite suppressants

Schedule IV

Pregnancy Category C

Indications

Treatment of obesity in patients with body mass index ≥30 kg/m^2 (or ≥27 kg/m^2 in patients with diabetes, hypertension, or other risk factors) in conjunction with other interventions (dietary restriction, exercise); used to produce and maintain weight loss.

Action

Acts as an inhibitor of the reuptake of serotonin, norepinephrine, and dopamine; increases the satiety-producing effects of serotonin. **Therapeutic Effects:** Decreased hunger with resultant weight loss in obese patients.

Pharmacokinetics

Absorption: 77% absorbed, then rapidly undergoes extensive first-pass hepatic metabolism (via the P450 3A4 metabolic pathway) to active metabolites (M1 and M2).

Distribution: Widely and rapidly distributed; high concentrations in liver and kidneys.

Metabolism and Excretion: Active metabolites are extensively metabolized to inactive metabolites that are mostly excreted by the kidneys.

Half-life: *M1 metabolite*—14 hr; *M2 metabolite*—16 hr.

TIME/ACTION PROFILE (appetite suppression/weight loss)

ROUTE	ONSET	PEAK	DURATION
PO	days	4 wk	unknown

Contraindications/Precautions

Contraindicated in: Hypersensitivity; Anorexia nervosa; Concurrent use of other centrally acting appetite suppressants, MAO inhibitors, SSRIs, sumatriptan, naratriptan, zolmitriptan, dihydroergotamine, dextromethorphan, meperidine, pentazocine, fentanyl, lithium, or tryptophan; Organic causes of obesity (untreated hypothyroidism); Severe hepatic/renal impairment; Uncontrolled/poorly controlled hypertension; History of coronary artery disease, CHF, arrhythmias, or stroke; Excessive consumption of alcohol; OB, Lactation: Pregnancy or lactation.

Use Cautiously in: History of seizures; Angle-closure glaucoma; Geri: Geriatric patients; Pedi: Children <16 yr (safety not established).

Adverse Reactions/Side Effects
CNS: NEUROLEPTIC MALIGNANT SYNDROME, SEIZURES, headache, insomnia, CNS stimulation, dizziness, drowsiness, emotional lability, mania, nervousness, psychosis. **EENT:** laryngitis/pharyngitis, rhinitis, sinusitis. **CV:** hypertension, palpitations, tachycardia, vasodilation. **GI:** anorexia, constipation, dry mouth, altered taste, dyspepsia, ↑ appetite, nausea. **GU:** dysmenorrhea. **Derm:** ↑ sweating, rash. **Misc:** SEROTONIN SYNDROME.

Interactions
Drug-Drug: Concurrent use of **other centrally acting appetite suppressants, MAO inhibitors, SSRIs, naratriptan, frovatriptan, rizatriptan, zolmitriptan, sumatriptan, dihydroergotamine, dextromethorphan, meperidine, pentazocine, fentanyl, lithium,** or **tryptophan** may result in potentially fatal "serotonin syndrome" (avoid concurrent use; allow 2 wk between use of MAO inhibitors and sibutramine). Concurrent use of **decongestants** may ↑ the risk of hypertension. **Drugs that affect the P450 3A4 enzyme system** may alter the effects of sibutramine. **Ketoconazole, cimetidine,** and **erythromycin** decrease metabolism and may ↑ blood levels and effects.

Route/Dosage
PO (Adults): 10 mg once daily; may be ↑ to 15 mg/day after 4 wk. Patients who do not tolerate an initial dose of 10 mg/day may be started on 5 mg/day.

Availability
Capsules: 5 mg, 10 mg, 15 mg.

NURSING IMPLICATIONS

Assessment
- Monitor patients for weight loss and adjust concurrent medications (antihypertensives, antidiabetics, lipid-lowering agents) as needed.
- Monitor blood pressure and heart rate regularly during therapy. Increases in blood pressure or heart rate, especially during early therapy, may require decrease in dose or discontinuation of sibutramine.
- Assess for serotonin syndrome (mental changes [agitation, hallucinations, coma], autonomic instability [tachycardia, labile blood pressure, hyperthermia], neuromuscular aberrations [hyper-reflexia, incoordination], and/or GI symptoms [nausea, vomiting, diarrhea]), especially in patients taking other serotonergic drugs (SSRIs, SNRIs, triptans).

Potential Nursing Diagnoses
Disturbed body image (Indications)
Imbalanced nutrition: more than body requirements (Indications)
Deficient knowledge, related to medication regimen (Patient/Family Teaching)

Implementation
- **PO:** Capsules should be taken once daily without regard to meals.

Patient/Family Teaching
- Instruct patient to take medication as directed and not to exceed dose recommended. Medication may need to be discontinued gradually. Advise patient to read *Patient Information* before taking and with each Rx refill, changes may occur.
- Advise patient to notify health care professional if signs of allergic reaction (rash, hives) or serotonin syndrome occur.
- Caution patient to avoid using other CNS depressants or excessive amounts of alcohol with this medication.
- Advise patient to consult health care professional before taking other Rx, OTC, or herbal products, especially weight-reducing agents, decongestants, antidepressants, cough suppressants, lithium, dihydroergotamine, triptans, or tryptophan.
- Emphasize the need for follow-up visits to monitor pulse and blood pressure.

Evaluation/Desired Outcomes
- Slow, consistent weight loss when combined with a reduced-calorie diet. If this does not occur, therapy should be re-evaluated. Loss of at least 10% of initial body weight should occur within 1 yr.

sildenafil (sil-den-a-fil)
Revatio, Viagra

sildenafil

Classification
Therapeutic: erectile dysfunction agents, vasodilators
Pharmacologic: phosphodiesterase type 5 inhibitors

Pregnancy Category B

Indications
Viagra: Erectile dysfunction. *Revatio:* Pulmonary arterial hypertension.

Action
Viagra: Enhances effects of nitric oxide released during sexual stimulation. Nitric oxide activates guanylate cyclase, which produces increased levels of cyclic guanosine monophosphate (cGMP). cGMP produces smooth muscle relaxation of the corpus cavernosum, which promotes increased blood flow and subsequent erection. cGMP also leads to vasodilation of the pulmonary vasculature. Sildenafil inhibits the enzyme phosphodiesterase type 5 (PDE5), PDE5 inactivates cGMP. *Revatio:* Produces vasodilation of the pulmonary vascular bed. **Therapeutic Effects:** *Viagra:* Enhanced blood flow to the corpus cavernosum and erection sufficient to allow sexual intercourse. Requires sexual stimulation. *Revatio:* Improved exercise tolerance and delay worsening of disease.

Pharmacokinetics
Absorption: Rapidly absorbed (41%) after oral administration.
Distribution: Widely distributed to tissues; negligible amount in semen.
Protein Binding: 96%.
Metabolism and Excretion: Mostly metabolized by the liver (by P450 3A4 enzyme system); one metabolite is active and accounts for 20% or more of drug effect. Metabolites excreted mostly (80%) in feces; 13% excreted in urine.
Half-life: 4 hr (for sildenafil and active metabolite).

TIME/ACTION PROFILE (vasodilation, ability to produce erection)

ROUTE	ONSET	PEAK	DURATION
PO	within 1 hr	30–120 min	up to 4 hr

Contraindications/Precautions
Contraindicated in: Hypersensitivity; Concurrent organic nitrate therapy (nitroglycerin, isosorbide mononitrate, isosorbide dinitrate), ritonavir, ketoconazole, and itraconazole; Pulmonary veno-occlusive disease; **Viagra:** OB, Pedi: Newborns, women, children.
Use Cautiously in: Serious underlying cardiovascular disease (including history of MI, stroke, or serious arrhythmia within 6 mo), cardiac failure, or coronary artery disease with unstable angina; History of CHF, coronary artery disease, uncontrolled hypertension (BP >170/110 mm Hg) or hypotension (BP <90/50 mm Hg), dehydration, autonomic dysfunction, or severe left ventricular outflow obstruction; Concurrent treatment with antihypertensives or glipizide; Renal impairment (CCr <30 mL/min, hepatic impairment; all result in ↑ blood levels; ↓ dose required with Viagra); Anatomic penile deformity (angulation, cavernosal fibrosis, Peyronie disease); Conditions associated with priapism (sickle cell anemia, multiple myeloma, leukemia); Bleeding disorders or active peptic ulceration; History of sudden severe vision loss or non-arteritic ischemic optic neuropathy (NAION); may ↑ risk of recurrence; Retinitis pigmentosa; Concurrent bosentan, erythromycin, or saquinavir (↓ dose recommended); Alpha adrenergic blockers (patients should be on stable dose of alpha blockers before starting sildenafil); Geri: ↑ blood levels and may require lower doses; consider age-related decrease in cardiac, hepatic, and renal function as well as concurrent drug therapy and chronic disease states; Lactation: Lactation; Pedi: *Revatio* Safe use in pediatric patients with pulmonary hypertension not established; May ↑ risk of bleeding with **warfarin**.

Adverse Reactions/Side Effects
CNS: headache, dizziness, insomnia. **EENT:** epistaxis, hearing loss, nasal congestion, vision loss. **CV:** MYOCARDIAL INFARCTION, SUDDEN DEATH, CARDIOVASCULAR COLLAPSE. **GI:** dyspepsia, diarrhea. **GU:** priapism, urinary tract infection. **Derm:** flushing, rash. **MS:** mylagia. **Neuro:** paresthesias.

Interactions
Drug-Drug: ↑ risk of hypotension with **nitrates** in any form or **ritonavir**; concurrent use is contraindicated because of the risk of serious and potentially fatal hypotension. Blood levels and effects, including the risk of hypotension may be ↑ by **enzyme inhibitors** including **cimetidine, erythromycin, tacrolimus, ketoconazole, itraconazole**, and **protease inhibitor antiretrovirals** including **nelfinavir, indinavir, saquinavir** (initial dose of sildenafil for erectile dysfunction should be ↓ to 25 mg). ↑ risk of hypotension with **alpha adrenergic blockers** and acute ingestion of **alcohol**. **Rifampin, bosentan, barbiturates, carbamazepine, phenytoin, efavirenz, nevirapine, rifampin** or **rifabutin** may ↓ blood levels and effects; dose adjustments may be necessary in the treat-

ment of pulmonary arterial hypertension. ↑ levels of **bosentan**. Use cautiously with **glipizide**.

Route/Dosage

Viagra (for erectile dysfunction)
PO (Adults): 50 mg taken 1 hr before sexual activity (range 25–100 mg taken 30 min–4 hr before sexual activity); not more than once daily; *Concurrent use with alpha-blocker antihypertensives*—do not use 50–100 mg dose within 4 hr of alpha blocker, 25-mg dose may be taken anytime.

PO (Geriatric Patients ≥65 yr or with concurrent enzyme inhibitors): 25 mg taken 1 hr before sexual activity (range 25–100 mg taken 30 min–4 hr before sexual activity); not more than once daily.

Hepatic/Renal Impairment
PO (Adults): 25 mg taken 1 hr before sexual activity (range 25–100 mg taken 30 min–4 hr before sexual activity); not more than once daily.

Revatio (for pulmonary arterial hypertension)
PO (Adults): 20 mg 3 times daily; dose adjustments may be necessary for concurrent bosentan, barbiturates, carbamazepine, phenytoin, efavirenz, nevirapine, rifampin, or rifabutin.

Availability
Tablets (Viagra): 25 mg, 50 mg, 100 mg. **Cost:** All strengths $115.99/10. **Tablets (Revatio):** 20 mg. **Cost:** $1,091.58/90.

NURSING IMPLICATIONS

Assessment
- **Viagra:** Determine erectile dysfunction before administration. Sildenafil has no effect in the absence of sexual stimulation.
- **Revatio:** Monitor hemodynamic parameters and exercise tolerance prior to and periodically during therapy.

Potential Nursing Diagnoses
Sexual dysfunction (Indications)
Risk for activity intolerance (Indications)

Implementation
- **PO:** Dose for *erectile dysfunction* is usually administered 1 hr before sexual activity. May be administered 30 min–4 hr before sexual activity.
- Dose for *pulmonary hypertension* is administered 3 times daily without regard to food. Doses should be spaced 4–6 hr apart.

Patient/Family Teaching
- Instruct patient to take sildenafil as directed. For *erectile dysfunction,* take approximately 1 hr before sexual activity and not more than once per day.
- Advise patient that *Viagra* is not indicated for use in women.
- Caution patient not to take sildenafil concurrently with alpha-adrenergic blockers (unless on a stable dose) or nitrates. If chest pain occurs after taking tadalafil, instruct patient to seek immediate medical attention. Advise patient taking sildenafil for pulmonary hypertension to consult health care professional prior to taking other Rx, OTC, or herbal products.
- Instruct patient to notify health care professional promptly if erection lasts longer than 4 hr or if experience sudden or decreased vision loss in one or both eyes or loss or decrease in hearing, ringing in the ears, or dizziness.
- Inform patient that sildenafil offers no protection against sexually transmitted diseases. Counsel patient that protection against sexually transmitted diseases and HIV infection should be considered.

Evaluation/Desired Outcomes
- Male erection sufficient to allow intercourse.
- Increased exercise tolerance.

---

silodosin (si-lo-do-sin)
Rapaflo

Classification
Therapeutic: benign prostatic hyperplasia (BPH) agents
Pharmacologic: alpha-adrenergic blockers

Pregnancy Category B

Indications
Treatment of the signs/symptoms or Benign Prostatic Hyperplasia (BPH).

Action
Blocks post synaptic alpha$_1$-adrenergic receptors. Decreases contractions in the smooth muscle of the prostatic capsule. **Therapeutic Effects:** Decreased signs and symptoms of BPH (urinary urgency, hesitancy, nocturia).

Pharmacokinetics
Absorption: 32% absorbed following oral administration.
Distribution: Unknown.

✦ = Canadian drug name. 🧬 = Genetic implication.
*CAPITALS indicates life-threatening; underlines indicate most frequent.

silodosin

Protein Binding: 97%.
Metabolism and Excretion: Extensively metabolized (CYP3A4, UGT2B7 and other metabolic pathways involved); 33.5% excreted in urine and 54.9% in feces.
Half-life: 13.3 hr.

TIME/ACTION PROFILE (effect on symptoms of BPH)

ROUTE	ONSET	PEAK	DURATION
PO	rapid	24 hr	24 hr*

*Following discontinuation.

Contraindications/Precautions
Contraindicated in: Not indicated for use in women or children; Severe renal impairment (CrCl less than 30 mL/min); Severe hepatic impairment (Child-Pugh score of 10 or greater); Concurrent use of strong CYP3A4 inhibitors or P-gp inhibitors.
Use Cautiously in: Moderate inhibitors of the CYP3A4 enzyme system; Cataract surgery (may cause Intraoperative Floppy Iris Syndrome); Moderate renal impairment (lower dose recommended); Geri: Increased risk of orthostatic hypotention; Pedi: Safety and effectiveness have not been established.

Adverse Reactions/Side Effects
CNS: dizziness, headache. **CV:** orthostatic hypotension. **GI:** diarrhea. **GU:** retrograde ejaculation.

Interactions
Drug-Drug: Strong inhibitors of CYP3A4 (including **ketoconazole**, **clarithromycin**, **itraconazole**, and **ritonavir**) ↓ metabolism, ↑ blood levels and risk of toxicity; concurrent use is contraindicated. Concurrent use with moderate **CYP3A4 inhibitors** (including **diltiazem**, **erythromycin**, and **verapamil**) may ↑ silodosin levels; use cautiously. Concurrent use with **antihypertensives** (including **calcium channel blockers** and **thiazides**), other **alpha blockers** and **phosphodiesterase type 5 inhibitors** (including **sildenafil** and **tadalafil**) ↑ the risk of dizziness and orthostatic hypotension. **P-glycoprotein (P-gp) inhibitors** including **cyclosporine**) may ↑ levels; concurrent use not recommended.

Route/Dosage
PO (Adults): 8 mg once daily.

Renal Impairment
PO (Adults CCr 30–50 mL/min): 4 mg once daily.

Availability
Capsules: 4 mg, 8 mg.

NURSING IMPLICATIONS
Assessment
- Assess patient for symptoms of benign prostatic hyperplasia (urinary hesitancy, feeling of incomplete bladder emptying, interruption of urinary stream, impairment of size and force of urinary stream, terminal urinary dribbling, straining to start flow, frequency, dysuria, nocturia, urgency) before and periodically during therapy.
- Assess patient for orthostatic reaction and syncope. Monitor BP (lying and standing) and during initial therapy and periodically thereafter.
- Rule out prostatic carcinoma before therapy; symptoms are similar.

Potential Nursing Diagnoses
Risk for injury (Side Effects)
Noncompliance (Patient/Family Teaching)

Implementation
- **PO:** Administer with food at the same meal each day.

Patient/Family Teaching
- Instruct patient to take medication with the same meal each day.
- May cause dizziness. Caution patient to avoid driving or other activities requiring alertness until response to the medication is known.
- Caution patient to avoid sudden changes in position to decrease orthostatic hypotension, especially patients with low blood pressure or concurrently taking antihypertensives.
- Advise patient to consult health care professional before taking any other Rx, OTC, or herbal products, especially cough, cold, or allergy remedies.
- Instruct patient to notify health care professional of medication regimen before any surgery. Patients planning cataract surgery should notify opthalmologist of silodosin therapy prior to surgery.
- Inform patient that silodosin may cause retrograde ejaculation (orgasm with reduced or no semen). This does not pose a safety concern and is reversible with discontinuation.
- Emphasize the importance of follow-up exams to evaluate effectiveness of medication.
- Geri: Assess risk for falls; implement fall prevention program and instruct patient and family in preventing falls at home.

Evaluation/Desired Outcomes
- Decreased symptoms of benign prostatic hyperplasia.

simethicone (si-meth-i-kone)

Degas, Extra Strength Gas-X, ✤Extra Strength Maalox GRF Gas Relief Formula, Flatulex, Gas-X, Genasyme, ✤Maalox GRF Gas Relief Formula, Maximum Strength Mylanta Gas, Mylanta Gas, Mylicon, ✤Ovol, ✤Ovol-40, Phazyme

Classification
Therapeutic: antiflatulent

Pregnancy Category UK

Indications
Relief of painful symptoms of excess gas in the GI tract that may occur postoperatively or as a consequence of: Air swallowing, Dyspepsia, Peptic ulcer, Diverticulitis.

Action
Causes the coalescence of gas bubbles. Does not prevent the formation of gas. **Therapeutic Effects:** Passage of gas through the GI tract by belching or passing flatus.

Pharmacokinetics
Absorption: No systemic absorption occurs.
Distribution: Not systemically distributed.
Metabolism and Excretion: Excreted unchanged in the feces.
Half-life: Unknown.

TIME/ACTION PROFILE (antiflatulent effect)

ROUTE	ONSET	PEAK	DURATION
PO	immediate	unknown	3 hr

Contraindications/Precautions
Contraindicated in: Not recommended for infant colic.
Use Cautiously in: Abdominal pain of unknown cause, especially when accompanied by fever; OB: Lactation: Has been used safely.

Adverse Reactions/Side Effects
None significant.

Interactions
Drug-Drug: None significant.

Route/Dosage
PO (Adults): 40–125 mg qid, after meals and at bedtime (up to 500 mg/day).
PO (Children 2–12 yr): 40 mg 4 times daily.
PO (Children <2 yr): 20 mg 4 times daily (up to 240 mg/day).

Availability (generic available)
Chewable tablets: 40 mg^{OTC}, 80 mg^{OTC}, 125 mg^{OTC}, 150 mg^{OTC}. **Tablets:** 60 mg^{OTC}, 80 mg^{OTC}, 95 mg^{OTC}. **Capsules:** ✤95 mg^{OTC}, 125 mg^{OTC}. **Drops:** 40 mg/0.6 mL^{OTC}, ✤40 mg/1 mL^{OTC}, ✤95 mg/1.425 mL^{OTC}. *In combination with:* antacids^{OTC}. See Appendix B.

NURSING IMPLICATIONS

Assessment
- Assess patient for abdominal pain, distention, and bowel sounds prior to and periodically throughout course of therapy. Frequency of belching and passage of flatus should also be assessed.

Potential Nursing Diagnoses
Acute pain (Indications)

Implementation
- **PO:** Administer after meals and at bedtime for best results. Shake liquid preparations well prior to administration. Chewable tablets should be chewed thoroughly before swallowing, for faster and more complete results.
- Drops can be mixed with 30 mL of cool water, infant formula, or other liquid as directed. Shake well before using.

Patient/Family Teaching
- Explain to patient the importance of diet and exercise in the prevention of gas. Also explain that this medication does not prevent the formation of gas.
- Advise patient to notify health care professional if symptoms are persistent.

Evaluation/Desired Outcomes
- Decrease in abdominal distention and discomfort.

---

simvastatin, See HMG-CoA REDUCTASE INHIBITORS (statins).

---

sirolimus (sir-oh-li-mus)
Rapamune

Classification
Therapeutic: immunosuppressants

Pregnancy Category C

Indications
Prevention of organ rejection in allogenic kidney transplantation (with corticosteroids and cyclosporine). Sirolimus is also eluted from the Cypher coronary stent used in angioplasty procedures.

Action
Inhibits T-lymphocyte activation/proliferation, which occurs as a response to antigenic and cytokine stimulation; antibody production is also inhibited. **Therapeutic Effects:** Decreased incidence and severity of organ rejection.

Pharmacokinetics
Absorption: Rapidly absorbed following oral administration (14% bioavailability).
Distribution: Concentrates in erythrocytes; distributes to heart, intestines, kidneys, liver, lungs, muscle, spleen, and testes in high concentrations.
Protein Binding: 92%.
Metabolism and Excretion: Extensively metabolized (some metabolism by P450 3A4 system); 91% excreted in feces.
Half-life: 62 hr.

TIME/ACTION PROFILE (blood levels)

ROUTE	ONSET	PEAK	DURATION
PO	rapid	1–2 hr	24 hr

Contraindications/Precautions
Contraindicated in: Hypersensitivity; Alcohol intolerance/sensitivity (solution contains ethanol); Concurrent ketoconazole, voriconazole, itraconazole, erythromycin, telithromycin, clarithromycin, rifampin, rifabutin, or grapefruit juice; Severe hepatic impairment; OB, Lactation: Pregnancy and lactation.
Use Cautiously in: Mild to moderate hepatic impairment; OB: Women with childbearing potential; Pedi: Children <13 yr (safety not established).

Adverse Reactions/Side Effects
Reflects combined therapy with corticosteroids and cyclosporine.
CNS: insomnia. **Resp:** interstitial lung disease. **CV:** edema, hypotension, pericardial effusion. **GI:** hepatic toxicity. **GU:** renal impairment. **Derm:** acne, rash, thrombocytopenic purpura. **F and E:** hypokalemia. **Hemat:** leukopenia, thrombocytopenia, anemia. **Metab:** hyperlipidemia. **MS:** arthralgias. **Neuro:** tremor. **Misc:** infection (including activation of latent viral infections such as BK virus-associated nephropathy), lymphocele, lymphoma, ↓ wound healing.

Interactions
Drug-Drug: Cyclosporine (modified) greatly ↑ blood levels (administer sirolimus 4 hr after cyclosporine). Drugs which inhibit the CYP3A4 enzyme system may be expected to ↑ blood levels and the risk of adverse reactions. **Ketoconazole**, **voriconazole**, **itraconazole**, **clarithromycin**, **erythromycin**, **telithromycin** significantly ↑ blood levels (concurrent use is contraindicated). Blood levels are also ↑ by **diltiazem** and **verapamil** (monitor sirolimus levels and adjust dose as necessary) and may be ↑ by **nicardipine**, **verapamil**, **clotrimazole**, **fluconazole**, **troleandomycin**, **metoclopramide**, **cimetidine**, **danazol**, and **protease inhibitor antiretrovirals**. **Rifampin** and **rifabutin** ↑ metabolism by stimulating the CYP3A4 enzyme system and significantly ↓ blood levels. Blood levels may also be ↓ by **carbamazepine**, **phenobarbital**, **phenytoin**, and **rifapentine**. Risk of renal impairment may be ↑ by concurrent use of other **nephrotoxic agents**. Concurrent use with **tacrolimus** and **corticosteroids** in lung transplantation may ↑ risk of anastomotic dehiscence; fatalites have been reported (not approved for this use). Concurrent use with **tacrolimus** and **corticosteroids** in liver transplantation may ↑ risk of hepatic artery thrombosis; fatalites have been reported (not approved for this use). May ↓ antibody response to and ↑ risk of adverse reactions to **live-virus vaccines** (avoid vaccination).
Drug-Natural Products: Concomitant use with **echinacea** and **melatonin** may interfere with immunosuppression. **St. John's wort** may ↑ blood levels and the risk of toxicity.
Drug-Food: Grapefruit juice ↓ CYP3A4 metabolism and ↑ levels; do not use as a diluent and avoid concurrent ingestion.

Route/Dosage
PO (Adults and Children ≥13 yr): 6-mg loading dose, followed by 2 mg/day maintenance dose. *Dosing following cyclosporine withdrawal*—Patients at low to moderate risk for rejection after transplantation may be withdrawn from cyclosporine over 4–8 wk beginning 2–4 mo after transplant. Thereafter, sirolimus dose should be titrated upward to maintain a whole blood trough level of 12–14 ng/mL. Clinical assessment should also be used to gauge dose. Dose changes can be made at 7–14 day intervals. The following formula may also be used: sirolimus maintenance dose = current dose x (target concentration/current concentration). If a large increase is needed, a loading dose may be given and blood levels reassessed 3–4 days later. Loading dose may be calculated by the following formula: sirolimus loading dose = 3 × (new maintenance

sirolimus 1157

dose-current maintenance dose). Loading doses >40 mg should be spread over 2 days.
PO (Adults and Children ≥13 yr and <40 kg): 3 mg/m² loading dose, followed by 1 mg/m²/day maintenance dose. *See adjustments above for doses following cyclosporine withdrawal.*

Hepatic Impairment
PO (Adults and Children ≥13 yr and <40 kg): ↓ maintenance dose by 33%; loading dose is unchanged.

Availability
Tablet: 1 mg, 2 mg. **Cost:** 1 mg $246.98/30.
Oral solution: 1 mg/mL in 60 mL bottles (with oral syringes). **Cost:** $480.95/60 mL.

NURSING IMPLICATIONS

Assessment
- Monitor blood pressure closely during therapy. Hypertension is a common complication of sirolimus therapy and should be treated.
- *Lab Test Considerations:* Monitor sirolimus blood levels when dose forms are changed and in patients likely to have altered drug metabolism, patients ≥13 yr who weigh <40 kg, patients with hepatic impairment, and during concurrent administration of drugs that may interact with sirolimus. Trough concentrations of ≥15 ng/mL are associated with an ↑ in adverse effects.
- Monitor patients for hyperlipidemia. May require additional interventions to treat hyperlipidemia.
- May cause anemia, leukopenia, thrombocytopenia, and hypokalemia.
- May cause ↑ AST, ↑ ALT, hypophosphatemia, and hyperglycemia.

Potential Nursing Diagnoses
Risk for infection (Adverse Reactions)

Implementation
- Therapy with sirolimus should be started as soon as possible post-transplant. Concurrent therapy with cyclosporine and corticosteroids is recommended. Sirolimus should be taken 4 hr after cyclosporine (MODIFIED, Neoral).
- Sirolimus should be ordered only by physicians skilled in immunosuppressive therapy, with the staff and facilities to manage renal transplant patients.
- Antimicrobial prophylaxis for *Pneumocystis jirovecii* pneumonia for 1 year and for cytomegalovirus protection for 3 months post-transplant are recommended.
- **PO:** Administer consistently with or without food. Do not administer with or mix with grapefruit juice.
- To dilute from bottle, use amber oral dose syringe to withdraw prescribed amount. Empty sirolimus from syringe into a glass or plastic container holding at least 2 oz (60 mL) of water or orange juice; do not use other liquids. Stir vigorously and drink at once. Refill container with at least 4 oz of additional liquid, stir vigorously, and drink at once.
- If using the pouch, empty entire contents of pouch into at least 2 oz of water or orange juice; do not use other liquids. Stir vigorously and drink at once. Refill container with at least 4 oz of additional liquid, stir vigorously, and drink at once.
- Store bottles and pouches in refrigerator. Solution may develop a slight haze when refrigerated; allow to stand at room temperature and shake gently until haze disappears. Sirolimus may remain in syringe at room temperature or refrigerated for up to 24 hr. Discard syringe after one use.

Patient/Family Teaching
- Instruct patient to take sirolimus at the same time each day, as directed. Advise patient to avoid taking with or diluting with grapefruit juice. Do not skip or double up on missed doses. Do not discontinue medication without advice of health care professional.
- Reinforce the need for lifelong therapy to prevent transplant rejection. Review symptoms of rejection for transplanted organ and stress need to notify health care professional immediately if they occur.
- Advise patient to wear sunscreen and protective clothing due to increased risk of skin cancer.
- Caution patient to notify health care professional if signs of infection occur.
- Advise patient of the risk of taking sirolimus during pregnancy. Caution women of childbearing yr to use effective contraception prior to, during, and for 12 wk following therapy.
- Emphasize the importance of repeated lab tests during sirolimus therapy.

Evaluation/Desired Outcomes
- Prevention of transplanted kidney rejection.

sitagliptin (sit-a-glip-tin)
Januvia

Classification
Therapeutic: antidiabetics
Pharmacologic: enzyme inhibitors

Pregnancy Category B

Indications
Adjunct to diet and exercise to improve glycemic control in patients with type 2 diabetes mellitus; may be used as monotherapy or combination therapy with metformin and a thiazolidinedione and/or a sulfonylurea.

Action
Inhibits the enzyme dipeptidyl peptidase-4 (DPP-4), which slows the inactivation of incretin hormones, resulting in increased levels of active incretin hormones. These hormones are released by the intestine throughout the day, and are involved in regulation of glucose homeostasis. Increased/prolonged incretin levels, increase insulin release and decrease glucagon levels.
Therapeutic Effects: Improved control of blood glucose.

Pharmacokinetics
Absorption: 87% absorbed following oral administration.
Distribution: Unknown.
Metabolism and Excretion: 79% excreted unchanged in urine, minor metabolism.
Half-life: 12.4 hr.

TIME/ACTION PROFILE

ROUTE	ONSET	PEAK	DURATION
PO	rapid	1–4 hr	24 hr

Contraindications/Precautions
Contraindicated in: Type 1 diabetes mellitus; Diabetic ketoacidosis; hypersensitivity.
Use Cautiously in: Renal impairment (dose ↓ required for CCr <50 mL/min; History of pancreatitis; OB: Use in pregnancy only if clearly needed. Lactation: Excretion into breast milk unknown; Pedi: Safety not established; Geri: Consider age-related ↓ in renal function when determining dose.

Adverse Reactions/Side Effects
CNS: headache. **GI:** PANCREATITIS, nausea, diarrhea. **Resp:** upper respiratory tract infection, nasopharyngitis. **Misc:** hypersensitivity reactions including anaphylaxis, angioedema, and exfoliative skin conditions (Stevens-Johnson syndrome), rash, urticaria.

Interactions
Drug-Drug: May slightly ↑ serum digoxin levels; monitoring recommended.

Route/Dosage
PO (Adults): 100 mg once daily.

Renal Impairment
PO (Adults): *CCr 30– <50ml/min*—50 mg once daily; *CCr <30 mL/min*—25 mg once daily.

Availability
Tablets: 25 mg, 50 mg, 100 mg. *In combination with:* metformin (Janumet) See Appendix B.

NURSING IMPLICATIONS

Assessment
- Observe patient for signs and symptoms of hypoglycemic reactions (abdominal pain, sweating, hunger, weakness, dizziness, headache, tremor, tachycardia, anxiety).
- Monitor for signs of pancreatitis (nausea, vomiting, anorexia, persistent severe abdominal pain, sometimes radiating to the back) during therapy. If pancreatitis occurs, discontinue sitagliptin and monitor serum and urine amylase, amylase/creatinine clearance ratio, electrolytes, serum calcium, glucose, and lipase.
- *Lab Test Considerations:* Monitor hemoglobin A1C prior to and periodically during therapy.
- Monitor renal function prior to and periodically during therapy.

Potential Nursing Diagnoses
Imbalanced nutrition: more than body requirements (Indications)
Noncompliance (Patient/Family Teaching)

Implementation
- Patients stabilized on a diabetic regimen who are exposed to stress, fever, trauma, infection, or surgery may require administration of insulin.
- PO: May be administered without regard to food.

Patient/Family Teaching
- Instruct patient to take sitagliptin as directed. Take missed doses as soon as remembered, unless it is almost time for next dose; do not double doses.
- Explain to patient that sitagliptin helps control hyperglycemia but does not cure diabetes. Therapy is usually long term.

sodium bicarbonate

- Instruct patient not to share this medication with others, even if they have the same symptoms; it may harm them.
- Encourage patient to follow prescribed diet, medication, and exercise regimen to prevent hyperglycemic or hypoglycemic episodes.
- Review signs of hypoglycemia and hyperglycemia with patient. If hypoglycemia occurs, advise patient to take a glass of orange juice or 2–3 tsp of sugar, honey, or corn syrup dissolved in water, and notify health care professional.
- Instruct patient in proper testing of blood glucose and urine ketones. These tests should be monitored closely during periods of stress or illness and health care professional notified if significant changes occur.
- Instruct patient to notify health care professional prior to taking any Rx, OTC, and herbal products.
- Advise patient to notify health care professional if pregnancy is planned or suspected or if breastfeeding.
- Advise patient to stop taking sitagliptin and notify health care professional promptly if symptoms of hypersensitivity reactions (rash; hives; swelling of face, lips, tongue, and throat; difficulty in breathing or swallowing) or pancreatitis occur.

Evaluation/Desired Outcomes
- Improved hemoglobin A1C, fasting plasma glucose and 2-hr post-prandial glucose levels.

---

sodium bicarbonate
(soe-dee-um bye-kar-boe-nate)
Baking Soda, Bell-Ans, Citrocarbonate, Neut, Soda Mint

Classification
Therapeutic: antiulcer agents
Pharmacologic: alkalinizing agents

Pregnancy Category C

Indications
PO, IV: Management of metabolic acidosis. **PO, IV:** Used to alkalinize urine and promote excretion of certain drugs in overdosage situations (phenobarbital, aspirin). **PO:** Antacid. **Unlabeled Use:** Stabilization of acid-base status in cardiac arrest and treatment of life-threatening hyperkalemia.

Action
Acts as an alkalinizing agent by releasing bicarbonate ions. Following oral administration, releases bicarbonate, which is capable of neutralizing gastric acid. **Therapeutic Effects:** Alkalinization. Neutralization of gastric acid.

Pharmacokinetics
Absorption: Following oral administration, excess bicarbonate is absorbed and results in metabolic alkalosis and alkaline urine.
Distribution: Widely distributed into extracellular fluid.
Metabolism and Excretion: Sodium and bicarbonate are excreted by the kidneys.
Half-life: Unknown.

TIME/ACTION PROFILE (PO = antacid effect; IV = alkalinization)

ROUTE	ONSET	PEAK	DURATION
PO	immediate	30 min	1–3 hr
IV	immediate	rapid	unknown

Contraindications/Precautions
Contraindicated in: Metabolic or respiratory alkalosis; Hypocalcemia; Hypernatremia; Excessive chloride loss; As an antidote following ingestion of strong mineral acids; Patients on sodium-restricted diets (oral use as an antacid only); Renal failure (oral use as an antacid only); Severe abdominal pain of unknown cause, especially if associated with fever (oral use as an antacid only).
Use Cautiously in: CHF; Renal insufficiency; Concurrent corticosteroid therapy; Chronic use as an antacid (may cause metabolic alkalosis and possible sodium overload); Pedi: May ↑ risk of cerebral edema in children with diabetic ketoacidosis.

Adverse Reactions/Side Effects
CV: edema. **GI:** PO—flatulence, gastric distention. **F and E:** <u>metabolic alkalosis</u>, hypernatremia, hypocalcemia, hypokalemia, sodium and water retention. **Local:** irritation at IV site. **Neuro:** tetany, cerebral hemorrhage (with rapid injection in infants).

Interactions
Drug-Drug: Following oral administration, may ↓ absorption of **ketoconazole**. Concurrent use with **calcium-containing antacids** may lead to milk-alkali syndrome. Urinary alkalinization may result in ↓ **salicylate** or **barbiturate** blood levels; ↑ blood levels of **quinidine**, **mexiletine**,

1160 sodium bicarbonate

flecainide, or **amphetamines**; ↑ risk of crystalluria from **fluoroquinolones**; ↓ effectiveness of **methenamine**. May negate the protective effects of **enteric-coated products** (do not administer within 1–2 hr of each other).

Route/Dosage
Contains 12 mEq of sodium/g.

Alkalinization of Urine
PO (Adults): 48 mEq (4 g) initially. Then 12–24 mEq (1–2 g) q 4 hr (up to 48 mEq q 4 hr) or 1 tsp of powder q 4 hr as needed.
PO (Children): 1–10 mEq/kg (84–840 mg/kg) per day in divided doses.
IV (Adults and Children): 2–5 mEq/kg as a 4–8 hr infusion.

Antacid
PO (Adults): *Tablets/powder*—325 mg–2 g 1–4 times daily or ½ tsp q 2 hr as needed. *Effervescent powder*—3.9–10 g in water after meals; patients >60 yr should receive 1.9–3.9 g after meals.

Systemic Alkalinization/Cardiac Arrest
IV (Adults and Children and Infants): *Cardiac arrest/urgent situations*—1 mEq/kg; may repeat 0.5 mEq/kg q 10 min. *Less urgent situations*—2–5 mEq/kg as a 4–8 hr infusion.

Renal Tubular Acidosis
PO (Adults): 0.5–2 mEq/kg/day in 4–5 divided doses.
PO (Children): 2–3 mEq/kg/day in 3–4 divided doses.

Availability (generic available)
Oral powder: (20.9 mEq Na/½ tsp) in 120-, 240-, 480-, and 2400-g containers[OTC]. **Tablets:** 325 mg (3.9 mEq Na/tablet)[OTC], ✤500 mg (6.0 mEq Na/tablet)[OTC], 520 mg (6.2 mEq Na/tablet)[OTC], 650 mg (7.7 mEq Na/tablet)[OTC]. **Solution for injection:** 4.2% (0.5 mEq/mL) in 2.5-, 5-, and 10-mL prefilled syringes, 5% (0.6 mEq/mL) in 500-mL containers, 7.5% (0.9 mEq/mL) in 50-mL vials and prefilled syringes and 200-mL vials, 8.4% (1 mEq/mL) in 10- and 50-mL vials and prefilled syringes. **Neutralizing additive solution for injection:** 4% (0.48 mEq/mL) in 5-mL vials, 4.2% (0.5 mEq/mL) in 6-mL vials.

NURSING IMPLICATIONS

Assessment
- **IV:** Assess fluid balance (intake and output, daily weight, edema, lung sounds) throughout therapy. Report symptoms of fluid overload (hypertension, edema, dyspnea, rales/crackles, frothy sputum) if they occur.
- Assess patient for signs of acidosis (disorientation, headache, weakness, dyspnea, hyperventilation), alkalosis (confusion, irritability, paresthesia, tetany, altered breathing pattern), hypernatremia (edema, weight gain, hypertension, tachycardia, fever, flushed skin, mental irritability), or hypokalemia (weakness, fatigue, U wave on ECG, arrhythmias, polyuria, polydipsia) throughout therapy.
- Observe IV site closely. Avoid extravasation, as tissue irritation or cellulitis may occur. If infiltration occurs, confer with physician or other health care professional regarding warm compresses and infiltration of site with lidocaine or hyaluronidase.
- **Antacid:** Assess patient for epigastric or abdominal pain and frank or occult blood in the stool, emesis, or gastric aspirate.
- *Lab Test Considerations:* Monitor serum sodium, potassium, calcium, bicarbonate concentrations, serum osmolarity, acid-base balance, and renal function prior to and periodically throughout therapy.
- Obtain arterial blood gases (ABGs) frequently in emergency situations and during parenteral therapy.
- Monitor urine pH frequently when used for urinary alkalinization.
- Antagonizes effects of pentagastrin and histamine during gastric acid secretion test. Avoid administration during the 24 hr preceding the test.

Potential Nursing Diagnoses
Impaired gas exchange (Indications)
Excess fluid volume (Side Effects)

Implementation
- This medication may cause premature dissolution of enteric-coated tablets in the stomach.
- **PO:** Tablets must be taken with a full glass of water.
- When used in treatment of peptic ulcers, may be administered 1 and 3 hr after meals and at bedtime.

IV Administration
- **Direct IV:** Used in cardiac arrest or urgent situations. *Diluent:* Use premeasured ampules or prefilled syringes to ensure accurate dose. *Rate:* Administer by rapid bolus. Flush IV line before and after administration to prevent incompatible medications used in arrest management from precipitating.
- **Continuous Infusion:** *Diluent:* May be diluted in dextrose, saline, and dextrose/saline combinations. Premixed infusions are already

sodium chloride (IV/oral) 1161

diluted and ready to use. *Rate:* May be administered over 4–8 hr.
- **Y-Site Compatibility:** acyclovir, amifostine, amikacin, aminophylline, asparaginase, atropine, aztreonam, bivalirudin, bumetanide, cefazolin, cefepime, ceftazidime, ceftizoxime, ceftriaxone, chloramphenicol, cimetidine, cladribine, clindamycin, cyclophosphamide, cyclosporine, cytarabine, daptomycin, daunorubicin, dexamethasone sodium phosphated-exmedetomidine, digoxin, docetaxel, doxorubicin, enalaprilat, ertapenem, erythromycin, esmolol, etoposide, etoposide phosphate, famotidine, fentanyl, filgrastim, fluconazole, fludarabine, furosemide, gallium nitrate, gemcitabine, gentamicin, granisetron, heparin, hydrocortisone sodium succinate, ifosfamide, indomethacin, insulin, ketorolac, labetalol, levofloxacin, lidocaine, linezolid, lorazepam, magnesium sulfate, melphalan, mesna, meperidine, methylprednisolone sodium succinate, metoclopramide, metoprolol, metronidazole, milrinone, morphine, nafcillin, nitroglycerin, nitroprusside, paclitaxel, palonosetron, pantoprazole, pemetrexed, penicillin G potassium, phenylephrine, phytonadione, piperacillin/tazobactam, potassium chloride, procainamide, propranolol, propofol, protamine, ranitidine, remifentanil, tacrolimus, teniposide, thiotepa, ticarcillin/clavulanate, tirofiban, tobramycin, tolazoline, vasopressin, vitamin B complex with C, voriconazole.
- **Y-Site Incompatibility:** allopurinol, amiodarone, amphotericin B, amphotericin B cholesteryl sulfate complex, ampicillin, anidulafungin, calcium chloride, calcium gluconate, caspofungin, cefotaxime, cefoxitin, cefuroxime, diazepam, diphenhydramine, dobutamine, doxorubicin liposome, doxycycline, epinephrine, fenoldopam, ganciclovir, haloperidol, hydroxyzine, idarubicin, imipenem/cilastatin, inamrinone, isoproterenol, lansoprazole, leucovorin, midazolam, nalbuphine, norepinephrine, ondansetron, phenytoin, prochlorperazine, promethazine, quinupristin/dalfopristin, sargramostim, trimethoprim/sulfamethoxazole, verapamil, vincristine, vinorelbine.
- **Solution Incompatibility:** Do not add to Ringer's solution, LR, or Ionosol products, as compatibility varies with concentration.

Patient/Family Teaching
- Instruct patient to take medication as directed. Take missed doses as soon as remembered unless almost time for next dose.
- Review symptoms of electrolyte imbalance with patients on chronic therapy; instruct patient to notify health care professional if these symptoms occur.
- Advise patient not to take milk products concurrently with this medication. Renal calculi or hypercalcemia (milk-alkali syndrome) may result.
- Emphasize the importance of regular follow-up examinations to monitor serum electrolyte levels and acid-base balance and to monitor progress.
- **Antacid:** Advise patient to avoid routine use of sodium bicarbonate for indigestion. Dyspepsia that persists >2 wk should be evaluated by a health care professional.
- Advise patient on sodium-restricted diet to avoid use of baking soda as a home remedy for indigestion.
- Instruct patient to notify health care professional if indigestion is accompanied by chest pain, difficulty breathing, or diaphoresis or if stools become dark and tarry.

Evaluation/Desired Outcomes
- Increase in urinary pH.
- Clinical improvement of acidosis.
- Enhanced excretion of selected overdoses and poisonings.
- Decreased gastric discomfort.

HIGH ALERT

sodium chloride (IV/oral)
(soe-dee-um klor-ide)
Slo-Salt

Classification
Therapeutic: mineral and electrolyte replacements/supplements

Pregnancy Category C

Indications
IV: Hydration and provision of NaCl in deficiency states. Maintenance of fluid and electrolyte status in situations in which losses may be excessive (excess diuresis or severe salt restriction). 0.45% ("half-normal saline") solution is most commonly used for hydration and the treatment of hyperosmolar diabetes (hypotonic). 0.9% ("normal

---

♦ = Canadian drug name. ᴳ = Genetic implication.
*CAPITALS indicates life-threatening; underlines indicate most frequent.

1162 sodium chloride (IV/oral)

saline") solution is used for: Replacement, Treatment of metabolic alkalosis, A priming fluid for hemodialysis, To begin and end blood transfusions. Small volumes of 0.9% NaCl (preservative-free or bacteriostatic) are used to reconstitute or dilute other medications. Hypertonic solution (3%, 5%) may be required in situations in which rapid replacement of sodium is necessary: Hyponatremia, Hypochloremia, Renal failure, Heart failure. **PO:** Prevention of or management of volume depletion due to salt restriction or heat prostration when excessive sweating occurs during exposures to high temperatures. **Irrigating Solutions:** 0.9% and 0.45% may be used as irrigating solutions. **Concentrated sodium chloride:** Used as an additive to parenteral fluid therapy in very specific situations.

Action
Sodium is a major cation in extracellular fluid and helps maintain water distribution, fluid and electrolyte balance, acid-base equilibrium, and osmotic pressure. Chloride is the major anion in extracellular fluid and is involved in maintaining acid-base balance. Solutions of NaCl resemble extracellular fluid. Reduces corneal edema by an osmotic effect. **Therapeutic Effects: IV, PO:** Replacement in deficiency states and maintenance of homeostasis.

Pharmacokinetics
Absorption: Well absorbed following oral administration. Replacement solutions of NaCl are administered IV only.
Distribution: Rapidly and widely distributed.
Metabolism and Excretion: Excreted primarily by the kidneys.
Half-life: Unknown.

TIME/ACTION PROFILE (various clinical effects†)

ROUTE	ONSET	PEAK	DURATION
PO	unknown	unknown	unknown
IV	rapid (min)	end of infusion	unknown

†PO, IV = electrolyte effects

Contraindications/Precautions
Contraindicated in: IV solution: Hypertonic (3%, 5%) solutions should not be used in patients with elevated, slightly decreased, or normal serum sodium; Fluid retention or hypernatremia.
Use Cautiously in: IV: Patients prone to metabolic, acid-base, or fluid and electrolyte abnormalities, including: geriatric patients, those with nasogastric suctioning, vomiting, diarrhea, diuretic therapy, glucocorticoid therapy, fistulas, CHF, severe renal failure, severe liver diseases (additional electrolytes may be required); Pedi: NaCl preserved with benzyl alcohol should not be used in neonates. **PO:** Inadequate hydration (water and other electrolytes must be replaced).

Adverse Reactions/Side Effects
Seen primarily during PO and IV use.
CV: CHF, PULMONARY EDEMA, edema. **F and E:** hypernatremia, hypervolemia, hypokalemia. **Local:** *IV*—extravasation, irritation at IV site.

Interactions
Drug-Drug: Excessive amounts of NaCl may partially antagonize the effects of **antihypertensives**. Use with **corticosteroids** may result in excess sodium retention.

Route/Dosage
IV (Adults): *0.9% NaCl (isotonic)*—1 L (contains 150 mEq sodium/L), rate and amount determined by condition being treated. *0.45% NaCl (hypotonic)*—1–2 L (contains 75 mEq sodium/L), rate and amount determined by condition being treated. *3%, 5% NaCl (hypertonic)*—100 mL over 1 hr (3% contains 50 mEq sodium per 100 mL; 5% contains 83.3 mEq sodium per 100 mL).
PO (Adults): 1–2 g 3 times daily.
PO, IV (Children and Infants): *Maintenance sodium requirements*—3–4 mEq/kg/day (maximum: 150 mEq/day).
PO, IV (Neonates): *Maintenance sodium requirements*—1–4 mEq/kg/day.

Availability (generic available)
IV solutions: 0.45%, 0.9%, 3%, 5%. **Diluents:** 0.9%. **Concentrate for dilution:** 14.6%, 23.4%. **Tablets:** 650 mg[OTC]. *In combination with:* potassium (Slo-Salt-K), dextrose, electrolytes.

NURSING IMPLICATIONS

Assessment
- Assess fluid balance (intake and output, daily weight, edema, lung sounds) throughout therapy.
- Assess patient for symptoms of hyponatremia (headache, tachycardia, lassitude, dry mucous membranes, nausea, vomiting, muscle cramps) or hypernatremia (edema, weight gain, hypertension, tachycardia, fever, flushed skin, mental irritability) throughout therapy. Sodium is measured in relation to its concentration to fluid in the body, and symptoms may change based on patient's hydration status.
- *Lab Test Considerations:* Monitor serum sodium, potassium, bicarbonate, and chloride

concentrations and acid-base balance periodically for patients receiving prolonged therapy with sodium chloride.
- Monitor serum osmolarity in patients receiving hypertonic saline solutions.

Potential Nursing Diagnoses
Deficient fluid volume (Indications)
Excess fluid volume (Side Effects)

Implementation
- **High Alert:** Accidental administration of hypertonic sodium chloride solutions (greater than 0.9%) have resulted in serious electrolyte imbalances. Do not confuse vials of concentrated sodium chloride (23.4%) with vials of sodium chloride flush solution (0.9%).
- Dose of NaCl depends on patient's age, weight, condition, fluid and electrolyte balance, and acid-base balance.
- Do not administer bacteriostatic NaCl containing benzyl alcohol as a preservative to neonates. This should not be used to reconstitute or to dilute solutions or to flush intravascular catheters in neonates.
- Infusion of 0.45% NaCl is hypotonic, 0.9% NaCl is isotonic, and 3% and 5% NaCl are hypertonic.

IV Administration
- **Intermittent Infusion:** Administer 3% or 5% NaCl via a large vein and prevent infiltration. After the first 100 mL, sodium, chloride, and bicarbonate concentrations should be re-evaluated to determine the need for further administration. **Rate:** Rate of hypertonic NaCl solutions should not exceed 100 mL/hr or 1 mEq/kg/hr.
- **Solution Compatibility:** D5W, D10W, Ringer's and lactated Ringer's injection, dextrose/Ringer's solution combinations, dextrose/LR combinations, dextrose/saline combinations, ⅙ M sodium lactate.

Patient/Family Teaching
- Explain to patient the purpose of the infusion.
- Advise patients at risk for dehydration due to exposure to extreme temperatures when and how to take NaCL tablets. Inform patients that undigested tablets may be passed in the stool; oral electrolyte solutions are preferable.

Evaluation/Desired Outcomes
- Prevention or correction of dehydration.
- Normalization of serum sodium and chloride levels.

- Prevention of heat prostration during exposure to high temperatures.

sodium citrate and citric acid
(soe-dee-um sye-trate and sit-rik as-id)
Bicitra, Oracit, ✦PMS-Dicitrate, Shohl's Solution modified

Classification
Therapeutic: antiurolithics, mineral and electrolyte replacements/supplements
Pharmacologic: alkalinizing agents

Pregnancy Category C

Indications
Management of chronic metabolic acidosis associated with chronic renal insufficiency or renal tubular acidosis. Alkalinization of urine. Prevention of cystine and urate urinary calculi. Prevention of aspiration pneumonitis during surgical procedures. Used as a neutralizing buffer.

Action
Converted to bicarbonate in the body, resulting in increased blood pH. As bicarbonate is renally excreted, urine is also alkalinized, increasing the solubility of cystine and uric acid. Neutralizes gastric acid. **Therapeutic Effects:** Provision of bicarbonate in metabolic acidosis. Alkalinization of the urine. Prevention of cystine and urate urinary calculi. Prevention of aspiration pneumonitis.

Pharmacokinetics
Absorption: Well absorbed following oral administration.
Distribution: Rapidly and widely distributed.
Metabolism and Excretion: Rapidly oxidized to bicarbonate, which is excreted primarily by the kidneys. Small amounts (<5%) excreted unchanged by the lungs.
Half-life: Unknown.

TIME/ACTION PROFILE (effects on serum pH)

ROUTE	ONSET	PEAK	DURATION
PO	rapid (min–hr)	unknown	4–6 hr

Contraindications/Precautions
Contraindicated in: Severe renal insufficiency; Severe sodium restriction; CHF, untreated hypertension, edema, or toxemia of pregnancy.

✦ = Canadian drug name. ⚜ = Genetic implication.
*CAPITALS indicates life-threatening; underlines indicate most frequent.

Use Cautiously in: OB: Lactation: Safety not established.

Adverse Reactions/Side Effects
GI: diarrhea. **F and E:** fluid overload, hypernatremia (severe renal impairment), hypocalcemia, metabolic alkalosis (large doses only). **MS:** tetany.

Interactions
Drug-Drug: May partially antagonize the effects of **antihypertensives**. Urinary alkalinization may result in ↓ **salicylate** or **barbiturate** levels or ↑ levels of **quinidine**, **flecainide**, or **amphetamines**.

Route/Dosage
Adjust dosage according to urine pH. Contains 1 mEq sodium and 1 mEq bicarbonate/mL solution.

Alkalinizer
PO (Adults): 10–30 mL solution diluted in water 4 times daily.
PO (Children): 5–15 mL solution diluted in water 4 times daily.

Antiurolithic
PO (Adults): 10–30 mL solution diluted in water 4 times daily.

Neutralizing Buffer
PO (Adults): 15–30 mL solution diluted in 15–30 mL of water.

Availability
Oral solution: 500 mg sodium citrate/334 mg citric acid/5 mL (Bicitra, PMS-Dicitrate), 490 mg sodium citrate/640 mg citric acid/5 mL (Oracit).

NURSING IMPLICATIONS

Assessment
- Assess patient for signs of alkalosis (confusion, irritability, paresthesia, tetany, altered breathing pattern) or hypernatremia (edema, weight gain, hypertension, tachycardia, fever, flushed skin, mental irritability) throughout therapy.
- Monitor patients with renal dysfunction for fluid overload (discrepancy in intake and output, weight gain, edema, rales/crackles, and hypertension).
- *Lab Test Considerations:* Prior to and every 4 mo throughout chronic therapy, monitor hematocrit, hemoglobin, electrolytes, pH, creatinine, urinalysis, and 24-hr urine for citrate.
- Monitor urine pH if used to alkalinize urine.

Potential Nursing Diagnoses
Deficient knowledge, related to medication regimen (Patient/Family Teaching)

Implementation
- **PO:** Solution is more palatable if chilled. Administer with 30–90 mL of chilled water. Administer 30 min after meals or as bedtime snack to minimize saline laxative effect.
- When used as preanesthetic, administer 15–30 mL of sodium citrate with 15–30 mL of chilled water.

Patient/Family Teaching
- Instruct patient to take as directed. Missed doses should be taken within 2 hr. Do not double doses.
- Instruct patients receiving chronic sodium citrate on correct method of monitoring urine pH, maintenance of alkaline urine, and the need to increase fluid intake to 3000 mL/day. When treatment is discontinued, pH begins to fall toward pretreatment levels.
- Advise patients receiving long-term therapy on need to avoid salty foods.

Evaluation/Desired Outcomes
- Correction of metabolic acidosis.
- Maintenance of alkaline urine with resulting decreased stone formation.
- Buffering the pH of gastric secretions, thereby preventing aspiration pneumonitis associated with intubation and anesthesia.

---

sodium ferric gluconate complex, See IRON SUPPLEMENTS.

---

sodium polystyrene sulfonate
(soe-dee-um po-lee-stye-reen sul-fon-ate)
Kalexate, Kayexalate, ✦ K-Exit, Kionex, ✦ PMS-Sodium Polystyrene Sulfonate, SPS

Classification
Therapeutic: hypokalemic, electrolyte modifiers
Pharmacologic: cationic exchange resins

Pregnancy Category C

Indications
Mild to moderate hyperkalemia (if severe, more immediate measures such as sodium bicarbonate IV, calcium, or glucose/insulin infusion should be instituted).

sodium polystyrene sulfonate 1165

Action
Exchanges sodium ions for potassium ions in the intestine (each 1 g is exchanged for 1 mEq potassium). **Therapeutic Effects:** Reduction of serum potassium levels.

Pharmacokinetics
Absorption: Distributed throughout the intestine but is nonabsorbable.
Distribution: Not distributed.
Metabolism and Excretion: Eliminated in the feces.
Half-life: Unknown.

TIME/ACTION PROFILE (decrease in serum potassium)

ROUTE	ONSET	PEAK	DURATION
PO	2–12 hr	unknown	6–24 hr
Rectal	2–12 hr	unknown	4–6 hr

Contraindications/Precautions
Contraindicated in: Life-threatening hyperkalemia (other, more immediate measures should be instituted); Hypersensitivity to saccharin or parabens (some products); Ileus; Known alcohol intolerance (suspension only).
Use Cautiously in: Geri: Geriatric patients; CHF, hypertension, edema; Sodium restriction; Constipation.

Adverse Reactions/Side Effects
GI: <u>constipation</u>, <u>fecal impaction</u>, anorexia, gastric irritation, nausea, vomiting. **F and E:** hypocalcemia, hypokalemia, sodium retention, hypomagnesemia.

Interactions
Drug-Drug: Administration with **calcium** or **magnesium-containing antacids** may ↓ resin-exchanging ability and ↑ risk of systemic alkalosis. Hypokalemia may enhance **digoxin** toxicity.

Route/Dosage
4 level tsp = 15 g (4.1 mEq sodium/g).
PO (Adults): 15 g 1–4 times daily in water or sorbitol (up to 40 g 4 times daily).
Rect (Adults): 30–50 g as a retention enema; repeat as needed q 6 hr.
PO, Rect (Children): 1 g/kg/dose q 6 hr.

Availability (generic available)
Suspension: 15 g sodium polystyrene sulfonate with 20 g sorbitol/60 mL, 15 g sodium polystyrene sulfonate with 14.1 g sorbitol/60 mL. **Powder:** 15 g/4 level tsp.

NURSING IMPLICATIONS

Assessment
- Monitor response of symptoms of hyperkalemia (fatigue, muscle weakness, paresthesia, confusion, dyspnea, peaked T waves, depressed ST segments, prolonged QT segments, widened QRS complexes, loss of P waves, and cardiac arrhythmias). Assess for development of hypokalemia (weakness, fatigue, arrhythmias, flat or inverted T waves, prominent U waves).
- Monitor intake and output ratios and daily weight. Assess for symptoms of fluid overload (dyspnea, rales/crackles, jugular venous distention, peripheral edema). Concurrent low-sodium diet may be ordered for patients with CHF (see Appendix M).
- In patients receiving concurrent digoxin, assess for symptoms of digoxin toxicity (anorexia, nausea, vomiting, visual disturbances, arrhythmias).
- Assess abdomen and note character and frequency of stools. Concurrent sorbitol or laxatives may be ordered to prevent constipation or impaction. Some products contain sorbitol to prevent constipation. Patient should ideally have 1–2 watery stools each day during therapy. Monitor for colonic necrosis if sorbitol is added.
- *Lab Test Considerations:* Monitor serum potassium daily during therapy. Notify health care professional when potassium ↓ to 4–5 mEq/L.
- Monitor renal function and electrolytes (especially sodium, calcium, bicarbonate, and magnesium) prior to and periodically throughout therapy.

Potential Nursing Diagnoses
Constipation (Side Effects)

Implementation
- Solution is stable for 24 hr when refrigerated.
- Consult health care professional regarding discontinuation of medications that may increase serum potassium (angiotensin-converting enzyme inhibitors, potassium-sparing diuretics, potassium supplements, salt substitutes).
- **PO:** An osmotic laxative (sorbitol) is usually administered concurrently to prevent constipation.
- For oral administration, shake commercially-available suspension well before use. When using powder, add prescribed amount to 3–4 mL

✦ = Canadian drug name. ◉ = Genetic implication.
*CAPITALS indicates life-threatening; <u>underlines</u> indicate most frequent.

water/g of powder. Shake well. Syrup may be ordered to improve palatability. Resin cookie or candy recipes are available; discuss with pharmacist or dietitian.
- **Retention Enema:** Precede retention enema with cleansing enema. Administer solution via rectal tube or 28-French Foley catheter with 30-mL balloon. Insert tube at least 20 cm and tape in place.
- For retention enema, add powder to 100 mL of prescribed solution (usually sorbitol or 20% dextrose in water). Shake well to dissolve powder thoroughly; should be of liquid consistency. Position patient on left side and elevate hips on pillow if solution begins to leak. Follow administration of medication with additional 50–100 mL of diluent to ensure administration of complete dose. Encourage patient to retain enema as long as possible, at least 30–60 min.
- After retention period, irrigate colon with 1–2 L of non–sodium-containing solution. Y-connector with tubing may be attached to Foley or rectal tube; cleansing solution is administered through one port of the Y and allowed to drain by gravity through the other port.

Patient/Family Teaching
- Explain purpose and method of administration of medication to patient.
- Advise patient to avoid taking antacids or laxatives during therapy, unless approved by health care professional; may cause systemic alkalosis.
- Inform patient of need for frequent lab tests to monitor effectiveness.

Evaluation/Desired Outcomes
- Normalization of serum potassium levels.

---

sodium salicylate, See SALICYLATES.

---

solifenacin (so-li-**fen**-a-sin)
VESIcare

Classification
Therapeutic: urinary tract antispasmodics
Pharmacologic: anticholinergics

Pregnancy Category C

Indications
Overactive bladder with symptoms (urge incontinence, urgency, frequency).

Action
Acts as a muscarinic (cholinergic) receptor antagonist; antagonizes bladder smooth muscle contraction. **Therapeutic Effects:** Decreased symptoms of overactive bladder.

Pharmacokinetics
Absorption: Well absorbed (90%).
Distribution: Unknown.
Protein Binding: 98%.
Metabolism and Excretion: Extensively metabolized by the CYP3A4 enzyme system. 69% excreted in urine as metabolites, 22% in feces.
Half-life: 45–68 hr.

TIME/ACTION PROFILE

ROUTE	ONSET	PEAK	DURATION
Oral	unknown	3–8 hr	24 hr

Contraindications/Precautions
Contraindicated in: Hypersensitivity; Urinary retention; Gastric retention; Uncontrolled angle-closure glaucoma; Severe hepatic impairment; Lactation: Lactation.
Use Cautiously in: Concurrent use of CYP3A4 inhibitors (use lower dose/clinical monitoring may be necessary); Moderate hepatic impairment (lower dose recommended); Renal impairment (dose should not exceed 5 mg/day if CCr < 30 mL/min); Bladder outflow obstruction; GI obstructive disorders, severe constipation or ulcerative colitis; Myasthenia gravis; Angle-closure glaucoma; OB: Use only if maternal benefit outweighs fetal risk; Pedi: Safety not established.

Adverse Reactions/Side Effects
EENT: blurred vision. **GI:** constipation, dry mouth, dyspepsia, nausea.

Interactions
Drug-Drug: Drugs that induce or inhibit the CYP3A4 enzyme system may significantly alter levels; **ketoconazole** ↑ levels and risk of toxicity (do not exceed 5 mg/day).

Route/Dosage
PO (Adults): 5 mg once daily, may be ↑ to 10 mg once daily; *hepatic impairment/severe renal impairment, concurrent use of ketoconazole or other inhibitors of CYP3A4*—dose should not exceed 5 mg/day.

Availability
Tablets: 5 mg, 10 mg.

NURSING IMPLICATIONS

Assessment
- Monitor voiding pattern and assess symptoms of overactive bladder (urinary urgency, urinary incontinence, urinary frequency) to and periodically during therapy.

Potential Nursing Diagnoses
Impaired urinary elimination (Indications)

Implementation
- **PO:** Administer once daily without regard to food. Tablets must be swallowed whole; do not break, crush, or chew.

Patient/Family Teaching
- Instruct patient to take solifenacin as directed. Advise patient to read the *Patient Information* before starting therapy and with each prescription refill. If a dose is missed, skip dose and take next day; do not take 2 doses in same day.
- Do not share solifenacin with others; may be dangerous.
- Inform patient of potential anticholinergic side effects (constipation, urinary retention, blurred vision, heat prostration in a hot environment).
- May cause dizziness and blurred vision. Caution patient to avoid driving and other activities that require alertness until response to medication is known.
- Advise patient to consult health care professional prior to taking Rx, OTC, or herbal products with solifenacin.

Evaluation/Desired Outcomes
- Decrease in symptoms of overactive bladder (urge urinary incontinence, urgency, frequency).

---

somatropin (recombinant), See GROWTH HORMONES.

---

sotalol (soe-ta-lole)
Betapace, Betapace AF, Sorine, ♦Sotacor

Classification
Therapeutic: antiarrhythmics (class III)

Pregnancy Category B

Indications
Management of life-threatening ventricular arrhythmias. **Betapace AF:** Maintenance of normal sinus rhythm in patients with highly symptomatic atrial fibrillation/atrial flutter (AF/AFL) who are currently in sinus rhythm.

Action
Blocks stimulation of beta$_1$ (myocardial) and beta$_2$ (pulmonary, vascular, and uterine) -adrenergic receptor sites. **Therapeutic Effects:** Suppression of arrhythmias.

Pharmacokinetics
Absorption: Well absorbed following oral administration (bioavailability 90–100%); IV administration results in complete bioavailability.
Distribution: Crosses the placenta; enters breast milk.
Metabolism and Excretion: Elimination is mostly renal.
Half-life: 12 hr (↑ in renal impairment).

TIME/ACTION PROFILE (antiarrhythmic effects)

ROUTE	ONSET	PEAK	DURATION
PO	hr	2–3 days	8–12 hr

Contraindications/Precautions
Contraindicated in: Hypersensitivity; Uncompensated CHF; Pulmonary edema; Asthma; Cardiogenic shock; Congenital or acquired long QT syndromes; Sinus bradycardia, 2nd- and 3rd-degree AV block (unless a functioning pacemaker is present); CCr <40 mL/min in patients who are being treated with Betapace AF.
Use Cautiously in: Renal impairment (↑ dosing interval recommended if CCr ≤60 mL/min for patients with ventricular arrhythmias); Hepatic impairment; Hypokalemia (↑ risk of arrhythmias); Geri: ↑ sensitivity to beta blockers; Diabetes mellitus (may mask signs of hypoglycemia); Thyrotoxicosis (may mask symptoms); Patients with a history of severe allergic reactions (intensity of reactions may be increased); OB, Lactation: Pedi: Safety not established; may cause fetal/neonatal bradycardia, hypotension, hypoglycemia, or respiratory depression.

Adverse Reactions/Side Effects
CNS: fatigue, weakness, anxiety, dizziness, drowsiness, insomnia, memory loss, mental depression, mental status changes, nervousness, nightmares. **EENT:** blurred vision, dry eyes, nasal stuffiness. **Resp:** bronchospasm, wheezing. **CV:** ARRHYTHMIAS, BRADYCARDIA, CHF, PULMONARY EDEMA, orthostatic hypotension, peripheral vasoconstriction. **GI:** constipation, diarrhea, nausea. **GU:** erectile dysfunction, decreased libido. **Derm:** itching, rashes. **Endo:** hyperglycemia, hypoglycemia. **MS:** arthralgia, back pain, muscle cramps. **Neuro:** paresthesia. **Misc:** drug-induced lupus syndrome.

1168 sotalol

Interactions
Drug-Drug: Concurrent use with other **class 1A antiarrhythmics** is not recommended due to ↑ risk of arrhythmias. **General anesthesia**, **IV phenytoin**, and **verapamil** may cause additive myocardial depression. Concurrent use with other **calcium channel blockers** may ↑ the risk of adverse cardiovascular reactions. Additive bradycardia may occur with **digoxin**. Additive hypotension may occur with other **antihypertensives**, acute ingestion of **alcohol**, or **nitrates**. Concurrent use with **amphetamines**, **cocaine**, **ephedrine**, **epinephrine**, **norepinephrine**, **phenylephrine**, or **pseudoephedrine** may result in unopposed alpha-adrenergic stimulation (excessive hypertension, bradycardia). Concurrent **thyroid hormone** administration may ↓ effectiveness. May alter the effectiveness of **insulin** or **oral hypoglycemic agents** (dose adjustments may be necessary). May ↓ the effectiveness of **beta-adrenergic bronchodilators** and **theophylline**. May ↓ the beneficial beta$_1$ cardiovascular effects of **dopamine** or **dobutamine**. Discontinuation of **clonidine** in patients receiving sotalol may result in excessive rebound hypertension. Use cautiously within 14 days of **MAO inhibitors** (may result in hypertension).

Route/Dosage

Ventricular Arrhythmias
PO (Adults): 80 mg twice daily; may be gradually ↑ (usual maintenance dose is 160–320 mg/day in 2–3 divided doses; some patients may require up to 480–640 mg/day).

IV (Adults): *Oral dose of 80 mg twice daily*—75 mg twice daily; *Oral dose of 120 mg twice daily*—112.5 mg twice daily; *Oral dose of 160 mg twice daily*—150 mg twice daily.

Renal Impairment
PO (Adults): *CCr 30–59 mL/min*—initial dose of 80 mg, with subsequent doses given q 24 hr; *CCr 10–29 mL/min*—initial dose of 80 mg, with subsequent doses given q 36–48 hr.

Renal Impairment
IV (Adults): *CCr 30–59 mL/min*—Administer q 24 hr; *CCr 10–29 mL/min*—Administer q 36–48 hr.

Atrial Fibrillation/Atrial Flutter
PO (Adults): 80 mg twice daily, may be ↑ during careful monitoring to 120 mg twice daily if necessary.

IV (Adults): *Oral dose of 80 mg twice daily*—75 mg twice daily; *Oral dose of 120 mg twice daily*—112.5 mg twice daily.

Renal Impairment
PO, IV (Adults): *CCr 40–60 mL/min*—Administer q 24 hr.

Availability (generic available)
Tablets: 80 mg, 120 mg, 160 mg, 240 mg. **Cost:** *Generic*—80 mg $204.95/180, 120 mg $304.99/180, 160 mg $359.41/180, 240 mg $366.44/180. **Tablets (Betapace AF):** 80 mg, 120 mg, 160 mg. **Solution for injection:** 15 mg/mL.

NURSING IMPLICATIONS

Assessment
- Monitor ECG prior to and periodically during therapy. May cause life threatening ventricular tachycardia associated with QT interval prolongation. Do not initiate sotalol therapy if baseline QTc is longer than 450 ms. If QT interval becomes ≥500 ms, reduce dose, prolong duration of infusion, or discontinue therapy.
- Monitor blood pressure and pulse frequently during dose adjustment period and periodically throughout therapy. Assess for orthostatic hypotension when assisting patient up from supine position.
- Monitor intake and output ratios and daily weight. Assess patient routinely for evidence of fluid overload (peripheral edema, dyspnea, rales/crackles, fatigue, weight gain, jugular venous distention).
- *Lab Test Considerations:* May cause increased BUN, serum lipoprotein, potassium, triglyceride, and uric acid levels.
- May cause increased ANA titers.
- May cause increase in blood glucose levels.
- *Toxicity and Overdose:* Monitor patients receiving beta blockers for signs of overdose (bradycardia, severe dizziness or fainting, severe drowsiness, dyspnea, bluish fingernails or palms, seizures). Notify health care professional immediately if these signs occur.
- Glucagon has been used to treat bradycardia and hypotension.

Potential Nursing Diagnoses
Decreased cardiac output (Side Effects)
Noncompliance (Patient/Family Teaching)

Implementation
- Patients should be hospitalized and monitored for arrhythmias during initiation of therapy and dose increases.
- Do not substitute Betapace for Betapace AF. Make sure patients transferred from Betapace to Betapace AF have enough Betapace AF upon leaving the hospital to allow for uninterrupted

therapy until Betapace AF prescription can be filled.
- **PO:** Take apical pulse prior to administering. If <50 bpm or if arrhythmia occurs, withhold medication and notify health care professional.
- Administer on an empty stomach, 1 hr before or 2 hr after meals. Administration with food, especially milk or milk products, reduces absorption by approximately 20%.
- Avoid administering antacids containing aluminum or magnesium within 2 hr before administration of sotalol.
- **IV:** IV formulation should only be used in patients who are NPO.

IV Administration

- **Intermittent Infusion:** *Diluent:* Dilute with 100–250 mL of 0.9% NaCl, D5W, or LR. *For 75 mg dose*, dilute with 114 mL or 294 mL for 100 mL or 250 mL volume, respectively. *For 112.5 mg dose*, dilute with 111 mL or 291 mL for 100 mL or 250 mL volume, respectively. *For 150 mg dose*, dilute with 108 mL or 288 mL for 100 mL or 250 mL volume, respectively. *Rate:* Infuse over 5 hr using a volumetric infusion pump to infuse intravenous at a constant rate.

Patient/Family Teaching

- Instruct patient to take medication as directed, at the same time each day, even if feeling well; do not skip or double up on missed doses. Take missed doses as soon as possible up to 8 hr before next dose. Abrupt withdrawal may precipitate life-threatening arrhythmias, hypertension, or myocardial ischemia.
- Advise patient to make sure enough medication is available for weekends, holidays, and vacations. A written prescription may be kept in wallet in case of emergency.
- Teach patient and family how to check pulse and blood pressure. Instruct them to check pulse daily and blood pressure biweekly. Advise patient to hold dose and contact physician or other health care professional if pulse is <50 bpm or if blood pressure changes significantly.
- May cause drowsiness or dizziness. Caution patients to avoid driving or other activities that require alertness until response to the drug is known.
- Advise patients to change positions slowly to minimize orthostatic hypotension, especially during initiation of therapy or when dose is increased.
- Caution patient that this medication may increase sensitivity to cold.
- Instruct patient to consult health care professional before taking any other Rx, OTC, or herbal products, especially cold preparations, concurrently with this medication.
- Diabetic patients should closely monitor blood glucose, especially if weakness, malaise, irritability, or fatigue occurs. Medication may mask tachycardia and increased blood pressure as signs of hypoglycemia, but dizziness and sweating may still occur.
- Advise patient to notify health care professional if fainting, slow pulse, difficulty breathing, wheezing, cold hands and feet, dizziness, confusion, depression, rash, fever, sore throat, unusual bleeding, bruising, or if pain or swelling at the infusion site occurs.
- Instruct patient to inform health care professional of medication regimen prior to treatment or surgery.
- Advise patient to carry identification describing disease process and medication regimen at all times.

Evaluation/Desired Outcomes
- Control of arrhythmias without appearance of detrimental side effects.

---

spironolactone, See DIURETICS (POTASSIUM-SPARING).

---

streptokinase, See THROMBOLYTIC AGENTS.

---

streptomycin, See AMINOGLYCOSIDES.

---

strong iodine solution, See IODINE, IODIDE.

---

sucralfate (soo-**kral**-fate)
Carafate, ✤ Sulcrate

Classification
Therapeutic: antiulcer agents
Pharmacologic: GI protectants

Pregnancy Category B

✤ = Canadian drug name. 🧬 = Genetic implication.
*CAPITALS indicates life-threatening; underlines indicate most frequent.

sucralfate

Indications
Short-term management of duodenal ulcers. Maintenance (preventive) therapy of duodenal ulcers. **Unlabeled Use:** Management of gastric ulcer or gastroesophageal reflux. Prevention of gastric mucosal injury caused by high-dose aspirin or other NSAIDs in patients with rheumatoid arthritis or in high-stress situations (e.g., intensive care unit). **Suspension:** Mucositis/stomatitis/rectal or oral ulcerations from various etiologies.

Action
Aluminum salt of sulfated sucrose reacts with gastric acid to form a thick paste, which selectively adheres to the ulcer surface. **Therapeutic Effects:** Protection of ulcers, with subsequent healing.

Pharmacokinetics
Absorption: Systemic absorption is minimal (<5%).
Distribution: Unknown.
Metabolism and Excretion: >90% is eliminated in the feces.
Half-life: 6–20 hr.

TIME/ACTION PROFILE (mucosal protectant effect)

ROUTE	ONSET	PEAK	DURATION
PO	1–2 hr	unknown	6 hr

Contraindications/Precautions
Contraindicated in: Hypersensitivity.
Use Cautiously in: Renal failure (accumulation of aluminum can occur).

Adverse Reactions/Side Effects
CNS: dizziness, drowsiness. **GI:** constipation, diarrhea, dry mouth, gastric discomfort, indigestion, nausea. **Derm:** pruritus, rashes.

Interactions
Drug-Drug: May decrease the absorption of **phenytoin**, **fat-soluble vitamins**, or **tetracycline**. Concurrent **antacids**, **cimetidine**, or **ranitidine** decrease the effectiveness of sucralfate. Decreases absorption of **fluoroquinolones** (separate administration by 2 hours).

Route/Dosage

Treatment of Ulcers
PO (Adults): 1 g qid, 1 hr before meals and at bedtime; or 2 g twice daily, on waking and at bedtime.

Prevention of Ulcers
PO (Adults): 1 g twice daily, 1 hr before a meal.

Gastroesophageal Reflux
PO (Adults): 1 g qid, 1 hr before meals and at bedtime (unlabeled).
PO (Children): 40–80 mg/kg/day divided q 6 hr, 1 hr before meals and at bedtime (unlabeled).

Stomatitis
PO (Adults and Children): 5–10 mL of suspension swish and spit or swish and swallow 4 times/day.

Proctitis
Rect (Adults): 2 g of suspension given as an enema once or twice daily.

Availability (generic available)
Tablets: 1 g. Oral suspension: 500 mg/5 mL.

NURSING IMPLICATIONS

Assessment
- Assess patient routinely for abdominal pain and frank or occult blood in the stool.

Potential Nursing Diagnoses
Acute pain (Indications)
Constipation (Side Effects)
Deficient knowledge, related to medication regimen (Patient/Family Teaching)

Implementation
- Do not confuse Carafate (sucralfate) with Cafergot (ergotamine/caffeine).
- **PO:** Administer on an empty stomach, 1 hr before meals and at bedtime. Tablet may be broken or dissolved in water before ingestion. Shake suspension well before administration.
- If nasogastric administration is required, consult pharmacist; protein-binding properties of sucralfate have resulted in formation of a bezoar when administered with enteral feedings and other medications.
- If antacids are also required for pain, administer 30 min before or after sucralfate dosage.

Patient/Family Teaching
- Advise patient to continue with course of therapy for 4–8 wk, even if feeling better, to ensure ulcer healing. If a dose is missed, take as soon as remembered unless almost time for next dose; do not double doses.
- Advise patient that increase in fluid intake, dietary bulk, and exercise may prevent drug-induced constipation.
- Emphasize the importance of routine examinations to monitor progress.

Evaluation/Desired Outcomes
- Decrease in abdominal pain.
- Prevention and healing of duodenal ulcers, seen by x-ray examination and endoscopy.

sulconazole, See **ANTIFUNGALS (TOPICAL).**

sulfasalazine
(sul-fa-**sal**-a-zeen)
Azulfidine, Azulfidine EN-tabs,
✤ PMS-Sulfasalazine, ✤ Salazopyrin,
✤ S.A.S

Classification
Therapeutic: antirheumatics (DMARD), gastrointestinal anti-inflammatories

Pregnancy Category B

Indications
Inflammatory bowel diseases including: Ulcerative colitis, Proctitis, Proctosigmoiditis. Rheumatoid arthritis unresponsive or intolerant to salicylates and/or NSAIDs.

Action
Locally acting anti-inflammatory action in the colon, where activity is probably a result of inhibition of prostaglandin synthesis. **Therapeutic Effects:** Reduction in the symptoms of inflammatory bowel disease.

Pharmacokinetics
Absorption: 10–15% absorbed after oral administration.
Distribution: Widely distributed; crosses the placenta and enters breast milk.
Protein Binding: 99%.
Metabolism and Excretion: Split by intestinal bacteria into sulfapyridine and 5-aminosalicylic acid. Some absorbed sulfasalazine is excreted by bile back into intestines; 15% excreted unchanged by the kidneys. Sulfapyridine also excreted mostly by the kidneys.
Half-life: 6 hr.

TIME/ACTION PROFILE (blood levels)

ROUTE	ONSET	PEAK	DURATION
PO	1 hr	1.5–6 hr	6–12 hr

Contraindications/Precautions
Contraindicated in: Hypersensitivity reactions to sulfonamides, salicylates, or sulfasalazine; Cross-sensitivity with furosemide, sulfonylurea hypoglycemic agents, or carbonic anhydrase inhibitors may exist; Glucose-6–phosphate dehydrogenase (G6PD) deficiency; Hypersensitivity to bisulfites (mesalamine enema only); Urinary tract or intestinal obstruction; Porphyria; Pedi: Children <2 yr (safety not established).
Use Cautiously in: Severe hepatic or renal impairment; History of porphyria; OB: Has been used safely; Lactation: Safety not established; may compete with bilirubin for binding sites on plasma proteins in the newborn and cause kernicterus.

Adverse Reactions/Side Effects
CNS: headache. **Resp:** pneumonitis. **GI:** anorexia, diarrhea, nausea, vomiting, drug-induced hepatitis. **GU:** crystalluria, oligospermia, orange-yellow discoloration of urine. **Derm:** rashes, exfoliative dermatitis, photosensitivity, yellow discoloration. **Hemat:** AGRANULOCYTOSIS, APLASTIC ANEMIA, blood dyscrasias, eosinophilia, megaloblastic anemia, thrombocytopenia. **Neuro:** peripheral neuropathy. **Misc:** *hypersensitivity reactions including*—SERUM SICKNESS and STEVENS-JOHNSON SYNDROME, fever.

Interactions
Drug-Drug: May ↑ action/risk of toxicity from **oral hypoglycemic agents**, **phenytoin**, **methotrexate**, **zidovudine**, or **warfarin**. ↑ risk of drug-induced hepatitis with other **hepatotoxic agents**. ↑ risk of crystalluria with **methenamine**. May ↓ metabolism and increase effects/toxicity of **mercaptopurine** or **thioguanine**.
Drug-Food: May ↓ **iron** and **folic acid** absorption.

Route/Dosage
Inflammatory bowel disease
PO (Adults): *Inflammatory bowel disease*—1 g q 6–8 hr (may start with 500 mg q 6–12 hr), followed by maintenance dose of 500 mg q 6 hr.
PO (Children >2 yr): *Initial*—6.7–10 mg/kg q 4 hr *or* 10–15 mg/kg q 6 hr *or* 13.3–20 mg/kg q 8 hr. *Maintenance*—7.5 mg/kg q 6 hr (not to exceed 2 g/day).

Rheumatoid arthritis
PO (Adults): 500 mg–1 g/day (as delayed-release tablets) for 1 wk, then ↑ by 500 mg/day q wk up to 2 g/day in 2 divided doses; if no benefit seen after 12 wk, increase to 3 g/day in 2 divided doses.
PO (Children ≥6 yr): 30–50 mg/kg/day in 2 divided doses (as delayed-release tablets); initiate therapy at ¼–⅓ of planned maintenance dose and increase q 7 days until maintenance dose is reached (not to exceed 2 g/day).

Availability (generic available)
Tablets: 500 mg. **Delayed-release (enteric-coated) tablets (Azulfidine EN-tabs):** 500 mg. **Oral suspension:** ✦ 250 mg/5 mL. **Rectal suspension:** ✦ 3 g.

NURSING IMPLICATIONS
Assessment
- Assess patient for allergy to sulfonamides and salicylates. Therapy should be discontinued if rash or fever occurs.
- Monitor intake and output ratios. Fluid intake should be sufficient to maintain a urine output of at least 1200–1500 mL daily to prevent crystalluria and stone formation.
- **Inflammatory Bowel Disease:** Assess abdominal pain and frequency, quantity, and consistency of stools at the beginning of and during therapy.
- **Rheumatoid Arthritis:** Assess range of motion and degree of swelling and pain in affected joints before and periodically during therapy.
- *Lab Test Considerations:* Monitor urinalysis, BUN, and serum creatinine before and periodically during therapy. May cause crystalluria and urinary cell calculi formation.
- *Lab Test Considerations:* Monitor CBC before and every 3–6 mo during prolonged therapy. Discontinue sulfasalazine if blood dyscrasias occur.

Potential Nursing Diagnoses
Acute pain (Indications)
Diarrhea (Indications)

Implementation
- Do not confuse sulfasalazine with sulfisoxazole.
- Varying dosing regimens of sulfasalazine may be used to minimize GI side effects.
- **PO:** Administer after meals or with food to minimize GI irritation, with a full glass of water. Do not crush or chew enteric-coated tablets. Shake oral suspension well before administration. Use a calibrated measuring device to measure liquid preparations.
- **Rect:** Patient should empty bowel before administration of rectal dose forms.
- Administer 60-mL retention enema once daily at bedtime. Solution should be retained for approximately 8 hr. Before administration of *rectal suspension*, shake bottle well and remove the protective cap. Have patient lie on left side with the lower leg extended and the upper leg flexed for support or place the patient in knee-chest position. Gently insert the applicator tip into the rectum, pointing toward the umbilicus. Squeeze the bottle steadily to discharge most of the preparation.

Patient/Family Teaching
- Instruct patient on the correct method of administration. Advise patient to take medication as directed, even if feeling better. Take missed doses as soon as remembered unless almost time for next dose.
- May cause dizziness. Caution patient to avoid driving or other activities that require alertness until response to medication is known.
- Advise patient to notify health care professional if skin rash, sore throat, fever, mouth sores, unusual bleeding or bruising, wheezing, fever, or hives occur.
- Caution patient to use sunscreen and protective clothing to prevent photosensitivity reactions.
- Inform patient that this medication may cause orange-yellow discoloration of urine and skin, which is not significant. May permanently stain contact lenses yellow.
- Instruct patient to notify health care professional if symptoms worsen or do not improve. If symptoms of acute intolerance (cramping, acute abdominal pain, bloody diarrhea, fever, headache, rash) occur, discontinue therapy and notify health care professional immediately.
- Inform patient that proctoscopy and sigmoidoscopy may be required periodically during treatment to determine response.
- Instruct patient to notify health care professional if symptoms do not improve after 1–2 mo of therapy.
- **Rect:** Instruct patient to use *rectal suspension* at bedtime and retain suspension all night for best results.

Evaluation/Desired Outcomes
- Decrease in diarrhea and abdominal pain.
- Return to normal bowel pattern in patients with inflammatory bowel disease. Effects may be seen within 3–21 days. The usual course of therapy is 3–6 wk.
- Maintenance of remission in patients with inflammatory bowel disease.
- Decrease in pain and inflammation, and increase in mobility in patients with rheumatoid arthritis.

HIGH ALERT

SULFONYLUREAS

glimepiride (glye-**me**-pye-ride)
Amaryl, ✦Apo-Glimepiride,
✦Co-Glimepiride

SULFONYLUREAS 1173

glipiZIDE (glip-i-zide)
Glucotrol, Glucotrol XL

glyBURIDE (glye-byoo-ride)
✦Apo-Glyburide, DiaBeta,
✦Dom-Glyburide, ✦Euglucon,
✦Gen-Glybe, Glynase PresTab

Classification
Therapeutic: antidiabetics
Pharmacologic: sulfonylureas

Pregnancy Category B (glyburide [Glynase PresTab]), **C** (glimepiride, glipizide, and glyburide [Diabeta])

Indications
Control of blood glucose in type 2 diabetes mellitus when diet therapy fails. Require some pancreatic function.

Action
Lower blood glucose by stimulating the release of insulin from the pancreas and increasing the sensitivity to insulin at receptor sites. May also decrease hepatic glucose production. **Therapeutic Effects:** Lowering of blood glucose in diabetic patients.

Pharmacokinetics
Absorption: All agents are well absorbed after oral administration.
Distribution: *Glyburide*—reaches high concentrations in bile and crosses the placenta.
Protein Binding: *Glimepiride*—99.5%, *glipizide*—99%, *glyburide*—99%.
Metabolism and Excretion: All agents are mostly metabolized by the liver. *Glimepiride*—converted to a metabolite with some hypoglycemic activity.
Half-life: *Glimepiride*—5–9.2; *glipizide*—2.1–2.6 hr; *glyburide*—10 hr.

TIME/ACTION PROFILE (hypoglycemic activity)

ROUTE	ONSET	PEAK	DURATION
Glimepiride	unknown	2–3 hr	24 hr
Glipizide	15–30 min	1–2 hr	up to 24 hr
Glyburide	45–60 min	1.5–3 hr	24 hr

Contraindications/Precautions
Contraindicated in: Hypersensitivity; Hypersensitivity with sulfonamides (cross-sensitivity may occur); Type 1 diabetes; Diabetic coma or ketoacidosis; Concurrent use of bosentan (glyburide only).

Use Cautiously in: Geri: ↑ sensitivity; dosage reduction may be required; Glucose 6-phosphate dehydrogenase deficiency (↑ risk of hemolytic anemia); Renal or hepatic dysfunction (↑ risk of hypoglycemia); Infection, trauma, or surgery (may alter requirements for control of blood glucose); Impaired pituitary, or adrenal function; Prolonged nausea or vomiting; Debilitated or malnourished patients (↑ risk of hypoglycemia); OB, Lactation: Safety not established; insulin recommended during pregnancy; Pedi: Safety and effectiveness not established.

Adverse Reactions/Side Effects
CNS: dizziness, drowsiness, headache, weakness. **GI:** constipation, cramps, diarrhea, drug-induced hepatitis, heartburn, ↑ appetite, nausea, vomiting. **Derm:** photosensitivity, rashes. **Endo:** hypoglycemia. **F and E:** hyponatremia. **Hemat:** APLASTIC ANEMIA, agranulocytosis, hemolytic anemia, leukopenia, pancytopenia, thrombocytopenia.

Interactions
Drug-Drug: ↑ risk of elevated liver enzymes when **bosentan** used with glyburide (avoid concurrent use). Effectiveness may be ↓ by concurrent use of **diuretics**, **corticosteroids**, **phenothiazines**, **oral contraceptives**, **estrogens**, **thyroid preparations**, **phenytoin**, **niacin**, **sympathomimetics**, and **isoniazid**. Alcohol, **androgens (testosterone)**, **chloramphenicol**, **clarithromycin**, **fluoroquinolones**, **MAO inhibitors**, **NSAIDs**, **salicylates**, **sulfonamides**, and **warfarin** may ↑ risk of hypoglycemia. Concurrent use with **warfarin** may alter the response to both agents (↑ effects of both initially, then ↓ activity); close monitoring recommended during any changes in dosage. **Beta blockers** may mask the signs and symptoms of hypoglycemia. May ↑ **cyclosporine** levels.

Route/Dosage

Glimepiride
PO (Adults): 1–2 mg once daily initially; may ↑ q 1–2 wk up to 8 mg/day (usual range 1–4 mg/day).
PO (Geriatric Patients): 1 mg/day initially.

Glipizide
PO (Adults): 5 mg/day initially, may be ↑ by 2.5–5 mg/day at weekly intervals as needed (maximum dose = 40 mg/day immediate-release), 20 mg/day (XL); XL dosage form is given once daily. Doses >15 mg/day should be given as

✦ = Canadian drug name. ☒ = Genetic implication.
*CAPITALS indicates life-threatening; underlines indicate most frequent.

2 divided doses of immediate-release tablets (not XL).
PO (Geriatric Patients): 2.5 mg/day initially.

Glyburide

The nonmicronized formulation (Diabeta) cannot be used interchangeably with the micronized formulation (Glynase PresTab)
PO (Adults): *DiaBeta(nonmicronized)*—2.5–5 mg once daily initially; may be ↑ by 2.5–5 mg/day at weekly intervals (range 1.25–20 mg/day). *Glynase PresTab (micronized)*—1.5–3 mg/day initially; may be ↑ by 1.5 mg/day at weekly intervals (range 0.75–12 mg/day; doses >6 mg/day should be given as divided doses).
PO (Geriatric Patients): *DiaBeta(nonmicronized)*—1.25 mg/day initially; may be ↑ by 2.5 mg/day at weekly intervals. *Glynase PresTab (micronized)*—0.75 mg/day; may be ↑ by 1.5 mg/day at weekly intervals.

Availability

Glimepiride (generic available)
Tablets: 1 mg, 2 mg, 4 mg. *In combination with:* pioglitazone (Duetact); rosiglitazone (Avandaryl); see Appendix B.

Glipizide (generic available)
Tablets: 5 mg, 10 mg. **Cost:** *Generic*—5 mg $16.65/100, 10 mg $12.22/100. **Extended-release tablets:** 2.5 mg, 5 mg, 10 mg. **Cost:** *Generic*—2.5 mg $32.97/90, 5 mg $32.97/90, 10 mg $59.97/90. *In combination with:* Metformin (Metaglip); see Appendix B.

Glyburide (generic available)
Tablets: 1.25 mg, 2.5 mg, 5 mg. **Micronized tablets:** 1.5 mg, 3 mg, 6 mg. *In combination with:* metformin (Glucovance); see Appendix B.

NURSING IMPLICATIONS

Assessment

- Observe for signs and symptoms of hypoglycemic reactions (sweating, hunger, weakness, dizziness, tremor, tachycardia, anxiety).
- Assess patient for allergy to sulfonamides.
- Patients on concurrent beta-blocker therapy may have very subtle signs of hypoglycemia.
- *Lab Test Considerations:* Monitor serum glucose and glycosylated hemoglobin periodically during therapy to evaluate effectiveness of treatment.
- Monitor CBC periodically during therapy. Report ↓ in blood counts promptly.
- May cause an ↑ in AST, LDH, BUN, and serum creatinine.

- *Toxicity and Overdose:* Overdose is manifested by symptoms of hypoglycemia. Mild hypoglycemia may be treated with administration of oral glucose. Severe hypoglycemia should be treated with IV D50W followed by continuous IV infusion of more dilute dextrose solution at a rate sufficient to keep serum glucose at approximately 100 mg/dL.

Potential Nursing Diagnoses
Imbalanced nutrition: more than body requirements (Indications)
Noncompliance (Patient/Family Teaching)

Implementation

- *High Alert:* Accidental administration of oral hypoglycemic agents to non-diabetic adults and children has resulted in serious harm or death. Before administering, confirm that patient has type 2 diabetes.
- *High Alert:* Several oral hypoglycemic agents are subject to sound-alike or look-alike confusion: Do not confuse glipizide with glyburide. Do not confuse Glucotrol with Glucotrol XL. Do not confuse micronase (glyburide) with Micro-K (potassium).
- Patients stabilized on a diabetic regimen who are exposed to stress, fever, trauma, infection, or surgery may require administration of insulin.
- To convert from other oral hypoglycemic agents, gradual conversion is not required. For insulin dosage of less than 20 units/day, change to oral hypoglycemic agents can be made without gradual dose adjustment. Patients taking 20 or more units/day should convert gradually by receiving oral agent and a 25–30% reduction in insulin dose every day or every 2nd day with gradual insulin dose reduction as tolerated. Monitor serum or urine glucose and ketones at least 3 times/day during conversion.
- **PO:** May be administered once in the morning with breakfast or divided into 2 doses.
- Administer *glipizide* 30 min before a meal.
- Do not administer *nonmicronized glyburide* with a meal high in fat. *Micronized glyburide* cannot be substituted for *nonmicronized glyburide*. These preparations are not equivalent.

Patient/Family Teaching

- Instruct patient to take medication at same time each day. Take missed doses as soon as remembered unless almost time for next dose. Do not take if unable to eat.
- Explain to patient that this medication controls hyperglycemia but does not cure diabetes. Therapy is long term.

- Review signs of hypoglycemia and hyperglycemia with patient. If hypoglycemia occurs, advise patient to take a glass of orange juice or 2–3 tsp of sugar, honey, or corn syrup dissolved in water or an appropriate number of glucose tablets and notify health care professional.
- Encourage patient to follow prescribed diet, medication, and exercise regimen to prevent hypoglycemic or hyperglycemic episodes.
- Instruct patient in proper testing of serum glucose and ketones. These tests should be closely monitored during periods of stress or illness and health care professional notified if significant changes occur.
- Concurrent use of alcohol may cause a disulfiram-like reaction (abdominal cramps, nausea, flushing, headaches, and hypoglycemia).
- May occasionally cause dizziness or drowsiness. Caution patient to avoid driving or other activities requiring alertness until response to medication is known.
- Caution patient to avoid other medications, especially alcohol, while on this therapy without consulting health care professional.
- Insulin is the recommended method of controlling blood glucose during pregnancy. Counsel female patients to use a form of contraception other than oral contraceptives and to notify health care professional promptly if pregnancy is planned or suspected.
- Caution patient to use sunscreen and protective clothing to prevent photosensitivity reactions.
- Advise patient to inform health care professional of medication regimen before treatment or surgery.
- Advise patient to carry a form of sugar (sugar packets, candy) and identification describing disease process and medication regimen at all times.
- Advise patient to notify health care professional promptly if unusual weight gain, swelling of ankles, drowsiness, shortness of breath, muscle cramps, weakness, sore throat, rash, or unusual bleeding or bruising occurs.
- Emphasize the importance of routine follow-up exams.

Evaluation/Desired Outcomes
- Control of blood glucose levels without the appearance of hypoglycemic or hyperglycemic episodes.

sulindac (soo-lin-dak)
✦ Apo-Sulin, Clinoril, ✦ Novo-Sundac

Classification
Therapeutic: antirheumatics, nonsteroidal anti-inflammatory agents

Pregnancy Category C

Indications
Management of inflammatory disorders, including: Rheumatoid arthritis, Osteoarthritis, Acute gouty arthritis, Bursitis.

Action
Inhibits prostaglandin synthesis. **Therapeutic Effects:** Suppression of pain and inflammation.

Pharmacokinetics
Absorption: Well absorbed from the GI tract after oral administration.
Distribution: Unknown. Enters breast milk in small amounts.
Metabolism and Excretion: Converted by the liver to active drug. Minimal amounts excreted unchanged by the kidneys.
Half-life: 7.8 hr (16.4 hr for active metabolite).

TIME/ACTION PROFILE

ROUTE	ONSET	PEAK	DURATION
PO (analgesic)	1–2 days	unknown	12 hr
PO (anti-inflammatory)	few days–1 wk	2 wk or more	unknown

Contraindications/Precautions
Contraindicated in: Hypersensitivity; Cross-sensitivity may occur with other NSAIDs, including aspirin; Active GI bleeding or ulcer disease; Peri-operative pain from coronary artery bypass graft (CABG) surgery; OB: May cause premature closure of ductus arteriosus in third trimester.
Use Cautiously in: Cardiovascular disease or risk factors for cardiovascular disease (may ↑ risk of serious cardiovascular thrombotic events, myocardial infarction, and stroke, especially with prolonged use); Severe renal, or hepatic disease (dosage modification recommended); History of ulcer disease; OB: Use in first and second trimester only if maternal benefit exceeds potential risks to fetus; Lactation, Pedi: Safety not established; Geri: May ↑ risk of GI bleeding.

✦ = Canadian drug name. ❚ = Genetic implication.
*CAPITALS indicates life-threatening; underlines indicate most frequent.

Adverse Reactions/Side Effects
CNS: dizziness, headache, drowsiness. **EENT:** blurred vision, tinnitus. **CV:** edema. **GI:** GI BLEEDING, DRUG-INDUCED HEPATITIS, constipation, diarrhea, discomfort, dyspepsia, nausea, vomiting, anorexia, flatulence, pancreatitis. **GU:** renal failure. **Derm:** EXFOLIATIVE DERMATITIS, STEVENS-JOHNSON SYNDROME, TOXIC EPIDERMAL NECROLYSIS, rashes, photosensitivity. **Hemat:** blood dyscrasias, prolonged bleeding time. **Misc:** allergic reactions including ANAPHYLAXIS and HYPERSENSITIVITY SYNDROME.

Interactions
Drug-Drug: Concurrent use of **aspirin** may ↓ effectiveness. ↑ risk of bleeding with **anticoagulants**, **thrombolytic agents**, **tirofiban**, **eptifibatide**, **clopidogrel**, **ticlopidine**, **cefoperazone**, **cefotetan**, or **valproic acid**. ↑ adverse GI side effects with **aspirin**, **corticosteroids**, and other **NSAIDs**. May ↓ response to **antihypertensives** or **diuretics**. May ↑ levels and risk of toxicity from **lithium**. May ↑ risk of hematologic toxicity from **antineoplastics** or **radiation therapy**. ↑ risk of adverse renal effects with **gold compounds**, **cyclosporine**, or chronic use of **acetaminophen**. **Antacids** ↓ levels and decrease effectiveness of sulindac. ↑ risk of photosensitivity reactions with other **photosensitizing medications**. ↑ risk of hypoglycemia with **insulins** or **oral hypoglycemic agents**. Should not be used concurrently with **dimethyl sulfoxide** because of ↑ risk of peripheral neuropathy and ↓ levels of sulindac and its metabolite.

Route/Dosage
PO (Adults): 150–200 mg twice daily (not to exceed 400 mg/day).

Availability (generic available)
Tablets: 150 mg, 200 mg.

NURSING IMPLICATIONS

Assessment
- Patients who have asthma, aspirin-induced allergy, and nasal polyps are at increased risk for developing hypersensitivity reactions. Monitor for rhinitis, asthma, and urticaria.
- Assess pain and range of movement before and after 1–2 wk of therapy.
- ***Lab Test Considerations:*** Evaluate BUN, serum creatinine, CBC, and liver function periodically in patients receiving prolonged therapy.
- Serum potassium, glucose, alkaline phosphatase, AST, and ALT may show ↑ levels.
- Bleeding time may be prolonged for 1 day after discontinuation of therapy.

Potential Nursing Diagnoses
Acute pain (Indications)
Impaired physical mobility (Indications)

Implementation
- Do not confuse Clinoril (sulindac) with Clozaril (clozapine).
- Administration in higher than recommended doses does not provide increased effectiveness but may cause increased side effects. Use lowest effective dose for shortest period of time.
- **PO:** May be administered with food, milk, or antacids to decrease GI irritation. Food slows but does not reduce the extent of absorption. Tablets may be crushed and mixed with fluids or food.

Patient/Family Teaching
- Advise patient to take this medication with a full glass of water and to remain in an upright position for 15–30 min after administration.
- Instruct patient to take medication as directed. Take missed doses as soon as remembered but not if almost time for the next dose. Do not double doses.
- May cause dizziness. Advise patient to avoid driving or other activities requiring alertness until response to the medication is known.
- Caution patient to avoid the concurrent use of alcohol, aspirin, NSAIDs, acetaminophen, or other OTC medications without consulting health care professional.
- Advise patient to inform health care professional of medication regimen before treatment or surgery.
- Advise patient to inform health care professional if pregnancy is planned or suspected.
- Advise patient to use sunscreen and protective clothing to prevent photosensitivity reactions.
- Advise patient to consult health care professional if rash, itching, visual disturbances, tinnitus, weight gain, edema, black stools, persistent headache, or influenza-like syndrome (chills, fever, muscle aches, pain) occurs.

Evaluation/Desired Outcomes
- Decreased pain and improved joint mobility. Partial arthritic relief may be seen within 7 days, but maximum effectiveness may require 2–3 wk of continuous therapy. Patients who do not respond to one NSAID may respond to another.

sumatriptan (soo-ma-**trip**-tan)
Imitrex, Imitrex STATdose, Sumavel DosePro

Classification
Therapeutic: vascular headache suppressants
Pharmacologic: 5-HT$_1$ agonists

Pregnancy Category C

Indications
Acute treatment of migraine attacks. **Subcut:** Acute treatment of cluster headache episodes.

Action
Acts as a selective agonist of 5-HT$_1$ at specific vascular serotonin receptor sites, causing vasoconstriction in large intracranial arteries. **Therapeutic Effects:** Relief of acute attacks of migraine.

Pharmacokinetics
Absorption: Well absorbed (97%) after subcut administration. Absorption after oral administration is incomplete and significant amounts undergo substantial hepatic metabolism, resulting in poor bioavailability (14%). Well absorbed after intranasal administration.
Distribution: Does not cross the blood-brain barrier. Remainder of distribution not known.
Metabolism and Excretion: Mostly metabolized (80%) by the liver.
Half-life: 2 hr.

TIME/ACTION PROFILE (relief of migraine)

ROUTE	ONSET	PEAK	DURATION
PO	within 30 min	2–4 hr	up to 24 hr
Subcut	30 min	up to 2 hr	up to 24 hr
Nasal	within 60 min	2 hr	unknown

Contraindications/Precautions
Contraindicated in: Hypersensitivity; Patients with ischemic heart disease or signs and symptoms of ischemic heart disease, Prinzmetal angina, or uncontrolled hypertension; Stroke or transient ischemic attack; Peripheral vascular disease (including, but not limited to, ischemic bowel disease); Concurrent MAO inhibitor therapy; Geri: Excessive risk of cardiovascular complications.
Use Cautiously in: Patients with childbearing potential; OB, Lactation: Pedi: Safety not established.
Exercise Extreme Caution in: Cardiovascular risk factors (hypertension, hypercholesterolemia, smoking, obesity, diabetes, family history, menopausal women or men >40 yr); use only if cardiovascular status has been evaluated and determined to be safe and 1st dose is administered under supervision.

Adverse Reactions/Side Effects
All adverse reactions are less common after oral administration.
CNS: <u>dizziness</u>, <u>vertigo</u>, anxiety, drowsiness, fatigue, feeling of heaviness, feeling of tightness, headache, malaise, strange feeling, tight feeling in head, weakness. **EENT:** alterations in vision, nasal sinus discomfort, throat discomfort. **CV:** MI, angina, chest pressure, chest tightness, coronary vasospasm, ECG changes, transient hypertension. **GI:** abdominal discomfort, dysphagia. **Derm:** <u>tingling</u>, <u>warm sensation</u>, burning sensation, cool sensation, flushing. **Local:** <u>injection site reaction</u>. **MS:** jaw discomfort, muscle cramps, myalgia, neck pain, neck stiffness. **Neuro:** numbness.

Interactions
Drug-Drug: The risk of vasospastic reactions may be ↑ by concurrent use of **ergotamine** or **dihydroergotamine** (avoid within 24 hr of each other). Concurrent use with **lithium**, **MAO inhibitors** (do not use within 2 wk of discontinuing MAO inhibitor), or **SSRI antidepressants** (may cause weakness, hyperreflexia, and incoordination). ↑ serotonin levels and serotonin syndrome may occur when used concurrently with **SSRI and SNRI antidepressants**.
Drug-Natural Products: ↑ risk of serotinergic side effects including serotonin syndrome with **St. John's wort** and **SAMe**.

Route/Dosage
PO (Adults): 25 mg initially; if response is inadequate at 2 hr, up to 100 mg may be given (initial doses of 25–50 mg may be more effective than 25 mg). If headache recurs, doses may be repeated q 2 hr (not to exceed 300 mg/day). If PO therapy is to follow subcut injection, additional PO sumatriptan may be taken q 2 hr (not to exceed 200 mg/day).
Subcut (Adults): 6 mg; may repeat after 1 hr (not to exceed 12 mg in 24 hr).
Intranasal (Adults): Single dose of 5, 10, or 20 mg in one nostril; may be repeated in 2 hr, not to exceed 40 mg/24 hr or treatment of >5 episodes/mo.

Hepatic Impairment
PO (Adults): 25 mg initially; if response is inadequate at 2 hr, up to 50 mg may be given (initial

doses of 25–50 mg may be more effective than 25 mg). If headache recurs, doses may be repeated q 2 hr (not to exceed 300 mg/day). If PO therapy is to follow subcut injection, additional PO sumatriptan may be taken q 2 hr (not to exceed 200 mg/day); no single oral dose should exceed 50 mg.

Availability (generic available)
Tablets: 25 mg, 50 mg, 100 mg. **Cost:** 25 mg $202.97/9, 50 mg $188.98/9, 100 mg $188.98/9. **Injection:** 4 mg/0.5-mL prefilled syringes (for use in STAT dose system), 6 mg/0.5-mL prefilled syringes (for use in STAT dose system), vials, or needle-free delivery system. **Cost:** 6 mg $117.15/2 prefilled syringes. **Nasal spray:** 5 mg/nasal spray device (delivers 5 mg/spray) (box of 6), 20 mg/nasal spray device (delivers 20 mg/spray) (box of 6). **Cost:** 5 mg $188.73/box, 20 mg $191.55/box. *In combination with:* naproxen (Treximet); see Appendix B.

NURSING IMPLICATIONS
Assessment
- Assess pain location, intensity, duration, and associated symptoms (photophobia, phonophobia, nausea, vomiting) during migraine attack.
- Give initial subcut dose under observation to patients with potential for coronary artery disease including postmenopausal women, men >40 yr, patients with risk factors for coronary artery disease such as hypertension, hypercholesterolemia, obesity, diabetes, smoking, or family history. Monitor blood pressure before and for 1 hr after initial injection. If angina occurs, monitor ECG for ischemic changes.
- Monitor for serotonin syndrome in patients taking SSRIs or SNRIs concurrently with sumatriptan.

Potential Nursing Diagnoses
Acute pain (Indications)

Implementation
- Do not confuse sumatriptan with zolmitriptan.
- **PO:** Tablets should be swallowed whole; do not crush, break, or chew. Tablets are film-coated to prevent contact with tablet contents, which have an unpleasant taste and may cause nausea and vomiting.
- **Subcut:** Administer as a single injection just below the skin. Solution is clear and colorless or pale yellow; do not use dark-colored or cloudy or if beyond expiration date.
- *Sumavel DosePro*: The snap-off tip should sit firmly on the end of the clear medication chamber; do not use if tip tilted or broken off upon removal from packaging. Administer only in abdomen or thigh.
- **Intranasal:** 10-mg dose may be administered as 2 sprays of 5 mg in one nostril or 1 spray in each nostril.

Patient/Family Teaching
- Inform patient that sumatriptan should be used only *during* a migraine attack. It is meant to be used for relief of migraine attacks but not to prevent or reduce the number of attacks.
- Instruct patient to administer sumatriptan as soon as symptoms of a migraine attack appear, but it may be administered at any time during an attack. If migraine symptoms return, a second injection may be used. Allow at least 1 hr between doses, and do not use more than two injections in any 24-hr period. Additional sumatriptan doses are not likely to be effective, and alternative medications may be used. If no relief from 1st dose, unlikely 2nd dose will provide relief. Advise patient to read *Patient Information* prior to using and with each Rx refill; new information may be available.
- Advise patient that lying down in a darkened room after sumatriptan administration may further help relieve headache.
- Caution patient not to use sumatriptan if pregnant, suspects pregnancy, or plans to become pregnant. Adequate contraception should be used during therapy.
- Advise patient to notify health care professional before next dose of sumatriptan if pain or tightness in chest occurs during use. If pain is severe or does not subside, notify health care professional immediately. If wheezing; heart throbbing; swelling of eyelids, face, or lips; skin rash; skin lumps; or hives occur, notify health care professional immediately, and do not take more sumatriptan without approval of health care professional. If usual dose fails to relieve three consecutive headaches, or if frequency and/or severity increases, notify health care professional. If feelings of tingling, heat, flushing, heaviness, pressure, drowsiness, dizziness, tiredness, or sickness develop, discuss with health care professional at next visit.
- Sumatriptan may cause dizziness or drowsiness. Caution patient to avoid driving or other activities requiring alertness until response to medication is known.
- Advise patient to avoid alcohol, which aggravates headaches, during sumatriptan use.
- Advise patient to consult health care professional before taking other Rx, OTC, or herbal

products concurrently with sumatriptan. Patients concurrently taking SSRI or SNRI antidepressants should notify health care professional promptly if signs of serotonin syndrome (mental status changes: agitation, hallucinations, coma; autonomic instability: tachycardia, labile blood pressure, hyperthermia; neuromuscular aberrations: hyper-reflexia, incoordination; and/or gastrointestinal symptoms: nausea, vomiting, diarrhea) occur.
- **Subcut:** Instruct patient on the proper technique for loading, administering, and discarding the autoinjector or for using *Sumavel DosePro*. Patient information pamphlet is provided. Instructional video is available from the manufacturer.
- Inform patient that pain or redness at the injection site usually lasts less than 1 hr.
- **Intranasal:** Instruct patient in proper technique for intranasal administration. Usual dose is a single spray in one nostril. If headache returns, a 2nd dose may be administered in ≥2 hr. Do not administer 2nd dose if no relief was provided by 1st dose without consulting health care professional.

Evaluation/Desired Outcomes
- Relief of migraine attack.

---

sunitinib (su-ni-ti-nib)
Sutent

Classification
Therapeutic: antineoplastics
Pharmacologic: kinase inhibitors

Pregnancy Category D

Indications
Gastrointestinal stromal tumor that has progressed or intolerance to imatinib. Advanced renal cell carcinoma.

Action
Inhibits multiple receptor tyrosine kinases, which are enzymes implicated in tumor growth, abnormal vascular growth, and tumor metastases.
Therapeutic Effects: Decreased tumor spread.

Pharmacokinetics
Absorption: Well absorbed following oral administration.
Distribution: Unknown.
Protein Binding: *Sunitinib*—95%; *primary active metabolite*—90%.
Metabolism and Excretion: Metabolized by the CYP3A4 enzyme system to its primary active metabolite. This metabolite is further metabolized by CYP3A4. Excretion is primarily fecal.
Half-life: *Sunitinib*—40–60 hr; *primary active metabolite*—80–110 hr.

TIME/ACTION PROFILE (blood levels)

ROUTE	ONSET	PEAK	DURATION
PO	unknown	6–12 hr	24 hr

Contraindications/Precautions
Contraindicated in: Hypersensitivity; OB, Lactation: Pregnancy, lactation; Concurrent use of ketoconazole or St. John's wort.
Use Cautiously in: Hepatic/renal impairment; OB: Childbearing potential; Pedi: Safety not established.

Adverse Reactions/Side Effects
CNS: <u>fatigue</u>, dizziness, headache. **CV:** CHF, hypertension, peripheral edema, QT interval prolongation, thromboembolic events. **GI:** <u>diarrhea</u>, dyspepsia, <u>nausea</u>, stomatitis, vomiting, altered taste, anorexia, constipation, ↑ lipase/amylase, ↑ liver enzymes, oral pain. **Derm:** alopecia, hand-foot syndrome, hair color change, rash, skin discoloration. **Endo:** adrenal insufficiency, hypothyroidism. **F and E:** dehydration, hypophosphatemia. **Hemat:** HEMORRHAGE, <u>anemia</u>, <u>lymphopenia</u>, neutropenia, thrombocytopenia. **Metab:** <u>hyperuricemia</u>. **MS:** arthralgia, back pain, limb pain, myalgia. **Misc:** <u>fever</u>.

Interactions
Drug-Drug: Ketoconazole and other **inhibitors of the CYP3A4 enzyme system** may ↑ levels and the risk of toxicity; dosage may need to be decreased (avoid ketoconazole). **Rifampin** and other **inducers of the CYP3A4 enzyme system** may ↓ levels and effectiveness; dose may need to be increased. ↑ risk of microangiopathic hemolytic anemia when used with bevacizumab (concurrent use not recommended).
Drug-Natural Products: St. John's wort may ↓ levels and effectiveness; avoid concurrent use.
Drug-Food: Blood levels and effects are ↑ by **grapefruit juice**; concurrent use should be avoided.

Route/Dosage
PO (Adults): 50 mg once daily for 4 wk, followed by 2-wk rest; alteration of dose is based on safety/tolerability and is made in 12.5-mg increments/decrements.

sunitinib

Availability
Capsules: 12.5 mg, 25 mg, 37.5 mg, 50 mg.

NURSING IMPLICATIONS
Assessment
- Monitor for signs of CHF (dyspnea, edema, jugular venous distention) during therapy. Assess left ventricular ejection fraction (LVEF) at baseline and periodically during therapy in patients with cardiac events in the previous 12 mo and a baseline ejection fraction in patients without cardiovascular risk factors. Discontinue sunitinib if signs of CHF occur.
- Monitor for hypertension and treat with standard antihypertensive therapy. If severe hypertension occurs, may discontinue sunitinib until controlled.
- Monitor ECG and electrolytes periodically during therapy; may cause QT prolongation and torsades de pointes.
- *Lab Test Considerations:* Monitor CBC with platelet count and serum chemistries including phosphate at the beginning of each treatment cycle. May cause neutropenia, lymphopenia, anemia, and thrombocytopenia. May cause ↑ creatinine, hypokalemia, hyperuricemia, and ↑ uric acid.
- May cause ↑ AST, ALT, alkaline phosphatase, total and indirect bilirubin, amylase and lipase.
- Monitor thyroid function in patients with symptoms of hypothyroidism. May be treated with standard medical practice.

Potential Nursing Diagnoses
Diarrhea (Adverse Reactions)
Nausea (Adverse Reactions)

Implementation
- **PO:** Administer once daily with or without food for 4 wk, then 2 wk off therapy.

Patient/Family Teaching
- Instruct patient to take sunitinib as directed for 4 wk, followed by 2 wk off. Take missed doses as soon as remembered, but not just before next dose. Take next dose at regular time. Do not take more than 1 dose at a time. Tell your health care professional about the missed dose.
- Advise patient to avoid grapefruit juice or grapefruit products during therapy.
- Advise patient that GI disorders (diarrhea, nausea, stomatitis, dyspepsia, vomiting) are common and may require antiemetic and antidiarrheal medications.
- Inform patient that sunitinib may cause discoloration (yellow) of skin and depigmentation of hair or skin.
- Advise women of childbearing potential to avoid becoming pregnant while receiving sunitinib.
- Advise patient to consult health care professional before taking other Rx, OTC, or herbal products during sunitinib therapy.
- Advise patient to notify health care professional if bleeding or swelling occur.

Evaluation/Desired Outcomes
- Decrease in tumor spread.

tacrine (tak-rin)
Cognex

Classification
Therapeutic: anti-Alzheimer's agents
Pharmacologic: cholinergics (cholinesterase inhibitors)

Pregnancy Category C

Indications
Mild to moderate dementia associated with Alzheimer's disease.

Action
Increases levels of acetylcholine in the CNS by inhibiting its breakdown. **Therapeutic Effects:** Improved cognitive function in patients with mild to moderate Alzheimer's disease. Does not cure the disease.

Pharmacokinetics
Absorption: Rapidly absorbed following oral administration, although bioavailability is low (17%).
Distribution: Unknown.
Metabolism and Excretion: Highly metabolized by the liver (mostly by the P450 enzyme system).
Half-life: 2–4 hr.

TIME/ACTION PROFILE (improvement in cognitive function)

ROUTE	ONSET	PEAK	DURATION
PO	within 6 wk	18–24 wk	unknown

Contraindications/Precautions
Contraindicated in: Hypersensitivity to tacrine or other acridines; Jaundice associated with previous courses of tacrine therapy.
Use Cautiously in: Patients with a history or risk of GI bleeding, including current therapy with NSAIDs.

Adverse Reactions/Side Effects
CNS: dizziness, headache. **CV:** bradycardia. **GI:** GI BLEEDING, anorexia, diarrhea, drug-induced hepatitis, dyspepsia, nausea, vomiting.

Interactions
Drug-Drug: Metabolized by the cytochrome P450 enzyme system; levels and effects may be altered by other drugs which increase/inhibit this system or drugs that may compete for this metabolic pathway. Increases **theophylline** levels and risk of toxicity (blood level monitoring recommended; dosage reduction may be required). Potentiates the effects of **succinylcholine** (increases neuromuscular blockade) during anesthesia; also potentiates the effects of other **cholinesterase inhibitors**. May potentiate the action of **cholinergics** (**bethanechol**). **Fluvoxamine** significantly increases blood levels and the risk of adverse reactions. **Cigarette smoking** decreases blood levels of tacrine. **Cimetidine** increases tacrine levels. May interfere with the action of **anticholinergics**. Concurrent use of **NSAIDs** may increase the risk of GI bleeding.
Drug-Food: Food decreases absorption of tacrine by 30–40%.

Route/Dosage
PO (Adults): 10 mg 4 times daily for 4 wk. If ALT remains unchanged, increase dose to 20 mg 4 times daily. Further increments may be made at 4-wk intervals as tolerated, up to 160 mg/day.

Availability
Capsules: 10 mg, 20 mg, 30 mg, 40 mg. **Cost:** 10 mg $147.01/120, 20 mg $147.01/120, 30 mg $147.01/120, 40 mg $147.01/120

NURSING IMPLICATIONS

Assessment
- Assess cognitive function (memory, attention, reasoning, language, ability to perform simple tasks) periodically throughout therapy.
- Monitor heart rate periodically during therapy. May cause bradycardia.
- *Lab Test Considerations:* May cause ALT elevations; monitor levels every other wk for the first 16 wk of therapy, monthly for 2 mo, and then every 3 mo throughout therapy. Biweekly monitoring should be resumed for at least 6 wk after any dose increase. If ALT levels are <3 times the upper limit of normal, continue dose titration; if levels are >3 to <5 times the upper limit of normal, decrease the dose of tacrine by 40 mg/day and resume dose titration when ALT returns to normal. Tacrine should be discontinued if ALT levels are >5 times the upper limit of normal. Levels usually return to normal 4–6 wk after discontinuation of therapy.
- Tacrine should be permanently discontinued and a new trial should not be attempted in patients with clinical jaundice and a total bilirubin >3 mg/dL.

TACROLIMUS

Potential Nursing Diagnoses
Disturbed thought process (Indications)
Risk for injury (Indications)
Impaired environmental interpretation syndrome (Indications)

Implementation
- **PO:** Administer at regular intervals between meals on an empty stomach. If GI upset occurs, may be administered with meals; however, plasma levels may be reduced by 30–40%.
- Tacrine capsules may be dissolved in any aqueous solution for patients with difficulty swallowing (orange juice best masks the bitter taste). Place intact capsule in liquid to avoid loss of medication by spillage.

Patient/Family Teaching
- Emphasize the importance of taking tacrine at regular intervals as directed. If a dose is missed, take as soon as possible unless within 2 hr of next dose; do not double doses or discontinue without consulting health care professional. Abrupt discontinuation of doses >80 mg/day may cause a decline in cognitive function and behavioral disturbances.
- Caution patient and caregiver that tacrine may cause dizziness, unsteadiness, and clumsiness.
- Advise patient and caregiver to notify health care professional if nausea, vomiting, diarrhea, rash, jaundice, or changes in the color of the stool occur or if new symptoms occur or previously noted symptoms increase in severity.
- Advise patient to notify health care professional of medication regimen prior to treatment or surgery.

Evaluation/Desired Outcomes
- Improvement in cognitive function (memory, attention, reasoning, language, ability to perform simple tasks) in patients with Alzheimer's disease.

TACROLIMUS
tacrolimus (oral, IV)
(ta-**kroe**-li-mus)
Prograf

tacrolimus (topical)
Protopic

Classification
Therapeutic: immunosuppressants

Pregnancy Category C

Indications
PO, IV: Prevention of organ rejection in patients who have undergone allogenic liver, kidney, or heart transplantation (used concurrently with corticosteroids) (used concurrently with azathioprine or mycophenolate mofetil in kidney or heart transplants). **Topical:** Moderate to severe atopic dermatitis in patients who do not respond to or cannot tolerate alternative, conventional therapies.

Action
Inhibit T-lymphocyte activation. **Therapeutic Effects:** Prevention of transplanted organ rejection. Improvement in signs/symptoms of atopic dermatitis.

Pharmacokinetics
Absorption: Absorption following oral administration is erratic and incomplete (bioavailability ranges 5–67%); minimal amounts absorbed following topical use.
Distribution: Cross the placenta and enter breast milk.
Protein Binding: 99%.
Metabolism and Excretion: 99% metabolized by the liver; <1% excreted unchanged in the urine.
Half-life: *Liver transplant patients*—11.7 hr; *healthy volunteers*—21.2 hr.

TIME/ACTION PROFILE (immunosuppression)

ROUTE	ONSET	PEAK	DURATION
PO	rapid	1.3–3.2 hr*	12 hr
IV	rapid	unknown	8–12 hr
topical†	unknown	1–2 wk	unknown

*Blood level
†Improvement in atopic dermatitis

Contraindications/Precautions
Contraindicated in: Hypersensitivity to tacrolimus or to castor oil (a component in the injection); Concurrent use with cyclosporine or sirolimus should be avoided; Lactation: Breastfeeding should be avoided; **Topical:** Weakened/compromised immune system; Malignant or premalignant skin condition; Pedi: Children <2 yr (safety not established).
Use Cautiously in: Renal or hepatic impairment (dose reduction may be required; if oliguria occurs, wait 48 hr before initiating tacrolimus); Exposure to sunlight/UV light (may ↑ risk of malignant skin changes); OB: Hyperkalemia and renal impairment may occur in the newborn; use only if benefit to mother justifies risk to the fetus; Pedi: Higher end of dosing range required to maintain adequate blood levels; **Topical:** Superficial skin infections.

TACROLIMUS 1183

Adverse Reactions/Side Effects
Noted primarily for PO and IV use.
CNS: SEIZURES, dizziness, headache, insomnia, tremor, abnormal dreams, agitation, anxiety, confusion, depression, emotional lability, hallucinations, posterior reversible encephalopathy syndrome, psychoses, somnolence. **EENT:** abnormal vision, amblyopia, sinusitis, tinnitus. **Resp:** cough, pleural effusion, asthma, bronchitis, pharyngitis, pneumonia, pulmonary edema. **CV:** hypertension, peripheral edema, QTc prolongation. **GI:** GI BLEEDING, abdominal pain, anorexia, ascites, constipation, diarrhea, dyspepsia, ↑ liver function tests, nausea, vomiting, cholangitis, cholestatic jaundice, dysphagia, flatulence, ↑ appetite, oral thrush, peritonitis. **GU:** nephrotoxicity, urinary tract infection. **Derm:** pruritus, rash, alopecia, herpes simplex, hirsutism, photosensitivity, sweating. **Endo:** hyperglycemia, hyperlipidemia. **F and E:** hyperkalemia, hypomagnesemia, hyperphosphatemia, hypocalcemia, hyponatremia, hypophosphatemia, metabolic acidosis, metabolic alkalosis. **Hemat:** anemia, leukocytosis, leukopenia, thrombocytopenia, coagulation defects. **Local:** *topical*—burning, stinging. **MS:** arthralgia, hypertonia, leg cramps, muscle spasm, myalgia, myasthenia, osteoporosis. **Neuro:** paresthesia, neuropathy. **Misc:** allergic reactions including ANAPHYLAXIS, generalized pain, abnormal healing, chills, fever, infection (including activation of latent viral infections such as BK virus-associated nephropathy), ↑ risk of lymphoma/skin cancer (topical).

Interactions
Noted primarily for PO and IV use, but should be considered for topical use.
Drug-Drug: Risk of nephrotoxicity is ↑ by concurrent use of **aminoglycosides**, **amphotericin B**, **cisplatin**, or **cyclosporine** (allow 24 hr to pass after stopping cyclosporine before starting tacrolimus). Concurrent use of **potassium-sparing diuretics**, **ACE inhibitors**, or **angiotensin II receptor blockers** ↑ risk of hyperkalemia. The following drugs ↑ tacrolimus blood levels: **azole antifungals**, **bromocriptine**, **calcium channel blockers**, **chloramphenicol**, **cimetidine**, **lansoprazole**, **clarithromycin**, **cyclosporine**, **danazol**, **erythromycin**, **magnesium/aluminum hydroxide methylprednisolone**, **omeprazole**, **nefazodone**, and **metoclopramide**, **protease inhibitors**, and **voriconazole**. **Phenobarbital**, **phenytoin**, **caspofungin**, **sirolimus carbamazepine**, and **rifamycins** may ↓ tacrolimus blood levels. **Vaccinations** may be less effective if given concurrently with tacrolimus (avoid use of live-virus vaccines). May ↑ levels of **mycophenolate mofetil** or **mycophenolic acid**.
Drug-Natural Products: Concomitant use with **astragalus**, **echinacea**, and **melatonin** may interfere with immunosuppression. **St John's wort** may ↓ tacrolimus blood levels.
Drug-Food: Food ↓ the rate and extent of GI absorption. **Grapefruit juice** ↑ absorption.

Route/Dosage
Because of the potential risk for anaphylaxis, the IV route of administration should be reserved for those patients unable to take the drug orally.

Kidney Transplantation
PO (Adults): *Initial dose (with azathioprine)*—0.2 mg/kg/day in 2 divided doses; titrate to achieve recommended whole blood trough concentration; *Initial dose (with mycophenolate mofetil and IL-2 antagonist)*—0.1 mg/kg/day in 2 divided doses; titrate to achieve recommended whole blood trough concentration.
PO (Children): 0.15–0.4 mg/kg/day in 2 divided doses; titrate to achieve recommended whole blood trough concentration.
IV (Adults): *Initial dose*—0.03–0.1 mg/kg/day as a continuous infusion; titrate dose to achieve recommended whole blood trough concentration.
IV (Children): 0.03–0.15 mg/kg/day.

Liver Transplantation
PO (Adults): *Initial dose*—0.1–0.15 mg/kg/day in two divided doses; titrate to achieve recommended whole blood trough concentration.
PO (Children): *Initial dose*—0.15–0.2 mg/kg/day in 2 divided doses; titrate to achieve recommended whole blood trough concentration.
IV (Adults and Children): Same as for kidney transplant.

Heart Transplantation
PO (Adults): *Initial dose*—0.075 mg/kg/day in two divided doses; titrate to achieve recommended whole blood trough concentration.
IV (Adults): *Initial dose*—0.01 mg/kg/day as a continuous infusion; titrate to achieve recommended whole blood trough concentration.

Atopic Dermatitis
Topical (Adults): Apply 0.03% or 0.1% ointment twice daily. Discontinue when signs/symptoms of atopic dermatitis resolve.

Topical (Children ≥2–15 yr): Apply 0.03% ointment twice daily. Discontinue when signs/symptoms of atopic dermatitis resolve.

Availability (generic available)
Capsules: 0.5 mg, 1 mg, 5 mg. **Cost:** 0.5 mg $359.96/180, 1 mg $694.46/180, 5 mg $3,645.61/180. **Injection:** 5 mg/mL. **Ointment:** 0.03%, 0.1%.

NURSING IMPLICATIONS
Assessment
- Assess for symptoms of posterior reversible encephalopathy syndrome [PRES] (headache, altered mental status, seizures, visual disturbances, hypertension) periodically during therapy. Confirm diagnosis by radiologic procedure. If PRES is suspected or diagnosed, maintain blood pressure control and immediately reduce immunosuppression. Symptoms are usually reversed on reduction or discontinuation of immunosuppression.
- **Prevention of Organ Rejection:** Monitor blood pressure closely during therapy. Hypertension is a common complication of tacrolimus therapy and should be treated.
- Observe patients receiving IV tacrolimus for the development of anaphylaxis (rash, pruritus, laryngeal edema, wheezing) for at least 30 min and frequently thereafter. If signs develop, stop infusion and initiate treatment.
- **Atopic Dermatitis:** Assess skin lesions prior to and periodically during therapy.
- Use only for short time, not continuously, and in the minimum dose possible to decrease risk of developing skin cancer.
- **Lab Test Considerations:** Tacrolimus blood level monitoring may be helpful in the evaluation of rejection and toxicity, dose adjustments, and assessment of compliance. For liver transplantation, most patients are stable when tacrolimus trough whole blood concentrations are maintained between 5–20 ng/mL. For kidney transplantation, during the first 3 mo, most patients maintained tacrolimus whole blood concentrations between 7–20 ng/mL and then between 5–15 ng/mL through 1 yr. For heart transplantation, from wk 1 to 3 mo, most patients maintained tacrolimus trough whole blood concentrations between 8–20 ng/mL and then between 6–18 ng/mL from 3–18 mo post-transplant.
- Monitor serum creatinine, potassium, and glucose closely. ↑ serum creatinine and ↓ urine output may indicate nephrotoxicity. May also cause insulin-dependent post-transplant diabetes mellitus (incidence is higher in African American and Hispanic patients).
- May also cause hyperuricemia, hypokalemia, hyperkalemia, hypomagnesemia, metabolic acidosis, metabolic alkalosis, hyperlipidemia, hyperphosphatemia, hypophosphatemia, hypocalcemia, and hyponatremia.
- Monitor CBC. May cause anemia, leukocytosis, and thrombocytopenia.

Potential Nursing Diagnoses
Risk for infection (Adverse Reactions)

Implementation
- Therapy with tacrolimus should be started no sooner than 6 hr post-transplantation. Concurrent therapy with corticosteroids is recommended in the early postoperative period.
- Tacrolimus should not be used concomitantly with cyclosporine. Tacrolimus or cyclosporine should be discontinued at least 24 hr before starting the other.
- Oral therapy is preferred because of the risk of anaphylactic reactions with IV tacrolimus. IV therapy should be replaced with oral therapy as soon as possible.
- Adults should be started at the lower end of the dose range; children require a higher doses to maintain blood trough concentrations similar to adults.
- **PO:** Oral doses can be initiated 8–12 hr after discontinuation of IV doses.
- **Topical:** Do not use continuously for a long time.

IV Administration
- **Continuous Infusion:** *Diluent:* Dilute in 0.9% NaCl or D5W. *Concentration:* 0.004–0.02 mg/mL. May be stored in polyethylene or glass containers for 24 hr following dilution. Do not store in PVC containers. *Rate:* Administer daily dose as a continuous infusion over 24 hr.
- **Y-Site Compatibility:** alfentanil, amifostine, amikacin, aminophylline, amiodarone, amphotericin B colloidal, amphotericin B liposome, anidulafungin, atracurium, aztreonam, benztropine, bivalirudin, bleomycin, bumetanide, buprenorphine, busulfan, butorphanol, calcium acetate, calcium chloride, calcium gluconate, carboplatin, carmustine, caspofungin, cefazolin, cefoperazone, cefotaxime, cefotetan, cefoxitin, ceftazidime, ceftizoxime, ceftriaxone, cefuroxime, chloramphenicol, chlorpromazine, cimetidine, ciprofloxacin, cisatracurium, cisplatin, clindamycin, cyclophosphamide, cyclosporine, cytarabine, dactinomycin, dapto-

mycin, dexamethasone, dexmedetomidine, dexrazoxane, digoxin, diltiazem, diphenhydramine, dobutamine, docetaxel, dolasetron, dopamine, doripenem, doxacurium, doxorubicin hydrochloride, doxycycline, droperidol, enalaprilat, ephedrine, epinephrine, epirubicin, ertapenem, erythromycin, esmolol, etoposide, etoposide phosphate, famotidine, fenoldopam, fentanyl, fluconazole, fludarabine, foscarnet, fosphenytoin, gemcitabine, gentamicin, glycopyrrolate, granisetron, haloperidol, heparin, hetastarch, hydralazine, hydrocortisone, hydromorphone, idarubicin, ifosfamide, imipenem/cilastatin, inamrinone, insulin, isoproterenol, ketorolac, labetalol, leucovorin, levofloxacin, levorphanol, lidocaine, linezolid, lorazepam, magnesium sulfate, mannitol, mechlorethamine, meperidine, meropenem, mesna, metaraminol, methotrexate, methyldopate, methylprednisolone, metoclopramide, metoprolol, metronidazole, micafungin, midazolam, milrinone, mitomycin, mitoxantrone, mivacurium, morphine, multivitamins, nafcillin, nalbuphine, naloxone, nesiritide, nicardipine, nitroglycerin, nitroprusside, norepinephrine, octreotide, ondansetron, oxacillin, oxaliplatin, oxytocin, paclitaxel, palonosetron, pancuronium, pemetrexed, penmicillin G, pentamidine, pentazocine, perphenazine, phentolamine, phenylephrine, piperacillin/tazobactam, potassium chloride, potassium phosphates, procainamide, prochlorperazine, promethazine, propranolol, quinapristin/dalfopristin, ranitidine, remifentanil, rocuronium, sodium acetate, sodium bicarbonate, sodium phosphates, streptozocin, succinylcholine, sufentanil, teniposide, theophylline, thiotepa, ticarcillin/clavulanate, tigecycline, tirofiban, tobramycin, tolazoline, trimethobenzamide, vancomycin, vasopressin, vecuronium, verapamil, vincristine, vinorelbine, voriconazole, zidovudine.

- **Y-Site Incompatibility:** acyclovir, allopurinol, azathioprine, cefepime, dantrolene, diazepam, diazoxide, esomeprazole, folic acid, ganciclovir, iron sucrose, levothyroxine, omeprazole, phenytoin, thiopental.

Patient/Family Teaching
- Instruct patient to take tacrolimus at the same time each day, as directed. Do not skip or double up on missed doses. Do not discontinue medication without advice of health care professional.
- Advise patient to avoid grapefruit and grapefruit juice during therapy.
- Reinforce the need for lifelong therapy to prevent transplant rejection. Review symptoms of rejection for transplanted organ and stress need to notify health care professional immediately if they occur.
- Emphasize the importance of repeated lab tests during tacrolimus therapy.
- Advise patient to avoid eating raw oysters or other shellfish; make sure they are fully cooked before eating.
- Instruct patient to notify health care professional if signs of diabetes mellitus (frequent urination, increased thirst or hunger) or PRES occur.
- Advise patient to wear protective clothing and sunscreen to avoid photosensitivity reactions.
- Instruct patient to avoid exposure to chicken pox, measles, mumps, and rubella. If exposed, see health care professional for prophylactic therapy.
- Advise patient of the risk of taking tacrolimus during pregnancy.
- Inform patient of the risk of lymphoma or skin cancer with tacrolimus therapy.
- **Topical:** Advise patients to contact health care professional if their symptoms do not improve after 6 wk of therapy, if their symptoms worsen, or they develop a skin infection.
- Instruct patient to use ointment only on areas of skin with atopic dermatitis.
- Advise patient to stop using the ointment when the signs/symptoms of atopic dermatitis go away.
- Advise patient to limit sun exposure during treatment.

Evaluation/Desired Outcomes
- Prevention of transplanted organ rejection.
- Management of atopic dermatitis.

tadalafil (ta-da-la-fil)
Adcirca, Cialis

Classification
Therapeutic: erectile dysfunction agents, vasodilators
Pharmacologic: phosphodiesterase type 5 inhibitors

Pregnancy Category B

Indications
Cialis: Erectile dysfunction. *Adcirca:* Pulmonary arterial hypertension.

Action
Increases cyclic guanosine monophosphate (cGMP) levels by inhibiting phosphodiesterase type 5 (PDE5) an enzyme responsible for the breakdown of cGMP. cGMP produces smooth muscle relaxation of the corpus cavernosum, which in turn promotes increased blood flow and subsequent erection. cGMP also leads to vasodilation of the pulmonary vasculature. **Therapeutic Effects:** *Cialis:* Enhanced blood flow to the corpus cavernosum and erection sufficient to allow sexual intercourse. Requires sexual stimulation. *Adcirca:* Improved exercise tolerance.

Pharmacokinetics
Absorption: Well absorbed following oral administration.
Distribution: Extensive tissue distribution; penetrates semen.
Protein Binding: 94%.
Metabolism and Excretion: Mostly metabolized by the liver (mainly CYP3A4 enzyme system); metabolites are excreted in feces (61%) and urine (36%).
Half-life: 17.5 hr.

TIME/ACTION PROFILE (vasodilation, improved erectile function)

ROUTE	ONSET	PEAK	DURATION
PO	rapid	0.5–6 hr	36

Contraindications/Precautions
Contraindicated in: Hypersensitivity; Concurrent use of nitrates; Unstable angina, recent history of stroke, life-threatening heart failure within 6 months, uncontrolled hypertension, arrhythmias, stroke within 6 months or MI within 90 days; Any other cardiovascular pathology precluding sexual activity; Known hereditary degenerative retinal disorders; Severe hepatic impairment; Severe renal impairment (Adcirca only); Congenital or acquired QT prolongation or concurrent use of Class IA or III antiarrhythmics; Concurrent use of ketoconazole, itraconazole, or rifampin (Adcirca only); Pedi: Women, children or newborns.
Use Cautiously in: Left ventricular outflow obstruction; Penile deformity; Renal impairment; Underlying conditions predisposing to priapism including sickle cell anemia, multiple myeloma or leukemia; Bleeding disorders or active peptic ulcer disease; Strong inhibitors of the CYP3A4 enzyme system; Alpha adrenergic blockers (patients should be on stable dose of alpha blockers before starting tadalafil); History of sudden severe vision loss or non arteritic ischemic optic neuropathy (NAION); may ↑ risk of recurrence; Geri: May experience more side effects.

Adverse Reactions/Side Effects
CNS: headache. **EENT:** HEARING LOSS, VISION LOSS, nasal congestion. **CV:** hypotension. **GI:** dyspepsia. **GU:** priapism. **Derm:** flushing. **MS:** back pain, limb pain, myalgia.

Interactions
Drug-Drug: Concurrent use of **nitrates** may cause serious, life threatening hypotension and is contraindicated. ↑ risk of hypotension with **alpha adrenergic blockers** and acute ingestion of **alcohol**. Strong inhibitors of CYP3A4 including **ritonavir**, **ketoconazole**, **itraconazole** ↑ effects and the risk of adverse reactions (dosage adjustments recommended; ketoconazole and itraconazole contraindicated with Adcirca). Similar effects may be expected of other **inhibitors of CY3A4**. CYP3A4 inducers may ↓ effects (**rifampin** contraindicated with Adcirca).

Route/Dosage
Cialis (for erectile dysfunction)
PO (Adults): 10 mg prior to sexual activity (range 5–20 mg; not to exceed one dose/24 hr) *or* 2.5 mg once daily (max: 5 mg/day); *Concurrent use of CYP3A4 inhibitors including itraconazole, ketoconazole and ritonavir*—single dose should not exceed 10 mg in any 72 hour period; for once daily dose regimen, daily dose should not exceed 2.5 mg.

Renal Impairment
PO (Adults): *CCr 31–50 mL/min*—Initial dose should not exceed 5 mg/day; maximum dose should not exceed 10 mg in 48 hr (no adjustment required for once daily use); *CCr <30 mL/min*—maximum dose 5 mg (once daily dose regimen not recommended).

Hepatic Impairment
PO (Adults): *Mild or moderate hepatic impairment (Child–Pugh class A or B)*—Daily dose should not exceed 10 mg (once daily dose regimen not recommended).

Adcirca (for pulmonary arterial hypertension)
PO (Adults): 40 mg once daily; *If receiving ritonavir for ≥1 wk*—start 20 mg once daily; may then ↑ to 40 mg once daily based on tolerability; *If initiating ritonavir while on Adcirca*—stop Adcirca ≥24 hr before starting ritonavir; may reinitiate Adcirca at 20 mg once daily after ≥1 wk

of therapy with ritonavir; may then ↑ to 40 mg once daily based on tolerability.

Renal Impairment
(Adults): *CCr 31–80 mL/min*—Start 20 mg once daily; may then ↑ to 40 mg once daily based on tolerability.

Hepatic Impairment
PO (Adults): *Mild or moderate hepatic impairment (Child–Pugh class A or B)*—Start with 20 mg once daily.

Availability
Tablets (Cialis): 2.5 mg, 5 mg, 10 mg, 20 mg. **Cost:** 5 mg $357.97/30, 10 mg $356.97/30, 20 mg $365.97/30. **Tablets (Adcirca):** 20 mg.

NURSING IMPLICATIONS

Assessment
- *Cialis:* Determine erectile dysfunction before administration. Tadalafil has no effect in the absence of sexual stimulation.
- *Adcirca:* Monitor hemodynamic parameters and exercise tolerance prior to and periodically during therapy.

Potential Nursing Diagnoses
Sexual dysfunction (Indications)
Risk for activity intolerance (Indications)

Implementation
- **PO:** Administer dose for *erectile dysfunction* at least 30 min prior to sexual activity; effectiveness may continue for 36 hr.
- Administer dose for *pulmonary hypertension* once daily.
- May be administered without regard to food.

Patient/Family Teaching
- Instruct patient to take tadalafil at least 30 min before sexual activity and not more than once per day. Inform patient that sexual stimulation is required for an erection to occur after taking tadalafil.
- Advise patient that tadalafil is not indicated for use in women.
- Caution patient not to take tadalafil concurrently with alpha adrenergic blockers (unless on a stable dose) or nitrates. If chest pain occurs after taking tadalafil, instruct patient to seek immediate medical attention.
- Advise patient to avoid excess alcohol intake (≥5 units) in combination with tadalafil; may increase risk of orthostatic hypotension, increased heart rate, decreased standing blood pressure, dizziness, headache.
- Instruct patient to notify health care professional promptly if erection lasts longer than 4 hr, if they are not satisfied with their sexual performance or develop unwanted side effects or if they experience sudden or decreased vision loss in one or both eyes or loss or decrease in hearing, ringing in the ears, or dizziness.
- Advise patient to consult health care professional before taking other Rx or OTC medications or herbal supplements that may interact with tadalafil.
- Inform patient that tadalafil offers no protection against sexually transmitted diseases. Counsel patient that protection against sexually transmitted diseases and HIV infection should be considered.

Evaluation/Desired Outcomes
- Male erection sufficient to allow intercourse.
- Increased exercise tolerance.

---

tamoxifen (ta-**mox**-i-fen)
✦ Alpha-Tamoxifen, ✦ Med Tamoxifen, Nolvadex-D, ✦ Novo-Tamoxifen, ✦ Tamofen, ✦ Tamone, ✦ Tamoplex

Classification
Therapeutic: antineoplastics
Pharmacologic: antiestrogens

Pregnancy Category D

Indications
Adjuvant therapy of breast cancer after surgery and radiation (delays recurrence). Palliative or adjunctive treatment of advanced breast cancer. Prevention of breast cancer in high-risk patients. Treatment of ductal carcinoma *in situ* following breast surgery and radiation.

Action
Competes with estrogen for binding sites in breast and other tissues. Reduces DNA synthesis and estrogen response. **Therapeutic Effects:** Suppression of tumor growth. Reduced incidence of breast cancer in high-risk patients.

Pharmacokinetics
Absorption: Absorbed after oral administration.
Distribution: Widely distributed.
Metabolism and Excretion: Mostly metabolized by the liver. Slowly eliminated in the feces. Minimal amounts excreted in the urine.

tamoxifen

Half-life: 7 days.

TIME/ACTION PROFILE (tumor response)

ROUTE	ONSET	PEAK	DURATION
PO	4–10 wk	several mo	several wk

Contraindications/Precautions
Contraindicated in: Hypersensitivity; Concurrent warfarin therapy with history of deep vein thrombosis (patients at high risk for breast cancer only); OB, Lactation: Pregnancy or lactation. **Use Cautiously in:** ↓ bone marrow reserve; Women with childbearing potential.

Adverse Reactions/Side Effects
CNS: confusion, depression, headache, weakness. **EENT:** blurred vision. **CV:** PULMONARY EMBOLISM, STROKE, edema. **GI:** nausea, vomiting. **GU:** UTERINE MALIGNANCIES, vaginal bleeding. **F and E:** hypercalcemia. **Hemat:** leukopenia, thrombocytopenia. **Metab:** hot flashes. **MS:** bone pain. **Misc:** tumor flare.

Interactions
Drug-Drug: **Estrogens** and **aminoglutethimide** may ↓ effectiveness of concurrently administered tamoxifen. Blood levels are ↑ by **bromocriptine**. May ↑ the anticoagulant effect of **warfarin**. Risk of thromboembolic events is ↑ by concurrent use of other **antineoplastics**.

Route/Dosage
Treatment of Breast Cancer
PO (Adults): 10–20 mg twice daily; doses of 20 mg/day may be taken as a single dose.

Prevention of Breast Cancer/Ductal Carcinoma *in situ*
PO (Adults): 20 mg once daily for 5 yr.

Availability (generic available)
Tablets: 10 mg, 20 mg. **Cost:** *Generic*—10 mg $39.97/90, 20 mg $49.97/90. **Enteric-coated tablets:** ✽ 20 mg.

NURSING IMPLICATIONS

Assessment
- Assess for an increase in bone or tumor pain. Confer with health care professional regarding analgesics. This transient pain usually resolves despite continued therapy.
- ***Lab Test Considerations:*** Monitor CBC, platelets, and calcium levels before and during therapy. May cause transient hypercalcemia in patients with metastases to the bone. An estrogen receptor assay should be assessed before initiation of therapy.
- Monitor serum cholesterol and triglyceride concentrations in patients with pre-existing hyperlipidemia. May cause ↑ concentrations.
- Monitor hepatic function tests and thyroxine (T$_4$) periodically during therapy. May cause ↑ serum hepatic enzyme and thyroxine concentrations.
- Gynecologic examinations should be performed regularly; may cause variations in Papanicolaou and vaginal smears.

Potential Nursing Diagnoses
Deficient knowledge, related to medication regimen (Patient/Family Teaching)

Implementation
- **PO:** Administer with food or fluids if GI irritation becomes a problem. Consult health care professional if patient vomits shortly after administration of medication to determine need for repeat dose.
- Do not crush, break, chew, or administer an antacid within 1–2 hr of enteric-coated tablet.

Patient/Family Teaching
- Instruct patient to take medication as directed. If a dose is missed, it should be omitted.
- If skin lesions are present, inform patient that lesions may temporarily increase in size and number and may have increased erythema.
- Advise patient to report bone pain to health care professional promptly. This pain may be severe. Inform patient that this may be an indication of the drug's effectiveness and will resolve over time. Analgesics should be ordered to control pain.
- Instruct patient to monitor weight weekly. Weight gain or peripheral edema should be reported to health care professional.
- This medication may induce ovulation and may have teratogenic properties. Advise patient to use a nonhormonal method of contraception during and for 1 mo after the therapy.
- Advise patient that medication may cause hot flashes. Notify health care professional if these become bothersome.
- Instruct patient to notify health care professional promptly if pain or swelling of legs, shortness of breath, weakness, sleepiness, confusion, nausea, vomiting, weight gain, dizziness, headache, loss of appetite, or blurred vision occurs. Patient should also report menstrual irregularities, vaginal bleeding, pelvic pain or pressure.

Evaluation/Desired Outcomes
- Decrease in the size or spread of breast cancer. Observable effects of therapy may not be seen for 4–10 wk after initiation.

---

tamsulosin (tam-**soo**-loe-sin)
Flomax

Classification
Therapeutic: none assigned
Pharmacologic: peripherally acting antiadrenergics

Pregnancy Category B

Indications
Management of outflow obstruction in male patients with prostatic hyperplasia.

Action
Decreases contractions in smooth muscle of the prostatic capsule by preferentially binding to alpha$_1$-adrenergic receptors. **Therapeutic Effects:** Decreased symptoms of prostatic hyperplasia (urinary urgency, hesitancy, nocturia).

Pharmacokinetics
Absorption: Slowly absorbed after oral administration.
Distribution: Widely distributed.
Protein Binding: 94–99%.
Metabolism and Excretion: Extensively metabolized by the liver; <10% excreted unchanged in urine.
Half-life: 14 hr.

TIME/ACTION PROFILE (↑ in urine flow)

ROUTE	ONSET	PEAK	DURATION
PO	unknown	2 wk	unknown

Contraindications/Precautions
Contraindicated in: Hypersensitivity.
Use Cautiously in: Patients at risk for prostate carcinoma (symptoms may be similar).

Adverse Reactions/Side Effects
CNS: dizziness, headache. **EENT:** rhinitis. **CV:** orthostatic hypotension. **GU:** retrograde/diminished ejaculation.

Interactions
Drug-Drug: Cimetidine may ↑ blood levels and the risk of toxicity. ↑ risk of hypotension with other peripherally acting anti-adrenergics (**doxazosin, prazosin, terazosin**); concurrent use should be avoided.

Route/Dosage
PO (Adults): 0.4 mg once daily after a meal; may be ↑ after 2–4 wk to 0.8 mg/day.

Availability
Capsules: 0.4 mg. **Cost:** $233.98/90.

NURSING IMPLICATIONS

Assessment
- Assess patient for symptoms of prostatic hyperplasia (urinary hesitancy, feeling of incomplete bladder emptying, interruption of urinary stream, impairment of size and force of urinary stream, terminal urinary dribbling, straining to start flow, dysuria, urgency) before and periodically during therapy.
- Assess patient for first-dose orthostatic hypotension and syncope. Incidence may be dose related. Observe patient closely during this period and take precautions to prevent injury.
- Monitor intake and output ratios and daily weight, and assess for edema daily, especially at beginning of therapy. Report weight gain or edema.
- Rectal exams prior to and periodically throughout therapy to assess prostate size are recommended.

Potential Nursing Diagnoses
Risk for injury (Side Effects)
Impaired urinary elimination (Indications)

Implementation
- Do not confuse Flomax (tamsulosin) with Fosamax (alendronate) or Volmax (albuterol).
- **PO:** Administer daily dose 30 min after the same meal each day. Swallow capsules whole; do not open, crush, or chew.
- If dose is interrupted for several days at either the 0.4-mg or 0.8-mg dose, restart therapy with the 0.4-mg/day dose.

Patient/Family Teaching
- Emphasize the importance of continuing to take this medication, even if feeling well. Instruct patient to take medication at the same time each day. If a dose is missed, take as soon as remembered unless almost time for next dose. Do not double doses.
- May cause dizziness. Advise patient to avoid driving or other activities requiring alertness until response to medication is known.
- Caution patient to change positions slowly to minimize orthostatic hypotension.

- Advise patient to consult health care professional before taking other Rx, OTC, or herbal products, especially cough, cold, or allergy remedies.
- Emphasize the importance of follow-up visits to determine effectiveness of therapy.

Evaluation/Desired Outcomes
- Decrease in urinary symptoms of benign prostatic hyperplasia.

---

tapentadol (ta-pen-ta-dol)
Nucynta

Classification
Therapeutic: analgesics (centrally acting), opioid analgesics
Pharmacologic: opioid agonists

Schedule II

Pregnancy Category C

Indications
Management of moderate to severe acute pain in patients ≥18 yr.

Action
Acts as μ-opioid receptor agonist. Also inhibits the reuptake of norepinephrine. **Therapeutic Effects:** Decrease in pain severity.

Pharmacokinetics
Absorption: 32% absorbed following oral administration.
Distribution: Widely distributed.
Metabolism and Excretion: Undergoes extensive first-pass hepatic metabolism (97%); metabolites have no analgesic activity; metabolized drug is 99% renally excreted.
Half-life: 4 hr.

TIME/ACTION PROFILE (analgesic effect)

ROUTE	ONSET	PEAK	DURATION
PO	unknown	1 hr	4–6 hr

Contraindications/Precautions
Contraindicated in: Significant respiratory depression in unmonitored settings or where resuscitative equipment is not readily available; Paralytic ileus; Severe hepatic impairment; Concurrent MAO inhibitors or use of MAO inhibitors in the preceding 2 wk; Lactation: Lactation; Pedi: Safe use in children <18 yr not established; not recommended.

Use Cautiously in: Conditions associated with hypoxia, hypercapnea, or decreased respiratory reserve including asthma, chronic obstructive pulmonary disease, cor pulmonale, extreme obesity, sleep apnea syndrome, myxedema, kyphoscoliosis, CNS depression, use of other CNS depressants or coma (↑ risk of further respiratory depression); use smallest effective dose; Geri: Elderly or debilitated patients (↑ risk of respiratory depression); consider age-related decrease in hepatic, renal, and cardiovascular function, concurrent disease states and drug therapy (initial dose should be lower); History of substance abuse or addiction disorder; History or ↑ risk of seizures; OB: Use in pregnancy only if potential benefit justifies potential risk to the fetus.

Adverse Reactions/Side Effects
CNS: SEIZURES, dizziness, headache, somnolence. **Resp:** RESPIRATORY DEPRESSION. **GI:** nausea, vomiting.

Interactions
Drug-Drug: Concurrent **MAO inhibitors** or use of MAO inhibitors in the preceding 2 wk can result in potentially life-threatening adverse cardiovascular reactions due to additive effects on norepinephrine levels. Concurrent use of other **CNS depressants** including **sedative/hypnotics, alcohol, antihistamines, antidepressants, phenothiazines,** and other **opioids** ↑ risk of further CNS depression; consider dose ↓ of one or both agents. ↑ risk of serotonin syndrome with **SNRIs, SSRIs, triptans, tricyclic antidepressants,** and **MAO inihibitors.**

Route/Dosage
PO (Adults): 50, 75, or 100 mg initially, then every 4–6 hr as needed and tolerated. If pain control is not achieved within first hour of first dose, additional dose may be given. Doses should not exceed 700 mg on the first day or 600 mg/day thereafter.

Hepatic Impairment
PO (Adults): *Moderate hepatic impairment—50 mg every 8 hr initially, then titrate to maintain analgesia without intolerable side effects.*

Availability
Immediate-release tablets: 50 mg, 75 mg, 100 mg.

NURSING IMPLICATIONS

Assessment
- Assess type, location, and intensity of pain before and 1 hr (peak) after administration.
- Assess blood pressure and respiratory rate before and periodically during administration. Monitor for respiratory depression especially during initial dosing and with patients at increased risk.

tapentadol 1191

- Assess bowel function routinely. Prevention of constipation should be instituted with increased intake of fluids and bulk and with laxatives to minimize constipating effects. Administer stimulant laxatives routinely if opioid use exceeds 2–3 days, unless contraindicated.
- Prolonged use may lead to physical and psychological dependence and tolerance, although these may be milder than with opioids. This should not prevent patient from receiving adequate analgesia. Most patients who receive tapentadol for pain do not develop psychological dependence.
- Monitor patient for seizures. May occur within recommended dose range. Risk is increased in patients with a history of seizures and in patients taking antidepressants (SSRIs, SNRIs, tricyclics) or other drugs that decrease the seizure threshold.
- Monitor for serotonin syndrome (mental-status changes [agitation, hallucinations, coma], autonomic instability [tachycardia, labile blood pressure, hyperthermia], neuromuscular aberrations [hyperreflexia, incoordination] and/or gastrointestinal symptoms [nausea, vomiting, diarrhea] in patients taking SSRIs, SNRIs, triptans, tricyclic antidepressants, or MAO inhibitors concurrently with tapentadol.
- *Toxicity and Overdose:* Overdose may cause respiratory depression. Naloxone (Narcan) may reverse some, but not all, of the symptoms of overdose. Treatment should be symptomatic and supportive. Maintain adequate respiratory exchange.

Potential Nursing Diagnoses
Acute pain (Indications)

Implementation
- Initial dose of 50 mg, 75 mg, or 100 mg is individualized based on pain severity, previous experience with similar drugs, and ability to monitor patient. Second dose may be administered as soon as 1 hr after first dose if adequate pain relief is not obtained with first dose.
- **PO:** Tapentadol may be administered without regard to meals.

Patient/Family Teaching
- Instruct patient on how and when to ask for and take pain medication and to take tapentadol as directed; do not adjust dose without consulting health care professional. Report breakthrough pain and adverse reactions to health care professional. Do not take tapentadol if pain is mild or can be controlled with other pain medications such as NSAIDs or acetaminophen. Do not stop abruptly; may cause withdrawal symptoms (anxiety, sweating, insomnia, rigors, pain, nausea, tremors, diarrhea, upper respiratory symptoms, hallucinations). Decrease dose gradually. Advise patient to read the *Medication Guide* prior to taking tapentadol and with each Rx refill, in case of new information.
- Do not share tapentadol with others, even it they have the same symptoms; may be dangerous.
- May cause dizziness and drowsiness. Caution patient to avoid driving or other activities requiring alertness until response to medication is known.
- Inform patient that tapentadol may cause seizures. Stop taking tapentadol and notify health care professional immediately if seizures occur.
- Advise patient to change positions slowly to minimize orthostatic hypotension.
- Caution patient to avoid concurrent use of alcohol or other CNS depressants with this medication.
- Advise patient to consult health care professional before taking other RX, OTC, or herbal products concurrently.
- Advise patient to notify health care professional if signs or serotonin syndrome occur.
- Advise female patients to notify health care professional if pregnancy is planned or suspected, or if breastfeeding.
- Encourage patient to turn, cough, and breathe deeply every 2 hr to prevent atelectasis.

Evaluation/Desired Outcomes
- Decrease in severity of pain without a significant alteration in level of consciousness or respiratory status.

---

telmisartan, See ANGIOTENSIN II RECEPTOR ANTAGONISTS.

✦ = Canadian drug name. ■ = Genetic implication.
*CAPITALS indicates life-threatening; underlines indicate most frequent.

temazepam (tem-az-a-pam)
Restoril

Classification
Therapeutic: sedative/hypnotics
Pharmacologic: benzodiazepines

Schedule IV

Pregnancy Category X

Indications
Short-term management of insomnia (<4 weeks).

Action
Acts at many levels in the CNS, producing generalized depression. Effects may be mediated by GABA, an inhibitory neurotransmitter. **Therapeutic Effects:** Relief of insomnia.

Pharmacokinetics
Absorption: Well absorbed after oral administration.
Distribution: Widely distributed; crosses blood-brain barrier. Probably crosses the placenta and enters breast milk. Accumulation of drug occurs with chronic dosing.
Protein Binding: 96%.
Metabolism and Excretion: Metabolized by the liver.
Half-life: 10–20 hr.

TIME/ACTION PROFILE (sedation)

ROUTE	ONSET	PEAK	DURATION
PO	30 min	2–3 hr	6–8 hr

Contraindications/Precautions
Contraindicated in: Hypersensitivity; Cross-sensitivity with other benzodiazepines may exist; Pre-existing CNS depression; Severe uncontrolled pain; Angle-closure glaucoma; Impaired respiratory function; Sleep apnea; OB: Neonates born to mothers taking temazepam may experience withdrawal effects; Lactation: Infants may become sedated. Discontinue drug or bottle feed.
Use Cautiously in: Pre-existing hepatic dysfunction; History of suicide attempt or drug addiction; Geri: Elderly patients have increased sensitivity to benzodiazepines. Appears on Beers list and is associated with increased risk of falls (↓ dose required).

Adverse Reactions/Side Effects
CNS: abnormal thinking, behavior changes, hangover, dizziness, drowsiness, hallucinations, lethargy, paradoxic excitation, sleep—driving. **EENT:** blurred vision. **GI:** constipation, diarrhea, nausea, vomiting. **Derm:** rashes. **Misc:** physical dependence, psychological dependence, tolerance.

Interactions
Drug-Drug: ↑ CNS depression with **alcohol**, **antidepressants**, **antihistamines**, **opioid analgesics**, and other **sedative/hypnotics**. May ↓ efficacy of **levodopa**. **Rifampin** or **smoking** ↑ metabolism and may ↓ effectiveness of temazepam. **Probenecid** may prolong effects of temazepam. Sedative effects may be ↓ by **theophylline**.
Drug-Natural Products: Concomitant use of **kava-kava**, **valerian**, **skullcap**, **chamomile**, or **hops** can ↑ CNS depression.

Route/Dosage
PO (Adults): 15–30 mg at bedtime initially if needed; some patients may require only 7.5 mg.
PO (Geriatric Patients or Debilitated Patients): 7.5 mg at bedtime.

Availability (generic available)
Capsules: 7.5 mg, 15 mg, 22.5 mg, 30 mg.

NURSING IMPLICATIONS

Assessment
- Assess mental status (orientation, mood, behavior) and potential for abuse prior to administering medication.
- Assess sleep patterns before and periodically throughout therapy.
- Prolonged high-dose therapy may lead to psychological or physical dependence. Restrict amount of drug available to patient, especially if patient is depressed or suicidal or has a history of addiction.
- Geri: Assess CNS effects and risk of falls. Institute falls prevention strategies.

Potential Nursing Diagnoses
Insomnia (Indications)
Risk for falls (Side Effects)

Implementation
- Do not confuse temazepam with flurazepam.
- Supervise ambulation and transfer of patients after administration. Remove cigarettes. Side rails should be raised and call bell within reach at all times.
- PO: Administer with food if GI irritation becomes a problem.

Patient/Family Teaching
- Instruct patient to take temazepam as directed. Teach sleep hygiene techniques (dark room, quiet, bedtime ritual, limit daytime napping, avoidance of nicotine and caffeine). If less ef-

fective after a few weeks, consult health care professional; do not increase dose.
- May cause daytime drowsiness or dizziness. Caution patient to avoid driving or other activities requiring alertness until response to medication is known. Geri: Instruct patient and family how to reduce falls risk at home.
- Advise patient to avoid the use of alcohol and other CNS depressants and to consult health care professional before using OTC preparations that contain antihistamines or alcohol.
- Advise patient to inform health care professional if pregnancy is planned or suspected.
- Emphasize the importance of follow-up appointments to monitor progress.
- Refer for psychotherapy if ineffective coping is basis for sleep pattern disturbance.
- Advise patient to take temazepam only if able to devote 8 hr to sleep.

Evaluation/Desired Outcomes
- Improvement in sleep pattern with decreased number of nighttime awakenings, improved sleep onset, and increased total sleep time, which may not be noticeable until the 3rd day of therapy.

tenecteplase, See THROMBOLYTIC AGENTS.

tenofovir (te-noe-fo-veer)
Viread

Classification
Therapeutic: antiretrovirals
Pharmacologic: nucleoside reverse transcriptase inhibitors

Pregnancy Category B

Indications
HIV infection (with other antiretrovirals). Chronic hepatitis B.

Action
Active drug (tenofovir) is phosphorylated intracellularly; tenofovir diphosphate inhibits HIV reverse transcriptase resulting in disruption of DNA synthesis. **Therapeutic Effects:** Slowed progression of HIV infection and decreased occurrence of sequelae. Increased CD4 cell count and decreased viral load. Decreased progression/sequelae of chronic hepatitis B infection.

Pharmacokinetics
Absorption: Tenofovir disoproxil fumarate is a prodrug, which is split into tenofovir, the active component.
Distribution: Absorption is enhanced by food.
Metabolism and Excretion: 70–80% excreted unchanged in urine by glomerular filtration and active tubular secretion.
Half-life: Unknown.

TIME/ACTION PROFILE (blood levels)

ROUTE	ONSET	PEAK	DURATION
PO	unknown	2 hr*	24 hr

*When taken with food

Contraindications/Precautions
Contraindicated in: Hypersensitivity; Lactation: HIV-infected women should not breast-feed.
Use Cautiously in: Co-infection with HIV and chronic hepatitis B; Obesity, women, prolonged nucleoside exposure (may be risk factors for lactic acidosis/hepatomegaly); Renal impairment (use cautiously if CCr <60 mL/min); History of pathologic bone fractures or at risk for osteopenia; OB: Has been used safely; Pedi: Safety not established.

Adverse Reactions/Side Effects
CNS: depression, headache, weakness. **GI:** HEPATOMEGALY, (with steatosis), diarrhea, nausea, abdominal pain, anorexia, vomiting, flatulence. **GU:** renal impairment. **F and E:** LACTIC ACIDOSIS, hypophosphatemia. **Derm:** rash. **MS:** ↓ bone mineral density.

Interactions
Drug-Drug: Concurrent use with **didanosine** results in ↑ blood levels of didanosine (tenofovir should be given 2 hours before or 1 hour after didanosine). Blood levels may be ↑ by **cidofovir**, **acyclovir**, **ganciclovir**, or **valganciclovir**. Risk of renal toxicity ↑ by other **nephrotoxic agents**. Combination therapy with **atazanavir** may lead to ↓ virologic response and possible resistance to atazanavir (small amounts of **ritonavir** may be added to boost blood levels); may also ↑ tenofovir levels. **Lopinavir/ritonavir** may ↑ levels. Concurrent use with **adefovir** for chronic hepatitis B infection should be avoided.

Route/Dosage
PO (Adults): 300 mg once daily.

Renal Impairment
PO (Adults): *CCr 30–49 mL/min*—300 mg every 48 hr; *CCr 10–29 mL/min*—300 mg every

72–96 hr; *Hemodialysis patients*—300 mg every 7 days following dialysis.

Availability
Tablets: 300 mg. *In combination with:* emtricitabine (Truvada); efavirenz and emtricitabine (Atripla). See Appendix B.

NURSING IMPLICATIONS

Assessment
- Monitor for change in severity of HIV symptoms and for symptoms of opportunistic infection before and during therapy.
- Monitor bone mineral density in patients who have a history of pathologic bone fracture or are at risk for osteopenia.
- *Lab Test Considerations:* Monitor viral load and CD4 count before and routinely during therapy to determine response.
- Monitor liver function tests and hepatitis B virus levels throughout and following therapy. If therapy is discontinued, may cause severe exacerbation of hepatitis B. May cause ↑ AST, ALT, alkaline phosphatase, creatine kinase, amylase, and triglyceride concentrations. Lactic acidosis may occur with hepatic toxicity causing hepatic steatosis; may be fatal, especially in women.
- May cause hypophosphatemia in patients with renal impairment.
- May cause hyperglycemia and glucosuria.

Potential Nursing Diagnoses
Risk for infection (Indications, Side Effects)
Risk for injury (Side Effects)

Implementation
- When tenofovir is administered concomitantly with didanosine, administer tenofovir 2 hr before or 1 hr after didanosine.
- **PO:** Administer once daily with a meal.

Patient/Family Teaching
- Instruct patient on the importance of taking tenofovir as directed, even if feeling better. Do not take more than prescribed amount and do not stop taking without consulting health care professional. Discontinuing therapy may lead to severe exacerbations. Take missed doses as soon as remembered; do not double doses. Caution patient not to share or trade this medication with others.
- Inform patient that tenofovir may cause hyperglycemia. Advise patient to notify health care professional if increased thirst or hunger; unexplained weight loss; increased urination; fatigue; or dry, itchy skin occurs.
- Advise patient to avoid taking other Rx, OTC, or herbal products, without consulting health care professional.
- Caution patient to avoid crowds and persons with known infections.
- Inform patient that tenofovir does not cure AIDS and does not reduce the risk of transmission of HIV to others through sexual contact or blood contamination. Caution patient to use a condom and avoid sharing needles or donating blood to prevent spreading HIV to others.
- Advise patient to notify health care professional immediately if symptoms of lactic acidosis (nausea, vomiting, unusual or unexpected stomach discomfort, and weakness) occur.
- Inform patient that changes in body fat distribution (increased fat in upper back and neck, breast, and trunk, and loss of fat from legs, arms, and face) may occur, but may not be related to drug therapy.
- Emphasize the importance of regular exams to monitor for side effects.

Evaluation/Desired Outcomes
- Decreased incidence of opportunistic infection and slowed progression of HIV infection.

---

terazosin (ter-ay-zoe-sin)
Hytrin

Classification
Therapeutic: antihypertensives
Pharmacologic: peripherally acting antiadrenergics

Pregnancy Category C

Indications
Mild to moderate hypertension (alone or with other agents). Urinary outflow obstruction in patients with prostatic hyperplasia.

Action
Dilates both arteries and veins by blocking postsynaptic alpha$_1$-adrenergic receptors. Decreases contractions in smooth muscle of the prostatic capsule. **Therapeutic Effects:** Lowering of blood pressure. Decreased symptoms of prostatic hyperplasia (urinary urgency, hesitancy, nocturia).

Pharmacokinetics
Absorption: Well absorbed after oral administration.
Distribution: Unknown.
Metabolism and Excretion: 50% metabolized by the liver. 10% excreted unchanged by the kid-

neys. 20% excreted unchanged in feces. 40% eliminated in bile.
Half-life: 12 hr.

TIME/ACTION PROFILE

ROUTE	ONSET†	PEAK‡	DURATION†
PO-hypertension	15 min	6–8 wk	24 hr
PO-prostatic hyperplasia	2–6 wk	unknown	unknown

†After single dose
‡After multiple oral dosing

Contraindications/Precautions
Contraindicated in: Hypersensitivity.
Use Cautiously in: Deyhdration, volume or sodium depletion (↑ risk of hypotension); OB, Lactation: Pedi: Safety not established; Patients undergoing cataract surgery (↑ risk of intraoperative floppy iris syndrome).

Adverse Reactions/Side Effects
CNS: dizziness, headache, weakness, drowsiness, nervousness. **EENT:** nasal congestion, blurred vision, conjunctivitis, intraoperative floppy iris syndrome, sinusitis. **Resp:** dyspnea. **CV:** first-dose orthostatic hypotension, arrhythmias, chest pain, palpitations, peripheral edema, tachycardia. **GI:** nausea, abdominal pain, diarrhea, dry mouth, vomiting. **GU:** erectile dysfunction, urinary frequency. **Derm:** pruritus. **Metab:** weight gain. **MS:** arthralgia, back pain, extremity pain. **Neuro:** paresthesia. **Misc:** fever.

Interactions
Drug-Drug: ↑ risk of hypotension with **sildenafil**, **tadalafil**, **vardenafil**, other **antihypertensives**, **nitrates**, or acute ingestion of **alcohol**. **NSAIDs**, **sympathomimetics**, or **estrogens** may ↓ effects of antihypertensive therapy.

Route/Dosage
The first dose should be taken at bedtime.

Hypertension
PO (Adults): 1 mg initially, then slowly ↑ up to 5 mg/day (usual range 1–5 mg/day); may be given as single dose or in 2 divided doses (not to exceed 20 mg/day).

Benign Prostatic Hyperplasia
PO (Adults): 1 mg at bedtime; gradually may be ↑ up to 5–10 mg/day.

Availability (generic available)
Tablets: 1 mg, 2 mg, 5 mg, 10 mg. **Cost:** *Generic*—1 mg $33.98/90, 2 mg $33.99/90, 5 mg $33.99/90, 10 mg $33.99/90.

NURSING IMPLICATIONS
Assessment
- Assess for first-dose orthostatic reaction (dizziness, weakness) and syncope. May occur 30 min–2 hr after initial dose and occasionally thereafter. Incidence may be dose related. Volume-depleted or sodium-restricted patients may be more sensitive. Observe patient closely during this period; take precautions to prevent injury. First dose may be given at bedtime to minimize this reaction.
- Monitor intake and output ratios and daily weight; assess for edema daily, especially at beginning of therapy.
- **Hypertension:** Monitor blood pressure and pulse frequently during initial dosage adjustment and periodically throughout therapy. Report significant changes.
- Monitor frequency of prescription refills to determine adherence.
- **Benign Prostatic Hyperplasia:** Assess patient for symptoms of prostatic hyperplasia (urinary hesitancy, feeling of incomplete bladder emptying, interruption of urinary stream, impairment of size and force of urinary stream, terminal urinary dribbling, straining to start flow, dysuria, urgency) before and periodically during therapy.
- Rule out prostatic carcinoma before therapy; symptoms are similar.

Potential Nursing Diagnoses
Risk for injury (Side Effects)
Noncompliance (Patient/Family Teaching)

Implementation
- May be used in combination with diuretics or beta blockers to minimize sodium and water retention. If these are added to terazosin therapy, reduce dose of terazosin initially and titrate to effect.
- **PO:** Administer daily dose at bedtime. If necessary, dose may be increased to twice daily.

Patient/Family Teaching
- Instruct patient to take medication at the same time each day. Take missed doses as soon as remembered. If not remembered until next day, omit; do not double doses.

✽ = Canadian drug name.   = Genetic implication.
*CAPITALS indicates life-threatening; underlines indicate most frequent.

- Advise patient to weigh self twice weekly and assess feet and ankles for fluid retention.
- May cause dizziness or drowsiness. Advise patient to avoid driving or other activities requiring alertness until response to the medication is known.
- Caution patient to avoid sudden changes in position to decrease orthostatic hypotension. Alcohol, CNS depressants, standing for long periods, hot showers, and exercising in hot weather should be avoided because of enhanced orthostatic effects.
- Advise patient to consult health care professional before taking any cough, cold, or allergy remedies.
- Instruct patient to notify health care professional of medication regimen before any surgery.
- Advise patient to notify health care professional if frequent dizziness, fainting, or swelling of feet or lower legs occurs.
- Emphasize the importance of follow-up exams to evaluate effectiveness of medication.
- **Hypertension:** Emphasize the importance of continuing to take this medication as directed, even if feeling well. Medication controls but does not cure hypertension.
- Encourage patient to comply with additional interventions for hypertension (weight reduction, low-sodium diet, smoking cessation, moderation of alcohol consumption, regular exercise, and stress management).
- Instruct patient and family on proper technique for blood pressure monitoring. Advise them to check blood pressure at least weekly and to report significant changes.

Evaluation/Desired Outcomes
- Decrease in blood pressure without appearance of side effects.
- Decreased symptoms of prostatic hyperplasia. May require 2–6 wk of therapy before effects are noticeable.

---

terbinafine (ter-bi-na-feen)
Lamisil

Classification
Therapeutic: antifungals (systemic)

Pregnancy Category B
For topical use, refer to Antifungals, Topical monograph

Indications
Onychomycosis (fungal nail infection). Tinea capitis.

Action
Interferes with fungal cell wall synthesis (ergosterol biosynthesis) by inhibiting the enzyme squalene epoxidase. **Therapeutic Effects:** Fungal cell death. **Spectrum:** Active against dermatophytes and other fungi.

Pharmacokinetics
Absorption: 70–80% absorbed after oral administration.
Distribution: Extensively distributed; penetrates dermis and epidermis; concentrates in stratum corneum, hair, scalp, and nails. Enters breast milk.
Protein Binding: 99%.
Metabolism and Excretion: Extensively metabolized by the liver.
Half-life: *Plasma*—22 days; longer from skin and nails.

TIME/ACTION PROFILE (antifungal tissue levels)

ROUTE	ONSET	PEAK	DURATION
PO	several days	days–wk	several wk

Contraindications/Precautions
Contraindicated in: Hypersensitivity; Chronic or active liver disease; CHF or left ventricular dysfunction.
Use Cautiously in: History of alcoholism; Renal impairment (dose ↓ recommended for CCr <50 mL/min); OB: Lactation: Safety not established.

Adverse Reactions/Side Effects
CNS: headache. **Resp:** cough, nasopharyngitis. **CV:** CHF. **GI:** HEPATOTOXICITY, anorexia, diarrhea, nausea, stomach pain, vomiting, altered taste, drug-induced hepatitis, taste disturbance. **Derm:** TOXIC EPIDERMAL NECROLYSIS, itching, rash. **Hemat:** neutropenia, pancytopenia. **Misc:** STEVENS-JOHNSON SYNDROME, pyrexia.

Interactions
Drug-Drug: Alcohol or other **hepatotoxic agents** may ↑ risk of hepatotoxicity. **Rifampin** and other **drugs that induce hepatic drug-metabolizing enzymes** may ↓ effectiveness. **Cimetidine** and other **drugs that inhibit hepatic drug-metabolizing enzymes** may ↑ effectiveness.
Drug-Natural Products: ↑ **caffeine** levels and side effects with caffeine-containing herbs (**cola nut**, **guarana**, **mate**, **tea**, **coffee**).

Route/Dosage
PO (Adults): 250 mg once daily for 6 wk for fingernail infection or 12 wk for toenail infection.

PO (Children ≥4 yr—≥35 kg): 250 mg/day for 6 wk.
PO (Children ≥4 yr—25–35 kg): 187.5 mg/day for 6 wk.
PO (Children ≥4 yr—<25 kg): 125 mg/day for 6 wk.

Availability (generic available)
Tablets: 250 mg. **Cost:** *Generic*—$140.99/90.
Oral granules: 125 mg packets, 187.5 mg packets.

NURSING IMPLICATIONS
Assessment
- Assess for signs and symptoms of infection (nail beds, scalp) before and periodically throughout therapy.
- Specimens for culture should be taken before instituting therapy. Therapy may be started before results are obtained.
- Monitor for skin rash. If progressive skin rash occurs, discontinue terbinafine.
- *Lab Test Considerations:* CBC should be monitored in patients receiving therapy for >6 wk. Discontinue if abnormal values occur.
- Monitor AST and ALT prior to, and periodically throughout, therapy. Terbinafine should be discontinued if symptomatic elevations occur.
- If signs of secondary infection occur, monitor neutrophil count. If <1000/mm³, discontinue treatment.
- May cause ↓ absolute lymphocyte count.
- Monitor serum potassium. May cause hypokalemia.

Potential Nursing Diagnoses
Risk for infection (Indications)
Noncompliance (Patient/Family Teaching)

Implementation
- Do not confuse with lamotrigine (Lamictal).
- **PO:** May be administered without regard to food.
- *Oral granules* should be taken with food and may be sprinkled on a spoonful of pudding or other soft, nonacidic food, such as mashed potatoes and swallowed in entirety. Applesauce or fruit-based foods should not be used.

Patient/Family Teaching
- Instruct patient to take medication as directed, for the full course of therapy, even if feeling better. Doses should be taken at the same time each day.
- Instruct patient to notify health care professional immediately if signs and symptoms of liver dysfunction (unusual fatigue, anorexia, nausea, vomiting, upper right abdominal pain, jaundice, dark urine, or pale stools) or rash occur. Terbinafine should be discontinued.
- Advise patient to consult health care professional before taking any Rx or OTC medications concurrently with terbinafine.

Evaluation/Desired Outcomes
- Resolution of clinical and laboratory indications of fungal nail infections. Inadequate period of treatment may lead to recurrence of active infection.
- Resolution of tinea capitis infection.

---

terbinafine, See ANTIFUNGALS (TOPICAL).

---

terbutaline (ter-byoo-ta-leen)

Classification
Therapeutic: bronchodilators
Pharmacologic: adrenergics

Pregnancy Category B

Indications
Management of reversible airway disease due to asthma or COPD; inhalation and subcut used for short-term control and oral agent as long-term control. **Unlabeled Use:** Management of preterm labor (tocolytic).

Action
Results in the accumulation of cyclic adenosine monophosphate (cAMP) at beta-adrenergic receptors. Produces bronchodilation. Inhibits the release of mediators of immediate hypersensitivity reactions from mast cells. Relatively selective for beta$_2$(pulmonary)-adrenergic receptor sites, with less effect on beta$_1$(cardiac)-adrenergic receptors. **Therapeutic Effects:** Bronchodilation.

Pharmacokinetics
Absorption: 35–50% absorbed following oral administration but rapidly undergoes first-pass metabolism. Well absorbed following subcut administration.
Distribution: Enters breast milk.
Metabolism and Excretion: Partially metabolized by the liver; 60% excreted unchanged by the kidneys following subcut administration.

✦ = Canadian drug name.   ▪ = Genetic implication.
*CAPITALS indicates life-threatening; underlines indicate most frequent.

terbutaline

Half-life: Unknown.

TIME/ACTION PROFILE (bronchodilation)

ROUTE	ONSET	PEAK	DURATION
PO	within 60–120 min	within 2–3 hr	4–8 hr
Subcut	within 15 min	within 0.5–1 hr	1.5–4 hr

Contraindications/Precautions
Contraindicated in: Hypersensitivity to adrenergic amines.
Use Cautiously in: Cardiac disease; Hypertension; Hyperthyroidism; Diabetes; Glaucoma; Geri: More susceptible to adverse reactions; may require dose ↓; Excessive use may lead to tolerance and paradoxical bronchospasm (inhaler); OB, Lactation: Pregnancy (near term) and lactation.

Adverse Reactions/Side Effects
CNS: nervousness, restlessness, tremor, headache, insomnia. **CV:** angina, arrhythmias, hypertension, tachycardia. **GI:** nausea, vomiting. **Endo:** hyperglycemia.

Interactions
Drug-Drug: Concurrent use with other **adrenergics** (sympathomimetic) will have additive adrenergic side effects. Use with **MAO inhibitors** may lead to hypertensive crisis. **Beta blockers** may negate therapeutic effect.
Drug-Natural Products: Use with caffeine-containing herbs (**cola nut**, **guarana**, **mate**, **tea**, **coffee**) ↑ stimulant effect.

Route/Dosage
PO (Adults and Children >15 yr): *Bronchodilation*—2.5–5 mg 3 times daily, given q 6 hr (not to exceed 15 mg/24 hr). *Tocolysis*—2.5–10 mg q 4–6 hr until delivery (unlabeled).

PO (Children 12–15 yr): *Bronchodilation*—2.5 mg 3 times daily (given q 6 hr) (not to exceed 7.5 mg/24 hr).

PO (Children <12 yr): *Bronchodilation*—0.05 mg/kg 3 times daily; may ↑ gradually (not to exceed 0.15 mg/kg 3–4 times daily or 5 mg/24 hr.

Subcut (Adults and Children ≥12 yr): *Bronchodilation*—250 mcg; may repeat in 15–30 min (not to exceed 500 mcg/4 hr).

Subcut (Children <12 yr): *Bronchodilation*—0.005–0.01 mg/kg; may repeat in 15–20 min.

IV (Adults): *Tocolysis*—2.5–10 mcg/min infusion; ↑ by 5 mcg/min q 10 min until contractions stop (not to exceed 30 mcg/min). After contractions have stopped for 30 min, ↓ infusion rate to lowest effective amount and maintain for 4–8 hr (unlabeled).

Availability (generic available)
Tablets: 2.5 mg, 5 mg. **Injection:** 1 mg/mL.

NURSING IMPLICATIONS
Assessment
- **Bronchodilator:** Assess lung sounds, respiratory pattern, pulse, and blood pressure before administration and during peak of medication. Note amount, color, and character of sputum produced, and notify health care professional of abnormal findings.
- Monitor pulmonary function tests before initiating therapy and periodically throughout therapy to determine effectiveness of medication.
- **Preterm Labor:** Monitor maternal pulse and blood pressure, frequency and duration of contractions, and fetal heart rate. Notify health care professional if contractions persist or increase in frequency or duration or if symptoms of maternal or fetal distress occur. Maternal side effects include tachycardia, palpitations, tremor, anxiety, and headache.
- Assess maternal respiratory status for symptoms of pulmonary edema (increased rate, dyspnea, rales/crackles, frothy sputum).
- Monitor mother and neonate for symptoms of hypoglycemia (anxiety; chills; cold sweats; confusion; cool, pale skin; difficulty in concentration; drowsiness; excessive hunger; headache; irritability; nausea; nervousness; rapid pulse; shakiness; unusual tiredness; or weakness) and mother for hypokalemia (weakness, fatigue, U wave on ECG, arrhythmias).
- **Lab Test Considerations:** May cause transient ↓ in serum potassium concentrations with higher than recommended doses.
- Monitor maternal serum glucose and electrolytes. May cause hypokalemia and hypoglycemia. Monitor neonate's serum glucose, because hypoglycemia may also occur in neonates.
- *Toxicity and Overdose:* Symptoms of overdose include persistent agitation, chest pain or discomfort, decreased blood pressure, dizziness, hyperglycemia, hypokalemia, seizures, tachyarrhythmias, persistent trembling, and vomiting.
- Treatment includes discontinuing beta-adrenergic agonists and symptomatic, supportive therapy. Cardioselective beta blockers are used cautiously, because they may induce bronchospasm.

Potential Nursing Diagnoses
Ineffective airway clearance (Indications)

Implementation
- **PO:** Administer with meals to minimize gastric irritation.
- Tablet may be crushed and mixed with food or fluids for patients with difficulty swallowing.
- **Subcut:** Administer subcut injections in lateral deltoid area. Do not use solution if discolored.

IV Administration
- **Continuous Infusion:** *Diluent:* May be diluted in D5W, 0.9% NaCl, or 0.45% NaCl. *Concentration:* 1 mg/mL (undiluted). *Rate:* Use infusion pump to ensure accurate dose. Begin infusion at 10 mcg/min. Increase dosage by 5 mcg every 10 min until contractions cease. Maximum dose is 80 mcg/min. Begin to taper dose in 5-mcg decrements after a 30–60 min contraction-free period is attained. Switch to oral dose form after patient is contraction-free 4–8 hr on the lowest effective dose.
- **Y-Site Compatibility:** insulin.

Patient/Family Teaching
- Instruct patient to take medication as directed. If on a scheduled dosing regimen, take a missed dose as soon as possible; space remaining doses at regular intervals. Do not double doses. Caution patient not to exceed recommended dose; may cause adverse effects, paradoxical bronchospasm, or loss of effectiveness of medication.
- Instruct patient to contact health care professional immediately if shortness of breath is not relieved by medication or is accompanied by diaphoresis, dizziness, palpitations, or chest pain.
- Advise patient to consult health care professional before taking any OTC medications or alcoholic beverages concurrently with this therapy. Caution patient also to avoid smoking and other respiratory irritants.
- **Preterm Labor:** Notify health care professional immediately if labor resumes or if significant side effects occur.

Evaluation/Desired Outcomes
- Prevention or relief of bronchospasm.
- Increase in ease of breathing.
- Control of preterm labor in a fetus of 20–36 wk gestational age.

---

terconazole, See ANTIFUNGALS (VAGINAL).

---

teriparatide (ter-i-**par**-a-tide)
Forteo

Classification
Therapeutic: hormones
Pharmacologic: parathyroid hormones (rDNA origin)

Pregnancy Category C

Indications
Treatment of osteoporosis in postmenopausal women at high risk for fractures. To increase bone mass in men with primary or hypogonadal osteoporosis at high risk for fractures. Treatment of osteoporosis in men and women with glucocorticoid-induced osteoporosis at high risk for fractures. Most useful for those have failed or are intolerant to other osteoporosis therapies.

Action
Regulates calcium and phosphate metabolism in bone and kidney by binding to specific cell receptors; stimulates osteoblastic activity. Increases serum calcium and decreases serum phosphorus. **Therapeutic Effects:** Increased bone mineral density with reduced risk of fractures.

Pharmacokinetics
Absorption: Extensively absorbed after subcut administration.
Distribution: Unknown.
Metabolism and Excretion: Metabolized by the liver; metabolites renally excreted.
Half-life: 1 hr (after subcut use).

TIME/ACTION PROFILE (effects on serum calcium)

ROUTE	ONSET	PEAK	DURATION
Subcut	2 hr	4–6 hr	16–24 hr

Contraindications/Precautions
Contraindicated in: Hypersensitivity; Paget's disease of the bone or other metabolic bone disease; Unexplained ↑ alkaline phosphatase; Pedi: Safety and efficacy not established; Previous radiation therapy, history of bone metastases, or skeletal malignancy; Pre-existing hypercalcemia; OB: Lactation: Pregnancy or lactation.
Use Cautiously in: Active or recent urolithiasis.

Adverse Reactions/Side Effects
CV: orthostatic hypotension. **MS:** muscle spasms.

Interactions
Drug-Drug: Transient hypercalcemia may ↑ the risk of **digoxin** toxicity.

Route/Dosage
Subcut (Adults): 20 mcg once daily.

Availability
Pre-filled pen delivery device (FORTEO pen): delivers 20 mcg/day.

NURSING IMPLICATIONS

Assessment
- Assess patient for bone mineral density before and periodically during therapy.
- *Lab Test Considerations:* Effects increase serum calcium and decrease serum phosphorus. Maximum effect is within 4–6 hr. By 16-hr post-dose, serum calcium has returned to near baseline. If hypercalcemia persists, discontinue teriparatide and evaluate cause of hypercalcemia.
- May asymptomatically increase serum uric acid concentrations.

Potential Nursing Diagnoses
Risk for injury (Indications)

Implementation
- Use of teriparatide should not continue more than 2 yr.
- **Subcut:** Administer subcut into thigh or abdominal wall once daily. May be administered at any time of day without regard to food. Solution should be clear and colorless. Do not use if solid particles appear, or if solution is cloudy or colored. Store pen in the refrigerator; do not freeze or use if it has been frozen. Minimize time out of refrigerator; use immediately and return to refrigerator. *Forteo* pen can be used for up to 28 days after the first injection. After the 28-day use period, discard the *Forteo* pen, even if it still contains some unused solution.

Patient/Family Teaching
- Advise patient to administer medication at same time each day. Administer missed doses as soon as remembered that day. Do not take more than one injection/day.
- Instruct patient on proper administration technique and disposal of needles. Patient should read *Medication Guide* and *User Manual* before starting therapy and re-read them each time prescription is refilled. User manual can be found at www.forteo.com/control/pen_user_manual. Caution patient to throw pen away after 28-day use period and not to share their pen with other patients.
- Discuss the importance of other treatments for osteoporosis (supplemental calcium and/or vitamin D, weight-bearing exercise, modification of behavioral factors such as smoking and/or alcohol consumption).
- May cause orthostatic hypotension during first several doses. Caution patient to administer medication in a lying or sitting position. If lightheadedness or palpitations occur, lie down until symptoms resolve. Notify health care professional if symptoms persist or worsen.
- Instruct patient to notify health care professional if persistent symptoms of hypercalcemia (nausea, vomiting, constipation, lethargy, muscle weakness) occur.
- Emphasize the importance of follow-up tests for bone mineral density.

Evaluation/Desired Outcomes
- Increased bone mineral density with reduced risk of fractures.

TESTOSTERONE
(tess-**toss**-te-rone)

testosterone buccal system, mucoadhesive
Striant

testosterone cypionate
Depo-Testosterone

testosterone enanthate
Delatestryl

testosterone pellets
Testopel

testosterone transdermal
Androderm

Classification
Therapeutic: hormones
Pharmacologic: androgens

Schedule III

Pregnancy Category X

Indications
Hypogonadism in androgen-deficient men. Delayed puberty in men (enanthate and pellets). Androgen-responsive breast cancer in post-menopausal women (palliative) (enanthate).

Action
Responsible for the normal growth and development of male sex organs. Maintenance of male

TESTOSTERONE 1201

secondary sex characteristics: Growth and maturation of the prostate, seminal vesicles, penis, scrotum, Development of male hair distribution, Vocal cord thickening, Alterations in body musculature and fat distribution. **Therapeutic Effects:** Correction of hormone deficiency in male hypogonadism: Initiation of male puberty. Suppression of tumor growth in some forms of breast cancer.

Pharmacokinetics

Absorption: Well absorbed from IM sites, through buccal mucosa, or through skin. Cypionate and enanthate salts are absorbed slowly.
Distribution: Cross the placenta.
Protein Binding: 98%.
Metabolism and Excretion: Metabolized by the liver. Absorption from buccal mucosa bypasses initial liver metabolism. 90% eliminated in urine as metabolites.
Half-life: *Buccal, enanthate, pellets*—10–100 min; *transdermal*—70 min; *cypionate*—8 days.

TIME/ACTION PROFILE (androgenic effects†)

ROUTE	ONSET	PEAK	DURATION
IM—cypionate, enanthate	unknown	unknown	2–4 wk
IM—propionate	unknown	unknown	1–3 days
Buccal	unknown	10–12 hr	12 hr
Pellets	unknown	unknown	3–6 mo
Transdermal	unknown	6–8 hr‡	24 hr§

†Response is highly variable among individuals; may take months
‡Plasma testosterone levels following applications of patch
§Following patch removal

Contraindications/Precautions

Contraindicated in: Hypersensitivity; Male patients with breast or prostate cancer; Severe liver, renal, or cardiac disease (propionate); Some products contain benzyl alcohol and should be avoided in patients with known hypersensitivity; Women (buccal, pellets, patch); OB, Lactation: Pregnancy or lactation.
Use Cautiously in: Diabetes mellitus; Coronary artery disease (enanthate); Pre-existing cardiac, renal, or liver disease; Benign prostatic hyperplasia (cypionate, pellets); Hypercalcemia (cypionate, enanthate, pellets); Sleep apnea (buccal); Obesity (buccal); Chronic lung disease (buccal); Pedi: Prepubertal males exposed to testosterone may experience premature development of secondary sexual characteristics, aggression, and other side effects; Geri: ↑ risk of prostatic hyperplasia/carcinoma.

Adverse Reactions/Side Effects

CNS: anxiety, confusion, depression, fatigue, headache, vertigo. **EENT:** deepening of voice. **CV:** edema. **GI:** abdominal cramps, changes in appetite, drug-induced hepatitis, nausea, vomiting; *buccal*-, bitter taste, ginigivitis, gum edema, gum tenderness. **GU:** menstrual irregularities, prostatic enlargement. **Endo:** *women*—change in libido, clitoral enlargement, ↓ breast size; *men*, acne, facial hair, gynecomastia, erectile dysfunction, oligospermia, priapism. **F and E:** hypercalcemia, hyperkalemia, hyperphosphatemia. **Derm:** male pattern baldness. **Local:** chronic skin irritation (transdermal), pain at injection/implantation site.

Interactions

Drug-Drug: May ↑ action of **warfarin**, **oral hypoglycemic agents**, and **insulin**. Concurrent use with **corticosteroids** may ↑ risk of edema formation.

Route/Dosage

Replacement Therapy

IM (Adults): 50–400 mg q 2–4 wk (enanthate or cypionate).
Transdermal (Adults): 5 mg applied q 24 hr (preferably in the evening); dosing range = 2.5–7.5 mg/day.
Buccal (Adults): 30 mg (one system) applied to gum region twice daily (in the morning and evening, spaced 12 hr apart).
Subcut (for subcutaneous implantation) (pellets) (Adults): 150–450 mg q 3–6 mo.

Delayed Male Puberty

IM (Children): 50–200 mg q 2–4 wk for up to 6 mo (enanthate).
Subcut (for subcutaneous implantation) (pellets) (Children): 150–450 mg q 3–6 mo.

Palliative Management of Breast Cancer

IM (Adults): 200–400 mg q 2–4 wk (enanthate).

Availability (generic available)

Testosterone cypionate injection (in oil): 100 mg/mL, 200 mg/mL. **Testosterone enanthate injection (in oil):** 200 mg/mL. **Testosterone transdermal patches:** 2.5 mg/day in packages of 60, 5 mg/day in packages of 60. **Testosterone buccal, mucoadhesive:** 30 mg/system in blister packs of 10 systems/pack. **Testosterone pellets:** 75 mg.

NURSING IMPLICATIONS
Assessment
- Monitor intake and output ratios, weigh patient twice weekly, and assess patient for edema. Report significant changes indicative of fluid retention.
- **Men:** Monitor for precocious puberty in boys (acne, darkening of skin, development of male secondary sex characteristics—increase in penis size, frequent erections, growth of body hair). Bone age determinations should be measured every 6 months to determine rate of bone maturation and effects on epiphyseal closure.
- Monitor for breast enlargement, persistent erections, and increased urge to urinate in men. Monitor for difficulty urinating in elderly men, because prostate enlargement may occur.
- **Women:** Assess for virilism (deepening of voice, unusual hair growth or loss, clitoral enlargement, acne, menstrual irregularity).
- In women with metastatic breast cancer, monitor for symptoms of hypercalcemia (nausea, vomiting, constipation, lethargy, loss of muscle tone, thirst, polyuria).
- *Lab Test Considerations:* Monitor hemoglobin and hematocrit periodically during therapy; may cause polycythemia.
- Monitor hepatic function tests, prostate specific antigen and serum cholesterol levels periodically during therapy. May cause ↑ serum AST, ALT, and bilirubin, ↑ cholesterol levels, and suppress clotting factors II, V, VII, and X.
- Monitor serum and urine calcium levels and serum alkaline phosphatase concentrations in women with metastatic breast cancer.
- Monitor serum sodium, chloride, potassium, and phosphate concentrations (may be ↑).
- Monitor blood glucose closely in patients with diabetes who are receiving oral hypoglycemic agents or insulin.
- *Transdermal:* Monitor serum testosterone concentrations 3–4 wk after starting therapy; these concentrations should be obtained in the morning (following application of patch during previous evening).
- *Buccal:* Monitor serum testosterone concentrations 4–12 wk after starting therapy.

Potential Nursing Diagnoses
Sexual dysfunction (Indications, Side Effects)

Implementation
- Do not confuse Virilon (testosterone) with Verelan (verapamil).
- Range-of-motion exercises should be done with all bedridden patients to prevent mobilization of calcium from the bone.
- **IM:** Administer IM deep into gluteal muscle. Crystals may form when vials are stored at low temperatures; warming and shaking vial will redissolve crystals. Use of a wet syringe or needle may cause solution to become cloudy but will not affect its potency.
- **Subcut:** Pellets are to be implanted subcutaneously by a health care professional.
- **Transdermal:** Apply patch to clean, dry, hairless skin on the back, abdomen, upper arms, or thighs. Do not apply to the scrotum. Also avoid application over bony prominences or a part of the body that may be subject to prolonged pressure during sleep or sitting. The patch does not need to be removed while swimming or taking a shower or bath.
- The sites of application should be rotated; once a patch is removed, the same site should not be used again for at least 1 wk.
- If skin irritation occurs, apply a small amount of OTC topical hydrocortisone cream after system removal or a small amount of 0.1% triamcinolone cream may be applied to the skin under the central drug reservoir of the Androderm system without affecting the absorption of testosterone. Ointment formulations should not be used for pretreatment because they may significantly reduce testosterone absorption.
- Patch should be removed if undergoing a magnetic resonance imaging (MRI) scan. The system contains aluminum and may predispose the patient to skin burns during the test.
- **Buccal:** Apply to gum region twice daily (about 12 hr apart), rotating sides with each dose.

Patient/Family Teaching
- Advise patient to report the following signs and symptoms promptly: in male patients, priapism (sustained and often painful erections) difficulty urinating, or gynecomastia; in female patients, virilism (which may be reversible if medication is stopped as soon as changes are noticed), or hypercalcemia (nausea, vomiting, constipation, and weakness); in male or female patients, edema (unexpected weight gain, swelling of feet), hepatitis (yellowing of skin or eyes and abdominal pain), or unusual bleeding or bruising.
- Explain rationale for prohibiting use of testosterone for increasing athletic performance. Testosterone is neither safe nor effective for

this use and has a potential risk of serious side effects.
- Instruct females to notify health care professional immediately if pregnancy is planned or suspected.
- Advise diabetic patients to monitor blood closely for alterations in blood glucose concentrations.
- Emphasize the importance of regular follow-up physical exams, lab tests, and x-ray exams to monitor progress.
- Radiologic bone age determinations should be evaluated every 6 mo in prepubertal children to determine rate of bone maturation and effects on epiphyseal centers.
- **Transdermal:** Advise patient to notify health care professional if their female sexual partner develops signs/symptoms of virilization (e.g. change in body hair distribution, significant increase in acne, deepening of voice, menstrual irregularities).
- Instruct patient that the protective plastic liner must be removed before applying the patch.
- Instruct patient to apply patch to a clean, dry area of skin on back, abdomen, upper arms, or thighs. The patch should not be applied to their genitals or over bony areas (e.g., upper shoulders or upper hip).
- Instruct patient to rotate the sites of application. Once a patch is removed, the site should not be used again for at least 1 week.
- Advise patient that the patch does not need to be removed while showering, bathing, or swimming.
- Advise patient that the patch should be removed prior to undergoing an MRI scan.
- If a patch falls off before noon, advise patient to replace it with a fresh patch which should be worn until a new patch is applied in the evening. If a patch falls off after noon, advise patient that it does not need to be replaced until a fresh patch is applied in the evening.
- **Buccal:** Instruct patient to place the rounded side surface of the buccal system in a comfortable position against the gum just above incisor tooth. Hold the system firmly in place with a finger over the lip and against the product for 30 seconds to ensure adhesion. Buccal system is designed to stay in position until removed; if it fails to adhere to the gum or falls off within the first 8 hr after application, remove original system and apply a new one (this counts as replacing the first dose; apply the next system ~12 hr after the original system was applied). If the buccal system falls off after 8 hr but before 12 hr, replace the original system (this replacement can serve as the second dose for that day).
- Advise patient to avoid dislodging buccal system and to check on placement after toothbrushing, use of mouthwash, eating or drinking. Do not chew or swallow buccal system. To remove, slide system downwards from gum toward tooth to avoid scratching the gum.

Evaluation/Desired Outcomes
- Resolution of the signs of androgen deficiency without side effects. Therapy is usually limited to 3–6 months followed by bone growth or maturation determinations.
- Decrease in the size and spread of breast malignancy in postmenopausal women. In antineoplastic therapy, response may require 3 months of therapy; if signs of disease progression appear, therapy should be discontinued.

tetracycline, See TETRACYCLINES.

TETRACYCLINES

doxycycline (dox-i-**sye**-kleen)
Adoxa, ✶Apo-Doxy, Doryx, Doxy, ✶Doxycin, ✶Doxytab, Monodox, ✶Novodoxylin, ✶Nu-Doxycycline, Oracea, Periostat, ✶PHL-Doxycycline, ✶PMS-Doxycycline, ✶Ratio-Doxycycline, Vibramycin, Vibra-Tabs

minocycline (min-oh-**sye**-kleen)
✶Apo-Minocycline, ✶DOM-Minocycline, Dynacin, ✶Enca, ✶Gen-Minocycline, Minocin, ✶Novo-Minocycline, ✶PMS-Minocycline, ✶Ratio-Minocycline, ✶Riva-Minocycline, Solodyn

tetracycline (te-tra-**sye**-kleen)
Sumycin

Classification
Therapeutic: anti-infectives
Pharmacologic: tetracyclines

Pregnancy Category D

Indications
Treatment of various infections caused by unusual organisms, including: *Mycoplasma, Chlamydia, Rickettsia, Borellia burgdorferi*. Treatment of gonorrhea and syphilis in penicillin-allergic patients. Prevention of exacerbations of chronic bronchitis. Treatment of inhalational anthrax (postexposure) and cutaneous anthrax (doxycycline only). Treatment of acne.

Action
Inhibits bacterial protein synthesis at the level of the 30S bacterial ribosome. **Therapeutic Effects:** Bacteriostatic action against susceptible bacteria. **Spectrum:** Includes activity against some gram-positive pathogens: *Bacillus anthracis, Clostridium perfringens, Clostridium tetani, Listeria monocytogenes, Nocardia, Propionibacterium acnes, Actinomyces israelii*. Active against some gram-negative pathogens: *Haemophilus influenzae, Legionella pneumophila, Yersinia enterocolitica, Yersinia pestis, Neisseria gonorrhoeae, Neisseria meningitidis*. Also active against several other pathogens, including: *Mycoplasma, Treponema pallidum, Chlamydia, Rickettsia, B. burgdorferi*.

Pharmacokinetics
Absorption: *Tetracycline*—60–80% absorbed following oral administration. *Doxycycline, minocycline*—well absorbed from the GI tract.
Distribution: Widely distributed, some penetration into CSF; cross the placenta and enter breast milk.
Metabolism and Excretion: *Doxycycline*—20–40% excreted unchanged by the urine; some inactivation in the intestine and some enterohepatic circulation with excretion in bile and feces. *Minocycline*—5–20% excreted unchanged by the urine; some metabolism by the liver with enterohepatic circulation and excretion in bile and feces. *Tetracycline*—Excreted mostly unchanged by the kidneys.
Half-life: *Doxycycline*—14–17 hr (↑ in severe renal impairment). *Minocycline*—11–26 hr. *Tetracycline*—6–12 hr.

TIME/ACTION PROFILE (blood levels)

ROUTE	ONSET	PEAK	DURATION
Doxycycline-PO	1–2 hr	1.5–4 hr	12 hr
Doxycycline-IV	rapid	end of infusion	12 hr
Minocycline-PO	rapid	2–3 hr	6–12 hr
Minocycline-PO extended-release	unknown	3.5–4 hr	24 hr
Tetracycline-PO	1–2 hr	2–4 hr	6–12 hr

Contraindications/Precautions
Contraindicated in: Hypersensitivity; Some products contain alcohol or bisulfites; avoid in patients with known hypersensitivity or intolerance; OB: Risk of permanent staining of teeth in infant if used during last half of pregnancy; Lactation: Lactation; Pedi: Children <8 yr (permanent staining of teeth); OB, Lactation: Pedi: Can be used in children and pregnant and lactating women for the treatment of anthrax (doxycycline only); Some products contain alcohol or bisulfites; avoid in patients with known hypersensitivity or intolerance; OB: Risk of permanent staining of teeth in infant if used during last half of pregnancy; Lactation: Lactation; Pedi: Children <8 yr (permanent staining of teeth); OB, Lactation: Pedi: Can be used in children and pregnant and lactating women for the treatment of anthrax (doxycycline only).
Use Cautiously in: Cachectic or debilitated patients; Renal disease; Hepatic impairment (doxycycline, minocycline); Nephrogenic diabetes insipidus.

Adverse Reactions/Side Effects
CNS: benign intracranial hypertension (higher in children); *minocycline*, dizziness. **EENT:** *minocycline*, vestibular reactions. **GI:** PSEUDOMEMBRANOUS COLITIS, diarrhea, nausea, vomiting, esophagitis, hepatotoxicity, pancreatitis. **Derm:** photosensitivity, rashes; *minocycline*, pigmentation of skin and mucous membranes. **Hemat:** blood dyscrasias. **Endo:** *minocycline*—thyroid disorders. **MS:** *minocycline*—lupus-like syndrome. **Local:** *doxycycline, minocycline*—phlebitis at IV site. **Misc:** hypersensitivity reactions, superinfection.

Interactions
Drug-Drug: May ↑ effect of **warfarin**. May ↓ effectiveness of **estrogen-containing hormonal contraceptives**. **Antacids, calcium, iron, zinc, aluminum,** and **magnesium** form insoluble compounds (chelates) and ↓ absorption of tetracyclines. **Sucralfate** may bind to tetracycline and ↓ its absorption from the GI tract. **Cholestyramine** or **colestipol** ↓ oral absorption of tetracyclines. **Adsorbent antidiarrheals** may ↓ absorption of tetracyclines. **Barbiturates, carbamazepine,** or **phenytoin** may ↓ activity of doxycycline.

TETRACYCLINES 1205

Drug-Food: Calcium in foods or **dairy products** ↓ absorption by forming insoluble compounds (chelates).

Route/Dosage
Doxycycline
PO (Adults and Children >8 yr and >45 kg): *Most infections*— 100 mg q 12 hr on the 1st day, then 100–200 mg once daily or 50–100 mg q 12 hr. *Gonorrhea*— 100 mg q 12 hr for 7 days or 300 mg followed 1 hr later by another 300-mg dose. *Malaria prophylaxis*— 100 mg once daily. *Lyme disease*— 100 mg twice daily. *Periodontitis*— 20 mg twice daily. *Anthrax*— 100 mg twice daily for 60 days.

PO (Children >8 yr and ≤45 kg): *Most infections*— 2–5 mg/kg/day in 1–2 divided doses (not to exceed 200 mg/day).

IV (Adults and Children >8 yr and >45 kg): 200 mg once daily or 100 mg q 12 hr on the 1st day, then 100–200 mg once daily or 50–100 mg q 12 hr. *Anthrax*— 100 mg q 12 hr change to oral when appropriate, for 60 days.

IV (Children >8 yr and ≤45 kg or ≤8 yr): 4.4 mg/kg once daily or 2.2 mg/kg q 12 hr on the 1st day, then 2.2–4.4 mg/kg/day given once daily or 1.1–2.2 mg/kg q 12 hr. *Anthrax*— 2.2 mg/kg q 12 hr, change to oral when appropriate, for 60 days.

Minocycline
Immediate-Release
PO (Adults): 100–200 mg initially, then 100 mg q 12 hr or 50 mg q 6 hr.

PO (Children ≥8 yr): 4 mg/kg initially, then 2 mg/kg q 12 hr.

Extended-Release
PO (Adults and Children ≥12 yr): *91–136 kg*— 135 mg once daily for 12 wk. *60–90 kg*-90 mg once daily for 12 wk. *45–59 kg*-45 mg once daily for 12 wk.

Tetracycline
PO (Adults): 250–500 mg q 6 hr or 500 mg–1 g q 12 hr. *Chronic treatment of acne*— 500 mg–2 g/day for 3 wk, then ↓ to 125 mg–1 g/day.

PO (Children ≥8 yr): 6.25–12.5 mg/kg q 6 hr or 12.5–25 mg/kg q 12 hr.

Availability
Doxycycline (generic available)
Tablets: 20 mg, 50 mg, 75 mg, 100 mg, 150 mg. **Delayed-release tablets:** 75 mg, 100 mg. **Capsules:** 50 mg, 100 mg. **Delayed-release capsules:** 40 mg. **Oral suspension (raspberry flavor):** 25 mg/5 mL in 60 mL bottles. **Syrup (apple-raspberry flavor):** 50 mg/5 mL in 473-mL bottles. **Powder for injection:** 100 mg/vial, 200 mg/vial.

Minocycline (generic available)
Capsules: 50 mg, 100 mg. **Tablets:** 50 mg, 75 mg, 100 mg. **Extended-release tablets:** 45 mg, 90 mg, 135 mg. **Oral suspension (custard flavor):** 50 mg/5 mL.

Tetracycline (generic available)
Capsules: 250 mg, 500 mg.

NURSING IMPLICATIONS
Assessment
- Assess for infection (vital signs; appearance of wound, sputum, urine, and stool; WBC) at beginning of and throughout therapy.
- Obtain specimens for culture and sensitivity before initiating therapy. First dose may be given before receiving results.
- Monitor bowel function. Diarrhea, abdominal cramping, fever, and bloody stools should be reported to health care professional promptly as a sign of pseudomembranous colitis. May begin up to several weeks following cessation of therapy.
- **IV:** Assess IV site frequently; may cause thrombophlebitis.
- *Lab Test Considerations:* Monitor renal and hepatic function and CBC periodically during long-term therapy.
- May cause ↑ AST, ALT, serum alkaline phosphatase, bilirubin, and amylase concentrations. Tetracyclines, except doxycycline, may cause ↑ serum BUN.

Potential Nursing Diagnoses
Risk for infection (Indications, Side Effects)
Noncompliance (Patient/Family Teaching)

Implementation
- Do not confuse doxycycline with doxepin.
- May cause yellow-brown discoloration and softening of teeth and bones if administered prenatally or during early childhood. Not recommended for children under 8 yr of age or

✦ = Canadian drug name. ■ = Genetic implication.
CAPITALS indicates life-threatening; underlines indicate most frequent.

TETRACYCLINES

during pregnancy or lactation unless used for the treatment of anthrax.
- **PO:** Administer around the clock. Administer at least 1 hr before or 2 hr after meals. *Doxycycline and minocycline* may be taken with food or milk if GI irritation occurs. Administer with a full glass of liquid and at least 1 hr before going to bed to avoid esophageal ulceration. Use calibrated measuring device for liquid preparations. Shake liquid preparations well. Do not administer within 1–3 hr of other medications.
- Avoid administration of calcium, zinc, antacids, magnesium- or aluminum-containing medications, sodium bicarbonate, or iron supplements within 1–3 hr of oral tetracyclines.

Doxycycline

- The *Oracea* product is only indicated for rosacea, not for infections.
- **PO:** To prepare doses for infants and children exposed to anthrax, place one 100 mg tablet in a small bowl and crush to a fine powder with a metal spoon, leaving no large pieces. Add 4 level teaspoons of lowfat milk, lowfat chocolate milk, regular chocolate milk, chocolate pudding, or apple juice. Mix food or drink and doxycycline powder until powder dissolves. Mixture is stable in a covered container for 24 hr if refrigerated (if made with milk or pudding) or at room temperature (if made with juice). Number of teaspoons to administer/dose is based on child's weight (0–12.5 lb—½ tsp; 12.5–25 lb—1 tsp; 25–37.5 lb—1½ tsp; 37.5–50 lb—2 tsp; 50–62.5 lb—2½ tsp; 62.5–75 lb—3 tsp; 75–87.5 lb—3½ tsp; 87.5–100 lb—4 tsp).
- Capsules may also be administered by carefully opening and sprinkling capsule contents on a spoonful of applesauce. The applesauce should be swallowed immediately without chewing and followed with a cool 8-ounce glass of water to ensure complete swallowing of the capsule contents. The applesauce should not be hot, and it should be soft enough to be swallowed without chewing. If mixture cannot be taken immediately, discard; do not store for later use.
- Do not open, break, crush or chew extended release capsules and tablets.

IV Administration

- **Intermittent Infusion:** *Diluent:* Dilute each 100 mg with 10 mL of sterile water or 0.9% NaCl for injection. Dilute further in 100–1000 mL of 0.9% NaCl, D5W, D5/LR, Ringer's, or lactated Ringer's solution. Solution is stable for 12 hr at room temperature and 72 hr if refrigerated. If diluted with D5/LR or lactated Ringer's solution, administer within 6 hr. Protect solution from direct sunlight. *Concentration:* Concentrations of less than 1 mcg/mL or greater than 1 mg/mL are not recommended. *Rate:* Administer over a minimum of 1–4 hr. Avoid rapid administration. Avoid extravasation.
- **Y-Site Compatibility:** acyclovir, alfentanyl, amifostine, amikacin, aminophylline, amiodarone, anidulafungin, ascorbic acid, atracurium, atropine, aztreonam, bivalirudin, bumetanide, buprenorphine, butorphanol, calcium chloride, calcium gulconate, carboplatin, caspofungin, cefonocid, cefotaxime, ceftriaxone, chlorpromazine, ciometidine, cisatracurium, cisplatin, clindamycin, codeine, cyanocobalamin, cyclophosphamide, cyclosporine, cytarabine, dactinomycin, daptomycin, dexmedetomidine, digoxin, diltiazem, diphenhydramine, dobutamine, docetaxel, dopamine, doxacurium, doxarubicin, enalapril, ephedrine, epinephrine, epirubicin, epoetin alfa, eftifibitide, ertapenem, esmolol, etoposide, etoposide phosphate, famotidine, fenoldopam, fentanyl, filgrastim, fluconazole, fludarabine, gemcitabine, gentamicin, glycopyrrolate, granisetron, hydromorphone, idarubicin, ifosfamide, imipenem/cilastatin, insulin, isoproterenol, labetalol, levofloxacin, lidocaine, linezolid, lorazepam, magnesium sulfate, mannitol, mechlorethamine, melphalan, meperidine, metaraminol, methoxamine, methyldopate, metoclopramide, metoprolol, metronidazole, miconazole, midazolam, milrinone, mitoxantrone, morphine, multivitamins, nalbuphine, naloxone, nesiritide, netilmicin, nitroglycerin, nitroprusside, norepinephrine, octreotide, ondansetron, oxaliplatin, oxytocin, paclitaxel, pancuronium, pantoprazole, papaverine, pentamidine, pentazocine, perphenazine, phentolamine, phenylephrine, phytonadione, potassium chloride, procainamide, prochlorperazine, promethazine, propofol, propranolol, protamine, pyridoxime, quinupristin/dalfopristin, ranitidine, remifentanil, ritodrine, rituximab, rocuronium, sargramostim, sodium acetate, streptokinase, succinylcholine, sufentanil, tacrolimus, teniposide, theophylline, thiamine, thiotepa, tirofiban, tobramycin, tolazoline, trastuzumab, trimetaphan, urokinase, vancomycin, vasopressin, vecuronium, verapamil, vincristine, vinorelbine, voriconazole.

- **Y-Site Incompatibility:** allopurinol, amphotericin B colloidal, amphotericin B liposome, ampicillin, ampicillin/sulbactam, azathioprine, cefazolin, cefoperazone, cefotetan, cefoxitin, ceftizoxime, cefuroxime, chloramphenicol, dantrolene, dexamethasone, diazepam, diazoxide, erythromycin, fluorouracil, folic acid, furosemide, ganciclovir, heparin, hydrocortisone, inamrinone, indomethacin, ketorolac, methotrexate, methylprednisolone, nafcillin, oxacillin, palonosetron, pemetrexed, penicillin G, pentobarbital, phenobarbital, phenytoin, piperacillin/tazobactam, sodium bicarbonate, trimethoprim/sulfamethoxazole.

Patient/Family Teaching

- Instruct patient to take medication around the clock and to finish the drug completely as directed, even if feeling better. Take missed doses as soon as possible unless it is almost time for next dose; do not double doses. Advise patient that sharing of this medication may be dangerous.
- Advise patient to avoid taking milk or other dairy products concurrently with oral tetracyclines. Also avoid taking antacids, zinc, calcium, magnesium- or aluminum-containing medications, sodium bicarbonate, and iron supplements within 1–3 hr of oral tetracyclines.
- Instruct patient to notify health care professional immediately if diarrhea, abdominal cramping, fever, or bloody stools occur and not to treat with antidiarrheals without consulting health care professionals.
- Advise female patient to use a nonhormonal method of contraception while taking tetracyclines and until next menstrual period.
- *Minocycline* commonly causes dizziness or unsteadiness. Caution patient to avoid driving or other activities requiring alertness until response to medication is known. Notify health care professional if these symptoms occur.
- Caution patient to use sunscreen and protective clothing to prevent photosensitivity reactions.
- Advise patient to report the signs of superinfection (black, furry overgrowth on the tongue; vaginal itching or discharge; loose or foul-smelling stools). Skin rash, pruritus, and urticaria should also be reported.
- Instruct patient to notify health care professional of medication regimen before treatment or surgery.
- Instruct patient to notify health care professional if symptoms do not improve within a few days for systemic preparations.
- Caution patient to discard outdated or decomposed tetracyclines; they may be toxic.
- **Malaria Prophylaxis:** Advise patient to avoid being bitten by mosquitoes by using protective measures, especially from dusk to dawn (e.g., staying in wellscreened areas, using mosquito nets, covering the body with clothing, and using an effective insect repellant). Doxycycline prophylaxis should begin 1-2 days before travel to the malarious area, continued daily while in the malarious area and after leaving the malarious area, should be continued for 4 more weeks to avoid development of malaria. Do not exceed 4 months.

Evaluation/Desired Outcomes

- Resolution of the signs and symptoms of infection. Length of time for complete resolution depends on the organism and site of infection.
- Decrease in acne lesions.
- Treatment of inhalation anthrax (post exposure) or treatment of cutaneous anthrax (doxycycline).
- Prevention of malaria.
- Reduction in inflammatory lesions associated with rosacea.

---

thalidomide (tha-lid-oh-mide)
Thalomid

Classification
Therapeutic: immunosuppressants

Pregnancy Category X

Indications

Cutaneous manifestations of moderate to severe erythema nodosum leprosum (ENL). Prevention (maintenance) and suppression of recurrent ENL. Newly diagnosed multiple myeloma (with dexamethasone). **Unlabeled Use:** Bechet's syndrome. HIV-associated wasting syndrome. Aphthous stomatitis (including HIV associated). Crohn's disease.

Action

May suppress excess levels of tumor necrosis factor-alpha (TNF-alpha) in patients with ENL and alter leukocyte migration by altering characteristics of cell surfaces. **Therapeutic Effects:** Decreased skin lesions in ENL and prevention of recurrence.

1208 thalidomide

Pharmacokinetics
Absorption: 67–93% absorbed following oral administration.
Distribution: Crosses the placenta; highly protein bound.
Protein Binding: Highly bound.
Metabolism and Excretion: Hydrolyzed in plasma to multiple metabolites.
Half-life: 5–7 hr.

TIME/ACTION PROFILE (dermatologic effects)

ROUTE	ONSET	PEAK	DURATION
PO	48 hr	1–2 mo	unknown

Contraindications/Precautions
Contraindicated in: Hypersensitivity; OB: Women with childbearing potential (unless specific conditions are met); Sexually mature men (unless specific conditions are met); Lactation: Potential for serious adverse reactions in the infant.
Use Cautiously in: Pedi: Children <12 yr (safety not established).

Adverse Reactions/Side Effects
CNS: dizziness, drowsiness. **CV:** bradycardia, edema, orthostatic hypotension, thromboembolic events (↑ risk with dexamethasone in multiple myeloma). **GI:** constipation. **Derm:** rash, photosensitivity. **Hemat:** neutropenia. **Neuro:** peripheral neuropathy. **Misc:** SEVERE BIRTH DEFECTS, hypersensitivity reactions, ↑ HIV viral load.

Interactions
Drug-Drug: ↑ CNS depression with concurrent use of **barbiturates**, **sedative/hypnotics**, **alcohol**, **chlorpromazine**, **reserpine**, or other **CNS depressants**. Concurrent use of **agents that may cause peripheral neuropathy** ↑ risk of peripheral neuropathy.
Drug-Natural Products: Concomitant use with **echinacea**, and **melatonin** may interfere with immunosuppression.

Route/Dosage
ENL
PO (Adults ≥50 kg): 100–300 mg/day initially; up to 400 mg/day has been used, depending on previous response. Every 3–6 mo, attempts should be made to taper and discontinue in decrements of 50 mg q 2–4 wk.

PO (Adults <50 kg): 100 mg/day initially; up to 400 mg/day has been used, depending on previous response. Every 3–6 mo, attempts should be made to taper and discontinue in decrements of 50 mg q 2–4 wk.

Multiple Myeloma
PO (Adults): 200 mg daily in 28-day treatment cycles. Dexamethasone 40 mg is administered on Days 1–4, 9–12, 17–20.

Availability
Capsules: 50 mg, 100 mg, 150 mg, 200 mg.

NURSING IMPLICATIONS
Assessment
- Assess patient monthly for initial 3 months and periodically during therapy to detect early signs of peripheral neuropathy (numbness, tingling, or pain in hands and feet). Commonly occurs with prolonged therapy, but has occurred following short-term use or following completion of therapy. May be severe and irreversible. Electrophysiologic testing may be done at baseline and every 6 mo to detect asymptomatic peripheral neuropathy. If symptoms occur, discontinue thalidomide immediately to limit further damage. Reinstate therapy only if neuropathy returns to baseline.
- Monitor for signs of hypersensitivity reaction (erythematous macular rash, fever, tachycardia, hypotension). May require discontinuation of therapy if severe. If reaction recurs when dosing is resumed, discontinue thalidomide.
- **Multiple Myeloma:** Assess for venous thromboembolism (dyspnea, chest pain, arm or leg swelling) periodically during therapy, especially in patients concurrently taking dexamethasone.
- Monitor for side effects (constipation, oversedation, peripheral neuropathy); may require discontinuation or dose reduction until side effects resolve.
- **Lab Test Considerations:** Monitor WBC with differential during therapy. May cause ↓ WBC. Do not initiate therapy with an ANC ≤750/mm³. If ANC ↓ to ≤750/mm³ during therapy, re-evaluate medication regimen; if neutropenia persists, consider discontinuing therapy.
- May cause ↑ viral load levels in patients with HIV.

Potential Nursing Diagnoses
Impaired skin integrity (Indications)
Risk for injury (Adverse Reactions)

Implementation
- Due to teratogenic effects, thalidomide may be prescribed only by prescribers registered in the System for Thalidomide Education and Prescribing Safety (STEPS) program. Thalidomide is started within 24 hr of a negative pregnancy

test with a sensitivity of at least 50 mIU/mL. Pregnancy testing must occur weekly during first month of therapy, then monthly thereafter in women with a regular menstrual cycle. For women with irregular menses, pregnancy testing should occur every 2 wk. If pregnancy occurs, thalidomide should be discontinued immediately. Any suspected fetal exposure must be reported to the FDA and the manufacturer, and patient should be referred to an obstetrician/gynecologist experienced in reproductive toxicity.

- If health care professionals or other caregivers are exposed to body fluids from patients receiving thalidomide, use appropriate precautions, such as wearing gloves to prevent the potential cutaneous exposure to thalidomide or washing the exposed area with soap and water.
- Corticosteroids may be used concurrently with thalidomide for patients with moderate to severe neuritis associated with a severe ENL reaction. Use of corticosteroids can be tapered and discontinued when neuritis resolves.
- **PO:** Administer once daily with water, preferably at bedtime and at least 1 hr after the evening meal. If divided doses are used, administer at least 1 hr after meals.

Patient/Family Teaching

- Instruct patient to take thalidomide as directed. Do not discontinue without notifying health care professional; dose should be tapered gradually.
- Advise patient that thalidomide should not be shared with others.
- Caution patient on the extreme importance of maintaining contraception for 1 month prior to, during, and for 1 mo following discontinuation of therapy. *For women of childbearing yr,* two methods of reliable contraception must be used unless complete abstinence is used. *For men,* a latex condom must be used, even if a successful vasectomy has been performed. Patients must meet *ALL* of the STEPS conditions: Understands and can follow instructions and is capable of complying with contraceptive measures, pregnancy testing, patient registration, and patient survey. Patients must receive verbal and written warnings of the potential teratogenicity of thalidomide and must acknowledge in writing their understanding and acceptance of these conditions.
- Advise patient to consult health care professional before using other RX, OTC, or herbal products. Concomitant use of HIV-protease inhibitors, modafinil, penicillins, rifampin, rifabutin, phenytoin, carbamazepine, or certain herbal supplements such as St. John's Wort with hormonal contraceptive agents may reduce the effectiveness of contraception during and for up to one month after discontinuation of these concomitant therapies. Therefore, women requiring treatment with one or more of these drugs must use two other effective or highly effective methods of contraception or abstain from heterosexual sexual contact while taking thalidomide.
- Frequently causes drowsiness or dizziness. Caution patient to avoid driving or other activities requiring alertness until response to medication is known.
- Advise patient to change positions slowly to minimize orthostatic hypotension.
- Caution patient to use sunscreen and protective clothing to prevent photosensitivity reactions.
- Instruct patient not to donate blood and male patients not to donate sperm while taking thalidomide.
- Advise patient to notify health care professional immediately if pain, numbness, tingling, or burning in hands or feet or shortness of breath, chest pain, swelling of arms or legs occur.

Evaluation/Desired Outcomes

- Resolution of the signs and symptoms of active ENL reaction. Usually requires at least 2 wk of therapy; then taper medication in 50 mg decrements every 2–4 wk.
- Prevention of recurrent ENL. Tapering off medication should be attempted every 3–6 mo in decrements of 50 mg every 2–4 wk.
- Decrease in serum and urine paraprotein measurements in patients with multiple myeloma.

---

theophylline, See BRONCHODILATORS (XANTHINES).

---

thiamine (thye-a-min)
♦ Betaxin, ♦ Bewon, Biamine, vitamin B1

Classification
Therapeutic: vitamins
Pharmacologic: water soluble vitamins

Pregnancy Category A

thiamine

Indications
Treatment of thiamine deficiencies (beriberi). Prevention of Wernicke's encephalopathy. Dietary supplement in patients with GI disease, alcoholism, or cirrhosis.

Action
Required for carbohydrate metabolism. **Therapeutic Effects:** Replacement in deficiency states.

Pharmacokinetics
Absorption: Well absorbed from the GI tract by an active process. Excessive amounts are not absorbed completely. Also well absorbed from IM sites.
Distribution: Widely distributed. Enters breast milk.
Metabolism and Excretion: Metabolized by the liver. Excess amounts are excreted unchanged by the kidneys.
Half-life: Unknown.

TIME/ACTION PROFILE (time for symptoms of deficiency—edema and heart failure—to resolve†)

ROUTE	ONSET	PEAK	DURATION
PO, IM, IV	hr	days	days–wk

†Confusion and psychosis take longer to respond

Contraindications/Precautions
Contraindicated in: Hypersensitivity; Known alcohol intolerance or bisulfite hypersensitivity (elixir only).
Use Cautiously in: Wernicke's encephalopathy (condition may be worsened unless thiamine is administered before glucose).

Adverse Reactions/Side Effects
Adverse reactions and side effects are extremely rare and are usually associated with IV administration or extremely large doses.
CNS: restlessness, weakness. **EENT:** tightness of the throat. **Resp:** pulmonary edema, respiratory distress. **CV:** VASCULAR COLLAPSE, hypotension, vasodilation. **GI:** GI bleeding, nausea. **Derm:** cyanosis, pruritus, sweating, tingling, urticaria, warmth. **Misc:** ANGIOEDEMA.

Interactions
Drug-Drug: None significant.

Route/Dosage

Thiamine Deficiency (Beriberi)
PO (Adults): 5–10 mg 3 times daily.
PO (Children): 10–50 mg/day in divided doses.
IM, IV (Adults): 5–100 mg 3 times daily.
IM, IV (Children): 10–25 mg/day.

Dietary Supplement
PO (Adults): 1–1.6 mg/day.
PO (Children 4–10 yr): 0.9–1 mg/day.
PO (Children birth–3 yr): 0.3–0.7 mg/day.

Availability (generic available)
Tablets: 5 mg^{OTC}, 10 mg^{OTC}, 25 mg^{OTC}, 50 mg^{OTC}, 100 mg^{OTC}, 250 mg^{OTC}, 500 mg^{OTC}. **Elixir:** ✹ 250 mcg/5 mL^{OTC}. **Injection:** 100 mg/mL in 1-mL ampules and prefilled syringes and 1-, 2-, 10-, and 30-mL vials. *In combination with:* other vitamins, minerals, and trace elements in multi-vitamin preparations^{OTC}.

NURSING IMPLICATIONS

Assessment
- Assess for signs and symptoms of thiamine deficiency (anorexia, GI distress, irritability, palpitations, tachycardia, edema, paresthesia, muscle weakness and pain, depression, memory loss, confusion, psychosis, visual disturbances, elevated serum pyruvic acid levels).
- Assess patient's nutritional status (diet, weight) prior to and throughout therapy.
- Monitor patients receiving IV thiamine for anaphylaxis (wheezing, urticaria, edema).
- *Lab Test Considerations:* May interfere with certain methods of testing serum theophylline, uric acid, and urobilinogen concentrations.

Potential Nursing Diagnoses
Imbalanced nutrition: less than body requirements (Indications)

Implementation
- Because of infrequency of single B-vitamin deficiencies, combinations are commonly administered.
- **IM, IV:** Parenteral administration is reserved for patients in whom oral administration is not feasible.
- **IM:** Administration may cause tenderness and induration at injection site. Cool compresses may decrease discomfort.

IV Administration

- **IV:** Sensitivity reactions and death have occurred from IV administration. An intradermal test dose is recommended in patients with suspected sensitivity. Monitor site for erythema and induration.
- **Direct IV:** *Concentration:* Administer undiluted at 100 mg/mL. *Rate:* Administer at a rate of 100 mg over 5 min.
- **Continuous Infusion:** *Diluent:* May be diluted in dextrose/Ringer's or LR combinations,

dextrose/saline combinations, D5W, D10W, Ringer's and LR injection, 0.9% NaCl, or 0.45% NaCl. Usually administered with other vitamins.
- **Y-Site Compatibility:** alfentanil, amikacin, ascorbic acid, atracurium, atropine, aztreonam, benztropine, bumetanide, buprenorphine, butorphanol, calcium chloride, calcium gluconate, cefazolin, cefonocid, cefotaxime, cefotetan, cefoxitin, ceftriaxone, cefuroxime, chlorpromazine, cimetidine, clindamycin, cyanocobalamin, cyclosporine, dexamethasone, digoxin, diphenhydramine, dobutamine, dopamine, doxycycline, enalaprilat, ephedrine, epinephrine, erythromycin, esmolol, famotidine, fentanyl, gentamicin, glycopyrrolate, heparin, insulin, isoproterenol, labetalol, lidocaine, magnesium sulfate, mannitol, meperidine, metaraminol, methoxamine, methyldopate, metoclopramide, metoprolol, morphine, multivitamins, nafcillin, nalbuphine, naloxone, nitroglycerin, nitroprusside, norepinephrine, oxacillin, oxytocin, papaverine, penicillin G, pentamidine, pentazocine, phentolamine, phenylephrine, phytonadione, potassium chloride, procainamide, prochlorperazine, promethazine, propranolol, protamine, pyridoxime, ranitidine, streptokinase, succinylcholine, sufentnail, theophylline, ticarcillin/clavulanate, tobramycin, tolazoline, trimetaphan, urokinase, vancomycin, vasopressin, verapamil.
- **Y-Site Incompatibility:** aminophylline, amphotericin B colloidal, azathioprine, cefoperazone, ceftazidime, ceftizoxime, chloramphenicol, dantrolene, diazepam, diazoxide, folic acid, furosemide, ganciclovir, hydrocortisone, imipemen/cilastatin, inamrinone, indomethacin, methylprednisolole, pentobarbital, phenobarbital, phenytoin, sodium bicarbonate, trimethoprim/sulfamethoxazole.
- **Additive Incompatibility:** Solutions with neutral or alkaline pH, such as carbonates, bicarbonates, citrates, and acetates.

Patient/Family Teaching
- Encourage patient to comply with dietary recommendations of health care professional. Explain that the best source of vitamins is a well-balanced diet with foods from the four basic food groups.
- Teach patient that foods high in thiamine include cereals (whole grain and enriched), meats (especially pork), and fresh vegetables; loss is variable during cooking.
- Caution patients self-medicating with vitamin supplements not to exceed RDA. The effectiveness of megadoses of vitamins for treatment of various medical conditions is unproved and may cause side effects.

Evaluation/Desired Outcomes
- Prevention of or decrease in the signs and symptoms of vitamin B deficiency.
- Decrease in the symptoms of neuritis, ocular signs, ataxia, edema, and heart failure may be seen within hours of administration and may disappear within a few days.
- Confusion and psychosis may take longer to respond and may persist if nerve damage has occurred.

---

thioridazine
(thye-oh-**rid**-a-zeen)

Classification
Therapeutic: antipsychotics
Pharmacologic: phenothiazines

Pregnancy Category C

Indications
Treatment of refractory schizophrenia. Considered second line treatment after failure with atypical antipsychotics.

Action
Alters the effects of dopamine in the CNS. Possesses significant anticholinergic and alpha-adrenergic blocking activity. **Therapeutic Effects:** Diminished signs and symptoms of psychoses.

Pharmacokinetics
Absorption: Absorption from tablets is variable; may be better with oral liquid formulations.
Distribution: Widely distributed, high concentrations in the CNS. Crosses the placenta and enters breast milk.
Protein Binding: ≥90%.
Metabolism and Excretion: Highly metabolized by the liver (primarily by CYP2D6 isoenzyme) and GI mucosa; the CYP2D6 enzyme system exhibits genetic polymorphism (~7% of population may be poor metabolizers and may have significantly ↑ thioridazine concentrations and an ↑ risk of adverse effects).
Half-life: 21–24 hr.

thioridazine

TIME/ACTION PROFILE (antipsychotic effects)

ROUTE	ONSET	PEAK	DURATION
PO	unknown	unknown	8–12 hr

Contraindications/Precautions
Contraindicated in: Hypersensitivity; Cross-sensitivity with other phenothiazines may exist; Angle-closure glaucoma; Bone marrow depression; Severe liver or cardiovascular disease; Known alcohol intolerance (concentrate only); Concurrent fluvoxamine, propranolol, pindolol, fluoxetine, other agents known to inhibit the CYP2D6 enzyme, or agents known to prolong the QTc interval (risk of life-threatening arrrhythmias); Hypokalemia (correct prior to use); QTc interval >450 msec.

Use Cautiously in: Debilitated patients; Glaucoma; Urinary retention; Diabetes mellitus; Patients with risk factors for electrolyte imbalance (dehydration, diuretic therapy); Respiratory disease; Prostatic hyperplasia; CNS tumors; Epilepsy; Intestinal obstruction; OB, Lactation: Safety not established. Recommend discontinue drug or bottle feed; Geri: May be at ↑ risk for extrapyramidal and CNS adverse effects; appears on Beers list; ↑ risk of mortality in elderly patients treated for dementia-related psychosis.

Adverse Reactions/Side Effects
CNS: NEUROLEPTIC MALIGNANT SYNDROME, sedation, extrapyramidal reactions, tardive dyskinesia. **EENT:** blurred vision, dry eyes, lens opacities, pigmentary retinopathy (high doses). **CV:** ARRHYTHMIAS, QTC PROLONGATION, hypotension, tachycardia. **GI:** constipation, dry mouth, anorexia, drug-induced hepatitis, ileus, weight gain. **GU:** urinary retention, priapism. **Derm:** photosensitivity, pigment changes, rashes. **Endo:** galactorrhea, amenorrhea. **Hemat:** AGRANULOCYTOSIS, leukopenia. **Metab:** hyperthermia. **Misc:** allergic reactions.

Interactions
Drug-Drug: Concurrent **fluvoxamine**, **propranolol**, **pindolol**, **fluoxetine**, other **agents known to inhibit the CYP450 2D6 enzyme**, or **agents known to prolong the QTc interval** ↑ risk of life-threatening arrhythmias. **Diuretics** ↑ the risk of electrolyte imbalance and arrhythmias. Additive hypotension with other **antihypertensives**, **nitrates**, and acute ingestion of **alcohol**. Additive CNS depression with other **CNS depressants**, including **alcohol**, **antihistamines**, **opioid analgesics**, **sedative/hypnotics**, and **general anesthetics**. Additive anticholinergic effects with other **drugs possessing anticholinergic properties**, including **antihistamines**, **antidepressants**, **atropine**, **haloperidol**, other **phenothiazines**, and **disopyramide**. **Lithium** ↓ blood levels of thioridazine. Thioridazine may mask early signs of **lithium** toxicity and ↑ the risk of extrapyramidal reactions. ↑ risk of agranulocytosis with **antithyroid agents**. Concurrent use with **epinephrine** may result in severe hypotension and tachycardia. May ↓ the effectiveness of **levodopa**.

Route/Dosage
PO (Adults and Children >12 yr): 50–100 mg 3 times daily initially; may be gradually ↑ to a maintenance dose of up to 800 mg/day.
PO (Children): 0.5 mg/kg/day in divided doses initially; may be gradually ↑ to a maintenance dose of up to 3 mg/kg/day.

Availability (generic available)
Tablets: 10 mg, 25 mg, 50 mg, 100 mg. **Concentrated oral solution:** 100 mg/mL.

NURSING IMPLICATIONS

Assessment
- Assess mental status (orientation, mood, behavior) before and periodically during therapy.
- Assess positive (delusions, hallucinations, agitation) and negative (social withdrawal) symptoms of schizophrenia.
- Assess weight and BMI initially and throughout theerapy.
- Monitor blood pressure (sitting, standing, lying), ECG, pulse, and respiratory rate before and frequently during the period of dose adjustment. May cause Q-wave and T-wave changes in ECG.
- Observe patient carefully when administering medication to ensure that medication is actually taken and not hoarded or cheeked.
- Assess patient for level of sedation after administration. Geri: Geriatric patients are more likely to become oversedated.
- Monitor intake and output ratios and daily weight. Report significant discrepancies.
- Monitor patient for onset of akathisia (restlessness or desire to keep moving) and extrapyramidal side effects (*parkinsonian*—difficulty speaking or swallowing, loss of balance control, pill rolling of hands, mask-like face, shuffling gait, rigidity, tremors; and *dystonic*—muscle spasms, twisting motions, twitching, inability to move eyes, weakness of arms or legs) every 2 mo during therapy and 8–12 wk after therapy has been discontinued. Report these symptoms; reduction in dosage or

discontinuation of medication may be necessary. Trihexyphenidyl, diphenhydramine, or benztropine may be used to control these symptoms. Benzodiazpines may alleviate akathisia.
- Monitor for tardive dyskinesia (uncontrolled rhythmic movement of mouth, face, and extremities; lip smacking or puckering; puffing of cheeks; uncontrolled chewing; rapid or worm-like movements of tongue, excessive eye blinking). Report immediately; may be irreversible.
- Monitor for development of neuroleptic malignant syndrome (fever, respiratory distress, tachycardia, seizures, diaphoresis, hypertension or hypotension, pallor, tiredness, severe muscle stiffness, loss of bladder control). Notify health care professional immediately if these symptoms occur.
- **Lab Test Considerations:** CBC, liver function tests, and ocular examinations should be evaluated periodically during therapy. May cause ↓ hematocrit, hemoglobin, leukocytes, granulocytes, platelets. May cause ↑ bilirubin, AST, ALT, and alkaline phosphatase. Agranulocytosis occurs between 4–10 wk of therapy with recovery 1–2 wk after discontinuation. May recur if medication is restarted. Liver function abnormalities may require discontinuation of therapy.
- May cause false-positive or false-negative pregnancy test results and false-positive urine bilirubin test results.
- May cause ↑ serum prolactin levels.

Potential Nursing Diagnoses
Disturbed thought process (Indications)
Sexual dysfunction (Side Effects)

Implementation
- To prevent contact dermatitis, avoid getting liquid preparations on hands, and wash hands thoroughly if spillage occurs.
- **PO:** Administer with food, milk, or full glass of water to minimize gastric irritation.
- Dilute concentrate in 120 mL of distilled or acidified tap water or fruit juice just before administration.

Patient/Family Teaching
- Advise patient to take medication as directed and not to skip doses or double up on missed doses. Take missed doses as soon as remembered unless almost time for the next dose. If more than 2 doses a day are ordered, the missed dose should be taken within 1 hr of the scheduled time or omitted. Abrupt withdrawal may lead to gastritis, nausea, vomiting, dizziness, headache, tachycardia, and insomnia.
- Inform patient of possibility of extrapyramidal symptoms and tardive dyskinesia. Instruct patient to report these symptoms immediately to health care professional.
- Advise patient to change positions slowly to minimize orthostatic hypotension.
- May cause drowsiness. Caution patient to avoid driving or other activities requiring alertness until response to medication is known.
- Advise patient to use sunscreen and protective clothing when exposed to the sun. Exposed surfaces may develop a blue-gray pigmentation, which may fade after discontinuation of the medication. Extremes in temperature should also be avoided, as this drug impairs body temperature regulation.
- Instruct patient to use frequent mouth rinses, good oral hygiene, and sugarless gum or candy to minimize dry mouth. Consult health care professional if dry mouth continues for >2 wk.
- Advise patient that increasing activity and bulk and fluids in the diet helps minimize the constipating effects of this medication.
- Caution patient to avoid taking alcohol or other CNS depressants concurrently with this medication.
- Advise patient not to take thioridazine within 2 hr of antacids or antidiarrheal medication.
- Inform patient that this medication may turn urine pink to reddish brown.
- Advise patient to notify health care professional of medication regimen before treatment or surgery.
- Instruct patient to notify health care professional promptly if sore throat, fever, unusual bleeding or bruising, rash, weakness, tremors, visual disturbances, dark-colored urine, or clay-colored stools occur.
- Emphasize the importance of routine follow-up exams to monitor response to medication and to detect side effects. Periodic ocular exams are indicated. Encourage continued participation in psychotherapy.

Evaluation/Desired Outcomes
- Decrease in positive symptoms (hallucinations, delusions, agitation) of schizophrenia.

THROMBOLYTIC AGENTS

HIGH ALERT

THROMBOLYTIC AGENTS

alteplase (**al**-te-plase)
Activase, ✶ Activase rt-PA, Cathflo Activase, tissue plasminogen activator, t-PA

reteplase (**re**-te-plase)
Retavase

streptokinase (strep-toe-**kye**-nase)
Streptase

tenecteplase (te-**nek**-te-plase)
TNKase

urokinase (yoor-oh-**kye**-nase)
Kinlytic

Classification
Therapeutic: thrombolytics
Pharmacologic: plasminogen activators

Pregnancy Category B (urokinase), C (alteplase, reteplase, streptokinase, tenecteplase)

Indications
Alteplase, reteplase, streptokinase, tenecteplase: Acute myocardial infarction (MI). **Alteplase, streptokinase, urokinase:** Acute massive pulmonary emboli. **Alteplase:** Acute ischemic stroke. **Streptokinase:** Acute deep vein thrombosis. **Streptokinase:** Acute arterial thrombi. **Streptokinase:** Occluded arteriovenous cannulae. **Alteplase:** Occluded central venous access devices.

Action
Convert plasminogen to plasmin, which is then able to degrade fibrin present in clots. Alteplase, reteplase, tenecteplase, and urokinase directly activate plasminogen. Streptokinase combines with plasminogen to form activator complexes, which then converts plasminogen to plasmin. **Therapeutic Effects:** Lysis of thrombi in coronary arteries, with preservation of ventricular function or improvement of ventricular function (and ↓ risk of CHF or death). Lysis of pulmonary emboli or deep vein thrombosis. Lysis of thrombi causing ischemic stroke, reducing risk of neurologic sequelae. Restoration of cannula or catheter patency and function.

Pharmacokinetics
Absorption: Complete after IV administration. Intracoronary administration or administration into occluded catheters or cannulae has a more localized effect.
Distribution: Streptokinase appears to cross the placenta minimally, if at all. Remainder of distribution for streptokinase or other agents is not known.
Metabolism and Excretion: *Alteplase, tenecteplase, urokinase*—Rapidly metabolized by the liver. *Reteplase*—Cleared primarily by the liver and kidneys. *Streptokinase*—Rapidly cleared from circulation by antibodies and other unknown mechanism.
Half-life: *Alteplase*—35 min; *reteplase*—13–16 min; *streptokinase*—initially 18 min (due to clearance by antibodies), then 83 min; *Tenecteplase*—20–24 min (initial phase), 90–130 min (terminal phase); *urokinase*—up to 20 min.

TIME/ACTION PROFILE (fibrinolysis)

ROUTE	ONSET	PEAK	DURATION
Alteplase IV	30 min	60 min	unknown
Reteplase IV	30 min	30–90 min	48 hr
Streptokinase IV	immediate	rapid	4 hr (up to 12 hr)
Tenecteplase IV	rapid	unknown	unknown
Urokinase IV	immediate	rapid	up to 12 hr

Contraindications/Precautions
Contraindicated in: Active internal bleeding; History of cerebrovascular accident; Recent (within 2 mo) intracranial or intraspinal injury or trauma; Intracranial neoplasm, AV malformation, or aneurysm; Severe uncontrolled hypertension; Known bleeding tendencies; Hypersensitivity; cross-sensitivity with other thrombolytics may occur.
Use Cautiously in: Recent (within 10 days) major surgery, trauma, GI or GU bleeding; Left heart thrombus; Severe hepatic or renal disease; Hemorrhagic ophthalmic conditions; Septic phlebitis; Previous puncture of a noncompressible vessel; Subacute bacterial endocarditis or acute pericarditis; Recent streptococcal infection or previous therapy with streptokinase (from 5 days–6 mo); may produce resistance because of antibody formation; ↑ dosage requirements may be encountered (streptokinase only); Geri: >75 yr; ↑ risk of intracranial bleeding; OB, Lactation: Pedi: Safety not established.
Exercise Extreme Caution in: Patients receiving concurrent anticoagulant therapy (↑ risk of intracranial bleeding).

Adverse Reactions/Side Effects
CNS: INTRACRANIAL HEMORRHAGE. **EENT:** epistaxis, gingival bleeding. **Resp:** bronchospasm,

THROMBOLYTIC AGENTS 1215

hemoptysis. **CV:** hypotension, reperfusion arrhythmias. **GI:** GI BLEEDING, RETROPERITONEAL BLEEDING, nausea, vomiting. **GU:** GU TRACT BLEEDING. **Derm:** ecchymoses, flushing, urticaria. **Hemat:** BLEEDING. **Local:** hemorrhage at injection sites, phlebitis at IV site. **MS:** musculoskeletal pain. **Misc:** allergic reactions including ANAPHYLAXIS, fever.

Interactions
Drug-Drug: Concurrent use of **aspirin**, other **NSAIDs**, **warfarin**, **heparin**, **low-molecular-weight heparins**, **direct thrombin inhibitors**, **abciximab**, **eptifibatide**, **tirofiban**, **clopidogrel**, **ticlopidine**, or **dipyridamole** may ↑ risk of bleeding, although these agents are frequently used together or in sequence. Effects may be ↓ by **antifibrinolytic agents**, including **aminocaproic acid** or **tranexamic acid**.
Drug-Natural Products: ↑ anticoagulant effect and bleeding risk with **anise**, **arnica**, **chamomile**, **clove**, **dong quai**, **fenugreek**, **feverfew**, **garlic**, **ginger**, **ginkgo**, **Panax ginseng**, **licorice**, and others.

Route/Dosage

Alteplase

Myocardial Infarction (Accelerated or Front-Loading Infusion)
IV (Adults): 15 mg bolus, then 0.75 mg/kg (up to 50 mg) over 30 min, then 0.5 mg/kg (up to 35 mg) over next 60 min; usually accompanied by heparin therapy.

Myocardial Infarction (3-Hour Infusion)
IV (Adults >65 kg): 60 mg over 1st hr (6–10 mg given as a bolus over first 1–2 min), 20 mg over the 2nd hr, and 20 mg over the 3rd hr for a total dose of 100 mg.
IV (Adults <65 kg): 0.75 mg/kg over 1st hr (0.075–0.125 mg/kg given as a bolus over first 1–2 min), 0.25 mg/kg over the 2nd hr, and 0.25 mg/kg over the 3rd hr for a total dose of 1.25 mg/kg (not to exceed 100 mg total).

Pulmonary Embolism
IV (Adults): 100 mg over 2 hr; follow with heparin.

Acute Ischemic Stroke
IV (Adults): 0.9 mg/kg (not to exceed 90 mg), given as an infusion over 1 hr, with 10% of the dose given as a bolus over the 1st min.

Occluded Venous Access Devices
IV (Adults and Children >30 kg): 2 mg/2 mL instilled into occluded catheter; if unsuccessful, may repeat once after 2 hr.
IV (Adults and Children <30 kg): 110% of the lumen volume (not to exceed 2 mg in 2 mL) instilled into occluded catheter; if unsuccessful, may repeat once after 2 hr.

Reteplase
IV (Adults): 10 units, followed 30 min later by an additional 10 units.

Streptokinase

Myocardial Infarction
IV (Adults): 1.5 million units given as a continuous infusion over up to 60 min.
Intracoronary (Adults): 20,000 unit bolus followed by 2000–4000 units/min infusion for 30–90 min.

Deep Vein Thrombosis, Pulmonary Emboli, Arterial Emboli, or Arterial Thromboses
IV (Adults): 250,000 unit loading dose over 30 min, followed by 100,000 unit/hr for 24 hr for pulmonary emboli or arterial thrombosis/embolism, 72 hr for deep vein thrombosis.

Tenecteplase
IV (Adults <60 kg): 30 mg.
IV (Adults ≥60 kg and <70 kg): 35 mg.
IV (Adults ≥70 kg and <80 kg): 40 mg.
IV (Adults ≥80 kg and <90 kg): 45 mg.
IV (Adults ≥90 kg): 50 mg.

Urokinase

Pulmonary Emboli
IV (Adults): 4400 unit/kg loading dose, followed by 4400 unit/kg/hr for 12 hr.

Availability

Alteplase
Powder for injection: 2 mg/vial, 50 mg/vial, 100 mg/vial.

Reteplase
Powder for injection: 10.8 units/vial.

Streptokinase
Powder for injection: 250,000 units/vial, 750,000 units/vial, 1,500,000 units/vial.

Tenecteplase
Powder for injection: 50 mg/vial.

THROMBOLYTIC AGENTS

Urokinase
Powder for injection: 250,000 units/vial.

NURSING IMPLICATIONS
Assessment
- Begin therapy as soon as possible after the onset of symptoms.
- Monitor vital signs, including temperature, continuously for coronary thrombosis and at least every 4 hr during therapy for other indications. Do not use lower extremities to monitor blood pressure. Notify health care professional if systolic BP >180 mm Hg or diastolic BP >110 mm Hg. Should not be given if hypertension is uncontrolled. Inform health care professional if hypotension occurs. Hypotension may result from the drug, hemorrhage, or cardiogenic shock.
- Assess patient carefully for bleeding every 15 min during the 1st hr of therapy, every 15–30 min during the next 8 hr, and at least every 4 hr for the duration of therapy. Frank bleeding may occur from sites of invasive procedures or from body orifices. Internal bleeding may also occur (decreased neurologic status; abdominal pain with coffee-grounds emesis or black, tarry stools; hematuria; joint pain). If uncontrolled bleeding occurs, stop medication and notify health care professional immediately.
- Inquire about previous reaction to streptokinase therapy. Assess patient for hypersensitivity reaction (rash, dyspnea, fever, changes in facial color, swelling around the eyes, wheezing). If these occur, inform health care professional promptly. Keep epinephrine, an antihistamine, and resuscitation equipment close by in the event of an anaphylactic reaction.
- Inquire about recent streptococcal infection. *Streptokinase* may be less effective if administered between 5 days and 6 mo of a streptococcal infection.
- Assess neurologic status throughout therapy. Altered sensorium or neurologic changes may be indicative of intracranial bleeding.
- **Myocardial Infarction:** Monitor ECG continuously. Notify health care professional if significant arrhythmias occur. Monitor cardiac enzymes. Radionuclide myocardial scanning and/or coronary angiography may be ordered 7–10 days after therapy to monitor effectiveness of therapy.
- Assess intensity, character, location, and radiation of chest pain. Note presence of associated symptoms (nausea, vomiting, diaphoresis). Notify health care professional if chest pain is unrelieved or recurs.
- Monitor heart sounds and breath sounds frequently. Inform health care professional if signs of CHF occur (rales/crackles, dyspnea, S_3 heart sound, jugular venous distention).
- **Acute Ischemic Stroke:** Assess neurologic status. Determine time of onset of stroke symptoms. Alteplase must be administered within 3–4.5 hr of onset (within 3 hr in patients older than 80 yr, those taking oral anticoagulants, those with a baseline National Institutes of Health Stroke Scale score 25, or those with both a history of stroke and diabetes).
- **Pulmonary Embolism:** Monitor pulse, blood pressure, hemodynamics, and respiratory status (rate, degree of dyspnea, ABGs).
- **Deep Vein Thrombosis/Acute Arterial Thrombosis:** Observe extremities and palpate pulses of affected extremities every hour. Notify health care professional immediately if circulatory impairment occurs. Computerized tomography, impedance plethysmography, quantitative Doppler effect determination, and/or angiography or venography may be used to determine restoration of blood flow and duration of therapy; however, repeated venograms are not recommended.
- **Cannula/Catheter Occlusion:** Monitor ability to aspirate blood as indicator of patency. Ensure that patient exhales and holds breath when connecting and disconnecting IV syringe to prevent air embolism.
- *Lab Test Considerations:* Hematocrit, hemoglobin, platelet count, fibrin/fibrin degradation product (FDP) titer, fibrinogen concentration, prothrombin time, thrombin time, and activated partial thromboplastin time (aPTT) may be evaluated before and frequently during therapy. Bleeding time may be assessed before therapy if patient has received platelet inhibitors.
- Obtain type and crossmatch and have blood available at all times in case of hemorrhage.
- Stools should be tested for occult blood loss and urine for hematuria periodically during therapy.
- ***Toxicity and Overdose: High Alert:*** If local bleeding occurs, apply pressure to site. If severe or internal bleeding occurs, discontinue infusion. Clotting factors and/or blood volume may be restored through infusions of whole blood, packed RBCs, fresh frozen plasma, or cryoprecipitate. Do not administer dextran; it has antiplatelet activity. Aminocaproic acid (Amicar) may be used as an antidote.

THROMBOLYTIC AGENTS 1217

Potential Nursing Diagnoses
Ineffective tissue perfusion (Indications)
Risk for injury (Side Effects)

Implementation
- **High Alert:** Overdosage and underdosage of thrombolytic medications have resulted in patient harm or death. Have second practitioner independently check original order, dosage calculations, and infusion pump settings. Do not confuse the abbreviation *t-PA* for alteplase (Activase) with the abbreviation *TNK t-PA* for tenecteplase (TNKase) and *r-PA* for reteplase (Retavase). Clarify orders that contain either of these abbreviations.
- Thrombolytic agents should be used only in settings in which hematologic function and clinical response can be adequately monitored.
- Starting two IV lines before therapy is recommended: one for the thrombolytic agent, the other for any additional infusions.
- Avoid invasive procedures, such as IM injections or arterial punctures, with this therapy. If such procedures must be performed, apply pressure to all arterial and venous puncture sites for at least 30 min. Avoid venipunctures at noncompressible sites (jugular vein, subclavian site).
- Acetaminophen may be ordered to control fever.

Alteplase

IV Administration

- **Intermittent Infusion:** *Diluent:* Vials are packaged with sterile water for injection (without preservatives) to be used as diluent. Do not use bacteriostatic water for injection. Reconstitute 20-mg vials with 20-mL and 50-mg vials with 50 mL using an 18-gauge needle. Avoid excess agitation during dilution; swirl or invert gently to mix. Solution may foam upon reconstitution. Bubbles will resolve upon standing a few min. Solution will be clear to pale yellow. Stable for 8 hr at room temperature. *Concentration:* May be administered as reconstituted (1 mg/mL) or may be further diluted immediately before use in an equal amount of 0.9% NaCl or D5W. *Rate:* Flush line with 20–30 mL of saline at completion of infusion to ensure entire dose is received. See Route and Dosage section for specific rates.
- **Y-Site Compatibility:** eptifibatide, lidocaine, metoprolol, propranolol.
- **Y-Site Incompatibility:** bivalirudin, dobutamine, dopamine, heparin, nitroglycerin.
- **Cathflo Activase:** Reconstitute by withdrawing 2.2 mL of sterile water (provided) and injecting into Cathflo Activase vial, directing diluent into powder for a concentration of 1 mg/mL. Allow slight foaming to dissipate by letting vial stand undisturbed. Do not use bacteriostatic water. Mix by gently swirling to dissolve; complete dissolution should occur within 3 min. Do not shake. Solution should be colorless to pale yellow. Use solution within 8 hr.
- Withdraw 2.0 mL of reconstituted solution and instill into occluded catheter. After 30 min dwell time, attempt to aspirate blood. If catheter remains occluded, allow 120 min dwell time. If catheter function is not restored after one dose, second dose may be instilled. If catheter function is restored, aspirate 4–5 mL of blood to remove Cathflo Activase and residual clot. Gently irrigate catheter with 0.9% NaCl.

Reteplase

IV Administration

- **Direct IV:** *Diluent:* Reconstitute using diluent, needle, syringe, and dispensing pin provided. Reconstitute only with sterile water for injection without preservatives. Solution is colorless. Do not administer solutions that are discolored or contain a precipitate. Slight foaming may occur; allow vial to stand undisturbed for several min to dissipate bubbles. Reconstitute immediately before use. Stable for 4 hr at room temperature. *Concentration:* Administer undiluted. *Rate:* Administer each bolus over 2 min into an IV line containing D5W; flush line before and after bolus.
- **Y-Site Incompatibility:** bivalirudin, heparin, No other medication should be infused or injected into line used for reteplase.

Streptokinase

IV Administration

- **Intracoronary:** Dilute 250,000 IU vial to a total volume of 125 mL with 0.9% NaCl or D5W. Administer 20,000 IU (10 mL) via bolus injection.
- **Rate:** Intracoronary bolus is administered over 15 sec–2 min.
- **Intermittent Infusion:** *Diluent:* Reconstitute with 5 mL of 0.9% NaCl or D5W (direct to sides of vial) and swirl gently; do not shake. Di-

✦ = Canadian drug name.   ❖ = Genetic implication.
*CAPITALS indicates life-threatening; underlines indicate most frequent.

lute further with 0.9% NaCl for a total volume of 45–500 mL (45 mL for MI, 90 mL for deep vein thrombosis or pulmonary embolism). Solution is slightly yellow in color. Administer through 0.8-micron pore–size filter. Use reconstituted solution within 24 hr. *Rate:* Administer dose for MI within 60 min.
- Intracoronary bolus should be followed by an intracoronary maintenance infusion of 2000 IU/min for 60 min.
- Loading dose for *deep vein thrombosis* or *pulmonary embolism* is administered over 30 min, followed by an infusion of 100,000 IU/hr.
- Use infusion pump to ensure accurate dose.
- **Y-Site Compatibility:** alfentanil, amikacin, aminophylline, ascorbic acid, atracurium, atropine, aztreonam, benztropine, bumetanide, buprenorphine, butorphanol, calcium chloride, calcium gluconate, cefazolin, cefonocid, cefoperazone, cefotaxime, cefotetan, cefoxitin, ceftazidime, ceftizoxime, ceftriaxone, cefuroxime, chloramphenicol, cimetidine, clindamycin, cyanocobalamin, cyclosporine, dexamethasone, digoxin, diphenhydramine, dobutamine, dopamine, doxycycline, enalaprilat, ephedrine, epinephrine, epoetin alfa, erythromycin, esmolol, famotidine, fentanyl, fluconazole, folic acid, furosemide, gentamicin, glycopyrrolate, heparin, hydrocortisone, imipenem/cilastatin, indomethacin, insulin, 'isoproterenol, ketorolac, labetalol, lidocaine, magnesium sulfate, mannitol, meperidine, methoxamine, methyldopate, methylprednisolone, metoclopramide, metoprolol, midazolam, morphine, multivitamins, nafcillin, naloxone, nitroglycerin, nitroprusside, norepinephrine, ondansetron, oxacillin, oxytocin, penicillin G, pentazocine, pentobarbital, phenobarbital, phentolamine, phenylephrine, phytonadione, potassium chloride, procainamide, propranolol, pyridoxine, ranitidine, sodium bicarbonate, succinylcholine, sufentanil, theophylline, thiamine, ticarcillin/clavulanate, tobramycin, trimetaphan, urokinase, verapamil.
- **Y-Site Incompatibility:** azathioprine, bivalirudin, chlorpromazine, dantrolene, diazepam, diazoxide, ganciclovir, hydroxyzine, nalbuphine, pentamidine, phenytoin, prochlorperazine, promethazine, trimethoprim/sulfamethoxazole, vancomycin.
- **Additive Incompatibility:** Do not admix with any other medication.
- **Cannula/Catheter Clearance:** Dilute 250,000 IU in 2 mL of 0.9% NaCl or D5W.
- *Rate:* Administer slowly, over 25–35 min, into each occluded limb of cannula, and then clamp for at least 2 hr. Aspirate contents carefully and flush lines with 0.9% NaCl.

Tenecteplase

IV Administration

- **Intermittent Infusion:** *Diluent:* Vials are packaged with sterile water for injection (without preservatives) to be used as diluent. Do not use bacteriostatic water for injection. Do not discard shield assembly. To reconstitute aseptically withdraw 10 mL of diluent and inject into the tenectplase vial, directing the stream into the powder. Slight foaming may occur; large bubbles will dissipate if left standing undisturbed for several minutes. Swirl gently until contents are completely dissolved; do not shake. *Concentration:* Solution containing 5 mg/mL is clear and colorless to pale yellow. Withdraw dose from reconstituted vial with the syringe and discard unused portion. Once dose is in syringe, stand the shield vertically on a flat surface (with green side down) and passively recap the red hub cannula. Remove the entire shield assembly, including the red hub cannula, by twisting counter clockwise. Shield assembly also contains the clear-ended blunt plastic cannula; retain for split septum IV access. Reconstitute immediately before use. May be refrigerated and administered within 8 hr. *Rate:* Administer as a single IV bolus over 5 seconds.
- **Y-Site Incompatibility:** Precipate forms in line when administered with dextrose-containing solutions. Flush line with saline-containing solution prior to and following administration of tenecteplase.
- **Additive Incompatibility:** Do not admix.

Urokinase

IV Administration

- **Intermittent Infusion:** *Diluent:* Reconstitute each 250,000 IU vial with 5 mL of sterile water for injection without preservatives (direct to sides of vial) and swirl gently; do not shake. Solution is light straw colored. Do not administer solutions that are discolored or contain a precipitate. Use reconstituted solution immediately after preparation. Infuse through a 0.45-micron filter.
- For *pulmonary embolism,* dilute the reconstituted solution further with 190 mL of 0.9% NaCl or D5W. *Rate:* For *pulmonary embolism,* administer loading dose over 10 min and follow with infusion of 4400 IU/kg/hr for 12 hr.
- Administer via infusion pump to ensure accurate dose.

- **Y-Site Compatibility:** alfentanil, amikacin, aminophylline, ascorbic acid, atracurium, atropine, aztreonam, benztropine, bumetanide, buprenorphine, butorphanol, calcium chloride, calcium gluconate, cefazolin, cefoperazone, cefotaxime, cefotetan, cefoxitin, ceftazidime, cefuroxime, chloramphenicol, cimetidine, clindamycin, cyanocobalamin, cyclosporine, dexamethasone, digoxin, diphenhydramine, dobutamine, dopamine, doxycycline, enalaprilat, ephedrine, epinephrine, epoetin, erythromycin, esmolol, famotidine, fentanyl, fluconazole, folic acid, furosemide, gentamicin, glycopyrrolate, heparin, hydrocortisone, imipenem/cilastatin, insulin, isoproterenol, ketorolac, labetalol, lidocaine, magnesium sulfate, mannitol, meperidine, metaraminol, methoxamine, methyldopa, metoclopramide, metoprolol, midazolam, morphine, multivitamins, nafcillin, nalbuphine, naloxone, nitroglycerin, nitroprusside, norepinephrine, ondansetron, oxytocin, papaverine, penicillin G, pentamidine, pentazocine, pentobarbital, phenobarbital, phenylephrine, phytonadione, potassium chloride, procainamide, propranolol, protamine, pyridoxime, ranitidine, sodium bicarbonate, streptokinase, succinylcholine, sufentanil, theophylline, thiamine, ticarcillin/clavulanate, tobramycin, tolazoline, trimetaphan, vasopressin, verapamil.
- **Y-Site Incompatibility:** amphotericin B colloidal, dantrolene, diazepam, diazoxide, hydralazine, inamrinone, phenytoin, prochlorperazine, promethazine, trimethoprim/sulfamethoxazole, vasopressin.

Patient/Family Teaching
- Explain purpose of medication and the need for close monitoring to patient and family. Instruct patient to report hypersensitivity reactions (rash, dyspnea) and bleeding or bruising.
- Explain need for bedrest and minimal handling during therapy to avoid injury. Avoid all unnecessary procedures such as shaving and vigorous tooth brushing.

Evaluation/Desired Outcomes
- Lysis of thrombi and restoration of blood flow.
- Prevention of neurologic sequelae in acute ischemic stroke.
- Cannula or catheter patency.

thyroid, See **THYROID PREPARATIONS**.

THYROID PREPARATIONS

levothyroxine
(lee-voe-thye-**rox**-een)
✤Eltroxin, ✤Euthyrox, Levo-T, Levothroid, Levoxyl, Synthroid, T_4, Unithroid

liothyronine
(lye-oh-**thye**-roe-neen)
Cytomel, l-triiodothyronine, T_3, Triostat

liotrix (**lye**-oh-trix)
T_3/T_4, Thyrolar

thyroid (**thye**-royd)
Armour thyroid, Westhroid

Classification
Therapeutic: hormones
Pharmacologic: thyroid preparations

Pregnancy Category A

Indications
Thyroid supplementation in hypothyroidism. Treatment or suppression of euthyroid goiters and thyroid cancer.

Action
Replacement of or supplementation to endogenous thyroid hormones. Principal effect is increasing metabolic rate of body tissues: Promote gluconeogenesis, Increase utilization and mobilization of glycogen stores, Stimulate protein synthesis, Promote cell growth and differentiation, Aid in the development of the brain and CNS. Contain T_3 (triiodothyronine) and T_4 (thyroxine) activity. **Therapeutic Effects:** Replacement in hypothyroidism to restore normal hormonal balance. Suppression of thyroid cancers.

Pharmacokinetics
Absorption: Levothyroxine is variably (40–80%) absorbed from the GI tract. Liothyronine and thyroid hormone are well absorbed.
Distribution: Distributed into most body tissues. Thyroid hormones do not readily cross the placenta; minimal amounts enter breast milk.
Metabolism and Excretion: Metabolized by the liver and other tissues. Thyroid hormone under-

1220 THYROID PREPARATIONS

goes enterohepatic recirculation and is excreted in the feces via the bile.

Half-life: T_3 *(liothyronine)* — 1–2 days; T_4 *(thyroxine)* — 6–7 days.

TIME/ACTION PROFILE (effects on thyroid function tests)

ROUTE	ONSET	PEAK	DURATION
Levothyroxine PO	unknown	1–3 wk	1–3 wk
Levothyroxine IV	6–8 hr	24 hr	unknown
Liothyronine PO	unknown	24–72 hr	72 hr
Liothyronine IV	unknown	unknown	unknown
Thyroid PO	days–wk	1–3 wk	days–wk

Contraindications/Precautions

Contraindicated in: Hypersensitivity; Recent MI; Hyperthyroidism.

Use Cautiously in: Cardiovascular disease (initiate therapy with lower doses); Severe renal insufficiency; Uncorrected adrenocortical disorders; Geri: Extremely sensitive to thyroid hormones; initial dose should be ↓ ; Pedi: Monitor neonates and infants for cardiac overload, arrhythmias, and aspiriation during first 2 wk of therapy (levothyroxine).

Adverse Reactions/Side Effects

Usually only seen when excessive doses cause iatrogenic hyperthyroidism.
CNS: nervousness, headache, insomnia, irritability. **CV:** angina pectoris, arrhythmias, hypotension, tachycardia. **GI:** cramps, diarrhea, vomiting; *levothyroxine tablets*, choking, gagging, dysphagia. **Derm:** hair loss (in children), sweating. **Endo:** hyperthyroidism, menstrual irregularities. **Metab:** heat intolerance, weight loss. **MS:** accelerated bone maturation in children.

Interactions

Drug-Drug: Bile acid sequestrants and orlistat ↓ absorption of orally administered thyroid preparations. May ↑ effects of warfarin. May ↑ requirement for insulin or oral hypoglycemic agents in diabetics. Concurrent estrogen therapy may ↑ thyroid replacement requirements. ↑ cardiovascular effects with adrenergics (sympathomimetics).
Drug-Food: Foods or supplements containing calcium, iron, magnesium, or zinc may bind levothyroxine and prevent complete absorption.

Route/Dosage

Levothyroxine

PO (Adults): *Hypothyroidism* — 50 mcg as a single dose initially; may be ↑ q 2–3 wk; usual maintenance dose is 75–125 mcg/day (1.5 mcg/kg/day).

PO (Geriatric Patients and Patients with Increased Sensitivity to Thyroid Hormones): 12.5–25 mcg as a single dose initially; may be ↑ q 6–8 wk; usual maintenance dose is 75 mcg/day.

PO (Children ≥12 yr): 2–3 mcg/kg/day (up to 150–200 mcg/day).

PO (Children 6–12 yr): 4–5 mcg/kg/day (100–125 mcg/day).

PO (Children 1–5 yr): 5–6 mcg/kg/day (75–100 mcg/day).

PO (Children 6–12 mo): 6–8 mcg/kg/day (50–75 mcg/day).

PO (Infants 3–6 mo): 8–10 mcg/kg/day (25–50 mcg/day).

PO (Infants 0–3 mo or Infants at Risk for Cardiac Failure): 10–15 mcg/kg/day or 25 mcg/day; may be ↑ after 4–6 wk to 50 mcg.

IM, IV (Adults): *Hypothyroidism* — 50–100 mcg/day as a single dose. *Myxedema coma/stupor* — 200–500 mcg IV; additional 100–300 mcg may be given on 2nd day, followed by daily administration of smaller doses.

IM, IV (Children): *Hypothyroidism* — ~50–80% of the oral dose.

Liothyronine

PO (Adults): *Mild hypothyroidism* — 25 mcg once daily; may ↑ by 12.5–25 mcg/day q 1–2 wk intervals; usual maintenance dose is 25–50 mcg/day. *Myxedema* — 2.5–5 mcg once daily initially; ↑ by 5–10 mcg/day q 1–2 wk up to 25 mcg/day, then ↑ by 12.5–25 mcg/day; usual maintenance dose is 25–50 mcg/day. *Simple goiter* — 5 mcg once daily initially; ↑ by 5–10 mcg/day q 1–2 wk up to 25 mcg/day, then ↑ by 12.5–25 mcg/day q wk until desired effect is obtained; usual maintenance dose is 50–100 mcg/day. *T_3 suppression test* — 75–100 mcg daily for 7 days. Radioactive ^{131}I is administered before and after 7-day course.

PO (Geriatric Patients or Patients with Cardiovascular Disease): 5 mcg/day initially; ↑ by no more than 5 mcg/day q 2 wk.

IV (Adults): *Myxedema coma* — 25–50 mcg initially (if cardiovascular disease is present, initial dose should be 10–20 mcg). Additional doses may be given, to a total of at least 65 mcg/

THYROID PREPARATIONS 1221

day (not to exceed 100 mcg/day). Doses should be at least 4 hr but not more than 12 hr apart.

Liotrix
Contains T_4 and T_3 in a ratio of 4:1.
PO (Adults): *Hypothyroidism*—Start with 50 mcg levothyroxine/12.5 mcg liothyronine; ↑ by 50 mcg levothyroxine/12.5 mcg liothyronine q 2–4 wk until desired effect is obtained; usual maintenance dose is 50–100 mcg levothyroxine/12.5–25 mcg liothyronine daily. *Myxedema/hypothyroidism with cardiovascular disease*—12.5 mcg levothyroxine/3.1 mcg liothyronine/day; ↑ by 12.5 mcg levothyroxine/3.1 mcg liothyronine q 2–4 wk until desired effect is obtained.
PO (Geriatric Patients): 12.5–25 mcg levothyroxine/3.1–6.2 mcg liothyronine/day; ↑ by 12.5–25 mcg levothyroxine/3.1–6.2 mcg liothyronine q 6–8 wk until desired effect is obtained.

Thyroid
Each 1 gr = 60 mg and is equivalent to 100 mcg or less of levothyroxine (T_4) or 25 mcg of liothyronine (T_3).
PO (Adults and Children): *Hypothyroidism*—60 mg/day; ↑ q 4 wk by 30 mg; usual maintenance dose is 60–120 mg/day. *Myxedema/hypothyroidism with cardiovascular disease*—15 mg/day initially; ↑ by 30 mg/day q 2 wk, then may ↑ by 30–60 mg q 2 wk; usual maintenance dose is 60–120 mg/day.
PO (Geriatric Patients): 7.5–15 mg/day initially; may double dose q 6–8 wk until desired effect is obtained.

Availability
Levothyroxine (generic available)
Tablets: 25 mcg, 50 mcg, 75 mcg, 88 mcg, 100 mcg, 112 mcg, 125 mcg, 137 mcg, 150 mcg, 175 mcg, 200 mcg, 300 mcg. **Cost:** *Levothroid*—50 mcg $22.95/90, 100 mcg $22.97/90; *Levoxyl*—50 mcg $31.97/90, 100 mcg $34.97/90; *Synthroid*—50 mcg $42.97/90, 100 mcg $46.97/90; *Unithroid*—50 mcg $31.97/90, 100 mcg $35.97/90; *Generic*—50 mcg $19.97/90, 100 mcg $25.97/90. **Powder for injection:** 200 mcg/vial, 500 mcg/vial.

Liothyronine (generic available)
Tablets: 5 mcg, 25 mcg, 50 mcg. **Solution for injection:** 10 mcg/mL.

Liotrix
Tablets: 12.5 mcg levothyroxine/3.1 mcg liothyronine, 25 mcg levothyroxine/6.25 mcg liothyronine, 50 mcg levothyroxine/12.5 mcg liothyronine, 100 mcg levothyroxine/25 mcg liothyronine, 150 mcg levothyroxine/37.5 mcg liothyronine.

Thyroid (generic available)
Tablets: 15 mg, 30 mg, 60 mg, 90 mg, 120 mg, 180 mg, 240 mg, 300 mg. **Cost:** 15 mg $15.97/90, 30 mg $22.97/90, 60 mg $22.97/90, 90 mg $28.97/90, 120 mg $34.97/90, 180 mg $49.97/90, 240 mg $65.97/90, 300 mg $75.92/90.

NURSING IMPLICATIONS

Assessment
- Assess apical pulse and blood pressure prior to and periodically during therapy. Assess for tachyarrhythmias and chest pain.
- **Children:** Monitor height, weight, and psychomotor development.
- ***Lab Test Considerations:*** Monitor thyroid function studies prior to and during therapy.
- Monitor TSH concentrations in adults 8–12 wk after changing from one brand to another.
- Monitor blood and urine glucose in diabetic patients. Insulin or oral hypoglycemic dose may need to be ↑.
- ***Toxicity and Overdose:*** Overdose is manifested as hyperthyroidism (tachycardia, chest pain, nervousness, insomnia, diaphoresis, tremors, weight loss). Usual treatment is to withhold dose for 2–6 days. Acute overdose is treated by induction of emesis or gastric lavage, followed by activated charcoal. Sympathetic overstimulation may be controlled by antiadrenergic drugs (beta blockers), such as propranolol. Oxygen and supportive measures to control symptoms such as fever are also used.

Potential Nursing Diagnoses
Deficient knowledge, related to medication regimen (Patient/Family Teaching)

Implementation
- Administer as a single dose, preferably before breakfast to prevent insomnia.
- Initial dose is low, especially in geriatric and cardiac patients. Dose is ↑ gradually, based on thyroid function tests. Side effects occur more rapidly with liothyronine because of its rapid onset of effect.
- For patients with difficulty swallowing, levothyroxine tablets can be crushed and placed in 5–10 mL of water and administered immediately via dropper or spoon; do not store suspension.

Levothyroxine

IV Administration

- **Direct IV:** *Diluent:* Reconstitute the 200-mcg and 500-mcg vials with 2 or 5 mL, respectively, of 0.9% NaCl without preservatives (diluent usually provided). Shake well to dissolve completely. Administer solution immediately after preparation; discard unused portion. ***Concentration:*** 100 mcg/mL. *Rate:* Administer at a rate of 100 mcg over 1 min. Do not add to IV infusions; may be administered through Y-tubing.
- **Y-Site Incompatibility:** Do not admix with other IV solutions or medications.

Liothyronine

IV Administration

- **IV:** Liothyronine injection is for IV use only. Do not give IM or subcut. Administer doses at least 4 hr and not more than 12 hr apart. Base doses on continuous monitoring of patient and response to therapy.
- Resume PO therapy as soon as patient is stable and able to take PO medication. When switching to PO therapy, discontinue IV liothyronine and initiate PO at low dose, increasing gradually according to patient's response.
- **Direct IV:** May be administered undiluted at 10 mcg/mL. *Rate:* Administer as a bolus.

Patient/Family Teaching

- Instruct patient to take medication as directed at the same time each day. Take missed doses as soon as remembered unless almost time for next dose. If more than 2–3 doses are missed, notify health care professional. Do not discontinue without consulting health care professional.
- Explain to patient that medication does not cure hypothyroidism; it provides a thyroid hormone. Therapy is lifelong.
- Caution patient not to change brands of thyroid preparations, as this may affect drug bioavailability.
- Advise patient to notify health care professional if headache, nervousness, diarrhea, excessive sweating, heat intolerance, chest pain, increased pulse rate, palpitations, weight loss >2 lb/wk, or any unusual symptoms occur.
- Caution patient to avoid taking other medications concurrently with thyroid preparations unless instructed by health care professional.
- Instruct patient to inform health care professional of thyroid therapy.
- Emphasize importance of follow-up exams to monitor effectiveness of therapy. Thyroid function tests are performed at least yearly.
- **Levothyroxine:** Advise patients to take Levoxyl tablets with water. Levoxyl tablets may rapidly swell and disintegrate resulting in choking, gagging, the tablet getting stuck in the throat, and difficulty swallowing. Taking with water usually prevents this.
- Pedi: Discuss with parents the need for routine follow-up studies to ensure correct development. Inform patient that partial hair loss may be experienced by children on thyroid therapy. This is usually temporary.

Evaluation/Desired Outcomes

- Resolution of symptoms of hypothyroidism and normalization of thyroid hormone levels.

---

tiagabine (tye-a-ga-been)
Gabitril

Classification
Therapeutic: anticonvulsants

Pregnancy Category C

Indications
Adjunctive treatment of partial seizures.

Action
Enhances the activity of gamma-aminobutyric acid, an inhibitory neurotransmitter. **Therapeutic Effects:** Decreased frequency of seizures.

Pharmacokinetics
Absorption: 90% absorbed following oral administration.
Distribution: Unknown.
Protein Binding: 96%.
Metabolism and Excretion: Mostly metabolized by the liver; 2% excreted unchanged in urine.
Half-life: *Without enzyme-inducing antiepileptic drugs*—7–9 hr; *with enzyme-inducing antiepileptic drugs*—4–7 hr.

TIME/ACTION PROFILE (blood levels)

ROUTE	ONSET	PEAK	DURATION
PO	unknown	45 min	unknown

Contraindications/Precautions
Contraindicated in: Hypersensitivity.
Use Cautiously in: All patients (may ↑ risk of suicidal thoughts/behaviors); Hepatic impairment (↓ dose/increased interval may be necessary); Patients receiving concurrent non–enzyme-inducing antiepileptic drug therapy such as valpro-

ates (may require lower doses and/or slower titration); Using tiagabine for off-label uses or other conditions leading to ↑ levels (may ↑ risk of new onset seizures); OB, Lactation: Pedi: Pregnancy, lactation, or children <12 yr (safety not established).

Adverse Reactions/Side Effects
CNS: SUICIDAL THOUGHTS, dizziness, drowsiness, nervousness, weakness, cognitive impairment, confusion, difficulty concentrating, hallucinations, headache, mental depression, personality disorder. **EENT:** abnormal vision, ear pain, tinnitus. **Resp:** dyspnea, epistaxis. **CV:** chest pain, edema, hypertension, palpitations, syncope, tachycardia. **GI:** abdominal pain, gingivitis, nausea, stomatitis. **GU:** dysmenorrhea, dysuria, metrorrhagia, urinary incontinence. **Derm:** alopecia, dry skin, rash, sweating. **Metab:** weight gain, weight loss. **MS:** arthralgia, neck pain. **Neuro:** ataxia, tremors. **Misc:** allergic reactions, chills, lymphadenopathy.

Interactions
Drug-Drug: Carbamazepine, phenytoin, primidone, and **phenobarbital** induce metabolism and ↓ blood levels; although concurrent therapy is usually necessary, adjustments may be required when altering regimens.

Route/Dosage
PO (Adults >18 yr): 4 mg once daily initially for 1 wk; may ↑ by 4–8 mg/day at weekly intervals, up to 56 mg/day in 2–4 divided doses.
PO (Children 12–18 yr): 4 mg once daily initially for 1 wk; may ↑ by 4 mg/day after 1 wk, then may ↑ by 4–8 mg/day at weekly intervals, up to 32 mg/day in 2–4 divided doses.

Availability
Tablets: 2 mg, 4 mg, 12 mg, 16 mg.

NURSING IMPLICATIONS

Assessment
- Assess location, duration, and characteristics of seizure activity.
- Assess mental status. May cause impaired concentration, speech or language problems, confusion, fatigue, and drowsiness. Symptoms may decrease with dose reduction or discontinuation.
- Monitor closely for notable changes in behavior that could indicate the emergence or worsening of suicidal thoughts or behavior or depression.
- *Toxicity and Overdose:* Therapeutic serum levels have not been determined. However, levels may be monitored prior to and following changes in the therapeutic regimen.

Potential Nursing Diagnoses
Risk for injury (Side Effects)

Implementation
- Do not confuse tiagabine with tizanidine.
- PO: Administer with food.
- Discontinue tiagabine gradually. Abrupt discontinuation may cause increase in seizure frequency.

Patient/Family Teaching
- Instruct patient to take medication as directed. Take missed doses as soon as possible unless almost time for next dose. Do not double doses. Do not discontinue abruptly; may cause increase in frequency of seizures. Instruct patient to read the *Medication Guide* before starting and with each Rx refill, changes may occur.
- Advise patient to notify health care professional immediately if frequency of seizures increases.
- May cause dizziness. Caution patient to avoid driving or activities requiring alertness until response to medication is known. Do not resume driving until physician gives clearance based on control of seizure disorder.
- Advise patient and family to notify health care professional if thoughts about suicide or dying, attempts to commit suicide; new or worse depression; new or worse anxiety; feeling very agitated or restless; panic attacks; trouble sleeping; new or worse irritability; acting aggressive; being angry or violent; acting on dangerous impulses; an extreme increase in activity and talking, other unusual changes in behavior or mood occur.
- Advise patient to notify health care professional if pregnancy is planned or suspected or if breastfeeding.
- Instruct patient to notify health care professional of medication regimen prior to treatment or surgery.
- Advise patient to carry identification describing disease process and medication regimen at all times.

Evaluation/Desired Outcomes
- Decrease in the frequency or cessation of seizures.

ticarcillin/clavulanate
(tye-kar-**sil**-in/klav-yoo-**la**-nate)
Timentin

Classification
Therapeutic: anti-infectives
Pharmacologic: extended spectrum penicillins

Pregnancy Category B

Indications
Treatment of: Skin and skin structure infections, Bone and joint infections, Septicemia, Lower respiratory tract infections, Intra-abdominal, gynecologic, and urinary tract infections.

Action
Binds to bacterial cell wall membrane, causing cell death. Addition of clavulanate enhances resistance to beta-lactamase, an enzyme that can inactivate penicillins. **Therapeutic Effects:** Bactericidal action. **Spectrum:** Similar to penicillin but extended to include several gram-negative aerobic pathogens, notably: *Pseudomonas aeruginosa, Escherichia coli, Citrobacter, Enterobacter, Haemophilus influenzae, Klebsiella, Serratia marcescens*. Active against some anaerobic bacteria, including bacteroides.

Pharmacokinetics
Absorption: IV administration results in complete bioavailability.
Distribution: Widely distributed. Enters CSF well when meninges are inflamed. Crosses the placenta; enters breast milk in low concentrations.
Metabolism and Excretion: 10% of ticarcillin is metabolized by the liver; 90% excreted unchanged by the kidneys. Clavulanate is metabolized by the liver.
Half-life: *Ticarcillin*—1.1 hr (↑ in renal impairment); *clavulanate*—1.1 hr.

TIME/ACTION PROFILE (blood levels)

ROUTE	ONSET	PEAK	DURATION
IV	rapid	end of infusion	4–6 hr

Contraindications/Precautions
Contraindicated in: Hypersensitivity to penicillins (cross-sensitivity with cephalosporins may occur).
Use Cautiously in: Renal impairment (dose ↓ and/or ↑ interval required if CCr <60 mL/min); Congestive heart failure (due to high sodium content); OB, Lactation: Safety not established; Pedi: Children <3 mo (safety not established).

Adverse Reactions/Side Effects
CNS: SEIZURES (high doses), confusion, lethargy. **CV:** CHF, arrhythmias. **GI:** PSEUDOMEMBRANOUS COLITIS, diarrhea, nausea. **GU:** hematuria (children only). **Derm:** rashes, urticaria. **F and E:** hypokalemia, hypernatremia. **Hemat:** bleeding, blood dyscrasias, ↑ bleeding time. **Local:** phlebitis. **Metab:** metabolic alkalosis. **Misc:** hypersensitivity reactions including ANAPHYLAXIS, superinfection.

Interactions
Drug-Drug: Probenecid ↓ renal excretion and ↑ blood levels.

Route/Dosage
Ticarcillin/clavulanate contains 4.51–6 mEq sodium/g and 0.15 mEq potassium/g of ticarcillin/clavulanate. 3 g ticarcillin plus 100 mg clavulanate labeled as 3.1 g combined potency. Dosing is based on ticarcillin component..

IV (Adults and Children >16 yr): 3 g ticarcillin q 4–6 hr.

IV (Children 3 mo–16 yr): *<60 kg*—Mild to moderate infection: 50 mg ticarcillin/kg q 6 hr; severe infection: 50 mg ticarcillin/kg q 4 hr. *≥60 kg*—Mild to moderate infection: 3 g ticarcillin q 6 hr; severe infection: 3 g ticarcillin q 4 hr.

Renal Impairment
IV (Adults): Give loading dose of 3 g ticarcillin × 1 dose, followed by maintenance dose based on CCr. *CCr 30–60 mL/min*—2 g ticarcillin q 4 hr; *10–30 mL/min*—2 g ticarcillin q 8 hr; *CCr <10 mL/min*—2 g ticarcillin q 12 hr; *CCr <10 mL/min with hepatic dysfunction*—2 g ticarcillin q 24 hr; *Peritoneal dialysis*—3 g ticarcillin q 12 hr; *Hemodialysis*—2 g ticarcillin q 12 hr supplemented with 3 g ticarcillin after each dialysis session.

Availability
Powder for injection: 3.1 g/vial, 31 g/vial. **Premixed infusion:** 3.1 g/100 mL.

NURSING IMPLICATIONS
Assessment
- Assess patient for infection (vital signs; appearance of wound, sputum, urine, and stool; WBC) at beginning of and throughout therapy.
- Obtain a history before initiating therapy to determine use of and reactions to penicillins or cephalosporins. Persons with a negative history of penicillin sensitivity may still have an allergic response.
- Obtain specimens for culture and sensitivity before initiating therapy. First dose may be given before receiving results.

- Observe patient for signs and symptoms of anaphylaxis (rash, pruritus, laryngeal edema, wheezing). Discontinue drug and notify physician immediately if these problems occur. Keep epinephrine, an antihistamine, and resuscitation equipment close by in case of anaphylactic reaction.
- **Lab Test Considerations:** Evaluate renal and hepatic function, CBC, serum potassium, and bleeding times prior to and routinely throughout therapy.
- May cause false-positive urine protein testing and increased BUN, creatinine, AST, ALT, serum bilirubin, alkaline phosphatase, LDH, and uric acid levels. May also cause ↑ bleeding time.
- May cause hypernatremia and hypokalemia with high doses.

Potential Nursing Diagnoses
Risk for infection (Indications, Side Effects)

Implementation

IV Administration

- **IV:** Change IV sites every 48 hr to prevent phlebitis.
- **Intermittent Infusion:** *Diluent:* Add 13 mL of sterile water for injection or 0.9% NaCl for injection to each 3.1-g vial, to provide a concentration of ticarcillin 200 mg/mL and clavulanic acid 6.7 mg/mL. Further dilute in 0.9% NaCl, D5W, or LR to achieve a concentration of 10–100 mg/mL. Reconstituted vials stable for 24 hr at room temperature or 72 hr if refrigerated. Infusion is stable for 24 hr at room temperature. If refrigerated, infusion is stable for 3 days (diluted in D5W) or 7 days (if diluted in 0.9% NaCl or LR). *Concentration:* 10–100 mg/mL. *Rate:* Infuse over 30 min.
- **Y-Site Compatibility:** allopurinol, amifostine, amikacin, anidulafungin, atropine, aztreonam, bivalirudin, bumetanide, cefazolin, cefepime, cefotaxime, cefoxitin, ceftazidime, ceftizoxime, ceftriaxone, cefuroxime, chloramphenicol , cimetidine, clindamycin, cyclophosphamide, cyclosporine, dexamethasone sodium phosphate, dexmedetomidine, digoxin, diltiazem, diphenhydramine, docetaxel, dopamine, doxorubicin liposome, doxycycline, enalaprilat, epinephrine, esmolol, etoposide phosphate, famotidine, fenoldopam, filgrastim, fluconazole, furosemide, gemcitabine, gentamicin, granisetron, heparin, hydrocortisone sodium succinate, hydromorphone, imipenem/cilastatin, insulin, isoproterenol, labetalol, levofloxacin, lidocaine, linezolid, lorazepam, melphalan, meperidine, methylprednisolone sodium succinate, metoclopramide, metoprolol, metronidazole, milrinone, morphine, nitroglycerin, nitroprusside, norepinephrine, ondansetron, palonosetron, pantoprazole, pemetrexed, penicillin G potassium, perphenazine, phenylephrine, procainamide, propofol, propranolol, ranitidine, remifentanil, sargramostim, sodium bicarbonate, tacrolimus, teniposide, theophylline, thiotepa, tirofiban, tobramycin, vasopressin, verapamil, vinorelbine, voriconazole.
- **Y-Site Incompatibility:** acyclovir, amphotericin B cholesteryl sulfate, azithromycin, caspofungin, diazepam, dobutamine, drotrecogin, erythromycin, ganciclovir, haloperidol, hydroxyzine, lansoprazole, phenytoin, promethazine, protamine, quinupristin/dalfopristin, trimethoprim/sulfamethoxazole. If aminoglycosides and penicillins must be administered concurrently, administer in separate sites at least 1 hr apart.

Patient/Family Teaching
- Advise patient to report signs of superinfection (black, furry overgrowth on the tongue; vaginal itching or discharge; loose or foul-smelling stools) and allergy.
- Caution patient to notify health care professional if fever and diarrhea occur, especially if stool contains blood, pus, or mucus. Advise patient not to treat diarrhea without consulting health care professional. May occur up to several weeks after discontinuation of medication.

Evaluation/Desired Outcomes
- Resolution of the signs and symptoms of infection. Length of time for complete resolution depends on the organism and site of infection.

---

ticlopidine (tye-cloe-pi-deen)

Classification
Therapeutic: antiplatelet agents
Pharmacologic: platelet aggregation inhibitors

Pregnancy Category B

Indications
Prevention of stroke in patients who have had a completed thrombotic stroke or precursors to

stroke and are unable to tolerate aspirin. **Unlabeled Use:** Prevention of subacute stent thrombosis in patients receiving intracoronary stents (given with aspirin).

Action
Inhibits platelet aggregation by altering the function of platelet membranes. Prolongs bleeding time. **Therapeutic Effects:** Decreased incidence of stroke in high-risk patients. Decreased incidence of subacute stent thrombosis.

Pharmacokinetics
Absorption: >80% absorbed after oral administration.
Distribution: Unknown.
Protein Binding: 98%.
Metabolism and Excretion: Extensively metabolized by the liver; minimal excretion of unchanged drug by the kidneys.
Half-life: *Single dose*—12.6 hr; *multiple dosing*—4–5 days.

TIME/ACTION PROFILE (effect on platelet function)

ROUTE	ONSET	PEAK	DURATION
PO	within 4 days	8–11 days	2 wk

Contraindications/Precautions
Contraindicated in: Hypersensitivity; Bleeding disorders; Active bleeding; Severe liver disease.
Use Cautiously in: Risk of bleeding (trauma, surgery, history of ulcer disease); Renal or hepatic impairment (dosage adjustments may be necessary); OB, Lactation: Pedi: Safety not established; Geri: Appears on Beers list. Geriatric patients have ↑ sensitivity.

Adverse Reactions/Side Effects
CNS: dizziness, headache, weakness. **EENT:** epistaxis, tinnitus. **GI:** diarrhea, abnormal liver function tests, anorexia, GI fullness, GI pain, nausea, vomiting. **GU:** hematuria. **Derm:** rashes, ecchymoses, pruritus, urticaria. **Hemat:** AGRANULOCYTOSIS, APLASTIC ANEMIA, INTRACEREBRAL BLEEDING, NEUTROPENIA, bleeding, thrombocytopenia. **Metab:** hypercholesterolemia, hypertriglyceridemia.

Interactions
Drug-Drug: **Aspirin** potentiates the effect of ticlopidine on platelets (concurrent use not recommended). ↑ risk of bleeding with **heparins**, **warfarin**, **tirofiban**, **eptifibatide**, or **thrombolytic agents**. **Cimetidine** ↓ metabolism of ticlopidine and may ↑ the risk of toxicity. Ticlopidine ↓ metabolism and ↑ the risk of toxicity of **theophylline**.
Drug-Food: Absorption ↑ by taking with **food**.

Route/Dosage
PO (Adults): 250 mg twice daily with food.

Availability (generic available)
Tablets: 250 mg.

NURSING IMPLICATIONS

Assessment
- Assess patient for symptoms of stroke periodically throughout therapy.
- *Lab Test Considerations:* Monitor bleeding time throughout therapy. Prolonged bleeding time (2–5 times the normal limit), which is time- and dose-dependent, is expected.
- Monitor CBC with differential and platelet count every 2 wk from the 2nd wk to the end of the 3rd mo of therapy; more frequently if absolute neutrophil count (ANC) is declining or <30% of baseline. If neutropenia occurs, ticlopidine should be discontinued. Neutrophil counts usually return to normal within 1–3 wk of discontinuation of therapy. After the first 3 mo of therapy, CBCs need to be obtained only for patients with signs and symptoms of infection.
- May cause thrombocytopenia, usually within 3–12 wk of initiation of therapy. If platelet count is <80,000/mm^3, discontinue ticlopidine.
- May cause ↑ serum total cholesterol and triglyceride levels. Levels usually increase 8–10% within the first mo and persist at that level.
- May cause ↑ alkaline phosphatase, bilirubin, AST, and ALT levels during the first 4 mo of therapy.
- *Toxicity and Overdose:* Prolonged bleeding time is normalized within 2 hr after administration of IV methylprednisolone. May also use platelet transfusions to reverse effects of ticlopidine on bleeding time.

Potential Nursing Diagnoses
Risk for injury (Indications, Side Effects)

Implementation
- **PO:** Administer with food or immediately after eating to minimize GI discomfort and increase absorption.

Patient/Family Teaching
- Instruct patient to take medication as directed. Missed doses should be taken as soon as possible unless almost time for next dose; do not double doses.
- Advise patient to notify health care professional promptly if fever, chills, sore throat, unusual bleeding or bruising, severe or persistent diarrhea, skin rash, jaundice, dark-colored urine, or light-colored stools occur.

tigecycline **1227**

- Advise patient to notify health care professional of medication regimen before treatment or surgery. Medication may need to be discontinued 10–14 days before surgery.
- Emphasize the importance of routine lab tests during the first 3 mo of therapy to monitor for side effects.

Evaluation/Desired Outcomes
- Prevention of stroke.

---

tigecycline (tye-gi-sye-kleen)
Tygacil

Classification
Therapeutic: anti-infectives
Pharmacologic: glycylcyclines

Pregnancy Category D

Indications
Complicated skin/skin structure infections, complicated intra-abdominal infections, or community-acquired bacterial pneumonia caused by susceptible bacteria.

Action
Inhibits bacterial protein synthesis by binding to the 30S ribosomal subunit. **Therapeutic Effects:** Resolution of infection. **Spectrum:** Active against the following Gram-positive bacteria: *Enterococcus faecalis* (vancomycin-susceptible strains only), *Staphylococcus aureus* (methicillin-sensitive and methicillin-resistant strains), *Streptococcus agalactiae*, *Streptococcus anginosus*, *Streptococcus pneumoniae*, and *Streptococcus pyogenes*. Also active against these Gram-positive organisms: *Citrobacter freundii*, *Enterobacter cloacae*, *Escherichia coli*, *Haemophilus influenzae* (beta-lactamase negative strains only), *Legionella pneumophila*, *Klebsiella oxytoca*, and *Klebsiella pneumoniae*. Additionally active against the following anaerobes: *Bacteroides fragilis*, *Bacteroides thetaiotaomicron*, *Bacteroides uniformis*, *Bacteroides vulgatus*, *Clostridium perfringens*, and *Peptostreptococcus micros*.

Pharmacokinetics
Absorption: IV administration results in complete bioavailability.
Distribution: Widely distributed with good penetration into gall bladder, lung, and colon; crosses the placenta.
Metabolism and Excretion: Minimal metabolism; primary route of elimination is biliary/fecal excretion of unchanged drug and metabolites (59%), 33% renal (22% unchanged).
Half-life: 27.1 hr (after 1 dose); 42.4 hr after multiple doses.

TIME/ACTION PROFILE (blood levels)

ROUTE	ONSET	PEAK	DURATION
IV	rapid	end of infusion	12 hr

Contraindications/Precautions
Contraindicated in: Hypersensitivity; Pedi: Children.
Use Cautiously in: Complicated intra-abdominal infections due to perforation; Severe hepatic impairment (↓ maintenance dose recommended); Geri: Older patients may be more sensitive to adverse effects; OB, Lactation: Use in pregnancy only when potential maternal benefit outweighs fetal risk; use cautiously during lactation.

Adverse Reactions/Side Effects
CNS: somnolence. **CV:** changes in heart rate, vasodilation. **GI:** PSEUDOMEMBRANOUS COLITIS, <u>nausea</u>, <u>vomiting</u>, altered taste, anorexia, dry mouth, hepatotoxicity, jaundice. **GU:** ↑ serum creatinine. **Endo:** hyperglycemia. **F and E:** hypocalcemia, hyponatremia. **Local:** injection site reactions. **Misc:** allergic reactions.

Interactions
Drug-Drug: May ↓ the effectiveness of **hormonal contraceptives**. Effects on **warfarin** are unknown (monitoring recommended).

Route/Dosage
IV (Adults >18 yr): 100 mg initially, then 50 mg every 12 hr for 5–14 days (skin/skin structure infections and intra-abdominal infections) or 7–14 days (pneumonia).

Hepatic Impairment
IV (Adults >18 yr): Child-Pugh C — 100 mg initially, then 25 mg every 12 hr.

Availability
Lyophilized powder for reconstitution: 50 mg.

NURSING IMPLICATIONS

Assessment
- Assess for infection (vital signs; appearance of wound, sputum, urine, and stool; WBC) at beginning of and throughout therapy.

♣ = Canadian drug name. ☒ = Genetic implication.
*CAPITALS indicates life-threatening; <u>underlines</u> indicate most frequent.

- Obtain specimens for culture and sensitivity before initiating therapy. 1st dose may be given before receiving results.
- Before initiating therapy, obtain a history of tetracycline hypersensitivity; may also have an allergic response to tigecycline.
- Monitor bowel function. Diarrhea, abdominal cramping, fever, and bloody stools should be reported to health care professional promptly as a sign of pseudomembranous colitis. May begin up to several weeks following cessation of therapy.
- **Lab Test Considerations:** May cause anemia, leukocytosis, and thrombocythemia.
- May cause ↑ serum alkaline phosphatase, amylase, bilirubin, LDH, AST, and ALT.
- May cause hyperglycemia, hypokalemia, hypoproteinemia, hypocalcemia, hyponatremia, and ↑ BUN level.

Potential Nursing Diagnoses
Risk for infection (Indications)

Implementation
- May cause yellow-brown discoloration and softening of teeth and bones if administered prenatally or during early childhood. Not recommended for children under 8 yr of age or during pregnancy or lactation unless used for the treatment of anthrax.

IV Administration
- **Intermittent Infusion:** Reconstitute each vial with 5.3 mL of 0.9% NaCl or D5W to achieve a concentration of 10 mg/mL. *Diluent:* Dilute further in 100 mL of D5W, LR, or 0.9% NaCl. Reconstituted solution should be yellow to orange in color. Do not administer solutions that are discolored or contain particulate matter. Infusion is stable for up to 24 hr at room temperature or for up to 48 hr if refrigerated. *Concentration:* Final concentration of infusion should be ≤1 mg/mL. *Rate:* Infuse over 30–60 min. Flush line before and after infusion with 0.9% NaCl or D5W.
- **Y-Site Compatibility:** acyclovir, alfentanil, allopurinol, amifostine, amikacin, aminocaproic acid, aminophylline, amphotericin B liposome, ampicillin, ampicillin/sulbactam, argatroban, azithromycin, aztreonam, bivalirudin, bumetanide, buprenorphine, butorphanol, calcium chloride, calcium gluconate, carboplatin, carmustine, caspofungin, cefazolin, cefepime, cefotaxime, cefotetan, cefoxitin, ceftazidime, ceftizoxime, ceftriaxone, cefuroxime, cimetidine, ciprofloxacin, cisatracurium, cisplatin, clindamycin, cyclophosphamide, cyclosporine, cytarabine, dacarbazine, dactinomycin, daptomycin, daunorubicin hydrochloride, dexamethasone, dexmedetomidine, dexrazoxane, digoxin, diltiazem, diphenhydramine, dobutamine, docetaxel, dolasetron, dopamine, doripenem, doxorubicin hydrochloride, doxorubicin liposome, droperidol, enalaprilat, epinephrine, eptifibatide, ertapenem, erythromycin, esmolol, etoposide, etoposide phosphate, famotidine, fenoldopam, fentanyl, fluconazole, fludarabine, fluorouracil, foscarnet, fosphenytoin, furosemide, ganciclovir, gemcitabine, gentamicin, glycopyrrolate, granisetron, haloperidol, heparin, hydrocortisone, hydromorphone, ifosfamide, imipenem/cilastatin, insulin, irinotecan, isoproterenol, ketorolac, labetalol, lansoprazole, lepirudin, leucovorin, levofloxacin, lidocaine, linezolid, lorazepam, magnesium sulfate, mannitol, mechlorethamine, melphalan, meperidine, meropenem, mesna, methohexital, methotrexate, methyldopa, metoclopramide, metoprolol, metronidazole, midazolam, milrinone, mitomycin, mitoxantrone, morphine, moxifloxacin, mycophenolate, nafcillin, nalbuphine, naloxone, nesiritide, nitroglycerin, nitroprusside, norepinephrine, octreotide, ondansetron, oxaliplatin, oxytocin, paclitaxel, palonosetron, pamidronate, pancuronium, pantoprazole, pemetrexed, pemtamidine, pentazocin, pentobarbital, phenobarbital, phenylephrine, piperacillin/tazobactam, potassium acetate, potassium chloride, potassium phosphate, procainamide, prochlorperazine, promethazine, propranolol, propofol, ranitidine, remifentanil, rocuronium, sodium acetate, sodium bicarbonate, sodium phosphate, streptozocin, succinylcholine, sufentanil, tacrolimus, teniposide, theophylline, thiopental, thiotepa, ticarcillin/clavulanate, tirofiban, tobramycin, topotecan, trimethoprim/sulfamethoxazole, vancomycin, vasopressin, vecuronium, vinblastine, vincristine, vinorelbine, zidovudine, zoledronic acid.
- **Y-Site Incompatibility:** amiodarone, amphotericin B colloidal, bleomycin, chloramphenicol, chlorpromazine, dantrolene, daunorubicin liposome, diazepam, epirubicin, hydralazine, idarubicin, nicardipine, phenytoin, quinapristin/dalfopristin, verapamil.

Patient/Family Teaching
- Advise patient that full course of therapy should be completed, even if feeling better. Skipping doses or not completing full course of therapy may result in decreased effectiveness and increased risk of bacterial resistance.

- Advise female patient to use a nonhormonal method of contraception while taking tigecycline and until next menstrual period.
- Instruct patient to notify health care professional if fever and diarrhea develop, especially if stool contains blood, pus, or mucus. Advise patient not to treat diarrhea without consulting health care professional.
- Advise patient to report the signs of superinfection (black, furry overgrowth on the tongue, vaginal itching or discharge, loose or foul-smelling stools). Skin rash, pruritus, and urticaria should also be reported.

Evaluation/Desired Outcomes
- Resolution of signs and symptoms of infection.

---

timolol† (tim-oh-lole)
Apo-Timol, Novo-Timol

Classification
Therapeutic: antihypertensives, vascular headache suppressants
Pharmacologic: beta blockers

Pregnancy Category C
†For ophthalmic use, see Appendix C

Indications
Hypertension (alone or with other agents). Prevention of MI. Prevention of migraine headaches. **Unlabeled Use:** Ventricular arrhythmias. Essential tremor. Anxiety.

Action
Blocks stimulation of beta$_1$(myocardial)- and beta$_2$(pulmonary, vascular, and uterine)-adrenergic receptor sites. **Therapeutic Effects:** Decreased heart rate and blood pressure. Prevention of MI. Decreased frequency of migraine headache.

Pharmacokinetics
Absorption: Well absorbed after oral administration.
Distribution: Enters breast milk.
Metabolism and Excretion: Extensively metabolized by the liver.
Half-life: 3–4 hr.

TIME/ACTION PROFILE (cardiovascular effects)

ROUTE	ONSET	PEAK	DURATION
PO	unknown	1–2 hr*	12–24 hr

*After single dose, full effect is not seen until several weeks of therapy

Contraindications/Precautions
Contraindicated in: Uncompensated CHF; Pulmonary edema; Cardiogenic shock; Bradycardia or heart block.
Use Cautiously in: Renal impairment; Hepatic impairment; Geri: May have ↑ sensitivity to beta blockers; initial dosage reduction recommended); Pulmonary disease (including asthma); Diabetes mellitus (may mask signs of hypoglycemia); Thyrotoxicosis (may mask symptoms); Patients with a history of severe allergic reactions (intensity of reactions may be increased); OB, Lactation: Pedi: Safety not established; may cause fetal/neonatal bradycardia, hypotension, hypoglycemia, or respiratory depression.

Adverse Reactions/Side Effects
CNS: fatigue, weakness, anxiety, depression, dizziness, drowsiness, insomnia, memory loss, mental status changes, nervousness, nightmares. **EENT:** blurred vision, dry eyes, nasal stuffiness. **Resp:** bronchospasm, wheezing. **CV:** ARRHYTHMIAS, BRADYCARDIA, CHF, PULMONARY EDEMA, orthostatic hypotension, peripheral vasoconstriction. **GI:** constipation, diarrhea, nausea. **GU:** erectile dysfunction, ↓ libido. **Derm:** itching, rashes. **Endo:** hyperglycemia, hypoglycemia. **MS:** arthralgia, back pain, muscle cramps. **Neuro:** paresthesia. **Misc:** ANAPHYLAXIS (rare).

Interactions
Drug-Drug: General anesthesia, IV phenytoin, and verapamil may ↑ myocardial depression. ↑ bradycardia may occur with digoxin. ↑ hypotension may occur with other antihypertensives, acute ingestion of alcohol, or nitrates. Concurrent use with amphetamines, cocaine, ephedrine, epinephrine, norepinephrine, phenylephrine, or pseudoephedrine may result in unopposed alpha-adrenergic stimulation (excessive hypertension, bradycardia). Concurrent thyroid administration may ↓ effectiveness. May alter the effectiveness of insulins or oral antidiabetics (dosage adjustments may be necessary). May ↓ effectiveness of bronchodilators and theophylline.
May ↓ beneficial cardiovascular effects of dopamine or dobutamine. Use cautiously within 14 days of MAO inhibitor therapy (may result in hypertension). Cimetidine may ↑ toxicity. Concurrent NSAIDs may ↓ antihypertensive action.

Route/Dosage
PO (Adults): *Antihypertensive*— 10 mg twice daily initially; may be ↑ q 7 days as needed

(usual maintenance dose is 10–20 mg twice daily; up to 60 mg/day). *Prevention of MI*— 10 mg twice daily, starting 1–4 wk after MI. *Prevention of vascular headache*— 10 mg twice daily initially, may be given as a single daily dose; may be ↑ up to 10 mg in the morning and 20 mg in the evening.

Availability (generic available)
Tablets: 5 mg, 10 mg, 20 mg.

NURSING IMPLICATIONS
Assessment
- Monitor blood pressure and pulse frequently during dose adjustment period and periodically during therapy. Assess for orthostatic hypotension when assisting patient up from supine position.
- Monitor intake and output ratios and daily weight. Assess patient routinely for evidence of fluid overload (peripheral edema, dyspnea, rales/crackles, fatigue, weight gain, jugular venous distention).
- **Hypertension:** Monitor frequency of prescription refills to determine adherence.
- **Vascular Headache Prophylaxis:** Assess frequency, severity, characteristics, and location of vascular headaches periodically during therapy.
- *Lab Test Considerations:* May cause ↑ BUN, serum lipoprotein, potassium, triglyceride, and uric acid levels.
- May cause ↑ ANA titers.
- May cause ↑ in blood glucose levels.
- ***Toxicity and Overdose:*** Monitor patients receiving beta blockers for signs of overdose (bradycardia, severe dizziness or fainting, severe drowsiness, dyspnea, bluish fingernails or palms, seizures). Notify health care provider immediately if these signs occur.
- Glucagon has been used to treat bradycardia and hypotension.

Potential Nursing Diagnoses
Decreased cardiac output (Side Effects)
Noncompliance (Patient/Family Teaching)

Implementation
- **PO:** Take apical pulse before administering. If <50 bpm or if arrhythmia occurs, withhold medication and notify health care professional.
- May be administered with food or on an empty stomach.
- Tablets may be crushed and mixed with food.

Patient/Family Teaching
- Instruct patient to take medication as directed, at the same time each day, even if feeling well; do not skip or double up on missed doses. Take missed doses as soon as possible up to 4 hr before next dose. Abrupt withdrawal may precipitate life-threatening arrhythmias, hypertension, or myocardial ischemia.
- Advise patient to make sure that enough medication is available for weekends, holidays, and vacations. A written prescription may be kept in wallet in case of emergency.
- Teach patient and family how to check pulse daily and blood pressure biweekly. Advise patient to hold dose and contact health care professional if pulse is <50 bpm or blood pressure changes significantly.
- May cause drowsiness or dizziness. Caution patients to avoid driving or other activities that require alertness until response to the drug is known.
- Advise patients to change positions slowly to minimize orthostatic hypotension, especially during initiation of therapy or when dose is increased.
- Caution patient that this medication may increase sensitivity to cold.
- Instruct patient to consult health care professional before taking other Rx, OTC, or herbal products, especially cold preparations, concurrently with this medication.
- Patients with diabetes should closely monitor blood glucose, especially if weakness, malaise, irritability, or fatigue occurs. Medication may mask tachycardia and increased blood pressure as signs of hypoglycemia, but dizziness and sweating may still occur.
- Advise patient to notify health care professional if slow pulse, difficulty breathing, wheezing, cold hands and feet, dizziness, confusion, depression, rash, fever, sore throat, unusual bleeding, or bruising occurs.
- Instruct patient to inform health care professional of medication regimen before treatment or surgery.
- Advise patient to carry identification describing disease process and medication regimen at all times.
- **Hypertension:** Reinforce the need to continue additional therapies for hypertension (weight loss, sodium restriction, stress reduction, regular exercise, moderation of alcohol consumption, and smoking cessation). Medication controls but does not cure hypertension.
- **Vascular Headache Prophylaxis:** Caution patient that sharing this medication may be dangerous.

Evaluation/Desired Outcomes
- Decrease in blood pressure.
- Prevention of MI.
- Prevention of vascular headaches.

---

tinidazole (ti-nid-a-zole)
Tindamax

Classification
Therapeutic: antiprotozoals
Pharmacologic: imidazoles

Pregnancy Category C

Indications
Bacterial vaginosis. Trichomoniasis. Giardiasis. Amebiasis.

Action
Interaction with protozoa results in release of a free nitro radical that has antiprotozoal activity.
Therapeutic Effects: Resolution of protozoal infections. **Spectrum:** Active against *Trichamonas vaginalis*, *Giardia duodenalis* (also known as *Giardia lamblia*), and *Entamoeba histolytica*.

Pharmacokinetics
Absorption: Rapidly and completely absorbed following oral administration.
Distribution: Extensively distributed; crosses placenta and blood-brain barrier, enters breast milk.
Metabolism and Excretion: Mostly metabolized (CYP3A4 enzyme system); 20–25% excreted unchanged in urine, 12% excreted in feces.
Half-life: 12–14 hr.

TIME/ACTION PROFILE (blood levels)

ROUTE	ONSET	PEAK	DURATION
PO	rapid	2 hr	24 hr

Contraindications/Precautions
Contraindicated in: Hypersensitivity; cross sensitivity with other imidazoles may occur; OB: First trimester of pregnancy; Lactation: Lactation.
Use Cautiously in: CNS pathology; History of blood dyscrasia; Hemodialysis (removes significant amount of tinidazole; supplement post-dialysis with additional 50% of dose); Hepatic impairment; Unrecognized candidiasis (requires concurrent antifungal therapy); Pedi: Children <3 yr (safety not established).

Adverse Reactions/Side Effects
CNS: dizziness, headache, malaise. **GI:** constipation, dyspepsia, metallic/bitter taste, vomiting. **Hemat:** transient leukopenia/neutropenia.

Interactions
Drug-Drug: ↑ risk of bleeding with **warfarin**. Disulfiram-like reaction may occur with **alcohol** or **propylene glycol**; **disulfiram** should be avoided for at least 2 weeks before tinidazole. May ↑ levels of **lithium, cyclosporine, tacrolimus, fluorouracil,** and **fosphenytoin** (observe/monitor for toxicity if administered concurrently). **Drugs that induce the CYP450 liver enzyme system (phenobarbital, rifampin, phenytoin or fosphenytoin)** may ↓ levels and effectiveness. **Drugs that inhibit the CYP450 liver enzyme system (cimetidine or ketoconazole)** may ↑ levels. Absorption is ↓ by **cholestyramine**; separate dosing.

Route/Dosage
PO (Adults): *Bacterial vaginosis*—1 g for 5 days; *Trichomoniasis and Giardiasis*—2 g single dose; *Intestinal amebiasis*—2 g/day for 3 days; *Amebic liver abscess*—2 g/day for 3–5 days.

PO (Children older than 3 yr): *Giardiasis*—50 mg/kg (up to 2 g) single dose; *Intestinal amebiasis*—50 mg/kg/day for 3 days; *Amebic liver abscess*—50 mg/kg/day for 3–5 days.

Availability
Tablets: 250 mg, 500 mg.

NURSING IMPLICATIONS

Assessment
- Assess patient for symptoms of infection (discharge, itching) prior to and during therapy.
- Monitor neurologic status during and after IV infusions. Inform health care professional if numbness, paresthesia, weakness, ataxia, or convulsions occur.
- **Giardiasis:** Monitor three stool samples taken several days apart, beginning 3–4 wk after treatment.
- *Lab Test Considerations:* May cause transient leukopenia and neutropenia. Monitor total and differential leukocyte counts if retreatment is necessary.
- May interfere with certain tests of serum chemistry values such as AST, ALT, LDH, triglycerides, and glucose hexokinase.

Potential Nursing Diagnoses
Risk for infection (Indications)
Diarrhea (Indications)

Implementation
- Symptoms of known or previously unrecognized candidiasis may become worse during therapy and require treatment with an antifungal agent.
- PO: Administer with food to decrease GI upset. May be crushed and prepared as a suspension in cherry syrup by pharmacist for patients unable to swallow tablets. Shake well before administering.

Patient/Family Teaching
- Instruct patient to take medication as directed, even if feeling better. Do not skip doses or double up on missed doses. If a dose is missed, take as soon as remembered if not almost time for next dose.
- Advise patients treated for trichomoniasis that sexual partners may be asymptomatic sources of reinfection and should be treated concurrently. Patient should also refrain from intercourse or use a condom to prevent reinfection.
- Caution patient to avoid intake of alcoholic beverages or preparations containing alcohol during and for at least 3 days after treatment with tinidazole. May cause a disulfiram-like reaction (flushing, nausea, vomiting, headache, abdominal cramps).
- May cause dizziness or drowsiness. Caution patient to avoid driving or other activities requiring alertness until response to medication is known.
- Inform patient that medication may cause an unpleasant metallic taste.
- Advise patient not to take Rx, OTC, or herbal products without consulting health care professional.
- Advise patient to inform health care professional if pregnancy is suspected before taking this medication.

Evaluation/Desired Outcomes
- Resolution of signs and symptoms of infection.

---

tinzaparin, See HEPARINS (LOW MOLECULAR WEIGHT).

---

tioconazole, See ANTIFUNGALS (VAGINAL).

---

tiotropium (tye-o-**trope**-ee-yum)
Spiriva

Classification
Therapeutic: bronchodilators
Pharmacologic: anticholinergics

Pregnancy Category C

Indications
Long-term maintenance treatment of bronchospasm due to COPD.

Action
Acts as anticholinergic by selectively and reversibly inhibiting M_3 receptors in smooth muscle of airways. **Therapeutic Effects:** Decreased incidence and severity of bronchospasm.

Pharmacokinetics
Absorption: 19.5% absorbed following inhalation.
Distribution: Extensive tissue distribution; due to route of administration ↑ concentrations occur in lung.
Metabolism and Excretion: 74% excreted unchanged in urine; 25% of absorbed drug is metabolized.
Half-life: 5–6 days.

TIME/ACTION PROFILE (bronchodilation)

ROUTE	ONSET	PEAK	DURATION
inhaln	rapid	5 min	24 hr

Contraindications/Precautions
Contraindicated in: Hypersensitivity to tiotropium, atropine of their derivatives; Concurrent ipratropium.
Use Cautiously in: Angle-closure glaucoma, prostatic hyperplasia, bladder neck obstruction (may worsen condition); CCr ≤50 mL/min (monitor closely); OB: Lactation: Pedi: Pregnancy, lactation, or children (safety not established).

Adverse Reactions/Side Effects
EENT: glaucoma. **Resp:** paradoxical bronchospasm. **CV:** tachycardia. **GI:** dry mouth, constipation. **GU:** urinary difficulty, urinary retention. **Misc:** hypersensitivity reactions including ANGIOEDEMA.

Interactions
Drug-Drug: Should not be used concurrently with **ipratropium** due to risk of additive anticholinergic effects.

Route/Dosage
Inhaln (Adults): 18 mcg once daily.

Availability

Dry powder capsules for inhalation: 18 mcg. Cost: $134.99/30 capsules.

NURSING IMPLICATIONS

Assessment
- **Inhaln:** Assess respiratory status (rate, breath sounds, degree of dyspnea, pulse) before administration and at peak of medication. Consult physician or other health care professional about alternative medication if severe bronchospasm is present; onset of action is too slow for patients in acute distress. If paradoxical bronchospasm (wheezing) occurs, withhold medication and notify physician or other health care professional immediately.

Potential Nursing Diagnoses
Ineffective airway clearance (Indications)
Risk for activity intolerance (Indications)

Implementation
- **Inhaln:** See Appendix D for administration of inhalation medications.

Patient/Family Teaching
- Instruct patient to take medication as directed. Capsules are for inhalation only and must not be swallowed. Take missed doses as soon as remembered unless almost time for the next dose; space remaining doses evenly during day. Do not double doses.
- Advise patient that tiotropium is not to be used for acute bronchospasm attacks, but may be continued during an acute exacerbation.
- Instruct patient in proper use and cleaning of the Handihaler inhaler. Review the *Patient's Instructions for Use* guide with patient. Capsules should be stored in sealed blisters; remove immediately before use or effectiveness of capsules is reduced. Tear blister strip carefully to expose only one capsule at a time. Discard capsules that are inadvertently exposed to air. *Spiriva* should be administered only via the Handihaler and the Handihaler should not be used with other medications. When disposing of capsule, tiny amount of powder left in capsule is normal.
- Advise patient that rinsing mouth after using inhaler, good oral hygiene, and sugarless gum or candy may minimize dry mouth; usually resolves with continued treatment.
- Advise patient to notify health care professional immediately if signs of glaucoma (eye pain or discomfort, blurred vision, visual halos or colored images in association with red eyes from conjunctival congestion and corneal edema) occur.
- Caution patient to avoid spraying medication in eyes; may cause blurring of vision and pupil dilation.
- Advise patient to inform health care professional if pregnancy is planned or suspected or if breastfeeding.
- Advise patient to consult health care professional before taking any Rx/OTC/herbal products, including eye drops.

Evaluation/Desired Outcomes
- Decreased dyspnea.
- Improved breath sounds.

HIGH ALERT

tirofiban (tye-roe-**fye**-ban)
Aggrastat

Classification
Therapeutic: antiplatelet agents
Pharmacologic: glycoprotein IIb/IIIa inhibitors

Pregnancy Category B

Indications
Treatment of acute coronary syndrome (unstable angina/non–Q-wave MI), including patients who will be managed medically and those who will undergo percutaneous transluminal angioplasty (PCTA) or atherectomy. Used concurrently with aspirin and heparin.

Action
Decreases platelet aggregation by reversibly antagonizing the binding of fibrinogen to the glycoprotein IIb/IIIa binding site on platelet surfaces. **Therapeutic Effects:** Inhibition of platelet aggregation resulting in decreased incidence of new MI, death, or refractory ischemia with the need for repeat cardiac procedures.

Pharmacokinetics
Absorption: IV administration results in complete bioavailability.
Distribution: Unknown.
Metabolism and Excretion: Excreted mostly unchanged by the kidneys (65%); 25% excreted unchanged in feces.
Half-life: 2 hr.

tirofiban

TIME/ACTION PROFILE (effects on platelet function)

ROUTE	ONSET	PEAK	DURATION
IV	rapid	30 min†	brief‡

†>90% inhibition of platelet aggregation at end of initial 30-min infusion
‡Inhibition is reversible following cessation of infusion

Contraindications/Precautions
Contraindicated in: Hypersensitivity; Active internal bleeding or history of bleeding within previous 30 days; History of intracranial hemorrhage, intracranial neoplasm, arteriovenous malformation or aneurysm; History of thrombocytopenia during previous tirofiban therapy; History of hemorrhagic stroke or other stroke within 30 days; Major surgical procedure or severe physical trauma within 30 days; History, symptoms, or other findings associated with aortic aneurysm; Severe hypertension (systolic BP >180 mm Hg and/or diastolic BP >110 mm Hg); Concurrent use of other glycoprotein IIb/IIIa receptor antagonists; Acute pericarditis; Lactation: Lactation.
Use Cautiously in: Platelet count <150,000/mm³; Hemorrhagic retinopathy; Female patients (↑ risk of bleeding); Severe renal insufficiency (↓ rate of infusion by 50% if CCr <30 mL/min); OB, Pedi: Safety not established; use in pregnancy only if clearly needed; Geri: ↑ risk of bleeding.

Adverse Reactions/Side Effects
Noted for patients receiving heparin and aspirin in addition to tirofiban.
CNS: dizziness, headache. **CV:** bradycardia, coronary dissection, edema, vasovagal reaction. **GI:** nausea. **Derm:** hives, rash. **Hemat:** bleeding, thrombocytopenia. **MS:** leg pain. **Misc:** fever, hypersensitivity reactions, pelvic pain, sweating.

Interactions
Drug-Drug: Concurrent use of **aspirin**, **NSAIDs**, **warfarin**, **heparin**, **heparin-like agents**, **abciximab**, **eptifibatide**, **clopidogrel**, **ticlopidine**, or **dipyridamole** may ↑ risk of bleeding, although these agents are frequently used together or in sequence. Risk of bleeding may be ↑ by concurrent use of **cefotetan**, **cefoperazone**, or **valproic acid**.
Drug-Natural Products: ↑ anticoagulant effect and bleeding risk with **anise**, **arnica**, **chamomile**, **clove**, **dong quai**, **fenugreek**, **feverfew**, **garlic**, **ginger**, **ginkgo**, **Panax ginseng**, **licorice**, and others.

Route/Dosage
IV (Adults): 0.4 mcg/kg/min for 30 min, then 0.1 mcg/kg/min, continued throughout angiography and for 12–24 hr after angioplasty or atherectomy.

Renal Impairment
IV (Adults): *CCr <30 mL/min*—0.2 mcg/kg/min for 30 min, then 0.05 mcg/kg/min, continued throughout angiography and for 12–24 hr after angioplasty or atherectomy.

Availability
Premixed solution for infusion: 5 mg/100 mL (50 mcg/mL) in 100-mL single-dose containers, 12.5 mg/250 mL (50 mcg/mL) in 250-mL single-dose containers.

NURSING IMPLICATIONS

Assessment
- Assess patient for bleeding. Most common is oozing from the arterial access site for cardiac catheterization. Arterial and venous punctures, IM injections, and use of urinary catheters, nasotracheal intubation, and nasogastric tubes should be minimized. Noncompressible sites for IV access should be avoided. If bleeding cannot be controlled with pressure, discontinue tirofiban and heparin immediately.
- During vascular access, avoid puncturing posterior wall of femoral artery. Maintain bedrest with head of bed elevated 30° and affected limb restrained in a straight position while the vascular sheath is in place. Heparin should be discontinued for 3–4 hr and activated clotting time (ACT) <180 sec or activated partial thromboplastin time (aPTT) <45 sec prior to pulling the sheath. Use compressive techniques to obtain hemostasis and monitor closely. Sheath hemostasis should be maintained for >4 hr before discharge from the hospital.
- Monitor for signs of thrombocytopenia (chills, low-grade fever) during therapy.
- *Lab Test Considerations:* Assess hemoglobin, hematocrit, and platelet count prior to tirofiban therapy, within 6 hr following loading infusion, and at least daily during therapy (more frequently if evidence of significant decline). May cause ↓ hemoglobin and hematocrit.
- If platelet count ↓ to <90,000/mm³, perform additional platelet counts to rule out pseudothrombocytopenia. If thrombocytopenia is confirmed, tirofiban and heparin should be discontinued and condition monitored and treated.
- To monitor unfractionated heparin, assess aPTT 6 hr after the start of heparin infusion. Adjust heparin to maintain aPTT at approximately 2 times control.

- May cause presence of urine and fecal occult blood.

Potential Nursing Diagnoses
Ineffective tissue perfusion (Indications)

Implementation
- **High Alert:** Use of antiplatelet medications has resulted in patient harm and/or death from internal hemorrhage or intracranial bleeding. Have second practitioner independently check original order, dosage calculations, and infusion pump settings.
- Most patients receive heparin and aspirin concurrently with tirofiban.
- Do not administer solutions that are discolored or contain particulate matter. Discard unused portion.

IV Administration
- **Intermittent Infusion:** *Diluent:* Tirofiban injection premix is ready for administration and dose not require any further dilution. *Concentration:* 50 mcg/mL. *Rate:* Based on patient's weight (see Route/Dosage section).
- **Y-Site Compatibility:** acyclovir, alfentanil, alopruinol, amifostine, amikacin, aminocaproic acid, aminophylline, amiodarone, ampicillin, ampicillin/sulbactam, anidulafungin, argatroban, arsenic trioxide, atracurium, atropine, azithromycin, aztreonam, bivalirudin, bleomycin, bumetanide, buprenorphine, butorphanol, calcium chloride, calcium gluconate, capreomycin, carboplatin, carmustine, caspofungin, cefazolin, cefepime, cefotaxime, cefotetan, cefoxitin, ceftazidime, ceftizoxime, ceftriaxone, cefuroxime, chloramphenicol, chlorpromazine, cimetidine, ciprofloxacin, cisatracurium, cisplatin, clindamycin, cyclophosphamide, cyclosporine, cytarabine, dactinomycin, daptomycin, dexamethasone, dexmedetomidine, dexrazoxane, digoxin, diltiazem, diphenhydramine, dobutamine, docetaxel, dolasetron, dopamine, doxacurium, doxorubicin, doxorubicin liposome, doxycycline, droperidol, enalaprilat, ephedrine, epinephrine, epirubicin, eptifibatide, ertapenem, erythromycin, esmolol, etoposide, etoposide phosphate, famotidine, fenoldopam, fentanyl, fluconazole, fludarabine, fluorouracil, foscarnet, fosphenytoin, furosemide, ganciclovir, gemcitabine, gentamicin, glycopyrrolate, granisetron, haloperidol, heparin, hydralazine, hydrocortisone, hydromorphone, idarubicin, ifosfamide, imipenem/cilastatin, insulin, irinotecan, isoproterenol, ketorolac, labetalol, leucovorin, lidocaine, linezolid, lorazepam, magnesium sulfate, mannitol, mechlorethamine, melphalan, meperidine, meropenem, mesna, methylhexital, methotrexate, methyldopate, methylprednisolone, metoclopramide, metoprolol, metronidazole, midazolam, milrinone, mitoxantrone, morphine, mycophenolate, nafcillin, nalbuphine, naloxone, nesiritide, nicardipine, nitroglycerin, nitroprusside, norepinephrine, octreotideondansetron, oxaliplatin, oxytocin, paclitaxel, palonosetron, pamidronate, pancuronium, pantoprazole, pemetrexed, pentobarbital, phenobarbital, phentolamine, phenylephrine, piperacillin/tazobactam, potassium acetate, potassium chloride, potassium phosphates, procainamide, prochlorperazine, promethazine, propranolol, quinupristin/dalfopristin, ranitidine, remifentanil, rocuronium, sodium acetate, sodium bicarbonate, streptozocin, succinylcholine, sufentanil, tacrolimus, teniposide, theophylline, thiopental, thiotepa, ticarcillin/clavulanate, tigecycline, tobramycin, topotecan, vancomycin, vasopressin, vecuronium, verapanil, vinblastine, vincristine, vinorelbine, voriconazole, zidovudine, zolendronic acid.
- **Y-Site Incompatibility:** amphotericin B colloidal, amphotericin B liposome, dantrolene, diazepam, phenytoin.

Patient/Family Teaching
- Inform patient of the purpose of tirofiban.
- Instruct patient to notify health care professional immediately if any bleeding is noted.

Evaluation/Desired Outcomes
- Inhibition of platelet aggregation resulting in decreased incidence of new MI, death, or refractory ischemia with the need for repeat cardiac procedures.

---

tizanidine (tye-zan-i-deen)
Zanaflex

Classification
Therapeutic: antispasticity agents (centrally acting)
Pharmacologic: adrenergics

Pregnancy Category C

Indications
Increased muscle tone associated with spasticity due to multiple sclerosis or spinal cord injury.

Action
Acts as an agonist at central alpha-adrenergic receptor sites. Reduces spasticity by increasing presynaptic inhibition of motor neurons. **Therapeutic Effects:** Decreased spasticity, allowing better function.

Pharmacokinetics
Absorption: Completely absorbed after oral administration but rapidly metabolized, resulting in 40% bioavailability.
Distribution: Widely distributed.
Metabolism and Excretion: 95% metabolized by the liver.
Half-life: 2.5 hr.

TIME/ACTION PROFILE (reduced muscle tone)

ROUTE	ONSET	PEAK	DURATION
PO	unknown	1–2 hr	3–6 hr

Contraindications/Precautions
Contraindicated in: Hypersensitivity.
Use Cautiously in: Renal impairment; Concurrent antihypertensive therapy; OB, Lactation: Pedi: Safety not established; Geri: Dose ↓ may be necessary due to ↓ clearance.
Exercise Extreme Caution in: Impaired hepatic function.

Adverse Reactions/Side Effects
CNS: anxiety, depression, dizziness, sedation, weakness, dyskinesia, hallucinations, nervousness. **EENT:** blurred vision, pharyngitis, rhinitis. **CV:** hypotension, bradycardia. **GI:** abdominal pain, diarrhea, dry mouth, dyspepsia, constipation, hepatocellular injury, ↑ liver enzymes, vomiting. **GU:** urinary frequency. **Derm:** rash, skin ulcers, sweating. **MS:** back pain, myasthenia, paresthesia. **Misc:** fever, speech disorder.

Interactions
Drug-Drug: Levels and effects ↑ by concurrent use of **hormonal contraceptives** or **alcohol**. ↑ risk of hypotension with **alpha$_2$-adrenergic agonist antihypertensives** (avoid concurrent use). ↑ CNS depression may occur with **alcohol** or other **CNS depressants** including some **antidepressants**, **sedative/hypnotics**, **antihistamines**, and **opioid analgesics**. Concurrent CYP1A2 inhbitors (**ciprofloxacin**, **fluvoxamine** and others) may ↑ levels and risk of hypotension and excessive sedation.

Route/Dosage
PO (Adults): 4 mg q 6–8 hr initially (no more than 3 doses/24 hr); ↑ by 2–4 mg/dose up to 8 mg/dose or 24 mg/day (not to exceed 36 mg/day). Some patients may tolerate twice-daily dosing.

Availability (generic available)
Tablets: 2 mg, 4 mg. **Cost:** *Generic*—2 mg $19.99/90, 4 mg $81.99/90. **Capsules:** 2 mg, 4 mg, 6 mg. **Cost:** 2 mg $159.70/90, 4 mg $216.37/90, 6 mg $300.35/90.

NURSING IMPLICATIONS
Assessment
- Assess muscle spasticity before and periodically during therapy.
- Monitor blood pressure and pulse, especially during dose titration. May cause orthostatic hypotension, bradycardia, dizziness, and, rarely, syncope. Effects are usually dose related.
- Observe patient for drowsiness, dizziness, and asthenia. A change in dose may alleviate these problems.
- *Lab Test Considerations:* Monitor liver function tests before and at 1, 3, and 6 mo of therapy. May cause ↑ in serum glucose, alkaline phosphatase, AST, and ALT levels.

Potential Nursing Diagnoses
Impaired physical mobility (Indications)
Risk for injury (Adverse Reactions)

Implementation
- Do not confuse tizanidine with tiagibine.
- Doses should be titrated carefully to prevent side effects.
- **PO:** May be taken without regard to meals.

Patient/Family Teaching
- Instruct patient to take tizanidine as directed. Tizanidine may need to be discontinued gradually.
- May cause dizziness and drowsiness. Advise patient to avoid driving or other activities requiring alertness until response to drug is known.
- Instruct patient to change positions slowly to minimize orthostatic hypotension.
- Advise patient to avoid concurrent use of alcohol or other CNS depressants while taking this medication.

Evaluation/Desired Outcomes
- Decrease in muscle spasticity with an increased ability to perform activities of daily living.

---

tobramycin, See AMINOGLYCOSIDES.

tolcapone (tole-ka-pone)
Tasmar

tolcapone

Classification
Therapeutic: antiparkinson agents
Pharmacologic: catechol-*O*-methyltransferase inhibitors

Pregnancy Category C

Indications
Management of Parkinson's disease with carbidopa/levodopa in patients without severe movement abnormalities who do not respond to other treatment.

Action
Acts as a selective and reversible inhibitor of the enzyme catechol-*O*-methyltransferase. Inhibition of this enzyme prevents the breakdown of levodopa, greatly increasing its availability to the CNS. **Therapeutic Effects:** Prolongs duration of response to levodopa without end-of-dose motor fluctuations. Decreased signs and symptoms of Parkinson's disease.

Pharmacokinetics
Absorption: Rapidly absorbed following oral administration with 65% bioavailability.
Distribution: Unknown.
Protein Binding: >99% bound to plasma proteins.
Metabolism and Excretion: Mostly metabolized by the liver; <0.5% excreted unchanged in urine.
Half-life: 2–3 hr.

TIME/ACTION PROFILE (blood levels)

ROUTE	ONSET	PEAK	DURATION
PO	unknown	1.7 hr	8 hr

Contraindications/Precautions
Contraindicated in: Hypersensitivity; Concurrent MAO inhibitor therapy; Clinical evidence of liver disease.
Use Cautiously in: Severe renal impairment (safety not established if CCr <25 mL/min); OB: Lactation: Safety not established.

Adverse Reactions/Side Effects
CNS: headache, sleep disorder, hallucinations, syncope, urges (gambling, sexual). **CV:** orthostatic hypotension. **GI:** HEPATOTOXICITY, HEPATIC FAILURE, constipation, diarrhea, anorexia, elevated liver enzymes, nausea, vomiting. **GU:** hematuria, yellow discoloration of urine. **Derm:** ↑ sweating, melanoma. **Neuro:** dyskinesia, dystonia.

Interactions
Drug-Drug: Concurrent use with **MAO inhibitors** is not recommended; both agents inhibit the metabolic pathways of catecholamines. May ↑ the effects of **methyldopa**, **apomorphine**, **dobutamine**, or **isoproterenol**; dose reduction may be necessary. ↑ the bioavailability of **levodopa** by two-fold; this is a desired effect.

Route/Dosage
PO (Adults): 100 mg 3 times daily; may be cautiously increased to 200 mg 3 times daily if benefit is justified.

Availability
Tablets: 100 mg, 200 mg.

NURSING IMPLICATIONS

Assessment
- Assess patient for signs and symptoms of Parkinson's disease (tremor, muscle weakness and rigidity, ataxic gait) prior to and throughout therapy.
- Assess blood pressure periodically during therapy.
- Monitor for signs and symptoms of liver dysfunction (persistent nausea, fatigue, lethargy, anorexia, jaundice, dark urine, pruritus, right upper quadrant tenderness) periodically during therapy.
- *Lab Test Considerations:* Monitor liver function tests before every 2–4 wk for the first 6 mo following initiation or dose increase and periodically thereafter. Discontinue tolcapone if liver function tests reach two times the upper limit of normal or if jaundice occurs; do not reinstate.

Potential Nursing Diagnoses
Impaired physical mobility (Indications)
Risk for injury (Indications, Side Effects)

Implementation
- **PO:** Administer 1st dose of the day of tolcapone together with carbidopa/levodopa. Administer subsequent doses 6 and 12 hr later.
- May be administered without regard to food.

Patient/Family Teaching
- Instruct patient to take medication as directed. Caution patient not to discontinue medication without consulting health care professional. Abrupt discontinuation or rapid dose reduction may result in neuroleptic malignant syndrome (elevated temperature, muscular rigidity, altered consciousness).

✽ = Canadian drug name. ❚ = Genetic implication.
*CAPITALS indicates life-threatening; underlines indicate most frequent.

- Caution patient to make position changes slowly to minimize orthostatic hypotension, especially at the beginning of therapy.
- May affect mental and/or motor performance. Caution patient to avoid driving or other activities requiring alertness until response to medication is known.
- Advise patient to avoid taking alcohol or other CNS depressants concurrently with tolcapone.
- Inform patient and caregiver that hallucinations, nausea, dyskinesia, or dystonia may occur during tolcapone therapy.
- Advise patient to notify health care professional if symptoms of liver failure (clay-colored stools, jaundice, fatigue, loss of appetite, lethargy), suspicious or unusual skin changes, hallucinations, or new or increased gambling, sexual, or other intense urges occur.
- Advise patient to notify health care professional if pregnancy is planned or suspected.
- Instruct patient to notify health care professional if persistent diarrhea occurs.
- Emphasize the importance of routine follow-up exams.

Evaluation/Desired Outcomes
- Decrease in signs and symptoms of Parkinson's disease.

---

tolnaftate, See ANTIFUNGALS (TOPICAL).

---

tolterodine (tol-ter-oh-deen)
Detrol, Detrol LA

Classification
Therapeutic: urinary tract antispasmodics
Pharmacologic: anticholinergics

Pregnancy Category C

Indications
Treatment of overactive bladder function that results in urinary frequency, urgency, or urge incontinence.

Action
Acts as a competitive muscarinic receptor antagonist resulting in inhibition of cholinergically mediated bladder contraction. **Therapeutic Effects:** Decreased urinary frequency, urgency, and urge incontinence.

Pharmacokinetics
Absorption: Well absorbed (77%) following oral administration.
Distribution: Unknown.
Protein Binding: 96.3%.
Metabolism and Excretion: Extensively metabolized by the liver (primarily by CYP2D6 isoenzyme) (the CYP2D6 enzyme system exhibits genetic polymorphism; ~7% of population may be poor metabolizers and may have significantly ↑ tolterodine concentrations and an ↑ risk of adverse effects); one metabolite (5-hydroxymethyltolterodine) is active; other metabolites are excreted in urine.
Half-life: *Tolterodine*—1.9–3.7 hr; *5-hydroxymethyltolterodine*—2.9–3.1 hr.

TIME/ACTION PROFILE (effects on bladder function)

ROUTE	ONSET	PEAK	DURATION
PO	unknown	unknown	12 hr

Contraindications/Precautions
Contraindicated in: Urinary retention; Gastric retention; Uncontrolled angle-closure glaucoma; Lactation: Lactation.
Use Cautiously in: GI obstructive disorders, including pyloric stenosis (↑ risk of gastric retention); Significant bladder outflow obstruction (↑ risk of urinary retention); Controlled angle-closure glaucoma; Myasthenia gravis; Significant hepatic impairment (lower doses recommended); Impaired renal function; OB: Safety not established; use only if potential maternal benefit justifies potential risk to fetus; Pedi: Safety not established.

Adverse Reactions/Side Effects
CNS: headache, dizziness. **EENT:** blurred vision, dry eyes. **GI:** dry mouth, constipation, dyspepsia.

Interactions
Drug-Drug: Erythromycin, **clarithromycin**, **ketoconazole**, **itraconazole**, and **miconazole** may inhibit metabolism and ↑ effects.

Route/Dosage
PO (Adults): 2 mg twice daily as tablets; may be lowered depending on response *or* 2–4 mg once daily as extended-release capsules.

PO (Adults with impaired hepatic function or concurrent enzyme inhibitors): 1 mg twice daily.

Availability
Tablets: 1 mg, 2 mg. **Cost:** 1 mg $359.59/180, 2 mg $359.96/180. **Extended-release capsules:** 2 mg, 4 mg. **Cost:** 2 mg $299.96/90, 4 mg $325.97/90.

NURSING IMPLICATIONS

Assessment
- Assess patient for urinary urgency, frequency, and urge incontinence periodically during therapy.

Potential Nursing Diagnoses
Impaired urinary elimination (Indications)
Urinary retention (Indications)

Implementation
- **PO:** Administer without regard to food.
- Extended-release capsules should be swallowed whole; do not open or chew.

Patient/Family Teaching
- Instruct patient to take tolterodine as directed.
- May cause dizziness and blurred vision. Caution patient to avoid driving or other activities requiring alertness until response to medication is known.

Evaluation/Desired Outcomes
- Decreased urinary frequency, urgency, and urge incontinence.

---

tolvaptan (tol-**vap**-tan)
Samsca

Classification
Therapeutic: electrolyte modifiers
Pharmacologic: vasopressin antagonists

Pregnancy Category C

Indications
Treatment of significant hypervolemic and euvolemic hyponatremia (serum sodium <125 mEq/L or less marked symptomatic hyponatremia that has resisted correction by fluid restriction), including patients with heart failure, cirrhosis, and Syndrome of Inappropriate Antidiuretic Hormone (SIADH).

Action
Acts as a selective vasopressin V2-receptor antagonist, resulting in increased renal water excretion and increased serum sodium. **Therapeutic Effects:** Correction of hyponatremia.

Pharmacokinetics
Absorption: 40% absorbed following oral administration.
Distribution: >99%.
Metabolism and Excretion: Extensively metabolized primarily by the CYP3A4 enzyme system; no renal elimination.

Half-life: 12 hr.

TIME/ACTION PROFILE

ROUTE	ONSET	PEAK	DURATION
PO	within 8 hr	2–4 hr†	7 days

† Blood level

Contraindications/Precautions
Contraindicated in: Urgent need to acutely raise serum sodium; Patients who cannot appropriately sense/respond to thirst; Hypovolemic hyponatremia; Concurrent use of strong CYP 3A inhibitors or moderate CYP 3A inhibitors; Anuria; Lactation: Avoid use during lactation.
Use Cautiously in: Severe malnutrition, alcoholism or advanced liver disease (↑ risk of osmotic demyelination; correct electrolyte abnormalities at a slower rates); Cirrhosis (↑ risk of GI bleeding, use only when the need to treat outweighs risk); Geri: May have increased sensitivity to effects; OB: Use during pregnancy only if the potential benefit justifies the potential risk to the fetus; Pedi: Safety and effectiveness in children has not been established.

Adverse Reactions/Side Effects
CNS: weakness. **GI:** constipation, dry mouth. **GU:** polyuria. **F and E:** thirst. **Metab:** hyperglycemia. **Neuro:** osmotic demyelination.

Interactions
Drug-Drug: Strong inhibitors of the CYP3A enzyme system including **ketoconazole**, **clarithromycin**, **itraconazole**, **telithromycin**, **saquinavir**, **nelfinavir**, **ritonavir**, and **nefazodone** ↑ levels and may ↑ effects and risk of toxicity; concurrent use should be avoided. **Moderate CYP 3A inhibitors** including **erythromycin**, **fluconazole**, **aprepitant**, **diltiazem**, and **verapamil** may have a similar effect and should also be avoided. **Inducers of the CYP3A enzyme system** including **rifampin** can ↓ blood levels and effectiveness; dosage adjustments may be necessary. Levels and risk of toxicity are also ↑ **P-gp inhibitors** including **cyclosporine**; dosage adjustments may be necessary. May ↑ **digoxin** levels; monitor carefully.
Drug-Food: **Grapefruit juice** ↑ levels and the risk of toxicity; avoid concurrent use. May ↑ risk of hyperkalemia with **angiotensin receptor blockers**, **ACE inhibitors**, and **potassium-sparing diuretics**.

✣ = Canadian drug name.   ▦ = Genetic implication.
*CAPITALS indicates life-threatening; underlines indicate most frequent.

Route/Dosage
PO (Adults): 15 mg once daily initially; may be increased at intervals of at least one day to 30 mg once daily, up to a maximum of 60 mg once daily.

Availability
Tablets: 15 mg, 30 mg.

NURSING IMPLICATIONS
Assessment
- Monitor neurologic status and assess for signs and symptoms of osmotic demyelination syndrome (trouble speaking, dysphagia, drowsiness, confusion, mood changes, involuntary movements, weakness, seizures), especially during initiation and after titration. If a rapid ↑ in sodium or symptoms occur, discontinue tolvaptan and consider administration of hypotonic fluid.
- Monitor fluid balance. If hypovolemia occurs interrupt or discontinue tolvaptan and provide supportive care (monitor vital signs, balance fluid and electrolytes).
- *Lab Test Considerations:* Monitor serum sodium levels frequently during initiation and dose titration and periodically during therapy. Too rapid correction of hyponatremia (>12 mEq/L/24 hr) can cause osmotic demyelination syndrome.
- Monitor serum potassium in patients with serum potassium >5 mEq/L or taking medication known to ↑ potassium.

Potential Nursing Diagnoses
Risk for imbalanced fluid volume (Indications)

Implementation
- Initiate and re-initiate therapy in a hospital.
- Avoid fluid restriction during first 24 hr of therapy.
- **PO:** Administer once daily without regard to meals.

Patient/Family Teaching
- Instruct patient to take tolvaptan as direct. Avoid drinking grapefruit juice during therapy; may cause ↑ levels. Take missed doses as soon as remembered, but not if just before next dose; do not double doses. Do not stop and restart therapy. Restarting therapy may require hospitalization.
- Inform patients they can continue fluid ingestion in response to thirst during therapy and should have water available to drink at all times during therapy. Following discontinuation of therapy, resume fluid restriction.
- Advise patient to notify health care professional before taking any other Rx, OTC, or herbal products.
- Advise patient to notify health care professional if signs of dehydration (vomiting, diarrhea, inability to drink normally, dizziness, feeling faint) or bleeding (vomiting bright red blood, dark blood clots, or coffee-ground-like material; black, tarry stools; bloody stools).
- Advise female patients to notify health care professional if pregnancy is planned or suspected or if breastfeeding.

Evaluation/Desired Outcomes
- Normalization of serum sodium levels.

---

topiramate (toe-peer-i-mate)
Topamax

Classification
Therapeutic: anticonvulsants, mood stabilizers

Pregnancy Category C

Indications
Seizures including: partial-onset, primary generalized tonic-clonic, seizures due to Lennox-Gastaut syndrome. Prevention of migraine headache in adults. **Unlabeled Use:** Adjunct in treatment of bipolar disorder. Infantile spasms.

Action
Action may be due to: Blockade of sodium channels in neurons, Enhancement of gamma-aminobutyrate (GABA), an inhibitory neurotransmitter, Prevention of activation of excitatory receptors. **Therapeutic Effects:** Decreased incidence of seizures. Decreased incidence/severity of migraine headache.

Pharmacokinetics
Absorption: Well absorbed (80%) after oral administration.
Distribution: Unknown.
Metabolism and Excretion: 70% excreted unchanged in urine.
Half-life: 21 hr.

TIME/ACTION PROFILE (blood levels†)

ROUTE	ONSET	PEAK	DURATION
PO	unknown	2 hr	12 hr

†After single dose

Contraindications/Precautions
Contraindicated in: Hypersensitivity; Lactation: Lactation.

topiramate

Use Cautiously in: All patients (may ↑ risk of suicidal thoughts/behaviors); Renal impairment (dose reduction recommended if CCr <70 mL/min/1.73 m²); Hepatic impairment; Dehydration; Patients predisposed to metabolic acidosis; Patients allergic to sulfa; OB: Use only if maternal benefit outweighs fetal risk; Pedi: Children are more prone to oligohydrosis and hyperthermia; safety in children <2 yr not established; Geri: Consider age-related ↓ in renal/hepatic impairment, concurrent disease states and drug therapy.

Adverse Reactions/Side Effects

CNS: INCREASED SEIZURES, SUICIDAL THOUGHTS, dizziness, drowsiness, fatigue, impaired concentration/memory, nervousness, psychomotor slowing, speech problems, sedation, aggressive reaction, agitation, anxiety, cognitive disorders, confusion, depression, malaise, mood problems. **EENT:** abnormal vision, diplopia, nystagmus, acute myopia/secondary angle closure glaucoma. **GI:** nausea, abdominal pain, anorexia, constipation, dry mouth. **GU:** kidney stones. **Derm:** oligohydrosis (↑ in children). **F and E:** hyperchloremic metabolic acidosis. **Hemat:** leukopenia. **Metab:** weight loss, hyperthermia (↑ in children). **Neuro:** ataxia, paresthesia, tremor. **Misc:** fever.

Interactions

Drug-Drug: Blood levels and effects may be ↓ by **phenytoin**, **carbamazepine**, or **valproic acid**. May ↑ blood levels and effects of **phenytoin** or **amitriptyline**. May ↓ blood levels and effects of **hormonal contraceptives**, **risperidone**, **lithium** or **valproic acid**. ↑ risk of CNS depression with **alcohol** or other **CNS depressants**. **Carbonic anhydrase inhibitors** (**acetazolamide**) may ↑ risk of kidney stones. Concurrent use with **valproic acid** may ↑ risk of hyperammonemia/encephalopathy.

Route/Dosage

Epilepsy (monotherapy)

PO (Adults and children ≥10 yr): *Seizures/migraine prevention*—50 mg/day initially, gradually ↑ over 6 wk to 400 mg/day in 2 divided doses.

Epilepsy (adjunctive therapy)

PO (Adults and Children ≥17 yr): 25–50 mg/day ↑ by 25–50 mg/day at weekly intervals up to 200–400 mg/day in 2 divided doses (200–400 mg/day in 2 divided doses for partial seizures and 400 mg/day in 2 divided doses for primary generalized tonic-clonic seizures); maximum dose: 1600 mg/day.

Renal Impairment

PO (Adults): *CCr<70 mL/min*—50% of the usual dose.

PO (Children 2–16 yr): *Partial onset seizures or Lennox–Gastaut syndrome*—Initial 1–3 mg/kg/day (maximum: 25 mg) nightly for 1 week then ↑ at 1–2 wk intervals up to 5–9 mg/kg/day in 2 divided doses. *Primary generalized tonic-clonic seizures*—Initial dose as above then gradually increase to 6 mg/kg/day over 8 wk.

Migraine prevention

PO (Adults): 25 mg at night initially, ↑ by 25 mg/day at weekly intervals up to target dose of 100 mg/day in 2 divided doses.

Availability (generic available)

Sprinkle capsules: 15 mg, 25 mg. **Cost:** 15 mg $114.19/60, 25 mg $139.96/60. **Tablets:** 25 mg, 50 mg, 100 mg, 200 mg. **Cost:** 25 mg $369.90/180, 50 mg $703.96/180, 100 mg $1,023.97/180, 200 mg $1,162.91/180.

NURSING IMPLICATIONS

Assessment

- Monitor closely for notable changes in behavior that could indicate the emergence or worsening of suicidal thoughts or behavior or depression.
- **Seizures:** Assess location, duration, and characteristics of seizure activity.
- **Migraines:** Assess pain location, intensity, duration, and associated symptoms (photophobia, phonophobia, nausea, vomiting) during migraine attack. Monitor frequency and intensity of pain on pain scale.
- **Bipolar Disorder:** Assess mental status (mood, orientation, behavior) and cognitive abilities before and periodically during therapy.
- *Lab Test Considerations:* Monitor CBC with differential and platelet count before therapy to determine baseline levels and periodically during therapy. Frequently causes anemia.
- Hepatic function should be monitored periodically throughout therapy. May cause ↑ AST and ALT levels.
- Evaluate serum bicarbonate prior to and periodically during therapy. If metabolic acidosis occurs, dosing taper or discontinuation may be necessary.

Potential Nursing Diagnoses
Risk for injury (Indications, Side Effects)
Disturbed thought process (Indications)

Implementation
- Implement seizure precautions.
- Do not confuse Topamax (topiramate) with Toprol (metoprolol).
- **PO:** May be administered without regard to meals.
- Do not break/crush tablets because of bitter taste.
- Contents of the sprinkle capsules can be sprinkled on a small amount (teaspoon) of soft food, such as applesauce, custard, ice cream, oatmeal, pudding, or yogurt. To open, hold the capsule upright so that you can read the word "TOP." Carefully twist off the clear portion of the capsule. It may be best to do this over the small portion of the food onto which you will be pouring the sprinkles. Sprinkle the entire contents of the capsule onto the food. Be sure the patient swallows the entire spoonful of the sprinkle/food mixture immediately without chewing. Follow with fluids immediately to make sure all of the mixture is swallowed. Never store a sprinkle/food mixture for use at another time.
- A 6 mg/mL oral suspension may be compounded by pharmacy for pediatric patients.

Patient/Family Teaching
- Instruct patient to take topiramate exactly as directed. Take missed doses as soon as possible but not just before next dose; do not double doses. Notify health care professional if more than 1 dose is missed. Medication should be gradually discontinued to prevent seizures and status epilepticus. Instruct patient to read the *Medication Guide* before starting and with each Rx refill, changes may occur.
- May cause decreased sweating and increased body temperature. Advise patients, especially parents of pediatric patients, to provide adequate hydration and monitoring, especially during hot weather.
- May cause dizziness, drowsiness, confusion, and difficulty concentrating. Caution patients to avoid driving or other activities requiring alertness until response to medication is known.
- Advise patient to maintain a fluid intake of 2000–3000 mL of fluid/day to prevent the formation of kidney stones.
- Instruct patient to notify health care professional immediately if periorbital pain or blurred vision occur. Medication should be discontinued if ocular symptoms occur. May lead to permanent loss of vision.
- Advise patient and family to notify health care professional if thoughts about suicide or dying, attempts to commit suicide; new or worse depression; new or worse anxiety; feeling very agitated or restless; panic attacks; trouble sleeping; new or worse irritability; acting aggressive; being angry or violent; acting on dangerous impulses; an extreme increase in activity and talking, other unusual changes in behavior or mood occur.
- Caution patient to make position changes slowly to minimize orthostatic hypotension.
- Advise patient not to take alcohol or other CNS depressants concurrently with this medication.
- Advise patient to use a nonhormonal form of contraception while taking topiramate.
- Instruct patient to notify health care professional of medication regimen before treatment or surgery.
- Advise patient to use sunscreen and wear protective clothing to prevent photosensitivity reactions.
- Advise patient to carry identification describing disease and medication regimen at all times.

Evaluation/Desired Outcomes
- Absence or reduction of seizure activity.
- Decrease in incidence and severity of migraine headaches.
- Remission of manic symptoms.

HIGH ALERT

topotecan (toe-poe-tee-kan)
Hycamtin

Classification
Therapeutic: antineoplastics
Pharmacologic: enzyme inhibitors

Pregnancy Category D

Indications
IV: Metastatic ovarian cancer that has not responded to previous chemotherapy. Small cell lung cancer unresponsive to first line therapy.
PO: Relapsed small cell lung cancer in patients with a complete or partial prior response and who are at least 45 days from the end of first-line chemotherapy. Stage IV-B persistent or recurrent cervical cancer not amenable to treatment with surgery or radiation (with cisplatin).

Action
Interferes with DNA synthesis by inhibiting the enzyme topoisomerase. **Therapeutic Effects:**

Death of rapidly replicating cells, particularly malignant ones.

Pharmacokinetics
Absorption: IV administration results in complete bioavailability.
Distribution: Unknown.
Metabolism and Excretion: 30% excreted in urine; small amounts metabolized by the liver.
Half-life: *PO*—3–6 hr; *IV*—2–3 hr.

TIME/ACTION PROFILE (effects on WBCs)

ROUTE	ONSET	PEAK	DURATION
PO	unknown	1–2 hr	24 hr
IV	within days	11 days	7 days

Contraindications/Precautions
Contraindicated in: Hypersensitivity; Pre-existing severe myelosuppression; OB, Lactation: Pregnancy or lactation.
Use Cautiously in: Impaired renal function (↓ dose if CCr <40 mL/min); Platelet count <25,000 cells/mm³ (↓ dose); Geri: May require dose ↓ due to age-related ↓ in renal function.

Adverse Reactions/Side Effects
CNS: headache, fatigue, weakness. **Resp:** dyspnea. **GI:** abdominal pain, diarrhea, nausea, vomiting, anorexia, constipation, ↑ liver enzymes, stomatitis. **Derm:** alopecia. **Hemat:** anemia, leukopenia, thrombocytopenia. **MS:** arthralgia.

Interactions
Drug-Drug: Neutropenia is prolonged by concurrent use of **filgrastim** (do not use until day 6; 24 hr following completion of topotecan). ↑ myelosuppression with other **antineoplastics** (especially **cisplatin**) or **radiation therapy**. May ↓ antibody response to and ↑ risk of adverse reactions from **live virus vaccines**.

Route/Dosage
PO (Adults): 2.3 mg/m²/day for 5 days repeated every 21 days (round calculated oral dose to nearest 0.25 mg and prescribe the minimum number of 1 mg and 0.25 mg capsules with the same number of capsules prescribed for each of the 5 days).
IV (Adults): *Ovarian and Small Cell Lung Cancer*—1.5 mg/m²/day for 5 days starting on day 1 of a 21-day course; *Cervical Cancer*—75 mg/m² on Days 1, 2, and 3 followed by cisplatin on Day 1 and repeated every 21 days.

Renal Impairment
PO (Adults): *Ovarian and Small Cell Lung Cancer*—CCr 30–49 mL/min—1.8 mg/m²/day starting on day 1 of a 21-day course.
IV (Adults): CCr 20–39 mL/min—0.75mg/m²/day for 5 days starting on day 1 of a 21-day course. *Cervical Cancer*—Administer at standard doses only if serum creatinine is ≤1.5 mg/dL. Do not administer if serum creatinine >1.5 mg/dL.

Availability
Capsules: 0.25 mg, 1 mg. **Powder for injection:** 4 mg/vial.

NURSING IMPLICATIONS
Assessment
- Monitor vital signs frequently during administration.
- Monitor for bone marrow depression. Assess for bleeding (bleeding gums, bruising, petechiae; guaiac stools, urine, and emesis) and avoid IM injections and taking rectal temperatures if platelet count is low. Apply pressure to venipuncture sites for 10 min. Assess for signs of infection during neutropenia. Anemia may occur. Monitor for increased fatigue, dyspnea, and orthostatic hypotension.
- Nausea and vomiting are common. Pretreatment with antiemetics should be considered.
- Assess IV site frequently for extravasation, which causes mild local erythema and bruising.
- *Lab Test Considerations:* Monitor CBC with differential and platelet count prior to administration and frequently during therapy. Baseline neutrophil count of ≥1500 cells/mm³ and platelet count of ≥100,000 cells/mm³ are required before first dose. The nadir of neutropenia occurs in 11 days, with a duration of 7 days. The nadir of thrombocytopenia occurs in 15 days, with a duration of 5 days. The nadir of anemia occurs in 15 days. Subsequent doses should not be administered until neutrophils recover to >1000 cells/mm³, platelets recover to >100,000 cells/mm³, and hemoglobin levels recover to 9.0 mg/dL. If severe neutropenia occurs during any course, subsequent doses should be reduced by 0.25 mg/m² or filgrastim may be administered following the subsequent course of therapy starting on day 6, 24 hr after the completion of topotecan.
- Monitor liver function. May cause transient ↑ in AST, ALT, and bilirubin concentrations.

Potential Nursing Diagnoses
Risk for infection (Adverse Reactions)

Implementation
- **High Alert:** Fatalities have occurred with chemotherapeutic agents. Before administering, clarify all ambiguous orders; double check single, daily, and course-of-therapy dose limits; have second practitioner independently double check original order, dose calculations and infusion pump settings.
- **PO:** May be taken without regard to food. Capsules must be swallowed whole; do not open, crush, or chew. If patient vomits after taking dose, do not replace dose.
- Solution should be prepared in a biologic cabinet. Wear gloves, gown, and mask while handling IV medication. Discard IV equipment in specially designated containers.

IV Administration
- **Intermittent Infusion:** *Diluent:* Reconstitute each vial with 4 mL of sterile water for injection. Dilute further in D5W or 0.9% NaCl. Infusion is stable for 24 hr at room temperature or up to 7 days if refrigerated. Solution is yellow to yellow-green. *Concentration:* 10–50 mcg/mL. *Rate:* Infuse over 30 min.
- **Y-Site Compatibility:** carboplatin, caspofungin, cimetidine, cisplatin, cyclophosphamide, dactinomycin, daptomycin, doxorubicin, ertapenem, etoposide, fenoldopam, gemcitabine, granisetron, ifosfamide, levofloxacin, methylprednisolone, metoclopramide, ondansetron, oxaliplatin, paclitaxel, palonosetron, prochlorperazine, teniposide, thiotepa, vincristine, voriconazole.
- **Y-Site Incompatibility:** dexamethasone sodium phosphate, fluorouracil, mitomycin, pantoprazole, pemetrexed, rituximab, trastuzumab.

Patient/Family Teaching
- Instruct patient to take as directed. If patient vomits after taking, do not replace dose; notify health care professional. Do not take missed doses; take next scheduled dose and notify health care professional. If any capsules are broken or leaking, do not touch with bare hands; dispose of capsules and wash hands with soap and water. Patient should be instructed to read the Patient Information guide prior to first dose and with each refill; new information may be available.
- May cause drowsiness or sleepiness during and for several days after therapy. Caution patient to avoid driving and other activities requiring alertness until response to medication is known.
- Instruct patient to notify health care professional if fever; chills; sore throat; signs of infection; bleeding gums; bruising; petechiae; blood in urine, stool, or emesis occurs. Caution patient to avoid crowds and persons with known infections. Instruct patient to use soft toothbrush and electric razor. Patient should be cautioned not to drink alcoholic beverages or take products containing aspirin or NSAIDs.
- May cause diarrhea. Advise patient to notify health care professional if diarrhea with fever or stomach pain or cramps or diarrhea that occurs more than 3 times/day.
- Advise patient to consult health care professional before taking other Rx, OTC, or herbal products with topotecan.
- Discuss with patient the possibility of hair loss. Explore methods of coping.
- Advise patient that this medication may have teratogenic effects. Contraception should be used during therapy.
- Instruct patient not to receive any vaccinations without advice of health care professional.
- Emphasize the need for periodic lab tests to monitor for side effects.

Evaluation/Desired Outcomes
- Decrease in size and spread of malignancy.

---

torsemide (tore-se-mide)
Demadex

Classification
Therapeutic: antihypertensives
Pharmacologic: loop diuretics

Pregnancy Category B

Indications
Edema due to: CHF, Hepatic or renal disease. Hypertension.

Action
Inhibits the reabsorption of sodium and chloride from the loop of Henle and distal renal tubule. Increases renal excretion of water, sodium, chloride, magnesium, hydrogen, and calcium. Effectiveness persists in impaired renal function.
Therapeutic Effects: Diuresis and subsequent mobilization of excess fluid (edema, pleural effusions). Decreased blood pressure.

Pharmacokinetics
Absorption: 80% absorbed after oral administration.

Distribution: Widely distributed.
Protein Binding: ≥99%.
Metabolism and Excretion: 80% metabolized by liver, 20% excreted in urine.
Half-life: 3.5 hr.

TIME/ACTION PROFILE (diuretic effect)

ROUTE	ONSET	PEAK	DURATION
PO	within 60 min	60–120 min	6–8 hr
IV	within 10 min	within 60 min	6–8 hr

Contraindications/Precautions
Contraindicated in: Hypersensitivity; Cross-sensitivity with thiazides and sulfonamides may occur; Hepatic coma or anuria.
Use Cautiously in: Severe liver disease (may precipitate hepatic coma; concurrent use with potassium-sparing diuretics may be necessary); Electrolyte depletion; Diabetes mellitus; Increasing azotemia; OB, Lactation: Pedi: Safety not established; Geri: May have ↑ risk of side effects, especially hypotension and electrolyte imbalance, at usual doses.

Adverse Reactions/Side Effects
CNS: dizziness, headache, nervousness. **EENT:** hearing loss, tinnitus. **CV:** hypotension. **GI:** constipation, diarrhea, dry mouth, dyspepsia, nausea, vomiting. **GU:** excessive urination. **Derm:** photosensitivity, rash. **Endo:** hyperglycemia, hyperuricemia. **F and E:** dehydration, hypocalcemia, hypochloremia, hypokalemia, hypomagnesemia, hyponatremia, hypovolemia, metabolic alkalosis. **MS:** arthralgia, muscle cramps, myalgia. **Misc:** ↑ BUN.

Interactions
Drug-Drug: ↑ hypotension with **antihypertensives**, **nitrates**, or acute ingestion of **alcohol**. ↑ risk of hypokalemia with other **diuretics**, **amphotericin B**, **stimulant laxatives**, and **corticosteroids**. Hypokalemia may ↑ risk of **digoxin** toxicity and ↑ risk of arrhythmia in patients taking drugs that prolong the QT interval. May ↑ risk of **lithium** toxicity. ↑ risk of ototoxicity with **aminoglycosides**. **NSAIDs** may ↓ effects. ↑ risk of **salicylate** toxicity (with use of high-dose **salicylate** therapy). **Cholestyramine** may ↓ absorption.

Route/Dosage
Congestive Heart Failure
PO, IV (Adults): 10–20 mg once daily; dose may be doubled until desired effect is obtained (maximum daily dose = 200 mg).

Chronic Renal Failure
PO, IV (Adults): 20 mg once daily; dose may be doubled until desired effect is obtained (maximum daily dose = 200 mg).

Hepatic Cirrhosis
PO, IV (Adults): 5–10 mg once daily (with aldosterone antagonist or potassium-sparing diuretic); dose may be doubled until desired effect is obtained (maximum daily dose = 40 mg).

Hypertension
PO, IV (Adults): 2.5–5 mg once daily, may be ↑ to 10 mg once daily after 4–6 wk (if still not effective, add another agent).

Availability (generic available)
Tablets: 5 mg, 10 mg, 20 mg, 100 mg. **Cost:** *Generic* — 5 mg $50.00/90, 10 mg $50.97/90, 20 mg $59.97/90, 100 mg $213.98/90. **Solution for injection:** 10 mg/mL.

NURSING IMPLICATIONS
Assessment
- Assess fluid status during therapy. Monitor daily weight, intake and output ratios, amount and location of edema, lung sounds, skin turgor, and mucous membranes. Notify physician or other health care provider if thirst, dry mouth, lethargy, weakness, hypotension, or oliguria occurs.
- Monitor blood pressure and pulse before and during administration. Monitor frequency of prescription refills to determine adherence in patients treated for hypertension.
- Assess patients receiving digoxin for anorexia, nausea, vomiting, muscle cramps, paresthesia, and confusion. Patients taking digoxin are at increased risk of digoxin toxicity due to potassium-depleting effect of the diuretic. Potassium supplements or potassium-sparing diuretics may be used concurrently to prevent hypokalemia.
- Assess patient for tinnitus and hearing loss. Audiometry is recommended for patients receiving prolonged high-dose IV therapy. Hearing loss is most common following rapid or high-dose IV administration in patients with decreased renal function or those taking other ototoxic drugs.
- Assess for allergy to sulfonamides.
- Geri: Diuretic use is associated with increased risk for falls in older adults. Assess falls risk and implement fall prevention strategies.

✸ = Canadian drug name. 🧬 = Genetic implication.
*CAPITALS indicates life-threatening; underlines indicate most frequent.

- **Lab Test Considerations:** Monitor electrolytes, renal and hepatic function, serum glucose, and uric acid levels before and periodically during therapy. May cause ↓ serum sodium, potassium, calcium, and magnesium concentrations. May also cause ↑ BUN, serum glucose, creatinine, and uric acid levels.

Potential Nursing Diagnoses
Excess fluid volume (Indications)
Risk for deficient fluid volume (Side Effects)

Implementation
- Administer medication in the morning to prevent disruption of sleep cycle.
- IV is preferred over IM for parenteral administration.
- **PO:** May be taken with food or milk to minimize gastric irritation.

IV Administration
- **Direct IV:** *Diluent:* Administer undiluted. *Concentration:* 10 mg/mL. *Rate:* Administer slowly over 2 min.
- May also be administered as a continuous infusion.
- **Y-Site Compatibility:** milrinone, nesiritide.

Patient/Family Teaching
- Instruct patient to take torsemide as directed. Take missed doses as soon as possible; do not double doses.
- Caution patient to change positions slowly to minimize orthostatic hypotension. Caution patient that the use of alcohol, exercise during hot weather, or standing for long periods during therapy may enhance orthostatic hypotension.
- Instruct patient to consult health care professional regarding a diet high in potassium (see Appendix M).
- Advise patient to contact health care professional if they gain more than 2–3 lb/day.
- Advise patient to consult health care professional before taking OTC medication or herbal products concurrently with this therapy.
- Instruct patient to notify health care professional of medication regimen prior to treatment or surgery.
- Caution patient to use sunscreen and protective clothing to prevent photosensitivity reactions.
- Advise patient to contact health care professional immediately if muscle weakness, cramps, nausea, dizziness, numbness, or tingling of extremities occurs.
- Advise diabetic patients to monitor blood glucose closely; may cause increased blood glucose levels.
- Emphasize the importance of routine follow-up examinations.
- **Hypertension:** Advise patients on antihypertensive regimen to continue taking medication even if feeling better. Torsemide controls but does not cure hypertension.
- Reinforce the need to continue additional therapies for hypertension (weight loss, exercise, restricted sodium intake, stress reduction, regular exercise, moderation of alcohol consumption, cessation of smoking).

Evaluation/Desired Outcomes
- Decrease in edema.
- Decrease in abdominal girth and weight.
- Increase in urinary output.
- Decrease in blood pressure.

tramadol (tra-ma-dol)
✽ Ralivia, Ryzolt, Ultram, Ultram ER

Classification
Therapeutic: analgesics (centrally acting)

Pregnancy Category C

Indications
Moderate to moderately severe pain (extended-release formulations indicated for patients who require around-the-clock pain management).

Action
Binds to mu-opioid receptors. Inhibits reuptake of serotonin and norepinephrine in the CNS.
Therapeutic Effects: Decreased pain.

Pharmacokinetics
Absorption: *Immediate-release*—75% absorbed after oral administration; *Extended-release (Ultram)*—85–90% (compared with immediate-release); *Extended-release (Ryzolt)*—95% (compared with immediate-release).
Distribution: Crosses the placenta; enters breast milk.
Metabolism and Excretion: Mostly metabolized by the liver; one metabolite has analgesic activity; 30% is excreted unchanged in urine.
Half-life: *Tramadol*—6–8 hr, *ER*—7.9 hr; *active metabolite*—7–9 hr; both are ↑ in renal or hepatic impairment.

TIME/ACTION PROFILE (analgesia)

ROUTE	ONSET	PEAK	DURATION
PO	1 hr	2–3 hr	4–6 hr
ER		12 hr	24 hr

Contraindications/Precautions
Contraindicated in: Hypersensitivity; Cross-sensitivity with opioids may occur; Patients who are

acutely intoxicated with alcohol, sedatives/hypnotics, centrally acting analgesics, opioid analgesics, or psychotropic agents; Patients who are physically dependent on opioid analgesics (may precipitate withdrawal); *Ryzolt only*—Acute or severe bronchial asthma or hypercapnia in unmonitored settings or in absence of resuscitative equipment; OB: Lactation: Pregnancy or lactation; *ER only*—CCr <30 mL/min or hepatic impairment.

Use Cautiously in: Geri:*Immediate-release*— Not to exceed 300 mg/day in patients >75 yr; *ER*—Use with extreme caution in patients >75 yr; Patients with a history of epilepsy or risk factors for seizures; Renal impairment (↑ dosing interval recommended if CCr <30 mL/min); Hepatic impairment (↑ dosing interval recommended in patients with cirrhosis); Patients receiving MAO inhibitors or CNS depressants; Patients who are suicidal; ↑ intracranial pressure or head trauma; Patients with a history of opioid dependence or who have recently received large doses of opioids; Pedi: Children <16 yr (safety not established).

Adverse Reactions/Side Effects

CNS: SEIZURES, dizziness, headache, somnolence, anxiety, CNS stimulation, confusion, coordination disturbance, euphoria, malaise, nervousness, sleep disorder, weakness. **EENT:** visual disturbances. **CV:** vasodilation. **GI:** constipation, nausea, abdominal pain, anorexia, diarrhea, dry mouth, dyspepsia, flatulence, vomiting. **GU:** menopausal symptoms, urinary retention/frequency. **Derm:** pruritus, sweating. **Neuro:** hypertonia. **Misc:** physical dependence, psychological dependence, tolerance.

Interactions

Drug-Drug: ↑ risk of CNS depression when used concurrently with other **CNS depressants**, including **alcohol, antihistamines, sedative/hypnotics, opioid analgesics, anesthetics**, or **psychotropic agents**. ↑ risk of seizures with high doses of **penicillins, cephalosporins, phenothiazines, opioid analgesics**, or **antidepressants**. **Carbamazepine** ↑ metabolism and ↓ effectiveness of tramadol (increased doses may be required). Use cautiously in patients who are receiving **MAO inhibitors** (↑ risk of adverse reactions). **Quinidine, fluoxetine, paroxetine, amitriptyline, ketoconazole,** and **erythromycin** may ↑ levels. ↑ risk of serotonin syndrome when used with **SSRI and SNRI antidepressants, TCAs, MAO inhibitors** and **5HT₁ agonists**.

Drug-Natural Products: Concomitant use of **kava-kava, valerian,** or **chamomile** can ↑ CNS depression. ↑ risk of serotonin syndrome when used with **St. Johns' wort**.

Route/Dosage
Immediate-release

PO (Adults ≥18 yr): *Rapid titration*—50–100 mg q 4–6 hr (not to exceed 400 mg/day or 300 mg in patients >75 yr). *Gradual titration*—25 mg/day initially, ↑ by 25 mg/day q 3 days to reach dose of 25 mg 4 times daily, then ↑ by 50 mg/day q 3 days to reach dose of 50 mg 4 times daily; may then use 50–100 mg q 4–6 hr (maximum dose = 400 mg/day).

Renal Impairment
PO (Adults): *CCr <30 mL/min*—increase dosing interval to q 12 hr (not to exceed 200 mg/day).

Hepatic Impairment
PO (Adults): 50 mg q 12 hr.

Extended-release

PO (Adults): *Ultram ER (not currently receiving immediate-release)*—100 mg once daily initially, may then titrate q 5 days up to 300 mg/day; *Ultram ER (currently receiving immediate-release)*—calculate 24-hr total dose of immediate-release product and give same dose (rounded down to next lowest 100-mg increment) of ER once daily (maximum dose = 300 mg/day); *Ryzolt (not currently receiving immediate-release)*—100 mg once daily initially, may then titrate by 100 mg/day q 2–3 days up to 300 mg/day; *Ryzolt (currently receiving immediate-release)*—Calculate 24-hr total dose of immediate-release product and give same dose (rounded down to next lowest 100-mg increment) of Ryzolt once daily (maximum dose = 300 mg/day).

Availability (generic available)
Tablets: 50 mg. **Cost:** *Generic*—$16.99/30 $85.25/100. **Extended-release tablets:** 100 mg, 200 mg, 300 mg. **Cost:** 100 mg $89.99/30, 200 mg $158.98/30, 300 mg $195.99/30. *In combination with:* acetaminophen (Ultracet). See Appendix B.

NURSING IMPLICATIONS
Assessment
- Assess type, location, and intensity of pain before and 2–3 hr (peak) after administration.
- Assess blood pressure and respiratory rate before and periodically during administration. Respiratory depression has not occurred with recommended doses.
- Assess bowel function routinely. Prevention of constipation should be instituted with increased intake of fluids and bulk and with laxatives to minimize constipating effects.
- Assess previous analgesic history. Tramadol is not recommended for patients dependent on opioids or who have previously received opioids for more than 1 wk; may cause opioid withdrawal symptoms.
- Prolonged use may lead to physical and psychological dependence and tolerance, although these may be milder than with opioids. This should not prevent patient from receiving adequate analgesia. Most patients who receive tramadol for pain do not develop psychological dependence. If tolerance develops, changing to an opioid agonist may be required to relieve pain.
- Monitor patient for seizures. May occur within recommended dose range. Risk is increased with higher doses and in patients taking antidepressants (SSRIs, SNRIs, tricyclics, or MAO inhibitors), opioid analgesics, or other drugs that decrease the seizure threshold. Also monitor for serotonin syndrome (mental-status changes (e.g., agitation, hallucinations, coma), autonomic instability (e.g., tachycardia, labile blood pressure, hyperthermia), neuromuscular aberrations (e.g., hyperreflexia, incoordination) and/or gastrointestinal symptoms (e.g., nausea, vomiting, diarrhea) in patients taking these drugs concurrently.
- **Lab Test Considerations:** May cause ↑ serum creatinine, elevated liver enzymes, decreased hemoglobin, and proteinuria.
- **Toxicity and Overdose:** Overdose may cause respiratory depression and seizures. Naloxone (Narcan) may reverse some, but not all, of the symptoms of overdose. Treatment should be symptomatic and supportive. Maintain adequate respiratory exchange. Hemodialysis is not helpful because it removes only a small portion of administered dose. Seizures may be managed with barbiturates or benzodiazepines; naloxone increases risk of seizures.

Potential Nursing Diagnoses
Acute pain (Indications)
Risk for injury (Side Effects)

Implementation
- Do not confuse tramadol with Toradol (ketorolac).
- Tramadol is considered to provide more analgesia than codeine 60 mg but less than combined aspirin 650 mg/codeine 60 mg for acute postoperative pain.
- For chronic pain, daily doses of 250 mg of tramadol provide pain relief similar to that of 5 doses/day of acetaminophen 300 mg/codeine 30 mg, 5 doses/day of aspirin 325 mg/codeine 30 mg, or 2–3 doses/day of acetaminophen 500 mg/oxycodone 5 mg.
- Explain therapeutic value of medication before administration to enhance the analgesic effect.
- Regularly administered doses may be more effective than prn administration. Analgesic is more effective if given before pain becomes severe.
- Tramadol should be discontinued gradually after long-term use to prevent withdrawal symptoms.
- **PO:** Tramadol may be administered without regard to meals. Extended-release tablets should be swallowed whole; do not crush, break, or chew.

Patient/Family Teaching
- Instruct patient on how and when to ask for pain medication.
- May cause dizziness and drowsiness. Caution patient to avoid driving or other activities requiring alertness until response to medication is known.
- Advise patient to change positions slowly to minimize orthostatic hypotension.
- Caution patient to avoid concurrent use of alcohol or other CNS depressants with this medication. Advise patient to notify health care professional before taking other RX, OTC, or herbal products concurrently.
- Advise female patients to notify health care professional if pregnancy is planned or suspected, or if breastfeeding.
- Advise patient to notify health care professional if seizures or if symptoms of serotonin syndrome occur.
- Encourage patient to turn, cough, and breathe deeply every 2 hr to prevent atelectasis.

Evaluation/Desired Outcomes
- Decrease in severity of pain without a significant alteration in level of consciousness or respiratory status.

trandolapril, See ANGIOTENSIN-CONVERTING ENZYME (ACE) INHIBITORS.

tranylcypromine, See MONOAMINE OXIDASE (MAO) INHIBITORS.

HIGH ALERT

trastuzumab
(traz-**too**-zoo-mab)
Herceptin

Classification
Therapeutic: antineoplastics
Pharmacologic: monoclonal antibodies

Pregnancy Category D

Indications
First-line treatment of metastatic breast cancer (with paclitaxel) that displays overexpression of the human epidermal growth factor receptor 2 (HER2) protein. Treatment of metastatic breast cancer (as monotherapy) that displays overexpression of the human epidermal growth factor receptor 2 (HER2) protein in patients who have already received other chemotherapy regimens. Adjuvant treatment of HER2 overexpressing node positive or node negative breast cancer (to be used with alone after multi-modality anthracycline-based therapy or as part of one of the following regimens: doxorubicin, cyclophosphamide, and either paclitaxel or docetaxel; with docetaxel and carboplatin).

Action
A monoclonal antibody that binds to HER2 sites in breast cancer tissue and inhibits proliferation of cells that overexpress HER2 protein. **Therapeutic Effects:** Regression of breast cancer and metastases.

Pharmacokinetics
Absorption: IV administration results in complete bioavailability.
Distribution: Binds to HER2 proteins.
Metabolism and Excretion: Unknown.
Half-life: 10-mg dose—1.7 days; 500-mg dose—12 days.

TIME/ACTION PROFILE (blood levels)

ROUTE	ONSET	PEAK	DURATION
IV	unknown	unknown	unknown

Contraindications/Precautions
Contraindicated in: None known.
Use Cautiously in: Pre-existing pulmonary conditions; Hypersensitivity to trastuzumab, Chinese hamster ovary cell proteins, or other components of the product; Hypersensitivity to benzyl alcohol (use sterile water for injection instead of bacteriostatic water, which accompanies the vial); Geri: May have ↑ risk of cardiac dysfunction; OB, Lactation: Use during pregnancy only if clearly needed; not recommended for use during lactation; Pedi: Safety not established.
Exercise Extreme Caution in: Patients with pre-existing cardiac dysfunction.

Adverse Reactions/Side Effects
CNS: dizziness, headache, insomnia, weakness, depression, . **Resp:** INTERSTITIAL PNEUMONITIS, PULMONARY EDEMA, PULMONARY FIBROSIS, dyspnea, increased cough, pharyngitis, rhinitis, sinusitis. **CV:** ARRHYTHMIAS, HF, hypertension, tachycardia. **GI:** abdominal pain, anorexia, diarrhea, nausea, vomiting. **Derm:** rash, acne, herpes simplex. **F and E:** edema. **Hemat:** anemia, leukopenia. **MS:** back pain, arthralgia, bone pain. **Neuro:** neuropathy, paresthesia, peripheral neuritis. **Misc:** HYPERSENSITIVITY REACTIONS, chills, fever, infection, pain, allergic reactions, flu-like syndrome.

Interactions
Drug-Drug: Concurrent **anthracycline** (**daunorubicin, doxorubicin,** or **idarubicin**) therapy may ↑ risk of cardiotoxicity. Blood levels are ↑ by concurrent **paclitaxel**.

Route/Dosage

Adjuvant Treatment of Breast Cancer
IV (Adults): *During and following paclitaxel, docetaxel, or docetaxel/carboplatin*—4 mg/kg initially, then 2 mg/kg weekly during chemotherapy for the first 12 wk (paclitaxel or docetaxel) or 18 wk (docetaxel/carboplatin); one wk after the last weekly dose, give 6 mg/kg q 3 wk; *As single agent within 3 wk following completion of multi-modality, anthracycline-based chemotherapy regimens*—8 mg/kg initially, then 6 mg/kg q 3 wk.

✽ = Canadian drug name. = Genetic implication.
*CAPITALS indicates life-threatening; underlines indicate most frequent.

1250 trastuzumab

Metastatic Breast Cancer
IV (Adults): 4 mg/kg initially, then 2 mg/kg weekly until disease progresses.

Availability
Lyophilized powder for injection: 440 mg/vial with 20 mL bacteriostatic water for injection (contains benzyl alcohol).

NURSING IMPLICATIONS
Assessment
- Assess for infusion-related symptoms (chills, fever, nausea, vomiting, pain [in some cases at tumor sites], headache, dizziness, dyspnea, hypotension, rash, and asthenia) following initial infusion. Severe reactions (bronchospasm, anaphylaxis, angioedema, hypoxia, severe hypotension) may occur during or immediately following the initial infusion. May be treated with epinephrine, corticosteroids, diphenhydramine, bronchodilators, and oxygen. Discontinue if dyspnea or severe hypotension occurs and discontinue permanently if severe reaction occurs.
- Assess for signs and symptoms of HF (dyspnea, increased cough, paroxysmal nocturnal dyspnea, peripheral edema, S_3 gallop, reduced ejection fraction) prior to and frequently during therapy. Baseline cardiac assessment of history, physical exam, and left ventricular ejection fraction (LVEF) with ECG or multiple gated acquisition (MUGA) scan. Monitor LVEF every 3 mo and at completion of therapy, every 6 mo for 2 yr. Withhold trastuzumab for ≥16% absolute decrease in LVEF from pre-treatment values or an LVEF value below institutional limits of normal and ≥10% absolute decrease in LVEF from pretreatment values. Repeat LVEF measures every 4 wk if dose is withheld. CHF associated with trastuzumab may be severe, resulting in cardiac failure, death, and stroke. Trastuzumab should be discontinued upon the development of significant CHF.
- Monitor patient for signs of pulmonary hypersensitivity reactions (dyspnea, pulmonary infiltrates, pleural effusion, noncardiogenic pulmonary edema, pulmonary insufficiency, hypoxia, acute respiratory distress syndrome). Patients with symptomatic pulmonary disease or extensive lung tumor involvement are at increased risk. Infusion should be discontinued if severe symptoms occur.
- ***Lab Test Considerations:*** HER2 protein overexpression is used to determine whether treatment with trastuzumab is indicated. HER2 protein overexpression is detected by HercepTest™ (IHC assay) and PathVysion™ (FISH assay).
- May cause anemia and leukopenia.

Potential Nursing Diagnoses
Diarrhea (Adverse Reactions)
Risk for infection (Adverse Reactions)

Implementation
- ***High Alert:*** Fatalities have occurred with chemotherapeutic agents. Before administering, clarify all ambiguous orders; double check single, daily, and course-of-therapy dose limits; have second practitioner independently double check original order, dose calculations and infusion pump settings.
- May be administered in the outpatient setting.

IV Administration
- **Intermittent Infusion:** Reconstitute each vial with 20 mL of bacteriostatic water for injection, directing the stream of diluent into lyophilized cake of trastuzumab. ***Concentration:*** 21 mg/mL. Swirl the vial gently; do not shake. May foam slightly; allow the vial to stand undisturbed for 5 min. Solution should be clear to slightly opalescent and colorless to pale yellow, without particulate matter. Label vial immediately in the area marked "Do not use after" with the date 28 days from the date of reconstitution. Stable for 24 hr at room temperature or 28 days if refrigerated. If patient is allergic to benzyl alcohol, use sterile water for injection for reconstitution. Use immediately and discard any unused portion. ***Diluent:*** Calculate to volume required for the desired dose, withdraw, and add it to an infusion containing 250 mL of 0.9% NaCl. Invert bag gently to mix. ***Rate:*** Infuse the 4 mg/kg loading dose over 90 min and the weekly 2 mg/kg dose over 30 min or 6 mg/kg over 90 min every 3 wk if the loading dose was well tolerated. Do not administer as an IV push or bolus.
- **Y-Site Compatibility:** acyclovir, amifostine, aminophylline, ampicillin, ampicillin/sulbactam, bleomycin, bumetanide, buprenorphine, busulfan, butorphanol, calcium gluconate, carboplatin, carmustine, cefazolin, ceftazidime, ceftizoxime, ceftriaxone, cefuroxime, cimetidine, ciprofloxacin, cisplatin, cyclophosphamide, cytarabine, dactinomycin, daunorubicin, dexamethasone, digoxin, diphenhydramine, dobutamine, docetaxel, dopamine, doxorubi-

cin, doxorubicin liposome, doxycycline, droperidol, enalaprilat, etoposide phosphate, famotidine, fentnayl, filgrastim, floxuridine, fluconazole, fluorouracil, ganciclovir, gemcitabine, gentamicin, gransietron, haloperidol, heparin, hydrocortisone, hydromorphone, ifosfamide, imipenem/cilastatin, leucovorin, lorazepam, magnesium sulfate, mannitol, meperidine, mesna, methotrexate, methylprednisolone, metoclopramide, metronidazole, mitomycin, mitoxantrone, paclitaxel, pentamidine, plicamycin, potassium chloride, prochlorperazine, promethazine, ranitidine, remifentanil, sargramostim, sodium bicarbonate, teniposide, theophylline, thiotepa, ticarcillin/clavulanate, tobramycin, trimethobenzamide, trimethoprim/sulfamethoxazole, vancomycin, vinblastine, vincristine, vinorelbine, zidovudine.
- **Y-Site Incompatibility:** aldesleukin, amikacin, amphotericin B colloidal, aztreonam, cefoperazone, cefotaxime, cefotetan, cefoxitin, chlorpromazine, clindamycin, cyclosporine, fludarabine, furosemide, idarubicin, irinotecan, levofloxacin, levorphanol, morphine, nalbuphine, ondansetron, piperacillin/tazobactam, streptozocin, topotecan.
- **Additive Incompatibility:** Do not dilute trastuzumab with or add to solutions containing dextrose. Do not mix or dilute with other drugs.

Patient/Family Teaching
- Instruct patient to notify health care professional promptly if new onset or worsening shortness of breath, cough, swelling of the ankles/legs, swelling of the face, palpitations, weight gain of more than 5 pounds in 24 hours, dizziness or loss of consciousness occur. Caution patient to avoid crowds and persons with known infections.
- May cause teratogenic effects. Caution patient to use contraception during and for at least 6 mo following completion of therapy.
- Advise patient not to receive any vaccinations without advice of health care professional.

Evaluation/Desired Outcomes
- Regression of breast cancer and metastases.

trazodone (traz-oh-done)

Classification
Therapeutic: antidepressants

Pregnancy Category C

Indications
Major depression. **Unlabeled Use:** Insomnia, chronic pain syndromes, including diabetic neuropathy, and anxiety.

Action
Alters the effects of serotonin in the CNS. **Therapeutic Effects:** Antidepressant action, which may develop only over several weeks.

Pharmacokinetics
Absorption: Well absorbed after oral administration.
Distribution: Widely distributed.
Protein Binding: 89–95%.
Metabolism and Excretion: Extensively metabolized by the liver (CYP3A4 enzyme system); minimal excretion of unchanged drug by the kidneys.
Half-life: 5–9 hr.

TIME/ACTION PROFILE (antidepressant effect)

ROUTE	ONSET	PEAK	DURATION
PO	1–2 wk	2–4 wk	wk

Contraindications/Precautions
Contraindicated in: Hypersensitivity; Recovery period after MI; Concurrent electroconvulsive therapy.
Use Cautiously in: Cardiovascular disease; Suicidal behavior; May ↑ risk of suicide attempt/ideation especially during early treatment or dose adjustment; Severe hepatic or renal disease (dose reduction recommended); Lactation: Discontinue drug or bottle feed; Pedi: Suicide risk may be greater in children and adolescents; safe use not established; Geri: Initial dose reduction recommended.

Adverse Reactions/Side Effects
CNS: SUICIDAL THOUGHTS, drowsiness, confusion, dizziness, fatigue, hallucinations, headache, insomnia, nightmares, slurred speech, syncope, weakness. **EENT:** blurred vision, tinnitus. **CV:** hypotension, arrhythmias, chest pain, hypertension, palpitations, QT interval prolongation, tachycar-

1252 trazodone

dia. **GI:** dry mouth, altered taste, constipation, diarrhea, excess salivation, flatulence, nausea, vomiting. **GU:** hematuria, erectile dysfunction, priapism, urinary frequency. **Derm:** rashes. **Hemat:** anemia, leukopenia. **MS:** myalgia. **Neuro:** tremor.

Interactions
Drug-Drug: May ↑ **digoxin** or **phenytoin** serum levels. ↑ CNS depression with other **CNS depressants**, including **alcohol**, **opioid analgesics**, and **sedative/hypnotics**. ↑ hypotension with **antihypertensives**, acute ingestion of **alcohol**, or **nitrates**. Concurrent use with **fluoxetine** ↑ levels and risk of toxicity from trazodone. **Drugs that inhibit the CYP3A4 enzyme system**, including **ritonavirindinavir** and **ketoconazole** ↑ levels and the risk of toxicity. **Drugs that induce the CYP3A4 enzyme system**, including **carbamazepine** ↓ levels and may decrease effectiveness. Do note use within 14 days of **MAOI** therapy. May ↑ prothrombin time (PT) with **warfarin**.
Drug-Natural Products: Concomitant use of **kava-kava**, **valerian**, or **chamomile** can ↑ CNS depression. ↑ risk of serotinergic side effects including serotonin syndrome with **St. John's wort** and **SAMe**.

Route/Dosage
PO (Adults): *Depression*—150 mg/day in 3 divided doses; ↑ by 50 mg/day q 3–4 days until desired response (not to exceed 400 mg/day in outpatients or 600 mg/day in hospitalized patients). *Insomnia*—25–100 mg at bedtime.
PO (Geriatric Patients): 75 mg/day in divided doses initially; may be ↑ q 3–4 days.

Availability (generic available)
Tablets: 50 mg, 100 mg, 150 mg, 300 mg.

NURSING IMPLICATIONS
Assessment
- Monitor blood pressure and pulse rate before and during initial therapy. Monitor ECGs in patients with pre-existing cardiac disease before and periodically during therapy to detect arrhythmias.
- Assess for possible sexual dysfunction.
- **Depression:** Assess mental status (orientation, mood, and behavior) frequently.
- Assess for suicidal tendencies, especially during early therapy. Restrict amount of drug available to patient. Risk may be increased in children, adolescents, and adults ≤24 yr. After starting therapy, children, adolescents, and young adults should be seen by health care professional at least weekly for 4 wk, every 3 wk for next 4 wk, and on advice of health care professional thereafter.
- **Pain:** Assess location, duration, intensity, and characteristics of pain before and periodically during therapy. Use pain scale to assess effectiveness of medicine.
- *Lab Test Considerations:* Assess CBC and renal and hepatic function before and periodically during therapy. Slight, clinically insignificant ↓ in leukocyte and neutrophil counts may occur.

Potential Nursing Diagnoses
Ineffective coping (Indications)
Sexual dysfunction (Side Effects)

Implementation
- **PO:** Administer with or immediately after meals to minimize side effects (nausea, dizziness) and allow maximum absorption of trazodone. A larger portion of the total daily dose may be given at bedtime to decrease daytime drowsiness and dizziness.

Patient/Family Teaching
- Instruct patient to take medication exactly as directed. If a dose is missed, take as soon as remembered. Do not take if within 4 hr of next scheduled dose; do not double doses. Consult health care professional before discontinuing medication; gradual dose reduction is necessary to prevent aggravation of condition.
- May cause drowsiness and blurred vision. Caution patient to avoid driving and other activities requiring alertness until response to drug is known.
- Caution patient to change positions slowly to minimize orthostatic hypotension.
- Advise patient to avoid concurrent use of alcohol or other CNS depressant drugs.
- Advise patient, family, and caregivers to look for suicidality, especially during early therapy or dose changes. Notify health care professional immediately if thoughts about suicide or dying, attempts to commit suicide, new or worse depression or anxiety, agitation or restlessness, panic attacks, insomnia, new or worse irritability, aggressiveness, acting on dangerous impulses, mania, or other changes in mood or behavior occur.
- Inform patient that frequent rinses, good oral hygiene, and sugarless candy or gum may diminish dry mouth. Health care professional should be notified if this persists >2 wk. An in-

crease in fluid intake, fiber, and exercise may prevent constipation.
- Advise patient to notify health care professional of medication regimen before treatment or surgery.
- Instruct patient to notify health care professional if priapism, irregular heartbeat, fainting, confusion, skin rash, or tremors occur or if dry mouth, nausea and vomiting, dizziness, headache, muscle aches, constipation, or diarrhea becomes pronounced.
- Emphasize the importance of follow-up exams to evaluate progress.

Evaluation/Desired Outcomes
- Resolution of depression.
- Increased sense of well-being.
- Renewed interest in surroundings.
- Increased appetite.
- Improved energy level.
- Improved sleep.
- Decrease in severity of pain in chronic pain syndromes. Therapeutic effects are usually seen within 1 wk, although 4 wk may be required to obtain significant therapeutic results.

---

triamcinolone, See CORTICOSTEROIDS (NASAL).

---

triamcinolone, See CORTICOSTEROIDS (SYSTEMIC).

---

triamcinolone, See CORTICOSTEROIDS (TOPICAL/LOCAL).

---

triamterene, See DIURETICS (POTASSIUM-SPARING).

---

triazolam (trye-az-oh-lam)
✽Apo-Triazo, ✽Gen-Triazolam, Halcion, ✽Novo-Triolam, ✽Nu-Triazo

Classification
Therapeutic: sedative/hypnotics
Pharmacologic: benzodiazepines

Schedule IV

Pregnancy Category X

Indications
Short-term management of insomnia.

Action
Acts at many levels in the CNS, producing generalized depression. Effects may be mediated by GABA, an inhibitory neurotransmitter. **Therapeutic Effects:** Relief of insomnia.

Pharmacokinetics
Absorption: Well absorbed following oral administration.
Distribution: Widely distributed, crosses blood-brain barrier. Probably crosses the placenta and enters breast milk.
Protein Binding: 89%.
Metabolism and Excretion: Metabolized by the liver.
Half-life: 1.6–5.4 hr.

TIME/ACTION PROFILE (sedation)

ROUTE	ONSET	PEAK	DURATION
PO	15–30 min	6–8 hr	unknown

Contraindications/Precautions
Contraindicated in: Hypersensitivity; Cross-sensitivity with other benzodiazepines may occur; Pre-existing CNS depression; Uncontrolled severe pain; OB: Lactation: Pedi: Safety not established.
Use Cautiously in: Pre-existing hepatic dysfunction (dose ↓ recommended); History of suicide attempt or drug addiction; Geri: Appears on Beers list and is associated with ↑ risk of falls (↓ dose required); ↑ sensitivity to benzodiazepines.

Adverse Reactions/Side Effects
CNS: abnormal thinking, behavior changes, <u>dizziness</u>, <u>excessive sedation</u>, hangover, <u>headache</u>, anterograde amnesia, confusion, hallucinations, sleep—driving, lethargy, mental depression, paradoxical excitation. **EENT:** blurred vision. **GI:** constipation, diarrhea, nausea, vomiting. **Derm:** rashes. **Misc:** physical dependence, psychological dependence, tolerance.

Interactions
Drug-Drug: **Cimetidine, erythromycin, fluconazole, itraconazole, ketoconazole, indinavir, nelfinavir, ritonavir,** or **saquinavir** may ↓ metabolism and enhance actions of triazolam; combination should be avoided. Additive CNS depression with **alcohol, antidepressants, antihistamines,** and **opioid analgesics**. May ↓ effectiveness of **levodopa**. May ↑ toxicity of

zidovudine. **Isoniazid** may ↓ excretion and ↑ effects of triazolam. Sedative effects may be ↓ by **theophylline**.
Drug-Natural Products: Concomitant use of **kava-kava**, **valerian**, **chamomile**, or **hops** can ↑ CNS depression.
Drug-Food: Grapefruit juice significantly ↑ blood levels and effects.

Route/Dosage
PO (Adults): 0.125–0.25 mg (up to 0.5 mg) at bedtime.
PO (Geriatric Patients or Debilitated Patients): 0.125 mg at bedtime initially; may be ↑ as needed.

Availability (generic available)
Tablets: 0.125 mg, 0.25 mg.

NURSING IMPLICATIONS
Assessment
- Assess sleep patterns prior to and periodically throughout therapy.
- Geri: Assess CNS effects and risk of falls. Institute falls prevention strategies.
- Prolonged high-dose therapy may lead to psychological or physical dependence. Restrict the amount of drug available to patient, especially if patient is depressed, suicidal, or has a history of addiction.

Potential Nursing Diagnoses
Insomnia (Indications)
Risk for injury (Side Effects)

Implementation
- Supervise ambulation and transfer of patients following administration. Remove cigarettes. Side rails should be raised and call bell within reach at all times.
- **PO:** Administer with food if GI irritation becomes a problem.

Patient/Family Teaching
- Instruct patient to take triazolam exactly as directed. Discuss the importance of preparing environment for sleep (dark room, quiet, avoidance of nicotine and caffeine). If less effective after a few weeks, consult health care professional; do not increase dose.
- May cause daytime drowsiness or dizziness. Caution patient to avoid driving or other activities requiring alertness until response to medication is known. Geri: Instruct patient and family how to reduce falls risk at home.
- Advise patient to avoid the use of alcohol and other CNS depressants and to consult health care professional prior to using OTC preparations that contain antihistamines or alcohol.
- Advise patient to inform health care professional if pregnancy is planned or suspected or if confusion, depression, or persistent headaches occur. Instruct family or caregiver to notify health care professional if personality changes occur.
- Instruct patient to notify health care professional if an increase in daytime anxiety occurs. May occur after as few as 10 days of therapy. May require discontinuation of triazolam.
- Emphasize the importance of follow-up appointments to monitor progress.

Evaluation/Desired Outcomes
- Improvement in sleep patterns, which may not be noticeable until the 3rd day of therapy.

---

tricalcium phosphate (39% Ca or 19.5 mEq/g), See CALCIUM SALTS.

---

trikates (potassium acetate/potassium bicarbonate/potassium citrate), See POTASSIUM SUPPLEMENTS.

---

trimethoprim/ sulfamethoxazole
(trye-**meth**-oh-prim/sul-fa-meth-**ox**-a-zole)
✤ Apo-Sulfatrim, ✤ Apo-Sulfatrim DS, Bactrim, Bactrim DS, ✤ Novo-Trimel, ✤ Novo-Trimel DS, ✤ Nu-Cotrimox, ✤ Nu-Cotrimox DS, ✤ Roubac, Septra, Septra DS, SMZ/TMP, Sulfatrim, TMP/SMX, TMP/SMZ

Classification
Therapeutic: anti-infectives, antiprotozoals
Pharmacologic: folate antagonists, sulfonamides

Pregnancy Category C

Indications
Treatment of: Bronchitis, *Shigella* enteritis, Otitis media, *Pneumocystis jirovecii* pneumonia (PCP), Urinary tract infections, Traveler's diarrhea. Prevention of PCP in HIV-positive patients.
Unlabeled Use: Biliary tract infections, osteomyelitis, burn and wound infections, chlamydial infections, endocarditis, gonorrhea, intra-abdominal infections, nocardiosis, rheumatic fever prophylaxis, sinusitis, eradication of meningococcal carriers, prophylaxis of urinary tract infec-

trimethoprim/sulfamethoxazole 1255

tions, and an alternative agent in the treatment of chancroid. Prevention of bacterial infections in immunosuppressed patients.

Action
Combination inhibits the metabolism of folic acid in bacteria at two different points. **Therapeutic Effects:** Bactericidal action against susceptible bacteria. **Spectrum:** Active against many strains of gram-positive aerobic pathogens including: *Streptococcus pneumoniae, Staphylococcus aureus,* Group A beta-hemolytic streptococci, *Nocardia, Enterococcus.* Has activity against many aerobic gram-negative pathogens, such as: *Acinetobacter, Enterobacter, Klebsiella pneumoniae, Escherichia coli, Proteus mirabilis, Shigella, Haemophilus influenzae,* including ampicillin-resistant strains. *P. jirovecii.* Not active against *Pseudomonas aeruginosa.*

Pharmacokinetics
Absorption: Well absorbed from the GI tract.
Distribution: Widely distributed. Crosses the blood-brain barrier and placenta and enters breast milk.
Metabolism and Excretion: Some metabolism by the liver (20%); remainder excreted unchanged by the kidneys.
Half-life: *Trimethoprim*—6–11 hr; *sulfamethoxazole*—9–12 hr, both prolonged in renal failure.

TIME/ACTION PROFILE (blood levels)

ROUTE	ONSET	PEAK	DURATION
PO	rapid	2–4 hr	6–12 hr
IV	rapid	end of infusion	6–12 hr

Contraindications/Precautions
Contraindicated in: Hypersensitivity to sulfonamides or trimethoprim; Megaloblastic anemia secondary to folate deficiency; Severe renal impairment; OB, Lactation: Pedi: Pregnancy, lactation, or children <2 mo (can cause kernicterus in neonates).
Use Cautiously in: Impaired hepatic or renal function (dosage ↓ required if CCr <30 mL/min); HIV-positive patients (↑ incidence of adverse reactions).

Adverse Reactions/Side Effects
CNS: fatigue, hallucinations, headache, insomnia, mental depression. **GI:** PSEUDOMEMBRANOUS COLITIS, HEPATIC NECROSIS, nausea, vomiting, diarrhea, stomatitis, hepatitis, cholestatic jaundice. **GU:** crystalluria. **Derm:** TOXIC EPIDERMAL NECROLYSIS, rashes, photosensitivity. **Hemat:** AGRANULOCYTOSIS, APLASTIC ANEMIA, hemolytic anemia, leukopenia, megaloblastic anemia, thrombocytopenia. **Local:** phlebitis at IV site. **Misc:** allergic reactions including ERYTHEMA MULTIFORME, STEVENS-JOHNSON SYNDROME, fever.

Interactions
Drug-Drug: May ↑ half-life, ↓ clearance, and exaggerate folic acid deficiency caused by **phenytoin**. May ↑ effects of **sulfonylurea oral antidiabetics, phenytoin, digoxin, thiopental** and **warfarin**. May ↑ toxicity of **methotrexate**. ↑ risk of thrombocytopenia from **thiazide diuretics** (↑ in geriatric patients). ↓ efficacy of **cyclosporine (decreases serum concentrations)** and ↑ risk of nephrotoxicity.

Route/Dosage
(TMP = trimethoprim; SMX = sulfamethoxazole). Dosing based on TMP content..

Bacterial Infections
PO, IV (Adults and Children >2 mo): *Mild-moderate infections*—6–12 mg TMP/kg/day divided q 12 hr; *Serious infection/Pneumocystis*—15–20 mg TMP/kg/day/divided q 6–8 hr.
PO (Adults): *Urinary tract infection/chronic bronchitis*—1 double strength tablet (160 mg TMP/800 mg SMX) q 12 hr for 10–14 days.

Urinary Tract Infection Prophylaxis
PO, IV (Adults and Children >2 mo): 2 mg TMP/kg/dose daily or 5 mg TMP/kg/dose twice weekly.

P. jirovecii Pneumonia (Prevention)
PO (Adults): 1 double strength tablet (160 mg TMP/800 mg SMX) daily (may also be given 3 times weekly).
PO (Children >1 mo): 150 mg TMP/m^2/day divided q 12 hr on 3 consecutive days/wk (not to exceed 320 mg TMP/1600 mg SMX per day).

Availability (generic available)
Tablets: ✸20 mg TMP/100 mg SMX, 80 mg TMP/400 mg SMX, 160 mg TMP/800 mg SMX. **Cost:** *Generic*—80 mg TMP/400 mg SMX $11.99/30, 160 mg TMP/800 mg SMX $12.99/30. **Oral suspension (cherry, grape flavors):** 40 mg TMP/200 mg SMX per 5 mL. **Cost:** *Generic*—$11.99/200 mL. **Solution for injection:** 16 mg TMP/80 mg SMX per mL in 5-, 10-, and 30-mL vials.

✸ = Canadian drug name. = Genetic implication.
*CAPITALS indicates life-threatening; underlines indicate most frequent.

NURSING IMPLICATIONS
Assessment
- Assess for infection (vital signs; appearance of wound, sputum, urine, and stool; WBC) at beginning of and during therapy.
- Obtain specimens for culture and sensitivity before initiating therapy. First dose may be given before receiving results.
- Inspect IV site frequently. Phlebitis is common.
- Assess patient for allergy to sulfonamides.
- Monitor intake and output ratios. Fluid intake should be sufficient to maintain a urine output of at least 1200–1500 mL daily to prevent crystalluria and stone formation.
- *Lab Test Considerations:* Monitor CBC and urinalysis periodically during therapy.
- May produce ↑ serum bilirubin, creatinine, and alkaline phosphatase.

Potential Nursing Diagnoses
Risk for infection (Indications, Side Effects)
Noncompliance (Patient/Family Teaching)

Implementation
- Do not confuse DS (double-strength) formulations with single-strength formulations.
- Do not administer medication IM.
- **PO:** Administer around the clock with a full glass of water. Use calibrated measuring device for liquid preparations.

IV Administration
- **Intermittent Infusion:** *Diluent:* Dilute each 5–mL of trimethoprim/sulfamethoxazole with 125 mL of D5W (stable for 24 hr at room temperature). May also dilute each 5-mL of drug with 75 mL of D5W if fluid restriction is required (stable for 6 hr at room temperature). Do not refrigerate. *Concentration:* Should not exceed 1.06 mg/mL. *Rate:* Infuse over 60–90 min.
- **Y-Site Compatibility:** acyclovir, aldesleukin, allopurinol, amifostine, amphotericin B cholesteryl, anidulafungin, atracurium, aztreonam, bivalirudin, cefepime, cisplatin, cyclophosphamide, cytarabine, daptomycin, dexmedetomidine, diltiazem, docetaxel, doxacurium, doxorubicin liposome, eptifibatide, ertapenem, etoposide, etoposide phosphate, fenoldopam, filgrastim, fludarabine, fluorouracil, gemcitabine, granisetron, hetastarch, hydromorphone, ifosfamide, levofloxacin, linezolid, lorazepam, magnesium sulfate, melphalan, methotrexate, metronidazole, milrinone, mitoxantrone, nicardipine, octreotide, oxaliplatin, paclitaxel, palonosetron, pancuronium, pantoprazole, pemetrexed, perphenazine, piperacillin/tazobactam, remifentanil, sargramostim, sodium acetate, teniposide, thiotepa, tigecycline, tirofiban, trastuzumab, vecuronium, vincristine, voriconazole, zidovudine.
- **Y-Site Incompatibility:** alfentanil, amikacin, aminophylline, amphotericin B colloidal, ampicillin, ampicillin/sulbactam, ascorbic acid, atropine, azathioprine, benztropine, bumetanide, buprenorphine, butorphanol, calcium chloride, calcium gluconate, caspofungin, cefazolin, cefotaxime, cefoxitin, ceftazidime, ceftriaxone, chloramphenicol, chlorpromazine, cimetidine, clindamycin, codeine, cyanocobalamin, cyclosporine, dantrolene, dexamethasone, diazepam, diazoxide, digoxin, diphenhydramine, dobutamine, dopamine, doxorubicin, doxycycline, ephedrine, epinephrine, epirubicin, epoetin alfa, erythromycin, famotidine, fentanyl, fluconazole, folic acid, furosemide, ganciclovir, gentamicin, glycopyrrolate, haloperidol, heparin, hydralazine, hydrocortisone, hydroxyzine, idarubicin, imipenem/cilastatin, inamrinone, indomethacin, insulin, isoproterenol, ketorolac, lidocaine, mannitol, mechlorethamine, metaraminol, methoxamine, methyldopate, methylprednisolone, metoclopramide, metoprolol, metronidazole, midazolam, multivitamins, nafcillin, nalbuphine, naloxone, nitroglycerin, nitroprusside, norepinephrine, ondansetron, oxacillin, oxytocin, papaverine, penicillin G, pentamidine, pentazocine, pentobarbital, phenobarbital, phentolamine, phenylephrine, phenytoin, phytonadione, potassium chloride, procainamide, prochlorperazine, promethazine, propranolol, protamine, quinupristin/dalfopristin, ranitidine, sodium bicarbonate, streptokinase, succinylcholine, sufentanil, thiamine, ticarcillin/clavulanate, tobramycin, tolazoline, trimetaphan, urokinase, vancomycin, verapamil, vinorelbine.

Patient/Family Teaching
- Instruct patient to take medication around the clock and to finish drug completely as directed, even if feeling well. Take missed doses as soon as remembered unless almost time for next dose. Advise patient that sharing of this medication may be dangerous.
- Instruct patient to notify health care professional if fever and diarrhea develop, especially if diarrhea contains blood, mucus, or pus. Advise patient not to treat diarrhea without consulting health care professional.
- Caution patient to use sunscreen and protective clothing to prevent photosensitivity reactions.

- Advise patient to notify health care professional if skin rash, sore throat, fever, mouth sores, or unusual bleeding or bruising occurs.
- Instruct patient to notify health care professional if symptoms do not improve within a few days.
- Emphasize importance of regular follow-up exams to monitor blood counts in patients on prolonged therapy.
- **Home Care Issues:** Instruct family or caregiver on dilution, rate, and administration of drug and proper care of IV equipment.

Evaluation/Desired Outcomes
- Resolution of the signs and symptoms of infection. Length of time for complete resolution depends on organism and site of infection.
- Resolution of symptoms of traveler's diarrhea.
- Prevention of Pneumocystis jirovecii pneumonia in patients with HIV.

---

trospium (tros-pee-yum)
Sanctura, Sanctura XR

Classification
Therapeutic: urinary tract antispasmodics
Pharmacologic: antimuscarinics

Pregnancy Category C

Indications
Overactive bladder with symptoms of urge urinary incontinence, urgency and urinary frequency.

Action
Antagonizes the effect of acetylcholine at muscarinic receptors in the bladder; this parasympatholytic action reduces bladder smooth muscle tone. **Therapeutic Effects:** Increased bladder capacity and decreased symptoms of overactive bladder.

Pharmacokinetics
Absorption: Less than 10% absorbed following oral administration; food significantly ↓ absorption.
Distribution: Mostly distributed to plasma.
Metabolism and Excretion: Of the 10% absorbed, 40% is metabolized. Unabsorbed drug is mainly excreted in feces. Of absorbed drug, 60% is eliminated in urine as unchanged drug via active tubular secretion.
Half-life: 20 hr.

TIME/ACTION PROFILE (anticholinergic effects)

ROUTE	ONSET	PEAK	DURATION
PO	unknown	5–6 hr	24 hr

Contraindications/Precautions
Contraindicated in: Hypersensitivity; Gastric or urinary retention, uncontrolled angle-closure glaucoma or risk for these conditions.
Use Cautiously in: Bladder outflow obstruction; Gastrointestinal obstructive disorders (ulcerative colitis, intestinal atony, myasthenia gravis); Controlled angle-closure glaucoma (use only if necessary and with careful monitoring); CCr <30 mL/min (dose ↓ recommended); Moderate to severe hepatic impairment; OB: Lactation: Use only if benefit justifies risks to fetus/newborn; Pedi: Safety not established; Geri: May have ↑ sensitivity to anticholinergic effects; ↓ dose may be required.

Adverse Reactions/Side Effects
CNS: headache, dizziness, drowsiness, fatigue. **EENT:** blurred vision. **GI:** constipation, dry mouth, dyspepsia. **GU:** urinary retention, urinary tract infection. **Misc:** fever, heat stroke.

Interactions
Drug-Drug: May interact with other **drugs that compete for tubular secretion**. ↑ risk of anticholinergic effects with other **drugs having anticholinergic properties**.

Route/Dosage
PO (Adults): 20 mg twice daily or 60 mg once daily (XR dose form).
PO (Adults ≥75 yr): Based on tolerability, dose may be ↓ to 20 mg once daily.

Renal Impairment
PO (Adults): *CCr <30 mL/min*— 20 mg once daily at bedtime.

Availability
Tablets: 20 mg. **Extended release tablets:** 60 mg.

NURSING IMPLICATIONS

Assessment
- Monitor voiding pattern and intake and output ratios.

Potential Nursing Diagnoses
Impaired urinary elimination (Indications)

trospium

Implementation
- **PO:** Administer 1 hr prior to meals or on an empty stomach.

Patient/Family Teaching
- Instruct patient to take as directed. If a dose is skipped, take next dose 1 hr prior to next meal.
- Caution patient that heat prostration (fever and heat stroke due to decreased sweating) may occur when trospium is taken in a hot environment.
- May cause drowsiness, dizziness, and blurred vision. Caution patient to avoid driving and other activities requiring alertness until response to medication is known. Advise patient to avoid alcohol; may increase drowsiness.

Evaluation/Desired Outcomes
- Increased bladder capacity and decreased symptoms of overactive bladder.

---

urokinase, See THROMBOLYTIC AGENTS.

valacyclovir
(val-ay-**sye**-kloe-veer)
Valtrex

Classification
Therapeutic: antivirals

Pregnancy Category B

Indications
Treatment of herpes zoster (shingles). Treatment/suppression of genital herpes. Reduction of transmission of genital herpes. Treatment of chickenpox. Treatment of herpes labialis (cold sores).

Action
Rapidly converted to acyclovir. Acyclovir interferes with viral DNA synthesis. **Therapeutic Effects:** Inhibited viral replication, decreased viral shedding, reduced time to healing of lesions. Reduced transmission of genital herpes.

Pharmacokinetics
Absorption: 54% bioavailable as acyclovir after oral administration of valacyclovir.
Distribution: CSF concentrations of acyclovir are 50% of plasma concentrations. Acyclovir crosses placenta; enters breast milk.
Metabolism and Excretion: Rapidly converted to acyclovir via intestinal/hepatic metabolism.
Half-life: 2.5–3.3 hr; up to 14 hr in renal impairment (acyclovir).

TIME/ACTION PROFILE (blood levels†)

ROUTE	ONSET	PEAK	DURATION
PO	unknown	1.5–2.5 hr	8–24 hr

†Acyclovir

Contraindications/Precautions
Contraindicated in: Hypersensitivity to valacyclovir or acyclovir.
Use Cautiously in: Renal impairment (dose ↓ / ↑ dosing interval recommended if CCr <50 mL/min); OB, Lactation: Pedi: Pregnancy, lactation, or children <2 yr (safety not established); Geri: Dose ↓ may be necessary due to ↑ risk of acute renal failure and CNS side effects.

Adverse Reactions/Side Effects
CNS: <u>headache</u>, dizziness, weakness. **GI:** <u>nausea</u>, abdominal pain, anorexia, constipation, diarrhea. **GU:** RENAL FAILURE, crystalluria. **Hemat:** THROMBOTIC THROMBOCYTOPENIC PURPURA/HEMOLYTIC UREMIC SYNDROME (very high doses in immunosuppressed patients).

Interactions
Drug-Drug: Probenecid and cimetidine ↑ blood levels; significant only in renal impairment. Concurrent use of other **nephrotoxic drugs** ↑ risk of adverse renal effects.

Route/Dosage
Herpes Zoster
PO (Adults): 1 g 3 times daily for 7 days.

Genital Herpes
PO (Adults): *Initial treatment*—1 g twice daily for 10 days. *Recurrence*—500 mg twice daily for 3 days. *Suppression of recurrence*—1 g once daily or 500 mg once daily in patients experiencing <10 recurrences/yr. *Suppression of recurrence in HIV-infected patients*—500 mg q 12 hr. *Reduction of transmission*—500 mg once daily for source partner.

Herpes Labialis
PO (Adults and Children ≥12 yr): 2 g then 2 g 12 hr later.

Chickenpox
PO (Children ≥2 yr): 20 mg/kg 3 times daily for 5 days (not to exceed 1 g 3 times daily).

Renal Impairment
PO (Adults): *CCr 30–49 mL/min*—1 g q 12 hr for herpes zoster treatment, no ↓ required for treatment of genital herpes; 1 g then 1 g 12 hr later for herpes labialis. *CCr 10–29 mL/min*—1 g q 24 hr for initial treatment of genital herpes, 500 mg q 24 hr for treatment of recurrent episodes of genital herpes, 500 mg q 48 hr for suppression of genital herpes in patients with 9 or fewer recurrences/yr, 500 mg q 24 hr for suppression of genital herpes in patients with ≥10 recurrences/yr or HIV-infected patients, 1 g q 24 hr for treatment of herpes zoster; 500 mg then 500 mg 12 hr later for herpes labialis. *CCr <10 mL/min*—500 mg q 24 hr for initial treatment of genital herpes, 500 mg q 24 hr for treatment of recurrent episodes of genital herpes, 500 mg q 48 hr for suppression of genital herpes in patients with 9 or fewer recurrences/yr, 500 mg q 24 hr for suppression of genital herpes in patients with ≥10 recurrences/yr or HIV-infected patients, 500 mg q 24 hr for treatment of herpes zoster; single 500 mg dose for herpes labialis.

Availability
Tablets: 500 mg, 1 g. **Cost:** 500 mg $177.99/30, 1 g $315.98/30500 mg $151.86/42, 1 g $103.24/20.

NURSING IMPLICATIONS
Assessment
- Assess lesions before and daily during therapy.
- Monitor patient for signs of thrombotic thrombocytic purpura/hemolytic uremic syndrome (thrombocytopenia, microangiopathic hemolytic anemia, neurologic findings, renal dysfunction, fever). Requires prompt treatment; may be fatal.

Potential Nursing Diagnoses
Risk for impaired skin integrity (Indications)
Risk for infection (Indications, Patient/Family Teaching)

Implementation
- **PO:** May be administered without regard to meals.
- **Herpes Zoster:** Implement valacyclovir therapy as soon as possible after the onset of signs or symptoms of herpes zoster; most effective if started within 48 hr of the onset of zoster rash. Efficacy of treatment started >72 hr after rash onset is unknown.
- **Genital Herpes and Herpes Labialis:** Implement treatment for genital herpes as soon as possible after onset of symptoms.
- **Chicken Pox:** Initiate therapy at the earliest sign or symptom; preferably within 24 hr of onset of rash.

Patient/Family Teaching
- Instruct patient to take valacyclovir exactly as directed for the full course of therapy. Take missed doses as soon as remembered if not just before next dose.
- Advise patient to maintain adequate hydration during therapy.
- **Herpes Zoster:** Inform patient that valacyclovir does not prevent the spread of infection to others. Precautions should be taken around others who have not had chickenpox or varicella vaccine, or are immunosuppressed, until all lesions have crusted.
- **Genital Herpes and Herpes Labialis:** Inform patient that valacyclovir does not prevent the spread of herpes labialis to others. Advise patient to avoid contact with lesions while lesions or symptoms are present. Valacyclovir reduces transmission of genital herpes to others. Advise patient to practice safe sex (avoid sexual intercourse when lesions are present and wear a condom made of latex or polyurethane during sexual contact).

Evaluation/Desired Outcomes
- Decrease in time to full crusting, loss of vesicles, loss of ulcers, and development of crusts in patients with acute herpes zoster (shingles).
- Decrease in time to full crusting, loss of vesicles, loss of ulcers, and development of crusts in patients with genital herpes.
- Decrease in frequency of outbreaks in patients with genital herpes.
- Decrease in time to full crusting, loss of vesicles, loss of ulcers, and development of crusts in patients with herpes labialis. Decrease in transmission of genital herpes.
- Treatment of chicken pox.

valganciclovir
(val-gan-**sye**-kloe-veer)
Valcyte

Classification
Therapeutic: antivirals

Pregnancy Category C

Indications
Treatment of cytomegalovirus (CMV) retinitis in patients with AIDS. Prevention of CMV disease in kidney, kidney/pancreas and heart transplant patients at risk.

Action
Valganciclovir is a prodrug which is rapidly converted to ganciclovir by intestinal and hepatic enzymes. CMV virus converts ganciclovir to its active form (ganciclovir phosphate) inside host cell, where it inhibits viral DNA polymerase. **Therapeutic Effects:** Antiviral effect directed preferentially against CMV-infected cells.

Pharmacokinetics
Absorption: 59.4% absorbed following oral administration, rapidly converted to ganciclovir.
Distribution: Unknown.
Metabolism and Excretion: Rapidly converted to ganciclovir; ganciclovir is mostly excreted by the kidneys.
Half-life: 4.1 hr (intracellular half-life of ganciclovir phosphate is 18 hr).

TIME/ACTION PROFILE (ganciclovir blood levels)

ROUTE	ONSET	PEAK	DURATION
PO	rapid	2 hr	12–24 hr

Contraindications/Precautions
Contraindicated in: Hypersensitivity to valganciclovir or ganciclovir; OB: Pregnancy or planned

valganciclovir **1261**

pregnancy; Lactation: Lactation; Hemodialysis; Patients undergoing liver transplantation.
Use Cautiously in: Renal impairment (dosage reduction recommended if CCr <60 mL/min); Pre-existing bone marrow depression; Previous or concurrent myelosuppressive drug therapy or radiation therapy; Geri: Age-related ↓ in renal function requires dosage reduction; Pedi: Children <4 mo (safety not established).

Adverse Reactions/Side Effects
CNS: SEIZURES, headache, insomnia, agitation, confusion, dizziness, hallucinations, psychosis, sedation. **GI:** abdominal pain, diarrhea, nausea, vomiting. **GU:** renal impairment. **Hemat:** NEUTROPENIA, THROMBOCYTOPENIA, anemia, aplastic anemia, bone marrow depression, pancytopenia. **Neuro:** ataxia, paresthesia, peripheral neuropathy. **Misc:** fever, hypersensitivity reactions, infections.

Interactions
Drug-Drug: ↑ risk of hematologic toxicity with **zidovudine**. Blood levels and effects may be ↑ by **probenecid**. Patients with renal impairment may experience accumulation of metabolites of **mycophenolate** and valganciclovir. ↑ blood levels and risk of toxicity from **didanosine**.
Drug-Food: Food ↑ absorption.

Route/Dosage
Treatment of CMV Disease
PO (Adults): *Induction*—900 mg twice daily for 21 days; *Maintenance treatment or patients with inactive CMV retinitis*—900 mg once daily.

Renal Impairment
CCr 40–59 mL/min (Adults): *Induction*—450 mg twice daily for 21 days; *Maintenance treatment or patients with inactive CMV retinitis*—450 mg once daily.

Renal Impairment
CCr 25–39 mL/min (Adults): *Induction*—450 mg once daily for 21 days; *Maintenance treatment or patients with inactive CMV retinitis*—450 mg every 2 days.

Renal Impairment
CCr 10–24 mL/min (Adults): *Induction*—450 mg every 2 days for 21 days; *Maintenance treatment or patients with inactive CMV retinitis*—450 mg twice weekly.

Prevention of CMV Disease in Transplant Patients
PO (Adults): *Kidney, kidney/pancreas, or heart transplant*—900 mg once daily, starting 10 days prior to transplant and continued for 100 days after.

Renal Impairment
PO (Adults): *CCr 40–59 mL/min*—450 mg once daily; *CCr 25–39 mL/min*—450 mg every 2 days; *CCr 12–24 mL/min*—450 mg twice weekly.

PO (Children 4 mo-16 yr): *Kidney or heart transplant*—Dose is based on body surface area (BSA) and CCr. Dose = $7 \times BSA \times CCr$ (see prescribing information for equations used for BSA and CCr); all calculated doses should be rounded to nearest 25 mg (max = 900 mg) and administered as oral solution; should be started 10 days prior to transplant and continued for 100 days after.

Renal Impairment
PO (Adults): *CCr 40–59 mL/min*—450 mg once daily; *CCr 25–39 mL/min*—450 mg every 2 days; *CCr 12–24 mL/min*—450 mg twice weekly.

Availability
Tablets: 450 mg. **Oral solution (tutti-frutti flavor):** 50 mg/mL.

NURSING IMPLICATIONS
Assessment
- Diagnosis of CMV retinitis should be determined by ophthalmoscopy prior to treatment with ganciclovir.
- Culture for CMV (urine, blood, throat) may be taken prior to administration. However, a negative CMV culture does not rule out CMV retinitis. If symptoms do not respond after several weeks, resistance to ganciclovir may have occurred. Ophthalmologic exams should be performed weekly during induction and every 2 wk during maintenance or more frequently if the macula or optic nerve is threatened. Progression of CMV retinitis may occur during or following ganciclovir treatment.
- Assess for signs of infection (fever, chills, cough, hoarseness, lower back or side pain, sore throat, difficult or painful urination). Notify health care professional if these symptoms occur.

✦ = Canadian drug name. ⚡ = Genetic implication.
*CAPITALS indicates life-threatening; underlines indicate most frequent.

- Assess for bleeding (bleeding gums, bruising, petechiae, or guaiac stools, urine, and emesis). Avoid IM injections and taking rectal temperatures. Apply pressure to venipuncture sites for 10 min.
- **Lab Test Considerations:** May cause granulocytopenia, anemia, and thrombocytopenia. Monitor neutrophil and platelet count closely throughout therapy. Do not administer if ANC <500/mm³, platelet count <25,000/mm³, or hemoglobin <8 g/dL. Recovery begins within 3–7 days of discontinuation of therapy.
- Monitor BUN and serum creatinine at least once every 2 wk throughout therapy. May cause ↑ in serum creatinine.

Potential Nursing Diagnoses
Risk for infection (Indications, Patient/Family Teaching)

Implementation
- Valganciclovir and ganciclovir are not interchangeable. Do not substitute.
- Valganciclovir tablets should be handled carefully. Do not break or crush. May be potentially teratogenic; avoid direct contact with broken or crushed tablets. If contact with the skin or mucous membranes occurs, wash thoroughly with soap and water and rinse eyes thoroughly with plain water.
- **PO:** Administer with food. Adults should take tablets, not oral solution.
- Valcyte for oral solution (50 mg/mL) must be prepared by the pharmacist prior to dispensing to the patient.

Patient/Family Teaching
- Instruct patient to take valganciclovir with food, exactly as directed.
- Inform patient that valganciclovir is not a cure for CMV retinitis. Progression of retinitis may continue in immunocompromised patients during and following therapy. Advise patients to have regular ophthalmic exams at least every 4–6 wk. Duration of therapy for CMV prevention is based on the duration and degree of immunosuppression.
- May cause seizures, sedation, dizziness, ataxia, and/or confusion. Caution patient not to drive or do other activities requiring alertness until response to medication is known.
- Advise patient to notify health care professional if fever; chills; sore throat; other signs of infection; bleeding gums; bruising; petechiae; or blood in urine, stool, or emesis occurs. Caution patient to avoid crowds and persons with known infections. Instruct patient to use soft toothbrush and electric razor. Patient should be cautioned not to drink alcoholic beverages or take products containing aspirin or NSAIDs.
- Advise patient that valganciclovir may have teratogenic effects. Women should use a nonhormonal and men a barrier method of contraception during and for at least 90 days following therapy.
- Caution patient to use sunscreen and protective clothing to prevent photosensitivity reactions.
- Emphasize the importance of frequent follow-up exams to monitor blood counts.

Evaluation/Desired Outcomes
- Management of the symptoms of CMV retinitis in patients with AIDS.

VALPROATES

divalproex sodium
(dye-val-**proe**-ex **soe**-dee-um)
✿ Apo-Divalproex, Depakote, Depakote ER, ✿ DOM-Divalproex, ✿ Epival, ✿ Gen-Divalproex, ✿ Novo-Divalproex, ✿ Nu-Divalproex, ✿ PHL-Divalproex, ✿ PMS-Divalproex

valproate sodium
(val-**proe**-ate **soe**-dee-um)
Depacon

valproic acid (val-**proe**-ik **as**-id)
✿ Apo-Valproic, Depakene, ✿ DOM-Valproic Acid, ✿ PHL-Valproic Acid, ✿ PMS-Valproic Acid, ✿ Ratio-Valprox, Stavzor

Classification
Therapeutic: anticonvulsants, vascular headache suppressants

Pregnancy Category D

Indications
Monotherapy and adjunctive therapy for simple and complex absence seizures. Monotherapy and adjunctive therapy for complex partial seizures. Adjunctive therapy for patients with multiple seizure types, including absence seizures. **Divalproex sodium only.** Manic episodes associated with bipolar disorder. Prevention of migraine headache.

Action
Increase levels of GABA, an inhibitory neurotransmitter in the CNS. **Therapeutic Effects:** Suppression of seizure activity. Decreased manic epi-

sodes. Decreased frequency of migraine headaches.

Pharmacokinetics

Absorption: Well absorbed following oral administration; divalproex is enteric-coated, and absorption is delayed. ER form produces lower blood levels. IV administration results in complete bioavailability.
Distribution: Rapidly distributed into plasma and extracellular water. Cross blood-brain barrier and placenta; enters breast milk.
Protein Binding: 80–90%, decreased in neonates, elderly, renal impairment, or chronic hepatic disease.
Metabolism and Excretion: Mostly metabolized by the liver; minimal amounts excreted unchanged in urine.
Half-life: Adults: 9–16 hr.

TIME/ACTION PROFILE (onset = anticonvulsant effect; peak = blood levels)

ROUTE	ONSET	PEAK	DURATION
PO—liquid	2–4 days	15–120 min	6–24 hr
PO—capsules	2–4 days	1–4 hr	6–24 hr
PO—delayed-release products	2–4 days	3–5 hr	12–24 hr
PO—extended-release products	2–4 days	7–14 hr	24 hr
IV	2–4 days	end of infusion	6–24 hr

Contraindications/Precautions

Contraindicated in: Hypersensitivity; Hepatic impairment; Known/suspected urea cycle disorders (may result in fatal hyperammonemic encephalopathy).
Use Cautiously in: All patients (may ↑ risk of suicidal thoughts/behaviors); Bleeding disorders; History of liver disease; Organic brain disease; Bone marrow depression; Renal impairment; Geri: ↑ risk of adverse effects; OB: Use during pregnancy is linked to congenital anomalies, neural tube defects, clotting abnormalities, and hepatic dysfunction in the neonate. Use with extreme caution. Lactation: Pass into breast milk. Consider discontinuing nursing when valproates are administered to the nursing mother; Pedi: Children, especially <2 yr (at ↑ risk for potentially fatal hepatotoxicity).

Adverse Reactions/Side Effects

CNS: SUICIDAL THOUGHTS, agitation, dizziness, headache, insomnia, sedation, confusion, depression. **CV:** peripheral edema. **EENT:** visual disturbances. **GI:** HEPATOTOXICITY, PANCREATITIS, abdominal pain, anorexia, diarrhea, indigestion, nausea, vomiting, constipation, increased appetite. **Derm:** alopecia, rashes. **Endo:** weight gain. **Hemat:** leukopenia, thrombocytopenia. **Metab:** HYPERAMMONEMIA. **Neuro:** HYPOTHERMIA, tremor, ataxia.

Interactions

Drug-Drug: ↑ risk of bleeding with **warfarin**. Blood levels and toxicity may be ↑ by **aspirin, carbamazepine, chlorpromazine, cimetidine, erythromycin,** or **felbamate**. ↑ CNS depression with other **CNS depressants**, including **alcohol, antihistamines, antidepressants, opioid analgesics, MAO inhibitors,** and **sedative/hypnotics**. **MAO inhibitors** and other **antidepressants** may ↓ seizure threshold and ↓ effectiveness of valproate. **Carbamazepine, meropenem, phenobarbital, phenytoin,** or **rifampin** may ↓ valproate blood levels. Valproate may ↑ toxicity of **carbamazepine, diazepam, amitriptyline, nortriptyline, ethosuximide, lamotrigine, phenobarbital, phenytoin, topiramate,** or **zidovudine**. Concurrent use with **topiramate** may ↑ risk of hypothermia. **Ertapenem, imipenem,** or **meropenem** may ↓ valproate blood levels.

Route/Dosage

Regular-release and delayed-release formulations usually given in 2–4 divided doses daily; extended-release formulation (Depakote ER) usually given once daily.

Anticonvulsant

PO (Adults and Children >10 yr): *Single-agent therapy (complex partial seizures)*—Initial dose of 10–15 mg/kg/day in 1–4 divided doses; ↑ by 5–10 mg/kg/day weekly until therapeutic response achieved (not to exceed 60 mg/kg/day); when daily dose exceeds 250 mg, give in divided doses. *Polytherapy (complex partial seizures)*—Initial dose of 10–15 mg/kg/day; ↑ by 5–10 mg/kg/day weekly until therapeutic response achieved (not to exceed 60 mg/kg/day); when daily dosage exceeds 250 mg, give in divided doses.

PO (Adults and Children >2 yr [>10 yr for Depakote ER and Stavzor]): *Simple and com-*

plex absence seizures—Initial dose of 15 mg/kg/day in 1–4 divided doses; ↑ by 5–10 mg/kg/day weekly until therapeutic response achieved (not to exceed 60 mg/kg/day); when daily dose exceeds 250 mg, give in divided doses.
IV (Adults and Children): Give same daily dose and at same frequency as was given orally; switch to oral formulation as soon as possible.
Rect (Adults and Children): Dilute syrup 1:1 with water for use as a retention enema. Give 17–20 mg/kg load, maintenance 10–15 mg/kg/dose q 8 hr.

Mood Stabilizer
PO (Adults): *Depakote and Stavzor*—Initial dose of 750 mg/day in divided doses initially, titrated rapidly to desired clinical effect or trough plasma levels of 50–125 mcg/mL (not to exceed 60 mg/kg/day). *Depakote ER*—Initial dose of 25 mg/kg once daily; titrated rapidly to desired clinical effect of trough plasma levels of 85–125 mcg/mL (not to exceed 60 mg/kg/day).

Migraine Prevention
PO (Adults and Children ≥16 yr): *Depakote and Stavzor*—250 mg twice daily (up to 1000 mg/day). *Depakote ER*—500 mg once daily for 1 wk, then ↑ to 1000 mg once daily.

Availability
Valproic Acid (generic available)
Capsules: 250 mg, ✤500 mg. **Cost:** *Generic*—$29.97/100. **Delayed-release capsules:** 125 mg, 250 mg, 500 mg. **Syrup:** 250 mg/5 mL. **Cost:** *Generic*—$17.99/150 mL.

Valproate Sodium (generic available)
Injection: 100 mg/mL in 5-mL vials.

Divalproex Sodium (generic available)
Delayed-release tablets (Depakote): 125 mg, 250 mg, 500 mg. **Cost:** 125 mg $85.85/100, 250 mg $159.98/100, 500 mg $296.66/100. **Capsules-sprinkle:** 125 mg. **Cost:** $83.31/100. **Extended-release tablets (Depakote ER):** 250 mg, 500 mg. **Cost:** 250 mg $134.97/90, 500 mg $225.97/90.

NURSING IMPLICATIONS

Assessment
- **Seizures:** Assess location, duration, and characteristics of seizure activity. Institute seizure precautions.
- **Bipolar Disorder:** Assess mood, ideation, and behavior frequently.
- **Migraine Prophylaxis:** Monitor frequency of migraine headaches.
- Geri: Assess geriatric patients for excessive somnolence.
- Assess for suicidal tendencies, especially during early therapy. Restrict amount of drug available to patient. Risk may be increased in children, adolescents, and adults ≤24 yr.
- **Lab Test Considerations:** Monitor CBC, platelet count, and bleeding time prior to and periodically during therapy. May cause leukopenia and thrombocytopenia.
- Monitor hepatic function (LDH, AST, ALT, and bilirubin) and serum ammonia concentrations prior to and periodically during therapy. May cause hepatotoxicity; monitor closely, especially during initial 6 mo of therapy; fatalities have occurred. Therapy should be discontinued if hyperammonemia occurs.
- May interfere with accuracy of thyroid function tests.
- May cause false-positive results in urine ketone tests.
- ***Toxicity and Overdose:*** Therapeutic serum levels range from 50–100 mcg/mL (50–125 mcg/mL for mania). Doses are gradually ↑ until a pre-dose serum concentration of at least 50 mcg/mL is reached. However, a good correlation among daily dose, serum level, and therapeutic effects has not been established. Monitor patients receiving near the maximum recommended 60 mg/kg/day for toxicity.

Potential Nursing Diagnoses
Risk for injury (Indications)

Implementation
- Do not confuse *Depakote ER* and regular dose forms. *Depakote ER* produces lower blood levels than *Depakote* dosing forms. If switching from *Depakote* to *Depakote ER*, increase dose by 8-20%.
- Single daily doses are usually administered at bedtime because of sedation.
- **PO:** Administer with or immediately after meals to minimize GI irritation. Extended-release and delayed-release tablets and capsules should be swallowed whole, do not open, break, or chew; will cause mouth or throat irritation and destroy extended release mechanism. Do not administer tablets with milk or carbonated beverages (may cause premature dissolution). Delayed-release divalproex sodium may cause less GI irritation than valproic acid capsules.
- Shake liquid preparations well before pouring. Use calibrated measuring device to ensure accurate dose. Syrup may be mixed with food or other liquids to improve taste.

- Sprinkle capsules may be swallowed whole or opened and entire capsule contents sprinkled on a teaspoonful of soft, cool food (applesauce, pudding). Do not chew mixture. Administer immediately; do not store for future use.
- To convert from valproic acid to divalproex sodium, initiate divalproex sodium at same total daily dose and dosing schedule as valproic acid. Once patient is stabilized on divalproex sodium, attempt administration 2–3 times daily.
- **Rect:** Dilute syrup 1:1 with water for use as a retention enema.

IV Administration

- **Intermittent Infusion:** *Diluent:* May be diluted in at least 50 mL of D5W, 0.9% NaCl, or LR. Solution is stable for 24 hr at room temperature. *Concentration:* 2 mg/mL. *Rate:* Infuse over 60 min (≤20 mg/min). Rapid infusion may cause increased side effects. Has been given as a one-time infusion of 1000 mg over 5–10 min @ 3 mg/kg/min up to 15 mg/kg in patients with no detectable valproate levels.
- **Y-Site Compatibility:** cefepime, ceftazidime.

Patient/Family Teaching

- Instruct patient to take medication as directed. If a dose is missed on a once-a-day schedule, take as soon as remembered that day. If on a multiple-dose schedule, take it within 6 hr of the scheduled time, then space remaining doses throughout the remainder of the day. Abrupt withdrawal may lead to status epilepticus.
- May cause drowsiness or dizziness. Caution patient to avoid driving or other activities requiring alertness until effects of medication are known. Tell patient not to resume driving until physician gives clearance based on control of seizure disorder.
- Caution patient to avoid taking alcohol, CNS depressants, OTC medications or herbal products concurrently with valproates without consulting health care professional.
- Advise patient and family to notify health care professional if thoughts about suicide or dying, attempts to commit suicide; new or worse depression; new or worse anxiety; feeling very agitated or restless; panic attacks; trouble sleeping; new or worse irritability; acting aggressive; being angry or violent; acting on dangerous impulses; an extreme increase in activity and talking, other unusual changes in behavior or mood occur.
- Instruct patient to notify health care professional of medication regimen prior to treatment or surgery.
- May cause teratogenic effects. Instruct female patients to notify health care professional immediately if pregnancy is planned or suspected or if breastfeeding. Advise pregnant patients taking valproates to enroll in the NAAED Pregnancy Registry by calling 1-888-233-2334; call must be made by patient. Registry Web site is www.aedpregnancyregistry.org.
- Advise patient to carry identification at all times describing medication regimen.
- Advise patient to notify health care professional if anorexia, abdominal pain, severe nausea and vomiting, yellow skin or eyes, fever, sore throat, malaise, weakness, facial edema, lethargy, unusual bleeding or bruising, pregnancy, or loss of seizure control occurs. Children <2 yr of age are especially at risk for fatal hepatotoxicity.
- Emphasize the importance of routine exams to monitor progress.

Evaluation/Desired Outcomes

- Decreased seizure activity.
- Decreased incidence of manic episodes in patients with bipolar disorders.
- Decreased frequency of migraine headaches.

---

valsartan, See ANGIOTENSIN II RECEPTOR ANTAGONISTS.

---

vancomycin (van-koe-**mye**-sin)
Vancocin

Classification
Therapeutic: anti-infectives

Pregnancy Category C

Indications

IV: Treatment of potentially life-threatening infections when less toxic anti-infectives are contraindicated. Particularly useful in staphylococcal infections, including: Endocarditis, Meningitis, Osteomyelitis, Pneumonia, Septicemia, Soft-tissue infections in patients who have allergies to penicillin or its derivatives or when sensitivity testing demonstrates resistance to methicillin. **PO:** Treat-

✦ = Canadian drug name. ❑ = Genetic implication.
*CAPITALS indicates life-threatening; underlines indicate most frequent.

vancomycin

ment of staphylococcal enterocolitis or pseudomembranous colitis due to *Clostridium difficile*.
IV: Part of endocarditis prophylaxis in high-risk patients who are allergic to penicillin.

Action
Binds to bacterial cell wall, resulting in cell death. **Therapeutic Effects:** Bactericidal action against susceptible organisms. **Spectrum:** Active against gram-positive pathogens, including: Staphylococci (including methicillin-resistant strains of *Staphylococcus aureus*), Group A beta-hemolytic streptococci, *Streptococcus pneumoniae*, *Corynebacterium*, *Clostridium difficile*, *Enterococcus faecalis*, *Enterococcus faecium*.

Pharmacokinetics
Absorption: Poorly absorbed from the GI tract.
Distribution: Widely distributed. Some penetration (20–30%) of CSF; crosses placenta.
Metabolism and Excretion: Oral doses excreted primarily in the feces; IV vancomycin eliminated almost entirely by the kidneys.
Half-life: Neonates: 6–10 hr; Children 3 mo–3 yr: 4 hr; Children >3 yr: 2–2.3 hr; Adults: 5–8 hr (↑ in renal impairment).

TIME/ACTION PROFILE (blood levels)

ROUTE	ONSET	PEAK	DURATION
IV	rapid	end of infusion	12–24 hr

Contraindications/Precautions
Contraindicated in: Hypersensitivity.
Use Cautiously in: Renal impairment (dosage reduction required if CCr ≤80 mL/min); Hearing impairment; Intestinal obstruction or inflammation (↑ systemic absorption when given orally); OB, Lactation: Safety not established.

Adverse Reactions/Side Effects
EENT: ototoxicity. **CV:** hypotension. **GI:** nausea, vomiting. **GU:** nephrotoxicity. **Derm:** rashes. **Hemat:** eosinophilia, leukopenia. **Local:** phlebitis. **MS:** back and neck pain. **Misc:** hypersensitivity reactions including ANAPHYLAXIS, chills, fever, "red man" syndrome (with rapid infusion), superinfection.

Interactions
Drug-Drug: May cause additive ototoxicity and nephrotoxicity with other **ototoxic** and **nephrotoxic drugs** (**aspirin**, **aminoglycosides**, **cyclosporine**, **cisplatin**, **loop diuretics**). May enhance neuromuscular blockade from **nondepolarizing neuromuscular blocking agents**.
↑ risk of histamine flush when used with **general anesthetics** in children.

Route/Dosage
Serious Systemic Infections
IV (Adults): 500 mg q 6 hr *or* 1 g q 12 hr (up to 4 g/day).
IV (Children >1 mo): 40 mg/kg/day divided q 6–8 hr *Staphylococcal CNS infection*—60 mg/kg/day divided q 6 hr, maximum dose: 1 g/dose.
IV (Neonates 1 wk–1 mo): <1200 g: 15 mg/kg/day q 24 hr. 1200–2000 g: 10–15 mg/kg/dose q 8–12 hr. >2000 g: 15–20 mg/kg/dose q 8 hr.
IV (Neonates <1 wk): <1200 g: 15 mg/kg/day q 24 hr. 1200–2000 g: 10–15 mg/kg/dose q 12–18 hr. >2000 g: 10–15 mg/kg/dose q 8–12 hr.
IT (Adults): 20 mg/day.
IT (Children): 5–20 mg/day.
IT (Neonates): 5–10 mg/day.

Endocarditis Prophylaxis in Penicillin-Allergic Patients
IV (Adults and Adolescents): 1-g single dose 1-hr preprocedure.
IV (Children): 20-mg/kg single dose 1-hr preprocedure.

Pseudomembranous Colitis
PO (Adults): 125–500 mg q 6 hr.
PO (Children): 40 mg/kg/day divided q 6 hr for 7–10 days (not to exceed 2 g/day).

Renal Impairment
IV (Adults): An initial loading dose of 750 mg–1 g (not less than 15 mg/kg); serum level monitoring is optimal for choosing maintenance dose in patients with renal impairment; these guidelines may be helpful. *CCr 50–80 mL/min*—1 g q 1–3 days; *CCr 10–50 mL/min*—1 g q 3–7 days; *CCr <10 mL/min*—1 g q 7–14 days.

Availability (generic available)
Capsules: 125 mg, 250 mg. **Injection:** 500-mg, 750-mg, 1-, 5-, 10-g vials.

NURSING IMPLICATIONS
Assessment
- Assess patient for infection (vital signs; appearance of wound, sputum, urine, and stool; WBC) at beginning of and throughout therapy.
- Obtain specimens for culture and sensitivity prior to initiating therapy. First dose may be given before receiving results.
- Monitor IV site closely. Vancomycin is irritating to tissues and causes necrosis and severe pain with extravasation. Rotate infusion site.
- Monitor blood pressure throughout IV infusion.

vancomycin

- Evaluate eighth cranial nerve function by audiometry and serum vancomycin levels prior to and throughout therapy in patients with borderline renal function or those >60 yr of age. Prompt recognition and intervention are essential in preventing permanent damage.
- Monitor intake and output ratios and daily weight. Cloudy or pink urine may be a sign of nephrotoxicity.
- Assess patient for signs of superinfection (black, furry overgrowth on tongue; vaginal itching or discharge; loose or foul-smelling stools). Report occurrence.
- Observe patient for signs and symptoms of anaphylaxis (rash, pruritus, laryngeal edema, wheezing). Discontinue drug and notify health care professional immediately if these problems occur. Keep epinephrine, an antihistamine, and resuscitation equipment close by in case of an anaphylactic reaction.
- **Pseudomembranous Colitis:** Assess bowel status (bowel sounds, frequency and consistency of stools, presence of blood in stools) throughout therapy.
- ***Lab Test Considerations:*** Monitor for casts, albumin, or cells in the urine or decreased specific gravity, CBC, and renal function periodically during therapy.
- May cause increased BUN levels.
- ***Toxicity and Overdose:*** Trough concentrations should not exceed 10 mcg/mL (mild-moderate infections) or 15–20 mcg/mL (for severe infections).

Potential Nursing Diagnoses
Risk for infection (Indications)
Disturbed sensory perception (auditory) (Side Effects)

Implementation
- **PO:** Use calibrated measuring device for liquid preparations. IV dose form may be diluted in 30 mL of water for oral or nasogastric tube administration. Resulting solution has bitter, unpleasant taste. May mix with a flavoring syrup to mask taste. Stable for 14 days if refrigerated.

IV Administration
- **Intermittent Infusion:** *Diluent:* To reconstitute, add 10 mL of sterile water for injection to 500-mg vial or 20 mL of sterile water for injection to 1-g vial for a concentration of 50 mg/mL. Dilute further with at least 100 mL of 0.9% NaCl, D5W, D5/0.9% NaCl, or LR for every 500 mg of vancomycin being administered. Reconstituted vials stable for 14 days if refrigerated. Infusion is stable for 96 hr if refrigerated. *Concentration:* ≤5 mg/mL. *Rate:* Infuse over at least 60 min (90 min for doses >1 g). Do not administer rapidly or as a bolus, to minimize risk of thrombophlebitis, hypotension, and "red-man (neck)" syndrome (sudden, severe hypotension; flushing and/or maculopapular rash of face, neck, chest, and upper extremities). May need to slow infusion further to 1.5–2 hr if red-man syndrome occurs.
- **IT:** *Diluent:* Dilute with preservative-free NS. *Concentration:* 1–5 mg/mL. *Rate:* Directly instill into ventricular cerebrospinal fluid.
- **Y-Site Compatibility:** acyclovir, aldesleukin, allopurinol, amifostine, aldesleukin, alfentanil, allopurinol, alprostadil, amifostine, amikacin, amiodarone, amsacrine, anidulafungin, atracurium, atropine, bumetanide, buprenorphine, butorphanol, calcium chloride, calcium gluconate, carboplatin, caspofungin, cefonicid, chlorpromazine, cimetidine, cisatracurium, cisplatin, clindamycin, cyanocobalamin, cyclophosphamide, cyclosporine, cytarabine, dactinomycin, dexamethasone, dexmedetomidine, digoxin, diltiazem, diphenhydramine, dobutamine, docetaxel, dopamine, doripenem, doxacurium, doxapram, doxorubicin hydrochloride, doxorubicin liposome, doxycycline, enalaprilat, ephedrine, epinephrine, epirubicin, ertapenem, erythromycin, esmolol, etoposide, etoposide phosphate, famotidine, fenoldopam, fentanyl, filgrastim, fluconazole, fludarabine, folic acid, gemcitabine, gentamicin, glycopyrrolate, granisetron, hetastarch, hydromorphone, ifosfamide, imipenem/cilastatin, insulin, isoproterenol, labetalol, levofloxacin, lidocaine, linezolid, lorazepam, magnesium sulfate, mannitol, mechlorethamine, melphalan, meperidine, meropenem, metaraminol, methoxamine, methyldopa, methylprednisolone, metoclopramide, metoprolol, metronidazole, midazolam, milrinonemitoxantrone, morphine, mycophenolate, nalbuphine, naloxone, nesiritide, nicardipine, nitroglycerin, nitroprusside, norepinephrine, octreotide, ondansetron, oxacillin, oxaliplatin, oxytocin, paclitaxel, palonosetron, pancuronium, papaverine, pemetrexed, penicillin G, pentamidine, pentazocine, pentobarbital, perphenazine, phenobarbital, phentolamine, phenylephrine, phytonadione, potassium chloride, procainamide,

prochlorperazine, promethazine, propranolol, protamine, pyridoxime, ranitidine, remifentanil, sodium acetate, sodium bicarbonate, sodium citrate, succinylcholine, sufentanil, tacrolimus, teniposide, theophylline, thiamine, thiotepa, tigecycline, tirofiban, tobramycin, tolazoline, trastuzumab, trimethaphan, vasopressin, vecuronium, verapamil, vincristine, vinorelbine, voriconazole, zidovudine.

- **Y-Site Incompatibility:** albumin, amphotericin B cholesteryl, amphotericin B colloidal, amphotericin B liposome, azithromycin, bivalirudin, cefoperazone, chloramphenicol, dantrolene, daptomycin, diazepam, diazoxide, drotrecogin, epoetin alfa, fluorouracil, furosemide, ganciclovir, heparin, idarubicin, indomethacin, ketorolac, pantoprazole, phenytoin, rituximab, streptokinase, trimethoprim/sulfamethoxazole, urokinase.

Patient/Family Teaching
- Advise patients on oral vancomycin to take as directed. Take missed doses as soon as remembered unless almost time for next dose; do not double dose.
- Instruct patient to report signs of hypersensitivity, tinnitus, vertigo, or hearing loss.
- Advise patient to notify health care professional if no improvement is seen in a few days.
- Patients with a history of rheumatic heart disease or valve replacement need to be taught importance of using antimicrobial prophylaxis prior to invasive dental or medical procedures.

Evaluation/Desired Outcomes
- Resolution of signs and symptoms of infection. Length of time for complete resolution depends on organism and site of infection.
- Endocarditis prophylaxis.

---

vardenafil (var-den-a-fil)
Levitra

Classification
Therapeutic: erectile dysfunction agents
Pharmacologic: phosphodiesterase type 5 inhibitors

Pregnancy Category C

Indications
Erectile dysfunction.

Action
Increases cyclic guanosine monophosphate (cGMP) levels by inhibiting phosphodiesterase type 5 (PDE5) an enzyme responsible for the breakdown of cGMP. cGMP produces smooth muscle relaxation of the corpus cavernosum, which in turn promotes increased blood flow and subsequent erection. **Therapeutic Effects:** Enhanced blood flow to the corpus cavernosum and erection sufficient to allow sexual intercourse. Requires sexual stimulation.

Pharmacokinetics
Absorption: 15% absorbed following oral administration; absorption is rapid.
Distribution: Extensive tissue distribution; penetrates semen.
Protein Binding: 95%.
Metabolism and Excretion: Mostly metabolized by the liver (mainly CYP3A4 enzyme system, minor metabolism by CYP2C). M1 metabolite has anti-erectile dysfunction activity. Parent drug and metabolites are mostly excreted in feces. 2–6% renally eliminated.
Half-life: 4–5 hr.

TIME/ACTION PROFILE

ROUTE	ONSET	PEAK	DURATION
PO	rapid	0.5–2 hr	4 hr

Contraindications/Precautions
Contraindicated in: Hypersensitivity; Concurrent use of nitrates or nitric oxide donors; Unstable angina, recent history of stroke, life-threatening arrhythmias, CHF or MI within 6 mo; End-stage renal disease requiring dialysis; Known hereditary degenerative retinal disorders; Severe hepatic impairment (Child-Pugh C); Congenital or acquired QT prolongation or concurrent use of Class IA or III antiarrhythmics; Pedi: Women, children or newborns.
Use Cautiously in: Other serious underlying cardiovascular disease or left ventricular outflow obstruction; Penile deformity; Underlying conditions predisposing to priapism including sickle cell anemia, multiple myeloma or leukemia; Bleeding disorders or active peptic ulcer diseases; History of sudden severe vision loss or non arteritic ischemic optic neuropathy (NAION); may ↑ risk of recurrence; Strong inhibitors of the CYP3A4 enzyme system; Alpha adrenergic blockers (patients should be on stable dose of alpha blockers before starting vardenafil); Geri: Have ↑ blood levels; ↓ dose required.

Adverse Reactions/Side Effects
CNS: headache, amnesia, dizziness. **EENT:** HEARING LOSS, VISION LOSS, rhinitis, sinusitis. **GI:** dyspepsia, nausea. **GU:** priapism. **Derm:** flushing. **Misc:** flu syndrome.

Interactions
Drug-Drug: Concurrent use of **nitrates** may cause serious, life-threatening hypotension and is contraindicated. Concurrent use of Class IA antiarrhythmics (such as **quindine** or **procainamide**) or **Class III antiarrhythmics** (such as **amiodarone** or **sotalol**) ↑ risk of serious arrhythmias and should be avoided. Concurrent use of alpha-adrenergic blockers may cause serious hypotension, lowest doses of each should be used initially. Strong inhibitors of CYP3A4 including **protease inhibitor antiretrovirals** (including **ritonavir**, **saquinavir**, and **indinavir**), **ketoconazole**, and **itraconazole** ↑ effects and the risk of adverse reactions (dosage adjustments recommended). Concurrent use of moderate inhibitors of CYP2C including **erythromycin** may also ↑ effects. ↑ risk of hypotension with **alpha adrenergic blockers** and acute ingestion of **alcohol**.

Route/Dosage
PO (Adults): 10 mg taken 1 hr prior to sexual activity (range 5–20 mg; not to exceed one dose/24 hr); *concurrent use of ritonavir*—single dose should not exceed 2.5 mg in any 72-hour period; *concurrent use of indinavir, ketoconazole 400 mg daily or itraconazole 400 mg daily*—single dose should not exceed 2.5 mg/24 hr; *concurrent use of ketoconazole or itraconazole 200 mg daily or erythromycin*—single dose should not exceed 5 mg/24 hr.
PO (Geriatric Patients >65 yr): 5 mg initial dose; titrate as tolerated.

Hepatic Impairment
PO (Adults): *Moderate hepatic impairment (Child-Pugh B)*—May start with 5 mg dose, subsequent dosing should not exceed 10.

Availability
Tablets: 2.5 mg, 5 mg, 10 mg, 20 mg. **Cost:** 2.5 mg $68.99/6, 5 mg $111.99/10, 10 mg $109.99/10, 20 mg $115.99/10.

NURSING IMPLICATIONS

Assessment
- Determine erectile dysfunction before administration. Vardenafil has no effect in the absence of sexual stimulation.

Potential Nursing Diagnoses
Sexual dysfunction (Indications)

Implementation
- **PO:** Dose is usually administered 1 hr before sexual activity. May be administered 30 min to 4 hr before sexual activity.
- May be administered without regard to food.

Patient/Family Teaching
- Instruct patient to take vardenafil approximately 1 hr before sexual activity and not more than once per day. Inform patient that sexual stimulation is required for an erection to occur after taking vardenafil.
- Advise patient that vardenafil is not indicated for use in women.
- Caution patient not to take tadalafil concurrently with alpha adrenergic blockers (unless on a stable dose) or nitrates. If chest pain occurs after taking tadalafil, instruct patient to seek immediate medical attention.
- Instruct patient to notify health care professional promptly if erection lasts longer than 4 hr, if they are not satisfied with their sexual performance or develop unwanted side effects or if they experience sudden or decreased vision loss in one or both eyes.
- Advise patient to consult health care professional before taking other Rx or OTC medications or herbal supplements that may interact with vardenafil.
- Inform patient that vardenafil offers no protection against sexually transmitted diseases. Counsel patient that protection against sexually transmitted diseases and HIV infection should be considered.

Evaluation/Desired Outcomes
- Male erection sufficient to allow intercourse.

---

varenicline (ver-en-i-cline)
Chantix

Classification
Therapeutic: smoking deterrents
Pharmacologic: nicotine agonists

Pregnancy Category C

Indications
Treatment of smoking cessation; in conjunction with nonpharmacologic support (educational materials/counseling).

Action
Selectively binds to alpha$_4$, beta$_2$ nicotinic acetylcholine receptors, acting as a nicotine agonist;

= Canadian drug name. = Genetic implication.
*CAPITALS indicates life-threatening; underlines indicate most frequent.

varenicline

prevents the binding of nicotine to receptors.
Therapeutic Effects: Decreased desire to smoke.

Pharmacokinetics
Absorption: 100% absorbed following oral administration.
Distribution: 24 hr.
Metabolism and Excretion: Minimally metabolized; 92% excreted in urine unchanged.
Half-life: 24 hr.

TIME/ACTION PROFILE

ROUTE	ONSET	PEAK	DURATION
PO	unknown	3–4 hr	24 hr

Contraindications/Precautions
Contraindicated in: Hypersensitivity; Lactation: Lactation; Pedi: Safety not established.
Use Cautiously in: Severe renal impairment (↓ dose recommended if CCr <30 mL/min); Psychiatric illness; Geri: Consider age-related ↓ in renal function; OB: Use only if maternal benefit outweighs fetal risk.

Adverse Reactions/Side Effects
CNS: SUICIDAL THOUGHTS/BEHAVIOR, ↓ attention span, anxiety, depression, insomnia, irritability, dizziness, restlessness, abnormal dreams, agitation, aggression, amnesia, disorientation, dissociation, hostility, migraine, psychomotor hyperactivity. **EENT:** blurred vision, visual disturbances. **CV:** syncope. **GI:** diarrhea, gingivitis, nausea, ↑ appetite, constipation, dyspepsia, dysphagia, enterocolitis, eructation, flatulence, gallbladder disorder, GI bleeding, ↑ liver function tests, vomiting. **Derm:** STEVENS-JOHNSON SYNDROME, flushing, hyperhydrosis, acne, dermatitis, dry skin. **Hemat:** anemia. **MS:** arthralgia, back pain, musculoskeletal pain, muscle cramps, myalgia, restless legs. **Misc:** ANGIOEDEMA, accidental injury, chills, fever, hypersensitivity, mild physical dependence.

Interactions
Drug-Drug: Smoking cessation may ↓ metabolism of **theophylline**, **warfarin**, and **insulin** resulting in ↑ effects; careful monitoring is recommended. Risk of adverse reactions (nausea, vomiting, dizziness, fatigue, headache) may be ↑ with **nicotine** replacement therapy (nicotine transdermal patches).

Route/Dosage
PO (Adults): Treatment is started one week prior to planned smoking cessation 0.5 mg once daily on the first three days, then 0.5 mg twice daily for the next 4 days, then 1 mg twice daily.

Renal Impairment
PO (Adults): *CCr <30 mL/min* — 0.5 mg daily, may ↑ to 0.5 mg twice daily.

Availability
Tablets: 0.5 mg, 1 mg.

NURSING IMPLICATIONS

Assessment
- Assess for desire to stop smoking.
- Assess for nausea. Usually dose-dependent. May require dose reduction.
- Assess mental status and mood changes, especially during initial few months of therapy and during dose changes. Risk may be increased in children, adolescents, and adults ≤24 yr. Inform health care professional if patient demonstrates significant increase in signs of depression (depressed mood, loss of interest in usual activities, significant change in weight and/or appetite, insomnia or hypersomnia, psychomotor agitation or retardation, increased fatigue, feelings of guilt or worthlessness, slowed thinking or impaired concentration, suicide attempt or suicidal ideation). Restrict amount of drug available to patient.
- *Lab Test Considerations:* May cause anemia.

Potential Nursing Diagnoses
Ineffective coping (Indications)

Implementation
- **PO:** Administer after eating with a full glass of water.

Patient/Family Teaching
- Instruct patient to take varenicline as directed. Set a date to stop smoking. Start taking varenicline 1 wk before quit date. Begin with 0.5 mg/day for the first 3 days, then for the next 4 days take one 0.5 mg tablet in the morning and in the evening. After first 7 days, increase to 1 mg tablet in the morning and evening.
- Encourage patient to attempt to quit, even if they had early lapses after quit day.
- Advise patient to stop taking varenicline and contact health care professional promptly if agitation, depressed mood, any changes in behavior that are not typical of nicotine withdrawal, or if suicidal thoughts or behavior occur.
- Provide patient with educational materials and counseling to support attempts to quit smoking.
- Caution patient not to share varenicline with others. May be harmful.
- May cause blurred vision, dizziness, and disturbance in attention. Caution patient to avoid

driving and other activities requiring alertness until response to medication is known.
- Inform patient that nausea and insomnia may occur and are usually transient. Advise patient to notify health care professional if these symptoms are persistent and bothersome; dose reduction may be considered.
- Advise patient to notify health care professional before taking Rx, OTC, or herbal products. Inform patient that some medications may require dose adjustments after quitting smoking.
- Advise patient to notify health care professional if pregnancy is planned or suspected or if breastfeeding.

Evaluation/Desired Outcomes
- Smoking cessation. Patients who have successfully stopped smoking at the end of 12 wk, should take an additional 12 wk course to increase the likelihood of long-term abstinence. Patients who do not succeed in stopping smoking during 12 wk of initial therapy or who relapse after treatment, should be encouraged to make another attempt once factors contributing to the failed attempt have been identified and addressed.

vasopressin (vay-soe-press-in)
Pitressin, ♣ Pressyn

Classification
Therapeutic: hormones
Pharmacologic: antidiuretic hormones

Pregnancy Category C

Indications
Central diabetes insipidus due to deficient antidiuretic hormone. **Unlabeled Use:** Management of pulseless VT/VF unresponsive to initial shocks, asystole, or pulseless electrical activity (PEA) (ACLS guidelines). Vasodilatory shock. Gastrointestinal hemorrhage.

Action
Alters the permeability of the renal collecting ducts, allowing reabsorption of water. Directly stimulates musculature of GI tract. In high doses acts as a nonadrenergic peripheral vasoconstrictor. **Therapeutic Effects:** Decreased urine output and increased urine osmolality in diabetes insipidus.

Pharmacokinetics
Absorption: IM absorption may be unpredictable.
Distribution: Widely distributed throughout extracellular fluid.
Metabolism and Excretion: Rapidly degraded by the liver and kidneys; <5% excreted unchanged by the kidneys.
Half-life: 10–20 min.

TIME/ACTION PROFILE (antidiuretic effect)

ROUTE	ONSET	PEAK	DURATION
IM, subcut	unknown	unknown	2–8 hr
IV	unknown	unknown	30–60 min

Contraindications/Precautions
Contraindicated in: Chronic renal failure with increased BUN; Hypersensitivity to beef or pork proteins.
Use Cautiously in: Perioperative polyuria (increased sensitivity to vasopressin); Comatose patients; Seizures; Migraine headaches; Asthma; Heart failure; Cardiovascular disease; Renal impairment; Pedi: Geri: ↑ sensitivity to vasopressin effects.

Adverse Reactions/Side Effects
CNS: dizziness, "pounding" sensation in head. **CV:** MI, angina, chest pain. **GI:** abdominal cramps, belching, diarrhea, flatulence, heartburn, nausea, vomiting. **Derm:** paleness, perioral blanching, sweating. **Neuro:** trembling. **Misc:** allergic reactions, fever, water intoxication (higher doses).

Interactions
Drug-Drug: Antidiuretic effect may be ↓ by concurrent administration of **alcohol**, **lithium**, **demeclocycline**, **heparin**, or **norepinephrine**. Antidiuretic effect may be ↑ by concurrent administration of **carbamazepine**, **chlorpropamide**, **clofibrate**, **tricyclic antidepressants**, or **fludrocortisone**. Vasopressor effect may be ↑ by concurrent administration of **ganglionic blocking agents**.

Route/Dosage
Diabetes insipidus
IM, Subcut (Adults): 5–10 units 2–4 times daily.
IM, Subcut (Children): 2.5–10 units 2–4 times daily.
IV (Adults and Children): 0.0005 units/kg/hr, double dosage q 30 min as needed to a maximum of 0.01 units/kg/hr.

Pulseless VT/VF, Asystole, or PEA (ACLS guidelines)
IV (Adults): 40 units as a single dose (unlabeled).
IV (Children): 0.4 units/kg after resuscitation and at least 2 doses of epinephrine.

Vasodilatory shock
IV (Adults): 0.01–0.1 units/min, titrate to effect.
IV (Infants and Children): 0.0003–0.002 units/kg/min, titrate to effect.

GI Hemorrhage
IV (Adults): 0.2–0.4 units/min then titrate to maximum dose of 0.9 units/min; if bleeding stops continue same dose for 12 hr then taper off over 24–48 hr.
IV (Children): 0.002–0.005 units/kg/min then titrate to maximum dose of 0.01 units/kg/min; if bleeding stops continue same dose for 12 hr then taper off over 24–48 hr.

Availability (generic available)
Injection: 20 units/mL in 0.5- and 1-mL ampules and vials.

NURSING IMPLICATIONS

Assessment
- Monitor BP, HR, and ECG periodically throughout therapy and continuously throughout cardiopulmonary resuscitation.
- **Diabetes Insipidus:** Monitor urine osmolality and urine volume frequently to determine effects of medication. Assess patient for symptoms of dehydration (excessive thirst, dry skin and mucous membranes, tachycardia, poor skin turgor). Weigh patient daily, monitor intake and output, and assess for edema.
- *Lab Test Considerations:* Monitor urine specific gravity throughout therapy.
- Monitor serum electrolyte concentrations periodically during therapy.
- *Toxicity and Overdose:* Signs and symptoms of water intoxication include confusion, drowsiness, headache, weight gain, difficulty urinating, seizures, and coma.
- Treatment of overdose includes water restriction and temporary discontinuation of vasopressin until polyuria occurs. If symptoms are severe, administration of mannitol, hypertonic dextrose, urea, and/or furosemide may be used.

Potential Nursing Diagnoses
Deficient fluid volume (Indications)
Excess fluid volume (Adverse Reactions)

Implementation
- Do not confuse Pitressin (vasopressin) with Pitocin (oxytocin).
- Aqueous vasopressin injection may be administered subcut or IM for diabetes insipidus.
- Administer 1–2 glasses of water at the time of administration to minimize side effects (blanching of skin, abdominal cramps, nausea).

IV Administration
- **Direct IV:** *Diluent:* Administer undiluted. *Concentration:* 20 units/mL. *Rate:* Administer over 1–2 sec during pulseless VT/VF, asystole, or PEA.
- **Continuous Infusion:** *Diluent:* Dilute 100 units of vasopressin in 250 mL of 0.9% NaCl or D5W. *Concentration:* 0.4 units/mL. *Rate:* See Route/Dosage section.
- **Y-Site Compatibility:** amiodarone, argatroban, ciprofloxacin, diltiazem, dobutamine, dopamine, drotrecogin, epinephrine, fluconazole, gentamicin, heparin, imipenem/cilastatin, insulin, lidocaine, linezolid, meropenem, metronidazole, milrinone, nitroglycerin, norepinephrine, pantoprazole, phenylephrine, procainamide, sodium bicarbonate.
- **Y-Site Incompatibility:** diazepam, phenytoin, trimethoprim/sulfamethoxazole.

Patient/Family Teaching
- Instruct patient to take medication as directed. Caution patient not to use more than prescribed amount. Take missed doses as soon as remembered, unless almost time for next dose.
- Advise patient to drink 1–2 glasses of water at time of administration to minimize side effects (blanching of skin, abdominal cramps, nausea). Inform patient that these side effects are not serious and usually disappear in a few minutes.
- Caution patient to avoid concurrent use of alcohol while taking vasopressin.
- Patients with diabetes insipidus should carry identification at all times describing disease process and medication regimen.

Evaluation/Desired Outcomes
- Decrease in urine volume.
- Relief of polydipsia.
- Increased urine osmolality in patients with central diabetes insipidus.
- Resolution of VT/VF.
- Improvement in signs of septic shock.

venlafaxine (ven-la-fax-een)
Effexor, Effexor XR

venlafaxine

Classification
Therapeutic: antidepressants, antianxiety agents
Pharmacologic: selective serotonin/norepinephrine reuptake inhibitors

Pregnancy Category C

Indications
Major depressive disorder. Generalized anxiety disorder (Effexor XR only). Social anxiety disorder (Effexor XR only). Panic disorder (Effexor XR only). **Unlabeled Use:** Premenstrual dysphoric disorder.

Action
Inhibits serotonin and norepinephrine reuptake in the CNS. **Therapeutic Effects:** Decrease in depressive symptomatology, with fewer relapses/recurrences. Decreased anxiety; Decrease in panic attacks.

Pharmacokinetics
Absorption: 92–100% absorbed after oral administration.
Distribution: Extensive distribution into body tissues.
Metabolism and Excretion: Extensively metabolized on first pass through the liver (primarily through CYP2D6 enzyme pathway). A small percentage of the population are poor metabolizers and will have higher blood levels with ↑ effects. One metabolite, O-desmethylvenlafaxine (ODV), has antidepressant activity; 5% of venlafaxine is excreted unchanged in urine; 30% of the active metabolite is excreted in urine.
Half-life: *Venlafaxine*—3–5 hr; *ODV*—9–11 hr (both are ↑ in hepatic/renal impairment).

TIME/ACTION PROFILE (antidepressant action)

ROUTE	ONSET	PEAK	DURATION
PO	within 2 wk	2–4 wk	unknown

Contraindications/Precautions
Contraindicated in: Hypersensitivity; Concurrent MAO inhibitor therapy.
Use Cautiously in: Cardiovascular disease, including hypertension; Hepatic impairment (↓ dose recommended); Impaired renal function (↓ dose recommended); History of seizures or neurologic impairment; History of mania; History of ↑ intraocular pressure or angle-closure glaucoma; History of drug abuse; OB: Use only if clearly required during pregnancy, weighing benefit to mother versus potential harm to fetus (potential for discontinuation syndrome or toxicity in the neonate when venlafaxine is taken during the 3rd trimester); Lactation: Potential for serious adverse reactions in infant; discontinue drug or discontinue breastfeeding; Pedi: ↑ risk of suicidal thinking and behavior (suicidality) in children and adolescents with major depressive disorder and other psychiatric disorders. Observe closely for suicidality and behavior changes.

Adverse Reactions/Side Effects
CNS: NEUROLEPTIC MALIGNANT SYNDROME, SEIZURES, SUICIDAL THOUGHTS, abnormal dreams, anxiety, dizziness, headache, insomnia, nervousness, weakness, abnormal thinking, agitation, confusion, depersonalization, drowsiness, emotional lability, worsening depression. **EENT:** rhinitis, visual disturbances, epistaxis, tinnitus. **CV:** chest pain, hypertension, palpitations, tachycardia. **GI:** abdominal pain, altered taste, anorexia, constipation, diarrhea, dry mouth, dyspepsia, nausea, vomiting, weight loss. **GU:** sexual dysfunction, urinary frequency, urinary retention. **Derm:** ecchymoses, itching, photosensitivity, skin rash. **Neuro:** paresthesia, twitching. **Misc:** SEROTONIN SYNDROME, chills, bleeding, yawning.

Interactions
Drug-Drug: Concurrent use with **MAO inhibitors** may result in serious, potentially fatal reactions (wait at least 2 wk after stopping MAO inhibitor before initiating venlafaxine; wait at least 1 wk after stopping venlafaxine before starting MAO inhibitors). Concurrent use with **alcohol** or other **CNS depressants**, including **sedatives/hypnotics**, **antihistamines**, and **opioid analgesics** in depressed patients is not recommended. Drugs that affect serotonergic neurotransmitter systems, including **linezolid**, **tramadol**, and **triptans**, ↑ risk of serotonin syndrome. **Lithium** may have ↑ serotonergic effects with venlafaxine; use cautiously in patients receiving venlafaxine. ↑ blood levels and may ↑ effects of **desipramine** and **haloperidol**. **Cimetidine** may ↑ the effects of venlafaxine (may be more pronounced in geriatric patients, those with hepatic or renal impairment, or those with pre-existing hypertension).
Ketoconazole may ↑ the effects of venlafaxine.
↑ risk of bleeding with **NSAIDS, aspirin, clopidogrel**, or **warfarin**.
Drug-Natural Products: Concomitant use of **kava-kava, valerian, chamomile**, or **hops** can ↑ CNS depression. ↑ risk of serotinergic side

effects including serotonin syndrome with **St. John's wort** and **SAMe**.

Route/Dosage
Major Depressive Disorder
PO (Adults): *Tablets*—75 mg/day in 2–3 divided doses; may ↑ by up to 75 mg/day every 4 days, up to 225 mg/day (not to exceed 375 mg/day in 3 divided doses); *Extended-release (XR) capsules*—75 mg once daily (some patients may be started at 37.5 mg once daily) for 4–7 days; may ↑ by up to 75 mg/day at intervals of not less than 4 days (not to exceed 225 mg/day).

General Anxiety Disorder
PO (Adults): *Extended-release (XR) capsules*—75 mg once daily (some patients may be started at 37.5 mg once daily) for 4–7 days; may ↑ by up to 75 mg/day at intervals of not less than 4 days (not to exceed 225 mg/day).

Social Anxiety Disorder
PO (Adults): *Extended-release (XR) capsules*—75 mg once daily.

Panic Disorder
PO (Adults): *Extended-release (XR) capsules*—37.5 mg once daily for 7 days; may then ↑ to 75 mg once daily; may then ↑ by 75 mg/day every 7 days (not to exceed 225 mg/day).

Hepatic Impairment
PO (Adults): ↓ daily dose by 50% in patients with mild-to-moderate hepatic impairment.

Renal Impairment
PO (Adults): *CCr 10–70 mL/min*— ↓ daily dose by 25–50%; *Hemodialysis*— ↓ daily dose by 50%.

Availability (generic available)
Tablets: 25 mg, 37.5 mg, 50 mg, 75 mg, 100 mg. **Cost:** *Generic*—25 mg $299.95/180, 37.5 mg $299.93/180, 50 mg $341.96/180, 75 mg $337.95/180, 100 mg $343.78/180. **Extended-release capsules:** 37.5 mg, 75 mg, 150 mg. **Cost:** 37.5 mg $275.97/90, 75 mg $318.99/90, 150 mg $355.97/90.

NURSING IMPLICATIONS

Assessment
- Assess mental status and mood changes. Inform health care professional if patient demonstrates significant increase in anxiety, nervousness, or insomnia.
- Assess suicidal tendencies, especially in early therapy. Restrict amount of drug available to patient. Risk may be increased in children, adolescents, and adults ≤24 yr.
- Monitor blood pressure before and periodically during therapy. Sustained hypertension may be dose-related; decrease dose or discontinue therapy if this occurs.
- Monitor appetite and nutritional intake. Weigh weekly. Report continued weight loss. Adjust diet as tolerated to support nutritional status.
- Assess for serotonin syndrome (mental changes [agitation, hallucinations, coma], autonomic instability [tachycardia, labile blood pressure, hyperthermia], neuromuscular aberrations [hyper-reflexia, incoordination], and/or GI symptoms [nausea, vomiting, diarrhea]), especially in patients taking other serotonergic drugs (SSRIs, SNRIs, triptans).
- *Lab Test Considerations:* Monitor CBC with differential and platelet count periodically during therapy. May cause anemia, leukocytosis, leukopenia, thrombocytopenia, basophilia, and eosinophilia.
- May cause an ↑ in serum alkaline phosphatase, bilirubin, AST, ALT, BUN, and creatinine.
- May also cause ↑ serum cholesterol.
- May cause electrolyte abnormalities (hyperglycemia or hypoglycemia, hyperkalemia or hypokalemia, hyperuricemia, hyperphosphatemia or hypophosphatemia, and hyponatremia).

Potential Nursing Diagnoses
Ineffective coping (Indications)
Risk for injury (Side Effects)

Implementation
- **PO:** Administer venlafaxine with food.
- Extended-release capsules should be swallowed whole; do not crush, break, or chew.
- Extended-release capsules may also be opened and contents sprinkled on a spoonful of applesauce. Take immediately and follow with a glass of water. Do not store mixture for later use.

Patient/Family Teaching
- Instruct patient to take venlafaxine as directed at the same time each day. Take missed doses as soon as possible unless almost time for next dose. Do not double doses or discontinue abruptly. Patients taking venlafaxine for >6 wk should have dose gradually decreased before discontinuation.
- Advise patient, family, and caregivers to look for suicidality, especially during early therapy or dose changes. Notify health care professional immediately if thoughts about suicide or dying, attempts to commit suicide; new or worse depression or anxiety; agitation or restlessness; panic attacks; insomnia; new or

worse irritability; aggressiveness; acting on dangerous impulses, mania, or other changes in mood or behavior or if symptoms of serotonin syndrome occur.
- May cause drowsiness or dizziness. Caution patient to avoid driving or other activities requiring alertness until response to the drug is known.
- Caution patient to avoid taking alcohol or other CNS-depressant drugs during therapy and not to take other Rx, OTC, or herbal products without consulting health care professional.
- Instruct female patients to inform health care professional if pregnancy is planned or suspected or if breastfeeding.
- Instruct patient to notify health care professional if signs of allergy (rash, hives) occur.
- Emphasize the importance of follow-up exams to monitor progress. Encourage patient participation in psychotherapy.

Evaluation/Desired Outcomes
- Increased sense of well-being.
- Renewed interest in surroundings. Need for therapy should be periodically reassessed. Therapy is usually continued for several months.
- Decreased anxiety.

verapamil (ver-ap-a-mil)
Calan, Calan SR, Covera-HS, Isoptin SR, ✦ Novo-Veramil, ✦ Nu-Verap, Verelan, Verelan PM

Classification
Therapeutic: antianginals, antiarrhythmics (class IV), antihypertensives, vascular headache suppressants
Pharmacologic: calcium channel blockers

Pregnancy Category C

Indications
Management of hypertension, angina pectoris, and/or vasospastic (Prinzmetal's) angina. Management of supraventricular arrhythmias and rapid ventricular rates in atrial flutter or fibrillation. **Unlabeled Use:** Prevention of migraine headache.

Action
Inhibits the transport of calcium into myocardial and vascular smooth muscle cells, resulting in inhibition of excitation-contraction coupling and subsequent contraction. Decreases SA and AV conduction and prolongs AV node refractory period in conduction tissue. **Therapeutic Effects:** Systemic vasodilation resulting in decreased blood pressure. Coronary vasodilation resulting in decreased frequency and severity of attacks of angina. Reduction of ventricular rate during atrial fibrillation or flutter.

Pharmacokinetics
Absorption: 90% absorbed after oral administration, but much is rapidly metabolized, resulting in bioavailability of 20–25%.
Distribution: Small amounts enter breast milk.
Protein Binding: 90%.
Metabolism and Excretion: Mostly metabolized by the liver.
Half-life: 4.5–12 hr.

TIME/ACTION PROFILE (cardiovascular effects)

ROUTE	ONSET	PEAK	DURATION
PO	1–2 hr	30–90 min†	3–7 hr
PO-ER	unknown	5–7 hr	24 hr
IV	1–5 min‡	3–5 min	2 hr‡

†Single dose; effects from multiple doses may not be evident for 24–48 hr

‡Antiarrhythmic effects; hemodynamic effects begin 3–5 min after injection and persist for 10–20 min

Contraindications/Precautions
Contraindicated in: Hypersensitivity; Sick sinus syndrome; 2nd- or 3rd-degree AV block (unless an artificial pacemaker is in place); Systolic BP <90 mm Hg; CHF, severe ventricular dysfunction, or cardiogenic shock, unless associated with supraventricular tachyarrhythmias; Concurrent IV beta blocker therapy.
Use Cautiously in: Severe hepatic impairment (dose ↓ recommended for most agents); History of serious ventricular arrhythmias or CHF; Geri: Dose ↓/slower IV infusion rates recommended (↑ risk of hypotension); OB, Lactation: Safety not established.

Adverse Reactions/Side Effects
CNS: abnormal dreams, anxiety, confusion, dizziness/lightheadedness, drowsiness, headache, jitteriness, nervousness, psychiatric disturbances, weakness. **EENT:** blurred vision, disturbed equilibrium, epistaxis, tinnitus. **Resp:** cough, dyspnea, shortness of breath. **CV:** ARRHYTHMIAS, CHF, bradycardia, chest pain, hypotension, palpitations, peripheral edema, syncope, tachycardia.

✦ = Canadian drug name. = Genetic implication.
*CAPITALS indicates life-threatening; underlines indicate most frequent.

GI: ↑ liver enzymes, anorexia, constipation, diarrhea, dry mouth, dysgeusia, dyspepsia, nausea, vomiting. **GU:** dysuria, nocturia, polyuria, sexual dysfunction, urinary frequency. **Derm:** dermatitis, erythema multiforme, flushing, photosensitivity, pruritus/urticaria, rash, sweating. **Endo:** gynecomastia, hyperglycemia. **Hemat:** anemia, leukopenia, thrombocytopenia. **Metab:** weight gain. **MS:** joint stiffness, muscle cramps. **Neuro:** paresthesia, tremor. **Misc:** STEVENS-JOHNSON SYNDROME, gingival hyperplasia.

Interactions
Drug-Drug: Additive hypotension may occur when used concurrently with **fentanyl**, other **antihypertensives**, **nitrates**, acute ingestion of **alcohol**, or **quinidine**. Antihypertensive effects may be ↓ by concurrent use of **NSAIDs**. Serum **digoxin** levels may be ↑. Concurrent use with **beta blockers**, **digoxin**, **disopyramide**, or **phenytoin** may result in bradycardia, conduction defects, or CHF. ↑ risk of hypotension and bradycardia with **erythromycin**, **clarithromycin**, or **telithromycin**. May ↓ metabolism of and ↑ risk of toxicity from **cyclosporine**, **prazosin**, **quinidine**, or **carbamazepine**. May ↓ effectiveness of **rifampin**. ↑ the muscle-paralyzing effects of **nondepolarizing neuromuscular-blocking agents**. Effectiveness may be ↓ by coadministration with **vitamin D compounds** and **calcium**. May alter serum **lithium** levels.
Drug-Natural Products: ↑ **caffeine** levels with caffeine-containing herbs (**cola nut**, **guarana**, **mate**, **tea**, **coffee**).
Drug-Food: Grapefruit juice ↑ serum levels and effect.

Route/Dosage
PO (Adults): 80–120 mg 3 times daily, ↑ as needed. *Patients with hepatic impairment or geriatric patients*—40 mg 3 times daily initially. *Extended-release preparations*—120–240 mg/day as a single dose; may be ↑ as needed (range 240–480 mg/day).
PO (Children up to 15 yr): 4–8 mg/kg/day in divided doses.
IV (Adults): 5–10 mg (75–150 mcg/kg); may repeat with 10 mg (150 mcg/kg) after 15–30 min.
IV (Children 1–15 yr): 2–5 mg (100–300 mcg/kg); may repeat after 30 min (initial dose not to exceed 5 mg; repeat dose not to exceed 10 mg).
IV (Children <1 yr): 0.75–2 mg (100–200 mcg/kg); may repeat after 30 min.

Availability (generic available)
Tablets: 40 mg, 80 mg, 120 mg. **Cost:** *Generic*—40 mg $44.96/270, 80 mg $44.96/270, 120 mg $34.45/270. **Extended-release tablets (Isoptin SR, Covera HS):** 120 mg, 180 mg, 240 mg. **Cost:** *Generic*—120 mg $49.97/90, 180 mg $27.97/90, 240 mg $35.97/90. **Extended-release capsules (Verelan PM):** 100 mg, 200 mg, 300 mg. **Cost:** 100 mg $166.01/90, 200 mg $213.02/90, 300 mg $308.52/90. **Extended-release capsules (Verelan):** 120 mg, 180 mg, 240 mg, 360 mg. **Cost:** *Generic*—120 mg $64.99/90, 180 mg $67.99/90, 240 mg $86.99/90, 360 mg $160.97/90. **Solution for injection:** 2.5 mg/mL. *In combination with:* trandolapril (Tarka); see Appendix B.

NURSING IMPLICATIONS

Assessment
- Monitor blood pressure and pulse before therapy, during dosage titration, and periodically throughout therapy. Monitor ECG periodically during prolonged therapy. Verapamil may cause prolonged PR interval.
- Monitor intake and output ratios and daily weight. Assess for signs of CHF (peripheral edema, rales/crackles, dyspnea, weight gain, jugular venous distention).
- Patients receiving digoxin concurrently with calcium channel blockers should have routine serum digoxin levels and be monitored for signs and symptoms of digoxin toxicity.
- **Angina:** Assess location, duration, intensity, and precipitating factors of patient's anginal pain.
- **Arrhythmias:** Monitor ECG continuously during administration. Notify health care professional promptly if bradycardia or prolonged hypotension occurs. Emergency equipment and medication should be available. Monitor blood pressure and pulse before and frequently during administration.
- *Lab Test Considerations:* Total serum calcium concentrations are not affected by calcium channel blockers.
- Monitor serum potassium periodically. Hypokalemia ↑ risk of arrhythmias and should be corrected.
- Monitor renal and hepatic functions periodically during long-term therapy. May cause ↑ hepatic enzymes after several days of therapy, which return to normal on discontinuation of therapy.

Potential Nursing Diagnoses
Decreased cardiac output (Indications)
Acute pain (Indications)

Implementation
- Do not confuse verapamil with Virilon (methyltestosterone). Do not confuse Covera (verapamil) with Provera (medroxyprogesterone).
- **PO:** Administer verapamil with meals or milk to minimize gastric irritation.
- Do not open, crush, break, or chew sustained-release capsules or tablets. Empty tablets that appear in stool are not significant.

IV Administration

- **IV:** Patients should remain recumbent for at least 1 hr after IV administration to minimize hypotensive effects.
- **Direct IV:** *Diluent:* Administer undiluted. *Concentration:* 2.5 mg/mL. *Rate:* Administer over 2 min. Geri: Administer over 3 min.
- **Y-Site Compatibility:** alfentanil, amikacin, argatroban, ascorbic acid, atracurium, atropine, aztreonam, bivalirudin, bumetanide, buprenorphine, butorphanol, calcium chloride, calcium gluconate, carboplatin, caspofungin, cefazolin, cefonocid, cefotaxime, cefotetan, cefoxitin, ceftizoxime, ceftriaxone, cefuroxime, chlorpromazine, cimetidine, ciprofloxacin, clindamycin, cyanocobalamin, cyclophosphamide, cyclosporine, cytarabine, dactinomycin, daptomycin, dexamethasone, dexmedetomidine, digoxin, diltiazem, diphenhydramine, dobutamine, docetaxel, dopamine, doxacurium, doxorubicin hydrochloride, doxycycline, enalaprilat, ephedrine, epinephrine, epirubicin, epotein alfa, eptifibatide, erythromycin, esmolol, etoposide, etoposide phosphate, famotidine, fenoldopam, fentanyl, fluconazole, fludarabine, gemcitabine, gentamicin, glycopyrrolate, granisetron, heparin, hetastarch, hydralazine, hydrocortisone sodium succinate, hydromorphone, ifosfamide, imipenem/cilastatin, inamrinone, insulin, isoproterenol, ketorolac, labetalol, levofloxacin, lidocaine, linezolid, lorazepam, magnesium sulfate, mannitol, mechlorethamine, meperidine, metaraminol, methotrexate, methoxamine, methyldopate, methylprednisolone sodium succinate, metoclopramide, metoprolol, metronidazole, miconazole, midazolam, milrinone, mitoxantrone, morphine, multivitamins, nalbuphine, naloxone, nesiritide, nitroglycerin, nitroprusside, norepinephrine, octreotide, ondansetron, oxaliplatin, oxytocin, paclitaxel, palonosetron, papaverine, pemetrexed, penicillin G, pentamidine, pentazocine, phentolamine, phenylephrine, phytonadione, piperacillin/tazobactam, potassium chloride, procainamide, prochlorperazine, promethazine, propranolol, protamine, pyridoxime, quinupristin/dalfopristin, ranitidine, rocuronium, sodium acetate, streptokinase, succinylcholine, sufentanil, tacrolimus, teniposide, theiphylline, thiamine, ticarcillin/clavulanate, tirofiban, tobramycin, tolazoline, trimethaphan, urokinase, vancomycin, vasopressin, vecuronium, vincristine, vinorelbine, voriconazole.
- **Y-Site Incompatibility:** acyclovir, albumin, aminophylline, amphotericin B cholesteryl, amphotericin B colloidal, amphotericin B liposome, ampicillin, ampicillin/sulbactam, azathioprine, cefoperazone, ceftazidime, chloramphenicol, dantrolene, diazepam, diazoxide, ertapenem, fluorouracil, folic acid, furosemide, ganciclovir, indomethacin, pantoprazole, pentobarbital, phenobarbital, phenytoin, piperacillin/tazobactam, propofol, sodium bicarbonate, thiotepa, tigecycline, trimethoprim/sulfamethoxazole.

Patient/Family Teaching
- Advise patient to take medication as directed, even if feeling well. Take missed doses as soon as possible unless almost time for next dose; do not double doses. May need to be discontinued gradually.
- Advise patient to avoid large amounts (6–8 glasses of grapefruit juice/day) during therapy.
- Instruct patient on correct technique for monitoring pulse. Instruct patient to contact health care professional if heart rate is <50 bpm.
- Caution patient to change positions slowly to minimize orthostatic hypotension.
- May cause drowsiness or dizziness. Advise patient to avoid driving or other activities requiring alertness until response to the medication is known.
- Instruct patient on importance of maintaining good dental hygiene and seeing dentist frequently for teeth cleaning to prevent tenderness, bleeding, and gingival hyperplasia (gum enlargement).
- Instruct patient to avoid concurrent use of alcohol or OTC medications, especially cold preparations, without consulting health care professional.

- Advise patient to notify health care professional if irregular heartbeats, dyspnea, swelling of hands and feet, pronounced dizziness, nausea, constipation, or hypotension occurs or if headache is severe or persistent.
- Caution patient to wear protective clothing and use sunscreen to prevent photosensitivity reactions.
- **Angina:** Instruct patient on concurrent nitrate or beta-blocker therapy to continue taking both medications as directed and use SL nitroglycerin as needed for anginal attacks.
- Advise patient to contact health care professional if chest pain does not improve, worsens after therapy, or occurs with diaphoresis; if shortness of breath occurs; or if severe, persistent headache occurs.
- Caution patient to discuss exercise restrictions with health care professional before exertion.
- **Hypertension:** Encourage patient to comply with other interventions for hypertension (weight reduction, low-sodium diet, smoking cessation, moderation of alcohol consumption, regular exercise, and stress management). Medication controls but does not cure hypertension.
- Instruct patient and family in proper technique for monitoring blood pressure. Advise patient to take blood pressure weekly and to report significant changes to health care professional.

Evaluation/Desired Outcomes
- Decrease in blood pressure.
- Decrease in frequency and severity of anginal attacks.
- Decrease in need for nitrate therapy.
- Increase in activity tolerance and sense of well-being.
- Suppression and prevention of atrial tachyarrhythmias.

HIGH ALERT

vinBLAStine (vin-blass-teen)
✱Velbe

Classification
Therapeutic: antineoplastics
Pharmacologic: vinca alkaloids

Pregnancy Category D

Indications
Combination chemotherapy of: Lymphomas, Nonseminomatous testicular carcinoma, Advanced breast cancer, Other tumors.

Action
Binds to proteins of mitotic spindle, causing metaphase arrest. Cell replication is stopped as a result (cell cycle–specific for M phase). **Therapeutic Effects:** Death of rapidly replicating cells, particularly malignant ones. Has immunosuppressive properties.

Pharmacokinetics
Absorption: Administered IV only, resulting in complete bioavailability.
Distribution: Does not cross the blood-brain barrier well.
Metabolism and Excretion: Converted by the liver to an active antineoplastic compound; excreted in the feces via biliary excretion, some renal elimination.
Half-life: 24 hr.

TIME/ACTION PROFILE (effects on white blood cell counts)

ROUTE	ONSET	PEAK	DURATION
IV	5–7 days	10 days	7–14 days

Contraindications/Precautions
Contraindicated in: Hypersensitivity; OB, Lactation: Pregnancy or lactation.
Use Cautiously in: Infection; ↓ bone marrow reserve; Patients with impaired hepatic function (↓ dose by 50% if serum bilirubin >3 mg/dL); OB: Instruct women of childbearing potential to avoid pregnancy during treatment.

Adverse Reactions/Side Effects
CNS: SEIZURES, mental depression, neurotoxicity, weakness. **Resp:** BRONCHOSPASM. **GI:** nausea, vomiting, anorexia, constipation, diarrhea, stomatitis. **GU:** gonadal suppression. **Derm:** alopecia, dermatitis, vesiculation. **Endo:** syndrome of inappropriate antidiuretic hormone (SIADH). **Hemat:** anemia, leukopenia, thrombocytopenia. **Local:** phlebitis at IV site. **Metab:** hyperuricemia. **Neuro:** neuritis, paresthesia, peripheral neuropathy.

Interactions
Drug-Drug: Additive bone marrow depression with other **antineoplastics** or **radiation therapy**. Bronchospasm may occur in patients who have been previously treated with **mitomycin**. May ↓ antibody response to **live-virus vaccines** and ↑ risk of adverse reactions. May ↓ **phenytoin** levels.

Route/Dosage
Doses may vary greatly, depending on tumor, schedule, condition of patient, and blood counts.

vinBLAStine

IV (Adults): *Initial*—3.7 mg/m² (100 mcg/kg), single dose; ↑ weekly as tolerated by 1.8 mg/m² (50 mcg/kg) to maximum of 18.5 mg/m² (usual dose is 5.5–7.4 mg/m²). *Maintenance*—10 mg 1–2 times/mo or one increment less than last dose q 7–14 days.

IV (Children): *Initial*—2.5 mg/m², single dose; ↑ weekly as tolerated by 1.25 mg/m² to maximum of 7.5 mg/m². *Maintenance*—one increment less than last dose q 7 days.

Availability (generic available)
Solution for injection: 1 mg/mL. **Powder for injection:** 10 mg/vial.

NURSING IMPLICATIONS

Assessment
- Monitor blood pressure, pulse, and respiratory rate during therapy. Notify physician immediately if respiratory distress occurs. Bronchospasm can be life-threatening and may occur at time of infusion or several hours to weeks later.
- Monitor for bone marrow depression. Assess for bleeding (bleeding gums, bruising, petechiae, guaiac stools, urine, and emesis) and avoid IM injections and taking rectal temperatures if platelet count is low. Apply pressure to venipuncture sites for 10 min. Assess for signs of infection during neutropenia. Anemia may occur. Monitor for increased fatigue, dyspnea, and orthostatic hypotension.
- May cause nausea and vomiting. Monitor intake and output, appetite, and nutritional intake. Prophylactic antiemetics may be used. Adjust diet as tolerated.
- Assess injection site frequently for redness, irritation, or inflammation. If extravasation occurs, infusion must be stopped and restarted elsewhere to avoid damage to subcut tissue. Standard treatment includes infiltration with hyaluronidase and application of heat.
- Monitor for symptoms of gout (increased uric acid, joint pain, edema). Encourage patient to drink at least 2 L of fluid per day. Allopurinol or alkalinization of urine may be used to decrease uric acid levels.
- *Lab Test Considerations:* Monitor CBC prior to and routinely throughout therapy. If WBC <2000, subsequent doses are usually withheld until WBC is ≥4000. The nadir of leukopenia occurs in 5–10 days and recovery usually occurs 7–14 days later. Thrombocytopenia may also occur in patients who have received radiation or other chemotherapy agents.
- Monitor liver function studies (AST, ALT, LDH, bilirubin) and renal function studies (BUN, creatinine) prior to and periodically throughout therapy.
- May cause ↑ uric acid. Monitor periodically during therapy.

Potential Nursing Diagnoses
Risk for infection (Adverse Reactions)
Imbalanced nutrition: less than body requirements (Adverse Reactions)

Implementation
- **High Alert:** Fatalities have occurred with chemotherapeutic agents. Before administering, clarify all ambiguous orders; double check single, daily, and course-of-therapy dose limits; have second practitioner independently double check original order, dose calculations, and infusion pump settings. Do not administer subcut, IM, or intrathecally (IT). IT administration is fatal. Vinblastine must be dispensed in an overwrap stating, "For IV use only." Overwrap should remain in place until immediately before administration.
- **High Alert:** Do not confuse vinblastine with vincristine.
- Solution should be prepared in a biologic cabinet. Wear gloves, gown, and mask while handling medication. Discard IV equipment in specially designated containers.
- Do not inject into extremities with impaired circulation; may cause thrombophlebitis.

IV Administration
- **Direct IV:** *Diluent:* Dilute each 10 mg with 10 mL of 0.9% NaCl for injection with phenol or benzyl alcohol. Solution is clear. Reconstituted medication is stable for 28 days if refrigerated. *Concentration:* 1 mg/mL. *Rate:* Administer each single dose over 1 min through Y-site injection of a free-flowing infusion of 0.9% NaCl or D5W.
- **Intermittent Infusion:** Dilution in large volumes (100–250 mL) or prolonged infusion (≥30 min) increases chance of vein irritation and extravasation.
- **Syringe Compatibility:** bleomycin, cisplatin, cyclophosphamide, droperidol, fluorouracil, leucovorin calcium, methotrexate, metoclopramide, mitomycin, vincristine.
- **Syringe Incompatibility:** furosemide.
- **Y-Site Compatibility:** allopurinol, amifostine, amphotericin B cholesteryl sulfate complex, az-

treonam, bleomycin, cisplatin, cyclophosphamide, doxorubicin, doxorubicin liposome, droperidol, etoposide phosphate, filgrastim, fludarabine, fluorouracil, gemcitabine, granisetron, heparin, leucovorin calcium, melphalan, methotrexate, metoclopramide, mitomycin, ondansetron, paclitaxel, pemetrexed, piperacillin/tazobactam, sargramostim, teniposide, thiotepa, vincristine, vinorelbine.
- **Y-Site Incompatibility:** cefepime, furosemide, lansoprazole.

Patient/Family Teaching
- Advise patient to notify health care professional if fever; chills; sore throat; signs of infection; bleeding gums; bruising; petechiae; or blood in urine, stool, or emesis occurs. Caution patient to avoid crowds and persons with known infections. Instruct patient to use soft toothbrush and electric razor. Caution patient not to drink alcoholic beverages or take products containing aspirin or NSAIDs.
- Instruct patient to inspect oral mucosa for redness and ulceration. Advise patient that, if ulceration occurs, to avoid spicy foods, use sponge brush, and rinse mouth with water after eating and drinking. Topical agents may be used if mouth pain interferes with eating. Stomatitis pain may require treatment with opioid analgesics.
- Instruct patient to report symptoms of neurotoxicity (paresthesia, pain, difficulty walking, persistent constipation).
- Advise patient that jaw pain, pain in organs containing tumor tissue, nausea, and vomiting may occur. Avoid constipation and report other adverse reactions.
- Advise patient that this medication may have teratogenic effects. Contraception should be used during and for at least 2 mo after therapy is concluded.
- Discuss with patient the possibility of hair loss. Explore coping strategies.
- Instruct patient not to receive any vaccinations without advice of health care professional.
- Emphasize need for periodic lab tests to monitor for side effects.

Evaluation/Desired Outcomes
- Regression of malignancy without the appearance of detrimental side effects.

HIGH ALERT

vinCRIStine (vin-kriss-teen)
Vincasar PFS

Classification
Therapeutic: antineoplastics
Pharmacologic: vinca alkaloids

Pregnancy Category D

Indications
Used alone and in combination with other treatment modalities (antineoplastics, surgery, or radiation therapy) in treatment of: Hodgkin's disease, Leukemias, Neuroblastoma, Malignant lymphomas, Rhabdomyosarcoma, Wilms' tumor, Other tumors.

Action
Binds to proteins of mitotic spindle, causing metaphase arrest. Cell replication is stopped as a result (cell cycle–specific for M phase). Has little or no effect on bone marrow. **Therapeutic Effects:** Death of rapidly replicating cells, particularly malignant ones. Has immunosuppressive properties.

Pharmacokinetics
Absorption: Administered IV only, resulting in complete bioavailability.
Distribution: Rapidly and widely distributed; extensively bound to tissues.
Metabolism and Excretion: Metabolized by the liver and eliminated in the feces via biliary excretion.
Half-life: 10.5–37.5 hr.

TIME/ACTION PROFILE (effects on blood counts†)

ROUTE	ONSET	PEAK	DURATION
IV	unknown	4 days	7 days

†Usually mild

Contraindications/Precautions
Contraindicated in: Hypersensitivity; OB, Lactation: Pregnancy or lactation.
Use Cautiously in: Infection; ↓ bone marrow reserve; Hepatic impairment (50% dose ↓ recommended if serum bilirubin >3 mg/dL); OB: Instruct women of childbearing potential to avoid pregnancy during treatment.

Adverse Reactions/Side Effects
CNS: agitation, insomnia, mental depression, mental status changes. **EENT:** cortical blindness, diplopia. **Resp:** bronchospasm. **GI:** <u>nausea</u>, <u>vomiting</u>, abdominal cramps, anorexia, constipation, ileus, stomatitis. **GU:** gonadal suppression, nocturia, oliguria, urinary retention. **Derm:** <u>alopecia</u>. **Endo:** syndrome of inappropriate antidiuretic hormone (SIADH). **Hemat:** anemia, leukopenia, thrombocytopenia (mild and brief). **Local:** <u>phlebitis</u> at IV site, tissue necrosis (from extravasa-

tion). **Metab:** hyperuricemia. **Neuro:** <u>ascending peripheral neuropathy</u>.

Interactions
Drug-Drug: Bronchospasm may occur in patients who have been previously treated with **mitomycin**. **L-asparaginase** may ↓ hepatic metabolism of vincristine (give vincristine 12–24 hr prior to asparaginase). May ↓ antibody response to **live-virus vaccines** and ↑ risk of adverse reactions.

Route/Dosage
Many other protocols are used.
IV (Adults): 10–30 mcg/kg (0.4–1.4 mg/m^2); may repeat weekly (not to exceed 2 mg/dose).
IV (Children >10 kg): 1.5–2 mg/m^2 single dose; may repeat weekly.
IV (Children <10 kg): 50 mcg/kg single dose; may repeat weekly.

Availability (generic available)
Solution for injection: 1 mg/mL.

NURSING IMPLICATIONS

Assessment
- Monitor blood pressure, pulse, and respiratory rate during therapy. Report significant changes.
- Monitor neurologic status. Assess for paresthesia (numbness, tingling, pain), loss of deep tendon reflexes (Achilles reflex is usually first involved), weakness (wrist drop or footdrop, gait disturbances), cranial nerve palsies (jaw pain, hoarseness, ptosis, visual changes), autonomic dysfunction (ileus, difficulty voiding, orthostatic hypotension, impaired sweating), and CNS dysfunction (decreased level of consciousness, agitation, hallucinations). Notify physician if these symptoms develop, as they may persist for months.
- Monitor intake and output ratios and daily weight; report significant discrepancies. Decreased urine output with concurrent hyponatremia may indicate SIADH, which usually responds to fluid restriction.
- Assess infusion site frequently for redness, irritation, or inflammation. If extravasation occurs, infusion must be stopped and restarted elsewhere to avoid damage to subcut tissue. Cellulitis and discomfort may be minimized by infiltration with hyaluronidase and application of moderate heat or by application of cold compresses.
- Assess nutritional status. An antiemetic may be used to minimize nausea and vomiting.
- Monitor for symptoms of gout (increased uric acid, joint pain, edema). Encourage patient to drink at least 2 liters of fluid per day. Allopurinol or alkalinization of urine may be used to decrease uric acid levels.
- *Lab Test Considerations:* Monitor CBC prior to and periodically throughout therapy. May cause slight leukopenia 4 days after therapy, which resolves within 7 days. Platelet count may ↑ or ↓.
- Monitor liver function studies (AST, ALT, LDH, bilirubin) and renal function studies (BUN, creatinine) prior to and periodically throughout therapy.
- May cause ↑ uric acid. Monitor periodically during therapy.

Potential Nursing Diagnoses
Risk for injury (Adverse Reactions)
Imbalanced nutrition: less than body requirements (Adverse Reactions)

Implementation
- *High Alert:* Fatalities have occurred with chemotherapeutic agents. Before administering, clarify all ambiguous orders; double check single, daily, and course-of-therapy dose limits; have second practitioner independently double check original order, dose calculations, and infusion pump settings. Do not administer subcut, IM, or intrathecally (IT). IT administration is fatal. Vincristine must be dispensed in an overwrap stating "For IV use only." Overwrap should remain in place until immediately before administration. Do not confuse vincristine with vinblastine.
- Solution should be prepared in a biologic cabinet. Wear gloves, gown, and mask while handling medication. Discard IV equipment in specially designated containers (see Appendix L).

IV Administration
- **Direct IV:** *Diluent:* Does not need to be reconstituted. *Concentration:* Administer undiluted at 1 mg/mL. *Rate:* Administer each dose direct IV push over 1 min through Y-site injection of a free-flowing infusion of 0.9% NaCl or D5W.
- **Syringe Compatibility:** bleomycin, cisplatin, cyclophosphamide, doxapram, doxorubicin, droperidol, fluorouracil, heparin, leucovorin calcium, methotrexate, metoclopramide, mitomycin, vinblastine.
- **Syringe Incompatibility:** furosemide.

vinorelbine

- **Y-Site Compatibility:** allopurinol, amifostine, amphotericin B cholesteryl sulfate complex, aztreonam, bleomycin, cisplatin, cyclophosphamide, doxorubicin, doxorubicin liposome, droperidol, etoposide phosphate, filgrastim, fludarabine, fluorouracil, gemcitabine, granisetron, heparin, leucovorin calcium, linezolid, melphalan, methotrexate, metoclopramide, mitomycin, ondansetron, oxaliplatin, paclitaxel, pemetrexed, piperacillin/tazobactam, sargramostim, teniposide, thiotepa, topotecan, vinblastine, vinorelbine.
- **Y-Site Incompatibility:** cefepime, furosemide, idarubicin, lansoprazole, sodium bicarbonate.

Patient/Family Teaching
- Instruct patient to notify health care professional immediately if redness, swelling, or pain at injection site occurs.
- Instruct patient to report symptoms of neurotoxicity (paresthesia, pain, difficulty walking, persistent constipation). Inform patient that increased fluid intake, dietary fiber, and exercise may minimize constipation. Stool softeners or laxatives may be used. Patient should inform health care professional if severe constipation or abdominal discomfort occurs, as this may be a sign of neuropathy.
- Advise patient to notify health care professional if fever; chills; sore throat; signs of infection; bleeding gums; bruising; petechiae; blood in urine, stool, or emesis; or mouth sores occur. Caution patient to avoid crowds and persons with known infections.
- Advise patient that this medication may have teratogenic effects. Contraception should be used during and for at least 2 mo after therapy is concluded.
- Discuss with patient the possibility of hair loss. Explore coping strategies.
- Instruct patient not to receive any vaccinations without advice of health care professional.
- Emphasize need for periodic lab tests to monitor for side effects.

Evaluation/Desired Outcomes
- Regression of malignancy without the appearance of detrimental side effects.

HIGH ALERT

vinorelbine (vine-oh-rel-been)
Navelbine

Classification
Therapeutic: antineoplastics
Pharmacologic: vinca alkaloids

Pregnancy Category D

Indications
Inoperable non–small-cell cancer of the lung in ambulatory patients (alone or with cisplatin).

Action
Binds to a protein (tubulin) of cellular microtubules, where it interferes with microtubule assembly. Cell replication is stopped as a result (cell cycle–specific for M phase). **Therapeutic Effects:** Death of rapidly replicating cells, particularly malignant ones.

Pharmacokinetics
Absorption: IV administration results in complete bioavailability.
Distribution: Highly bound to platelets and lymphocytes.
Metabolism and Excretion: Mostly metabolized by the liver. At least one metabolite is active. Large amounts eliminated in feces; 11% excreted unchanged by the kidneys.
Half-life: 28–44 hr.

TIME/ACTION PROFILE (effect on WBCs)

ROUTE	ONSET	PEAK	DURATION
IV	unknown	7–10 days	7–15 days

Contraindications/Precautions
Contraindicated in: Hypersensitivity; Active infections; ↓ bone marrow reserve; OB, Lactation: Pregnancy or lactation.
Use Cautiously in: Impaired hepatic function (dose ↓ recommended if total bilirubin >2 mg/dL); Debilitated patients (↑ risk of hyponatremia); Granulocytopenic patients (temporarily discontinue or reduce dose); Pedi: Safety not established; OB: Instruct women of childbearing potential to avoid pregnancy during treatment.

Adverse Reactions/Side Effects
CNS: fatigue. **Resp:** shortness of breath. **CV:** chest pain. **GI:** constipation, nausea, abdominal pain, anorexia, diarrhea, transient ↑ in liver enzymes, vomiting. **Derm:** alopecia, rashes. **F and E:** hyponatremia. **Hemat:** anemia, neutropenia, thrombocytopenia. **Local:** irritation at IV site, skin reactions, phlebitis. **MS:** arthralgia, back pain, jaw pain, myalgia. **Neuro:** neurotoxicity. **Misc:** pain in tumor-containing tissue.

Interactions
Drug-Drug: ↑ bone marrow depression with other **antineoplastics** or **radiation therapy**.

vinorelbine 1283

Concurrent use with **cisplatin** ↑ risk and severity of bone marrow depression. Concurrent use with **mitomycin** or **chest radiation** ↑ risk of pulmonary reactions.

Route/Dosage
IV (Adults): 30 mg/m² once weekly.

Hepatic Impairment
IV (Adults): *Total bilirubin 2.1–3 mg/dL*—15 mg/m² once weekly; *total bilirubin ≥3 mg/dL*—7.5 mg/m² once weekly.

Availability (generic available)
Solution for injection: 10 mg/mL.

NURSING IMPLICATIONS

Assessment
- Monitor blood pressure, pulse, and respiratory rate during therapy. Note significant changes. Acute shortness of breath and severe bronchospasm may occur infrequently shortly after administration. Treatment with corticosteroids, bronchodilators, and supplemental oxygen may be required, especially in patients with a history of pulmonary disease.
- Assess frequently for signs of infection (sore throat, temperature, cough, mental status changes), especially when nadir of granulocytopenia is expected.
- Monitor neurologic status. Assess for paresthesia (numbness, tingling, pain), loss of deep tendon reflexes (Achilles reflex is usually first involved), weakness (wrist drop or footdrop, gait disturbances), cranial nerve palsies (jaw pain, hoarseness, ptosis, visual changes), autonomic dysfunction (constipation, ileus, difficulty voiding, orthostatic hypotension, impaired sweating), and CNS dysfunction (decreased level of consciousness, agitation, hallucinations). These symptoms may persist for months. The incidence of neurotoxicity associated with vinorelbine is less than that of other vinca alkaloids.
- Monitor intake and output and daily weight for significant discrepancies.
- Assess nutritional status. Mild to moderate nausea is common. An antiemetic may be used to minimize nausea and vomiting.
- Monitor for symptoms of gout (increased uric acid, joint pain, edema). Encourage patient to drink at least 2 L of fluid/day. Allopurinol and alkalinization of urine may decrease uric acid levels.
- *Lab Test Considerations:* Monitor CBC prior to each dose and routinely during therapy. The nadir of granulocytopenia usually occurs 7–10 days after vinorelbine administration and recovery usually follows within 7–15 days. If granulocyte count is <1500/mm³, dose reduction or temporary interruption of vinorelbine may be warranted. If repeated episodes of fever and/or sepsis occur during granulocytopenia, future dose of vinorelbine should be modified. May also cause mild to moderate anemia. Thrombocytopenia rarely occurs.
- Monitor liver function studies (AST, ALT, LDH, bilirubin) and renal function studies (BUN, creatinine) prior to and periodically during therapy. May cause ↑ uric acid; monitor periodically during therapy.

Potential Nursing Diagnoses
Risk for injury (Adverse Reactions)
Risk for infection (Adverse Reactions)

Implementation
- **High Alert:** Fatalities have occurred with chemotherapeutic agents. Before administering, clarify all ambiguous orders; double check single, daily, and course-of-therapy dose limits; have second practitioner independently double check original order, dose calculations, and infusion pump settings.
- Solution should be prepared in a biologic cabinet. Wear gloves, gown, and mask while handling medication. Discard IV equipment in specially designated containers.
- Assess infusion site frequently for redness, irritation, or inflammation. Vinorelbine is a vesicant. If extravasation occurs, infusion must be stopped and restarted elsewhere to avoid damage to subcut tissue. Treatment of extravasation includes application of warm compresses applied over the area immediately for 30–60 min, then alternating on/off every 15 min for 1 day to increase systemic absorption of the drug. Hyaluronidase 150 units diluted in 1–2 mL of 0.9% NaCl, 1 mL for each mL extravasated, should be injected through existing IV cannula or subcut if the needle has been removed to enhance absorption and dispersion of the extravasated drug.

IV Administration
- **Direct IV:** *Diluent:* Dilute vinorelbine with 0.9% NaCl or D5W. *Concentration:* 1.5–3 mg/mL. *Rate:* Infuse over 6–10 min into Y-

VITAMIN B₁₂ PREPARATIONS

site closest to bag of a free-flowing IV or into a central line.
- Flush vein with at least 75–125 mL of 0.9% NaCl or D5W administered over 10 min or more following administration of vinorelbine.
- **Intermittent Infusion:** *Diluent:* Dilute vinorelbine with 0.9% NaCl, D5W, 0.45% NaCl, D5/0.45% NaCl, Ringer's or lactated Ringer's injection. Solution should be colorless to pale yellow. Do not administer solutions that are discolored or contain particulate matter. Diluted solution is stable for 24 hr at room temperature. *Concentration:* 0.5–2 mg/mL. *Rate:* Infuse over 6–10 min (up to 30 min) into Y-site closest to bag of a free-flowing IV or into a central line.
- Flush vein with at least 75–125 mL of 0.9% NaCl or D5W administered over 10 min or more following administration of vinorelbine.
- **Y-Site Compatibility:** amikacin, aztreonam, bleomycin, bumetanide, buprenorphine, butorphanol, calcium gluconate, carboplatin, carmustine, cefotaxime, ceftazidime, ceftizoxime, chlorpromazine, cimetidine, cisplatin, clindamycin, cyclophosphamide, cytarabine, dacarbazine, dactinomycin, daunorubicin, dexamethasone sodium phosphate, diphenhydramine, doxorubicin, doxorubicin liposome, doxycycline, droperidol, enalaprilat, etoposide, famotidine, filgrastim, floxuridine, fluconazole, fludarabine, gemcitabine, gentamicin, granisetron, haloperidol, hydrocortisone, hydromorphone, idarubicin, ifosfamide, imipenem/cilastatin, lorazepam, mannitol, mechlorethamine, melphalan, meperidine, mesna, methotrexate, metoclopramide, metronidazole, mitoxantrone, morphine, nalbuphine, ondansetron, oxaliplatin, potassium chloride, prochlorperazine, promethazine, ranitidine, streptozocin, teniposide, ticarcillin/clavulanate, tobramycin, vancomycin, vinblastine, vincristine, zidovudine.
- **Y-Site Incompatibility:** acyclovir, allopurinol, aminophylline, amphotericin B, amphotericin B cholesteryl sulfate, ampicillin, cefazolin, ceftriaxone, cefuroxime, fluorouracil, furosemide, ganciclovir, lansoprazole, methylprednisolone, mitomycin, sodium bicarbonate, thiotepa, trimethoprim/sulfamethoxazole.

Patient/Family Teaching
- Instruct patient to report symptoms of neurotoxicity (paresthesia, pain, difficulty walking, persistent constipation).
- Inform patient that increased fluid intake, dietary fiber, and exercise may minimize constipation. Stool softeners or laxatives may be necessary. Patient should be advised to report severe constipation or abdominal discomfort, as this may be a sign of ileus, which may occur as a consequence of neuropathy.
- Advise patient to notify health care professional if fever; chills; sore throat; signs of infection; bleeding gums; bruising; petechiae; blood in urine, stool, or emesis; or mouth sores occur.
- Caution patient to avoid crowds and persons with known infections.
- Advise patient that this medication may have teratogenic effects. Contraception should be used during and for at least 2 mo after therapy is concluded.
- Discuss with patient the possibility of hair loss and explore coping strategies.
- Instruct patient not to receive any vaccinations without advice of health care professional.
- Emphasize the need for periodic lab tests to monitor for side effects.

Evaluation/Desired Outcomes
- Decrease in the size or spread of malignancy without detrimental side effects.

VITAMIN B₁₂ PREPARATIONS

cyanocobalamin
(sye-an-oh-koe-**bal**-a-min)
Nascobal, Rubramin PC

hydroxocobalamin
(hye-drox-oh-koe-**bal**-a-min)
Cyanokit

Classification
Therapeutic: antianemics, vitamins
Pharmacologic: water soluble vitamins

Pregnancy Category C

Indications
Vitamin B₁₂ deficiency (parenteral product or nasal spray should be used when deficiency is due to malabsorption). Pernicious anemia (only parenteral products should be used for initial therapy; nasal or oral products are not indicated until patients have achieved hematologic remission following parenteral therapy and have no signs of CNS involvement). Part of the Schilling test (vitamin B₁₂ absorption test) (diagnostic). Cyanide poisoning (Cyanokit only).

Action
Necessary coenzyme for metabolic processes, including fat and carbohydrate metabolism and protein synthesis. Required for cell production

and hematopoiesis. **Therapeutic Effects:** Corrects manifestations of pernicious anemia (megaloblastic indices, GI lesions, and neurologic damage). Corrects vitamin B_{12} deficiency. Reverses symptoms of cyanide toxicity (Cyanokit only).

Pharmacokinetics
Absorption: Oral absorption in GI tract requires intrinsic factor and calcium; well absorbed after IM, subcut and nasal administration.
Distribution: Stored in the liver and bone marrow; crosses placenta, enters breast milk.
Metabolism and Excretion: Primarily excreted unchanged in urine.
Half-life: *Cyanocobalamin*—6 days (400 days in liver); *Hydroxocobalamin*—26–31 hr.

TIME/ACTION PROFILE (reticulocytosis)

ROUTE	ONSET	PEAK	DURATION
Cyanocobalamin IM, subcut, nasal	unknown	3–10 days	unknown
Hydroxocobalamin IM	unknown	unknown	unknown

Contraindications/Precautions
Contraindicated in: Hypersensitivity; Pedi: Avoid using preparations containing benzyl alcohol in premature infants (associated with fatal "gasping syndrome").
Use Cautiously in: Hereditary optic nerve atrophy (accelerates nerve damage); Uremia, folic acid deficiency, concurrent infection, iron deficiency (response to B_{12} will be impaired); Renal dysfunction (when using aluminum-containing products); Pedi: *Cyanokit*—Safety and effectiveness not established.

Adverse Reactions/Side Effects
CNS: headache; *Cyanokit*, dizziness, memory impairment, restlessness. **CV:** heart failure; *Cyanokit*, hypertension, chest pain, tachycardia. **EENT:** *Cyanokit*—dry throat, eye redness, eye swelling. **GI:** diarrhea; *Cyanokit*, abdominal discomfort, dyspepsia, dysphagia, hematochezia, nausea, vomiting. **Derm:** itching; *Cyanokit*, erythema, rash. **F and E:** hypokalemia. **GU:** *Cyanokit*—red urine. **Hemat:** thrombocytosis. **Resp:** pulmonary edema; *Cyanokit*, dyspnea. **Local:** pain at IM site. **Misc:** hypersensitivity reactions including ANAPHYLAXIS.

Interactions
Drug-Drug: Chloramphenicol and **antineoplastics** may ↓ hematologic response to vitamin B_{12}. **Colchicine, aminosalicylic acid, cimetidine**, and excess intake of **alcohol**, or **vitamin C** may ↓ oral absorption/effectiveness of vitamin B_{12}.

Route/Dosage

Cyanocobalamin (oral products are usually not recommended due to poor absorption and should be used only if patient refuses the IM, deep subcutaneous, or intranasal route of administration)

PO (Adults and Children): *Vitamin B_{12} deficiency*—amount depends on deficiency (up to 1000 mcg/day have been used).

PO (Adults): *Pernicious anemia (for hematologic remission only)*—1000–2000 mcg/day.

IM, Subcut (Adults): *Vitamin B_{12} deficiency*—30 mcg/day for 5–10 days, then 100–200 mcg/month. *Pernicious anemia*—100 mcg/day for 6–7 days; if improvement, give same dose every other day for 7 doses, then every 3–4 days for 2–3 wk; once hematologic values return to normal (remission), can give maintenance dose of 100 mcg/month (doses up to 1000 mcg have been used for maintenance) (could alternatively use oral or intranasal formulations below for maintenance at specified doses). *Schilling test*—Flushing dose is 1000 mcg.

IM, Subcut (Children): *Vitamin B_{12} deficiency*—0.2 mcg/kg for 2 days, then 1000 mcg/day for 2–7 days, then 100 mcg/week for 1 month. *Pernicious anemia*-30–50 mcg/day for 2 or more weeks (to a total dose of 1000–5000 mcg), then give maintenance dose of 100 mcg/month (doses up to 1000 mcg have been used for maintenance).

Intranasal (Adults): *Vitamin B_{12} deficiency*—500 mcg (one spray) in one nostril once weekly. *Pernicious anemia (for hematologic remission only)*—500 mcg (one spray) in one nostril once weekly.

Hydroxocobalamin

IM (Adults): *Vitamin B_{12} deficiency*—30 mcg/day for 5–10 days, then 100–200 mcg/month. *Pernicious anemia*—100 mcg/day for 6–7 days; if improvement, give same dose every other day for 7 doses, then every 3–4 days for 2–3 wk; once hematologic values return to normal (remis-

sion), give maintenance dose of 100 mcg/month. *Schilling test*—Flushing dose is 1000 mcg.
IM (Children): *Vitamin B_{12} deficiency*—100 mcg/day for 2 or more weeks (to achieve total dose of 1000–5000 mcg), then 30–50 mcg/month. *Pernicious anemia*—30–50 mcg/day for 2 or more weeks (to achieve total dose of 1000–5000 mcg), then 100 mcg/month.
IV (Adults): *Cyanide poisoning (Cyanokit only)*—5 g over 15 min; another 5 g dose may be infused over 15–120 min depending upon severity of poisoning (maximum cumulative dose = 10 g).

Availability

Cyanocobalamin (generic available)
Tablets: 50 mcg^OTC, 100 mcg^OTC, 250 mcg^OTC, 500 mcg^OTC, 1000 mcg^OTC, 5000 mcg^OTC. **Extended-release tablets:** 1000 mcg^OTC, 1500 mcg^OTC. **Sublingual tablets:** 2500 mcg^OTC. **Lozenges:** 100 mcg^OTC, 250 mcg^OTC, 500 mcg^OTC. **Nasal spray:** 500 mcg/0.1 mL actuation (8 sprays/bottle). **Injection:** 1000 mcg/mL in 1-, 10- and 30-mL vials.

Hydroxocobalamin (generic available)
Injection: 1000 mcg/mL in 30-mL vials. **Powder for injection (Cyanokit):** 2.5 g/vial (2 vials in each kit).

NURSING IMPLICATIONS

Assessment
- Assess patient for signs of vitamin B_{12} deficiency (pallor; neuropathy; psychosis; red, inflamed tongue) before and periodically during therapy.
- *Lab Test Considerations:* Monitor plasma folic acid, vitamin B_{12}, and iron levels, hemoglobin, hemtaocrit, and reticulocyte count before treatment, 1 mo after the start of therapy, and then every 3–6 mo. Evaluate serum potassium level in patients receiving vitamin B_{12} for pernicious anemia for hypokalemia during the first 48 hr of treatment. Serum potassium and platelet counts should be monitored routinely during the course of therapy.
- **Cyanokit:** Management of cyanide poisoning should also include establishment of airway, ensuring adequate oxygenation and hydration, cardiovascular support, and seizure management. Monitor BP and HR continuously during and after infusion and immediately report significant changes. The maximal ↑ in BP usually occurs toward the end of the infusion. BP usually returns to baseline within 4 hr of drug administration.

Potential Nursing Diagnoses
Imbalanced nutrition: less than body requirements (Indications)
Activity intolerance (Indications)

Implementation
- Usually administered in combination with other vitamins; solitary vitamin B_{12} deficiencies are rare.
- Administration of vitamin B_{12} by the oral route is useful only for nutritional deficiencies. Patients with small-bowel disease, malabsorption syndrome, or gastric or ileal resections require parenteral administration.
- **PO:** Administer with meals to increase absorption.
- May be mixed with fruit juices. Administer immediately after mixing; ascorbic acid alters stability.
- **Intranasal:** Dose should not be administered within 1 hr of hot food or liquids (these substances may result in the formation of nasal secretions which may result in ↓ effectiveness of nasal spray).
- **IM, Subcut:** Vials should be protected from light.
- If subcutaneous route used, deep subcutaneous administration is preferred.

IV Administration
- **IV:** IV route should only be used with Cyanokit.
- **Intermittent Infusion:** *Diluent:* Dilute each Cyanokit vial with 100 mL of 0.9% NaCl, D5W, or LR. Gently invert the vial for at least 30 sec prior to infusion. Reconstituted vial can be hung for infusion and is stable for 6 hr at room temperature. Discard any unused solution after 6 hr. *Rate:* Administer initial 5-g dose over 15 min. Administer additional 5-g dose over 15–120 min.
- **Y-Site Incompatibility:** ascorbic acid, blood products, sodium nitrite, sodium thiosulfate.
- **Additive Incompatibility:** diazepam, dobutamine, dopamine, fentanyl, nitroglycerin, pentobarbital, propofol, thiopental.

Patient/Family Teaching
- Encourage patient to comply with diet recommendations of health care professional. Explain that the best source of vitamins is a well-balanced diet with foods from the four basic food groups.
- Foods high in vitamin B_{12} include meats, seafood, egg yolk, and fermented cheeses; few vitamins are lost with ordinary cooking.
- Patients self-medicating with vitamin supplements should be cautioned not to exceed RDA.

Effectiveness of megadoses for treatment of various medical conditions is unproved and may cause side effects.
- Inform patients with pernicious anemia of the lifelong need for vitamin B_{12} replacement.
- Emphasize the importance of follow-up exams to evaluate progress.
- **Intranasal:** Instruct patient in proper administration technique. Review *Patient Information Sheet* and demonstrate use of actuator. Unit must be primed with 3 strokes upon using for the first time. Unit must be primed with 1 stroke before each of the remaining doses. Advise patient to clear nose, then place tip approximately 1 inch into nostril and press pump once, firmly and quickly. After dose, remove unit from nose and massage dosed nostril gently for a few seconds. Vial delivers 8 doses. Unit should be stored at room temperature and protected from light.
- **Intermittent Infusion:** Advise patient that skin redness may last up to 2 wk and that their urine may remain red for up to 5 wk after drug administration. Instruct patient to avoid sun exposure while their skin is red. Advise patient to contact health care professional if skin or urine redness persist after these time periods. Advise patient that a rash may develop from 7–28 days after drug administration. It will usually resolve without treatment within a few weeks. Advise patient to contact health care professional if rash persists after this time period.

Evaluation/Desired Outcomes
- Resolution of the symptoms of vitamin B_{12} deficiency.
- Increase in reticulocyte count.
- Improvement in manifestations of pernicious anemia.
- Resolution of symptoms of cyanide poisoning.

VITAMIN D COMPOUNDS

calcitriol (kal-si-**trye**-ole)
1,25-dihydroxycholecalciferol, Calcijex, Rocaltrol, vitamin D_3 (active)

cholecalciferol
Delta-D, vitamin D_3 (inactive)

doxercalciferol
(**dox**-er-kal-**sif**-e-role)
Hectorol, vitamin D_2

ergocalciferol
(**er**-goe-kal-**sif**-e-role)
Drisdol, ✦Ostoforte, vitamin D_2

paricalcitol (par-i-**kal**-si-tole)
Zemplar

Classification
Therapeutic: vitamins
Pharmacologic: fat-soluble vitamins

Pregnancy Category B (doxercalciferol), C (calcitriol, cholecalciferol, ergocalciferol, paricalcitol)

Indications
Calcitriol: Management of hypocalcemia in chronic renal dialysis (IV and PO). Treatment of hypocalcemia in patients with hypoparathyroidism or pseudohypoparathyroidism (PO only). Management of secondary hyperparathyroidism and resulting metabolic bone disease in predialysis patients with moderate to severe renal insufficiency (CCr 15–55 mL/min) (PO only). **Cholecalciferol:** Treatment or prevention of vitamin D deficiency. **Doxercalciferol:** Treatment of secondary hyperparathyroidism in patients undergoing chronic renal dialysis (IV and PO). Treatment of secondary hyperparathyroidism in patients with Stage 3 or 4 chronic kidney disease (PO only). **Ergocalciferol:** Treatment of familial hypophosphatemia. Treatment of hypoparathyroidism. Treatment of vitamin D-resistant rickets. **Paricalcitol:** Prevention and treatment of secondary hyperparathyroidism in patients with Stage 3 or 4 (PO) or Stage 5 (PO and IV) chronic kidney disease.

Action
Cholecalciferol requires activation in the liver and kidneys to create the active form of vitamin D_3 (calcitriol). Doxercalciferol and ergocalciferol require activation in the liver to create the active form of vitamin D_2. Paricalcitol is a synthetic analogue of calcitriol. Vitamin D: Promotes the absorption of calcium and ↓ parathyroid hormone concentration. **Therapeutic Effects:** Treatment and prevention of deficiency states, particularly bone manifestations. Improved calcium and phosphorous homeostasis in patients with chronic kidney disease.

Pharmacokinetics
Absorption: *Calcitriol, doxercalciferol, ergocalciferol, paricalcitol*—Well absorbed follow-

ing oral administration. *Calcitriol, doxercalciferol, paricalcitol*—IV administration results in complete bioavailability.
Distribution: Calcitriol and paricalcitol cross the placenta; calcitriol also enters breast milk.
Protein Binding: *Calcitriol and paricalcitol*—99.9%.
Metabolism and Excretion: *Calcitriol*—Undergoes enterohepatic recycling and is excreted mostly in bile. *Cholecalciferol*—Converted by the liver and kidneys to calcitriol (active form of vitamin D_3. *Ergocalciferol*—Converted to active form of vitamin D_2 by sunlight, the liver, and the kidneys. *Doxercalciferol*—Converted by the liver to the active form of vitamin D_2. *Paricalcitol*—mostly metabolized by the liver and excreted via hepatobiliary elimination.
Half-life: *Calcitriol*—5–8 hr. *Cholecalciferol*—14 hr. *Doxercalciferol*—32–37 hr (up to 96 hr). *Paricalcitol*—14–20 hr.

TIME/ACTION PROFILE (effects on serum calcium)

ROUTE	ONSET	PEAK	DURATION
Calcitriol-PO	2–6 hr	2–6 hr	3–5 days
Calcitriol-IV	unknown	unknown	unknown
Cholecalciferol-PO	unknown	unknown	unknown
Doxercalciferol PO	unknown	8 wk	1 wk
Doxercalciferol-IV	unknown	8 wk	1 wk
Ergocalciferol-PO	12–24 hr	unknown	up to 6 mo
Paricalcitol-PO	unknown	2–4 wk	unknown
Paricalitol IV	unknown	up to 2 wk	unknown

Contraindications/Precautions
Contraindicated in: Hypersensitivity; Hypercalcemia; Vitamin D toxicity; Lactation: Potential for serious adverse reactions in infant; Concurrent use of magnesium-containing antacids or other vitamin D supplements; **Ergocalciferol**: Known intolerance to tartrazine; **Cholecalciferol and ergocalciferol**: Malabsorption problems.
Use Cautiously in: Calcitriol, doxercalciferol, paricalcitol: Patients receiving digoxin; OB: Pregnancy (safety not established).

Adverse Reactions/Side Effects
Seen primarily as manifestations of toxicity (hypercalcemia).
CNS: headache, somnolence, weakness; *doxercalciferol,* dizziness, malaise. **EENT:** conjunctivitis, photophobia, rhinorrhea. **Resp:** *doxercalciferol and ergocalciferol*—dyspnea. **CV:** arrhythmias, edema, hypertension; *doxercalciferol,* bradycardia; *paricalcitol,* palpitations. **GI:** PANCREATITIS, abdominal pain, anorexia, constipation, dry mouth, liver function test elevation, metallic taste, nausea, polydipsia, vomiting, weight loss. **GU:** albuminuria, azotemia, decreased libido, nocturia, polyuria. **Derm:** pruritus. **F and E:** hypercalcemia. **Metab:** hyperthermia. **MS:** bone pain, muscle pain; *doxercalciferol,* arthralgia; *paricalcitol,* metastatic calcification. **Local:** pain at injection site. **Misc:** *calcitriol*—allergic reactions, chills, fever.

Interactions
Drug-Drug: Cholestyramine, colestipol, or **mineral oil** ↓ absorption of vitamin D analogues. Use with **thiazide diuretics** may result in hypercalcemia. **Corticosteroids** ↓ effectiveness of vitamin D analogues. Using calcitriol, doxercalciferol, or paricalcitol with **digoxin** may ↑ risk of arrhythmias. Vitamin D requirements ↓ by **phenytoin** and other **hydantoin anticonvulsants, sucralfate, barbiturates,** and **primidone**. Concurrent use with **magnesium-containing drugs** may lead to hypermagnesemia. Concurrent use of **calcium-containing drugs** may ↑ risk of hypercalcemia. Concurrent use of other **Vitamin D supplements** may ↑ risk of hypercalcemia. **Agents that induce liver enzymes (phenobarbital, rifampin)** and **agents that inhibit liver enzymes (atazanavir, clarithromycin, erythromycin, indinavir, itraconazole, ketoconazole, nefazodone, nelfinavir, ritonavir, saquinavir, verapamil, voriconazole)** may alter requirements for doxercalciferol and paricalcitol (monitoring of calcium and phosphorus recommended).
Drug-Food: Ingestion of **foods high in calcium content** (see Appendix M) may lead to hypercalcemia.

Route/Dosage
Calcitriol
PO (Adults): *Hypocalcemia during dialysis*—0.25 mcg/day or every other day; if needed, may ↑ by 0.25 mcg/day at 4–8 wk intervals (typical dosage = 0.5–1 mcg/day). *Hypoparathyroidism*—0.25 mcg/day initially; if needed, may ↑ dose by 0.25 mcg/day at 2–4 wk intervals (typical dosage = 0.5–2 mcg/day). *Predialysis patients*—0.25 mcg/day (up to 0.5 mcg/day).
PO (Children): *Hypocalcemia during dialysis*—0.25–2 mcg/day. *Hypoparathyroidism (children ≥6 yr)*—0.25 mcg/day initially; if needed, may ↑ dose by 0.25 mcg/day at 2–4 wk intervals (typical dosage = 0.5–2 mcg/day). *Hypoparathyroidism (children 1–5 yr)*—0.25–

VITAMIN D COMPOUNDS

0.75 mcg/day. *Hypoparathyroidism (children <1 yr)*—0.04–0.08 mcg/kg/day. *Predialysis patients (children ≥3 yr)*—0.25 mcg/day (up to 0.5 mcg/day). *Predialysis patients (children <3 yr)*—10–15 ng/kg/day.

IV (Adults): *Hypocalcemia during dialysis*—0.5 mcg (0.01 mcg/kg) 3 times weekly. May be increased by 0.25–0.5 mcg/dose at 2-4 wk intervals (typical maintenance dose = 0.5–3.0 mcg 3 times weekly [0.01–0.05 mcg/kg 3 times weekly]).

IV (Children): *Hypocalcemia during dialysis*-0.01–0.05 mcg/kg 3 times weekly.

Cholecalciferol
PO (Adults): 400–1000 units daily.

Doxercalciferol
PO (Adults): *Dialysis patients*—10 mcg 3 times weekly (at dialysis); dose may be adjusted by 2.5 mcg at 8-wk intervals based on intact PTH concentrations (maximum dose = 20 mcg 3 times weekly). *Non-dialysis patients*—1 mcg/day; dose may be adjusted by 0.5 mcg at 2 wk intervals based on intact PTH concentrations (maximum dose = 3.5 mcg/day).

IV (Adults): 4 mcg 3 times weekly at the end of dialysis; dose may be adjusted by 1–2 mcg at 8-wk intervals based on intact PTH concentrations (maximum dose = 6 mcg 3 times weekly).

Ergocalciferol
PO (Adults): *Vitamin D–resistant rickets*—12,000–500,000 units/day (to be used with phosphate supplement). *Familial hypophosphatemia*—10,000–80,000 units/day (with phosphorus 1–2 g/day). *Hypoparathyroidism*—50,000–200,000 units/day (to be used with calcium supplement).

PO (Children): *Vitamin D–resistant rickets*—40,000–80,000 units/day (to be used with phosphate supplement). *Familial hypophosphatemia*—10,000–80,000 units/day (with phosphorus 1–2 g/day). *Hypoparathyroidism*—50,000–200,000 units/day (to be used with calcium supplement).

Paricalcitol

Stage 3 or 4 Chronic Kidney Disease
PO (Adults): *Baseline intact PTH concentration ≤500 pg/mL*—Initiate with 1 mcg/day or 2 mcg 3 times weekly; dose can be adjusted at 2–4 wk intervals based on intact PTH, calcium, and phosphate concentrations. *Baseline intact PTH concentration >500 pg/mL*—Initiate with 2 mcg/day or 4 mcg 3 times weekly; dose can be adjusted at 2–4 wk intervals based on intact PTH, calcium, and phosphate concentrations.

Stage 5 Chronic Kidney Disease
PO (Adults): Initial dose (in mcg) is based on following equation: baseline intact PTH concentration (pg/mL)/80; dose should be given 3 times weekly; dose can be adjusted at 2–4 wk intervals based on intact PTH, calcium, and phosphate concentrations.

IV (Adults and Children ≥5 yr): 0.04–0.1 mcg/kg 3 times weekly during dialysis; dose can be adjusted by 2–4 mcg at 2–4 wk intervals based on intact PTH, calcium, and phosphate concentrations (doses up to 0.24 mcg/kg have been used).

Availability

Calcitriol (generic available)
Capsules: 0.25 mcg, 0.5 mcg. **Oral solution:** 1 mcg/mL. **Solution for injection:** 1 mcg/mL.

Cholecalciferol
Tablets: 400 units[OTC], 1000 units[OTC]. *In combination with:* alendronate (Fosamax Plus D), see Appendix B.

Doxercalciferol
Capsules: 0.5 mcg, 1 mcg, 2.5 mcg. **Solution for injection:** 2 mcg/mL.

Ergocalciferol (generic available)
Liquid: 8000 units/mL[Rx, OTC]. **Capsules:** 50,000 units.

Paricalcitol
Capsules: 1 mcg, 2 mcg, 4 mcg. **Solution for injection:** 2 mcg/mL, 5 mcg/mL.

NURSING IMPLICATIONS

Assessment
- Assess for symptoms of vitamin deficiency prior to and periodically during therapy.
- Assess patient for bone pain and weakness prior to and during therapy.
- Observe patient carefully for evidence of hypocalcemia (paresthesia, muscle twitching, laryngospasm, colic, cardiac arrhythmias, and Chvostek's or Trousseau's sign). Protect symptomatic patient by raising and padding side rails; keep bed in low position.
- Pedi: Monitor height and weight; growth arrest may occur in prolonged high-dose therapy.

VITAMIN D COMPOUNDS

- **Rickets/Osteomalacia:** Assess patient for bone pain and weakness prior to and during therapy.
- **Lab Test Considerations:** During *calcitriol* therapy, serum calcium and phosphate concentrations should be drawn twice weekly initially. Serum calcium, magnesium, alkaline phosphatase, and intact PTH should then be monitored at least monthly. During *cholecalciferol* therapy, serum calcium, phosphate, and alkaline phosphatase concentrations should be monitored periodically. During *doxercalciferol* therapy, serum ionized calcium, phosphate, and intact PTH concentrations should be monitored prior to initiation of therapy, and then weekly during the first 12 wk of therapy, then periodically. Alkaline phosphatase should be monitored periodically. During *ergocalciferol* therapy, serum calcium and phosphate concentrations should be monitored every 2 wk. During oral *paricalcitol* therapy, serum calcium, phosphate, and intact PTH concentrations should be monitored at least every 2 wk for the first 3 mo of therapy or after any dosage adjustment, then monthly for 3 mo, then every 3 mo. During IV *paricalcitol* therapy, serum calcium and phosphate concentrations should be monitored twice weekly initially until dosage stabilized, and then at least monthly. Serum intact PTH concentrations should be monitored every 3 mo.
- The serum calcium × phosphate product (Ca × P) should not exceed 70 mg^2/dL^2 (55 mg^2/dL^2 for doxercalciferol) (patients may be at ↑ risk of calcification).
- Calcitriol may cause false ↑ cholesterol levels.
- **Toxicity and Overdose:** Toxicity is manifested as hypercalcemia, hypercalciuria, and hyperphosphatemia. Assess patient for appearance of nausea, vomiting, anorexia, weakness, constipation, headache, bone pain, and metallic taste. Later symptoms include polyuria, polydipsia, photophobia, rhinorrhea, pruritus, and cardiac arrhythmias. Notify health care professional immediately if these signs of hypervitaminosis D occur. Treatment usually consists of discontinuation of calcitriol, a low-calcium diet, use of low-calcium dialysate in peritoneal dialysis patients, and administration of a laxative. IV hydration and loop diuretics may be ordered to increase urinary excretion of calcium. Hemodialysis may also be used.

Potential Nursing Diagnoses
Imbalanced nutrition: less than body requirements (Indications)

Implementation
- Do not confuse Calciferol (ergocalciferol) with calcitriol.
- **PO:** May be administered without regard to meals. Measure solution accurately with calibrated dropper provided by manufacturer. May be mixed with juice, cereal, or food, or dropped directly into mouth. Calcitriol capsules or solution should be protected from light.

IV Administration
- **Direct IV:** Administer *calcitriol, doxercalciferol, and paracalcitol* undiluted by rapid injection through the catheter at the end of a hemodialysis period.

Patient/Family Teaching
- Advise patient to take medication as directed. Take missed doses as soon as remembered that day, unless almost time for next dose; do not double up on doses.
- Review diet modifications with patient. See Appendix M for foods high in calcium and vitamin D. Renal patients must still consider renal failure diet in food selection. Health care professional may order concurrent calcium supplement.
- Encourage patient to comply with dietary recommendations of health care professional. Explain that the best source of vitamins is a well-balanced diet with foods from the 4 basic food groups and the importance of sunlight exposure. See Appendix M for foods high in vitamin D.
- Patients self-medicating with vitamin supplements should be cautioned not to exceed RDA. The effectiveness of megadoses for treatment of various medical conditions is unproved and may cause side effects.
- Advise patient to avoid concurrent use of antacids containing magnesium.
- Review symptoms of overdosage and instruct patient to report these promptly to health care professional.
- Emphasize the importance of follow-up exams to evaluate progress.

Evaluation/Desired Outcomes
- Normalization of serum calcium and parathyroid hormone levels.
- Resolution or prevention of vitamin D deficiency.
- Improvement in symptoms of vitamin D–resistant rickets.

vitamin E (vye-ta-min E)
alpha tocopherol, Amino-Opti-E, Aquasol E, E-200, E-400, E-1000, E-Complex-600, E-Vitamin, Liqui-E, Pheryl-E, Vita Plus E, ✺Webber Vitamin E

Classification
Therapeutic: vitamins
Pharmacologic: fat-soluble vitamins

Pregnancy Category A (doses within RDA), C (doses >RDA)

Indications
PO: Used as a dietary supplement. Used in low-birth-weight infants to prevent and treat hemolysis due to vitamin E deficiency. **Topical:** Treatment of irritated, chapped, or dry skin.

Action
Prevents the oxidation (antioxidant) of other substances. Protects RBC membranes against hemolysis, especially in low-birth-weight neonates.
Therapeutic Effects: Prevention and treatment of deficiency in high-risk patients.

Pharmacokinetics
Absorption: 20–80% absorbed following oral administration. Absorption requires fat and bile salts.
Distribution: Widely distributed, stored in adipose tissue (4-yr supply).
Metabolism and Excretion: Metabolized by the liver, excreted in bile.
Half-life: Unknown.

TIME/ACTION PROFILE

ROUTE	ONSET	PEAK	DURATION
PO	unknown	unknown	unknown

Contraindications/Precautions
Contraindicated in: Hypersensitivity to ingredients in preparations (parabens, propylene, glycol).
Use Cautiously in: Anemia due to iron deficiency; Vitamin K deficiency (may ↑ risk of bleeding); Pedi: Oral administration may cause necrotizing enterocolitis in low-birth-weight infants.

Adverse Reactions/Side Effects
Seen primarily with large doses over long periods of time.
CNS: fatigue, headache, weakness. **EENT:** blurred vision. **GI:** NECROTIZING ENTEROCOLITIS (oral administration in low-birth-weight infants), cramps, diarrhea, nausea. **Derm:** rash. **Endo:** gonadal dysfunction.

Interactions
Drug-Drug: Cholestyramine, colestipol, orlistat, mineral oil, and **sucralfate** ↓ absorption. May ↓ hematologic response to **iron supplements**. May ↑ the risk of bleeding with **warfarin** or **aspirin**.
Drug-Natural Products: ↑ bleeding risk with **anise, arnica, chamomile, clove, dong quai, fenugreek, feverfew, garlic, ginger, ginkgo, Panax ginseng, licorice,** and others.

Route/Dosage
Other dosing regimens may be used.
PO (Adults and Children): Determined by nutritional intake or degree of deficiency.
Topical (Adults and Children): Apply to affected areas as needed.

Availability
Capsules: 100 units^OTC, 200 units^OTC, 400 units^OTC, 600 units^OTC, ✺800 units^OTC, 1000 units^OTC. **Oral solution:** 26.6 units/mL^OTC, 50 units/mL^OTC, 77 units/mL^OTC. **Tablets:** 100 units^OTC, 200 units^OTC, 400 units^OTC, 500 units^OTC, 800 units^OTC. **Chewable tablets:** 400 units^OTC. **Ointment:** ^OTC. **Cream:** ^OTC. **Lotion:** ^OTC. **Oil:** ^OTC.

NURSING IMPLICATIONS

Assessment
- Assess patient for signs of vitamin E deficiency (*neonates*—irritability, edema, hemolytic anemia, creatinuria; *adults/children [rare]*—muscle weakness, ceroid deposits, anemia, creatinuria) prior to and periodically throughout therapy.
- Assess nutritional status through 24-hr diet recall. Determine frequency of consumption of vitamin E–rich foods.
- *Lab Test Considerations:* Large doses may increase cholesterol, triglyceride, and CPK levels.

Potential Nursing Diagnoses
Imbalanced nutrition: less than body requirements (Indications)

Implementation
- **PO:** Administer with or after meals.
- Chewable tablets should be chewed well or crushed before swallowing. Solution may be dropped directly into mouth or mixed with ce-

real, fruit juice, or other food. Use calibrated dropper supplied by manufacturer to measure solution accurately.

Patient/Family Teaching
- Instruct patient to take medication as directed. If a dose is missed, it should be omitted, because fat-soluble vitamins are stored in the body for long periods.
- Encourage patient to comply with diet recommendations of health care professional. Explain that the best source of vitamins is a well-balanced diet with foods from the four basic food groups.
- Foods high in vitamin E include vegetable oils, wheat germ, whole-grain cereals, egg yolk, and liver. Vitamin E content is not markedly affected by cooking.
- Patients self-medicating with vitamin supplements should be cautioned not to exceed RDA. The effectiveness of megadoses for treatment of various medical conditions is unproved, and this may cause side effects and toxicity.
- Review symptoms of overdosage (blurred vision, flu-like symptoms, headache, breast enlargement). Instruct patient to report these promptly to health care professional.
- Mineral oil may interfere with the absorption of fat-soluble vitamins and should not be used concurrently.

Evaluation/Desired Outcomes
- Prevention of or decrease in the symptoms of vitamin E deficiency.
- Control of dry or chapped skin.

---

voriconazole
(vor-i-**kon**-a-zole)
VFEND

Classification
Therapeutic: antifungals

Pregnancy Category D

Indications
Serious systemic fungal infections including candidemia, esophageal candidiasis, candidal deep tissue and skin infections, abdominal, kidney, bladder wall and wound infections, and aspergillosis.

Action
Inhibits fungal ergosterol synthesis leading to production of abnormal fungal plasma membrane.
Therapeutic Effects: Antifungal activity.

Pharmacokinetics
Absorption: Well absorbed following oral administration (96%); IV administration results in complete bioavailability.
Distribution: Extensive tissue distribution.
Metabolism and Excretion: Highly metabolized by the hepatic P450 enzymes (CYP2C19, CYP2C9, CYP3A4); <2% excreted unchanged in urine. Much individual variation in metabolism; metabolites are inactive. The CYP2C19 enzyme system exhibits genetic polymorphism; 15–20% of Asian patients and 3–5% of Caucasian and Black patients may be poor metabolizers and may have significantly ↑ voriconazole concentrations and an ↑ risk of adverse effects.
Half-life: Dose-dependent; increased in hepatic impairment.

TIME/ACTION PROFILE (blood levels)

ROUTE	ONSET	PEAK	DURATION
PO	rapid	1–2 hr	12 hr
IV	rapid	end of infusion	12 hr

Contraindications/Precautions
Contraindicated in: Concurrent use of ritonavir, rifampin, rifabutin, St. John's wort, carbamazepine, and phenobarbital (decrease antifungal activity); Concurrent use of sirolimus, pimozide, quinidine, ergotamine, and dihydroergotamine (↑ risk of toxicity of these agents); Tablets contain lactose and should be avoided in patients with galactose intolerance, Lapp lactase deficiency, or glucose-galactose malabsorption.
Use Cautiously in: Mild to moderate liver disease (Child-Pugh Class A and B); maintenance dose reduction recommended; Renal impairment (CCr <50 mL/min); use only if justified by risk/benefit assessment (IV form should be avoided, use oral form only); OB, Lactation: Use only if benefits justify risk; Pedi: Children <12 yr (safety not established).

Adverse Reactions/Side Effects
CNS: dizziness, hallucinations, headache. **EENT:** visual disturbances, eye hemorrhage. **CV:** changes in blood pressure, tachycardia, peripheral edema, tachycardia. **GI:** HEPATOTOXICITY, abdominal pain, diarrhea, nausea, pancreatitis, vomiting. **Derm:** photosensitivity, rash. **F and E:** hypokalemia, hypomagnesemia. **Misc:** allergic reactions including STEVENS-JOHNSON SYNDROME, chills, fever, infusion reactions.

Interactions
Drug-Drug: Voriconazole is a substrate and inhibitor of the **CYP3A4**, **CYP2C9**, and **CYP2C19**

enzyme systems. **Carbamazepine, ritonavir, phenobarbital, St. John's wort, rifabutin,** and **rifampin** ↑ metabolism and ↓ antifungal activity of voriconazole; concurrent use is contraindicated. **Efavirenz** ↑ metabolism and ↓ antifungal activity of voriconazole; voriconazole also ↓ metabolism and ↑ risk of toxicity of **efavirenz**; if used together, ↑ dose of voriconazole to 400 mg q 12 hr and ↓ dose of efavirenz to 300 mg daily. ↓ metabolism and ↑ risk of toxicity from **dihydroergotamine, ergotamine, pimozide, rifabutin, quinidine,** and **sirolimus**; concurrent use is contraindicated. ↓ metabolism and ↑ risk of toxicity from **cyclosporine, HMG-CoA reductase inhibitors,** some **benzodiazepines (alprazolam, midazolam, triazolam),** some **calcium channel blockers, sulfonylureas (glipizide, glyburide, tolbutamine), alfentanil, tacrolimus, warfarin, vinca alkaloids (vincristine, vinblastine);** careful monitoring required during concurrent use. **Phenytoin** ↑ metabolism and ↓ antifungal activity of voriconazole; voriconazole ↑ **phenytoin** levels and may cause toxicity; careful monitoring required during concurrent use. ↑ blood levels of **omeprazole**; ↓ omeprazole dose by 50% during concurrent use. Similar effects may occur with other **proton-pump inhibitors**. May ↓ metabolism and ↑ blood levels and effects of **protease-inhibitor antiretrovirals** and **non-nucleoside reverse transcriptase inhibitor antiretrovirals**; frequent monitoring recommended. **Non-nucleoside reverse transcriptase inhibitor antiretrovirals**; may induce or inhibit the metabolism of voriconazole; frequent monitoring recommended.

Route/Dosage
IV (Adults and children >12 yr): *Loading dose*—6 mg/kg every 12 hour for 2 doses, followed by *maintenance dosing*—3–4 mg/kg every 12 hours. IV then switched to oral dosing when possible. If intolerance occurs, dose may be ↓ to 3 mg/kg every 12 hr. If phenytoin is coadministered, ↑ maintenance dose to 5 mg/kg every 12 hr.
PO (Adults and children >12 yr and >40 kg): *Most infections*— (following IV loading dose) 200 mg every 12 hr; may be increased to 300 mg every 12 hr if response if inadequate. If phenytoin is coadministered, ↑ maintenance dose to 400 mg every 12 hr; *esophageal candidiasis*—200 mg every 12 hr for 14 days or 7 days following symptom resolution.
PO (Adults and children >12 yr and <40 kg): *Most infections*— (following IV loading dose) 100 mg every 12 hr; may be increased to 150 mg every 12 hr if response is inadequate. If phenytoin is coadministered, ↑ maintenance dose to 200 mg every 12 hr; *esophageal candidiasis*—100 mg every 12 hr for 14 days or 7 days following symptom resolution.

Hepatic Impairment
IV (Adults and Children >12 yr): Use standard loading dose, ↓ maintenance dose by 50%.

Availability
Tablets: 50 mg, 200 mg. **Oral suspension (orange):** 40 mg/mL. **Powder for injection (requires reconstitution):** 200 mg/vial.

NURSING IMPLICATIONS

Assessment
- Monitor for signs and symptoms of fungal infections prior to and during therapy.
- Obtain specimens for culture and histopathology prior to therapy to isolate and identify organism. Therapy may be started before results are received.
- Monitor visual function including visual acuity, visual field, and color perception in patients receiving more than 28 days of therapy. Vision usually returns to normal within 14 days after discontinuation of therapy.
- Monitor for allergic reactions during infusion of voriconazole (flushing, fever, sweating, tachycardia, chest tightness, dyspnea, faintness, nausea, pruritus, rash). Symptoms occur immediately upon start of infusion. May require discontinuation.
- Monitor patients with risk factors for acute pancreatitis (recent chemotherapy, hematopoietic stem cell transplantation [HSCT]) for the signs of pancreatitis (abdominal pain, ↑ serum amylase and lipase).
- ***Lab Test Considerations:*** Monitor liver function tests prior to and during therapy. If abnormal liver function tests occur, monitor for development of severe hepatic injury. Discontinue therapy if clinical signs and symptoms of liver disease develop.
- Monitor renal function (serum creatinine) during therapy.

Potential Nursing Diagnoses
Risk for infection (Indications)

Implementation
- Once patient can tolerate oral medication, PO voriconazole may be used.
- Correct electrolyte disturbances (hypokalemia, hypomagnesemia, hypocalcemia) prior to initiation therapy.
- **PO:** Administer 1 hr before or 1 hr after a meal.

IV Administration
- **Intermittent Infusion:** Reconstitute each 200-mg vial with 19 mL of sterile water for injection to achieve concentration of 10 mg/mL. Calculate volume of 10 mg/mL solution required for patient dose. *Diluent:* Withdraw and discard equal volume of diluent from infusion bag or bottle to be used. Withdraw required volume of voriconazole solution from vial(s) and add to appropriate volume of 0.9% NaCl, LR, D5/LR, D5/0.45% NaCl, D5W, 0.45% NaCl, or D5/0.9% NaCl. Reconstituted solution stable for 24 hr if refrigerated. Discard partially used vials. *Concentration:* Final concentration of infusion should be 0.5–5 mg/mL. *Rate:* Infuse over 1–2 hr at a rate not to exceed 3 mg/kg/hr.
- **Y-Site Compatibility:** acyclovir, alfentanil, allopurinol, amifostine, amikacin, aminocaproic acid, aminophylline, amiodarone, amphotericin B liposome, ampicillin, ampicillin/sulbactam, anidulafungin, azithromycin, aztreonam, bivalirudin, bleomycin, bumetanide, buprenorphine, butorphanol, calcium acetate, calcium chloride, calcium gluconate, carboplatin, carmustine, caspofungin, cefazolin, cefotaxime, cefotetan, cefoxitin, ceftazidime, ceftizoxime, ceftriaxone, chloramphenicol, chlorpromazine, cimetidine, ciprofloxacin, cisatracurium, cisplatin, clindamycin, cyclophosphamide, cytarabine, dacarbazine, dactinomycin, daptomycin, daunorubicin, dexamethasone, dexmedetomidine, dexrazoxane, digoxin, diltiazem, diphenhydramine, dobutamine, docetaxel, dolasetron, dopamine, doripenem, doxacurium, doxycycline, droperidol, enalaprilat, ephedrine, epinephrine, epirubicin, ertapenem, erythromycin, esmolol, etoposide, etoposide phosphate, famotidine, fenoldopam, fentanyl, fluconazole, fludarabine, fluorouracil, foscarnet, fosphenytoin, furosemide, ganciclovir, gemcitabine, gentamicin, glycopyrrolate, granisetron, haloperidol, heparin, hydralazine, hydrocortisone, ifosfamide, imipenem/cilastatin, inamrinone, insulin, irinotecan, isoproterenol, ketorolac, labetalol, leucovorin, levofloxacin, lidocaine, linezolid, lorazepam, magnesium sulfate, mannitol, mechlorethamine, melphalan, meperidine, meropenem, mesna, metaraminol, methohexital, methotrexate, methyldopate, methylprednisolole, metioclopramide, metoprolol, metronidazole, midazolam, milrinone, mitomycin, morphine, nafcillin, nalbuphine, naloxone, nicardipine, nitroglycerin, norepinephrine, octreotide, ondansetron, oxaliplatin, oxytocin, paclitaxel, pamidronate, pancuronium, pentamidine, pentazocine, pentobarbital, phenobarbital, phentolamine, phenylephrine, piperacillin/tazobactam, potassium chloride, potassium phosphates, procainamide, promethazine, propranolol, quinupristin/dalfopristin, remifentanil, rocuronium, sodium acetate, sodium bicarbonate, sodium phosphates, streptozocin, succinylcholine, sufentanil, tacrolimus, teniposide, theophylline, thiotepa, ticarcillin/clavulanate, tirofiban, tobramycin, topotecan, trimethobenzamide, trimethoprim/sulfamethoxazole, vancomycin, vasopressin, vecuronium, verapamil, vinblastine, vincristine, vinorelbine, zidovudine.
- **Y-Site Incompatibility:** amphotericin B colloidal, busulfan, cefepime, cyclosporine, dantrolene, diazepam, doxorubicin, idarubicin, mitoxantrone, nitroprusside, pantoprazole, phenytoin, thiopental.

Patient/Family Teaching
- May cause blurred vision, photophobia, and dizziness. Caution patient to avoid driving and other activities requiring alertness until response to medication is known. Also advise patient to avoid driving at night during voriconazole therapy.
- Advise patient to avoid direct sunlight during voriconazole therapy.

Evaluation/Desired Outcomes
- Resolution of fungal infections.

HIGH ALERT

warfarin (war-fa-rin)
Coumadin, Jantoven, ✽Warfilone

Classification
Therapeutic: anticoagulants
Pharmacologic: coumarins

Pregnancy Category X

Indications
Prophylaxis and treatment of: Venous thrombosis, Pulmonary embolism, Atrial fibrillation with embolization. Management of myocardial infarction: Decreases risk of death, Decreases risk of subsequent MI, Decreases risk of future thromboembolic events. Prevention of thrombus formation and embolization after prosthetic valve placement.

Action
Interferes with hepatic synthesis of vitamin K-dependent clotting factors (II, VII, IX, and X). **Therapeutic Effects:** Prevention of thromboembolic events.

Pharmacokinetics
Absorption: Well absorbed from the GI tract after oral administration.
Distribution: Crosses the placenta but does not enter breast milk.
Protein Binding: 99%.
Metabolism and Excretion: Metabolized by the liver.
Half-life: 42 hr.

TIME/ACTION PROFILE (effects on coagulation tests)

ROUTE	ONSET	PEAK	DURATION
PO, IV	36–72 hr	5–7 days†	2–5 days‡

† At a constant dose
‡ After discontinuation

Contraindications/Precautions
Contraindicated in: Uncontrolled bleeding; Open wounds; Active ulcer disease; Recent brain, eye, or spinal cord injury or surgery; Severe liver or kidney disease; Uncontrolled hypertension; OB: Crosses placenta and may cause fatal hemorrhage in the fetus. May also cause congenital malformation.
Use Cautiously in: Malignancy; Patients with history of ulcer or liver disease; History of poor compliance; Women with childbearing potential; Asian patients or those who carry the CYP2C9*2 allele and/or the CYP2C9*3 allele, or with the VKORC1 AA genotype (↑ risk of bleeding with standard dosing; lower initial doses should be considered); Pedi: Has been used safely but may require more frequent PT/INR assessments; Geri: Due to greater than expected anticoagulant response, initiate and maintain at lower doses.

Adverse Reactions/Side Effects
GI: cramps, nausea. **Derm:** dermal necrosis. **Hemat:** BLEEDING. **Misc:** fever.

Interactions
Drug-Drug: **Abciximab**, **androgens**, **capecitabine**, **cefotetan**, **chloral hydrate**, **chloramphenicol**, **clopidogrel**, **disulfiram**, **fluconazole**, **fluoroquinolones**, **itraconazole**, **metronidazole** (including vaginal use), **thrombolytics**, **eptifibatide**, **tirofiban**, **ticlopidine**, **sulfonamides**, **quinidine**, **quinine**, **NSAIDs**, **valproates**, and **aspirin** may ↑ the response to warfarin and ↑ the risk of bleeding. Chronic use of **acetaminophen** may ↑ the risk of bleeding. Chronic **alcohol** ingestion may ↓ action of warfarin; if chronic **alcohol** abuse results in significant liver damage, action of warfarin may be ↑ due to ↓ production of clotting factor. Acute **alcohol** ingestion may ↑ action of warfarin. **Barbiturates**, **carbamazepine**, **rifampin**, and **hormonal contraceptives containing estrogen** may ↓ the anticoagulant response to warfarin. **Many other drugs** may affect the activity of warfarin.
Drug-Natural Products: St. John's wort ↓ effect. ↑ bleeding risk with **anise**, **arnica**, **chamomile**, **clove**, **dong quai**, **fenugreek**, **feverfew**, **garlic**, **ginger**, **ginkgo**, **Panax ginseng**, **licorice**, and others.
Drug-Food: Ingestion of large quantities of **foods high in vitamin K content** (see list in Appendix M) may antagonize the anticoagulant effect of warfarin.

Route/Dosage
PO, IV (Adults): 2–5 mg/day for 2–4 days; then adjust daily dose by results of INR. Initiate therapy with lower doses in geriatric or debilitated patients or in Asian patients or those with CYP2C9*2 and/or CYP2C9*3 alleles or VKORC1 AA genotype.

PO, IV (Children >1 mo): Initial loading dose—0.2 mg/kg (maximum dose: 10 mg) for 2–4 days then adjust daily dose by results of INR, use 0.1 mg/kg if liver dysfunction is present. Maintenance dose range—0.05–0.34 mg/kg/day.

✽ = Canadian drug name.   = Genetic implication.
*CAPITALS indicates life-threatening; underlines indicate most frequent.

warfarin

Availability (generic available)
Tablets: 1 mg, 2 mg, 2.5 mg, 3 mg, 4 mg, 5 mg, 6 mg, 7.5 mg, 10 mg. **Cost:** *Coumadin*—5 mg $85.00/90; *Jantoven*—5 mg $58.14/90; *Generic*—5 mg $34.99/90. **Injection:** 5 mg/vial.

NURSING IMPLICATIONS
Assessment
- Assess for signs of bleeding and hemorrhage (bleeding gums; nosebleed; unusual bruising; tarry, black stools; hematuria; fall in hematocrit or blood pressure; guaiac-positive stools, urine, or nasogastric aspirate).
- Assess for evidence of additional or increased thrombosis. Symptoms depend on area of involvement.
- **Geri:** Patients over 60 yr exhibit greater than expected PT/INR response. Monitor for side effects at lower therapeutic ranges.
- **Pedi:** Achieving and maintaining therapeutic PT/INR ranges may be more difficult in the pediatric patient. Assess PT/INR levels more frequently.
- **Lab Test Considerations:** Monitor PT, INR and other clotting factors frequently during therapy. Therapeutic PT ranges 1.3–1.5 times greater than control; however, the INR, a standardized system that provides a common basis for communicating and interpreting PT results, is usually referenced. Normal INR (not on anticoagulants) is 0.8–1.2. An INR of 2.5–3.5 is recommended for patients at very high risk of embolization (for example, patients with mitral valve replacement and ventricular hypertrophy). Lower levels are acceptable when risk is lower. Heparin may affect the PT/INR; draw blood for PT/INR in patients receiving both heparin and warfarin at least 5 hr after the IV bolus dose, 4 hr after cessation of IV infusion, or 24 hr after subcut heparin injection. Asian patients and those who carry the CYP2C9*2 allele and/or the CYP2C9*3 allele, or those with VKORC1 AA genotype may require more frequent monitoring and lower doses.
- Monitor hepatic function and CBC before and periodically throughout therapy.
- Monitor stool and urine for occult blood before and periodically during therapy.
- ***Toxicity and Overdose:*** Withholding 1 or more doses of warfarin is usually sufficient if INR is excessively elevated or if minor bleeding occurs. If overdose occurs or anticoagulation needs to be immediately reversed, the antidote is vitamin K (phytonadione, AquaMEPHYTON). Administration of whole blood or plasma also may be required in severe bleeding because of the delayed onset of vitamin K.

Potential Nursing Diagnoses
Ineffective tissue perfusion (Indications)
Risk for injury (Side Effects)

Implementation
- ***High Alert:*** Medication errors involving anticoagulants have resulted in serious harm or death from internal or intracranial bleeding. Before administering, evaluate recent INR or PT results and have second practitioner independently check original order.
- Because of the large number of medications capable of significantly altering warfarin's effects, careful monitoring is recommended when new agents are started or other agents are discontinued. Interactive potential should be evaluated for all new medications (Rx, OTC, and natural products).
- Administer medication at same time each day.
- **PO:** Medication requires 3–5 days to reach effective levels; usually begun while patient is still on heparin.
- Do not interchange brands; potencies may not be equivalent.

IV Administration
- **Direct IV:** Reconstitute each 5-mg vial with 2.7 mL of sterile water for injection. Reconstituted solution is stable for 4 hr at room temperature. ***Diluent:*** No further dilution needed before administration. ***Concentration:*** 2 mg/mL. ***Rate:*** Administer over 1–2 min.
- **Y-Site Compatibility:** amikacin, ascorbic acid, cefazolin, ceftriaxone, dopamine, epinephrine, heparin, lidocaine, metaraminol, morphine, nitroglycerin, oxytocin, potassium chloride, ranitidine.
- **Y-Site Incompatibility:** aminophylline, ceftazidime, cimetidine, ciprofloxacin, dobutamine, esmolol, gentamicin, labetalol, metronidazole.

Patient/Family Teaching
- Instruct patient to take medication as directed. Take missed doses as soon as remembered that day; do not double doses. Inform health care professional of missed doses at time of checkup or lab tests. Inform patients that anticoagulant effect may persist for 2–5 days following discontinuation. Advise patient to read *Medication Guide* before starting therapy and with each Rx refill.
- Review foods high in vitamin K (see Appendix M). Patient should have consistent limited intake of these foods, as vitamin K is the

antidote for warfarin, and alternating intake of these foods will cause PT levels to fluctuate. Advise patient to avoid cranberry juice or products during therapy.
- Caution patient to avoid IM injections and activities leading to injury. Instruct patient to use a soft toothbrush, not to floss, and to shave with an electric razor during warfarin therapy. Advise patient that venipunctures and injection sites require application of pressure to prevent bleeding or hematoma formation.
- Advise patient to report any symptoms of unusual bleeding or bruising (bleeding gums; nosebleed; black, tarry stools; hematuria; excessive menstrual flow) and pain, color, or temperature change to any area of your body to health care professional immediately. Patients with a deficiency in protein C and/or S mediated anticoagulant response may be at greater risk for tissue necrosis.
- Instruct patient not to drink alcohol or take other Rx, OTC, or herbal products, especially those containing aspirin or NSAIDs, or to start or stop any new medications during warfarin therapy without advice of health care professional.
- Advise patient to notify health care professional if pregnancy is planned or suspected or if breastfeeding.
- Instruct patient to carry identification describing medication regimen at all times and to inform all health care personnel caring for patient on anticoagulant therapy before lab tests, treatment, or surgery.
- Emphasize the importance of frequent lab tests to monitor coagulation factors.

Evaluation/Desired Outcomes
- Prolonged PT (1.3–2.0 times the control; may vary with indication) or INR of 2–4.5 without signs of hemorrhage.

zafirlukast (za-feer-loo-kast)
Accolate

Classification
Therapeutic: antiasthmatics, bronchodilators
Pharmacologic: leukotriene antagonists

Pregnancy Category B

Indications
Long-term control agent in the management of asthma.

Action
Antagonizes the effects of leukotrienes, which are components of slow-reacting substance of anaphylaxis (SRSA). These substances mediate the following: Airway edema, Smooth muscle constriction, Altered cellular activity. Result is decreased inflammatory process that is part of asthma. **Therapeutic Effects:** Decreased frequency and severity of asthma.

Pharmacokinetics
Absorption: Rapidly absorbed after oral administration.
Distribution: Enters breast milk.
Protein Binding: 99%.
Metabolism and Excretion: Mostly metabolized by the liver; 10% excreted unchanged by the kidneys.
Half-life: 10 hr.

TIME/ACTION PROFILE (improved symptoms of asthma)

ROUTE	ONSET	PEAK	DURATION
PO	unknown	1 wk	unknown

Contraindications/Precautions
Contraindicated in: Hypersensitivity; Lactation: Lactation.
Use Cautiously in: Acute attacks of asthma; Patients >55 yr (↑ risk of infection); Hepatic impairment (may need lower doses); Geri: May need lower doses to avoid side effects; OB, Pedi: Pregnancy or children <7 yr (safety not established).

Adverse Reactions/Side Effects
CNS: SUICIDAL THOUGHTS, headache, agitation, aggression, anxiety, depression, dizziness, dream abnormalities, hallucinations, insomnia, irritability, restlessness, tremor, weakness. **GI:** HEPATOTOXICITY, abdominal pain, diarrhea, dyspepsia, nausea, vomiting. **MS:** arthralgia, back pain, myalgia. **Misc:** CHURG-STRAUSS SYNDROME, fever, infection (geriatric patients), pain.

Interactions
Drug-Drug: Levels are ↑ by **aspirin**. Levels are ↓ by **erythromycin** and **theophylline**. ↑ effects and risk of bleeding with **warfarin**.
Drug-Food: Food (especially high-fat or high-protein meal) ↓ absorption.

Route/Dosage
PO (Adults and Children ≥12 yr): 20 mg twice daily.
PO (Children 7–11 yr): 10 mg twice daily.

Availability
Tablets: 10 mg, 20 mg.

NURSING IMPLICATIONS

Assessment
- Assess lung sounds and respiratory function before and periodically during therapy.
- Monitor closely for changes in behavior that could indicate the emergence or worsening of depression or suicidal thoughts.
- **Lab Test Considerations:** Monitor liver function periodically during therapy. May cause ↑ ALT concentrations. If liver dysfunction occurs, zafirlukast should be discontinued.

Potential Nursing Diagnoses
Ineffective airway clearance (Indications)
Deficient knowledge, related to medication regimen (Patient/Family Teaching)

Implementation
- **PO:** Administer at regular intervals on an empty stomach, 1 hr before or 2 hr after meals.

Patient/Family Teaching
- Instruct patient to take medication on an empty stomach as directed, at evenly spaced intervals, even if not experiencing symptoms of asthma. Take missed doses as soon as remembered unless almost time for next dose. Do not double doses. Do not discontinue therapy without consulting health care professional.
- Instruct patient not to discontinue or reduce other asthma medications without consulting health care professional.
- Advise patient that zafirlukast is not used to treat acute asthma attacks but may be continued during an acute exacerbation.
- Advise patient to notify health care professional of behavioral changes or thoughts of suicide.

- Advise patient to notify health care professional if symptoms of Churg-Strauss syndrome (generalized flu-like syndrome, fever, muscle aches and pain, weight loss, worsening respiratory symptoms) occur. Occurs rarely but may be life-threatening. More likely to occur when weaning from systemic corticosteroids.

Evaluation/Desired Outcomes
- Prevention of and reduction in symptoms of asthma.

zaleplon (za-lep-lon)
Sonata

Classification
Therapeutic: sedative/hypnotics

Schedule IV

Pregnancy Category C

Indications
Short-term management of insomnia in patients unable to get at least 4 hr of sleep; especially useful in sleep initiation disorders.

Action
Produces CNS depression by binding to GABA receptors in the CNS. Has no analgesic properties.
Therapeutic Effects: Sedation and induction of sleep.

Pharmacokinetics
Absorption: Rapidly absorbed following oral administration.
Distribution: Enters breast milk.
Metabolism and Excretion: Extensively metabolized in the liver (mostly by aldehyde oxidase and some by CYP 450 3A4 enzymes).
Half-life: Unknown.

TIME/ACTION PROFILE

ROUTE	ONSET	PEAK	DURATION
PO	within min	unknown	3–4 hr

Contraindications/Precautions
Contraindicated in: Hypersensitivity; Severe hepatic impairment; OB, Lactation: Pregnancy or lactation.
Use Cautiously in: Mild to moderate hepatic impairment, weight ≤50 kg, or concurrent cimetidine therapy (initiate therapy at lowest dose); Impaired respiratory function; History of suicide attempt; Pedi: Safety not established; Geri: ↑ risk of cognitive impairment. If used, start at lowest dose.

Adverse Reactions/Side Effects
CNS: abnormal thinking, amnesia, anxiety, behavior changes, depersonalization, dizziness, drowsiness, hallucinations, headache, impaired memory (briefly following dose), impaired psychomotor function (briefly following dose), malaise, sleep—driving, vertigo, weakness. **EENT:** abnormal vision, ear pain, epistaxis, hearing sensitivity, ocular pain, altered sense of smell. **CV:** peripheral edema. **GI:** abdominal pain, anorexia, colitis, dyspepsia, nausea. **GU:** dysmenorrhea. **Derm:** photosensitivity. **Neuro:** hyperesthesia, paresthesia, tremor. **Misc:** fever.

Interactions
Drug-Drug: Cimetidine ↓ metabolism and ↑ effects (initiate therapy at a lower dose). Additive CNS depression with other **CNS depressants** including **alcohol**, **antihistamines**, **opioid analgesics**, other **sedative/hypnotics**, **phenothiazines**, and **tricyclic antidepressants**. Effects may be ↓ by drugs that induce the CYP 450 3A4 enzyme system including **rifampin**, **phenytoin**, **carbamazepine**, and **phenobarbital**.
Drug-Natural Products: Concomitant use of **kava-kava**, **valerian**, **chamomile**, or **hops** can ↑ CNS depression.
Drug-Food: Concurrent ingestion of a **high-fat meal** slows the rate of absorption.

Route/Dosage
PO (Adults <65 yr): 10 mg (range 5–20 mg) at bedtime.
PO (Geriatric Patients or Patients <50 kg): Initiate therapy at 5 mg at bedtime (not to exceed 10 mg at bedtime).

Hepatic Impairment
PO (Adults): Initiate therapy at 5 mg at bedtime (not to exceed 10 mg at bedtime).

Availability (generic available)
Capsules: 5 mg, 10 mg. **Cost:** 5 mg $106.99/30, 10 mg $103.99/90.

NURSING IMPLICATIONS

Assessment
- Assess mental status, sleep patterns, and potential for abuse prior to administering this medication. Prolonged use of >7–10 days may lead to physical and psychological dependence. Limit amount of drug available to the patient.
- Assess alertness at time of peak effect. Notify health care professional if desired sedation does not occur.
- Assess patient for pain. Medicate as needed. Untreated pain decreases sedative effects.

Potential Nursing Diagnoses
Insomnia (Indications)
Risk for injury (Side Effects)

Implementation
- Before administering, reduce external stimuli and provide comfort measures to increase effectiveness of medication.
- Protect patient from injury. Supervise ambulation and transfer of patients after administration. Remove cigarettes. Side rails should be raised and call bell within reach at all times.
- **PO:** Tablets should be swallowed whole with full glass of water immediately before bedtime or after going to bed and experiencing difficulty falling asleep. Do not administer with or immediately after a high-fat or heavy meal.

Patient/Family Teaching
- Instruct patient to take zaleplon as directed. Do not take more than the amount prescribed because of the habit-forming potential. Not recommended for use longer than 7–10 days. Rebound insomnia (1–2 nights) may occur when stopped. If used for 2 wk or longer, abrupt withdrawal may result in dysphoria, insomnia, abdominal or muscle cramps, vomiting, sweating, tremors, and seizures.
- Because of rapid onset, advise patient to go to bed immediately after taking zaleplon.
- May cause daytime drowsiness or dizziness. Advise patient to avoid driving or other activities requiring alertness until response to this medication is known.
- Inform patient that amnesia may occur, but can be avoided if zaleplon is only taken when patient is able to get >4 hr sleep.
- Caution patient to avoid concurrent use of alcohol or other CNS depressants.

Evaluation/Desired Outcomes
- Relief of insomnia.

---

zanamivir (za-**na**-mi-veer)
Relenza

Classification
Therapeutic: antivirals
Pharmacologic: neuramidase inhibitors

Pregnancy Category C

Indications
Treatment of uncomplicated acute illness caused by influenza virus in patients ≥7 yr who have been symptomatic ≤2 days. Prevention of influenza in patients ≥5 yr.

Action
Inhibits the enzyme neuramidase, which may alter virus particle aggregation and release. **Therapeutic Effects:** Reduced duration or prevention of flu-related symptoms.

Pharmacokinetics
Absorption: 4–17% of inhaled dose is systemically absorbed.
Distribution: Unknown.
Protein Binding: <10%.
Metabolism and Excretion: Mainly excreted by kidneys as unchanged drug; unabsorbed drug is excreted in feces.
Half-life: 2.5–5.1 hr.

TIME/ACTION PROFILE (blood levels)

ROUTE	ONSET	PEAK	DURATION
Inhalation	rapid	1–2 hr	12 hr

Contraindications/Precautions
Contraindicated in: Hypersensitivity to zanamivir or lactose.
Use Cautiously in: Chronic obstructive pulmonary disease or asthma (increased risk of decreased lung function and/or bronchospasm); OB, Lactation: Safety not established; Pedi: Children <7 yr (for treatment) or <5 yr (for prophylaxis) (safety not established; children may be at ↑ risk for neuropsychiatric events).

Adverse Reactions/Side Effects
CNS: SEIZURES, abnormal behavior, agitation, delirium, hallucinations, nightmares. **Resp:** bronchospasm. **Misc:** allergic reactions.

Interactions
Drug-Drug: None noted.

Route/Dosage

Treatment
Inhaln (Adults and children ≥7 yr): 10 mg (given as 2 inhalations of 5 mg each) twice daily for 5 days.

Prophylaxis
Inhaln (Adults and children ≥5 yr): 10 mg (given as 2 inhalations of 5 mg each) daily for 10 days (for household setting) (28 days for community outbreaks).

Availability
Powder for inhalation: 5 mg/blister.

✦ = Canadian drug name. = Genetic implication.
*CAPITALS indicates life-threatening; underlines indicate most frequent.

1302　ziconotide

NURSING IMPLICATIONS
Assessment
- Assess patient for signs and symptoms of influenza (fever, headache, myalgia, cough, sore throat) before administration. Determine duration of symptoms. Indicated for patients who have been symptomatic for up to 2 days.

Potential Nursing Diagnoses
Risk for infection (Indications)

Implementation
- Consider available information on influenza drug susceptibility patterns and treatment effects before using zanamivir for prophylaxis.
- **Inhaln:** Administer 2 doses on the first day of treatment whenever possible; must have at least 2 hours between doses. Doses should be administered 12 hr apart on subsequent days.

Patient/Family Teaching
- Instruct patient to use zanamivir exactly as directed and to finish entire 5-day course, even if feeling better.
- Instruct patient in the use of the DISKHALER. Patient should read the accompanying Patient Instructions for Use.
- Advise patients that zanamivir is not a substitute for a flu shot. Patients should receive annual flu shot according to immunization guidelines.
- Patients with a history of asthma should be advised to have a fast-acting inhaled bronchodilator available in case of bronchospasm following zanamivir administration. If using bronchodilator and zanamivir concurrently, administer bronchodilator first.
- Advise patients to report behavioral changes (hallucinations, delirium, and abnormal behavior) to health care professional immediately.

Evaluation/Desired Outcomes
- Reduced duration or prevention of flu-related symptoms.

---

ziconotide (zi-ko-no-tide)
Prialt

Classification
Therapeutic: analgesics
Pharmacologic: n-type calcium channel blockers

Pregnancy Category C

Indications
Management of severe chronic pain when conventional therapies (analgesics or other adjunctive measures) have failed.

Action
Blocks spinal N-channel calcium channels, decreasing transmission of pain signals to the brain. Has no effect on opioid receptors. **Therapeutic Effects:** Decrease in severe pain.

Pharmacokinetics
Absorption: IT administration results in complete bioavailability in the CSF. Minimal plasma distribution.
Distribution: Distributes in entire CSF volume.
Metabolism and Excretion: Degraded by enzymes in tissues and fluids.
Half-life: 4.6 hr (in CSF).

TIME/ACTION PROFILE

ROUTE	ONSET	PEAK	DURATION
IT	rapid	2–3 days	unknown

Contraindications/Precautions
Contraindicated in: Hypersensitivity; History of psychosis; Infection at microinfusion injection site; Uncontrolled bleeding; Spinal cord obstruction; Lactation: Can cause sedation and side effects in the infant.
Use Cautiously in: History of suicidal ideation/psychiatric disorder; Pedi: Safety not established; OB: Pregnancy; Geri: ↑ susceptibility to adverse CNS effects.

Adverse Reactions/Side Effects
CNS: MENINGITIS, confusion, dizziness, drowsiness, headache, impaired memory, weakness, aphasia, ↓ alertness/responsiveness, cognitive impairment, hallucinations, memory impairment, psychiatric symptoms, speech disorder. **CV:** changes in blood pressure. **EENT:** nystagmus, abnormal vision. **GI:** nausea, anorexia, vomiting. **Local:** catheter/injection site reactions. **MS:** hypertonia, urinary retention, ↑ creatine kinase. **Neuro:** abnormal gait, ataxia. **Misc:** fever.

Interactions
Drug-Drug: ↑ risk of CNS depression with other **CNS depressants** including **anticonvulsants, phenothiazines, antipsychotics, antihistamines, opioids, sedatives,** or **diuretics**.

Route/Dosage
IT (Adults): up to 2.4 mcg/day initially (0.1 mcg/hr), may be gradually ↑ 2–3 times/wk in increments of 2.4 mcg/day up to a maximum of 19.2 mcg/day (0.8 mcg/hr) over 21 days.

Availability
Solution for intrathecal use: 25 mcg/mL, 100 mcg/mL.

zidovudine **1303**

NURSING IMPLICATIONS
Assessment
- Assess level of pain prior to and periodically during therapy.
- Assess mental status during therapy. If psychiatric symptoms (cognitive impairment, hallucinations, changes in mood or level of consciousness) or neurological impairment. Discontinuation of therapy may be required, but other causes should be considered. Ziconotide may be discontinued abruptly without withdrawal symptoms.
- Monitor for signs of meningitis (fever, headache, stiff neck, altered mental status, nausea, vomiting, seizures) frequently during therapy. May occur within 24 hr of breach in sterility. If meningitis occurs, obtain CSF cultures and institute antibiotic therapy. Usually requires removal of microinfusion system, catheter, and any other foreign body within the IT space.
- *Lab Test Considerations:* Monitor serum CK levels every other week for the first month, monthly thereafter, and if neuromuscular symptoms (myalgias, myasthenia, muscle cramps, asthenia, reduction in physical activity) occur. May cause ↑ CK levels. If symptoms continue and CK remains ↑ or continues to rise, dose reduction or discontinuation may be required.

Potential Nursing Diagnoses
Chronic pain (Indications)

Implementation
- Ziconotide is not an opioid and cannot prevent or relieve symptoms of opioid withdrawal. Do not discontinue opioids abruptly. For withdrawal from IT opioid, gradually taper opioid IT infusion over several weeks, and replace with an equianalgesic dose of oral opioids. Ziconotide does not potentiate opioid-induced respiratory depression.
- Ziconotide should be administered under the direction of a physician experienced in IT therapy. Do not administer IV.
- **IT:** IT dose is delivered using a programmable implanted variable-rate microinfusion device or an external microinfusion device and catheter. Ziconotide may be administered undiluted (25 mcg/mL in 20-mL vial) or diluted (100 mg/mL in 1-, 2-, or 5-mL vials). Dilute with 0.9% NaCl (preservative—free) using aseptic technique. 100 mg/mL formulation may be administered undiluted once an appropriate dose is established. Refrigerate, but do not freeze, after preparation; administer within 24 hr. Discard solution if discolored or containing particulate matter or any unused portion in vial. Pump refills should be done every 40 days if diluted solution is used or every 60 days if solution is undiluted. Pump should be rinsed and filled according to manufacturer's directions.
- *Rate:* Dose should be adjusted according to patient's severity of pain, response to therapy, and occurrence of side effects.

Patient/Family Teaching
- Instruct patient on correct technique for care of equipment.
- May cause dizziness and drowsiness. Caution patient to avoid driving and other activities requiring alertness until response to ziconotide is known.
- Advise patient to avoid taking alcohol and other CNS depressants during ziconotide therapy. Consult health care professional prior to taking Rx, OTC, or herbal products during therapy.
- Instruct patient and caregiver to contact health care professional immediately if changes in mental status (lethargy, confusion, disorientation, decreased alertness), changes in mood or perception (hallucinations, including unusual tactile sensations in oral cavity), symptoms of depression or suicidal ideation, or nausea, vomiting, seizures, fever, headache, or still neck occur; may be symptoms of developing meningitis.
- Advise patient to consult health care professional if new or worsening muscle pain, soreness, or weakness with or without darkened urine occur.

Evaluation/Desired Outcomes
- Decrease in pain intensity.

---

zidovudine (zye-**doe**-vue-deen)
✤Apo-Zidovudine, azidothymidine, AZT, ✤Novo-AZT, Retrovir

Classification
Therapeutic: antiretrovirals
Pharmacologic: nucleoside reverse transcriptase inhibitors

Pregnancy Category C

Indications
HIV infection (with other antiretrovirals). Reduction of maternal/fetal transmission of HIV. **Unla-**

zidovudine

beled Use: Chemoprophylaxis after occupational exposure to HIV.

Action
Following intracellular conversion to its active form, inhibits viral RNA synthesis by inhibiting the enzyme DNA polymerase (reverse transcriptase). Prevents viral replication. **Therapeutic Effects:** Virustatic action against selected retroviruses. Slowed progression and decreased sequelae of HIV infection. Decreased viral load and improved CD4 cell counts. Decreased transmission of HIV to infants born to HIV-infected mothers.

Pharmacokinetics
Absorption: Well absorbed following oral administration.
Distribution: Widely distributed; enters the CNS. Crosses the placenta.
Metabolism and Excretion: Mostly (75%) metabolized by the liver; 15–20% excreted unchanged by the kidneys.
Half-life: 1 hr.

TIME/ACTION PROFILE (blood levels)

ROUTE	ONSET	PEAK	DURATION
PO	unknown	0.5–1.5 hr	4 hr
IV	rapid	end of infusion	4 hr

Contraindications/Precautions
Contraindicated in: Hypersensitivity; Lactation: Breastfeeding not recommended in HIV-infected patients.
Use Cautiously in: ↓ bone marrow reserve (dose ↓ required for anemia or granulocytopenia); Severe hepatic or renal disease (dose modification may be required); Geri: Select dose carefully due to potential for age-related ↓ in hepatic, renal, or cardiac function.

Adverse Reactions/Side Effects
CNS: SEIZURES, headache, weakness, anxiety, confusion, ↓ mental acuity, dizziness, insomnia, mental depression, restlessness, syncope. **GI:** HEPATOMEGALY (with steatosis), PANCREATITIS, abdominal pain, diarrhea, nausea, anorexia, drug-induced hepatitis, dyspepsia, oral mucosa pigmentation, vomiting. **F and E:** LACTIC ACIDOSIS. **Derm:** nail pigmentation. **Endo:** fat redistribution, gynecomastia. **Hemat:** anemia, granulocytopenia, pure red-cell aplasia, thrombocytosis. **MS:** back pain, myopathy. **Neuro:** tremor.

Interactions
Drug-Drug: ↑ bone marrow depression with other **agents having bone marrow–depressing properties**, antineoplastics, radiation therapy, or **ganciclovir**. ↑ neurotoxicity may occur with **acyclovir**. Toxicity may be ↑ by concurrent administration of **probenecid** or **fluconazole**. Levels are ↓ by **clarithromycin**.

Route/Dosage
Management of HIV Infection
PO (Adults): 100 mg q 4 hr while awake or 200 mg 3 times daily or 300 mg twice daily (depends on combination and clinical situation).
PO (Children 6 wk–<12 yr): *4–8.9 kg*–12 mg/kg 2 times daily or 8 mg/kg 3 times daily; *9–29.9 kg*–9 mg/kg 2 times daily or 6 mg/kg 3 times daily; *≥30 kg*–300 mg 2 times daily or 200 mg 3 times daily.
IV (Adults and Children >12 yr): 1 mg/kg infused over 1 hr q 4 hr. Change to oral therapy as soon as possible.
IV (Children): 120 mg/m² q 6 hr (not to exceed 160 mg/dose) or 20 mg/m²/hr as a continuous infusion.

Prevention of Maternal/Fetal Transmission of HIV Infection
PO (Adults >14 wk Pregnant): 100 mg 5 times daily until onset of labor.
IV (Adults during Labor and Delivery): 2 mg/kg over 1 hr, then continuous infusion of 1 mg/kg/hr until umbilical cord is clamped.
IV (Infants): 1.5 mg/kg q 6 hr until able to take PO.
PO (Infants): 2 mg/kg q 6 hr, started within 12 hr of birth and continued for 6 wk.
PO (Neonates premature <30 wk gestational age at birth): 2 mg/kg q 12 hr then ↑ to q 8 hr at 4 wk of age.
PO (Neonates premature ≥30 wk gestational age at birth): 2 mg/kg q 12 hr then ↑ to q 8 hr at 2 wk of age.
IV (Neonates premature <30 wk gestational age at birth): 1.5 mg/kg q 12 hr then ↑ to q 8 hr at 4 wk of age.
IV (Neonates premature ≥30 wk gestational age at birth): 1.5 mg/kg q 12 hr then ↑ to q 8 hr at 2 wk of age.

Availability (generic available)
Capsules: 100 mg. **Tablets:** 300 mg. **Oral syrup:** 50 mg/5 mL. **Solution for injection:** 10 mg/mL. *In combination with:* lamivudine (Combivir; see Appendix B).

NURSING IMPLICATIONS
Assessment
- Assess patient for change in severity of symptoms of HIV and for symptoms of opportunistic infections during therapy.
- *Lab Test Considerations:* Monitor viral load and CD4 counts prior to and periodically during therapy.
- Monitor CBC every 2 wk during the first 8 wk of therapy in patients with advanced HIV disease, and decrease to every 4 wk after the first 2 mo if zidovudine is well tolerated or monthly during the first 3 mo and every 3 mo thereafter unless indicated in patients who are asymptomatic or have early symptoms. Commonly causes granulocytopenia and anemia. Anemia may occur 2–4 wk after initiation of therapy. Anemia may respond to epoetin administration (see epoetin monograph). Granulocytopenia usually occurs after 6–8 wk of therapy. Consider dose reduction, discontinuation of therapy, or blood transfusions if hemoglobin is <7.5 g/dL or reduction of >25% from baseline and/or granulocyte count is <750/mm³ or reduction of >50% from baseline. Therapy may be gradually resumed when bone marrow recovery is evident.
- May cause ↑ serum AST, ALT, and alkaline phosphatase levels. Lactic acidosis may occur with hepatic toxicity, causing hepatic steatosis; may be fatal, especially in women.
- Monitor serum amylase, lipase, and triglycerides periodically during therapy. Elevated serum levels may indicate pancreatitis and require discontinuation.

Potential Nursing Diagnoses
Risk for infection (Indications, Side Effects)

Implementation
- Do not confuse Retrovir (zidovudine) with Ritonavir.
- Administer doses around the clock.
- **IV:** Patient should receive the IV infusion only until oral therapy can be administered.

IV Administration
- **Intermittent Infusion:** *Diluent:* Remove calculated dose from the vial and dilute with D5W or 0.9% NaCl. Do not use solutions that are discolored. Stable for 8 hr at room temperature or 24 hr if refrigerated. *Concentration:* Not to exceed 4 mg/mL. *Rate:* Infuse at a constant rate over 1 hr or over 30 min in neonates. Avoid rapid infusion or bolus injection.
- **Continuous Infusion:** Has also been administered via continuous infusion.
- **Y-Site Compatibility:** acyclovir, allopurinol, amifostine, amikacin, amphotericin B, amphotericin B cholesteryl sulfate, amphotericin B colloidal, amphotericin B liposome, aztreonam, bivalirudin, carboplatin, caspofungin, cefepime, ceftazidime, ceftriaxone, cimetidine, cisatracurium, cisplatin, clindamycin, cyclophosphamide, cytarabine, dactinomycin, dexamethasone sodium phosphate, dexmedetomidine, diltiazem, dobutamine, docetaxel, dopamine, doripenem, doxacurium, doxorubicin hydrochloride, doxorubicin liposome, epirubicin, ertapenem, erythromycin lactobionate, etoposide, etoposide phosphate, fenoldopam, filgrastim, fluconazole, fludarabine, fluorouracil, gemcitabine, gentamicin, granisetron, heparin, hydromorphone, ifosfamide, imipenem/cilastatin, levofloxacin, linezolid, lorazepam, mechlorethamine, melphalan, meperidine, methotrexate, metoclopramide, metronidazole, milrinone, mitoxantrone, morphine, nafcillin, nesiritide, octreotide, ondansetron, oxacillin, oxaliplatin, oxytocin, paclitaxel, palonosetron, pantoprazole, pemetrexed, pentamidine, phenylephrine, piperacillin/tazobactam, potassium chloride, quinapristin/dalfopristin, ranitidine, remifentanil, rituxumab, rocuronium, sargramostim, sodium acetate, tacrolimus, teniposide, thiotepa, tigecycline, tirofiban, tobramycin, trimethoprim/sulfamethoxazole, trastuzumab, trimetrexate, vancomycin, vasopressin, vecuronium, vincristine, vinorelbine, voriconazole.
- **Y-Site Incompatibility:** lansoprazole.
- **Additive Incompatibility:** blood products or protein solutions.

Patient/Family Teaching
- Instruct patient to take zidovudine as directed, around the clock, even if sleep is interrupted. Emphasize the importance of compliance with therapy, not taking more than prescribed amount, and not discontinuing without consulting health care professional. Take missed doses as soon as remembered unless almost time for next dose; do not double doses. Inform patient that long-term effects of zidovudine are unknown at this time.
- Instruct patient that zidovudine should not be shared with others.

- Zidovudine may cause dizziness or fainting. Caution patient to avoid driving or other activities requiring alertness until response to medication is known.
- Inform patient that zidovudine does not cure HIV and does not reduce the risk of transmission of HIV to others through sexual contact or blood contamination. Caution patient to use a condom during sexual contact and avoid sharing needles or donating blood to prevent spreading the AIDS virus to others.
- Instruct patient to notify health care professional promptly if fever, sore throat, signs of infection, muscle weakness, or shortness of breath occurs. Caution patient to avoid crowds and persons with known infections. Instruct patient to use soft toothbrush, to use caution when using toothpicks or dental floss, and to have dental work done prior to therapy or deferred until blood counts return to normal. Patient should also notify health care professional if shortness of breath, muscle aches, symptoms of hepatitis or pancreatitis, or other unexpected reactions occur.
- Advise patient to avoid taking any RX, OTC, or herbal products without consulting health care professional.
- Inform patient that redistribution and accumulation of body fat may occur, causing central obesity, dorsocervical fat enlargement (buffalo hump), peripheral wasting, breast enlargement, and cushingoid appearance. The cause and long-term effects are not known.
- Advise patients not to breastfeed during therapy.
- Emphasize the importance of regular follow-up exams and blood counts to determine progress and monitor for side effects.

Evaluation/Desired Outcomes
- Decrease in viral load and increase in CD4 counts in patients with HIV.
- Delayed progression of AIDS and decreased opportunistic infections in patients with HIV.
- Reduction of maternal/fetal transmission of HIV.

zinc sulfate (zink sul-fate)
Orazinc, ✤PMS Egozinc, Verazinc, Zinc 220, Zincate, Zinkaps

Classification
Therapeutic: mineral and electrolyte replacements/supplements
Pharmacologic: trace metals

Pregnancy Category C (parenteral)

Indications
Replacement and supplementation therapy in patients who are at risk for zinc deficiency, including patients on long-term parenteral nutrition.
Unlabeled Use: Management of impaired wound healing due to zinc deficiency.

Action
Serves as a cofactor for many enzymatic reactions. Required for normal growth and tissue repair, wound healing, and senses of taste and smell.
Therapeutic Effects: Replacement in deficiency states.

Pharmacokinetics
Absorption: Poorly absorbed from the GI tract (20–30%).
Distribution: Widely distributed. Concentrates in muscle, bone, skin, kidney, liver, pancreas, retina, prostate, RBCs, and WBCs.
Metabolism and Excretion: 90% excreted in feces, remainder lost in urine and sweat.
Half-life: Unknown.

TIME/ACTION PROFILE (blood levels)

ROUTE	ONSET	PEAK	DURATION
PO	unknown	2 hr	unknown
IV	unknown	unknown	unknown

Contraindications/Precautions
Contraindicated in: Hypersensitivity or allergy to any components in formulation; Pregnancy or lactation (supplemental amounts >RDA for pregnant or lactating patients); Preparations containing benzyl alcohol should not be used in neonates.
Use Cautiously in: Renal failure.

Adverse Reactions/Side Effects
GI: gastric irritation (oral use only), nausea, vomiting.

Interactions
Drug-Drug: Oral zinc may ↓ absorption of **tetracyclines** or **fluoroquinolones**.
Drug-Food: Caffeine, dairy products, and **bran** may ↓ absorption of orally administered zinc.

Route/Dosage
RDA = 15 mg. Doses expressed in mg of elemental zinc unless otherwise noted. Zinc sulfate contains 23% zinc.

Deficiency

PO (Adults): *Prevention of deficiency*—15–19 mg/day; *treatment of deficiency*—must be individualized; based on degree of deficiency.

IV Nutritional Supplementation—Metabolically Stable Patients

IV (Adults): 2.5–4 mg/day; up to 12 mg/day in patients with excessive losses.

IV (Infants and Children ≤5 yr): 100 mcg/kg/day.

IV (Infants up to 3 kg): 300 mcg/kg/day.

Availability (generic available)

Tablets: 66 mg^OTC, 110 mg^OTC. **Capsules:** 220 mg^OTC. **Injection:** 1 mg/mL in 10- and 30-mL vials, 5 mg/mL in 5- and 10-mL vials.

NURSING IMPLICATIONS

Assessment

- Monitor progression of zinc deficiency symptoms (impaired wound healing, growth retardation, decreased sense of taste, decreased sense of smell) during therapy.
- ***Lab Test Considerations:*** Serum zinc levels may not accurately reflect zinc deficiency.
- Long-term high-dose zinc therapy may cause ↓ serum copper concentrations.
- Monitor serum alkaline phosphatase concentrations monthly; may ↑ with zinc therapy.
- Monitor HDL concentrations monthly in patients on long-term high-dose zinc therapy. Serum concentrations may be ↓.

Potential Nursing Diagnoses

Imbalanced nutrition: less than body requirements (Indications)

Implementation

- **PO:** Administer oral doses with food to decrease gastric irritation. Administration with caffeine, dairy products, or bran may impair absorption.
- **IV:** Zinc is often included as a trace mineral in total parenteral nutrition solution prepared by pharmacist.

Patient/Family Teaching

- Encourage patient to comply with diet recommendations of health care professional. Explain that the best source of vitamins is a well-balanced diet with foods from the four basic food groups. Foods high in zinc include seafood, organ meats, and wheat germ.
- Patients self-medicating with vitamin supplements should be cautioned not to exceed RDA. The effectiveness of megadoses for treatment of various medical conditions is unproved and may cause side effects.
- Instruct patients receiving oral zinc to notify health care professional if severe nausea or vomiting, abdominal pain, or tarry stools occur.
- Emphasize the importance of follow-up exams to evaluate progress.

Evaluation/Desired Outcomes

- Improved wound healing.
- Improved senses of taste or smell. 6–8 wk of therapy may be required before full effect is seen.

---

ziprasidone (zi-pra-si-done)
Geodon

Classification
Therapeutic: antipsychotics, mood stabilizers
Pharmacologic: piperazine derivatives

Pregnancy Category C

Indications

Schizophrenia; IM form is reserved for control of acutely agitated patients. Bipolar mania (acute manic and manic/mixed episodes).

Action

Effects probably mediated by antagonism of dopamine type 2 (D2) and serotonin type 2 (5-HT$_2$). Also antagonizes α_2 adrenergic receptors. **Therapeutic Effects:** Diminished schizophrenic behavior.

Pharmacokinetics

Absorption: 60% absorbed following oral administration; 100% absorbed from IM sites.
Distribution: Unknown.
Protein Binding: 99%; potential for drug interactions due to drug displacement is minimal.
Metabolism and Excretion: 99% metabolized by the liver; <1% excreted unchanged in urine.
Half-life: *PO*—7 hr; *IM*—2–5 hr.

TIME/ACTION PROFILE (blood levels)

ROUTE	ONSET	PEAK	DURATION
PO	within hours	1–3 days†	unknown
IM	rapid	60 min	unknown

†Steady state achieved following continuous use

✦ = Canadian drug name. = Genetic implication.
*CAPITALS indicates life-threatening; underlines indicate most frequent.

Contraindications/Precautions

Contraindicated in: Hypersensitivity; History of QT prolongation (persistent QTc measurements >500 msec), arrhythmias, recent MI or uncompensated heart failure; Concurrent use of other drugs known to prolong the QT interval including quinidine, dofetilide, sotalol, other class Ia and III antiarrhythmics, pimozide, sotalol, thioridazine, chlorpromazine, pentamidine, arsenic trioxide, mefloquine, dolasetron, tacrolimus, droperidol, and moxifloxacin; Hypokalemia or hypomagnesemia; Lactation: Discontinue drug or bottle feed.

Use Cautiously in: Concurrent diuretic therapy or diarrhea (may ↑ the risk of hypotension, hypokalemia, or hypomagnesemia); Significant hepatic impairment; History of cardiovascular or cerebrovascular disease; Hypotension, concurrent antihypertensive therapy, dehydration, or hypovolemia (may ↑ risk of orthostatic hypotension); OB: Use only if potential benefit outweighs potential risk to the fetus; Pedi: Safety not established; Geri: Alzheimer's dementia or age >65 yr (may ↑ risk of seizures). Geriatric patients (may require ↓ doses; ↑ risk of mortality in elderly patients treated for dementia-related psychosis); Patients at risk for aspiration pneumonia; History of suicide attempt.

Adverse Reactions/Side Effects

CNS: NEUROLEPTIC MALIGNANT SYNDROME, seizures, dizziness, drowsiness, restlessness, extrapyramidal reactions, syncope, tardive dyskinesia. **Resp:** cough/runny nose. **CV:** PROLONGED QT INTERVAL, orthostatic hypotension. **GI:** constipation, diarrhea, nausea, dysphagia. **GU:** amenorrhea, impotence. **Hemat:** AGRANULOCYTOSIS, leukopenia, neutropenia. **Endo:** galactorrhea. **Derm:** rash, urticaria.

Interactions

Drug-Drug: Concurrent use of **quinidine**, **dofetilide**, **other class Ia and III antiarrhythmics**, **pimozide**, **sotalol**, **thioridazine**, **chlorpromazine**, **pentamidine**, **arsenic trioxide**, **mefloquine**, **dolasetron**, **tacrolimus**, **droperidol**, **moxifloxacin**, or other agents that prolong the QT interval may result in potentially life-threatening adverse drug reactions (concurrent use contraindicated). Additive CNS depression may occur with **alcohol**, **antidepressants**, **antihistamines**, **opioid analgesics**, or **sedative/hypnotics**. Blood levels and effectiveness may be ↓ by **carbamazepine**. Blood levels and effects may be ↑ by **ketoconazole**.

Route/Dosage

PO (Adults): *Schizophrenia*—20 mg twice daily initially; dose increments may be made at 2- day intervals up to 80 mg twice daily; *Mania*—40 mg twice on first day, then 60 or 80 mg twice daily on second day, then 40–80 mg twice daily.

IM (Adults): 10–20 mg as needed up to 40 mg/day; may be given as 10 mg every 2 hr or 20 mg every 4 hr.

Availability

Capsules: 20 mg, 40 mg, 60 mg, 80 mg. **Cost:** 20 mg $974.88/180, 40 mg $975.96/180, 60 mg $1,172.00/180, 80 mg $1,172.00/180. **Lyophilized powder for injection (requires reconstitution):** 20 mg/vial.

NURSING IMPLICATIONS

Assessment

- Monitor patient's mental status (orientation, mood, behavior) prior to and periodically during therapy.
- Assess weight and BMI initially and throughout therapy.
- Monitor blood pressure (sitting, standing, lying) and pulse rate prior to and frequently during initial dose titration. Patients found to have persistent QTc measurements of >500 msec should have ziprasidone discontinued. Patients who experience dizziness, palpitations, or syncope may require further evaluation (i.e., Holter monitoring).
- Assess for rash during therapy. May be treated with antihistamines or corticosteroids. Usually resolves upon discontinuation of ziprasidone. Medication should be discontinued if no alternative etiology for rash is found.
- Observe carefully when administering medication to ensure medication is actually taken and not hoarded or cheeked.
- Monitor for onset of akathisia (restlessness or desire to keep moving) and extrapyramidal side effects (*parkinsonian*—difficulty speaking or swallowing, loss of balance control, pill rolling of hands, mask-like face, shuffling gait, rigidity, tremors and dystonic muscle spasms, twisting motions, twitching, inability to move eyes, weakness of arms or legs) every 2 mo during therapy and 8–12 wk after therapy has been discontinued. Notify health care professional if these symptoms occur, as reduction in dose or discontinuation of medication may be necessary. Trihexyphenidyl or benztropine may be used to control these symptoms.
- Although not yet reported for ziprasidone, monitor for possible tardive dyskinesia (uncontrolled rhythmic movement of mouth, face, and extremities, lip smacking or puckering, puffing of cheeks, uncontrolled chewing, rapid

or worm-like movements of tongue). Report these symptoms immediately; may be irreversible.
- Monitor frequency and consistency of bowel movements. Increasing bulk and fluids in the diet may help to minimize constipation.
- Ziprasidone lowers the seizure threshold. Institute seizure precautions for patients with history of seizure disorder.
- Monitor for development of neuroleptic malignant syndrome (fever, respiratory distress, tachycardia, seizures, diaphoresis, hypertension or hypotension, pallor, tiredness). Notify health care professional immediately if these symptoms occur.
- Monitor for symptoms related to hyperprolactinemia (menstrual abnormalities, galactorrhea, sexual dysfunction).
- *Lab Test Considerations:* Monitor serum potassium and magnesium prior to and periodically during therapy. Patients with low potassium or magnesium should have levels treated and check prior to resuming therapy. Obtain fasting blood glucose and cholesterol levels initially and throughout therapy.
- Monitor CBC frequently during initial months of therapy in patients with pre-existing or history of low WBC. May cause leukopenia, neutropenia, or agranulocytosis. Discontinue therapy if this occurs.
- Monitor serum prolactin prior to and periodically during therapy. May cause ↑ serum prolactin levels.

Potential Nursing Diagnoses
Risk for other-directed violence (Indications)
Disturbed thought process (Indications)
Imbalanced nutrition: risk for more than body requirements (Side Effects)

Implementation
- Dose adjustments should be made at intervals of no less than 2 days. Usually patients should be observed for several weeks before dose titration.
- Patients on parenteral therapy should be converted to oral doses as soon as possible.
- **PO:** Administer capsules with food or milk to decrease gastric irritation. Capsules should be swallowed whole; do not open.
- **IM:** Add 1.2 mL of Sterile Water for Injection to the vial; shake vigorously until all drug is dissolved for a concentration of 20 mg/mL. Discard unused portion. Do not mix with other products or solutions. Do not administer solutions that are discolored or contain particulate matter.

Patient/Family Teaching
- Instruct patient to take medication as directed. Do not discontinue medication without discussing with health care professional, even if feeling well. Patients on long-term therapy may need to discontinue gradually.
- Inform patient of possibility of extrapyramidal symptoms. Instruct patient to report these symptoms immediately.
- Advise patient to change positions slowly to minimize orthostatic hypotension.
- May cause seizures and drowsiness. Caution patient to avoid driving or other activities requiring alertness until response to medication is known.
- Caution patient to avoid concurrent use of alcohol, other CNS depressants, Rx, OTC and herbal products without consulting health care professional.
- Advise patient to notify health care professional of medication regimen prior to treatment or surgery.
- Instruct patient to notify health care professional promptly if dizziness, loss of consciousness, palpitations, menstrual abnormalities, galactorrhea or sexual dysfunction occur or if pregnancy is planned or suspected.
- Advise female patients to notify health care professional if pregnancy is planned or suspected, or if breastfeeding or planning to breastfeed.
- Advise patient of need for continued medical follow-up for psychotherapy, eye exams, and laboratory tests.

Evaluation/Desired Outcomes
- Decrease in acute excited, manic behavior.
- Decrease in positive (delusions, hallucinations) and negative symptoms (social withdrawal, flat, blunted affect) of schizophrenia.

---

zoledronic acid
(zoe-led-**dron**-ic **as**-id)
Reclast, Zometa

Classification
Therapeutic: bone resorption inhibitors, electrolyte modifiers, hypocalcemics
Pharmacologic: biphosphonates

Pregnancy Category C

zoledronic acid

Indications
Hypercalcemia of malignancy (Zometa only). Multiple myeloma and metastatic bone lesions from solid tumors (Zometa only). Paget's disease (Reclast only). Treatment of osteoporosis in men (Reclast only). Treatment and prevention of osteoporosis in postmenopausal women (Reclast only). Treatment and prevention of glucocorticoid-induced osteoporosis in patients expected to be on glucocorticoids for at least 12 months (Reclast only).

Action
Inhibits bone resorption. Inhibits increased osteoclast activity and skeletal calcium release induced by tumors. **Therapeutic Effects:** Decreased serum calcium. Decreased serum alkaline phosphatase. Decreased fractures, radiation/surgery to bone, or spinal cord compression in patients with multiple myeloma or metastatic bone lesions. Decreased hip, vertebral, or non-vertebral osteoporosis-related fractures in postmenopausal women. Increased bone mass in men, postmenopausal women, and patients on prolonged corticosteroid therapy.

Pharmacokinetics
Absorption: IV administration results in complete bioavailability.
Distribution: Unknown.
Metabolism and Excretion: Mostly excreted unchanged by the kidneys.
Half-life: 167 hr.

TIME/ACTION PROFILE (effect on serum calcium)

ROUTE	ONSET	PEAK	DURATION
IV	within 4 days	4-7 days	30 days

Contraindications/Precautions
Contraindicated in: Hypersensitivity to zoledronic acid or other bisphosphonates.
Use Cautiously in: Severe renal impairment (not recommended if CCr <35 mL/min); History of aspirin-induced asthma; Concurrent use of loop diuretics or dehydration (↑ risk of renal impairment; correct deficits prior to use); Concurrent use of nephrotoxic drugs; Dental surgery (may ↑ risk of jaw osteonecrosis); OB, Lactation: Pedi: Safety not established.

Adverse Reactions/Side Effects
CNS: agitation, anxiety, confusion, insomnia. **EENT:** conjunctivitis. **CV:** hypotension, chest pain, leg edema. **GI:** abdominal pain, constipation, diarrhea, nausea, vomiting, dysphagia. **GU:** renal impairment/failure. **Derm:** pruritus, rash. **F and E:** hypophosphatemia, hypocalcemia, hypokalemia, hypomagnesemia. **Hemat:** anemia. **MS:** musculoskeletal pain, osteonecrosis (primarily of jaw). **Misc:** fever, flu-like syndrome.

Interactions
Drug-Drug: Concurrent use of **loop diuretics** or **aminoglycosides** ↑ risk of hypocalcemia. Concurrent use of **NSAIDs** may ↑ risk of nephrotoxicity.

Route/Dosage
Reclast
IV (Adults): *Paget's disease*—5 mg as a single dose (information regarding retreatment unknown); *Treatment of osteoporosis in men or postmenopausal women, treatment/prevention of glucocorticoid-induced osteoporosis*—5 mg once early; *Prevention of osteoporosis in postmenopausal women*—5 mg every 2 yr.

Zometa
IV (Adults): *Hypercalcemia of malignancy*—4 mg; may be repeated after 7 days; *Multiple myeloma and bone metastases from solid tumors*—4 mg q 3–4 wk (has been used for up to 15 mo).

Availability
Solution for IV infusion (Zometa): 4 mg/5-mL vial. Solution for IV infusion (premixed) (Reclast): 5 mg/100 mL.

NURSING IMPLICATIONS

Assessment
- Monitor intake and output ratios. Initiate a vigorous saline hydration promptly and maintain a urine output of 2 L/day during therapy. Patients should be adequately hydrated, but avoid overhydration. Do not use diuretics prior to treatment of hypovolemia.
- Assess for acute-phase reaction (fever, mylagia, flu-like symptoms, headache, arthralgia). Usually occur within 3 days of dose and resolve within 3 days of onset, but may take 7–14 days to resolve; incidence decreases with repeat dosing.
- **Hypercalcemia:** Monitor symptoms of hypercalcemia (nausea, vomiting, anorexia, weakness, constipation, thirst, cardiac arrhythmias).
- Observe for evidence of hypocalcemia (paresthesia, muscle twitching, laryngospasm, Chvostek's or Trousseau's sign).
- **Paget's Disease:** Assess for symptoms of Paget's disease (bone pain, headache, decreased visual and auditory acuity, increased skull size) periodically during therapy.

zoledronic acid

- **Osteoporosis:** Assess patients via bone density study for low bone mass before and periodically during therapy.
- **Lab Test Considerations:** Monitor serum creatinine prior to each treatment. Patients with a normal serum creatinine prior to treatment, who develop an increase of 0.5 mg/dL within 2 wk of next dose should have next dose withheld until serum creatinine is within 10% of baseline value. Patients with an abnormal serum creatinine prior to treatment who have an increase of 1.0 mg/dL within 2 wk of next dose should have next dose withheld until serum creatinine is within 10% of baseline value.
- Assess serum calcium, phosphate, and magnesium before and periodically during therapy. If hypocalcemia, hypophosphatemia, or hypomagnesemia occur, temporary supplementation may be required.
- Monitor CBC with differential and hemoglobin and hematocrit closely during therapy.
- *Paget's Disease:* Monitor serum alkaline phosphatase prior to and periodically during therapy to monitor effectiveness.

Potential Nursing Diagnoses
Risk for injury (Indications)

Implementation
- Vigorous saline hydration alone may be sufficient to treat mild, asymptomatic hypercalcemia. Adequate rehydration is required prior to administration.
- Patients on long-term therapy should have 1200 mg of oral calcium and 800–1000 units of Vitamin D each day.
- Patients treated for *Paget's disease* should receive 1500 mg elemental calcium and 800 IU of vitamin D daily, particularly during the 2 wk after dosing. Patients with osteoporosis should take 1200 mg of calcium and 800–1000 IU of Vitamin D daily.
- Administration of acetaminophen or ibuprofen following administration may reduce the incidence of acute-phase reaction symptoms.

IV Administration
- **Intermittent Infusion: *Diluent:*** Reconstitute *Zometa* by adding 5 mL of sterile water for injection to each vial for a solution containing 4 mg of zoledronic acid. Medication must be completely dissolved prior to withdrawal of solution. Dilute 4-mg dose further with 100 mL of 0.9% NaCl or D5W. If not used immediately, may be refrigerated for up to 24 hr. *Reclast* comes ready to use 5 mg in 100-mL solution. If refrigerated, allow solution to reach room temperature prior to administration. Do not administer solution that is discolored or contains particulate matter. ***Rate:*** Administer as a single infusion over at least 15 min. Rapid infusions increase risk of renal deterioration and renal failure.
- **Y-Site Compatibility:** bivalirudin, daptomycin, ertapenem, octreotide, oxytocin, tigecycline, tirofiban.
- **Y-Site Incompatibility:** Manufacturer recommends administration as a single infusion in a line separate from all other drugs. Calcium-containing solutions.
- **Additive Incompatibility:** Do not mix with solutions containing calcium, such as Lactated Ringer's solution.

Patient/Family Teaching
- Explain the purpose of zoledronic acid to patient. Advise patient to read medication guide prior to administration.
- Advise patients of the importance of adequate hydration. Patient should be instructed to drink at least two glasses of water prior to receiving dose.
- Advise patient to notify health care professional before taking any Rx, OTC, or herbal products with zoledronic acid.
- Advise patient to eat a balanced diet and consult health care professional about the need for supplemental calcium and vitamin D.
- Inform patient that severe musculoskeletal pain may occur within days, months, or yr after starting zoledronic acid. Symptoms may resolve completely after discontinuation or slow or incomplete resolution may occur. Notify health care professional if severe pain occurs.
- Encourage patient to participate in regular exercise and to modify behaviors that increase the risk of osteoporosis (stop smoking, reduce alcohol consumption).
- Advise patient to inform health care professional of zoledronic acid therapy prior to dental surgery.
- Advise patient to notify health care professional if pregnancy is planned or suspected or if breastfeeding.
- Emphasize the importance of lab tests to monitor progress.

Evaluation/Desired Outcomes
- Decrease in serum calcium.
- Decrease in serum alkaline phosphatase and the progression of Paget's disease.
- Reversal of the progression of osteoporosis with decreased fractures and other sequelae.

---

zolmitriptan (zole-mi-trip-tan)
Zomig, Zomig-ZMT

Classification
Therapeutic: vascular headache suppressants
Pharmacologic: 5-HT$_1$ agonists

Pregnancy Category C

Indications
Acute treatment of migraine headache.

Action
Acts as an agonist at specific 5-HT$_1$ receptor sites in intracranial blood vessels and sensory trigeminal nerves. **Therapeutic Effects:** Cranial vessel vasoconstriction with resultant decrease in migraine headache.

Pharmacokinetics
Absorption: Well absorbed (40%) following oral and intranasal administration.
Distribution: Unknown.
Metabolism and Excretion: Mostly metabolized by the liver; some conversion to metabolites that are more active than zolmitriptan. 8% excreted unchanged in urine.
Half-life: 3 hr (for zolmitriptan and active metabolite).

TIME/ACTION PROFILE (relief of headache)

ROUTE	ONSET	PEAK	DURATION
PO	unknown	1.5 hr*	unknown
Intranasal	unknown	3 hr	unknown

*3 hr for orally disintegrating tablets

Contraindications/Precautions
Contraindicated in: Hypersensitivity; Significant underlying heart disease (including ischemic heart disease, history of MI, coronary artery vasospasm, uncontrolled hypertension); Stroke or transient ischemic attack; Peripheral vascular disease (including, but not limited to ischemic bowel disease); Concurrent (or within 24 hr) use of other 5-HT agonists, ergotamine, or ergot-type medications; Concurrent (or within 2 wk) use of MAO inhibitors; Hemiplegic or basilar migraine; Symptomatic Wolff-Parkinson-White syndrome or other arrhythmias.

Use Cautiously in: Cardiovascular risk factors (hypertension, hypercholesterolemia, cigarette smoking, obesity, diabetes, strong family history, menopausal females or males >40 yr [use only if cardiovascular status has been evaluated and determined to be safe and 1st dose is administered under supervision]); Hepatic impairment (use lower doses); OB, Lactation: Pedi: Safety not established.

Adverse Reactions/Side Effects
CNS: dizziness, drowsiness, vertigo, weakness. **EENT:** throat pain/tightness/pressure. **CV:** MI, angina, chest pain/pressure/tightness/heaviness, hypertension, palpitations. **GI:** dry mouth, dyspepsia, dysphagia, nausea. **Derm:** sweating, warm/cold sensation. **MS:** myalgia, myasthenia. **Neuro:** hypesthesia, paresthesia. **Misc:** feeling of heaviness, pain.

Interactions
Drug-Drug: Because of ↑ risk of cerebral vasospasm, avoid concurrent use of other **5-HT agonists** (**naratriptan**, **sumatriptan**, **rizatriptan**) and/or **ergot-type preparations** (**dihydroergotamine**). Concurrent use of **MAO inhibitors** ↑ blood levels and risk of toxicity (avoid use within 2 wk of MAO inhibitors). Blood levels may be ↑ by **hormonal contraceptives**. **Cimetidine** ↑ half-life of zolmitriptan and its active metabolite. Concurrent use with **SSRI antidepressants** may result in weakness, hyperreflexia and incoordination. ↑ serotonin levels and serotonin syndrome may occur when used concurrently with **SSRI and SNRI antidepressants**.
Drug-Natural Products: ↑ risk of serotinergic side effects including serotonin syndrome with **St. John's wort** and **SAMe**.

Route/Dosage
PO (Adults): 2.5 mg or less initially; if headache returns, dose may be repeated after 2 hr (not to exceed 10 mg/24 hr).
Intranasal (Adults): single 5-mg dose; may be repeated after 2 hr (not to exceed 10 mg/24 hr).

Availability
Tablets: 2.5 mg, 5 mg. **Orally disintegrating tablets:** 2.5 mg, 5 mg. **Nasal spray:** 5 mg/100 mcL unit-dose spray device (package of 6).

NURSING IMPLICATIONS

Assessment
- Assess pain location, intensity, duration, and associated symptoms (photophobia, phonophobia, nausea, vomiting) during migraine attack.

- Monitor for serotonin syndrome in patients taking SSRIs or SNRIs concurrently with zolmitriptan.

Potential Nursing Diagnoses
Acute pain (Indications)

Implementation
- Do not confuse zolmitriptan with sumatriptan.
- **PO:** Initial dose is 2.5 mg. Lower doses can be achieved by breaking 2.5-mg tablet.
- Orally disintegrating tablets should be left in the package until use. Remove from the blister pouch. Do not push tablet through the blister; peel open the blister pack with dry hands and place tablet on tongue. Tablet will dissolve rapidly and be swallowed with saliva. No liquid is needed to take the orally disintegrating tablet.
- **Intranasal:** Remove cap from nasal spray. Hold upright and block one nostril. Tilt head slightly back, insert device into opposite nostril, and depress plunger. May repeat in 2 hr.

Patient/Family Teaching
- Inform patient that zolmitriptan should be used only during a migraine attack. It is meant to be used to relieve migraine attack but not to prevent or reduce the number of attacks.
- Instruct patient to administer zolmitriptan as soon as symptoms appear, but it may be administered any time during an attack. If migraine symptoms return, a 2nd dose may be used. Allow at least 2 hr between doses, and do not use more than 10 mg in any 24-hr period.
- If dose does not relieve headache, additional zolmitriptan doses are not likely to be effective; notify health care professional.
- Advise patient that lying down in a darkened room following zolmitriptan administration may further help relieve headache.
- May cause dizziness or drowsiness. Caution patient to avoid driving or other activities requiring alertness until response to medication is known.
- Advise patient to notify health care professional prior to next dose of zolmitriptan if pain or tightness in the chest occurs during use. If pain is severe or does not subside, notify health care professional immediately. If wheezing; heart throbbing; swelling of eyelids, face, or lips; skin rash; skin lumps; or hives occur, notify health care professional immediately and do not take more zolmitriptan without approval of health care professional. If feelings of tingling, heat, flushing, heaviness, pressure, drowsiness, dizziness, tiredness, or sickness develop, discuss with health care professional at next visit.
- Advise patient to avoid alcohol, which aggravates headaches, during zolmitriptan use.
- Advise patient to consult health care professional before taking other Rx, OTC, or herbal products concurrently with sumatriptan. Patients concurrently taking SSRI or SNRI antidepressants should notify health care professional promptly if signs of serotonin syndrome (mental status changes: agitation, hallucinations, coma; autonomic instability: tachycardia, labile blood pressure, hyperthermia; neuromuscular aberrations: hyper-reflexia, incoordination; and/or gastrointestinal symptoms: nausea, vomiting, diarrhea) occur.
- Caution patient not to use zolmitriptan if pregnancy is planned or suspected or if breastfeeding. Adequate contraception should be used during therapy.

Evaluation/Desired Outcomes
- Relief of migraine attack.

---

zolpidem (zole-pi-dem)
Ambien, Ambien CR, Edluar, Zolpimist

Classification
Therapeutic: sedative/hypnotics

Schedule IV

Pregnancy Category C

Indications
Insomnia.

Action
Produces CNS depression by binding to GABA receptors. Has no analgesic properties. **Therapeutic Effects:** Sedation and induction of sleep.

Pharmacokinetics
Absorption: Rapidly absorbed following oral administration. Controlled-release formulation releases 10 mg immediately, then another 2.5 mg later.
Distribution: Minimal amounts enter breast milk; remainder of distribution not known.
Metabolism and Excretion: Converted to inactive metabolites, which are excreted by the kidneys.
Half-life: 2.5–3 hr (↑ in geriatric patients and patients with hepatic impairment).

✺ = Canadian drug name.　✇ = Genetic implication.
*CAPITALS indicates life-threatening; underlines indicate most frequent.

zolpidem

TIME/ACTION PROFILE (sedation)

ROUTE	ONSET	PEAK*	DURATION
PO	rapid	30 min–2 hr	6–8 hr
PO-ER	rapid	2–4 hr	6–8 hr
PO-Spray	rapid	unknown	unknown
SL	rapid	unknown	unknown

*Food delays peak levels and effects

Contraindications/Precautions
Contraindicated in: Hypersensitivity; Sleep apnea.
Use Cautiously in: History of previous psychiatric illness, suicide attempt, drug or alcohol abuse; Hepatic impairment (initial dose reduction recommended); Geri: Geriatric patients (initial dose ↓ recommended); Pulmonary disease; OB, Lactation: Pedi: Pregnancy, lactation, or children (safety not established).

Adverse Reactions/Side Effects
CNS: daytime drowsiness, dizziness, abnormal thinking, amnesia, behavior changes, "drugged" feeling, hallucinations, sleep-driving. **GI:** diarrhea, nausea, vomiting. **Misc:** ANAPHYLACTIC REACTIONS, hypersensitivity reactions, physical dependence, psychological dependence, tolerance.

Interactions
Drug-Drug: CNS depression may ↑ with **sedatives/hypnotics**, **alcohol**, **phenothiazines**, **tricyclic antidepressants**, **opioid analgesics**, or **antihistamines**.
Drug-Natural Products: Concomitant use of **kava-kava**, **valerian**, or **chamomile** can ↑ CNS depression.
Drug-Food: Food ↓ and delays absorption.

Route/Dosage
PO, SL (Adults): *Tablets, spray, or SL tablets*—10 mg at bedtime; *Extended-release tablets*—12.5 mg at bedtime.
PO, SL (Geriatric Patients, Debilitated Patients, or Patients with Hepatic Impairment): *Tablets, spray or SL tablets*—5 mg at bedtime initially; *Extended-release tablets*—6.25 mg at bedtime.

Availability (generic available)
Tablets: 5 mg, 10 mg. **Cost:** *Generic*—5 mg $15.99/30, 10 mg $17.99/30. **Extended-release tablets:** 6.25 mg, 12.5 mg. **Cost:** 6.25 mg $109.99/30, 12.5 mg $110.99/30. **Sublingual tablets (Edluar):** 5 mg, 10 mg. **Oral spray (Zolpimist):** 5 mg/spray (60 sprays/container).

NURSING IMPLICATIONS
Assessment
- Assess mental status, sleep patterns, and potential for abuse prior to administration. Prolonged use of >7–10 days may lead to physical and psychological dependence. Limit amount of drug available to the patient.
- Assess alertness at time of peak effect. Notify health care professional if desired sedation does not occur.
- Assess patient for pain. Medicate as needed. Untreated pain decreases sedative effects.

Potential Nursing Diagnoses
Insomnia (Indications)
Risk for injury (Side Effects)

Implementation
- Before administering, reduce external stimuli and provide comfort measures to increase effectiveness of medication.
- Protect patient from injury. Raise bed side rails. Assist with ambulation. Take patient's cigarettes.
- **PO:** Tablets should be swallowed whole with full glass of water. For faster onset of sleep, do not administer with or immediately after a meal.
- Swallow extended-release tablets whole; do not crush, break, or chew.
- **SL:** To open the blister pack, separate the individual blisters at the perforations. Peel off top layer of paper and push tablet through foil. Place the tablet under the tongue, allow to disintegrate; do not swallow or take with water.
- **Oral Spray:** Do not take with or immediately after a meal. Spray is a clear, colorless, and cherry-flavor solution.

Patient/Family Teaching
- Instruct patient to take zolpidem as directed. Advise patient not to take zolpidem unless able to stay in bed a full night (7–8 hours) before being active again. Do not take more than the amount prescribed because of the habit-forming potential. Not recommended for use longer than 7–10 days. If used for 2 wk or longer, abrupt withdrawal may result in fatigue, nausea, flushing, light-headedness, uncontrolled crying, vomiting, GI upset, panic attack, or nervousness. Instruct patient to read *Patient Information* for correct product before taking and with each Rx refill, changes may occur.
- Because of rapid onset, advise patient to go to bed immediately after taking zolpidem.
- May cause daytime drowsiness or dizziness. Advise patient to avoid driving or other activi-

ties requiring alertness until response to this medication is known.
- Caution patient that complex sleep-related behaviors (sleep-driving) may occur while asleep.
- Advise patient to notify health care professional immediately if signs of anaphylaxis (swelling of the tongue or throat, trouble breathing, and nausea and vomiting) occur.
- Caution patient to avoid concurrent use of alcohol or other CNS depressants.
- **Oral Spray:** To prime, patients should be told to point the black spray opening away from their face and other people and spray 5 times. For administration, hold container upright with the black spray opening pointed directly into the mouth. Press down fully on pump to make sure a full dose (5 mg) is sprayed directly into mouth over tongue. For 10-mg dose, a second spray should be administered. If not used for 14 days, re-prime with 1 spray.

Evaluation/Desired Outcomes
- Relief of insomnia.

---

zonisamide (zoe-**niss**-a-mide)
Zonegran

Classification
Therapeutic: anticonvulsants
Pharmacologic: sulfonamides

Pregnancy Category C

Indications
Partial seizures in adults.

Action
Raises the threshold for seizures and reduces duration of seizures probably by action on sodium and calcium channels. **Therapeutic Effects:** Decreased frequency of partial seizures.

Pharmacokinetics
Absorption: Well absorbed following oral administration.
Distribution: Binds extensively to red blood cells.
Metabolism and Excretion: Mostly metabolized by the liver; 35% excreted unchanged in urine. Some metabolism occurs via CYP3A4 enzyme system.
Half-life: 63 hr (plasma).

TIME/ACTION PROFILE (blood levels†)

ROUTE	ONSET	PEAK	DURATION
PO	unknown	2–6 hr	24 hr

†Requires 2 weeks of dosing to achieve steady-state blood levels

Contraindications/Precautions
Contraindicated in: Hypersensitivity to zonisamide or sulfonamides.
Use Cautiously in: All patients (may ↑ risk of suicidal thoughts/behaviors); Hepatic or renal disease (may require slower titration/more frequent monitoring; ↑ risk of metabolic acidosis with renal impairment); Patients with respiratory disorders, diarrhea, or undergoing surgery (↑ risk of metabolic acidosis); OB, Lactation: Use only if potential benefit justifies risk to fetus/infant; Pedi: Children ≤16 yr (safety not established; ↑ risk of oligohydrosis, hyperthermia, and/or metabolic acidosis).

Adverse Reactions/Side Effects
CNS: SUICIDAL THOUGHTS, drowsiness, fatigue, agitation/irritability, depression, dizziness, psychomotor slowing, psychosis, weakness. **EENT:** amblyopia, tinnitus. **Resp:** cough, pharyngitis. **GI:** anorexia, nausea, vomiting. **F and E:** metabolic acidosis. **GU:** kidney stones. **Derm:** oligohydrosis (↑ in children), rash. **Metab:** hyperthermia (↑ in children). **Neuro:** abnormal gait, hyperasthesia, incoordination, tremor. **Misc:** ALLERGIC REACTIONS INCLUDING STEVENS-JOHNSON SYNDROME.

Interactions
Drug-Drug: Drugs that induce or inhibit CYP3A4 may alter blood levels and effects of zonisamide. Blood levels and effects may be ↓ by **phenytoin**, **carbamzepine**, **phenobarbital**, or **valproate**.

Route/Dosage
PO (Adults and Children >16 yr): 100 mg once daily initially for 2 wk, then ↑ to 200 mg daily for 2 wk; with subsequent increments of 100 mg made at 2-wk intervals as required (range 100–600 mg/day). Can be given as a single daily dose or in 2 divided doses.

Availability (generic available)
Capsules: 25 mg, 50 mg, 100 mg.

NURSING IMPLICATIONS

Assessment
- Monitor closely for notable changes in behavior that could indicate the emergence or wors-

= Canadian drug name. = Genetic implication.
*CAPITALS indicates life-threatening; underlines indicate most frequent.

ening of suicidal thoughts or behavior or depression.
- Monitor frequency, duration, and characteristics of seizures.
- Monitor patient frequently for development of skin rash. Unexplained rash may require discontinuation of therapy.
- Assess patient for allergy to sulfa drugs.
- ***Lab Test Considerations:*** Monitor renal function periodically during therapy. May cause ↑ creatinine and BUN.
- Measure serum bicarbonate before starting and periodically during therapy. Metabolic acidosis may be more frequent and severe in younger patients.
- May cause ↑ in serum alkaline phosphatase.

Potential Nursing Diagnoses
Risk for injury (Adverse Reactions)

Implementation
- **PO:** May be administered with or without meals. Capsules should be swallowed whole.

Patient/Family Teaching
- Instruct patient to take zonisamide as directed, even if feeling well. Consult health care professional if a dose is missed. Do not discontinue abruptly without consulting health care professional; may cause seizures. Instruct patient to read the *Medication Guide* before starting and with each Rx refill, changes may occur.
- Instruct patient to contact health care professional immediately if skin rash occurs or seizures worsen. Patient should also contact health care professional if a child taking zonisamide is not sweating as usual, with or without a fever, or if they develop fever, sore throat, oral ulcers, easy bruising, depression, unusual thoughts, speech or language problems.
- May cause drowsiness. Caution patient to avoid driving or other activities requiring alertness until cleared by physician and effects of medication is known.
- Advise patient to increase fluid intake to at least 6–8 glasses of water/day to minimize risk of kidney stones. Instruct patient to contact health care professional if symptoms of kidney stones (sudden back pain, abdominal pain, blood in urine) occur.
- Advise patient and family to notify health care professional if thoughts about suicide or dying, attempts to commit suicide; new or worse depression; new or worse anxiety; feeling very agitated or restless; panic attacks; trouble sleeping; new or worse irritability; acting aggressive; being angry or violent; acting on dangerous impulses; an extreme increase in activity and talking, other unusual changes in behavior or mood occur.
- Instruct patient to consult health care professional prior to taking other Rx, OTC, or herbal products.
- May have teratogenic effects. Advise women of childbearing age to use effective contraception throughout therapy. Instruct patient to notify health care professional if pregnancy is planned or suspected or if planning to breast feed.

Evaluation/Desired Outcomes
- Decrease in frequency and duration of partial seizures.

Less Commonly Used Drugs

acamprosate calcium
(a-**cam**-pro-sate)
Campral

Classification
Therapeutic: alcohol abuse therapy adjuncts
Pharmacologic: gamma aminobutyric acid (GABA) analogues

Pregnancy Category C

Indications
Maintenance of alcohol abstinence; part of a comprehensive alcohol abstinence program.

Contraindications/Precautions
Contraindicated in: Hypersensitivity; CCr 30 mL/min or less.
Use Cautiously in: CCr 30–50 mL/min (dose reduction necessary); History of depression or suicide attempt; OB: Use only if potential maternal benefit outweighs fetal risk; Lactation, Pedi: Safety not established.

Adverse Reactions/Side Effects
CNS: abnormal thinking, anxiety, depression, drowsiness, headache. **EENT:** abnormal vision. **Resp:** cough, dyspnea, pharyngitis, rhinitis. **CV:** palpitations, peripheral edema, syncope, vasodilation. **GI:** abdominal pain, anorexia, constipation, diarrhea, flatulence, ↑ appetite, nausea, taste perversion, vomiting. **GU:** ↓ libido, erectile dysfunction. **Derm:** rash. **Metab:** weight gain. **MS:** arthralgia, back pain, myalgia. **Neuro:** tremor.

Route/Dosage
PO (Adults): Two 333-mg tablets (666 mg/dose) three times daily. Lower doses may be effective in some patients.

Renal Impairment
PO (Adults): *CCr 30–50 mL/min*—One 333-mg tablet three times daily.

activated charcoal
Acta-Char Liquid-A, Actidose-Aqua, ✤ Aqueous Charcodote, ✤ Charac-50, CharcoAid 2000, ✤ Charcodote, Insta-Char, Insta-Char Aqueous Suspension, Liqui-Char, SuperChar Aqueous

Classification
Therapeutic: antidotes
Pharmacologic: adsorbents

Pregnancy Category C

Indications
Acute management of many oral poisonings following emesis/lavage.

Contraindications/Precautions
Contraindicated in: No known contraindications.
Use Cautiously in: Poisonings due to cyanide, corrosives, ethanol, methanol, petroleum distillates, organic solvents, mineral acids, or iron; Endoscopic examination (observation will be obscured).

Adverse Reactions/Side Effects
GI: black stools, constipation, diarrhea, vomiting.

Route/Dosage
Antidote
PO (Adults): 25–100 g (may be repeated q 4–6 hr).
PO (Children 1–12 yr): 25–50 g (may be repeated q 4–6 hr).
PO (Children <1 yr): 1 g/kg (may be repeated q 4–6 hr).

aldesleukin (al-dess-**loo**-kin)
interleukin-2, IL-2, Proleukin

Classification
Therapeutic: antineoplastics
Pharmacologic: interleukins

Pregnancy Category C

Indications
Management of metastatic renal cell carcinoma.

Contraindications/Precautions
Contraindicated in: Hypersensitivity to aldesleukin or mannitol; Cross-sensitivity to *Escherichia coli*—derived proteins may occur; Patients with any history of cardiac or pulmonary disease as assessed by abnormal thallium stress

1317

testing or abnormal pulmonary function testing; Patients who have experienced any of the following toxicities during previous courses of aldesleukin—sustained ventricular tachycardia (≥5 beats), angina pectoris or MI as indicated by ECG changes, respiratory problems requiring more than 72 hr of intubation, pericardial tamponade, renal toxicity requiring more than 72 hr of dialysis, CNS dysfunction consisting of more than 48 hr of coma or psychosis, intractable seizures, bowel perforation or ischemia, GI bleeding requiring surgical intervention; Patients who have had allograft organ transplantation (increased risk of rejection).

Use Cautiously in: Patients with a history of cardiovascular, respiratory, hepatic, or renal disease; Patients with a history of seizures or suspected CNS metastases (symptoms may be exaggerated and seizures may occur); Patients with child-bearing potential; OB, Lactation: Pedi: Safety not established.

Adverse Reactions/Side Effects
Resp: APNEA, RESPIRATORY FAILURE, dyspnea, pulmonary congestion, pulmonary edema, hemoptysis, pleural effusion, pneumothorax, tachypnea, wheezing. **CV:** CARDIAC ARREST, CHF, MI, STROKE, arrhythmias, hypotension, tachycardia, myocardial ischemia, pericardial effusion, thrombosis. **GI:** BOWEL PERFORATION, diarrhea, jaundice, nausea, stomatitis, vomiting, ascites, hepatomegaly. **GU:** oliguria/anuria, proteinuria, dysuria, hematuria, renal failure. **Derm:** EXFOLIATATIVE DERMATITIS, pruritus. **F and E:** acidosis, hypocalcemia, hypokalemia, hypomagnesemia, hypophosphatemia, alkalosis, hyperkalemia, hyperuricemia, hyponatremia. **Hemat:** anemia, coagulation disorders, leukopenia, thrombocytopenia, eosinophilia, leukocytosis. **Misc:** CAPILLARY LEAK SYNDROME, chills, fever, weight gain, weight loss.

Route/Dosage
IV (Adults): 600,000 IU/kg (0.037 mg/kg) every 8 hr for 14 doses. Cycle is repeated once after a 9-day rest period to a total of 28 doses. After a rest period of 7 wk, patients who have had a beneficial response may be evaluated for additional courses.

alitretinoin (a-li-tret-i-noyn)
Panretin

Classification
Therapeutic: antineoplastics
Pharmacologic: retinoids

Pregnancy Category D

Indications
Topical treatment of cutaneous lesions from AIDS-related Kaposi's sarcoma (KS).

Contraindications/Precautions
Contraindicated in: Hypersensitivity to retinoids; OB: Potential for birth defects; Lactation: Use breast milk alternative.
Use Cautiously in: Patients with childbearing potential; Pedi: Safety not established.

Adverse Reactions/Side Effects
Local: pain, pruritus, rash, edema, exfoliative, dermatitis, paresthesia.

Route/Dosage
Topical (Adults): Apply generous coating twice daily to KS lesions initially; application may be increased to 3–4 times daily.

amoxapine (a-mox-a-peen)
Asendin

Classification
Therapeutic: antidepressants

Pregnancy Category C

Indications
Treatment of various types of depression. **Unlabeled Use:** Anxiety, insomnia, neuropathic and chronic pain syndromes.

Contraindications/Precautions
Contraindicated in: Angle-closure glaucoma; Recent MI; Prolongation of QTc interval; Cardiac arrhythmia; Heart failure.
Use Cautiously in: Pre-existing cardiovascular disease; Prostatic hyperplasia (increased susceptibility to urinary retention); History of seizures (threshold may be lowered); May ↑ risk of suicide attempt/ideation especially during dose early treatment or dose adjustment; OB: Use only if clearly needed and maternal benefits outweigh risk to fetus; Lactation: May result in sedation in infant; discontinue drug or bottle feed; Pedi: Suicide risk, especially at initiation of therapy, may be greater in children and adolescents; Geri: May be more susceptible to adverse effects; dosage reduction required.

Adverse Reactions/Side Effects
CNS: NEUROLEPTIC MALIGNANT SYNDROME, fatigue, sedation, extrapyramidal reactions, tardive dyskinesia. **EENT:** blurred vision, dry eyes, dry mouth. **CV:** ARRHYTHMIAS, hypotension, ECG changes. **GI:** constipation, increased appetite, weight gain, paralytic ileus. **GU:** testicular swelling, urinary retention. **Derm:** photosensitivity, rash. **Endo:**

gynecomastia, sexual dysfunction. **Hemat:** blood dyscrasias. **Misc:** fever.

Route/Dosage
PO (Adults): 50 mg 2–3 times daily, increase to 100 mg 2–3 times daily by end of 1 week (not to exceed 300 mg daily in outpatients, 600 mg daily in divided doses in hospitalized patients). Once optimal dose is achieved, may be given as a single bedtime dose; no single dose to exceed 300 mg.

PO (Geriatric Patients): 25 mg 2–3 times daily, may be increased to 50 mg 2–3 times daily (not >300 mg/day).

---

arsenic trioxide
(ar-sen-ik trye-ox-ide)
Trisenox

Classification
Therapeutic: antineoplastics
Pharmacologic: heavy metals

Pregnancy Category D

Indications
Induction of remission and consolidation in patients with acute promyelocytic leukemia (APL) who do not respond to or tolerate retinoid and anthracycline chemotherapy and whose disease is associated with the presence of the t(15; 17) translocation or PML/RAR-alpha gene expression.

Contraindications/Precautions
Contraindicated in: Hypersensitivity to arsenic; OB: Can cause fetal injury; Lactation: Excreted in breast milk.
Use Cautiously in: Renal impairment.
Exercise Extreme Caution in: Pre-existing electrolyte abnormalities (correct prior to administration); concurrent use of drugs known to prolong QT interval, concurrent use of potassium wasting diuretics or amphotericin; Pedi: Safety not established in children <5 yr.

Adverse Reactions/Side Effects
CNS: fatigue, headache, insomnia, weakness. **Resp:** hypoxia, dyspnea, pleural effusion. **CV:** QT PROLONGATION, COMPLETE AV BLOCK, atrial arrhythmias. **GI:** abdominal pain, constipation, increase liver enzymes. **GU:** renal failure. **Derm:** dermatitis. **Endo:** hyperglycemia, hypoglycemia. **F and E:** acidosis, hypocalcemia, hyperkalemia, hypokalemia, hypomagnesemia. **Hemat:** NEUTROPENIA, APL DIFFERENTIATION SYNDROME, DISSEMINATED INTRAVASCULAR COAGULATION, THROMBOCYTOPENIA, hyperleukocytosis, anemia, leukocytosis. **MS:** back pain, arthralgia, bone pain, neck pain, limb pain, myalgia. **Misc:** allergic reactions, fever, infection/sepsis.

Route/Dosage
IV (Adults and Children ≥5 yr): *Induction*—0.15 mg/kg/day until bone marrow remission (not to exceed 60 doses); *consolidation*—starting 3–6 wk after completion of induction; 0.15 mg/kg/day for 25 doses over a period of 5 wk.

---

ascorbic acid
(as-kor-bik as-id)
✤Apo-C, Ascorbicap, Cebid, Cecon, Cecore-500, Cemill, Cenolate, Cetane, Cevalin, Cevi-Bid, Flavorcee, Mega-C/A Plus, Ortho/CS, Sunkist

Classification
Therapeutic: vitamins
Pharmacologic: water soluble vitamins

Pregnancy Category C

Indications
Treatment and prevention of vitamin C deficiency (scurvy) with dietary supplementation. Supplemental therapy in some GI diseases during long-term parenteral nutrition or chronic hemodialysis. States of increased requirements such as: Pregnancy, Lactation, Stress, Hyperthyroidism, Trauma, Burns, Infancy. **Unlabeled Use:** Prevention of the common cold.

Contraindications/Precautions
Contraindicated in: Tartrazine hypersensitivity (some products contain tartrazine—FDC yellow dye #5).
Use Cautiously in: Recurrent kidney stones; OB: Avoid chronic use of large doses in pregnant women.

Adverse Reactions/Side Effects
CNS: drowsiness, fatigue, headache, insomnia. **GI:** cramps, diarrhea, heartburn, nausea, vomiting. **GU:** kidney stones. **Derm:** flushing. **Hemat:** deep vein thrombosis, hemolysis (in G6PD deficiency), sickle cell crisis. **Local:** pain at subcut or IM sites.

Route/Dosage
PO (Adults): *Scurvy*—500 mg/day for at least 14 days. *Prevention of deficiency*—50–100 mg/day.
PO (Children): *Scurvy*—100–300 mg/day for at least 14 days. *Prevention of deficiency*—30–45 mg/day.
IM (Adults): *Scurvy*—100–500 mg/day for at least 14 days.
IM (Children): *Scurvy*—100–300 mg/day for at least 14 days.
IV (Adults and Children): *Prevention of deficiency*—determined by need.

bethanechol (be-than-e-kole)
Duvoid, Urabeth, Urecholine

Classification
Therapeutic: urinary tract stimulants
Pharmacologic: cholinergics

Pregnancy Category C

Indications
Postpartum and postoperative nonobstructive urinary retention or urinary retention caused by neurogenic bladder.

Contraindications/Precautions
Contraindicated in: Hypersensitivity; Mechanical obstruction of the GI or GU tract.
Use Cautiously in: History of asthma; Ulcer disease; Cardiovascular disease; Epilepsy; Hyperthyroidism; Sensitivity to cholinergic agents or effects; OB: Lactation, Pedi: Safety not established.

Adverse Reactions/Side Effects
CNS: headache, malaise. **EENT:** lacrimation, miosis. **Resp:** bronchospasm. **CV:** HEART BLOCK, SYNCOPE/CARDIAC ARREST, bradycardia, hypotension. **GI:** abdominal discomfort, diarrhea, nausea, salivation, vomiting. **GU:** urgency. **Misc:** flushing, sweating, hypothermia.

Route/Dosage
PO (Adults): 25–50 mg 3 times daily. Dose may be determined by administering 5–10 mg q 1–2 hr until response is obtained or total of 50 mg administered *or* by starting with 10 mg, giving 25 mg 6 hr later, then, if needed, 50 mg 6 hr later.
PO (Children): 0.2 mg/kg 3 times daily or 0.15 mg/kg 4 times daily.
Subcut (Adults): 5 mg 3–4 times daily. Dose may be determined by administering 2.5 mg q 15–30 min until response is obtained or total of 4 doses administered.

Subcut (Children): 0.06 mg/kg 3 times daily or 0.05 mg/kg 4 times daily.

biperiden (by-per-i-den)
Akineton

Classification
Therapeutic: antiparkinson agents
Pharmacologic: anticholinergics

Pregnancy Category C

Indications
Adjunctive treatment of all forms of Parkinson's disease, including drug-induced extrapyramidal effects and acute dystonic reactions.

Contraindications/Precautions
Contraindicated in: Hypersensitivity; Angle-closure glaucoma; Bowel obstruction; Megacolon; Tardive dyskinesia.
Use Cautiously in: Prostatic enlargement; Seizure disorders; Cardiac arrhythmias; OB, Lactation: Safety not established; Geri: Increased risk of adverse reactions; lower doses may be necessary.

Adverse Reactions/Side Effects
CNS: confusion, depression, dizziness, hallucinations, headache, sedation, weakness. **EENT:** blurred vision, dry eyes, mydriasis. **CV:** arrhythmias, hypotension, palpitations, tachycardia. **GI:** constipation, dry mouth, ileus, nausea. **GU:** hesitancy, urinary retention. **Misc:** decreased sweating.

Route/Dosage
Parkinsonism
PO (Adults): 2 mg 3–4 times daily initially (not to exceed 16 mg/day).

Extrapyramidal Reactions
PO (Adults): 2 mg 1–3 times daily.
IM, IV (Adults): 2 mg, may repeat q 30 min (not to exceed 8 mg or 4 doses/24 hr).
IM (Children): 40 mcg (0.04 mg)/kg or 1.2 mg/m^2, may repeat q 30 min (not to exceed 4 doses/24 hr).

botulism immune globulin
(**bot**yoo-lism im-**yoon glob**-yoo-lin)
BabyBIG

LESS COMMONLY USED DRUGS 1321

Classification
Therapeutic: vaccines/immunizing agents
Pharmacologic: immune globulins

Pregnancy Category UK

Indications
Infant botulism caused by type A or B toxin in children <1 yr.

Contraindications/Precautions
Contraindicated in: History of severe reactions to other immunoglobulins; Selective immunoglobulin A deficiency.
Use Cautiously in: Pre-existing renal impairment, diabetes mellitus, volume depletion, sepsis, paraproteinemia, concurrent nephrotoxic agents (↑ risk of adverse renal reactions; use lowest concentration and slowest infusion rate).

Adverse Reactions/Side Effects
Derm: rash. **Misc:** infusion reactions.

Route/Dosage
IV (Children <1 yr): 1 mL/kg (50 mg/kg) as a single infusion.

---

bromocriptine
(broe-moe-**krip**-teen)
✦Alti-Bromocriptine, ✦Apo-Bromocriptine, Cycloset, Parlodel

Classification
Therapeutic: antiparkinson agents, antidiabetics
Pharmacologic: dopamine agonists

Pregnancy Category B

Indications
Adjunct to levodopa in the treatment of parkinsonism (Parlodel only). Treatment of hyperprolactinemia (amenorrhea/galactorrhea), including associated female infertility (Parlodel only). Treatment of prolactin-secreting adenomas (Parlodel only). Treatment of acromegaly (Parlodel only). Treatment of type 2 diabetes (as adjunct to diet and exercise) (Cycloset only). **Unlabeled Use:** Management of neuroleptic malignant syndrome.

Contraindications/Precautions
Contraindicated in: Hypersensitivity to bromocriptine, ergot alkaloids, or bisulfites; Severe cardiovascular disease or peripheral vascular disease; History of syncopal migraines (↑ risk of syncope) (Cycloset only); Lactation; Concurrent use of dopamine antagonists (e.g., clozapine, olanzapine, ziprasidone) or other dopamine agonists (e.g., ropinirole); Type 1 diabetes (Cycloset only); Diabetic ketoacidosis (Cycloset only).
Use Cautiously in: Cardiac disease; Mental disturbances; May restore fertility (additional contraception may be required if pregnancy is undesirable); Hepatic impairment; Concurrent antihypertensive therapy (↑ risk of hypotension); OB, Pedi: Safety not established.

Adverse Reactions/Side Effects
CNS: dizziness, drowsiness, confusion, hallucinations, headache, insomnia, nightmares. **EENT:** burning eyes, nasal stuffiness, visual disturbances. **Resp:** PULMONARY FIBROSIS, effusions, pulmonary infiltrates. **CV:** MI, orthostatic hypotension. **GI:** nausea, abdominal pain, anorexia, dry mouth, metallic taste, vomiting. **Derm:** urticaria. **MS:** leg cramps. **Misc:** digital vasospasm (acromegaly only).

Route/Dosage

Parkinsonism
PO (Adults): 1.25 mg 1–2 times daily, ↑ by 2.5 mg/day in 2–4 wk intervals (range is 2.5–100 mg/day in divided doses; up to 40 mg/day have been used).

Hyperprolactinemia
PO (Adults): 1.25–2.5 mg/day initially, may be gradually ↑ q 3–7 days up to 2.5 mg 2–3 times daily.

Acromegaly
PO (Adults): 1.25–2.5 mg/day for 3 days, ↑ by 1.25–2.5 mg q 3–7 days until optimal response is obtained (usual range 10–30 mg/day; up to 100 mg/day).

Pituitary Adenomas
PO (Adults): 1.25 mg 2–3 times daily, may be ↑ over several weeks (range 2.5–20 mg/day).

Type 2 Diabetes (Cycloset only)
PO (Adults): 0.8 mg once daily (within 2 hr of arising in morning); may be ↑ by 0.8 mg q 7 days (range 1.6–4.8 mg/day).

Neuroleptic Malignant Syndrome (Unlabeled)
PO (Adults): 5 mg once daily initially, dose increased as required up to 20 mg/day.

✦ = Canadian drug name. ❖ = Genetic implication.
*CAPITALS indicates life-threatening; underlines indicate most frequent.

brompheniramine
(brome-fen-**ir**-a-meen)
Bromfenac, Dimetapp Allergy, Nasahist B, ❋ Dimetane

Classification
Therapeutic: allergy, cold, and cough remedies, antihistamines

Pregnancy Category B

Indications
Symptomatic relief of allergic symptoms (rhinitis, urticaria) caused by histamine release.

Contraindications/Precautions
Contraindicated in: Hypersensitivity; Acute attacks of asthma; Known alcohol intolerance (some elixirs); Lactation: Potential for adverse reaction in nursing infants.
Use Cautiously in: Angle-closure glaucoma; Liver disease; OB: Safety not established; Geri: More susceptible to adverse reactions; use lower initial dose; Pedi: Children <4 yr (OTC cough and cold products containing this medication should be avoided).

Adverse Reactions/Side Effects
CNS: drowsiness, sedation, dizziness, excitation (in children). **EENT:** blurred vision. **CV:** hypertension, arrhythmias, hypotension, palpitations. **GI:** dry mouth, constipation, obstruction. **GU:** retention, urinary hesitancy. **Derm:** sweating.

Route/Dosage
PO (Adults and Children ≥12 yr): 4 mg q 4–6 hr daily as needed (not to exceed 24 mg/day).
PO (Children 6–12 yr): 2 mg q 4–6 hr as needed (not to exceed 12 mg/day).
PO (Children 4–6 yr): 1 mg q 4–6 hr as needed (not to exceed 6 mg/day).

chlorambucil
(klor-**am**-byoo-sill)
Leukeran

Classification
Therapeutic: antineoplastics, immunosuppressants
Pharmacologic: alkylating agents

Pregnancy Category D

Indications
Management of chronic lymphocytic leukemia, malignant lymphoma, and Hodgkin's disease (alone and in combination with other agents).

Contraindications/Precautions
Contraindicated in: Hypersensitivity; Previous resistance; OB, Lactation: Can cause fetal or neonatal harm; avoid becoming pregnant; do not breastfeed.
Use Cautiously in: Infection; Other chronic debilitating diseases; Geri: More sensitive to effects.

Adverse Reactions/Side Effects
Resp: pulmonary fibrosis. **GI:** nausea, stomatitis (rare), vomiting. **GU:** decreased sperm count, sterility. **Derm:** alopecia (rare), dermatitis, rash. **Hemat:** LEUKOPENIA, anemia, thrombocytopenia. **Metab:** hyperuricemia. **Misc:** allergic reactions, risk of second malignancy.

Route/Dosage
PO (Adults): 0.1–0.2 mg/kg/day (3–6 mg/m^2/day) (usual range 4–10 mg/day as a single dose or in divided doses), then adjust dose on basis of blood counts; *or* 0.4 mg/kg (12 mg/m^2) twice weekly, increased by 0.1 mg/kg (3 mg/m^2) q 2 wk, then adjusted as necessary.
PO (Geriatric Patients): Initial dose should not be more than 2–4 mg/day.
PO (Children): 0.1–0.2 mg/kg/day (4.5 mg/m^2/day) single dose or in divided doses.

clomiPRAMINE
(kloe-**mip**-ra-meen)
Anafranil

Classification
Therapeutic: antiobsessive agents
Pharmacologic: tricyclic antidepressants

Pregnancy Category C

Indications
Obsessive-Compulsive Disorder (OCD). **Unlabeled Use:** Depression, neuropathic pain/chronic pain.

Contraindications/Precautions
Contraindicated in: Hypersensitivity; Angle-closure glaucoma; Recent myocardial infarction; History of QTc prolongation; Cardiac arrythmias; Heart failure; Concurrent MAO inhibitor or clonidine use (avoid if possible); OB: Potential for fetal harm or neonatal withdrawal syndrome; Lactation: Discontinue drug or bottle feed.
Use Cautiously in: History of seizures (threshold may be lowered); Patients with pre-existing cardiovascular disease; Older men with prostatic hyperplasia (may be more susceptible to urinary retention); Hyperthyroidism (increased risk of arrhythmias); May ↑ risk of suicide attempt/ide-

ation especially during dose early treatment or dose adjustment; risk may be greater in children or adolescents; Pedi: Safety not established in children <10 yr; Geri: ↑ risk of arrhythmias.

Adverse Reactions/Side Effects
CNS: SEIZURES, lethargy, sedation, weakness, aggressive behavior. **EENT:** blurred vision, dry eyes, dry mouth, vestibular disorder. **CV:** ARRHYTHMIAS, ECG changes, orthostatic hypotension. **GI:** constipation, nausea, vomiting, weight gain, eructation. **GU:** male sexual dysfunction, urinary retention. **Derm:** dry skin, photosensitivity. **Endo:** gynecomastia. **Hemat:** anemia. **MS:** muscle weakness. **Neuro:** extrapyramidal reactions. **Misc:** hyperthermia.

Route/Dosage
PO (Adults): *Antiobsessive*—25 mg/day, increased over 2-wk period to 100 mg/day in divided doses. May be further increased over several weeks up to 250–300 mg/day in divided doses. Once stabilizing dose is reached, entire daily dose may be given at bedtime. *Antidepressant*—25 mg 3 times daily, may be increased as needed (unlabeled).
PO (Geriatric Patients): 20–30 mg/day initially, may be increased as needed.
PO (Children >10–17 yr): 25 mg/day initially, increased over 2-wk period to 3 mg/kg/day or 100 mg/day (whichever is smaller) in divided doses. May be further increased to 3 mg/kg/day or 200 mg/day (whichever is smaller) in divided doses. Once stabilizing dose is reached, entire daily dose may be given at bedtime.

cytomegalovirus immune globulin
(site-oh-**meg**-a-loe-vye-rus)
CMVIG, CytoGam

Classification
Therapeutic: vaccines/immunizing agents
Pharmacologic: immune globulins

Pregnancy Category C

Indications
Prevention of cytomegalovirus (CMV) disease associated with transplantation of kidney, lung, liver, pancreas, or heart (if transplant is other than kidney from CMV-positive donors to CMV-negative recipient, then concurrent ganciclovir should be considered).

Contraindications/Precautions
Contraindicated in: Hypersensitivity to immune globulins or albumin; Selective IgA deficiency.
Use Cautiously in: OB: Lactation: Pregnancy or lactation (safety not established); Renal insufficiency or predisposition to acute renal failure.

Adverse Reactions/Side Effects
CNS: headache, tremor, anxiety, seizures. **Hemat:** pancytopenia, hemolysis, leukopenia. **Resp:** wheezing, dyspnea, pulmonary edema. **CV:** hypotension, thromboembolism. **GI:** nausea, vomiting, hepatic dysfunction. **Derm:** flushing, rash. **GU:** oliguria, anuria, acute renal failure. **MS:** back pain, muscle cramps. **Misc:** allergic reactions including chills, fever, ANAPHYLAXIS.

Route/Dosage

Kidney Transplant
IV (Adults): 150 mg/kg within 72 hr of transplantation, followed by 100 mg/kg at 2, 4, 6, and 8 wk, then 50 mg/kg at 12 and 16 wk post-transplantation.

Liver, Pancreas, Lung, or Heart Transplant
IV (Adults): 150 mg/kg within 72 hr of transplantation, and at 2, 4, 6, and 8 wk, then 100 mg/kg after at 12 and 16 wk post-transplantation.
IV (Children): Safety and efficacy has not been established in pediatrics, however adult doses have been used in children.

danazol (da-na-zole)
♣Cyclomen, Danocrine

Classification
Therapeutic: hormones
Pharmacologic: androgens

Pregnancy Category X

Indications
Treatment of moderate endometriosis that is unresponsive to conventional therapy. Palliative therapy of fibrocystic breast disease. Prophylaxis of hereditary angioedema.

Contraindications/Precautions
Contraindicated in: Hypersensitivity; Male patients with breast or prostate cancer; Hypercalcemia; Severe hepatic, renal, or cardiac disease; Pregnancy or lactation.

♣ = Canadian drug name. = Genetic implication.
*CAPITALS indicates life-threatening; underlines indicate most frequent.

Use Cautiously in: Previous history of liver disease; History of porphyria; Coronary artery disease; Prepubertal boys.

Adverse Reactions/Side Effects
CNS: emotional lability. **EENT:** deepening of voice. **CV:** edema. **GI:** hepatitis (cholestatic jaundice). **GU:** amenorrhea, clitoral enlargement, testicular atrophy. **Derm:** acne, hirsutism, oiliness. **Endo:** amenorrhea, anovulation, decreased breast size (women), decreased libido. **Metab:** weight gain.

Route/Dosage
PO (Adults and Adolescents): *Endometriosis*—400 mg twice daily (for milder cases may initiate therapy with 100–200 mg twice daily). *Fibrocystic breast disease*—50–200 mg twice daily. *Hereditary angioedema*—200 mg 2–3 times daily. Attempt to decrease dosage by 50% or less q 1–3 mo. If acute attack occurs, increase dose by up to 200 mg/day.

---

didanosine (dye-dan-oh-seen)
ddI, dideoxyinosine, Videx, Videx EC

Classification
Therapeutic: antiretrovirals
Pharmacologic: nucleoside reverse transcriptase inhibitors

Pregnancy Category B

Indications
HIV infection (with other antiretrovirals).

Contraindications/Precautions
Contraindicated in: Hypersensitivity; Lactation: Lactation; Concurrent use of ribavirin or allopurinol.
Use Cautiously in: History of gout; Renal impairment (dosage modification required if CCr <60 mL/min; ↑ risk of pancreatitis); History of seizures; Diabetes mellitus; Pedi: ↑ risk of pancreatitis.

Adverse Reactions/Side Effects
CNS: SEIZURES, headache, dizziness, insomnia, lethargy, pain, weakness. **EENT:** rhinitis, ear pain, epistaxis, optic neuritis, parotid gland enlargement, photophobia, retinal depigmentation, sialoadenitis. **Resp:** cough, asthma. **CV:** arrhythmias, edema, hypertension, vasodilation. **GI:** HEPATOMEGALY (WITH STEATOSIS), LIVER FAILURE, PANCREATITIS, anorexia, diarrhea, liver function abnormalities, nausea, vomiting, abdominal pain, constipation, dry mouth, dyspepsia, flatulence, stomatitis. **GU:** urinary frequency. **Derm:** alopecia, ecchymoses, rash. **Endo:** fat redistribution, hyperglycemia. **Hemat:** granulocytopenia, anemia, bleeding, leukopenia. **Metab:** LACTIC ACIDOSIS, hyperlipidemia, hyperuricemia, weight loss. **MS:** RHABDOMYOLYSIS, arthritis, myalgia. **Neuro:** peripheral neuropathy, poor coordination. **Misc:** chills, fever, anaphylactoid reactions.

Route/Dosage
PO (Adults ≥60 kg): *Oral solution*—200 mg bid; *Videx EC capsules*—400 mg once daily; *with tenofovir*—250 mg once daily.
PO (Adults <60 kg): *Oral solution*—125 mg bid; *Videx EC capsules*—250 mg once daily; *with tenofovir*—200 mg once daily.
PO (Children 2 wk-8 mo): *Oral solution*—100 mg/m² q 12 hr.
PO (Children >8 mo): *Oral solution*—120 mg q 12 hr.
PO (Children 6–18 yr and ≥20 kg): *Videx EC capsules*—20–24.9 kg: 200 mg once daily; 25–59.9 kg: 250 mg once daily; ≥60 kg: 400 mg once daily.

Renal Impairment
PO (Adults >60 kg): *CCr 30–59 mL/min*—*Oral solution*—100 mg q 12 hr or 200 mg once daily; *Videx EC capsules*—200 mg once daily; *CCr 10–29 mL/min*—*Oral solution*–150 mg once daily; *Videx EC capsules*—125 mg once daily; *CCr <10 mL/min*—*Oral solution*–100 mg once daily *Videx EC capsules*—125 mg once daily.
PO (Adults <60 kg): *CCr 30–59 mL/min*—*Oral solution*—75 mg q 12 hr or 150 mg once daily; *Videx EC capsules*—125 mg once daily; *CCr 10–29 mL/min*—*Oral solution*—100 mg once daily; *Videx EC capsules*—125 mg once daily; *CCr <10 mL/min*—*Oral solution*—75 mg once daily; *Videx EC capsules*—not to be used.

---

disulfiram (di-sul-fir-am)
Antabuse

Classification
Therapeutic: alcohol abuse therapy adjuncts
Pharmacologic: enzyme inhibitors

Pregnancy Category C

Indications
Management of chronic alcoholism in patients who require or desire an enforced state of sobriety, which may allow for additional supportive and psychotherapeutic treatment.

Contraindications/Precautions
Contraindicated in: Hypersensitivity to disulfiram or other thiurams (including those used in rubber vulcanization and pesticides); Significant cardiovascular disease; Psychosis; Concurrent or recent use of metronidazole, paraldehyde, alcohol or alcohol-containing products; Lactation.
Use Cautiously in: Diabetes; Hyperthyroidism; Epilepsy; Cerebral damage; Hepatic or renal impairment or pathology; Pregnancy or children (safety not established).

Adverse Reactions/Side Effects
CNS: drowsiness, fatigue, headache, psychoses. **EENT:** optic neuritis. **GI:** HEPATIC TOXICITY, metallic/garlic-like taste. **GI:** erectile dysfunction. **Derm:** acneiform eruptions, allergic dermatitis. **Neuro:** peripheral neuritis/neuropathy, polyneuritis.

Route/Dosage
PO (Adults): 500 mg/day for 1–2 wk, then 250 mg/day (up to 500 mg/day).

---

eflornithine (topical)
(ee-**flor**-ni-theen)
Vaniqa

Classification
Therapeutic: facial hair removers (topical)

Pregnancy Category C

Indications
Reduction of unwanted facial hair in women.

Contraindications/Precautions
Contraindicated in: Hypersensitivity.
Use Cautiously in: Pregnancy, lactation or children <12 yr (safety not established).

Adverse Reactions/Side Effects
Local: burning, rash, stinging, tingling.

Route/Dosage
Topical (Adults): Apply a thin layer to affected areas of the face and adjacent involved areas under the chin and rub in thoroughly. Do not wash for 4 hr following application. Use twice daily at least 8 hr apart.

---

enfuvirtide (en-**foo**-veer-tide)
Fuzeon

Classification
Therapeutic: antiretrovirals
Pharmacologic: fusion inhibitors

Pregnancy Category B

Indications
Management of HIV infection in combination with other antiretrovirals in patients with evidence of progressive HIV-1 replication despite ongoing treatment.

Contraindications/Precautions
Contraindicated in: Hypersensitivity; Lactation: Breastfeeding not recommended for HIV-infected mothers.
Use Cautiously in: OB: Use only if clearly indicated; Pedi: Safety not established in children <6 yr.

Adverse Reactions/Side Effects
CNS: fatigue. **EENT:** conjunctivitis. **Resp:** cough, pneumonia, sinusitis. **GI:** diarrhea, nausea, abdominal pain, anorexia, dry mouth, pancreatitis, weight loss. **Local:** injection site reactions. **MS:** myalgia, limb pain. **Misc:** hypersensitivity reactions, herpes simplex.

Route/Dosage
Subcut (Adults): 90 mg twice daily.
Subcut (Children 6–16 yr): 2 mg/kg twice daily (not to exceed 90 mg/dose).

---

flutamide (floo-ta-mide)
Eulexin

Classification
Therapeutic: antineoplastics
Pharmacologic: antiandrogens

Pregnancy Category D

Indications
Treatment of prostate carcinoma in conjunction with luteinizing hormone–releasing hormone (LHRH) analogues such as leuprolide.

Contraindications/Precautions
Contraindicated in: Hypersensitivity; Severe hepatic impairment.
Use Cautiously in: Severe cardiovascular disease.

Adverse Reactions/Side Effects
Side effects primarily caused by LHRH antagonist. **CNS:** anxiety, confusion, drowsiness, mental depression, nervousness. **CV:** edema, hypertension.

GI: HEPATOTOXICITY, diarrhea, nausea, vomiting. **GU:** erectile dysfunction, loss of libido. **Derm:** photosensitivity, rash. **Endo:** gynecomastia. **Misc:** hot flashes.

Route/Dosage
PO (Adults): 250 mg q 8 hr; given concurrently with leuprolide.

guanfacine (gwahn-fa-seen)
Intuniv, Tenex

Classification
Therapeutic: antihypertensives
Pharmacologic: centrally acting antiadrenergics

Pregnancy Category B

Indications
Hypertension (with thiazide-type diuretics) (immediate-release). Attention-deficit hyperactivity disorder (ADHD) (extended-release).

Contraindications/Precautions
Contraindicated in: Hypersensitivity.
Use Cautiously in: Severe coronary artery disease or recent myocardial infarction; Geri: May have ↑ sensitivity, especially those with hepatic, cardiac, or renal dysfunction; Cerebrovascular disease; Severe renal or liver disease; History of hypotension, heart block, bradycardia, or cardiovascular disease; OB, Lactation: Pedi: Pregnancy, lactation, or children <6 yr (safety not established).

Adverse Reactions/Side Effects
CNS: drowsiness, headache, weakness, depression, dizziness, fatigue, insomnia, irritability. **EENT:** tinnitus. **Resp:** dyspnea. **CV:** bradycardia, chest pain, hypotension, palpitations, rebound hypertension. **GI:** constipation, dry mouth, abdominal pain, nausea. **GU:** erectile dysfunction.

Route/Dosage
Immediate-release and extended-release tablets should not be interchanged.

Hypertension
PO (Adults): 1 mg daily given at bedtime, may be ↑ if necessary at 3–4 wk intervals up to 2 mg/day; may also be given in 2 divided doses.

ADHD
PO (Adults and Children ≥6 yr): 1 mg daily in morning; may be ↑ by 1 mg/day at weekly intervals to achieve dose of 1–4 mg/day.

hydroxyurea (hye-drox-ee-yoor-ee-a)
Droxia, Hydrea, Mylocel

Classification
Therapeutic: antineoplastics
Pharmacologic: antimetabolites

Pregnancy Category D

Indications
Treatment of head and neck carcinoma. Treatment of ovarian carcinoma. Treatment of resistant chronic myelogenous leukemia. Treatment of melanoma. Reduction of painful crises in sickle cell anemia and decreased need for transfusions in adult patients with a history of recurrent moderate to severe crises (at least 3 in the preceding yr). **Unlabeled Use:** Used as part of antiretroviral therapy in patients with HIV infection.

Contraindications/Precautions
Contraindicated in: Hypersensitivity; Pregnancy or lactation; Some products contain tartrazine (FDC yellow dye #5) and should be avoided in patients with known hypersensitivity.
Use Cautiously in: Patients with childbearing potential; Renal impairment (close monitoring of hematologic parameters recommended, dosage reduction may be necessary); Hepatic impairment (close monitoring of hematologic parameters recommended); Myeloproliferative disorders (may increase risk of vasculitic ulcerations and gangrene); Active infections; Decreased bone marrow reserve; Other chronic debilitating illness; Geriatric patients (may be more sensitive to effects, lower doses may be required); Obese patients or patients with edema (dose should be determined using ideal body weight).

Adverse Reactions/Side Effects
CNS: drowsiness (large doses). **GI:** anorexia, diarrhea, nausea, vomiting, constipation, hepatitis, stomatitis. **GU:** dysuria, infertility, renal tubular dysfunction. **Derm:** alopecia, exacerbation of post-radiation erythema, erythema, pruritus, rashes. **Hemat:** leukopenia, anemia, thrombocytopenia. **Metab:** hyperuricemia. **Misc:** chills, fever, malaise.

Route/Dosage

Head and Neck Cancer, Ovarian Cancer, Malignant Melanoma
PO (Adults): 60–80 mg/kg (2–3 g/m^2) as a single daily dose q 3 days or 20–30 mg/kg/day

as a single dose. Therapy should be initiated 7 days prior to radiation and continued.

Resistant Chronic Myelogenous Leukemia
PO (Adults): 20–30 mg/kg/day in 1–2 divided doses.

Sickle Cell Anemia
PO (Adults and Children): 15 mg/kg/day as a single dose, may increase by 5 mg/kg/day q 12 wk up to 35 mg/kg/day.

iloprost (eye-lo-prost)
Ventavis

Classification
Therapeutic: vasodilators
Pharmacologic: prostacyclins

Pregnancy Category C

Indications
Management of New York Class III/IV symptoms of pulmonary hypertension, where there is marked limitation of physical activity.

Contraindications/Precautions
Contraindicated in: Hypersensitivity; Systolic BP <85 mm Hg; Lactation: Lactation.
Use Cautiously in: Concurrent use of drugs or coexisting medical conditions that may ↑ risk of syncope; COPD, asthma, or acute pulmonary infection (may ↑ risk of bronchospasm); Pedi: Safety not established; OB: Use only if maternal benefit outweighs fetal risk.

Adverse Reactions/Side Effects
CNS: dizziness, fainting, headache, insomnia. **EENT:** epistaxis. **Resp:** ↑ cough, bronchospasm, dyspnea, hemoptysis, wheezing. **CV:** CHF, vasodilation, chest pain, hypotension, peripheral edema, supraventricular tachycardia. **GI:** diarrhea, gingival bleeding, nausea, vomiting. **GU:** renal failure. **Derm:** facial flushing. **MS:** back pain, jaw-muscle spasm, muscle cramps.

Route/Dosage
Inhaln (Adults): 2.5 mcg initially, then 5 mcg/dose 6–9 times daily; not more than every 2 hr.

indinavir (in-din-a-veer)
Crixivan

Classification
Therapeutic: antiretrovirals
Pharmacologic: protease inhibitors

Pregnancy Category C

Indications
HIV infection (with other antiretrovirals). **Unlabeled Use:** Prevention of HIV infection after known exposure (with other antiretrovirals).

Contraindications/Precautions
Contraindicated in: Hypersensitivity; Dehydration; Concurrent amiodarone, alprazolam, dihydroergotamine, ergotamine, ergonovine, methylergonovine, midazolam, pimozide, rifampin, triazolam, lovastatin, simvastatin, rosuvastatin, atazanavir, or St. John's wort.
Use Cautiously in: Hepatic impairment (dose ↓ recommended in moderate to severe hepatic insufficiency caused by cirrhosis); Hemophilia (↑ risk of bleeding); Diabetes mellitus; Lactation, Pedi: Safety not established; breastfeeding not recommended in HIV-infected patients.

Adverse Reactions/Side Effects
CNS: dizziness, drowsiness, fatigue, headache, insomnia, weakness. **GI:** abdominal pain, acid regurgitation, altered taste, asymptomatic hyperbilirubinemia, diarrhea, nausea, vomiting. **GU:** nephrolithiasis. **Endo:** hyperglycemia. **F and E:** KETOACIDOSIS. **MS:** back pain, flank pain. **Misc:** redistribution of body fat.

Route/Dosage
PO (Adults): 800 mg q 8 hr.

mebendazole (me-**ben**-da-zole)
Vermox

Classification
Therapeutic: antihelmintics

Pregnancy Category C

Indications
Treatment of: Whipworm (trichuriasis), Pinworm (enterobiasis), Roundworm (ascariasis), Hookworm (uncinariasis) infections, Drug of choice for capillariasis.

Contraindications/Precautions
Contraindicated in: Hypersensitivity.
Use Cautiously in: Impaired liver function; Crohn's ileitis; Ulcerative colitis; Pregnancy, lac-

tation, or children <2 yr (safety not established; may be used in first trimester only if benefit justifies potential risk to fetus).

Adverse Reactions/Side Effects
Most side effects and adverse reactions are seen with high-dose therapy only. **CNS:** SEIZURES (rare), dizziness, headache. **EENT:** tinnitus. **GI:** abdominal pain, diarrhea, increased liver enzymes (high dose, long-term therapy), nausea, vomiting. **Derm:** rash, urticaria, alopecia. **Hemat:** agranulocytosis, reversible myelosuppression (leukopenia, thrombocytopenia). **Neuro:** numbness. **Misc:** fever.

Route/Dosage

Enterobiasis
PO (Adults and Children >2 yr): 100 mg as a single dose; repeat in 2–3 wk.

Trichuriasis, Ascariasis, Hookworm, or Mixed Infections
PO (Adults and Children >2 yr): 100 mg twice daily for 3 days. If not cured in 3–4 wk, a 2nd course is given.

Capillariasis
PO (Adults and Children >2 yr): 200 mg twice daily for 20 days.

---

mechlorethamine
(me-klor-**eth**-a-meen)
Mustargen, nitrogen mustard

Classification
Therapeutic: antineoplastics
Pharmacologic: alkylating agents

Pregnancy Category D

Indications
Part of combination therapy of Hodgkin's disease and malignant lymphomas. Used palliatively in: Bronchogenic carcinoma, Leukemias. Administered into cavities (pleural, peritoneal) to prevent reaccumulation of malignant effusions.

Contraindications/Precautions
Contraindicated in: Hypersensitivity; Pregnancy; Lactation.
Use Cautiously in: Infections; Decreased bone marrow reserve; Previous radiotherapy or chemotherapy (dose reduction required); Obesity or severe edema (dose should be based on ideal dry body weight); Geri: Geriatric patients or patients with chronic debilitating illnesses; Patients with childbearing potential.

Adverse Reactions/Side Effects
CNS: SEIZURES, drowsiness, headache, vertigo, weakness. **GI:** nausea, vomiting, anorexia, diarrhea. **GU:** infertility. **Derm:** rashes, alopecia. **Hemat:** LEUKOPENIA, THROMBOCYTOPENIA, anemia. **Local:** tissue necrosis, phlebitis at IV site. **Metab:** hyperuricemia. **Misc:** reactivation of herpes zoster.

Route/Dosage
IV (Adults and Children): 0.4 mg/kg as single dose or divided over 2–4 days (not to exceed 0.2–0.3 mg/kg in patients who have received previous chemotherapy or radiation therapy); *as part of MOPP regimen for Hodgkin's lymphoma in adults*—6 mg/m^2 on days 1 and 8 of 28-day cycle; doses in subsequent cycles are determined by blood counts.
Intracavitary (Adults): 0.4 mg/kg.
Intrapericardial (Adults): 0.2 mg/kg.

---

mercaptopurine
(mer-kap-toe-**pyoor**-een)
Purinethol

Classification
Therapeutic: antineoplastics
Pharmacologic: antimetabolites

Pregnancy Category D

Indications
Leukemias (with other agents), including: Acute lymphocytic leukemia, Acute myelogenous leukemia. **Unlabeled Use:** Treatment of: Some lymphomas, Polycythemia vera, Crohn's disease, Psoriatic arthritis.

Contraindications/Precautions
Contraindicated in: Hypersensitivity; OB, Lactation: Pregnancy or lactation; Severe liver disease.
Use Cautiously in: Infections; ↓ bone marrow reserve; Patients with TPMT enzyme deficiency (substantial dosage reductions are required to avoid hematologic adverse events); Geri: ↑ risk of adverse reactions; Other chronic debilitating illnesses; OB: Patients with childbearing potential.

Adverse Reactions/Side Effects
CNS: weakness. **GI:** HEPATOTOXICITY, anorexia, diarrhea, nausea, vomiting. **Derm:** alopecia, hyperpigmentation. **Endo:** gonadal suppression, oligospermia. **Hemat:** anemia, leukopenia, thrombocytopenia. **Metab:** hyperuricemia. **Misc:** fever.

Route/Dosage
PO (Adults): *Initial dose*—2.5 mg/kg (80–100 mg/m^2)/day as a single dose or divided doses; after 4 wk, if necessary, dose may be slowly ↑ to 5 mg/kg/day (dose should be rounded to the nearest 25 mg); *maintenance dose*—1.5–2.5 mg/kg (50–100 mg/m^2)/day.
PO (Children): 2.5 mg/kg/day (75 mg/m^2) single dose or divided doses (dose should be rounded to the nearest 25 mg).

minoxidil (systemic)
(mi-**nox**-i-dill)

Classification
Therapeutic: antihypertensives
Pharmacologic: vasodilators

Pregnancy Category C

Indications
Severe symptomatic hypertension or hypertension associated with end-organ damage that has failed to respond to combinations of more conventional therapy.

Contraindications/Precautions
Contraindicated in: Hypersensitivity; Pheochromocytoma.
Use Cautiously in: Recent MI; Severe renal impairment (can be used in moderate renal impairment); Geri: May be more sensitive to effects; consider age-related ↓ in body mass and hepatic/renal/cardiovascular function; OB, Lactation: Safety not established.

Adverse Reactions/Side Effects
CNS: headache. **Resp:** PULMONARY EDEMA. **CV:** CHF, ECG changes (alteration in T waves), tachycardia, angina, pericardial effusion. **GI:** nausea. **Derm:** hypertrichosis, pigment changes, rashes. **Endo:** gynecomastia, menstrual irregularities. **F and E:** sodium and water retention. **Misc:** intermittent claudication.

Route/Dosage
PO (Adults and Children >12 yr): *Hypertension*—5 mg once daily or in 2 divided doses; may double at 3-day intervals; usual range 10–40 mg/day (for rapid control with careful monitoring, doses may be adjusted q 6 hr; up to 100 mg/day have been used).
PO (Children <12 yr): *Hypertension*—0.2 mg/kg/day (5 mg maximum) as a single dose or 2 divided doses; may be gradually ↑ at 3-day intervals in increments of 50–100% until response is obtained; usual range 0.25–1 mg/kg/day (for rapid control, doses may be adjusted q 6 hr; not to exceed 50 mg/day).

nelfinavir (nell-**finn**-a-veer)
Viracept

Classification
Therapeutic: antiretrovirals
Pharmacologic: protease inhibitors

Pregnancy Category B

Indications
HIV infection (with other antiretrovirals).

Contraindications/Precautions
Contraindicated in: Hypersensitivity; Concurrent amiodarone, ergot derivatives, midazolam, quinidine, rifampin, pimozide, simvastatin, lovastatin, St. John's wort, or triazolam; Lactation: Breastfeeding should be avoided by HIV-infected patients.
Use Cautiously in: Hemophiliacs (↑ risk of bleeding); Diabetes mellitus (may exacerbate condition); Hepatic impairment.

Adverse Reactions/Side Effects
CNS: SEIZURES, anxiety, depression, dizziness, drowsiness, emotional lability, headache, hyperkinesia, insomnia, malaise, migraine headache, sleep disorders, suicidal ideation, weakness.
EENT: acute iritis, pharyngitis, rhinitis, sinusitis.
Resp: dyspnea. **GI:** diarrhea, anorexia, dyspepsia, ↑ liver function tests, epigastric pain, flatulence, GI bleeding, hepatitis, nausea, oral ulcerations, pancreatitis, vomiting. **GU:** nephrolithiasis, sexual dysfunction. **Derm:** pruritus, rash, sweating, urticaria. **Endo:** fat redistribution, hyperglycemia. **F and E:** dehydration. **Hemat:** anemia, leukopenia, thrombocytopenia. **Metab:** hyperlipidemia, hyperuricemia. **MS:** arthralgia, arthritis, back pain, myalgia, myopathy. **Neuro:** myasthenia, paresthesia. **Misc:** allergic reactions, fever.

Route/Dosage
PO (Adults and Children >13 yr): 750 mg 3 times daily *or* 1250 mg twice daily.
PO (Children 2–13 yr): 20–30 mg/kg 3 times daily (not to exceed 750 mg 3 times daily).

pegaptanib (peg-**apt**-i-nib)
Macugen

1330 LESS COMMONLY USED DRUGS

Classification
Therapeutic: ocular agents
Pharmacologic: vascular endothelial growth-factor antagonists

Pregnancy Category B

Indications
Neovascular (wet) age-related macular degeneration.

Contraindications/Precautions
Contraindicated in: Ocular/periocular infections.
Use Cautiously in: OB: Use only if maternal benefit outweighs fetal risk; Lactation, Pedi: Safety not established.

Adverse Reactions/Side Effects
EENT: cataract, blurred vision, conjunctival bleeding, irritation/pain, ↑ intraocular pressure, ocular inflammation, infection (rare), retinal detachment (rare), traumatic cataract formation (rare). **Misc:** Anaphylaxis, angioedema.

Route/Dosage
Intravitreal (Adults): 0.3 mg every 6 wk.

---

penicillamine
(pen-i-**sill**-a-meen)
Cuprimine, Depen

Classification
Therapeutic: antidotes, antirheumatics (DMARD), antiurolithics
Pharmacologic: chelating agents

Pregnancy Category D

Indications
Progressive rheumatoid arthritis resistant to conventional therapy. Management of copper deposition in Wilson's disease. Management of recurrent cystine calculi. **Unlabeled Use:** Adjunct in the treatment of heavy metal poisoning.

Contraindications/Precautions
Contraindicated in: Hypersensitivity; Cross-sensitivity with penicillin may exist; Patients currently receiving gold salts, antimalarials, antineoplastics, oxyphenbutazone, or phenylbutazone; Concurrent use of iron supplements; OB: Pregnancy (penicillamine should be avoided in pregnant patients with rheumatoid arthritis or cystinuria); OB: Lactation.
Use Cautiously in: Renal impairment (increased risk of adverse renal reactions in patients with rheumatoid arthritis); History of aplastic anemia due to penicillamine; Patients requiring surgery (may impair wound healing); Geri: Geriatric patients (increased risk of hematologic toxicity, skin rash and taste abnormality; dose reduction recommended); OB: Pregnancy (for patients with Wilson's disease, limit daily dose to <1 g. If cesarean section is planned, decrease daily dose to 250 mg for last 6 wk of pregnancy and until incision is healed).

Adverse Reactions/Side Effects
EENT: blurred vision, eye pain. **Resp:** coughing, shortness of breath, wheezing. **GI:** altered taste, anorexia, cholestatic jaundice, diarrhea, drug-induced pancreatitis, dyspepsia, epigastric pain, hepatic dysfunction, nausea, oral ulceration, vomiting. **GU:** proteinuria. **Derm:** pemphigus, ecchymoses, hives, itching, rashes, wrinkling. **Hemat:** APLASTIC ANEMIA, anemia, eosinophilia, leukopenia, thrombocytopenia, thrombocytosis. **MS:** arthralgia, migratory polyarthritis. **Neuro:** myasthenia gravis syndrome. **Misc:** GOODPASTURE'S SYNDROME (GLOMERULONEPHRITIS AND INTRA-ALVEOLAR HEMORRHAGE), allergic reactions, fever, lymphadenopathy, systemic lupus erythematosus-like syndrome.

Route/Dosage
PO (Adults): *Antirheumatic*—125–250 mg/day as a single dose; may be slowly ↑ up to 1.5 g/day. *Chelating agent (Wilson's disease)*—250 mg qid. *Antiurolithic*—500 mg 4 times daily.
PO (Children >6 mo): *Chelating agent (Wilson's disease)*—250 mg/day as a single dose; older children may receive the adult dose. *Antiurolithic*—7.5 mg/kg 4 times daily.

---

pentobarbital
(pen-toe-**bar**-bi-tal)
Nembutal, ✤ Novopentobarb, ✤ Nova Rectal

Classification
Therapeutic: anticonvulsants, sedative/hypnotics
Pharmacologic: barbiturates

Schedule II (oral and parenteral), III (rectal)

Pregnancy Category D

Indications
Hypnotic agent (short-term). Preoperative sedation and other situations in which sedation is required. Treatment of seizures. **Unlabeled Use: IV:** Induction of coma in selected patients with

cerebral ischemia and management of increased intracranial pressure (high doses).

Contraindications/Precautions
Contraindicated in: Hypersensitivity; Some products contain tartrazine, alcohol, or propylene glycol and should be avoided in patients with known hypersensitivity or intolerance; Comatose patients or those with pre-existing CNS depression (unless used to induce coma); Uncontrolled severe pain; Pregnancy or lactation.
Use Cautiously in: Hepatic dysfunction; Severe renal impairment; Patients who may be suicidal or who may have been addicted to drugs previously; Geriatric or debilitated patients (initial dosage reduction recommended); Hypovolemic shock; Hypnotic use should be short-term (chronic use may lead to dependence).

Adverse Reactions/Side Effects
CNS: drowsiness, hangover, lethargy, delirium, excitation, mental depression, vertigo. **Resp:** respiratory depression. *IV*, LARYNGOSPASM, bronchospasm. **CV:** *IV*—hypotension. **GI:** constipation, diarrhea, nausea, vomiting. **Derm:** rashes, urticaria. **Local:** phlebitis at IV site. **MS:** arthralgia, myalgia, neuralgia. **Misc:** hypersensitivity reactions including ANGIOEDEMA and SERUM SICKNESS, physical dependence, psychological dependence.

Route/Dosage
PO (Adults): *Sedative*—20 mg 3–4 times daily. *Hypnotic/preoperative sedative*—100 mg.
PO (Children): *Sedative*—2–6 mg/kg/day. *Preoperative sedative*—2–6 mg/kg (up to 100 mg/dose).
IM (Adults): *Hypnotic/preoperative sedative*—150–200 mg.
IM (Children): *Sedative*—2–6 mg/kg/day in divided doses. *Preoperative sedative*—2–6 mg/kg (up to 100 mg/dose).
IV (Adults): *Hypnotic/anticonvulsant*—100 mg initially; additional small doses may be given q min up to 500 mg total. *Induction of coma*—5–7 mg/kg, then 3–4 mg/kg q 3–4 hr dose adjusted by serum level (unlabeled).
IV (Children): *Sedative*—1–3 mg/kg to a maximum of 100 mg until asleep. *Conscious sedation*—Initial 2 mg/kg, may repeat q 5–10 min with 1–2 mg/kg until adequate sedation acheived. Maximum total dose 6 mg/kg or 150–200 mg. *Induction of coma*—10–15 mg/kg slowly over 1–2 hr, followed by a maintenance infusion of 1–3 mg/kg/hr.
Rect (Adults): *Sedative*—30 mg 2–4 times daily. *Hypnotic*—120–200 mg at bedtime.
Rect (Children): *Sedative*—2 mg/kg (60 mg/m²) 3 times daily.
Rect (Children 12–14 yr): *Preoperative sedative/hypnotic*—60–120 mg.
Rect (Children 5–12 yr): *Preoperative sedative/hypnotic*—60 mg.
Rect (Children 1–4 yr): *Preoperative sedative/hypnotic*—30–60 mg.
Rect (Children 2 mo–1 yr): *Preoperative sedative/hypnotic*—30 mg.

polycarbophil
(pol-i-**kar**-boe-fil)
Bulk Forming Fiber Laxative, Equalactin, FiberCon, Fiber-Lax, Konsyl Fiber, Mitrolan

Classification
Therapeutic: antidiarrheals, laxatives
Pharmacologic: bulk-forming agents

Pregnancy Category UK

Indications
Treatment of constipation or diarrhea that may be associated with diverticulosis or irritable bowel syndrome.

Contraindications/Precautions
Contraindicated in: Hypersensitivity; Abdominal pain; Nausea or vomiting (especially when associated with fever or other signs of acute abdomen); Serious intra-abdominal adhesions; Dysphagia.
Use Cautiously in: Pregnancy or lactation (has been used safely).

Adverse Reactions/Side Effects
GI: abdominal fullness.

Route/Dosage
PO (Adults): 1 g 1–4 times daily or as needed (not to exceed 6 g/24 hr); for severe diarrhea, may repeat q 30 min.
PO (Children 6–12 yr): 500 mg 1–3 times daily or as needed (not to exceed 3 g/24 hr); for severe diarrhea, may repeat q 30 min.
PO (Children 2–6 yr): 500 mg 1–2 times daily or as needed (not to exceed 1.5 g/24 hr); for severe diarrhea, may repeat q 30 min.

POTASSIUM PHOSPHATES
(poe-**tass**-ee-um **foss**-fates)

monobasic potassium phosphate
K-Phos Original

potassium phosphates
Neutra-Phos-K

potassium phosphate

Classification
Therapeutic: antiurolithics, mineral and electrolyte replacements/supplements

Pregnancy Category C

Indications
Treatment and prevention of phosphate depletion in patients who are unable to ingest adequate dietary potassium. Adjunct therapy of urinary tract infections with methenamine hippurate or mandelate (potassium and sodium phosphates or monobasic potassium phosphate). Prevention of calcium urinary stones (potassium and sodium phosphates or monobasic potassium phosphate). Phosphate salts of potassium may be used in hypokalemic patients with metabolic acidosis or coexisting phosphorus deficiency.

Contraindications/Precautions
Contraindicated in: Hyperkalemia; Hyperphosphatemia; Hypocalcemia; Severe renal impairment; Untreated Addison's disease; Severe tissue trauma; Hyperkalemic familial periodic paralysis.
Use Cautiously in: Hyperparathyroidism; Cardiac disease; Renal impairment.

Adverse Reactions/Side Effects
Related to hyperphosphatemia, unless otherwise indicated. **CNS:** confusion, listlessness, weakness. **CV:** ARRHYTHMIAS, CARDIAC ARREST, ECG changes (absent P waves, widening of the QRS complex with biphasic curve), hypotension, *hyperkalemia*, ARRHYTHMIAS, ECG changes (prolonged PR interval, ST segment depression, tall-tented T waves). **GI:** diarrhea, abdominal pain, nausea, vomiting. **F and E:** hyperkalemia, hyperphosphatemia, hypocalcemia, hypomagnesemia. **Local:** irritation at IV site, phlebitis. **MS:** *hyperkalemia*—muscle cramps; *hypercalcemia*—tremors. **Neuro:** flaccid paralysis, heaviness of legs, paresthesias.

Route/Dosage
Monobasic Potassium Phosphate
PO (Adults and Children >4 yr): 1 g (7.4 mmol) in water 4 times daily.
PO (Children <4 yr): 200 mg (6.4 mmol) in water 4 times daily.

Potassium Phosphates
PO (Adults and Children >4 yr): 1.45 g (8 mmol) 4 times daily.
PO (Children <4 yr): 200 mg (6.4 mmol) phosphorus 4 times daily.
IV (Adults): 10 mmol phosphorus/day as an infusion.
IV (Infants): 1.5–2 mmol phosphorus/day as an infusion.

ranibizumab
(ran-i-**bi**-zoo-mab)
Lucentis

Classification
Therapeutic: ocular agents
Pharmacologic: monoclonal antibodies

Pregnancy Category C

Indications
Treatment of neovascular (wet) macular degeneration.

Contraindications/Precautions
Contraindicated in: Hypersensitivity; Ocular/periocular infections.
Use Cautiously in: OB: Use only in pregnancy if clearly needed, use cautiously during lactation; Pedi: Safe use in children not established.

Adverse Reactions/Side Effects
EENT: conjunctival hemorrhage, eye pain, ↑ intraocular pressure, intraocular inflammation, vitreal floaters, endophthalmitis, retinal detachment. **CV:** arterial thromboembolic events.

Route/Dosage
Intravitreal (Adults): 0.5 mg (0.05 ml) once monthly; after 4 months, injections may be given every 1–3 months.

riboflavin (rye-boe-flay-vin)
vitamin B$_2$

Classification
Therapeutic: vitamins
Pharmacologic: water soluble vitamins

Pregnancy Category A

Indications
Treatment and prevention of riboflavin deficiency, which may be associated with poor nutritional status or chronic debilitating illnesses.

Contraindications/Precautions
Contraindicated in: No known contraindications.
Use Cautiously in: No known precautions.

Adverse Reactions/Side Effects
GU: yellow discoloration of urine (large doses only).

Route/Dosage
Treatment of Deficiency
PO (Adults): 5–10 mg/day.

---

rifapentine (rif-a-**pen**-teen)
Priftin

Classification
Therapeutic: agents for amyotrophic lateral sclerosis, antituberculars

Pregnancy Category C

Indications
Treatment of pulmonary tuberculosis: Must be used in combination with other agents.

Contraindications/Precautions
Contraindicated in: Hypersensitivity to rifapentine or other rifamycins (rifampin or rifabutin).
Use Cautiously in: History of liver disease; Pregnancy, lactation, or children <12 yr (safety not established).
Exercise Extreme Caution in: Concurrent protease inhibitor therapy.

Adverse Reactions/Side Effects
CNS: dizziness, headache. **Resp:** hemoptysis. **CV:** hypertension. **GI:** PSEUDOMEMBRANOUS COLITIS, anorexia, diarrhea, dyspepsia, increased liver enzymes, nausea, vomiting. **GU:** hematuria, proteinuria, pyuria, urinary casts. **Derm:** acne, pruritus, rash. **Hemat:** anemia, leukopenia, lymphopenia, neutropenia, thrombocytosis. **MS:** arthralgia. **Misc:** pain.

Route/Dosage
Must be used in combination with other antituberculars.
PO (Adults): *Intensive phase*—600 mg twice weekly (not less than 72 hr between doses) for 2 months; *continuation phase*—600 mg once weekly for 4 months.

---

saquinavir (sa-**kwin**-a-vir)
Invirase

Classification
Therapeutic: antiretrovirals
Pharmacologic: protease inhibitors

Pregnancy Category B

Indications
HIV infection with ritonavir (may also add other antiretrovirals).

Contraindications/Precautions
Contraindicated in: Hypersensitivity; Concurrent dihydroergotamine (or other ergot derivatives), midazolam, rifabutin, rifampin, lovastatin, simvastatin, and triazolam; Lactation: Breastfeeding not recommended in HIV-infection.
Use Cautiously in: Diabetes mellitus (may exacerbate hyperglycemia; hyperglycemia may progress to ketoacidosis); Hemophilia (↑ risk of bleeding); Hepatic impairment (may exacerbate liver dysfunction caused by hepatitis B or C or other causes); OB, Pedi: Pregnancy or children <16 yr (safety not established).

Adverse Reactions/Side Effects
CNS: SEIZURES, confusion, headache, mental depression, psychic disorders, weakness. **CV:** thrombophlebitis. **GI:** abdominal discomfort, diarrhea, ↑ liver enzymes, jaundice, nausea. **Derm:** photosensitivity, severe cutaneous reactions. **Endo:** hyperglycemia. **Hemat:** acute myeloblastic leukemia, hemolytic anemia, thrombocytopenia. **Neuro:** ataxia. **Misc:** STEVENS-JOHNSON SYNDROME.

Route/Dosage
PO (Adults): 600 mg 3 times daily within 2 hr of a meal *or* 1000 mg twice daily.

---

sodium phosphate (**soe**-dee-um **foss**-fate)

Classification
Therapeutic: mineral and electrolyte replacements/supplements
Pharmacologic: phosphate supplements

Pregnancy Category C

Indications
Treatment and prevention of phosphate depletion in patients who are unable to ingest adequate dietary phosphates.

= Canadian drug name. = Genetic implication.
*CAPITALS indicates life-threatening; underlines indicate most frequent.

Contraindications/Precautions
Contraindicated in: Hyperphosphatemia; Hypocalcemia; Severe renal impairment.
Use Cautiously in: Hyperparathyroidism; Cardiac disease; Hypernatremia; Hypertension.

Adverse Reactions/Side Effects
Related to hyperphosphatemia, unless otherwise indicated. **CNS:** confusion, listlessness, weakness. **Resp:** *hypernatremia*—shortness of breath. **CV:** ARRHYTHMIAS, CARDIAC ARREST, ECG changes (absent P waves, widening of the QRS complex with biphasic curve), hypotension; *hypernatremia*—edema. **GI:** diarrhea, abdominal pain, nausea, vomiting. **F and E:** hyperkalemia, hypernatremia, hyperphosphatemia, hypocalcemia, hypomagnesemia. **Local:** irritation at IV site, phlebitis. **MS:** *hypocalcemia*—tremors. **Neuro:** flaccid paralysis, heaviness of legs, paresthesias of extremities.

Route/Dosage
IV (Adults): 12–15 mmol phosphorus/liter of parenteral nutrition.
IV (Children): *Hypophosphatemia*–0.08–0.36 mmol/kg over 6 hr; *Maintenance*—<25 kg: 0.5–1.5 mmol/kg/day; 25–45 kg: 0.5–1 mmol/kg/day.
IV (Neonates): *Maintenance*—0.8–1.5 mmol/kg/day (infused as part of parenteral nutrition).

---

stavudine (stav-yoo-deen)
d4T, Zerit, Zerit XR

Classification
Therapeutic: antiretrovirals
Pharmacologic: nucleoside reverse transcriptase inhibitors

Pregnancy Category C

Indications
HIV infection unresponsive or intolerant to conventional therapy.

Contraindications/Precautions
Contraindicated in: Hypersensitivity.
Use Cautiously in: Patients with a history of alcohol abuse; Patients with a history of liver disease or hepatic impairment; Renal impairment (dose reduction and/or increased dosing interval recommended if CCr <50 mL/min); History of peripheral neuropathy; OB, Lactation: Safety not established; avoid breastfeeding by HIV-infected mothers because of transmission of the virus in breast milk; concurrent use with didanosine during pregnancy may ↑ the risk of fetal lactic acidosis.

Adverse Reactions/Side Effects
CNS: headache, insomnia, weakness. **GI:** HEPATOMEGALY (WITH STEATOSIS), HEPATIC TOXICITY, PANCREATITIS, anorexia, diarrhea. **F and E:** LACTIC ACIDOSIS. **Hemat:** anemia. **MS:** arthralgia, myalgia. **Endo:** fat redistribution. **Neuro:** peripheral neuropathy.

Route/Dosage
PO (Adults ≥60 kg): 40 mg q 12 hr.
PO (Adults <60 kg): 30 mg q 12 hr.
PO (Children ≥30 kg): 30 mg q 12 hr.
PO (Children at least 14 days old and <30 kg): 1 mg/kg q 12 hr (not to exceed 40 mg q 12 hr).
PO (Infants birth–13 days): 0.5 mg/kg q 12 hr.

Renal Impairment
PO (Adults ≥60 kg): *CCr 26–50 mL/min*—20 mg q 12 hr; *CCr 10–25 mL/min*—20 mg q 24 hr.
PO (Adults <60 kg): *CCr 26–50 mL/min*—15 mg q 12 hr; *CCr 10–25 mL/min*—15 mg q 24 hr.

---

succimer (sux-i-mer)
Chemet

Classification
Therapeutic: antidotes
Pharmacologic: chelating agents

Pregnancy Category C

Indications
Treatment of lead poisoning in children with blood lead levels >45 mcg/dL.

Contraindications/Precautions
Contraindicated in: Hypersensitivity or allergy to succimer; Lactation (should be discouraged during succimer therapy).
Use Cautiously in: Renal failure (chelates are not dialyzable); Children (increased risk of bradyarrhythmias); Children with skeletal muscle myopathy (more prone to rare, but serious, adverse reactions); Geriatric patients (use lower doses to adjust for decreased renal, hepatic, and cardiac function); Pregnancy or children <1 yr (safety not established).

Adverse Reactions/Side Effects
CNS: dizziness, drowsiness, headache. **EENT:** cloudy film in eye, otitis media, plugged ears, watery eyes. **Resp:** cough, nasal congestion, rhinorrhea, sore throat. **CV:** arrhythmias. **GI:** nausea, vomiting, abdominal cramps, anorexia, diarrhea,

elevated liver function tests, hemorrhoidal symptoms, metallic taste. **GU:** oliguria, proteinuria, voiding difficulty. **Derm:** mucocutaneous eruptions, pruritus, rashes. **Hemat:** eosinophilia, thrombocytosis. **MS:** back, rib, flank pain; leg pain. **Neuro:** paresthesia, sensorimotor neuropathy. **Misc:** chills, fever, flu-like syndrome, moniliasis.

Route/Dosage
PO (Adults and Children): 10 mg/kg (350 mg/m^2) q 8 hr for 5 days, then reduce to 10 mg/kg (350 mg/m^2) q 12 hr for 2 more wk. Repeated courses should follow a 2-wk rest period.

tegaserod (te-gas-er-od)
Zelnorm

Classification
Therapeutic: anti-irritable bowel syndrome agents
Pharmacologic: 5-HT$_4$ antagonists

Pregnancy Category B

Indications
Short-term treatment of irritable bowel syndrome (IBS) in women whose primary symptom is constipation in patients <55 yr. Chronic idiopathic constipation in patients <55 yr for whom no other treatment has provided satisfactory relief and/or who had satisfactory improvement previously with tegaserod. Only available under an emergency invesitgational new drug (IND) process. To qualify, patients must have a condition characterized as immediately life-threatening or requiring hospitalization. Physicians would need to make the request for emergency use through the FDA.

Contraindications/Precautions
Contraindicated in: Hypersensitivity; Moderate to severe hepatic impairment; Severe renal impairment; History of bowel obstruction, gallbladder disease, sphincter of Oddi dysfunction, or intra-abdominal adhesions; Concurrent or frequent diarrhea; Exclusion criteria for emergency access include: History, current diagnosis, or symptoms of CV disease, Presence of CV risk factors, Uncompensated depression or anxiety, Suicidal ideation or behavior.
Use Cautiously in: Mild hepatic impairment; Geri: Safety not established; OB: Pregnancy, lactation or children <18 yr (safety not established).

Adverse Reactions/Side Effects
CNS: headache. **GI:** diarrhea.

Route/Dosage
PO (Adults): 6 mg twice daily before meals.

temsirolimus
(tem-si-**ro**-li-mus)
Torisel

Classification
Therapeutic: antineoplastics
Pharmacologic: enzyme inhibitors, kinase inhibitors

Pregnancy Category D

Indications
Advanced renal cell carcinoma.

Contraindications/Precautions
Contraindicated in: OB: Pregnancy and lactation.
Use Cautiously in: Hypersensitivity to temsirolimus, sirolimus or polysorbate 80; Perioperative patients (may impair wound healing); OB: Patients which child-bearing potential; Pedi: Safe use in children not established.

Adverse Reactions/Side Effects
CNS: weakness. **EENT:** conjunctivitis. **CV:** hypertension, venous thromboembolism. **Resp:** INTERSTITIAL LUNG DISEASE. **GI:** BOWEL PERFORATION, anorexia, ↑ liver enzymes, mucositis, nausea. **GU:** RENAL FAILURE. **Derm:** rash, abnormal wound healing. **Endo:** hyperglycemia. **F and E:** edema, hypophosphatemia. **Hemat:** anemia, leukopenia, lymphopenia, thrombocytopenia. **Metab:** hyperlipidemia, hypertriglyceridemia. **Misc:** hypersensitivity reactions including ANAPHYLAXIS, ↑ risk of infections.

Route/Dosage
IV (Adults): 25 mg once weekly; dose modification is required for bone marrow toxicity or concurrent use of agents affecting the CYP 3A4 enzyme system (pre-treatment with antihistamine is recommended).

thioguanine
(thye-oh-**gwon**-een)
6-thioguanine, ✦ Lanvis

✦ = Canadian drug name. ☒ = Genetic implication.
*CAPITALS indicates life-threatening; underlines indicate most frequent.

1336 LESS COMMONLY USED DRUGS

Classification
Therapeutic: antineoplastics
Pharmacologic: antimetabolites

Pregnancy Category D

Indications
Induction and consolidation of remission in acute nonlymphocytic leukemia (in combination with other agents).

Contraindications/Precautions
Contraindicated in: Hypersensitivity; OB, Lactation: Pregnancy or lactation; Tumors with demonstrated resistance to thioguanine or mercaptopurine (usually complete cross-resistance).
Use Cautiously in: Patients with childbearing potential; Infections; ↓ bone marrow reserve; Other chronic debilitating illnesses; ⚡ Patients with TPMT enzyme deficiency (substantial dosage reductions are required to avoid hematologic adverse events).

Adverse Reactions/Side Effects
EENT: loss of vibratory sense. **GI:** diarrhea, hepatotoxicity, jaundice, nausea, stomatitis, vomiting, anorexia, hepatic veno-occlusive disease. **GU:** gonadal suppression. **Derm:** dermatitis, rash. **Hemat:** anemia, leukopenia, thrombocytopenia, pancytopenia. **Metab:** hyperuricemia. **Neuro:** unsteady gait.

Route/Dosage
Many other protocols are used.
PO (Adults and Children): *Induction*—2 mg/kg (75–100 mg/m^2) per day, rounded off to nearest 20 mg given as single dose; after 4 wk may ↑ to 3 mg/kg. *Maintenance*—2–3 mg/kg (100 mg/m^2) per day.

---

tiludronate (tye-loo-droe-nate)
Skelid

Classification
Therapeutic: bone resorption inhibitors
Pharmacologic: biphosphanates

Pregnancy Category C

Indications
Management of Paget's disease of the bone in patients with: Serum alkaline phosphatase ≥2 times the upper limit of normal, Symptoms, Risk for complications.

Contraindications/Precautions
Contraindicated in: Hypersensitivity; Severe renal impairment (CCr <30 mL/min).
Use Cautiously in: Dental surgery (may ↑ risk of jaw osteonecrosis); OB, Lactation: Pedi: Safety not established.

Adverse Reactions/Side Effects
CNS: anxiety, drowsiness, fatigue, insomnia, nervousness, syncope, vertigo, weakness. **EENT:** cataracts, conjunctivitis, glaucoma, pharyngitis, rhinitis, sinusitis. **Resp:** bronchitis. **CV:** chest pain, dependent edema, hypertension, peripheral edema. **GI:** abdominal pain, anorexia, constipation, diarrhea, dry mouth, dysphagia, esophageal ulcer, esophagitis, flatulence, gastric ulcer, gastritis, nausea, tooth disorder, vomiting. **GU:** urinary tract infection. **Derm:** flushing, increased sweating, pruritus, rash, skin disorder. **Endo:** hyperparathyroidism. **F and E:** hypocalcemia. **MS:** musculoskeletal pain, arthrosis, involuntary muscle contractions, osteonecrosis (primarily of jaw), pathological fractures. **Neuro:** paresthesia. **Misc:** infection.

Route/Dosage
PO (Adults): 400 mg/day taken with 8 oz of plain water only, for 3 mo.

---

tipranavir (ti-pran-a-veer)
Aptivus

Classification
Therapeutic: antiretrovirals
Pharmacologic: protease inhibitors

Pregnancy Category C

Indications
Advanced HIV disease resistant to more than one protease inhibitor (must be used with ritonavir).

Contraindications/Precautions
Contraindicated in: Hypersensitivity; Moderate to severe hepatic impairment (Child-Pugh Class B or C); Concurrent use of some antiarrhythmics (amiodarone, flecainide, propafenone, quinidine), ergot derivatives, midazolam (oral), or triazolam.
Use Cautiously in: Known sulfonamide allergy (contains sulfa moiety); Pre-existing liver disease (may ↑ risk of hepatotoxicity); History of or risk factors for diabetes (may cause hyperglycemia); Hemophilia (may ↑ risk of bleeding); Patients at ↑ risk for bleeding.

Adverse Reactions/Side Effects
CV: INTRACRANIAL HEMORRHAGE, fatigue, headache. **GI:** HEPATOTOXICITY, abdominal pain, diarrhea, nausea, vomiting. **Derm:** rash (↑ in

women and peds). **Endo:** hyperglycemia. **Metab:** ↑ cholesterol, ↑ triglycerides. **Misc:** allergic reactions, bleeding, fat redistribution, fever, immune reconstitution syndrome.

Route/Dosage
PO (Adults): 500 mg twice daily with ritonavir 200 mg twice daily.

PO (Children ≥2 yr): 14 mg/kg (max: 500 mg/dose) twice daily with ritonavir 6 mg/kg (max: 200 mg/dose) twice daily; if intolerance develops, may ↓ dose to tipranavir 12 mg/kg twice daily with ritonavir 5 mg/kg twice daily.

---

tolmetin (tole-met-in)
Tolectin, Tolectin DS, ✱ Novo-Tolmetin

Classification
Therapeutic: antirheumatics, nonsteroidal anti-inflammatory agents

Pregnancy Category UK

Indications
Management of inflammatory disorders including: Rheumatoid arthritis, Juvenile rheumatoid arthritis, Osteoarthritis.

Contraindications/Precautions
Contraindicated in: Hypersensitivity; Cross-sensitivity may exist with other NSAIDs, including aspirin; Active GI bleeding or ulcer disease; Perioperative pain from coronary artery bypass graft (CABG) surgery.

Use Cautiously in: Cardiovascular disease or risk factors for cardiovascular disease (may ↑ risk of serious cardiovascular thrombotic events, myocardial infarction, and stroke, especially with prolonged use); Severe renal, or hepatic disease; History of ulcer disease; Severe hepatic or renal impairment (dosage reduction recommended); Geri: Geriatric patients (↑ risk of GI bleeding; **OB, Pedi:** Pregnancy and lactation (safety not established; avoid use during 2nd and 3rd trimesters).

Adverse Reactions/Side Effects
CNS: dizziness, headache, drowsiness, mental depression, sleep disturbances. **EENT:** tinnitus, visual disturbances. **CV:** edema, hypertension. **GI:** DRUG-INDUCED HEPATITIS, GI BLEEDING, diarrhea, discomfort, dyspepsia, nausea, vomiting, constipation, flatulence. **GU:** renal failure. **Derm:** EXFOLIATIVE DERMATITIS, STEVENS-JOHNSON SYNDROME, TOXIC EPIDERMAL NECROLYSIS, rashes.

LESS COMMONLY USED DRUGS **1337**

Hemat: prolonged bleeding time. **MS:** muscle weakness. **Misc:** allergic reactions including ANAPHYLAXIS.

Route/Dosage
PO (Adults): 400 mg 3 times daily initially, followed by maintenance dose of 600–1800 mg/day in 3–4 divided doses (not to exceed 2000 mg/day).

PO (Children >2 yr): 20 mg/kg/day in 3–4 divided doses initially, followed by maintenance dose of 15–30 mg/kg/day in 3–4 divided doses.

---

trifluoperazine
(trye-floo-oh-**pair**-a-zeen)
✱Apo-Trifluoperazine, ✱ Novo-Flurazine, ✱ PMS-Trifluoperazine, ✱ Solazine, ✱ Terfluzine

Classification
Therapeutic: antipsychotics (conventional)
Pharmacologic: phenothiazines

Pregnancy Category C

Indications
Schizophrenia, nonpsychotic anxiety. Considered second-line treatment after failure with atypical antipsychotics. **Unlabeled Use:** Other psychotic disorders; bipolar disorder.

Contraindications/Precautions
Contraindicated in: Hypersensitivity; Cross-sensitivity with other phenothiazines may exist; Hypersensitivity to bisulfites (oral concentrate only); Angle-closure glaucoma; Bone marrow depression; Severe liver or cardiovascular disease; Lactation: Discontinue drug or bottle feed.

Use Cautiously in: Geri: Geriatric or debilitated patients (dose reduction recommended); ↑ risk of mortality in elderly patients treated for dementia-related psychosis; OB: Safety not established; may cause adverse effects in the newborn; Diabetes mellitus; Respiratory disease; Prostatic hyperplasia; CNS tumors; Epilepsy; Intestinal obstruction.

Adverse Reactions/Side Effects
CNS: NEUROLEPTIC MALIGNANT SYNDROME, extrapyramidal reactions, sedation, tardive dyskinesia. **EENT:** dry eyes, blurred vision, lens opacities. **CV:** hypotension, tachycardia. **GI:** constipation, anorexia, dry mouth, hepatitis, ileus. **GU:** urinary retention, priapism. **Derm:** photosensitivity, pigment changes, rashes. **Endo:** galactorrhea,

---

✱ = Canadian drug name. ᗉ = Genetic implication.
*CAPITALS indicates life-threatening; underlines indicate most frequent.

amenorrhea. **Hemat:** AGRANULOCYTOSIS, leukopenia. **Metab:** hyperthermia. **Misc:** allergic reactions.

Route/Dosage
PO (Adults): *Psychoses*—2–5 mg 1–2 times daily (up to 40 mg/day). *Anxiety*—1–2 mg bid (not to exceed 6 mg/day or treatment longer than 12 wk).
PO (Children 6–12 yr): 1 mg once or twice daily (up to 15 mg/day).
IM (Adults): 1–2 mg q 4–6 hr (up to 10 mg/day).
IM (Children): 1 mg once or twice daily.

trihexyphenidyl
(trye-hex-ee-**fen**-i-dill)
✦Apo-Trihex, Artane, ✦PMS-Trihexyphenidyl, Trihexane, Trihexy

Classification
Therapeutic: antiparkinson agents
Pharmacologic: anticholinergics

Pregnancy Category C

Indications
Adjunct in the management of parkinsonian syndrome of many causes, including drug-induced parkinsonism.

Contraindications/Precautions
Contraindicated in: Hypersensitivity; Angle-closure glaucoma; Acute hemorrhage; Tachycardia secondary to cardiac insufficiency; Thyrotoxicosis; Known alcohol intolerance (elixir only).
Use Cautiously in: Geriatric and very young patients (increased risk of adverse reactions); Intestinal obstruction or infection; Prostatic hyperplasia; Chronic renal, hepatic, pulmonary, or cardiac disease; Pregnancy, lactation, or children (safety not established).

Adverse Reactions/Side Effects
CNS: dizziness, nervousness, confusion, drowsiness, headache, psychoses, weakness. **EENT:** blurred vision, mydriasis. **CV:** orthostatic hypotension, tachycardia. **GI:** dry mouth, nausea, constipation, vomiting. **GU:** urinary hesitancy, urinary retention. **Derm:** decreased sweating.

Route/Dosage
PO (Adults): 1–2 mg/day initially; increase by 2 mg q 3–5 days. Usual maintenance dose is 6–10 mg/day in 3 divided doses (up to 15 mg/day). Extended-release (Artane Sequels) preparations may be given q 12 hr after daily dose has been determined using conventional tablets or liquid.

trimipramine
(trye-**mip**-ra-meen)
Surmontil

Classification
Therapeutic: antidepressants
Pharmacologic: tricyclic antidepressants

Pregnancy Category C

Indications
Treatment of depression, often in conjunction with psychotherapy.

Contraindications/Precautions
Contraindicated in: Hypersensitivity; cross-sensitivity may occur with other tricyclic antidepressants; Recovery phase following MI; Concurrent MAO inhibitor therapy; wait 2 wk following cessation to initiate trimipramine in lower doses initially; Angle-closure glaucoma.
Use Cautiously in: History or symptoms compatible with bipolar disease (may precipitate mixed/manic episodes; May ↑ risk of suicide attempt/ideation especially during early treatment or dose adjustment; Pedi: risk may be greater in children and adolescents; Prostatic hyperplasia (↑ risk of urinary retention); History of seizures (may ↓ threshold); Hepatic impairment; Electroshock therapy (may ↑ risk of adverse reactions); Increased intraocular pressure; Hyperthyroidism (↑ risk of cardiovascular toxicity); OB: Use only if clearly needed and maternal benefits outweigh risks to fetus; Lactation: May cause sedation in infant; Pedi: Safety not established; Geri: ↑ risk of adverse reactions, including falls secondary to sedative and anticholinergic affects.
Exercise Extreme Caution in: Pre-existing cardiovascular disease.

Adverse Reactions/Side Effects
CNS: lethargy, sedation. **EENT:** blurred vision, dry eyes, dry mouth. **CV:** arrhythmias, hypotension, ECG changes. **GI:** constipation, hepatitis, paralytic ileus, increased appetite, weight gain. **GU:** urinary retention, ↓ libido. **Derm:** photosensitivity. **Endo:** changes in blood glucose, gynecomastia. **Hemat:** blood dyscrasias.

Route/Dosage
PO (Adults): 75 mg/day in divided doses or as a single daily dose at bedtime; may be increased up to 150 mg/day; not to exceed 200 mg/day (300 mg/day in hospitalized patients). *Adolescent and elderly patients*—50 mg/day, may gradually increase up to 100 mg/day.

triptorelin (trip-to-**rel**-in)
Trelstar Depot

Classification
Therapeutic: antineoplastics
Pharmacologic: hormones

Pregnancy Category X

Indications
Palliative treatment of advanced prostate cancer when orchiectomy or estrogen administration are contraindicated or unacceptable.

Contraindications/Precautions
Contraindicated in: Hypersensitivity to triptorelin or similar agents; Pregnancy, lactation, or children.
Use Cautiously in: Metastatic vertebral lesions and/or upper or lower urinary tract obstruction (symptoms may transiently worsen following initiation of therapy); Renal or hepatic impairment (may need dosage adjustment).

Adverse Reactions/Side Effects
CNS: dizziness, emotional lability, fatigue, headache, insomnia. **CV:** hypertension. **GI:** diarrhea, vomiting. **GU:** erectile dysfunction, urinary retention, urinary tract infection. **Derm:** pruritus. **Hemat:** anemia. **Local:** injection site pain. **MS:** musculoskeletal pain. **Misc:** allergic reactions including ANAPHYLAXIS and ANGIOEDEMA.

Route/Dosage
IM (Adults): 3.75 mg monthly.

verteporfin (ver-te-**por**-fin)
Visudyne

Classification
Therapeutic: none assigned
Pharmacologic: photodynamic agents

Pregnancy Category C

Indications
Treatment of age-related macular degeneration in patients with predominantly classic subfoveal choroidal neovascularization.

Contraindications/Precautions
Contraindicated in: Hypersensitivity; Porphyria; Exposure to direct sunlight.
Use Cautiously in: Moderate/severe hepatic impairment; Pregnancy, lactation or children (safety not established).

Adverse Reactions/Side Effects
CNS: headache, weakness. **EENT:** visual disturbances, cataracts, conjunctivitis/conjunctival injection, dry eyes, ocular itching, severe vision loss, subconjunctival/subretinal/vitreous hemorrhage. **Derm:** photosensitivity. **Local:** injection site reactions including extravasation and rashes. **MS:** back pain (during infusion). **Misc:** fever, flu-like syndrome.

Route/Dosage
IV (Adults): 6 mg/m^2 infused over 10 min, followed by appropriate laser light delivery initiated 15 min after the start of the infusion.

zileuton (zye-**loo**-ton)
Zyflo CR

Classification
Therapeutic: bronchodilators
Pharmacologic: leukotriene antagonists

Pregnancy Category C

Indications
Long-term control agent in the management of asthma.

Contraindications/Precautions
Contraindicated in: Hypersensitivity; Active liver disease or transaminases ≥3 times upper limit of normal.
Use Cautiously in: Acute attacks of asthma; History of liver disease or alcohol consumption; OB, Lactation: Pedi: Pregnancy, lactation, or children <12 yr (safety not established).

Adverse Reactions/Side Effects
CNS: SUICIDAL THOUGHTS, headache, agitation, aggression, anxiety, depression, dizziness, dream abnormalities, hallucinations, insomnia, irritability, malaise, nervousness, restlessness, somnolence, tremor, weakness. **EENT:** conjunctivitis. **CV:** chest pain. **GI:** abdominal pain, constipation, dyspepsia, flatulence, ↑ liver enzymes, nausea, vomiting. **GU:** urinary tract infection, vaginitis. **Derm:** pruritus. **MS:** arthralgia, myalgia, neck pain. **Neuro:** hypertonia. **Misc:** fever, lymphadenopathy.

Route/Dosage
PO (Adults and Children ≥12 yr): 1200 mg twice daily.

✦ = Canadian drug name. ❚ = Genetic implication.
*CAPITALS indicates life-threatening; underlines indicate most frequent.

Natural/Herbal Products

The following monographs introduce some commonly used natural products. Because the amounts of active ingredients in these agents are not standardized or currently subject to FDA guidelines for medicines, *Davis's Drug Guide for Nurses*, although respectful of patients' right to choose from a variety of therapeutic options, does not endorse their routine use unless supervised by a knowledgeable health care professional. Users should take into account the possibility of adverse reactions and interactions and consider the relative lack of data supporting widespread use of these products. Doses are poorly standardized, and individuals are advised to read package labels carefully to ensure safe and efficacious use.

aloe (al-oh)

Other Name(s):
Aloe vera, Cape aloe, Aloe latex, Burn plant, Curacao aloe

Classification
Therapeutic: laxatives, wound/ulcer/decubiti healing agent

Common Uses
PO: Cathartic laxative. **Topical:** Use on burns/sunburns, wounds, irritated skin, psoriasis; topical anti-infective.

Action
PO: Exerts a laxative effect by increasing colonic motility, reducing water absorption from the bowel and stimulating bowel, chloride secretion and water content. **Topical:** May help accelerate wound healing through inhibition of thromboxane A2 and increased microcirculation, although the evidence is inconsistent. May have some activity against gram-positive, gram-negative bacteria and yeast. **Therapeutic Effects:** Relief of constipation. Improved wound healing.

Pharmacokinetics
Absorption: Unknown.
Distribution: Unknown.
Metabolism and Excretion: Unknown.
Half-life: Unknown.

TIME/ACTION PROFILE

ROUTE	ONSET	PEAK	DURATION
PO, Topical	unknown	unknown	unknown

Contraindications/Precautions
Contraindicated in: Intestinal obstruction; Inflammatory intestinal diseases (including Crohn's disease); Appendicitis and abdominal pain of unknown origin; OB: Safety not established; Pedi: Oral aloe not appropriate for children <12 yr.
Use Cautiously in: Renal disease; Fluid or electrolyte abnormalities; Diabetes; Alcohol containing products should be used cautiously in patients with known intolerance or liver disease; Pedi: Cautious use in children >12 yr old.

Adverse Reactions/Side Effects
Derm: Contact dermatitis, skin irritation. **Endo:** hypoglycemia. **F and E:** HYPOKALEMIA, dehydration. **GI:** Cramping, diarrhea, laxative dependence (chronic use). **GU:** hematuria.

Interactions
Natural Product-Drug: Combining oral aloe with potassium-wasting drugs (e.g., **diuretics**, other **laxatives**, **corticosteroids**, **cisplatin**, **amphotericin B**) may worsen hypokalemia. Hypokalemia may ↑ risk of toxicity from **digoxin** and some **antiarrhythmics**. May have additive effects with **antidiabetic** agents. May ↑ bleeding risk with **warfarin**. **Alcohol**-containing preparations may interact with **disulfiram** and **metronidazole**.
Natural-Natural: ↑ hypokalemia risk with **licorice** and **horsetail**. Additive effects with stimulant laxative herbs and herbs with hypoglycemic potential.

Route/Commonly Used Doses
PO (Adults): *Constipation*—100–200 mg aloe or 50 mg of aloe extract taken in the evening. Do not use for >1–2 wk without medical advice; *Juice*—1 teaspoonful tid after meals.
Topical (Adults): Aloe gel can be applied liberally to affected areas 3–5 times daily.

Availability
Alone or in combination with other herbal medicinals[OTC]**; Capsules**[OTC]**; Juice**[OTC]**; Tincture (1:10 in 50% alcohol)**[OTC]**; Topical or gel or applied directly from cut plant.**

NURSING IMPLICATIONS

Assessment
- **Constipation:** Assess for abdominal distention, presence of bowel sounds, and usual pattern of elimination.
- Assess color, consistency, and amount of stool produced.
- **Topical:** Perform baseline skin assessment prior to applying aloe to minor wounds, burns, and abrasions. Observe the size, character, and location of the affected area prior to the application of aloe.
- Note topical response assessing for increased inflammation, drainage, pain, warmth, and/or pruritus.
- *Lab Test Considerations:* Monitor serum potassium in patients with chronic use and CBC in patients who self medicate and experience bloody diarrhea or have ulcerative colitis or Crohn's disease.

Potential Nursing Diagnoses
Constipation (Indications)
Risk for impaired skin integrity
Deficient knowledge, related to medication regimen

Implementation
- **PO:** Administer laxative at bedtime to induce a bowel movement in the morning.
- **Topical:** Wash hands and then apply liberally to affected area of skin. Cover broken areas of skin with a light nonadhering dressing (e.g., band-aid dressing with *Telfa* lining) to facilitate keeping area clean. Do not apply an occlusive dressing over site of application.

Patient/Family Teaching
- **Constipation:** Instruct patients with preexisting intestinal disorders (e.g., ulcerative colitis, Crohn's disease, irritable bowel syndrome) not to take aloe juice without the advice of a health care professional.
- Counsel patients that the oral juice should not be taken if they are experiencing abdominal pain, nausea, vomiting, or fever.
- Inform patients that occasional constipation may not be an issue but persistent constipation may represent a more serious health problem and to consult their health care professional.
- Advise patients to expect laxative response to the oral juice in 8–12 hr.
- Caution patients that the cathartic effects may be dramatic and that accompanying dehydration and electrolyte imbalances may occur. If severe diarrhea occurs or persists, seek out treatment from their health care professional.
- Advise patients other than those with spinal cord injury that laxatives should only be used for short-term therapy. Although this is considered by some to be a natural way of correcting constipation it still carries the risk of electrolyte imbalance and dependency with chronic use.
- Encourage patients to use other forms of bowel regulation: increasing bulk in the diet, increasing fluid intake, and increasing mobility, as appropriate. Normal bowel habits are individualized and may vary from 3 times/day to 3 times/wk.
- Advise patients to consume a 1500–2000 mL/day during therapy to prevent dehydration.
- Direct patients with a known cardiac history not to take this herbal supplement without the advice of their health care professional because of the risk of hypokalemia worsening arrhythmias.
- Caution patients with cardiac history to avoid straining during bowel movements (Valsalva maneuver).
- **Topical:** Advise patients that topical applications should only be used for minor burns, abrasions, or wounds. Wounds of larger size or more serious burns should be treated by a health care professional.
- Instruct patients using topical application on a nonintact skin surface about signs and symptoms of infection (milky or discolored drainage, redness, warmth, swelling, pain) and to promptly seek out treatment of a health care professional if this occurs.
- Counsel patients that if improvement in the wound is not occurring or it worsens, stop treatment with aloe vera and seek the advice of a health care professional.
- Warn patients with risk factors for delayed wound healing (e.g., diabetic patients, vascular disease) not to self-medicate with aloe vera without the approval of their health care professional.

Evaluation
- A soft, formed bowel movement.
- Evacuation of the colon.
- Relief of sunburn pain.
- Wound healing in small localized burns or abrasions.

*CAPITALS indicates life-threatening; underlines indicate most frequent.

arnica (ar-ni-cuh)

Other Name(s):
Arnica montana, leopard's bane, mountain tobacco, mountain snuff, wolf's bane

Classification
Therapeutic: immune stimulant, anti-inflammatory

Common Uses
Topical treatment of insect bites, bruises, acne, boils, sprains, muscle, and joint pain.

Action
Polysaccharides in arnica may produce a slight anti-inflammatory and analgesic effect. Some antibacterial effects are seen, in addition to a counterirritant effect, which may aid in wound healing. **Therapeutic Effects:** Decreased inflammation. Pain relief.

Pharmacokinetics
Absorption: Systemic absorption may occur following topical application to broken skin.
Distribution: Unknown.
Metabolism and Excretion: Unknown.
Half-life: Unknown.

TIME/ACTION PROFILE

ROUTE	ONSET	PEAK	DURATION
Topical	unknown	unknown	unknown

Contraindications/Precautions
Contraindicated in: Not for oral use (except in highly diluted homeopathic preparations); Arnica allergy; Avoid use on broken skin; Infectious or inflammatory GI conditions; OB: Pregnancy and lactation.
Use Cautiously in: Infectious or inflammatory GI conditions; Surgery (discontinue use 2 wk prior to procedure due to antiplatelet effects).

Adverse Reactions/Side Effects
GI: abdominal pain, vomiting, diarrhea (if taken orally). **Derm:** edematous dermatitis with pustules (chronic treatment of damaged skin), eczema (prolonged use). **Misc:** local allergic reactions.

Interactions
Natural Product-Drug: Alcohol-containing preparations may interact with **disulfuram** and **metronidazole**. Potential for reduced effectiveness of **antihypertensives** has been noted. May potentiate the effects of **anticoagulants** and **antiplatelet agents**, increasing the risk of bleeding.
Natural-Natural: May increase risk of bleeding with **clove**, **garlic**, **ginger**, **ginkgo**, and **ginseng**.

Route/Commonly Used Doses
Topical (Adults): *Topical*—rub or massage arnica tincture, cream or gel onto injured area. Do not apply to broken skin; *Compress*—dilute 1 tablespoon of arnica tincture in ½ L water. Wet a gauze pad with solution and apply to affected area for 15 min. For use in poultices, dilute tincture 3 to 10 times with water.

Availability
Cream, tincture, salve, ointment, gel, and oil[OTC]; **Topical (preparations should contain not more than 20-25% arnica tincture or 15% arnica oil)**[OTC]; **Homeopathic preparations**[OTC].

NURSING IMPLICATIONS

Assessment
- Inspect skin for breaks prior to application to ensure arnica is applied only to an intact surface. Note the size, character, and location of affected area prior to application of arnica.
- After application, assess the affected area for signs of allergic response.
- *Toxicity and Overdose:* Systemic absorption may result in nausea, vomiting, organ damage, hypertension, cardiotoxicity, arrhythmias, muscular weakness, collapse, vertigo, renal dysfunction, coma and death. If ingested orally, induce emesis and gastric lavage to remove undigested contents. Supportive care may be necessary. Do not take orally or apply to nonintact skin to avoid systemic absorption.

Potential Nursing Diagnoses
Acute pain (Indications)

Implementation
- Clean skin with a non-alcohol containing cleanser prior to applying arnica. Apply topically to affected area, or site of injury ensuring skin is intact.
- Do not take orally or apply to an open wound because of potential for systemic absorption with toxicity.

Patient/Family Teaching
- Teach patients to inspect the affected area for breaks in the skin and not to apply arnica to any areas where the skin is broken.

*CAPITALS indicates life-threatening; underlines indicate most frequent.

- Warn patients that use on nonintact skin and oral ingestion may cause life-threatening toxicity.
- Advise patients that arnica should only be used for short period of time in the treatment of minor aches and pains associated with local muscle, joint, or skin pain. Prolonged use may cause allergic/hypersensitivity reactions to develop.
- Instruct patients taking antihypertensive agents to avoid concurrent use of arnica.
- Advise female patients to notify health care professional if pregnancy is planned or suspected. Arnica should be avoided during pregnancy.

Evaluation
- Relief of, or improvement in, minor aches and pains associated with muscle or joint overuse, or sprains and/or local skin irritation from insect bites, bruises, boils, or acne.

bilberry

Other Name(s):
Vaccinium myrtillus

Classification
Therapeutic: ocular agents

Common Uses
Visual acuity improvement, atherosclerosis, venous insufficiency, varicose veins, diabetes mellitus, diarrhea, hemorrhoids, peptic ulcer disease, osteoarthritis, and chronic fatigue syndrome.

Action
Anthocyanidins in bilberry have a variety of effects including increased glycosaminoglycans synthesis, decreasing vascular permeability, reducing membrane thickness, redistribution of microvascular blood flow and formation of interstitial fluid. **Therapeutic Effects:** Decreased inflammation. Decreased edema. Decreased blood glucose. Improved circulation.

Pharmacokinetics
Absorption: Unknown.
Distribution: Unknown.
Metabolism and Excretion: Eliminated by the kidneys.
Half-life: Unknown.

TIME/ACTION PROFILE

	ONSET	PEAK	DURATION
PO	Unknown	Unknown	Unknown

Contraindications/Precautions
Contraindicated in: Hypersensitivity or allergy to bilberry; Leaves are potentially toxic with chronic use of 1.5 g/kg/day.
Use Cautiously in: Diabetic patients; Patients at risk for bleeding; OB: Avoid use in pregnancy due to lack of safety data.

Adverse Reactions/Side Effects
Endo: low blood sugar. **GI:** diarrhea, upset stomach. **Hemat:** bleeding, bruising.

Interactions
Natural Product-Drug: May ↑ effects of **anticoagulants and antiplatelet drugs** and ↓ platelet activity. May ↑ effects of **antidiabetic agents** and cause hypoglycemia.
Natural-Natural: Avoid use with chromium-containing herbs and supplements (bilberry contains chromium). Avoid use with herbs with hypoglycemic properties.

Route/Commonly Used Doses
PO (Adults): 80-480 mg of bilberry extract daily in 2-3 divided doses.

Availability
Liquid extract; Tablets; Softgel capsules.

NURSING IMPLICATIONS

Assessment
- Monitor blood pressure periodically during therapy, coagulation panel, blood glucose.
- *Lab Test Considerations:* Monitor coagulation studies in patients on anticoagulants and antiplatelet agents.
- Monitor blood glucose periodically during therapy. May cause hypoglycemia.

Potential Nursing Diagnoses
Activity intolerance (Indications)
Diarrhea (Indications)

Implementation
- Administer without regard to food.

Patient/Family Teaching
- Instruct patient to take bilberry as directed.

Evaluation
- Improvement in vascular insufficiency.
- Decrease in diarrhea.

black cohosh (blak coe-hosh)
Remifemin

Other Name(s):
baneberry, black snakeroot, bugbane,

phytoestrogen, rattle root, rattleweed, rattle top, squawroot

Classification
Therapeutic: none assigned

Do not confuse black cohosh with blue or white cohosh

Common Uses
Management of menopausal symptoms. Premenstrual discomfort. Dysmenorrhea. Mild sedative. Rheumatism.

Action
Therapeutic effects are produced by glycosides isolated from the fresh or dried rhizome with attached roots. Mechanism of action is unclear.
Therapeutic Effects: May decrease symptoms of menopause, including hot flashes, sweating, sleep disturbance, and anxiety. Has no effect on vaginal epithelium.

Pharmacokinetics
Absorption: Unknown.
Distribution: Unknown.
Metabolism and Excretion: Unknown.
Half-life: Unknown.

TIME/ACTION PROFILE

ROUTE	ONSET	PEAK	DURATION
PO	unknown	unknown	unknown

Contraindications/Precautions
Contraindicated in: OB: Pregnancy and lactation.
Use Cautiously in: Breast cancer (may increase risk of metastasis); Hormone-sensitive cancers; Protein S deficiency (increased risk for thrombosis); Liver disease.

Adverse Reactions/Side Effects
Neuro: SEIZURES (in combination with evening primrose and chasteberry), headache, dizziness. **GI:** GI upset, hepatotoxicity. **Derm:** rash. **Misc:** weight gain, cramping, breast tenderness, vaginal spotting/bleeding.

Interactions
Natural Product-Drug: Unknown effects when combined with hormone replacement therapy and **antiestrogens** (e.g., **tamoxifen**). Concurrent use with **hepatotoxic drugs** may ↑ risk of liver damage. **Alcohol-containing preparations** may interact with **disulfiram** and **metronidazole**. May ↓ cytotoxic effects of **cisplatin**.

May precipitate hypotension when used in combination with **antihypertensives**.
Natural-Natural: May ↑ risk of hepatotoxicity when used with **chaparral**, **comfrey**, **kava**, and **niacin**.

Route/Commonly Used Doses
PO (Adults): *Tablets (Remifemin®)* — 20 mg bid. *Liquid extract* — 0.3–2 mL bid-tid. *Tincture* — 2–4 mL bid–tid. *Dried rhizome* — 0.3–2 g tid. Do not use for more than 6 mo.

Availability
Alone or in combination with other herbal medicinals^{OTC}; **Tablets (Remifemin® 20 mg [best studied black cohosh product])**^{OTC}; **Liquid extract (1:1 in 90% alcohol)**^{OTC}; **Tincture (1:10 in 60% alcohol)**^{OTC}; **Dried rhizome**.

NURSING IMPLICATIONS

Assessment
- Assess frequency and severity of menopausal symptoms.
- Monitor blood pressure for patients on antihypertensive drugs; may increase effects and cause hypotension.
- Assess for history of seizures or liver disease.

Potential Nursing Diagnoses
Sleep deprivation (Indications)

Implementation
- Administration with food may help to minimize nausea.

Patient/Family Teaching
- Advise patient to notify health care professional if pregnancy is planned or suspected. Avoid use during pregnancy; may induce a miscarriage.
- Patients with seizures, liver dysfunction, excessive alcohol intake, cancer, or other medical problems should be advised to consult their health care professional prior to initiating self-therapy with this herb.
- Advise patient to consult health care professional before taking with other estrogen replacements.
- Emphasize the importance of continued medical supervision for Pap smears, mammograms, pelvic examinations, and blood pressure monitoring at the intervals indicated by health care professional.

Evaluation
- Resolution of menopausal vasomotor symptoms.

*CAPITALS indicates life-threatening; underlines indicate most frequent.

chondroitin (konn-**droy**-tinn)

Other Name(s):
chondroitin polysulfate, CPS, CDS

Classification
Therapeutic: nonopioid analgesics

Common Uses
Osteoarthritis. Ischemic heart disease. Hyperlipidemia. Osteoporosis. **Ophth:** In combination with sodium hyaluronate, for use as a surgical aid in cataract extraction or lens implantation, and as a lubricant.

Action
May serve as a building block of articular cartilage. May protect cartilage against degradation. May have antiatherogenic properties. **Therapeutic Effects:** Improvement in osteoarthritis symptoms.

Pharmacokinetics
Absorption: 8–18% is absorbed orally.
Distribution: Unknown.
Metabolism and Excretion: Unknown.
Half-life: Unknown.

TIME/ACTION PROFILE

ROUTE	ONSET	PEAK	DURATION
PO	unknown	unknown	unknown

Contraindications/Precautions
Contraindicated in: OB: Pregnancy and lactation.
Use Cautiously in: Asthma (may exacerbate symptoms); Clotting disorders (may ↑ risk of bleeding); Prostate cancer (may ↑ risk of metastasis or recurrence).

Adverse Reactions/Side Effects
GI: heartburn, nausea, diarrhea. **Hemat:** bleeding (antiplatelet effect). **Misc:** allergic reactions, edema, hair loss.

Interactions
Natural Product-Drug: Use of chondroitin with **anticoagulant** and **antiplatelet** drugs, **thrombolytics, NSAIDs**, some **cephalosporins**, and **valproates** may ↑ risk of bleeding.
Natural-Natural: Herbs with anticoagulant or antiplatelet properties may ↑ bleeding risk when combined with chondroitin, including: **anise, arnica, chamomile, clove, dong quai, fenugreek, feverfew, ginger, ginkgo, Panax ginseng, licorice,** and others.

Route/Commonly Used Doses
PO (Adults): *Osteoarthritis*— 200–400 mg 2–3 times daily or 1000–1200 mg once daily. *Prevention of recurrent myocardial infarction*— 10 grams daily in 3 divided doses for 3 months followed by 1.5 grams daily in 3 divided doses as maintenance therapy.
IM (Adults): *Osteoarthritis*— 50 mg twice weekly for 8 wk every 4 mo.

Availability
Tablets[OTC]; Capsules[OTC]; Injection (not available in US); Ophthalmic Drops Rx in combination with sodium hyaluronate (Viscoat).

NURSING IMPLICATIONS

Assessment
- Evaluate drug profile before starting therapy with this herbal supplement. If the patient is taking anticoagulants or antiplatelet drugs, avoid use of this herb.
- Monitor pain (type, location, and intensity) and range of motion on an ongoing basis as an indicator of drug efficacy.
- Evaluate gastric discomfort and instruct patient to seek out the advice of a health care professional if persistent gastric discomfort occurs.
- Assess for signs of bleeding and discontinue herbal supplement promptly and seek out health care professional for follow-up.

Potential Nursing Diagnoses
Chronic pain (Indications)
Impaired physical mobility (Indications)

Implementation
- Administer with food.

Patient/Family Teaching
- Advise patients that this herbal supplement is usually taken with glucosamine.
- Caution patients who take aspirin or NSAIDs or other nonprescription medications not to take this herbal supplement without conferring with their health care professional.
- Advise female patients to notify health care professional if pregnancy is planned or suspected or if breastfeeding; avoid use.
- Instruct patients that this medication works by building up cartilage and that this requires that the medication be taken consistently over a period of time. It is not recommended as a supplemental pain medication.

*CAPITALS indicates life-threatening; underlines indicate most frequent.

Evaluation
- Improvement in pain and range of motion.
- Reduced need for supplemental or breakthrough pain medication.

Crataegus Species, see hawthorn.

---

dong quai (don kwi)

Other Name(s):
Angelica sinensis, Chinese Angelica, Dang Gui, Danggui, Don Quai, Ligustilides, Phytoestrogen, Radix angelicae gigantis, Tang Kuei, Tan Kue Bai Zhi

Classification
Therapeutic: none assigned

Common Uses
Premenstrual syndrome. Various uses as a blood purifier. Topically in combination with other ingredients for premature ejaculation.

Action
May have vasodilating and antispasmodic properties. Binds to estrogen receptors. **Therapeutic Effects:** Improved ejaculatory latency.

Pharmacokinetics
Absorption: Unknown.
Distribution: Unknown.
Metabolism and Excretion: Unknown.
Half-life: Unknown.

TIME/ACTION PROFILE

ROUTE	ONSET	PEAK	DURATION
PO	unknown	unknown	unknown

Contraindications/Precautions
Contraindicated in: Allergy to carrot, celery, mugwort or other members of the Apiaceae family; OB: Pregnancy and lactation.
Use Cautiously in: Hormone sensitive cancers and conditions (may exacerbate effects or stimulate growth of cancer cells); Protein S deficiency (↑ risk for thrombosis); Surgery (discontinue 2 wk prior to procedure).

Adverse Reactions/Side Effects
Derm: photosensitivity. **GI:** diarrhea. **Misc:** Some constituents are carcinogenic and mutagenic.

Interactions
Natural Product-Drug: Alcohol-containing preparations may interact with **disulfiram** and **metronidazole**. Use of dong quai with **anticoagulant** and **antiplatelet** drugs, **thrombolytics**, **NSAIDs**, some **cephalosporins**, and **valproates** may increase risk of bleeding.
Natural-Natural: Herbs with antiplatelet or anticoagulant properties may increase bleeding risk when combined with dong quai including: **angelica, clove, danshen, garlic, ginger, ginkgo, panax ginseng,** and **willow**.

Route/Commonly Used Doses
PO (Adults): *Bulk herb*—3–4.5 g per day in divided doses with meals; *Extract*—1 ml (20–40 drops) three times daily.

Availability
Bulk herb[OTC]; Extract[OTC].

NURSING IMPLICATIONS

Assessment
- Assess pain and menstrual patterns prior to and following menstrual cycle to determine effectiveness of this herbal supplement.
- Assess for pregnancy prior to recommending use of the herbal supplement and warn women not to take this herb if pregnancy is planned or suspected.
- Assess for history of hormone sensitive cancers or conditions and warn against use.
- Assess medication profile including prescription and over the counter use of products such as aspirin and ibuprofen-based products to treat menstrual pain.

Potential Nursing Diagnoses
Acute pain (Indications)
Deficient knowledge, related to medication regimen (Patient/Family Teaching)

Implementation
- Take with meals.

Patient/Family Teaching
- Warn patients not to take this medication if pregnant or breastfeeding.
- Inform patients to avoid use of aspirin or other NSAIDs concurrently because of the risk of bleeding.
- Notify patients that there are no studies supporting the use of this herbal supplement for treatment of menopausal symptoms.
- Tell patients to consult their health care professional if taking prescription medications before taking Dong Quai.

---

*CAPITALS indicates life-threatening; underlines indicate most frequent.

1348 NATURAL/HERBAL PRODUCTS

- Discontinue the herbal supplement if diarrhea or excessive bleeding occurs and contact a health care provider if symptoms do not resolve.
- Instruct patients that photosensitivity may occur and to wear sun screen and protective clothing if sun exposure is anticipated.

Evaluation
- Reduction in menstrual pain and cramping and regular periods with normal flow.

---

echinacea (Echinacea Purpurea) (ek-i-nay-sha)

Other Name(s):
American coneflower, black sampson, black susan, brauneria angustifolia, kansas snakeroot, purple coneflower, red sunflower, rudbeckia, sampson root, scurvy root

Classification
Therapeutic: immune stimulants

Common Uses
Bacterial and viral infections. Prevention and treatment of colds, coughs, flu, and bronchitis. Fevers. Wounds and burns. Inflammation of the mouth and pharynx. Urinary tract infections. Vaginal candidiasis.

Action
Medicinal parts derived from the roots, leaves, or whole plant of perennial herb (Echinacea). *Echinacea purpurea herba* has been reported to promote wound healing, which may be due to an increase in white blood cells, spleen cells, and increased activity of granulocytes, as well as an increase in helper T cells and cytokines. *E. purpurea radix* has been shown to have antibacterial, antiviral, anti-inflammatory, and immune-modulating effects. **Therapeutic Effects:** Resolution of respiratory and urinary tract infections. Decreased duration and intensity of common cold. Improved wound healing. Stimulates phagocytosis; inhibits action of hyaluronidase (secreted by bacteria), which helps bacteria gain access to healthy cells. Externally, has antifungal and bacteriostatic properties.

Pharmacokinetics
Absorption: Unknown.
Distribution: Unknown.
Metabolism and Excretion: Unknown.
Half-life: Unknown.

TIME/ACTION PROFILE

ROUTE	ONSET	PEAK	DURATION
PO	unknown	unknown	unknown

Contraindications/Precautions
Contraindicated in: Multiple sclerosis, leukosis, collagenoses, AIDS, tuberculosis, auto-immune diseases; Hypersensitivity and cross-sensitivity in patients allergic to plants in Asteraceae/Compositae plant family (daisies, chrysanthemums, marigolds, etc.); OB: Pregnancy and lactation.
Use Cautiously in: Diabetes; Pedi: May increase risk of rash in children; Tinctures should be used cautiously in alcoholics or patients with liver disease; Do not take longer than 8 wk—may suppress immune function.

Adverse Reactions/Side Effects
CNS: dizziness, fatigue, headache, somnolence. **EENT:** tingling sensation on tongue, sore throat. **GI:** nausea, vomiting, heartburn, constipation, abdominal pain, diarrhea. **Derm:** allergic reaction, rash (more common in children). **Misc:** fever.

Interactions
Natural Product-Drug: May possibly interfere with **immunosuppressants** because of its immunostimulant activity. May ↑ risk for hepatotoxicity from **anabolic steroids**, **methotrexate**, or **ketoconazole** when taken with echinacea. May ↑ **midazolam** availability.
Natural-Natural: May ↑ risk for hepatotoxicity when taken with **kava**.

Route/Commonly Used Doses
PO (Adults): *Tablets*—6.78 mg tablets, take 2 tabs 3 times daily. *Capsules*—500–1000 mg 3 times a day for 5–7 days. *Fluid extract*—1–2 mL tid; solid form (6.5:1)—150–300 mg tid. Should not be used for more than 8 wk at a time. *Tea*—½ tsp comminuted drug, steeped and strained after 10 min, 1 cup 5–6 times daily on the first day, titrating down to 1 cup daily over the next 5 days. *Echinacea purpuren herb juice*—6-9 mL/day. *Liquid*—20 drops every 2 hr for the first day of symptoms, then 3 times daily for up to 10 days.
Topical (Adults): *Ointment, lotion, tincture used externally*—1.5–7.5 mL tincture, 2–5 g dried root.

Availability
Capsules[OTC]**; Tablets; Dried Root**[OTC]**: The dried root can be steeped and strained in

*CAPITALS indicates life-threatening; underlines indicate most frequent.

boiling water and taken as a tea; **Liquid extract**[OTC]: 1:1 in 45% alcohol. **Tincture**[OTC]: 1:5 in 45% alcohol. **Blended teas**[OTC]; **Echinacea purpuren herb juice**[OTC].

NURSING IMPLICATIONS

Assessment
- Assess wound for size, appearance, and drainage prior to the start of and periodically during therapy.
- Assess frequency of common mild illnesses (such as a cold) in response to use.

Potential Nursing Diagnoses
Risk for impaired skin integrity (Indications)

Implementation
- Tinctures may contain significant concentrations of alcohol and may not be suitable for children, alcoholics, patients with liver disease, or those taking disulfiram, metronidazole, some cephalosporins, or sulfonylurea oral antidiabetic agents.
- Prolonged use of this agent may cause overstimulation of the immune system, and use beyond 8 wk is not recommended. Therapy of 10–14 days is usually considered sufficient.
- May be taken without regard to food.

Patient/Family Teaching
- Herb is more effective for treatment than prevention of colds. Take at first sign of symptoms.
- Advise patient to seek immediate treatment for an illness that does not improve after taking this herb.
- Instruct patient that the usual course of therapy is 10–14 days and 8 wk is the maximum.
- Inform patient that use of this herb is not recommended in severe illnesses (e.g., AIDS, tuberculosis) or autoimmune diseases (e.g., multiple sclerosis, collagen diseases, etc.).
- Caution patient that prolonged use of this herb may result in overstimulation of the immune system, possibly with subsequent immunosuppression.
- Warn pregnant or breastfeeding women not to use this herb.
- Instruct patient to consult health care professional before taking any prescription or OTC medications concurrently with echinacea.
- Keep tincture in a dark bottle away from sunlight. Should be taken several times a day.
- Store herb in airtight container away from sunlight.

Evaluation
- Improved wound healing.
- Infrequent common illnesses.
- Illnesses of shorter duration and less severity.

---

feverfew (fee-vurr-fyoo)

Other Name(s):
Altamisa, Bachelor's Button, Chrysanthemum parethenium, Featerfoiul, Featherfew, Featherfoil, Flirtwort Midsummer Daisy, Pyrethrum parthenium, Santa Maria, Tanaceti parthenii, Wild chamomile, Wild quinine

Classification
Therapeutic: vascular headache suppressants

Common Uses
PO: Migraine headache prophylaxis. **Topical:** Toothaches and as an antiseptic.

Action
The sesquiterpene lactone, parthenolide, may provide feverfew's migraine prophylaxis effects. Feverfew may also have antiplatelet and vasodilatory effects and block prostaglandin synthesis.
Therapeutic Effects: May reduce the symptoms and frequency of migraine headaches.

Pharmacokinetics
Absorption: Unknown.
Distribution: Unknown.
Metabolism and Excretion: Unknown.
Half-life: Unknown.

TIME/ACTION PROFILE

ROUTE	ONSET	PEAK	DURATION
PO	2–4 mo	unknown	unknown

Contraindications/Precautions
Contraindicated in: OB: Pregnancy and lactation; Feverfew hypersensitivity or allergy to Asteraceae/Compositae family plants, including ragweed, chrysanthemums, daisies, and marigolds.
Use Cautiously in: Use >4 mo (safety and efficacy not established).

Adverse Reactions/Side Effects
CNS: "Post-Feverfew Syndrome" (anxiety, headache, insomnia, muscle and joint aches). **CV:** *with long-term use*—tachycardia. **GI:** nausea, vomiting, diarrhea, heartburn, mouth ulceration and soreness (from chewing fresh leaves).
Derm: contact dermatitis (when used topically).

*CAPITALS indicates life-threatening; underlines indicate most frequent.

Interactions
Natural Product-Drug: Use of feverfew with **anticoagulant** and **antiplatelet** drugs, **thrombolytics**, **NSAIDs**, some **cephalosporins**, and **valproates** may increase risk of bleeding. Concomitant use with **NSAIDs** may also reduce feverfew effectiveness.

Natural-Natural: Use with **anise**, **arnica**, **chamomile**, **clove**, **dong quai**, **fenugreek**, **garlic**, **ginger**, **ginkgo**, **licorice**, and **Panax ginseng** may increase anticoagulant potential of feverfew.

Route/Commonly Used Doses
PO (Adults): 50–100 mg feverfew extract daily (standardized to 0.2–0.35% parthenolide) or 50–125 mg freeze-dried leaf daily with or after food.

Availability
Feverfew extract, standardized to 0.2-0.35% parthenolide[OTC]. **Freash leaf** [OTC]; **Freeze-dried leaf** [OTC].

NURSING IMPLICATIONS
Assessment
- Monitor frequency, intensity, and duration of migraine headaches prior to and during ongoing therapy.
- Assess for mouth ulcers or skin ulcerations during therapy.

Potential Nursing Diagnoses
Acute pain (Indications)
Deficient knowledge, related to medication regimen (Patient/Family Teaching)

Implementation
- Take with food or on a full stomach.

Patient/Family Teaching
- Instruct patients to take this medication on a consistent basis to prevent migraine headaches. This herbal supplement is not for treatment of migraines.
- Warn patients about mouth ulcers and sores and that if this occurs to seek the advice of a health care professional. Encourage proper oral hygiene.
- Advise patients not to abruptly stop this product because of the possibility of post-feverfew syndrome. Tell patients that anxiety, headache, insomnia, and muscle aches may indicate withdrawal. Feverfew should be gradually tapered.
- Review dietary and medication profile of patient to identify potential interactions. Instruct patient about other herbs that may interact with feverfew.
- Counsel patients on anticoagulants not to take feverfew except as directed by their health care provider.
- Advise patients to avoid using NSAIDs as this may reduce the effectiveness of feverfew.
- Instruct patients to look for signs of bleeding such as unusual bruising or inability to clot after a cut and to seek the advice of a health care professional if this occurs.
- Inform patients that feverfew should reduce the number of migraines and severity of symptoms but that duration of the migraine may not be affected.

Evaluation
- Reduction in the frequency and severity of migraine headaches.

garlic (gar-lik)
Other Name(s):
Alli sativa bulbus, Allium sativum

Classification
Therapeutic: lipid-lowering agents

Common Uses
PO: Hypertension, hyperlipidemia, cardiovascular disease prevention, colorectal and gastric cancer prevention. **Topical:** Dermal fungal infections including tinea corporis, cruris, and pedis.

Action
May have HMG-CoA inhibitor properties in lowering cholesterol, but less effectively than statin drugs; vasodilatory and antiplatelet properties.
Therapeutic Effects: Decreased cholesterol levels. Decreased platelet aggregation.

Pharmacokinetics
Absorption: Garlic oil is well absorbed.
Distribution: Unknown.
Metabolism and Excretion: Kidney and lungs.
Half-life: Unknown.

TIME/ACTION PROFILE

ROUTE	ONSET	PEAK	DURATION
PO	4–25 wk	unknown	unknown

Contraindications/Precautions
Contraindicated in: Bleeding disorders. Discontinue use 1-2 wk prior to surgery.

*CAPITALS indicates life-threatening; underlines indicate most frequent.

Use Cautiously in: Diabetes, gastrointestinal infection or inflammation.

Adverse Reactions/Side Effects
CNS: dizziness. **GI:** Irritation of the mouth, esophagus, and stomach, nausea, bad breath, vomiting, flatulence, diarrhea. **Derm:** Contact dermatitis and other allergic reactions (asthma, rash, anaphylaxis [rare]), Diaphoresis. **Hemat:** Chronic use or excessive dose may lead to ↓ hemoglobin production and lysis of RBCs, platelet dysfunction, prolonged bleeding time. **Misc:** body odor.

Interactions
Natural Product-Drug: Use of garlic with **anticoagulants**, **antiplatelet agents**, and **thrombolytics** may ↑ risk of bleeding. May ↓ the effectiveness of **contraceptive drugs** and **cyclosporine**. May ↓ plasma concentrations of **saquinavir**, **nevirapine**, **delavirdine**, and **efavirenz**. May ↓ **isoniazid** levels by 65%. **Natural-Natural:** Herbs with anticoagulant or antiplatelet properties may increase bleeding risk when combined with garlic, including: **angelica, anise, asafoetida, bogbean, boldo, capsicum, celery, chamomile, clove, danshen, dong quai, fenugreek, feverfew, ginger, ginkgo, Panax ginseng, horse chestnut, horseradish, licorice, meadowsweet, prickly ash, onion, papain, passionflower, poplar, quassia, red clover, turmeric, wild carrot, wild lettuce, willow,** and others.

Route/Commonly Used Doses
PO (Adults): 200–400 mg tid of standardized garlic powder extract with 1.3% allin. *Fresh garlic*—1–7 cloves per day. One clove contains approximately 4 grams of garlic.
Topical (Adults): *Tinea infections*—0.4% cream, 0.6% gel, or 1% gel applied bid × 7 days.

Availability
Capsules^OTC; Tablets^OTC; Topical cream; Topical gel; Fresh garlic^OTC.

NURSING IMPLICATIONS

Assessment
- Elicit from patients their usual dietary intake especially in regard to fat consumption.
- Assess patient's reason for using this herbal remedy and knowledge about hyperlipidemia.
- Ascertain the amount of garlic the patient consumes on a regular basis.

Potential Nursing Diagnoses
Deficient knowledge, related to medication regimen (Patient/Family Teaching)
Noncompliance (Patient/Family Teaching)

Implementation
- Take orally as fresh clove, capsule, or tablet.
- Do not exceed recommended dose.

Patient/Family Teaching
- Instruct patients about the need to follow a healthy diet (low in fat and high in vegetables and fruits) in conjunction with garlic. Other lipid reducing strategies, such as exercise and smoking cessation, should also be employed.
- Inform patients that there are other more effective agents for lipid reduction available.
- Emphasize the need for follow-up exams with a health care professional to assess effectiveness of the regimen.
- Warn patients about the potential for bleeding and not to take this herbal remedy without notifying their health care provider if they are on other medications. Instruct patients undergoing elective surgery to stop using garlic 2 weeks prior to surgery and to notify the surgeon that they are taking garlic in the event of emergent surgery.
- Notify patients that allergies may occur and to discontinue use if symptoms develop.

Evaluation
- Normalization of lipid profile.
- Prevention of cardiac disease.

ginger (Zingiber Officinale)
(jin-jer)

Other Name(s):
Calicut, cochin, gengibre, ginger root, imber, ingwerwurzel, ingwer, Jamaica ginger, jenjibre, jiang, kankyo, zen-zero, zingiber

Classification
Therapeutic: antianemics

Common Uses
Prevention and treatment of nausea and vomiting associated with motion sickness, loss of appetite, pregnancy, surgery, and chemotherapy. Prevention of postoperative nausea and vomiting. May be used for dyspepsia, flatulence, relief of joint pain in rheumatoid arthritis, cramping, and diarrhea. Tonic (toning/strengthening agent) in gout, gas, respiratory infections, anti-inflammatory,

*CAPITALS indicates life-threatening; underlines indicate most frequent.

stimulant (tones the gut, increases saliva and gastric juices, acts as anticoagulant, decreases blood cholesterol).

Action
Antiemetic effect due to increasing GI motility and transport; may act on serotonin receptors. Shown to be hypoglycemic, hypotensive or hypertensive, and positive inotropic agent. Inhibits prostaglandins and platelets, lowers cholesterol, and improves appetite and digestion. **Therapeutic Effects:** Decreased nausea and vomiting due to motion sickness, surgery, and chemotherapy. Decreased joint pain and improvement of joint motion in rheumatoid arthritis. Antioxidant.

Pharmacokinetics
Absorption: Unknown.
Distribution: Unknown.
Metabolism and Excretion: Unknown.
Half-life: Unknown.

TIME/ACTION PROFILE

ROUTE	ONSET	PEAK	DURATION
PO	unknown	unknown	unknown

Contraindications/Precautions
Contraindicated in: Pregnancy and lactation (if using large amounts); Gallstones.
Use Cautiously in: Patients with increased risk of bleeding; Diabetes; Anticoagulant therapy; Cardiovascular disease.

Adverse Reactions/Side Effects
GI: minor heartburn. **Derm:** dermatitis (when used topically).

Interactions
Natural Product-Drug: May increase risk of bleeding when used with **anticoagulants**, **antiplatelet agents**, and **thrombolytics**. May have additive effects with **antidiabetic agents** (causing hypoglycemia) and **calcium channel blockers** (causing hypotension).
Natural-Natural: May theoretically increase risk of bleeding when used with other **herbs** that have anticoagulant or antiplatelet activities.

Route/Commonly Used Doses
PO (Adults): *Motion sickness*— 1000 mg dried ginger root taken 30 min–4 hr before travel or 250 mg qid. *Postoperative nausea prevention*— 1000 mg ginger taken 1 hr before induction or anesthesia. *Chemotherapy–induced nausea*— 2-4 g/day. Up to 2 g freshly powdered drug has been used as an antiemetic (not to exceed 4 g/day). *Osteoarthritis*— 170 mg tid or 225 mg bid of ginger extract. *Whole root rhizome*— 0.25–1 g for other illnesses. *Tea*— pour 150 mL boiling water over 0.5–1 g of ginger and strain after 5 min. *Tincture*— 0.25-3 mL.

Availability
Alone or in combination with other herbal medicinals[OTC]; **Dried powdered root**[OTC]; **Syrup**[OTC]; **Tincture**[OTC]; **Tablets**[OTC]; **Capsules (≥550 mg)**[OTC]; **Spice**[OTC]; **Tea**[OTC].

NURSING IMPLICATIONS

Assessment
- Assess patient for nausea, vomiting, abdominal distention, and pain prior to and after administration of the herb when used as an antiemetic agent.
- Assess pain, swelling, and range of motion in affected joints prior to and after administration when used in the treatment of arthritis.
- Assess patient for epigastric pain prior to and after administration when used as a gastroprotective agent.
- Monitor blood pressure in patients with cardiovascular disease including hypertension.

Potential Nursing Diagnoses
Acute pain (Indications)
Deficient knowledge, related to medication regimen (Patient/Family Teaching)

Implementation
- Administer ginger prior to situations where nausea or vomiting is anticipated (e.g., motion sickness).
- Dosage form and strengths vary with each disease state. Ensure that proper formulation and dose are administered for the indicated use.
- Give to increase peristalsis.

Patient/Family Teaching
- Instruct patients receiving anticoagulants not to take this herb without the advice of health care professional (increased risk of bleeding).
- Tell patient to stop the herb immediately if palpitations occur and contact health care professional.
- Advise patient to observe for easy bruising or other signs of bleeding. If they occur, stop the herb immediately and contact health care professional.
- Warn patients with a history of gallbladder disease to use this herb only under the supervision of health care professional.
- Instruct patient to consult health care professional before taking any prescription or OTC medications concurrently with ginger.

*CAPITALS indicates life-threatening; underlines indicate most frequent.

NATURAL/HERBAL PRODUCTS

- Herb is meant to be used as a tonic, not for long-term use.

Evaluation
- Prevention of nausea and vomiting.
- Relief of epigastric pain.
- Improved joint mobility and relief of pain.

ginkgo (ging-ko)

Other Name(s):
Bai guo ye, fossil tree, ginkgo folium, Japanese silver apricot, kew tree, maidenhair-tree, salisburia adiantifolia, yinhsing

Classification
Therapeutic: antiplatelet agents, central nervous system stimulants

Common Uses
Symptomatic relief of organic brain dysfunction (dementia syndromes, short-term memory deficits, inability to concentrate, depression). Intermittent claudication. Vertigo and tinnitus of vascular origin. Improvement of peripheral circulation. Premenstrual syndrome.

Action
Improves tolerance to hypoxemia, especially in cerebral tissue. Inhibits development of cerebral edema and accelerates its regression. Improves memory, blood flow (microcirculation), compensation of disequilibrium, and rheological properties of blood. Inactivates toxic oxygen radicals. Antagonizes platelet-activating factor. Interferes with bronchoconstriction and phagocyte chemotaxis. **Therapeutic Effects:** Symptomatic relief of dementia syndromes. Inhibits arterial spasm, decreases capillary fragility and blood viscosity. Improves venous tone, relaxes vascular smooth muscle.

Pharmacokinetics
Absorption: 70–100% absorption.
Distribution: Unknown.
Metabolism and Excretion: Unknown.
Half-life: Unknown.

TIME/ACTION PROFILE

ROUTE	ONSET	PEAK	DURATION
PO	unknown	unknown	unknown

Contraindications/Precautions
Contraindicated in: Hypersensitivity; Pregnancy and lactation.

Use Cautiously in: Bleeding disorders; Children (fresh seeds have caused seizures and death); Diabetes; Epilepsy Surgery (discontinue use 2 wk prior).

Adverse Reactions/Side Effects
CNS: CEREBRAL BLEEDING, dizziness, headache, vertigo, seizure. **CV:** palpitations. **GI:** flatulence, stomach upset. **Derm:** allergic skin reaction. **Hemat:** bleeding. **Misc:** hypersensitivity reactions.

Interactions
Natural Product-Drug: Theoretically may potentiate effects of **anticoagulants**, **thrombolytics**, **antiplatelet agents**, and **MAO inhibitors**. May also ↑ risk of bleeding with some **cephalosporins**, **valproic acid**, and **NSAIDs**. May ↓ effectiveness of **anticonvulsants**. May alter **insulin** metabolism requiring dose adjustments of antidiabetic drugs.
Natural-Natural: May ↑ risk of bleeding when used with other **herbs** with antiplatelet effects (including **angelica**, **arnica**, **chamomile**, **feverfew**, **garlic**, **ginger**, and **licorice**).

Route/Commonly Used Doses

Organic Brain Syndromes
PO (Adults): 120–240 mg ginkgo leaf extract daily in 2 or 3 doses.

Intermittent Claudication
PO (Adults): 120–240 mg ginkgo leaf extract daily in 2 or 3 doses.

Vertigo and Tinnitus
PO (Adults): 120–160 mg ginkgo leaf extract daily in 2 or 3 doses.

Cognitive Function Improvement
PO (Adults): 120–600 mg per day.

Premenstrual Syndrome
PO (Adults): 80 mg BID starting on the 16th day of the menstrual cycle until the 5th day of the next cycle.

Availability
Ginkgo leaf extract (acetone/water): 22–27% flavonoid glycosides, 5–7% terpene lactones, 2.6–3.2% bilobalide, <5 ppm of ginkgolic acids.

NURSING IMPLICATIONS

Assessment
- Exclude other treatable causes of dementia prior to instituting treatment with ginkgo.

*CAPITALS indicates life-threatening; underlines indicate most frequent.

- Assess cognitive function (memory, attention, reasoning, language, ability to perform simple tasks) periodically throughout therapy.
- Assess frequency, duration, and severity of muscle cramps (claudication) experienced by the patient prior to and periodically throughout therapy.
- Assess for headache and neurosystem changes (thromboembolism).

Potential Nursing Diagnoses
Disturbed thought process (Indications)
Acute pain (Indications)
Deficient knowledge, related to medication regimen (Patient/Family Teaching)

Implementation
- Start dose at 120 mg per day and increase as needed to minimize side effects.
- Administration for a minimum of 6–8 wk of 80 mg (tid) (not <6 wk) is required to determine response.
- May be administered without regard to food.
- Use of dried leaf preparations in the form of a tea is not recommended because of insufficient quantity of active ingredients.
- Advise patients to avoid crude ginkgo plant parts which can cause severe allergic reactions.
- Take this herb at the same time daily.
- Keep this herb out of the reach of children as seizures may occur with increased doses of ginkgo seeds.

Patient/Family Teaching
- Advise patient to observe for easy bruising and other signs of bleeding and report to health care professional if they occur.
- Caution patient to keep this herb out of the reach of children because ingestion has been associated with seizures.
- Warn patient to avoid handling the pulp or seed coats because of the risk of contact dermatitis. Wash skin under free-flowing water promptly if contact does occur.
- Instruct patient not to exceed recommended doses because large doses may result in toxicity (restlessness, diarrhea, nausea and vomiting, headache).
- Notify patients receiving anticoagulant or antiplatelet therapy not to take this medication without approval of health care professional and frequent monitoring.
- Instruct patient to consult health care professional before taking any prescription or OTC medications concurrently with ginkgo.

Evaluation
- Improvement in walking distances pain-free.
- Improvement in tinnitus and vertigo.
- Improvement in short-term memory, attention span, and ability to perform simple tasks.
- Improvement in sexual function.
- Decreased symptoms of premenstrual syndrome.

ginseng (Panax Ginseng)
(jin-seng)

Other Name(s):
Asian ginseng, Chinese ginseng, hong shen, Japanese ginseng, Korean ginseng, red ginseng, renshen, white ginseng

Classification
Therapeutic: none assigned

Common Uses
Improving physical and mental stamina. General tonic to energize during times of fatigue and inability to concentrate. Sedative, sleep aid, antidepressant. Diabetes. Enhanced sexual performance/aphrodisiac. Increased longevity. Adjunctive treatment of cancer. Increased immune response. Increased appetite.

Action
Main active ingredient is ginsenoside from the dried root. Serves as CNS stimulant and depressant. Enhances immune function. Interferes with platelet aggregation and coagulation. Has analgesic, anti-inflammatory, and estrogen-like effects.
Therapeutic Effects: Improves mental and physical ability. May improve appetite, memory, sleep pattern. May reduce fasting blood glucose level in diabetic patients.

Pharmacokinetics
Absorption: Unknown.
Distribution: Unknown.
Metabolism and Excretion: Unknown.
Half-life: Unknown.

TIME/ACTION PROFILE

ROUTE	ONSET	PEAK	DURATION
PO	unknown	unknown	unknown

Contraindications/Precautions
Contraindicated in: Pregnancy (androgenization of fetus); Lactation; Children; Manic-depressive disorders and psychosis; Hypertension;

*CAPITALS indicates life-threatening; underlines indicate most frequent.

Asthma; Infection; Organ transplant recipients (can interfere with immunosuppressive therapy); Hormone-sensitive cancers.
Use Cautiously in: Autoimmune diseases; Cardiovascular disease; Diabetics (may have hypoglycemic effects); Patients receiving anticoagulants; Bleeding disorders; Schizophrenia (may cause agitation).

Adverse Reactions/Side Effects
CNS: agitation, depression, dizziness, euphoria, headaches, <u>insomnia</u>, nervousness. **CV:** hypertension, tachycardia. **GI:** diarrhea. **GU:** amenorrhea, vaginal bleeding. **Derm:** skin eruptions. **Endo:** estrogen-like effects. **Misc:** fever, mastalgia, STEVENS-JOHNSON SYNDROME.

Interactions
Natural Product-Drug: May ↓ anticoagulant activity of **warfarin**. May interfere with **MAO inhibitors** treatment and cause headache, tremulousness, and manic episodes. May enhance blood glucose lowering effects of **oral hypoglycemics** and **insulin**. May interfere with **immunosuppressant** therapy. Use with caution when taking **estrogens**.
Natural-Natural: May ↑ risk of bleeding when used with **herbs** that have antiplatelet or anticoagulant activities. May prolong the QT interval when used with **bitter orange**, **country mallow** and **ephedra** and ↑ risk of life-threatening arrhythmias. May ↑ risk of hypoglycemia when used with herbs with hypoglycemic potential.
Natural-Food: May potentiate effects of **caffeine** in **coffee** or **tea** and CNS stimulant effects of **mate**.

Route/Commonly Used Doses
PO (Adults): *Capsule*—200–600 mg/day; *extract*—100–300 mg 3 times daily; *crude root*—1–2 g/day; *infusion—tea*—1–2 g root daily (½ tbsp/cup water) up to 3 times daily (P. ginseng tea bag usually contains 1500 mg of ginseng root). Do not use for longer than 3 months. *Cold/flu prevention*—100 mg daily 4 wk prior to influenza vaccination and continued for 8 wk; *Chronic bronchitis*—100 mg BID for 9 days combined with antibiotic therapy; *Erectile dysfunction*—900 mg TID; *Type 2 diabetes*—200 mg daily.

Availability (generic available)
Root powder[OTC]; **Extract in alcohol**[OTC]; **Capsules**[OTC]; **Tea bags**[OTC].

NURSING IMPLICATIONS
Assessment
- Assess level of energy, attention span, and fatigue person is experiencing prior to initiating and periodically during therapy.
- Assess appetite; sleep duration; and perceived quality, emotional lability, and work efficiency prior to and during therapy.
- Patients with chronic medical problems should not use this herb without the advice of health care professional.
- Assess for ginseng toxicity (nervousness, insomnia, palpitations, and diarrhea).
- Monitor patients with diabetes more frequently for hypoglycemia until response to the agent is ascertained.
- Assess for the development of ginseng abuse syndrome (occurs when large doses of the herb are taken concomitantly with other psychomotor stimulants such as coffee and tea. May present as diarrhea, hypertension, restlessness, insomnia, skin eruptions, depression, appetite suppression, euphoria, and edema).

Potential Nursing Diagnoses
Energy field disturbance (Indications)
Insomnia (Indications)

Implementation
- May be taken without regard to food.
- Take at the same time daily and do not increase dose above the recommended amount because of potential toxic effects.

Patient/Family Teaching
- Warn patients with cardiovascular disease, hypertension or hypotension, or on steroid therapy to avoid the use of this herb.
- Caution pregnant or breastfeeding women not to use this herb.
- Instruct patient in the symptoms of ginseng toxicity and to reduce dose or stop use of the herb if they occur.
- Inform patient to limit the amount of caffeine consumed.
- Advise patients with diabetes to monitor blood sugar levels until response to this agent is known.
- Inform patient that the recommended course of therapy is 3 wk. A repeated course is feasible. Do not use for longer than 3 mo.
- Teach patient about the signs and symptoms of hepatitis (yellow skin or whites of eyes, dark urine, light colored stools, lack of appetite for

*CAPITALS indicates life-threatening; <u>underlines</u> indicate most frequent.

several days or longer, nausea, abdominal pain) and to stop use of the herb and promptly contact health care professional if they occur. (This herb is hepatoprotectant at low doses, but hepatodestructive at high doses.)
- Caution patient not to exceed recommended doses because of potential side effects and toxicity.
- If diarrhea develops, stop herb.
- Instruct patient to consult health care professional before taking any Rx or OTC medications concurrently with ginseng.

Evaluation
- Improved energy level and sense of well-being.
- Improved quality of sleep.
- Improved concentration and work efficiency.
- Improved appetite.
- May need to take for several weeks before seeing results.

glucosamine
(glew-**kos**-ah-meen)

Other Name(s):
2-amino-2-deoxyglucose sulfate, chitosamine

Classification
Therapeutic: antirheumatics

Common Uses
Osteoarthritis. Temporomandibular joint (TMJ) arthritis. Glaucoma.

Action
May stop or slow osteoarthritis progression by stimulating cartilage and synovial tissue metabolism. **Therapeutic Effects:** Decreased pain and improved joint function.

Pharmacokinetics
Absorption: 0.9% absorbed.
Distribution: Unknown.
Metabolism and Excretion: 74% eliminated via first-pass metabolism.
Half-life: Unknown.

TIME/ACTION PROFILE

ROUTE	ONSET	PEAK	DURATION
PO	unknown	unknown	unknown

Contraindications/Precautions
Contraindicated in: Shellfish allergy (glucosamine is often derived from marine exoskeletons); Pregnancy and lactation.

Use Cautiously in: Diabetes (may worsen glycemic control); Asthma (may exacerbate symptoms).

Adverse Reactions/Side Effects
GI: nausea, heartburn, diarrhea, constipation. **CNS:** headache, drowsiness. **Derm:** skin reactions.

Interactions
Natural Product-Drug: May antagonize the effects of **antidiabetics**. May induce resistance to some chemotherapy drugs such as **etoposide**, **teniposide**, and **doxorubicin**.
Natural-Natural: None known.

Route/Commonly Used Doses
PO (Adults): 500 mg three times daily.
Topical (Adults): use cream as needed for up to 8 wk.

Availability
Tablets[OTC]; Capsules[OTC]; Topical cream, 30 mg/g in combination with other ingredients[OTC].

NURSING IMPLICATIONS

Assessment
- Evaluate for shellfish allergy prior to initiating therapy.
- Monitor pain (type, location, and intensity) and range of motion on an ongoing basis as an indicator of drug efficacy.
- Assess glucose levels via home monitoring device for patients with diabetes until response is ascertained.
- Evaluate gastric discomfort and instruct patient to seek out the advice of a health care provider if persistent gastric discomfort occurs.
- Assess bowel function and symptomatically treat constipation with improved fluid intake and bulk in diet and bulk laxatives if necessary.

Potential Nursing Diagnoses
Acute pain (Indications)
Impaired physical mobility (Indications)

Implementation
- Take prior to meals.

Patient/Family Teaching
- Warn patients with a shellfish allergy that this herbal supplement should not be used.
- Instruct patients that the effects of this drug come from stimulating cartilage and synovial tissue metabolism and that the supplement must be taken on a regular basis to achieve

benefit. It should not be used as an intermittent pain medication.
- Contact a health care provider if gastric discomfort develops and persists.
- Caution diabetics to monitor glucose values to ascertain impact on glycemic control.

Evaluation
- Improvement in pain and range of motion.

grape seed extract

Other Name(s):
Vitis vinifera, Vitis coignetiae, Oligomeric Proanthocyanidins (OPCs)

Classification
Therapeutic: cardioprotective agents

Common Uses
Chronic venous insufficiency, edema, diabetic retinopathy, varicose veins, cancer prevention, atherosclerosis, cirrhosis, prevention of collagen breakdown, vision problems, constipation, antioxidant, wound healing.

Action
Grape flavonoids have a wide range of effects including antioxidant, vasodilatory, antiplatelet, decreased superoxide production, free-radical removal and inhibition of collagenase.
Therapeutic Effects: Reduced risk of coronary disease. Decreased skin and vasculature breakdown.

Pharmacokinetics
Absorption: unknown.
Distribution: unknown.
Metabolism and Excretion: unknown.
Half-life: unknown.

TIME/ACTION PROFILE

ROUTE	ONSET	PEAK	DURATION
PO	Unknown	Unknown	Unknown

Contraindications/Precautions
Contraindicated in: Hypersensitivity or allergy to grape seed extract; Patients with bleeding disorders or receiving anticoagulant therapy.
Use Cautiously in: OB: Avoid use in pregnancy due to lack of safety data.

Adverse Reactions/Side Effects
CV: hypertension. **CNS:** dizziness, headache. **Derm:** dry skin. **EENT:** sore throat, cough. **GI:** nausea, diarrhea. **Hemat:** ↑ risk of bleeding.

Interactions
Natural Product-Drug: May ↑ anticoagulant effects of **warfarin**. May ↓ plasma levels of CYP1A2 substrates.
Natural-Natural: May inhibit the growth of **lactobacillus acidophilus**. May ↑ BP in hypertensive patients also taking **vitamin C**.

Route/Commonly Used Doses
PO (Adults): 75–300 mg daily.

Availability
Tablets; Capsules.

NURSING IMPLICATIONS

Assessment
- Monitor blood pressure periodically during therapy.
- *Lab Test Considerations:* Monitor serum cholesterol levels periodically during therapy.

Potential Nursing Diagnoses
Activity intolerance (Indications)

Implementation
- Administer as directed. Doses may vary.

Patient/Family Teaching
- Advise patient not to take grape seed extract with Vitamin C; may cause increase in blood pressure.
- Advise female patients to notify health care professional if pregnancy is planned or suspected.

Evaluation
- Decrease in cholesterol.
- Decrease in blood pressure.

green tea (green tee)

Other Name(s):
Camellia sinensis

Classification
Therapeutic: central nervous system stimulants

Common Uses
Bladder, esophageal, ovarian and pancreatic cancer risk reduction, mental alertness, hypotension, cervical dysplasia associated with human papillomavirus infection, hyperlipidemia, weight loss, protection of the skin from sun damage, genital warts, dental caries, Parkinson's disease.

Action
Caffeine in green tea stimulates the CNS and cardiovascular system through adenosine receptor

*CAPITALS indicates life-threatening; underlines indicate most frequent.

blockade and phosphodiesterase inhibition.
Therapeutic Effects: Improved cognitive performance and mental alertness.

Pharmacokinetics
Absorption: Unknown.
Distribution: Unknown.
Metabolism and Excretion: Unknown.
Half-life: Unknown.

TIME/ACTION PROFILE

ROUTE	ONSET	PEAK	DURATION
PO	Unknown	Unknown	Unknown

Contraindications/Precautions
Contraindicated in: Allergy/hypersensitivity; Pregnancy and lactation (doses >200 mg/day due to caffeine content).
Use Cautiously in: Patients with caffeine sensitivity. Long-term use of doses >250 mg/day may produce tolerance, psychological dependence, tachyarrhythmias, and sleep disturbances; Iron deficiency anemia (may worsen); Diabetes (may impair glucose control); Cardiac conditions (may induce arrhythmias in sensitive individuals); Bleeding disorders.

Adverse Reactions/Side Effects
CV: arrhythmia, tachycardia. **CNS:** agitation, dizziness, excitement, insomnia, tremors. **GI:** nausea, vomiting, diarrhea, hepatotoxicity, abdominal pain. **F and E:** hypokalemia. **Endo:** hyperglycemia. **Hemat:** prolonged bleeding time.

Interactions
Natural Product-Drug: Green tea may ↓ effects of **adenosine**. ↑ risk of bleeding with **anticoagulants** or **antiplatelet** agents. ↑ effects of **CNS stimulants**. May impair glucose control from **antidiabetic** agents. Abrupt withdrawal can ↑ **lithium** levels. May ↓ **dipyridamole**—induced vasodilation. **Verapamil** can ↑ caffeine concentrations by 25%. Additive effects with **methylxanthines**.
Natural-Natural: ↑ risk of adverse cardiovascular effects with **bitter orange**. ↑ risk of hepatotoxicity with hepatotoxic herbs or supplements. ↑ risk of seizures, hypertension, or stroke with **ephedra** and **creatine**.

Route/Commonly Used Doses
PO (Adults): Range: 1–10 cups/day. One cup provides approximately 60 mg of caffeine.

Availability
Tea leaves.

NURSING IMPLICATIONS
Assessment
- Monitor blood pressure and heart rate periodically during therapy.
- **Lab Test Considerations:** Monitor serum glucose, homocysteine and uric acid levels periodically during therapy.
- Monitor liver and kidney function periodically during therapy.

Potential Nursing Diagnoses
Impaired memory (Indications)

Implementation
- May be taken as tea or as an extract in capsules.

Patient/Family Teaching
- Advise women who may be pregnant or who are breastfeeding to limit green tea due to the caffeine content.

Evaluation
- Improvement in memory.

---

hawthorne (Crataegus Species)
(haw-thorn)

Other Name(s):
aubepine, cum flore, hagedorn, maybush, whitehorn

Classification
Therapeutic: antihypertensives, inotropics

Common Uses
Hypertension. Mild to moderate CHF. Angina. Spasmolytic. Sedative.

Action
Active compounds in hawthorn include flavonoids and procyanidins. Increase coronary blood flow. Positive inotropic and chronotropic effects because of increased permeability to calcium and inhibition of phosphodiesterase. **Therapeutic Effects:** Increased cardiac output. Decreased blood pressure, myocardial workload, and oxygen consumption.

Pharmacokinetics
Absorption: Unknown.
Distribution: Unknown.
Metabolism and Excretion: Unknown.
Half-life: Unknown.

*CAPITALS indicates life-threatening; underlines indicate most frequent.

TIME/ACTION PROFILE

ROUTE	ONSET	PEAK	DURATION
PO	unknown	6-8 wk	unknown

Contraindications/Precautions
Contraindicated in: Pregnancy (potential uterine activity); Lactation.
Use Cautiously in: Concurrent use with ACE inhibitors and digoxin; Do not discontinue use abruptly.

Adverse Reactions/Side Effects
CNS: agitation, dizziness, fatigue, vertigo, headache, sedation (high dose), sleeplessness, sweating. **CV:** hypotension (high dose), palpitations. **GI:** nausea.

Interactions
Natural Product-Drug: May potentiate effects of **digoxin**, **calcium channel blockers**, and **beta blockers**. Concurrent use with **theophylline**, **caffeine**, **epinephrine**, **phosphodiesterase-5 inhibitors** (**sildenafil**, **tadalafil**, **vardenafil**) and **nitrates** may potentiate adverse cardiovascular effects. May cause additive CNS depression when used with other **CNS depressants**.
Natural-Natural: Additive effect with other cardiac glycoside–containing **herbs** (**digitalis leaf**, **black hellebore**, **oleander leaf**, and others). Additive hypotensive effects with herbs than lower blood pressure such as **ginger**, **panax ginseng**, and **valerian**. Additive effect with other cardioactive herbs (**devil's claw**, **fenugreek**, and others).

Route/Commonly Used Doses
PO (Adults): *Heart failure*— 160–1800 mg standardized hawthorn leaf with flower extract in 2–3 divided doses daily. *Hawthorn fluid extract (1:1 in 25% alcohol)*—0.5–1 mL tid; *hawthorn fruit tincture (1:5 in 45% alcohol)*—1–2 mL tid; *dried hawthorn berries*—300–1000 mg tid.

Availability (generic available)
Dried fruit[OTC]; Liquid extract of the fruit or leaf [OTC]; Tincture of the fruit or leaf [OTC].

NURSING IMPLICATIONS

Assessment
- Auscultate lung sounds for signs of heart failure (rales, crackles, wheezing).
- Assess weight daily and look for signs of fluid overload (swelling of ankles, shortness of breath, sleeping with multiple pillows).
- Assess blood pressure periodically throughout therapy.
- Assess pulse for rate and regularity of rhythm.

Potential Nursing Diagnoses
Decreased cardiac output (Indications)
Deficient knowledge, related to medication regimen (Patient/Family Teaching)

Implementation
- Administered as 2–3 divided doses daily at the same time.
- May be taken without regard to food.

Patient/Family Teaching
- Advise patients that there are other proven therapies available for treatment of heart failure. These therapies should be employed prior to initiating treatment with hawthorn.
- Tell patient not to take hawthorn without the advice of health care professional.
- Instruct patients in the symptoms of a heart attack (pain in the region of the heart, jaw, arm, or upper abdomen; sweating; chest tightness) and heart failure (shortness of breath, chest tightness, dizziness, sweating) and to promptly contact health care professional if they occur.
- Advise patient to report weight gain or persistent swelling of the feet to health care professional.
- Warn patients who self-medicate to consult health care professional if there is no improvement in symptoms in 6-8 wk. Effects may not be seen for 3 mo.
- Teach patient to make position changes slowly to minimize the risk of orthostatic hypotension.
- Caution patient not to combine with other cardiac and BP medications unless under supervision of health care professional because of possible additive effects.
- This herb may cause drowsiness. Patients should avoid driving or other activities that require mental alertness until response to herb is known.
- Avoid alcohol and other CNS depressants while taking hawthorn unless under supervision of health care professional.
- Profuse sweating and dehydration under extreme heat may increase the BP-lowering properties of hawthorn, leading to severe hypotension. Warn patients to avoid exertion in hot weather to minimize the risk of side effects.
- Instruct patients that hawthorn helps control the symptoms of heart failure but does not

*CAPITALS indicates life-threatening; underlines indicate most frequent.

1360 NATURAL/HERBAL PRODUCTS

cure the disease. Lifestyle changes (salt restriction, weight management, exercise as tolerated, adherence to medication regimens) still need to be followed.
- Although hawthorn has been studied in Europe for management of heart failure, there are no conclusive studies to recommend use of this herb.
- Instruct patient to consult health care professional before taking any prescription or OTC medications concurrently with hawthorn.

Evaluation
- Decrease in symptoms of CHF.
- Improved cardiac output as evidenced by improved activity tolerance.

Hypericum Perforatum, see St. John's wort

kava-kava (Piper Methysticum)
(ka-va-ka-va)

Other Name(s):
Ava pepper, intoxicating pepper, kao, kew, tonga, wurzelstock, yagona

Classification
Therapeutic: antianxiety agents, sedative/hypnotics

Common Uses
Anxiety, stress, restlessness, insomnia, benzodiazepine withdrawal. Mild muscle aches and pains. Menstrual cramps and PMS.

Action
Alters the limbic system modulation of emotional processes. Shown to have centrally-acting skeletal muscle relaxant properties activated. **Therapeutic Effects:** Relief of anxiety. Sedation.

Pharmacokinetics
Absorption: Peak plasma level occurs about 1.8 hr after an oral dose.
Distribution: Enters breast milk.
Metabolism and Excretion: Elimination occurs primarily by renal excretion (both unchanged and metabolites) and in the feces. Metabolized by the liver (reduction or demethylation).
Half-life: Approximately 9 hr.

TIME/ACTION PROFILE

ROUTE	ONSET	PEAK	DURATION
PO	1.8 hr	unknown	8 hr

Contraindications/Precautions
Contraindicated in: Pregnancy (may affect uterine tone) and lactation; Patients with endogenous depression (may increase risk of suicide); Children under 12 yr of age; Hepatitis or other liver disease.
Use Cautiously in: Concurrent use of other hepatotoxic agents; Depression and Parkinson's disease (may worsen symptoms); Should not be used for more than 3 mo to prevent psychological addiction.

Adverse Reactions/Side Effects
CNS: dizziness, headache, drowsiness, sensory disturbances, extrapyramidal effects. **EENT:** Pupil dilation, red eyes, visual accommodation disorders. **GI:** HEPATIC TOXICITY, gastrointestinal complaints. **Derm:** allergic skin reactions, yellow discoloration of skin, pellagroid dermopathy. **Hemat:** decreased lymphocytes, decreased platelets. **Metab:** weight loss (long-term, high dose). **Neuro:** ataxia, muscle weakness.

Interactions
Natural Product-Drug: Additive effect when used with **alprazolam**. Potentiates effect of **CNS depressants** (**ethanol, barbiturates, benzodiazepines, opioid analgesics**). Has decreased the effectiveness of **levodopa** in few cases. Theoretically, may have additive effects with **antiplatelet agents**.
Natural-Natural: Concurrent use with other hepatotoxic products such as **DHEA, coenzyme Q-10** (high doses), and **niacin** can increase the risk of liver damage. Theoretically, may have additive sedative effects when used with other **herbs** with sedative properties.

Route/Commonly Used Doses
PO (Adults): *Antianxiety*—100 mg (70 mg kavalactones) 3 times daily; *Benzodiazepine withdrawal*—50–300 mg/day over one week while tapering benzodiazepine over 2 wk (use 70% kavalactone extract). *Insomnia*—180–210 mg kavalactones. Typically taken as a tea by simmering the root in boiling water and then straining.

Availability (generic available)
Dried root extracts (alcohol or acetone based) containing 30–70% kavapyrones.

*CAPITALS indicates life-threatening; underlines indicate most frequent.

NURSING IMPLICATIONS
Assessment
- Assess muscle spasm, associated pain, and limitations of movement prior to and periodically throughout therapy.
- Assess degree of anxiety and level of sedation (visual disturbances and changes in motor reflexes are side effects) prior to and periodically throughout therapy.
- Assess sleep patterns and level of sedation upon arising.
- Prolonged use may lead to depression of platelet and lymphocyte counts.

Potential Nursing Diagnoses
Anxiety (Indications)
Impaired physical mobility (Adverse Reactions)
Risk for injury (Side Effects)

Implementation
- Prepared as a drink from pulverized roots, tablets, capsules, or extract.

Patient/Family Teaching
- Inform patient that significant, serious side effects may occur with prolonged use. Use for longer than 1 mo is not recommended without supervision of health care professional.
- Caution patient to not use alcohol or other CNS depressants while taking this herb because the combination potentiates the herb's sedative effect.
- Advise patients that driving a car or performing other activities requiring mental alertness should be avoided until response to therapy is determined.
- Warn patients to stop use of the herb immediately if shortness of breath or signs of liver disease (yellowing of the skin or whites of the eyes, brown urine, nausea, vomiting, light-colored stools, unusual tiredness, weakness, stomach or abdominal pain, loss of appetite) occur and contact health care professional.
- Advise patients who have liver disease or liver problems, or persons who are taking drug products that can affect the liver, to consult health care professional before using kava-containing supplements.
- Inform patient that although there is no evidence of physiological dependence, the risk of psychological dependence still exists.
- Counsel pregnant and breastfeeding women not to use this herb.
- Instruct patient to consult health care professional before taking any prescription or OTC medications concurrently with kava-kava.

Evaluation
- Decrease in anxiety level.
- Decrease in muscle spasms.
- Relief of insomnia.

milk thistle (milk this-ul)

Other Name(s):
Holy thistle, Lady's thistle, Mary Thistle, Silybin, Silymarin

Classification
Therapeutic: antidotes

Common Uses
Cirrhosis, chronic hepatitis, gallstones, psoriasis, liver cleansing and detoxification, treatment of liver toxicity due to alcohol, Amanita mushroom poisoning (European IV formulation) and chemicals.

Action
The active component, silymarin, has antioxidant and hepatoprotectant actions. Silymarin helps prevent toxin penetration and stimulates hepatocyte regeneration.

Pharmacokinetics
Absorption: 23–47% absorbed after oral administration.
Distribution: Unknown.
Metabolism and Excretion: Hepatic metabolism by cytochrome P450 3A4.
Half-life: 6 hr.

TIME/ACTION PROFILE

ROUTE	ONSET	PEAK	DURATION
PO	5–30 days or more	unknown	unknown

Contraindications/Precautions
Contraindicated in: Pregnancy and lactation (insufficient information available); Allergy to chamomile, ragweed, asters, chrysanthemums and other members of the family Compositae.
Use Cautiously in: Hormone sensitive cancers/conditions (milk thistle plant parts may have estrogenic effects).

Adverse Reactions/Side Effects
GI: Laxative effect, nausea, bloating, anorexia.
Misc: Allergic reactions.

Interactions
Natural Product-Drug: In vitro, milk thistle extract inhibited the drug-metabolizing enzyme cy-

*CAPITALS indicates life-threatening; underlines indicate most frequent.

1362 NATURAL/HERBAL PRODUCTS

tochrome P450 3A4. Interactions have not been reported in humans, but milk thistle should be used cautiously with other drugs metabolized by 3A4, such as **cyclosporine, carbamazepine, HMG-CoA inhibitors, ketoconazole,** and **alprazolam.**
Natural-Natural: None known.

Route/Commonly Used Doses
PO (Adults): *Hepatic cirrhosis*—420 mg/day of extract containing 70–80% silymarin; *Chronic active hepatitis*—240 mg bid of silibinin; *Tea*—3–4 times daily 30 minutes before meals. Tea is not recommended as silymarin is not sufficiently water soluble.
IV (Adults): 20–50 mg/kg over 24 hr, 48 hr post mushroom ingestion (IV formulation not available in US).

Availability
Capsules^{OTC}; Tablets^{OTC}; Crude drug^{OTC}; Tea^{OTC}; Extract^{OTC}.

NURSING IMPLICATIONS

Assessment
- Assess patients for signs of liver failure such as jaundice, mental status changes, abdominal distention (ascites) and generalized edema.
- Monitor liver function tests periodically throughout therapy.
- Evaluate consistency and frequency of bowel movements.

Potential Nursing Diagnoses
Deficient knowledge, related to medication regimen (Patient/Family Teaching)

Implementation
- Orally as an extract, capsule, tablets or as a dried fruit as a single daily dose or divided into three doses.
- Tea is not recommended as Milk Thistle is not water-soluble.

Patient/Family Teaching
- Inform patient of the symptoms of liver failure; advise patient to report worsening symptomotolgy promptly to health care professional.
- Emphasize the need for blood tests to monitor liver function tests.
- Advise patients to abstain from alcohol and to follow a diet consistent with the liver or gallbladder disease being treated.

Evaluation
- Normalization of liver function tests.
- Reduction in jaundice, abdominal distention, fatigue, and other symptoms associated with liver disease.

Panax Ginseng, see **ginseng.**

Piper Methysticum, see **kava-kava.**

SAMe (sam-ee)

Other Name(s):
Ademetionine, S-adenosylmethionine,

Classification
Therapeutic: antidepressants

Pregnancy Category UK

Common Uses
Treatment of depression. Has also been used to manage: osteoarthritis, fibromyalgia, liver disease, migraine headaches.

Action
May aid in the production, activation, and metabolism of various amines, phospholipids, hormones, and neurotransmitters. May stimulate articular cartilage growth and repair. **Therapeutic Effects:** Decreased depression. Anti-inflammatory and analgesic effects improve symptoms of osteoarthritis.

Pharmacokinetics
Absorption: Rapidly and extensively metabolized following oral administration.
Distribution: Unknown.
Metabolism and Excretion: Actively metabolized by the liver.
Half-life: 100 min.

TIME/ACTION PROFILE (antidepressant action)

ROUTE	ONSET	PEAK	DURATION
PO (depression)	1–2 wk	unknown	unknown
PO (osteoarthritis)	30 days	unknown	unknown

Contraindications/Precautions
Contraindicated in: Hypersensitivity; Bipolar disorder.

---

*CAPITALS indicates life-threatening; underlines indicate most frequent.

Use Cautiously in: Pregnancy, lactation, or children (safety not established); Bipolar disorder (can induce mania); Parkinson's disease (may worsen symptoms).

Adverse Reactions/Side Effects
CNS: agitation, dizziness, mild insomnia, manic reactions (in patients with bipolar disorder). **GI:** vomiting, diarrhea, flatulence.

Interactions
Natural Product-Drug: Avoid use with **antidepressants**, **meperidine**, **pentazocine**, **tramadol**, and **dextromethorphan** (additive serotinergic effects may occur). May reduce the effectiveness of **levodopa** and worsen Parkinsonian symptoms. Should not be used concurrently with **MAO inhibitors**. Avoid use of SAMe within 2 wk of using an **MAO inhibitor**.
Natural-Natural: Avoid use with natural products that increase serotonin levels such as **l-tryptophan** and **St. John's wort**.

Route/Commonly Used Doses
PO (Adults): *Depression*— 200 mg once or twice daily, adjusted upward over 2 wk (range 400–1600 mg/day); *Liver disorders*— 1200–1600 mg/day; *Osteoarthritis*— 200 mg tid; *Fibromyalgia*— 800 mg/day.

Availability
Tablets: 100 mg, 200 mg, 400 mg^{OTC}.

NURSING IMPLICATIONS

Assessment
- Assess mental status for symptoms of depression prior to and periodically during therapy; advise patients with depression to be evaluated by a health care professional.
- Assess symptoms of pain and fatigue prior to and periodically during therapy.

Potential Nursing Diagnoses
Ineffective coping (Indications)
Deficient knowledge, related to medication regimen (Patient/Family Teaching)

Implementation
- Only enteric-coated formulations are recommended due to bioavailability problems.
- **PO:** Initial dose should be 200 mg once or twice daily to minimize GI disturbances. Dose may be adjusted upward over 1–2 wk depending on response and tolerance.

Patient/Family Teaching
- Instruct patient to take SAMe according to directions.

- The SAMe butanedisulfonate salt may be preferable due to greater stability.

Evaluation
- Decrease in symptoms of depression.
- Improvement in osteoarthritis symptoms.

---

saw palmetto

Other Name(s):
American Dwarf Palm Tree, Cabbage Palm, Ju-Zhong, Palmier Nain, Sabal, Sabal Fructus, Saw Palmetto Berry, Serenoa repens

Classification
Therapeutic: benign prostatic hyperplasia (BPH) agents

Common Uses
Benign prostatic hyperplasia.

Action
Exerts antiandrogenic, anti-inflammatory, and antiproliferative properties in prostate tissue resulting in improvement in BPH symptoms such as frequent urination, hesitancy, urgency, and nocturia. Comparable in efficacy to finasteride but may be less effective than prazosin. **Therapeutic Effects:** Decreased urinary symptoms of BPH.

Pharmacokinetics
Absorption: Unknown.
Distribution: Unknown.
Metabolism and Excretion: Unknown.
Half-life: Unknown.

TIME/ACTION PROFILE

ROUTE	ONSET	PEAK	DURATION
PO	1–2 mo	unknown	48 wk (longest studied treatment duration)

Contraindications/Precautions
Contraindicated in: Pregnancy and lactation.
Use Cautiously in: Prior to surgery (discontinue 2 weeks before to prevent bleeding).

Adverse Reactions/Side Effects
CNS: dizziness, headache. **GI:** nausea, vomiting, constipation, and diarrhea.

Interactions
Natural Product-Drug: Hormonal action may interfere with other hormonal therapies (**testosterone**, **hormonal contraceptives**). Avoid use

---

*CAPITALS indicates life-threatening; underlines indicate most frequent.

with **antiplatelet** or **anticoagulant drugs** (may ↑ bleeding risk).
Natural-Natural: Concomitant use with herbs that affect platelet aggregation such as **ginger, garlic, ginkgo,** and **ginseng** may ↑ bleeding risk.

Route/Commonly Used Doses
PO (Adults): *Lipophilic extract (80–90% fatty acids)* — 160 mg twice daily or 320 mg once daily. *Whole berries* — 1–2 g daily. *Liquid extract from berry pulp* — 1–2 mL three times daily. *Tea (efficacy is questionable due to lipophilicity of active constituents)* — 1 cup three times daily. Tea is prepared by steeping 0.5–1 g dried berry in 150 mL boiling water for 5–10 minutes.

Availability
Lipophilic extract (80-90% fatty acids)^{OTC}; **Whole berries**^{OTC}; **Liquid extract**^{OTC}.

NURSING IMPLICATIONS
Assessment
- Assess patient for symptoms of benign prostatic hypertrophy (BPH) (urinary hesitancy, feeling of incomplete bladder emptying, interruption in urinary stream, impairment in size and force of urinary stream, terminal urinary dribbling, straining to start flow, dysuria, urgency) before and periodically during therapy.
- Rectal exams prior to and periodically throughout therapy to assess prostate size are recommended.

Potential Nursing Diagnoses
Impaired urinary elimination (Indications)
Deficient knowledge, related to medication regimen (Patient/Family Teaching)

Implementation
- Take on a full stomach to minimize GI effects.

Patient/Family Teaching
- Advise patients to start therapy with this herbal supplement only after evaluation by a health care professional who will provide continued follow-up care.
- Inform patients that saw palmetto does not alter the size of the prostate but still should relieve the symptoms associated with BPH.
- Tell patients that taking this herbal supplement with food should reduce the GI effects and make it easier to tolerate.

Evaluation
- Decrease in urinary symptoms of BPH.

St. John's wort (Hypericum perforatum) (saynt jonz wort)

Other Name(s):
Amber, Demon chaser, Goatweed, Hardhay, Klamath weed, Rosin rose, Tipton weed

Classification
Therapeutic: antidepressants

Common Uses
PO: Management of mild to moderate depression and obsessive compulsive disorder (OCD). (Not effective for major depression.) **Topical:** Inflammation of the skin, blunt injury, wounds, and burns. Other uses are for capillary strengthening, decreasing uterine bleeding, and reducing tumor size.

Action
Derived from *Hypericum perforatum*; the active component is *hypericin*. **PO:** Antidepressant action may be due to ability to inhibit reuptake of serotonin and other neurotransmitters. **Topical:** Anti-inflammatory, antifungal, antiviral, and antibacterial properties. **Therapeutic Effects: PO:** Decreased signs and symptoms of depression. **Topical:** Decreased inflammation of burns or other wounds.

Pharmacokinetics
Absorption: Unknown.
Distribution: Unknown.
Metabolism and Excretion: Unknown.
Half-life: *Hypericum constituents* — 24.8–26.5 hr.

TIME/ACTION PROFILE

ROUTE	ONSET	PEAK	DURATION
PO	10–14 days	within 4–6 wk	unknown

Contraindications/Precautions
Contraindicated in: Pregnancy, lactation, or children.
Use Cautiously in: History of phototoxicity; Surgery (discontinue 2 wk prior to surgical procedures); Alzheimer's disease (may induce psychosis); Patients undergoing general anesthesia (may cause cardiovascular collapse); History of suicide attempt, severe depression, schizophrenia or bipolar disorder (can induce hypomania or psychosis).

*CAPITALS indicates life-threatening; underlines indicate most frequent.

Adverse Reactions/Side Effects
CNS: dizziness, restlessness, sleep disturbances. **CV:** hypertension. **Endo:** hypoglycemia. **GI:** abdominal pain, bloating, diarrhea, dry mouth, feeling of fullness, flatulence, nausea, vomiting. **Neuro:** neuropathy. **Derm:** allergic skin reactions (hives, itching, skin rash), phototoxicity. **Misc:** serotonin syndrome.

Interactions
Natural Product-Drug: Concurrent use with **alcohol** or other **antidepressants** (including **SSRIs** and **MAO inhibitors**) may ↑ risk of adverse CNS reactions. May ↓ the effectiveness and serum concentrations of **digoxin**, **alprazolam**, **amitriptyline**, **imatinib**, **irinotecan**, **warfarin**, and **protease inhibitors**. Use with **MAO inhibitors**, **tramadol**, **pentazocine**, and **selective serotonin agonists** could result in serotonin syndrome. May ↓ effectiveness of **oral contraceptives**. May ↓ plasma **cyclosporine** and **tacrolimus** levels by 30–70% and cause acute transplant rejection. May ↑ metabolism of **phenytoin** and **phenobarbital** and cause loss of seizure control. Avoid use of St. John's wort and **MAO inhibitors** within 2 wk of each other. **Natural-Natural:** May ↑ risk of serotonin syndrome when taken with **tryptophan** and **SAM-e**.

Route/Commonly Used Doses
PO (Adults): *Mild Depression*—300 mg of St. John's wort (standardized to 0.3% hypericin) 3 times daily or 250 mg twice daily of 0.2% hypericin extract. *OCD*-450 mg twice daily of extended release preparation.
Topical (Adults): 0.2–1 mg total hypericin daily.

Availability

Preparations for Oral Use
Dried herb^OTC; Dried (hydroalcoholic) extract^OTC; Oil^OTC; Tincture^OTC.

Preparations for Topical Application
Liquid^OTC; Semisolid^OTC.

NURSING IMPLICATIONS

Assessment
- **Depression:** Assess patient for depression periodically during therapy.
- **Inflammation:** Assess skin or skin lesions periodically during therapy.

Potential Nursing Diagnoses
Ineffective coping (Indications)
Anxiety (Indications)
Deficient knowledge, related to medication regimen (Patient/Family Teaching)

Implementation
- **PO:** Tea can be prepared by mixing 2-4 dried herb in 150 mL of boiling water and steeping for 10 min.

Patient/Family Teaching
- Instruct patient to take St. John's wort as directed.
- Patients with depression should be evaluated by health care professional. Standard therapy may be of greater benefit for moderate to severe depression.
- Advise patient to notify health care professional of medication regimen prior to treatment or surgery.
- Caution patients to avoid sun exposure and use protective sunscreen to reduce the risk of photosensitivity reactions.
- Inform patient to purchase herbs from a reputable source and that products and their contents vary among different manufacturers.
- Caution patient not to use alcohol while taking St. John's wort.
- Warn patients that St. John's wort may reduce the therapeutic effectiveness of several drugs.
- May potentiate effect of sedatives and side effects of other antidepressants. Do not take within 2 wk of MAO inhibitor therapy.
- Instruct patient to consult health care professional before taking other Rx, OTC, or herbal products concurrently with St. John's wort.
- Inform patient that St. John's wort is usually taken for a period of 4–6 wk. If no improvement is seen, another therapy should be considered.

Evaluation
- Decrease in signs and symptoms of depression or anxiety.
- Improvement in skin inflammation.

valerian (vuh-lare-ee-en)

Other Name(s):
Amantilla, All-Heal, Baldrian, Baldrianwurzel, Belgium Valerian, Common Valerian, Fragrant Valerian, Garden Heliotrope, Garden Valerian, Indian Valerian, Mexican Valerian, Pacific Valerian, Tagara, Valeriana, Valeriana officinalis, Valerianae radix, Valeriana rhizome, Valeriane

*CAPITALS indicates life-threatening; underlines indicate most frequent.

NATURAL/HERBAL PRODUCTS

Classification
Therapeutic: antianxiety agents, sedative/hypnotics

Common Uses
Insomnia. Anxiety.

Action
May increase concentrations of the inhibitory CNS transmitter GABA. **Therapeutic Effects:** Improvement in sleep quality.

Pharmacokinetics
Absorption: Unknown.
Distribution: Unknown.
Metabolism and Excretion: Unknown.
Half-life: Unknown.

TIME/ACTION PROFILE

ROUTE	ONSET	PEAK	DURATION
PO	30–60 min	2 hr	unknown

Contraindications/Precautions
Contraindicated in: Pregnancy and lactation.
Use Cautiously in: Alcohol use (may have additive sedative effects).

Adverse Reactions/Side Effects
CNS: drowsiness, headache. **Misc:** Benzodiazepine-like withdrawal symptoms with discontinuation after long-term use.

Interactions
Natural Product-Drug: Additive CNS depression with **alcohol**, **antihistamines**, **sedative hypnotics** and other **CNS depressants**. Alcohol-containing preparations may interact with **disulfuram** and **metronidazole**.
Natural-Natural: Additive sedative effects can occur when used with herbal supplements with sedative properties such as **kava**, **l-tryptophan**, **melatonin**, **SAMe**, and **St. John's wort**.

Route/Commonly Used Doses
PO (Adults): *Tea*—1 cup tea 1–5 times daily. Tea is made by steeping 2–3 g root in 150 mL boiling water for 5–10 min then straining. *Tincture*—1–3 mL 1–5 times daily. *Extract*—400–900 mg up to 2 hr before bedtime or 300–450 mg divided tid.

Availability
Capsules[OTC]; Extract[OTC]; Tea[OTC]; Tincture[OTC].

NURSING IMPLICATIONS

Assessment
- Assess degree of anxiety and level of sedation prior to and periodically throughout therapy.
- Assess sleep patterns.
- Assess response in the elderly population where drowsiness and loss of balance may pose a significant risk for injury.

Potential Nursing Diagnoses
Anxiety (Indications)
Risk for injury (Side Effects)

Implementation
- Take 1 to 2 hr before bedtime if used for nighttime hypnotic.
- Administer orally three to five times daily to control anxiety.

Patient/Family Teaching
- Warn patients to avoid use of other medications or herbals that have a sedative effect, as the combination will increase drowsiness and sedation.
- Warn patients against driving or operating heavy machinery after taking valerian.
- Inform patients not to take this herbal supplement if pregnant or breastfeeding.
- Counsel patients to avoid activities requiring mental alertness until response to this supplement is known.
- Notify patients that dependence with withdrawal symptoms may develop with prolonged use.
- Instruct patients to avoid consuming alcohol while taking this herbal supplement.
- Encourage patients to eliminate stimulants such as caffeine and to provide an environment that promotes restful sleep.

Evaluation
- Decreased anxiety level.
- Improvement in sleep with a feeling of restfulness without drowsiness upon awakening.

Zingiber Officinale, see **ginger**.

---

*CAPITALS indicates life-threatening; underlines indicate most frequent.

APPENDICES

Appendix A. Recent Drug Approvals.. **1369**

Appendix B. Combination Drugs **1378**

Appendix C. Ophthalmic Medications **1397**

Appendix D. Medication Administration Techniques.. **1404**

Appendix E. Formulas Helpful for Calculating Doses... **1407**

Appendix F. Body Surface Area Nomograms **1409**

Appendix G. Normal Values of Common Laboratory Tests.. **1411**

Appendix H. Commonly Used Abbreviations **1414**

Appendix I. Pregnancy Categories.. **1416**

Appendix J. Controlled Substances Schedules **1417**

Appendix K. Equianalgesic Dosing Guidelines **1418**

Appendix L. Recommendations for the Safe Handling of Hazardous Drugs **1421**

Appendix M. Food Sources for Specific Nutrients... **1423**

Appendix N. Insulins and Insulin Therapy **1425**

Appendix O. Canadian and U.S. Pharmaceutical Practices **1427**

Appendix P. Routine Pediatric and Adult Immunizations.. **1429**

Appendix Q. Administering Medications to Children **1436**

Appendix R. Pediatric Dosage Calculations... **1437**

Appendix S. Pediatric Fluid and Electrolyte Requirements **1438**

Appendix T. Early Management of Anaphylactic Reactions **1439**

Appendix U. The Cytochrome P450 System **1440**

APPENDIX A
Recent Drug Approvals

To view full-text monographs of drugs that have been recently released from the FDA or to learn about changes to dosage forms, please visit www.DrugGuide.com.

benzyl alcohol
(**ben**-zill **al**-ko-hol)
Ulesfia

Classification
Therapeutic: pediculocides

Pregnancy Category B

Indications
Topical treatment of head lice in patients ≥6 mo.

Contraindications/Precautions
Contraindicated in: None noted; Pedi: Children <6 mo (safety not established; risk of gasping syndrome in neonates).
Use Cautiously in: OB: Lactation.

Adverse Reactions/Side Effects
EENT: ocular irritation. **Derm:** contact dermatitis, erythema, pruritus, pyoderma. **Local:** application site anesthesia, application site hypoesthesia, application site irritation, pain.

Route/Dosage
Topical (Adults and Children ≥6 mo): *Short hair 0–2 in long*—apply 4–6 oz (½–¾ bottle), repeat in 7 days; *Short hair 2–4 in long*—apply 6–8 oz (¾–1 bottle), repeat in 7 days; *Medium hair 4–8 in long*—apply 8–12 oz (1–1 ½ bottles), repeat in 7 days; *Medium hair 8–16 in long*—apply 12–24 oz (1 ½–3 bottles), repeat in 7 days; *Long hair 16–22 in long*—apply 24–32 oz (3–4 bottles), repeat in 7 days; *Long hair >22 in long*—apply 32–48 oz (4–6 bottles), repeat in 7 days.

ciclesonide (inhalation)
(si-**kless**-o-nide)
Alvesco

Classification
Therapeutic: antiasthmatics
Pharmacologic: corticosteroids (inhalation)

Pregnancy Category C

Indications
Maintenance treatment of asthma as preventive therapy in patients ≥12 yr. Not for acute treatment of bronchospasm.

Contraindications/Precautions
Contraindicated in: Hypersensitivity to ciclesonide or any other ingredients in the formulation; Acute asthma/status asthmaticus.
Use Cautiously in: Geri: Consider age-related ↓ in cardiac, renal and hepatic function, concurrent disease state and drug therapy; consider lower initial dose; OB: ↓ dose may be sufficient; Lactation: Many corticosteroids enter breast milk, hypercorticism may be seen with ↑ maternal doses; Pedi: Safety and effectiveness in children <12 has not been established.

Adverse Reactions/Side Effects
CNS: headache. **EENT:** *candida* infection of mouth and pharynx, nasal congestion, nasopharyngitis, pharyngolaryngeal pain, cataracts, ↑ intraocular pressure. **Endo:** adrenal suppression (↑ dose, long term therapy), ↓ growth (children). **MS:** arthralgia, back pain, ↓ bone mineral density (↑ dose, long term therapy), extremity pain. **Misc:** worsening of infections.

Route/Dosage
Inhaln (Adults ≥12 yr): *Previous therapy with bronchodilators alone*—80 mcg twice daily, may be ↑ to 160 mcg twice daily; *Previous therapy with inhaled corticosteroids*—80 mcg twice daily, may be ↑ to 320 mcg twice daily; *Previous therapy with oral corticosteroids*—320 mcg twice daily.

dalfampridine
(dal-**fam**-pri-deen)
Ampyra

Classification
Therapeutic: anti-multiple sclerosis agents
Pharmacologic: potassium channel blockers

Pregnancy Category C

1369

Indications
Treatment of multiple sclerosis, to improve walking speed.

Contraindications/Precautions
Contraindicated in: History of seizures; Moderate/severe renal impairment (↑ risk of seizures); Lactation: Avoid use during lactation.
Use Cautiously in: Geri: Consider age-related ↓ in renal function; OB: Use during pregnancy only if potential benefit justifies potential risk to fetus; Pedi: safety and effectiveness in children <18 yr not established.

Adverse Reactions/Side Effects
CNS: dizziness, headache, insomnia, weakness. **EENT:** nasopharyngitis, pharyngolaryngeal pain. **GI:** constipation, dyspepsia, nausea. **GU:** urinary tract infection. **MS:** back pain. **Neuro:** balance disorder, multiple sclerosis relapse, paresthesia.

Route/Dosage
PO (Adults): 10 mg twice daily.

---

everolimus (e-ve-ro-li-mus)
Afinitor

Classification
Therapeutic: antineoplastics
Pharmacologic: kinase inhibitors

Pregnancy Category D

Indications
Advanced renal cell carcinoma which has failed treatment with sunitinib or sorafenib.

Contraindications/Precautions
Contraindicated in: Hypersensitivity to everolimus or other rapamycins; Severe hepatic impairment (Child-Pugh class C); OB: May cause fetal harm, avoid use during pregnancy; Lactation: Avoid breastfeeding.
Use Cautiously in: Moderate hepatic impairment (Child-Pugh class B); dose reduction required; Geri: Elderly patients may be more sensitive to drug effects; consider age-related ↓ in hepatic function, concurrent disease states and drug therapy; Pedi: Safe use in children has not been established.

Adverse Reactions/Side Effects
CNS: fatigue, weakness, headache. **Resp:** PNEUMONITIS, cough, dyspnea. **GI:** anorexia, diarrhea, mucositis, mouth ulcers, nausea, stomatitis, vomiting, dysgeusia. **F and E:** peripheral edema. **Derm:** dry skin, pruritus, rash. **Hemat:** anemia, leukopenia, thrombocytopenia. **Metab:** hyperglycemia, hyperlipidemia, hypertriglyceridemia. **MS:** extremity pain. **Misc:** INFECTIONS, hypersensitivity reactions including ANAPHYLAXIS, fever.

Route/Dosage
PO (Adults): 10 mg once daily; *Concurrent use of strong inducers of CYP3A4*—↑ dose in 5 mg increments up to 20 mg/daily.

Hepatic Impairment
PO (Adults): *Moderate hepatic impairment*—5 mg once daily.

---

fosaprepitant (injection)
(fos-a-**prep**-i-tant)
Emend

Classification
Therapeutic: antiemetics
Pharmacologic: neurokinin antagonists

Pregnancy Category B

Indications
Prevention of nausea and vomiting associated with emetogenic chemotherapy.

Contraindications/Precautions
Contraindicated in: Hypersensitivity; Concurrent use with pimozide (risk of life-threatening adverse cardiovascular reactions); Lactation: May cause unwanted effects in nursing infants.
Use Cautiously in: OB: Use only if clearly needed; Pedi: Safety not established.

Adverse Reactions/Side Effects
CNS: dizziness, fatigue, weakness. **GI:** diarrhea. **Misc:** hiccups.

Route/Dosage
IV (Adults): 115 mg 30 min prior to chemotherapy on day 1.

---

fospropofol (foss-**pro**-po-fol)
Lusedra

Classification
Therapeutic: general anesthetics

Pregnancy Category B

Indications
Monitored anesthesia care (MAC) in adults undergoing diagnostic/therapeutic procedures.

Contraindications/Precautions
Contraindicated in: None noted.
Use Cautiously in: Compromised cardiac function, reduced vascular tone or reduced intravascular volume (↑ risk of hypotension); Hepatic impairment; Renal impairment (safety not established for CCr <30 mL/min); Geri: Patients ≥65 yr or those with severe systemic disease (dose reduction required); OB, Lactation: Not recommended for use during labor, delivery or lactation (may cause neonatal respiratory and cardiovascular depression); Pedi: Children <18 yr (safety not established, use not recommended).

Adverse Reactions/Side Effects
Resp: RESPIRATORY DEPRESSION, cough, hypoxemia. **CV:** hypotension. **Derm:** pruritus. **Neuro:** paresthesia. **Misc:** loss of purposeful responsiveness.

Route/Dosage
Patients weighing >90 kg should be dosed as if they are 90 kg; patients weighing <60 kg should be dosed as if they are 60 kg.
IV (Adults): 6.5 mg/kg (not to exceed 16.5 mL) initially, followed by supplemental doses of 1.6 mg/kg (not to exceed 4 mL or more frequently that every 4 min) as needed.

---

lacosamide (la-**kose**-a-mide)
Vimpat

Classification
Therapeutic: anticonvulsants
Schedule V

Pregnancy Category C

Indications
Adjunctive therapy of partial-onset seizures.

Contraindications/Precautions
Contraindicated in: Hypersensitivity; Severe hepatic impairment; Lactation: Lactation.
Use Cautiously in: CCr <30 mL/min (use lower daily dose); All patients (may ↑ risk of suicidal thoughts/behaviors); Mild to moderate hepatic impairment; titrate dose carefully, use lower daily dose; Known cardiac conduction problems or severe cardiac disease (MI or CHF); OB: Use during pregnancy only if potential benefit justifies risk to the fetus; Pedi: Children <17 yr (safety and effectiveness not established); Geri: Titrate dose carefully.

Adverse Reactions/Side Effects
CNS: SUICIDAL THOUGHTS, dizziness, headache, syncope, vertigo. **EENT:** diplopia. **CV:** PR interval prolongation. **GI:** nausea, vomiting. **Neuro:** ataxia. **Misc:** physical dependence, psychological dependence, multiorgan hypersensitivity reactions (Drug Reaction with Eosinophilia and Systemic Symptoms—DRESS).

Route/Dosage
PO, IV (Adults): 50 mg twice daily; may be ↑ weekly by 100 mg/day in two divided doses up to a maintenance dose of 200–400 mg/day given in two divided doses.

Hepatic/Renal Impairment
PO, IV (Adults): *CCr ≤30 mL/min or mild to moderate hepatic impairment*—daily dose should not exceed 300 mg.

---

liraglutide (lir-**ah**-gloo-tide)
Victoza

Classification
Therapeutic: antidiabetics
Pharmacologic: glucagon-like peptide-1 (GLP-1) receptor agonists

Pregnancy Category C

Indications
Adjunct treatment to diet and exercise to improve glycemic control in adults with type 2 diabetes mellitus; not recommended as first line therapy.

Contraindications/Precautions
Contraindicated in: Personal or family history of Medullary Thyroid Carcinoma (MTC)/Multiple Endocrine Neoplasia syndrome type 2 (MEN 2); Lactation: Avoid use during lactation; Pedi: Not recommended in children.
Use Cautiously in: History of pancreatitis; Hepatic/renal impairment; OB: Use during pregnancy only if potential benefit justifies potential risk to fetus.

Adverse Reactions/Side Effects
CNS: headache. **GI:** diarrhea, nausea, vomiting, constipation, pancreatitis. **Local:** injection site reactions.

Route/Dosage
Subcut (Adults): 0.6 mg once daily initially, may be ↑ at weekly intervals up to 1.8 mg/day.

---

ofatumumab (oh-fa-**too**-moo-mab)
Azerra

Classification
Therapeutic: antineoplastics
Pharmacologic: monoclonal antibodies

Pregnancy Category C

Indications
Chronic lymphocytic leukemia (CLL) refractory to fludarabine and alemtuzumab.

Contraindications/Precautions
Contraindicated in: None noted.
Use Cautiously in: History of hepatitis B infection (may reactivate); OB: Use during pregnancy only if potential benefit to mother justifies potential risk to fetus; Lactation: Use cautiously during lactation; Pedi: safe and effectiveness in children has not been established.

Adverse Reactions/Side Effects
CNS: weakness. **CV:** peripheral edema. **GI:** INTESTINAL OBSTRUCTION, REACTIVATION OF HEPATITIS B. **Derm:** sweating. **Hemat:** anemia, neutropenia, thrombocytopenia. **MS:** back pain, muscle spasm. **Neuro:** PROGRESSIVE MULTIFOCAL LEUKOENCEPHALOPATHY (PML). **Misc:** INFECTIONS, INFUSION REACTIONS, chills, fever.

Route/Dosage
IV (Adults): 300 mg initial initially, followed 1 wk later by 2000 mg weekly for 7 doses, followed 4 wk later by 2000 mg every 4 wk for 4 doses (total regimen is 12 doses).

---

romidepsin (roe-mi-**dep**-sin)
ISTODAX

Classification
Therapeutic: antineoplastics
Pharmacologic: enzyme inhibitors, histone deacetylase (HDAC) inhibitors

Pregnancy Category D

Indications
Treatment of cutaneous T-cell lymphoma (CTCL) that has not responded to at least one prior systemic therapy.

Contraindications/Precautions
Contraindicated in: OB: Pregnancy (may cause fetal harm); Lactation: Avoid use.
Use Cautiously in: Congenital long QT syndrome, history of significant cardiovascular disease, and concurrent antiarrhythmic or other medications that cause significant QT prolongation (↑ risk of arrhythmias); Electrolyte abnormalities (correct magnesium and potassium abnormalities prior to use); Moderate to severe hepatic impairment or end-stage renal disease; Geri: Elderly patients may be more sensitive to drug effects; Pedi: safe and effective use in children has not been established.

Adverse Reactions/Side Effects
CNS: fatigue. **CV:** ECG changes. **GI:** anorexia, nausea, vomiting. **Hemat:** anemia, leukopenia, thrombocytopenia.

Route/Dosage
IV (Adults): 14 mg/m^2 on days 1, 8, and 15 of a 28-day cycle, cycle may be repeated every 28 days depending on benefit and patient tolerance; dose may be ↓ to 10 mg/m^2 if adverse reactions occur.

---

rufinamide (roo-**fin**-a-mide)
Banzol

Classification
Therapeutic: anticonvulsants
Pharmacologic: triazoles

Pregnancy Category C

Indications
Adjunctive treatment of seizures associated with Lennox-Gastaut syndrome in patients >4 yr.

Contraindications/Precautions
Contraindicated in: Hypersensitivity; Familial short QT syndrome; Severe hepatic impairment.
Use Cautiously in: All patients (may ↑ risk of suicidal thoughts/behaviors); Mild to moderate hepatic impairment.

Adverse Reactions/Side Effects
CNS: SUICIDAL THOUGHTS, dizziness, fatigue, headache, somnolence. **EENT:** diplopia. **CV:** QT prolongation. **GI:** nausea, changes in appetite. **GU:** urinary frequency. **Derm:** rash. **Hemat:** anemia. **Neuro:** ataxia, coordination abnormalities, gait disturbances. **Misc:** MULTI-ORGAN HYPERSENSITIVITY REACTIONS, hypersensitivity reactions (↑ children).

Route/Dosage
PO (Adults): 400–800 mg/day in two divided doses, ↑ by 400–800 mg every 2 days until a maximum daily dose of 3200 mg/day (1600 mg twice daily) is reached.
PO (Children ≥4 yr): 10 mg/kg/day in two divided doses, ↑ by 10 mg/kg every 2 days until a maximum daily dose of 45 mg/kg/day or 3200 mg/day given in 2 divided doses, whichever is less, is reached.

telavancin (tel-a-**van**-sin)
Vibativ

Classification
Therapeutic: anti-infectives
Pharmacologic: lipoglycopeptides

Pregnancy Category C

Indications
Treatment of complicated skin/skin structure infections caused by susceptible bacteria.

Contraindications/Precautions
Contraindicated in: Congenital long QT syndrome, known prolongation of the QTc interval, uncompensated heart failure, or severe left ventricular hypertrophy (risk of fatal arrhythmias); OB: do not use during pregnancy unless potential maternal benefit outweighs potential risk to fetus.
Use Cautiously in: Renal impairment (efficacy may be reduced; dose reduction recommended for CCr ≤50 mL/min); Geri: Consider age-related ↓ in renal function, adjust dose accordingly (↑ risk of adverse renal reactions); Lactation: Use cautiously during breastfeeding; Pedi: Safety and effectiveness in children have not been established.

Adverse Reactions/Side Effects
CNS: dizziness. **CV:** QTc prolongation. **GI:** PSEUDOMEMBRANOUS COLITIS, taste disturbance, nausea, vomiting, abdominal pain. **GU:** foamy urine, nephrotoxicity. **Misc:** infusion reactions.

Route/Dosage
IV (Adults): 10 mg/kg ever 24 hr for 7–14 days.

Renal Impairment
IV (Adults): *CCr 30–50 mL/min*—7.5 mg/kg every 24 hr; *CCr 10–≤30 mL/min*—10 mg/kg every 48 hr.

▓ tetrabenazine
(te-tra-**ben**-a-zeen)
Xenazine

Classification
Therapeutic: antichoreas
Pharmacologic: reversible monoamine depleters

Pregnancy Category C

Indications
Treatment of chorea due to Huntington's Disease.

Contraindications/Precautions
Contraindicated in: Hepatic impairment; Concurrent use of reserpine or MAO inhibitors; Patients who are actively suicidal or have untreated depression; Lactation: Lactation.
Use Cautiously in: History of/propensity for depression or history of psychiatric illness; history of suicidality; ▓ Poor CYP2D6 metabolizers; initial dose reduction required; Concurrent use of CYP2D6 inhibitors; dose modification required; Recent history of myocardial infarction or unstable heart disease; OB: Use during pregnancy only when potential benefit justifies potential risk to the fetus; Pedi: Safety and efficacy not established.

Adverse Reactions/Side Effects
CNS: anxiety, fatigue, insomnia, depression, sedation/somnolence, cognitive defects, dizziness, headache. **Resp:** shortness of breath. **CV:** hypotension, QTc prolongation. **GI:** nausea, dysphagia. **Neuro:** akathisia, balance difficulty, dysarthria, Parkinsonism, unsteady gait. **Misc:** NEUROLEPTIC MALIGNANT SYNDROME.

Route/Dosage
PO (Adults): 12.5 mg/day for one wk initially, ↑ by 12.5 weekly up to 37.5–50 mg/day in three divided doses; *concurrent use of strong inhibitors or CYP2D6 or poor CYP2D6 metabolizers*—start with initial dose of 6.25 mg, titrate carefully.

✷ = Canadian drug name. ▓ = Genetic implication.
*CAPITALS indicates life-threatening; underlines indicate most frequent.

tocilizumab
(toe-si-**liz**-oo-mab)
Actemra

Classification
Therapeutic: antirheumatics, immunosuppressants
Pharmacologic: interleukin antagonists

Pregnancy Category C

Indications
Treatment of adults with moderately-to severely-active rheumatoid arthritis who have not responded to one or more TNF antagonist therapies. May be used alone or with methotrexate or other DMARDs.

Contraindications/Precautions
Contraindicated in: Serious infections; Patients at risk for GI perforation, including patients with diverticulitis; Active hepatic disease/impairment; Absolute neutrophil count (ANC) <2000/mm³ (<500/mm³ while on therapy) or platelet count below 100,000/mm³ (<50,000/mm³ while on therapy); Lactation: Not recommended during lactation.
Use Cautiously in: Renal or hepatic impairment; Patients with tuberculosis risk factors; Geri: ↑ risk of adverse reactions; OB: Use during pregnancy only if potential benefit justifies potential risk to fetus; Pedi: Safe and effective use in children has not been established.

Adverse Reactions/Side Effects
CNS: headache, dizziness. **EENT:** nasopharyngitis. **Resp:** upper respiratory tract infections. **CV:** hypertension. **GI:** GASTROINTESTINAL PERFORATION, ↑ liver enzymes. **Derm:** rash. **Hemat:** NEUTROPENIA, THROMBOCYTOPENIA. **Metab:** ↑ lipids. **Misc:** SERIOUS INFECTIONS INCLUDING TUBERCULOSIS, DISSEMINATED FUNGAL INFECTIONS AND INFECTIONS WITH OPPORTUNISTIC PATHOGENS, hypersensitivity reactions including ANAPHYLAXIS, infusion reactions.

Route/Dosage
PO (Adults): 4 mg/kg may be ↑ to 8 mg/kg based on clinical response; dosage reductions are recommended for elevated liver enzymes, neutropenia, and thrombocytopenia.

vigabatrin (vye-**gah**-bat-rin)
Sabril

Classification
Therapeutic: anticonvulsants, none assigned

Pregnancy Category C

Indications
Management (adjunctive) of refractory Complex Partial Seizures in Adults in patients who have responded inadequately to several alternative treatments; not a first-line treatment. Management of infantile spasms (IS) in patients 1 mo-2 yr.

Contraindications/Precautions
Contraindicated in: History or high risk of other types of irreversible vision loss unless benefits of treatment clearly outweigh risks; OB: Use during pregnancy only if the potential benefit justifies the potential risk to the fetus (may cause fetal harm); Lactation: Enters breast milk; breastfeeding should be avoided.
Use Cautiously in: Renal impairment (dose modification recommended for CCr <50 mL/min); History of suicidal ideation; Geri: Consider age-related ↓ in renal function adjust dose accordingly (↑ risk of sedation/confusion); Pedi: abnormal MRI signal changes have been seen in infants.

Adverse Reactions/Side Effects
CNS: SUICIDAL THOUGHTS, confusional state, memory impairment, drowsiness, fatigue. **CV:** edema. **EENT:** blurred vision, nystagmus, vision loss. **Hemat:** anemia. **Metab:** weight gain. **MS:** arthralgia. **Neuro:** abnormal coordination, tremor, peripheral neuropathy.

Route/Dosage
PO (Adults): 500 mg twice daily initially, may be ↑ in 500 mg increments every 7 days depending on response up to 1.5 g twice daily.

Renal Impairment
PO (Adults): *CCr >50 –80 mL/min*— ↓ dose by 25%; *CCr >30–50 mL/min*— ↓ dose by 50%; *CCr >10– <30 mL/min*— ↓ dose by 75%.
PO (Children 1 mo–2 yr): 50 mg/kg/day given in 2 divided doses initially, increasing by 25–50 mg/kg/day increments every 3 days up to a maximum of 150 mg/kg/day; dosage adjustments are necessary for renal impairment.

Recent Drug Approvals 1375

NEW DOSAGE FORMS

Generic Name (Brand Name)	New Dosage Form
acyclovir/hydrocortisone (Lipsovir)	Topical cream for early treatment of coldsores.
alpha$_1$-proteinase inhibitor (Prolastin-C)	More concentrated form allows ↓ infusion volume and time.
amlodipine/telmisartan (Twynsa)	Combination calcium channel blocker/angiotensin receptor blocker for hypertension.
aztreonam (Cayston)	75 mg inhalation solution for cystic fibrosis.
calcitriol (Vectical)	3 mcg/g ointment for plaque psoriasis.
capsaicin (Qutenza)	8% capsaicin for postherpetic neuralgia pain.
ciprofloxacin (Cetraxal)	0.2% otic solution for acute otitis externa.
clonidine	Once daily extended-release tablet and oral suspension formulation for hypertension.
colesevelam (Welchol)	1.875 g and 3.75 g single-dose packets for oral suspension for LDL and glucose control.
dexamethasone (Ozurdex)	0.7 mg intravitreal implant for macular edema.
diclofenac (Pennsaid)	1.5% topical solution for osteoarthritis of the knee.
estradiol (Vagifem)	10 mcg vaginal tablet, a lower dose for atrophic vaginitis.
ganciclovir (Zirgan)	0.015% ophthalmic gel for acute herpetic keratitis.
human papillomavirus vaccine, bivalent (Types 16 and 18), recombinant (Cervarix)	IM Injection for prevention of some diseases caused by oncogenic human papillomavirus (HPV) types 16 and 18.
hydromorphone (Exalgo)	Extended-release tablets 8 mg, 12 mg, and 16 mg for once-daily dosing.
levonorgestrel (Plan B One-Step)	1.5 mg tablet single-dose emergency contraceptive.
meningococcal vaccine, quadravalent (Menveo)	For routine immunization of adolescents 11–18 yr and other high risk groups.
olanzapine (Zyprexa Relprevv)	210 mg, 300 mg, and 405 mg extended-release injection for schizophrenia.
omeprazole/sodium bicarbonate (Zegerid OTC)	20 mg omeprazole/1100 mg sodium bicarbonate for over-the-counter treatment of heartburn.
pneumococcal 13-valent conjugate vaccine (Prevnar 13)	Replacement vaccine for Prevnar, a 7-valent vaccine for infants/young children ages 6 wk–5 yr for the prevntion of invasive pneumococcal disease (IPD) and otitis media; adds six additional types of bacteria.
pramipexole (Mirapex ER)	0.375 mg, 0.75 mg, 1.5 mg, 3 mg, and 4.5 mg extended-release tablets for treatment of early Parkinson's disease.
pregabalin (Lyrica)	20 mg/ml oral solution for treatment of various painful syndromes and as an adjunct anticonvulsant.
ritonavir (Norvir)	100 mg tablets, no refrigeration needed, must be taken with meals.
sildenafil (Revatio)	10 mg injectable formulation for pulmonary hypertension.
tranexamic acid (Lysteda)	650 mg tablets for menorrhagia.
trazodone (Oleptro)	150 mg and 300 mg extended-release tablets for major depression.

RECENT LABELING CHANGES (New Warnings/Indications)

Generic Name (Brand Name)	Labeling Change
bismuth subsalicylate (Maalox Total Relief)	Manufacturer will rename trade name in September 2010 to avoid confusion with other Maalox products that do not contain bismuth subsalicylate.
bortezomib (Velcade)	New dosing guidelines for patients with hepatic impairment.
colesevelam (Welchol)	New indication for treatment of hypercholesterolemia in children 10–17 yr.

RECENT LABELING CHANGES (New Warnings/Indications) (continued)

deferasirox (Exjade)	New warning regarding risk of GI hemorrhage, contraindications in renal impairment, drug interaction with cholestyramine and co-morbidities for cytopenias, renal and hepatic adverse reactions.
desipramine (Norpramin)	New warning regarding use of extreme caution in patients who have cardiovascular history.
didanosine (Videx)	New warning regarding risk of non-cirrhotic portal hypertension.
duloxetine (Cymbalta)	New indication for maintenance treatment of depression.
exenatide (Byetta)	New warning regarding development of renal failure.
ERYTHROPOIESIS-STIMULATING AGENTS (ESAs) (Epogen, ✻ EPO, Procrit) **darbepoetin** (Aranesp)	Mandatory participation in ongoing risk management program to monitor and evaluation ↑ tumor growth and shortened survival in cancer patients and risk of thromboembolic phenomenon in other patient populations.
fondaparinux (Arixtra)	New Cautions for low weight patients (< 50 kg) and those with renal impairment
human papillomavirus vaccine (Gardasil)	New indication for prevention of genital warts in boys and men.
LONG-ACTING BETA-AGONISTS (LABAs), aformoterol (Brovana), **formoterol** (Foradil), **salmeterol** (Serevent)	New warning: LABAs are contraindicated without an asthma controller medication and only be used long-term when asthma cannot be adequately controlled on asthma controller medications. LABAs should be discontinued once asthma control is achieved. Pediatric/adolescent patients who need a LABA in addition to an inhaled corticosteroid should use a combination product containing both an inhaled corticosteroid such as Advair (fluticasone/salmeterol) or Symbicort (budesonide/formoterol).
natalizumab (Tysabri)	New warning: risk of progressive multifocal leukoencephalopathy (PML) ↑ with ↑ number of infusions.
olanzapine (Zyprexa)	New indication for use in adolescents 13–17 yr: New warning: Consider long term effects of hyperlipidemia and weight gain in adolescents.
quetiapine (Seroquel XR)	New indication as adjunctive treatment of major depression.
olmesartan (Benicar)	New indication for the treatment of hypertension in pediatric patients aged 6–16 yr.
rasagiline (Azilect)	New reduced restrictions on medications and foods.
riluzole (Rilutek)	New warning regarding interstitial lung disease as an adverse effect.
ritonavir (Norvir)	New warning regarding possible adverse cardiovascular interaction with saquinavir (Invirase); may possibly prolong QT or PR intervals and ↑ the risk for abnormal heart rhythms, including torsades de pointes. Avoid combined use with medications known to cause QT interval prolongation such as Class IA (such as quinidine,) or Class III (such as amiodarone) antiarrhythmic drugs; or in patients with a history of QT interval prolongation.
rituximab (Rituxan)	New indication, in combination with fludarabine and cyclophosphamide for chronic lymphocytic leukemia (CLL).
rosuvastatin (Rosuvastatin)	New indications for primary prevention of cardiovascular disease in patients at risk of a cardiac event and for treatment of hypercholesterolemia in children 10–17 yr.
sibutramine (Meridia)	New warnings/contraindications regarding ↑ risk of heart attack/stroke in high risk patients.
sirolimus (Rapamune)	New warning regarding blood level determinations; assay methods may vary.
zanamavir (Relenza)	Inhaln powder.

Recent Drug Approvals

DISCONTINUED DRUGS

Generic Name (Brand Name)	Reason for Discontinuation
aminoglutethimide (Cytadren)	Adrenal suppression and the need for steroid therapy.
carteolol (Cartrol)	Oral product discontinued by manufacturer; ophthalmic product still available.
cloxacillin (Tegopen)	Discontinued by manufacturer.
daunorubicin lipsome (DaunoXome)	Discontinued by manufacturer.
efalizumab (Raptiva)	Potential risk of progressive multifocal leukencephalopathy (PML).
gonadorelin acetate (Lutrepulse Kit)	Discontinued by manufacturer.
gonadorelin hydrochloride (Factrel)	Discontinued by manufacturer.
molindone (Moban)	Discontinued by manufacturer.
ritodrine (Yutopar)	Discontinued by manufacturer.
trimetrexate (Neutrexin)	Discontinued by manufacturer.

APPENDIX B
Combination Drugs

Note: The drugs listed in this section are in alphabetical order according to trade names. If the trade name does not specify dose form, the dose form is either a tablet or capsule. Following each trade name are the generic names and doses of the active ingredients contained in each preparation. For information on these drugs, look up each generic name in the combination. For inert ingredients, see drug label. (**OTC**) signifies "over-the-counter" or nonprescription medication.

A-200 Shampoo—0.33% pyrethrins + 4% piperonyl butoxide (**OTC**)
Acanya Topical Gel—1.2% clindamycin + 2.5% benzoyl peroxide
Accuretic 10/12.5—quinapril 10 mg + hydrochlorothiazide 12.5 mg
Accuretic 20/12.5—quinapril 20 mg + hydrochlorothiazide 12.5 mg
Accuretic 20/25—quinapril 20 mg + hydrochlorothiazide 25 mg
Actifed Cold and Allergy—chlorpheniramine 4 mg + phenylephrine 10 mg (**OTC**)
Activella Tablets 0.5/0.1—estradiol 0.5 mg + norethindrone 0.1 mg
Activella Tablets 1/0.5—estradiol 1 mg + norethindrone 0.5 mg
Actoplus Met 15/500—pioglitazone 15 mg + metformin 500 mg
Actoplus Met 15/850—pioglitazone 15 mg+ metformin 850 mg
Actoplus Met XR 15/1000—pioglitazone 15 mg + metformin extended-release 1000 mg
Actoplus Met XR 30/1000—pioglitazone 30 mg + metformin extended-release 1000 mg
Adderall 5 mg—dextroamphetamine sulfate 1.25 mg + dextroamphetamine saccharate 1.25 mg + amphetamine aspartate 1.25 mg + amphetamine sulfate 1.25 mg
Adderall 7.5 mg—dextroamphetamine sulfate 1.875 mg + dextroamphetamine saccharate 1.875 mg + amphetamine aspartate 1.875 mg + amphetamine sulfate 1.875 mg
Adderall 10 mg—dextroamphetamine sulfate 2.5 mg + dextroamphetamine saccharate 2.5 mg + amphetamine aspartate 2.5 mg + amphetamine sulfate 2.5 mg
Adderall 12.5 mg—dextroamphetamine sulfate 3.125 mg + dextroamphetamine saccharate 3.125 mg + amphetamine aspartate 3.125 mg + amphetamine sulfate 3.125 mg
Adderall 15 mg—dextroamphetamine sulfate 3.75 mg + dextroamphetamine saccharate 3.75 mg + amphetamine aspartate 3.75 mg + amphetamine sulfate 3.75 mg
Adderall 20 mg—dextroamphetamine sulfate 5 mg + dextroamphetamine saccharate 5 mg + amphetamine aspartate 5 mg + amphetamine sulfate 5 mg
Adderall 30 mg—dextroamphetamine sulfate 7.5 mg + dextroamphetamine saccharate 7.5 mg + amphetamine aspartate 7.5 mg + amphetamine sulfate 7.5 mg
Adderall XR 5 mg—dextroamphetamine saccharate 1.25 mg + dextroamphetamine sulfate 1.25 mg + amphetamine aspartate monohydrate 1.25 mg + amphetamine sulfate 1.25 mg
Adderall XR 10 mg—dextroamphetamine saccharate 2.5 mg + dextroamphetamine sulfate 2.5 mg + amphetamine aspartate monohydrate 2.5 mg + amphetamine sulfate 2.5 mg
Adderall XR 15 mg—dextroamphetamine saccharate 3.75 mg + dextroamphetamine sulfate 3.75 mg + amphetamine aspartate monohydrate 3.75 mg + amphetamine sulfate 3.75 mg
Adderall XR 20 mg—dextroamphetamine saccharate 5 mg + dextroamphetamine sulfate 5 mg + amphetamine aspartate monohydrate 5 mg + amphetamine sulfate 5 mg
Adderall XR 25 mg—dextroamphetamine saccharate 6.25 mg + dextroamphetamine sulfate 6.25 mg + amphetamine aspartate monohydrate 6.25 mg + amphetamine sulfate 6.25 mg
Adderall XR 30 mg—dextroamphetamine saccharate 7.5 mg + dextroamphetamine sulfate 7.5 mg + amphetamine aspartate monohydrate 7.5 mg + amphetamine sulfate 7.5 mg
Advair Diskus 100—(per actuation) fluticasone 100 mcg + salmeterol 50 mcg
Advair Diskus 250—(per actuation) fluticasone 250 mcg + salmeterol 50 mcg

Combination Drugs 1379

Advair Diskus 500—(per actuation) fluticasone 500 mcg + salmeterol 50 mcg
Advair HFA 45—(per actuation) fluticasone 45 mcg + salmeterol 21 mcg
Advair HFA 115—(per actuation) fluticasone 115 mcg + salmeterol 21 mcg
Advair HFA 230—(per actuation) fluticasone 230 mcg + salmeterol 21 mcg
Advicor 500/20—extended-release niacin 500 mg + lovastatin 20 mg
Advicor 750/20—extended-release niacin 750 mg + lovastatin 20 mg
Advicor 1000/20—extended-release niacin 1000 mg + lovastatin 20 mg
Advicor 1000/40—extended-release niacin 1000 mg + lovastatin 40 mg
Advil Cold & Sinus—pseudoephedrine 30 mg + ibuprofen 200 mg (OTC)
Advil Multi-Symptom Cold—chlorpheniramine 2 mg + pseudoephedrine 30 mg + ibuprofen 200 mg (OTC)
Advil PM Liquigels—diphenhydramine 25 mg + ibuprofen 200 mg (OTC)
Aggrenox—aspirin 25 mg + extended-release dipyridamole 200 mg
Alavert Allergy and Sinus—loratadine 5 mg + pseudoephedrine 120 mg (OTC)
Aldactazide 25/25—hydrochlorothiazide 25 mg + spironolactone 25 mg
Aldactazide 50/50—hydrochlorothiazide 50 mg + spironolactone 50 mg
Alesse—levonorgestrel 0.1 mg + ethinyl estradiol 20 mcg
Aleve-D Sinus & Cold—naproxen 220 mg + extended-release pseudoephedrine 120 mg (OTC)
Alka-Seltzer Effervescent, Original—citric acid 1000 mg + sodium bicarbonate 1916 mg + aspirin 325 mg (OTC)
Alka-Seltzer Effervescent, Extra-Strength—citric acid 1000 mg + sodium bicarbonate 1985 mg + aspirin 500 mg (OTC)
Alka-Seltzer Plus Cold & Cough Liqui-Gels—dextromethorphan 10 mg + phenylephrine 5 mg + chlorpheniramine 2 mg + acetaminophen 325 mg (OTC)
Alka-Seltzer Plus Night Cold Formula Liquid Gels—acetaminophen 325 mg + doxylamine 6.25 mg + dextromethorphan 10 mg + phenylephrine 5 mg (OTC)
Alka-Seltzer Plus Sinus Formula—phenylephrine 7.8 mg + aspirin 325 mg (OTC)
Allegra-D 12 Hour—fexofenadine 60 mg + extended-release pseudoephedrine 120 mg
Allegra-D 24 Hour—fexofenadine 180 mg + extended-release pseudoephedrine 240 mg
Allerfrim Syrup—(per 5 ml) triprolidine 1.25 mg + pseudoephedrine 30 mg (OTC)
Amoclan 200 Suspension—(per 5 ml) amoxicillin 200 mg + clavulanate potassium 28.5 mg
Amoclan 400 Suspension—(per 5 ml) amoxicillin 400 mg + clavulanate potassium 57 mg
Amoclan 600 Suspension—(per 5 ml) amoxicillin 600 mg + clavulanate potassium 42.9 mg
Anacin—aspirin 400 mg + caffeine 32 mg (OTC)
Anacin Max Strength—aspirin 500 mg + caffeine 32 mg (OTC)
Analpram Topical Cream—1% hydrocortisone + 1% pramoxine
Analpram Topical Lotion—2.5% hydrocortisone + 1% pramoxine
Anaplex DM Syrup—(per 5 ml) brompheniramine 4 mg + dextromethorphan 30 mg + pseudoephedrine 60 mg
Anexsia 5/325—hydrocodone 5 mg + acetaminophen 325 mg
Anexsia 5/500—hydrocodone 5 mg + acetaminophen 500 mg
Anexsia 7.5/325—hydrocodone 7.5 mg + acetaminophen 325 mg
Anexsia 7.5/650—hydrocodone 7.5 mg + acetaminophen 650 mg
Anexsia 10/750—hydrocodone 10 mg + acetaminophen 750 mg
Angeliq—drosperinone 0.5 mg + estradiol 1 mg
Apri—desogestrel 0.15 mg + ethinyl estradiol 30 mcg
Aranelle
   Phase I—norethindrone 0.5 mg + ethinyl estradiol 35 mcg
   Phase II—norethindrone 1 mg + ethinyl estradiol 35 mcg
   Phase III—norethindrone 0.5 mg + ethinyl estradiol 35 mcg
Arthrotec 50/200—diclofenac 50 mg + misoprostol 200 mcg
Arthrotec 75/200—diclofenac 75 mg + misoprostol 200 mcg
Atacand HCT 16/12.5—candesartan 16 mg + hydrochlorothiazide 12.5 mg
Atacand HCT 32/12.5—candesartan 32 mg + hydrochlorothiazide 12.5 mg
Atacand HCT 32/25—candesartan 32 mg + hydrochlorothiazide 25 mg

1380 APPENDIX B

✧ **Atacand Plus**—candesartan 16 mg + hydrochlorothiazide 12.5 mg
Atripla—efavirenz 600 mg + emtricitabine 200 mg + tenofovir 300 mg
Augmentin 250—amoxicillin 250 mg + clavulanate potassium 125 mg
Augmentin 500—amoxicillin 500 mg + clavulanate potassium 125 mg
Augmentin 875—amoxicillin 875 mg + clavulanate potassium 125 mg
Augmentin XR—amoxicillin 1000 mg + clavulanate potassium 62.5 mg
Augmentin 125 Chewable—amoxicillin 125 mg + clavulanate potassium 31.25 mg
Augmentin 200 Chewable—amoxicillin 200 mg + clavulanate potassium 28.5 mg
Augmentin 250 Chewable—amoxicillin 250 mg + clavulanate potassium 62.5 mg
Augmentin 400 Chewable—amoxicillin 400 mg + clavulanate potassium 57 mg
Augmentin 125 mg Suspension—(per 5 ml) amoxicillin 125 mg + clavulanate potassium 31.25 mg
Augmentin 200 mg Suspension—(per 5 ml) amoxicillin 200 mg + clavulanate potassium 28.5 mg
Augmentin 250 mg Suspension—(per 5 ml) amoxicillin 250 mg + clavulanate potassium 62.5 mg
Augmentin 400 mg Suspension—(per 5 ml) amoxicillin 400 mg + clavulanate potassium 57 mg
Augmentin ES-600 Suspension—(per 5 ml) amoxicillin 600 mg + clavulanate potassium 42.9 mg
Avalide 150/12.5—irbesartan 150 mg + hydrochlorothiazide 12.5 mg
Avalide 300/12.5—irbesartan 300 mg + hydrochlorothiazide 12.5 mg
Avalide 300/25—irbesartan 300 mg + hydrochlorothiazide 25 mg
Avandamet 2/500—rosiglitazone 2 mg + metformin 500 mg
Avandamet 2/1000—rosiglitazone 2 mg + metformin 1000 mg
Avandamet 4/500—rosiglitazone 4 mg + metformin 500 mg
Avandamet 4/1000—rosiglitazone 4 mg + metformin 1000 mg
Avandaryl 4/1—rosiglitazone 4 mg + glimepiride 1 mg
Avandaryl 4/2—rosiglitazone 4 mg + glimepiride 2 mg
Avandaryl 4/4—rosiglitazone 4 mg + glimepiride 4 mg
Avandaryl 8/2—rosiglitazone 8 mg + glimepiride 2 mg
Avandaryl 8/4—rosiglitazone 8 mg + glimepiride 4 mg
Aviane—levonorgestrel 0.1 mg + ethinyl estradiol 20 mcg
Azor 5/20—amlodipine 5 mg + olmesartan 20 mg
Azor 5/40—amlodipine 5 mg + olmesartan 40 mg
Azor 10/20—amlodipine 10 mg + olmesartan 20 mg
Azor 10/40—amlodipine 10 mg + olmesartan 40 mg
Bactrim—trimethoprim 80 mg + sulfamethoxazole 400 mg
Bactrim DS—trimethoprim 160 mg + sulfamethoxazole 800 mg
Balziva—norethindrone 0.4 mg + ethinyl estradiol 35 mcg
Bayer Back & Body—aspirin 500 mg + caffeine 32.5 mg (OTC)
Bayer PM—aspirin 500 mg + diphenhydramine 38.3 mg (OTC)
Benadryl-D Allergy & Sinus Tablets—phenylephrine 10 mg + diphenhydramine 25 mg (OTC)
Benicar HCT 20/12.5—olmesartan 20 mg + hydrochlorothiazide 12.5 mg
Benicar HCT 40/12.5—olmesartan 40 mg + hydrochlorothiazide 12.5 mg
Benicar HCT 40/25—olmesartan 40 mg + hydrochlorothiazide 25 mg
BenzaClin Topical Gel—1% clindamycin + 5% benzoyl peroxide
Benzamycin Topical Gel—5% benzoyl peroxide + 3% erythromycin
Bicitra Solution—(per 5 ml) sodium citrate 500 mg + citric acid 334 mg
Bidil—isosorbide dinitrate 20 mg + hydralazine 37.5 mg
Blephamide Ophthalmic Suspension/Ointment—0.2% prednisolone + 10% sodium sulfacetamide
Brevicon—norethindrone 0.5 mg + ethinyl estradiol 35 mcg
Bromfed DM Liquid—(per 5 mL) brompheniramine 2 mg + dextromethorphan 10 mg + pseudoephedrine 30 mg
Bronkaid Dual Action—ephedrine 25 mg + guaifenesin 400 mg (OTC)
Bufferin—aspirin 325 mg + calcium carbonate 158 mg + magnesium oxide 63 mg + magnesium carbonate 34 mg (OTC)
Butapap 50/325—butalbital 50 mg + acetaminophen 325 mg
Butapap 50/650—butalbital 50 mg + acetaminophen 650 mg
Caduet 2.5/10—amlodipine 2.5 mg + atorvastatin 10 mg

Caduet 2.5/20—amlodipine 2.5 mg + atorvastatin 20 mg
Caduet 2.5/40—amlodipine 2.5 mg + atorvastatin 40 mg
Caduet 5/10—amlodipine 5 mg + atorvastatin 10 mg
Caduet 5/20—amlodipine 5 mg + atorvastatin 20 mg
Caduet 5/40—amlodipine 5 mg + atorvastatin 40 mg
Caduet 5/80—amlodipine 5 mg + atorvastatin 80 mg
Caduet 10/10—amlodipine 10 mg + atorvastatin 10 mg
Caduet 10/20—amlodipine 10 mg + atorvastatin 20 mg
Caduet 10/40—amlodipine 10 mg + atorvastatin 40 mg
Caduet 10/80—amlodipine 10 mg + atorvastatin 80 mg
Cafergot—ergotamine 1 mg + caffeine 100 mg
Caltrate 600+D—vitamin D 200 IU + calcium 600 mg (OTC)
Capozide 25/15—captopril 25 mg + hydrochlorothiazide 15 mg
Capozide 25/25—captopril 25 mg + hydrochlorothiazide 25 mg
Capozide 50/15—captopril 50 mg + hydrochlorothiazide 15 mg
Capozide 50/25—captopril 50 mg + hydrochlorothiazide 25 mg
Cesia
  Phase I—desogestrel 0.1 mg + ethinyl estradiol 25 mcg
  Phase II—desogestrel 0.25 mg + ethinyl estradiol 25 mcg
  Phase III—desogestrel 0.15 mg + ethinyl estradiol 25 mcg
Cetacaine Topical Spray—14% benzocaine + 2% tetracaine + 2% butamben + 0.005% cetyl dimethyl ethyl ammonium bromide
Cheracol Cough Syrup—(per 5 mL) codeine 10 mg + guaifenesin 100 mg
Children's Advil Cold Liquid—(per 5 mL) ibuprofen 100 mg + pseudoephedrine 15 mg (OTC)
Chlor-Trimeton 4 Hour Relief—pseudoephedrine 60 mg + chlorpheniramine 4 mg (OTC)
Chlor-Trimeton 12 Hour Relief—pseudoephedrine 120 mg + chlorpheniramine 8 mg (OTC)
Ciprodex Otic Suspension—0.3% ciprofloxacin + 0.1% dexamethasone
Cipro HC Otic Suspension—0.2% ciprofloxacin + 1% hydrocortisone
Clarinex-D 12 Hour—desloratadine 2.5 mg + pseudoephedrine 120 mg
Clarinex-D 24 Hour—desloratadine 5 mg + pseudoephedrine 120 mg
Claritin-D 12 Hour—loratadine 5 mg + pseudoephedrine 120 mg (OTC)
Claritin-D 24-Hour—loratadine 10 mg + pseudoephedrine 240 mg (OTC)
✳ **Clavulin 500**—amoxicillin 500 mg + clavulanic acid 125 mg
✳ **Clavulin 875**—amoxicillin 875 mg + clavulanic acid 125 mg
✳ **Clavulin 125 Suspension**—(per 5 mL) amoxicillin 125 mg + clavulanic acid 31.25 mg
✳ **Clavulin 200 Suspension**—(per 5 mL) amoxicillin 200 mg + clavulanic acid 28.5 mg
✳ **Clavulin 250 Suspension**—(per 5 mL) amoxicillin 250 mg + clavulanic acid 62.5 mg
✳ **Clavulin 400 Suspension**—(per 5 mL) amoxicillin 400 mg + clavulanic acid 57 mg
ClimaraPro Transdermal Patch (release per day)—estradiol 0.045 mg + levonorgestrel 0.015 mg
Clorpres 15/0.1—chlorthalidone 15 mg + clonidine 0.1 mg
Clorpres 15/0.2—chlorthalidone 15 mg + clonidine 0.2 mg
Clorpres 15/0.3—chlorthalidone 15 mg + clonidine 0.3 mg
Co-Gesic—acetaminophen 500 mg + hydrocodone 5 mg
Codimal—pseudoephedrine 30 mg + chlorpheniramine 2 mg + acetaminophen 325 mg (OTC)
Codimal DH Syrup—(per 5 mL) hydrocodone 1.66 mg + phenylephrine 5 mg + pyrilamine 8.33 mg
Codimal DM Syrup—(per 5 mL) phenylephrine 5 mg + pyrilamine 8.33 mg + dextromethorphan 10 mg (OTC)
Codimal-L.A.—chlorpheniramine 8 mg + pseudoephedrine 120 mg
Codimal PH Syrup—(per 5 mL) codeine 10 mg + phenylephrine 5 mg + pyrilamine 8.33 mg
Col-Probenecid—probenecid 500 mg + colchicine 0.5 mg
Coly-Mycin S Otic Suspension—1% hydrocortisone + neomycin base 3.3 mg/mL + colistin 3 mg/mL + 0.05% thonzonium bromide
Colyte—PEG 3350 240 g + sodium sulfate 22.72 g + sodium bicarbonate 6.72 g + sodium chloride 5.84 g + potassium chloride 2.98 g
Combigan Ophthalmic Solution—0.2% brimonidine + 0.5% timolol

CombiPatch 0.05/0.14—estradiol 0.05 mg/day + norethindrone 0.14 mg/day
CombiPatch 0.05/0.25—estradiol 0.05 mg/day + norethindrone 0.25 mg/day
Combivent—(per actuation) ipratropium bromide 18 mcg + albuterol 103 mcg
Combivir—lamivudine 150 mg + zidovudine 300 mg
Combunox—oxycodone 5 mg + ibuprofen 400 mg
Congestac—guaifenesin 400 mg + pseudoephedrine 60 mg (OTC)
Contac Cold & Flu Maximum Strength Caplets—chlorpheniramine 2 mg + phenylephrine 5 mg + acetaminophen 500 mg (OTC)
Contac Cold & Flu Non-Drowsy Maximum Strength Caplets—phenylephrine 5 mg + acetaminophen 500 mg (OTC)
Coricidin HBP Chest Congestion and Cough—dextromethorphan 10 mg + guaifenesin 200 mg (OTC)
Coricidin HBP Cold and Flu—acetaminophen 325 mg + chlorpheniramine 2 mg (OTC)
Coricidin HBP Cough and Cold—chlorpheniramine 4 mg + dextromethorphan 30 mg (OTC)
Coricidin HBP Maximum Strength Flu—acetaminophen 500 mg + chlorpheniramine 2 mg + dextromethorphan 15 mg (OTC)
Cortisporin Otic Solution/Suspension—(per mL) neomycin 3.5 mg + polymyxin B 10,000 units + hydrocortisone 10 mg
Cortisporin Topical Cream—(per g) neomycin 3.5 mg + polymyxin B 10,000 units + hydrocortisone 5 mg
Corzide 40/5—nadolol 40 mg + bendroflumethiazide 5 mg
Corzide 80/5—nadolol 80 mg + bendroflumethiazide 5 mg
Cosopt Ophthalmic Solution—2% dorzolamide + 0.5% timolol
✽ **Coversyl Plus**—perindopril 4 mg + indapamide 1.25 mg
✽ **Coversyl Plus LD**—perindopril 2 mg + indapamide 0.625 mg
Creon—lipase 6000 units + amylase 30,000 units + protease 19,000 units
Creon—lipase 12,000 units + amylase 60,000 units + protease 38,000 units
Creon—lipase 24,000 units + amylase 120,00 units + protease 76,000 units
Cryselle—norgestrel 0.3 mg + ethinyl estradiol 30 mcg
Cyclessa
  Phase I—desogestrel 0.1 mg + ethinyl estradiol 25 mcg
  Phase II—desogestrel 0.125 mg + ethinyl estradiol 25 mcg
  Phase III—desogestrel 0.15 mg + ethinyl estradiol 25 mcg
Cyclomydril Ophthalmic Solution—0.2% cyclopentolate + 1% phenylephrine
Dallergy Caplets—chlorpheniramine 8 mg + phenylephrine 20 mg + methscopolamine 2.5 mg
Dallergy Extended Release—phenylephrine 20 mg + chlorpheniramine 12 mg + methscopolamine 2.5 mg
Dallergy-JR Capsules—phenylephrine 20 mg + chlorpheniramine 4 mg
Dallergy Syrup—(per 5 mL) chlorpheniramine 2 mg + phenylephrine 8 mg + methscopolamine 0.75 mg
Dallergy Tablets—chlorpheniramine 4 mg + phenylephrine 10 mg + methscopolamine 1.25 mg
Damason-P—hydrocodone 5 mg + aspirin 500 mg
Darvocet A500—propoxyphene napsylate 100 mg + acetaminophen 500 mg
Darvocet-N 50—propoxyphene napsylate 50 mg + acetaminophen 325 mg
Darvocet-N 100—propoxyphene napsylate 100 mg + acetaminophen 650 mg
Dayquil Cold & Flu Relief Liquid—(per 5 mL) acetaminophen 325 mg + dextromethorphan 10 mg + phenylephrine 5 mg (OTC)
Dayquil Sinus Liquicaps—acetaminophen 325 mg + phenylephrine 5 mg (OTC)
Deconamine—pseudoephedrine 60 mg + chlorpheniramine 4 mg
Deconamine SR—pseudoephedrine 120 mg + chlorpheniramine 8 mg
Deconamine Syrup—(per 5 mL) pseudoephedrine 30 mg + chlorpheniramine 2 mg
Desogen—ethinyl estradiol 30 mcg + desogestrel 0.15 mg
Difil-G Forte Liquid—(per 5 mL) dyphylline 100 mg + guaifenesin 100 mg
Difil-G Tablets—dyphylline 200 mg + guaifenesin 300 mg
Dilex-G Syrup—(per 5 mL) dyphylline 100 mg + guaifenesin 200 mg
Dilex G Tablets—dyphylline 200 mg + guaifenesin 400 mg

Combination Drugs 1383

Dimetapp Cold & Allergy Elixir—(per 5 mL) phenylephrine 2.5 mg + brompheniramine 1 mg (OTC)
Dimetapp Cough & Cold DM Elixir—(per 5 mL) phenylephrine 2.5 mg + brompheniramine 1 mg + dextromethorphan 5 mg (OTC)
Dimetapp Long-Acting Cough Plus Cold Elixir—(per 5 mL) chlorpheniramine 1 mg + dextromethorphan 7.5 mg (OTC)
Dimetapp Cold & Congestion Elixir—(per 5 mL) diphenhydramine 6.25 mg + phenylephrine 2.5 mg (OTC)
Diovan HCT 80/12.5—valsartan 80 mg + hydrochlorothiazide 12.5 mg
Diovan HCT 160/12.5—valsartan 160 mg + hydrochlorothiazide 12.5 mg
Diovan HCT 160/25—valsartan 160 mg + hydrochlorothiazide 25 mg
Diovan HCT 320/12.5—valsartan 320 mg + hydrochlorothiazide 12.5 mg
Diovan HCT 320/25—valsartan 320 mg + hydrochlorothiazide 25 mg
Donnatal—phenobarbital 16.2 mg + hyoscyamine 0.1037 mg + atropine 0.0194 mg + scopolamine 0.0065 mg
Donnatal Elixir—(per 5 mL) phenobarbital 16.2 mg + hyoscyamine 0.1037 mg + atropine 0.0194 mg + scopolamine 0.0065 mg + 23% alcohol
Donnatal Extentabs—phenobarbital 48.6 mg + hyoscyamine 0.3111 mg + atropine 0.0582 mg + scopolamine 0.0195 mg
Dristan Cold Multi-Symptom Formula—acetaminophen 325 mg + phenylephrine 5 mg + chlorpheniramine 2 mg (OTC)
Duac CS Topical Gel—1% clindamycin + 5% benzoyl peroxide
Duetact 2/30—glimepiride 2 mg + pioglitazone 30 mg
Duetact 4/30—glimepiride 4 mg + pioglitazone 30 mg
DuoNeb—(per 3 mL) albuterol sulfate 2.5 mg + ipratropium bromide 0.5 mg inhalation solution
Dyazide—hydrochlorothiazide 25 mg + triamterene 37.5 mg
Elixophyllin-GG Liquid—(per 15 mL) guaifenesin 100 mg + theophylline 100 mg
Embeda 20/0.8—morphine sulfate 20 mg + naltrexone 0.8 mg
Embeda 30/1.2—morphine sulfate 30 mg + naltrexone 1.2 mg
Embeda 50/2—morphine sulfate 50 mg + naltrexone 2 mg
Embeda 60/2.4—morphine sulfate 60 mg + naltrexone 2.4 mg
Embeda 80/3.2—morphine sulfate 80 mg + naltrexone 3.2 mg
Embeda 100/4—morphine sulfate 100 mg + naltrexone 4 mg
EMLA Topical Cream—2.5% lidocaine + 2.5% prilocaine
Empresse
   Phase I—levonorgestrel 0.05 mg + ethinyl estradiol 30 mcg
   Phase II—levonorgestrel 0.075 mg + ethinyl estradiol 40 mcg
   Phase III—levonorgestrel 0.125 mg + ethinyl estradiol 30 mcg
Endocet 5/325—oxycodone 5 mg + acetaminophen 325 mg
Endocet 7.5/325—oxycodone 7.5 mg + acetaminophen 325 mg
Endocet 7.5/500—oxycodone 7.5 mg + acetaminophen 500 mg
Endocet 10/325—oxycodone 10 mg + acetaminophen 325 mg
Endocet 10/650—oxycodone 10 mg + acetaminophen 650 mg
Endodan—oxycodone 4.88 mg + aspirin 325 mg
Enlon Plus—edrophonium 10 mg/mL + atropine 0.14 mg/mL
Enpresse 28
   Phase I—levonorgestrel 0.05 mg + ethinyl estradiol 30 mcg
   Phase II—levonorgestrel 0.075 mg + ethinyl estradiol 40 mcg
   Phase III—levonorgestrel 0.125 mg + ethinyl estradiol 30 mcg
Epifoam Aerosol Foam—1% hydrocortisone + 1% pramoxine
Epzicom—abacavir 600 mg + lamivudine 300 mg
Esgic—butalbital 50 mg + acetaminophen 325 mg + caffeine 40 mg
Esgic-Plus—butalbital 50 mg + acetaminophen 500 mg + caffeine 40 mg
Estrostep Fe
   Phase I—norethindrone 1 mg + ethinyl estradiol 20 mcg
   Phase II—norethindrone 1 mg + ethinyl estradiol 30 mcg

Phase III—norethindrone 1 mg + ethinyl estradiol 35 mcg
Phase IV—ferrous fumarate 75 mg
Excedrin Back and Body—acetaminophen 250 mg + aspirin 250 mg (OTC)
Excedrin Extra Strength—acetaminophen 250 mg + aspirin 250 mg + caffeine 65 mg (OTC)
Excedrin Migraine—aspirin 250 mg + acetaminophen 250 mg + caffeine 65 mg (OTC)
Excedrin P.M.—acetaminophen 500 mg + diphenhydramine citrate 38 mg (OTC)
Excedrin Sinus Headache—phenylephrine 5 mg + acetaminophen 325 mg (OTC)
Excedrin Tension Headache—acetaminophen 500 mg + caffeine 65 mg (OTC)
Exforge 5/160—amlodipine 5 mg + valsartan 160 mg
Exforge 5/320—amlodipine 5 mg + valsartan 320 mg
Exforge 10/160—amlodipine 10 mg + valsartan 160 mg
Exforge 10/320—amlodipine 10 mg + valsartan 320 mg
Fansidar—sulfidoxine 500 mg + pyrimethamine 25 mg
Femcon Fe—norethindrone 0.4 mg + ethinyl estradiol 35 mcg + ferrous fumarate 75 mg
Femhrt 0.5/2.5—norethindrone 0.5 mg + ethinyl estradiol 2.5 mcg
Femhrt 1/5—norethindrone 1 mg + ethinyl estradiol 5 mcg
Ferro-Sequels—docusate sodium 100 mg + ferrous fumarate 150 mg (OTC)
Fioricet—acetaminophen 325 mg + caffeine 40 mg + butalbital 50 mg
Fioricet with codeine—acetaminophen 325 mg + caffeine 40 mg + butalbital 50 mg + codeine 30 mg
Fiorinal—aspirin 325 mg + caffeine 40 mg + butalbital 50 mg
Fiorinal with codeine—aspirin 325 mg + caffeine 40 mg + butalbital 50 mg + codeine 30 mg
Fosamax Plus D 70/2800—alendronate 70 mg + cholecalciferol 2800 IU
Fosamax Plus D 70/5600—alendronate 70 mg + cholecalciferol 5600 IU
FML-S Ophthalmic Suspension—0.1% fluorometholone + 10% sulfacetamide
Gas-Ban—calcium carbonate 300 mg + simethicone 40 mg (OTC)
Gaviscon Extra Strength—magnesium carbonate 105 mg + aluminum hydroxide 160 mg (OTC)
Gaviscon Extra-Strength Liquid—(per 5 mL) aluminum hydroxide 254 mg + magnesium carbonate 237.5 mg (OTC)
Gaviscon Liquid—(per 5 mL) aluminum hydroxide 31.7 mg + magnesium carbonate 119.3 mg (OTC)
Gaviscon Regular Strength—magnesium trisilicate 14.2 mg + aluminum hydroxide 80 mg (OTC)
Gelusil—aluminum hydroxide 200 mg + magnesium hydroxide 200 mg + simethicone 25 mg (OTC)
Genac Tablets—triprolidine 2.5 mg + pseudoephedrine 60 mg (OTC)
Genatuss DM Syrup—(per 5 mL) guaifenesin 100 mg + dextromethorphan 10 mg (OTC)
Glucovance 1.25/250—glyburide 1.25 mg + metformin 250 mg
Glucovance 2.5/500—glyburide 2.5 mg + metformin 500 mg
Glucovance 5/500—glyburide 5 mg + metformin 500 mg
Golytely—PEG 3350 236 g + sodium sulfate 22.74 g + sodium bicarbonate 6.74 g + sodium chloride 5.86 g + potassium chloride 2.97 g
Golytely Packets—PEG 3350 227.1 g + sodium sulfate 21.5 g + sodium bicarbonate 6.36 g + sodium chloride 5.53 g + potassium chloride 2.82 g
Granulex Topical Aerosol—(per 0.8 mL) trypsin 0.12 mg + Balsam Peru 87 mg + castor oil 788 mg
Guaituss AC Syrup—(per 5 mL) codeine 10 mg + guaifenesin 100 mg
Helidac—bismuth subsalicylate 262.4-mg tablets plus metronidazole 250-mg tablets plus tetracycline 500-mg capsules in a compliance package
Humalog Mix 50/50—insulin lispro protamine suspension 50% + insulin lispro solution 50%
Humalog Mix 75/25—insulin lispro protamine suspension 75% + insulin lispro solution 25%
Hycomine Compound—chlorpheniramine 2 mg + acetaminophen 250 mg + phenylephrine 10 mg + hydrocodone 5 mg + caffeine 30 mg
Hycotuss Expectorant—(per 5 mL) guaifenesin 100 mg + hydrocodone 5 mg + 10% alcohol
Hydromet Syrup—(per 5 mL) hydrocodone 5 mg + homatropine 1.5 mg
Hyzaar 50/12.5—losartan 50 mg + hydrochlorothiazide 12.5 mg
Hyzaar 100/12.5—losartan 100 mg + hydrochlorothiazide 12.5 mg
Hyzaar 100/25—losartan 100 mg + hydrochlorothiazide 25 mg

Ibudone 5/200—hydrocodone 5 mg + ibuprofen 200 mg
Ibudone 10/200—hydrocodone 10 mg + ibuprofen 200 mg
Imodium Multi-Symptom Relief—loperamide 2 mg + simethicone 125 mg (OTC)
Inderide 40/25—propranolol 40 mg + hydrochlorothiazide 25 mg
IsonaRif—isoniazid 150 mg + rifampin 300 mg
Janumet 50/500—sitagliptin 50 mg + metformin 500 mg
Janumet 50/1000—sitagliptin 50 mg + metformin 1000 mg
Jolessa—levonorgestrel 0.15 mg + ethinyl estradiol 30 mcg
Junel 1/20—norethindrone 1 mg + ethinyl estradiol 20 mcg
Junel 1.5/30—norethindrone 1.5 mg + ethinyl estradiol 30 mcg
Junel Fe 1/20—norethindrone 1 mg + ethinyl estradiol 20 mcg with 7 tablets of ferrous fumarate 75 mg per container
Junel Fe 1.5/30—norethindrone 1.5 mg + ethinyl estradiol 30 mcg with 7 tablets of ferrous fumarate 75 mg per container
Kaletra 100/25 capsules—lopinavir 100 mg + ritonavir 25 mg
Kaletra 200/50 capsules—lopinavir 200 mg + ritonavir 50 mg
Kaletra solution—(per mL) lopinavir 80 mg + ritonavir 20 mg
Kariva—desogestrel 0.15 mg + ethinyl estradiol 20 mcg/10 mcg
Kelnor—ethinyl estradiol 35 mcg + ethynodiol 1 mg
Lactinex—mixed culture of *Lactobacillus acidophilus* and *L. bulgaricus* (OTC)
Leena
    Phase I—norethindrone 0.5 mg + ethinyl estradiol 35 mcg
    Phase II—norethindrone 1 mg + ethinyl estradiol 35 mcg
    Phase III—norethindrone 0.5 mg + ethinyl estradiol 35 mcg
Lessina—levonorgestrel 0.1 mg + ethinyl estradiol 20 mcg
Levlen—levonorgestrel 0.15 mg + ethinyl estradiol 30 mcg
Levlite—levonorgestrel 0.1 mg + ethinyl estradiol 20 mcg
Levora—levonorgestrel 0.15 mg + ethinyl estradiol 30 mcg
Librax—chlordiazepoxide 5 mg + clidinium 2.5 mg
Lida-Mantle-HC Topical Cream—0.5% hydrocortisone + 3% lidocaine
Limbitrol 5/12.5—chlordiazepoxide 5 mg + amitriptyline 12.5 mg
Limbitrol DS 10/25—chlordiazepoxide 10 mg + amitriptyline 25 mg
Loestrin 1/20—norethindrone 1 mg + ethinyl estradiol 20 mcg
Loestrin 1.5/30—norethindrone 1.5 mg + ethinyl estradiol 30 mcg
Loestrin Fe 1/20—norethindrone 1 mg + ethinyl estradiol 20 mcg with 7 tablets of ferrous fumarate 75 mg per container
Loestrin Fe 1.5/30—norethindrone 1.5 mg + ethinyl estradiol 30 mcg with 7 tablets of ferrous fumarate 75 mg per container
Lomotil—diphenoxylate 2.5 mg + atropine 0.025 mg
Lomotil Liquid—(per 5 mL) diphenoxylate 2.5 mg + atropine 0.025 mg
Lonox—diphenoxylate 2.5 mg + atropine 0.025 mg
Lo/Ovral—ethinyl estradiol 30 mcg + norgestrel 0.3 mg
Lopressor HCT 50/25—metoprolol tartrate 50 mg + hydrochlorothiazide 25 mg
Lopressor HCT 100/25—metoprolol tartrate 100 mg + hydrochlorothiazide 25 mg
Lopressor HCT 100/50—metoprolol tartrate 100 mg + hydrochlorothiazide 50 mg
Lorcet 10/650—hydrocodone 10 mg + acetaminophen 650 mg
Lorcet-HD—hydrocodone 10 mg + acetaminophen 500 mg
Lorcet Plus—hydrocodone 7.5 mg + acetaminophen 650 mg
Lortab 5/500—hydrocodone 5 mg + acetaminophen 500 mg
Lortab 7.5/500—hydrocodone 7.5 mg + acetaminophen 500 mg
Lortab 10/500—hydrocodone 10 mg + acetaminophen 500 mg
Lortab Elixir—(per 5 mL) hydrocodone 2.5 mg + acetaminophen 167 mg
LoSeasonique—levonorgestrel 0.1 mg + ethinyl estradiol 20 mcg
✤ **Losec 1-2-3 A**—omeprazole 20 mg (14 doses), clarithromycin 500 mg (14 doses), amoxicillin 1 g (14 doses) in a convenience package

✤ **Losec 1-2-3 M**—omeprazole 20 mg (14 doses), clarithromycin 250 mg (14 doses), metronidazole 500 mg (14 doses) in a convenience package
Lotensin HCT 5/6.25—benazepril 5 mg + hydrochlorothiazide 6.25 mg
Lotensin HCT 10/12.5—benazepril 10 mg + hydrochlorothiazide 12.5 mg
Lotensin HCT 20/12.5—benazepril 20 mg + hydrochlorothiazide 12.5 mg
Lotensin HCT 20/25—benazepril 20 mg + hydrochlorothiazide 25 mg
Lotrel 2.5/10—amlodipine 2.5 mg + benazepril 10 mg
Lotrel 5/10—amlodipine 5 mg + benazepril 10 mg
Lotrel 5/20—amlodipine 5 mg + benazepril 20 mg
Lotrel 5/40—amlodipine 5 mg + benazepril 40 mg
Lotrel 10/20—amlodipine 10 mg + benazepril 20 mg
Lotrel 10/40—amlodipine 10 mg + benazepril 40 mg
Lotrisone Topical Cream/Lotion—0.05% betamethasone + 1% clotrimazole
Low-Ogestrel—norgestrel 0.3 mg + ethinyl estradiol 30 mcg
Lufyllin-GG Elixir—(per 15 mL) dyphylline 100 mg + guaifenesin 100 mg
Lufyllin-GG Tablets—dyphylline 200 mg + guaifenesin 200 mg
Lutera—levonorgestrel 0.1 mg + ethinyl estradiol 20 mcg
Lybrel—levonorgestrel 0.09 mg + ethinyl estradiol 20 mcg
Maalox Advanced Maximum Strength Chewables—calcium carbonate 1000 mg + simethicone 60 mg (OTC)
Maalox Advanced Maximum Strength Liquid—(per 5 mL) aluminum hydroxide 400 mg + magnesium hydroxide 400 mg + simethicone 40 mg (OTC)
Maalox Advanced Regular Strength Liquid—(per 5 mL) aluminum hydroxide 200 mg + magnesium hydroxide 200 mg + simethicone 20 mg (OTC)
Magnacet 2.5/400—oxycodone 2.5 mg + acetaminophen 400 mg
Magnacet 5/400—oxycodone 5 mg + acetaminophen 400 mg
Magnacet 7.5/400—oxycodone 7.5 mg + acetaminophen 400 mg
Magnacet 10/400—oxycodone 10 mg + acetaminophen 400 mg
Malarone—atovaquone 250 mg + proguanil 100 mg
Malarone Pediatric—atovaquone 62.5 mg + proguanil 25 mg
Mapap Multi-Symptom Cold—acetaminophen 325 mg + phenylephrine 5 mg + dextromethorphan 10 mg (OTC)
Marvelon—ethinyl estradiol 30 mcg + desogestrel 0.15 mg
Maxitrol Ophthalmic Suspension/Ointment—(per g) neomycin 3.5 mg + 0.1% dexamethasone + polymyxin B 10,000 units
Maxzide—hydrochlorothiazide 50 mg + triamterene 75 mg
Maxzide-25—hydrochlorothiazide 25 mg + triamterene 37.5 mg
Metaglip 2.5/250—glipizide 2.5 mg + metformin 250 mg
Metaglip 2.5/500—glipizide 2.5 mg + metformin 500 mg
Metaglip 5/500—glipizide 5 mg + metformin 500 mg
Micardis HCT 40/12.5—telmisartan 40 mg + hydrochlorothiazide 12.5 mg
Micardis HCT 80/12.5—telmisartan 80 mg + hydrochlorothiazide 12.5 mg
Micardis HCT 80/25—telmisartan 80 mg + hydrochlorothiazide 25 mg
Microgestin 1/20—norethindrone 1 mg + ethinyl estradiol 20 mcg
Microgestin 1.5/30—norethindrone 1.5 mg + ethinyl estradiol 30 mcg
Microgestin Fe 1/20—norethindrone 1 mg + ethinyl estradiol 20 mcg per tablet with 7 tablets of ferrous fumarate 75 mg per container
Microgestin Fe 1.5/30—norethindrone 1.5 mg + ethinyl estradiol 30 mcg per tablet with 7 tablets of ferrous fumarate 75 mg per container
Midol Menstrual Complete—acetaminophen 500 mg + caffeine 60 mg + pyrilamine 15 mg (OTC)
Midol Teen Formula—acetaminophen 500 mg + pamabrom 25 mg (OTC)
Midrin—isometheptene 65 mg + acetaminophen 325 mg + dichloralphenazone 100 mg
Migergot Suppositories—ergotamine 2 mg + caffeine 100 mg
Mircette—desogestrel 0.15 mg + ethinyl estradiol 20 mcg/10 mcg
Modicon—norethindrone 0.5 mg + ethinyl estradiol 35 mcg

Combination Drugs 1387

❖ **Moduret**—amiloride 5 mg + hydrochlorothiazide 50 mg
Mononessa—ethinyl estradiol 35 mcg + norgestimate 0.25 mg
Motofen—difenoxin 1 mg + atropine 0.025 mg
Motrin Children's Cold Suspension—(per 5 mL) ibuprofen 100 mg + pseudoephedrine 15 mg (OTC)
Mucinex Cold Liquid—(per 5 mL) guaifenesin 100 mg + phenylephrine 2.5 mg (OTC)
Mucinex Cough Mini-Melts—guaifenesin 100 mg + dextromethorphan 5 mg (OTC)
Mucinex Cough Liquid—(per 5 mL) guaifenesin 100 mg + dextromethorphan 5 mg (OTC)
Mucinex D—guaifenesin 600 mg + pseudoephedrine 60 mg (OTC)
Mucinex D Maximum Strength—guaifenesin 1200 mg + pseudoephedrine 120 mg (OTC)
Mucinex DM—guaifenesin 600 mg + dextromethorphan 30 mg (OTC)
Mucinex DM Maximum Strength—guaifenesin 1200 mg + dextromethorphan 60 mg (OTC)
Murocoll-2 Ophthalmic Solution—0.3% scopolamine + 10% phenylephrine
Mylanta Regular Strength Liquid—(per 5 mL) aluminum hydroxide 200 mg + magnesium hydroxide 200 mg + simethicone 20 mg (OTC)
Mylanta Maximum Strength Liquid—(per 5 mL) aluminum hydroxide 400 mg + magnesium hydroxide 400 mg + simethicone 40 mg (OTC)
Mylanta Supreme Liquid—(per 5 mL) calcium carbonate 400 mg + magnesium hydroxide 135 mg (OTC)
Mylanta Ultimate Strength Chewables—calcium carbonate 700 mg + magnesium hydroxide 300 mg (OTC)
Mylanta Ultimate Strength Liquid—(per 5 mL) aluminum hydroxide 500 mg + magnesium hydroxide 500 mg (OTC)
Naphcon-A Ophthalmic Solution—0.025% naphazoline + 0.3% pheniramine (OTC)
Nasatab LA—guaifenesin 500 mg + pseudoephedrine 120 mg
Necon 0.5/35—norethindrone 0.5 mg + ethinyl estradiol 35 mcg
Necon 1/35—norethindrone 1 mg + ethinyl estradiol 35 mcg
Necon 7/7/7
  Phase I—norethindrone 0.5 mg + ethinyl estradiol 35 mcg
  Phase II—norethindrone 0.75 mg + ethinyl estradiol 35 mcg
  Phase III—norethindrone 1 mg + ethinyl estradiol 35 mcg
Necon 10/11-28
  Phase I—norethindrone 0.5 mg + ethinyl estradiol 35 mcg
  Phase II—norethindrone 1 mg + ethinyl estradiol 35 mcg
Neosporin Antibiotic Topical Ointment—(per g) neomycin 3.5 mg + bacitracin 400 units + polymyxin B 5000 units (OTC)
Neosporin G.U. Irrigant—(per mL) neomycin 40 mg + polymyxin B 200,000 units
Neosporin Ophthalmic Solution—(per mL) polymyxin B 10,000 units + neomycin 1.75 mg + gramicidin 0.025 mg
Neosporin + Pain Relief Antibiotic Topical Cream—(per g) neomycin 3.5 mg + polymyxin B 10,000 units + pramoxine 10 mg (OTC)
Neosporin + Pain Relief Antibiotic Topical Ointment—(per g) neomycin 3.5 mg + polymyxin B 10,000 units + bacitracin 500 units + pramoxine 10 mg (OTC)
Niferex-150 Forte—ferrous sulfate 150 mg + vitamin B12 25 mcg + folic acid 1 mg
Norco 5/325—hydrocodone 5 mg + acetaminophen 325 mg
Norco 7.5/325—hydrocodone 7.5 mg + acetaminophen 325 mg
Norco 10/325—hydrocodone 10 mg + acetaminophen 325 mg
Nordette—levonorgestrel 0.15 mg + ethinyl estradiol 30 mcg
Norgesic—orphenadrine 25 mg + caffeine 30 mg + aspirin 385 mg
Norgesic Forte—orphenadrine 50 mg + caffeine 60 mg + aspirin 770 mg
Norinyl 1/35—norethindrone 1 mg + ethinyl estradiol 35 mcg
Norinyl 1/50—norethindrone 1 mg + mestranol 50 mcg
Nortrel 0.5/35—norethindrone 0.5 mg + ethinyl estradiol 35 mcg
Nortrel 1/35—norethindrone 1 mg + ethinyl estradiol 35 mcg

Nortrel 7/7/7
  Phase I—norethindrone 0.5 mg + ethinyl estradiol 35 mcg
  Phase II—norethindrone 0.75 mg + ethinyl estradiol 35 mcg
  Phase III—norethindrone 1 mg + ethinyl estradiol 35 mcg
NuLytely—PEG 3350 420 g + sodium bicarbonate 5.72 g + sodium chloride 11.2 g + potassium chloride 1.48 g
Nuvaring—etonogestrel 0.12 mg/day + ethinyl estradiol 15 mcg/day
Nyquil Children's Liquid—(per 15 mL) dextromethorphan 15 mg + chlorpheniramine 2 mg (OTC)
Nyquil Cold & Flu Relief Liquicaps—acetaminophen 325 mg + dextromethorphan 15 mg + doxylamine 6.25 mg (OTC)
Nyquil Cold & Flu Symptom Relief Plus Vitamin C Caplets—acetaminophen 325 mg + dextromethorphan 15 mg + doxylamine 6.25 mg + ascorbic acid 100 mg (OTC)
Nyquil Cold & Flu Relief Liquid—(per 15 mL) acetaminophen 500 mg + dextromethorphan 15 mg + doxylamine 6.25 mg (OTC)
Nyquil Cough Liquid—(per 15 mL) dextromethorphan 15 mg + doxylamine 6.25 mg (OTC)
Nyquil D Liquid—(per 15 mL) acetaminophen 500 mg + dextromethorphan 15 mg + doxylamine 6.25 mg + pseudoephedrine 30 mg (OTC)
Nyquil Less Drowsy Cold & Flu Relief Liquid—(per 15 mL) acetaminophen 325 mg + dextromethorphan 15 mg + chlorpheniramine 2 mg (OTC)
Nyquil Sinus Liquicaps—acetaminophen 325 mg + doxylamine 6.25 mg + phenylephrine 5 mg (OTC)
Ocella—drosperinone 3 mg + ethinyl estradiol 30 mcg
Ogestrel—norgestrel 0.5 mg + ethinyl estradiol 50 mcg
Opcon-A Ophthalmic Solution—0.027% naphazoline + 0.3% pheniramine (OTC)
Optase Topical Gel—(per g) trypsin 0.12 mg + Balsam Peru 87 mg + castor oil 788 mg
Oraqix Periodontal Gel—2.5% lidocaine + 2.5% prilocaine
Ornex—pseudoephedrine 30 mg + acetaminophen 325 mg (OTC)
Ornex Maximum Strength—pseudoephedrine 30 mg + acetaminophen 500 mg (OTC)
Ortho-Cept—ethinyl estradiol 30 mcg + desogestrel 0.15 mg
Ortho-Cyclen—ethinyl estradiol 35 mcg + norgestimate 0.25 mg
Ortho-Evra—norelgestromin 150 mcg/day + ethinyl estradiol 20 mcg/day
Ortho-Novum 1/35—norethindrone 1 mg + ethinyl estradiol 35 mcg
Ortho-Novum 1/50—norethindrone 1 mg + mestranol 50 mcg
Ortho-Novum 10/11–28
  Phase I—norethindrone 0.5 mg + ethinyl estradiol 35 mcg
  Phase II—norethindrone 1 mg + ethinyl estradiol 35 mcg
Ortho-Novum 7/7/7–28
  Phase I—norethindrone 0.5 mg + ethinyl estradiol 35 mcg
  Phase II—norethindrone 0.75 mg + ethinyl estradiol 35 mcg
  Phase III—norethindrone 1 mg + ethinyl estradiol 35 mcg
Ortho-Prefest—estradiol 1 mg (15 tablets) and estradiol 1 mg + norgestimate 0.09 mg (15 tablets) in a 30-tablet blister package
Ortho Tri-Cyclen
  Phase I—norgestimate 0.18 mg + ethinyl estradiol 35 mcg
  Phase II—norgestimate 0.215 mg + ethinyl estradiol 35 mcg
  Phase III—norgestimate 0.25 mg + ethinyl estradiol 35 mcg
Ortho Tri-Cyclen Lo
  Phase I—norgestimate 0.18 mg + ethinyl estradiol 25 mcg
  Phase II—norgestimate 0.215 mg + ethinyl estradiol 25 mcg
  Phase III—norgestimate 0.25 mg + ethinyl estradiol 25 mcg
Ovcon-35—ethinyl estradiol 35 mcg + norethindrone 0.4 mg
Ovcon-50—ethinyl estradiol 50 mcg + norethindrone 1 mg
P-V-Tussin—hydrocodone 5 mg + pseudoephedrine 60 mg
Pamprin Cramp—acetaminophen 250 mg + pamabrom 25 mg + magnesium salicylate 250 mg (OTC)
Pamprin Max—acetaminophen 250 mg + aspirin 250 mg + caffeine 65 mg (OTC)
Pamprin Multi-Symptom—acetaminophen 500 mg + pamabrom 25 mg + pyrilamine 15 mg (OTC)

Combination Drugs 1389

Pancrease MT 4—lipase 4000 units + amylase 12,000 units + protease 12,000 units
Pancrease MT 10—lipase 10,000 units + amylase 30,000 units + protease 30,000 units
Pancrease MT 16—lipase 16,000 units + amylase 48,000 units + protease 48,000 units
Pancrease MT 20—lipase 20,000 units + amylase 56,000 units + protease 44,000 units
Parcopa 10/100—carbidopa 10 mg + levodopa 100 mg
Parcopa 25/100—carbidopa 25 mg + levodopa 100 mg
Parcopa 25/250—carbidopa 25 mg + levodopa 250 mg
Pediacare Children's Allergy & Cold Liquid—(per 5 mL) phenylephrine 5 mg + diphenhydramine 12.5 mg (OTC)
Pediacare Children's Multisymptom Cold Liquid—(per 5 mL) phenylephrine 2.5 mg + dextromethorphan 5 mg (OTC)
Pepcid Complete—calcium carbonate 800 mg + magnesium hydroxide 165 mg + famotidine 10 mg (OTC)
Percocet 2.5/325—oxycodone 2.5 mg + acetaminophen 325 mg
Percocet 5/325—oxycodone 5 mg + acetaminophen 325 mg
Percocet 7.5/325—oxycodone 7.5 mg + acetaminophen 325 mg
Percocet 7.5/500—oxycodone 7.5 mg + acetaminophen 500 mg
Percocet 10/325—oxycodone 10 mg + acetaminophen 325 mg
Percocet 10/650—oxycodone 10 mg + acetaminophen 650 mg
Percodan—oxycodone 4.88 mg + aspirin 325 mg
Percogesic—phenyltoloxamine 30 mg + acetaminophen 325 mg (OTC)
Peri-Colace—docusate sodium 50 mg + sennosides 8.6 mg (OTC)
Phrenilin—butalbital 50 mg + acetaminophen 325 mg
Phrenilin Forte—butalbital 50 mg + acetaminophen 650 mg
Polycitra Syrup—(per 5 mL) potassium citrate 550 mg + sodium citrate 500 mg + citric acid 334 mg
Poly-Hist DM Syrup—(per 5 mL) phenylephrine 7.5 mg + pyrilamine 8.33 mg + dextromethorphan 10 mg
Polysporin Topical Ointment/Powder—(per g) polymyxin B 10,000 units + bacitracin 500 units (OTC)
Polytrim Ophthalmic Solution—(per mL) polymyxin B 10,000 units + trimethoprim 1 mg
Portia—levonorgestrel 0.15 mg + ethinyl estradiol 30 mcg
Pramosone Topical Cream/Lotion/Ointment—1% pramoxine + 1% hydrocortisone
Pramosone Topical Cream/Lotion/Ointment—1% pramoxine + 2.5% hydrocortisone
PrandiMet 1/500—repaglinide 1 mg + metformin 500 mg
PrandiMet 2/500—repaglinide 2 mg + metformin 500 mg
Premphase—conjugated estrogens 0.625 mg + medroxyprogesterone 5 mg (14 tablets) plus conjugated estrogens 0.625 mg (14 tablets) in a compliance package
✤ **Premplus 0.625/2.5**—conjugated estrogens 0.625 mg + medroxyprogesterone 2.5 mg
✤ **Premplus 0.625/5**—conjugated estrogens 0.625 mg + medroxyprogesterone 5 mg
Prempro 0.3/1.5—conjugated estrogens 0.3 mg + medroxyprogesterone 1.5 mg (28 tablets) in a compliance package
Prempro 0.45/1.5—conjugated estrogens 0.45 mg + medroxyprogesterone 1.5 mg (28 tablets) in a compliance package
Prempro 0.625/2.5—conjugated estrogens 0.625 mg + medroxyprogesterone 2.5 mg (28 tablets) in a compliance package
Prempro 0.625/5—conjugated estrogens 0.625 mg + medroxyprogesterone 5 mg (28 tablets) in a compliance package
Previfem—ethinyl estradiol 35 mcg + norgestimate 0.25 mg
Prevpac—amoxicillin 500-mg capsules + clarithromycin 500-mg tablets + lansoprazole 30-mg capsules in a compliance package
Primalev 2.5/300—oxycodone 2.5 mg + acetaminophen 300 mg
Primalev 5/300—oxycodone 5 mg + acetaminophen 300 mg
Primalev 7.5/300—oxycodone 7.5 mg + acetaminophen 300 mg
Primalev 10/300—oxycodone 10 mg + acetaminophen 300 mg

Primatene Tablets—ephedrine 12.5 mg + guaifenesin 200 mg (OTC)
Primaxin 250 mg I.V. For Injection—imipenem 250 mg + cilastatin sodium 250 mg
Primaxin 500 mg I.V. For Injection—imipenem 500 mg + cilastatin sodium 500 mg
Prinzide 10/12.5—lisinopril 10 mg + hydrochlorothiazide 12.5 mg
Prinzide 20/12.5—lisinopril 20 mg + hydrochlorothiazide 12.5 mg
Prinzide 20/25—lisinopril 20 mg + hydrochlorothiazide 25 mg
Proctofoam-HC Rectal Foam—1% hydrocortisone + 1% pramoxine
✽ **Protrin**—trimethoprim 80 mg + sulfamethoxazole 400 mg
✽ **Protrin DF**—trimethoprim 160 mg + sulfamethoxazole 800 mg
Pylera—bismuth subcitrate potassium 140 mg + metronidazole 125 mg + tetracycline 125 mg
Quasense—levonorgestrel 0.15 mg + ethinyl estradiol 30 mcg
Quinaretic 10/12.5—quinapril 10 mg + hydrochlorothiazide 12.5 mg
Quinaretic 20/12.5—quinapril 20 mg + hydrochlorothiazide 12.5 mg
Quinaretic 20/25—quinapril 20 mg + hydrochlorothiazide 25 mg
Rebetron—interferon alfa-2b (Intron A) + oral ribavirin (Rebetrol) 200 mg
Reclipsen—desogestrel 0.15 mg + ethinyl estradiol 30 mcg
Reprexain 2.5/200—hydrocodone 2.5 mg + ibuprofen 200 mg
Reprexain 5/200—hydrocodone 5 mg + ibuprofen 200 mg
Reprexain 7.5/200—hydrocodone 7.5 mg + ibuprofen 200 mg
Reprexain 10/200—hydrocodone 10 mg + ibuprofen 200 mg
Respahist—pseudoephedrine 60 mg + brompheniramine 6 mg
Respaire-60 SR—guaifenesin 200 mg + pseudoephedrine 60 mg
Respaire-120 SR—guaifenesin 250 mg + pseudoephedrine 120 mg
RID Maximum Strength Shampoo—0.33% pyrethrins + 4% piperonyl butoxide (OTC)
Rifamate—isoniazid 150 mg + rifampin 300 mg
Rifater—rifampin 120 mg + isoniazid 50 mg + pyrazinamide 300 mg
✽ **Robaxacet-8**—methocarbamol 400 mg + acetaminophen 325 mg + codeine 8 mg
✽ **Robaxacet**—methocarbamol 400 mg + acetaminophen 325 mg
✽ **Robaxacet Extra Strength**—methocarbamol 400 mg + acetaminophen 500 mg
Robitussin Children's Cough & Cold CF Liquid—(per 5 mL) guaifenesin 50 mg + phenylephrine 2.5 mg + dextromethorphan 5 mg (OTC)
Robitussin Children's Cough & Cold Long-Acting Liquid—(per 5 mL) chlorpheniramine 1 mg + dextromethorphan 7.5 mg (OTC)
Robitussin Cough & Cold CF Liquid—(per 5 mL) guaifenesin 100 mg + phenylephrine 5 mg + dextromethorphan 10 mg (OTC)
Robitussin Cough & Cold D Liquid—(per 5 mL) pseudoephedrine 30 mg + guaifenesin 200 mg + dextromethorphan 15 mg (OTC)
Robitussin Cough & Cold Long-Acting Liquid—(per 5 mL) chlorpheniramine 2 mg + dextromethorphan 15 mg (OTC)
Robitussin Cough & Chest Congestion DM Liquid—(per 5 mL) guaifenesin 100 mg + dextromethorphan 10 mg (OTC)
Robitussin Cough & Chest Congestion DM Max Liquid—(per 5 mL) guaifenesin 200 mg + dextromethorphan 10 mg (OTC)
Robitussin Cough, Cold & Flu Liquid—(per 5 mL) acetaminophen 160 mg + chlorpheniramine 1 mg + phenylephrine 2.5 mg + dextromethorphan 5 mg (OTC)
Robitussin Nighttime Cough & Cold Liquid—(per 5 mL) phenylephrine 2.5 mg + diphenhydramine 6.25 mg (OTC)
Rolaids Extra Strength Tablets—calcium carbonate 675 mg + magnesium hydroxide 135 mg (OTC)
Rolaids Multi-Symptom Tablets—calcium carbonate 675 mg + magnesium hydroxide 135 mg + simethicone 60 mg (OTC)
Rolaids Regular Tablets—calcium carbonate 550 mg + magnesium hydroxide 110 mg (OTC)
Rondec DM Drops—(per 1 mL) phenylephrine 3.5 mg + chlorpheniramine 1 mg + dextromethorphan 3 mg
Rondec DM Syrup—(per 5 mL) phenylephrine 12.5 mg + chlorpheniramine 4 mg + dextromethorphan 15 mg

Combination Drugs 1391

Rondec Oral Drops—(per 1 mL) phenylephrine 3.5 mg + chlorpheniramine 1 mg
Rondec Syrup—(per 5 mL) chlorpheniramine 4 mg + phenylephrine 12.5 mg
Roxicet 5/500—oxycodone 5 mg + acetaminophen 500 mg
Roxicet—oxycodone 5 mg + acetaminophen 325 mg
Roxicet Oral Solution—(per 5 mL) acetaminophen 325 mg + oxycodone 5 mg
Ru-Tuss DM Syrup—(per 5 mL) guaifenesin 100 mg + pseudoephedrine 45 mg + dextromethorphan 15 mg (OTC)
Rynatan—phenylephrine 25 mg + chlorpheniramine 9 mg
Rynatan Pediatric Suspension—(per 5 mL) phenylephrine 5 mg + chlorpheniramine 4.5 mg
Rynatuss—ephedrine 10 mg + carbetapentane 60 mg + chlorpheniramine 5 mg + phenylephrine 10 mg
Scot-Tussin DM Maximum Strength Liquid—(per 5 mL) chlorpheniramine 2 mg + dextromethorphan 15 mg (OTC)
Scot-Tussin Original Liquid—(per 5 mL) phenylephrine 4 mg + pheniramine 13 mg + sodium salicylate 83 mg + caffeine citrate 25 mg (OTC)
Scot-Tussin Senior Liquid—(per 5 mL) guaifenesin 200 mg + dextromethorphan 15 mg (OTC)
Seasonale—levonorgestrel 0.15 mg + ethinyl estradiol 30 mcg
Seasonique—levonorgestrel 0.15 mg + ethinyl estradiol 30 mcg/10 mcg
Sedapap—acetaminophen 650 mg + butalbital 50 mg
Semprex-D—acrivastine 8 mg + pseudoephedrine 60 mg
Senokot-S—sennosides 8.6 mg + docusate sodium 50 mg (OTC)
Seno Sol-SS—sennosides 8.6 mg + docusate sodium 50 mg (OTC)
Septra—trimethoprim 80 mg + sulfamethoxazole 400 mg
Septra DS—trimethoprim 160 mg + sulfamethoxazole 800 mg
Silafed Syrup—(per 5 mL) pseudoephedrine 30 mg + triprolidine 1.25 mg (OTC)
Simcor 500/20—niacin 500 mg + simvastatin 20 mg
Simcor 750/20—niacin 750 mg + simvastatin 20 mg
Simcor 1000/20—niacin 1000 mg + simvastatin 20 mg
Sinemet 10/100—carbidopa 10 mg + levodopa 100 mg
Sinemet 25/100—carbidopa 25 mg + levodopa 100 mg
Sinemet 25/250—carbidopa 25 mg + levodopa 250 mg
Sinemet CR 25-100—carbidopa 25 mg + levodopa 100 mg
Sinemet CR 50-200—carbidopa 50 mg + levodopa 200 mg
Sine-Off Severe Cold—phenylephrine 5 mg + acetaminophen 325 mg + guaifenesin 200 mg (OTC)
Sine-Off Non-Drowsy Maximum Strength—phenylephrine 5 mg + acetaminophen 500 mg (OTC)
Sine-Off Sinus/Cold Medicine—phenylephrine 5 mg + chlorpheniramine 2 mg + acetaminophen 500 mg (OTC)
Solage Topical Liquid—2% mequinol + 0.01% tretinoin
Solia—desogestrel 0.15 mg + ethinyl estradiol 30 mcg
Soma Compound—aspirin 325 mg + carisoprodol 200 mg
Sprintec—norgestimate 0.25 mg + ethinyl estradiol 35 mcg
Sronyx—levonorgestrel 0.1 mg + ethinyl estradiol 20 mcg
Stalevo 50—carbidopa 12.5 mg + entacapone 200 mg + levodopa 50 mg
Stalevo 75—carbidopa 12.5 mg + entacapone 200 mg + levodopa 75 mg
Stalevo 100—carbidopa 25 mg + entacapone 200 mg + levodopa 100 mg
Stalevo 125—carbidopa 25 mg + entacapone 200 mg + levodopa 125 mg
Stalevo 150—carbidopa 37.5 mg + entacapone 200 mg + levodopa 150 mg
Stalevo 200—carbidopa 25 mg + entacapone 200 mg + levodopa 200 mg
Suboxone N2—buprenorphine 2 mg + naloxone 0.5 mg
Suboxone N8—buprenorphine 8 mg + naloxone 2 mg
Sudafed PE Children's Cough & Cold Liquid—(per 5 mL) dextromethorphan 5 mg + phenylephrine 2.5 mg (OTC)
Sudafed PE Cough & Cold—phenylephrine 5 mg + guaifenesin 100 mg + acetaminophen 325 mg + dextromethorphan 10 mg (OTC)

Sudafed PE Nighttime Cold—phenylephrine 5 mg + diphenhydramine 25 mg + acetaminophen 325 mg (OTC)
Sudafed PE Non-Drying Sinus—guaifenesin 200 mg + pseudoephedrine 30 mg (OTC)
Sudafed PE Severe Cold Formula—phenylephrine 5 mg + diphenhydramine 12.5 mg + acetaminophen 325 mg (OTC)
Sudafed PE Sinus & Allergy—phenylephrine 10 mg + chlorpheniramine 4 mg (OTC)
Sudafed PE Sinus Headache—phenylephrine 5 mg + acetaminophen 325 mg (OTC)
Sudafed PE Triple Action—phenylephrine 5 mg + guaifenesin 200 mg + acetaminophen 325 mg (OTC)
Sudafed Sinus & Pain 12 Hour—pseudoephedrine 120 mg + naproxen 220 mg (OTC)
Sudafed Sinus Liquicaps—guaifenesin 200 mg + pseudoephedrine 30 mg (OTC)
Sudafed Triple Action—pseudoephedrine 30 mg + guaifenesin 200 mg + acetaminophen 325 mg (OTC)
Sudal 12—pseudoephedrine 30 mg + chlorpheniramine 4 mg
Sulfacet-R Topical Lotion—10% sodium sulfacetamide + 5% sulfur
Symbicort 80/4.5—(per actuation) budesonide 80 mcg + formoterol 4.5 mcg
Symbicort 160/4.5—(per actuation) budesonide 160 mcg + formoterol 4.5 mcg
Symbyax 3/25—olanzapine 3 mg + fluoxetine 25 mg
Symbyax 6/25—olanzapine 6 mg + fluoxetine 25 mg
Symbyax 6/50—olanzapine 6 mg + fluoxetine 50 mg
Symbyax 12/25—olanzapine 12 mg + fluoxetine 25 mg
Symbyax 12/50—olanzapine 12 mg + fluoxetine 50 mg
Synalgos-DC—aspirin 356.4 mg + caffeine 30 mg + dihydrocodeine 16 mg
Synercid Powder for Injection—quinupristin 150 mg + dalfopristin 350 mg
Taclonex Topical Ointment/Suspension—0.005% calcipotriene + 0.064% betamethasone
Talacen—acetaminophen 650 mg + pentazocine 25 mg
Talwin NX—pentazocine 50 mg + naloxone 0.5 mg
Tarka 1/240—trandolapril 1 mg (immediate release) + verapamil 240 mg (sustained release)
Tarka 2/180—trandolapril 2 mg (immediate release) + verapamil 180 mg (sustained release)
Tarka 2/240—trandolapril 2 mg (immediate release) + verapamil 240 mg (sustained release)
Tarka 4/240—trandolapril 4 mg (immediate release) + verapamil 240 mg (sustained release)
✤ **Tazocin for Injection 2.25 g**—piperacillin 2 g + tazobactam 0.25 g
✤ **Tazocin for Injection 3.375 g**—piperacillin 3 g + tazobactam 0.375 g
✤ **Tazocin for Injection 4.5 g**—piperacillin 4 g + tazobactam 0.5 g
Tekturna HCT 150/12.5—aliskiren 150 mg + hydrochlorothiazide 12.5 mg
Tekturna HCT 150/25—aliskiren 150 mg + hydrochlorothiazide 25 mg
Tekturna HCT 300/12.5—aliskiren 300 mg + hydrochlorothiazide 12.5 mg
Tekturna HCT 300/25—aliskiren 300 mg + hydrochlorothiazide 25 mg
Tenoretic 50—chlorthalidone 25 mg + atenolol 50 mg
Tenoretic 100—chlorthalidone 25 mg + atenolol 100 mg
Terra-Cortril Ophthalmic Suspension—1.5% hydrocortisone acetate + 0.5% oxytetracycline
Terramycin with Polymyxin B Sulfate Ophthalmic Ointment—(per g) polymyxin B 10,000 units + oxytetracycline 5 mg
Teveten HCT 600/12.5—eprosartan 600 mg + hydrochlorothiazide 12.5 mg
Teveten HCT 600/25—eprosartan 600 mg + hydrochlorothiazide 25 mg
Thera-Flu Cold & Cough Hot Liquid—(per packet) phenylephrine 10 mg + dextromethorphan 20 mg + pheniramine 20 mg (OTC)
Thera-Flu, Cold & Sore Throat Hot Liquid—(per packet) phenylephrine 10 mg + pheniramine 20 mg + acetaminophen 325 mg (OTC)
Thera-Flu Daytime Severe Cold & Cough Caplets—phenylephrine 5 mg + dextromethorphan 10 mg + acetaminophen 325 mg (OTC)
Thera-Flu Daytime Severe Cold & Cough Hot Liquid—(per packet) acetaminophen 650 mg + phenylephrine 10 mg + dextromethorphan 20 mg (OTC)
Thera-Flu Flu & Chest Congestion Hot Liquid—(per packet) guaifenesin 400 mg acetaminophen 650 mg (OTC)

Combination Drugs

Thera-Flu Flu & Sore Throat Hot Liquid—(per packet) phenylephrine 10 mg + pheniramine 20 mg + acetaminophen 650 mg (OTC)
Thera-Flu Nighttime Severe Cold & Cough Caplets—phenylephrine 5 mg + dextromethorphan 10 mg + chlorpheniramine 2 mg + acetaminophen 325 mg (OTC)
Thera-Flu Nighttime Severe Cold & Cough Hot Liquid—(per packet) phenylephrine 10 mg + diphenhydramine 25 mg + acetaminophen 650 mg (OTC)
Thera-Flu Warming Relief Cold & Chest Congestion Syrup—(per 15 mL) guaifenesin 200 mg + acetaminophen 325 mg + phenylephrine 5 mg (OTC)
Thera-Flu Warming Relief Daytime Severe Cough & Cold Syrup—(per 15 mL) phenylephrine 5 mg + dextromethorphan 10 mg + acetaminophen 325 mg (OTC)
Thera-Flu Warming Relief Flu & Sore Throat Syrup—(per 15 mL) phenylephrine 5 mg + diphenhydramine 12.5 mg + acetaminophen 325 mg (OTC)
Thera-Flu Warming Relief Nighttime Severe Cold & Cough Syrup—(per 15 mL) phenylephrine 5 mg + diphenhydramine 12.5 mg + acetaminophen 325 mg (OTC)
Tilia Fe
  Phase I—norethindrone 1 mg + ethinyl estradiol 20 mcg
  Phase II—norethindrone 1 mg + ethinyl estradiol 30 mcg
  Phase III—norethindrone 1 mg + ethinyl estradiol 35 mcg
  Phase IV—ferrous fumarate 75 mg
Timentin for Injection—ticarcillin 3 g + clavulanic acid 0.1 g
Titralac Plus—calcium carbonate 420 mg + simethicone 21 mg (OTC)
TobraDex Ophthalmic Suspension/Ointment—0.1% dexamethasone + 0.3% tobramycin
Treximet—sumatriptan 85 mg + naproxen 500 mg
Triacin-C Cough Syrup—(per 5 mL) codeine 10 mg + pseudoephedrine 30 mg + triprolidine 1.25 mg
Tri—Legest Fe
  Phase I—norethindrone 1 mg + ethinyl estradiol 20 mcg
  Phase II—norethindrone 1 mg + ethinyl estradiol 30 mcg
  Phase III—norethindrone 1 mg + ethinyl estradiol 35 mcg
  Phase IV—ferrous fumarate 75 mg
Tri-Levlen
  Phase I—levonorgestrel 0.05 mg + ethinyl estradiol 30 mcg
  Phase II—levonorgestrel 0.075 mg + ethinyl estradiol 40 mcg
  Phase III—levonorgestrel 0.125 mg + ethinyl estradiol 30 mcg
Triaminic Chest & Nasal Congestion Liquid—(per 5 mL) guaifenesin 50 mg + phenylephrine 2.5 mg (OTC)
Triaminic Cold & Allergy Liquid—(per 5 mL) chlorpheniramine 1 mg + phenylephrine 2.5 mg (OTC)
Triaminic Cough & Sore Throat Liquid—(per 5 mL) acetaminophen 160 mg + dextromethorphan 5 mg (OTC)
Triaminic–D Multi-Symptom Cold Liquid—(per 5 mL) pseudoephedrine 15 mg + dextromethorphan 7.5 mg + chlorpheniramine 1 mg (OTC)
Triaminic Day Time Cold & Cough Liquid—(per 5 mL) phenylephrine 2.5 mg + dextromethorphan 5 mg (OTC)
Triaminic Day Time Thin Strips Cold & Cough—phenylephrine 2.5 mg + dextromethorphan 5 mg (OTC)
Triaminic Multi-Symptom Fever Liquid—(per 5 mL) acetaminophen 160 mg + dextromethorphan 7.5 mg + chlorpheniramine 1 mg (OTC)
Triaminic Night Time Cold & Cough Liquid—(per 5 mL) phenylephrine 2.5 mg + diphenhydramine 6.25 mg (OTC)
Triaminic Night Time Thin Strips Cold & Cough—phenylephrine 5 mg + diphenhydramine 12.5 mg (OTC)
Triaminic Softchews Cough & Runny Nose—chlorpheniramine 1 mg + dextromethorphan 5 mg (OTC)
Triaminic Softchews Cough & Sore Throat—acetaminophen 160 mg + dextromethorphan 5 mg (OTC)

Tri-Lo-Sprintec
  Phase I—norgestimate 0.18 mg + ethinyl estradiol 25 mcg
  Phase II—norgestimate 0.215 mg + ethinyl estradiol 25 mcg
  Phase III—norgestimate 0.25 mg + ethinyl estradiol 25 mcg
Tri-Luma Topical Cream—0.01% fluocinolone + 4% hydroquinone + 0.05% tretinoin
TriLyte—PEG 3350 420 g + sodium bicarbonate 5.72 g + sodium chloride 11.2 g + potassium chloride 1.48 g
TriNessa
  Phase I—norgestimate 0.18 mg + ethinyl estradiol 35 mcg
  Phase II—norgestimate 0.215 mg + ethinyl estradiol 35 mcg
  Phase III—norgestimate 0.25 mg + ethinyl estradiol 35 mcg
Tri-Norinyl
  Phase I—norethindrone 0.5 mg + ethinyl estradiol 35 mcg
  Phase I—norethindrone 1 mg + ethinyl estradiol 35 mcg
  Phase I—norethindrone 0.5 mg + ethinyl·estradiol 35 mcg
Triphasil
  Phase I—levonorgestrel 0.05 mg + ethinyl estradiol 30 mcg
  Phase II—levonorgestrel 0.075 mg + ethinyl estradiol 40 mcg
  Phase III—levonorgestrel 0.125 mg + ethinyl estradiol 30 mcg
Tri-Previfem
  Phase I—norgestimate 0.18 mg + ethinyl estradiol 35 mcg
  Phase I—norgestimate 0.215 mg + ethinyl estradiol 35 mcg
  Phase I—norgestimate 0.25 mg + ethinyl estradiol 35 mcg
Tri-Sprintec
  Phase I—norgestimate 0.18 mg + ethinyl estradiol 35 mcg
  Phase I—norgestimate 0.215 mg + ethinyl estradiol 35 mcg
  Phase I—norgestimate 0.25 mg + ethinyl estradiol 35 mcg
✽ **Trisulfa**—trimethoprim 80 mg + sulfamethoxazole 400 mg
✽ **Trisulfa DS**—trimethoprim 160 mg + sulfamethoxazole 800 mg
Trivora
  Phase I—levonorgestrel 0.05 mg + ethinyl estradiol 30 mcg
  Phase II—levonorgestrel 0.075 mg + ethinyl estradiol 40 mcg
  Phase III—levonorgestrel 0.125 mg + ethinyl estradiol 30 mcg
Trizivir—abacavir 300 mg + lamivudine 150 mg + zidovudine 300 mg
Truvada—emtricitabine 200 mg + tenofovir 300 mg
TussiCaps 5/4—hydrocodone 5 mg + chlorpheniramine 4 mg
TussiCaps 10/8—hydrocodone 10 mg + chlorpheniramine 8 mg
Tussigon—hydrocodone 5 mg + homatropine 1.5 mg
Tussionex Suspension—(per 5 mL) chlorpheniramine 8 mg + hydrocodone 10 mg
Tussi-Organidin NR Liquid—(per 5 mL) codeine 10 mg + guaifenesin 300 mg
Tussi-Organidin DM NR Liquid—(per 5 mL) guaifenesin 300 mg + dextromethorphan 10 mg
Tylenol Allergy Multisymptom Gelcaps—acetaminophen 325 mg + chlorpheniramine 2 mg + phenylephrine 5 mg (**OTC**)
Tylenol Allergy Multisymptom Nighttime Caplets—acetaminophen 325 mg + diphenhydramine 25 mg + phenylephrine 5 mg (**OTC**)
Tylenol Children's Plus Cold & Allergy Liquid—(per 5 mL) acetaminophen 160 mg + diphenhydramine 12.5 mg + phenylephrine 2.5 mg (**OTC**)
Tylenol Children's Plus Cold & Cough Liquid—(per 5 mL) acetaminophen 160 mg + dextromethorphan 5 mg + phenylephrine 2.5 mg (**OTC**)
Tylenol Children's Plus Cold & Stuffy Nose Liquid—(per 5 mL) acetaminophen 160 mg + phenylephrine 2.5 mg (**OTC**)
Tylenol Children's Plus Cold Liquid—(per 5 mL) acetaminophen 160 mg + chlorpheniramine 1 mg + phenylephrine 2.5 mg (**OTC**)
Tylenol Children's Plus Cough & Runny Nose Liquid—(per 5 mL) acetaminophen 160 mg + chlorpheniramine 1 mg + dextromethorphan 5 mg (**OTC**)

Combination Drugs 1395

Tylenol Children's Plus Cough & Sore Throat Liquid—(per 5 mL) acetaminophen 160 mg + dextromethorphan 5 mg (OTC)
Tylenol Children's Plus Flu Liquid—(per 5 mL) acetaminophen 160 mg + chlorpheniramine 1 mg + dextromethorphan 5 mg + phenylephrine 2.5 mg (OTC)
Tylenol Children's Plus Multi-Symptom Cold Liquid—(per 5 mL) acetaminophen 160 mg + dextromethorphan 5 mg + chlorpheniramine 1 mg + phenylephrine 2.5 mg (OTC)
Tylenol Cold Head Congestion Daytime Caplets—acetaminophen 325 mg + phenylephrine 5 mg + dextromethorphan 10 mg (OTC)
Tylenol Cold Head Congestion Nighttime Caplets—acetaminophen 325 mg + phenylephrine 5 mg + dextromethorphan 10 mg + chlorpheniramine 2 mg (OTC)
Tylenol Cold Head Congestion Severe Caplets—acetaminophen 325 mg + phenylephrine 5 mg + dextromethorphan 10 mg + guaifenesin 200 mg (OTC)
Tylenol Cold Multi-Symptom Daytime Caplets—acetaminophen 325 mg + phenylephrine 5 mg + dextromethorphan 10 mg (OTC)
Tylenol Cold Multi-Symptom Daytime Liquid—(per 15 mL) acetaminophen 325 mg + phenylephrine 5 mg + dextromethorphan 10 mg (OTC)
Tylenol Cold Multi-Symptom Nighttime Caplets—acetaminophen 325 mg + phenylephrine 5 mg + dextromethorphan 10 mg + chlorpheniramine 2 mg (OTC)
Tylenol Cold Multi-Symptom Nighttime Liquid—(per 15 mL) acetaminophen 325 mg + phenylephrine 5 mg + dextromethorphan 10 mg + doxylamine 6.25 mg (OTC)
Tylenol Cold Multi-Symptom Severe Caplets—acetaminophen 325 mg + guaifenesin 200 mg + phenylephrine 5 mg + dextromethorphan 10 mg (OTC)
Tylenol Cold Multi-Symptom Severe Liquid—(per 15 mL) acetaminophen 325 mg + guaifenesin 200 mg + phenylephrine 5 mg + dextromethorphan 10 mg (OTC)
Tylenol Cold Severe Congestion Daytime Caplets—acetaminophen 325 mg + pseudoephedrine 30 mg + dextromethorphan 15 mg + guaifenesin 200 mg (OTC)
Tylenol Cough & Severe Congestion Daytime Liquid—(per 15 mL) acetaminophen 325 mg + phenylephrine 5 mg + dextromethorphan 10 mg + guaifenesin 200 mg (OTC)
Tylenol Cough & Sore Throat Daytime Liquid—(per 15 mL) acetaminophen 500 mg + dextromethorphan 15 mg (OTC)
Tylenol Cough & Sore Throat Nighttime Liquid—(per 15 mL) acetaminophen 500 mg + dextromethorphan 15 mg + doxylamine 6.25 mg (OTC)
Tylenol PM—acetaminophen 500 mg + diphenhydramine 25 mg (OTC)
Tylenol Severe Allergy Caplets—diphenhydramine 12.5 mg + acetaminophen 500 mg (OTC)
Tylenol Sinus Congestion & Pain Daytime Gelcaps—acetaminophen 325 mg + phenylephrine 5 mg (OTC)
Tylenol Sinus Congestion & Pain Nighttime Caplets—acetaminophen 325 mg + chlorpheniramine 2 mg + phenylephrine 5 mg (OTC)
Tylenol Sinus Congestion & Pain Severe Caplets—acetaminophen 325 mg + guaifenesin 200 mg + phenylephrine 5 mg (OTC)
Tylenol Sinus Severe Congestion Daytime Caplets—acetaminophen 325 mg + guaifenesin 200 mg + pseudoephedrine 30 mg (OTC)
Tylenol with codeine No. 3—acetaminophen 300 mg + codeine 30 mg
Tylenol with codeine No. 4—acetaminophen 300 mg + codeine 60 mg
Tylox 5/500—oxycodone 5 mg + acetaminophen 500 mg
Ultracet—tramadol 37.5 mg + acetaminophen 325 mg
Unasyn for Injection 1.5 g—ampicillin 1 g + sulbactam 0.5 g
Unasyn for Injection 3 g—ampicillin 2 g + sulbactam 1 g
Uniretic 7.5/12.5—moexipril 7.5 mg + hydrochlorothiazide 12.5 mg
Uniretic 15/12.5—moexipril 15 mg + hydrochlorothiazide 12.5 mg
Uniretic 15/25—moexipril 15 mg + hydrochlorothiazide 25 mg
Valturna 150/160—aliskiren 150 mg + valsartan 160 mg
Valturna 300/320—aliskiren 300 mg + valsartan 320 mg
Vanoxide HC Lotion—0.5% hydrocortisone + 5% benzoyl peroxide 320 mg

Vanquish Extra Strength Pain Reliever—aspirin 227 mg + acetaminophen 194 mg + caffeine 33 mg (OTC)
Vaseretic 5/12.5—enalapril 5 mg + hydrochlorothiazide 12.5 mg
Vaseretic 10/25—enalapril 10 mg + hydrochlorothiazide 25 mg
Vasocidin Ophthalmic Solution—0.23% prednisolone + 10% sulfacetamide
Vasocon-A Ophthalmic Solution—0.05% naphazoline + 0.5% antazoline (OTC)
Velivet
  Phase I—desogestrel 0.1 mg + ethinyl estradiol 25 mcg
  Phase II—desogestrel 0.125 mg + ethinyl estradiol 25 mcg
  Phase III—desogestrel 0.15 mg + ethinyl estradiol 25 mcg
Vicks 44 Custom Care Chesty Cough Liquid—(per 15 mL) guaifenesin 200 mg + dextromethorphan 20 mg (OTC)
Vicks 44 Custom Care Congestion Liquid—(per 15 mL) phenylephrine 10 mg + dextromethorphan 20 mg (OTC)
Vicks 44 Custom Care Cough & Cold PM Liquid—(per 15 mL) acetaminophen 650 mg + dextromethorphan 30 mg + chlorpheniramine 4 mg (OTC)
Vicks Pediatric Formula 44E Cough & Chest Congestion Relief Liquid—(per 15 mL) dextromethorphan 10 mg + guaifenesin 100 mg (OTC)
Vicks Pediatric Formula 44M Cough & Cold Relief Liquid—(per 15 mL) chlorpheniramine 2 mg + dextromethorphan 15 mg (OTC)
Vicodin—hydrocodone 5 mg + acetaminophen 500 mg
Vicodin ES—hydrocodone 7.5 mg + acetaminophen 750 mg
Vicodin HP—hydrocodone 10 mg + acetaminophen 660 mg
Vicoprofen— hydrocodone 7.5 mg + ibuprofen 200 mg
Visine-A Ophthalmic Solution—0.025% naphazoline + 0.3% pheniramine (OTC)
Vusion Topical Ointment—0.25% miconazole + 15% zinc oxide
Vytorin 10/10—ezetimibe 10 mg + simvastatin 10 mg
Vytorin 10/20—ezetimibe 10 mg + simvastatin 20 mg
Vytorin 10/40—ezetimibe 10 mg + simvastatin 40 mg
Vytorin 10/80—ezetimibe 10 mg + simvastatin 80 mg
Xenaderm Topical Ointment—(per g) trypsin 90 USP units + Balsam Peru 87 mg + castor oil 788 mg
Yasmin—drosperinone 3 mg + ethinyl estradiol 30 mcg
Yaz—drosperinone 3 mg + ethinyl estradiol 20 mcg
Zenchent—norethindrone 0.4 mg + ethinyl estradiol 35 mcg
Zestoretic 10/12.5—lisinopril 10 mg + hydrochlorothiazide 12.5 mg
Zestoretic 20/12.5—lisinopril 20 mg + hydrochlorothiazide 12.5 mg
Zestoretic 20/25—lisinopril 20 mg + hydrochlorothiazide 25 mg
Ziac 2.5/6.25—bisoprolol 2.5 mg + hydrochlorothiazide 6.25 mg
Ziac 5/6.25—bisoprolol 5 mg + hydrochlorothiazide 6.25 mg
Ziac 10/6.25—bisoprolol 10 mg + hydrochlorothiazide 6.25 mg
Ziana Topical Gel—1.2% clindamycin + 0.025% tretinoin
Zosyn for Injection 2.25 g—piperacillin 2 g + tazobactam 0.25 g
Zosyn for Injection 3.375 g—piperacillin 3 g + tazobactam 0.375 g
Zosyn for Injection 4.5 g—piperacillin 4 g + tazobactam 0.5 g
Zovia 1/35—ethynodiol 1 mg + ethinyl estradiol 35 mcg
Zovia 1/50—ethynodiol 1 mg + ethinyl estradiol 50 mcg
Zydone 5/400—hydrocodone 5 mg + acetaminophen 400 mg
Zydone 7.5/400—hydrocodone 7.5 mg + acetaminophen 400 mg
Zydone 10/400—hydrocodone 10 mg + acetaminophen 400 mg
Zylet Ophthalmic Suspension—0.5% loteprednol + 0.3% tobramycin
Zyrtec-D Allergy & Congestion—cetirizine 5 mg + pseudoephedrine 120 mg (OTC)

APPENDIX C
Ophthalmic Medications

General Info: See Appendix D for administration techniques for ophthalmic agents.
Consult health care professional regarding:
Concurrent use of contact lenses (medication or additives may be absorbed by the lens).
Concurrent administration of other ophthalmic agents (order and spacing may be important).
ADRs = adverse reactions.

DRUG NAME	DOSE	NOTES

Anesthetics

Uses: Provide brief local anesthesia to allow measurement of intraocular pressure, removal of foreign bodies, or other superficial procedures.
CAUTIONS: Repeated use may result in increased risk of CNS and cardiovascular toxicity; cross-sensitivity with some local anesthetics may occur.

Drug	Dose	Notes
proparacaine (Alcaine, Ophthaine, Ophthetic, Paracaine, ✺ Diocaine)	**Adults and children:** 1–2 drops of 0.5% solution (single dose)	• Does not interact with ophthalmic cholinesterase inhibitors • ADRs: ophthalmic—irritation; systemic—irregular heartbeat, CNS depression
tetracaine (Altracaine, Pontocaine, Tetcaine, ✺ Minims Tetracaine)	**Adults:** 1–2 drops of 0.5% solution (single dose)	• May interact with ophthalmic cholinesterase inhibitors, resulting in increased duration of action and risk of toxicity • ADRs: ophthalmic—irritation; systemic—irregular heartbeat, CNS depression

Antihistamines
Uses: Various forms of allergic conjunctivitis.

Drug	Dose	Notes
azelastine (Optivar)	**Adults and children ≥3 yr:** 1 drop of 0.05% solution twice daily	• ADRs: transient burning/stinging, headache, bitter taste
bepotastine (Bepreve)	**Adults and children ≥2 yr:** 1 drop of 1.5% solution twice daily	• ADRs: taste disturbance, headache, local irritation
emedastine (Emadine)	**Adults and children ≥3 yr:** 1 drop of 0.05% solution up to 4 times daily	• ADRs: headache, drowsiness, malaise, local irritation
epinastine (Elestat)	**Adults and children ≥3 yr:** 1 drop of 0.05% solution twice daily	• ADRs: headache, local irritation
ketotifen (Alaway, Claritin Eye, Zaditor, Zyrtec Itchy Eye)	**Adults and children ≥3 yr:** 1 drop of 0.025% solution twice daily (given 6–8 hr apart)	• OTC • ADRs: local irritation
olopatadine (Pataday, Patanol)	**Adults and children ≥3 yr:** *Patanol*—1 drop of 0.1% solution twice daily (given 6–8 hr apart); *Pataday*—1 drop of 0.2% solution twice daily	• Small amounts are absorbed; excreted in urine • ADRs: headache, conjunctival irritation

Anti-infectives/Antifungals/Antivirals
Uses: Localized superficial ophthalmic infections (e.g., bacterial conjunctivitis).
CAUTIONS: small amounts may be absorbed and result in hypersensitivity reactions.

Drug	Dose	Notes
azithromycin (AzaSite)	**Adults and children ≥1 yr:** 1 drop of 1% solution twice daily (given 8–12 hr apart) for 2 days, then once daily for 5 more days	• ADRs: eye irritation • When used to treat ocular chlamydial infections, concurrent systemic therapy is required
bacitracin	**Adults and children:** ¼–½-in ribbon q 3–4 hr for acute infections or 2–3 times daily for mild-moderate infections	• ADRs: eye irritation

APPENDIX C

DRUG NAME	DOSE	NOTES
besifloxacin (Besivance)	**Adults and children ≥1 yr:** 1 drop of 0.6% suspension 3 times daily (given 4–12 hr apart) for 7 days	• ADRs: headache, eye irritation
ciprofloxacin (Ciloxan)	**Adults and children >1 yr:** *Bacterial conjunctivitis*—Solution: 1–2 drops q 2 hr while awake for 2 days, then q 4 hr while awake for 5 days; Ointment: ½" ribbon 3 times daily for 2 days, then twice daily for 5 days; *Corneal ulcers*—Solution: 1–2 drops q 15 min for 6 hr, then q 30 min while awake for rest of day, then q 1 hr while awake for next 24 hr, then q 4 hr while awake for next 12 days or longer if re-epithelialization does not occur.	• May cause harmless white crystalline precipitate that resolves over time • ADRs: altered taste, systemic allergic reactions, photophobia, discomfort
erythromycin (Romycin)	**Adults and children:** *Treatment of infections*—½-in ribbon 2–6 times daily **Infants:** *Prophylaxis of ophthalmia neonatorum*—thin strip in each eye as a single dose	• ADRs: irritation
gatifloxacin (Zymar)	**Adults and children ≥1 yr:** 1 drop of 0.3% solution q 2 hr while awake (up to 8 times/day) for 2 days, then 4 times daily for 5 more days	• ADRs: irritation, headache, ↓ visual acuity, taste disturbance
gentamicin (Genoptic, Gentak, Gentesol, ✽ Alcomicin)	**Adults and children:** *Solution*—1–2 drops of 0.3% solution q 2–4 hr; *Ointment*—½-in ribbon q 8–12 hr	• ADRs: irritation, burning, stinging, blurred vision (ointment)
levofloxacin (Iquix, Quixin)	**Adults and children ≥1 yr:** *Quixin (bacterial conjunctivitis)*—1–2 drops q 2 hr while awake for 2 days (up to 8 times/day); then every 4 hr while awake for 5 more days (up to 4 times/day); *Iquix (conjunctival ulcers)*—1–2 drops q 30 min–2 hr while awake and 4–6 hr after retiring for 3 days, then 1–2 drops q 1–4 hr while awake.	• ADRs: altered taste, systemic allergic reactions, photophobia
moxifloxacin (Vigamox)	**Adults and children ≥1 yr:** 1 drop of 0.5% solution 3 times daily for 7 days.	• ADRs: irritation, ↓ visual acuity
ofloxacin (Ocuflox)	**Adults and children ≥1 yr:** *Bacterial conjunctivitis*—1–2 drops of 0.3% solution q 2–4 hr while awake for 2 days, then 4 times daily for 5 more days; *Corneal ulcer*—1–2 drops of 0.3% solution q 30 min while awake and q 4–6 hr after retiring for 2 days, then q hr while awake for 4–6 more days, then 4 times daily until cured.	• ADRs: altered taste, systemic allergic reactions, photophobia
sulfacetamide (Bleph-10, Ocu-Sulf 10, ✽ Sulfex)	**Adults and children >2 mo:** 1–2 drops of 10% solution q 2–3 hr while awake (less frequently at night)	• Cross-sensitivity with other sulfonamides (including thiazides) may occur • ADRs: local irritation
tobramycin (AK-Tob, Tobrex)	**Adults and children ≥2 mo:** *Solution*—1–2 drops of 0.3% solution q 1–4 hr depending on severity of infection; *Ointment*—thin strip q 8–12 hr	• Ointment may retard corneal wound healing • ADRs: irritation, burning, stinging, blurred vision (ointment)

Antifungal

DRUG NAME	DOSE	NOTES
natamycin (Natacyn)	**Adults:** 1 drop of 5% suspension q 1–2 hr for 3–4 days, then 6–8 times/day for 2–3 wk	• ADRs: irritation, swelling

Ophthalmic Medications

DRUG NAME	DOSE	NOTES
Antivirals		
trifluridine (Viroptic)	**Adults and children ≥6 yr:** 1 drop of 1% solution q 2 hr (up to 9 drops/day) while awake until cornea re-epithelializes, then q 4 hr for 7 more days (not to exceed 21 days)	• ADRs: burning, stinging; keratopathy

Artificial Tears/Ocular Lubricants (sterile buffered isotonic solutions/ointments)

Uses: Artificial tears—keep the eyes moist with isotonic solutions and wetting agents in the management of dry eyes due to lack of tears; also provide lubrication for artificial eyes. Ocular lubricants—provide lubrication and protection in a variety of conditions including exposure keratitis, decreased corneal sensitivity, corneal erosions, keratitis sicca, during/following ocular surgery or removal of a foreign body.

DRUG NAME	DOSE	NOTES
Artificial tears (Adsorbotear, Akwa Tears, Aquasite, Artificial Tears Plus, Cellufresh, Celluvisc, Comfort Tears, Dakrina, Dry Eye Therapy, Dry Eyes Duratears Naturale, Dwelle, Eye-Lube-A, Genteal Lubricant Eye Gel, HypoTears, HypoTears PF, Isopto Alkaline, Isopto Plain, Just Tears, Lacril, Lacri-Lube NP, Lacri-Lube S.O.P., Lacrisert, Liquifilm Forte, Liquifilm Tears, LubriTears, Moisture Drops, Murine Solution, Murocel, Nature's Tears, Nu-Tears, Nu-Tears II, Nutra Tear, Paralube, Refresh, Refresh PM, Tear Drop, TearGard, Teargen, Tearisol, Tears Naturale, Tears Naturale Free, Tears Naturale II, Tears Plus, Tears Renewed, Ultra Tears, Vit-A-Drops, Viva-Drops)	**Adults and children:** *Artificial tears*—Solution: 1–2 drops 3–4 times daily; Insert: 1 insert 1–2 times daily; *Ocular lubricants*—small amount instilled into conjunctiva several times daily	• May alter effects of other concurrently administered ophthalmic medications • ADRs: photophobia, lid edema stinging (insert only), transient blurred vision, eye discomfort

Beta Blockers

Uses: Management of chronic open-angle glaucoma and other forms of ocular hypertension (↓ the formation of aqueous humor).
CAUTIONS: Systemic absorption is minimal but may occur. Systemic absorption may result in additive adverse cardiovascular effects (bradycardia, hypotension), especially when used with other cardiovascular agents (antihypertensives, antiarrhythmics). Other systemic adverse reactions may occur, including bronchospasm or delirium (geriatric patients). Concurrent use with ophthalmic epinephrine may decrease effectiveness.

DRUG NAME	DOSE	NOTES
betaxolol (Betoptic, Betoptic S)	**Adults:** *Solution*—1–2 drops of 0.5% solution twice daily; *Suspension*—1 drop of 0.25% suspension twice daily	• ADRs: conjunctivitis, ↓ visual acuity, ocular burning, rash (may be less likely than others to cause bronchospasm if systemically absorbed)
carteolol	**Adults:** 1 drop of 1% solution twice daily	• ADRs: ocular burning, ↓ visual acuity
levobunolol (AKBeta, Betagan)	**Adults:** 1 drop of 0.25% solution 1–2 times daily or 1 drop of 0.5% solution once daily	• ADRs: conjunctivitis, ↓ visual acuity, ocular burning, rash
metipranolol (OptiPranolol)	**Adults:** 1 drop of 0.3% solution twice daily	• Lasts up to 24 hr • Can be used safely with pilocarpine, epinephrine, and acetazolamide • ADRs: conjunctivitis, ↓ visual acuity, ocular burning, rash
timolol (Betimol, Istalol, Timoptic, Timoptic-XE, ✸ Apo-Timop)	**Adults:** *Solution*—1 drop of 0.25–0.5% solution 1–2 times daily; *Gel-forming solution*—1 drop of 0.25–0.5% solution once daily	• Lasts up to 24 hr • ADRs: conjunctivitis, ↓ visual acuity, ocular burning, rash

Carbonic Anhydrase Inhibitor

Uses: Management of open-angle glaucoma or other forms of ocular hypertension (↓ formation of aqueous humor).
CAUTIONS: May exacerbate kidney stones; should not be used in patients with CCr <30 mL/min; may have cross-sensitivity with sulfonamides.

DRUG NAME	DOSE	NOTES
brinzolamide (Azopt)	**Adults:** 1 drop of 1% suspension into each affected eye 3 times daily	• ADRs: burning, stinging, unusual taste

DRUG NAME	DOSE	NOTES
dorzolamide (Trusopt)	**Adults:** 1 drop of 2% solution 3 times daily	• ADRs: bitter taste, ocular irritation or allergy

Cholinergics (direct-acting)

Uses: Treatment of open-angle glaucoma (facilitates the outflow of aqueous humor); also used to facilitate miosis after ophthalmic surgery or before examination (to counteract mydriatics).
CAUTIONS: Conditions in which pupillary constriction occurs should be avoided. If significant systemic absorption occurs, bronchospasm, sweating, ↑ urination and salivation may occur.

DRUG NAME	DOSE	NOTES
acetylcholine (Miochol-E)	**Adults:** 0.5–2 mL instilled into anterior chamber before or after securing one or more sutures	• ADRs: corneal edema, corneal clouding
carbachol (Isopto Carbachol, Miostat)	**Adults and children:** 1–2 drops of 0.01–3% solution 1–3 times daily	• ADRs: blurred vision, altered vision, stinging, eye pain
pilocarpine (Isopto Carpine, Ocusert Pilo, Pilopine HS, ✺ Miocarpine, ✺ Spersacarpine)	**Adults:** *Glaucoma*—Solution: 1–2 drops of 0.5–4% solution up to 6 times daily; Gel: ½-in. strip of 4% gel at bedtime; *Counteracting mydriatic sympathomimetics*—1 drop of 1% solution (may be repeated prior to surgery)	• ADRs: blurred vision, altered vision, stinging, eye pain, headache

Cholinergics (cholinesterase inhibitors)

Uses: Management of glaucoma not controlled with short-acting miotics or other agents; also used in varying doses for accommodative esotropia (diagnosis and treatment).
CAUTIONS: Enhance neuromuscular blockade from succinylcholine; intensify the actions of cocaine and some other local anesthetics; additive toxicity with antimyasthenics, anticholinergics, and cholinesterase inhibitors (including some pesticides). Use cautiously in patients with history or risk of retinal detachment.

DRUG NAME	DOSE	NOTES
echothiophate (Phospholine Iodide)	**Adults:** 1 drop 1–2 times daily	• Irreversible cholinesterase inhibitor • May cause hyperactivity in patients with Down syndrome • ADRs: blurred vision, change in vision, brow ache, miosis, eyelid twitching, watering eyes

Corticosteroids

Uses: Management of inflammatory eye conditions including allergic conjunctivitis, nonspecific superficial keratitis, infectious conjunctivitis (with anti-infectives); management of corneal injury; suppression of graft rejection following keratoplasty; prevention of postoperative inflammation.
CAUTIONS: Infectious ocular processes (avoid in herpes simplex keratitis), especially fungal and viral ocular infections (may mask symptoms); diabetes, glaucoma, or epithelial compromise

DRUG NAME	DOSE	NOTES
dexamethasone (Maxidex, ✺ Diodex, ✺ PMS Dexamethasone, ✺ RO-Dexasone, ✺ Spersadex)	**Adults and children:** *Solution*—1–2 drops of 0.1% solution q 1 hr during the day and q 2 hr during the night, gradually ↓ the dose to q 3–4 hr, then to 3–4 times daily; *Suspension*—1–2 drops of 0.1% suspension up to 4–6 times daily	• As condition improves, ↓ frequency of administration • ADRs: corneal thinning, ↑ intraocular pressure, irritation
difluprednate (Durezol)	**Adults:** 1 drop of 0.05% emulsion 4 times daily beginning 24 hr after surgery and continued for 2 wk, then 2 times daily for 1 wk, then taper	• As condition improves, ↓ frequency of administration • ADRs: blepharitis, photophobia, ↓ visual acuity
fluorometholone (FML, FML Forte, Flarex, Fluor-Op)	**Adults and children >2 yr:** *Suspension*—1–2 drops 2–4 times daily (up to 1–2 drops q 2–4 hr during initial 24–48 hr); *Ointment*—½-in strip 1–3 times daily (up to q 4 hr during initial 24–48 hr)	• As condition improves, ↓ frequency of administration • ADRs: blurred vision (ointment), corneal thinning, ↑ intraocular pressure, irritation
loteprednol (Alrex, Lotemax)	**Adults:** *Alrex*—1 drop 4 times daily; *Lotemax*—1–2 drops 4 times daily (up to 1 drop every hr)	• Alrex (0.2% suspension) used for seasonal allergic conjunctivitis • Lotemax (0.5% suspension) used for steroid-responsive inflammatory conditions and postoperatively • ADRs: corneal thinning, ↑ intraocular pressure, irritation

Ophthalmic Medications

DRUG NAME	DOSE	NOTES
prednisolone (Omnipred, Pred Forte, Pred Mild)	**Adults and children:** 1–2 drops of 0.12–1% solution/suspension q 1 hr during the day and q 2 hr during the night until favorable response, then 1 drop q 4 hr	• As condition improves, ↓ frequency of administration • ADRs: corneal thinning, ↑ intraocular pressure, irritation
rimexolone (Vexol)	**Adults:** 1–2 drops of 1% suspension 2–4 times daily (up to q 4 hr) (may use q 1–2 hr during first 1–2 days)	• As condition improves, ↓ frequency of administration • ADRs: corneal thinning, ↑ intraocular pressure, irritation

Cycloplegic Mydriatics

Uses: Preparation for cycloplegic refraction; management of uveitis (not tropicamide).
CAUTIONS: Use cautiously in patients with a history of glaucoma; systemic absorption may cause anticholinergic effects such as confusion, unusual behavior, flushing, hallucinations, slurred speech, drowsiness, swollen stomach (infants), tachycardia, dry mouth.

DRUG NAME	DOSE	NOTES
atropine (Atropine-Care, Isopto Atropine)	**Adults:** *Cycloplegic refraction*—1–2 drops of 1% solution 1 hr before procedure; *Uveitis*—Solution: 1–2 drops of 1% solution 1–2 times daily (up to 4 times daily); Ointment: 0.3–0.5 cm of 1% ointment up to 3 times daily	• Effects on accommodation may last 6 days; mydriasis may last 12 days • ADRs: irritation, blurred vision, photophobia
cyclopentolate (AK-Pentolate, Cyclogyl, Cylate, Pentolair, ✹ Minims)	**Adults:** 1 drop of 0.5–2% solution; may repeat in 5 min **Children:** 1 drop of 0.5–2% solution; may be followed 5–10 min later by 1 drop of 0.5–1% solution **Premature and small infants:** 1 drop of 0.5% solution single dose	• Peak of cycloplegia is within 25–75 min and lasts 6–24 hr • Peak of mydriasis is within 30–60 min and may last several days • 2% solution used for heavily pigmented iris • ADRs: irritation, blurred vision, photophobia
homatropine (Isopto Homatropine, ✹ Minims Homatropine)	**Adults and children:** *Cycloplegic refraction*—1 drop of 2–5% solution, may repeat in 5–10 min for 2–3 more doses; *Uveitis*—1–2 drops of 2–5% solution 2–3 times daily (up to q 3–4 hr in adults)	• Cycloplegia and mydriasis may persist for 24–72 hr • ADRs: irritation, blurred vision, photophobia
scopolamine (Isopto Hyoscine)	**Adults and children:** *Cycloplegic refraction*—1–2 drops of 0.25% solution 1 hr before procedure (repeat twice daily for 2 days in children); *Uveitis*—1 drop of 0.25% solution up to 4 times daily	• Shorter duration than atropine, but mydriasis and cycloplegia may persist for 3–7 days • ADRs: irritation, blurred vision, photophobia
tropicamide (Mydral, Mydriacyl, Tropicacyl, ✹ Minims Tropicamide)	**Adults and children:** 1–2 drops of 0.5–1% solution	• Stronger solution/repeated dosing may be required in patients with dark irides • Peak effect occurs in 20–40 min • Cycloplegia lasts 2–6 hr; mydriasis lasts up to 7 hr • ADRs: irritation, blurred vision, photophobia

Immunomodulators

Uses: To ↑ tear production when the cause of dry eye is inflammation secondary to keratoconjunctivitis sicca.
CAUTIONS: Tear production is not ↑ during concurrent use of ophthalmic NSAIDs or punctal plugs.

DRUG NAME	DOSE	NOTES
cyclosporine (Restasis)	**Adults:** 1 drop of 0.05% ophthalmic emulsion in each eye twice daily	• Emulsion should be inverted to obtain uniform opaque appearance prior to use. • ADRs: irritation, blurred vision

Mast Cell Stabilizers

Uses: Vernal keratoconjunctivitis.
CAUTIONS: Require several days of treatment before effects are seen.

DRUG NAME	DOSE	NOTES
cromolyn (Crolom, ✹ Opticrom)	**Adults and children >4 yr:** 1–2 drops of 4% solution 4–6 times daily	• Do not wear contact lenses concurrently • ADRs: irritation

DRUG NAME	DOSE	NOTES
lodoxamide (Alomide)	Adults and children ≥2 yr: 1–2 drops of 0.1% solution 4 times daily for up to 3 mo	• ADRs: blurred vision, foreign body sensation, irritation
nedocromil (Alocril)	Adults and children ≥3 yr: 1–2 drops of 2% solution in each eye twice daily throughout period of exposure	• Avoid concurrent use of contact lenses • ADRs: headache, ocular burning, unpleasant taste, nasal congestion
pemirolast (Alamast)	Adults and children >3 yr: 1–2 drops of 0.1% solution in each affected eye 4 times daily	• Symptoms may improve within a few days, but optimal response may take up to 4 wk • ADRs: discomfort, dry eyes, foreign body sensation

Nonsteroidal Anti-inflammatory Drugs

Uses: Management of pain/inflammation following surgery (bromfenac, diclofenac, ketorolac, nepafenac), allergic conjunctivitis (ketorolac), inhibition of perioperative miosis (flurbiprofen).
CAUTIONS: Cross-sensitivity with systemic NSAIDs may occur; concurrent use of anticoagulants, other NSAIDs, thrombolytics, some cephalosporins, and valproates may ↑ the risk of bleeding. May slow/delay healing. Avoid contact lens use.

DRUG NAME	DOSE	NOTES
bromfenac (Xibrom)	Adults: 1 drop of 0.09% solution in affected eye(s) twice daily starting 24 hr after surgery and for 2 wk following	• Contains sulfites • Avoid contact lenses • ADRs: irritation, headache
diclofenac (Voltaren)	Adults: 1 drop of 0.1% solution starting 24 hr after surgery and for 2 wk following	• Do not wear hydrocel contact lenses concurrently • ADRs: irritation, allergic reactions
flurbiprofen (Ocufen)	Adults: 1 drop of 0.03% solution q 30 min, beginning 2 hr prior to surgery (4 drops total in each eye)	• ADRs: irritation, allergic reactions
ketorolac (Acular, Acular Preservative Free, Acular LS, Acuvail)	Adults and children >3 yr: *Allergic conjunctivitis*—Acular: 1 drop 4 times daily (Acular); *Postoperative*—Acular: 1 drop 4 times daily in operated eye starting 24 hr after cataract surgery and for 2 wk following; Acular LS: 1 drop 4 times daily in operated eye after corneal refractive surgery for up to 4 days; Acuvail: 1 drop twice daily prior to cataract surgery and for 2 wk following; Preservative–free solution: 1 drop 4 times daily in operated eye after incisional refractive surgery for up to 3 days	• ADRs: irritation, allergic reactions
nepafenac (Nevanac)	Adults and Children >10 yr: 1 drop of 0.1% suspension into affected eye(s) 3 times daily starting one day prior to cataract removal and for 2 wk following surgery	• ADRs: irritation, photophobia, headache, hypertension, nausea/vomiting

Ocular Decongestants/Vasoconstrictors

Uses: ↓ ocular congestion due to irritation by vasoconstricting conjunctival blood vessels; stronger solutions have mydriatic effects.
CAUTIONS: Systemic absorption may result in adverse cardiovascular effects; excessive/prolonged use may produce rebound hyperemia; use caution in patients at risk for acute angle-closure glaucoma; cardiovascular effects may be exaggerated by MAO inhibitors and dose adjustment may be required within 21 days of MAO inhibitors; ↑ risk of arrhythmias with inhalation anesthetics.

DRUG NAME	DOSE	NOTES
naphazoline (Albalon, Allerest, Allergy Drops, Clear Eyes Lubricating Eye Redness Reliever, Comfort Eye Drops, Degest 2, Estivin II, Nafazair, Naphcon, Ocu-Zoline, VasoClear, Vasocon, ❋ AK-Con)	Adults: 1–2 drops of 0.012–0.025% solution 4 times daily as needed (for up to 3 days) or 1–2 drops of 0.1% solution q 3–4 hr as needed	• ADRs: ophthalmic-rebound hyperemia; systemic-dizziness, headache, nausea, sweating, weakness
oxymetazoline (OcuClear, Visine LR)	Adults and children ≥6 yr: 1–2 drops of 0.025% solution q 6 hr as needed	• ADRs: ophthalmic-rebound hyperemia; systemic-headache, insomnia, nervousness, tachycardia

Ophthalmic Medications

DRUG NAME	DOSE	NOTES
phenylephrine (AK-Dilate, AK-Nefrin, Dilatair, I-Phrine, Isopto Frin, Mydfrin, Ocu-Phrin, Prefrin, ✻ Minims Phenylephrine, ✻ Spersaphrine)	**Adults:** *Decongestant*—1–2 drops of 0.12% solution up to 4 times daily as needed (for up to 3 days); *Mydriasis*—1 drop of 2.5 solution, may repeat in 10–60 min as needed **Children:** *Mydriasis*—1 drop of 2.5% solution, may repeat in 10–60 min as needed	• ADRs: ophthalmic-blurred vision, irritation; systemic-dizziness, tachycardia, hypertension, paleness, sweating, trembling
tetrahydrozoline (Eyesine, Geneye, Murine Plus, Optigene 3, Visine)	**Adults:** 1–2 drops of 0.05% solution 2–4 times daily	• ADRs: ophthalmic—irritation; systemic—tachycardia, hypertension

Osmotics
Uses: ↓ superficial edema of the cornea prior to examination.

glycerin (Ophthalgan)	**Adults:** 1–2 drops prior to exam	• Avoid using in patients with hypersensitivity to chlorobutanol

Prostaglandin Agonist
Uses: Management of open-angle glaucoma (↑ outflow of aqueous humor).
CAUTIONS: May change eye color to brown; will form precipitate with thimerosal-containing products; can be used with other agents to ↓ intraocular pressure.

bimatoprost (Lumigan)	**Adults:** 1 drop of 0.03% solution once daily in the evening	• ADRs: local irritation, foreign body sensation, ↑ eyelash growth, ↑ brown pigmentation in iris
latanoprost (Xalatan)	**Adults:** 1 drop of 0.005% solution once daily	• ADRs: local irritation, foreign body sensation, ↑ eyelash growth, ↑ brown pigmentation in iris
travoprost (Travatan, Travatan Z)	**Adults:** 1 drop of 0.004% solution once daily in the evening	• ADRs: local irritation, foreign body sensation, ↑ eyelash growth, ↑ brown pigmentation in iris

Sympathomimetics
Uses: Management of glaucoma (↓ formation of aqueous humor).
CAUTIONS: Systemic absorption may result in adverse cardiovascular and CNS reactions (especially in patients with cardiovascular disease); avoid use in patients predisposed to acute angle-closure glaucoma.

apraclonidine (Iopidine)	**Adults:** *Postoperative reduction of intraocular pressure*—1–2 drops of 0.5% solution 3 times daily or 1 drop of 1% solution 1 hr before surgery and upon completion of surgery	• A selective alpha-adrenergic agonist • Monitor pulse and blood pressure • Avoid concurrent use with MAO inhibitors • ADRs: ophthalmic-irritation, mydriasis; systemic-allergic reactions, arrhythmias, bradycardia, drowsiness, dry nose, fainting, headache, nervousness, weakness
brimonidine (Alphagan P)	**Adults:** 1 drop 3 times daily (8 hr apart)	• A selective alpha-adrenergic agonist • Avoid concurrent use with MAO inhibitors • Tricyclic antidepressants may ↓ effectiveness; additive CNS depression may occur with other CNS depressants, additive adverse cardiovascular effects with other cardiovascular agents • ADRs: ophthalmic—irritation; systemic—drowsiness, dizziness, dry mouth, headache, weakness, muscular pain
dipivefrin (Propine)	**Adults:** 1 drop of 0.1% solution q 12 hr	• Converted to epinephrine in the eye • Wait 15 min before inserting soft contact lenses • ADRs: ophthalmic—local irritation, macular edema (aphakic patients); systemic—arrhythmias, hypertension

APPENDIX D
Medication Administration Techniques

Subcutaneous Injection Sites

Administration of Ophthalmic Medications

For instillation of ophthalmic solutions, instruct patient to lie down or tilt head back and look at ceiling. Pull down on lower lid, creating a small pocket, and instill solution into pocket. With systemically acting drugs, apply pressure to the inner canthus for 1–2 min to minimize systemic absorption. Instruct patient to gently close eye. Wait 5 min before instilling second drop or any other ophthalmic solutions.

For instillation of ophthalmic ointment, instruct patient to hold tube in hand for several minutes to warm. Squeeze a small amount of ointment (¼–½ in.) inside lower lid. Instruct patient to close eye gently and roll eyeball around in all directions with eye closed. Wait 10 min before instilling any other ophthalmic ointments.

Do not touch cap or tip of container to eye, fingers, or any surface.

Administration of Medications with Metered-Dose Inhalers

Instruct patient on the proper use of the metered-dose inhaler. There are 3 methods of using a metered-dose inhaler. Shake inhaler well. (1) Take a drink of water to moisten the throat; place the inhaler mouthpiece 2 finger-widths away from mouth; tilt head back slightly. While activating the inhaler, take a slow, deep breath for 3–5 sec; hold the breath for 10 sec; and breathe out slowly. (2) Exhale and close lips firmly around mouthpiece. Administer during second half of inhalation, and hold breath for as long as possible to ensure deep instillation of medication. (3) Use of spacer. Consult health care professional to determine method desired prior to instruction. Allow 1–2 min between inhalations. Rinse mouth with

Medication Administration Techniques **1405**

water or mouthwash after each use to minimize dry mouth and hoarseness. Wash inhalation assembly at least daily in warm running water.

For use of dry powder inhalers, turn head away from inhaler and exhale (do not blow into inhaler). Do not shake. Close mouth tightly around the mouthpiece of the inhaler and inhale rapidly.

Steps for Using Your Inhaler*
1. Remove the cap and hold inhaler upright.
2. Shake the inhaler.
3. Tilt your head back slightly and breathe out slowly.
4. Position the inhaler in one of the following ways (A or B is optimal, but C is acceptable for those who have difficulty with A or B. C is required for breath-activated inhalers):

A. Open mouth with inhaler 1 to 2 inches away.

B. Use space/holding chamber (this is recommended especially for young children and for people using corticosteroids).

C. In the mouth. Do not use for corticosteroids.

D. NOTE: Inhaled dry powder capsules require a different inhalation technique. To use a dry powder inhaler, it is important to close the mouth tightly around the mouthpiece of the inhaler and to inhale rapidly.

5. Press down on the inhaler to release medication as you start to breathe in slowly.
6. Breathe in slowly (3 to 5 sec).
7. Hold your breath for 10 sec to allow the medicine to reach deeply into your lungs.
8. Repeat puff as directed. Waiting 1 minute between puffs may permit second puff to penetrate your lungs better.
9. Spacers/holding chambers are useful for all patients. They are particularly recommended for young children and older adults and for use with **inhaled corticosteroids**. Avoid common inhaler mistakes. Follow these inhaler tips:

- Breathe out before pressing your inhaler.
- Inhale slowly.
- Breathe in through your mouth, not your nose.
- Press down on your inhaler at the start of inhalation (or within the first second of inhalation).
- Keep inhaling as you press down on inhaler.
- Press your inhaler only once while you are inhaling (one breath for each puff).
- Make sure you breathe in evenly and deeply.
- If you are using a short-acting bronchodilator inhaler and a corticosteroid inhaler, use the bronchodilator first, and allow 5 min to elapse before using the corticosteroid.

Other inhalers have become available in addition to the one illustrated here. Different types of inhalers may require different techniques.

Administration of Medications by Nebulizer

Administer in a location where patient can sit comfortably for 10–15 min. Plug in compressor. Mix medication as directed, or empty unit-dose vials into nebulizer. Do not mix different types of medications

---

*Source: Expert Panel Report 2: Guidelines for the Diagnosis and Management of Asthma. National Asthma Education and Prevention Program, National Heart, Lung, and Blood Institute, 1997.

APPENDIX D

without checking with health care professional. Assemble mask or mouthpiece and connect tubing to port on compressor. Have patient sit in a comfortable upright position. Make sure that mask fits properly over nose and mouth and that mist does not flow into eyes, or put mouthpiece into mouth. Turn on compressor. Instruct patient to take slow deep breaths. If possible, patient should hold breath for 10 sec before slowly exhaling. Continue this process until medication chamber is empty. Wash mask in hot soapy water; rinse well and allow to air dry before next use.

Administration of Nasal Sprays

Clear nasal passages of secretions prior to use. If nasal passages are blocked, use a decongestant immediately prior to use to ensure adequate penetration of the spray. Keep head upright. Breathe in through nose during administration. Sniff hard for a few minutes after administration.

Intramuscular Injection Sites

The dorsogluteal site is associated with sciatic nerve injury. The deltoid and ventrogluteal sites are the preferred sites for adults; the vastus lateralis site is preferred in children under 2 yr of age.

APPENDIX E
Formulas Helpful for Calculating Doses

Ratio and Proportion

A ratio is the same as a fraction and can be expressed as a fraction (½) or in the algebraic form (1:2). This relationship is stated as *one is to two*.

A proportion is an equation of equal fractions or ratios.

$$\frac{1}{2} = \frac{4}{8}$$

To calculate doses, begin each proportion with the two known values, for example 15 grains = 1 gram (known equivalent) or 10 milligrams = 2 milliliters (dosage available) on one side of the equation. Next, make certain that the units of measure on the opposite side of the equation are the same as the units of the known values and are placed on the same level of the equation.

Problem A:
$$\frac{15 \text{ gr}}{1 \text{ g}} = \frac{10 \text{ gr}}{x \text{ g}}$$

Problem B:
$$\frac{10 \text{ mg}}{2 \text{ mL}} = \frac{5 \text{ mg}}{x \text{ mL}}$$

Once the proportion is set up correctly, cross-multiply the opposing values of the proportion.

Problem A:
$$\frac{15 \text{ gr}}{1 \text{ g}} \times \frac{10 \text{ gr}}{x \text{ g}}$$

$$15x = 10$$

Problem B:
$$\frac{10 \text{ mg}}{2 \text{ mL}} \times \frac{5 \text{ mg}}{x \text{ mL}}$$

$$10x = 10$$

Next, divide each side of the equation by the number with the *x* to determine the answer. Then, add the unit of measure corresponding to *x* in the original equation.

Problem A:
$$\frac{15x}{15} = \frac{10}{15}$$

$$x = \frac{2}{3} \text{ or } 0.6 \text{ g}$$

Problem B:
$$\frac{10x}{10} = \frac{10}{10}$$

$$x = 1 \text{ mL}$$

Calculation of IV Drip Rate

To calculate the drip rate for an intravenous infusion, 3 values are needed:
  I. The amount of solution and corresponding time for infusion. May be ordered as:

$$1000 \text{ mL over 8 hr}$$

or

$$125 \text{ mL/hr}$$

  II. The equivalent in time to convert hr to min.

$$1 \text{ hr} = 60 \text{ min}$$

  III. The drop factor or number of drops that equal 1 mL of fluid. (This information can be found on the IV tubing box.)

$$10 \text{ gtt} = 1 \text{ mL}$$

Set up the problem by placing each of the 3 values in a proportion.

$$\frac{125 \text{ mL}}{1 \text{ hr}} \times \frac{1 \text{ hr}}{60 \text{ min}} \times \frac{10 \text{ gtt}}{1 \text{ mL}}$$

Units of measure can be canceled out from the upper and lower levels of the equation.
The units cancel, leaving:

$$\frac{125}{1} \times \frac{1}{60 \text{ min}} \times \frac{10 \text{ gtt}}{1}$$

Next, multiply each level across and divide the numerator by the denominator for the answer.

$$\frac{125}{1} \times \frac{1}{6 \text{ min}} \times \frac{1 \text{ gtt}}{1}$$

$$125/6 = 20.8 \text{ or } 21 \text{ gtt/min}$$

Calculation of Creatinine Clearance (CCr) in Adults from Serum Creatinine

$$\text{Men: CCr} = \frac{\text{ideal body weight (kg)} \times (140 - \text{age})}{72 \times \text{serum creatinine (mg/dL)}}$$

$$\text{Women: CCr} = 0.85 \times \text{calculation for men}$$

Calculation of Body Surface Area (BSA) in Adults and Children

Dubois method:

$$\text{SA (cm}^2) = \text{wt (kg)}^{0.425} \times 71.84$$

$$\text{SA (m}^2) \; K \times \sqrt[3]{\text{wt}^2 \text{ (kg)}} \; \text{(common K value 0.1 for toddlers, 0.103 for neonates)}$$

Simplified method:

$$\text{BSA (m}^2) = \sqrt{\frac{\text{ht (cm)} \times \text{wt (kg)}}{3600}}$$

Body Mass Index

$$\text{BMI} = \text{wt (kg)/ht (m}^2)$$

APPENDIX F
Body Surface Area Nomograms

ESTIMATING BODY SURFACE AREA IN CHILDREN

For pediatric patients of average size, body surface area may be estimated with the scale on the left. Match weight to corresponding surface area. For other pediatric patients, use the scale on the right. Lay a straightedge on the correct height and weight points for your patient, and observe the point where it intersects on the surface area scale at center.

Reproduced from *Nelson Textbook of Pediatrics*, 16th edition. Courtesy W.B. Saunders Co., Philadelphia, PA.

APPENDIX F

ESTIMATING BODY SURFACE AREA IN ADULTS

Use a straightedge to connect the patient's height in the left-hand column to weight in the right-hand column. The intersection of this line with the center scale estimates the body surface area.

Source: Dubois D, Dubois EF. A formula to estimate the appropriate surface area if height and weight be known. *Archives of Internal Medicine*. 1916:17;863-71. Copyright © 2009, American Medical Association. All rights reserved.

APPENDIX G
Normal Values of Common Laboratory Tests

SERUM TESTS

HEMATOLOGIC	MEN	WOMEN
Hemoglobin	13.5–18 g/dL	12–16 g/dL
Hematocrit	40–54%	38–47%
Red blood cells (RBC)	4.6–6.2 million/mm^3	4.2–5.4 million/mm^3
Mean corpuscular volume (MCV)	76–100 (micrometer)^3	76–100 (micrometer)^3
Mean corpuscular hemoglobin (MCH)	27–33 picogram	27–33 picogram
Mean corpuscular hemoglobin concentration (MCHC)	33–37 g/dL	33–37 g/dL
Erythrocyte sedimentation rate (ESR)	≤20 mm/hr	≤30 mm/hr
Leukocytes (WBC)	5000–10,000/mm^3	5000–10,000/mm^3
Neutrophils	54–75% (3000–7500/mm^3)	54–75% (3000–7500/mm^3)
Bands	3–8% (150–700/mm^3)	3–8% (150–700/mm^3)
Eosinophils	1–4% (50–400/mm^3)	1–4% (50–400/mm^3)
Basophils	0–1% (25–100/mm^3)	0–1% (25–100/mm^3)
Monocytes	2–8% (100–500/mm^3)	2–8% (100–500/mm^3)
Lymphocytes	25–40% (1500–4500/mm^3)	25–40% (1500–4500/mm^3)
T lymphocytes	60–80% of lymphocytes	60–80% of lymphocytes
B lymphocytes	10–20% of lymphocytes	10–20% of lymphocytes
Platelets	150,000–450,000/mm^3	150,000–450,000/mm^3
Prothrombin time (PT)	9.6–11.8 sec	9.5–11.3 sec
Partial thromboplastin time (PTT)	30–45 sec	30–45 sec
Bleeding time (duke)	1–3 min	1–3 min
(ivy)	3–6 min	3–6 min
(template)	3–6 min	3–6 min

CHEMISTRY	MEN	WOMEN
Sodium	135–145 mEq/L	135–145 mEq/L
Potassium	3.5–5.0 mEq/L	3.5–5.0 mEq/L
Chloride	95–105 mEq/L	95–105 mEq/L
Bicarbonate (HCO$_3$)	19–25 mEq/L	19–25 mEq/L
Total calcium	9–11 mg/dL or 4.5–5.5 mEq/L	9–11 mg/dL or 4.5–5.5 mEq/L
Ionized calcium	4.2–5.4 mg/dL or 2.1–2.6 mEq/L	4.2–5.4 mg/dL or 2.1–2.6 mEq/L
Phosphorus/phosphate	2.4–4.7 mg/dL	2.4–4.7 mg/dL
Magnesium	1.8–3.0 mg/dL or 1.5–2.5 mEq/L	1.8–3.0 mg/dL or 1.5–2.5 mEq/L
Glucose	65–99 mg/dL	65–99 mg/dL
Osmolality	285–310 mOsm/kg	285–310 mOsm/kg
Ammonia (NH$_3$)	10–80 mcg/dL	10–80 mcg/dL
Amylase	≤130 U/L	≤130 U/L
Creatine phosphokinase total (CK, CPK)	<150 U/L	<150 U/L
Creatine kinase isoenzymes, MB fraction	>5% in MI	>5% in MI
Lactic dehydrogenase (LDH)	50–150 U/L	50–150 U/L
Protein, total	6–8 g/d	6–8 g/d
Albumin	4–6 g/dL	4–6 g/dL

HEPATIC	MEN	WOMEN
AST	8–46 U/L	7–34 U/L
ALT	10–30 IU/mL	10–30 IU/mL
Total bilirubin	0.3–1.2 mg/dL	0.3–1.2 mg/dL
Conjugated bilirubin	0.0–0.2 mg/dL	0.0–0.2 mg/dL
Unconjugated (indirect) bilirubin	0.2–0.8 mg/dL	0.2–0.8 mg/dL
Alkaline phosphatase	20–90 U/L	20–90 U/L

APPENDIX G

RENAL	MEN	WOMEN
BUN	6–20 mg/dL	6–20 mg/dL
Creatinine	0.6–1.3 mg/dL	0.5–1.0 mg/dL
Uric acid	4.0–8.5 mg/dL	2.7–7.3 mg/dL

ARTERIAL BLOOD GASES	MEN	WOMEN
pH	7.35–7.45	7.35–7.45
Po_2	80–100 mm Hg	80–100 mm Hg
Pco_2	35–45 mm Hg	35–45 mm Hg
O_2 saturation	95–97%	95–97%
Base excess	+2–(−2)	+2–(−2)
Bicarbonate (HCO_3^-)	22–26 mEq/L	22–26 mEq/L

URINE TESTS

URINE	MEN	WOMEN
pH	4.5–8.0	4.5–8.0
Specific gravity	1.010–1.025	1.010–1.025

DRUG LEVELS, THERAPEUTIC AND TOXIC CONVENTIONAL (US SYSTEM OF MEASUREMENTS)

DRUG	THERAPEUTIC LEVEL	TOXIC LEVEL
acetaminophen	10–30 mcg/mL	>200 mcg/mL at 4 hr or 50 mcg/mL at 12 hr after ingestion
amikacin	peak: 20–30 mcg/mL trough: <8 mcg/mL	peak: >40 mcg/mL trough: >10 mcg/mL
amiodarone	0.5–2.5 mg/L	>2.5 mg/L
amitriptyline	0.5–2.5 mcg/mL	>2.5 mcg/mL
amoxapine	120–150 ng/mL	>500 ng/mL
carbamazepine	4–12 mcg/mL	>15 mcg/mL
chloramphenicol	peak: 10–25 mcg/mL trough: 5–15 mcg/mL	peak: >40 mcg/mL trough: >15 mcg/mL
chlordiazepoxide	0.1–3 mcg/mL	>25 mcg/mL
chlorpromazine	50–300 ng/mL	>750 ng/mL
clonazepam	20–80 ng/mL	>80 ng/mL
cyclosporine	100–400 ng/mL	>400 ng/mL
desipramine	50–300 ng/mL	>300 ng/mL
diazepam	0.2–1.5 mcg/mL	>1.5 mcg/mL
digoxin	0.5–2 ng/mL	>2.5 ng/mL
disopyramide	2.8–7.5 mcg/mL	>7.5 mcg/mL
doxepin	110–250 ng/mL	>500 ng/mL
ethosuximide	40–100 mcg/mL	>100 mcg/mL
flecainide	0.2–1 mcg/mL	>1 mcg/mL
gentamicin	peak: 6–10 mcg/mL trough: <1 mcg/mL	trough: >1 mcg/mL
haloperidol	5–20 ng/mL	>42 ng/mL
imipramine	150–250 ng/mL	>500 ng/mL
kanamycin	peak: 15–30 mcg/mL trough: 5–10 mcg/mL	peak: >35 mcg/mL trough: >10 mcg/mL
lidocaine	1.5–5 mcg/mL	>6 mcg/mL
lithium	0.6–1.2 mEq/L	>1.5 mEq/L
meperidine	70–500 ng/mL	>1000 ng/mL
mexiletine	0.5–2 mcg/mL	>2 mcg/mL
morphine	65–80 ng/mL	>200 ng/mL
nortriptyline	50–150 ng/mL	>500 ng/mL
phenobarbital	15–40 mcg/mL	>40 mcg/mL
phenytoin	10–20 mcg/mL	>30 mcg/mL
primidone	5–12 mcg/mL	>15 mcg/mL
procainamide	procainamide: 4–10 mcg/mL	procainamide: >10 mcg/mL

Normal Values of Common Laboratory Tests

	N-acetylprocainamide (NAPA): 15–25 mcg/mL	
propranolol	50–100 ng/mL	>150 ng/mL
quinidine	2–5 mcg/mL	>6 mcg/mL
salicylate	100–400 mcg/mL	>400 mcg/mL
theophylline	10–20 mcg/mL	>20 mcg/mL
tobramycin	peak: 6–10 mcg/mL trough: <1 mcg/mL	trough: >1 mcg/mL
trazadone	0.5–2.5 mcg/mL	>2.5 mcg/mL
valproic acid	50–125 mcg/mL	>125 mcg/mL
vancomycin	trough: 10–20 mcg/mL	trough: >20 mcg/mL

APPENDIX H
Commonly Used Abbreviations

ABGs arterial blood gases
ac before meals
ACE angiotensin-converting enzyme
ADH antidiuretic hormone
A-G ratio albumin-globulin ratio
AHF antihemolytic factor
ALT alanine aminotransferase
ANA antinuclear antibodies
ANC absolute neutrophil count
AST aspartate aminotransferase
ATP adenosine triphosphate
AV atrioventricular
bid two times a day
BMI body mass index
BP blood pressure
bpm beats per minute
BSA body surface area
BUN blood urea nitrogen
cap capsule
CBC complete blood count
CCr creatinine clearance
CHF congestive heart failure
COMT catechol-O-methyltransferase
CNS central nervous system
CPK creatine phosphokinase
CR controlled-release
CSF colony-stimulating factor; cerebrospinal fluid
CT computed tomography
CV cardiovascular
CVP central venous pressure
D5/LR 5% dextrose and lactated Ringer's solution
D5/0.9% NaCl 5% dextrose and 0.9% NaCl; 5% dextrose and normal saline
D5/0.25% NaCl 5% dextrose and 0.25% NaCl; 5% dextrose and quarter normal saline
D5/0.45% NaCl 5% dextrose and 0.45% NaCl; 5% dextrose and half normal saline
D5W 5% dextrose in water
D10W 10% dextrose in water
Derm dermatologic
dL deciliter
DMARD disease-modifying antirheumatic drug
DNA deoxyribonucleic acid
DVT deep vein thrombosis
ECG electrocardiogram
ECMO extracorporeal membrane oxygenation
EENT eye, ear, nose, and throat
Endo endocrine
ER extended-release
ESRD end-stage renal disease
F and E fluid and electrolyte
g gram(s)
GABA gamma-aminobutyric acid
GERD gastroesophageal reflux disease
GFR glomerular filtration rate
GI gastrointestinal
G6PD glucose-6-phosphate dehydrogenase
gt(t) drop(s)
GTT glucose tolerance test
GU genitourinary
Hb A_{1c} hemoglobin A_{1c}, glycosylated hemoglobin
HDL high-density lipoproteins
Hemat hematologic
HF heart failure
hr(s) hour(s)
HR heart rate
HRT hormone replacement therapy
IA intra-articular
IL intralesional
IM intramuscular
Inhaln inhalation
INR international normalized ratio
IPPB intermittent positive-pressure breathing
IS intrasynovial
IT intrathecal
IV intravenous
K potassium
KCl potassium chloride
kg kilogram
L liter
LA long-acting
LDH lactic dehydrogenase
LDL low-density lipoproteins
LR lactated Ringer's solution
M molar

Commonly Used Abbreviations

MAOI	monoamine oxidase inhibitor	**PVC**	premature ventricular contraction
mcg	microgram(s)	**q**	every
MDI	metered dose inhaler	**qid**	four times a day
mEq	milliequivalent	**q 2 hr**	every 2 hours
Metab	metabolic	**q 3 hr**	every 3 hours
mg	milligram(s)	**q 4 hr**	every 4 hours
min(s)	minute(s)	**RBC**	red blood cell count
Misc	miscellaneous	**Rect**	rectally or rectal
mL	milliliter(s)	**REM**	rapid eye movement
mM	millimole	**Resp**	respiratory
MRI	magnetic resonance imaging	**RTU**	ready to use
MS	musculoskeletal	**Rx**	prescription
MUGA	multiple-gated (image) acquisition (analysis)	**SA**	sinoatrial
Na	sodium	**subcut**	subcutaneous
NaCl	sodium chloride	**sec(s)**	second(s)
0.9% NaCl	0.9% sodium chloride, normal saline	**SL**	sublingual
		SR	sustained-release
Neuro	neurologic	**SSRI(s)**	selective serotonin reuptake inhibitor(s)
NPO	nothing by mouth		
NS	sodium chloride, normal saline (0.9% NaCl)	**stat**	immediately
		supp	suppository
NSAIDs	nonsteroidal anti-inflammatory drugs	**tab**	tablet
		tbsp	tablespoon(s)
OCD	obsessive-compulsive disorder	**tid**	three times a day
Oint	ointment	**Top**	topically or topical
Ophth	ophthalmic	**tsp**	teaspoon(s)
OTC	over-the-counter	**UK**	unknown
pc	after meals	**Vag**	vaginal
PCA	patient-controlled analgesia	**VF**	ventricular fibrillation
PO	by mouth, orally	**VLDL**	very low-density lipoproteins
prn	as needed	**VT**	ventricular tachycardia
PT	prothrombin time	**WBC**	white blood cell count
PTT	partial thromboplastin time	**wk(s)**	week(s)
		yr(s)	year(s)

APPENDIX I
Pregnancy Categories

Category A

Adequate, well-controlled studies in pregnant women have not shown an increased risk of fetal abnormalities.

Category B

Animal studies have revealed no evidence of harm to the fetus, however, there are no adequate and well-controlled studies in pregnant women. **or** Animal studies have shown an adverse effect, but adequate and well-controlled studies in pregnant women have failed to demonstrate a risk to the fetus.

Category C

Animal studies have shown an adverse effect and there are no adequate and well-controlled studies in pregnant women. **or** No animal studies have been conducted and there are no adequate and well-controlled studies in pregnant women.

Category D

Studies, adequate well-controlled or observational, in pregnant women have demonstrated a risk to the fetus. However, the benefits of therapy may outweigh the potential risk.

Category X

Studies, adequate well-controlled or observational, in animals or pregnant women have demonstrated positive evidence of fetal abnormalities. The use of the product is contraindicated in women who are or may become pregnant.

Note: The designation UK is used when the pregnancy category is unknown.

APPENDIX J
Controlled Substances Schedules

Classes or schedules are determined by the Drug Enforcement Agency (DEA), an arm of the United States Justice Department, and are based on the potential for abuse and dependence liability (physical and psychological) of the medication. Some states may have stricter prescription regulations. Physicians, dentists, podiatrists, and veterinarians may prescribe controlled substances. Nurse practitioners and physician's assistants may prescribe controlled substances with limitations that vary from state to state.

Schedule I (C-I)

Potential for abuse is so high as to be unacceptable. May be used for research with appropriate limitations. Examples are LSD and heroin.

Schedule II (C-II)

High potential for abuse and extreme liability for physical and psychological dependence (amphetamines, opioid analgesics, dronabinol, certain barbiturates). Outpatient prescriptions must be in writing. In emergencies, telephone orders may be acceptable if a written prescription is provided within 72 hr. No refills are allowed.

Schedule III (C-III)

Intermediate potential for abuse (less than C-II) and intermediate liability for physical and psychological dependence (certain nonbarbiturate sedatives, certain nonamphetamine CNS stimulants, and certain opioid analgesics). Outpatient prescriptions can be refilled 5 times within 6 mo from date of issue if authorized by prescriber. Telephone orders are acceptable.

Schedule IV (C-IV)

Less abuse potential than Schedule III with minimal liability for physical or psychological dependence (certain sedative/hypnotics, certain antianxiety agents, some barbiturates, benzodiazepines, chloral hydrate, pentazocine, and propoxyphene). Outpatient prescriptions can be refilled 6 times within 6 mo from date of issue if authorized by prescriber. Telephone orders are acceptable.

Schedule V (C-V)

Minimal abuse potential. Number of outpatient refills determined by prescriber. Some products (cough suppressants with small amounts of codeine, antidiarrheals containing paregoric) may be available without prescription to patients >18 yr of age.

APPENDIX K
Equianalgesic Dosing Guidelines

OPIOID ANALGESICS STARTING ORAL DOSE COMMONLY USED FOR SEVERE PAIN

NAME	EQUIANALGESIC DOSE ORAL*	EQUIANALGESIC DOSE PARENTERAL†	STARTING ORAL DOSE ADULTS	STARTING ORAL DOSE CHILDREN	COMMENTS	PRECAUTIONS AND CONTRAINDICATIONS
a. Morphine-like agonists (mu agonists)						
morphine	30 mg	10 mg	15–30 mg	0.3 mg/kg	Standard of comparison for opioid analgesics. Sustained release preparations (MS Contin, OramorphSR) release over 8–12 hr. Other formulations (Kadian and Avinza) last 12–24 hr. Generic sustained release morphine preparations are now available.)	For all opioids, caution in patients with impaired ventilation, bronchial asthma, increased intracranial pressure, liver failure.
hydromorphone (Dilaudid)	7.5 mg	1.5 mg	4–8 mg	0.06 mg/kg	Slightly shorter duration than morphine.	
fentanyl		0.1 mg				
oxycodone	20 mg	—	10–20 mg	0.3 mg/kg		
methadone	10 mg	5 mg	5–10 mg	0.2 mg/kg	Good oral potency, long plasma half-life (24–36 hr).	Accumulates with repeated dosing, requiring decreases in dose size and frequency, especially on days 2–5. Use with caution in older adults.
levorphanol (Levodromoran)	4 mg (acute), 1 mg (chronic)	2 mg (acute), 1 mg (chronic)	2–4 mg	0.04 mg/kg	Long plasma half-life (12–16 hr, but may be as long as 90–120 hr after one wk of dosing).	Accumulates on days 2 and 3. Use with caution in older adults.
oxymorphone (Opana)	10 mg	1 mg	—		5 mg rectal suppository ~5 mg morphine parenteral.	Like parenteral morphine.

1418

Equianalgesic Dosing Guidelines

NAME	EQUIANALGESIC DOSE ORAL*	EQUIANALGESIC DOSE PARENTERAL†	STARTING ORAL DOSE ADULTS	STARTING ORAL DOSE CHILDREN	COMMENTS	PRECAUTIONS AND CONTRAINDICATIONS
meperidine (Demerol)	Not recommended	Not recommended	Not Recommended		Slightly shorter acting than morphine accumulates with repetitive dosing causing CNS excitation; avoid in children with impaired renal function or who are receiving monoamine oxidase inhibitors.‡	Use with caution. Normeperidine (toxic metabolite) accumulates with repetitive dosing causing CNS excitation and a high risk of seizure. Avoid in children, renal impairment and patients on monoamine oxidase inhibitors.‡
b. Mixed agonists—antagonists (kappa agonists)						
nalbuphine (Nubain)	—	10 mg	—	—	Not available orally, not scheduled under Controlled Substances Act.	Incidence of psychotomimetic effects lower than with pentazocine; may precipitate withdrawal in opioid-dependent patients.
butorphanol (Stadol)	—	2 mg	—	—	Like nalbuphine. Also available in nasal spray.	Like nalbuphine.
pentazocine (Talwin)	50 mg	30 mg	—	—		
c. Partial agonist						
buprenorphine (Buprenex)	—	0.4 mg	—	—	Lower abuse liability than morphine; does not produce psychotomimetic effects. Sublingual tablets now available both plain and with naloxone for opioid-dependent patient management for specially certified physicians. These tablets are not approved as analgesics.	May precipitate withdrawal in narcotic-dependent patients; not readily reversed by naloxone; avoid in labor.

*Starting dose should be lower for older adults.
†These are standard parenteral doses for acute pain in adults and can also be used to convert doses for IV infusions and repeated small IV boluses. For single IV boluses, use half the IM dose. IV doses for children > 6 mo. = parenteral equianalgesic dose times weight (kg)/100.
‡Irritating to tissues with repeated IM injections.
Modified from American Pain Society, *Principles of Analgesic Use in the Treatment of Acute Pain and Cancer Pain*, ed.6. American Pain Society, 2008.

GUIDELINES FOR PATIENT-CONTROLLED INTRAVENOUS OPIOID ADMINISTRATION FOR ADULTS WITH ACUTE PAIN

DRUG	USUAL STARTING DOSE AFTER LOADING	USUAL DOSE RANGE	USUAL LOCKOUT (MIN)	USUAL LOCKOUT RANGE (MIN)
Morphine (1 mg/mL)	1 mg	0.5–2.5 mg	8	5–10
Hydromorphone (0.2 mg/mL)	0.2 mg	0.05–0.4 mg	8	5–10
Fentanyl (50 mcg/mL)	20 mcg	10–50 mcg	6	5–8

*Standard concentrations for most PCA machines are listed in parentheses.
Modified from *American Pain Society, Principles of Analgesic Use in the Treatment of Acute Pain and Cancer Pain*, ed.6. American Pain Society, 2008.

FENTANYL TRANSDERMAL DOSE BASED ON DAILY MORPHINE DOSE

ORAL 24-HR MORPHINE (mg/day)	TRANSDERMAL FENTANYL (mg/day)	FENTANYL TRANSDERMAL (mcg/hr)
30–90	0.6	25
91–150	1.2	50
151–210	1.8	75
211–270	2.4	100
271–330	3.0	125
331–390	3.6	150
391–450	4.2	175
451–510	4.8	200
511–570	5.4	225
571–630	6.0	250
631–690	6.6	275
691–750	7.2	300
For each additional 60 mg/day	+0.6	+25

*A 10-mg IM or 60-mg oral dose of morphine every 4 hr for 24 hr (total of 60 mg/day IM or 360 mg/day oral) was considered approximately equivalent to fentanyl transdermal 100 mcg/hr.

APPENDIX L
Recommendations for the Safe Handling of Hazardous Drugs*

Hazardous Drugs (HDs) have toxic, carcinogenic, mutagenic, and/or teratogenic potential, may cause irritation to the skin, eyes, and mucous membranes, and may cause ulceration and necrosis of tissue. For these obvious reasons, health care workers must minimize their exposure to these chemicals. The U.S. Department of Labor, Occupational Safety & Health Administration (OSHA) has laid out very specific recommendations called Guidelines for the Safe Handling of Hazardous Drugs, which can be found at http://www.osha.gov/dts/osta/otm/otm _ vi/otm _ vi _ 2.html. Refer to this document and your facility's policy and procedure manuals for detailed recommendations.

Means of Exposure

Exposure to HDs occurs during preparation and administration of these drugs or during patient care. Inhalation of aerosolized particles, accidental exposure to skin and eyes, and handling contaminated linens or equipment are the primary potential routes of exposure. Even when great care is taken, splattering, spraying, and aerosolization of HDs can occur when withdrawing the needle from a drug vial, opening an ampule, or expelling air from a syringe. Blood, body fluids, and excreta can contain HDs and expose staff to potentially dangerous amounts of hazardous drugs.

Protecting Against Exposure

Preparation of HDs should occur in a specified area called a Biological Safety Cabinet (BSC). If a BSC is not available, the nurse or other staff member preparing an HD should wear a respirator with a high-efficiency filter and full face coverage or partial face coverage with splash goggles and a respirator. Staff should also wear protective gowns and don two sets of latex gloves. Tuck gloves in at the wrist (inner glove under cuff, outer glove over cuff).

Use aseptic technique when preparing the drug for administration and handle equipment carefully to prevent dripping, spraying, or other exposure. Once prepared, wipe bags or bottles with moist gauze to remove spray or spills and swab entry ports with alcohol. Label all syringes and IV bags with a warning label and standard labeling. If being transported, the bag, bottle, or vial should be packaged in a sealed plastic bag and placed inside a secure container. Excess solution should be discarded in a covered disposable container.

Administration of HDs

Wear the same personal protective equipment (PPE) (gown, gloves, splash goggles) for administering the HD as for preparing it. Always wear a respirator when administering aerosolized drugs. In addition to wearing PPE, obtain the following equipment to use during administration: gauze for cleanup, alcohol wipes, disposable plastic-backed absorbent liner, puncture-resistant container (for needles/syringes), resealable plastic bag with warning label and other accessory warning labels.

---

*Controlling occupational exposure to hazardous drugs. OSHA Technical Manual. Section VI: Chapter 2. Available at http://www.osha.gov/dts/osta/otm/otm _ vi _ 2.html. Accessed December 17, 2007.

Caring for Patients Receiving HDs

The following precautions are recommended:

- Observe standard precautions.
- Wear gown and gloves when in the patient's room for 48 hr following administration of a hazardous drug.
- Wear eye protection if splashing is possible.
- Wear a gown and gloves when handling contaminated laundry. Bag contaminated linens separately.

Managing Spills

Have spill kits available in areas where HDs are handled. The kit should include splash goggles, 2 pairs of gloves, utility gloves, gown, 2 sheets of absorbent material, spill-control pillows (2 sizes), "sharps" container, and 2 large HD disposal bags.

- Clean up spills only when properly protected and using the facility's procedure.
- Report area of spill to administrative staff.
- For small spills (less than 5 mL or 5 g), mop up liquids with absorbent gauze or use damp gauze to pick up solid contaminated material. Broken fragments should be picked up with a scoop and disposed in a sharps container. Wash the area three times with detergent followed by water.
- Isolate large spill areas and use absorbent sheets or spill-control pads. Use damp cloths if a powder is spilled. Spills greater than 150 mL (or 1 vial) require decontamination.

If Exposure Occurs

Risk of injury can be minimized by following these steps:

- Immediately remove gloves and gown.
- Immediately wash the affected skin with soap and water.
- Flood eyes at eyewash fountain or flush with water or isotonic eyewash for at least 15 min.
- Obtain medical attention and follow protocols for specific exposure.
- Document exposure.

APPENDIX M
Food Sources for Specific Nutrients

Potassium-Rich Foods

- artichoke
- avocados
- bananas
- cantaloupe
- cassava
- dried fruits
- grapefruit
- honey dew
- jack fruit
- kiwi
- kohlrabi
- lima beans
- mango
- meats
- milk
- dried peas and beans
- nuts
- oranges/orange juice
- papaya
- peaches
- pears
- plantains
- pomegranate
- potatoes (white and sweet)
- prunes/prune juice
- pumpkin
- rhubarb
- salt substitute
- spinach
- sunflower seeds
- Swiss chard
- tomatoes/tomato juice
- vegetable juice
- winter squash

Sodium-Rich Foods

- baking mixes (pancakes, muffins)
- barbecue sauce
- buttermilk
- butter/margarine
- canned chili
- canned seafood
- canned soups
- canned spaghetti sauce
- cured meats
- dry onion soup mix
- "fast" foods
- frozen dinners
- macaroni and cheese
- microwave dinners
- Parmesan cheese
- pickles
- potato salad
- pretzels, potato chips
- salad dressings (prepared)
- salt
- sauerkraut
- tomato ketchup

Calcium-Rich Foods

- broccoli
- canned salmon/sardines
- clams
- cream soups
- greens: collard and turnip
- molasses (blackstrap)
- oysters
- refried beans
- spinach
- tofu

Vitamin K-Rich Foods

- asparagus
- beans
- broccoli
- brussel sprouts
- cabbage
- cauliflower
- collards
- green tea
- kale
- milk
- mustard greens
- spinach
- swiss chard
- turnips
- yogurt

Low-Sodium Foods

- baked or broiled poultry
- canned pumpkin
- cooked turnips
- egg yolk
- fresh vegetables
- fruit
- grits (not instant)
- honey
- jams and jellies
- lean meats
- low-calorie mayonnaise
- macaroons
- potatoes
- puffed wheat and rice
- red kidney and lima beans
- sherbet
- unsalted nuts
- whiskey

Foods That Acidify Urine

- cheeses
- corn
- cranberries
- eggs
- fish
- grains (breads and cereals)
- lentils
- meats
- nuts (Brazil, filberts, walnuts)
- pasta
- plums
- poultry
- prunes
- rice

Foods That Alkalinize Urine

- all fruits except cranberries, prunes, plums
- all vegetables (except corn)
- milk
- nuts (almonds, chesnuts)

Foods Containing Tyramine

- aged cheeses (blue, Boursault, brick, Brie, Camembert, cheddar, Emmenthaler, Gruyère, mozzarella, Parmesan, Romano, Roquefort, Stilton, Swiss)
- American processed cheese
- avocados (especially over-ripe)
- bananas
- bean curd
- beer and ale
- caffeine-containing beverages (coffee, tea, colas)
- caviar
- chocolate
- distilled spirits
- fermented sausage (bologna, salami, pepperoni, summer sausage)
- liver
- meats prepared with tenderizer
- miso soup
- over-ripe fruit
- peanuts
- raisins
- raspberries
- red wine (especially Chianti)
- sauerkraut
- sherry
- shrimp paste
- smoked or pickled fish
- soy sauce
- vermouth
- yeasts
- yogurt

Iron-Rich Foods

- cereals
- clams
- dried beans and peas
- dried fruit
- leafy green vegetables
- lean red meats
- molasses (blackstrap)
- organ meats

Vitamin D-Rich Foods

- canned salmon, sardines, tuna
- cereals
- fish
- fish liver oils
- fortified milk
- nonfat dry milk

APPENDIX N
Insulins and Insulin Therapy

The goal of therapy for diabetic patients is to provide insulin coverage that most closely resembles endogenous insulin production and results in the best glycemic control without hypoglycemia. Although daytime control of hyperglycemia may be accomplished with bolus doses of rapid-acting insulin analogs, elevations in fasting glucose may remain a problem. If fasting blood glucose levels remain elevated, the basal insulin dose (intermediate or long-acting) may have to be adjusted.

Most insulins used today are recombinant DNA human insulins. Produced through genetic engineering, synthetic human insulin is "manufactured" by yeast or nonpathogenic *E. coli*. In recent years, pharmaceutical companies have developed several new types and formulations of insulin.

Different insulins are distinguished by how quickly they are absorbed, the time and length of peak activity, and overall duration of action. Onset, peak, and duration of action times are approximate and vary according to individual factors such as injection site, blood supply, concurrent illnesses, lifestyle, and exercise level. These factors can vary from patient to patient and can vary in any patient from day to day.

There are 4 kinds of insulins: rapid-acting, short-acting, intermediate-acting, and long-acting and premixed combinations.

Rapid-Acting Insulins

Rapid-acting insulins are analogs of regular insulin. An analog is a chemical structure very similar to another but differing in one component. Humalog (lispro), Apidra (glulisine), and Novolog (aspart) are rapid-acting insulin analogs. The amino acid sequences of these analogs are nearly identical to human insulin. They differ in the positioning of certain proteins, which allow them to enter the bloodstream rapidly—within 10 min of subcutaneous injection. This closely mimics the body's own insulin response and allows greater flexibility in eating schedules for diabetic patients. Also, because these insulins leave the bloodstream quickly, the risk of hypoglycemic episodes several hours after the meal is lessened. The peak time for rapid-acting insulins is 1–2 hr and the duration is 3–4 hr. Rapid-acting insulin solutions are clear. Both insulin aspart and insulin glulisine can be given intravenously.

Short-Acting Insulin

Regular insulin is short-acting insulin and is available commercially as Humulin R or Novolin R. The onset of regular insulin is 0.5–1 hr; its peak activity occurs 2–3 hr after subcutaneous injection and its duration of action is 6–8 hr. This time/action profile makes rigid meal scheduling necessary, as the patient must estimate that a meal will occur within 45 min of injection. Short-acting insulin solutions are clear. Regular insulin can be given intravenously.

Intermediate-Acting Insulins

Intermediate-acting insulin contain protamine, which delays onset, peak, and duration of action to provide basal insulin coverage. Basal insulins are given to control blood glucose levels throughout the day when not eating. Commercially, intermediate-acting insulins are available as Humulin N or Novolin N. (The "N" stands for NPH). Action starts between 1 and 4 hr after injecting. Peak activity occurs between 6 and 12 hr. Duration of action lasts 18–24 hr. The addition of protamine causes the cloudy appearance of intermediate-acting insulins and results in the formulation being a suspension rather than a solution. This is why these insulins must be gently mixed before administering. Intermediate-acting insulins can be mixed with short- or rapid-acting insulins to provide both basal and bolus coverage.

Long-Acting Insulins

Long-acting insulins have the most delayed onset and the longest duration of all insulins. Products include Lantus (insulin glargine), and Levemir (insulin detemir). Peaks are not as prominent in long-acting insulins. In fact, insulin glargine has no real peak action because it forms slowly dissolving crystals in the subcutaneous tissue. The onset of action of insulin glargine is 1 hr after subcutaneous injection. Full activity occurs within 4 to 5 hr and remains constant for 24 hr. Even though insulin glargine and insulin detemir are clear solutions, neither can be diluted or mixed with any other insulin or solution. Mixing insulin glargine or insulin detemir with other insulin products can alter the onset of action and time to peak effect. If bolus insulin is to be given at the same time as insulin glargine or insulin detemir, two separate syringes and injection sites must be used.

Combination Insulins

Various combinations of premixed insulins are available, containing fixed proportions of two different insulins, usually a short- and an intermediate-acting insulin. Typically the intermediate-acting insulin makes up 70% to 75% of the mixture, with rapid- or short- acting insulin making up the remainder. Onset, peak, and duration vary according to each specific product. Brand names of these products include Humulin 70/30 (70% NPH, 30% regular), Humalog Mix 75/25 (75% insulin lispro protamine suspension and 25% insulin lispro), Humalog Mix 50/50 (50% insulin lispro protamine suspension and 50% insulin lispro), and Novolin 70/30 (70% NPH, 30% regular), or Novolog 70/30 (70% insulin aspart protamine suspension and 30% insulin aspart).

BRAND NAME	GENERIC NAME	TYPE OF INSULIN	ONSET/PEAK/DURATION
Apidra	insulin glulisine	Rapid-acting	<15 min/1–2 hr/3–4 hr
Humalog	insulin lispro	Rapid-acting	<15 min/1–2 hr/3–4 hr
Novolog	insulin aspart	Rapid-acting	<15 min/1–2 hr/3–4 hr
Humulin R	regular insulin	Short-acting	½–1 hr/2–3 hr/3–6 hr
Novolin R	regular insulin	Short-acting	½–1 hr/2–3 hr/3–6 hr
Humulin N	NPH	Intermediate-acting	2–4 hr/4–10 hr/10–16 hr
Novolin N	NPH	Intermediate-acting	2–4 hr/4–10 hr/10–16 hr
Levemir	insulin detemir	Long-acting	minimal peak; lasts up to 24 hr
Lantus	insulin glargine	Long-acting	no peak; lasts up to 24 hr

APPENDIX O
Canadian and U.S. Pharmaceutical Practices

In the United States and Canada, most drugs are prescribed and used similarly. However, certain processes and actions of the U.S. and Canadian pharmaceutical industries differ in significant ways, affecting both consumers and health care providers. Safety, marketing, and availability are three of these issues.

Safety

Controversy related to the importation of medications from Canada by U.S. consumers has sometimes raised concerns about the safety of these drugs. These fears are unfounded; in fact, the Canadian approval and manufacturing processes are very similar to U.S. processes. Both countries have pharmaceutical-related standards, laws, and policies to ensure that chemical entities marketed for human diseases and conditions are safe and effective. The process of taking a new drug from the laboratory to the pharmacy shelves includes:

Scientific development. The process begins with research. Scientists develop a new molecular entity targeted at a specific disease, symptom, or condition.

Patenting. The manufacturer applies for a patent, which prevents other drug companies from manufacturing a chemically identical drug. Patent protection lasts 17 years in the United States and 20 years in Canada. After the patent expires, any manufacturer can make generic versions of the chemical; generics typically cost much less than the brand-name drug.

Pre-clinical testing. Before the drug is taken by human subjects, pre-clinical testing of the chemical is performed on animals. Testing helps identify drug action, toxicity effects, side effects, adverse reactions, dosage amounts and routes, and administration procedures. This phase can take 3 to 5 years.

Permission to begin clinical testing. Once the drug is found to have demonstrable positive health effects and to be safe for animals, the manufacturer applies for permission to begin clinical studies on human subjects. In the United States, this is called New Drug Application (NDA) and is administered by the Food and Drug Administration (FDA). In Canada, this is called a Clinical Trial Application (CTA) and is administered by Health Canada.

Clinical trials. Clinical trials are initiated to establish the potential benefits and risks for humans. Several sub-phases are required in the clinical trials phase whereby increasingly larger sample sizes are used.

Phase 0: A new designation for first-in-human trials, which are designed to assess whether the drug affects humans in the manner expected.

Phase I: Between 20 and 80 healthy volunteers are recruited to assess safety, tolerance, dosage ranges, pharmacokinetics, and pharmacodynamics.

Phase II: Up to 300 patients with the disease are enrolled to assess efficacy and toxicity. Variables from Phase I trials may also be assessed.

Phase III: Between 1000 and 3000 patients are entered into a randomized, double-blind study designed to confirm effectiveness, compare the new treatment with existing treatments, and study side effects further.

Phase IV: Ongoing surveillance of the drug after it receives approval and is marketed to assess for rare or long-term effects.

Approval. The results of the clinical studies are reviewed by Health Canada in Canada and by the FDA in the United States. These regulatory bodies assess every aspect of the drug, including the labeling. The approval process has been deemed excessively long by physicians and patients anxious to try new remedies for refractory or terminal diseases, and efforts have been made to shorten the process in both countries. Although approval times for new drugs were found to be significantly longer in Canada, it has been noted that significantly fewer drugs have been pulled from the market for safety reasons. Statistically, Canadians remove 2% of new drugs for safety reasons, whereas 3.6% of new drugs are taken off the market in the United States.[1]

Marketing. Once a drug has been approved, it can be prescribed to consumers or, if it does not require a prescription, purchased by them.

Post-Marketing Surveillance. More clinical data become available when the drug is marketed and used by many people for longer periods of time. Pharmacovigilance is the term used to refer to the process of ongoing assessment of a drug's safety and effectiveness during this phase.

Differences Between Canadian and U.S. Drug Pricing and Marketing

One major difference between the two countries is pricing. In Canada, the Patented Medicine Prices Review Board (PMPRB) regulates the prices manufacturers can charge for prescription and nonprescription medicines. This is to ensure that prices are not excessive. No such controls exist in the United States, which is why many citizens purchase their medications from Canadian online pharmacies. One study found that U.S. citizens can save approximately 24% if they buy their medications from Canadian pharmacies rather than from a U.S. chain pharmacy.[2]

Another difference is in advertising. In the United States, manufacturers can market drugs directly, and forcefully, to consumers, a controversial privilege that has resulted in consumers requesting specific medications despite not necessarily understanding the complete risks and benefits. In Canada, such advertising is limited and subject to the approval of the Advertising Standards Canada (ASC) agency and the Pharmaceutical Advertising Advisory Board (PAAB). To address this issue in the United States, the Institute of Medicine (IOM) has recommended that the FDA ban direct-to-consumer advertising for the first 2 years after a drug is marketed. Such a delay may help to prevent large numbers of people experiencing side effects not observed in the clinical trials, such as occurred with sildenafil (Viagra) when several patients died or developed vision problems in the first months after marketing began.

Drug Schedule, Availability, and Pregnancy Category Differences

Most Canadian provinces (with the exception of Québec) use drug schedules similar to U.S. schedules of controlled substances. Canada uses four categories, whereas the United States uses five (see Appendix J for controlled substance schedules). The Canadian drug schedules are:

- **Schedule I:** Available only by prescription and provided by a pharmacist.
- **Schedule II:** Available only from a pharmacist; must be kept in an area with no public access.
- **Schedule III:** Available via open access in a pharmacy (over-the-counter).
- **Unscheduled:** Can be sold in any store without professional supervision.

Another difference is in availability. Some potentially dangerous drugs—such as heparin, insulin, and codeine-containing cough medicines—are available only with a prescription in the United States but are available over-the-counter in Canada. Similarly, some Canadian drugs are available in combinations not found in the United States (see Appendix B for new Canadian combination drugs).

Although Canada currently does not have pregnancy categories like the United States, it is developing them. Canadian prescribers practice under the premise that no drug should be given to a pregnant woman unless the benefits to the mother clearly outweigh the potential risks to the fetus. Canadian health care providers may refer to a drug's FDA pregnancy category for guidance (see Appendix I).

SOURCES CITED

1. Rawson N. "Canadian and U.S. Drug Approval Times and Safety Considerations." Ann Pharmacother. 37(10):1403–1408, 2003. Published Online, August 1, 2003. http://www.theannals.com. DOI 10.1345/aph.1D110 (accessed 15 December 2007).
2. Quon B., Firszt R., Eisenberg M. "A Comparison of Brand-Name Drug Prices Between Canadian-Based Internet Pharmacies and Major U.S. Drug Chain Pharmacies. Ann Intern Med. 143(6):397–403, 2005. http://www.annals.org/cgi/content/abstract/143/6/397 (accessed 10 December 2007).

ADDITIONAL REFERENCES

Canadian Pharmacists Association. "From Research Lab to Pharmacy Shelf." http://www.pharmacists.ca/content/hcp/resource_centre/drug_therapeutic_info/pdf/DrugApprovalProcess.pdf (accessed 15 December 2007).

Health Canada. http://www.hc-sc.gc.ca/ahc-asc/index_e.html (accessed 15 December 2007).

Tomalin A. "Drugs Used in Pregnancy: The Regulatory Process." Can J Clin Pharmacol. 14(1):e5–e9, 2007. http://www.cjcp.ca/pdf/CJCP2007_e5_e9.pdf (accessed 10 December 2007).

U.S. Food and Drug Administration. http://www.fda.gov (accessed 15 December 2007).

APPENDIX P
Routine Pediatric and Adult Immunizations

Immunization recommendations change frequently. For the latest recommendations see http://www.cdc.gov/nip.

ROUTINE PEDIATRIC IMMUNIZATIONS (0–18 yr)

GENERIC NAME (BRAND NAMES)	ROUTE/DOSAGE	CONTRAINDICATIONS/ PRECAUTIONS	ADVERSE REACTIONS/SIDE EFFECTS	NOTES
Diphtheria toxoid, tetanus toxoid, and acellular pertussis vaccine (DTaP, Daptacel, Infanrix, Tripedia)	0.5 mL IM at 2, 4, 6, 15–18 mo and 4–6 yr (1st dose may be given as early as age 6 wk; 4th dose may be given at 12 mo).	Acute infection; previous CNS damage; convulsions.	Redness, tenderness, induration at site; fever; malaise; myalgia; urticaria; hypotension; neurologic reactions; allergic reactions (all less than with DTwP).	Individual components may be given as separate injections if unusual reactions occur.
Tetanus toxoid, **reduced** diphtheria toxoid, and acellular pertussis vaccine absorbed (Tdap, Adacell, Boostrix)	0.5 mL IM given at age 11–12 yr if 5 yr have elapsed since last dose of DTaP; one-time dose may be given to all adolescents who have not received previous Tdap.	Previous reactions to DTaP; progressive neurological disease; recent (within 7 days) CNS pathology.	Fatigue, headache, gastrointestinal symptoms, pain at injection site.	Pertussis protection in addition to diphtheria and tetanus designed to protect against older children becoming ill with pertussis from passing it on to very young unprotected children in whom the disease has heightened morbidity.
Polio vaccine, inactivated (IPV, IPOL, Poliovax)	0.5 mL IM or subcut at 2, 4, and 6–18 mo and at 4–6 yr (1st dose may be given as early as age 6 wk).	Hypersensitivity to neomycin, streptomycin, or polymyxin B; acute febrile illness; pregnancy.	Erythema, induration, pain at injection site; fever.	Oral polio vaccine (OPV) is no longer recommended for use in the United States.
Measles, mumps, and rubella vaccines (M-M-R II)	0.5 mL subcut at 12–15 mo and at 4–6 yr.	Allergy to egg, gelatin, or neomycin; active infection; severe immunosuppression (in the absence of severe immunosuppression, HIV is not a contraindication); pregnancy.	Burning, stinging, pain at injection site; arthritis/arthralgia; fever; encephalitis; allergic reactions.	If unusual reactions occur, individual components may be given as separate injections. Immunosuppression may ↓ antibody response to injection and ↑ the risk of viral transmission.

1429

GENERIC NAME (BRAND NAMES)	ROUTE/DOSAGE	CONTRAINDICATIONS/ PRECAUTIONS	ADVERSE REACTIONS/SIDE EFFECTS	NOTES
Haemophilus b conjugate vaccine (Hib, PedvaxHIB, ActHIB, Hiberix)	*ActHIB*—0.5 mL IM at 2, 4, and 6 mo, with a booster at 12–15 mo; *PedvaxHIB*—0.5 mL IM at 2 and 4 mo, with a booster dose at 12–15 mo; *Hiberix*—can only be used for the booster dose (any of the products can be used for the booster dose).	If co-administered with other immunizations, consider contraindications of all products.	Induration, erythema, tenderness at injection site; fever.	
Hepatitis B vaccine (HepB, Engerix-B, Recombivax HB)	0.5 mL IM at 0, 1–2, and 6–18 mo. Dose is same for patients age 0–19 yr. *Infants born to HBsAg-positive mothers:* Administer 0.5 mL of hepatitis B immune globulin IM and 1st dose of hepatitis B vaccine; give 2nd and 3rd doses of hepatitis B vaccine at 1 mo and 6 mo, respectively.	Hypersensitivity to yeast.	Local soreness.	A 2-dose series (separated by ≥4 mo) of the adult formulation (Recombivax HB) can be used in children 11–15 yr.
Meningococcal conjugate vaccine (MCV4, Menactra)	0.5 mL IM single dose at 11-12 yr or at age 13–18 yr if not previously vaccinated.	Hypersensitivity to any components.	Fatigue, malaise, anorexia, pain at injection site.	Routine vaccination with meningococcal vaccine also is recommended for college freshmen living in dormitories who are previously unvaccinated and children ≥2 yr who are at high risk (anatomic or functional asplenia; persistent complement component deficiency; travel or reside in areas in which meningococcal disease is hyperendemic or epidemic).
Varicella vaccine (Var, Varivax)	0.5 mL subcut at 12–15 mo and at 4–6 yr (2nd dose may be given earlier if ≥3 mo have elapsed since the 1st dose); for persons 7–18 yr who have not been vaccinated or without a history of chickenpox, 2 doses should be given (≥3 mo apart if 7–12 yr or ≥28 days apart if ≥13 yr).	Allergy to gelatin or neomycin; active infection; immunosuppression (including HIV); pregnancy.	Local soreness, fever.	Given to children and adolescents who do not have evidence of immunity. immunosuppression may ↓ antibody response to injection and ↑ the risk of viral transmission.

Routine Pediatric and Adult Immunizations

GENERIC NAME (BRAND NAMES)	ROUTE/DOSAGE	CONTRAINDICATIONS/ PRECAUTIONS	ADVERSE REACTIONS/SIDE EFFECTS	NOTES
Hepatitis A vaccine (HepA, Havrix, Vaqta)	Should be given to all children age 12–23 mo; give a total of 2 doses of pediatric formulation (each 0.5 mL) IM at least 6 mo apart.	Acute febrile illness	Local reactions, headache.	Also recommended in children ≥2 yr who live in areas with high rates of hepatitis A or are in other high-risk groups (e.g., chronic liver disease, clotting factor disorders, illicit drug users).
Pneumococcal conjugate vaccine (7–valent) (PCV, Prevnar)	0.5 mL IM at 2, 4, 6, and 12–15 mo.	Hypersensitivity to all components including diphtheria toxoid; moderate to severe febrile illness.	Erythema induration, tenderness, nodule formation at injection site, fever.	One dose may also be given to previously unvaccinated healthy children age 24–59 mo. For high-risk children (e.g., sickle cell disease; anatomic or functional asplenia; chronic cardiac, pulmonary, or renal disease; diabetes; HIV; immunosuppression; cochlear implant) age 24–59 mo, give 2 doses (≥8 wk apart) if previously received <3 doses or 1 dose if previously received 3 doses.
Pneumococcal polysaccharide vaccine (PPSV, Pneumovax 23)	0.5 mL IM or subcut ≥8 wk after final dose of PCV in high-risk children ≥2 yr (see Notes section for pneumococcal conjugate vaccine for definition of high risk).	Hypersensitivity to all components including diphtheria toxoid; moderate to severe febrile illness.	Erythema induration, tenderness, nodule formation at injection site, fever.	A 2nd dose may be given 5 yr later in children with immunosuppression, sickle cell disease, or anatomic/functional asplenia.
Influenza vaccine *injection (trivalent inactivated)*: (Afluria, Fluarix, FluLaval, Fluvirin, Fluzone; *intranasal (live attenuated)*: (FluMist)	*Injection*: *Age 6–35 mo*: 2 doses of 0.25 mL IM given 4 wk apart for initial season, then one dose annually. *Age 3–8 yr*: 2 doses of 0.5 mL IM given 4 wk apart for initial season, then one dose annually. *Age ≥9 yr*: 0.5 mL IM single dose annually. **Intranasal:** *Age 2–8 yr*: If not previously vaccinated with influenza vaccine—2 doses of 0.2 mL (given as 0.1 mL in each nostril) 4 wk apart, then one dose annually. If previously vaccinated with influenza vaccine—1 dose of 0.2 mL (given as 0.1 mL in each nostril) annually. *Age ≥9 yr*: 1 dose of 0.2 mL (given as 0.1 mL dose in each nostril) annually.	Hypersensitivity to eggs/egg products. Hypersensitivity to thimerosal (injection only). Avoid use in patients with acute neurologic compromise. Fluvirin should only be used in children ≥4 yr. FluMist should be avoided in pregnancy; chronic pulmonary (including asthma), cardiovascular (not hypertension), renal, hepatic, neurological, hematologic, or metabolic (including diabetes) disorders; immunosuppression (including HIV); chronic salicylate therapy (children 6 mo–18 yr).	*Injection*: local soreness, fever, myalgia, possible neurologic toxicity. *Intranasal*: upper respiratory congestion, malaise.	Immunosuppression may ↓ antibody response to injection and ↑ the risk of viral transmission with intranasal route.

GENERIC NAME (BRAND NAMES)	ROUTE/DOSAGE	CONTRAINDICATIONS/ PRECAUTIONS	ADVERSE REACTIONS/SIDE EFFECTS	NOTES
Human papillomavirus vaccine (HPV, Gardasil)	0.5 mL IM in males and females age 9–26 yr, repeat at 2 and 6 mo after 1st dose.	Hypersensitivity to yeast; pregnancy.	Headache, dizziness, fever, nausea, diarrhea, syncope, local soreness.	Used to prevent cervical, vulvar, and vaginal cancer caused by HPV types 16 and 18 in females and to prevent genital warts caused by HPV types 6 and 11 in males and females. Series should not be started in infants older than 15 wk.
Rotavirus vaccine (RV, Rotarix [RV1], RotaTeq [RV5])	*Rotarix*—1 mL PO at 2 and 4 mo; *RotaTeq*—2 mL PO at 2, 4, and 6 mo. First dose of either product may be given as early as age 6 wk; final dose should be given no later than age 8 mo.	History of uncorrected congenital malformation of GI tract (Rotarix).	Fever, irritability, diarrhea, vomiting.	

Nursing Implications:

Assessment
Assess previous immunization history and history of hypersensitivity.
Assess for history of latex allergy. Some prefilled syringes may use latex components and should be avoided in those with hypersensitivity.

Potential Nursing Diagnoses
Infection, risk for (Indications).
Knowledge, deficient, related to medication regimen (Patient/Family Teaching).

Implementation
Measles, mumps, and rubella vaccine; trivalent oral poliovirus vaccine; and diphtheria toxoid, tetanus toxoid, and pertussis vaccine may be given concomitantly.
Do not administer FluMist concurrently with other vaccines, or in patients who have received a live virus vaccine within 1 mo or an inactivated vaccine within 2 wk of vaccination.
Administer each immunization by appropriate route:
PO: Rotavirus.
Subcut: measles, mumps, rubella, polio, varicella, pneumococcal polysaccharide.
IM: diphtheria, tetanus toxoid, pertussis, polio, Haemophilus b, hepatitis B, meningococcal conjugate, hepatitis A, pneumococcal conjugate, pneumococcal polysaccharide, influenza injection, human papillomavirus.
Intranasal: FluMist.

Patient/Family Teaching
Inform parent of potential and reportable side effects of immunization. Notify health care professional if patient develops fever higher than 39.4°C (103°F); difficulty breathing; hives; itching; swelling of eyes, face, or inside of nose; sudden, severe tiredness or weakness; or convulsions.
Review next scheduled immunization with parent.

Evaluation
Prevention of diseases through active immunity.

ROUTINE ADULT IMMUNIZATIONS

GENERIC NAME (BRAND NAMES)	INDICATIONS	DOSAGE/ROUTE	CONTRAINDICATIONS	ADVERSE REACTIONS/SIDE EFFECTS
Hepatitis A vaccine (Hepa, Havrix, Vaqta*)	High-risk groups (e.g., chronic liver disease, clotting factor disorders, illicit drug users, men who have sex with men, some health care workers, food handlers); travel to endemic areas; recent (<2 wk) exposure to HepA (if ≤40 yr).	1 mL IM, followed by 1 mL IM 6–18 mo later (adult dose form).	Hypersensitivity to alum or 2-phenoxyethanol.	Local reactions, headache.
Hepatitis B vaccine (HepB, Engerix-B, Recombivax HB)	High-risk patients (e.g., household contacts or sex partners of HBsAg-positive persons, IV drug users, sexually active persons not in a monogamous relationship, men who have sex with men, HIV, STDs, hemodialysis, health care workers, inmates); chronic liver disease; all unvaccinated adolescents.	3 doses of 1 mL IM, given at 0, 1–2, and 4–6 mo.	Anaphylactic allergy to yeast.	Local soreness.
Human papillomavirus vaccine (HPV, Gardasil)	All previously unvaccinated women through age 26 yr. Also recommended for males through age 26 yr for prevention of genital warts caused by HPV types 6 and 11.	0.5 mL IM, repeat at 2 and 6 mo after initial dose.	Hypersensitivity to yeast; pregnancy.	Headache, dizziness, fever, nausea, diarrhea, syncope, local soreness.
Influenza vaccine *injection (trivalent inactivated)*: (Afluria, Fluarix, FluLaval, Fluvirin, Fluzone); *intranasal (live attenuated)*: (FluMist)	All adults.	*Injection*: 0.5 mL IM annually. *Intranasal (for adults <50 yr)*: Single 0.2 mL dose (given as 0.1 mL in each nostril) annually.	Hypersensitivity to eggs/egg products. Hypersensitivity to thimerosal (injection only). Patients with acute neurologic compromise. FluMist should be avoided in pregnancy; chronic pulmonary (including asthma), cardiovascular (not hypertension), renal, hepatic, neurological, hematologic, or metabolic (including diabetes) disorders; immunosuppression (including HIV); age ≥50 yr.	*Injection*: local soreness, fever myalgia, possible neurologic toxicity. *Intranasal*: upper respiratory congestion, malaise. Immunosuppression may ↓ antibody response to injection and ↑ the risk of viral transmission with intranasal route.

GENERIC NAME (BRAND NAMES)	INDICATIONS	DOSAGE/ROUTE	CONTRAINDICATIONS	ADVERSE REACTIONS/SIDE EFFECTS
Measles, mumps, and rubella vaccines (M-M-R II)	Adults born in 1957 or later with unreliable history of MMR illness or immunization; high-risk groups (e.g., health care workers, college students, international travelers); women of childbearing age (with no evidence of rubella immunity or immunization).	0.5 mL subcut, 1 or 2 doses in adults born in 1957 or later with unreliable history; high-risk groups should receive a total of 2 doses given 1 mo apart.	Allergy to egg, gelatin, or neomycin; active infection; severe immunosuppression (in the absence of severe immunosuppression, HIV is not a contraindication); pregnancy (also avoid becoming pregnant for 4 wk after immunization).	Burning, stinging, pain at injection site; arthritis/arthralgia; fever; encephalitis; allergic reactions. Immunosuppression may ↓ antibody response to injection and ↑ the risk of viral transmission.
Meningococcal conjugate vaccine (MCV4, Menactra)	College freshmen living in dormitories who are previously unvaccinated; anatomic or functional asplenia; persistent complement component deficiency; travel or reside in areas in which meningococcal disease is hyperendemic or epidemic.	0.5 mL IM single dose. Revaccination with MCV4 is indicated in patients previously vaccinated with MCV4 or meningococcal polysaccharide vaccine (MPSV4) and who also remain at ↑ risk for infection (revaccinate after 5 yr of previous dose)	Hypersensitivity to any components.	Fatigue, malaise, anorexia, pain at injection site.
Pneumococcal polysaccharide vaccine (PPSV, Pneumovax 23)	All adults ≥65 yr; high-risk patients (e.g., chronic cardiac or pulmonary disease [including asthma], chronic liver disease, alcoholism, diabetes, cigarette smoker, anatomic or functional asplenia, sickle cell disease; immunosuppression (including HIV), cochlear implants).	0.5 mL IM or subcut; one-time revaccination should also be given ≥5 yr after 1st dose to those ≥65 yr (if 1st dose was given before age 65) and to high-risk patients.	Hypersensitivity to all components including diphtheria toxoid.	Erythema induration, tenderness, nodule formation at injection site, fever.
Tetanus toxoid, **reduced** diphtheria toxoid and acellular pertussis vaccine absorbed (Tdap, Adacell, Boostrix)	Single dose should be given instead of Td in adults (19–64 yr) if they received their last dose of Td ≥10 yr ago (and did not previously receive a dose of Tdap).	0.5 mL IM to replace one dose of DTaP.	Previous reactions to DTaP; progressive neurological disease; recent (within 7 days) CNS pathology.	Fatigue, headache, gastrointestinal symptoms, pain at injection site

GENERIC NAME (BRAND NAMES)	INDICATIONS	DOSAGE/ROUTE	CONTRAINDICATIONS	ADVERSE REACTIONS/SIDE EFFECTS
Tetanus-diphtheria (Td, Decavac)	All adults who lack written documentation of a primary series consisting of ≥3 doses of tetanus– and diphtheria–toxoid–containing vaccine; booster dose should be given to all adults every 10 yr above regarding use of Tdap to replace one dose of Td in booster series).	*Unimmunized:* 2 doses 0.5 mL IM 1–2 mo apart, then a 3rd dose 6–12 mo later; *immunized:* 0.5 mL IM booster every 10 yr.	Neurologic or severe hypersensitivity reaction to prior dose.	Local pain and swelling.
Varicella vaccine (Var, Varivax)	Any adult without a history of chickenpox or herpes zoster (shingles), a history of receiving 2 doses of varicella vaccine, or laboratory evidence of immunity. Health care workers and pregnant women born in U.S. before 1980 who do not meet the above criteria should be tested for immunity.	0.5 mL subcut; repeated 4–8 wk later.	Allergy to gelatin or neomycin; active infection; immunosuppression (including HIV); pregnancy (also avoid becoming pregnant for 4 wk after immunization).	Local soreness, fever. Immunosuppression may → antibody response to injection and ↑ the risk of viral transmission.
Zoster vaccine (Zos, Zostavax)	All adults ≥60 yr (regardless of previous history of chickenpox or herpes zoster).	0.65 mL subcut single dose.	Allergy to gelatin or neomycin; active infection; immunosuppression (including HIV); pregnancy.	Local soreness, fever. Immunosuppression may → antibody response to injection and ↑ the risk of viral transmission.

*Less commonly used vaccines are not included.
SOURCE: Adapted from the recommendations of the National Immunization Program: http://www.cdc.gov/nip.

APPENDIX Q
Administering Medications to Children

General Guidelines

Medication administration to a pediatric patient can be challenging. Prescribers should order dosage forms that are age appropriate for their patients. If a child is unable to take a particular dosage form, ask the pharmacist if another form is available or for other options.

Oral Liquids

Pediatric liquid medicines may be given with plastic medicine cups, oral syringes, oral droppers, or cylindrical dosing spoons. Parents should be taught to use these calibrated devices rather than using household utensils. If a medicine comes with a particular measuring device, do not use it with another product. For young children, it is best to squirt a little of the dose at a time into the side of the cheek away from the bitter taste buds at the back of the tongue.

Eye Drops/Ointments

Tilt the child's head back and gently press the skin under the lower eyelid and pull the lower lid away slightly until a small pouch is visible. Insert the ointment or drop (1 at a time) and close the eye for a few minutes to keep the medicine in the eye.

Ear Drops

Shake otic suspensions well before administration. For children <3 yr, pull the outer ear outward and downward before instilling drops. For children ≥3 yr, pull the outer ear outward and upward. Keep child on side for 2 min and instill a cotton plug into ear.

Nose Drops

Clear nose of secretions prior to use. A nasal aspirator (bulb syringe) or a cotton swab may be used in infants and young children. Ask older children to blow their nose. Tilt child's head back over a pillow and squeeze dropper without touching the nostril. Keep child's head back for 2 min.

Suppositories

Keep refrigerated for easier administration. Wearing gloves, moisten the rounded end with water or petroleum jelly prior to insertion. Using your pinky finger for children <3 yr and your index finger for those ≥3 yr, insert the suppository into the rectum about ½ to 1 inch beyond the sphincter. If the suppository slides out, insert it a little farther than before. Hold the buttocks together for a few minutes and have the child hold their position for about 20 min, if possible.

Topicals

Clean affected area and dry well prior to application. Apply a thin layer to the skin and rub in gently. Do not apply coverings over the area unless instructed to do so by the prescriber.

Metered-Dose Inhalers

Generally the same principles apply in children as in adults, except the use of spacers is recommended for young children (see Appendix D).

APPENDIX R
Pediatric Dosage Calculations

Most drugs in children are dosed according to body weight (mg/kg) or body surface area (BSA) (mg/m^2). Care must be taken to properly convert body weight from pounds to kilograms (1 kg = 2.2 lb) before calculating doses based on body weight. Doses are often expressed as mg/kg/day or mg/kg/dose, therefore orders written "mg/kg/d" which is confusing, *require further clarification from the prescriber*.

Chemotherapeutic drugs are commonly dosed according to body surface area which requires an extra verification step (BSA calculation) prior to dosing. Medications are available in multiple concentrations, therefore *orders written in "mL" rather than "mg" are not acceptable and require further clarification*.

Dosing also varies by indication, therefore diagnostic information is helpful when calculating doses. The following examples are typically encountered when dosing medication in children.

Example 1.

Calculate the dose of amoxicillin suspension in mLs for otitis media for a 1-yr-old child weighing 22 lb. The dose required is 40 mg/kg/day divided BID and the suspension comes in a concentration of 400 mg/5 mL.

Step 1. Convert pounds to kg:	22 lb × 1 kg/2.2 lb = 10 kg
Step 2. Calculate the dose in mg:	10 kg × 40 mg/kg/day = 400 mg/day
Step 3. Divide the dose by the frequency:	400 mg/day ÷ 2 (BID) = 200 mg/dose BID
Step 4. Convert the mg dose to mL:	200 mg/dose ÷ 400 mg/5 mL = **2.5 mL BID**

Example 2.

Calculate the dose of ceftriaxone in mLs for meningitis for a 5-yr-old weighing 18 kg. The dose required is 100 mg/kg/day given IV once daily and the drug comes pre-diluted in a concentration of 40 mg/mL.

Step 1. Calculate the dose in mg:	18 kg × 100 mg/kg/day = 1800 mg/day
Step 2. Divide the dose by the frequency:	1800 mg/day ÷ 1 (daily) = 1800 mg/dose
Step 3. Convert the mg dose to mL:	1800 mg/dose ÷ 40 mg/mL = **45 mL once daily**

Example 3.

Calculate the dose of vincristine in mLs for a 4-yr-old with leukemia weighing 37 lb and is 97 cm tall. The dose required in 2 mg/m^2 and the drug comes in 1 mg/mL concentration.

Step 1. Convert pounds to kg:	37 lb × 1 kg/2.2 lb = 16.8 kg
Step 2. Calculate BSA (see Appendix F):	$\sqrt{16.8 \text{ kg} \times 97 \text{ cm}/3600}$ = 0.67 m^2
Step 3. Calculate the dose in mg:	2 mg/m^2 × 0.67 m^2 = 1.34 mg
Step 4. Calculate the dose in mL:	1.34 mg ÷ 1 mg/mL = **1.34 mg**

APPENDIX S
Pediatric Fluid and Electrolyte Requirements

How to calculate maintenance fluid requirements in children:

1. **Body Surface Area Method** (commonly used in children >10 kg):

$$1500-2000 \text{ mL/m}^2/\text{day} \div 24 = \text{fluid rate in mL/hr}$$

Example: Calculate maintenance fluids in mL/hr for a child with a BSA = 0.8 m².

Answer: 1500 mL/m²/day × 0.8 m² = 1200 mL/day ÷ 24 hr = 50 mL/hr
2000 mL/m²/day × 0.8 m² = 1600 mL/day ÷ 24 hr = 66.6 mL/hr

Range: 50–66.6 mL/hr.

2. **Body Weight Method**

<10 kg	100 mL/kg/day
11–20 kg	1000 mL + 50 mL/kg for each kg >10
>20 kg	1500 mL + 20 mL/kg for each kg >20

Example: Calculate maintenance fluids in mL/hr for a child weighing 25 kg.

Answer: 1500 mL + 20 mL/kg × 5 kg = 1500 mL + 100 mL = 1600 mL
1600 mL ÷ 24 hr = 66.6 mL/hr

Daily Electrolyte Requirements in Children

Sodium	2–6 mEq/kg/day
Potassium	2–4 mEq/kg/day
Calcium	1–4 mEq/kg/day*
Magnesium	0.3–0.5 mEq/kg/day
Phosphorous	0.5–2 mmol/kg/day*

*Neonates may require the higher end of the calcium and phosphorous dosage range due to rapid bone development.

Conditions that May Alter Fluid Requirements in Children

Fever
Hyperventilation
Sweating
Hyperthyroidism
Renal failure
Diarrhea

Oral Rehydration Therapy (ORT)

ORT is as effective as IV therapy in managing fluid and electrolytes in children with mild to moderate dehydration due to diarrhea. Commercially available premixed ORT solutions typically contain low concentrations of glucose (2–3%), 45–75 mEq/L sodium, 20–25 mEq/L potassium, 30–35 mEq/L of citrate (bicarbonate source). Low sugar content provides little caloric support but facilitates intestinal sodium and water absorption. All commercially available ORT solutions are equally safe and effective, and are preferred over household remedies (e.g., colas, juices, chicken broth) which are not formulated based on the physiology of acute diarrhea.

APPENDIX T
Early Management of Anaphylactic Reactions

1. **Discontinue suspected drug.**
   (stop IV, tourniquet IM or subcut site.)

2. **Maintain airway.**
   Aminophylline or other bronchodilators may be required for severe respiratory distress.

3. **Administer *epinephrine*.**
   IM, Subcut (Adults): 0.3–0.5 mg, may repeat q 5–15 min
   IM, Subcut (Children): 0.01 mg/kg, or 0.1 mg may repeat q 5–15 min
   IV (Adults): 0.1 mg over 5 min or 1–4 mcg/min infusion
   IV (Children): 0.01 mg/kg/dose or 0.1–0.2 mg over 5 min, may repeat q 30 min or 0.1–1.5 mcg (maximum)/kg/min infusion

4. **Administer *antihistamines*.**
   May prevent recurrence and decrease intensity of reaction.
   diphenhydramine (Benadryl)
   IM, IV (Adults): 50–100 mg single dose, may follow with 50 mg every 6 hr for 1–2 days
   IM, IV (Children): 5 mg/kg/day in divided doses q 6–8 hr (not to exceed 300 mg/day), may follow with oral therapy for 1–2 days
   cimetidine (Tagamet)
   IV (Adults): 300 mg q 6 hr
   IV (Children): 25–30 mg/kg/day in 6 divided doses

5. **Support blood pressure.**
   If necessary, use fluids and/or vasopressors. Patients receiving beta blockers may be resistant to the effects of vasopressers.

6. **Administer *corticosteroids*.**
   (may decrease intensity of reaction.)
   hydrocortisone (Solu-Cortef)
   IV (Adults and Children): 100–1000 mg, may follow with 7 mg/kg/day IV or oral therapy for 1–2 days.

7. **Document reaction.**
   in medical record, inform patient/family to carry identification.

1439

APPENDIX U
The Cytochrome P450 System: What Is It and Why Should I Care?[1]

Looking beyond the obvious takes time, energy, insight, and fortitude; yet this is what we are called to do. We are nurses—tireless care providers. Yet, when the subject of the liver's enzyme system, also called the cytochrome P450 system, is discussed, we feel the urge to run the other way...or better yet, to just ignore the conversation. Yet, can we do this as the tireless care provider? The answer to this question is clear and simple: no, we cannot. This is because numerous medications, nutrients, and herbal therapies are metabolized through the cytochrome P450 (CYP450) enzyme system. This system can be inhibited or induced by drugs, and once altered can be clinically significant in the development of drug-drug interactions that may cause unanticipated adverse reactions or therapeutic failures. This article will review the basic concepts of the CYP450 system and relate these concepts to clinically significant altered responses.

The CYP450 enzymes are essential for the production of numerous agents including cholesterol and steroids. Additionally, these enzymes are necessary for the detoxification of foreign chemicals and the metabolism of drugs. CYP450 enzymes are so named because they are bound to membranes within a cell (cyto) and contain a heme pigment (chrome and P) that absorbs light at a wavelength of 450 nm when exposed to carbon monoxide.[2] There are more than 50 CYP450 enzymes, but the CYP1A2, CYP2C19, CYP2D6, CYP1A2, CYP3A4, and CYP3A5 enzymes are responsible for metabolizing 45% of drug metabolism. The CYP2D6 (20–30%), the CYP2C9 (10%) and the CYP2E1 and CYP1A2 (5%) complete this enzyme system.[3]

Drugs that cause CYP450 drug interactions are referred to as either inhibitors or inducers. An inducing agent can increase the rate of another drug's metabolism by as much as two- to threefold which develops over a period of a week. When an inducing agent is prescribed with another medication, the dosage of the other medication may need to be adjusted since the rate of metabolism is increased and the effect of the medication reduced. This can lead to a therapeutic failure of the medication. Conversely, if a medication is taken with an agent that inhibits it metabolism, then the drug level can rise and possibly result in a harmful or adverse effect. Information regarding a drug's CYP450 metabolism and its potential for inhibition or induction can be found on the drug label and accessed through the U.S. Food and Drug Administration (FDA) or manufacturer's websites.[2]

When we assess our patients and provide management modalities, these are implemented within a framework of the patient's heritage, race, and culture. This is also true in pharmacology as well (i.e., "pharmacogenetics"). This concept is important to examine since we know that there exists genetic variability, which may influence a patient's response to commonly prescribed drug classes. This genetic variability can be defined as polymorphism. Seven percent of Caucasians and two to seven percent of African Americans are poor metabolizers of drugs dependent on CYP2D6, which metabolizes many beta blockers, antidepressants, and opioids. This is because the drug's metabolism via CYP450 enzymes exhibits genetic variability.[2]

Recently, researchers have studied the genetic variability in metabolism among women who were prescribed tamoxifen and medications that inhibit the CYP2D6 enzyme. To review, tamoxifen is biotransformed to the potent anti-estrogen, endoxifen, by this enzyme. CYP2D6 genetic variation (individuals considered extensive metabolizers versus poor metabolizers) and inhibitors of the enzyme markedly reduce endoxifen plasma concentrations in tamoxifen-treated patients.

The researchers concluded that CYP2D6 metabolism is an "independent predictor of breast cancer outcome in post-menopausal women receiving tamoxifen for early breast cancer. Determination of CYP2D6 genotype may be of value in selecting adjuvant hormonal therapy and it appears CYP2D6 inhibitors should be avoided in tamoxifen-treated women".[4] Do oncology patients come to us with only their cancer and its treatment? No, they come with multifaceted dimensions and co-morbid conditions such as hypertension, dyslipidemia, depression, seizure disorders, etc. For example, several antidepressants (paroxetine [Paxil] and fluoxetine [Prozac]) are inhibitors of metabolism when given with drugs metabolized through the CYP2D6 enzyme, such as haloperidol (Haldol), metoprolol (Lopressor), and hydrocodone. Thus, the therapeutic response can be accentuated. Medications that inhibit the CYP3A4 enzyme such as amiodarone and antifungals, can affect the therapeutic response of fentanyl, alprazolam (Xanax), and numerous statins; as a result, the effect of these drugs can be enhanced leading to potential toxic levels.[5]

At times, these CYP 450 inducers and inhibitors are commonly ingested items such grapefruit juice and tobacco. In the case of grapefruit juice, there are numerous medications known to interact with grapefruit juice including statins, antiarrhythmic agents, immunosuppressive agents, and calcium channel blockers. Furthermore, the inhibition of the enzyme system seems to be dose dependent; thus, the more a patient drinks, the more the inhibition that occurs. Additionally, the effects can last for several days if grapefruit juice is consumed on a regular basis. Luckily, the effect of this is not seen with other citrus juices.

Hopefully, this brief review has opened the door to your inquisitive nature on how the liver's enzyme system is effected by numerous medications and why some patients experience clinically significant unanticipated adverse reactions or therapeutic failures.

CYP1A2

Substrates	Inhibitors	Inducers
Alosetron, Amitriptyline, Clozapine, Cyclobenzaprine, Desipramine, Diazepam, Fluvoxamine, Imipramine, Mexiletine, Mirtazapine, Olanzapine, Propranolol, Ropinirole, Theophylline, (R)-Warfarin	Cimetidine, Ciprofloxacin, Fluvoxamine, Ketoconazole, Lidocaine, Mexiletine	Carbamazepine, Cigarette smoke, Phenobarbital, Rifampin

CYP2C9

Substrates	Inhibitors	Inducers
Celecoxib, Glimepiride, Glipizide, Losartan, Montelukast, Nateglinide, Phenytoin, Sulfamethoxazole, Voriconazole, (S)-Warfarin	Amiodarone, Delavirdine, Efavirenz, Fluconazole, Fluvastatin, Ketoconazole, Sulfamethoxazole, Zafirlukast	Carbamazepine, Phenobarbital, Phenytoin, Rifampin

CYP2C19

Substrates	Inhibitors	Inducers
Citalopram, Diazepam, Escitalopram, Esomeprazole, Imipramine, Lansoprazole, Nelfinavir, Omeprazole, Pantoprazole, Phenytoin, Rabeprazole, Voriconazole	Delavirdine, Efavirenz, Esomeprazole, Fluoxetine, Fluvoxamine, Lansoprazole, Omeprazole, Rabeprazole, Sertraline, Ticlopidine	Carbamazepine, Phenytoin, Rifampin

CYP2D6

Substrates	Inhibitors	Inducers
Amitriptyline, Aripiprazole, Atomoxetine, Codeine, Desipramine, Dextromethorphan, Flecainide, Fluoxetine, Haloperidol, Imipramine, Lidocaine, Metoprolol, Mexiletine, Mirtazapine, Nefazodone, Nortriptyline, Oxycodone, Paroxetine, Propafenone, Propranolol, Risperidone, Ritonavir, Tramadol. Venlafaxine	Amiodarone, Cimetidine, Clozapine, Delavirdine, Desipramine, Fluoxetine, Haloperidol, Lidocaine, Methadone, Paroxetine, Pimozide, Quinidine, Ritonavir, Sertraline, Ticlopidine	None

CYP3A Substrates	Inhibitors	Inducers
Alprazolam, Amiodarone, Aprepitant, Aripiprazole, Atorvastatin, Buspirone, Calcium channel blockers, Carbamazepine, Cilostazol, Citalopram, Clarithromycin, Clonazepam, Cyclosporine, Dapsone, Delavirdine, Diazepam, Disopyramide, Efavirenz, Ergot derivatives, Erlotinib, Erythromycin, Escitalopram, Estrogens, Fentanyl, Geftinib, Glucocorticoids, Imatinib, Indinavir, Irinotecan, Itraconazole, Ketoconazole, Lansoprazole, Lidocaine, Losartan, Lovastatin, Methadone, Midazolam, Mirtazapine, Montelukast, Nateglinide, Nefazodone, Nelfinavir, Nevirapine, Ondansetron, Paclitaxel, Pimozide, Protease inhibitors, Quetiapine, Quinidine, Repaglinide, Rifabutin, Sibutramine, Sildenafil, Simvastatin, Sirolimus, Tacrolimus, Tadalafil, Tamoxifen, Theophylline, Tiagabine, Ticlopidine, Vardenafil, (R)-Warfarin, Zolpidem, Zonisamide	Amiodarone, Aprepitant, Cimetidine, Clarithromycin, Cyclosporine, Delavirdine, Diltiazem, Efavirenz, Erythromycin, Fluconazole, Grapefruit juice, Imatinib, Indinavir, Itraconazole, Ketoconazole, Metronidazole, Nefazodone, Nelfinavir, Quinidine, Ritonavir, Saquinavir, Sertraline, Verapamil, Voriconazole	Carbamazepine, Efavirenz, Nevirapine, Phenobarbital, Phenytoin, Rifabutin, Rifampin, St. John's wort

1. Jamison T. (Winter 2008). Oncology Nursing Society, Metro Detroit Chapter Newsletter, Volume XXIII, Issue 1.
2. Lynch, T. & Price, A (2007). The effect of P450 metabolism on drug response, interactions, and adverse effects. American Family Physician, 76(3), 391–397.
3. Arcangelo, V. P. & Peterson, A. M. (2006). Pharmacotherapeutics for Advanced Practice: A Practical Approach. (2nd ed). Philadelphia: Lippincott Williams and Wilkins.
4. Goetz, M., Knox, S, Suman, V., & Rae, J. (2007). The impact of cytochrome P450 2D6 metabolism in women receiving adjuvant tamoxifen. Breast Cancer Research and Treatment. 101(1), 113–122.
5. Lehne, R. (2007). Pharmacology: for Nursing Care (6th edition). St Louis, MO: Saunders, Elsevier.

BIBLIOGRAPHY

AHFS Drug Information BOOK ONLINE. Jackson, WY: Teton Data Systems, 2007. Based on: Gerald K. McEvoy, editor. AHFS Drug Information (2007). Bethesda, MD: American Society of Health-System Pharmacists, Inc.; 2007. STAT!Ref Medical Reference Library. Accessed November 1, 2007.

American Hospital Formulary Service: Drug Information 2009. American Society of Hospital Pharmacists, Bethesda, MD, 2009.

American Pain Society: Principles of Analgesic Use in the Treatment of Acute Pain and Cancer Pain, ed 6. American Pain Society, Skokie, IL, 2008.

Blumenthal, M, et al: The Complete German Commission E Monographs: Therapeutic Guide to Herbal Medicines. Integrative Medical Communications, Boston, 1998.

DRUGDEX® System [intranet database]. Version 5.1. Greenwood Village, Colo: Thomson Healthcare. Accessed November 1, 2009.

Drug Facts and Comparisons On-line, version 4.0. Facts and Comparisons, a Wolters Kluwer Company, St. Louis, 2009.

Fetrow, CW and Avila, JR: Professional's Handbook of Complementary & Alternative Medicines, ed. 3. Lippincott Williams & Wilkins, Philadelphia, PA, 2004.

IV INDEX® System [intranet database]. Version 5.1. Greenwood Village, Colo: Thomson Healthcare. Accessed August 30, 2009.

Jonas, WB, and Levin, JS (eds): Essentials of Complementary and Alternative Medicine. Lippincott Williams & Wilkins, a Wolters Kluwer Company, Baltimore and Philadelphia, 1999.

Kemp, SF, deShazo, RD: Prevention and treatment of anaphylaxis. Clin Allergy Immunol 2008;21:477–498.

Kuhn, MA, Winston, D: Herbal Therapy and Supplements: A Scientific and Traditional Approach. Lippincott, Philadelphia, 2001.

Van Leeuwen, A.M., Kranpitz, T, Smith, L: Davis's Comprehensive Handbook of Laboratory and Diagnostic Tests with Nursing Implications, ed 2. FA Davis Company, Philadelphia, PA, 2006.

Lexi-Comp, Inc: (Lexi-Drugs [Comp + Specialties]). Lexi-Comp, Inc.; Accessed December 1, 2009.

McCaffery, M, and Pasero, C: Pain: Clinical Manual, ed 2. Mosby-Yearbook, St Louis, 1999.

National Institutes of Health Warren Grant Magnuson Clinical Center: Drug—Nutrient Interactions, Bethesda, MD, 2005. http://www.cc.nih.gov/ccc/supplements/intro.html.

National Kidney Foundation: A-Z Guide for High Potassium Foods, National Kidney Foundation, 2005.

PDR for Herbal Medicines, ed 4. Thomson Healthcare, 2009.

Pennington, JAT, Douglass, JS: Bowes and Church's Food Values of Portions Commonly Used. ed 18. Philadelphia: Lippincott Williams & Wilkins, 2004. 1–496.

Phelps, SJ, Hak, EB, Crill, CM: Pediatric Injectable Drugs, ed. 8. American Society of Health-System Pharmacists, Bethesada, 2007.

Physicians' Desk Reference (PDR): Thomson Healthcare, Montvale, NJ, 2009.

Polovich, M, White, JM, and Kelleher, LO: Chemotherapy and Biotherapy Guidelines and Recommendations for Practice, ed. 2. Oncology Nursing Society, Pittsburgh, 2005.

Taketomo CK, Hodding JH, and Kraus DM: Pediatric Dosage Handbook, ed 14. Lexi-Comp, 2007–2008.

Trissel, LA: Handbook on Injectable Drugs, ed 14. American Society of Hospital Pharmacists, Bethesda, 2007.

USP Dispensing Information (USP-DI): Drug Information for the Health Care Professional, Volume 1, ed 27. Micromedex, Rockville, MD, 2007.

http://www.fda.gov/cder/index.html Accessed November 1, 2009.

http://www.ons.org/news.shtml.

http://www.accessdata.fda.gov/scripts/cder/drugsatfda/.

COMPREHENSIVE INDEX*

1–Day, 190
🌀 2-amino-2-deoxyglucose sulfate, 1356
40 Winks, 450

A

A-200 Shampoo, 1378
🧬 abacavir, **109**, 23, 67
abarelix, 23
Abelcet, 165, C8
🍁 Abenol, 112
Abilify, 195
abobotulinum toxin A, 23
Abraxane, 975
Abreva, 465
acamprosate calcium, 1317
Acanya Topical Gel, 1378
acarbose, 110, 46
Accolate, 1299
Accuneb, 126
Accupril, 176
Accuretic 10/12.5, 1378
Accuretic 20/12.5, 1378
Accuretic 20/25, 1378
acebutolol, C7
ACE INHIBITORS, 53, C7. *See* ANGIOTENSIN-CONVERTING ENZYME (ACE) INHIBITORS
acellular pertussis vaccine, 1429
Aceon, 176
Acephen, 112
Aceta, 112
Acetadote, 116
acetaminophen, 112, 65, 96. *See also* butalbital, acetaminophen; butalbital acetaminophen, Caffeine; hydrocodone/acetaminophen; oxycodone; acetaminophen; propoxyphene napsylate/acetaminophen.
🍁 Acetazolam, 114
acetaZOLAMIDE, 114, 42, 85, C4, C8, C9, C15
acetohexamide, C8, C11
acetylcholine, 1400
acetylcysteine, 116
🍁 Acid Control, 660
Aciphex, 1095
Aclovate, 380

Acta-Char Liquid-A, 1317
Actemra, 1374
ActHIB, 1430
Acticin, 1012
Acticort, 381
Actidose-Aqua, 1317
Actifed Cold and Allergy, 1378
🍁 Actiprofen, 688
Actiq, 564, 22, C15
Activase, 1214
🍁 Activase rt-PA, 1214
activated charcoal, 1317
ACTIVE FACTOR X INHIBITORS, 40
Activella Tablets 1/0.5, 1378
Activella Tablets 0.5/0.1, 1378
Actonel, 1114
Actoplus Met 15/850, 1378
Actoplus Met 15/500, 1378
Actoplus Met/Actoplus Met XR, 22
Actoplus Met XR 15/1000, 1378
Actoplus Met XR 30/1000, 1378
Actos, 1030, 22
Acular, 1402
Acular LS, 1402
Acular Preservative Free, 1402
Acuvail, 1402
acyclovir, 118, 73, C2, C4
acyclovir/hydrocortisone, 1375
Adacell, 1429, 1434
Adalat, C6
Adalat CC, 921, C14
🍁 Adalat PA, 921
🍁 Adalat XL, 921
adalimumab, 121, 68
Adcirca, 1185
Adderall, 163
Adderall 10 mg, 1378
Adderall 20 mg, 1378
Adderall 30 mg, 1378
Adderall 5 mg, 1378
Adderall 7.5 mg, 1378
Adderall 12.5 mg, 1378
Adderall 15 mg, 1378
Adderall XR, 163
Adderall XR 10 mg, 1378
Adderall XR 20 mg, 1378
Adderall XR 30 mg, 1378
Adderall XR 5 mg, 1378
Adderall XR 15 mg, 1378

Adderall XR 25 mg, 1378
🌀 Ademetionine, 1362
Adenocard, 123
Adenoscan, 123
adenosine, 123, 35, C4
Adipex-P, 1017
Adoxa, 1203
Adrenalin, 504
ADRENERGICS, **53, 78**
Adriamycin, C15
Adriamycin PFS, 479
Adriamycin RDF, 479
Adsorbotear, 1399
Advair, C8
Advair Diskus 250, 1378
Advair Diskus 100, 1378
Advair Diskus 500, 1379
Advair Diskus/HFA, 22
Advair HFA 45, 1379
Advair HFA 115, 1379
Advair HFA 230, 1379
Advicor, C8
Advicor 750/20, 1379
Advicor 500/20, 1379
Advicor 1000/20, 1379
Advicor 1000/40, 1379
Advil, 688
Advil Cold & Sinus, 1379
Advil Migraine Liqui-Gels, 688
Advil Multi-Symptom Cold, 1379
Advil PM Liquigels, 1379
AeroBid, 366
AeroBid-M, 366
Aeroseb-HC, 381
Aerospan, 366
Afeditab CR, 921, C6
Afinitor, 1370
Afluria, 1431, 1433
aformoterol, 1376
Aggrastat, 1233
Aggrenox, 1379
AKBeta, 1399
🍁 AK-Con, 1402
AK-Dilate, 1403
Akineton, 1320
AK-Nefrin, 1403
Akne-Mycin, 523
AK-Pentolate, 1401
AK-Tob, 1398
Akwa Tears, 1399
Ala-Cort, 381
Alamag, 803

---

*Entries for **generic** names appear in **boldface type.** Trade names appear in regular type, with Canadian trade names preceded by a maple leaf icon (🍁). CLASSIFICATIONS appear in **BOLDFACE SMALL CAPS**. *Combination Drugs* appear in *italics*, herbal products are preceded by a yin-yang icon (🌀) and drugs with genetic implications are preceded by a double-helix icon (🧬).

1445

Alamast, 1402
Ala-Scalp, 381
Alavert, 798
Alavert Allergy and Sinus, 1379
Alaway, 1397
Albalon, 1402
Albuminar, 125
albumin (human), 125
Albutein, 125
albuterol, 126, 37, 78
Alcaine, 1397
alclometasone, 380, 83
🍁Alcomicin, 1398
Aldactazide 25/25, 1379
Aldactazide 50/50, 1379
Aldactone, 456
Aldara, 705
aldesleukin, 16, 1317
ALDOSTERONE ANTAGONISTS, 53
alemtuzumab, 128, 16, 59
alendronate, 130, 77
Alesse, 1379
Aleve, 900, C6
Aleve-D Sinus & Cold, 1379
Alfen Jr, 648
Alferon N, 724
alfuzosin, 132
Alimta, 999
aliskiren, 133, 54
alitretinoin, 16, 1318
ALKALINIZING AGENTS, 92
Alka-Mints, 265
Alka-Seltzer Effervescent, Extra-Strength, 1379
Alka-Seltzer Effervescent, Original, 1379
Alka-Seltzer Plus Cold & Cough Liqui-Gels, 1379
Alka-Seltzer Plus Night Cold Formula Liquid Gels, 1379
Alka-Seltzer Plus Sinus Formula, 1379
Alkeran, 817
ALKYLATING AGENTS, 59
Allegra, 575
Allegra-D 12 Hour, 1379
Allegra-D 24 Hour, 1379
Aller-Chlor, 316
🍁Allerdryl, 450
Alerest, 1402
Allerfrim Syrup, 1379
Allergy, 316
Allergy Drops, 1402
Allergy Medication, 450
AllerMax, 450
AllerNaze, 369
🌐All-Heal, 1365
Alli, 954
🌐Alli sativa bulbus, 1350
🌐Allium sativum, 1350
Alloprim, 134
allopurinol, 134, C4

almotriptan, 136, 106
Alocril, 1402
🌐aloe, 94, 1341
🌐Aloe latex, 1341
🌐Aloe vera, 1341
Alomide, 1402
Alora, 532
alosetron, 23, 1441
Aloxi, 981
ALPHA-ADRENERGIC BLOCKERS, 106
Alphaderm, 381
Alphagan P, 1403
ALPHA-GLUCOSIDASE INHIBITORS, 46
alpha₁-proteinase inhibitor, 1375
🍁Alpha-Tamoxifen, 1187
alpha tocopherol, 1291
alprazolam, 138, 34, 1442, C6, C7, C15
Alramucil, 1079
Alrex, 1400
Altace, 176
🌐Altamisa, 1349
Altarussin, 648
alteplase, 1214, 104
AlternaGEL, 140
🍁Alti-Bromocriptine, 1321
🍁Alti-MPA, 812
Altoprev, 666
Altracaine, 1397
Alu-Cap, 140
🍁Alugel, 140
Aluminet, 140
aluminum hydroxide, 140, 72. *See also* magnesium hydroxide/aluminum hydroxide
Alu-Tab, 140
Alvesco, 1369
alvimopan, 23
🌐Amantilla, 1365
Amaryl, 1172, C16
🌐Amber, 1364
Ambien, 1313
Ambien CR, 1313
AmBisome, 165, C8
ambrisentan, 23
amcinonide, 380, 83
Amerge, 902
🌐American coneflower, 1348
🌐American Dwarf Palm Tree, 1363
A-Methapred, 372
Amicar, 143
Amigesic, 1131
amikacin, 145, 55, C2, C4
amiloride, 456, 85
aminocaproic acid, 143, C4
Aminofen, 112
aminoglutethimide, 1377

AMINOGLYCOSIDES, 145, 55
Amino-Opti-E, 1291
aminophylline, 240, 37, 78, C4
amiodarone, 151, 16, 35, 1441–1442, C2–C3, C6
Amitone, 265
amitriptyline, 154, 44, 1441, C6
amlodipine, 157, 54, 80
amlodipine/telmisartan, 1375
Amnesteem, 744
Amnesteem/Claravis/Sotret, 22
Amoclan, 160
Amoclan 200 Suspension, 1379
Amoclan 400 Suspension, 1379
Amoclan 600 Suspension, 1379
amoxapine, 44, 1318
amoxicillin, 158, 56, 72
amoxicillin/clavulanate, 160, 56, C15
Amoxil, 158
amphetamine mixtures, 163, 81, C6
Amphetamine Salt, 163
Amphojel, 140
Amphotec, 165, C8
amphotericin B, C4, C8
amphotericin B cholesteryl sulfate, 165, 50
amphotericin B colloidal, C2, C4
amphotericin B cholesteryl sulfate/lipid complex/liposome, 16
amphotericin B deoxycholate, 165, 50
amphotericin B lipid complex, 165, 50
amphotericin B liposome, 165, 50, C2, C4
ampicillin, 169, 56, C2, C4
ampicillin/sulbactam, 172, 56, C2, C4
🍁Ampicin, 169
Ampyra, 1369
Amrix, 383, C6
Anacin, 1379
Anacin Max Strength, 1379
Anaflex, 1131
Anafranil, 1322
Ana-Guard, 504
anakinra, 174, 68
Analpram Topical Cream, 1379
Analpram Topical Lotion, 1379
Anaplex DM Syrup, 1379
Anaprox, 900, C6

Anaprox DS, 900
Anaspaz, 684, C6
anastrazole, 59
anastrozole, 175, 59
🍁Ancalixir, 1015
Ancef, 291
Androderm, 1200
Androgel/Testim, 22
Android, C6
Anestacon, 784
🍁Anexate, 587
Anexsia 5/325, 1379
Anexsia 7.5/325, 1379
Anexsia, 675
Anexsia 7.5/650, 1379
Anexsia 5/500, 1379
Anexsia 10/750, 1379
☯Angelica sinensis, 1347
Angeliq, 1379
Angiomax, 234
🧬**ANGIOTENSIN-CONVERTING ENZYME (ACE) INHIBITORS, 176**
🧬**ANGIOTENSIN II RECEPTOR ANTAGONISTS, 182, 53, C7**
anidulafungin, 186, 50, C2, C4
ANOREXIC AGENTS, C6
Antabuse, 1324
ANTACIDS, 72
Antara, 559
ANTHRACYCLINES, 59
ANTI-ALZHEIMER'S AGENTS, 29
ANTIANDROGENS, 59
ANTIANEMICS, 30
ANTIANGINALS, 31
ANTIANXIETY AGENTS, 32
ANTIARRHYTHMICS, 34, C7
　CLASS IA, 35
　CLASS IB, 35
　CLASS IC, 35
　CLASS II, 35
　CLASS III, 35
　CLASS IV, 35
ANTIASTHMATICS, 36
ANTICHOLINERGICS, 37, 61, 78
ANTICOAGULANTS, 39
ANTICONVULSANTS, 40, C7
ANTIDEPRESSANTS, 42, C7
ANTIDIABETICS, 44
ANTIDIARRHEALS, 46
ANTIEMETICS, 47
ANTIESTROGENS, 59
ANTIFUNGALS, 49
　TOPICAL, 187
　VAGINAL, 190
ANTIHISTAMINES, 50, C7
ANTIHYPERTENSIVES, 52

ANTI-INFECTIVES, 54
ANTIMETABOLITES, 59
ANTINAUSEANTS, C7
ANTINEOPLASTICS, 56
ANTIPARKINSON AGENTS, 60, C7
ANTIPLATELET AGENTS, 61
ANTIPSYCHOTICS, 62, C7
ANTIPYRETICS, 65
ANTIRETROVIRALS, 66
ANTIRHEUMATICS, 67
ANTITHROMBOTICS, 40
ANTITUBERCULARS, 69
ANTITUMOR ANTIBIOTICS, 59
ANTIULCER AGENTS, 70
Antivert, 811
ANTIVIRALS, 72
Anusol HC, 381
ANXIOLYTICS, C7
Anzemet, 469
Apacet, 112
APAP, 112
Apidra, 721
Aplenzin, 249, 22
🍁Apo-Acetaminophen, 112
🍁Apo-Acetazolamide, 114
🍁Apo-Allopurinol, 134
🍁Apo-Alpraz, 138
🍁Apo-Amiloride, 456
🍁Apo-Amitriptyline, 154
🍁Apo-Amoxi, 158
🍁Apo-Ampi, 169
🍁Apo-ASA, 1131
🍁Apo-ASEN, 1131
🍁Apo-Atenolol, 204
🍁Apo-Benztropine, 225
🍁Apo-Bromocriptine, 1321
🍁Apo-C, 1319
🍁Apo-Cal, 265
🍁Apo-Carbamazepine, 272
🍁Apo-Cephalex, 291
🍁Apo-Chlordiazepoxide, 314
🍁Apo-Chlorthalidone, 458
🍁Apo-Cimetidine, 660
🍁Apo-Ciproflox, 589
🍁Apo-Clorazepate, 347
🍁Apo-Diazepam, 431
🍁Apo-Diclo, 435
🍁Apo-Diltiaz, 445
🍁Apo-Dipyridamole, 454
🍁Apo-Divalproex, 1262
🍁Apo-Doxy, 1203
🍁Apo-Erythro-EC, 523
🍁Apo-Erythro-ES, 523
🍁Apo-Famotidine, 660
🍁Apo-Ferrous Gluconate, 736
🍁Apo-Ferrous Sulfate, 736
🍁Apo-Fluphenazine, 600
🍁Apo-Flurazepam, 603
🍁Apo-Folic, 606

🍁Apo-Furosemide, 620
🍁Apo-Glimepiride, 1172
🍁Apo-Glyburide, 1173
🍁Apo-Haloperidol, 651
🍁Apo-Hydro, 458
🍁Apo-Hydroxyzine, 682
🍁Apo-Ibuprofen, 688
🍁Apo-Imipramine, 703
🍁Apo-Indomethacin, 708
🍁Apo-ISDN, 742
🍁Apo-ISMN, 742
🍁Apo-K, 1041
🍁Apo-Keto, 754
🍁Apo-Keto-E, 754
🍁Apo-Lorazepam, 799
🍁Apo-Methyldopa, 840
🍁Apo-Metoclop, 847
🍁Apo-Metronidazole, 854
🍁Apo-Minocycline, 1203
🍁Apo-Napro-Na, 900
🍁Apo-Naproxen, 900
🍁Apo-Nifed, 921
🍁Apo-Nitrofurantoin, 928
🍁Apo-Nizatidine, 660
🍁Apo-Norfloxacin, 589
🍁Apo-Ofloxacin, 589
🍁Apo-Oxazepam, 961
🍁Apo-Pen VK, 1002
🍁Apo-Piroxicam, 1034
🍁Apo-Propranolol, 1071
🍁Apo-Quin-G, 1089
🍁Apo-Quinidine, 1089
🍁Apo-Ranitidine, 660
🍁Apo-Salvent, 126
Apo-Selegiline, 1141
🍁Apo-Sulfatrim, 1254
🍁Apo-Sulfatrim DS, 1254
🍁Apo-Sulin, 1175
🍁Apo-Theo LA, 240
🍁Apo-Timol, 1229
🍁Apo-Timop, 1399
🍁Apo-Triazo, 1253
🍁Apo-Trifluoperazine, 1337
🍁Apo-Trihex, 1338
🍁Apo-Valproic, 1262
🍁Apo-Zidovudine, 1303
apraclonidine, 1403
aprepitant, 191, 49, 1442
Apresoline, 671
Apri, 1379
Apri 28, 358
Apriso, 825
Aptivus, 1336
Aquachloral, 312
Aquasite, 1399
Aquasol E, 1291
🍁Aqueous Charcodote, 1317
Ara-C, 392
Aranelle, 359

Aranesp, 403, 1376
Arava, 771
Aredia, 983
argatroban, 193, 16, 40
Argatroban, 193
Aricept, 470
Aricept ODT, 470
Arimidex, 175
aripiprazole, 195, 64, 1441–1442
Aristospan, 372
Arixtra, 608, 1376
Armour thyroid, 1219, C6
🍁 arnica, 94, 1343
Arnica montana, 1343
AROMATASE INHIBITORS, 59
arsenic trioxide, 16, 59, 1319
Artane, 1338
🍁 Arthrinol, 1131
🍁 Arthrisin, 1131
Arthropan, 1131
Arthrotec 75/200, 1379
Arthrotec 50/200, 1379
Artificial tears, 1399
Artificial Tears Plus, 1399
🍁 Artria S.R, 1131
ASA, 1131
Asacol, 825
Asacol HD, 825
🍁 Asaphen, 1131
ascorbic acid, 107, 1319
Ascorbicap, 1319
Ascriptin, 1131
asenapine, 197, 64
Asendin, 1318
🍁 Asian ginseng, 1354
Asmanex, 366
asparaginase, 199, 16, 59
A-Spas S/L, 684
Aspercin, 1131
Aspergum, 1131
aspirin, 1131, 65, 95. *See also* butalbital, aspirin, caffeine; hydrocodone/ aspirin; oxycodone/aspirin; propxyphene napsylate/ aspirin; propoxyphene/ aspirin/caffeine
Aspirin Free Anacin, 112
Aspirin Free Pain Relief, 112
Aspirtab, 1131
AsthmaHaler Mist, 504
AsthmaNefrin (racepinephrine), 504
Astramorph, 880
Astramorph PF, 880
🍁 Astrin, 1131
Atacand, 182
Atacand HCT 16/12.5, 1379
Atacand HCT 32/12.5, 1379
Atacand HCT 32/25, 1379
🍁 *Atacand Plus, 1380*

Atarax, 682
atazanavir, 201, 67
atenolol, 204, 32, 54, 75
Ativan, 799
atomoxetine, 205, 1441
atorvastatin, 666, 91, 1442
atovaquone, 207
Atripla, 1380
Atro-Pen, 208
atropine, 208, 35, 38, 1401, C1, C2, C4. *See also* difenoxin/atropine; diphenoxylate/atropine; Isopto Atropine.
Atropine-Care, 1401
Atrovent, 732
Atrovent HFA, 732
🍁 aubepine, 1358
Augmentin, 160
Augmentin 875, 1380
Augmentin 250, 1380
Augmentin 500, 1380
Augmentin 200 Chewable, 1380
Augmentin 400 Chewable, 1380
Augmentin 200 mg Suspension, 1380
Augmentin 400 mg Suspension, 1380
Augmentin 250 Chewable, 1380
Augmentin 250 mg Suspension, 1380
Augmentin 125 Chewable, 1380
Augmentin ES, 160
Augmentin ES-600 Suspension, 1380
Augmentin 125 mg Suspension, 1380
Augmentin XR, 160, 1380
Augmentir, C15
Avalide 150/12.5, 1380
Avalide 300/12.5, 1380
Avalide 300/25, 1380
Avandamet, 22
Avandamet 2/500, 1380
Avandamet 4/500, 1380
Avandamet 2/1000, 1380
Avandamet 4/1000, 1380
Avandaryl 4/1, 1380
Avandaryl 4/2, 1380
Avandaryl 4/4, 1380
Avandaryl 8/2, 1380
Avandaryl 8/4, 1380
Avandaryl, 22
Avandia, 1128, C8
🍁 Ava pepper, 1360
Avapro, 182
Avastin, 226
Avelox, 589, 22
Aventyl, 936

Aviane, 1380
Aviane-28, 358
Avinza, 880, C8
🍁 Avirax, 118
Avodart, 492
Avonex, 728
Axert, 136
Axid, 660
Axid AR, 660
Axocet, 255
🍁 Axsam, 271
azacitidine, 210, 16, 59
Azasan, 212
AzaSite, 1397
azathioprine, 212, 17, 89
azelastine, 52, 1397
Azerra, 1372
azidothymidine, 1303
Azilect, 1100, 1376
azithromycin, 214, 56, 1397, C2, C4
Azopt, 1399
Azor 5/20, 1380
Azor 5/40, 1380
Azor 10/20, 1380
Azor 10/40, 1380
Azo-Standard, 1014
AZT, 1303, 17
aztreonam, 1375, C2, C4
Azulfidine, 1171
Azulfidine EN-tabs, 1171

B

BabyBIG, 1320
🍁 Bachelor's Button, 1349
bacitracin, 56, 1397
baclofen, 219, 102
Bactine, 381
Bactocill, 1005
Bactrim, 1254, 1380
Bactrim DS, 1254, 1380
Bactroban, 885
Bactroban Nasal, 885
🍁 Bai guo ye, 1353
Baking Soda, 1159
🍁 Baldrian, 1365
🍁 Baldrianwurzel, 1365
🍁 Balminil Decongestant Syrup, 1077
🍁 Balminil DM, 430
Balziva, 1380
Balziva-28, 358
🍁 baneberry, 1344
Banobese, 1017
Banophen, 450
Banzel, 22
Banzol, 1372
Baraclude, 500
BARBITURATES, 42, 101, C6
Baridium, 1014
🍁 Barriere-HC, 381
Basalgel, 140

COMPREHENSIVE INDEX 1449

basiliximab, 220, 89
Bayer Aspirin, 1131
Bayer Back & Body, 1380
Bayer PM, 1380
BCNU, 281
becaplermin, 222
beclomethasone, 365, 369, 37, 83
Beconase AQ, 369
Beesix, 1083
Belgium Valerian, 1365
BELLADONNA ALKALOIDS, C6
Bell-Ans, 1159
✤Beloc, 851
Beloc-ZOK, 851
Benadryl, 450, C6
Benadryl Allergy, 450
Benadryl-D Allergy & Sinus Tablets, 1380
Benadryl Dye-Free Alergy, 450
benazepril, 176, 53
bendamustine, 223, 16, 59
Benicar, 182, 1376
Benicar HCT 20/12.5, 1380
Benicar HCT 40/12.5, 1380
Benicar HCT 40/25, 1380
Bentyl, 438, C6
✤Bentylol, 438
Benylin Adult, 430
✤Benylin-E, 648
Benylin Pediatric, 430
BenzaClin Topical Gel, 1380
Benzamycin Topical Gel, 1380
benzathine penicillin G, 1002, 56
BENZODIAZEPINES, 34, 42, 101, C7
benztropine, 225, 38, 61
benzyl alcohol, 1369
bepotastine, 52, 1397
Bepreve, 1397
besifloxacin, 56, 1398
Besivance, 1398
BETA BLOCKERS, 32, 73, 106, C7
  NONSELECTIVE, 54, 75
  SELECTIVE, 54, 75
✤Betachron E-R, 1071
✤Betacort, 380
✤Betaderm, 380
Betagan, 1399
✤Bataloc Durules, 851
✤Betaloc-ZOK, 851
betamethasone, 372, 380, 37, 68, 83
Betapace, 1167
Betapace AF, 1167
Betaseron, 728
Beta-Val, 380

✤Betaxin, 1209
betaxolol, 75, 1399
bethanechol, 1320
Betimol, 1399
✤Betnelan, 372
✤Betnesol, 372
✤Betnovate, 380
Betoptic, 1399
Betoptic S, 1399
bevacizumab, 226, 16, 59
✤Bewon, 1209
Biamine, 1209
Biaxin, 334
Biaxin XL, 334
bicalutamide, 228, 59
Bicillin L-A, 1002
Bicitra, 1163
Bicitra Solution, 1380
BiCNU, 281
Bidil, 1380
BiDil, 673
BIGUANIDES, 46
☯bilberry, 1344
BILE ACID SEQUESTRANTS, 91
☯billberry, 94
bimatoprost, 229, 1403
BioCal, 265
☯Bio-Hydrochlorothiazide, 458
biperiden, 61, 1320
BIPHOSPHONATES, 77
Bisac-Evac, 230
bisacodyl, 230, 90, C6
✤Bisaco-Lax, 230
✤Bisacolax, 230
Bismatrol, 231
bismuth subsalicylate, 231, 1375, 47, 72
bisoprolol, 233, 54, 75
bivalirudin, 234, 16, 40
☯black cohosh, 94, 1344
Black-Draught, 1145
☯black sampson, 1348
☯black snakeroot, 1344
☯black susan, 1348
Blenoxane, 236
bleomycin, 236, 16, 59
Bleph-10, 1398
Blephamide Ophthalmic Suspension/Ointment, 1380
✤Bonamine, 811
BONE RESORPTION INHIBITORS, 76
Bonine, 811
Boniva, 687
Boostrix, 1429, 1434
bortezomib, 239, 1375, 16, 59
bosentan, 23
Botox/Botox Cosmetic, 22

botulism immune globulin, 105, 1320
☯brauneria angustifolia, 1348
Breonesin, 648
Brevibloc, 528
Brevicon, 1380
Brevicon-28, 358
brimonidine, 1403
brinzolamide, 1399
Bromfed DM Liquid, 1380
Bromfenac, 1322
bromfenac, 97, 1402
bromocriptine, 61, 1321
brompheniramine, 52, 1322
BRONCHODILATORS, 37, 77
  XANTHINES, 240
✤Broncho-Grippol-DM, 430
Bronkaid Dual Action, 1380
Brovana, 1376
Bucet, Bupap, 255
Budeprion SR, 249
Budeprion XL, 249
budesonide, 365, 369, 372, 23, 37, 68, 83
Bufferin, 1131, 1380
☯bugbane, 1344
BULK-FORMING AGENTS, 90
Bulk Forming Fiber Laxative, 1331
bumetanide, 244, 85, C2, C4
Bumex, 244
Buminate, 125
bupivacaine, 502
Buprenex, 246, 1419
buprenorphine, 246, 16, 99, 1419, C1
bupropion, 249, 22, 44, C11, C12
✤Burinex, 244
☯Burn plant, 1341
BuSpar, 251, C12
buspirone, 1442, C11
busPIRone, 251, 34, C11, C12
busulfan, 252, 16, 59
Busulfex, 252
butalbital, acetaminophen, 255
butalbital, acetaminophen, caffeine, 255
butalbital, aspirin, caffeine, 255
BUTALBITAL COMPOUND, 255
butalbital compounds, 96
Butapap 50/325, 1380
Butapap 50/650, 1380
butenafine, 187, 50

---

*Entries for **generic** names appear in **boldface type**. Trade names appear in regular type, with Canadian trade names preceded by a maple leaf icon (✤). **CLASSIFICATIONS** appear in **BOLDFACE SMALL CAPS**. *Combination Drugs* appear in *italics*, herbal products are preceded by a yin-yang icon (☯) and drugs with genetic implications are preceded by a double-helix icon (𝌀).

1450 COMPREHENSIVE INDEX

Butex Forte, 255
butoconazole, 190, 50
butorphanol, 257, 16, 99, 1419, C1, C2
Byetta, 550, 1376
Bystolic, 905

C

🌐 Cabbage Palm, 1363
cabergoline, 261
Caduet 2.5/10, 1380
Caduet 2.5/20, 1381
Caduet 2.5/40, 1381
Caduet 5/10, 1381
Caduet 5/20, 1381
Caduet 5/40, 1381
Caduet 5/80, 1381
Caduet 10/10, 1381
Caduet 10/20, 1381
Caduet 10/40, 1381
Caduet 10/80, 1381
Cafcit, 262
Cafergot, 1381
caffeine citrate, 262, 81, C4
Calan, 1275
Calan SR, 1275
Calcarb, 265
Calci-Chew, 265
Calciday, 265
Calcijex, 1287
Calcilac, 265
✤ Calcilean, 654
Calci-Mix, 265
✤ Calciparine, 654
✤ Calcite, 265
CALCITONIN, 263
  rDNA, 263
  salmon, 263, 87
Cal-Citrate 250, 265
calcitriol, 1287, 1375, 107, C4
calcium acetate (25% Ca or 12.6 mEq/g), 265, 92
calcium carbonate (40% Ca or 20 mEq/g), 265, 92
CALCIUM CHANNEL BLOCKERS, 32, 54, 78, C7
calcium chloride, C2–C3, C4
calcium chloride (27% Ca or 13.6 mEq/g), 265, 92
calcium citrate (21% Ca or 12 mEq/g), 265, 92
calcium gluconate, C2–C3, C4
calcium gluconate (9% Ca or 4.5 mEq/g), 265, 92
calcium lactate (13% Ca or 6.5 mEq/g), 265, 92
CALCIUM SALTS, 265, 92
CaldeCORT Anti-Itch, 381

Caldolor, 688
✤ Calglycine, 265
🌐 Calicut, 1351
Cal-Lac, 265
✤ Calmylin #1, 430
✤ Calmylin Expectorant, 648
Cal-Plus, 265
✤ Calsan, 265
Caltrate, 265
Caltrate 600+D, 1381
Cambia, 435, 22
🌐 Camellia sinensis, 1357
Camila, 359
Campath, 128
Campral, 1317
Camptosar, 734
Canasa, 825
Cancidas, 285
candesartan, 182, 53
✤ Canesten, 187, 190
🌐 Cape aloe, 1341
capecitabine, 269, 16, 59
Capex, 380
Capoten, 176
Capozide 25/15, 1381
Capozide 25/25, 1381
Capozide 50/15, 1381
Capozide 50/25, 1381
capsaicin, 271, 1375, 96
Capsin, 271
captopril, 176, 53
Capzasin-P, 271
Carac, 594
Carafate, 1169
carbachol, 1400
carbamazepine, 272, 42, 1441–1442
CARBAPENEMS, 55
Carbatrol, 272
Carbex, 1141
carbidopa/levodopa, 275, 61
✤ Carbolith, 792
CARBONIC ANHYDRASE INHIBITORS, 85
carbonyl iron, 736, 31
carboplatin, 277, 16, 59
Cardene, 915
Cardene IV, 915
Cardene SR, 915
Cardiazem CD, 445
Cardizem, 445, C15
Cardizem LA, 445
Cardizem SR, 445
Cardura, 475, C6, C8
Cardura XL, 475
carisoprodol, 280, 102, C6
Carmol HC, 381
carmustine, 281, 16, 59
Caroid, 230
carteolol, 1377, 75, 1399
Carter's Little Pills, 230
Cartia XT, 445

Cartrol, 1377
carvedilol, 283, 54, 75
Casodex, 228
caspofungin, 285, 50, C2, C4
castor oil, C6
Cataflam, 435
Catapres, 343, C6
Catapres-TTS, 343
CATECHOL-*O*-METHYLTRANSFERASE INHIBITORS, 61
Cathflo Activase, 1214
Cayston, 1375
CCR5 CO-RECEPTOR ANTAGONISTS, 67
🌐 CDS, 1346
Cebid, 1319
Cecon, 1319
Cecore-500, 1319
Cedax, 300
✤ Cedocard-SR, 742
cefaclor, 294, 55
cefadroxil, 291, 55
cefazolin, 291, 55, C2, C4
cefdinir, 300, 55
cefditoren, 300, 55
cefepime, 287, 56, C2, C4
cefixime, 300, 56
Cefizox, 300
cefoperazone, 300, 56
cefotaxime, 300, 56, C2, C4
cefotetan, 294, 55
cefoxitin, 294, 55, C2, C4
cefpodoxime, 300, 56
cefprozil, 294, 55
ceftazidime, 300, 56, C2, C4
ceftibuten, 300, 56
Ceftin, 294
ceftizoxime, 300, 56, C2
ceftriaxone, 300, 56, C2, C4
cefuroxime, 294, 55, C2, C4
Cefzil, 294
Celebrex, 290, C8
celecoxib, 290, 69, 95, 97, 1441
✤ Celestoderm, 380
Celestone, 372
Celexa, 330, C8
CellCept, 887
Cellufresh, 1399
Celluvisc, 1399
Cemill, 1319
Cenafed, 1077
Cena-K, 1041
Cenestin, 535
Cenolate, 1319
CENTRALLY-ACTING, 102
CENTRALLY ACTING ANTIADRENERGICS, 54
CENTRAL NERVOUS SYSTEM STIMULANTS, 80
cephalexin, 291, 55

CEPHALOSPORINS
FIRST GENERATION, 291
SECOND GENERATION, 294
THIRD GENERATION, 300
Cerebyx, 616, C8
certolizumab pegol, 308, 22, 68
Cerubidine, 408
Cervarix, 1375
Cervidil Vaginal Insert, 448
🍁 C.E.S., 535
Cesia, 359
Cetacaine Topical Spray, 1381
Cetacort, 381
Cetane, 1319
cetirizine, 309, 52
Cetraxal, 1375
cetuximab, 311, 16, 59
Cevalin, 1319
Cevi-Bid, 1319
Chantix, 1269
🍁 Charac-50, 1317
CharcoAid 2000, 1317
🍁 Charcodote, 1317
Chemet, 1334
Cheracol Cough Syrup, 1381
Children's Advil, 688
Children's Advil Cold Liquid, 1381
Children's Hold, 430
Children's Loratidine, 798
Children's Motrin, 688
Children's Pain Reliever, 112
☯ Chinese Angelica, 1347
☯ Chinese ginseng, 1354
☯ chitosamine, 1356
Chlo-Amine, 316
chloralhydrate, 16
chloral hydrate, 312, 101
chlorambucil, 16, 59, 1322
Chlorate, 316
chlordiazepoxide, 314, 34, 101, C6
chlordiazepoxide-amitriptyline, C6
Chloromag, 804
chlorothiazide, 458, 54, 85
chlorpheniramine, 316, 52, C6
🍁 Chlorpromanyl, 318
chlorproPAMIDE, C11, C12
chlorpropamide, C6, C11
chlorpromazine, 17
chlorproMAZINE, 318, 48, 64, C1, C2, C4, C11, C12
chlorthalidone (thiazide-like), 458, 54, 85
Chlor-Trimeton, 316, C6

Chlor-Trimeton Allergy 4 Hour, 316
Chlor-Trimeton Allergy 8 Hour, 316
Chlor-Trimeton Allergy 12 Hour, 316
Chlor-Trimeton 4 Hour Relief, 1381
Chlor-Trimeton 12 Hour Relief, 1381
🍁 Chlor-Tripolon, 316
chlorzoxazone, 321, 102, C6
Cholac, 761
cholecalciferol, 1287
cholestyramine, 322, 91
choline and magnesium salicylates, 1131, 65, 95
choline salicylate, 1131, 65, 95
☯ chondroitin, 94, 1346
☯ chondroitin polysulfate, 1346
Chooz, 265
☯ Chrysanthemum parethenium, 1349
Cialis, 1185
ciclesonide, 369, 37, 83
inhalation, 1369
ciclopirox, 187, 50
cidofovir, 324, 73
🍁 Cidomycin, 145
Cillium, 1079
cilostazol, 326, 62, 1442
Ciloxan, 1398
cimetidine, 660, 72, 1441–1442, C6
Cimzia, 308, 22
cinacalcet, 326
Cipro, 589
Ciprodex Otic Suspension, 1381
ciprofloxacin, 589, 1375, 22, 56, 1398, 1441, C2, C4
Cipro HC Otic Suspension, 1381
Cipro/Proquin XR, 22
Cipro XR, 589
cisplatin, 328, 16, 59
citalopram, 330, 44, 1441–1442
Citrate of Magnesia, 804
Citrical, 265
Citrical Liquitab, 265
Citrocarbonate, 1159
Citroma, 804
🍁 Citromag, 804
cladribine, 332, 16, 59
Claforan, 300

Claravis, 744, 22
Clarinex, 417
Clarinex-D 12 Hour, 1381
Clarinex-D 24 Hour, 1381
clarithromycin, 334, 56, 72, 1442
Claritin, 798
Claritin-D 12 Hour, 1381
Claritin-D 24-Hour, 1381
Claritin Eye, 1397
Claritin Hives Relief, 798
Claritin 24-Hour Allergy, 798
Claritin Reditabs, 798
🍁 Clavulin, 160
🍁 *Clavulin 875, 1381*
🍁 *Clavulin 500, 1381*
🍁 *Clavulin 200 Suspension, 1381*
🍁 *Clavulin 400 Suspension, 1381*
🍁 *Clavulin 250 Suspension, 1381*
🍁 *Clavulin 125 Suspension, 1381*
Clear-Atadine, 798
Clear Eyes Lubricating Eye Redness Reliever, 1402
Cleocin, 337
Cleocin T, 337
clevidipine, 336, 54, 80
Cleviprex, 336
clidinium-chlordiazepoxide, C6
Climara, 532
ClimaraPro Transdermal Patch (release per day), 1381
Clinda-Derm, 337
Clindagel, 337
ClindaMax, 337
clindamycin, 337, 56, C2, C4
Clindesse, 337
Clindets, 337
Clinoril, 1175
clobetasol, 380, 83
Clobex, 380
clocortolone, 380, 83
Cloderm, 380
clofarabine, 340, 16, 59
Clolar, 340
clomiPHENE, C11, C12
clomiPRAMINE, 1322, C11, C12
clonazepam, 341, 42, 1442
clonidine, 343, 1375, 53, C6, C8
clopidogrel, 346, 62

*Entries for **generic** names appear in **boldface type**. Trade names appear in regular type, with Canadian trade names preceded by a maple leaf icon (🍁). **CLASSIFICATIONS** appear in **BOLDFACE SMALL CAPS**. *Combination Drugs* appear in *italics*, herbal products are preceded by a yin-yang icon (☯) and drugs with genetic implications are preceded by a double-helix icon (🧬).

clorazepate, 347, 42, 101, C6
Clorpres 15/0.1, 1381
Clorpres 15/0.2, 1381
Clorpres 15/0.3, 1381
Clotrimaderm, 187, 190
clotrimazole, 187, 190, 50
cloxacillin, 1377
clozapine, 349, 22, 64, 1441
Clozaril, 349
Clozaril/Fazaclo ODT, 22
CMT, 1131
CMVIG, 1323
cochin, 1351
codeine, 351, 16, 99, 1441
Codimal, 1381
Codimal DH Syrup, 1381
Codimal DM Syrup, 1381
Codimal-L.A., 1381
Codimal PH Syrup, 1381
Cogentin, 225
Co-Gesic, 675, 1381
Co-Glimepiride, 1172
Cognex, 1181
Colace, 466
colchicine, 354, 16, 22
Colcrys, 354, 22
colesevelam, 356, 1375, 91
Colestid, 357
colestipol, 357, 91
Col-Probenecid, 1381
Coly-Mycin S Otic Suspension, 1381
Colyte, 1036, 1381
Combigan Ophthalmic Solution, 1381
CombiPatch 0.05/0.14, 1382
CombiPatch 0.05/0.25, 1382
Combivent, 1382
Combivir, 1382
Combunox, 967, 1382
Comfort Eye Drops, 1402
Comfort Tears, 1399
Commit, 918
Common Valerian, 1365
Compazine, 17
Compoz, 450
Compoz Nighttime Sleep Aid, 450
Compro, 1056
Comtan, 499
concentrated regular insulin, 46
Concerta, 844
Congest, 535
Congestac, 1382
Congestaid, 1077
Co-Norfloxacin, 589
Constilac, 761
Constulose, 761
Contac Cold & Flu Maximum Strength Caplets, 1382

Contac Cold & Flu Non-Drowsy Maximum Strength Caplets, 1382
CONTRACEPTIVES, HORMONAL, 358, 87
Copegus, 1107
Cordarone, 151, C6
Cordran, 380
Cordran-SP, 380
Coreg, 283
Coreg CR, 283
Corgard, 892
Coricidin HBP Chest Congestion and Cough, 1382
Coricidin HBP Cold and Flu, 1382
Coricidin HBP Cough and Cold, 1382
Coricidin HBP Maximum Strength Flu, 1382
Corlopam, 562
Cormax, 380
Coronex, 742
Correctol Stool Softener Soft Gels, 466
Cortacet, 381
Cortaid, 381
Cortate, 381
Cort-Dome, 381
Cortef, 372
Cortef Feminine Itch, 381
Cortenema, 372
Corticaine, 381
CORTICOSTEROIDS, 37, 68, 82
INHALATION, 365, 83
NASAL, 369, 83
OPHTHALMIC, 83
SYSTEMIC, 372, 83
TOPICAL/LOCAL, 380, 83
Corticreme, 381
Cortifair, 381
Cortifoam, 381
cortisone, 372, 37, 68, 83
Cortisporin Otic Solution/Suspension, 1382
Cortisporin Topical Cream, 1382
Cortizone, 381
Cortone, 372
Corvert, 691
Coryphen, 1131
Corzide 40/5, 1382
Corzide 80/5, 1382
Cosopt Ophthalmic Solution, 1382
Coumadin, 1295, C8, C16
COUMARINS, 40
Covera-HS, 1275
Coversyl, 176
Coversyl Plus, 1382
Coversyl Plus LD, 1382
Cozaar, 182
CPS, 1346

CPZ, 17
Creon, 985, 1382
Creon/Zenpap, 22
Creo-Terpin, 430
Crestor, 666
Crinone, 1060
Crixivan, 1327
Crolom, 1401
cromolyn, 1401
Cruex, 187
Cryselle, 358, 1382
Crystapen, 1002
C/T/S, 337
Cubicin, 401
cum flore, 1358
Cuprimine, 1330
Curacao aloe, 1341
Cutivate, 380
cyanocobalamin, 1284, 31, 107
Cyanokit, 1284
Cyclessa, 359
cyclobenzaprine, 383, 102, 1441, C6
Cyclocort, 380
Cyclogyl, 1401
Cyclomen, 1323
Cyclomydril Ophthalmic Solution, 1382
cyclopentolate, 1401
cyclophosphamide, 384, 16, 59, 89
cycloSERINE, C11
Cycloset, 1321
cyclosporine, C4, C11
cycloSPORINE, 387, 69, 89, C11, C15
Cylate, 1401
Cymbalta, 490, 1376
CYP1A2, 1441
CYP3A, 1442
CYP2C19, 1441
CYP2C9, 1441
CYP2D6, 1441
cyproheptadine, 390, 52, C6
Cystospaz, 684
Cystospaz-M, 684
Cytadren, 1377
cytarabine, 392, 16, 59
CytoGam, 1323
cytomegalovirus immune globulin, 105, 1323
Cytomel, 1219
Cytosar, 392
Cytosar-U, 392
cytosine arabinoside, 392
Cytotec, 869
Cytovene, 626

D

dacarbazine, 397, 16, 59
Dacodyl, 230

COMPREHENSIVE INDEX 1453

Dacogen, 410
Dakrina, 1399
🍁 Dalacin C, 337
🍁 Dalacin T, 337
dalfampridine, 1369
Dallergy Caplets, 1382
Dallergy Extended Release, 1382
Dallergy-JR Capsules, 1382
Dallergy Syrup, 1382
Dallergy Tablets, 1382
Dalmane, 603, C6
dalteparin, 657, 40
Damason-P, 1382
danazol, 87, 1323
☯ Dang Gui, 1347
☯ Danggui, 1347
Danocrine, 1323
Dantrium, 398
dantrolene, 398, 102
Dapacin, 112
dapsone, 1442
Daptacel, 1429
daptomycin, 401, 56, C2
Daraprim, 1085
darbepoetin, 403, 1376, 31, 87
darifenacin, 405, 38
darunavir, 406, 67
Darvocet, C8
Darvocet A500, 1068, 1382
Darvocet-N 50, 1068, 1382
Darvocet-N 100, 1068, 1382
Darvon, 1068, C6
Darvon/Darvon-N/Darvocet-N, 22
Darvon N, 1068
DAUNOrubicin hydrochloride, 408, 16, 59, C11
daunorubicin lipsome, 1377, C8
DaunoXome, 1377
Daypro, 959, C6
Dayquil Cold & Flu Relief Liquid, 1382
Dayquil Sinus Liquicaps, 1382
Daytrana, 844
DC Softgels, 466
DDAVP, 418
DDAVP Rhinal Tube, 418
DDAVP Rhinyle Drops, 418
ddI, 1324
Decavac, 1435
decitabine, 410, 16, 60
Decofed, 1077
Deconamine, 1382
Deconamine SR, 1382
Deconamine Syrup, 1382

deferasirox, 1376
deferoxamine, 412
Deficol, 230
Degas, 1155
Degest 2, 1402
Delatestryl, 1200
delavirdine, 1441–1442
Delestrogen, 532
Delsym, 430
Delta-D, 1287
Demadex, 1244
Demerol, 820, 1419, C6
☯ Demon chaser, 1364
Denavir, 1001
Depacon, 1262
Depakene, 1262
Depakote, 1262
Depakote ER, 1262
Depen, 1330
DepoCyt, 392
DepoDur, 880
Depo-Estradiol, 532
Depo-Medrol, 372
Depo-Provera, 359, 812
Depo-subQ Provera 104, 359
Depo-Sub Q Provera 104, 812
Depo-Testosterone, 1200
Dermabet, 380
Dermacort, 381
Derma-Smoothe/FS, 380
Dermatop, 381
DermiCort, 381
🍁 Dermovate, 380
Dermtex HC, 381
Desferal, 412
desipramine, 413, 1376, 44, 1441
desirudin, 415, 40
desloratadine, 417, 52
desmopressin, 418, 87
Desogen, 358, 1382
Desonate, 380
desonide, 380, 83
DesOwen, 380
desoximetasone, 380, 83
desvenlafaxine, 420, 44, 69
Detrol, 1238
Detrol LA, 1238
DexAlone, 430
dexamethasone, 372, 1375, 37, 68, 83, 1400, C2, C4
dexchlorpheniramine, C6
Dexedrine, 428
DexFerrum, 736
Dexilant, 422
dexlansoprazole, 422, 72
dexmedetomidine, 423, 101
dexmethylphenidate, 424, 81

DexPak, 372
dexrazoxane, 426
dextroamphetamine, 428, 81
dextromethorphan, 430, 1441
D.H.E. 45, 518
DiaBeta, 1173, C8, C13
Diabetic Tussin, 648
Diabinese, C6
Dialume, 140
Diamox, 114
Diamox Sequels, 114
Diar-aid Caplets, 794
Diastat, 431
🍁 Diazemuls, 431
diazepam, 431, 34, 42, 101–102, 1441–1442, C1, C2, C4, C6
diazoxide, C4
Dicarbosil, 265
diclofenac, 435, 1375, 97, 1402
diclofenac epolamine (topical patch), 435
diclofenac potassium, 435, 22, 95, 97
diclofenac sodium, 435, 95, 97
diclofenac sodium (topical gel), 435
diclofenac topical, 97
dicloxacillin, 1005, 56
dicyclomine, 438, 38, C6
didanosine, 1376, 67, 1324
dideoxyinosine, 1324
🍁 Didrocal, 542
Didronel, 542
difenoxin/atropine, 453, 38, 47
Difil-G Forte Liquid, 1382
Difil-G Tablets, 1382
diflorasone, 380, 83
Diflucan, 581, C8
difluprednate, 83, 1400
Digibind, 443
DigiFab, 443
digoxin, 439, 16, 35, C2, C4, C6
digoxin immune Fab, 443
dihydroergotamine, 518, 106
1,25-dihydroxycholecalciferol, 1287
Dilacor XR, 445
Dilantin, 1020
Dilatair, 1403
Dilatrate-SR, 742
Dilaudid, 677, 1418

1454 COMPREHENSIVE INDEX

Dilaudid-HP, 677
Dilex-G Syrup, 1382
Dilex G Tablets, 1382
Diltia XT, 445
diltiazem, 445, 32, 35, 54, 80, 1442, C2–C3, C15
dimenhyDRINATE, C11, C13
🍁 Dimetane, 1322
Dimetapp Allergy, 1322
Dimetapp Children's ND Non-Drowsy Allergy, 798
Dimetapp Cold & Allergy Elixir, 1383
Dimetapp Cold & Congestion Elixir, 1383
Dimetapp Cough & Cold DM Elixir, 1383
Dimetapp Decongestant Pediatric, 1077
Dimetapp Long-Acting Cough Plus Cold Elixir, 1383
Dimetapp Maximum Strength 12–Hour Non-Drowsy Extentabs, 1077
dinoprostone, 448
🍁 Diocane, 1397
Diocto, 466
Dioctocal, 466
🍁 Diodex, 1400
Diovan, 182
Diovan HCT 80/12.5, 1383
Diovan HCT 160/12.5, 1383
Diovan HCT 160/25, 1383
Diovan HCT 320/12.5, 1383
Diovan HCT 320/25, 1383
🍁 Diovol Ex, 803
Dipentum, 946
DIPEPTIDYL PEPTIDASE-4 INHIBITORS, 46
Diphen AF, 450
Diphen Cough, 450
Diphenhist, 450
diphenhydrAMINE, 450, 52, C11, C13
diphenhydramine, C1, C2, C4, C6, C11, C12
diphenoxylate/atropine, 453, 38, 47
Diphtheria toxoid, 1429
dipivefrin, 1403
Dipridacot, 454
Diprivan, 1066, C8
Diprolene, 380
Diprolene AF, 380
dipyridamole, 454, 62, C6
DIRECT-ACTING, 102
Disalcid, 1131
disopyramide, 1442, C6
DisperMox, 158
disulfiram, 1324
Ditropan, 964, C6
Ditropan XL, 964

DIURETICS, 84, C7
  POTASSIUM-SPARING, 456
  THIAZIDE, 458
Diuril, 458
divalproex sodium, 1262, 42, 106
Divigel, 532
🍁 Dixarit, 343
DMARDS, 68. *See* **DISEASE-MODIFYING ANTIRHEUMATIC DRUGS**
🍁 DM Syrup, 430
🍁 Doan's Backache Pills, 1131
Doan's Regular Strength Tablets, 1131
DOBUTamine, 461, 16, C2–C3, C11, C13
Dobutrex, 461
docetaxel, 462, 16, 59
docosanol, 465, 73
Docu, 466
DOCUSATE, 466
docusate calcium, 466, 90
docusate sodium, 466, 90
Docusoft S, 466
🍁 Dodd's Extra Strength, 1131
🍁 Dodd's Pills, 1131
dofetilide, 467, 23, 35
DOK, 466
dolasetron, 469, 48
Dolgic, 255
Dolorac, 271
🍁 DOM-Cephalexin, 291
🍁 Dom-Cimetidine, 660
🍁 DOM-Divalproex, 1262
🍁 Dom-Glyburide, 1173
🍁 DOM-Hydrochlorothiazide, 458
🍁 DOM-Minocycline, 1203
🍁 Dom-Nizatidine, 660
🍁 Dom-Ranitidine, 660
🍁 DOM-Valproic Acid, 1262
donepezil, 470, 30
🍂 dong quai, 1347
🍂 dongquai, 94
Donnamar, 684
Donnatal, 1383, C6
Donnatal Elixir, 1383
Donnatal Extentabs, 1383
🍂 Don Quai, 1347
🍁 Dopamet, 840
DOPamine, 471, 16, C2–C3, C11, C13
DOPAMINE AGONISTS, 61
Doral, C6
Doribax, 473
doripenem, 473, 55, C2
Dormin, 450
Doryx, 1203
dorzolamide, 1400
DOS, 466
DOSS, 466
DOS Softgels, 466
doxazosin, 475, 54, C6

doxepin, 476, 34, 44, 52, C6
doxercalciferol, 1287, 107
Doxil, 482
Doxine, 1083
DOXOrubicin, 479, 59, C11, C15
doxorubicin, C8, C11
DOXOrubicin, liposomal, 482, C8
DOXOrubicin liposome, 59
Doxy, 1203
🍁 Doxycin, 1203
doxycycline, 1203, 56, C2, C4
🍁 Doxytab, 1203
Dramamine Less Drowsy Formula, 811
🍁 Drenison, 380
Drisdol, 1287
Dristan Cold Multi-Symptom Formula, 1383
Drixoral 12 Hour Non-Drowsy Formula, 1077
Drixoral Liquid Cough Caps, 430
dronedarone, 485, 23, 35
droperidol, 487, 101, C1, C2
drotrecogin, 489, 56
Droxia, 1326
Dry Eyes Duratears Naturale, 1399
Dry Eye Therapy, 1399
DSS, 466
d4T, 1334
DTaP, 1429
🍁 DTIC, 397
DTIC-Dome, 397
Duac CS Topical Gel, 1383
Duetact, 23
Duetact 2/30, 1383
Duetact 4/30, 1383
Dulcagen, 230
Dulcolax, 230, C6
Dulcolax Magnesia Tablets, 804
Dulcolax Stool Softener, 466
duloxetine, 490, 1376, 44
DuoNeb, 1383
Duraclon, 343, C6
Duragesic, 570
🍁 Duralith, 792
Duramorph, 880
Durezol, 1400
Duricef, 291
dutasteride, 492
Duvoid, 1320
Dwelle, 1399
Dyazide, 1383
Dynacin, 1203
DynaCirc, 746
DynaCirc CR, 746
Dyrenium, 456
Dysport, 23

COMPREHENSIVE INDEX

E

E-200, 1291
E-400, 1291
E-1000, 1291
Easprin, 1131
☯echinacea, 94
☯echinacea (Echinacea Purpureas), 1348
ECHINOCANDINS, 50
echothiophate, 1400
EC-Naprosyn, 900
econazole, 187, 50
Ecotrin, 1131
✤ Ectosone, 380
eculizumab, 23
Edecrin, C6
ED-IN-SOL, 736
Edluar, 1313, 23
ED-SPAZ, 684
Edur-Acin, 914
E.E.S., 523
efalizumab, 1377
efavirenz, 495, 67, 1441–1442
Effer-K, 1041
Effer-Syllium, 1079
Effexor, 1272, C8
Effexor/Effexor XR, 23
Effexor XL, C8
Effexor XR, 1272
Effient, 1048, 23
Efidac 24, 1077
eflornithine (topical), 1325
Efudex, 594
✤ Elavil, 154
Eldepryl, 1141
Elestat, 1397
Elestrin, 532
eletriptan, 496, 106
Elidel, 1029
Eligard, 778
Elimite, 1012
Elitek, 1102
Elixophyllin-GG Liquid, 1383
ElixSure Children's Cough Syrup, 430
Ellence, 508
✤ Elocom, 381
Elocon, 381
Eloxatin, 957
Elspar, 199
✤ Eltor 120, 1077
eltrombopag, 23
✤ Eltroxin, 1219
Emadine, 1397
Embeda, 880, 23
Embeda 30/1.2, 1383

Embeda 50/2, 1383
Embeda 60/2.4, 1383
Embeda 80/3.2, 1383
Embeda 20/0.8, 1383
Embeda 100/4, 1383
Embeline, 380
Embeline E, 380
emedastine, 52, 1397
Emend, 191, 1370
✤ Emex, 847
EMLA, 787
EMLA Topical Cream, 1383
✤ Emo-Cort, 381
Emsam, 1143
emtricitabine, 498, 67
Emtriva, 498
E-Mycin, 523
Enablex, 405
⚕ **enalapril/enalaprilat, 176, 53, C2, C4**
Enbrel, 539, 23
✤ Enca, 1203
Endocet 5/325, 1383
Endocet 7.5/325, 1383
Endocet, 966
Endocet 10/325, 1383
Endocet 7.5/500, 1383
Endocet 10/650, 1383
Endocodone, 966
Endodan, 966, 1383
Endolor, 255
Endometrin, 1060
enfuvirtide, 67, 1325
Engerix-B, 1430, 1433
Enjuvia, 535
Enlon Plus, 1383
enoxaparin, 657, 40
Enpresse, 359
entacapone, 499, 61
entecavir, 500, 73
Entereg, 23
Entocort EC, 372
✤ Entrophen, 1131
Enulose, 761
Enzymase-16, 985
ENZYME INHIBITORS, 46, 59
ENZYMES, 59
ephedrine, C8
EPIDURAL LOCAL ANESTHETICS, 502
Epifoam Aerosol Foam, 1383
✤ Epimorph, 880
epinastine, 52, 1397
epinephrine, 504, 16, 37, 78, C8
EpiPen, 504
epirubicin, 508, 16, 59
Epitol, 272
✤ Epival, 1262

Epivir, 762
Epivir-HBV, 762
eplerenone, 511, 53
EPO, 512, 1376
epoetin, 512, 31, 87
Epogen, 512, 1376
✤ Eprex, 512
⚕ **eprosartan, 182, 53**
epsilon aminocaproic acid, 143
eptifibatide, 515, 16, 62
Epzicom, 23, 1383
Equalactin, 1331
Equetro, 272
Equilet, 265
Eraxis, 186
Erbitux, 311
ergocalciferol, 1287, 107
ergoloid mesylates, C6
Ergomar, 518
ergometrine, 517
ergonovine, 517
ergotamine, 518, 106
Ergotrate, 517
erlotinib, 520, 16, 59, 1442
Errin, 359
Ertaczo, 1146
ertapenem, 522, 55, C2
✤ Erybid, 523
Eryc, 523
Erygel, 523
EryPed, 523
Ery-Tab, 523
Erythrocin, 523
✤ Erythromid, 523
erythromycin, 56, 1398, 1442, C4
ERYTHROMYCIN, 523
erythromycin base, 523
erythromycin ethylsuccinate, 523
erythromycin lactobionate, 523, C2
erythromycin stearate, 523
erythromycin (topical), 523
ERYTHROPOIESIS-STIMULATING AGENTS (ESAs), 1376
erythropoietin, 512
escitalopram, 526, 44, 1441–1442
Esedrix, 458
Esgic, 255, 1383
Esgic-Plus, 255, 1383
Eskalith, 792
esmolol, 528, 16, 35, 75
esomeprazole, 530, 72, 1441
Estivin II, 1402
Estrace, 532

---

*Entries for **generic** names appear in **boldface type**. Trade names appear in regular type, with Canadian trade names preceded by a maple leaf icon (✤). **CLASSIFICATIONS** appear in **BOLDFACE SMALL CAPS**. *Combination Drugs* appear in *italics*, herbal products are preceded by a yin-yang icon (☯) and drugs with genetic implications are preceded by a double-helix icon (⚕).

COMPREHENSIVE INDEX

Estraderm, 532
ESTRADIOL, 532
estradiol, 1375
estradiol acetate, 532, 87
estradiol cypionate, 532, 87
estradiol topical emulsion, 532, 87
estradiol topical gel, 532, 87
estradiol transdermal spray, 532, 87
estradiol transdermal system, 532, 87
estradiol vaginal ring, 532, 87
estradiol vaginal tablet, 532, 87
estradiol valerate, 532, 87
Estrasorb, 532
Estring, 532
EstroGel, 532
estrogens, 1442, C6
estrogens, conjugated (equine), 535, 87
estrogens, conjugated (synthetic, A), 535, 87
estrogens, conjugated (synthetic, B), 535, 87
Estrostep, 359
Estrostep Fe, 359
eszopiclone, 538, 101
etanercept, 539, 23, 68
ethacrynic acid, C4, C6
ethambutol, 541, 70
ethinyl estradiol/ desogestrel, 358–359, 87
ethinyl estradiol/ drospirenone, 358, 87
ethinyl estradiol/ethynodiol, 358, 87
ethinyl estradiol/ etonogestrel, 359, 87
ethinyl estradiol/ levonergestrel, 87
ethinyl estradiol/ levonorgestrel, 358–359
ethinyl estradiol/ norelgestromin, 359, 87
ethinyl estradiol/ norethindrone, 358–359, 87
ethinyl estradiol/ norgestimate, 358–359, 87
ethinyl estradiol/norgestrel, 358, 87
Ethyol, 141
✸Etibi, 541
etidronate, 542, 77
etodolac, 544, 69, 95
etonorgestrel, 359
Etopophos, 546

etoposide, 546, 59
etoposide phosphate, 546, 59
etoposides, 16
ETOPOSIDES, 546
etravirine, 548, 67
✸Euglucon, 1173
Eulexin, 1325
✸Euthyrox, 1219
EvaMist, 532
everolimus, 1370, 60
Evista, 1096, C8
E-Vitamin, 1291
Evoclin, 337
Exalgo, 1375
Excedrin Back and Body, 1384
Excedrin Extra Strength, 1384
Excedrin IB, 688
Excedrin Migraine, 1384
Excedrin P.M., 1384
Excedrin Sinus Headache, 1384
Excedrin Tension Headache, 1384
Exelderm, 187
Exelon, 1123
exenatide, 550, 1376, 46
Exforge 5/160, 1384
Exforge 5/320, 1384
Exforge 10/160, 1384
Exforge 10/320, 1384
Exjade, 1376
Ex-Lax, 1145
Ex-Lax Chocolated, 1145
Ex-Lax Stool Softener, 466
Extavia, 23
EXTENDED SPECTRUM PENICILLINS, 56
Extina, 187
Extra Strength Dynafed (Billups, P.J.), 112
Extra Strength Dynafed E.X., 112
Extra Strength Gas-X, 1155
✸Extra Strength Maalox GRF Gas Relief Formula, 1155
Eye-Lube-A, 1399
Eyesine, 1403
ezetimibe, 552, 91
✸Ezetrol, 552

F

Factive, 589, 23
Factrel, 1377
famciclovir, 555, 73
famotidine, 660, 72, C2, C4
Famvir, 555
Fanapt, 696
Fansidar, 1384
Fastin, 1017
FAT-SOLUBLE VITAMINS, 107

FazaClo, 349
Fe50, 736
◐Featerfoiul, 1349
◐Featherfew, 1349
◐Featherfoil, 1349
febuxostat, 556
Feen-a-Mint, 230
Feldene, 1034, C6
felodipine, 557, 32, 54, 80
Femara, 775
Femcon Fe, 358, 1384
Fembrt 1/5, 1384
Fembrt 0.5/2.5, 1384
Femiron, 736
✸Femogex, 532
Femring, 532
Femtrace, 532
fenofibrate, 559, 91
fenofibric acid, 561, 23, 91
Fenoglide, 559
fenoldopam, 562, 54
fentanyl, 1418, 1420, 1442, C2–C3, C4
fentanyl, buccal, 16
fentanyl (buccal soluble film), 23
fentanyl buccal/ transmucosal, 564, 99, C16
fentanyl, parenteral, 567, 16, 99
FENTANYL TRANSDERMAL, 570, 1420, 16, 99, C16
fentanyl (transmucosal), 16, 22, C15
Fentora, 564, C16
Feosol, 736, C6
Feostat, 736
Feraheme, 573
Feratab, 736
Fer-gen-sol, 736
Fergon, 736
Fer-In-Sol, 736
Fer-Iron, 736
✸Fero-Grad, 736
Ferralet, 736
Ferrlecit, 737
Ferro-Sequels, 1384
ferrous fumarate, 736, 31
ferrous gluconate, 736, 31
ferrous sulfate, 736, 31, C6
✸Fertinic, 736
ferumoxytol, 573, 31
fesoterodine, 574, 38
Feverall, 112
◐feverfew, 94, 1349
Fexmid, C6
fexofenadine, 575, 52
Fiberall, 1079
FiberCon, 1331
Fiber-Lax, 1331
Fibrepur, 1079
filgrastim, 576

COMPREHENSIVE INDEX

finasteride, 578
Fioricet, 255, 1384
Fioricet with codeine, 1384
Fiorinal, 255, 1384
Fiorinal with codeine, 1384
Fiortal, 255
FIRST-GENERATION CEPHALOSPORINS, 55
Flagyl, 854
Flagyl ER, 854
Flarex, 1400
Flatulex, 1155
Flavorcee, 1319
flecainide, 579, 35, 1441
Flector, 435
Fleet Enema, 1025
Fleet Laxative, 230
Fleet Sof-Lax, 466
Fletchers' Castoria, 1145
Flexeril, 383, C6
☯ Flirtwort Midsummer Daisy, 1349
Flomax, 1189
Flonase, 369
Flovent Diskus, 366
Flovent HFA, 366
Floxin, 589
Fluarix, 1431, 1433
fluconazole, 581, 50, 1441–1442, C2, C4
Fludara, 583
fludarabine, 583, 16, 59
fludrocortisone, 586, 87
FluLaval, 1431, 1433
flumazenil, 587, C4
FluMist, 1431, 1433
flunisolide, 366, 369, 37, 83
☯ fluocinolone, 380, 83
fluocinonide, 380, 83
✦ Fluoderm, 380
✦ Fluolar, 380
✦ Fluonide, 380
fluorometholone, 83, 1400
Fluor-Op, 1400
Fluoroplex, 594
FLUOROQUINOLONES, 589, 56
fluorouracil, 594, 16, 59
fluoxetine, 597, 23, 44, 1441, C6
fluphenazine, 600, 64
flurandrenolide, 380, 83
flurazepam, 603, 101, C6
flurbiprofen, 97, 1402
flutamide, 59, 1325
fluticasone, 366, 369, 380, 22, 37, 83
fluvastatin, 666, 91, 1441
Fluvirin, 1431, 1433

fluvoxamine, 604, 44, 1441
Fluzone, 1431, 1433
FML, 1400
FML Forte, 1400
FML-S Ophthalmic Suspension, 1384
Focalin, 424
Focalin XR, 424
FoilleCort, 381
folate, 606
folic acid, 606, 31, 108, C8
folinic acid, 776, C8
Folvite, 606
fondaparinux, 608, 1376, 16, 40
Foradil, 610, 1376
formoterol, 610, 1376, 23, 37, 78
✦ Formulex, 438
Fortamet, 829
Fortaz, 300
Forteo, 1199, 23
Fortical, 263
Fosamax, 130
Fosamax Plus D 70/2800, 1384
Fosamax Plus D 70/5600, 1384
fosamprenavir, 612, 67
fosaprepitant (injection), 1370, 31
foscarnet, 614, 73, C4
⚕ **fosinopril, 176, 53**
fosphenytoin, 616, 35, 42, C4
fospropofol, 1370
Fosrenol, 769
☯ fossil tree, 1353
Fragmin, 657
☯ Fragrant Valerian, 1365
Frova, 618
frovatriptan, 618, 106
5-FU, 594
Fumasorb, 736
Fumerin, 736
✦ Fungizone, 165
Fungoid, 187
Furadantin, 928, C6
furosemide, 620, 85, C2–C3, C4
FUSION INHIBITORS, 67
Fuzeon, 1325

G

gabapentin, 623, 42
Gabitril, 1222
galantamine, 624, 30

gamma benzene hexachloride, 788
ganciclovir, 626, 1375, 73, C2, C4
Ganidin NR, 648
Garamycin, 145
Gardasil, 670, 1376, 1432–1433
☯ Garden Heliotrope, 1365
☯ Garden Valerian, 1365
☯ garlic, 94, 1350
Gas-Ban, 1384
Gastrosed, 684
Gas-X, 1155
gatifloxacin, 56, 1398, C2
Gaviscon Extra Strength, 1384
Gaviscon Extra-Strength Liquid, 1384
Gaviscon Liquid, 1384
Gaviscon Regular Strength, 1384
✦ GBH, 788
G-CSF, 576
gefitinib, 628, 16, 59
geftinib, 1442
Gelnique, 964, C6
Gelusil, 1384
✦ Gelusil Extra Strength, 803
gemcitabine, 629, 16, 59
gemfibrozil, 632, 91
gemifloxacin, 589, 23, 56
gemtuzumab ozogamicin, 633, 16, 59
Gemzar, 629
Genacote, 1131
Genac Tablets, 1384
Genafed, 1077
Genahist, 450
Genapap, 112
Genasyme, 1155
Genatuss DM Syrup, 1384
Gencalc, 265
✦ Gen-Cimetidine, 660
✦ Gen-Divalproex, 1262
Genebs, 112
Generlac, 761
Geneye, 1403
✦ Gen-Famotidine, 660
☯ gengibre, 1351
✦ Gen-Glybe, 1173
Gengraf, 387
Gen-K, 1041
✦ Gen-Medroxy, 812
✦ Gen-Minocycline, 1203
✦ Gen-Nizatidine, 660
Genoptic, 1398
Genotropin, 645
Genpril, 688
✦ Gen-Ranitidine, 660

---

*Entries for **generic** names appear in **boldface type**. Trade names appear in regular type, with Canadian trade names preceded by a maple leaf icon (✦). **CLASSIFICATIONS** appear in **BOLDFACE SMALL CAPS**. *Combination Drugs* appear in *italics*, herbal products are preceded by a yin-yang icon (☯) and drugs with genetic implications are preceded by a double-helix icon (⚕).

COMPREHENSIVE INDEX

Gen-Salbutamol, 126
Gen-Selegiline, 1141
Gentak, 1398
gentamicin, 145, 55, 1398, C2, C4
Genteal Lubricant Eye Gel, 1399
Gentesol, 1398
Gen-Triazolam, 1253
Gen-XENE, 347
Geodon, 1307
ginger, 94
ginger root, imber, 1351
ginger (Zingiber Officinale), 1351
ginkgo, 94, 1353
ginkgo folium, 1353
Gin Pain Pills, 1131
ginseng, 94
ginseng (Panax Ginseng), 1354
Gleevec, 698
Gliadel, 281
glimepiride, 1172, 22–23, 46, 1441, C16
glipizide, 1441
glipiZIDE, 1173, 46, C11, C13
GlucaGen, 634
glucagon, 634, 87
GLUCAGON-LIKE PEPTIDE-1 (GLP-1) RECEPTOR AGONISTS, 46
glucocorticoids, 1442
Gluconorm, 1103
Glucophage, 829
Glucophage XR, 829
glucosamine, 94, 1356
Glucotrol, 1173, C13
Glucotrol XL, 1173, C13
Glucovance 1.25/250, 1384
Glucovance 2.5/500, 1384
Glucovance 5/500, 1384
Glumetza, 829
glyBURIDE, 1173, 46, C11, C12
glycerin, 1403
GlycoLax, 1036
GLYCOPROTEIN IIB/IIIA INHIBITORS, 62
glycopyrrolate, 636, 38, C1, C2, C4
Glynase PresTab, 1173
Glyset, 863
G-Mycin, 145
Goatweed, 1364
golimumab, 638, 23, 68
Golytely, 1384
GoLYTELY, 1036
Golytely Packets, 1384
gonadorelin acetate, 1377
gonadorelin hydrochloride, 1377
goserelin, 640, 59, 87
granisetron, 48, C2, C4

granisetron (oral and IV), 642
granisetron (transdermal), 642
Granulex Topical Aerosol, 1384
granulocyte colony stimulating factor, 576
grape seed extract, 94, 1357
green tea, 94, 1357
GROWTH HORMONES, 645
guaifenesin, 648
Guaituss AC Syrup, 1384
guanfacine, 54, 1326
Guiatuss, 648
Gynecort, 381
Gyne-Lotrimin-3, 190
Gynezole-1, 190

H

Haemophilus b conjugate vaccine, 1430
hagedorn, 1358
halcinonide, 380, 83
Halcion, 1253, C6
Haldol, 651
Haldol Decanoate, 651
Haldol LA, 651
Halenol, 112
Halfprin, 1131
halobetasol, 380, 83
Halofed, 1077
Halog, 380
haloperidol, 651, 64, 1441, C1, C2
Haltran, 688
Hardhay, 1364
Havrix, 1431, 1433
hawthorne, 94
hawthorne (Crataegus Species), 1358
HCl, 17
HCT, 17
HCTZ, 17
Headache Tablets, 1131
Healthprin, 1131
Hectorol, 1287
Helidac, 1384
Hemocyte, 736
Hemril-HC, 381
HepA, 1431, 1433
Hepalean, 654
heparin, 654, 16, 40, C2–C3, C8
Heparin Leo, 654
HEPARINS (LOW MOLECULAR WEIGHT), 657, 16, 40
Hepatitis A vaccine, 1431, 1433
Hepatitis B vaccine, 1430, 1433
HepB, 1430, 1433

Hep-Lock, 654
Hep-Lock U/P, 654
Herceptin, 1249
Hespan, C8
Hexit, 788
Hib, 1430
Hiberix, 1430
Hi-Cor, 381
HISTAMINE H₂ ANTAGONISTS, 660, 72
Histantil, 1061
HMG-CoA REDUCTASE INHIBITORS (statins), 666, 91
Hold, 430
Holy thistle, 1361
homatropine, 1401
hong shen, 1354
HORMONE, 46
HORMONES, 31, 59, 86–87
HPV, 1432–1433
5-HT₁ AGONISTS, 106
5-HT₃ ANTAGONISTS, 48
Humalog, 721, C8
Humalog Mix 75/25, 712, 1384
Humalog Mix 50/50, 712, 1384
human papillomavirus vaccine, 670, 1375, 1376, 1432, 1433, 105
Humatrope, 645
Humira, 121
Humulin 70/30, 712, C8
Humulin N, 717
Humulin R, 714
Humulin R U-500 (concentrated), 714
Hycamtin, 1242
Hycodan, 675
Hycomine Compound, 1384
Hycort, 381
Hycotuss Expectorant, 1384
HYDANTOINS, 42
Hydergine, C6
Hyderm, 381
hydrALAZINE, 671, 54, C11, C13
hydralazine, C2, C4, C8, C11
hydralazine/isosorbide dinitrate, 673
Hydrea, 1326
hydrochloric acid, 17
hydrochlorothiazide, 458, 17, 54, 85
Hydrocil, 1079
hydrocodone, 675, 16, 99, C8
hydrocodone/ acetaminophen, 675
hydrocodone/ibuprofen, 675

COMPREHENSIVE INDEX 1459

hydrocortisone, 372, 381, 17, 37, 68, 83, C3
hydrocortisone sodium, C4
Hydromet Syrup, 1384
hydromorphone, 677, 1375, 16, 99, 1418, C1, C2–C3, C8
Hydromorphone, 1420, C3
Hydrostat IR, 677
Hydro-Tex, 381
hydroxocobalamin, 1284, 31, 108
hydroxychloroquine, 680, 68
hydroxyurea, 16, 59, 1326
hydrOXYzine, 682, 34, 52, 101, C11, C13
hydroxyzine, C1, C6, C8, C11
hyoscyamine, 684, 38, C6
HyperRHO S/D Full Dose, 1105
HyperRHO S/D Mini-Dose, 1105
hypoglycemic agents, oral, 16
HypoTears, 1399
HypoTears PF, 1399
Hyrexin-50, 450
Hytinic, 736
Hytone, 381
Hytrin, 1194
Hytuss, 648
Hytuss-2X, 648
Hyzaar 50/12.5, 1384
Hyzaar 100/12.5, 1384
Hyzaar 100/25, 1384
Hyzine-50, 682

I

ibandronate, 687, 77
Ibudone, 675
Ibudone 5/200, 1385
Ibudone 10/200, 1385
ibuprofen, 69. See also hydrocodone/ibuprofen
ibuprofen (injection), 688
ibuprofen, oral, 688, 65, 95, 97
ibutilide, 691, 35
Icar, 736
Idamycin, 692
idarubicin, 692, 16, 59, C8
Ifex, 694
ifosfamide, 694, 16, 59
IL-2, 1317
iloperidone, 696, 64
iloprost, 1327
Ilozyme, 985

imatinib, 698, 16, 59, 1442
IMDUR, 742
imipenem/cilastatin, 700, 55, C3, C5
imipramine, 703, 44, 1441
imiquimod, 705, 73
Imitrex, 1177
Imitrex STATdose, 1177
IMMUNE GLOBULINS, 105
IMMUNOSUPPRESSANTS, 87
Imodium, 794
Imodium A-D, 794
Imodium Multi-Symptom Relief, 1385
Implanon, 359
♣ Impril, 703
Imuran, 212
inamrinone, C5
Inapsine, 487
INCRETRIN MIMETIC AGENT, 46
♣ Indameth, 708
indapamide, 706, 54, 85
Inderal, 1071, 17
Inderal LA, 1071
Inderide 40/25, 1385
☯ Indian Valerian, 1365
indinavir, 67, 1327, 1442
♣ Indocid, 708
Indocin, 708
Indocin I.V, 708
♣ Indocin PDA, 708
Indocin SR, 708
indomethacin, 708, 69, 97, C5
Infanrix, 1429
Infant's Pain Reliever, 112
InFeD, 736
Infergen, 23
infliximab, 710, 68
Influenza vaccine, 1431, 1433
Infumorph, 880
☯ ingwer, 1351
☯ ingwerwurzel, 1351
INH, 741
Innohep, 657
InnoPran XL, 1071
♣ Insomnal, 450
Inspra, 511
Insta-Char, 1317
Insta-Char Aqueous Suspension, 1317
insulin, 17
insulin aspart protamine suspension/insulin aspart injection mixtures, rDNA origin, 712
insulin aspart protamine suspension/insulin aspart

solution mixtures, rDNA origin, 46, 87
insulin aspart, rDNA origin, 721, 46, 87
insulin detemir, 719, 46, 87
insulin glargine, 719, 46, 87
insulin glulisine, 721, 46, 87
insulin lispro/protamine insulin lispro mixture, rDNA origin, 46
insulin lispro protamine suspension/insulin lispro injection mixtures, rDNA origin, 712
insulin lispro protamine suspension/insulin lispro solution mixtures, rDNA origin, 46, 87
insulin lispro, rDNA origin, 721, 46, 87
INSULIN (mixtures), 712, 16
insulin, regular (injection, concentrated), 714, 46, 87, 17, C2–C3
INSULINS, 46, 87
  intermediate-acting, 717, 16
  long-acting, 719, 16
  rapid acting, 721, 16
  short acting, 714, 16
♣ Insulin-Toronto, 714
inteferon beta-1a, 728
Integrilin, 515
Intelence, 548
interferon alfa-2a, 23
interferon alfacon-1, 23
interferon alpha-2b, 724
interferon alpha-n3, 724
interferon beta-1b, 728, 23
INTERFERONS, ALPHA, 724
INTERFERONS, BETA, 728
interleukin-2, 1317
INTERLEUKIN ANTAGONISTS, 67
☯ intoxicating pepper, 1360
Intron A, 724, 23
Intropin, 471
Intuniv, 1326
Invanz, 522
Invega, 979
Invega Sustenna, 979
Invirase, 1333
IODINE, IODIDE, 730
Ionamin, 1017
Iopidine, 1403
I-Phrine, 1403
IPOL, 1429

---

*Entries for **generic** names appear in **boldface type.** Trade names appear in regular type, with Canadian trade names preceded by a maple leaf icon (♣). **CLASSIFICATIONS** appear in **BOLDFACE SMALL CAPS.** *Combination Drugs* appear in *italics,* herbal products are preceded by a yin-yang icon (☯) and drugs with genetic implications are preceded by a double-helix icon (⚕).

1460 COMPREHENSIVE INDEX

ipratropium, 732, 37–38, 78
Iprivask, 415
IPV, 1429
Iquix, 1398
■ **irbesartan, 182, 53**
Iressa, 628
irinotecan, 734, 16, 59, 1442
iron dextran, 736, 31
iron polysaccharide, 736, 31
iron sucrose, 736, 31
IRON SUPPLEMENTS, **736, 31**
Isentress, 1097
ISMO, 742
isocarbazid, 876, 44
IsonaRif, 1385
isoniazid, 741, 70
Isoptin SR, 1275
Isopto Alkaline, 1399
Isopto Atropine, 1401
Isopto Carbachol, 1400
Isopto Carpine, 1400
Isopto Frin, 1403
Isopto Homatropine, 1401
Isopto Hyoscine, 1401
Isopto Plain, 1399
Isordil, 742
ISOSORBIDE, 742
isosorbide dinitrate, 742, 32
isosorbide mononitrate, 742, 32
✤ Isotamine, 741
isotretinoin, 744, 22
isradipine, 746, 32, 54, 80
Istalol, 1399
ISTODAX, 1372
itraconazole, 748, 50, 1442
ixabepilone, 750, 16, 60
Ixempra, 750

J

◐ Jamaica ginger, 1351
Jantoven, 1295
Janumet 50/500, 1385
Janumet 50/1000, 1385
Januvia, 1158
◐ Japanese ginseng, 1354
◐ Japanese silver apricot, 1353
Jenamicin, 145
◐ jenjibre, 1351
◐ jiang, kankyo, zenzero, 1351
Jolessa, 359, 1385
Jolivette, 359
Junel 1/20, 1385
Junel 1.5/30, 1385
Junel 21 1/20, 358
Junel 21 1.5/20, 358
Junel Fe 1/20, 358, 1385
Junel Fe 1.5/30, 358, 1385

Junior Strength Advil, 688
Just Tears, 1399
◐ Ju-Zhong, 1363

K

K+ 10, 1041
Kadian, 880
Kalcinate, 265
Kaletra, 795, 23
Kaletra 200/50 capsules, 1385
Kaletra 100/25 capsules, 1385
Kaletra solution, 1385
Kalexate, 1164
✤ Kalium Durules, 1041
kanamycin, 145, 55, C5
◐ kansas snakeroot, 1348
◐ kao, 1360
Kaochlor, 1041
Kaochlor Eff, 1041
Kaochlor S-F, 1041
Kaon, 1041
Kaon-Cl, 1041
Kaopectate, 231
Kaopectate II Caplets, 794
Kao-Tin, 231
Kapectolin, 231
✤ Karacil, 1079
Kariva, 358, 1385
◐ kava-kava, 94
◐ kava-kava (Piper Methysticum), 1360
Kay Ciel, 1041
Kayexalate, 1164
Kaylixir, 1041
K+ Care, 1041
K+Care ET, 1041
KCl, 1041, 17
K-Dur, 1041
Keflex, 291
K-Electrolyte, 1041
Kelnor, 1385
Kelnor 1/35, 358
Kemstro, 219
Kenalog, 372, 381
Kepivance, 978
Keppra, 782
Keppra/Keppra XR, 23
Keppra XR, 782
Ketamine, C5
ketoconazole, 187, 50, 1441–1442
ketoconazole (systemic), 753, 50
ketoprofen, 754, 65, 69, 95, 97
ketorolac, 756, 95, 97, 1402, C1, C3, C5
ketotifen, 52, 1397
◐ kew, 1360
◐ kew tree, 1353
✤ K-Exit, 1164
K-G Elixir, 1041

K-Ide, 1041
Kid Kare, 1077
✤ Kidrolase, 199
Kineret, 174
Kinlytic, 1214
Kionex, 1164
◐ Klamath weed, 1364
✤ Klean-Prep, 1036
K-Lease, 1041
✤ K-Long, 1041
Klonopin, 341, C8
K-Lor, 1041
Klor-Con, 1041
Klor-Con/EF, 1041
Klorvess Liquid, 1041
Klotrix, 1041
K-Lyte, 1041
K-Lyte/Cl, 1041
K-Lyte/Cl Powder, 1041
K-Lyte DS, 1041
K-Med, 1041
K-Norm, 1041
✤ Koffex, 430
Kolyum, 1041
Konsyl, 1079
Konsyl Fiber, 1331
◐ Korean ginseng, 1354
K-Phos M.F, 1039
K-Phos Neutral, 1039
K-Phos No. 2, 1039
K-Phos Original, 1332
Kristalose, 761
K-Sol, 1041
K-Tab, 1041
Kuric, 187
K-Vescent, 1041
Kytril, 642

L

labetalol, 759, 16, 32, 54, 75, C3, C5
lacosamide, 1371, 23, 42
Lacril, 1399
Lacri-Lube NP, 1399
Lacri-Lube S.O.P., 1399
Lacrisert, 1399
LactiCare-HC, 381
Lactinex, 1385
lactulose, 761, 90
◐ Lady's thistle, 1361
Lamictal, 764, 23
Lamisil, 1196
Lamisil AT, 187
lamivudine, 762, 23, 67, 73, C8
lamotrigine, 764, 23, 42, C8
Lanacort 9-1-1, 381
Lanoxicaps, 439
Lanoxin, 439, C6
lansoprazole, 767, 72, 1441–1442, C5
lanthanum carbonate, 769

COMPREHENSIVE INDEX 1461

Lantus, 719
✤ Lanvis, 1335
lapatinib, 770, 16, 59
✤ Largactil, 318
Lariam, 23
Lasix, 620
✤ Lasix Special, 620
latanoprost, 1403
Latisse, 229
LAXATIVES, 89
✤ Laxit, 230
Leena, 359
leflunomide, 771, 68
Lemoderm, 381
lenalidomide, 23
☯leopard's bane, 1343
lepirudin (rDNA), 773, 16, 40
Lescol, 666
Lescol XL, 666
Lessina, 1385
Lessina-28, 358
Letairis, 23
letrozole, 775, 59
leucovorin calcium, 776, C8
Leukeran, 1322, C8
Leukine, 1136
LEUKOTRIENE ANTAGONISTS, 37, 78
leuprolide, 778, 59, 87
Leustatin, 332
levalbuterol, 780, 37, 78
Levaquin, 589, 23
✤ Levate, 154
Levbid, 684
Levemir, 719
levetiracetam, 782, 23, 42
Levitra, 1268
Levlen, 1385
Levlen-28, 358
Levlite, 1385
levobunolol, 75, 1399
levocarnitine, C5
Levodromoran, 1418
levofloxacin, 589, 23, 56, 1398, C3
levonorgestrel, 359, 1375, 87
levonorgestrel/ethinyl estradiol, 87
Levophed, 934
Levora, 1385
Levora-28, 358
levorphanol, 99, 1418
Levo-T, 1219
Levothroid, 1219
levothyroxine, 1219, 87, C3, C5
Levoxyl, 1219

Levsin, 684, C6
Levsinex, 684
Lexapro, 526
Lexiva, 612
L-hyoscyamine, 684
Lialda, 825
Librax, 1385, C6
Libritabs, 314
Librium, 314, C6
Lida-Mantle-HC Topical Cream, 1385
✤ Lidemol, 380
Lidex, 380
Lidex-E, 380
lidocaine, 16, 35, 1441–1442, C2–C3
lidocaine (local anesthetic), 784
lidocaine (mucosal), 784
lidocaine (parenteral), 784
lidocaine patch, 784
lidocaine/prilocaine, 787
lidocaine (topical), 784
Lidoderm, 784
LidoPen, 784
☯Ligustilides, 1347
Limbitrol 5/12.5, 1385, C6
Limbitrol DS 10/25, 1385
lindane, 788
linezolid, 790, 56, C3, C5
Lioresal, 219
liothyronine, 1219, 87
liotrix, 1219, 87
Lipidil Micro, 559
✤ *Lipidil Supra, 559*
LIPID-LOWERING AGENTS, 90
Lipitor, 666
Lipofen, 559
LIPOGLYCOPEPTIDES, 54
Lipsovir, 1375
Liqui-Cal, 265
Liqui-Char, 1317
Liquid Cal-600, 265
Liqui-E, 1291
Liquifilm Forte, 1399
Liquifilm Tears, 1399
Liquiprin, 112
liraglutide, 1371, 46
⛨ **lisinopril, 176, 53**
lithium, 792
✤ Lithizine, 792
Lithobid, 792
Little Colds Cough Formula Drops, 430
Livalo, 666
L-M-X 4, 784
L-M-X 5, 784
LoCHOLEST, 322
LoCHOLEST Light, 322

Locoid, 381
Lodine, 544
Lodine XL, 544
lodoxamide, 1402
Loestrin 1/20, 1385
Loestrin 1.5/30, 1385
Loestrin 21 1/20, 358
Loestrin 21 1.5/30, 358
Loestrin Fe 1/20, 358, 1385
Loestrin Fe 1.5/30, 358, 1385
Lofibra, 559
Logen, 453
Lomanate, 453
Lomotil, 453, 1385
Lomotil Liquid, 1385
LONG-ACTING BETA-AGONISTS (LABAs), 1376
Lonox, 453, 1385
LOOP DIURETICS, 54, 85
Lo/Ovral, 1385
Lo/Ovral 28, 358
loperamide, 794, 47
Lopid, 632
lopinavir, 23
lopinavir/ritonavir, 795, 67
✤ Lopresor, 851
✤ Lopresor SR, 851
Lopressor, 851
Lopressor HCT 50/25, 1385
Lopressor HCT 100/25, 1385
Lopressor HCT 100/50, 1385
Loprox, 187
Lopurin, 134
loratadine, 798, 52
lorazepam, 799, 34, 101, C2–C3, C5, C8
Lorcet 10/650, 1385
Lorcet-HD, 675, 1385
Lorcet Plus, 1385
Lortab, 675
Lortab 5/500, 1385
Lortab 7.5/500, 1385
Lortab 10/500, 1385
Lortab Elixir, 1385
losartan, 182, 53, 1441–1442
LoSeasonique, 359, 1385
✤ Losec, 950
✤ *Losec 1-2-3 A, 1385*
✤ *Losec 1-2-3 M, 1386*
Lotemax, 1400
Lotensin, 176
Lotensin HCT 5/6.25, 1386
Lotensin HCT 10/12.5, 1386
Lotensin HCT 20/12.5, 1386
Lotensin HCT 20/25, 1386
loteprednol, 83, 1400
Lotrel 2.5/10, 1386
Lotrel 5/10, 1386

---

*Entries for **generic** names appear in **boldface type**. Trade names appear in regular type, with Canadian trade names preceded by a maple leaf icon (✤). **CLASSIFICATIONS** appear in **BOLDFACE SMALL CAPS**. *Combination Drugs* appear in *italics*, herbal products are preceded by a yin-yang icon (☯) and drugs with genetic implications are preceded by a double-helix icon (⛨).

1462 COMPREHENSIVE INDEX

Lotrel 5/20, 1386
Lotrel 5/40, 1386
Lotrel 10/20, 1386
Lotrel 10/40, 1386
✺Lotriderm, 187
Lotrimin AF, 187
Lotrimin Ultra, 187
Lotrisone Topical Cream/Lotion, 1386
Lotronex, 23
lovastatin, 666, 91, 1442
Lovaza, 949
Lovenox, 657
Low-Ogestrel, 1386
Low-Ogestrel 28, 358
✺Lozide, 706
L-PAM, 817
l-triiodothyronine, 1219
LubriTears, 1399
Lucentis, 1332
Lufyllin-GG Elixir, 1386
Lufyllin-GG Tablets, 1386
Lugol's solution, 730
Lumigan, 1403
Luminal, 1015
Lunesta, 538
Lupron, 778
Lupron Depot, 778
Lupron Depot-3 Month, 778
Lupron Depot-4 Month, 778
Lupron Depot-Ped, 778
Lusedra, 1370
Lutera, 358, 1386
Lutrepulse Kit, 1377
Luvox, 604
Luvox CR, 604
Luxiq, 380
Lybrel, 359, 1386
✺Lyderm, 380
Lyrica, 1051, 1375, 23
Lysteda, 1375

M

Maalox, 803
Maalox Advanced Maximum Strength Chewables, 1386
Maalox Advanced Maximum Strength Liquid, 1386
Maalox Advanced Regular Strength Liquid, 1386
Maalox Antacid Caplets, 265
Maalox Antidiarrheal Caplets, 794
✺Maalox GRF Gas Relief Formula, 1155
Maalox Total Relief, 1375
Macrobid, 928, C6
Macrodantin, 928
MACROLIDES, 56
Macugen, 1329
magaldrate, 803, 72
Magan, 1131

Magnacet, 966
Magnacet 2.5/400, 1386
Magnacet 5/400, 1386
Magnacet 7.5/400, 1386
Magnacet 10/400, 1386
MAGNESIUM AND ALUMINUM SALTS, 803
magnesium chloride, 90
magnesium chloride (12% Mg; 9.8 mEq Mg/g), 804, 92
magnesium citrate, 90
magnesium citrate (16.2% Mg; 4.4 mEq Mg/g), 804, 92
magnesium gluconate, 90
magnesium gluconate (5.4 % Mg; 4.4 mEq/g), 804, 92
magnesium hydroxide, 90
magnesium hydroxide/aluminum hydroxide, 803, 72
magnesium hydroxide (41.7% Mg; 34.3 mEq Mg/g), 804, 92
magnesium oxide, 90
magnesium oxide (60.3% Mg; 49.6 mEq Mg/g), 804, 93
magnesium salicylate, 1131, 65, 95
MAGNESIUM SALTS, 92
MAGNESIUM SALTS (ORAL), 804
magnesium sulfate, 17
magnesium sulfate (IV, parenteral), 806, 16, 93, C2–C3, C5
Magonate, 804
Mag-Ox 400, 804
Magtrate, 804
🌿maidenhair-tree, 1353
Malarone, 1386
Malarone Pediatric, 1386
Mallamint, 265
mannitol, 808, 85, C3
Mapap, 112
Mapap Multi-Symptom Cold, 1386
Maranox, 112
maraviroc, 810, 67
Marcaine, 502
Marcillin, 169
Margesic, 255
Marplan, 876
Marten-Tab, 255
Marthritic, 1131
Marvelon, 1386
🌿Mary Thistle, 1361
Matulane, 1054
Mavik, 176
Maxalt, 1125

Maxalt-MLT, 1125
✺Maxeran, 847
Maxidex, 1400
Maximum Relief Ex-Lax, 1145
Maximum Strength Mylanta Gas, 1155
Maximum Strength Nytol, 450
Maximum Strength Sleepinal, 450
Maxipime, 287
Maxitrol Ophthalmic Suspension/Ointment, 1386
Maxzide, 1386
Maxzide-25, 1386
🌿maybush, 1358
MCV4, 1430, 1434
Measles, mumps, and rubella vaccines, 1429, 1434
mebendazole, 1327
mechlorethamine, 16, 59, 1328
meclizine, 811, 49, 52
Meda, 112
Medi-First Sinus Decongestant, 1077
Medigesic, 255
Medipren, 688
Mediquell, 430
Medrol, 372, C14
medroxyPROGESTERone, 812, 59, 87, C11, C14
medroxyprogesterone, 359, 87, C11
✺Med Tamoxifen, 1187
mefloquine, 23
Mefoxin, 294
Mega-C/A Plus, 1319
Megace, 814
megestrol, 814, 59, 87
MEGLITINIDES, 46
meloxicam, 815, 95, 97
melphalan, 817, 16, 59
memantine, 819, 30
Menactra, 1430, 1434
Menadol, 688
Meningococcal conjugate vaccine, 1430, 1434
meningococcal vaccine, quadravalent, 1375
Menostar, 532
Mentax, 187
Menveo, 1375
meperidine, 820, 16, 99, 1419, C1, C2–C3, C5, C6
Mephyton, 1026
meprobamate, C6
Mepron, 207
mercaptopurine, 59, 1328
Meridia, 1150, 1376
meropenem, 823, 55, C5
Merrem, 823

COMPREHENSIVE INDEX 1463

mesalamine, 825
✤ M-Eslon, 880
mesna, 826
Mesnex, 826
Mestinon, 1081
✤ Mestinon SR, 1081
Mestinon Timespan, 1081
mestranol/norethindrone, 358, 87
Metadate CD, 844
Metadate ER, 844
✤ Metaderm, 380
Metaglip 2.5/250, 1386
Metaglip 2.5/500, 1386
Metaglip 5/500, 1386
Metamucil, 1079
metaproterenol, C6
metaxalone, 828, 102
metformin, 829, 22, 46, C8
methadone, 831, 16, 99, 1418, 1441–1442
Methadose, 831
Methergine, 842
methimazole, 834
methocarbamol, 835, 102, C6
methotrexate, 836, 16–17, 59, 68, 89
methyldopa, 840, 54, C6
methyldopa-hydrochlorothiazide, C6
methylergonovine, 842
Methylin, 844
Methylin ER, 844
methylnaltrexone, 843, 90
methylphenidate, 844, 81
methylPREDNISolone, 372, 37, 68, 83, C3, C5, C11, C14
methylTESTOSTERone, C6, C11, C14
metipranolol, 75, 1399
metoclopramide, 847, 23, 49, C1, C3, C5
metolazone, 850, 54, 85
✤ Metoprol, 851
metoprolol, 851, 16, 32, 54, 75, 1441, C3
Metozolv ODT, 847
Metozolv ODT/Reglan, 23
MetroCream, 854
MetroGel, 854
MetroGel-Vaginal, 854
Metro IV, 854
MetroLotion, 854
metronidazole, 854, 56, 72, 1442, C3, C5, C8
Mevacor, 666
☯ Mexican Valerian, 1365

mexiletine, 1441
MgSO4, 17
Miacalcin, 263
micafungin, 857, 50, C3, C5
Micardis, 182
Micardis HCT 40/12.5, 1386
Micardis HCT 80/12.5, 1386
Micardis HCT 80/25, 1386
Micatin, 187
miconazole, 187, 190, 50
✤ Micozole, 187
MICRhoGAM, 1105
Microdantin, C6
Microgestin, 358
Microgestin 1/20, 1386
Microgestin 1.5/30, 1386
Microgestin Fe 1/20, 358, 1386
Microgestin Fe 1.5/30, 1386
Micro-K, 1041
Micro-K ExtenCaps, 1041
Micro-LS, 1041
microNefrin, 504
Micronor, 359
Microzide, 458
✤ Midamor, 456
midazolam, 858, 16, 34, 101, 1442, C1, C2–C3, C5
Midol Maximum Strength Cramp Formula, 688
Midol Menstrual Complete, 1386
Midol PM, 450
Midol Teen Formula, 1386
Midrin, 1386
Mifeprex, 862, 23
mifepristone, 862, 23
Migergot Suppositories, 1386
miglitol, 863, 46
Migranal, 518
Miles Nervine, 450
☯ milk thistle, 94, 1361
milnacipran, 864, 23
milrinone, 866, 16, C2–C3, C5
mineral oil, C6
MINERALS/ELECTROLYTES/PH MODIFIERS, 91
Mini-Gamulin R, 1105
✤ Minims, 1401
✤ Minims Homatropine, 1401
✤ Minims Phenylephrine, 1403
✤ Minims Tetracaine, 1397
✤ Minims Tropicamide, 1401
Minipress, 1049
Minitran, 929
Minocin, 1203
minocycline, 1203, 56

minoxidil, 1329, 54
✤ Miocarpine, 1400
Miochol-E, 1400
Miostat, 1400
MiraLax, 1036
Mirapex, 1044
Mirapex ER, 1375
Mircette, 358, 1386
Mirena, 359
mirtazapine, 867, 44, 1441–1442
misoprostol, 869, 72
mitomycin, 870, 16, 59
mitoxantrone, 872, 16–17, 59
✤ Mitran, 314
Mitrolan, 1331
M-M-R II, 1429, 1434
Moban, 1377
Mobic, 815
Mobidin, 1131
modafinil, 874, 81
Modane, 230
Modane Bulk, 1079
Modane Soft, 466
✤ Modecate Concentrate, 600
Modicon, 358, 1386
✤ Moduret, 1387
☒ **moexipril, 176**, 53
Moisture Drops, 1399
molindone, 1377
MOM, 804
mometasone, 366, 369, 381, 37, 83
Monistat-1, 190
Monistat-3, 190
Monistat-7, 190
Monistat-1Day, 190
MONOAMINE OXIDASE (MAO) INHIBITORS, 876, 44
MONOAMINE OXIDASE TYPE B INHIBITORS, 61
monobasic potassium phosphate, 93, 1332
MONOCLONAL ANTIBODIES, 37, 59
Monocor, 233
Monodox, 1203
Mono-Gesic, 1131
Monoket, 742
Mononessa, 1387
MonoNessa, 358
Monopril, 176
montelukast, 879, 37, 78, 1441–1442
morphine, 880, 16, 99, 1418, 1420, C1, C2–C3, C5, C8
✤ Morphine H.P., 880

---

*Entries for **generic** names appear in **boldface type**. Trade names appear in regular type, with Canadian trade names preceded by a maple leaf icon (✤). **CLASSIFICATIONS** appear in **BOLDFACE SMALL CAPS**. *Combination Drugs* appear in *italics*, herbal products are preceded by a yin-yang icon (☯) and drugs with genetic implications are preceded by a double-helix icon (☒).

COMPREHENSIVE INDEX

morphine non-concentrated oral liquid, C8
morphine oral liquid concentrate, C8
morphine sulfate, 17, 23
✹ Morphitec, 880
✹ M.O.S, 880
✹ M.O.S.-S.R, 880
Motofen, 453, 1387
Motrin, 688
Motrin Children's Cold Suspension, 1387
Motrin Drops, 688
Motrin IB, 688
Motrin Junior Strength, 688
Motrin Migraine Pain, 688
🍁 mountain snuff, 1343
🍁 mountain tobacco, 1343
MoviPrep, 1036
Moxatag, 158
moxifloxacin, 589, 22, 56, 1398, C3
M-Oxy, 966
MS, 17
MS Contin, 880, 1418, C8
✹ MS-IR, 880
MSIR, 880
MSO4, 17
MTX, 17
Mucinex, 648
Mucinex Cold Liquid, 1387
Mucinex Cough Liquid, 1387
Mucinex Cough Mini-Melts, 1387
Mucinex D, 1387
Mucinex DM, 1387
Mucinex D Maximum Strength, 1387
Mucinex DM Maximum Strength, 1387
✹ Mucomyst, 116
Multaq, 485, 23
✹ Multipax, 682
mupirocin, 885, 56
Murine Plus, 1403
Murine Solution, 1399
Murocel, 1399
Murocoll-2 Ophthalmic Solution, 1387
muromonab-CD3, 886, 89
Mustargen, 1328
Mutamycin, 870
Myambutol, 541
Mycamine, 857
Mycelex, 187
Mycelex-3, 190
Mycelex-7, 190
Mycobutin, 1110
mycophenolate mofetil, 887, 89
mycophenolic acid, 887, 89
Mycostatin, 187, 190, 938
Mydfrin, 1403

Mydral, 1401
Mydriacyl, 1401
Myfortic, 887
✹ Mylanta, 803
Mylanta Gas, 1155
✹ Mylanta Lozenges, 265
Mylanta Maximum Strength Liquid, 1387
Mylanta Natural Fiber Supplement, 1079
Mylanta Regular Strength Liquid, 1387
Mylanta Supreme Liquid, 1387
Mylanta Ultimate Strength Chewables, 1387
Mylanta Ultimate Strength Liquid, 1387
Myleran, 252
Mylicon, 1155
Mylocel, 1326
Mylotarg, 633
Myobloc, 23

N

nabumetone, 891, 69, 97
nadolol, 892, 32, 54, 75
✹ Nadostine, 187, 938
nafarelin, 894, 87
Nafazair, 1402
nafcillin, 1005, 56, C3, C5
naftifine, 187, 50
Naftin, 187
nalbuphine, 895, 16, 99, 1419, C1, C3
naloxone, 898, C5
naltrexone, 23
Namenda, 819
naphazoline, 1402
Naphcon, 1402
Naphcon-A Ophthalmic Solution, 1387
Naprelan, 900
Naprosyn, 900, C6
✹ Naprosyn-E, 900
✹ Naprosyn-SR, 900
naproxen, 900, 65, 95, 97, C6
naproxen sodium, 23
naratriptan, 902, 106
Nardil, 876
Naropin, 502
Nasacort AQ, 369
Nasahist B, 1322
NASAL, 52
Nasarel, 369
Nasatab LA, 1387
Nascobal, 1284
Nasonex, 369
Natacyn, 1398
natalizumab, 1376, 23
natamycin, 50, 1398

nateglinide, 903, 16, 46, 1441–1442
Natrecor, 910
✹ Natulan, 1054
Naturacil Caramels, 1079
NATURAL/HERBAL PRODUCTS, 93
✹ Natural Source Fibre Laxative, 1079
Nature's Tears, 1399
Navelbine, 1282
✹ Naxen, 900
Nebcin, 145
nebivolol, 905, 54, 75
NebuPent, 1007
Necon 1/35, 358, 1387
Necon 7/7/7, 359
Necon 0.5/35, 358, 1387
Necon 1/50, 358
Necon 10/11, 359
nedocromil, 1402
nefazodone, 906, 44, 1441–1442
nelfinavir, 67, 1329, 1441–1442
Nembutal, 1330
Neo-Diaral, 794
🍁 Neo-DM, 430
Neo-Fer, 736
Neo-Fradin, 145
🍁 Neo-K, 1041
neomycin, 145, 55
Neopap, 112
Neoral, 387
Neosporin Antibiotic Topical Ointment, 1387
Neosporin G.U. Irrigant, 1387
Neosporin Ophthalmic Solution, 1387
Neosporin + Pain Relief Antibiotic Topical Cream, 1387
Neosporin + Pain Relief Antibiotic Topical Ointment, 1387
neostigmine, 908
nepafenac, 97, 1402
Nephro-Calci, 265
✹ Nephro-Fer, 736
Nephron, 504
nesiritide, 910, 16
Nestrex, 1083
Neulasta, 998
Neumega, 953
Neupogen, 576
NEUROKININ ANTAGONISTS, 31
Neurontin, 623
Neut, 1159
Neutra-Phos, 1039
Neutra-Phos-K, 1332
Neutrexin, 1377
Nevanac, 1402
nevirapine, 912, 23, 67, 1442

Nexium, 530
Nexterone, 151
Nia-Bid, 914
Niac, 914
Niacels, 914
niaciamide, 108
niacin, 914, 91, 108
niacinamide, 914, 91
Niacor, 914
Niaspan, 914
niCARdipine, 915, 32, 54, 80, C11, C14
nicardipine, C11
Nico-400, 914
Nicobid, 914
Nicoderm CQ, 918
Nicolar, 914
Nicorette, 918
nicotinamide, 914
NICOTINE, 918
nicotine chewing gum, 918
nicotine inhaler, 918
nicotine lozenge, 918
nicotine nasal spray, 918
nicotine transdermal, 918
Nicotinex, 914
nicotinic acid, 914
Nicotrol Inhaler, 918
Nicotrol NS, 918
✸ Nidagel, 854
Nifedical XL, 921
NIFEdipine, 921, 32, 54, 80, C11, C14
nifedipine, C6, C11
Niferex, 736
Niferex-150 Forte, 1387
Nighttime Sleep Aid, 450
nilotinib, 923, 16, 59
Nilstat, 938
nimodipine, 925, 80
Niravam, 138, C6
nisoldipine, 926, 54, 80
NITRATES, 32
Nitrek, 929
Nitro-Bid, 929
Nitro-Bid IV, 929
Nitro drip, 17
Nitro-Dur, 929
nitrofurantoin, 928, 56, C6
✸ Nitrogard SR, 929
nitrogen mustard, 1328
nitroglycerin, 929, 17, 32, C2–C3
Nitrolingual, 929
Nitromist, 929
Nitropress, 932
nitroprusside, 932, 16–17, 54, C2–C3
NitroQuick, 929

Nitrostat, 929
Nitro-Time, 929
Nix, 1012
nizatidine, 660, 72
Nizoral, 187, 753
Nizoral A-D, 187
✸ Nolvadex-D, 1187
Non-Drowsy Allergy Relief for Kids, 798
NON-NUCLEOSIDE REVERSE TRANSCRIPTASE INHIBITORS, 67
NONOPIOID ANALGESICS, 94
NONSTEROIDAL ANTI-INFLAMMATORY AGENTS, 95–97
No Pain-HP, 271
Norco 5/325, 1387
Norco 7.5/325, 1387
Norco, 675
Norco 10/325, 1387
Nordette, 1387
Nordette-28, 358
Nordiflex, 645
Norditropin, 645
norepinephrine, 934, 16, C2–C3
norethindrone, 359, 87
norethindrone/ethinyl acetate, 359, 87
Norethin 1/35E, 358
Norflex, C6
Norflex, 17
Norflox, 17
norfloxacin, 589, 17, 23, 56
Norfranil, 703
Norgesic, 1387
Norgesic Forte, 1387
norgestimate/ethinyl estradiol, 87
norgestrel, 87. See also ethinyl estradiod/norgestrel
Norinyl 1/35, 1387
Norinyl 1+ 35, 358
Norinyl 1/50, 1387
Norinyl 1+50, 358
Noritate, 854
normal human serum albumin, 125
Noroxin, 589, 23
Norpace, C6
Norpramin, 413, 1376
Nor-Q D, 359
Nortrel 1/35, 358, 1387
Nortrel 7/7/7, 359
Nortrel 0.5/35, 358, 1387
nortriptyline, 936, 44, 1441
Norvasc, 157
Norvir, 1119, 1375–1376
✸ Novamedopa, 840

✸ Novamoxin, 158
Novantrone, 872
✸ Nova Rectal, 1330
✸ Novasen, 1131
✸ Novo-Alprazol, 138
✸ Novo-Ampicillin, 169
✸ Novo-Atenolol, 204
✸ Novo-AZT, 1303
✸ Novobetamet, 380
✸ Novo-Carbamaz, 272
✸ Novo-Chlorhydrate, 312
✸ Novo-Chlorpromazine, 318
✸ Novo-Cimetine, 660
✸ Novo-Clopate, 347
✸ Novo-Diltazem, 445
✸ Novodipam, 431
✸ Novodipiradol, 454
✸ Novo-Divalproex, 1262
✸ Novodoxylin, 1203
✸ Novo-Famotidine, 660
✸ Novoferrogluc, 736
✸ Novoferrosulfa, 736
✸ Novoflupam, 603
✸ Novo-Flurazine, 1337
✸ Novofolacid, 606
✸ Novofumar, 736
✸ Novo-Gesic, 112
✸ Novo-Hydrazide, 458
✸ Novohydrocort, 381
✸ Novohydroxyzin, 682
✸ Novo-Hylazin, 671
✸ Novo-Levofloxacin, 589
✸ Novolin, C8
Novolin 70/30, 712, C8
✸ Novolin ge NPH, 717
Novolin N, 717
Novolin R, 714
Novolog, 721, C8
NovoLog Mix 70/30, 712, C8
NovoLog Mix 50/50, 712
✸ Novo-Lorazem, 799
✸ Novo-Medrone, 812
✸ Novo-Metformin, 829
✸ Novo-Methacin, 708
✸ Novo-metoprol, 851
✸ Novo-Minocycline, 1203
✸ Novo-Naprox, 900
✸ Novo-Naprox Sodium DS, 900
✸ Novo-Niacin, 914
✸ Novonidazol, 854
✸ Novo-Nifedin, 921
✸ Novo-Nizatidine, 660
✸ Novo-Norfloxacin, 589
✸ Novopentobarb, 1330
✸ Novo-Pen-VK, 1002
✸ Novo-Peridol, 651
✸ Novo-Pheniram, 316
✸ Novo-Pirocam, 1034
✸ Novopoxide, 314

---

*Entries for **generic** names appear in **boldface type**. Trade names appear in regular type, with Canadian trade names preceded by a maple leaf icon (✸). **CLASSIFICATIONS** appear in **BOLDFACE SMALL CAPS**. *Combination Drugs* appear in *italics*, herbal products are preceded by a yin-yang icon (☯) and drugs with genetic implications are preceded by a double-helix icon (⚕).

1466 COMPREHENSIVE INDEX

Novopramine, 703
Novopranol, 1071
Novo-Profen, 688
Novo-Ranitidine, 660
Novo-rythro, 523
Novo-Salmol, 126
Novo-Selegiline, 1141
Novosemide, 620
Novosorbide, 742
Novospiroton, 456
Novo-Sundac, 1175
Novo-Tamoxifen, 1187
Novo-Theophyl SR, 240
Novo-Timol, 1229
Novo-Tolmetin, 1337
Novo-Trimel, 1254
Novo-Trimel DS, 1254
Novo-Triolam, 1253
Novo-Veramil, 1275
Novoxapam, 961
Noxafil, 1037
NPH insulin (isophane insulin suspension), 717, 46, 87
NPH/regular insulin mixtures, 712, 46, 87
Nplate, 23
NSAIDs, 69. *See also* **NONSTEROIDAL ANTI-INFLAMMATORY AGENTS**
Nu-Alpraz, 138
Nu-Amoxi, 158
Nu-Ampi, 169
Nubain, 895, 1419
Nu-Cal, 265
Nu-Cephalex, 291
Nu-Cimet, 660
NUCLEOSIDE REVERSE TRANSCRIPTASE INHIBITORS, 67
Nu-Cotrimox, 1254
Nu-Cotrimox DS, 1254
Nucynta, 1190, 23
Nu-Diltiaz, 445
Nu-Divalproex, 1262
Nu-Doxycycline, 1203
Nu-Famotidine, 660
Nu-Furosemide, 620
Nu-Hydro, 458
Nu-Ibuprofen, 688
Nu-Indo, 708
Nu-Iron, 736
NuLev, 684
Nu-Loraz, 799
NuLytely, 1036, 1388
Nu-Medopa, 840
Nu-Naprox, 900
Nu-Nifed, 921
Nu-Pen-VK, 1002
Nu-Pirox, 1034
Nuprin, 688
Nu-Ranitidine, 660
Nu-Selegiline, 1141
Nu-Tears, 1399

Nu-Tears II, 1399
Nutracort, 381
Nutra Tear, 1399
Nu-Triazo, 1253
Nutropin, 645
Nutropin AQ, 645
Nuvaring, 1388
NuvaRing, 359
Nu-Verap, 1275
Nyaderm, 187
Nyquil Children's Liquid, 1388
Nyquil Cold & Flu Relief Liquicaps, 1388
Nyquil Cold & Flu Relief Liquid, 1388
Nyquil Cold & Flu Symptom Relief Plus Vitamin C Caplets, 1388
Nyquil Cough Liquid, 1388
Nyquil D Liquid, 1388
Nyquil Less Drowsy Cold & Flu Relief Liquid, 1388
Nyquil Sinus Liquicaps, 1388
nystatin, 187, 190, 938, 50
Nystop, 187
Nytol, 450

O

Obi-Nix, 1017
OBY-CAP, 1017
Ocella, 358, 1388
octreotide, 941, 47, 87
OcuClear, 1402
Ocufen, 1402
Ocuflox, 1398
Ocu-Phrin, 1403
Ocusert Pilo, 1400
Ocu-Sulf 10, 1398
Ocu-Zoline, 1402
ofatumumab, 1372, 59
ofloxacin, 589, 56, 1398
Oforta, 583
Ogestrel, 1388
Ogestrel 28, 358
olanzapine, 943, 1375–1376, 23, 64, 1441
Oleptro, 1375
Oligomeric Proanthocyanidins (OPCs), 1357
olmesartan, 182, 1376, 54
olopatadine, 946, 1397, 52
olsalazine, 946
Olux, 380
Olux-E, 380
omalizumab, 948, 23, 37
omega-3-acid ethyl esters, 949, 91
omeprazole, 950, 72, 1441
omeprazole/sodium bicarbonate, 1375
Omnaris, 369
Omnicef, 300

Omnipen, 169
Omnipred, 1401
Omnitrope, 645
onabotulinum toxin A, 22
Oncaspar, 996
ondansetron, 951, 48, 1442, C1, C3, C5
Onglyza, 1138
Onsolis, 564, 23
Onxol, 975
Opana, 969, 1418
Opana ER, 969
Opcon-A Ophthalmic Solution, 1388
Ophthaine, 1397
Ophthalgan, 1403
OPHTHALMIC NSAIDS, 97
OPHTHALMICS, 50, 52, 75
Ophthetic, 1397
OPIOID AGONISTS, 99
OPIOID AGONISTS/ANTAGONISTS, 99
OPIOID ANALGESICS, 97, C7
OPIOID ANTAGONISTS, 90
oprelvekin, 953
Optase Topical Gel, 1388
Opticrom, 1401
Optigene 3, 1403
OptiPranolol, 1399
Optivar, 1397
Orabase-HCA, 381
Oracea, 1203
Oracit, 1163
OramorphSR, 1418
Oramorph SR, 880
Oraphen-PD, 112
Orapred, 372, C14
Orapred ODT, 372
Oraqix Periodontal Gel, 1388
Oraverse, 1018
Orazinc, 1306
Oretic, 458
Organidin NR, 648
orlistat, 954, 108
Ornex, 1388
Ornex·DM, 430
Ornex Maximum Strength, 1388
orphenadrine, C6
orphenadrine, 17
Ortho-Cept, 358, 1388
Orthoclone OKT3, 886
Ortho/CS, 1319
Ortho-Cyclen, 358, 1388
Ortho-Evra, 1388
Ortho Evra, 359
Ortho-Novum 1/35, 358, 1388
Ortho-Novum 7/7/7, 359
Ortho-Novum 1/50, 1388
Ortho-Novum 10/11, 359
Ortho-Prefest, 1388
Ortho Tri-Cyclen, 359
Ortho Tri-Cyclen Lo, 359
Orudis-E, 754

COMPREHENSIVE INDEX 1467

🍁 Orudis-SR, 754
Os-Cal, 265
oseltamivir, 956, 73
Osmitrol, 808
OsmoPrep, 1025
Osmoprep/Visicol, 23
OSMOTIC DIURETICS, 85
OSMOTICS, 90
🍁 Ostoforte, 1287
Ovcon-35, 1388
Ovcon 35, 358
Ovcon-50, 1388
Ovcon 50, 358
🍁 Ovol, 1155
🍁 Ovol-40, 1155
oxacillin, 1005, 56, C5
oxaliplatin, 957, 16, 59–60
oxaprozin, 959, 69, 97, C6
oxazepam, 961, 34, 101, C6
oxcarbazepine, 962, 42
oxiconazole, 187, 50
Oxistat, 187
OXYBUTYNIN, 964, 38, C6
Oxycet, 966
🍁 Oxycodan, 966
oxycodone, 966, 99, 1418, 1441, C8
oxycodone (immediate-release), C8
oxycodone/acetaminophen, 966
oxycodone/aspirin, 966
oxycodone compound, 16
oxycodone/ibuprofen, 966
Oxycontin, 966, C8
Oxycontin (controlled-release), C8
OxyFAST, 966
OxyIR, 966
oxymetazoline, 1402
oxymorphone, 969, 16, 99, 1418
oxytocin, 972, 16–17, 87, C2–C3
Oxytrol, 964, C6
Oysco, 265
Oyst-Cal, 265
Oystercal, 265
Ozurdex, 1375

P

Pacerone, 151, C6
☯ Pacific Valerian, 1365
paclitaxel, 975, 16, 59, 1442
paclitaxel protein-bound particles (albumin-bound), 975

Pain Doctor, 271
Pain-X, 271
🍁 Palafer, 736
palifermin, 978
paliperidone, 979, 64
☯ Palmier Nain, 1363
palonosetron, 981, 48
Pamelor, 936
pamidronate, 983, 77
Pamprin Cramp, 1388
Pamprin Max, 1388
Pamprin Multi-Symptom, 1388
Panadol, 112
Pancrease MT 4, 985, 1389
Pancrease MT 16, 985, 1389
Pancrease MT 10, 985, 1389
Pancrease MT 20, 985, 1389
Pancrebarb MS-8, 985
pancrelipase, 985, 22
pancuronium, 986, 16, C5
Pandel, 381
panitumumab, 988, 16, 59
Panixine, 291
Panretin, 1318
🍁 Pantoloc, 990
pantoprazole, 990, 72, 1441, C3, C5
Paracaine, 1397
paracetamol, 112
Parafon Forte DSC, 321, C6
Paralube, 1399
Paraplatin, 277
🍁 Paraplatin-AQ, 277
Parcopa, 275
Parcopa 25/250, 1389
Parcopa 25/100, 1389
Parcopa 10/100, 1389
paricalcitol, 1287, 107
🍁 Pariet, 1095
Parlodel, 1321
Parnate, 876
paroxetine, 1441
  hydrochloride, 992, 34, 44
  mesylate, 992, 34, 44
🍁 Parvolex, 116
Pataday, 1397
Patanase, 946
Patanol, 1397
🍁 Paveral, 351
Paxil, 992
Paxil CR, 992
pazopanib, 994, 16, 23, 60
PCA, 17
PCE, 523
PCV, 1431
PediaCare Allergy Formula, 316

Pediacare Children's Allergy & Cold Liquid, 1389
PediaCare Children's Fever, 688
Pediacare Children's Multisymptom Cold Liquid, 1389
PediaCare Infants' Decongestant Drops, 1078
Pediapred, 372
Pediatric Nasal Decongestant, 1078
PediCare Infant's Long Acting Cough Drops, 430
PedvaxHIB, 1430
pegaptanib, 1329
pegaspargase, 996, 16, 59
Pegasys, 724, 23
pegfilgrastim, 998
peginterferon alfa-2a, 23
peginterferon alfa-2b, 23
peginterferon alpha-2a, 724
peginterferon alpha-2b, 724
Pegintron, 724
PegIntron, 23
PEG-L-asparaginase, 996
pemetrexed, 999, 16, 59
pemirolast, 1402
Penbritin, 169
penciclovir, 1001, 73
Penecort, 381
penicillamine, 68, 1330
🍁 Penicilline V, 1002
penicillin G, 1002, 56, C5
penicillin G potassium, C3
PENICILLINS, 1002, 56
PENICILLINS, PENICILLINASE RESISTANT, 1005
penicillin V, 1002, 56
Penlac, 187
Pennsaid, 1375
Pentam 300, 1007
pentamidine, 1007, C5
Pentasa, 825
pentazocine, 1010, 16, 99, 1419, C6
pentobarbital, 42, 101, 1330, C1, C3, C5
Pentolair, 1401
Pepcid, 660
Pepcid AC, 660
Pepcid Complete, 1389
Peptic Relief, 231
Pepto-Bismol, 231
Pepto Diarrhea Control, 794
Percocet 2.5/325, 1389
Percocet 5/325, 1389
Percocet 7.5/325, 1389
Percocet, 966, C8

---

*Entries for **generic** names appear in **boldface type**. Trade names appear in regular type, with Canadian trade names preceded by a maple leaf icon (🍁). **CLASSIFICATIONS** appear in **BOLDFACE SMALL CAPS**. Combination Drugs appear in *italics*, herbal products are preceded by a yin-yang icon (☯) and drugs with genetic implications are preceded by a double-helix icon (🧬).

Percocet 10/325, 1389
Percocet 7.5/500, 1389
Percocet 10/650, 1389
Percodan, 966, 1389
Percogesic, 1389
Percolone, 966
Perdiem, 1079
Perforomist, 610
Periactin, 390
Peri-Colace, 1389
Peridol, 651
perindopril, 176, 53
Periostat, 1203
PERIPHERALLY ACTING ANTIADRENERGICS, 54
Permapen, 1002
permethrin, 1012
Persantine, 454, C6
Persantine IV, 454
Pertofrane, 413
Pertussin Cough Suppressant, 430
Pertussin CS, 430
Pertussin ES, 430
Pexeva, 992
Pfizerpen, 1002
Pharma-Cort, 381
Phazyme, 1155
Phenazo, 1014
phenazopyridine, 1014, 96
phenelzine, 876, 44
Phenetron, 316
phenobarbital, 1015, 42, 101, 1441–1442, C5
PHENOTHIAZINES, 48, 64
Phentercot, 1017
phentermine, 1017, 108
phentolamine, 1018
Phentride, 1017
phenylalanine mustard, 817
phenylephrine, 1403, C3
Phenytek, 1020
phenytoin, 1020, 35, 42, 1441–1442, C3, C5
Pheryl-E, 1291
Philliips Liqui-Gels, 466
Phillips Magnesia Tablets, 804
Phillips Milk of Magnesia, 804
PHL-Divalproex, 1262
PHL-Doxycycline, 1203
PHL-Hydrochlorothiazide, 458
PHL-Nizatidine, 660
PHL-Ranitidine, 660
PHL-Valproic Acid, 1262
PhosLo, 265
phosphate/biphosphate, 1025, 90
Phospholine Iodide, 1400
Phrenilin, 255, 1389
Phrenilin Forte, 255, 1389
Phyllocontin, 240
phytoestrogen, 1345
Phytoestrogen, 1347

phytonadione, 1026, 107, C5
pilocarpine, 1028, 1400
Pilopine HS, 1400
Pima, 730
pimecrolimus, 1029, 89
pimozide, 1441–1442
pioglitazone, 1030, 22–23, 46
piperacillin, C5
piperacillin/tazobactam, 1032, 56, C3, C5
piroxicam, 1034, 69, 97, C6
PIT, 17
pitavastatin, 666, 91
Pitocin, 972, 17
Pitressin, 1271, 17
Pitrex, 187
Plan B, 359
Plan B One-Step, 1375
Plaquenil, 680
Plasbumin, 125
PLATELET ADHESION INHIBITORS, 62
PLATELET AGGREGATION INHIBITORS, 62
Platinol, 328
Platinol-AQ, 328
Plavix, 346
Plenaxis, 23
Pletal, 326
PMS-ASA, 1131
PMS-Cephalexin, 291
PMS-Chloral Hydrate, 312
PMS-Cimetidine, 660
PMS-Cyproheptadine, 390
PMS Dexamethasone, 1400
PMS-Diazepam, 431
PMS-Dicitrate, 1163
PMS-Divalproex, 1262
PMS-Doxycycline, 1203
PMS Egozinc, 1306
PMS Ferrous Sulfate, 736
PMS-Fluphenazine, 600
PMS-Furosemide, 620
PMS Haloperidol, 651
PMS-Hydrochlorothiazide, 458
PMS Hydromorphone, 677
PMS Isoniazid, 741
PMS-Isosorbide, 742
PMS Lindane, 788
PMS-Methylphenidate, 844
PMS-Minocycline, 1203
PMS-Nizatidine, 660
PMS-Norfloxacin, 589
PMS-Nystatin, 938
PMS-Piroxicam, 1034
pms Propranolol, 1071
PMS Pyrazinamide, 1080
PMS-Ranitidine, 660
PMS-Sodium Polystyrene Sulfonate, 1164
PMS-Sulfasalazine, 1171

PMS-Theophylline, 240
PMS-Trifluoperazine, 1337
PMS-Trihexyphenidyl, 1338
PMS-Valproic Acid, 1262
Pneumococcal conjugate vaccine (7–valent), 1431
Pneumococcal polysaccharide vaccine, 1431, 1434
pneumococcal 13-valent conjugate vaccine, 1375
Pneumovax 23, 1431, 1434
Podactin, 187
PODOPHYLLOTOXIN DERIVATIVES, 59
Polio vaccine, inactivated, 1429
Poliovax, 1429
polycarbophil, 47, 1331
Polycillin, 169
Polycitra Syrup, 1389
polyethylene glycol, 1036, 90
polyethylene glycol/ electrolyte, 1036, 90
Poly-Hist DM Syrup, 1389
Polysporin Topical Ointment/ Powder, 1389
Polytrim Ophthalmic Solution, 1389
Pontocaine, 1397
Portia, 1389
Portia-28, 358
posaconazole, 1037, 50
Posture, 265
Potasalan, 1041
potassium acetate, 1041, 93
potassium and sodium phosphates, 1039, 93
potassium bicarbonate, 1041, 93
potassium bicarbonate/ potassium chloride, 1041, 93
potassium bicarbonate/ potassium citrate, 1041, 93
potassium chloride, 1041, 17, 93, C2–C3, C5
potassium chloride/ potassium bicarbonate/ potassium citrate, 1041, 93
potassium gluconate, 1041, 93
potassium gluconate/ potassium chloride, 1041, 93
potassium gluconate/ potassium citrate, 1041, 93
potassium iodide, 730

COMPREHENSIVE INDEX

potassium phosphate, 93, 1332, C3
potassium phosphates, 16, 93, 1332
POTASSIUM PHOSPHATES, 93, 1332
✤ Potassium-Rougier, 1041
POTASSIUM SALTS, 93
✤ Potassium Sandoz, 1041
POTASSIUM-SPARING DIURETICS, 85
potassium supplements, 16
POTASSIUM SUPPLEMENTS, 1041
✤ Poxi, 314
PPSV, 1431, 1434
pramipexole, 1044, 1375, 61
pramlintide, 1046, 16, 46, 87
Pramosone Topical Cream/ Lotion/Ointment, 1389
PrandiMet 1/500, 1389
PrandiMet 2/500, 1389
Prandin, 1103
prasugrel, 1048, 23, 62
Pravachol, 666
⚕ **pravastatin,** 666, 91
prazosin, 1049, 54
Precedex, 423
Precose, 110
Pred Forte, 1401
Pred Mild, 1401
prednicarbate, 381, 83
predniSOLONE, 372, 1401, 37, 68, 83, C11, C14
predniSONE, 372, 37, 68, 83, C11, C14
Prefrin, 1403
pregabalin, 1051, 1375, 23, 42, 96
Prelone, 372
Premarin, 535
Premphase, 1389
✤ *Premplus 0.625/2.5, 1389*
✤ *Premplus 0.625/5, 1389*
Prempro 0.3/1.5, 1389
Prempro 0.45/1.5, 1389
Prempro 0.625/2.5, 1389
Prempro 0.625/5, 1389
Prepidil Endocervical Gel, 448
✤ Pressyn, 1271
Prevacid, 767
Prevacid 24 Hr, 767
Prevalite, 322
✤ Prevex, 380
Prevex HC, 381
Previfem, 358, 1389
Prevnar 13, 1375
Prevnar, 1431

Prevpac, 1389
Prezista, 406
Prialt, 1302
Priftin, 1333
Prilosec, 950, C8
Prilosec OTC, 950
Primacor, 866
Primalev, 966
Primalev 2.5/300, 1389
Primalev 5/300, 1389
Primalev 7.5/300, 1389
Primalev 10/300, 1389
Primatene, 504
Primatene Tablets, 1390
Primaxin, 700
Primaxin 500 mg I.V. For Injection, 1390
Primaxin 250 mg I.V. For Injection, 1390
Principen, 169
Prinivil, 176
Prinzide 10/12.5, 1390
Prinzide 20/12.5, 1390
Prinzide 20/25, 1390
Pristiq, 420
Proair HFA, 126
procainamide, 1052, 17, 35
procaine penicillin G, 1002, 56
Pro-Cal-Sof, 466
procarbazine, 1054, 16, 59
Procardia, 921, C6
Procardia XL, 921
Prochieve, 1060
prochlorperazine, 1056, 17, 48, 64, C1, C3
Procrit, 512, 1376
Proctocort, 381
Proctofoam-HC Rectal Foam, 1390
✤ Procytox, 384
✤ Prodiem, 1079
Prodium, 1014
progesterone, 1060, 87
PROGESTINS, 59
Prograf, 1182
Prolastin-C, 1375
Pro-Lax, 1079
Proleukin, 1317
Prolixin, 600
Prolixin Decanoate, 600
Promacta, 23
Promethacon, 1061
promethazine, 1061, 16, 48, 52, 101, C1, C5, C6
Promethegan, C6
Prometrium, 1060

propafenone, 1064, 35, 1441
propantheline, C6
proparacaine, 1397
Propecia, 578
Propine, 1403
propofol, 1066, 16
propoxyphene, 22, 99, C6
propoxyphene hydrochloride, 1068
propoxyphene hydrochloride/ acetaminophen, 1068
propoxyphene napsylate, 1068
propoxyphene napsylate/ acetaminophen, 1068
propranolol, 1071, 16, 32, 35, 54, 75, 106, 1441, C5
propylthiouracil, 1074
✤ Propyl-Thyracil, 1074
Proquin XR, 589
Proscar, 578
Prostigmin, 908
Prostin E Vaginal Suppository, 448
protamine, C5
protamine sulfate, 1076
PROTEASE INHIBITORS, 67
Protonix, 990
Protonix IV, 990
PROTON-PUMP INHIBITORS, 72
Protopic, 1182
✤ *Protrin, 1390*
✤ *Protrin DF, 1390*
Proventil HFA, 126
Provera, 812, C14
✤ Provera Pak, 812
Provigil, 874
Prozac, 597, C6, C8
Prozac Weekly, 597
pseudoephedrine, 1077
Psorcon, 380
psyllium, 1079, 90
PTU, 1074
Pulmicort Flexhaler, 365
Pulmicort Respules, 365
✤ Pulmophylline, 240
Purinethol, 1328
✤ Purinol, 134
☯ purple coneflower, 1348
P-V-Tussin, 1388
Pylera, 1390
pyrazinamide, 1080, 70
☯ Pyrethrum parthenium, 1349
Pyri, 1083
Pyridium, 1014
Pyridium Plus, 1014

---

*Entries for **generic** names appear in **boldface type**. Trade names appear in regular type, with Canadian trade names preceded by a maple leaf icon (✤). **CLASSIFICATIONS** appear in **BOLDFACE SMALL CAPS**. *Combination Drugs* appear in *italics*, herbal products are preceded by a yin-yang icon (☯) and drugs with genetic implications are preceded by a double-helix icon (⚕).

pyridostigmine, 1081
pyridoxine, 1083, 108
pyrimethamine, 1085

Q

Qualaquin, 1091
Quasense, 359, 1390
quazepam, C6
Questran, 322
Questran Light, 322
quetiapine, 1087, 1376, 64, 1442
Quibron-T, 240
quinapril, 176, 53
Quinaretic 10/12.5, 1390
Quinaretic 20/12.5, 1390
Quinaretic 20/25, 1390
quinidine, 1089, 1441–1442
quinidine gluconate, 1089, 35
quinidine sulfate, 1089, 35
quinine, 1091
quinupristin/dalfopristin, 1093, 56
Quixin, 1398
Qutenza, 1375
QVAR, 365

R

rabeprazole, 1095, 72, 1441
Radix angelicae gigantis, 1347
Ralivia, 1246
raloxifene, 1096, 77
raltegravir, 1097, 60
ramelteon, 1098, 23, 101
ramipril, 176, 53
Ranexa, 1099
ranibizumab, 1332
Raniclor, 294
ranitidine, 660, 72, C5
ranolazine, 1099, 32
Rapaflo, 1153
Rapamune, 1155, 1376
Raptiva, 1377
rasagiline, 1100, 1376
rasagline, 61
rasburicase, 1102
Ratio-Diltiazem CD, 445
Ratio-Doxycycline, 1203
Ratio-Minocycline, 1203
Ratio-MPA, 812
Ratio-Ranitidine, 660
Ratio-Valprox, 1262
rattle root, 1345
rattle top, 1345
rattleweed, 1345
Razadyne, 624
Razadyne ER, 624
Rebetol, 1107

Rebetron, 1390
Rebif, 728
Reclast, 1309
Reclipsen, 358, 1390
Recombivax HB, 1430, 1433
red ginseng, 1354
red sunflower, 1348
Redutemp, 112
Refludan, 773
Refresh, 1399
Refresh PM, 1399
Regitine, 1018
Reglan, 847
Regonol, 1081
Regranex, 222
regular insulin (insulin injection), 46
Regulax-SS, 466
Regulex, 466
Reguloid Natural, 1079
Relafen, 891
Relenza, 1301, 1376
Reliable Gentle Laxative, 230
Relistor, 843
Relpax, 496
Remeron, 867
Remeron Soltabs, 867
Remicade, 710
Remifemin, 1344
Renagel, 1149
Renedil, 557
RENIN INHIBITORS, 54
renshen, 1354
Renvela, 1149
repaglinide, 1103, 16, 46, 1442
Repan, 255
Repap CF, 255
Reprexain, 675
Reprexain 2.5/200, 1390
Reprexain 5/200, 1390
Reprexain 7.5/200, 1390
Reprexain 10/200, 1390
Requip, 1126
Requip XL, 1126
reserpine, C6
Respbaist, 1390
Respaire-60 SR, 1390
Respaire-120 SR, 1390
Restasis, 1401
Restoril, 1192, C6
Resectisol, 808
Resyl, 648
Retavase, 1214
reteplase, 1214, 104
Retrovir, 1303, C8
Revatio, 1151, 1375
Revimine, 471
Revlimid, 23
Reyataz, 201
R-Gel, 271
Rheumatrex, 836
Rhinalar, 369

Rhinocort Aqua, 369
Rh₀(D) globulin IV, 105
Rh₀(D) globulin microdose IM, 105
Rh₀(D) IMMUNE GLOBULIN, 1105
Rh₀(D) immune globulin IV, 1105
Rh₀(D) immune globulin microdose IM, 1105
Rh₀(D) immune globulin microdose IM, IV, 1105
Rh₀(D) immune globulin standard dose IM, 1105, 105
Rhodis, 754
RhoGAM, 1105
Rhophylac, 1105
rHu GM-CSF (recombinant human granulocyte/macrophage colony-stimulating factor), 1136
Rhulicort, 381
ribavirin, 1107, 73
riboflavin, 108, 1332
Rid·a·Pain·HP, 271
Ridenol, 112
RID Maximum Strength Shampoo, 1390
rifabutin, 1110, 1442
Rifadin, 1112
Rifamate, 1390
rifampin, 1112, 70, 1441–1442, C5
rifapentine, 1333
Rifater, 1390
rifaximin, 1114, 56
Rilutek, 1376
riluzole, 1376
rimabotulinum toxin B, 23
Rimactane, 1112
rimexolone, 83, 1401
Riomet, 829
Riopan Plus, 803
Riopan Plus Double Strength, 803
Riphenidate, 844
risedronate, 1114, 77
Risperdal, 1116
Risperdal Consta, 1116
Risperdal M-TAB, 1116
risperidone, 1116, 64, 1441
Ritalin, 844
Ritalin LA, 844
Ritalin-SR, 844
ritodrine, 1377
ritonavir, 1119, 1375–1376, 23, 67, 1441–1442, C8
Rituxan, 1121, 1376
rituximab, 1121, 1376, 16, 59
Riva-Minocycline, 1203

COMPREHENSIVE INDEX 1471

- ✹ Rivanase AQ, 369
- ✹ Riva-Norfloxacin, 589
- ✹ Riva-Ranitidine, 660
- ✹ Rivasa, 1131
- **rivastigmine, 1123, 30**
- ✹ Rivotril, 341
- **rizatriptan, 1125, 106**
- ✹ *Robaxacet-8, 1390*
- ✹ *Robaxacet, 1390*
- ✹ *Robaxacet Extra Strength, 1390*
- Robaxin, 835, C6
- ✹ Robidex, 430
- ✹ Robidrine, 1078
- Robinul, 636
- Robinul-Forte, 636
- Robitussin, 648
- *Robitussin Children's Cough & Cold CF Liquid, 1390*
- *Robitussin Children's Cough & Cold Long-Acting Liquid, 1390*
- Robitussin Cough Calmers, 430
- *Robitussin Cough & Chest Congestion DM Liquid, 1390*
- *Robitussin Cough & Chest Congestion DM Max Liquid, 1390*
- *Robitussin Cough & Cold CF Liquid, 1390*
- *Robitussin Cough & Cold D Liquid, 1390*
- *Robitussin Cough, Cold & Flu Liquid, 1390*
- *Robitussin Cough & Cold Long-Acting Liquid, 1390*
- Robitussine CoughGels, 430
- Robitussin Maximum Strength Cough Suppressant, 430
- *Robitussin Nighttime Cough & Cold Liquid, 1390*
- Robitussin Pediatric, 430
- Rocaltrol, 1287
- Rocephin, 300
- Rodex, 1083
- ✹ RO-Dexasone, 1400
- ✹ Rofact, 1112
- ✹ Rogitine, 1018
- Rolaids Calcium Rich, 265
- *Rolaids Extra Strength Tablets, 1390*
- *Rolaids Multi-Symptom Tablets, 1390*
- *Rolaids Regular Tablets, 1390*
- Romazicon, 587
- **romidepsin, 1372, 59**
- **romiplostim, 23**
- Romycin, 1398

- *Rondec DM Drops, 1390*
- *Rondec DM Syrup, 1390*
- *Rondec Oral Drops, 1391*
- *Rondec Syrup, 1391*
- **ropinirole, 1126, 61, 1441**
- **ropivacaine, 502**
- **rosiglitazone, 1128, 22, 46**
- ☯ Rosin rose, 1364
- ⛓ **rosuvastatin, 666, 1376, 91**
- Rosuvastatin, 1376
- Rotarix [RV1], 1432
- RotaTeq [RV5], 1432
- **Rotavirus vaccine, 1432**
- ✹ Roubac, 1254
- Rowasa, 825
- Roxanol, 880
- Roxanol Rescudose, 880
- Roxanol-T, 880
- *Roxicet, 966, 1391*
- *Roxicet 5/500, 1391*
- *Roxicet Oral Solution, 1391*
- Roxicodone, 966
- Roxilox, 966
- Roychlor, 1041
- Rozerem, 1098, 23
- Rubex, 479
- Rubramin PC, 1284
- ☯ rudbeckia, 1348
- **rufinamide, 1372, 22, 42**
- Rulox, 803
- Rum-K, 1041
- *Ru-Tuss DM Syrup, 1391*
- RV, 1432
- *Rynatan, 1391*
- *Rynatan Pediatric Suspension, 1391*
- *Rynatuss, 1391*
- Rythmol, 1064
- Rythmol SR, 1064
- Ryzolt, 1246

S

- S-2, 504
- ☯ Sabal, 1363
- ☯ Sabal Fructus, 1363
- Sabril, 1374, 23
- **sacrosidase, 23**
- ☯ S-adenosylmethionine, 1362
- Saizen, 645
- Salagen, 1028
- ✹ Salazopyrin, 1171
- Salflex, 1131
- Salgesic, 1131
- **SALICYLATES, 1131, 95**
- **SALINES, 90**
- ☯ salisburia adiantifolia, 1353
- **salmeterol, 1134, 1376, 22, 37, 78**

- ✹ Salofalk, 825
- **salsalate, 1131, 65, 95**
- Salsitab, 1131
- ☯ SAMe, 94, 1362
- ☯ sampson root, 1348
- Samsca, 1239, 23
- Sanctura, 1257
- Sanctura XR, 1257
- Sancuso, 642
- Sandimmune, 387
- Sandostatin, 941
- Sandostatin LAR, 941
- ✹ Sans-Acne, 523
- ☯ Santa Maria, 1349
- Saphris, 197
- **saquinavir, 67, 1333, 1442**
- Sarafem, 597
- **sargramostim, 1136**
- ✹ S.A.S, 1171
- Savella, 864, 23
- ☯ saw palmetto, 94, 1363
- ☯ Saw Palmetto Berry, 1363
- **saxagliptin, 1138, 46**
- Scopace, 1139
- **scopolamine, 1139, 38, 49, 1401, C1**
- Scot-Tussin Allergy DM, 450
- *Scot-Tussin DM Maximum Strength Liquid, 1391*
- Scot-tussin Expectorant, 648
- *Scot-Tussin Original Liquid, 1391*
- *Scot-Tussin Senior Liquid, 1391*
- ☯ scurvy root, 1348
- SD-Deprenyl, 1141
- *Seasonale, 359, 1391*
- *Seasonique, 359, 1391*
- **SECOND-GENERATION CEPHALOSPORINS, 55**
- Sedapap, 255, 1391
- **SEDATIVE/HYPNOTICS, 99**
- ✹ Sedatuss, 430
- **SELECTIVE ESTROGEN RECEPTOR MODULATORS, 77**
- **SELECTIVE SEROTONIN REUPTAKE INHIBITORS (SSRIS), 17, 34, 44**
- **selegiline, 1141, 44, 61**
- ✹ Selestoject, 372
- ✹ Seloken-ZOK, 851
- Selzentry, 810
- *Semprex-D, 1391*
- Sena-Gen, 1145
- Senexon, 1145
- **sennosides, 1145, 90**
- Senokot, 1145
- *Senokot-S, 1391*

---

*Entries for **generic** names appear in **boldface type**. Trade names appear in regular type, with Canadian trade names preceded by a maple leaf icon (✹). **CLASSIFICATIONS** appear in **BOLDFACE SMALL CAPS**. *Combination Drugs* appear in *italics*, herbal products are preceded by a yin-yang icon (☯) and drugs with genetic implications are preceded by a double-helix icon (⛓).

1472 COMPREHENSIVE INDEX

SenokotXTRA, 1145
Seno Sol-SS, 1391
Sensipar, 326
Sensorcaine, 502
Septra, 1254, 1391
Septra DS, 1254, 1391
Serax, 961, C6
● Serenoa repens, 1363
Serevent, 1376
Serevent Diskus, 1134
Seroquel, 1087
Seroquel XR, 1087, 1376
Serostim, 645
Serostim LQ, 645
sertaconazole, 1146, 50
sertraline, 1147, 44, 1441–1442, C16
Serutan, 1079
sevelamer, 1149
Shohl's Solution modified, 1163
Siblin, 1079
sibutramine, 1150, 1376, 108, 1442
Silace, 466
Siladril, 450
Silafed Syrup, 1391
Silapap, 112
sildenafil, 1151, 1375, 1442
Silfedrine, 1078
silodosin, 1153
Silphen, 450
Siltussin DAS, 648
Siltussin SA, 648
● Silybin, 1361
● Silymarin, 1361
Simcor 750/20, 1391
Simcor 500/20, 1391
Simcor 1000/20, 1391
simethicone, 1155
Simply Cough, 430
Simply Stuffy, 1078
Simponi, 638, 23
Simron, 736
Simulect, 220
simvastatin, 666, 91, 1442
Sinemet, 275
Sinemet 25/250, 1391
Sinemet 25/100, 1391
Sinemet 10/100, 1391
Sinemet CR, 275
Sinemet CR 25-100, 1391
Sinemet CR 50-200, 1391
Sine-Off Non-Drowsy Maximum Strength, 1391
Sine-Off Severe Cold, 1391
Sine-Off Sinus/Cold Medicine, 1391
Sinequan, 476
Singulair, 879
Sinustop, 1078
sirolimus, 1155, 1376, 89, 1442
sitagliptin, 1158, 46

Skelaxin, 828, C6
SKELETAL MUSCLE RELAXANTS, CENTRALLY ACTING, 101, C7
Skelid, 1336
Sleep-Eze 3, 450
Sleepwell 2-night, 450
Slo-Mag, 804
Slo-Niacin, 914
Slo-Salt, 1161
Slow FE, 736
Slow-K, 1041
SMZ/TMP, 1254
Snooze Fast, 450
Soda Mint, 1159
sodium bicarbonate, 1159, 72, 92, C2–C3
sodium chloride, 1161, 16, 93
sodium citrate and citric acid, 1163, 92
Sodium Diuril, 458
sodium ferric gluconate complex, 737, 31
sodium oxybate, 23
sodium phosphate, 1333, C3
sodium phosphate, dibasic anhydrous, 23
sodium phosphate, monobasic, monohydrate, 23
sodium polystyrene sulfonate, 1164
sodium salicylate, 1131, 65, 95
Soflax, 466
Solage Topical Liquid, 1391
Solaraze, 435
Solarcaine Aloe Extra Burn Relief, 784
✺ Solazine, 1337
Solfoton, 1015
Solia, 358, 1391
solifenacin, 1166, 38
Soliris, 23
Solodyn, 1203
Solu-Cortef, 372
Solu-Medrol, 372
Soma, 280, C6
Soma Compound, 1391
somatropin (recombinant), 645, 87
Sominex, 450
✺ Somnol, 603
Sonata, 1300
Sorine, 1167
✺ Sotacor, 1167
sotalol, 1167, 35, 75
Sotret, 744
Span-FF, 736
✺ Spasmoban, 438
Spectracef, 300
✺ Spersacarpine, 1400

✺ Spersadex, 1400
✺ Spersaphrine, 1403
Spiriva, 1232
spironolactone, 456, 85
Sporanox, 748
Sprintec, 358, 1391
SPS, 1164
● squawroot, 1345
Sronyx, 358, 1391
SSKI, 730
SSRI, 17
Stadol, 257, 1419
Stadol NS, 257
Stalevo 75, 1391
Stalevo 125, 1391
Stalevo 50, 1391
Stalevo 150, 1391
Stalevo 100, 1391
Stalevo 200, 1391
Starlix, 903
✺ Statex, 880
stavudine, 67, 1334
Stavzor, 1262
Stelara, 23
✺ Stemetil, 1056
Sterapred, 372
✺ Stieprox, 187
Stimate, 418
STIMULANT LAXATIVES, 90
● St. John's wort, 94, 1442
● St. John's wort (Hypericum perforatum), 1364
St. Joseph Adult Chewable Aspirin, 1131
Stool Softener, 466
STOOL SOFTENERS, 90
Strattera, 205
Streptase, 1214
streptokinase, 1214, 104
streptomycin, 145, 55
Striant, 1200
strong iodine solution, 730
Sublimaze, 567
Suboxone N2, 1391
Suboxone N8, 1391
Subutex, 246
succimer, 1334
succinate, C4
Sucraid, 23
sucralfate, 1169, 72
Sucrets Cough Control Formula, 430
Sudafed, 1078
Sudafed Childrens's Non-Drowsy, 1078
Sudafed 12 Hour, 1078
Sudafed Non-Drowsy Maximum Strength, 1078
Sudafed PE Children's Cough & Cold Liquid, 1391
Sudafed PE Cough & Cold, 1391

Sudafed PE Nighttime Cold, 1392
Sudafed PE Non-Drying Sinus, 1392
Sudafed PE Severe Cold Formula, 1392
Sudafed PE Sinus & Allergy, 1392
Sudafed PE Sinus Headache, 1392
Sudafed PE Triple Action, 1392
Sudafed Sinus Liquicaps, 1392
Sudafed Sinus & Pain 12 Hour, 1392
Sudafed Triple Action, 1392
Sudal 12, 1392
Sudodrin, 1078
Sular, 926
sulconazole, 187, 50
✻ Sulcrate, 1169
sulfacetamide, 56, 1398
Sulfacet-R Topical Lotion, 1392
sulfADIAZINE, C11
sulfamethoxazole, 1441
sulfasalazine, 1171, 69
Sulfatrim, 1254
✻ Sulfex, 1398
sulfiSOXAZOLE, C11, 69
Sulfolax, 466
SULFONYLUREAS, 1172, 46
sulindac, 1175, 69, 97
sumatriptan, 1177, 23, 106
Sumavel DosePro, 1177
Sumycin, 1203
sunitinib, 1179, 16, 60
Sunkist, 1319
SuperChar Aqueous, 1317
✻ Supeudol, 966
Suprax, 300
Surfak, 466
Surmontil, 1338
Surpass, 265
Surpass Extra Strength, 265
Sus-Phrine, 504
Sustiva, 495
Sutent, 1179
Syllact, 1079
Symbicort, 23
Symbicort 80/4.5, 1392
Symbicort 160/4.5, 1392
Symbyax 3/25, 1392
Symbyax 6/25, 1392
Symbyax 12/25, 1392
Symbyax, 23
Symbyax 6/50, 1392
Symbyax 12/50, 1392

Symlin, 1046
Synacort, 381
Synalar, 380
Synalgos-DC, 1392
✻ Synamol, 380
Synarel, 894
✻ Syn-Clonazepam, 341
✻ Syn-Diltiazem, 445
Synercid, 1093
Synercid Powder for Injection, 1392
✻ Synflex, 900
✻ Synflex DS, 900
✻ Syn-Nadolol, 892
Synthroid, 1219
✻ Syntocinon, 972
SYSTEMIC, 50, 52

T

T₄, 1219
T₃, 1219
✻ 642 Tab, 1068
Taclonex Topical Ointment/ Suspension, 1392
tacrine, 1181, 30
🧬 **TACROLIMUS, 1182, 1442, 89, C5**
tadalafil, 1185, 1442
Tagamet, 660, C6
Tagamet HB, 660
☯ Tagara, 1365
Talacen, 1392
Talwin, 1010, 1419, C6
Talwin NX, 1010, 1392
Tambocor, 579
Tamiflu, 956
✻ Tamofen, 1187
✻ Tamone, 1187
✻ Tamoplex, 1187
tamoxifen, 1187, 1442, 59
tamsulosin, 1189
☯ Tanaceti parthenii, 1349
☯ Tang Kuei, 1347
☯ Tan Kue Bai Zhi, 1347
Tapanol, 112
Tapazole, 834
tapentadol, 1190, 23, 99
Tarceva, 520
Tarka 1/240, 1392
Tarka 2/180, 1392
Tarka 2/240, 1392
Tarka 4/240, 1392
Tasigna, 923
Tasmar, 1236
Tavist ND, 798
TAXOIDS, 59
Taxol, 975
Taxotere, 462

Tazicef, 300
✻ *Tazocin for Injection 2.25 g, 1392*
✻ *Tazocin for Injection 3.375 g, 1392*
✻ *Tazocin for Injection 4.5 g, 1392*
Taztia XT, 445
3TC, 762
Td, 1435
Tdap, 1429, 1434
T-Diet, 1017
Tear Drop, 1399
TearGard, 1399
Teargen, 1399
Tearisol, 1399
Tears Naturale, 1399
Tears Naturale Free, 1399
Tears Naturale II, 1399
Tears Plus, 1399
Tears Renewed, 1399
✻ Tebrazid, 1080
Tecnal, 255
tegaserod, 1335
Tegopen, 1377
Tegretol, 272
✻ Tegretol CR, 272
Tegretol-XR, 272
Tekturna, 133
Tekturna HCT 150/12.5, 1392
Tekturna HCT 150/25, 1392
Tekturna HCT 300/12.5, 1392
Tekturna HCT 300/25, 1392
telavancin, 1373, 23, 54
telbivudine, 23
Teldrin, 316
Telechlor, 316
🧬 **telmisartan, 182, 54**
✻ Telzir, 612
temazepam, 1192, 101, C6
Temovate, 380
Temovate E, 380
Tempra, 112
temsirolimus, 16, 56, 1335
Tencon, 255
tenecteplase, 1214, 104
Tenex, 1326
Ten-K, 1041
tenofovir, 1193, 67
Tenoretic 50, 1392
Tenoretic 100, 1392
Tenormin, 204
Teramine, 1017
Terazol-3, 190
Terazol-7, 190
terazosin, 1194, 54
terbinafine, 187, 1196, 50

---

*Entries for **generic** names appear in **boldface type**. Trade names appear in regular type, with Canadian trade names preceded by a maple leaf icon (✻). **CLASSIFICATIONS** appear in **BOLDFACE SMALL CAPS**. *Combination Drugs* appear in *italics*, herbal products are preceded by a yin-yang icon (☯) and drugs with genetic implications are preceded by a double-helix icon (🧬).

1474 COMPREHENSIVE INDEX

terbutaline, 1197, 37, 78, C5
terconazole, 190, 50
✱ Terfluzine, 1337
Teril, 272
teriparatide, 1199, 23, 87
Terra-Cortril Ophthalmic Suspension, 1392
Terramycin with Polymyxin B Sulfate Ophthalmic Ointment, 1392
Testopel, 1200
TESTOSTERONE, 1200, 22
testosterone buccal system, mucoadhesive, 1200, 87
testosterone cypionate, 1200, 87
testosterone enanthate, 1200, 87
testosterone pellets, 1200, 87
testosterone transdermal, 1200, 87
Testred, C6
Tetanus-diphtheria, 1435
tetanus toxoid, 1429
Tetanus toxoid, reduced diphtheria toxoid, and acellular pertussis vaccine absorbed, 1429
Tetanus toxoid, reduced diphtheria toxoid and acellular pertussis vaccine absorbed, 1434
Tetcaine, 1397
tetrabenazine, 1373, 23
tetracaine, 1397
TETRACYCLIC ANTIDEPRESSANTS, 44
TETRACYCLINES, 1203, 56
tetrahydrozoline, 1403
Teveten, 182
Teveten HCT 600/12.5, 1392
Teveten HCT 600/25, 1392
Tev-Tropin, 645
Texacort, 381
thalidomide, 1207, 16, 23, 89
Thalitone, 458
Thalomid, 1207, 23
Theo-24, 240
Theochron, 240
theophylline, 240, 37, 78, 1441–1442
Thera-Flu Cold & Cough Hot Liquid, 1392
Thera-Flu, Cold & Sore Throat Hot Liquid, 1392
Thera-Flu Daytime Severe Cold & Cough Caplets, 1392

Thera-Flu Daytime Severe Cold & Cough Hot Liquid, 1392
Thera-Flu Flu & Chest Congestion Hot Liquid, 1392
Thera-Flu Flu & Sore Throat Hot Liquid, 1393
Thera-Flu Nighttime Severe Cold & Cough Caplets, 1393
Thera-Flu Nighttime Severe Cold & Cough Hot Liquid, 1393
TheraFlu Thin Strips Long Acting Cough, 430
Thera-Flu Warming Relief Cold & Chest Congestion Syrup, 1393
Thera-Flu Warming Relief Daytime Severe Cough & Cold Syrup, 1393
Thera-Flu Warming Relief Flu & Sore Throat Syrup, 1393
Thera-Flu Warming Relief Nighttime Severe Cold & Cough Syrup, 1393
Theralax, 230
Therevac SB, 466
thiamine, 1209, 108
THIAZIDE DIURETICS, 54, 85
THIAZIDE-LIKE DIURETICS, 54, 85
THIAZOLIDINEDIONES, 46
THIENOPYRIDINES, 62
thioguanine, 16, 56, 1335
6-thioguanine, 1335
thioridazine, 1211, 64, C6
THIRD-GENERATION CEPHALOSPORINS, 55
Thorazine, 17
Thrive, 918
THROMBIN INHIBITORS, 40
THROMBOLYTIC AGENTS, 1214, 16
THROMBOLYTICS, 102
thyroid, 1219, 87
THYROID PREPARATIONS, 1219
Thyrolar, 1219
ThyroSafe, 730
ThyroShield, 730
tiagabine, 1222, 42, 1442, C8
Tiazac, 445
ticarcillin, C5
ticarcillin/clavulanate, 1224, 56, C3, C5
ticlopidine, 1225, 62, 1441–1442, C6
Tigan, C6
tigecycline, 1227, 56, C3
Tikosyn, 467, 23
Tilia Fe, 359

tiludronate, 1336
Timentin, 1224
Timentin for Injection, 1393
timolol, 1229, 54, 75, 106, 1399
Timoptic, 1399
Timoptic-XE, 1399
Tinactin, 187
Tindamax, 1231
Ting, 187
tinidazole, 1231
tinzaparin, 657, 40
tioconazole, 190, 50
tiotorpium, 38
tiotropium, 1232, 37, 78
Tipramine, 703
tipranavir, 67, 1336
✱ Tipton weed, 1364
tirofiban, 1233, 16, 62
tissue plasminogen activator, 1214
Titralac, 265
Titralac Plus, 1393
tizanidine, 1235, C8
TMP/SMX, 1254
TMP/SMZ, 1254
TNKase, 1214
TOBI, 145
TobraDex Ophthalmic Suspension/Ointment, 1393
tobramycin, 145, 55, 1398, C3, C5
Tobrex, 1398
tocilizumab, 1374, 67
Tofranil, 703
Tofranil PM, 703
tolcapone, 1236, 61
TOLAZamide, C11, C14
TOLBUTamide, C11, C14
Tolectin, 1337
Tolectin DS, 1337
tolmetin, 97, 1337
tolnaftate, 187, 50
tolterodine, 1238, 38
tolvaptan, 1239, 23, 93
✱ tonga, 1360
Topamax, 1240, 23, C8
Topicort, 380
Topicort-LP, 380
✱ Topilene, 380
topiramate, 1240, 23, 42
✱ Topisone, 380
topotecan, 1242, 16
Toprol-XL, 851, C8
✱ Topsyn, 380
✱ Toradol, 756
Torisel, 1335
torsemide, 1244, 54, 85
Totacillin, 169
Totect, 426
Toviaz, 574
t-PA, 1214

COMPREHENSIVE INDEX

Tracleer, 23
tramadol, 1246, 1441, C8
Trandate, 759
trandolapril, 176, 53
tranexamic acid, 1375
TRANSDERMAL FENTANYL, 1420
Transderm-Scop, 1139
✤ Transderm-V, 1139
Tranxene, 347, C6
Tranxene-SD, 347
tranylcypromine, 876, 44
trastuzumab, 1249, 16, 59
Travatan, 1403
Travatan Z, 1403
travoprost, 1403
trazodone, 1251, 1375, 44, C8
Treanda, 223
Trelstar Depot, 1339
Trexall, 836
Treximet, 23, 1393
Triacin-C Cough Syrup, 1393
Triad, 255
✤ Triadapin, 476
✤ Triaderm, 381
triamcinolone, 369, 372, 381, 37, 68, 83
Triaminic Allergy Congestion Softchews, 1078
Triaminic Chest & Nasal Congestion Liquid, 1393
Triaminic Cold & Allergy Liquid, 1393
Triaminic Cough & Sore Throat Liquid, 1393
Triaminic Day Time Cold & Cough Liquid, 1393
Triaminic Day Time Thin Strips Cold & Cough, 1393
Triaminic–D Multi-Symptom Cold Liquid, 1393
Triaminic Multi-Symptom Fever Liquid, 1393
Triaminic Night Time Cold & Cough Liquid, 1393
Triaminic Night Time Thin Strips Cold & Cough, 1393
Triaminic Softchews Cough & Runny Nose, 1393
Triaminic Softchews Cough & Sore Throat, 1393
Triaminic Thin Strips Long Acting Cough, 430
triamterene, 456, 85
✤ Trianide, 381
Triaprin, 255
triazolam, 1253, 101, C6

tricalcium phosphate (39% Ca or 19.5 mEq/g), 265, 92
Tricor, 559
Tricosal, 1131
TRICYCLIC ANTIDEPRESSANTS, 44
Triderm, 381
Tridil, 929
trifluoperazine, 64, 1337
trifluridine, 73, 1399
Triglide, 559
Trihexane, 1338
Trihexy, 1338
trihexyphenidyl, 61, 1338
Tri-K, 1041
✤ Trikacide, 854
trikates (potassium acetate/ potassium bicarbonate/ potassium citrate), 1041, 93
Tri-Legest Fe, 359
Trileptal, 962
Tri-Levlen, 359
Tri-Lipix, 561
Trilipix, 23
Trilisate, 1131
Tri-Lo-Sprintec, 359
Tri-Luma Topical Cream, 1394
TriLyte, 1036, 1394
trimethobenzamide, C6
trimethoprim/ sulfamethoxazole, 1254, 56, C3, C5
trimetrexate, 1377
trimipramine, 44, 1338
Trimox, 158
Tri-Nessa, 359
Tri-Norinyl, 359
Triostat, 1219
Tripedia, 1429
Tri-Previfem, 359
triptorelin, 59, 1339
Trisenox, 1319
Tri-Sprintec, 359
✤ *Trisulfa, 1394*
✤ *Trisulfa DS, 1394*
✤ Trivagizole-3, 190
Trivaris, 372
Trivora 28, 359
Trizivir, 23, 1394
Tropicacyl, 1401
tropicamide, 1401
trospium, 1257
Truphylline, 240
Trusopt, 1400
Truvada, 1394
T_3/T_4, 1219
Tums, 265

Tums E-X, 265
TussiCaps 5/4, 1394
TussiCaps 10/8, 1394
Tussigon, 1394
Tussigon (U.S. antitussive formulations contain homatropine), 675
Tussionex Suspension, 1394
Tussi-Organidin DM NR Liquid, 1394
Tussi-Organidin NR Liquid, 1394
Tusstat, 450
Twilite, 450
Twin-K, 1041
Twynsta, 1375
Tygacil, 1227
Tykerb, 770
Tylenol, 112
Tylenol Allergy Multisymptom Gelcaps, 1394
Tylenol Allergy Multisymptom Nighttime Caplets, 1394
Tylenol Children's Plus Cold & Allergy Liquid, 1394
Tylenol Children's Plus Cold & Cough Liquid, 1394
Tylenol Children's Plus Cold Liquid, 1394
Tylenol Children's Plus Cold & Stuffy Nose Liquid, 1394
Tylenol Children's Plus Cough & Runny Nose Liquid, 1394
Tylenol Children's Plus Cough & Sore Throat Liquid, 1395
Tylenol Children's Plus Flu Liquid, 1395
Tylenol Children's Plus Multi-Symptom Cold Liquid, 1395
Tylenol Cold Head Congestion Daytime Caplets, 1395
Tylenol Cold Head Congestion Nighttime Caplets, 1395
Tylenol Cold Head Congestion Severe Caplets, 1395
Tylenol Cold Multi-Symptom Daytime Caplets, 1395
Tylenol Cold Multi-Symptom Daytime Liquid, 1395
Tylenol Cold Multi-Symptom Nighttime Caplets, 1395
Tylenol Cold Multi-Symptom Nighttime Liquid, 1395
Tylenol Cold Multi-Symptom Severe Caplets, 1395
Tylenol Cold Multi-Symptom Severe Liquid, 1395

---

*Entries for **generic** names appear in **boldface type**. Trade names appear in regular type, with Canadian trade names preceded by a maple leaf icon (✤). **CLASSIFICATIONS** appear in **BOLDFACE SMALL CAPS**. *Combination Drugs* appear in *italics*, herbal products are preceded by a yin-yang icon (☯) and drugs with genetic implications are preceded by a double-helix icon (⚎).

Tylenol Cold Severe Congestion Daytime Caplets, 1395
Tylenol Cough & Severe Congestion Daytime Liquid, 1395
Tylenol Cough & Sore Throat Daytime Liquid, 1395
Tylenol Cough & Sore Throat Nighttime Liquid, 1395
Tylenol PM, 1395
Tylenol Severe Allergy Caplets, 1395
Tylenol Sinus Congestion & Pain Daytime Gelcaps, 1395
Tylenol Sinus Congestion & Pain Nighttime Caplets, 1395
Tylenol Sinus Congestion & Pain Severe Caplets, 1395
Tylenol Sinus Severe Congestion Daytime Caplets, 1395
Tylenol with codeine No. 3, 1395
Tylenol with codeine No. 4, 1395
Tylox, 966
Tylox 5/500, 1395
Tysabri, 1376, 23
Tyzeka, 23

U

✱Ulcidine, 660
Ulesfia, 1369
Uloric, 556
Ultracet, 1395
Ultram, 1246
Ultram ER, 1246
Ultrase MT 12, 985
Ultrase MT 20, 985
Ultra Tears, 1399
Ultravate, 380
Unasyn, 172
Unasyn for Injection 1.5 g, 1395
Unasyn for Injection 3 g, 1395
Uni-Ace, 112
✱Unicort, 381
Unifed, 1078
Uniphyl, 240
Uniretic 7.5/12.5, 1395
Uniretic 15/12.5, 1395
Uniretic 15/25, 1395
Unisom Nighttime Sleep-Aid, 450
Unithroid, 1219
Univasc, 176
Urabeth, 1320
Urecholine, 1320

urokinase, 1214, 104
Uro-KP Neutral, 1039
Uro-Mag, 804
✱Uromitexan, 826
Uroxatral, 132
✱Urozide, 458
ustekinumab, 23
UTI Relief, 1014

V

VACCINES/IMMUNIZING AGENTS, 104
☘Vaccinium myrtillus, 1344
Vagifem, 532, 1375
Vagistat-3, 190
Vagistat-1, 190
valacyclovir, 1259, 73
Valcyte, 1260
☘valerian, 94, 1365
☘Valeriana, 1365
☘Valerianae radix, 1365
☘Valeriana officinalis, 1365
☘Valeriana rhizome, 1365
☘Valeriane, 1365
valganciclovir, 1260, 73
Valium, 431, C6
Valnac, 380
VALPROATES, 1262, 42
valproate sodium, 1262, 42, 106, C5
valproic acid, 1262, 42, 106
valsartan, 182, 54
Valtrex, 1259
Valturna 150/160, 1395
Valturna 300/320, 1395
Vanadom, 280
Vancocin, 1265
vancomycin, 1265, 56, C3, C5
Vandazole, 854
Vaniqa, 1325
Vanos, 380
Vanoxide HC Lotion, 1395
Vanquish Extra Strength Pain Reliever, 1396
Vantin, 300
Vaqta, 1431, 1433
Var, 1430, 1435
vardenafil, 1268, 1442
varenicline, 1269
Varicella vaccine, 1430, 1435
Varivax, 1430, 1435
VASCULAR HEADACHE SUPPRESSANTS, 105
Vaseretic 5/12.5, 1396
Vaseretic 10/25, 1396
Vasocidin Ophthalmic Solution, 1396
VasoClear, 1402
Vasocon, 1402

Vasocon-A Ophthalmic Solution, 1396
VASODILATORS, 54, C7
vasopressin, 1271, 17, 87, C2–C3, C5
Vasotec, 176
Vasotec IV, 176
Vectibix, 988
Vectical, 1375
✱Velbe, 1278
Velcade, 239, 1375
Velivet, 359
venlafaxine, 1272, 23, 34, 44, 1441
Venofer, 736
Ventavis, 1327
✱Ventodisk, 126
Ventolin HFA, 126
✱Ventolin nebules, 126
VePesid, 546
Veramyst, 369
verapamil, 1275, 32, 35, 54, 80, 106, 1442, C3, C5
Verazinc, 1306
Verdeso, 380
Verelan, 1275
Verelan PM, 1275
Vermox, 1327
Versed, 858
verteporfin, 1339
VESIcare, 1166
Vexol, 1401
VFEND, 1292
Viagra, 1151
Vibativ, 1373, 23
Vibramycin, 1203
Vibra-Tabs, 1203
Vicks 44 Cough Relief, 430
Vicks 44 Custom Care Chesty Cough Liquid, 1396
Vicks 44 Custom Care Congestion Liquid, 1396
Vicks 44 Custom Care Cough & Cold PM Liquid, 1396
Vicks Formula 44 Pediatric Formula, 430
Vicks Pediatric Formula 44E Cough & Chest Congestion Relief Liquid, 1396
Vicks Pediatric Formula 44M Cough & Cold Relief Liquid, 1396
Vicodin, 675, 1396
Vicodin ES, 1396
Vicodin HP, 1396
Vicoprofen, 675, 1396
Victoza, 1371
Vidaza, 210
Videx, 1376, 1324
Videx EC, 1324
vigabatrin, 1374, 23, 40
Vigamox, 1398

COMPREHENSIVE INDEX 1477

Vimpat, 1371, 23
vinBLAStine, 1278, 16, 59, C8, C11
VINCA ALKALOIDS, **59**
Vincasar PFS, 1280
vinCRIStine, 1280, 16, 59, C8, C11, C16
vinorelbine, 1282, 16, 59
Viokase, 985
Viracept, 1329
Viramune, 912, 23
Virazole, 1107
Viread, 1193
Virilon, C6
Viroptic, 1399
Visicol, 1025
Visine, 1403
Visine-A Ophthalmic Solution, 1396
Visine LR, 1402
Vistaril, 682, C6
Vistide, 324
Visudyne, 1339
Vitabee 6, 1083
Vit-A-Drops, 1399
Vitalax, 1079
vitamin B, 606, 914
vitamin B$_2$, 1332
vitamin B$_6$, 1083
vitamin B1, 1209
VITAMIN B$_{12}$ PREPARATIONS, 1284
vitamin D$_2$, 1287
vitamin D$_3$ (active), 1287
VITAMIN D COMPOUNDS, 1287
vitamin D$_3$ (inactive), 1287
vitamin E, 1291, 107
vitamin K, 1026
VITAMINS, **31, 107**
Vita Plus E, 1291
☯ Vitis coignetiae, 1357
☯ Vitis vinifera, 1357
Vitrasert, 626
Viva-Drops, 1399
Vivelle-Dot, 532
🍁 Vivol, 431
V-Lax, 1079
Voltaren, 435, 1402
Voltaren Gel, 435
Voltaren XR, 435
voriconazole, 1292, 50, 1441–1442, C3, C5
VoSpire ER, 126
Votrient, 994, 23
VP-16, 546
Vusion Topical Ointment, 1396

Vytorin 10/10, 1396
Vytorin 10/20, 1396
Vytorin 10/40, 1396
Vytorin 10/80, 1396

W

warfarin, 1295, 16, 40, 1441–1442, C16
🍁 Warfilone, 1295
WATER SOLUBLE VITAMINS, **107**
🍁 Webber Vitamin E, 1291
WEIGHT CONTROL AGENTS, **108**
Welchol, 356, 1375
Wellbutrin, 249, C12
Wellbutrin SR, 249, C8
Wellbutrin XL, 249, C8
Westcort, 381
Westhroid, 1219
☯ white ginseng, 1354
☯ whitehorn, 1358
☯ Wild chamomile, 1349
☯ Wild quinine, 1349
WinRho SDF, 1105
☯ wolf's bane, 1343
Women's Gentle Laxative, 230
☯ wurzelstock, 1360
Wycillin, 1002

X

Xalatan, 1403
Xanax, 138, C6, C8, C15
Xanax XR, 138, C15
XANTHINES, **78**
Xeloda, 269
Xenaderm Topical Ointment, 1396
Xenazine, 1373, 23
Xenical, 954
Xibrom, 1402
Xifaxan, 1114
Xigris, 489
Xolair, 948, 23
Xolegel, 187
Xopenex, 780
Xopenex HFA, 780
Xylocaine, 784
Xylocaine Viscous, 784
🍁 Xylocard, 784
Xyrem, 23

Y

☯ yagona, 1360
Yasmin, 358, 1396
Yaz, 358, 1396
☯ yinhsing, 1353
Yutopar, 1377

Z

Zaditor, 1397
zafirlukast, 1299, 37, 78, 1441
zaleplon, 1300, 101
Zanaflex, 1235
zanamavir, 1376
zanamivir, 1301, 73
Zantac, 660, C8
Zantac 75, 660
Zantac 150, 660
Zantac EFFERdose, 660
Zantryl, 1017
Zaroxolyn, 850
Zeasorb-AF, 187
Zebeta, 233, C8
Zebet-A, C8
Zegerid OTC, 1375
Zelapar, 1141
Zelnorm, 1335
Zemplar, 1287
Zenchant, 358
Zenchent, 1396
Zenpap, 22
Zenpep, 985
Zerit, 1334
Zerit XR, 1334
Zestoretic 10/12.5, 1396
Zestoretic 20/12.5, 1396
Zestoretic 20/25, 1396
Zestril, 176, C8
Zetia, 552, C8
Ziac 2.5/6.25, 1396
Ziac 5/6.25, 1396
Ziac 10/6.25, 1396
Ziagen, 109, 23
Ziana Topical Gel, 1396
ziconotide, 1302
zidovudine, 1303, 17, 23, 67, C5
Zilactin-L, 784
zileuton, 1339
Zinacef, 294
Zinc 220, 1306
Zincate, 1306
zinc sulfate, 1306, 93
Zinecard, 426
☯ zingiber, 1351
Zinkaps, 1306
ziprasidone, 1307, 64
Zipsor, 435
Zirgan, 1375
Zithromax, 214
Zmax, 214
Zocor, 666, C8
Zofran, 951
Zofran ODT, 951
Zoladex, 640

---

*Entries for **generic** names appear in **boldface type**. Trade names appear in regular type, with Canadian trade names preceded by a maple leaf icon (🍁). CLASSIFICATIONS appear in BOLDFACE SMALL CAPS. *Combination Drugs* appear in *italics*, herbal products are preceded by a yin-yang icon (☯) and drugs with genetic implications are preceded by a double-helix icon (🧬).

zoledronic acid, 1309, 77
zolmitriptan, 1312, 106
Zoloft, 1147, C16
zolpidem, 1313, 23, 101, 1442
Zolpimist, 1313, 23
Zometa, 1309
Zomig, 1312
Zomig-ZMT, 1312
Zonalon, 476, C6
Zonegran, 1315, 23
zonisamide, 1315, 23, 42, 1442
Zorbtive, 645
ZORprin, 1131
Zos, 1435

Zostavax, 1435
Zoster vaccine, 1435
Zostrix, 271
Zostrix-HP, 271
Zosyn, 1032
Zosyn for Injection 2.25 g, 1396
Zosyn for Injection 3.375 g, 1396
Zosyn for Injection 4.5 g, 1396
Zovia 1/35, 358, 1396
Zovia 1/50, 358, 1396
Zovirax, 118
Zyban, 249, C12
Zydone, 675
Zydone 5/400, 1396

Zydone 7.5/400, 1396
Zydone 10/400, 1396
Zyflo CR, 1339
Zylet Ophthalmic Suspension, 1396
Zyloprim, 134
Zymar, 1398
Zyprexa, 943, 1376, C8
Zyprexa Relprevv, 1375
Zyprexa Zydis, 943
Zyprexa/Zyprexa Zydis, 23
Zyrtec, 309, C8
Zyrtec-D Allergy & Congestion, 1396
Zyrtec Itchy Eye, 1397
Zyvox, 790

Measurement Conversion Table

Metric System Equivalents

1 gram (g) = 1000 milligrams (mg)
1000 grams = 1 kilogram (kg)
.001 milligram = 1 microgram (mcg)
1 liter (L) = 1000 milliliters (ml)
1 milliliter = 1 cubic centimeter (cc)
1 meter = 100 centimeters (cm)
1 meter = 1000 millimeters (mm)

Conversion Equivalents

Volume

1 milliliter = 15 minims (M) = 15 drops (gtt)

5 milliliters = 1 fluidram = 1 teaspoon (tsp)

15 milliliters = 4 fluidrams = 1 tablespoon (T)

30 milliliters = 1 ounce (oz) = 2 tablespoons

500 milliliters = 1 pint (pt)

1000 milliliters = 1 quart (qt)

Weight

1 kilogram = 2.2 pounds (lb)
1 gram (g) = 1000 milligrams = 15 grains (gr)
0.6 gram = 600 milligrams = 10 grains
0.5 gram = 500 milligrams = 7.5 grains
0.3 gram = 300 milligrams = 5 grains
0.06 gram = 60 milligrams = 1 grain

Length

2.5 centimeters = 1 inch

Centigrade/Fahrenheit Conversions

$C = (F - 32) \times 5/9$
$F = (C \times 9/5) + 32$

PUPIL SCALE mm: 1 2 3 4 5 6 7 8

DAVIS'S
DRUG GUIDE
for NURSES® TWELFTH EDITION

SAFETY FIRST!

Powerful Learning and Teaching Resources
Online at DavisPlus

FREE for STUDENTS & PRACTITIONERS
- **NEW!** Interactive Flash Cards
- **NEW!** Audio podcasts
- Video clips
- Animations
- Interactive Case Studies
- Select Tutorials from the CD-ROM, with multiple-choice questions for each topic
- And more!

FREE for INSTRUCTORS
Upon Adoption
- **NEW!** Test Bank
- **UPDATED!** Case Studies
- **UPDATED!** PowerPoints
- **UPDATED!** Drug Search Installer
- **UPDATED!** Drug Guide Scavenger Hunt
- And more!

www.DrugGuide.com

FREE Monthly Updates
Sign up at www.DrugGuide.com, powered by Unbound Medicine®, to receive e-mail alerts on important, new information.

- Search for **medications**, including the latest **FDA-approved drugs**.
- Access the latest drug updates.
- And more!